Thieme

Atlas of 360 Degree Skull Base Surgery

Narayan Jayashankar, DORL, DNB (ENT), MNAMS
Consultant Otorhinolaryngologist and Skull Base Surgeon
Nanavati Superspeciality Hospital
Mumbai, Maharashtra, India

Prepageran Narayanan, FRCSEd, FRCS (Glasg), MS (Distinction) UM, AM, FAMM, DPT, DPMP
Senior Professor and Consultant
Department of Otorhinolaryngology Head & Neck Surgery
Faculty of Medicine
University Malaya
Kuala Lumpur, Malaysia

2907 Illustrations

Thieme
Delhi • Stuttgart • New York • Rio de Janeiro

Publishing Director: Ritu Sharma
Senior Development Editor: Dr Nidhi Srivastava
Director-Editorial Services: Rachna Sinha
Project Manager: Apoorva Goel
Vice President Sales and Marketing: Arun Kumar Majji
Managing Director & CEO: Ajit Kohli

Thieme Medical and Scientific Publishers Private Limited.
A - 12, Second Floor, Sector - 2, Noida - 201 301,
Uttar Pradesh, India, +911204556600
Email: customerservice@thieme.in
www.thieme.in

Cover design: Thieme Publishing Group
Cover images: Courtesy of Narayan Jayashankar and Prepageran Narayanan
Page make-up by RECTO Graphics, India

Printed in India by EIH Limited- Unit Printing Press

5 4 3 2 1

ISBN: 978-93-86293-39-8
eISBN: 978-93-90553-14-3

I dedicate this book to my parents, my wife Geetha, and children Shreya and Rishabh.

Narayan Jayashankar

Dedicated to the Divine Mother, Atuk, my parents, Uncle Chandran, my wife Nitha,
and my boys Thessvin and Tharvin.
To all my teachers, colleagues, and students in this journey.
To our patients for having faith and trusting their lives in our hands.

Prepageran Narayanan

Contents

Foreword

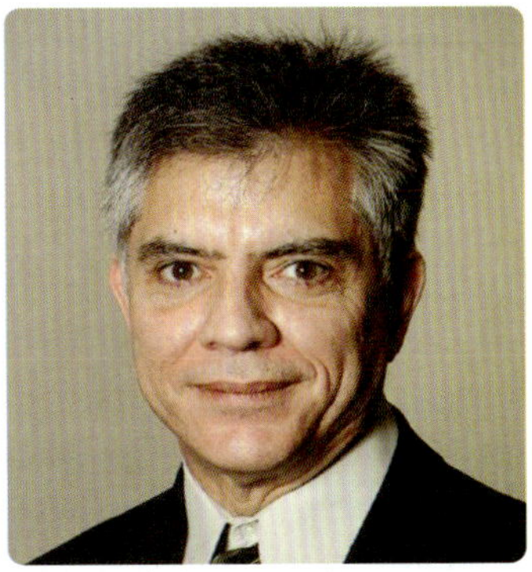

"Anatomy is to physiology as geography is to history; it describes the theatre of events."

—Jean Fernel

I am greatly honored to write the foreword on the request of Drs. Jayashankar and Narayanan for their opus *Atlas of 360 Degree Skull Base Surgery*. As the title implies, this compendium offers the opportunity to examine the anatomical features encountered when one approaches lesions of the skull base from multiple points of view around its circumference. Historically, the direction of surgical corridors was limited majorly by the training and degree of familiarity of the surgeon; thus, having a 360° perspective is a relatively new concept that deserves the insightful consideration afforded by this noteworthy publication.

One cannot overemphasize that anatomy, or "the theatre of events," is the foundation of surgery, providing the blueprint and guidance for the three main components of any procedure, namely, the approach, the surgical management of a lesion, and the final repair. This premise has been considered gospel ever since the humble beginnings of surgery and will remain so, regardless of new technologies and techniques. In fact, novel techniques and technological advances have a symbiotic relationship with anatomy, as the former cannot be designed or used without comprehending the latter, and yet their adoption contributes to its understanding.

Skull base surgery fully illustrates these concepts, as its current state is the result of the evolution of techniques, which were catapulted by engineering advancements in surgical instrumentation and devices; in turn, new procedures triggered the need for further innovation. Similar to other aspects of our daily life, the past 30 years have brought a significant acceleration of progress. A field that was previously dominated by traditional open techniques that required the sacrifice or mobilization of large volume of normal structures, even when using microscopic assistance, is now complemented by various minimally-invasive and minimal-access techniques that use alternative means of visualization, such as endoscopes and exoscopes. In addition, current surgeons may be assisted by robotic systems, surgical navigation devices, virtual reality projections, intraoperative MR, CT and ultrasound imaging, intrinsic or induced tissue fluorescence, spectral imaging, among other existing and developing improvements. All these strategies strive to further the surgeon's anatomical understanding of the surgical field.

Anatomy is constant; however, our perception depends on our brain processing the surgical field. Thus, it is highly dependent on our fund of knowledge, prior experiences, and image recognition. Visualization technologies aid the surgeon in the latter respect but cannot be a substitute for the surgeon's judgement. As mentioned previously, technical and technological advances have facilitated the possibility of approaching and managing skull base problems using routes and corridors that would not have been possible or acceptable using traditional techniques, prompting surgeons to learn the intricacies of the skull base surgical anatomy from unconventional perspectives.

This exhaustive book, containing 76 chapters, including multiple subthemes in over 1000 pages, will help us to comprehend the anatomical complexities of the skull base in its 360° and should be part of the library of any modern skull base surgeon. I highly commend the editors for bringing together this extensive and far-reaching anthology, written by a brilliant and diverse array of authors, who present their perspectives and knowledge on this most consequential subject.

Ricardo L. Carrau, MD
Professor
Department of Otolaryngology—Head & Neck Surgery
Director of the Comprehensive Skull Base Surgery Program
The Ohio State University Medical Center
Columbus, Ohio, USA

Foreword

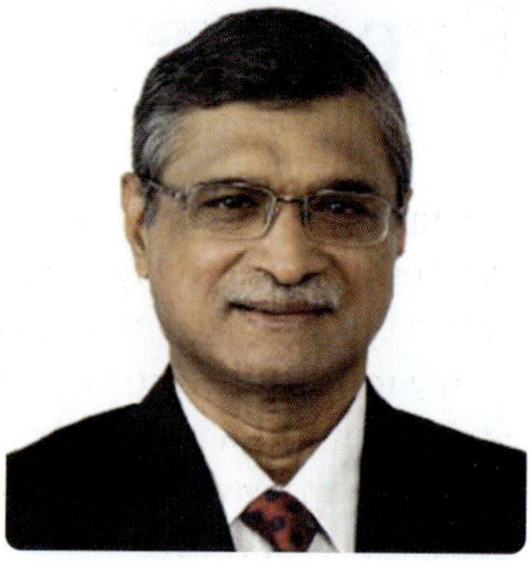

It is a privilege to write a foreword for the *Atlas of 360 Degree Skull Base Surgery* by Dr. Narayan Jayashankar and Dr. Prepagaran Narayanan.

Addressing lesions of the skull base has been a challenging task. With the evolution of endoscopes, specialized instruments, and navigation systems, surgery has become safer and has allowed the surgeon to tackle lesions which till now were considered out of bounds. This is one aspect of surgery where teamwork is essential, and the team usually would consist of a neurosurgeon, a rhinologist, an otologist, and a head and neck surgeon. Over a period of time, these roles may fuse into each other as they gain more and more expertise to overlap the dissection each one is capable of doing.

Dr. Narayan Jayashankar and Dr. Prepagaran Narayanan are dedicated ENT surgeons who have trained themselves, and have excelled in surgery of skull base lesions. This atlas is a result of the tremendous experience that these two surgeons and their colleagues have pooled together.

The text in the atlas is enhanced by over 2,000 beautiful illustrations whose quality and clarity help the reader easily understand the various concepts that the authors describe. The authors have addressed the various lesions to be dealt with in a very systematic manner, dividing the text into 29 sections which deal with the different aspects of transnasal, transorbital, and lateral skull base surgical techniques. I feel this atlas will be an invaluable guide to the practicing surgeons dealing with lesions of skull base, and also to postgraduate students training in different aspects of otorhinolaryngology and skull base surgery. I would like to compliment the editors and the various authors for sharing their experience in this atlas.

Milind Kirtane, MS (ENT), DORL, Dsc (Hon)
Professor Emeritus
The Seth G.S. Medical College
KEM Hospital
Mumbai, Maharashtra, India

Preface

The foundation of skull base surgery was strengthened by the close cooperation between otorhinolaryngologists and neurosurgeons and a plethora of innovative ideas that helped improve the existing approaches as well as develop new approaches. This was aided by the tremendous innovations in various equipments and instruments developed for skull base surgery.

My foray into practicing skull base surgery started as a neurotologist and a lateral skull base surgeon in 1999 and subsequently extended to endoscopic transnasal skull base surgery in 2005. For this, I thank my teachers in India and abroad who have shaped my mind and helped me harness my skills. I was also fortunate to work with neurosurgical colleagues who were extremely cooperative and helped me grow with their continued support. The value of countless hours spent in the anatomy dissection hall cannot be overemphasized.

I met Prepageran around 2006 and our friendship blossomed. I have always been very impressed with his amicable personality and excellent surgical skills. It dawned on us that we were, at that time, among very few otorhinolaryngologists who could work all around the skull base, whether it be transtemporal, endonasal, or open approaches. As our experience grew, we decided to pass on our knowledge to the next generation through this Atlas. This book has been developed to explain in detail, pictorially, the various approaches, their indications, and the subtle surgical nuances that help in achieving good results. Covering every possible approach in literature is beyond the scope of this project. However, we have tried to cover the most common topics. We have also invited illustrious colleagues in India and abroad to write certain chapters that bear their stamp of excellence due to their tremendous experience in the subject. This was done with the genuine intent of giving the reader a rich insight into various topics.

I would specifically like to thank Prepageran and his colleagues for their excellent cooperation in this project. I thank all the contributors for their respective chapters in this book. Being the masters in their fields, their chapters are pearls of wisdom, which have greatly enhanced the quality of this book. I thank my parents for an excellent upbringing with strong values. A very special thanks to my wife and children who have always been very supportive of my academic pursuits. I would also like to thank my residents over the years who have assisted me in various procedures. It has also been a great experience collaborating with the editorial and marketing teams at Thieme who are helping this book to reach out to numerous colleagues and young minds.

Narayan Jayashankar, DORL, DNB (ENT), MNAMS

Preface

Skull base surgery has recently evolved into a subspecialty of its own, involving multidisciplinary teamwork to provide the best care for patients. In otorhinolaryngology, few surgeons perform the whole range of skull base surgeries encompassing endoscopic transnasal, posterolateral, and open skull base approaches as both the editors of this manual do. This manual of 360-degree skull base was written with the collaboration of esteemed colleagues worldwide to provide comprehensive skull base surgical approaches in a step-by-step manner as performed by the authors. We hope this manual will be useful and informative for the future 360-degree skull base surgeons.

Prepageran Narayanan, FRCSEd, FRCS (Glasg), MS (Distinction) UM, AM, FAMM, DPT, DPMP

About the Authors

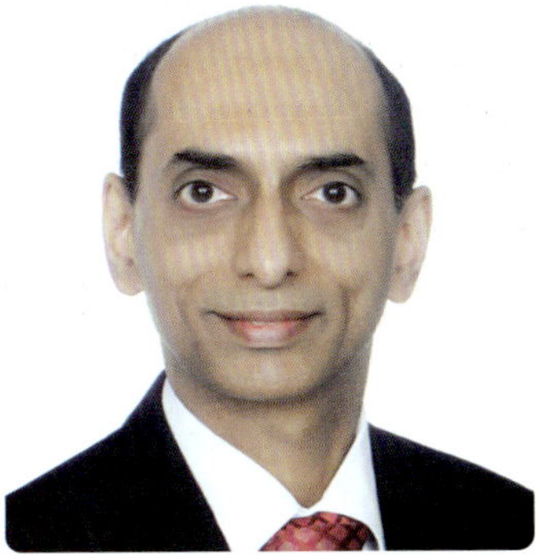

Narayan Jayashankar is a leading surgeon in the fields of neurotology, lateral skull base surgery, and endoscopic transnasal skull base surgery in India. His excellent surgical skills and command over the subject have made him a prominent, sought-after name in the fields of otorhinolaryngology and skull base surgery. He has been practicing in Mumbai, India, for the past 20 years, propagating the possibilities and reach of these fields. His knack for simplifying the most complex of topics, employing clean dissection skills, and coming up with excellent surgical results have entailed numerous invitations to lectures, live demonstrations, and cadaveric dissections at various institutions in India and abroad. He has been a guest faculty for over 250 workshops across the country and worldwide and has been invited as a speaker at world congresses. He has published articles in peer-reviewed journals and is also a reviewer for prestigious indexed journals. He has authored *Atlas of Neurotology and Lateral Skull Base Surgery*, published by Thieme, and has also contributed chapters to various textbooks. He is a board-certified teacher for postgraduate course in otorhinolaryngology in India.

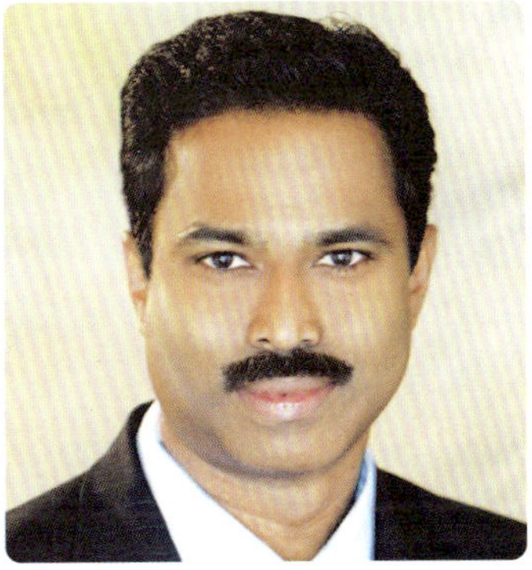

Prepageran Narayanan has achieved international prominence in endoscopic skull base, posterolateral skull base, otology, as well as cochlear implants surgery. His leadership qualities and international fame are demonstrated through the leading roles he plays in international committees and editorial boards. His continual innovations, peer-reviewed publications, and lectures are a reflection of his years of expertise in the field and reinforce his recent appointment as the President of the 9th World Congress of Endoscopic Surgery of the Skull Base, Brain, and Spine, to be held in 2022. His academic excellence often entails invitations to workshops, surgeries, live dissections, and lectures across continents—Asia, Europe, Australia, Africa, North America, and South America—where he shares his surgical expertise. His global reputation and passion to teach has attracted many fellows from all over the world to train under his wings at the University of Malaya where he mentors 360 degree skull base fellowships. He has also written more than 220 peer-reviewed publications and more than 20 books or dissection manuals till date.

Contributors

A. B. Zulkiflee, MBBS (Mal), M Surg ORL-HNS (Mal), FRCS (Glasgow), AM (Mal)
Professor
Department of Otorhinolaryngology
Faculty of Medicine
University of Malaya
Kuala Lumpur, Malaysia

Achala Kamath, MS (ENT)
Consultant ENT Surgeon
Mumbai, Maharashtra, India

Adam Jadczak, MD
Consultant
Department of Radiology
Division of Neuroradiology
University Hospital Basel, University of Basel
Petersgraben, Switzerland

Adzreil Bakri, MBBChBAO (Ireland), MRCSEd (ENT), MORL-HNS (UM)
Senior Physician
Faculty of Medicine
University of Malaya
Kuala Lumpur, Malaysia

Alexandre B. Todeschini, MD
Fellow at the Department of Neurological Surgery
Wexner Medical Center
The Ohio State University College of Medicine
Columbus, Ohio, USA

Amol Patil, DORL, DNB
ENT Consultant
Nanavati Superspeciality Hospital
Mumbai, Maharashtra, India

Amol Raheja, MBBS, MCh
Assistant Professor
Department of Neurosurgery
All India Institute of Medical Sciences
New Delhi, India

Amr Mohamed, MBBCh, MSc, MRCS, FRCS (SN)
Consultant Neurosurgeon
University Hospital Wales
Cardiff, London, UK

Anagha Joshi, MS (ENT), DNB, DORL
Associate Professor
Department of Otorhinolaryngology
Lokmanya Tilak Municipal Medical College and General Hospital
Mumbai, India;
Visiting Consultant
H N Reliance Hospital
Mumbai, Maharashtra, India

Ananth Chintapalli, MS
Senior Resident
Department of ENT—Head & Neck Surgery
Kamineni Academy of Medical Sciences and Research Center
Hyderabad, Telangana, India;
Fellowship in Rhinology & Skull Base Surgery – Vancouver, BC, Canada;
Consultant Rhinologist – Medikeri's Superspeciality
ENT Center
Bangalore, India

Ankit S. Shah, MBBS, MS, MCh
Fellow in Skull Base & Cerebrovascular Neurosurgery
Department of Neurosurgery
All India Institute of Medical Sciences
New Delhi, India

Ashish R. Sharma, MBBS, MS, MCh
Postdocotoral Fellow
Department of Neurosurgery
Sanjay Gandhi Postgraduate Institute of Medical Sciences
Lucknow, Uttar Pradesh, India

Ashish Suri, MBBS, MCh, DNB, FAMS, FNASc
Professor
Department of Neurosurgery
All India Institute of Medical Sciences
New Delhi, India

Asiya Kamber Zaidi, MBBS, MS ENT (Gold Medal), FWAMS
Fellowship in Endoscopic Ear Surgery (India);
Fellowship in Advanced Otorhinolaryngology and Skull Base Surgery (Malaysia);
Senior Registrar
Mahatma Gandhi Memorial Medical College and Maharaja Yashwant Rao Hospital
Indore, Madhya Pradesh, India

Benjamin S. Bleier, MD, FACS, FARS
Associate Professor
Claire and John Bertucci Chair in OHNS;
Director of Translational Research
Director of Endoscopic Skull Base Surgery
Director (Co) of Center for Orbital Surgery
Department of Otolaryngology
Massachusetts Eye and Ear Infirmary
Harvard Medical School
Boston, USA

Bradley A. Otto, MD
Associate Professor
Department of Otolaryngology—Head & Neck Surgery
The Ohio State University Wexner Medical Center
Columbus, Ohio, USA

Daniel M. Prevedello, MD, FACS
Professor
Department of Neurological Surgery;
Director
Minimally Invasive Cranial Surgery Program;
Co-Director
Comprehensive Skull Base Center at The James;
Director
Pituitary Surgery Program
The Wexner Medical Center
The Ohio State University
Columbus, Ohio, USA

Dominik Cordier, MD
Assistant Professor and Senior Consultant
Department of Neurosurgery
University Hospital Basel, University of Basel
Basel, Switzerland

Eugene Hung Chih Wong, MBChB, MRCS (Gen), MRCS (ENT), MPhil, MS (ORL-HNS)
Otorhinolaryngologist/Lecturer
Department of Surgery
Faculty of Medicine and Health Sciences
University Malaysia Sabah
Kota Kinabalu, Sabah, Malaysia

Fintan Sheerin, MA, MB Bchir, MRCP, FRCR
Head of Department of Neuroradiology
Oxford University Hospitals
Oxford, UK

Gaurav Shankar Medikeri, MS (ENT)
Consultant Rhinologist
Medikeri Superspeciality ENT Centre
Bangalore, Karnataka, India;
Program Director
Skull Base Unit
HCG Group of Hospitals
Fellowship in Rhinology and Anterior Skull Base
Vancouver, Canada;
Fellowship in Rhinology and Skull Base Surgery
Liverpool, UK;
Fellowship in Rhinoplasty and Facial Cosmetic Surgery
Shimmian Rhinoplasty Clinic
Seoul, Korea

Ing Ping Tang, MD, MS (ORLHNS), FRCS
Professor & Senior Consultant
Head of Department ORL-HNS
Faculty of Medicine & Health Sciences
Universiti Malaysia Sarawak
Sarawak, Malaysia

Jacques Magnan, MD
Professor Emeritus
University of Aix-Marseille (F)
Head of the ORL and Head & Neck Surgery
Hôpital Nord
Marseille, France

Jash Patel, B MedSci (Hons), MB ChB, FRCS (England), MD, FRCS (SN)
Consultant Neurosurgeon
John Radcliffe Hospital, Oxford University Hospitals
University of Oxford (Anatomy)
Neurovascular Research Lead of the Academic Committee of the Society of British Neurological Surgeons
Intercollegiate (JCIE) and International (JSCFE) Examiner in Neurosurgery
Oxford, UK

Jeyaganesh V., MBBS MMed Anaesthesia
Anesthesiologist
Department of Anesthesiology
Faculty of Medicine
University of Malaya
Kuala Lumpur, Malaysia

Jeyanthi Kulasegarah, FRCS, MD, DOHNS, MRCS, MB, BCh, BAO, NUI
Medical Lecturer
Department of Otorhinolaryngology
Faculty of Medicine, University of Malaya
Kuala Lumpur, Malaysia

John Clemente de Leon, MD
Department of Neurological Surgery
Fujita Health University
Aichi, Japan

Jonathan Rychen, MD
Junior Consultant
Department of Neurosurgery
University Hospital Basel, University of Basel
Spitalstrasse, Basel, Switzerland

Jun Muto, MD, PhD
Senior Assistant Professor
Department of Neurological Surgery
Fujita Health University
Aichi, Japan

Jürgen Hench, MD
Assistant Professor and Senior Consultant
Institute of Pathology, Divisions of Neuropathology and Molecular Pathology
University Hospital Basel, University of Basel
Spitalstrasse, Switzerland

Kamlesh Singh Bhaisora, MBBS, MS, MCh
Assistant Professor
Department of Neurosurgery
Sanjay Gandhi Postgraduate Institute of Medical Sciences
Lucknow, Uttar Pradesh, India

K. P. Morwani, MS (ENT)
Otorhinolaryngologist & Skull Base Surgeon
HOD Fortis Hiranandani Hospital
HOD Raheja Hospital
Nanavati Superspeciality Hospital
Mumbai, Maharashtra, India

Kanu Lal Saha, FCPS (Otolaryngology)
Associate Professor
Otology Division
Department of Otolaryngology—Head and Neck Surgery
Bangabandhu Sheik Mujib Medical University
Shahbag, Dhaka, Bangladesh

Kashmira Chavan, DNB (ENT)
Consultant ENT Surgeon
Dr L Hiranandani Hospital
Mumbai, Maharashtra, India

Kein Seong Mun, MBBS, MPath
Associate Professor
Department of Pathology
University Malaya Specialist Centre
Jalan University
Kuala Lumpur, Malaysia

Kong Yew Liew, MORL-HNS
Consultant ENT, Head and Neck Surgeon
Department of Otorhinolaryngology
University of Malaya
Kuala Lumpur, Malaysia

Kuntal Kanti Das, MBBS, MS, MCh
Associate Professor
Department of Neurosurgery
Sanjay Gandhi Postgraduate Institute of Medical Sciences
Lucknow, Uttar Pradesh, India

Kyle VanKoevering, MD
Assistant Professor
Department of Otolaryngology—Head and Neck Surgery
Ohio State University Wexner Medical Center
Columbus, Ohio, USA

Liew Yiew Toong, MRCS (Mal), MRCS (Ireland), MOrl (Head & Neck Surgery)
Medical Lecturer
Department of Otorhinolaringology
Faculty of Medicine
University of Malaya
Kuala Lumpur, Malaysia

Luigi Mariani, MD
Professor and Chair
Department of Neurosurgery
University Hospital Basel, University of Basel
Spitalstrasse, Switzerland

Madhuri Mehta, MS (ENT)
Director
Department of ENT and Head and Neck Surgery
N. C. Jindal Institute of Medical Sciences and Research
Hisar, Haryana, India

Madhu Sudhan V, MS (ENT), DNB
ENT Consultant
Pristyn Care ENT Clinic
Bangalore, India

Malik Ibrahim Malik, MD
Assistant Professor
Department of Otolaryngology—Head and Neck Surgery
Oumdurman Islamic University, Sudan;
Rhinology and Anterior Skull Base Surgery Fellow
University Malaya
Ibn Sina Specialized Hospital
Khartoum, Sudan

Michel Roethlisberger, MD
Assistant Professor and Senior Consultant
Department of Neurosurgery, University Hospital Basel
University of Basel
Spitalstrasse, Basel, Switzerland;
Endoscopic and Lateral Skullbase Surgery Fellow
Department of Neurosurgery
Department of Oto-Rhino-Laryngology
University of Malaya Specialist Center (UMSC)
Jalan Universiti
Kuala Lumpur, Selangor, Malaysia

Milind Kirtane, MS (ENT), DORL, Dsc (Hon)
Professor Emeritus
The Seth G.S. Medical College
KEM Hospital
Mumbai, Maharashtra, India

Mohan Kameswaran, DSc, MS, FRCS (Ed), FAMS, FICS, DLO
Managing Director and Chief Senior Consultant
Department of Neurotology, Implants, and Skull Base Surgery
Madras ENT Research Foundation
Raja Annamalaipuram
Chennai, Tamil Nadu, India

Narayan Jayashankar, DORL, DNB (ENT), MNAMS
Consultant Otorhinolaryngologist and Skull Base Surgeon
Nanavati Superspeciality Hospital
Mumbai, Maharashtra, India

Neelesh Tiwari, MS (ENT)
Fellow
Skull Base Surgery
Department of Head Neck Surgical Oncology
Tata Memorial Hospital
Mumbai, Maharashtra, India

Nishit J. Shah, MS (ENT), DNB, DORL
Honorary Consultant
Department of ENT
Bombay Hospital and Medical Research Centre;
Breach Candy Hospital
Mumbai, Maharashtra, India

Nyall London, MD, PhD
Assistant Professor
Department of Otolaryngology—Head and Neck Surgery
Johns Hopkins University
Baltimore, Maryland, USA

Prashik Waghmare, DNB (Neurosurgery)
Consultant Neurosurgeon
Jeevan Jyot Hospital
Ambikapur, India

Prathamesh S. Pai, MS (ENT), DNB, DORL, MNAMS
Professor and Consultant Surgeon
Department of Head & Neck Surgical Oncology
Tata Memorial Hospital
Mumbai, Maharashtra, India

Prepageran Narayanan, FRCSEd, FRCS (Glasg), MS (Distinction) UM, AM, FAMM, DPT, DPMP
Senior Professor and Consultant
Department of Otorhinolaryngology Head & Neck Surgery
Faculty of Medicine
University Malaya
Kuala Lumpur, Malaysia

R. Chandra Shekar Reddy, MS (ENT)
Fellow in Skull Base Surgery
Nanavati Superspeciality Hospital
Mumbai, Maharashtra, India

Rafael Uribe, MD, MHS
Endoscopic Skull Base and Pituitary Surgery Fellow
Department of Neurological Surgery
Weill Cornell Medical Center – New York Presbyterian Hospital
New York, New York, USA

Raghu Nandhan, MS, DNB, MRCS (Ed), DOHNS (Eng), FRCS (ORL-HNS), MCh (UK), PhD
Consultant ENT Surgeon
Department of Neurotology, Implants and Skull Base Surgery
Madras ENT Research Foundation, Raja Annamalaipuram
Chennai, Tamil Nadu, India

Rajan Shah, MCh (Neurosurgery)
Head
Department of Neurosurgery
Nanavati Superspeciality Hospital
Mumbai, Maharashtra, India

Raphael Guzman, MD
Professor and Vice Chair
Department of Neurosurgery
Chief of Pediatric Neurosurgery
University Hospital Basel, University of Basel
Spitalstrasse, Switzerland

Renuka Bradoo, MS, DORL
Professor and Head of Department
Department of ENT & Head, Neck Surgery
Lokmanya Tilak Municipal Medical College & General Hospital
Mumbai, Maharashtra, India

Revadi Govindaraju, MD, MS (ORL-H&N Surgery)
Fellowship in Rhinology
Clinical Specialist/Senior Lecturer
Department of Otorhinolaryngology
University Malaya Medical Centre
Jalan Universiti
Kuala Lumpur, Malaysia

Ricardo L. Carrau, MD
Professor
Department of Otolaryngology—Head & Neck Surgery;
Director of the Comprehensive Skull Base Surgery Program
The Ohio State University Medical Center
Columbus, Ohio, USA

Robert Iorga, MD, FEBNS, FRCS (SN)
Consultant Neurosurgeon
St George's Hospital
London, UK

Saif Al-Zahid, MBBCh, MPhil, FRCS (ORL-HNS)
Otology Fellow
ENT Department
Sir Charles Gairdener Hospital
Nedlands, Western Australia, Australia

Sampath Chandra Prasad Rao, MS, DNB, FEB-ORLHNS
Consultant
Department of ENT—Skull Base Surgery
Manipal Hospital, Old HAL Road, Bangalore, India

Samuel MacKeith, MB ChB, FRCS (ORL-HNS), MPhil
Consultant ENT Surgeon
Department of Otolaryngology
Oxford University Hospitals
Oxford, UK

Sanjeeva Jeyaretna, MD, FRCS (SN)
Consultant Neurosurgeon
Director for Skull Base Surgery
Oxford University Hospitals
Oxford, UK

Sanjay Behari, MBBS, MS, MCh, DNB, FAANS
Professor and Head
Department of Neurosurgery
Sanjay Gandhi Postgraduate Institute of Medical Sciences
Lucknow, Uttar Pradesh, India

Sarina K. Mueller, MD
Consultant
Department of Otolaryngology—Head and Neck Surgery
Friedrich- Alexander- Universität Erlangen- Nürnberg (FAU)
Erlangen, Germany

Satish Jain, MBBS, MS (ENT)
Director
Jain ENT Hospital
Jaipur, Rajasthan, India

Sien Hui Tan, MBBS (UK), MRCS (Ireland), DOHNS (UK), MS (ORL-HNS) (UM)
Consultant
Department of Otorhinolaryngology
Faculty of Medicine, University of Malaya
Kuala Lumpur, Selangor, Malaysia

Sudhendoo Babhulkar, DNB (Neuro)
Jr Consultant
Department of Neurosurgery
Nanavati Superspeciality Hospital
Mumbai, Maharashtra, India

Suresh Sankhla, DNB, FICS
Head
Department of Neurosurgery
Global Hospital
Mumbai, Maharashtra, India

Swati Kodur Patil, DLO, DNB (ENT)
Senior Resident
Department of Otorhinolaryngology
Nanavati Superspeciality Hospital
Mumbai, Maharashtra, India

Tejal Patel, MS (ENT)
Speciality Medical Officer
Department of ENT
Lokmanya Tilak Municipal Medical College & General Hospital
Mumbai, Maharashtra, India

Theodore H. Schwartz, MD, FACS
David and Ursel Barnes Professor of Minimally Invasive Neurosurgery;
Director
Anterior Skull Base and Pituitary Surgery;
Director
Epilepsy Research Laboratory
Departments of Neurological Surgery, Otolaryngology, and Neuroscience
Weill Cornell Medical Center – New York Presbyterian Hospital
New York, New York, USA

Vicknes Waran, MBBS, FRCSEd, FRCS
Senior Professor and Consultant
Neurosurgery Division
Faculty of Medicine
University of Malaya
Kuala Lumpur, Malaysia

Vijay K. Anand, MD
Clinical Professor of Otolaryngology
Department of Otolaryngology, Head and Neck Surgery
Weill Cornell Medical Center – New York Presbyterian Hospital
New York, USA

Viraj J. Kaluskar, DNB-ENT
Honorary Consultant (ENT)
Criticare Hospital, Paramount Hospital, and Jeevan Vikas Kendra Hospital
Mumbai, Maharashtra, India

Warren O. Bennett, MBBS, MA (Oxon), DOHNS, FRCS (ORL-HNS)
Advanced Rhinology and Anterior Skull Base Fellow
Queen Elizabeth University Hospital
Glasgow, UK

Wong HT, MBBS (University Malaya), Master in Otorhinolaryngology, Head & Neck Surgery (University Malaya), MRCS (Ireland)
Medical Lecturer
Department of Otorhinolaryngology
Faculty of Medicine
University of Malaya
Kuala Lumpur, Malaysia

Yuichi Hirose, MD, PhD
Professor and Chair
Department of Neurosurgery
Fujita Health University
Aichi, Japan

Yves Brand, MD
Assistant Professor and Chair
Department of Oto-Rhino-Laryngology
Cantonal Hospital Graubünden
Loëstrasse, Switzerland

Abbreviations

3D FSPGR: three-dimensional fast spoiled gradient echo
3rdCP: choroid plexus of the third ventricle
AA: arch of atlas
ABIs: auditory brainstem implants
ABR: auditory brainstem response
ACA: anterior cerebral artery
ACFDL: anterior cranial fossa dura
aChA: anterior choroidal artery
AComA: anterior communicating artery
ACP: anterior clinoid process
ACS: anterior wall of the cavernous sinus
ACTH: adrenocorticotrophic hormone
AD: arachnoidal dura
ADH: antidiuretic hormone
AEA: anterior ethmoidal artery
AEC: anterior ethmoidal canal
AEPs: acoustic evoked potentials
AFD: anterior cranial fossa dura
AFD: anterior fossa dura
Ag: anterior genu
AHL: asymmetrical hearing loss
AICA: anterior inferior cerebellar artery
AL: apical ligament
ALL: anterior longitudinal ligament
ALT-VISION: Anatomical Laboratory for Visuospatial Innovations in Otolaryngology and Neurosurgery
AOL: atlanto-occipital ligament
AOM: atlanto-occipital membrane
APC: adenomatous polyposis coli
aPG: anterior pituitary gland
ApL: apical ligament
AR: anterior recess
aSS: accessory dividing septum
AWSS: anterior wall of sphenoid sinus
atPG: anterior pituitary gland
AVHT: auditory verbal habilitation therapy
AW: anterior wall
AZ: annulus of Zinn
BA: basilar artery
BAER: brainstem auditory evoked response
BAHA: bone-anchored hearing aid
BC: blood clot
BCIs: bone conduction implants
BF: biodegradable foams
BMI: body mass index
BP: basilar plexus
BPF: basiopharyngeal fascia
BPPV: benign paroxysmal positional vertigo
BSP basisphenoid
BS: bony septum
BSNS: biphenotypic sinonasal sarcoma
C: clivus
C1 FT: foramen transversarium of the atlas
C1N: C1 nerve root
C2N: C2 nerve root
CA: carotid artery
CAEP: cortical auditory evoked potentials
CaHA: calcium hydroxylapatite
CAP: categories of auditory performance
CB: carotid bifurcations
CC: chiasmatic cistern
CCa: clival carotid
CCAP: cochlear compound action potential
CCJ: craniocervical junction
CCL: caroticoclinoid ligament
CEA: carcinoembryonic antigen
CG: cholesterol granuloma
ChS: chiasmatic sulcus
cICA: cavernous internal carotid artery
cICA: clinoidal internal carotid artery
CIGS: camera for image-guided surgery
CIs: cochlear implants
CMC: carboxymethylcellulose
CN III: oculomotor nerve
CN V1: trigeminal nerve
CN: cochlear nerve
CN6: abducent nerve
CN7: facial nerve
CN8: vestibulocochlear nerve
CNS: central nervous system
CNs: cranial nerves
CNV3: mandibular branch of the trigeminal nerve
COD: cemento-osseous dysplasia
CeP: cerebral peduncle
ChP: choroid plexus
CP: cribriform plate
CPA: cerebellopontine angle
CPAP: continuous positive airway pressure
CPDB: classical Paget's disease of bone
CPR: cardiopulmonary resuscitation
CR: clival ridge

CRH: corticotropin-releasing hormone
CrL: cruciate ligament
CROS: contralateral routing of signal
CRP: C-reactive protein
CS: cavernous sinus
CSF: cerebrospinal fluid
CT: computed tomography
CTA: computed tomography angiography
CUSA: cavitational ultrasonic aspirator
D PICA: distal posterior inferior cerebellar artery
DB: debrider
DDR: distal dural ring
DI: diabetes insipidus
DKFZ: German Cancer Research Centre
DL: dentate ligaments
DM: dura mater
DNAP: dorsal nucleus action potential
DPS: dura of planum sphenoidale
DR: dural ring
D: diaphragma sellae
DS: dorsum sellae
DST: dura of sella turcica
DT: dural tail
DTI: diffusion tension imaging
DTS: dura of tuberculum sellae
DWI: diffusion-weighted imaging
EABR: evoked auditory brainstem response
EAC: external auditory canal
EAM: external acoustic meatus
EB: ethmoidal bulla
EBV: Epstein–Barr virus
EC: ethmoidal crest
ECD: extracapsular dissection
ECG: electrocardiography
ED: endolymphatic duct
EEA: endoscopic endonasal approach
EETN: endoscopic endonasal transpterygoid nasopharyngectomy
EF: extraconal fat
ELTC: extreme lateral transcondylar (approach)
EM: monitor for the endoscope
EMLRs: early midlatency responses
ENKTLNT: extranodal natural killer (NK)/T-cell lymphoma nasal type
ENT: ear, nose, and throat surgeon
EOP: external occipital protuberance
ER: estrogen receptor
ES: endolymphatic sac
ESR: erythrocyte sedimentation rate
ET: eustachian tube
EVD: external ventricular drainage
F: fornix
FAP: familial adenomatous polyposis
FB: foreign body
FD: fibrous dysplasia
FDA: Food and Drug Administration
FEES: fiberoptic evaluation of swallowing
FESS: functional endoscopic sinus surgery
FFMT: functioning free muscle transfer
FFPE: formalin-fixed, paraffin-embedded
FG: fat graft
FIAC: fundus of the IAC
FIESTA: fast imaging employing steady-state acquisition
FISH: fluorescence in situ hybridization
FaL: falciform ligament
FLG: fascia lata graft
FL: foramen lacerum
FLAIR: flow-attenuated inversion recovery scan
FM: foramen of Monro
FN: facial nerve
FNAC: fine-needle aspiration cytology
FO: foramen ovale
FOL: fibro-osseous lesions
FR: foramen rotundum
FS: frontal sinus
FSE: fast spin-echo
FSH: follicle-stimulating hormone
FT: foramen transversarium
FTOZ: frontotemporal orbitozygomatic craniotomy
GAN: great auricular nerve
GCF: gantry control frame
GF: Gelfoam
GFAP: glial filament acidic protein
GG: gasserian ganglion
GH: growth hormone
GHRH: growth hormone–releasing hormone
GNAS1: guanine nucleotide-binding protein alpha-stimulating activity polypeptide 1
GnRH: gonadotropin-releasing hormone
GPP: pterygopalatine ganglion
GRASP: golden-angle radial sparse parallel
GSPN: greater (medial) superficial petrosal nerves
GTR: gross total resection
GWS: greater wing of sphenoid
H&E: hematoxylin and eosin
HA: hyaluronic acid
HB2: Hadad–Bassagasteguy 2
HBF: Hadad–Bassagasteguy (nasoseptal) flap
HBNPF: Hadad–Bassagasteguy nasoseptal pedicle flap

HC: hyaline crystal
HcICA: horizontal segment of the cavernous internal carotid artery
HEI: House Ear Institute
HPE: histopathological examination
HPV: human papillomavirus
HRCT: high-resolution computed tomography
HT: hypothalamus
IAC: internal auditory canal
IAM: internal acoustic meatus
IC: inferior clivus
ICA: internal carotid artery
ICD: implanted cardioverter defibrillator
ICL: interclinoid ligament
icON: intracanalicular optic nerve
ICS: intercavernous sinus
IcS: intraconal space
icT: intracranial component of the tumor
ICV: internal cerebral vein
IF: intraconal fat
IGF-1: insulin-like growth factor 1
IGF-2: insulin-like growth factor 2
IGS: image-guided surgery
IHA: inferior hypophyseal artery
IIPV: intermittent positive pressure ventilation
IJV: internal jugular vein
IL: injection laryngoplasty
ILAC: infralabyrinthine air cells
ILT: inferolateral trunk
IMA: internal maxillary artery
iMRI: intraoperative magnetic resonance imaging
IMRT: intensity-modulated radiotherapy
INF: interferon
IOF: inferior orbital fissure
ION: intraconal optic nerve
ioON: intraorbital optic nerve
IPC: interpeduncular cistern
IPH: intraparenchymal hemorrhage
IPL: inferior parasellar ligament
IPS: inferior petrosal sinus
IRM: inferior rectus muscle
IS: infundibular stalk
IT: inferior turbinate
ITAC: intestinal-type adenocarcinoma
ITE: in-the-ear (model)
ITF: infratemporal fossa
IUD: intrauterine device
IV: intravenous
IVH: intraventricular hemorrhage
JF: jugular foramen
JNA: juvenile nasopharyngeal angiofibroma
JOF: juvenile ossifying fibroma
KSCC: keratinizing squamous cell carcinoma
LaB: lamella of the bulla
LaMT: lamella of the middle turbinate
LAR: laryngeal adductor response
LaUP: lamella of the uncinate process
LC: longus colli
LcICA: lacerum segment of the petrous internal carotid artery
LCNs: lower cranial nerves
LCS: lateral wall of the cavernous sinus
LCSC: lateral compartment of the cavernous sinus
LH: luteinizing hormone
LM: Liliequist's membrane
LMCA: lateral meningeal clival artery
LMWCK: low-molecular weight cytokeratin
LOCR: lateral opticocarotid recess
LP: lamina papyracea
LPP: lateral pterygoid plate
LRM: lateral rectus muscle
LSCC: lateral semicircular canal
LT: lamina terminalis
LtA1: left proximal anterior cerebral artery
LtA2: left distal anterior cerebral artery
LtAH: left recurrent arteries of Heubner
LTBR: lateral temporal bone resection
LtcICA: left cavernous internal carotid artery
LtCN3: left third cranial nerve
LtCN6: left sixth cranial nerve
LtCS: left cavernous sinus
LtFM: left foramen of Monro
LtFPB: left frontopolar branch
LtFS: left frontal sinus
LtGR: left rectal gyrus
LtHT: left hypothalamic wall
LtICV: left internal cerebral vein
LtiHA: left inferior hypophyseal artery
LtITF: left infratemporal fossa
LtLOCR: left lateral optico-carotid recess
LtM: left lateral tubercular portion of the meningioma
LtMS: left maxillary sinus
LtMT: left middle turbinate
LtNFS: left contralateral nasoseptal flap
LtNSF: left nasoseptal flap
LtNSF: left pedicled nasoseptal flap
LtOA: left ophthalmic artery
LtOAp: left medial orbital apex wall
LtOCR: left opticocarotid recess

LtON: left optic nerve
LtOT: left optic tract
LtPCA: left posterior cerebral artery
LtPEA: left posterior ethmoid artery
LtpICA: left paraclival internal carotid artery
LtSCA: left superior cerebellar artery
LtscICA: left supraclinoid internal carotid artery
LtSO: left sphenoid ostium
LtSV: left septal vein
LtT: left thalamus
LtTC: left lateral tumor capsule
LtTS: left lateral aspect of the tuberculum sellae
LtTV: left thalamic vein
LV: lateral ventricles
LVCP: choroid plexus of the lateral ventricles
LWCS: lateral wall of the cavernous sinus
LWS: lesser wing of the sphenoid
MA: mastoid antrum
MB: mammillary body
MBSS: modified barium swallow study
mC: midclivus
MC: mucocele
MCA: middle cerebral artery
MCF: middle cranial fossa
MCS: medial wall of the cavernous sinus
MCW: mucocele wall
MD: microdebrider
MDT: multidisciplinary team
ME: meningoencephalocele
MEPs: motor evoked potentials
MFD: middle fossa dura
MHT: meningohypophyseal trunk
MIGS: monitor for image-guided surgery
MM: Muller's muscle
MMA: middle meningeal artery
MMCA: medial meningeal clival artery
MOCR: medial opticocarotid recess
MOW: medial orbital walls
MP: mastoid process
MPF: mucoperichondrial flap
MPR: multiplanar reconstruction
MPT: maximum phonation time
MR: median raphe
MRA: magnetic resonance angiography
MRI: magnetic resonance imaging
MRM: medial rectus muscle
MRV: magnetic resonance venography
MS: maxillary sinus
MSA: muscle-specific actin
mSS: main dividing septum
MST: maxillary strut
MT: middle turbinate
MTF: middle turbinate flap
MTL: mesial temporal lobe
MV: mandibulovidian artery
MVD: microvascular decompression
MWCS: medial wall of the cavernous sinus
NB: nasal bone
NF KappaB: nuclear factor kappa-B
NF: nasal floor
NF2: neurofibromatosis type 2
NIBP: noninvasive blood pressure
NIRS: near-infrared spectroscopy
NKSCC: nonkeratinizing squamous cell carcinoma
NMES: neuromuscular electrical stimulation
NOS: not otherwise specified
NPS: nasopharyngectomy specimen
NP: nasopharynx
NPC: nasopharyngeal carcinoma
NS: nasal septum
NSF: nasoseptal flap
OA: ophthalmic artery
OB: left orbit
OC: optic canal
OCh: optic chiasm
OCR: opticocarotid recess
OD: outer dura
OFo: optic foramina
OF: orbital floor
ON: optic nerve
ONB: olfactory neuroblastoma
OP: odontoid process/peg
OPPB: orbital process of the palatine bone
ONS: optic nerve sheath
OS: optic strut
OSAS: obstructive sleep apnea syndrome
OT: orbital tumor
OTE/BTE: over-the-ear/behind-the-ear (model)
O-Zy: orbitozygomatic
P PICA: proximal posterior inferior cerebellar artery
PA: petrous apex
PiA: pituitary adenoma
PyA: pyriform aperture
PBF: pharyngobasilar fascia
PC: posterior choana
PCA: posterior cerebral artery
PCF: petroclival fissure
pcICA: paraclinoid internal carotid artery
pcICA: paraclival internal carotid artery
pCom: posterior communicating artery

PCP: posterior clinoid process
PCSC: posterior compartment of the cavernous sinus
PDGF-B: platelet-derived growth factor subunit B
PDR: proximal dural ring
PE: posterior ethmoidal cells
PEA: posterior ethmoid artery
pEAC: posterior external auditory canal wall
PEC: posterior ethmoidal canal
peICA: petrous internal carotid artery
PES: pharyngeal electrical stimulation
PET: positron emission tomography
PET-CT: positron emission tomography computed tomography
PF: pituitary fossa
PFD: posterior fossa dura
PG: pituitary gland
Pg: posterior genu
pICA: paraclival internal carotid artery
PICA: posterior inferior cerebellar artery
PL: pituitary ligaments
PLNA: posterior lateral nasal artery
PNO: pneumo-orbita
PNS: paranasal sinus
PO: periorbita
POTS: petro-occipital transsigmoid approach
PP: perpendicular plate
PPF: pterygopalatine fossa
pPG: posterior pituitary gland
PR: posterior recess
PRL: prolactin
PSt: pituitary stalk
PS: planum sphenoidale
PrC: prepontine cistern
PSA: prostate-specific antigen
PSCC: posterior semicircular canal
PsJOF: psammomatoid variant of juvenile ossifying fibroma
PSM: pharyngeal squeeze maneuver
PTA: posttraumatic amnesia
ptPG: posterior pituitary gland
PVA: polyvinyl alcohol
PW: posterior wall
QOL: quality of life
RaH: recurrent artery of Heubner
RAPD: relative afferent pupillary defect
Rca: rectus capitis anterior muscle
RC: Rathke's cleft cyst
RCC: renal cell carcinoma
REZ: root exit zone
RG: rectal gyri
RISA: retrosigmoid intradural suprameatal approach
RLN: recurrent laryngeal nerve
RO: roof of the orbit
rON: right optic nerve
RS: rostrum sphenoidale
RSC: retrosigmoid craniotomy
RtA1: right proximal anterior cerebral artery
RtA2: right distal anterior cerebral artery
RtAC: right anterior clinoid process
RtAH: right recurrent arteries of Heubner
RtcICA: right cavernous internal carotid artery
RtCN3: right third cranial nerve
RtCN6: right sixth cranial nerve
RtCS: right cavernous sinus
RtFM: right foramen of Monro
RtFPB: right frontopolar branch
RtFS: right frontal sinus
RtGR: right rectal gyrus
RtHT: right hypothalamic wall
RticON: right intra-canalicular optic nerve
RtICV: right internal cerebral vein
RtiHA: right inferior hypophyseal artery
RtioON: right intraorbital nerve
RtIT: right inferior turbinectomy
RtLOCR: right lateral optico-carotid recess
RtLV: right lateral ventricle
RtM: right lateral tubercular portion of the meningioma
RtMO: right medial orbit
RtMT: right middle turbinate
RtNSF: right nasoseptal flap
RtOA: right ophthalmic artery
RtOAp: right medial orbital apex wall
RtOCR: right opticocarotid recess
RtON: right optic nerve
RtOT: right olfactory tract
RtPCA: right posterior cerebral artery
RT-PCR: reverse transcription polymerase chain reaction
RtpICA: right paraclival internal carotid artery
RtSCA: right superior cerebellar artery
RtscICA: right supraclinoid internal carotid artery
RtSO: right sphenoid ostium
RtsPEA: right posterior ethmoid artery
RtSV: right septal vein
RtT: right thalamus
RtTC: right lateral tumor capsule
RtTS: right lateral aspect of the tuberculum sellae

RtTV: right thalamic vein
SAH: subarachnoid hemorrhage
SAS: accessory sphenoid septum
SB: septal bone
SC: sphenoid cavity
SCA: superior cerebellar artery
SCC: semicircular canals
SCL: superior longitudinal band of the cruciform ligament
StCM: sternocleidomastoid muscle
SCM: superior constrictor muscles
SCSC: superior compartment of the cavernous sinus
SD: sella dura
sD: sphenoid divider
SDA: sinodural angle
SEPs: sensory evoked potentials
SER: sphenoethmoid recess
SF: sellar floor
SF1: steroidogenic factor 1
SH: seromucinous hamartoma
sHA: superior hypophyseal artery
SIADH: syndrome of inappropriate antidiuretic hormone secretion
SIR: Speech Intelligibility Rating
SK: sphenoid keel
sLM: sellar Liliequist membrane
SMA: smooth muscle actin
SMAS: superficial musculoaponeurotic system
SMG: submandibular gland
SN: sympathetic nerve
SNECs: sinonasal neuroendocrine carcinomas
SNUCs: sinonasal undifferentiated carcinomas
SO: sphenoid ostium/ostia
SOM: superior oblique muscle
SOF: superior orbital fissure
SP: soft palate
SyP: sympathetic plexus
SPA: sphenopalatine artery
sPA: superior petrous apex
SPF: sphenopalatine foramen
SPL: superior parasellar ligament
SpS: sphenoid sinus
SPS: superior petrosal sinus
SR: sphenoid rostrum
SRM: superior rectus muscle
SRS: stereotactic radiosurgery
SS: sigmoid sinus
SSCC: superior semicircular canal
SSD: single-sided deafness
SSF: sphenoid sinus floor
SSLR: sphenoid sinus lateral recess
SSTR: somatostatin receptors
ST: sella turcica
sT: superior turbinates
STH: somatotropic hormone
STIR: short tau inversion recovery
STR: subtotal resection
SV: septal vein
SV: short vertical
SVS: sphenovomerine suture
SW: sphenoid wall
SWM: sphenoid wing meningioma
T1W1: T1-weighted imaging
T2W1: T2-weighted imaging
TC: tumor capsule
TCAs: transcranial approaches
TCL: transverse band of the cruciform ligament
TF: temporal fossa
TFB: temporal fossa bone
TFD: temporal fossa dura
TFL: tensor fascia lata
TG: tissue glue
TGG: trigeminal ganglion
TGF-β1: transforming growth factor β1
TH: thalamus
TL: temporal lobe
TLD: temporal lobe dura
TM: tectorial membrane
TN: trigeminal neuralgia
TNFRSF11A: tumor necrosis factor receptor superfamily member-11A
TOF: time-of-flight
TPC: tumor pseudocapsule
TRANSSPHER: transsphenoidal nonfunctioning pituitary adenoma surgery
TrJOF: trabecular variant of juvenile ossifying fibroma
TSa Taming Sari
TSi: transverse sinus
TS: tuberculum sellae
TSH: thyroid-stimulating hormone
TSH-Oma: thyroid-stimulating hormone-producing adenoma
TSJ: transverse-sigmoid junction
TSM: tuberculum sellae meningioma
TT: tegmen tympani
TV: thalamic vein
UA: ultrasonic aspirator
UP: uncinate process

UPMC: University of Pittsburgh Medical Center
UPSIT: University of Pennsylvania smell identification test
V2: maxillary nerve
V3: mandibular nerve
VA: vertebral artery
VC: vidian canal
VCP: valosin-containing protein
VEGF: vascular endothelial growth factor
VFSS: videofluroscopic swallowing study
VHI: voice handicap index
VMAT: volumetric modulated arc therapy
VN: vestibular nerve
VP: venous plexus
Vp Vicryl patch
VPI: velopharyngeal incompetence
VT: trigeminal vein
WHO: World Health Organization

Section I

Pituitary Gland Tumors

Chapter 1

Pathologies of the Sellar Region

Michel Roethlisberger, Revadi Govindaraju, Jonathan Rychen, Adam Jadczak, Yves Brand, Jeyaganesh V., Kein Seong Mun, Jürgen Hench, Luigi Mariani, Prepageran Narayanan, and Vicknes Waran

Introduction to the Sellar Region

The sellar region contains numerous essential structures, which embryologically arise in a complex manner, resulting in tight neighborship of otherwise unrelated tissues. As the prime example, the pituitary gland contains epithelial structures, arising from the future oral cavity, differentiates into neuroendocrine cells, has a dedicated vascular network facilitating hormone release and at the same time comprises a direct junction to the central nervous system (CNS). Besides the pituitary gland, the sellar region also lies within the former anterior neuropore where germ cell progenitors are located in the embryo and at the same time is close to the anterior end of the former notochord, a cartilage-like structure still present in the early human embryo and evolution's first attempt toward bilateral symmetric creatures with a spinal cord that would later evolve into vertebrates and ultimately humans. Such a potpourri of highly specialized and very different progenitor cell lineages explains the often-confusing morphological appearance of tumors that most likely arise from these structures that typically have a midline orientation. Besides lesions caused by nonresident cell populations or external factors, such as meningiomas, metastases, apoplexy, or abscesses, the sellar region is highly enriched in rare, locoregionally specific neoplasms of extremely diverse cell-of-origin lineage.

Introduction to the Pituitary Gland

The anterior lobe of the pituitary gland or adenohypophysis integrates the hormonal signals controlling thyroid, adrenal, reproductive, and growth functions and is controlled by complex central and peripheral neuronal signals. These lead to trophic hormone secretion and reversible plastic changes in cell growth. Secreted hormones by the pituicytes are prolactin (PRL), growth hormone (GH), adrenocorticotropic hormone (ACTH), follicle-stimulating hormone (FSH), luteinizing hormone (LH), and thyroid-stimulating hormone (TSH). The posterior lobe of the pituitary gland, also named neurohypophysis, is a neural structure mainly involved in the secretion of antidiuretic hormone (ADH) and oxytocin. It is furthermore the interface between the CNS and endocrine system.

The pituitary gland is anatomically embedded within the sella turcica, contains remaining ectodermal as well as mesenchymal and stromal tissue and is highly vascularized. Hence, a broad variety of pituitary and non-pituitary neoplasms can arise from the sellar and parasellar regions. There is a broad variation in clinical manifestations, diagnostic evaluation, and treatment patterns between the different entities.

This chapter provides a comprehensive overview of common lesions of the pituitary gland. We present our institutional experience in treating these lesions with the endonasal endoscopic approach. We further describe the institution's principle with a tailored approach and zonal dissection of the base of skull adjusted to the individual characteristics of the lesion treated. Different variations and extensions of the transseptal transsphenoidal approach are described and demonstrated with a collection of surgical cases.

Pathologies and Its Variants

Diagnostic Approaches in Neuropathology

For about a century, histology represented the mainstay of neuropathological diagnostics. In contrast to general surgical pathology, where tumors are often diagnosed in a stepwise bioptic approach, neuropathologists are often forced to make their preliminary diagnosis within minutes based on intraoperative smears or touch-prep specimens, followed by hematoxylin and eosin (H&E)-stained cryosections of typically millimeter-sized specimens. Such a procedure is able to differentiate between neoplasia and reactive changes, and, in addition, frequently allows to significantly narrow down clinical differential diagnosis. While subsequent paraffin embedding of the biopsy tissue still represents the standard approach in many neuropathological laboratories, increasing awareness of robust molecular distinction systems has led to significant changes to the World Health Organization (WHO) tumor classifications.[1–3] While sequencing approaches alone are usually unable to define particular neoplasms, epigenetic mapping has, within only about 5 years, added an entirely novel layer to neuropathological routine diagnostics.[4] This approach is, since the introduction of light microscopy in pathological work-up in the 19th century, the first modality that is able to diagnose CNS-related tumors with higher granularity than an expert interpretation of histological slides. In fact, an overall misclassification rate of approximately 12% has been observed in a large, international, retrospective study.[4] The result of these efforts is an artificial intelligence–based system that is able to recognize the vast majority of all CNS-related tumors currently acknowledged by the WHO. The so-called classifier algorithm is publicly available for free. The underlying DNA methylation analysis works with both native and fixed tissue from which nucleic acids are extracted. Generally, a high content of vital lesional cells is required in the biopsy, and this aim can be achieved by close collaboration of the neurosurgeon and neuropathologist. Necrotic tissue, cauterized regions, or areas with very low tumor cell content are typically unsuited for methylome analysis. During intraoperative cryosection examination, the neurosurgeon can be advised to obtain an alternative specimen should the examined one be unsuitable. In addition, DNA extraction from native specimens leads to higher yield in DNA than from formalin-fixed, paraffin-embedded (FFPE) tissue. Hence, keeping intraoperatively frozen biopsies in their native state and using a few sections of those for DNA extraction is not only the fastest but also the most successful way of performing methylome analysis. Besides tumor classification, methylome analysis also reveals the genomic copy number profile of the sample at no extra cost, which can contain diagnostic, prognostic, and predictive information. Hence, from our experience, it is almost imperative for neurosurgeons and neuropathologists to make use of this timely approach of morphomolecular diagnostics. Still, immunohistochemistry plays its role, for example, in estimating proliferation fraction of a particular lesion, but its diagnostic yield has by far been superseded by methylomics. Still, many neuropathological institutions are not yet equipped to perform methylome analysis but affordable, even mobile options to subject specimens to this technique have been developed to achieve molecular tumor classification within approximately 6 hours (**Fig. 1.1**).[5] In the following sections, we will always refer to this map. To summarize, methylome testing allows for an optimized recognition of all lesions discussed in the following.

Pituitary Adenomas

The pathogenesis of pituitary adenomas is still under debate. Tumors emerging from this tissue are the result of a monoclonal outgrowth because of genetic alterations,[6–8] in combination with regulatory factors and epigenetic processes participating as part of the tumorigenesis.[9] Most likely a potential "secondary hit" leads to a monoclonal expansion of these cells.[10] This might be supported by the fact that incidental findings of pituitary microadenomas are extensively more frequent than the diagnosed disease itself.[10,11]

The current WHO classification recognizes eight types of pituitary adenomas (**Table 1.1**).[1–4,12] By contrast, recent classification based on DNA methylation patterns has so far allowed separation of seven adenoma types, several of which correspond to those histological entities.[4] The current WHO classification has currently dropped the previous concept of so-called atypical pituitary adenomas, which used to be the term to describe tumors with increased proliferation rate and nuclear p53 accumulation.[1–4,12] This has been toned down to "the Ki-67 proliferation index that can be used as a parameter for prognostic evaluation of individual adenomas," which leaves us with no more grading scheme. In addition, the WHO has introduced a series of more or less specific immunohistochemical parameters aiming at the differentiation of eight major adenoma cell lineages, the majority of which contains several subgroups.[1–4,12] These novel entity designations partially match unbiased lineage distinction by methylation profiling, while some subtypes bear a significant ambiguity risk upon histological examination. In sum, endocrinological blood testing should remain the standard of care to clinically define adenoma. Histological examination can reveal significantly increased proliferation rates and to some extent tumor types that tend to be more aggressive. Finally, methylation profiling should be used to make hard distinctions between tumor types, which, in addition, feature type-specific copy number profiles. Local aggressiveness is currently best assessed by macroscopic appearance (radiographically or intraoperatively), while the rare case of pituitary carcinoma depends on unambiguous metastatic spread, hence remaining a clinical distinction.

The prevalence of all pituitary adenomas per 100,000 was recently reported to be as high as 77.6 in an epidemiological study from England and has most likely been underestimated in older studies.[13] Standardized incidence rates per 100,000 for all pituitary adenomas are reported as 4 in a population-based study in Northern Finland from cases diagnosed between 1992 and 2007.[14]

Clinically confirmed prognostic factors for pituitary adenomas are as follows:

- *Tumor size*: Anatomical extension of the tumor is usually determined by magnetic resonance imaging (MRI). Pituitary adenomas are generally divided into "micro" (<10 mm), "macro" (>10 mm), and "giant" (≥40 mm) adenomas.
- *Invasiveness*: MRI determines the invasive behavior of pituitary adenoma. Described correlates are cavernous sinus, sphenoid or ethmoid bone invasion. Cavernous sinus invasion is prognostically relevant and has initially been described by Knosp et al. (**Table 1.2**).[15]

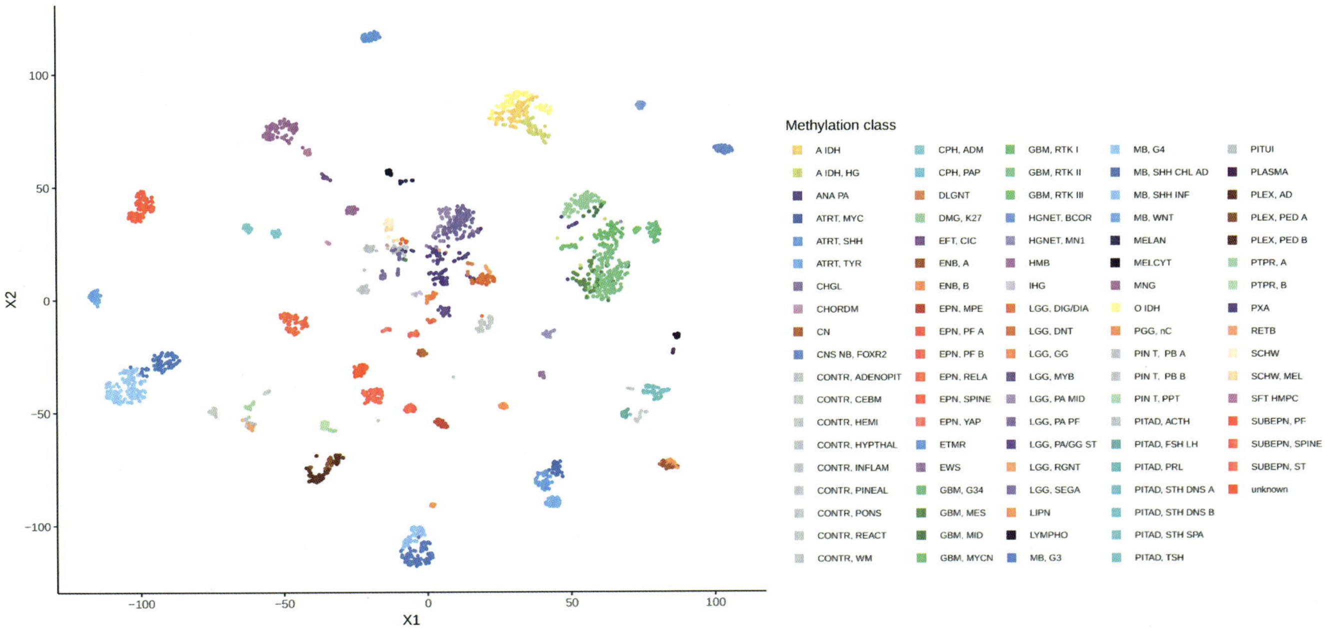

Fig. 1.1 *t-SNE plot of the Brain Tumor Classifier Reference* Cohort: UMAP/t-SNE contains the currently approved epigenetic landscape of CNS-related tumors and locoregional tissues.[4,5] Each dot represents the methylome dataset of a single specimen. Coloring indicates the methylation class. Of note, dimension reduction algorithms are able to distinguish these methylomes in an entity-specific way. The respective methylation classes have been defined by the German Cancer Research Centre (DKFZ) and their abbreviations are shown in the legend. The full descriptions of these molecular tumor entities can be viewed at http://www.molecularneuropathology.org. This is a public service provided free of charge. This plot was created with nanoDx.[5]

- *Proliferation rate*: Prior to the current WHO classification, morphological criteria of pituitary adenoma were assessed in FFPE, H&E, and silver-stained resection specimens, augmented by immunohistochemistry. These criteria were used to classify the tumors. Proliferative activity was determined with the mitotic count, proliferative fraction/Ki-67 labeling index, and p53[1,8,16–20] and have more clinical value nowadays. Absolute cutoff values have been removed from the current WHO classification.[1–4,12]
- *Extrasellar extension*: Pituitary adenomas extending beyond the sella turcica have to be distinguished clinically.[21] Wilson et al. initially described this relevant morphological criterion (**Table 1.3**).[22] Besides this, nodular extensions seem to be relevant for the surgical outcome, as recently described by Mooney et al. (**Table 1.4**).[23]

A gray zone of pituitary adenomas exhibiting aggressive behaviors remains. They distinguish themselves with rapid growth, early and frequent recurrence, and resistance to conventional treatment.[24] Those lesions never develop metastasis but show a clearly worse outcome and higher retreatment rates than regular pituitary adenomas.

Currently, the morphology of FFPE, H&E, and silver-stained resection specimens, augmented by immunohistochemistry for Ki-67 (MIB-1), p53 cytokeratins, synaptophysin, and peptide hormones, primarily aids in discriminating these tumors from non-pituitary gland lesions.[10–15] To date, there is no neuropathological procedure to make solid statements about aggressiveness.[25]

Infrequently, pituitary adenomas extend beyond their anatomical limits and invade surrounding structures.[26] Despite extensive clinical, histological, and molecular workup, it is currently impossible to predict their potential outcome, that is a more invasive phenotype, which would likely be associated with disease relapse.[21] Patients at high risk for a more aggressive behavior would potentially profit from tighter surveillance, prophylactic measures, and earlier interventions.[26] Indeed, recent data suggest diverging, subtype-specific pathogenic pathways, which, if identified beforehand, might supersede the current classification based on histology and immunohistochemistry.[1,16,27]

Because of the fact that despite a lower grade such tumors exhibit a more aggressive behavior, newer studies suggest an adaption of a more clinically useful terminology. Hence, the WHO morphofunctional as opposed to the DNA

Table 1.1 The various morphofunctional pituitary adenoma types are compared to lineage-specific methylation patterns that correlate with biological tumor entities[1–5,12]

Adenoma type	Immunophenotype	Transcription factors	Methylation class
Somatotroph adenomas			
Densely granulated somatotroph adenoma	GH ± PRL ± alpha subunit, LMWCK: perinuclear or diffuse	PIT1	*Pituitary adenomas, STH producing, densely granulated:* Two distinct methylation classes (group A and B) of unknown clinical significance. STH densely granulated, group A: Tumors with the histological diagnosis pituitary adenoma (STH producing, densely granulated). Median age is 45 years (range 37–59). Additional characteristic molecular features of this class are not known. Numeric whole chromosome changes are frequent in this class, with gains of chromosomes 3, 5, 7, 8, 9, 12, and 20 and loss of chromosomes 15 and 22 in over 50% of cases. STH densely granulated, group B: Tumors with the histological diagnosis pituitary adenoma (STH producing, densely granulated) but also single cases with different histological diagnosis. Median age is 47.5 years (range 18–75). Additional characteristic molecular features of this class are not known. While some cases show chromosomal imbalances in copy number analysis, highly recurrent chromosomal alterations are not observed.
Sparsely granulated somatotroph adenoma	GH ± PRL, LMWCK: dot-like (fibrous bodies)	PIT1	*Pituitary adenoma, STH sparsely granulated* Tumors with the histological diagnosis pituitary adenoma (STH producing, sparsely granulated) but also single cases with different histological diagnosis. Median age is 48 years (range 30–71). Additional characteristic molecular features of this class are not known. While some cases show chromosomal imbalances in copy number analysis, highly recurrent large chromosomal alterations are not observed.
Mammosomatotroph adenoma	GH + PRL (in same cell) ± alpha subunit	PIT1, ER-alpha	–
Mixed somatotroph and lactotroph adenoma	GH + PRL (in different cells) ± alpha subunit	PIT1, ER-alpha	–
Lactotroph adenomas			
Sparsely granulated lactotroph adenoma	PRL	PIT1, ER-alpha	*Pituitary adenoma, prolactin* Tumors with the histological diagnosis pituitary adenoma (prolactin producing) and "atypical" pituitary adenoma. Median age is 57 years (range 12–78). Additional characteristic molecular features of this class are not known. Numeric whole chromosome changes are frequent in this class, with gain of chromosomes 3, 5, 7, 8, 9, 12, 14, and 19 in over 60% of cases.
Densely granulated lactotroph adenoma	PRL	PIT1, ER-alpha	
Acidophilic stem cell adenoma	PRL, GH (focal and inconstant), LMWCK: fibrous bodies (inconstant)		
Thyrotroph adenoma			
	TSH-beta, alpha subunit	PIT1, GATA2	*Pituitary adenoma, TSH* Tumors with the histological diagnosis pituitary adenoma (TSH producing). Median age is 43 years (range 23–69). Additional characteristic molecular features of this class are not known. Numeric whole chromosome changes are frequent in this class, with gains of chromosomes 7 and 14 and loss of chromosomes 1p and 11 in over 50% of cases.

Adenoma type	Immunophenotype	Transcription factors	Methylation class
Corticotroph adenomas			
Densely granulated corticotroph adenoma	ACTH, LMWCK: diffuse pattern	TPIT	*Pituitary adenoma, ACTH* Tumors with the histological diagnosis pituitary adenoma (ACTH producing). Median age is 46 years (range 19–67). Additional characteristic molecular features of this class are not known. While some cases show chromosomal imbalances in copy number analysis, highly recurrent chromosomal alterations are not observed.
Sparsely granulated corticotroph adenoma	ACTH, LMWCK: diffuse pattern	TPIT	
Crooke cell adenoma	ACTH, LMWCK: ring-like pattern	TPIT	
Gonadotroph adenoma			
Sparsely granulated gonadotroph adenoma	FSH-beta, LH-beta, alpha subunit (various combinations)	SF1, GATA2, ER-alpha (variable)	*Pituitary adenoma, FSH/LH* Tumors with the histological diagnosis gonadotropin-producing pituitary adenoma and to a lesser extent "atypical" pituitary adenomas. Median age is 65 years (range 18–79). Additional characteristic molecular features of this class are not known. Large recurrent chromosomal alterations are not observed and most cases show a flat profile in copy number analysis.
Null cell adenoma			
	No markers	None	–
Plurihormonal adenomas			
Plurihormonal PIT1-positive adenoma	GH, PRL, TSH-beta ± alpha subunit	PIT1	–
Adenomas with unusual immunohistochemical combinations	Various combinations	Other transcription factors (variable)	–
Double adenomas			
Distinct adenomas	Usually PRL and ACTH, respectively	PIT1 and TPIT, respectively	–

Abbreviations: ACTH, adrenocorticotropin hormone; ER, estrogen receptor; FSH, follicle-stimulating hormone; GH, growth hormone; LH, luteinizing hormone; LMWCK, low-molecular weight cytokeratin; PRL, prolactin; SF1, steroidogenic factor 1; STH, somatotropic hormone; TSH, thyroid-stimulating hormone.

Note: Morphofunctional descriptions modified from WHO classification 61 and methylation classes adapted from brain tumor classifier version v11b4 63.[1–5,12] Note that in particular, those morphofunctional types that have ambiguous immunohistochemical staining patterns do not form distinct methylation classes. In general, the overlap between methylation patterns, combined with entity-specific chromosomal aberrations, is negligible.

Table 1.2 Knosp grading system for the parasellar extension of pituitary macroadenoma defined by invasion of the cavernous sinus on the basis of MRI.[15] The Knosp grade 3 can be subdivided as proposed by Micko et al.[330]

Grade	Parasellar extension
0	Adenoma does not extend the medial carotid line
1	Adenoma crosses the medial line not extending past the intercarotid line
2	Adenoma extends beyond the intercarotid line but not laterally to the cavernous carotid artery
3	Adenoma extends laterally to the cavernous carotid artery
3A	Adenoma extends superiorly to the lateral line
3B	Adenoma extends inferiorly to the lateral line
4	Cavernous carotid artery is completely encased by adenoma

Table 1.3 Wilson's grading system for the extrasellar extension of pituitary adenomas[22]

Stage	Suprasellar extension
O	No suprasellar extension
A	Extension into suprasellar cistern only
B	Extension into anterior recess of the third ventricle
C	Obliteration of anterior recess and deformation of floor of third ventricle
D	Intradural extension into anterior, middle, or posterior fossa
E	Extradural invasion into cavernous sinus

Table 1.4 The TRANSSPHER grading system for independent predictors of gross total resection in a prospective multicenter trial of transsphenoidal pituitary surgery for nonfunctioning pituitary adenomas

Point	Nonfunctioning pituitary adenoma characteristic	
1	Tumor diameter > 40 mm in any plane	
1	Knosp's grades 3–4	
1	Nodular extension	
Sum	Likelihood of achieving gross total resection (%)	
	Multicenter cohort	**Combined multicenter and validation cohort**
0	90	89
1	63	54
2	33	25
3	0	17

Note: The TRANSSPHER-grading system is based on readily measurable characteristics that predict the likelihood of achieving gross total resection after transsphenoidal surgery.
Source: Adapted from Mooney et al.[23]

methylation-based classification does have similarities and discrepancies (**Table 1.1**).

In a more clinical approach, Dai et al.[28] proposed the designation "refractory pituitary adenoma" to define this subgroup with the following:

- High Ki-67 index/rapid growth
- Early and high frequency of recurrence
- Resistance to conventional treatments and/or salvage treatment
- Poor prognosis
- Lack of cerebrospinal fluid (CSF) or systemic metastases

Recently Raverot et al. integrated the criteria of invasiveness and proliferative activity in a grading system for sporadic pituitary adenomas (**Table 1.5**).[29]

Pituitary Carcinoma

The current WHO classification distinguishes a clinical-pathological entity termed pituitary carcinoma, defined solely by confirmed metastatic spread.[30] While pituitary adenomas are frequent lesions, the latter is extraordinarily rare.[8] Radiological and neurosurgical work-up, and, to a minimal extent, neuropathological examination of the resection specimen can only give hints about a potential invasive component.[31] The presence of metastases that spread into other organs including brain and even CSF dissemination is suggestive for this entity.[1,16,32]

Null Cell Adenoma

This entity describes benign pituitary tumors without any clinical or immunohistochemical evidence of hormonal production usually presenting as pituitary macroadenomas (**Table 1.1**).[33]

Pituitary Hyperplasia

Underlying extracranial diseases may influence the trophic activity of the pituitary gland and lead to hyperplasia presenting as sellar mass. Most commonly, a lactotroph hyperplasia during pregnancy is seen. Primary hypothyroidism[34,35]

Table 1.5 Grading system for sporadic pituitary adenomas based on invasiveness and proliferative activity

Grade	Invasiveness and proliferative activity
1a	Noninvasive tumor
1b	Noninvasive and proliferative tumor
2a	Invasive tumor
2b	Invasive and proliferative tumor
3	Metastatic tumor (cerebrospinal or systemic metastases)

Source: Adapted from Raverot et al. 2014.[29]

and hypogonadism[36] are associated with thyrotroph and gonadotroph hyperplasia, while ectopic secretion of GH-releasing hormone leads to somatotroph hyperplasia.[37,38] However, from a neuropathological point of view, the hypothesis of hyperplasia has to be rejected in case of clonal expansion of cells sharing the same genomic aberration.

Nonpituitary Lesions of the Sellar and Parasellar Region

The sellar and parasellar region can be the site of other neoplastic and nonneoplastic mass lesions that should be considered in the differential diagnosis of pituitary adenomas (**Table 1.6**).

Craniopharyngioma

Craniopharyngiomas are solid or partially cystic tumors originating along the vestiges of the stomodeal diverticulum. They are encountered most commonly in the region of the infundibular stalk where remnant epithelial tissue forms Rathke's pouch. Specific features are addressed in Chapter 7.

Meningioma

Meningiomas originate in the parasellar leptomeninges. They can involve the sella either as isolated intrasellar lesion or as part of meningiomas arising from the tuberculum sella, the planum sphenoidale, the diaphragma sella, and rarely the anterior clinoid process. Larger meningioma of the skull base arising from the sphenoid wing or the petroclival region can involve the sella and parasellar region as well. Specific features are addressed in Chapter 11.

Chordoma

Chordomas are locally aggressive or malignant midline tumors originating from notochordal elements with a characteristic slow growth pattern. They are mainly of parasellar location in the region of the clivus or the craniocervical junction. Specific features are addressed in Chapter 15.

Germ Cell Tumors

These are midline tumors that are diagnosed within the first three decades of life. They represent 1% of all intracranial tumors in adults and approximately 6% in children.[33] They are most frequently encountered in the pineal gland region, but may appear in the sella as well. Bifocal synchronous lesions have been described.[39]

Metastases

They can radiographically mimic any locoregional tumor type; however, metastasis of the sellar region does feature distinctive histological and molecular characteristics typical of the respective primary tumor.[40,41]

Cystic Lesions of the Sella

Many lesions that are found within the sella may be cystic in nature, for example, craniopharyngioma, meningioma, pituitary adenoma, and metastases. Also, nonneoplastic and reactive changes, such as Rathke's cleft cyst (RCC), can appear cystic. In the case of only reactive and resorptive residual tissue, the term xanthogranuloma of the sellar region is used[33,42–46] (**Table 1.6**).

Cystic Pituitary Adenoma

Pituitary adenomas may be cystic in nature. These cysts develop because of necrosis, hemorrhage, or cystic degeneration.[46–48]

Cystic Craniopharyngioma

Craniopharyngioma can appear as isolated cystic intrasellar masses.[46–48] Specific features are addressed in Chapter 7.

Cystic Meningioma

Suprasellar meningiomas have been described to develop a cystic configuration in rare occasions.[46] The latter may be the result of necrosis, intratumoral hemorrhage, or entrapped CSF.[49,50]

Table 1.6 Nonpituitary lesions of the sella and differential diagnosis of cystic intrasellar lesions

Benign tumors	
	Craniopharyngioma
	Meningioma
	Neurohypophyseal gangliocytoma
	Neurohypophyseal glioma
	Granular cell tumor
	Spindle cell oncocytoma
Malignant tumors	
Primary	Germ cell tumor (ectopic pinealoma)
	Sarcoma
	Chordoma and other soft tissue and bone tumors
	Neurohypophyseal high-grade glioma
Secondary	Lung carcinoma
	Breast carcinoma
Pituitary hyperplasia	
	Lactotroph hyperplasia (during pregnancy)
	Thyrotroph and gonadotroph hyperplasia
	Somatotroph hyperplasia because of ectopic GHRH
Cysts	
	Cystic pituitary adenoma
	Cystic craniopharyngioma
	Rathke's cleft cyst
	Arachnoid cyst
	Cystic meningioma
	Sphenoid sinus mucocele
	Cystic epidermoid and dermoid
	Cystircercosis
	Pituitary abscess
	Giant aneurysm
	Aneurysmal bone cysts of the sphenoid
Empty sella syndrome	
Vascular lesions	
	Saccular aneurysm
	Carotid arteriovenous fistula
	Cavernous malformation
Inflammatory lesions	
	Lymphocytic hypophysitis
	Granulomatous hypophysitis

Abbreviation: GHRH, growth hormone–releasing hormone.
Sources: Adapted from Louis et al. 2016 and Snyder et al. 2008.[2,46]

Rathke's Cleft Cyst

RCCs are thought to originate from the embryonic remnants of Rathke's pouch.[46,51] The development of RCC occurs when a rostral outpouching of the primitive oral cavity occurring at the third or fourth week of gestation meets a downward projection from the diencephalon.[42,52] Normally small Rathke's cleft remnant cysts exist in the pars intermedia.[53] The unilocular cysts are between the anterior and posterior pituitary lobes and have a watery to proteinaceous content. The cyst wall is composed of cuboidal and ciliated cells, with occasional goblet cells and metaplastic squamous epithelium (**Fig. 1.2**). CSF-like fluid or more proteinaceous, mucoid fluid with high protein concentration, cholesterol, or methemoglobin can be found.[48]

Intrasellar Arachnoid Cyst

Arachnoid cysts can develop anywhere in the subarachnoid space and therefore rarely be the cause of an intrasellar cystic lesion.[44–46] Small defects in the diaphragma sellae might allow arachnoid tissue to herniate into the sella. If separated, they might appear as intrasellar lesions.[44,45] Another theory suggests small arachnoid remnants below the diaphragma sellae as origin of these lesions.[43,54]

Epidermoid and Dermoid Cysts

These are developmental lesions from misplaced squamous or dermoid tissue during neural tube closure. They are most commonly encountered as extra- or intradural masses and contain white waxy material.[46] When arising in the sella or the parasellar region, these lesions are located paramedian.[55] Dermoid cysts on the contrary are typically found in the midline and contain desquamated epithelium, sebaceous material, and dermal appendages[55] (**Fig. 1.3**). Intraoperatively, they appear white and flaky.[46] Strictly speaking, distinction of a mature monodermal teratoma and a dysontogenetic lesion is only possible on the basis of genomic sequencing, and hence not made in daily routine diagnostics, since such distinction is of very little clinical relevance.

Mucoceles

Mucoceles originating in the paranasal sinuses are defined as nonneoplastic epithelial-lined cystic masses containing mucinous secretions with inflammatory reaction.[56,57] Mucoceles share features of pseudostratified ciliated respiratory mucosa (**Fig. 1.4**). They most commonly occur in the frontal and ethmoid sinuses.[58,59] Mucoceles arising from the sphenoid sinus comprise only 1 to 2% of all cases.[59,60] The underlying pathomechanism might be the obstruction of the sphenoid sinus ostium.[46] Intracranial involvement is described in the literature with 12 to 20%, involving the sellar floor or clivus.[57,61] Pure intrasellar mucoceles are extremely rare and are encountered postoperatively after transsphenoidal surgeries.[62,63]

Synchronous Lesions of the Sellar Region

The body of literature reveals a variety of pathologies coexisting in the sellar and parasellar region.[64,65] The presence of a so-called concurrent or synchronous tumor is confirmed by colocalization of two morphologically distinct tumors arising within the sellar and parasellar region.[66] A collision tumor is present, when two tumor types are growing into one another, which has to be differentiated from tumor-to-tumor metastasis.[67]

Pituitary Adenoma as Part of Synchronous Lesions

Pituitary adenomas as most frequent sellar lesions vary from nonfunctioning to functioning adenomas, while the second lesions have a broad variety of entities.[40,41,64,65,68–81] Reported synchronous lesions consist of second pituitary adenoma entity,[68] Rathke's cleft cyst,[64] meningioma,[66,69–75] craniopharyngioma,[77] neurosarcoidosis,[64] gangliocytoma,[64,78] schwannoma,[64] metastasis,[40,41] esthesioneuroblastoma,[79] and vascular lesions[80,81] among others.

Pituitary Adenoma and Meningioma

Predominantly, GH-secreting pituitary adenomas are reported in coexistence with meningiomas.[66,69–71] A syndromic entity or obvious pathophysiological connection has not been found to date,[65,82] when the history of radiotherapy is absent.[83] Several pathophysiological mechanisms are discussed in the literature including secretion of growth factor that initiates the growth of another lesion.[65] Especially the case of GH-producing pituitary adenoma inducing arachnoid cap cell transformation to meningioma is discussed, as this synchronous tumor seems to be the most frequently reported entity.[66,69–74,82,84,85]

Pituitary Abscess

Abscesses involving the sellar region are rare. Smaller series demonstrate that neither clinical signs nor imaging studies including computed tomography (CT) and MRI were sufficiently reliable in diagnosing abscesses preoperatively and distinguishing them from pituitary adenomas. The patients did present more frequently with locoregional mass symptoms instead of classical features including fever, leukocytosis, and meningism.[86]

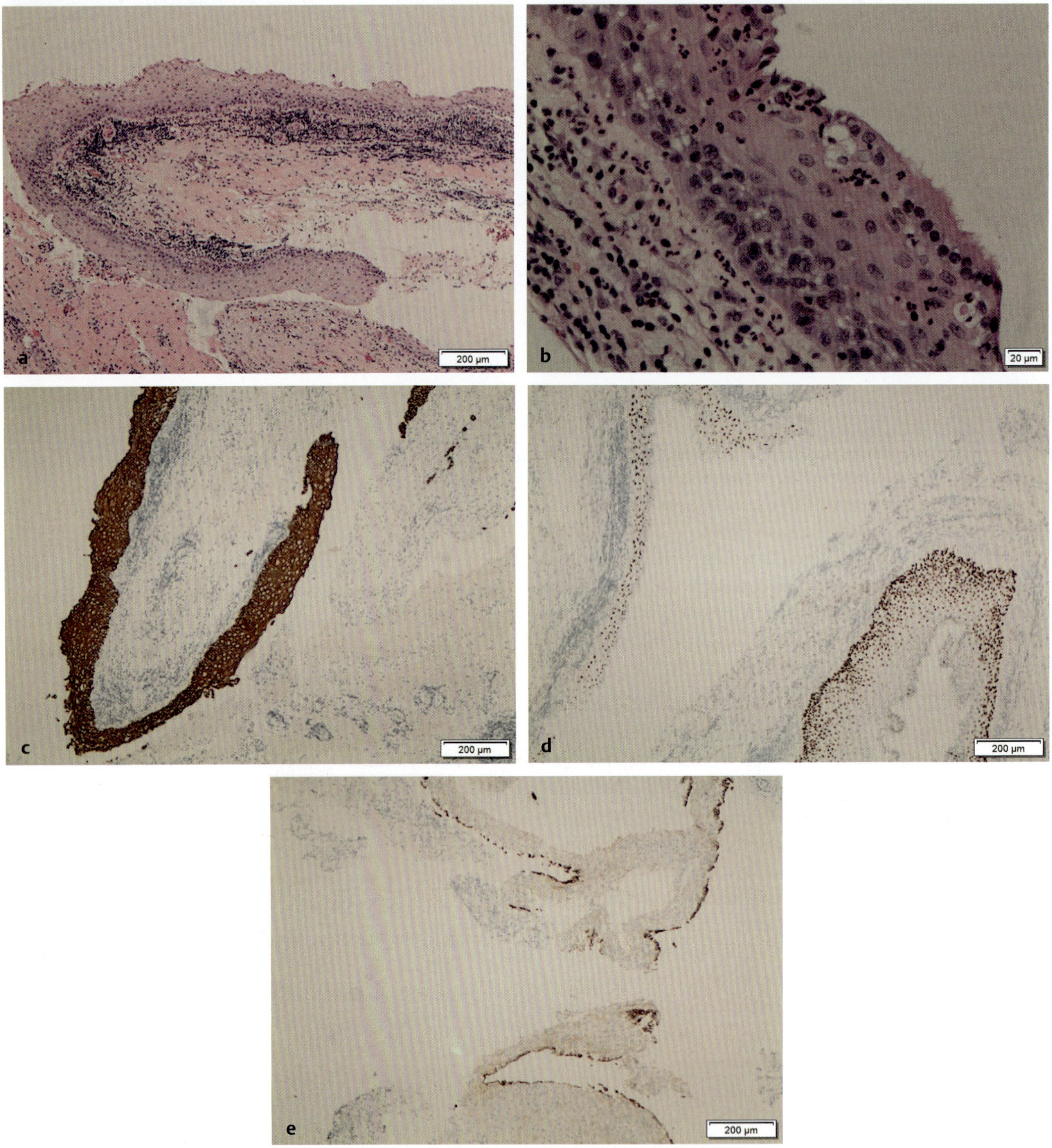

Fig. 1.2 Histomorphological features of a Rathke's cleft cyst with squamous metaplasia. The lesion shows a fibrocollagenous cyst wall with foci of inflammation (predominantly chronic). The cyst wall is lined by mainly stratified squamous epithelium, which in focal areas show remnant superficial ciliated columnar cell layers. Clusters of foamy macrophages are also seen. No pituitary tissue, dysplasia, increase in mitosis, or any evidence of malignancy is present. Immunohistochemistry: The epithelium is positive for MNF116, with the glandular component staining EMA-positive and the squamoid component staining p63-positive. **(a)** Sheets of the cyst wall show inflamed fibrous tissue lined by stratified squamous epithelium (hematoxylin & eosin, original magnification × 40). **(b)** Focal areas of the cyst wall lining show a remnant ciliated columnar cell layer. Scattered foamy macrophages are also seen (hematoxylin & eosin, original magnification × 200). The epithelial lining is positive for **(c)** MNF116, **(d)** p63, and **(e)** EMA (original magnification × 40). The correlating radiological and intraoperative features of the same case are demonstrated in **Fig. 1.34**.

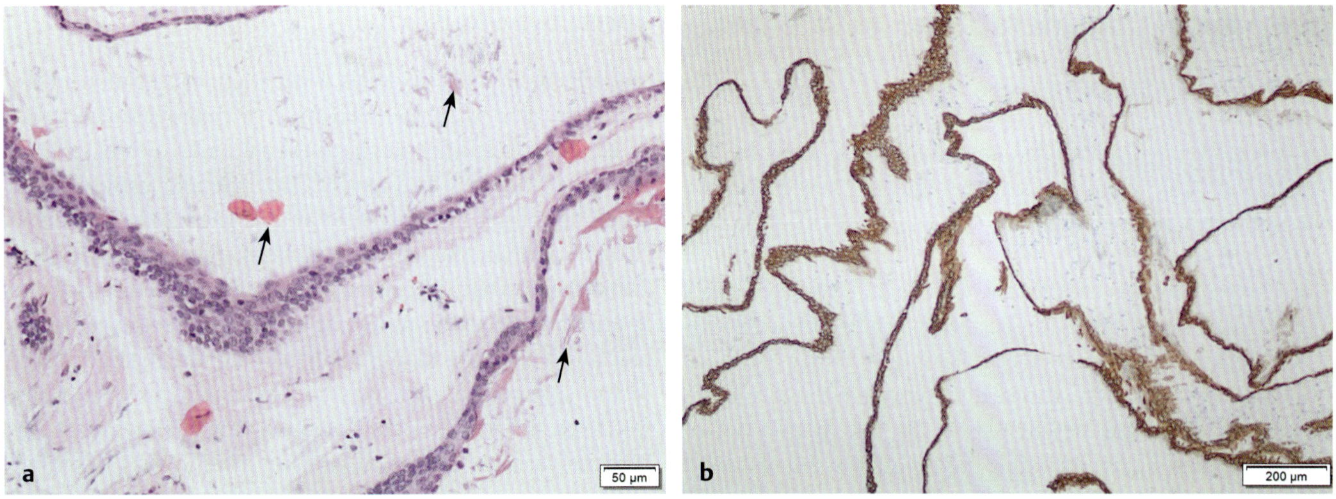

Fig. 1.3 Histomorphological features of an epidermoid cyst. The morphology presents itself as a cystic lesion with thin fibrous walls lined by keratinizing squamous epithelium and containing clumps of amorphous grayish material as well as scattered anucleate squames. No skin adnexae or immature/malignant elements are seen. The lining cells are strongly positive for MNF116, focally positive for EMA, and negative for GFAP. **(a)** The cyst wall is lined by stratified nonkeratinizing squamous epithelium with loose squames (*arrows*) (hematoxylin & eosin, original magnification × 100). **(b)** The lining epithelium is strongly positive for MNF116 (MNF116 antibody, original magnification × 40).

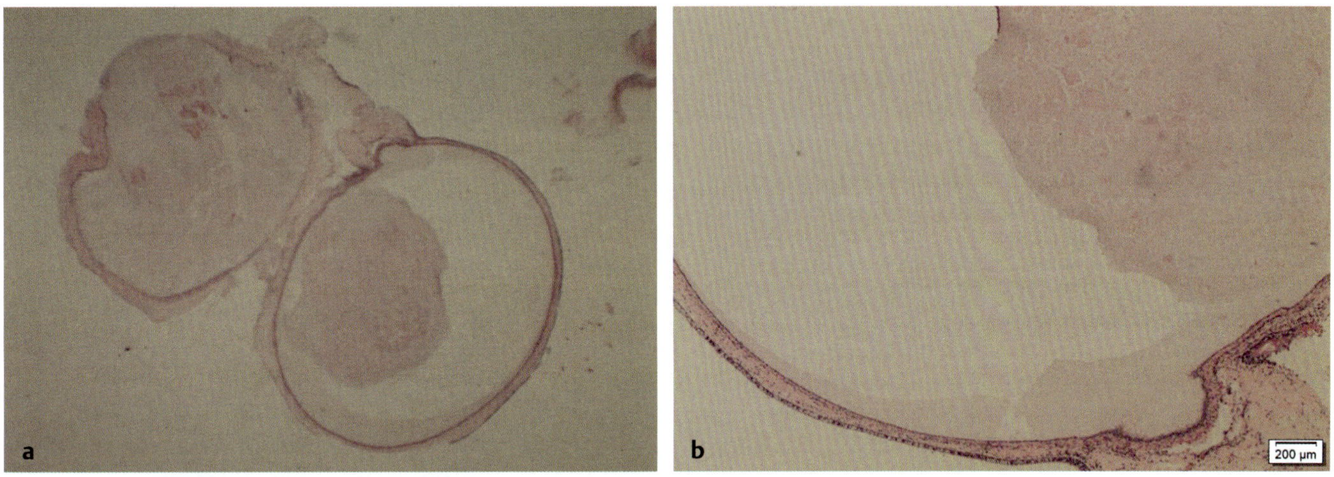

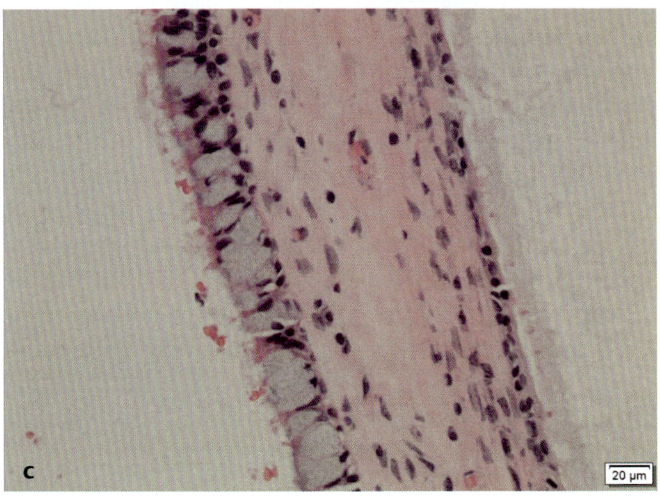

Fig. 1.4 Histomorphological features of a paranasal sinus mucocele. The lesion shows two cystic structures with thin fibrous tissue walls lined and covered by benign respiratory-type epithelium with goblet cells and cilia. Other areas of the cyst are lined by attenuated low cuboidal, focally ciliated, epithelium. The contents are pinkish mucoid secretions. Also present are fragments of inflamed fibrous tissue, lined in areas by respiratory epithelium and admixed with bits of lamellar bone. No malignancy seen. **(a)** Two intact cysts with thin walls, containing pale pinkish secretions (hematoxylin & eosin, original magnification × 4). **(b)** Thin fibrous wall lined by single-layered benign epithelium (hematoxylin & eosin, original magnification × 20). **(c)** Left surface shows ciliated respiratory type epithelial lining with goblet cells, right surface is lined by single layered benign cuboidal cells (hematoxylin & eosin, original magnification × 200). The correlating radiological and intraoperative features of the same case are demonstrated in (**Fig. 1.38**).

Anatomical Considerations

The Base of Skull Regions

The base of skull is a complex anatomical area that can be divided into four main anatomical regions. These defined areas require a tailored approach concept, if they need to be approached surgically:[87,88]

- *Anterior midline skull base*: The region between the frontal sinus and the posterior ethmoidal arteries (**Fig. 1.5a–c**).
- *Middle skull base*: The region between the planum sphenoidale and the sellar floor (**Fig. 1.6a, b**).
- *Parasellar region*: Including the cavernous sinuses and Meckel's cave areas (**Fig. 1.7**).
- *Posterior midline skull base*: The region between the clivus and the craniovertebral junction (**Fig. 1.8** and **Fig. 1.9**).

This anatomical orientation in the sagittal and coronal plane allows access to different pathologies of the base of skull. The most common pathologies in the sagittal plane are pituitary macroadenoma, CSF leak, meningocele or encephalocele, meningioma, craniopharyngioma, Rathke's cleft cyst, esthesioneuroblastoma, chondrosarcoma, chordoma, craniovertebral invagination, and inflammatory pannus. The most common pathologies in the coronal plane are inverted papilloma, sinonasal tumors, trigeminal schwannoma, cholesterol granuloma, cholesteatoma, hemangioma, and extensive nasopharyngeal tumors.[87,88]

Endonasal Landmarks

The first identifiable structures when entering either the right or the left nostril are the inferior turbinate, the middle turbinate, and the nasal septum. When the middle turbinate is mobilized medially, the uncinate process and the ethmoidal bulla enclosing the semilunar hiatus are identifiable located in the middle nasal cavity. When the head of the middle turbinate is dislocated laterally, the space between the middle turbinate and the nasal septum is widened. This allows posterior exposition of the middle nasal cavity to reach the anterior wall of the sphenoid sinus in a transnasal approach.[89–91]

The tail of the inferior turbinate extends posteriorly and limits the choana laterally, while the vomer defines the medial and the floor of the sphenoid sinus its superior limitation. It forms the roof of the choana followed by the sphenoethmoidal recess, and the sphenoid ostium, which is usually located approximately 1.5 cm superiorly[87,88] (**Fig. 1.10**).

Sphenoid Sinus

The sphenoid sinus occupies a geographical location in the skull base and is surrounded by vital neurovascular structures. Various studies describe the superior turbinate to be the best landmark to identify the sphenoid ostium.[89–93] A study performed by Halawi et al. analyzed 202 CT scans of patients without history of paranasal sinus surgery.[94] They found that the natural ostium of the sphenoid sinus is located approximately at the midpoint of the sphenoid face. When measured from the planum sphenoidale, the mean distance to the sphenoid ostium was approximately 11 mm (range 4–19), or 45.5% of the total sphenoid height. However, a significant variable degree of pneumatization was described in the study, and the ostium was closer to the base of skull with lesser degree of pneumatization. In detail, the sphenoid ostium was closer to the planum sphenoidale when a sellar or presellar pneumatization was present, compared to sinuses with postsellar pneumatization.[94]

While the sphenoid ostia are the main landmark in the anterior wall of the sphenoid sinus, the posterior wall is dominated by several bony protuberances and depressions formed by the critical neurovascular structures of the base of skull.[87,88] Shape and extent of these landmarks vary according to the extent of pneumatization.[95]

Sella Turcica and Diaphragma Sellae

The sella turcica, a symmetric depression in the posteromedian aspect of the posterior sphenoid wall, is the main midline landmark. The anterior margin is formed by the tuberculum sellae in the midline and by the opticocarotid recesses and anterior clinoid processes bilaterally (**Fig. 1.11**). The posterior margin is formed by the dorsum sellae in the midline and by the posterior clinoid processes bilaterally (**Fig. 1.12**). The sellar floor is usually a thin layer of bone.[87,88,95]

The roof of the sella turcica is formed by the diaphragma sellae, a dural membrane that lies in continuation with the tentorium cerebelli, and provides the entry point for the infundibular stalk and the supplying vascular structures.[96] It is composed of two layers of dura mater and shows a remarkable variation in morphology of the diaphragmal opening.[96] The diaphragma sellae lies between the superior aspect of the pituitary gland and defines the inferior limitation of the suprasellar cistern.[97] A cadaveric study performed by Campero et al. described an average anteroposterior distance of 7.2 mm (range 3–11 mm) and the average lateral-to-lateral distance of 7.33 mm (range 4–14 mm). It is postulated

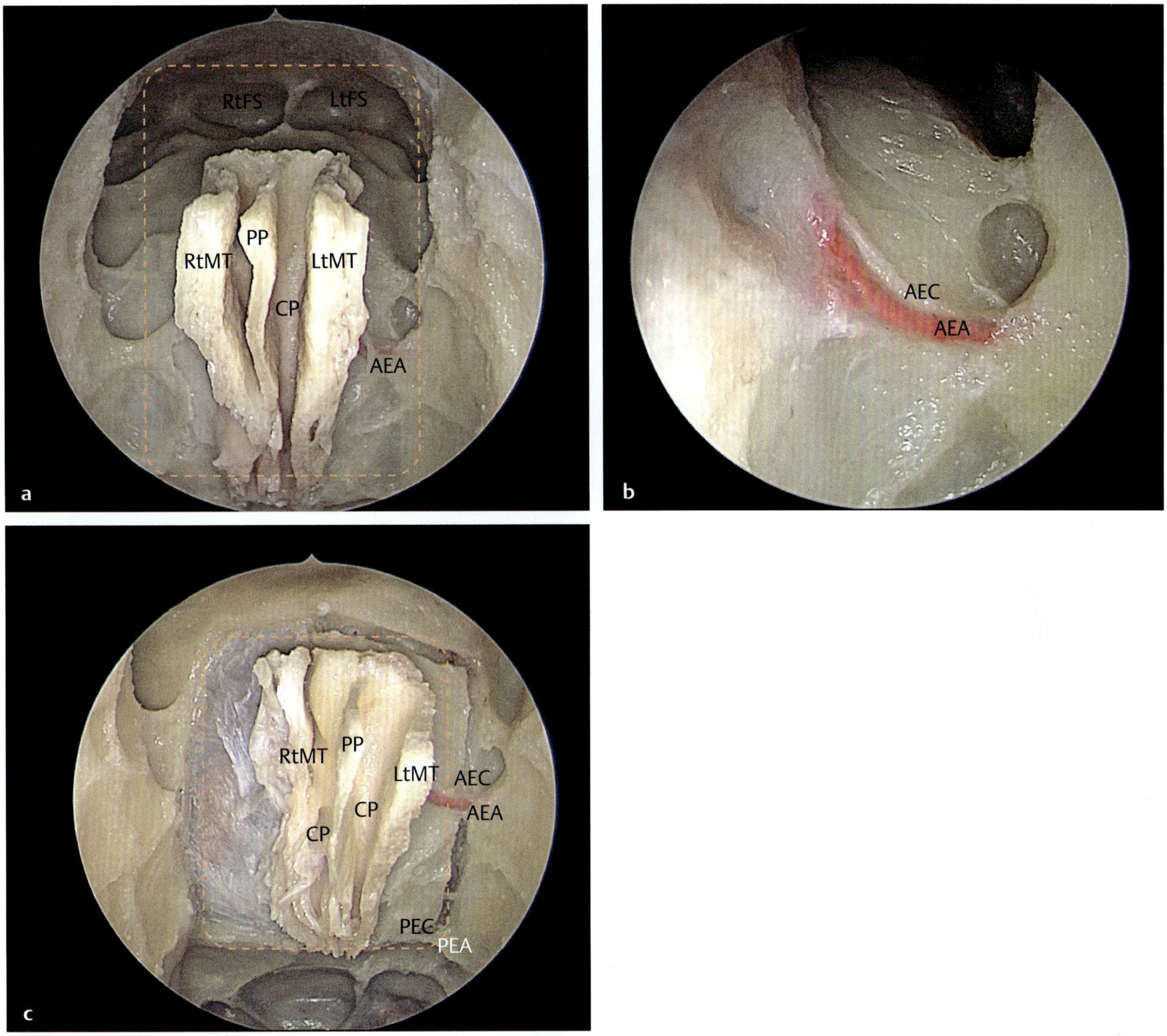

Fig. 1.5 The anterior midline skull base (*orange square*) extends from the left (LtFS) and right (RtFS) frontal sinuses to the posterior ethmoidal arteries. **(a)** Exposition of the anterior midline skull base with the midline defined by the perpendicular plate (PP) of ethmoid, and the insertion of the left (LtMT) and right (RtMT) middle turbinates into the base of skull. In between, the cribriform plate (CP) is visible. **(b)** A close-up view of the anterior ethmoidal artery (AEA) with the accompanying nerve, coursing posterolaterally from the orbit, then anteromedially towards the cribriform plate. It is one of the terminal branches of the ophthalmic artery, the main arterial supply of the orbit. The ophthalmic artery courses below the optic nerve in the optic canal, crosses to the lateral side at the orbital apex, and continues from lateral to medial above the nerve. The other arterial branches of the ophthalmic artery are the central retinal, the lacrimal, ciliary, the posterior ethmoidal arteries, the supraorbital, the dorsal nasal arteries, and several muscular branches. **(c)** The anterior (AEA) and posterior (PEA) ethmoidal arteries arise from the ophthalmic artery in the medial third of the orbit and enter anterior midline skull base (*orange square*) via the anterior (AEC) and posterior (PEC) ethmoidal canals. The opening of the ethmoidal canals on the orbital side are found at the junction of the roof and medial wall of the orbit, where the frontoethmoid suture is formed by the medial edge of the orbital plate of the frontal bone above the perpendicular plate, which is a part of the ethmoidal bone below. These distal segments of the arteries define the anterior and posterior end of the lateral edge of the cribriform plate (CP).

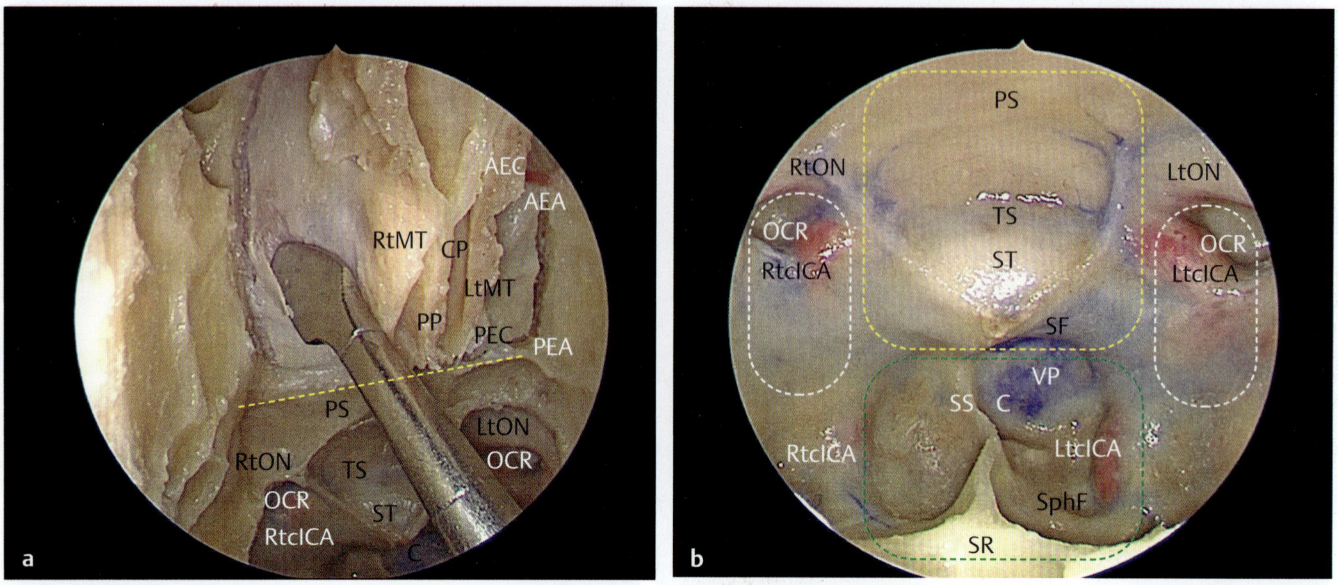

Fig. 1.6 (a) The middle skull base (*yellow line*) extends from the posterior limit of the cribriform plate (CP) defined by the posterior ethmoidal artery (PEA) and canal (PEC), and extends from the posteriorly extending planum sphenoidale (PS) to the floor of the sella turcica (ST). **(b)** The middle skull base (*yellow square*) consists of the planum sphenoidale (PS), the tuberculum sellae (TS), and the sella turcica (ST), with the sellar floor (SF) being the most posterior limitation. Laterally, the parasellar region (*white square*) is located, defined by the cavernous sinuses and Meckel's cave. Posteriorly, the posterior midline skull base (*green square*) continues consisting of the clivus (C) and the craniovertebral junction.

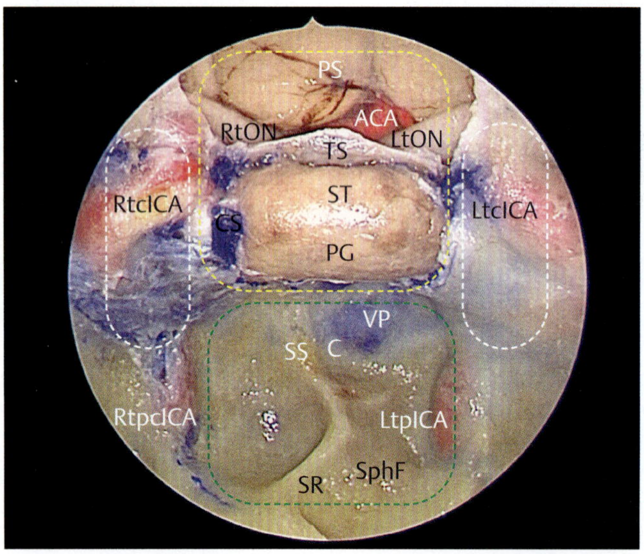

Fig. 1.7 The parasellar region (*white square*) is defined by the cavernous sinus (CS) and Meckel's cave, and contains the left (LtcICA) and right (RtcICA) cavernous internal carotid arteries with the cavernous arterial branches, the abducens nerve medially, and the oculomotor nerve, the trochlear nerve, and the ophthalmic division, and maxillary division of the trigeminal nerve in the lateral wall of the CS. The Meckel's cave contains the Gasser ganglion, which divides into the ophthalmic, maxillary, and mandibular division of the trigeminal nerve. Middle skull base (*yellow square*), posterior midline skull base (*green square*).

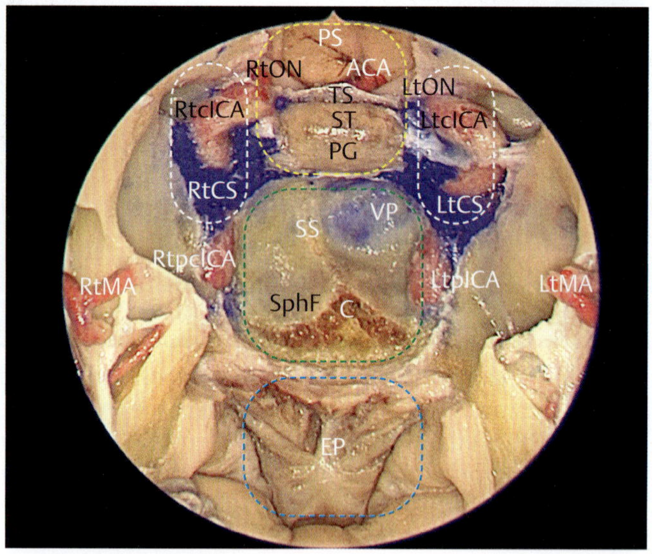

Fig. 1.8 The posterior midline skull base (*green square*) extends from the clivus (C) to the craniovertebral junction (*blue square*). Middle skull base (*yellow square*), parasellar region (*white square*).

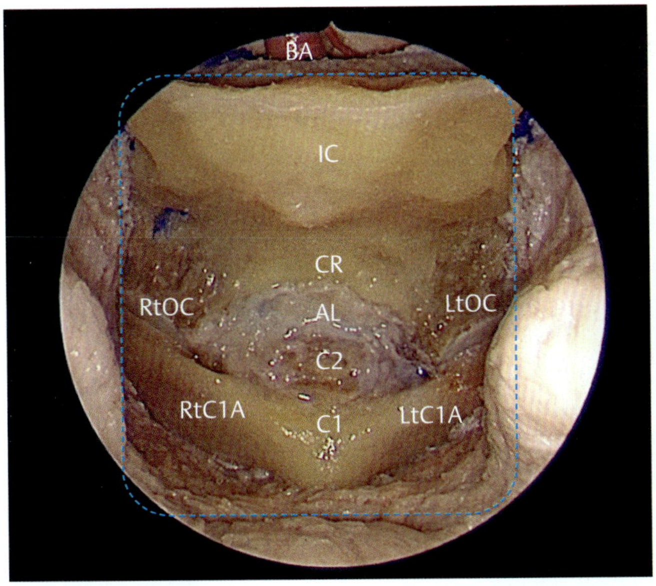

Fig. 1.9 Exposition of the craniovertebral junction (*blue square*), with the anterior longitudinal ligament, the anterior atlanto-occipital ligament, and the tectorial membrane removed that connect the inferior clivus (IC) and the atlas (C1) along the right (RtC1A) and left (LtC1A) arch of C1. The apical ligament (AL) extends from the most inferior clival ridge (CR) to the odontoid apex (C2).

that this anatomical variability might be a prerequisite for different growth patterns in pituitary tumors toward either the cavernous sinus or the suprasellar region.[96]

The inferior hypophyseal artery, a branch of the cavernous segment of the internal carotid artery (ICA), supplies the posterior pituitary gland (neurohypophysis).[98]

Cavernous Sinus

The lateral margins of the sella are defined by the medial wall of the cavernous sinuses on each side.[87,88,95] These extradural venous sinuses extend from the superior orbital fissure back to the petrous apex on each side and drain blood from the following:

- Ophthalmic veins
- Middle and inferior cerebral veins
- Sphenoparietal sinuses

The cavernous sinuses drain from anterior to posterior and enter the following:

- Superior petrosal sinus to the transverse sinus
- Inferior petrosal sinus to the internal jugular vein

Tumors with cavernous sinus invasion represent a neurosurgical challenge, as already described by Knosp et al.[15] Newer anatomical studies with special focus for the endonasal endoscopic anatomical orientation describe four compartments with distinct boundaries based on their spatial relationship with the cavernous ICA:[99]

- Superior compartment: Interclinoid ligament and oculomotor nerve
- Posterior compartment: Gulfar segment of the abducens nerve and inferior hypophyseal artery
- Inferior compartment: Sympathetic nerve and distal cavernous abducens nerve
- Lateral compartment: All cavernous cranial nerves and the inferolateral arterial trunk

The same study by Fernandez-Miranda et al. including pre- and postoperative MRI studies of 98 subjects with intraoperatively confirmed cavernous sinus invasion by a pituitary adenoma was analyzed according to this anatomical compartmentalization.[99] Twenty-nine out of 98 patients (29.6%) had a single compartment invaded, while 69 out of 98 (70.4%) had multiple compartments affected. The superior compartment (79 out of 98, 80.6%) was most commonly affected, followed by the posterior (64 out of 98, 65.3%), inferior (45 out of 98, 45.6%), and lateral (23 out of 98, 23.5%) compartments. The authors additionally reported residual tumor rates by compartment, being most frequently located in the lateral (80%), and less frequently in the posterior, superior, and the inferior compartment.[99]

A network of intercommunicating sinuses beneath the diaphragma sellae also connects the cavernous sinuses to each other, namely the anterior and posterior intercavernous sinuses (**Fig. 1.11**).

The medial wall of the cavernous sinus is formed by the sphenoid periosteum, and is often invaded by pituitary adenomas.[15,100,101] Surgical mobilization and/or removal of the medial wall has been described when radical resection of functional tumors is warranted, but remains a surgical challenge.[100,101] In an anatomical cadaveric study of 20 human heads by Truong et al., the medial wall of the cavernous sinus was found to form an intact single layer of dura. This layer is distinguishable from the capsule of the pituitary gland and the periosteal layer that forms the anterior wall of the cavernous sinus (**Fig. 1.13a**).[101] In approximately one-third of specimens, the medial wall of the cavernous sinus was indented or well adhered to the cavernous ICA.

The cavernous segment of the ICA occupies the inferomedial aspect of the cavernous sinus. Labib et al. classified the ICA following important landmarks in endonasal endoscopic surgery based on anatomical correlations and described six distinct segments.[102] The parasellar ICA can further be divided into a cavernous and a paraclinoid segment: (**Fig. 1.13b**)[99,102]

- *Parapharyngeal ICA segment*: Carotid bifurcation to ICA foramen
- *Petrous ICA segment*: Carotid canal to posterolateral aspect of the foramen lacerum

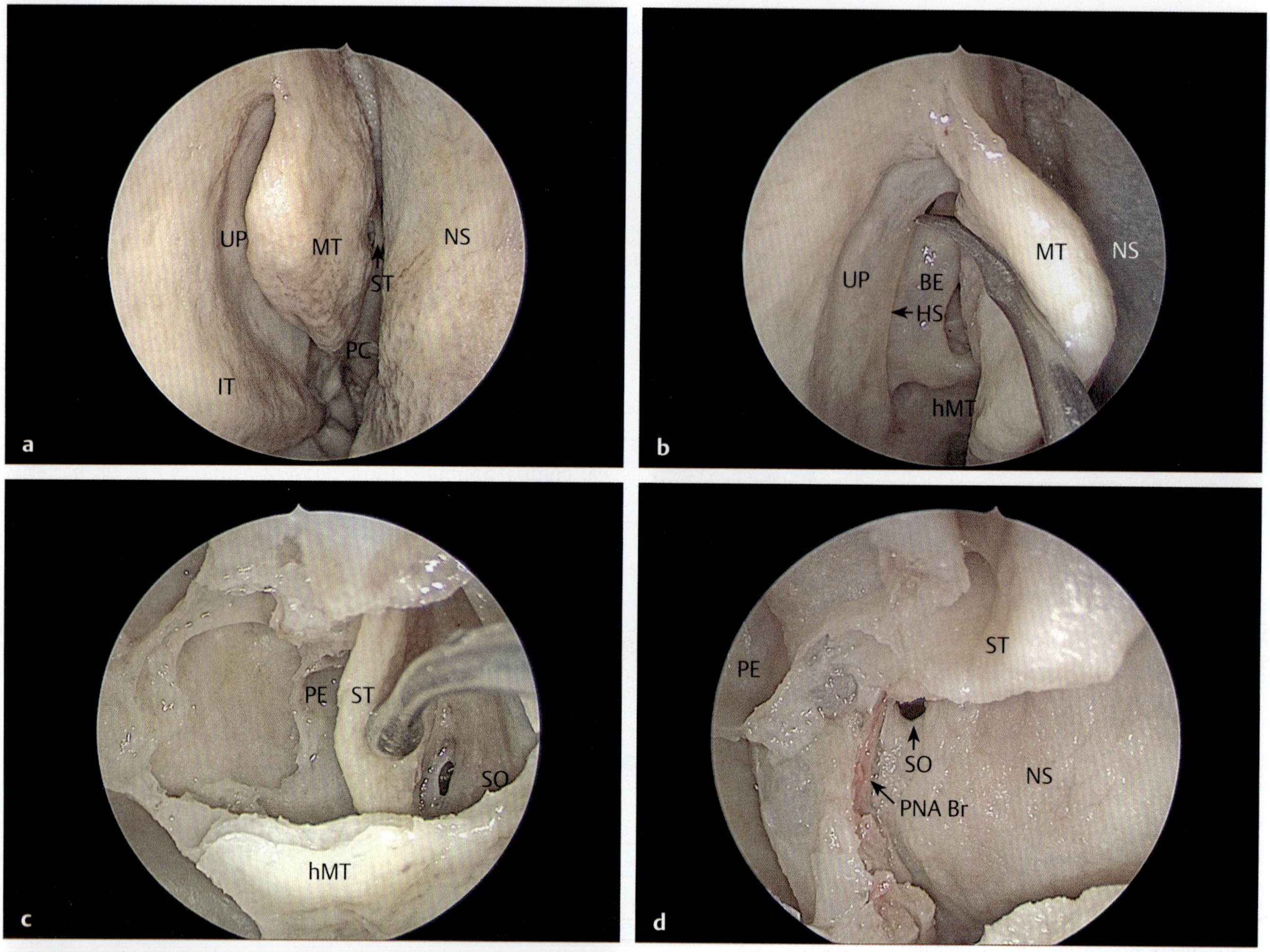

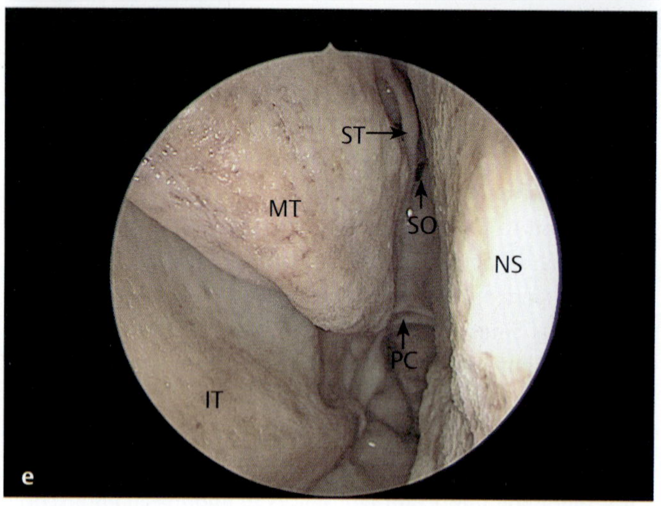

Fig. 1.10 Endoscopic view of the right nasal cavity in a cadaveric specimen. **(a)** Middle turbinate and the septum are important landmarks for endoscopic endonasal surgery. **(b)** In a transethmoidal approach, the uncinate process bulla and ethmoidalis are identified, followed by complete ethmoidectomy and partial middle turbinectomy. **(c)** The superior turbinate comes into view as the posterior ethmoidal cells are cleared. **(d)** The sphenoid ostia is often situated medial to the superior turbinate; in this specimen the superior turbinate has been resected in its inferior third and the vertical branch of the posterior septal artery can be identified. **(e)** Transsphenoidal surgical access can also be acquired via a transnasal approach in which the sphenoid ostia is identified medial to the superior turbinate and superior to posterior choana without an ethmoidectomy done as an initial step.

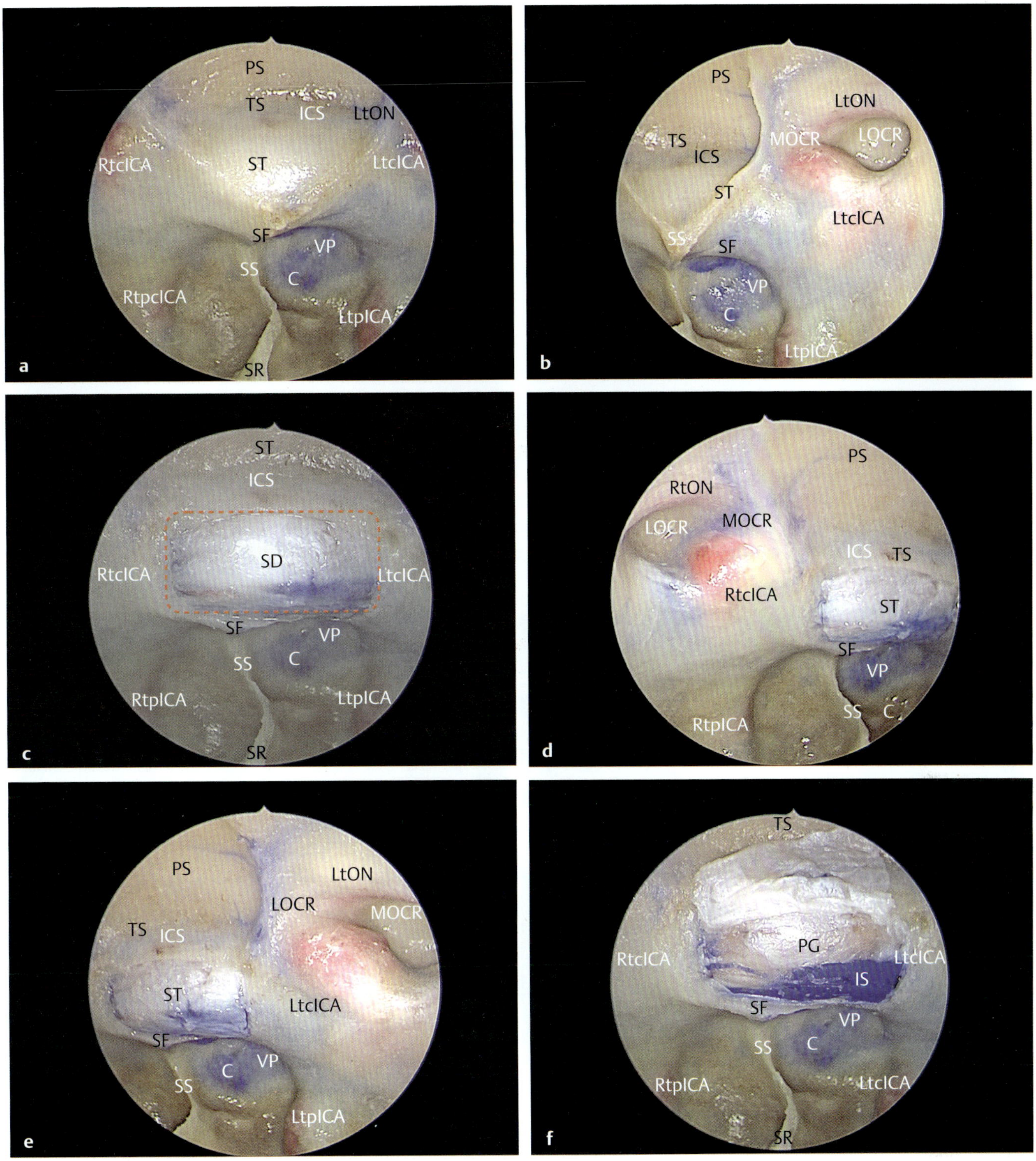

Fig. 1.11 Endonasal endoscopic view of the sella turcica and the posteromedial end of the optic canal within the sphenoid cavity in a cadaveric specimen. **(a, b)** The preforaminal segment of the optic canal is estimated to lie between the medial opticocarotid recess (MOCR) and the most posteromedial part of the lateral opticocarotid recess (LOCR). The intracanalicular segment lies from the posterior part of LOCR and extends anteriorly. **(c–f)** Transsellar approach (*orange square*) in a cadaveric specimen. The double-layered nature of the dura covering the sellar floor can be appreciated.

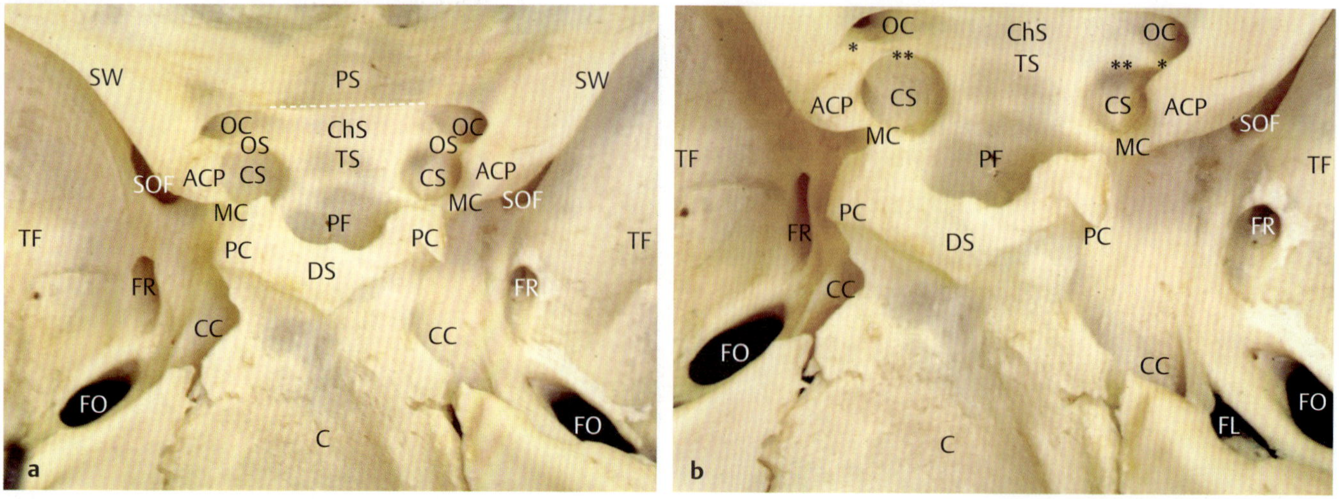

Fig. 1.12 (a, b) Superior oblique view of the intracranial aspect to demonstrate the topoanatomical relationship of the pituitary fossa (PF) to the adjacent anatomical sites in a dry bone specimen. The optic strut (OS) and the anterior clinoid process (ACP) represent bony structures that are closely related to significant anatomical structures including the cavernous sinus, the internal carotid artery, the optic nerve, and the pituitary gland. The OS has a neural-facing aspect (*) related to structures passing along the superior orbital fissure (SOF) and optic canal (OC) and a vascular-facing aspect (**) related to the internal carotid artery. The attachment of the falciform ligament covering the optic nerves when entering the OC is lateral to the ACP and medial to the limbus sphenoidale (*white line*).

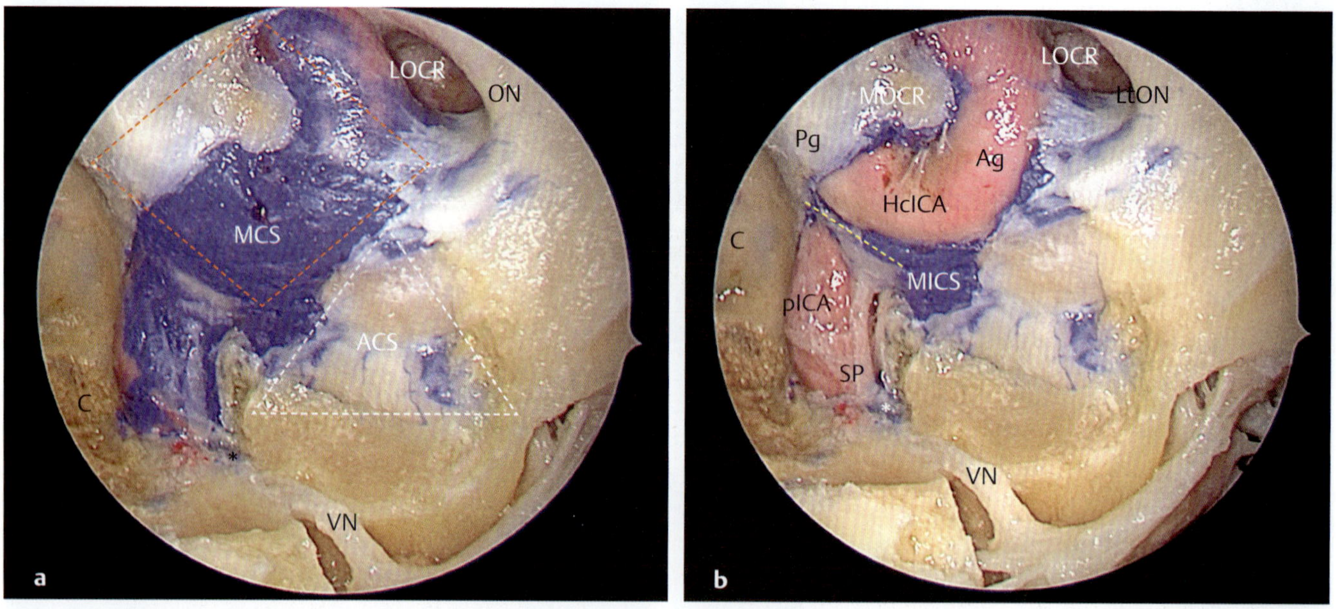

Fig. 1.13 Endonasal endoscopic anatomical dissection of the cavernous sinus in a cadaveric specimen with emphasis on the Amin Kassam classification.[103] **(a)** Endoscopic anteroinferior view of the medial wall of the cavernous sinus (MCS) with the periosteal layer of the anterior cavernous sinus wall (*white triangle*) removed.[100,101] The outer dura (periosteal) layer to the sellar floor transforms to the anterior wall of the cavernous sinus (ACS) (*white triangle*). The inner dural layer transforms to the diaphragm and forms the medial wall of the cavernous sinus (*orange square*). **(b)** The MCS has been removed and segments of the ICA can be appreciated. The parasellar ICA is a continuation of the paraclival internal carotid artery (pICA) (*yellow line*), and is divided into a cavernous internal carotid artery (cICA) and a paraclinoidal internal carotid artery.[100–103] The cICA can further be divided into a short vertical segment, a posterior genu (Pg), a horizontal segment (HcICA), and an anterior genu (Ag). The petro-occipital venous plexus (*), also known as internal carotid artery venous plexus of Rektorzik, consists of small veins surrounding the petrous segment of the internal carotid artery. It communicates with the cavernous sinus antero-superiorly, the inferior petro-occipital vein and the anterior condylar confluence posteriorly, and the clival diploic veins medially.

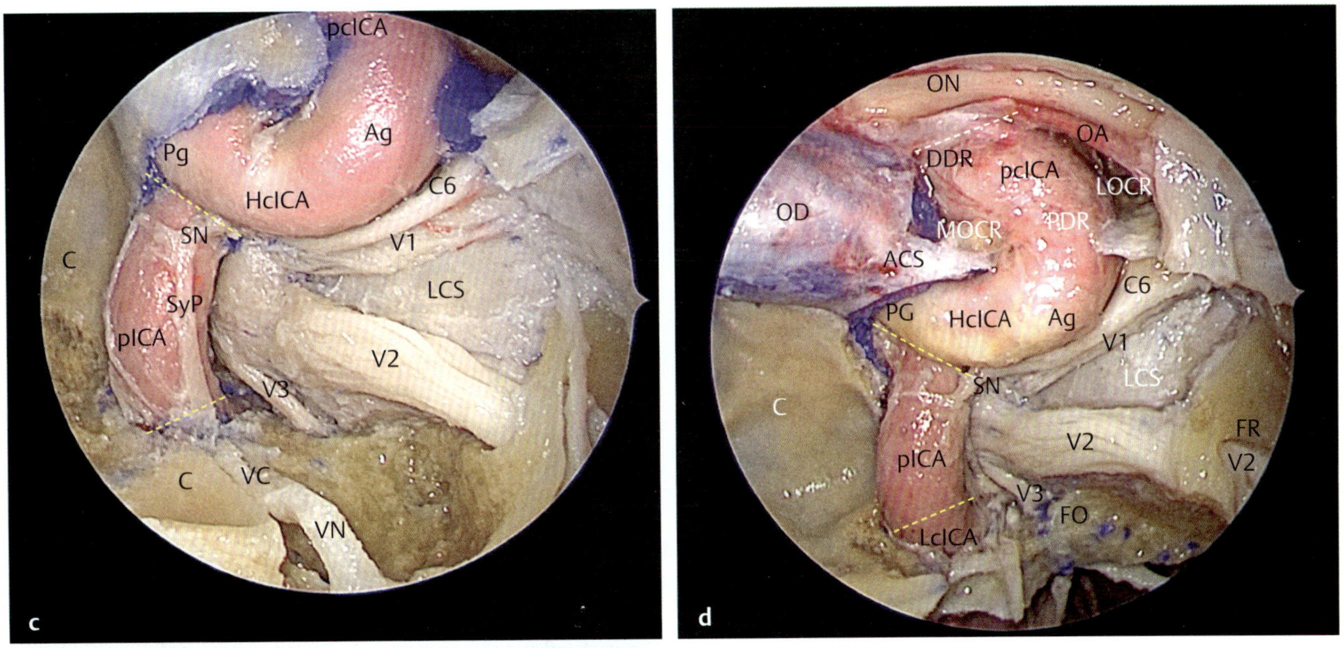

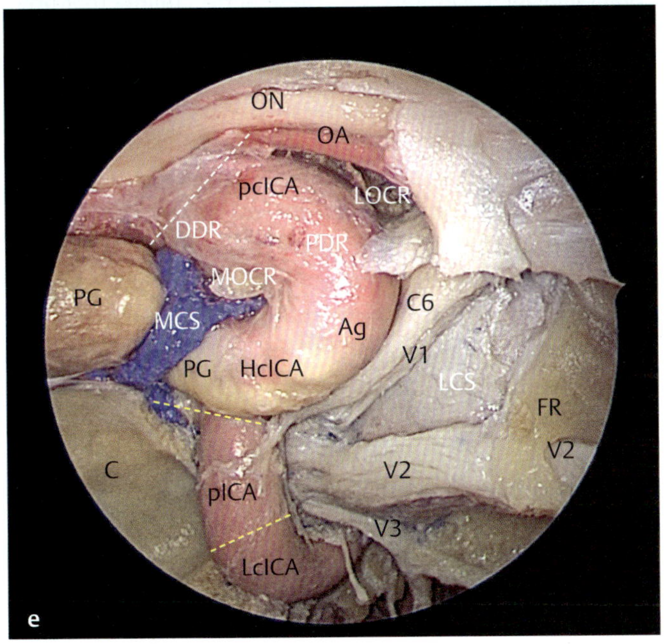

Fig. 1.13 *(Continued)* **(c)** The venous plexus of the cavernous sinus has been removed, along with the vidian canal (VC). The vidian nerve (VN) as its content serves as a landmark to the petroclival junction and the petrous ICA at the point of transition from the horizontal petrous ICA to the vertical paraclival segment (pICA) at the level of the foramen lacerum (*inferior yellow line*).[104,105] The sympathetic plexus (SyP) along the pICA can be appreciated. The Pg, the HcICA, the Ag of the cavernous internal carotid artery, and the paraclinoidal internal carotid artery (pcICA) can be appreciated. The lateral compartment of the cavernous sinus and its lateral wall (LCS) are visible, along with the cavernous cranial nerves. The inferolateral trunk is located within this compartment. **(d, e)** The vidian canal and nerve have been removed. The horizontal lacerum segment of the petrous internal carotid artery (peICA) changes into the vertical paraclival internal carotid artery (pICA) at the level of the foramen lacerum (*inferior yellow line*). The cavernous internal carotid artery (cICA) is a continuation of the paraclival internal carotid artery (pICA) that changes into the short vertical segment of the cavernous internal carotid artery (*superior yellow line*). The Pg, the HcICA, and the Ag of the cavernous internal carotid artery can be appreciated. The abducens nerve (cranial nerve VI) (C6) lies at the inferolateral aspect of the cavernous carotid artery. The paraclinoidal ICA (pcICA) is located within the clinoidal triangle in the cavernous sinus roof and is the continuation of the Ag of the cavernous ICA. Its proximal extent (*inferior white line*) is defined by the proximal dural ring (PDR), the distal extent (*superior white line*) is demarcated by the distal dural ring (DDR). The bone of the medial opticocarotid recess (MOCR) has been left and its topo-anatomical relationship to the internal carotid artery is visible. The same accounts for the lateral opticocarotid recess (LOCR). The double-layered nature of the dura covering the sellar floor can be appreciated. The outer dura (OD) periosteal layer to the sellar floor transforms to the anterior wall of the cavernous sinus (D). The inner dural layer transforms to the diaphragm and forms the medial wall of the cavernous sinus (mCS) (E).

- *Paraclival ICA segment*: Posterolateral foramen lacerum to the superomedial aspect of the petrous apex
- *Cavernous ICA segment*: Superomedial petrous apex to the proximal dural ring
  - *Short vertical segment*: Continuation of the paraclival ICA
  - Horizontal segment
  - Anterior genu
  - *Posterior genu*: Transition between the short vertical and the horizontal segments
- *Paraclinoid ICA segment*: Proximal to the distal dural ring
- *Intradural ICA segment*: Distal ring to ICA bifurcation

Consecutively, important surgical landmarks that correlate with the above-described ICA segments in the context of endonasal endoscopic surgical anatomy have been described and confirmed in cadaveric and surgical studies by several groups (**Fig. 1.13c–e**):[102–106]

- *Parapharyngeal ICA segment*: Eustachian tube, fossa of Rosenmuller, and levator veli palatini
- *Petrous ICA segment*: Vidian canal and mandibular segment of the trigeminal nerve (V3)
- *Paraclival ICA segment*: Fibrocartilage of foramen lacerum, foramen rotundum, maxillary strut, lingular process of the sphenoid bone, and the paraclival protuberance
- *Cavernous ICA segment*: Sellar floor and petrous apex
- *Paraclinoid ICA segment*: Medial and lateral opticocarotid recess, lateral tubercular recesses, and the distal osseous arch of the carotid sulcus

The use of the vidian canal and its content as a surgical landmark to the petroclival junction and petrous ICA is an important concept. This was highlighted by Kassam et al. while describing approaches to the middle third of the clivus, the petrous bone, the middle cranial fossa, the inferior and superior portions of the cavernous sinus, and the medial portion of the infratemporal fossa through a series of five modular approaches.[103] These can further be divided into two categories relative to the horizontal segment of the petrous ICA:[104]

- *Infrapetrous* category (below the plane of the horizontal ICA):
  - *Zone 1*: Infrapetrous medial petrous apex approach
  - *Zone 2*: Infrapetrous petroclival approach
- *Suprapetrous* category (above the plane of the horizontal ICA):
  - *Zone 3*: Suprapetrous quadrangular Meckel's cave approach
  - *Zone 4*: Suprapetrous superior cavernous sinus approach
  - *Zone 5*: Transpterygoid and infratemporal approach

A series of cadaveric studies have confirmed this relationship and correlated the results with intraoperative findings. Hence, the vidian canal provides a reliable landmark for the point of transition from the horizontal petrous ICA to the vertical paraclival segment of the ICA at the level of the foramen lacerum (**Fig. 1.13c–e**).[102,104,105,107]

The lateral wall of the cavernous sinus is formed by dura extending from the petrous apex to the superior orbital fissure. The anterior border of the lateral wall is the tentorium cerebelli. The cavernous cranial nerves are located within the superior and lateral compartment of the cavernous sinus and its lateral wall. The oculomotor nerve (cranial nerve III) is located within the superior compartment along with the interclinoid ligament.[99] The trochlear nerve (cranial nerve IV), the ophthalmic division of the trigeminal nerve (cranial nerve V1), and the maxillary division of the trigeminal nerve (V2) are located within the lateral compartment of the cavernous sinus along with the inferolateral trunk, a cavernous branch of the cavernous ICA. These nerves follow that order from superior to inferior.[99] At the posterior aspect of the cavernous sinus, near the petrous apex, the dural Dorello canal contains the abducens nerve (cranial nerve VI) before entering the cavernous sinus, along with the sympathetic nerve. The abducens nerve lies at the inferolateral aspect of the cavernous carotid artery and is located more medially when compared to the other cavernous cranial nerves.[99] The posterior aspect of the cavernous sinus is further related to the Meckel cave, which contains the gasserian cistern and the trigeminal ganglion. At the anterior aspect of the cavernous sinus, the cranial nerves III, IV, V1, and VI enter the orbit via the superior orbital fissure. The maxillary nerve (V2) passes anteriorly through the foramen rotundum where it crosses the pterygopalatine fossa with the pterygopalatine ganglion before entering the infraorbital canal (**Fig. 1.14**).

Medial and Lateral Opticocarotid Recess

The lateral opticocarotid recess is a more or less pneumatized negative imprint of the optic strut, the bony part of the anterior clinoid process that separates the optic canal from the superior orbital fissure.[102,108,109] The superior border of the lateral opticocarotid recess is covered by a thickening of the dura and an arciform course of the periosteum.[110,111] These ligamentous strands form the distal dural ring, which separates the optic nerve and the paraclinoid segment of the ICA from the clinoid segment of the ICA (**Fig. 1.13e** and **Fig. 1.15**).[101,110] Accordingly, the inferior border of the lateral opticocarotid recess consists of thickened dura and periosteum forming the proximal dural ring enveloping the oculomotor nerve (third cranial nerve) within the cavernous sinus toward the superior orbital fissure (**Fig. 1.15**). The lateral

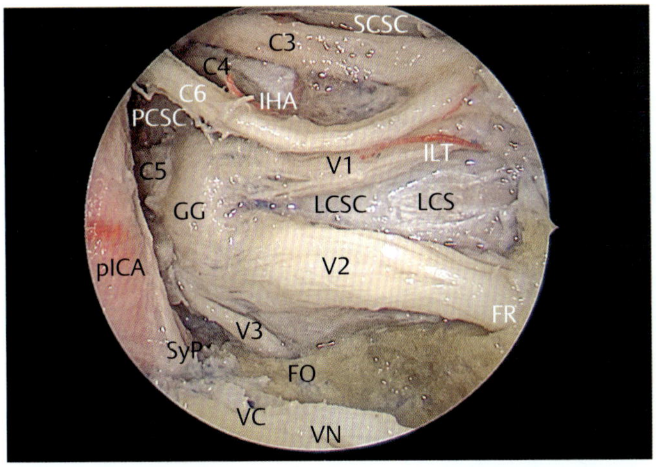

Fig. 1.14 The cavernous internal carotid artery has been dissected and medialized to expose the four compartments and the lateral wall of the cavernous sinus (LCS). The oculomotor nerve (cranial nerve III) (C3) is related to the superior compartment of the cavernous sinus (SCSC) in relationship with the interclinoid ligament. The abducens nerve (cranial nerve VI) (C6) lies at the inferolateral aspect of the cavernous carotid artery. The gulfar segment of the abducens nerve (C6) is located within the posterior compartment of the cavernous sinus (PCSC) together with the inferior hypophyseal artery (IHA). The distal cavernous segment of the abducens nerve is located in the inferior compartment of the cavernous sinus along with the sympathetic nerve (SN). The other cavernous cranial nerves are located within the lateral compartment of the cavernous sinus (LCSC) along with the inferolateral trunk (ILT), namely the trochlear nerve (cranial nerve IV) (C4), the ophthalmic division of the trigeminal nerve (V1), and the maxillary division of the trigeminal nerve (V2), the latter leaving the cavernous sinus via the foramen rotundum (FR). The nerves follow that order from superior to inferior. The pterygopalatine ganglion is a parasympathetic ganglion found in the pterygopalatine fossa close to the sphenopalatine foramen, mainly innervated by the greater petrosal nerve, a branch of the facial nerve (cranial nerve VII). It is responsible for the innervation of the lacrimal gland and the nasal mucosa. The pterygopalatine ganglion is associated with the maxillary division of the trigeminal nerve (V2), which can be identified and followed back via the foramen rotundum (FR) to the gasserian ganglion (GG). The vidian nerve passes through the vidian canal and is in close relationship with transition zone of the horizontal lacerum segment of the petrous internal carotid artery (LcICA) to the vertical paraclival internal carotid artery (pICA) at the level of the foramen lacerum. These two nerves are not accounted as cavernous cranial nerves.

opticocarotid recess is located inferior to the optic nerve and lateral to the carotid artery and is a useful landmark for identifying the position of the medial opticocarotid recess.[110,111] The medial opticocarotid recess correlates intracranially with the medial clinoid process, a bony structure only present in approximately 50% of patients. The bony prominences of the cavernous ICA and the optic nerve in combination with the lateral opticocarotid recess are useful landmarks to locate the medial opticocarotid recess (**Fig. 1.13e** and **Fig. 1.15**).[110,111]

Parasellar Ligaments

Truong et al. classified several parasellar ligaments according to the anatomical landmarks where these fibrous structures anchor to the medial wall of the cavernous sinus (**Fig. 1.15**):[101]

- *Caroticoclinoid ligament*: Strongest and largest fan-like arranged group of ligaments from the middle clinoid toward the clinoid ICA segment and anterior clinoid process. Present in most specimens (97.7%).
- *Superior parasellar ligament*: Horizontal cavernous ICA and/or lateral wall of the cavernous sinus. Present in approximately half of the specimens.
- *Inferior parasellar ligament*: Anterior wall of the cavernous sinus or anterior surface of the short vertical segment of the cavernous ICA. Present in most specimens (95%).
- *Posterior parasellar ligament*: Short vertical segment of the cavernous ICA and/or the posterior carotid sulcus. Present in approximately half of the specimens.

Pituitary Gland

The pituitary gland, also named hypophysis cerebri, is embedded within the sella turcica and connected with a loose reticular ligament to the medial wall of the cavernous sinus.[112–114] The pituitary gland has a larger anterior lobe, also named adenohypophysis, and a smaller posterior lobe, also named neurohypophysis. The intermediate lobe, known as pars intermedia, is embedded in between these two lobes.[7,114,115] Embryologically, only the neurohypophysis is derived from the diencephalic neuroectoderm and is a "neural structure." The adenohypophysis and pars intermedia are derived from the stomodeal ectoderm that aligns the anterior and posterior walls of the Rathke's pouch, respectively.[42,114,116] From an anatomical standpoint of view, the pars distalis of the pituitary gland consists of the anteriorly located adenohypophysis within the pituitary fossa. The pars tuberalis is a thin cranial extension of the pars distalis located at the anterior margin, where the infundibular stem

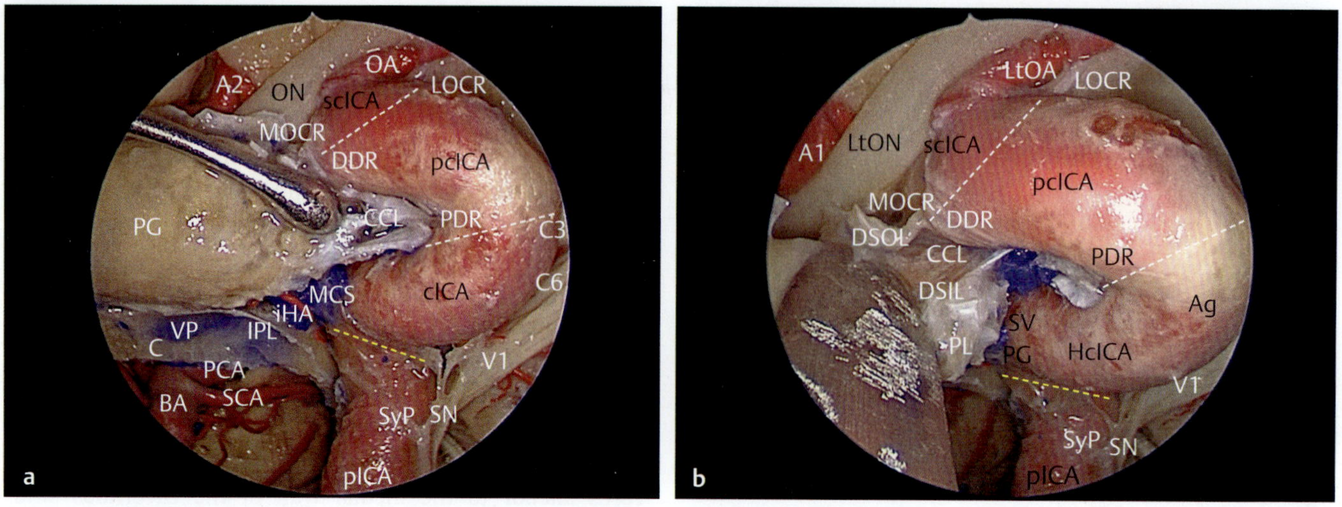

Fig. 1.15 (a) Topoanatomical relationships between the proximal (PDR) and distal (DDR) dural ring and the medial (MOCR) and lateral (LOCR) opticocarotid recess. The PDR (*light white line*) has been removed in the anterior aspect of the cavernous internal carotid artery (cICA), its lateral continuation is in relationship with the oculomotor nerve (third cranial nerve) (C3). The DDR (*dashed white line*) demarks the border between the cavernous (cICA) and the paraclinoidal (pcICA) internal carotid artery. **(b)** Endonasal endoscopic view of the upper sellar and paraclinoid region. The pituitary gland (PG) is wrapped inside a thin and transparent pituitary capsule. Loose connections, the so-called pituitary ligaments (PL), connect the pituitary capsule to the medial wall of the cavernous sinus (MCS).[101] The clinoid space is opened and inner (DSIL) and the outer (DSOL) layer of the diaphragma sellae are dissected apart from each other.[101] The layers of the diaphragma sellae are in continuity with the MCS. The caroticoclinoid ligament (CCL) is a bundle of fibers from the PDR via the middle clinoid and from the MCS, where the DSIL inserts.[101] The DSOL is in continuation with the DDR. The CCL consists of fibrous bundles from the PDR, middle clinoid, and the upper portion of the MCS.[101] The CCL loops posterior to the anterior genu (Ag) of the cavernous internal carotid artery, merges with the interclinoid ligament more posteriorly and inserts at the anterior clinoid process at its inferior aspect.[101]

enters the pituitary gland.[112–114] Proximal to the infundibular stem, the median eminence is a small bulge rostral to the tuber cinereum, which is formed by the gray matter of the hypothalamus posteriorly to the optic chiasm and anteriorly to the mamillary bodies. These structures form the floor of the third ventricle.[112–114] The portion of the neurohypophysis that lies within the posterior aspect of the pituitary fossa is called the pars nervosa. The pars nervosa is contiguous with the infundibulum, which extends superiorly through a defect in the diaphragma sellae in continuation with the median eminence of the hypothalamus.[112–114] The inferior hypophyseal artery, a branch of the cavernous segment of the ICA, provides the arterial blood supply of the neurohypophysis. Accordingly, the superior hypophyseal artery feeds a network of fenestrated capillaries, the so-called "hypophyseal portal system," responsible for the arterial supply of the adenohypophysis. The lack of a blood–brain barrier is crucial for the intravascular diffusion of the pituitary hormones.[112–114]

Suprasellar Region

Historically, the suprasellar space was reached by surgical opening of the diaphragma sellae when an enlarged sella was present in case of a sellar tumorous mass. This microsurgical maneuver was referred to as a transsellar transdiaphragmatic approach.[110,117,118] Based on this experience, the midline microscopic and endoscopic transsphenoidal transsellar approaches have been extended to reach the suprasellar region. The removal of the tuberculum sellae (transtuberculum approach) and the posterior portion of the planum sphenoidale (transplanum approach) have since been described extensively[110,111,119–126] (**Fig. 1.16**). The development of new imaging modalities and the widespread use of techniques such as image-guided surgery profoundly influenced the extended indication for suprasellar lesions including pituitary adenomas with mainly suprasellar extension, giant pituitary adenomas, Rathke's cleft cysts, craniopharyngiomas, and tuberculum sellae meningiomas.[110,111,123–127] With the knowledge of the median suprasellar endonasal endoscopic anatomy, brain retraction - that is necessary when using transcranial approaches - can be avoided. However, the topoanatomical relationship of the suprasellar neurovascular structures has to be appreciated from the opposite side, when compared to the well-known bilateral subfrontal approach.[110,128,129]

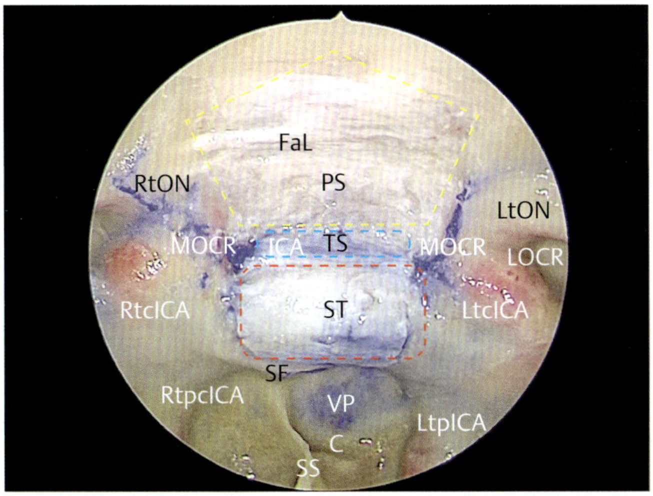

Fig. 1.16 Transtuberculum (*blue square*) and transplanum (*yellow pentagon*) approach in a cadaveric specimen after a performed transsellar approach (*orange square*). Endonasal endoscopic transsphenoidal anteroinferior view in a cadaveric specimen after removal of the bone covering the sella turcica (ST), the tuberculum sellae (TS), and the planum sphenoidale (PS) up to the falciform ligament (FaL).

Four corridors to reach the suprasellar cisterns have been described in the literature:[110,111,128]

- *First corridor*: Anterior to the optic chiasm
- *Second corridor*: Superior to the optic chiasm and inferior to the anterior communicating artery
- *Third corridor*: Inferior to the optic chiasm and superior to the pituitary gland
- *Fourth corridor*: Inferior or lateral to the pituitary gland

Suprachiasmatic Region

By removing the bone covering the planum sphenoidale (transplanum approach) and tuberculum sellae (transtuberculum approach), the suprachiasmatic region can be exposed (**Fig. 1.16**). After opening the corresponding dura, the chiasmatic cistern and the lamina terminalis cistern are the topoanatomical regions of interest (**Fig. 1.17a**). From an endonasal endoscopic perspective, exposition of the chiasmatic cistern reveals the anterior aspect of the optic chiasm and the medial aspects of both optic nerves. By removing the arachnoid membranes of the lamina terminalis cistern, the pre- and postcommunicating segments of the anterior cerebral arteries and its collateralization by the anterior communicating artery forming the "H-complex" are visible. The recurrent artery of Heubner, usually arising from the postcommunicating segments of the anterior cerebral arteries, as well as the H-complex itself, do show a remarkable amount of anatomical variation among individuals.[130–133] These variations can regularly be observed when performing surgery on lesions involving the chiasmatic and lamina terminalis cistern.[110,111,128] The lamina terminalis itself can be found within the space between the optic chiasm and the anterior communicating artery (**Fig. 1.17b, c**).

Subchiasmatic Region

By removing the bone and opening the dura covering the sella turcica, (transsellar approach) the infundibular stalk inferior to the optic chiasm and the superior surface of the pituitary gland along with the diaphragma sellae are identifiable. The superior hypophyseal artery, a branch of the supraclinoid segment of the ICA, supplies the median eminence and the infundibular stalk.[112–114] Along with this vessel, small perforating branches for the inferior surface of the optic chiasm and optic nerves are usually present (**Fig. 1.18a**).[110,111,128] Arising from the clinoid segment of the ICA, the ophthalmic arteries are located inferiorly to the optic nerves and are identifiable within the subchiasmatic cistern (**Fig. 1.18b**).[110,111,128]

Retrosellar Region

When the anatomical dissection is continued in a superior posterior direction between the pituitary stalk and the ICA superior to the dorsum sellae, the retrosellar region can be exposed[110,111,128] (**Fig. 1.19a, b**). The Liliequist membrane is located under the floor of the third ventricle, anteriorly extending from the dorsum sellae to the mammillary bodies. The lateral insertion of the Liliequist membrane has been studied in anatomical cadaveric dissections and is along or adjacent to the oculomotor nerves or corresponding arachnoid sheaths.[134–136] It consists of a single or double arachnoid layer and is usually divided into three segments:

- *Sellar segment*: Most frequently seen on imaging
- *Diencephalic sheet*: Less frequently isolated in cadaveric studies
- *Mesencephalic sheet*: Less frequently isolated in cadaveric studies

When dissecting through the mesencephalic sheet of the Liliequist membrane, the upper third of the basilar artery located ventrally to the pons cerebri, the perforating pontine branches, the superior cerebellar arteries, the posterior cerebral arteries, and the oculomotor nerve (third cranial nerve) in between are visible within the prepontine cistern[134–136] (**Fig. 1.19c**).

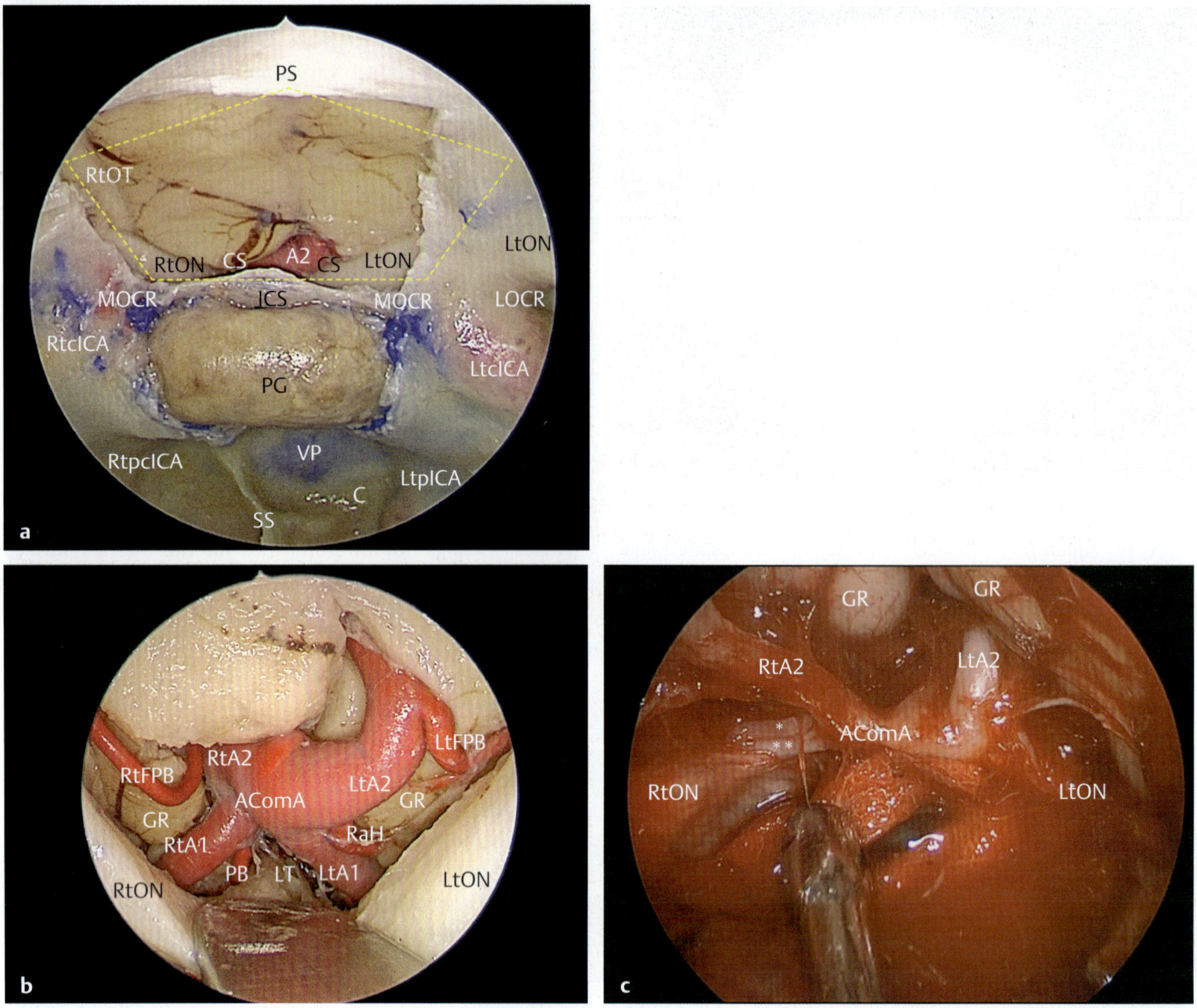

Fig. 1.17 **(a)** The suprachiasmatic region is exposed after removal of the dura mater covering the planum sphenoidale and the tuberculum sellae (*yellow pentagon*). The chiasmatic cistern (CCS), the anterior margin of the optic chiasm (OCh), and the medial portions of the left (LtON) and right (RtON) optic nerves are visible along with the postcommunicating segment of the anterior cerebral artery (A2). The medial aspect of the right olfactory tract (RtOT) can be appreciated passing superiorly to the RtON along the olfactory groove anteriorly. **(b)** The arachnoid of the lamina terminalis cistern has been removed, and the precommunicating segments of the right (RtA1) and left (LtA1) anterior cerebral arteries are visible, interconnected by the anterior communicating artery (AComA). A perforating branch (PB) arising from the RtA1 can be appreciated. The right (RtA2) and left (LtA2) postcommunicating segments of the anterior cerebral arteries are rotated to the left. The LtA2 gives origin to a recurrent artery of Heubner (RaH). The left (LtFPB) and right (RtFPB) frontopolar branches have their origin from the postcommunicating segments of the anterior cerebral arteries, respectively. The space between the optic chiasm and the AComA reveals the lamina terminalis (LT). **(c)** Intraoperative visualization of the of the suprachiasmatic region after resection of a pediatric craniopharyngioma with suprasellar extension. The precommunicating anterior cerebral arteries are covered by a cottonoid. The AComA and the LtA2 and RtA2 are visible. A right recurrent artery of Heubner (*) and a perforating branch (**) are visible.

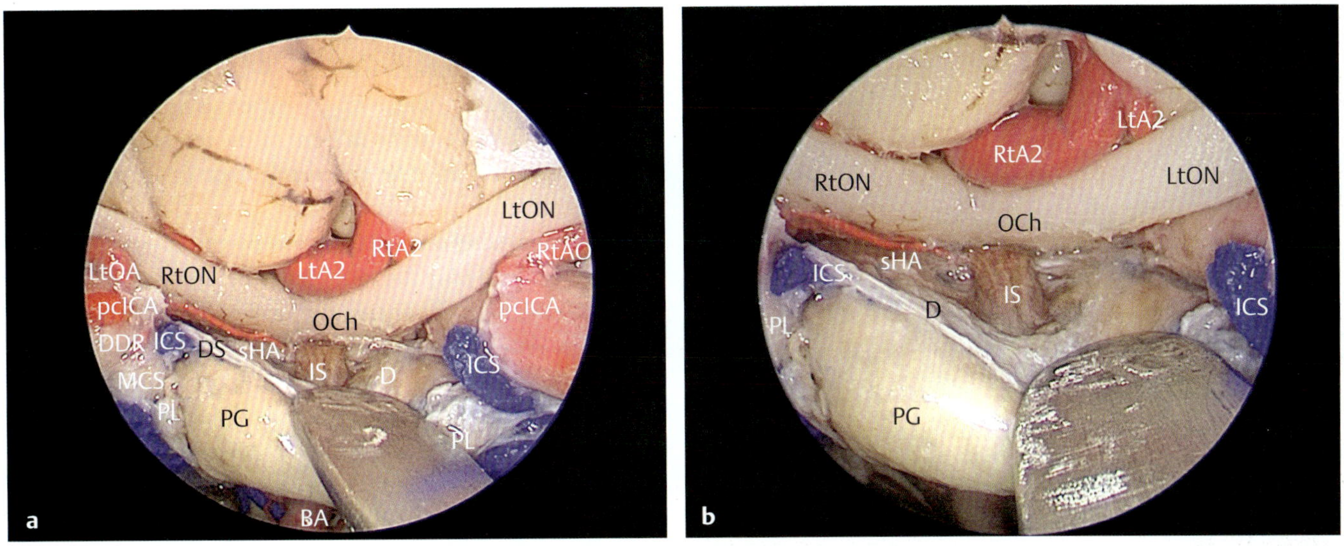

Fig. 1.18 Exposition of the subchiasmatic region after removal of the dural covering of the tuberculum sellae, the intercavernous sinus (ICS), and the dura covering the sella turcica in a cadaveric specimen. **(a, b)** The infundibular stalk (IS) is located below the optic chiasm (OCh) and passes through the diaphragma sellae (D). The superior hypophyseal artery (sHA) and the perforating branches for the inferior surface of the optic chiasm are visible. The left (LtOA) and right (RtOA) ophthalmic arteries arising superiorly to the distal dural ring (DDR) from the paraclinoid internal carotid artery (pcICA), respectively, are located below the left (LtON) and right (RtON) optic nerve.

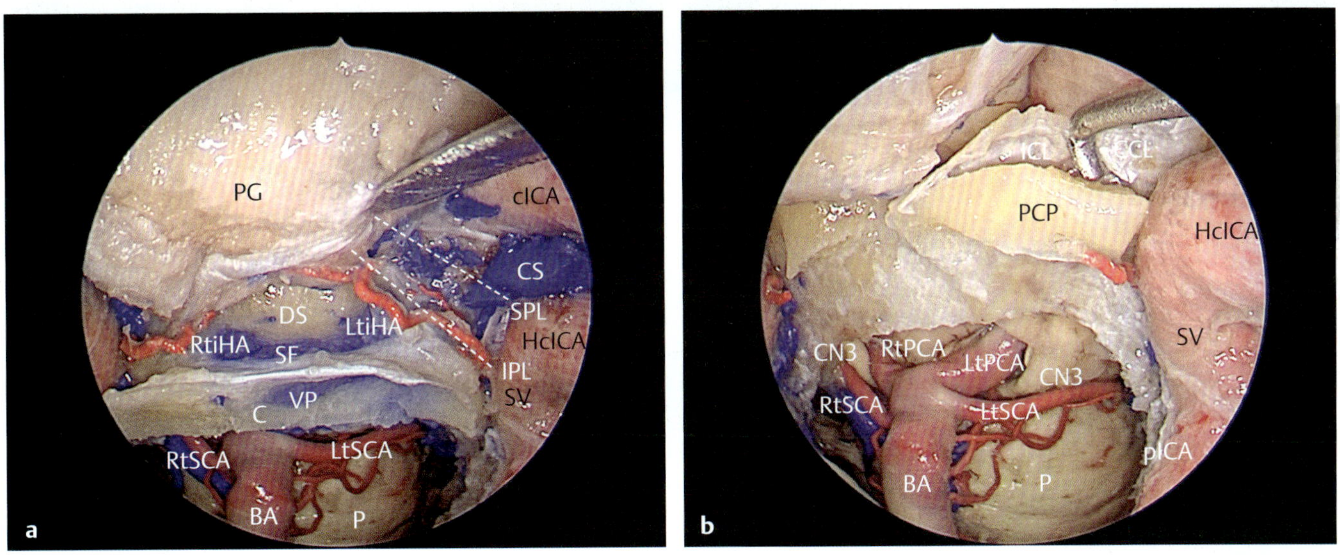

Fig. 1.19 Endonasal endoscopic inferosuperior view toward the retrosellar region in a cadaveric specimen. **(a)** The pituitary gland (PG) is elevated cranially, and the sellar floor (SF) as well as the dorsum sellae (DS) are visible. The thin and fan-like superior parasellar ligament (SPL) originates from the superoposterior aspect of the medial wall of the cavernous sinus approximately at the same level as the caroticoclinoid ligament (CCL) and interconnects the medial wall of the cavernous sinus with the horizontal portion of the cavernous ICA (cICA) and/or the lateral wall of the cavernous sinus.[101] The inferior parasellar ligament (IPL) connects the medial wall of the cavernous sinus to the anterior wall of the cavernous sinus and/or the short vertical portion of the cavernous internal carotid artery (SVcICA).[101] The left (LtiHA) and right (RtiHA) inferior hypophyseal arteries are identifiable. Below the SF, the upper third of the basilar artery (BA), the pons (P), and the left (LtSCA) and right (RtSCA) superior cerebellar arteries are visible. **(b)** After removal of the sellar floor and the dorsum sellae, the posterior clinoid process (PCP) is mobilized. The CCL loops behind the anterior genu of the ICA and merges with the interclinoid ligament (ICL) posteriorly.[101] The upper third of the BA, the P, the LtSCA and RtSCA, the oculomotor nerve (third cranial nerve) (C3), and the left (LtPCA) and right (RtPCA) posterior cerebral arteries are identifiable. *(Continued)*

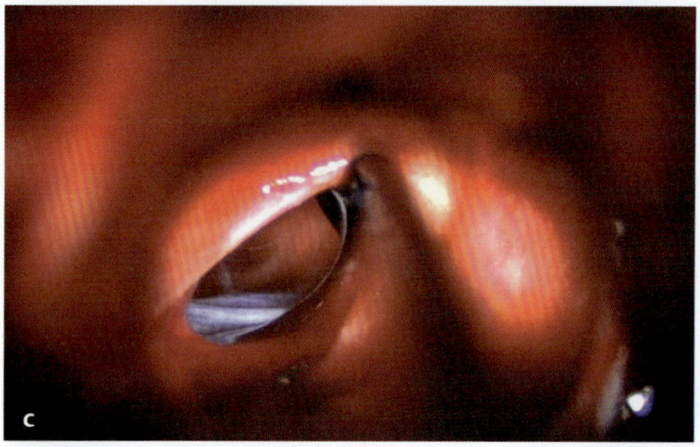

Fig. 1.19 *(Continued)* **(c)** intraoperative visualization of the Liliequist's membrane (LM) in the retrosellar space during surgical marsupialization of an intrasellar arachnoid cyst between the dorsum sellae and the diaphragma sellae (D). The prepontine cistern (PrC) as part of the retrosellar space.

Ventricular Region

Superior to the prepontine cistern, when dissecting through the mesencephalic sheet of the Liliequist membrane, the floor of the third ventricle in front of the mammillary bodies can be visualized.[110,111,128] When the floor is opened, access into the third ventricle is provided. Usually, this route is in continuation with the sellar region by the tumorous lesion itself, when following the tumor into the suprasellar space, as it is the case in craniopharyngioma extending into the third ventricle. When the resection of a lesion in this area is possible through an endonasal endoscopic approach, a panoramic view of the ventricular cavity is possible (**Fig. 1.20a**). The walls of the third ventricle, which are formed by the hypothalamic walls inferiorly and the medial portions of the thalami bilaterally, are interconnected by the interthalamic commissure (**Fig. 1.20b**). The third ventricle continues to the lateral ventricles via the foramina of Monro bilaterally (**Fig. 1.20c**).

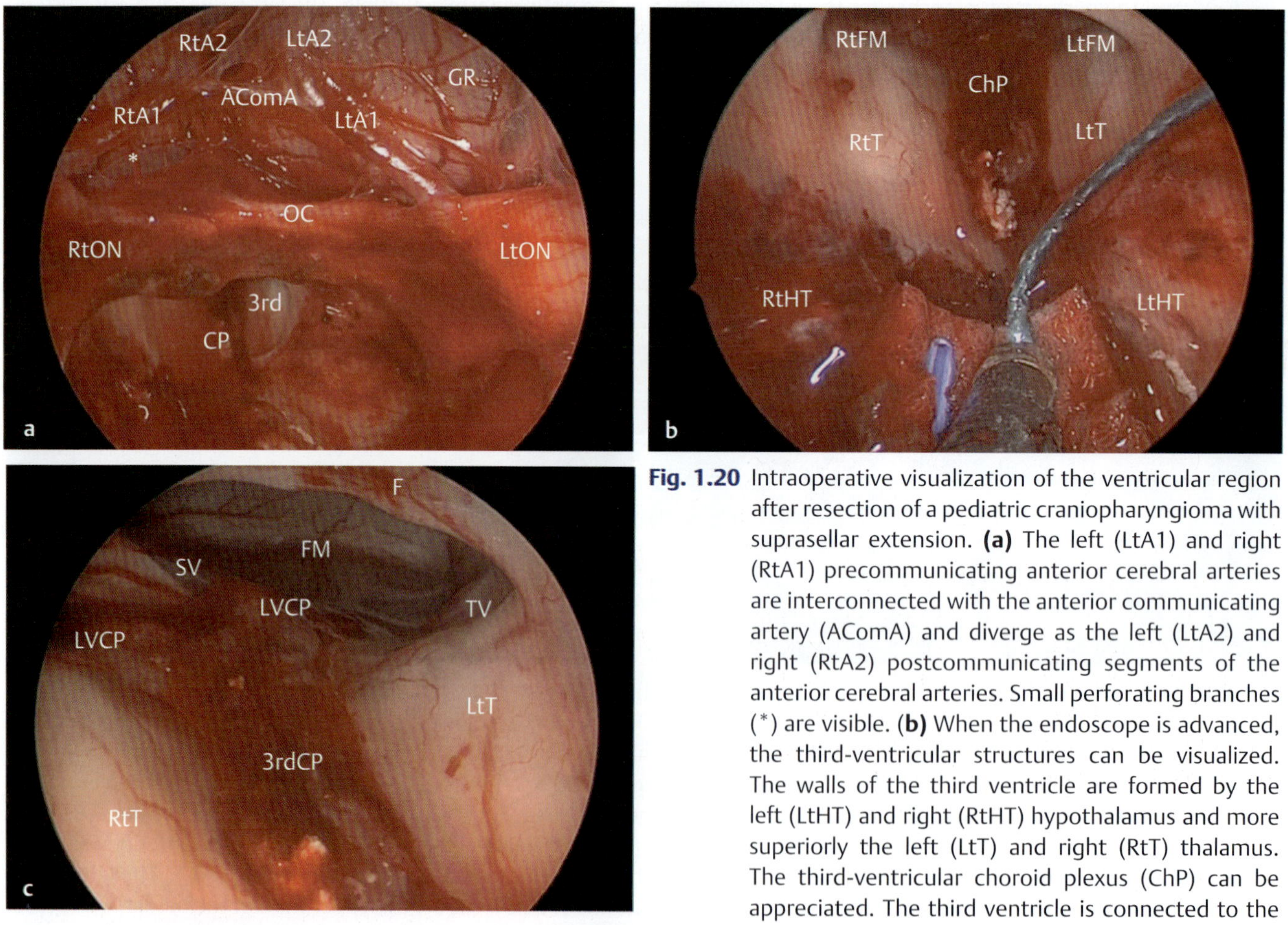

Fig. 1.20 Intraoperative visualization of the ventricular region after resection of a pediatric craniopharyngioma with suprasellar extension. **(a)** The left (LtA1) and right (RtA1) precommunicating anterior cerebral arteries are interconnected with the anterior communicating artery (AComA) and diverge as the left (LtA2) and right (RtA2) postcommunicating segments of the anterior cerebral arteries. Small perforating branches (*) are visible. (**b**) When the endoscope is advanced, the third-ventricular structures can be visualized. The walls of the third ventricle are formed by the left (LtHT) and right (RtHT) hypothalamus and more superiorly the left (LtT) and right (RtT) thalamus. The third-ventricular choroid plexus (ChP) can be appreciated. The third ventricle is connected to the lateral ventricles via the left (LtFM) and right (RtFM) foramen of Monro. **(c)** Detailed visualization of the foramen of Monro (FM) via the endonasal endoscopic suprasellar approach. The LtT and RtT form the superolateral aspect of the third ventricle and the inferior border of the FM. The septal vein (SV) and the thalamic vein (TV) merge to form the internal cerebral vein within the tela choroidea. The choroid plexus of the lateral ventricles (LVCP) is attached to the tela choroidea and merges to form the choroid plexus of the third ventricle (3rdCP). The superior border of the FM is formed by the fornix (F).

More posteriorly, the pineal and suprapineal recesses, the posterior commissure, the habenular commissure, the habenular trigone, and the aqueduct might even be visualized.[110,111,128]

Clinical Considerations

Sellar pathologies are clinically significant and generally present as an incidental finding on MRI. Neurological symptoms include visual impairment and mass effect symptoms (e.g., headaches). The clinical presentation of a pituitary adenoma does not only correlate with the size of the tumor causing locoregional symptoms. Abnormalities related to under- or oversecretion of hormones classify the tumor as nonfunctioning or functioning pituitary adenomas, the latter being more likely to be detected earlier and with smaller sizes because of their well-known distinct clinical endocrinological syndromes.[137]

Nonfunctioning Pituitary Adenomas

Nonfunctioning pituitary adenomas are the most common tumors of the sella with an estimated prevalence of 15 to 20% (22.2 per 100,000) (**Table 1.1**).[14,138] Estimation of the true incidence and prevalence remains difficult due to a high frequency of clinical occult and incidental lesions.[138] The northern Finnish study revealed a standardized incidence rate of 1.0 per 100,000 persons.[13]

Common presenting symptom in an endocrine-inactive tumor is a gradual visual disturbance over months or even years. Occasional headaches might occur most likely because of the expansion of the sellar dura.[22,33,137] Suprasellar extension of the tumor leads to compression of the optic chiasm and consecutive bitemporal hemianopia. Diminished visual acuity occurs with progressive compression of the optic apparatus. Lateral extension of the pituitary adenoma can correlate with diplopia, when the ocular nerves are involved within the cavernous sinus, and trigeminal neuralgia in rare occasions. Another rare presentation includes spontaneous CSF rhinorrhea when the lesion erodes the bone of the sphenoid sinus. Nonfunctioning pituitary macroadenomas can lead to hypopituitarism because of compression of the normal pituitary gland and the pituitary stalk. As more than 80% of these tumors are gonadotroph adenoma, hypopituitarism is the most common endocrinological abnormality found within this subgroup, resulting in secondary hypogonadism in men and women.[139,140] Hypogonadism presents with amenorrhea in women and with infertility and decreased libido in both sexes. Deficiency in GH leads to growth disorders in children and reduced general condition and metabolic syndrome in the adult. Hypothyroidism leads among others to weight gain, cold intolerance, fatigue, dry skin, and depression. Deficiency in ACTH can lead to weakness, orthostatic hypotension, and to adrenal crisis. Many patients with a nonfunctional adenoma will have a mild elevation of PRL upon laboratory examination (values between 20 and 200 ng/mL). This is explained with a reduced physiological inhibitory stimulus of dopamine on lactotroph cells when the pituitary stalk is compressed by the tumorous mass, the so-called "stalk effect."[141]

Functioning Pituitary Adenoma

About 65% of pituitary adenomas are functioning adenomas. Functioning pituitary adenomas are more likely to be microadenomas than nonfunctioning pituitary adenomas, probably because of the early manifestation of hormone-mediated signs and symptoms. If hormonal hypersecretion is present, a detected sellar mass is by definition a pituitary adenoma. The most common hormone-producing adenomas are prolactinomas, followed by GH-, ACTH-, FSH-, LH-, and TSH-secreting tumors with associated clinical syndromes.[33] Hypersecreting tumors are challenging lesions, as total tumor removal is critical to achieve physiological hormonal levels.

Prolactin-Producing Adenoma (Lactotroph Adenoma or Prolactinoma)

These prolactin-secreting benign pituitary tumors originate from the PRL adenohypophyseal cells (**Table 1.1**). This entity can present as microadenoma but may reach extensively large sizes. Prolactinomas are the most common pituitary adenoma,[33,142,143] with an estimated prevalence of 44.4 per 100,000 and a standardized incidence rate of 2.2 per 100,000.[13,14] Prolactinomas usually cause hyperprolactinemia with associated hypogonadism in women and men.

Hyperprolactinemia leads to hypogonadotropic hypogonadism and may cause amenorrhea and galactorrhea in women, gynecomastia in men, and decreased libido in both sexes. A serum PRL concentration of more than 200 ng/mL is considered diagnostic for this adenoma subgroup. Detected values between 20 and 200 ng/mL are known to be caused by compression of the infundibular stalk and consecutive impairment of the dopaminergic inhibitions, and might therefore be present in non-lactotroph sellar masses. When there is a high clinical suspicion for a prolactinoma but the initial PRL values are low, it is important to obtain serum dilutions because of the "hook effect," which leads to falsely low prolactin values. With modern laboratory techniques, this issue has been resolved.[141]

ACTH-Producing Adenoma (Corticotroph Adenoma)

ACTH-producing benign primary pituitary tumors do originate from corticotroph cells secreting propriomelanocortin, from which ACTH and beta-endorphin are cleaved (**Table 1.1**). Several other peptides are byproducts of this secretion process. Corticotroph adenomas usually present as microadenomas and are associated with Cushing's disease.[33] This entity has a reported prevalence of 1.2 per 100,000 with a standardized incidence rate of 0.17 per 100,000.[13,14]

Overproduction of ACTH from a pituitary adenoma leads to Cushing's disease and may cause diabetes, hypertension, osteoporosis, purple striae, truncal obesity, moon facies, amenorrhea, impotence, and general weakness. Initial work-up demonstrates elevated 24-hour urine cortisol excretion and elevated late-night salivary cortisol values. The ACTH concentration is typically high-normal or high. A positive corticotropin-releasing hormone (CRH)-stimulation test and a positive high-dose dexamethasone suppression test indicate a pituitary source of hypercortisolism. The majority (90%) of pituitary adenomas in Cushing's disease are microadenomas. If they are not visible on MRI and/or the biochemical constellation is unclear, an inferior petrosal sinus sampling can be performed to confirm the pituitary origin of the Cushing's syndrome.[144]

Growth Hormone-Producing Adenoma (Somatotroph Adenomas)

These GH-producing benign primary pituitary tumors with excessive secretion of GH are derived from the somatotroph cells of the adenohypophysis (**Table 1.1**). This entity presents as micro- or macroadenoma and is associated with gigantism (young patients) and acromegaly (adults).[33] The prevalence per 100,000 is reported to be 8.6 with a standardized incidence rate of 0.34 per 100,000.[13] Excessive secretion of GH causes acromegaly in adults (with coarsening of facial features, growth of hands and feet, carpal tunnel syndrome, frontal bossing, macroglossia, joint pain, fatigue, and obstructive sleep apnea) and gigantism in children. The measurement of the serum insulin-like growth factor-1 (IGF-1) is recommended as the first diagnostic step, followed by serum GH levels after an oral glucose load. Inadequate suppression of serum GH after a glucose load confirms the diagnosis.[145]

TSH-Producing Adenoma (Thyrotroph Adenoma, TSH-Oma)

These TSH-producing benign pituitary lesions are rare and account for about 1% of pituitary adenomas (**Table 1.1**).[33,146] The tumors clinically present with hyperthyroidism when secretion of intact TSH is present. The majority of them only secrete TSH-alpha or -beta subunits and hence are clinically nonfunctioning.[147,148] Thyrotroph adenomas are generally diagnosed as macroadenomas and are found to be invasive at the time of surgery.[149,150]

This rare functioning adenoma entity causes secondary hyperthyroidism, clinically apparent with weight loss, heat intolerance, fine hair, moist skin, anxiety, tachycardia and tachyarrhythmia, muscle weakness, fatigue, and menstrual changes. Laboratory work-up demonstrates elevation of free serum thyroxine (T4) and triiodothyronine (T3) with normal or elevated serum TSH levels, as compared to primary hyperthyroidism, where decreased TSH levels are expected.[149,150]

LH- and FSH-Producing Adenoma (Gonadotroph Adenoma)

These benign gonadotropin-producing primary pituitary tumors generally present as clinically silent nonfunctioning sellar masses (**Table 1.1**). Some patients have clinical and chemical signs of gonadal dysfunction, most probably because of the locoregional mass effect.[33]

Plurihormonal Adenoma

This subgroup includes benign pituitary tumors with coexpression of pituitary hormones without a common cellular origin.[33] The lactotroph and somatotroph adenoma secretes both PRL and GH and is the most frequently reported plurihormonal tumor of the pituitary gland, although any combination is possible (**Table 1.1**). Exclusive secretion of FSH and LH is rare and clinically silent. FSH and LH secretions are usually found in plurihormonal tumors.[151]

Pituitary Apoplexy

Pituitary apoplexy is a clinical syndrome characterized by the abrupt onset of headache, nausea, visual disturbance, and ophthalmoplegia, in association with hemorrhage or infarction within the pituitary fossa (**Fig. 1.21**).[33,152] Pituitary apoplexy is slightly more common in males (60 vs. 40%) than in females, with a mean age of onset of 50 years.[152–158] Pathophysiologically, larger tumors' size outgrowing their blood supply has been postulated, leading to infarction followed by secondary hemorrhage in certain cases. Another theory proposes that larger tumors compress their own blood supply leading to infarction and secondary hemorrhage.[152,159,160] Several comorbid conditions, procedures, and drugs have been associated and described as predisposing factors.[152] An extensive amount of case reports and small series has been published on pituitary apoplexy. Because of its rare condition, and sudden onset in the absence of prior suspicion for a pituitary pathology, studies

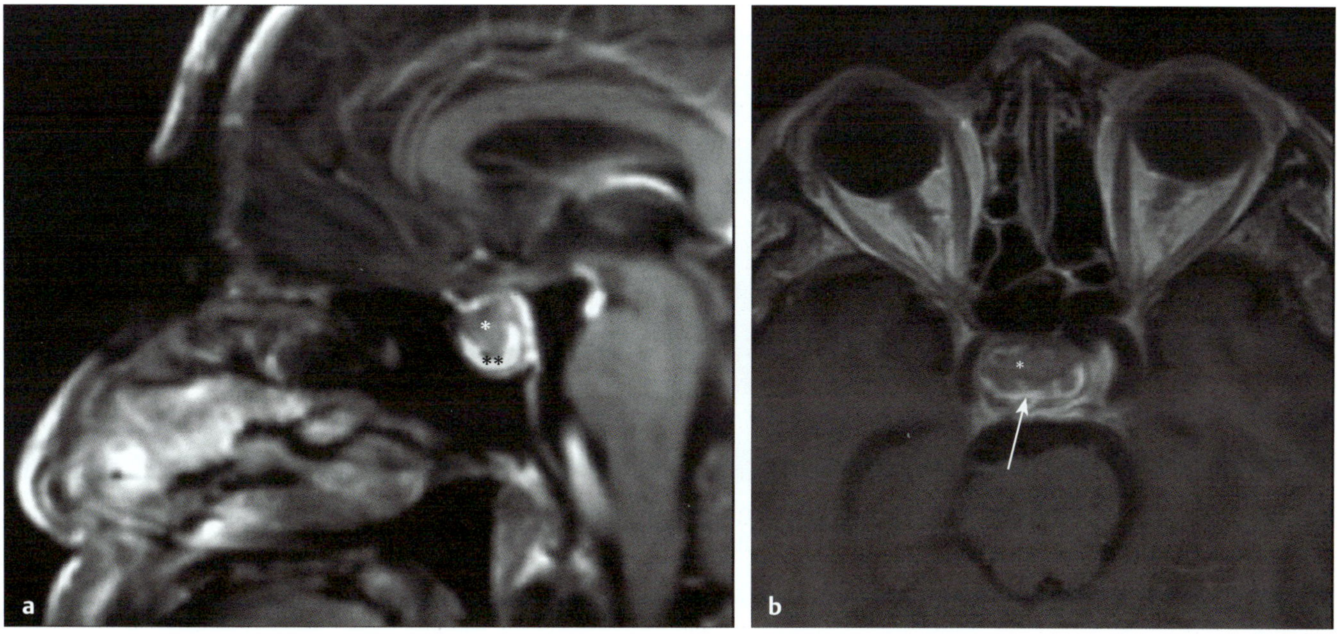

Fig. 1.21 Radiological diagnosis of a pituitary apoplexia in a 51-year-old patient presenting with 2 weeks history of headache and vomiting. Neurocranial MRI revealed a sellar mass. **(a)** Sagittal T1-weighted noncontrast-enhanced, **(b)** axial T1-weighted gadolinium-enhanced MRI sections demonstrating a mixed signal hyper- (*arrow*) and hypointense (*) sellar lesion with focal strong contrast enhancement (**). A pituitary apoplexia was most likely to be present.

remain scarce. In a larger series of patients with surgically treated pituitary adenoma, approximately 5% presented with a classical apoplexy.[152–158] It is important to distinguish the term "apoplexia" from the incidental finding of pituitary hemorrhage or infarction, that are found in an additional 5% of patients,[152,157,158] and microhemorrhage and signal-shortening that are frequently seen in pituitary macroadenomas.[48,161] The majority of apoplexy cases (approximately 80%) are found in association with a preexisting pituitary tumor that has not been known previous to the sudden event.[152,156,162] A reported tendency for apoplexy to occur more frequently in nonfunctioning pituitary adenoma could either be based on inherent differences in tumor biology, or because of enhanced preliminary detection of secreting tumors.[152] Larger size as a risk factor for apoplexia in nonfunctioning pituitary adenoma is difficult to extract methodologically because of the fact that tumor size prior to the ictal event is impossible to asses when only the imaging after the hemorrhage is available.[152,163,164]

Pituitary apoplexia is an emergency situation that warrants surgical therapy as the primary treatment option to quickly decompress the optic apparatus and the cranial nerves (**Fig. 1.22, Fig. 1.23, Fig. 1.24,** and **Fig. 1.25**) with the goal of recovery and preservation of neurological function, especially visual recovery.[154,156] Reported recovery rates for visual acuity deficits were 100%, and approximately two-thirds for visual field defects and ocular paresis, when surgery is performed within a week. A significantly worse outcome has been found, when the intervention was performed later than a week after the ictus.[152,154,156] A subset of patients might be managed with an expectant strategy, but based on the selected cohorts, this cannot be applied to an unselected cohort of pituitary apoplexia patients.[165–167] As important as the surgical intervention is hormone replacement therapy to prevent adrenal crisis.[152] With appropriate diagnosis within a timely fashion and appropriate management, death by pituitary insufficiency (e.g., Addison's crisis or diabetes insipidus) should be avoidable and permanent neurological complications such as blindness or permanent ophthalmoplegia can be significantly reduced.[152] Hence, based on the available evidence, rapid surgical decompression within 7 days is recommended in the case of a newly diagnosed pituitary apoplexia.[152] Potential candidates for medical management might be patients with only ocular palsy. Another subgroup reported are patients with a mild and nonprogressive visual loss responsive to steroid treatment.[165–167] Concerning endocrine outcome, a complete evaluation of anterior pituitary hormone is recommended approximately 6 weeks after presentation with or without surgical intervention. Many patients are left with permanent endocrine deficits requiring long-term hormone replacement and management after the ictus,[152] with reported rates up to approximately 90% for at least one anterior pituitary hormone.[152,153] Recommendations for an optimal imaging schedule remain scant. Repeat imaging in about 6 months after the pituitary apoplexia seems to be appropriate, followed by annual repetitions.[152]

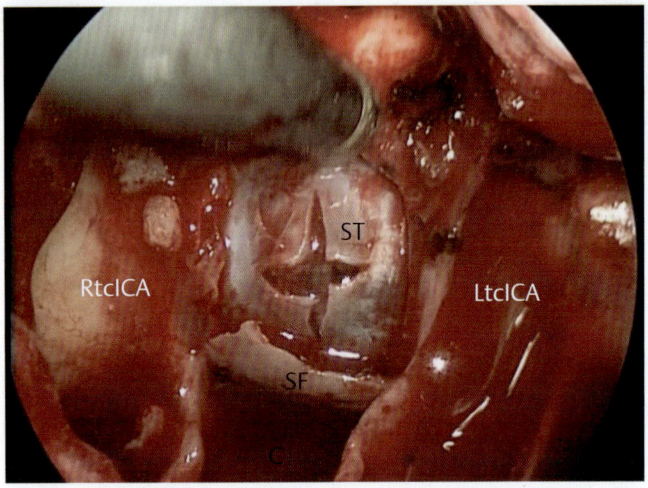

Fig. 1.22 Pituitary apoplexia emergency surgery. Endonasal endoscopic view of the sella turcica (ST) with a cruciate incision using a blade or scissors.

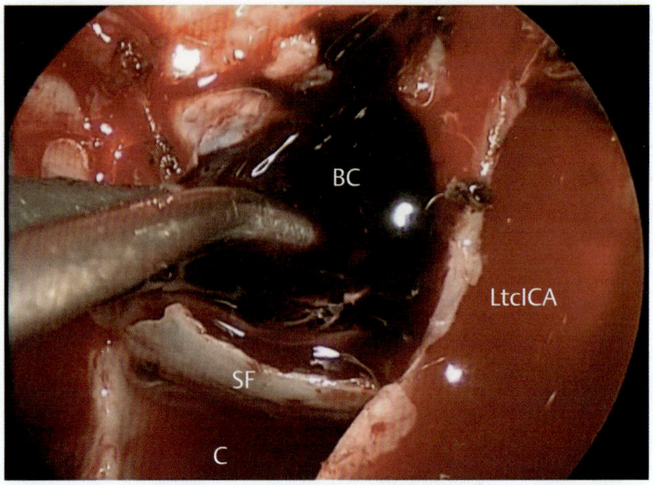

Fig. 1.23 Pituitary apoplexia emergency surgery. The liquified sellar blood clot (BC) and parts of the hemorrhagic pituitary adenoma are being evacuated under pressure using ring curette and suction.

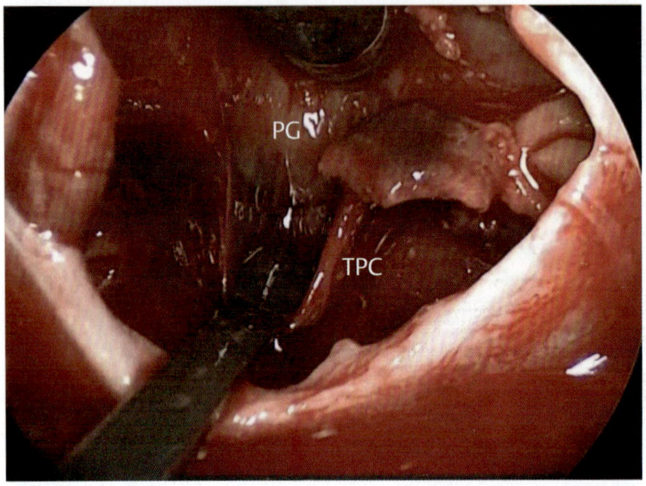

Fig. 1.24 Pituitary apoplexia emergency surgery. After hematoma and tumor resection, the tumor pseudocapsule (TPC) is dissected from the pituitary gland (PG) and removed.

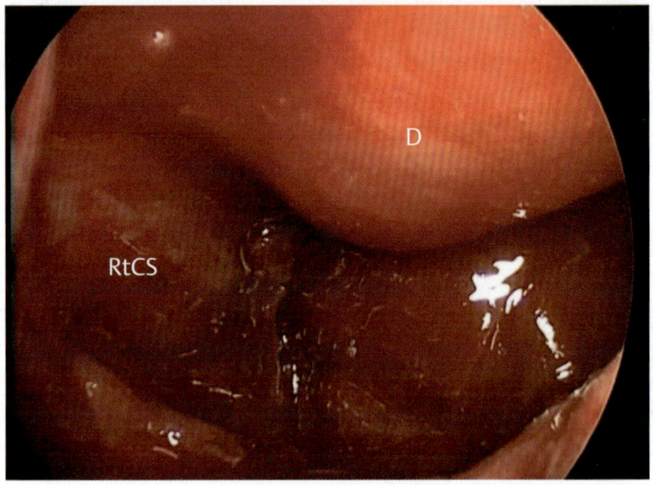

Fig. 1.25 Pituitary apoplexia emergency surgery. Endonasal endoscopic view showing the right (RtCS) and left (LtCS) cavernous sinus after tumor removal and the diaphragma sellae (D) dropping into the sella turcica.

Cystic Lesions of the Sella

Cystic lesions of the sella demonstrate similarities in their clinical manifestation as compared to nonfunctioning pituitary adenoma and solid cystic craniopharyngioma.

Cystic Pituitary Adenoma

These lesions typically present with nonspecific locoregional features such as headache, visual disturbance, or hypopituitarism, the latter being more frequent if a previous surgery was performed.[44–46,48]

Cystic Craniopharyngioma

At any age, patients with cystic craniopharyngioma present with headache, vision loss, and hypopituitarism.[168] Memory loss and cognitive deficits are described.[44] In the pediatric population, growth and sexual retardation, obesity, and hydrocephalus are the most common presenting symptoms.[169,170] In 6 to 38% of presenting cases, diabetes insipidus is diagnosed.[168,171]

Rathke's Cleft Cyst

Rathke's cleft cysts might reach significant enlargement and generate symptoms of optic chiasm compression and hypopituitarism within all age groups. The presentation peaks at the age of 40 to 60 years.[46,172,173] The most common presenting sign in patients with Rathke's cleft cysts is headache, hyperprolactinemia, or visual disturbance.[172–175]

Intrasellar Arachnoid Cyst

Symptomatic arachnoid cysts in adults most typically present with headache followed by decreased visual acuity and less commonly hypopituitarism.[43,46] An attempt to identify factors aiding the differential diagnosis of cystic craniopharyngioma, Rathke's cleft cyst, and arachnoid cysts was attempted by Shin et al.[44] Although only 52 patients were included in this study, some clinical inferences could be made. Patients with arachnoid cysts tended to be older at the time of initial diagnosis when compared to the other lesions. All three cystic lesions had the typical locoregional mass effect symptoms in common (visual field disturbances and headaches). However, neuropsychological deficits including reduced short-term memory favored the diagnosis of a craniopharyngioma.[44]

Epidermoid and Dermoid Cysts

Epidermoid tumors typically present in middle-aged patients with symptoms of mass effect, such as headache and vision loss.[45,46] Some reports have also described an uncommon clinical presentation mimicking that of a pituitary apoplexy.[45]

Mucoceles

The tendency of mucoceles to expand and erode into the adjacent tissue poses potential complications. Typically, they may present with headache, anosmia, nasal symptoms, and ophthalmoplegia.[56,57]

Radiological Considerations

MRI is the mainstay modality for imaging of the pituitary gland, the sella turcica and the parasellar region and is considered to be the gold standard. The role of CT mainly lies in the assessment of the endonasal and paranasal anatomy and the preoperative approach planning, but also for the evaluation of bony changes and calcifications. Analysis of the radiology films preoperatively prepares the surgeon for variations in anatomy as well as extension of the tumor.

Endonasal Anatomy

Nasal cavity: The study of the MRI and CT films should include septal deviations and concha bullosa as well as the presence of Onodi cells (sphenoethmoidal air cells) (**Fig. 1.26**).

Sphenoid bone: The sphenoid bone is of central importance for endoscopic neurosurgical and otorhinological skull base surgery while treating neoplastic lesions as well as CSF leakage. The sphenoid cavity provides a safe and natural approach to crucial structures including the sella turcica, optic nerve, planum sphenoidale, tuberculum sellae, and the sellar orbital junction.[176] A broad anatomical variability of these structures has been reported, putting patients at risk while removal of bony structures within the sphenoid sinus cavity is performed during surgery.[177]

Sphenoid sinus: Renn and Rhoton et al. performed extensive anatomical studies. Topographically, the sphenoid sinus separates the cavernous sinuses harboring both intracavernous carotid arteries as well as the optic, extraocular, and trigeminal nerves. Anteroposteriorly, it separates the pituitary gland from the nasal cavity. The depth is defined as

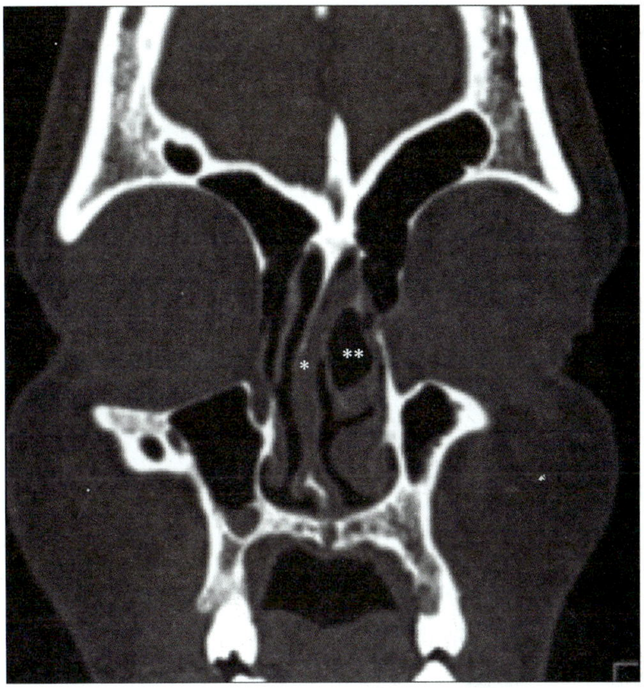

Fig. 1.26 Bone-weighted computed tomography images of the paranasal sinus and its relevance for transsphenoidal surgery. A deviated nasal septum (*) and left concha bullosa (**) are seen on a coronal plane.

the distance from the sphenoid ostium to the closest part of the sella and is 17 mm (12–23 mm).[94,176,178] Variation in size, shape, and the degree of pneumatization of the sphenoid sinus is very common.[179]

Based on its pneumatization, three types of sphenoid sinus configurations have been defined (**Table 1.7**).[180–182] The thickness of the anterior sellar wall ranges from 0.1 to 0.7 mm, with the highest diameter identified at the clivus and tuberculum sellae and the smallest along the anterior sellar wall. The intrinsic surface of the sphenoid sinus is covered by bone, 1 mm of diameter, and periosteum, separating the ICAs together with mucosa. Bone can be absent between soft tissue and the arteries, a variation commonly known as "dehiscent" ICA.[179,180,183] The ICAs run in the lateral aspect of the sphenoid bone, and their course is marked by a typical groove.[178–180] The optic canals protrude into the superolateral portion of the sinus, again potentially lacking bone that separates the optic sheath and sinus mucosa. In this case, a "dehiscent" optic nerve is present. In nearly 80% of the studied optic canals, less than 0.5 mm of bone separated the optic nerve and sheath from the sinus.[179,184] As a central landmark for transsphenoidal endoscopic skull base surgery, a pneumatized recess extending laterally into the optic strut between the optic canal and the prominence overlying the ICA and superior orbital fissure can be identified, defined as the lateral optico-carotid recess.[179,184]

Intersinus septum: Especially the intersinus septum varies greatly in symmetry, shape, thickness, location, and completeness. Posterior termination is related to the sellar floor (48%), the opticocarotid recess, the bony covering of the ICA (34%), or the lateral walls of the sinus anterior to the ICA (25%). The main septum might often be located off the midline crossing the anterior wall of the sella and bifurcating posteriorly (9%), or present as two distinct septae (3%). The most common type of sphenoid sinus has multiple small cavities within large paired sinuses. A single major septum separating the sinus into two large cavities is found in 68%, and even in these cases, the septae are often located off the midline (>8 mm) or are deflected to one side. No major septum is found in 28%, a major septum well off midline in 47%. The smaller cavities are separated by septae oriented in all directions.[176,179,180]

In our experience, a systematic assessment of the intersinus septum anatomy in preoperative MRI (T2 and T1 sequences with adequate contrast) is sufficient. CT, if available, should involve the coronal, sagittal, and axial plane to create a three-dimensional impression of the individual septal anatomy. Surgically relevant are shelfs, dividers, and walls (**Fig. 1.27, Fig. 1.28,** and **Fig. 1.29; Table 1.8**).

Preoperative planning for transsphenoidal surgery: The high variability has a direct impact on surgical planning for endoscopic skull base cases,[176] exposing surrounding

Table 1.7 Pneumatization of the sphenoid sinus

Main type	Subtype	Frequency (%)	Anatomical extension of pneumatization
Sellar		76	Air cavity extends into the body of sphenoid below the sella and as far as:
	Sellar	54.7	Below the sella
	Postsellar	22.3	Posteriorly as the clivus
Presellar		24	Air cavity does not penetrate beyond the anterior sellar wall
Conchal		Rare	Area below the sella is a solid block (>10 mm) without an air cavity

Sources: Adapted from Hamberger et al.[180,181] and Hamid et al.[182]

Table 1.8 Description of intersinus septum in MRI T1 with appropriate contrast, MRI T2, and CT bone in all planes

Sphenoid intersinus septum	Plane	Imaging modality	Imitation of anatomical landmark
Shelf	Axial	MRI (T1, T2), CT	Planum sphenoidale, sella turcica
Divider	Sagittal	MRI (T1, T2), CT	Skewing of the anatomical midline toward one side (cavernous or paraclinoidal carotid, opticocarotid recess)
Wall	Horizontal	MRI (T1, T2), CT	Anterior wall of sphenoid sinus, sella turcica
Mucosa	Any	MRI (T1, T2)	

Abbreviations: CT, computed tomography; MRI, magnetic resonance imaging.

Note: This classification is relevant when approaching the sphenoid sinus in endonasal endoscopic surgery, as they might skew or imitate important landmarks of the base of skull.

Sources: Adapted from Roethlisberger et al. 2020 and Waran et al. 2013.[212]

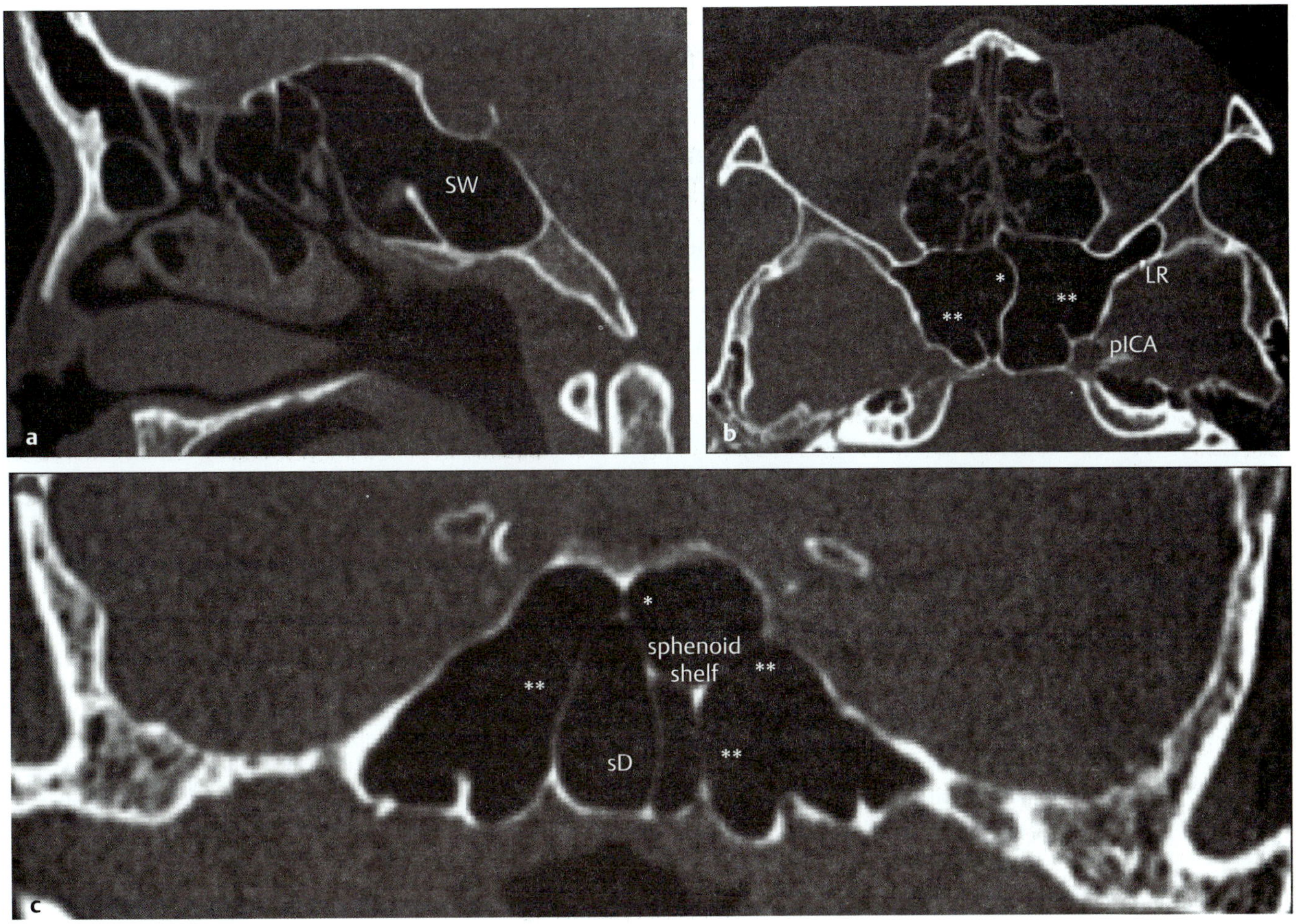

Fig. 1.27 Bone-weighted computed tomography images of the sphenoid sinus and its relevance for transsphenoidal surgery. **(a)** Sellar type pneumatization in a sagittal CT section of the sphenoid sinus, which is the most frequently detected variation of sphenoid pneumatization. A sphenoid wall (SW) type intersinus septum, which is oriented in the coronal plane, can be seen. **(b)** A main sphenoidal intersinus septum (*) and two accessory septae (**) in an axial CT section are present, one of which inserts into the left paraclival internal carotid artery (pICA). A lateral recess (LR) of the sphenoid sinus is seen on the left side. **(c)** Coronal CT section of a multichambered sphenoid sinus. The main sphenoidal intersinus septum (*) and three accessory septae (**) are present and act as sphenoid divider (sD) type intersinus septae. A sphenoid shelf type intersinus septum, which is oriented in the axial plane, is also present.

structures including the optic, vidian, maxillary, oculomotor, trochlear, and abducent nerves, and the ICA.[185–187] Additionally, intrasellar pathologies significantly change sellar morphology presenting during surgery.[177] CT and MRI provide information on the insertion site of the intersinus septae at the base of skull necessary for transsphenoidal surgery.[177,179,180]

Preoperative assessment of neuroimaging studies is therefore mandatory. Until today, it remains unclear, whether MRI and CT are necessary for each case of transsphenoidal surgery, or if predictors can be identified in MRI where a CT might yield more information for the surgeon in the preoperative planning.

Imaging for Pituitary Adenoma

MRI of the sella is indispensable when assessing pituitary adenomas.[188] Typical imaging protocols include T1-weighted spin-echo (SE) precontrast and postcontrast and fast-SE (FSE) T2-weighted sequences mainly in coronal orientation. Also, acquisition of dynamic postcontrast images is brightly recommended, though the technical options available show some variety. Usually, a small field of view (20 × 25 cm), thin slices (≤3 mm), and high-resolution matrix (256 × 512) are favorable.[189] Also, a half dose contrast injection will be recommended by many authors to decrease the "overshining" effect of the pituitary gland.[190] Fluid-attenuated inversion

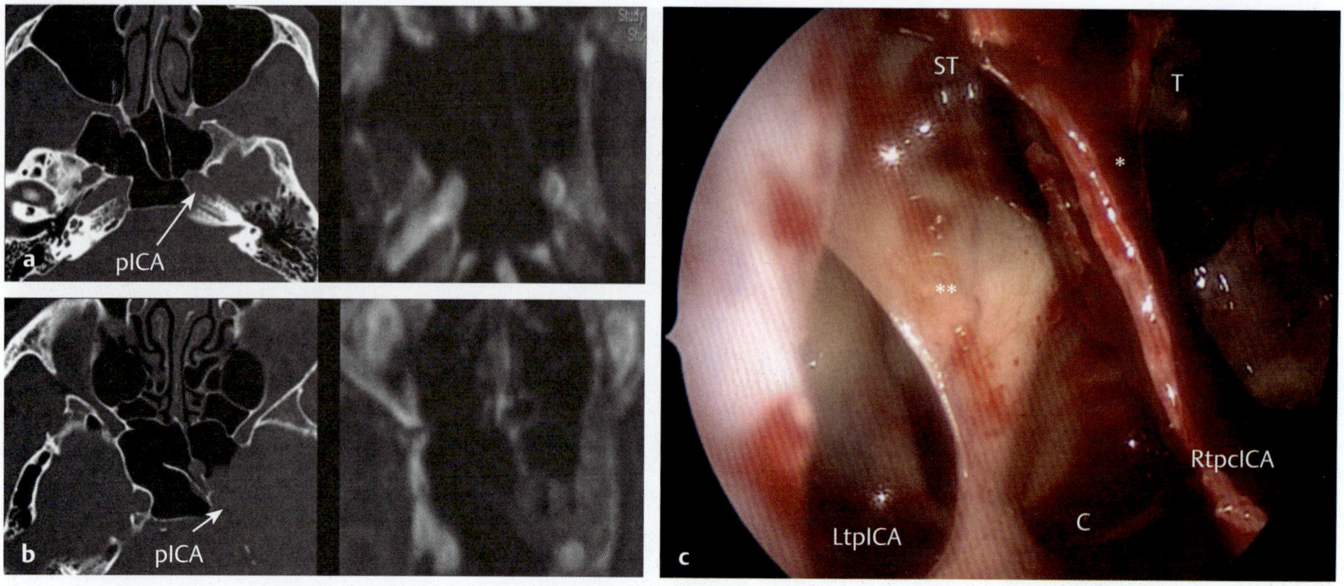

Fig. 1.28 Sphenoidal septations inserting into the paraclival (pCIA) or cavernous (cICA) internal carotid artery may also be seen on high-quality images of MRI scan, with focus on T2 and T1 with adequate contrast enhancement. **(a)** Axial section of a high-resolution CT confirming a main and an accessory intersinus septum attaching to the left paraclival ICA (*left*). An axial T1-weighted postcontrast MRI sequence reveals the same two intersinus septum inserting into the left paraclival ICA (*right*). **(b)** Axial section of a high-resolution CT confirming a main and an accessory intersinus septum attaching to the left paraclival ICA (*left*). Axial T1-weighted postcontrast MRI sequence shows one main septum and a second small intrasinusal septum going into the direction of the left paraclival ICA, disturbed by the pathological process of an invasive pituitary adenoma (*right*). **(c)** Intraoperative confirmation of a main (*) and an accessory (**) intersinus septum deviating to the left with probable insertion into the left paraclival ICA (LtpICA) inferiorly. The right paraclival ICA (RtpcICA) is not involved by a sphenoid septum. The tumor is visible in the upper left part of the picture (T). The clivus (C) is exposed in the middle part of the picture.

recovery (FLAIR) and diffusion-weighted imaging (DWI) are helpful adjuncts for certain differential diagnosis. For the vascular structures, sequences for MR angiography (MRA) and venography (MRV) are well described,[188] but the latter is mostly of no further use in the evaluation of pathologies of the pituitary gland.

Though benign, pituitary tumors are located in a critical area adjacent to the cavernous sinus, the ICAs, the optic nerve, and the optic chiasm.[188] Hence, the tumor may invade the following regions:

- *Parasellar region*: Involvement of the cavernous ICA and the cavernous cranial nerves (**Table 1.2; Fig. 1.30** and **Fig. 1.31**).
- *Subchiasmatic region*: Compression and dislocation of the optic chiasm and the optic nerves (**Table 1.3; Fig. 1.30** and **Fig. 1.31**).
- *Suprasellar region*: Encasement of intracranial arteries such as the ICA bifurcation, the middle and anterior cerebral artery, and even reach the ventricular region (**Table 1.3**; **Fig. 1.30** and **Fig. 1.31**).
- *Inferior compartment*: Sphenoid and ethmoid sinuses and the clivus with erosion of bone that can be appreciated in bone-weighted CT scans (**Fig. 1.30**).

Solid Pituitary Adenoma

Microadenoma: Pituitary microadenomas are less than 10 mm in size. They present as ovoid, flattened, or triangular intrasellar lesions with hypo- or isointensity on T1-weighted sequences.[188,190] Depending on their hormonal activity, they tend to be in specific locations within the adenohypophysis (**Table 1.9**). T2-weighted sequences vary between the different subtypes.[188]

Early-phase dynamic contrast-enhanced sequences are used to identify small microadenomas, with typical delayed enhancement when compared with the surrounding pituitary gland tissue.[188,191] Newer methods like FSE, high-resolution 3D gradient echo, and golden-angle radial sparse parallel (GRASP) sequences were recently proposed to overcome the limitations of current methods and improve sensitivity.[161,192]

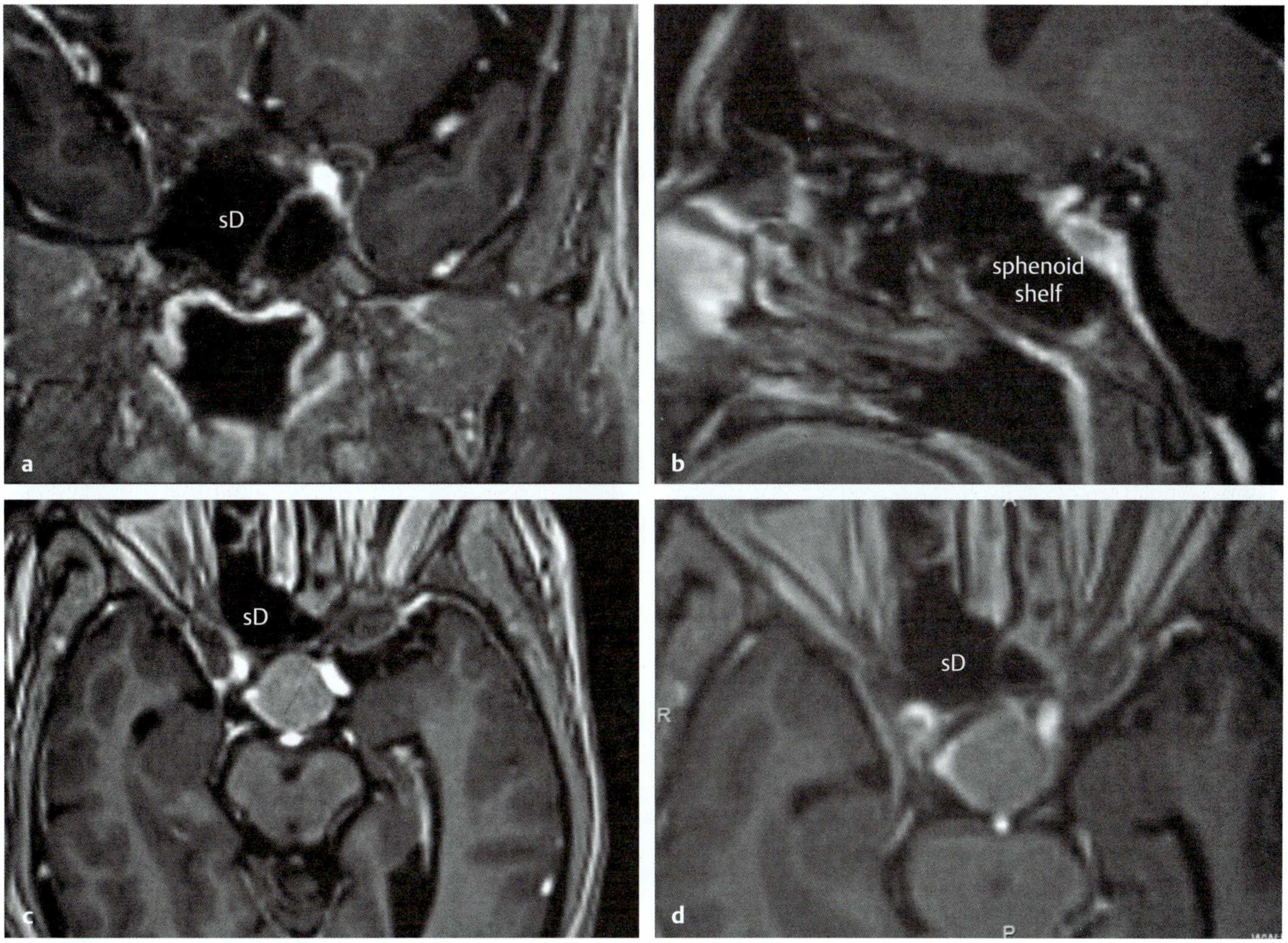

Fig. 1.29 T1-weighted postcontrast MRI sequences demonstrating the different orientation of sphenoid intersinus septae. **(a)** Coronal MRI sequence showing a sphenoid divider (sD) type intersinus septum oriented in the sagittal plane. **(b)** Sagittal MRI sequence showing a sphenoid shelf type intersinus septum oriented in the axial plane. **(c, d)** Axial MRI sequence showing an sD type intersinus septum oriented in the sagittal plane.

Table 1.9 **Description of the regional distribution of hormone-secreting microadenomas within the pituitary gland in neuroimaging**

Pituitary microadenomas	Location within the adenohypophysis	T2-weighted sequence appearance
Prolactin-producing adenoma (lactotroph adenomas or prolactinomas)	Inferolateral	Hyperintense in more than 80%
ACTH-producing adenoma	Central	
Growth hormone–producing adenoma	Lateral	Iso- or hypointensity in more than 67%
Thyroid-stimulating hormone-producing adenoma (TSH-Oma)	Central	

Abbreviation: ACTH, adrenocorticotropic hormone.

Sources: Adapted from Lysack et al.[188] and Bonneville et al.[190]

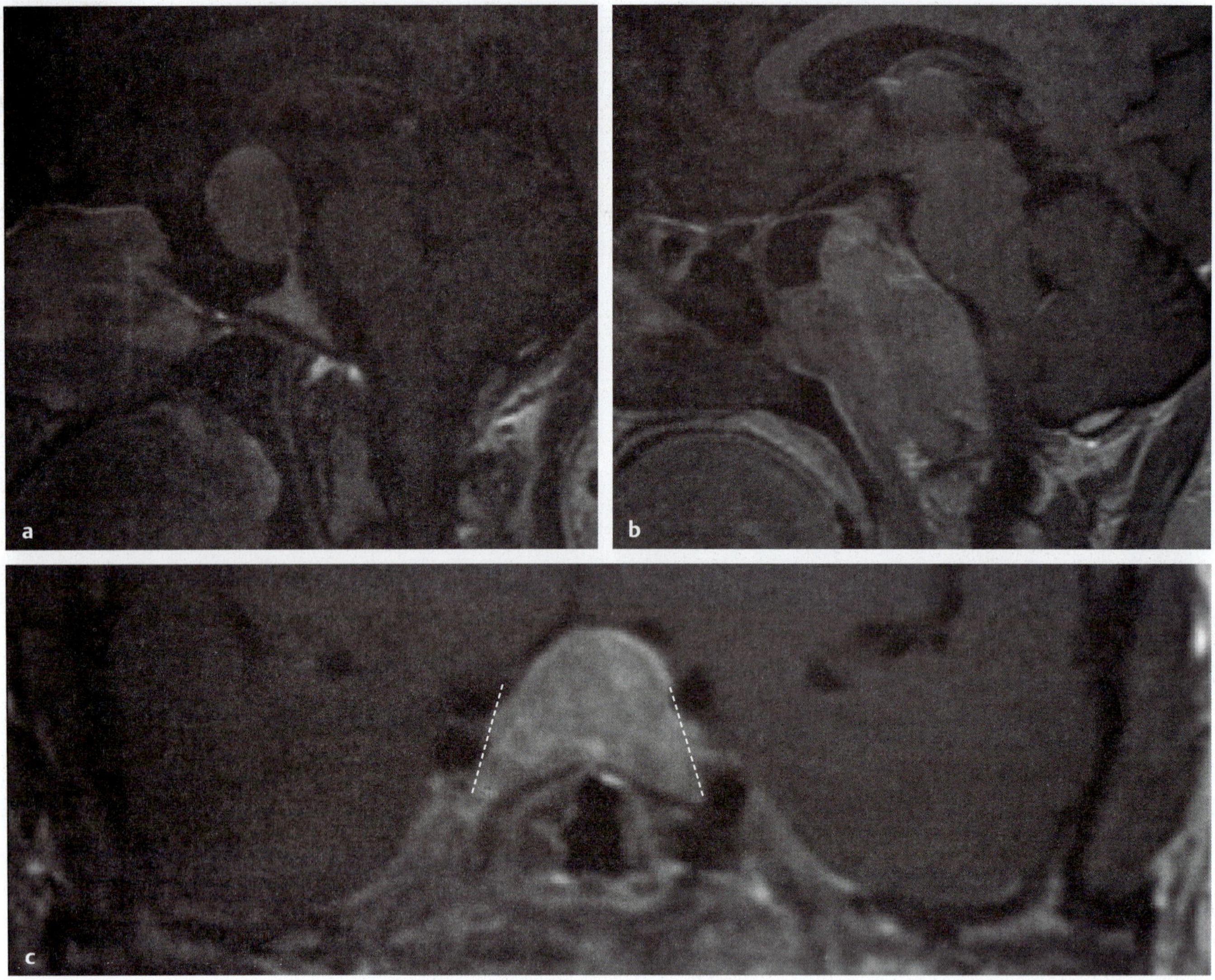

Fig. 1.30 T1-weighted contrast-enhanced MRI sections demonstrating parasellar extensions of a pituitary tumor. **(a)** Sagittal MRI section demonstrating the suprasellar extension. **(b)** Sagittal MRI section demonstrating tumorous invasion into the sphenoid sinus and erosion of the clivus. **(c)** Cavernous sinus invasion is measured in coronal T1-weighted contrast-enhanced MRI sections using the Knosp grading score (**Table 1.2**). In the present example, a Knosp grade 1 invasion on the right side and a Knosp grade 2 invasion on the left side are present (*white lines*).

Macroadenoma: Pituitary macroadenomas have a size larger than 10 mm and are considered as "giant" when reaching a diameter more than 40 mm. These tumors usually are nonfunctioning adenomas because of the lack of hormone-mediated signs and symptoms. Hence, locoregional mass effect symptoms lead to diagnostic imaging, when the tumors extend beyond the sellar borders to the suprasellar and parasellar region. Remodeling of the sella with enlargement and bony erosion is present, when compared to microadenomas.[188,193] The normal pituitary gland is compressed and might appear as circumferential hyperintense rim ("pseudocapsule") mostly above or behind the lesion with higher signal intensity when compared with the lesion itself[48,161] (**Table 1.10**).

Distinguishing compression or invasion of the medial cavernous sinus wall by a macroadenoma is a challenging feature in neuroimaging.[15,190,194–196] The prevalence of the medial cavernous sinus wall has been described to be up to 43% radiographically and 18% when compared intraoperatively.[197] Dhandapani et al. gave a comprehensive overview for the different radiological approaches.[197] In sum, inferolateral venous compartment obliteration and Knosp grades 3 and 4 revealed the highest correlation with intraoperative cavernous sinus invasion and the lowest correlation with gross total resection.[197]

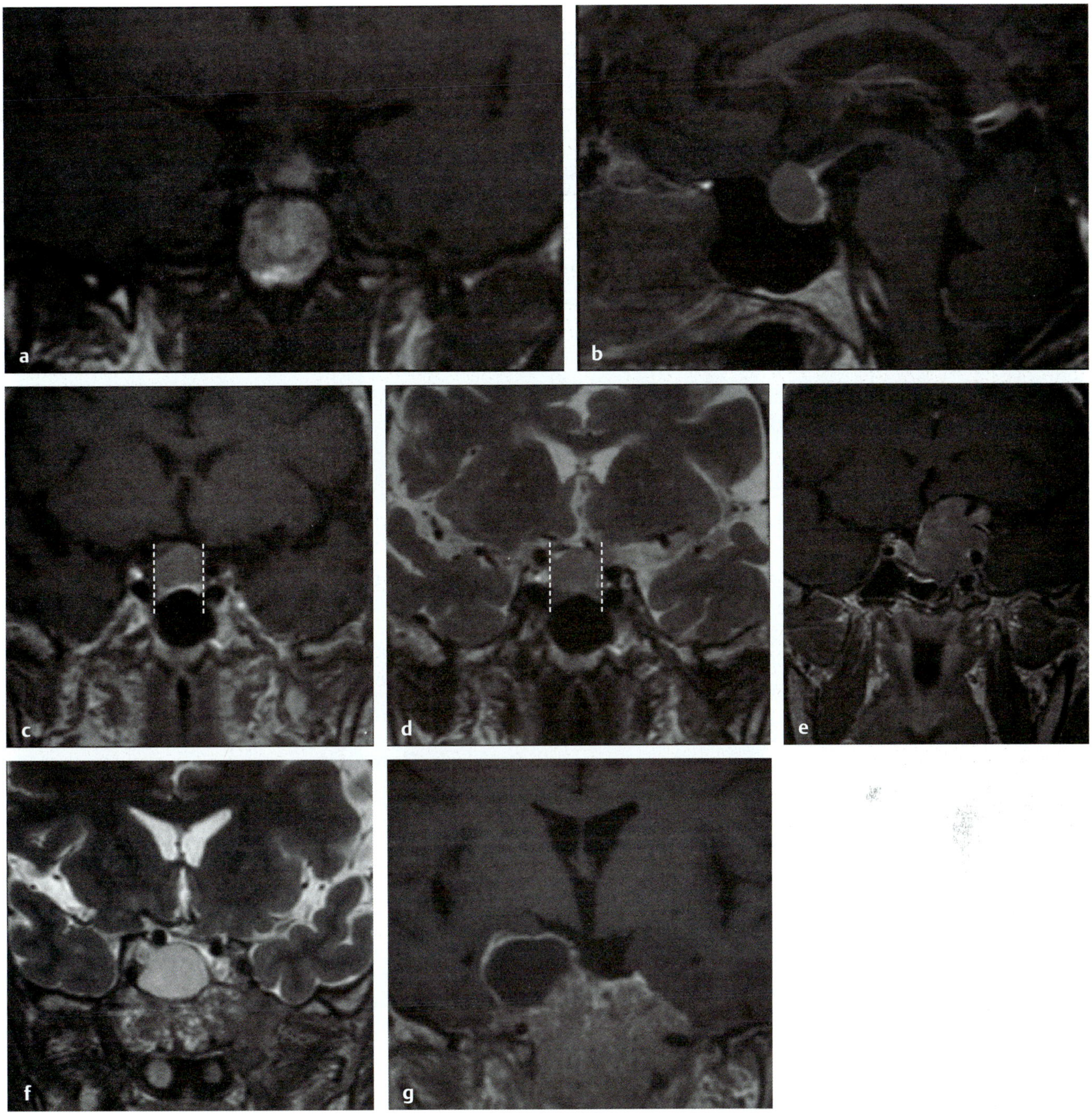

Fig. 1.31 T2- and T1 contrast-enhanced MRI sections demonstrating the variable appearance of pituitary adenomas. **(a)** Coronal, **(b)** sagittal dynamic T1 contrast-enhanced MRI section showing a sellar mass in the anterior lobe of the pituitary gland with delayed enhancement with normal signal behavior of the posterior pituitary gland. **(c, d)** Coronal T2- and T1-weighted noncontrast-enhanced MRI sections showing a hyperintense sellar mass compressing the left optic nerve. The optic chiasm and the cavernous sinus are not affected by this lesion (Knosp grade 0 [*white line*]). **(e)** Coronal T1-weighted contrast-enhanced MRI section demonstrating a sellar mass with significant suprasellar extension and encasement of the left cavernous (cICA) and clinoidal (cICA) internal carotid artery. **(f, g)** Coronal T2 FRFSE- and T1 contrast-enhanced MRI sections showing a cystic pituitary macroadenoma with an intrasellar and a parasellar cystic component on the superolateral side. Pituitary adenoma cysts appear hypointense in T1-weighted sequences with a thick wall enhancement.

Table 1.10 Description of typical radiological features of pituitary macroadenomas in neuroimaging with MRI

Pituitary macroadenoma		Radiological features
T1-weighted precontrast		Isointense to normal pituitary gland tissue, high signal if there are areas of focal hemorrhages
T1-weighted postcontrast		Homogenously hypoenhancing
	Noninvasive	Interposition of normal pituitary tissue between tumor and the medial cavernous sinus wall
		Less than 25% encasement of the cavernous carotid artery
	Invasive	Greater than 67% encasement of the cavernous carotid artery
		Complete encasement of the cavernous carotid artery
T2 weighted		Low signal with calcification and diffuse iron deposition; high signal intensity if there are areas of cystic change
T2-weighted gradient echo		Acute and old hemorrhage appear as areas of low signal intensity
T2-weighted flow-attenuated inversion recovery scan (FLAIR)		Cyst shows higher signal intensity compared to solid tumor

Sources: Adapted from Lysack et al. 2008[188] and Patronas et al. 2014.[161]

Cystic Lesions of the Sella

The radiological differentiation of cystic sellar masses based on their entity may be complex. Radiographic findings are heterogeneous. The differential diagnosis of cystic lesions located in the sellar and parasellar region is summarized in **Table 1.6**.

Cystic Pituitary Adenoma

Cystic pituitary adenomas may appear as heterogeneous hypodense lesions on CT scan, occasionally with erosion into the sphenoid bone[48]. Generally, cystic pituitary adenomas are hypointense in T1-weighted sequences. They frequently present with a thick wall enhancement.[48,198] The topographical relation of the pituitary stalk to the cystic lesions has been proposed to allow differentiation between a cystic pituitary adenoma and a Rathke's cleft cyst. The cystic pituitary adenoma leads to a posterior deviation of the stalk, while the Rahtke cleft cyst pushes the latter anteriorly[46,199] (**Fig. 1.32**).

Cystic Craniopharyngioma

In general, calcification or solid components favor the diagnosis of a craniopharyngioma.[44] The cystic components are, depending on type and age, often greater in volume than the solid components.[45,46,200] Calcifications on CT are more frequent in pediatric cases as well as for the adamantinomatous subtype, adding up to 60% of cases[200] (**Fig. 1.33**). Specific features are addressed in Chapter 7.

Cystic Meningioma

Visualization of a dural attachment and the dural "tail" might rise the suspicion of a meningioma.[46] As meningioma tends to calcify, differentiation from a craniopharyngioma can be difficult in cystic cases.[49,50]

Rathke's Cleft Cyst

Rathke's cleft cysts appear as well-circumscribed, spherical, or ovoid intrasellar radiological finding. The normal pituitary gland may be circumferential if the cyst arises within the gland ("claw sign"). Signal behavior depends on the variable content of the cysts.[44–46] A low intensity on T1-weighted sequences with a high intensity on T2-weighted sequences is suggestive for cysts filled with thin, CSF-like fluid. Cysts with more proteinaceous, mucoid fluid correlate with higher intensity on both T1- and T2-weighted sequences or a high intensity on T1-weighted sequences with a low intensity on T2-weighted sequences.[44–46] A small nonenhancing intracystic nodule is considered a pathognomonic finding. It should appear hyperintense to surrounding fluid on T1 and hypointense on T2. Depending on the signal of the surrounding fluid, it may be inapparent on one sequence or the other[201] (**Fig. 1.34**).

Intrasellar Arachnoid Cyst

Arachnoid cysts are commonly found intracranially and are typically recognized on MRI by a cyst-filled cavity with identical imaging characteristics to CSF.[43,44,46] Altered MRI

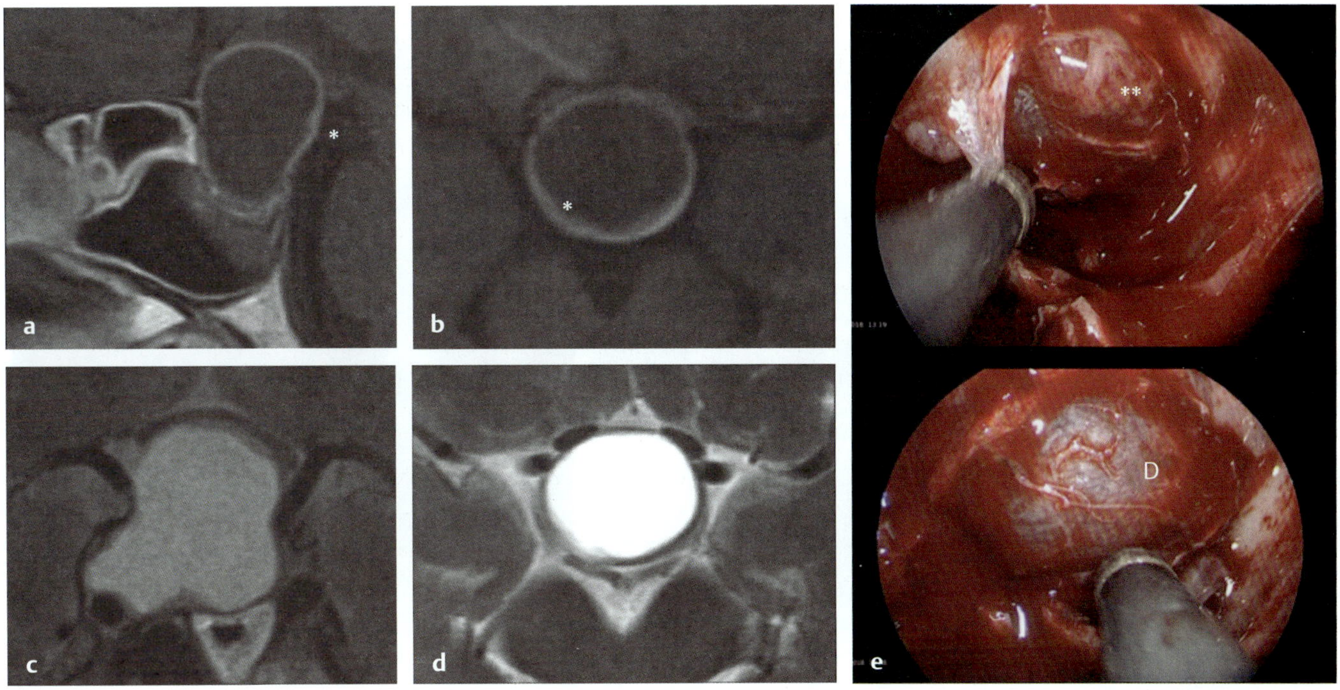

Fig. 1.32 **(a)** Sagittal, **(b)** axial T1-weighted contrast-enhanced, **(c)** coronal, and **(d)** Axial T2-weighted MRI sections of a cystic pituitary adenoma. Cystic pituitary adenoma appears hypointense in T1-weighted sequences with a thick wall enhancement and hyperintense in T2 with an isointense wall signal. The cystic pituitary adenoma leads to a posterior deviation of the stalk and neurohypophysis (*). **(e)** Intraoperative visualization of a cystic pituitary adenoma revealing typical granular pituitary adenoma tissue (**) after evacuation of the cyst, along the prolapsing diaphragma sellae (D).

signaling is found with higher protein content or evidence of hemorrhage.[202] Isolated intrasellar arachnoid cysts are rare (**Fig. 1.35**).

Epidermoid and Dermoid Cysts

Standard CT and MR have been reported to be unreliable to definitively diagnose epidermoid or dermoid tumors.[45] They present as nonenhancing lesions on CT, sometimes with the density of fat. Hypo- or hyperintensity on T1-weighted sequences and hypo- or hyperintensity on T2- (**Fig. 1.36**) as well as diffusion-weighted sequences (diffusion restriction) (**Fig. 1.37**) are suggestive for these lesions,[203] the latter one usually seen with the epidermoid. Hyperintensity in T1-weighted sequences is only seen if the lesion has a high lipid component,[46] but may also be seen with blood products and calcifications.

Mucoceles

Mucoceles are described as nonenhancing cystic lesions with potential bony erosion and/or remodeling in CT. A bright cystic cavity on T2-weighted sequences can be aknowledged[43,46,204] (**Fig. 1.38**).

Synchronous Lesions of the Sella

The radiological differentiation between a pituitary macroadenoma and a sellar/parasellar meningioma can be difficult if coexistence is present.[205–207] However, the differentiation of a pituitary adenoma with supra-/parasellar extension from a pituitary adenoma with a colliding supra/parasellar meningioma is of crucial importance, as treatment strategies vary among these pathologies.[73,74,122]

Surgical Considerations

Pituitary surgery has seen a remarkable shift from transcranial approaches (TCAs) within the past decades. The use of a rigid endoscope in skull base surgeries started with the transsphenoidal approach to the skull base for pituitary lesions, where Gerard Guiot was the first neurosurgeon. However, routine use of this method was abandoned because

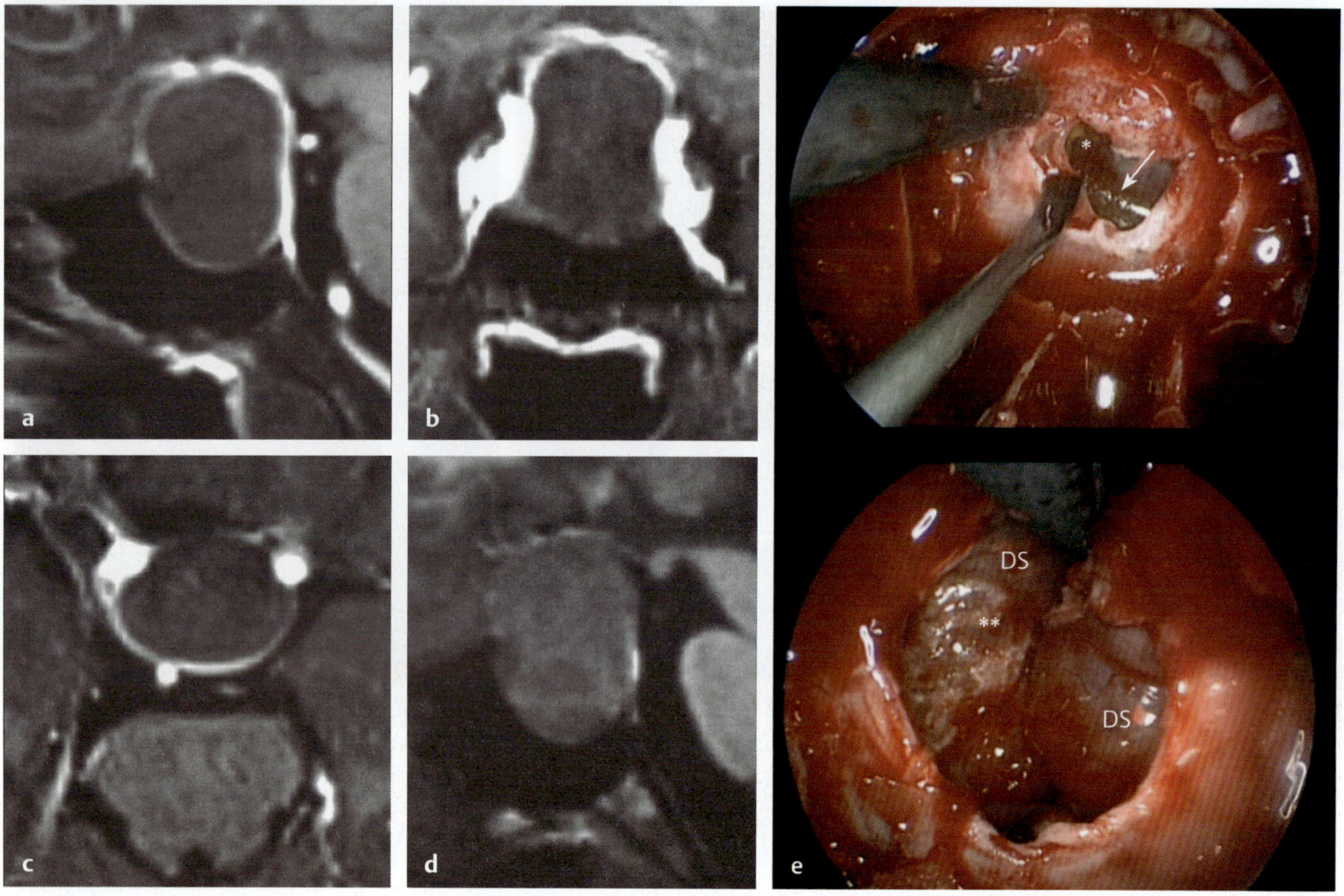

Fig. 1.33 **(a)** Sagittal, **(b)** coronal, **(c)** axial T1-weighted contrast-enhanced, **(d)** sagittal coronal T1-weighted noncontrast-enhanced MRI section of a solitary cystic intra- and suprasellar craniopharyngioma. In T1-weighted sequences, the cystic craniopharyngioma can be of high to intermediate to low intensity depending on the content of the cyst. The cyst wall enhances vividly in T1 contrast-enhanced images. The cystic elements of adamantinomatous craniopharyngioma are of high intensity on T1-weighted and high or mixed intensity on T2-weighted images. Cysts of the solid–cystic papillary subtype are of low intensity on T1-weighted and high intensity on T2-weighted images. **(e)** Intraoperative visualization of a solitary cystic intra- and suprasellar craniopharyngioma. Typical yellowish tumor tissue (*) and cholesterol crystals within the cyst fluid content (*white arrow*) as well as firmer calcified tumor parts (**) along the diaphragma sellae (D) can be identified.

of inadequate visualization of the surgical field. In the late 1970s, the endoscope was reintroduced.[208] Nowadays, transsphenoidal surgery is the preferred operative corridor for treating symptomatic pituitary adenoma. TCAs for supra-/parasellar extra-axial lesions include pterional, transsylvian, subfrontal, or supraorbital corridors. Microscopic transsphenoidal surgery includes endonasal or sublabial approaches.[121,122]

Nowadays, fully endoscopic transsphenoidal surgery is getting more common.[209–211] The route to the sphenoid sinus through which the surgery is performed is variable among surgeons according to their personal preferences and includes the transseptal, transnasal, and transethmoidal approach. In our institution, the preferred access for surgery is via a **transseptal transsphenoidal** route. This technique was initially used with the assistance of a modified speculum, which was abandoned in the later years.[212–214]

The superiority of the endoscopic transsphenoidal technique when compared to the transsphenoidal microscopic technique has been a subject of long and intensive debate. In general, the use of an endoscope for the transnasal transsphenoidal approach brings certain advantages and disadvantages, when compared to the classic microscopic technique. The comparison of both techniques remains somewhat limited due to the lack of prospective randomized trials. Comparisons are therefore based on prospective trials (TRANSSPHER Study) and reviews and meta-analyses of studies of the individual techniques.[215] The majority of

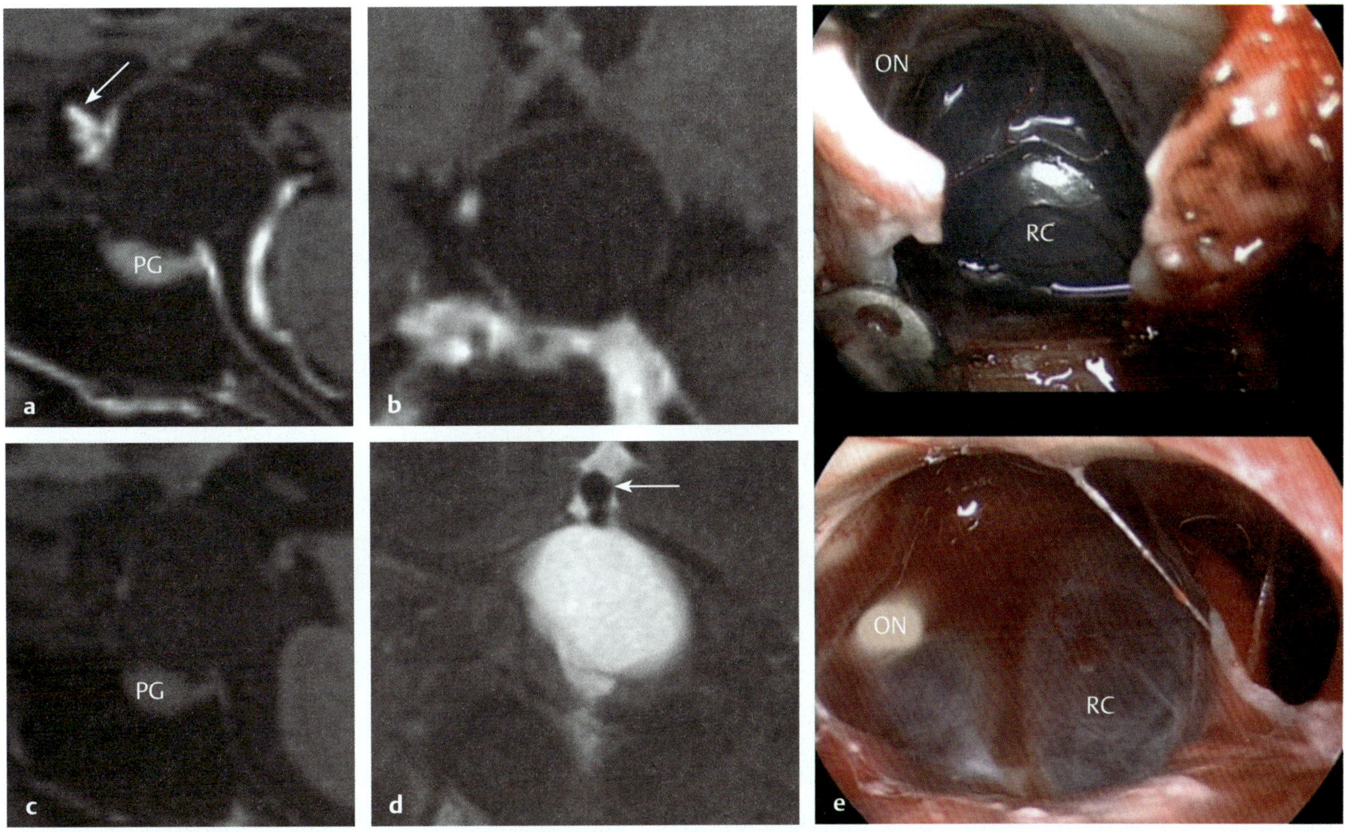

Fig. 1.34 **(a)** Sagittal, **(b)** coronal, **(c)** axial T1-weighted contrast-enhanced, **(d)** axial T2-weighted MRI section of a Rathke's cleft cyst. This cystic lesion appears as well-circumscribed, spherical, or ovoid intrasellar mass. A low intensity on T1-weighted sequences with a high intensity on T2-weighted sequences is suggestive for cysts filled with thin, CSF-like fluid. In this particular case, the incidental finding of a cerebral arterial aneurysm arising from the anterior communicating artery is present (*white arrow*). **(e)** Intraoperative visualization of a Rathke's cleft cyst (RC). The cyst wall is homogenous and there is no obvious tumor tissue associated with the cyst wall. The cyst fluid content is CSF-like.

reports included in the systematic reviews and metaanalyses are retrospective and nonrandomized or controlled trials. Only one meta-analysis by Bastos et al. included two randomized and three prospective nonrandomized trials; however, the low number of patients is a major limitation to draw conclusions in terms of gross total resection (GTR) and complications between the two groups.[216]

Potential Advantages of the Endonasal Endoscopic Approach

The use of the endonasal endoscopic approach avoids external incisions and preserves neurological, visual, and masticatory functions in well-selected patients.[217] In our institution, the minimally invasive fully endoscopic approach is performed in collaboration between the neurosurgeon and the rhinologist.[218,219] The ENT surgeon provides the endonasal access for the neurosurgeon and subsequently assists during the osteodural exposure and further intradural tumor resection. Thus, the neurosurgeon is able to perfom bimanual dissection and a third hand is provided for more complex maneuvers. This highlights the importance of a true team approach with consecutive advancement of endoscopic skull base surgery, resulting in the development of the extended endoscopic approaches.

- *Visualization of the surgical field*: With the rigid rod lens telescope, a panoramic view of the sellar floor and the surrounding structures of critical importance is achieved. Because of better illumination, there is an improved view for intrasellar and extrasellar extensions. This provides a better visualization of corners not seen with the microscope.[220–223]
- *Approach-related morbidity*: Because of the minimal invasiveness, lower nasal morbidity and a faster recovery period postoperatively has been described.[209,224] The concurrent use of an image-guided surgery (IGS) system as adjunct allows the exact localization of the lesion and the anatomical limitations. This allows for a tailored approach planning as well as a zonal dissection of the skull base.[219]

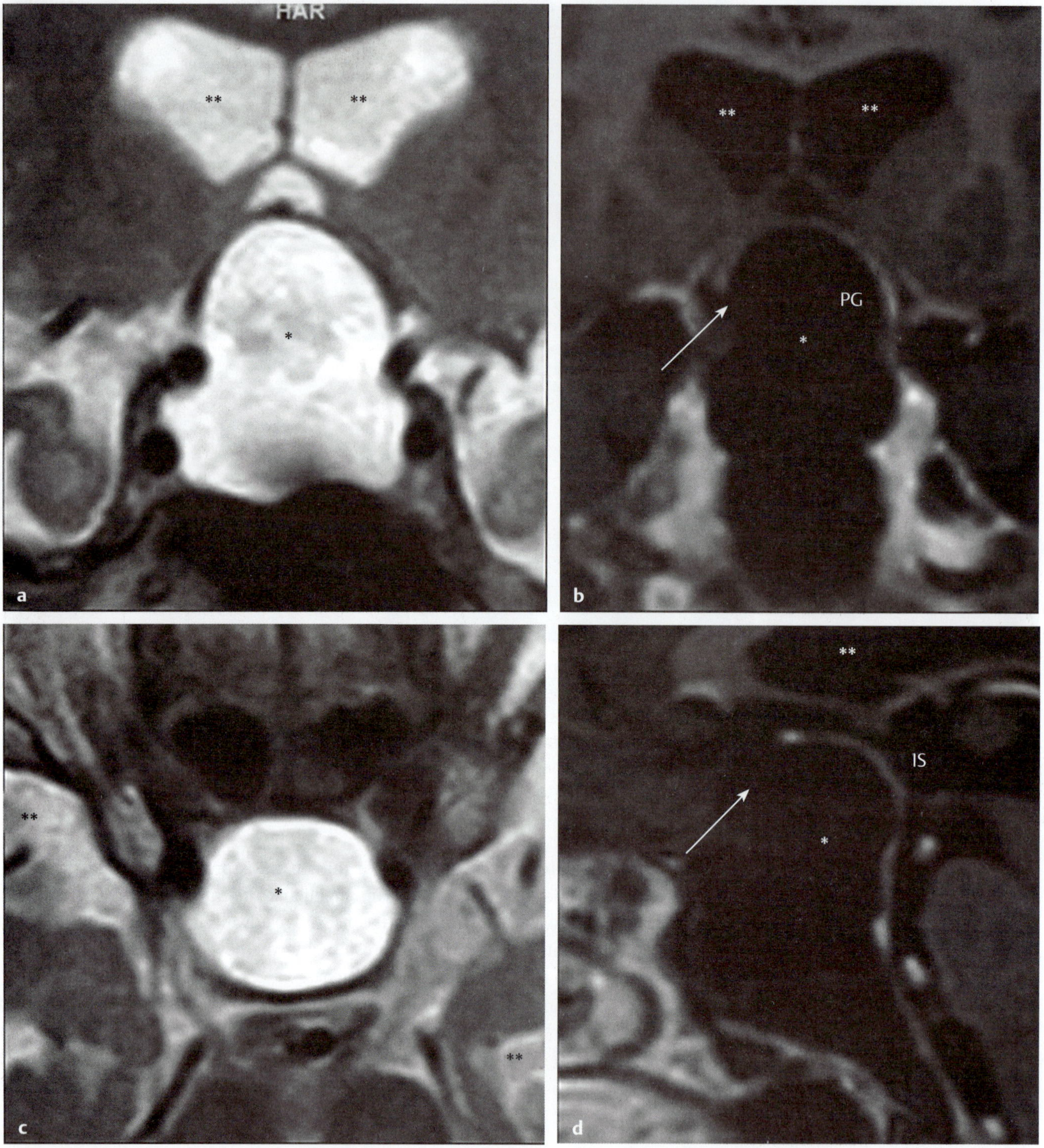

Fig. 1.35 **(a)** Coronal T1-weighted contrast-enhanced, **(b)** coronal T2-weighted, **(c)** axial T2-weighted, **(d)** sagittal T1-weighted contrast-enhanced MRI section of an intrasella arachnoid cyst. Arachnoid cysts are typically recognized on MRI by a cyst-filled cavity (*) with identical imaging characteristics to CSF (**) without contrast enhancement of the cyst wall (*white arrow*). The infundibular stalk (IS) and the pituitary gland (PG) , however, do enhance and are dislocated by the lesion.

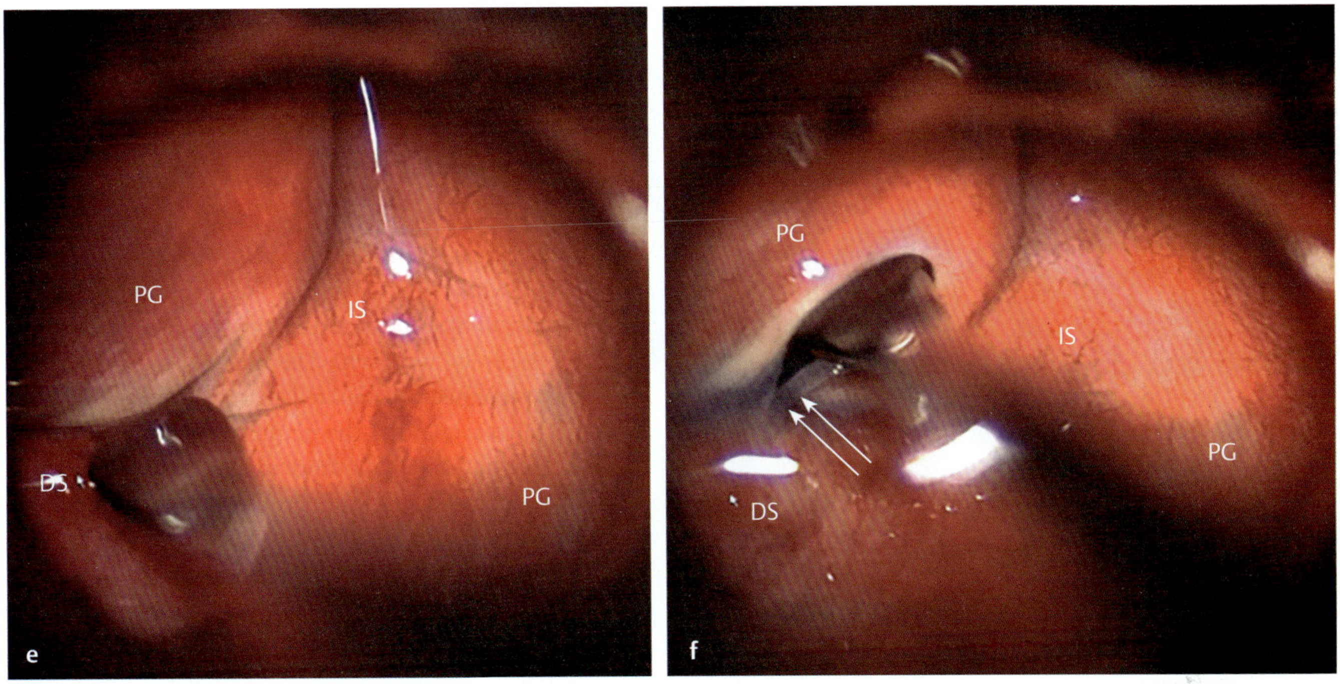

Fig. 1.35 *(Continued)* (**e** and **f**) Intraoperative visualization of an intrasellar arachnoid cyst with the flattened pituitary gland (PG) and infundibular stalk (IS) along the cystic and the protruding diaphragma sella. The dorsum sellae (DS) is visible. The arachnoid cyst wall (*double arrow*) is visible between the DS and the diaphragma sellae.

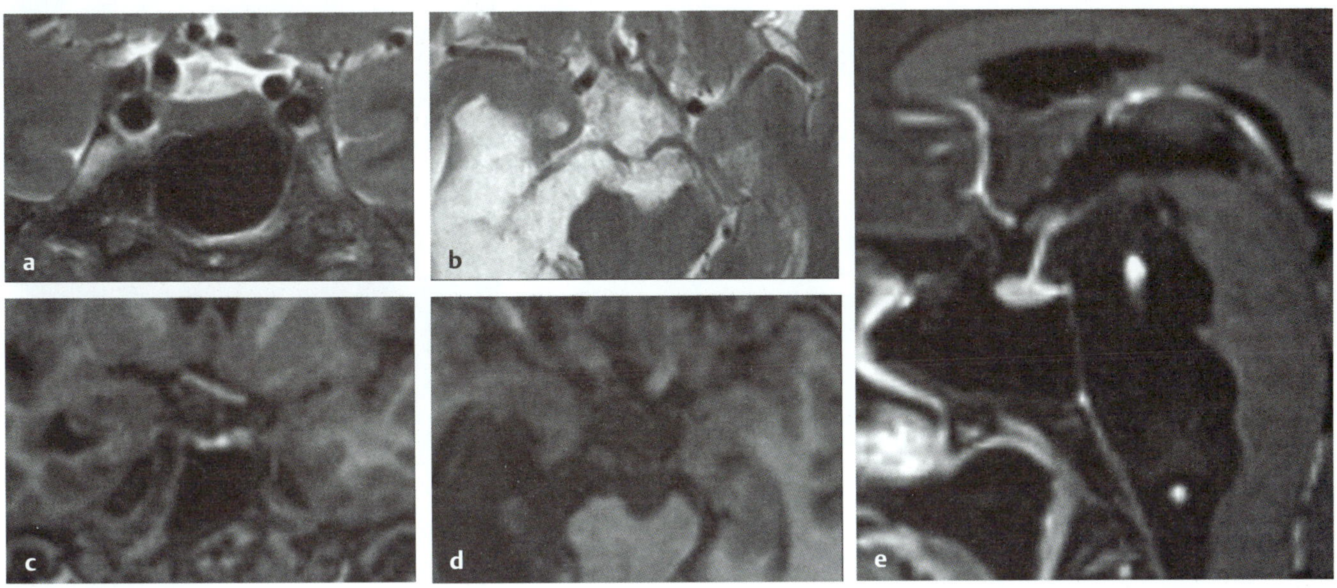

Fig. 1.36 **(a)** Coronal and **(b)** axial T2-weighted, **(c)** coronal and **(d)** axial T1-weighted noncontrast-enhanced, **(e)** sagittal T1-weighted contrast-enhanced MRI sections demonstrating an anterior, middle, and posterior fossa epidermoid cyst. Hypo- or hyperintensity on T1-weighted sequences and hypo- or hyperintensity on T2 are suggestive for these lesions.

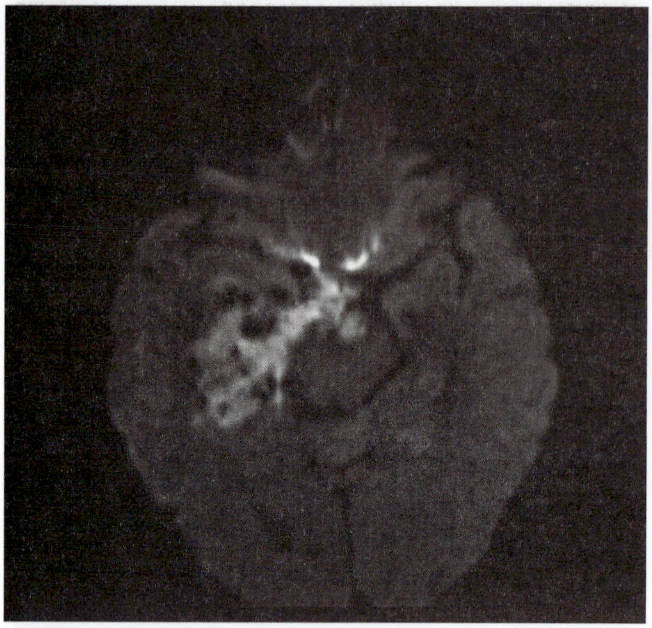

Fig. 1.37 Axial diffusion-weighted sequences show a diffusion restriction within the anterior, middle, and posterior fossa epidermoid cysts.

- *Surgical training*: The endonasal endoscopic approach serves as a platform for surgeons to develop their skill for more advanced parasellar and suprasellar lesions.

Potential Disadvantages of the Endonasal Endoscopic Approach

- *Visualization of the surgical field*: A two-dimensional vision, with the lack of accurate depth perception, is described when comparing this technique with the microscopic approach. The endoscope provides a monocular view compared to the binocular view of the microscope that the neurosurgeon is accustomed to. Therefore, compensatory maneuvers are necessary to overcome the lack of depth perceptions, including bimanual dissection with one hand constantly in the field and providing gentle palpation with a suction tip. Besides that, the surgeons can also move the endoscope to provide a dynamic visualization of the surgical field.[217] During surgery, the endoscope and its light path have to be kept clear and clean.

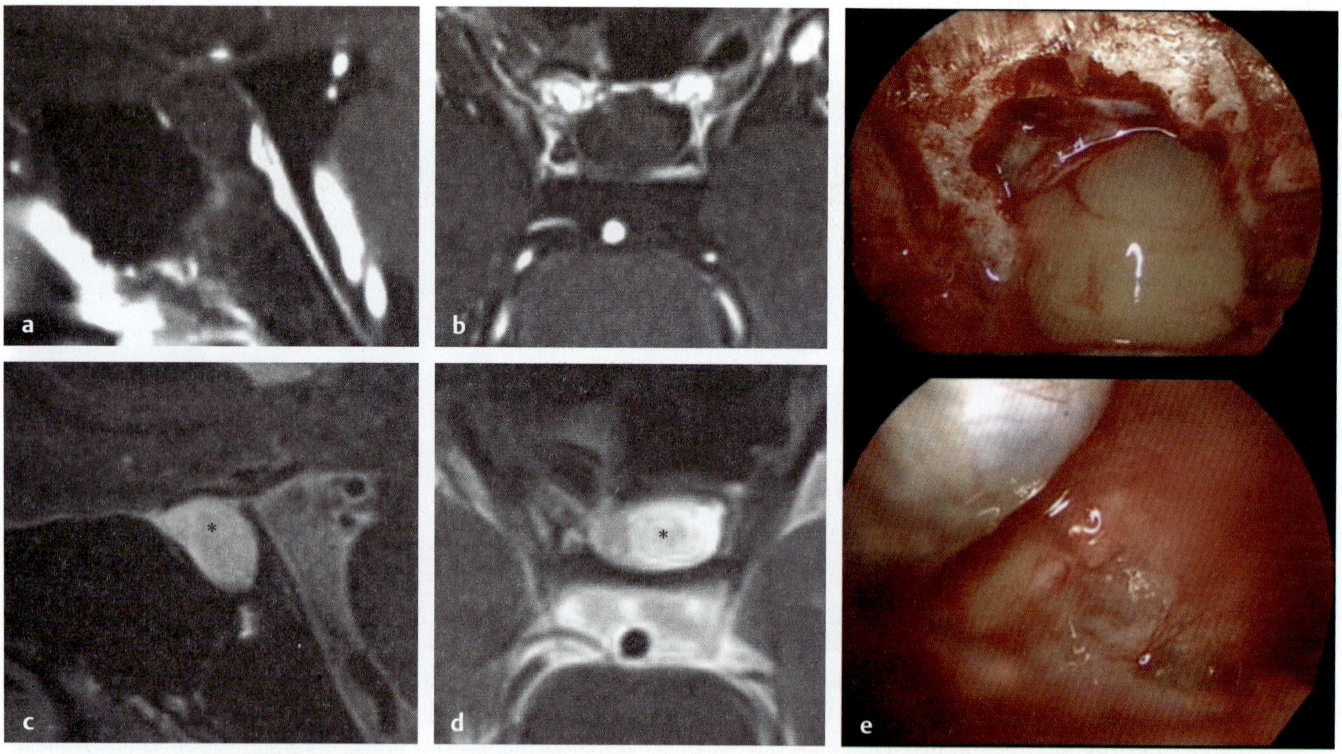

Fig. 1.38 **(a)** Coronal and **(b)** axial T1-weighted contrast-enhanced, **(c)** sagittal and **(d)** axial T2-weighted MRI section of an intrasellar mucocele. They present as nonenhancing cystic lesions. A bright cystic cavity (*) on T2-weighted sequences can be acknowledged. **(e)** Intraoperative visualization of an intrasellar mucocele. The cyst content is thickened and consists of mucus; there is no evidence of cholesterol crystals, old hemorrhage, or CSF-like fluid. Along the cyst cavity, no tumorous tissue or a capsule can be appreciated, as it would be recognizable in other cystic sellar lesions (e.g., cystic pituitary adenoma, cystic craniopharyngioma, Rathke's cleft cyst).

- *Surgical training*: The endoscopic technique potentially brings bring technical unfamiliarities for surgeons who are used to operate with a microscope. However, learning curves have been reported in the literature when institutions change to endoscopic surgery.[225–228] Experienced surgeons using the microscopic technique are very efficient and have low morbidities in resecting pituitary lesions.[19,97] Retrospective comparisons between both techniques therefore inherit a selection bias with limited power. For more complex maneuvers and bimanual microneurosurgical dissection by the neurosurgeon, an assistant and an endoscope holder are necessary.[220–223] This so-called "two-nostril four-hands technique" has been described for different approaches to the sellar region.[229,230]

Proven Advantages of the Endonasal Endoscopic Approach

Proven advantages of the endonasal endoscopic approach are the lack of external incisions, the avoidance of translocation of the maxillofacial skeleton, preservation of neurovascular structures, and the avoidance of brain retraction. However, the extent of resection of endonasal structures and bony coverage of the base of skull and dura is not automatically "minimally invasive," and this term can only be used when extended transcranial approaches for certain skull base pathologies are taken into account. The endonasal endoscopic approach is associated with less trauma to the normal soft tissue and facial skeleton, resulting in shorter recovery time as well as shorter delay between surgery and the start of adjuvant treatment compared to open approaches in anterior skull base malignancies.[231] Generally, and especially for pituitary adenoma surgery, important outcomes are the extent of resection, surgical complications, and endonasal outcomes.

Approach-Related Morbidity and Mortality

- *Effectiveness and outcome*: A meta-analysis of 1,014 patients with pituitary adenomas in 15 studies performed by Gao et al. did demonstrate superiority of the endoscopic transsphenoidal approach in effectiveness and outcome when compared with the microscopic technique.[23,209,232–246]
- *Approach-related morbidity* (*nasal outcome*): The rate of septal perforation was found to be less frequent when using the endonasal endoscopic approach, while there was no difference in postoperative epistaxis.[209] This finding was confirmed in a recent meta-analysis performed by Li et al., where EEA was associated with a lower incidence of septal perforations in patients with pituitary adenoma.[247]
- *Length of hospital stay*: Purely endoscopic surgery was superior in terms of the length of postoperative hospital stay, however, no differences in terms of length of operation, rate of meningitis, diabetes insipidus, CSF leakage or hypopituitarism were found.[209]
- *Complications*: A pooled data meta-analysis of radiological criteria and comparison of endoscopic and microscopic surgery by Dhandapani et al. revealed carotid injury and cranial nerve deficits with the endonasal endoscopic approach in 0.9 and 5%, respectively.[197] A systematic review of effects and complications between the endoscopic endonasal approach and the microscopic technique was recently published by Li et al. The authors evaluated 13 reports and found no statistical significant difference for visual outcome, complication rate, GTR, CSF leakage, electrolyte disturbances and endocrinological outcomes, and infectious complications (e.g., meningitis) between the two groups of comparison. Again, longer hospitalization time was found to be associated with the microscopic approach.[248]

Extent of Resection

In general, several meta-analyses have found no clear difference in terms of effectiveness for pituitary adenoma removal when comparing the endonasal endoscopic to the microscopic approach. Systematic literature reviews by Rotenberg et al., Strychowsky et al., and a meta-analysis by Goudakos et al. were the first to confirm these findings.[249–251] A meta-analysis by Ammirati et al. included 24 reports using the endoscopic endonasal approach in 2,125 patients and 22 reports using the microscopic approach in 3,518 patients. GTR rates were similar between the groups of comparison with 70% and 65%, respectively.[252] In a subsequent meta-analysis of 1,014 patients with pituitary adenomas in 15 studies performed by Gao et al., however, the endonasal endoscopic approach was superior in terms of GTR.[209] This was also reported in a recent systematic review and meta-analysis performed by Li et al. (2017), where EEA was associated with a higher GTR rate in patients with pituitary adenoma.[247] On the other hand, a recent analysis of extent-of-resection data from a prospective multicenter study in transsphenoidal nonfunctioning pituitary adenoma surgery (TRANSSPHER) did not demonstrate a difference in GTR between the two techniques.[23] Little et al. and the TRANSSPHER Study group further compared the two techniques in a prospective multicenter controlled study comparing surgical outcomes (TRANSPHER Study).[215] Experienced surgeons who performed microscopic surgery and less experienced surgeons who performed endoscopic surgery achieved similar extents of tumor resection and quality outcomes in patients with nonfunctioning pituitary adenomas.[215] Nevertheless, institutions already utilizing the technique are expanding its indication as the operative skills improve and better instrumentations allow for better visualization of previously inaccessible spaces.[111,120,253] Among endoscopic series with medial cavernous sinus wall invasion, a pooled data meta-analysis of radiological criteria and comparison of endoscopic and microscopic surgery by Dhandapani et al. revealed a significant correlation of the extent of resection with the number of patients but no correlation with complications. These findings indicate the relative safety of the endonasal endoscopic approach in experienced hands for removing tumors with medial cavernous sinus wall invasion.[197]

Tumor size, infra-, supra-, and parasellar extension have been found to predict the extent of persistent disease.[15,197,254,255]

- *Tumor size*: A prospective multicenter study in transsphenoidal surgery for nonfunctioning pituitary adenoma (TRANSSPHER-Grade) by Mooney et al. analyzed 222 patients from 7 centers treated by 15 surgeons, where approximately one-fifth of patients had residual disease. They found that a maximum tumor diameter greater than 40 mm was an independent predictor for incomplete resection (**Table 1.4**).[23] In functioning adenoma, tumors greater than 15 mm in diameter had higher probability of not being cured in patients with acromegaly.[254,255]
- *Infrasellar extension*: Infrasellar extension, including the invasion of the clivus and the sphenoid bone, increased the risk of persistent disease in patients with acromegaly.[254,255]
- *Suprasellar extension*: Wilson et al. initially described suprasellar extension in their series (**Table 1.3**).[22] Specifically, nodular extensions seem to be relevant for surgical outcome, as recently described by Mooney et al. (**Table 1.4**).[23] In studies for functioning adenomas, suprasellar extension had a higher probability of not being cured in patients with acromegaly.[254,255]
- *Parasellar extension*: Knosp et al. proposed a grading system, where surgically proven invasion of the cavernous sinus space was present in all grade 4 and grade 3 cases and in all but one of the grade 2 cases, while no invasion was present in grade 0 and grade 1 cases (**Table 1.2**).[15] They further demonstrated a statistically higher proliferation rate in the surgically observed invasive grades when compared to noninvasive grades.[15] The Knosp grading system remains a reliable predictor for persisting disease to date and has been integrated in newer proposed classifications such as the TRANSSPHER Grade (**Table 1.4**).[23,195,197,242,256]
- A pooled data meta-analysis of radiological criteria and comparison of endoscopic and microscopic surgery by Dhandapani et al. demonstrated significantly overestimated intraoperative medial cavernous sinus wall invasion for each Knosp grade with microscopy when compared with the endonasal endoscopic approach.[197] The latter had significantly higher rates of GTR (47 vs. 21%), particularly for Knosp grades 3 and 4. In functioning adenoma, invasiveness according to MRI staging increased the risk of persistent disease in patients with acromegaly.[254,255]

Comparison of Mononostril versus Binostril Endonasal Endoscopic Approach

In most instances, the instruments and the endoscope are channeled via a **single nostril** to perform surgery. If the view is limited or the working channel space is too crowded, a **binostril technique** is utilized. A small retrospective clinical and cadaver study by Conrad et al. compared the binostril to the mononostril endonasal endoscopic approach and the surgical techniques involved in 40 patients and 10 cadavers. The binostril technique was superior for the resection of larger tumors with parasellar and suprasellar expansion and tumors requiring extended approaches, because of a better maneuverability of instruments and a wider exposure of the sphenoid sinus. The mononostril technique was feasible for tumors with limited extension in the intra- and suprasellar area. Endocrinological and ophthalmological outcome, residual tumor rate, and adverse events, such as CSF leaks and diabetes insipidus, were similar between both techniques.[214]

A systematic literature review and meta-analysis performed by Wen et al. included 30 studies involving 4,805 patients. The rates of GTR, endocrinological and ophthalmological outcomes, postoperative CSF leakage, permanent diabetes insipidus, and infectious complications were similar between both the techniques. However, the binostril group had less temporary diabetes insipidus (2.9 vs. 5.3%), less anterior pituitary insufficiency (2.3 vs. 6.4%), and fewer hospitalization days (3.2 vs. 4.4 days) than the mononostril group. Patients in the mononostril group had less rate of epistaxis (0.4 vs. 1.5%) than patients in the binostril group. For invasive macroadenomas, the binostril group seems to demonstrate a tendency toward better outcomes though there was no subgroup analysis between the two groups.[213]

Preoperative Considerations

The treatment and management of patients with pituitary lesions are interdisciplinary. In larger institutions, the preoperative work-up of these patients involves endocrinologists, ophthalmologists, neurosurgeons, ENT surgeons, and neuroradiologists. Usually, patients are evaluated by multidisciplinary consensus at regularly held tumor boards.

Endocrinological Assessment

Hypothalamic–pituitary hormonal function and excess hormone should be evaluated, if a pituitary adenoma is present: serum prolactin, total or free T4, TSH, LH and FSH, free testosterone, estrogen and progesterone, morning cortisol 24-hour urinary free cortisol, insulin-like growth factor.

Ophthalmological Assessment

Visual acuity and visual field using Goldman's perimetry as well as optometry in cases of double vision are mandatory.

Neurological Assessment

Focal neurological deficits and neuropsychological changes in large lesions with extrasellar extension and hypothalamic or frontal or temporal lobe involvement can be present on admission.

Rhinological Assessment

Endoscopic examination of the nose should be performed to rule out signs of infection, synechiae, or congenital anomalies. Any active bacterial sinusitis should be adequately treated prior to undergoing an endoscopic skull base surgery.

Radiological Investigations

High-resolution MRI brain with sellar and IGS protocol, and a high-resolution CT scan of the paranasal sinuses, if indicated, are mandatory prior surgery.

Preoperative Radiological Considerations

The surgeon should systematically assess available imaging. This is of special importance when selecting surgical modalities and variations of the available approached and tailoring the surgical corridor to reach the region of interest:

- *Nasal anatomy*: Signs of upper airway infection, septal deviations, signs of trauma.
- *Sphenoid anatomy*: Three-dimensional orientation (shelf, divider, wall) and insertion site (cavernous or paraclinoid ICA, opticocarotid recess, or optic nerves) of the sphenoid septations, mucosa, pneumatization pattern (sellar, presellar, or postsellar type), and bone thickness.
- *Cavernous carotid artery*: Space between carotid siphon (intercarotid distance), probable dehiscence, bulging into the sphenoid cavity.
- *Lesion*: Tumor size in the three planes. The firmness of the lesion can be appreciated with its appearance in MRI T2-weighted sequences. Hyperintensity is suggestive for a softer tumor. Cavernous invasion (Knosp grading) (**Table 1.2**), suprasellar extension, nodular extensions, relationship to tuberculum and planum sphenoidale, intra- versus suprasellar ratio, presence and location of a cystic component with respect to the solid component (especially superior vs. inferior). Erosion of adjacent structures, for example clivus or lateral sphenoid bone, and indentation of the temporal lobes. Extension into the sphenoid cavity or posterior ethmoidal cells should be acknowledged.
- *Neurovascular structures*: Normal pituitary gland (rim enhancement, posterior lobe) and location of the infundibular stalk. Dislocation and compression of the optic chiasm and the optic nerves. Branches of the anterior cerebral artery (frontopolar branches, H-complex). Aberrations in the course of the para- and supraclinoidal ICA and intracerebral aneurysms (**Fig. 1.34**).
- *Recurrent cases*: The presence or absence of endonasal structures, the presence of scar tissue, adhesions and synechias should be anticipated. Mucosal flaps over the surgical site or a fat graft from the previous surgery might be recognizable on preoperative imaging. Branches of the anterior cerebral artery might have migrated near the sella and the tumor residual because of scarring (sagittal plane T1 contrast enhanced).

Selection of the Surgical Approach

The main principle of the endonasal endoscopic approach is the use of preexisting airspaces to gain access to the base of skull. A wide surgical corridor has to be created to allow adequate visualization and instrumentation. This can be achieved with customized removal of the bony coverage of the skull base (osteodural exposure). When this osteodural exposure is adapted to the extension of the treated pathology, a tailored zonal dissection of the skull base is possible.

An optimal skull base approach:

- Allows adequate access to the lesion of interest.
- Facilitates the extent of resection with the goal of GTR.
- Minimizes brain retraction.
- Allows identification and minimizes manipulation of crucial neurovascular structures.
- Allows an optimal skull base defect repair.

Operative routes to access pituitary adenoma consist of transcranial and transsphenoidal microscopic and endoscopic approaches with potential expansion of the corridors along the skull base.[121,122]

When to Prefer a Transcranial Approach for Lesions of the Pituitary Gland

Several factors have to be considered to evaluate if an endonasal endoscopic approach is suitable. Besides the biological characteristics and the vascularity of the lesion, the location of the lesion in relation to critical anatomical structures has to be taken into account. Hence, the endonasal endoscopic approach generally is less feasible for lesions that extend laterally beyond the critical neurovascular structures, with the exception of cystic or soft lesions or if the goal of the operation is subtotal resection (STR) rather than GTR of the tumor.[217] Therefore, although the transsphenoidal route is an established working horse for pituitary lesions, certain configurations might still be an indication for primary transcranial approaches or second-stage transcranial resection after transsphenoidal debulking:

- Suprasellar posterior to the infundibulum (pterional).
- Extensive suprasellar extension (subfrontal, pterional).
- Involvement of the third ventricle (transcallosal approaches).

Several nuances of the endonasal endoscopic approach have been described in the literature and can be used when treating lesions of the pituitary gland. In our experience, a tailored approach with zonal dissection of the base of skull based on the anatomical extent of the lesions can be followed.

In the modern era of endoscopic skull base approaches, IGS is established and broadly used.[257,258] When following the principle of tailoring approaches for zonal dissection, IGS is a very helpful tool. However, certain general aspects have to be considered:

- Intraoperative IGS has to be regarded as an adjunct to the surgeon's anatomical knowledge.
- It is of crucial importance to match the preoperative sphenoid anatomy as well as the relevant landmarks of the skull base with the surgeon's view of the field with the aid of intraoperative IGS.
- Sphenoid shelves can imitate the planum sphenoidale and mislead a correct dissection of the skull base.
- Sphenoid dividers can skew the midline and mislead the surgeon's view of the exposed skull base.
- The cavernous carotid arteries and the optic nerves should be identified using common anatomical landmarks (opticocarotid recess, carotid-clival window) with the aid of intraoperative IGS.
- The paraclival carotids should be identified and a clear midline view available before starting the opening of the skull base.

In general, the endonasal endoscopic transseptal transsphenoidal approach consists of a nasal phase (tailored approach), the osteodural exposure of the skull base (zonal dissection), the intradural (resection of the lesion), and the closure of the dural skull base defect. The following sections describe different variations of the endonasal endoscopic transseptal transsphenoidal approach to the sella with detailed information on each surgical step.

Presurgical Phase

The evolution of skull base surgeries, intraoperative monitoring, and intraoperative imaging has produced unique problems and concerns for the neuroanesthesiologist. The main primary concerns are airway management, patient positioning, blood loss, electrolyte imbalances, and certain aspects during intraoperative monitoring and imaging. Because of anatomical anomalies, the airway management may be difficult in patients with acromegaly and Cushing's disease. Airway evaluation using the usual metrics may be misleading in patients with acromegaly. It may be advisable to pretreat patients with medical therapy for a few months prior to surgery, in order to minimize airway edema and complications during intubation.[259] In most of the cases, the airway is not shared with the skull base surgeon. Exceptions are known for transoral, transmandibular, or transmaxillary approaches. In these special scenarios, evaluation of the applicability for an oral intubation is necessary or a tracheostomy has to be considered.[260] Upper airway edema may occur if long surgical time is expected and the patient must be put on regular dose of dexamethasone.[260]

In endonasal endoscopic skull base surgery, patient positioning is important as most patients will have their head pinned and there will be no room for movement. The anesthesiologist must ensure that the tube is well secured and not kinked. Further on, jugular venous kinking, caused by neck flexion or rotation, has to be avoided. A poorly positioned patient may develop intraoperative complications such as rising carbon dioxide and brain swelling.[261] If high risk of venous air embolism is expected, a central venous catheter should be installed. It is relevant to pad pressure points sufficiently to avoid peripheral nerve injuries.

The major skull base surgeries may be associated with significant blood loss. Therefore, the overall goal is to maintain normal intravascular volume, replace losses slowly with crystalloid solution and blood. The neuroanesthesiologists' main goal is to maintain blood pressure normotensive or slightly hypotensive. A sudden surge in blood pressure should be avoided as this may increase intraoperative bleeding.

Like any other surgeries, preoperative electrolyte levels should be corrected. Patients with intracranial pathologies may present with electrolyte derangement. Hence, an early referral to an endocrine physician may be helpful. Intraoperative regular arterial blood gases may also help to guide and allow correction.

Intraoperative neurophysiological monitoring is used to improve postoperative outcomes especially if cranial nerves are involved. Depending on the type of monitoring used, anesthetic agent need to be tailored. The use of neuromuscular blocking agent is avoided if motor nerve monitoring is used, as for example for motor evoked potentials. In our institution, any muscle relaxant is repeated after the initial intubating dose of rocuronium. If other monitoring modalities like brainstem auditory evoked potentials or sensory evoked potentials are used, an adjustment of inhalation gases' concentration is necessary. Other physiological parameters like temperature and blood pressure will also affect the monitoring, and these parameters need to be maintained within normal ranges.

Lastly, new modalities like intraoperative imaging (e.g., intraoperative MRI and CT) influence the way the authors deliver anesthesia in their institution. In our case of an intraoperative MRI with a two-room solution, the tubes and wires need to be MRI compatible and the patient needs be transferred to the MRI suite under general anesthesia. Therefore, proper guidelines and checklists are mandatory and have to be used previous to each surgery to prevent any problems with metallic objects and noncompatible material[262] (**Table 1.11a, b**).

Anesthesia for skull base surgeries like any other complex surgeries will need a good communication and team work between the anesthetist and surgeons. General anesthesia with orotracheal intubation and throat pack in situ is standard. Prophylactic antibiotic should be given at induction of the anesthesia. Generally, bladder catheterization is recommended and should be kept postoperatively to monitor urine output in the first days.

Patient Positioning

The patient's head is placed neutrally with a supine neck in a slightly extended position (**Fig. 1.39**). According to the anatomical region that is surgically addressed, the head can be either slightly extended to reach the anterior skull base in a more direct trajectory (transcribriform approach), or slightly flexed to reach the posterior fossa (transclivus or craniocervical junction).[87,88] In our institution, the head is fixed within a NORAS frame for intraoperative MRI (**Fig. 1.40**).

Equipment

The evolution of endonasal endoscopic approaches has produced a paradigm shift in skull base surgery. Specialized instrumentation, such as bipolar forceps, microdebrider, high-speed drills, computer-assisted surgical navigation, and Doppler ultrasound probes, are some of the technological adjuncts that contributed to this remarkable evolution. A certain armamentarium of surgical instruments and tools is relevant when performing endoscopic endonasal surgical approaches to the skull base. These are necessary to ensure a safe and effective performance such as bimanual microdissection using a narrow surgical window.[263]

- Rigid rod lens telescope (0 and 30 degrees), 18 cm in length and 4 mm in diameter (Karl Storz Endoscopy, Tuttlingen, Germany), without a working channel.
- Monitor
- Image guided surgery system—either mobile or fixed installed in the operation theater.
- Suction (big, small, maxillary J-sucker)
- Monopolar suction
- Endoscopic bipolar forceps
- Hemostatic agents and delivery system (Taming Sari)[264,265]
- Hemostatic agents
- Bone wax
- Prepare abdomen for fat graft

Ergonomical Aspects

To perform the two-surgeon four-hand technique, certain ergonomical aspects have to be considered.[229] To allow a more flexible handling of instruments for mononostril and binostril approaches, the two surgeons in our institution stand on either side of the patient (**Fig. 1.41**). The ENT surgeon stabilizes the endoscope either on the upper or the lower edge of the naris. This allows a certain degree of angulation (**Fig. 1.42**). The ENT surgeon can insert instruments and assist the tumor resection, the so-called **two-surgeon** three- and **four-hands procedures** (**Fig. 1.43**). There is further advantage of this position in extended cases with longer duration of the operation, where the surgeons' position in relation to the video screen is relevant. The screen is placed between both surgeons at the level of the patient's head. This allows a natural posture and full view of the screen for both surgeons (**Fig. 1.44**). The camera for the IGS should be placed ipsilateral to the installed reference point system (**Fig. 1.44**).

Table 1.11a Preoperative checklist for intraoperative MRI

No.	Patient's items	Yes ✓	No ×	Comment/details
1	Cardiac/brain pacemaker			
2	Aneurysm clips			
3	Metallic surgical objects, e.g., spinal implant etc.			
4	Implanted cardioverter defibrillator (ICD)			
5	Electronic implant or device			
6	Magnetically activated implant or device			
7	Neurostimulation system			
8	Spinal cord stimulator			
9	Internal electrodes or wires			
10	Cochlear, otologic, or other ear implant			
11	Programmable shunt			
12	Any metallic fragment or foreign body			
13	Any external or internal metallic object, e.g., metal jewelry			
14	Hearing aid			
15	Dentures/braces			
16	Other implant			
17	Other device			
18	Any type of prosthesis (breast, eye, limb, etc.)			
19	Stent (cardiac)			
20	Joint replacement (hip, knee, etc.)			
21	IUD or diaphragm			
All metals objects are noncompatible with MRI				

Abbreviation: IUD, intrauterine device.

Note: This checklist has to be carried out at ward by the operating surgeons when taking operation/procedure consent and has to be rechecked by the nurses when the patient is passed over at the operation theater reception (University Malaya Medical Centre, intraoperative MRI checklist, Centre for Image Guided and Minimally Invasive Therapy 1 [CIGMIT 1]).

Table 1.11b Anesthetic induction checklist for intraoperative MRI

No.	Details	Yes ✓	No ×	Comment
1	Patient particulars and consent			
2	Patient position confirmed			
3	Ventilator/circuits/monitors—in OT checked			
4	Ventilator/circuits/monitors—in MRI room checked			
5	O2 trolley, O2 cylinder, regulator, self-inflating bag, and connectors are in good function, enough pressure (cylinder) and MRI compatible			
6	MRI compatible ECG dots/leads/SpO2 probe cables available and easily identified			
7	Plain tracheal tube only			
8	Check no ferromagnetic items on canvas prior to transfer			
9	Insert ear plugs			

Note: This checklist has to be carried out on bed/trolley prior to the transfer on the operation table by the responsible anesthetist. Patient intubation and lines have to be done before transfer on the operation table (University Malaya Medical Centre, intraoperative MRI checklist, Centre for Image Guided and Minimally Invasive Therapy 1 [CIGMIT 1]).

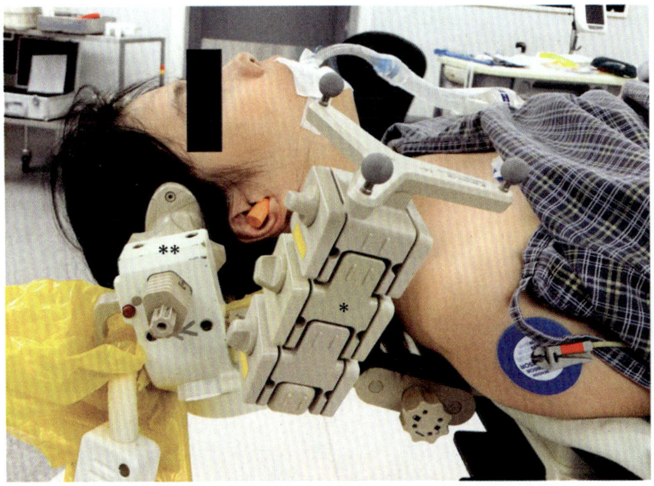

Fig. 1.39 Positioning of the patient prior to an endonasal endoscopic transsphenoidal surgery. The neck of the patient is slightly extended and minimal contralateral lateroflexion of the head might provide some ergonomical advantages for the neurosurgeon standing on the right side of the patient. The reference arm for the image-guided surgery system (*) is fixed on a NORAS frame (**) for intraoperative acquisition of magnetic resonance imaging (iMRI) for extent of resection control.

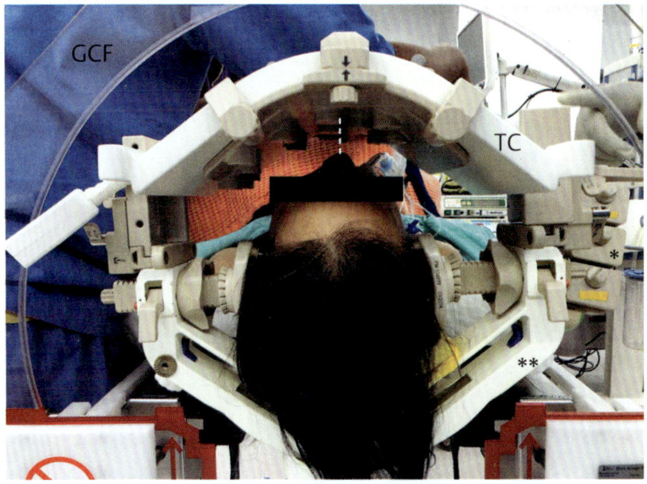

Fig. 1.40 Patient fixation and installation prior to an endonasal endoscopic transsphenoidal surgery with intraoperative acquisition of magnetic resonance imaging for extent of resection control. The reference arm for the image-guided surgery system (*) is fixed on a NORAS frame (**). The top-coil for the intraoperative MRI is installed over the patient's head without contact to avoid pressure points during image acquisition (*white line*). The whole installation has to be controlled by using a gantry control frame (GCF), which represents the gantry of the MRI, to avoid spatial problems when entering the MRI tube.

Intraoperative MRI for Extent of Resection

There has been a remarkable amount of literature supporting intraoperative MRI (iMRI) to achieve a greater extent of resection in a variety of intracranial tumors.[66,266,267] Especially, the advantages of iMRI to control the extent of resection of pituitary adenoma is well described.[256] The application of iMRI has shown overall improved rates of gross total excision in selected publications.[266–269] Several authors have argued that with the use of endonasal endoscopic techniques and hence better visualization of the sella, a gross total excision may be achieved through the endoscopic approach alone, and iMRI might lose its benefit when compared to the microscopic approach. However, iMRI revealed residual disease despite the surgeon's prediction, necessitating further excision using an updated image guidance in several publications.[267] Zaidi et al. reported improved gross total excision rates with iMRI (80%) when compared to cases where iMRI was not used (60%).[266] When gross total excision is achieved and confirmed by iMRI, postoperative routine imaging might not be necessary and further follow-up can be adapted. Serious complications such as postoperative hematoma can be identified early and addressed prior to closure.[270] A study conducted by Coburger et al. demonstrated a higher progression-free survival after 2 years in cases where iMRI was used when compared to cases without iMRI.[267] These aspects do ensure better surgical outcomes and might reduce the need of subsequent revision surgeries. A relevant setback in the utility of iMRI is a significant prolongation of the surgical time, as dictated by previous authors in the literature.[267] Expenses involving the installation and use of an iMRI unit together with dedicated and trained staff for an efficient workflow might be a relevant limitation for smaller centers.[266] This is why, in our institution, the MRI unit is used for routine diagnostic work and is not exclusively used for intraoperative scanning.[66] The interpretation of iMRI scans remains challenging, as the differentiation of blood products from devascularized residual disease is difficult in some cases. This harbors the potential risk of overtreatment.[271]

With dedicated imaging teams, iMRI acquisition in our institution reached an average time of 22 to 25 minutes.[66] The use of a standardized workflow protocol with trained staff and standardized preoperative checklists for anesthesia prior to the surgery and prior to patient transfer into

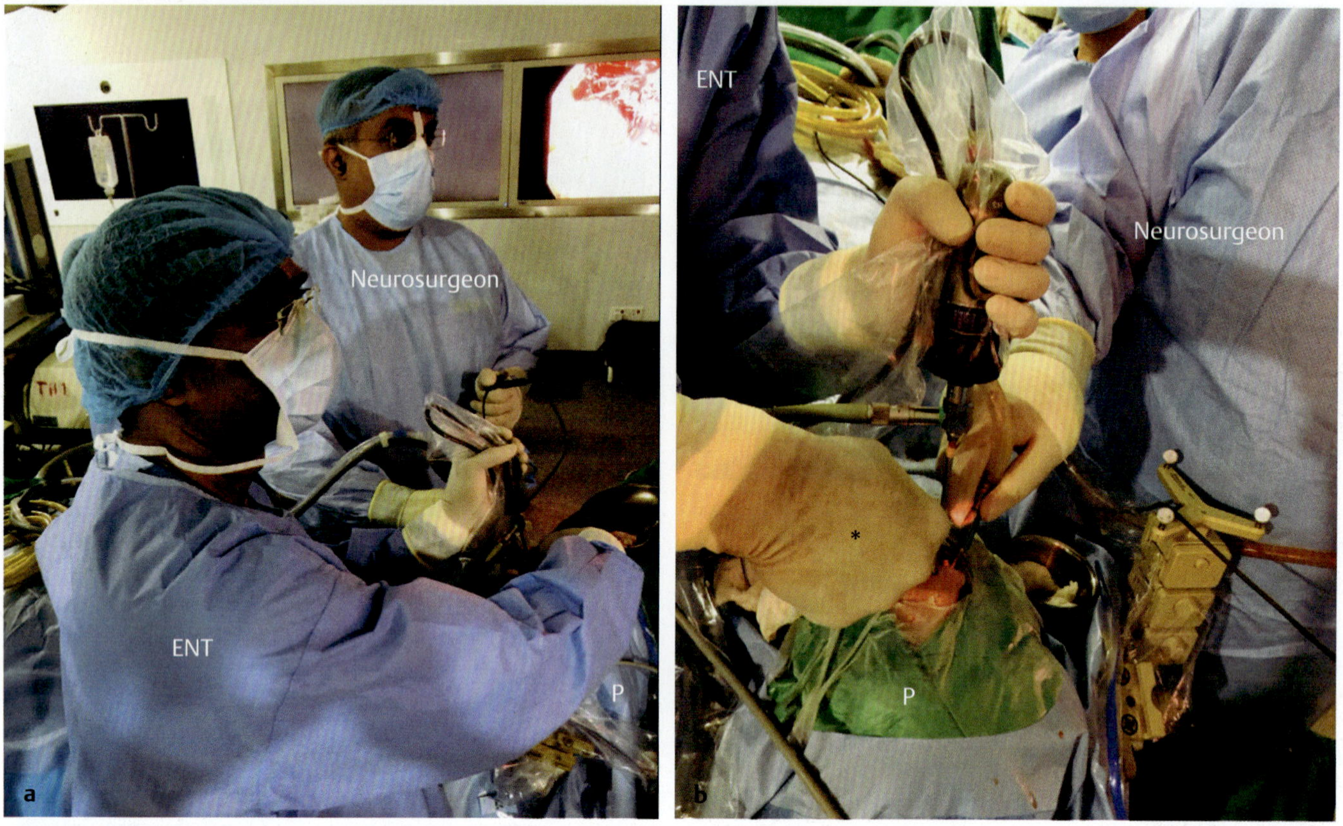

Fig. 1.41 Institutional experience in ergonomical aspects concerning the surgeons' position during endonasal endoscopic skull base surgeries. **(a)** For the two-surgeon four-hand technique, the neurosurgeon stands on the left, and the ENT surgeon (ENT) stands on the right side of the patient's head (P). **(b)** The ENT surgeon, on the patient's left side, holds and stabilizes the endoscope and can assist the neurosurgeon with a third hand (*) in more complex maneuvers.

the MRI tube is mandatory and is of crucial importance to maintain highest patient safety when acquiring iMRI images (**Table 1.11c–f**).

Nasal Phase (Tailored Approach)

Endoscopic Endonasal Mononostril Transseptal Transsphenoidal Approach

This variation can be used for primary surgery of small- to medium-sized pituitary adenomas or intrasellar lesions suggestive to be a pituitary adenoma.

- The nose is sprayed with cophenylcaine (lignocaine 5% and phenylephrine 0.5% spray) prior to packing performed with cottonoids soaked with adrenaline 1:1,000. Nasal packing is performed along the nasal floor and in between septum and middle turbinate.
- The midface is prepared and draped with modified towels/drapes to allow placement of the IGS tracking system instruments. Additionally, the abdomen is also routinely prepared for later fat graft harvest (if required).
- The preliminary packing is removed and the nose is again inspected with a 0-degree nasal endoscope and the whole surgery is recorded in digital media.
- Both the sphenoethmoidal recesses are packed with cottonoids/neuropatties soaked in adrenaline 1:1,000.
- The osteocartilaginous junction is infiltrated with a mixture of mepivacaine and adrenaline 1:100,000 on both sides of the septum (**Fig. 1.45a, b**).
- A bipolar diathermy is used to cauterize the site of incision followed by a vertical incision at the osteocartilaginous junction (**Fig. 1.46**).
- The mucoperichondrial flap is elevated on one side of the septum. The elevation of the ipsilateral mucoperichondrial flap is continued posteriorly until the sphenoid rostrum is identified (**Fig. 1.47a–c**).
- The mucoperichondrial flap elevation is extended to the sphenovomerine suture and the sphenoid ostium is located while at the same time taking care not to damage the posterior septal artery (**Fig. 1.48a**).

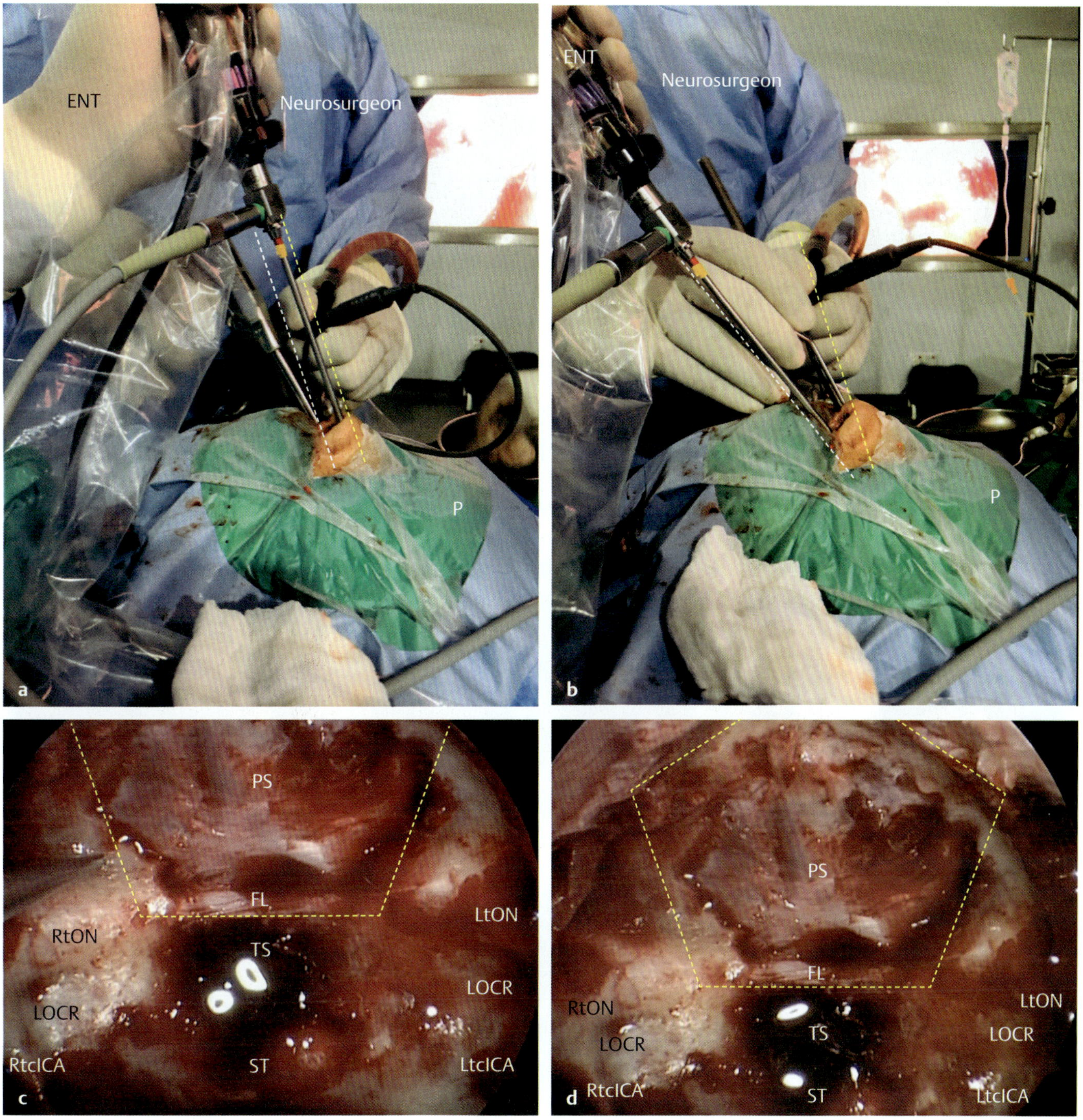

Fig. 1.42 Institutional experience in ergonomical aspects and arm positioning during the two-surgeon four-hand binostril technique. The ENT surgeon (ENT) must position his or her left hand and arm, the light and the camera cable ergonomically and comfortably to provide a tangential parallel working trajectory for the neurosurgeon. **(a)** Angulation of the endoscope during the two-surgeon four-hand binostril technique. The ENT surgeon anchors the endoscope in the nasal tip (apical). This provides the normal zero-degree view for both surgeons**. (b)** The ENT surgeon anchors the endoscope on the floor of the nasal aperture (caudal) and points the camera upward. This angulation almost provides a 30-degree view. **(c)** Zero-degree view while defining the lateral extent of the osteodural exposure of a tuberculum sellae meningioma. **(d)** 30-degree view while defining the lateral extent of the osteodural exposure of a tuberculum sellae meningioma. *(Continued)*

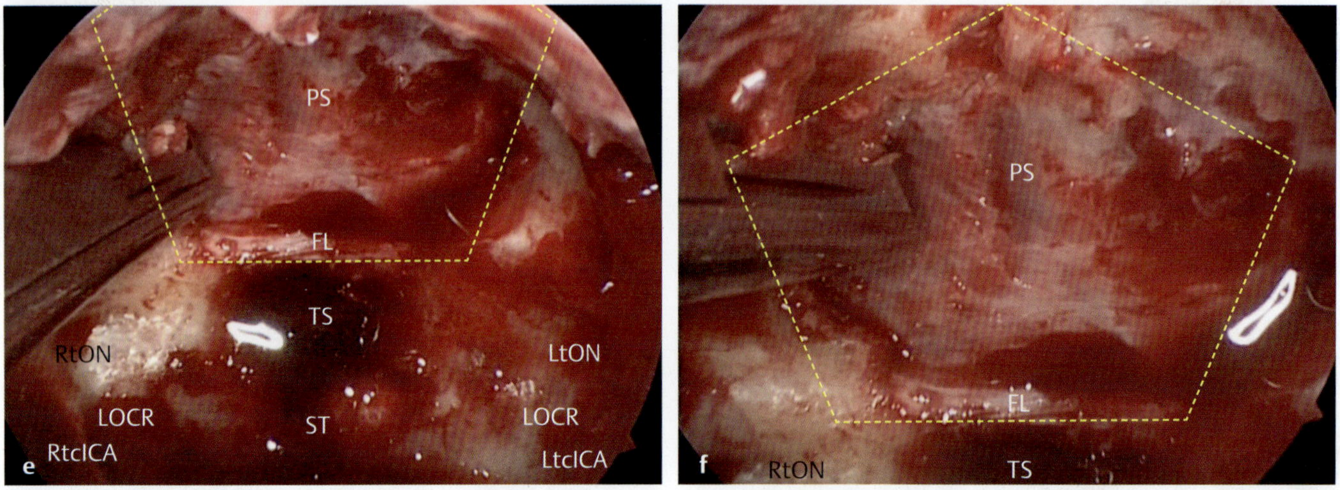

Fig. 1.42 *(Continued)* **(e)** Zero-degree view while removing bone covering the lateral planum sphenoidale (PS). **(f)** A 30-degree view while removing bone covering the lateral PS.

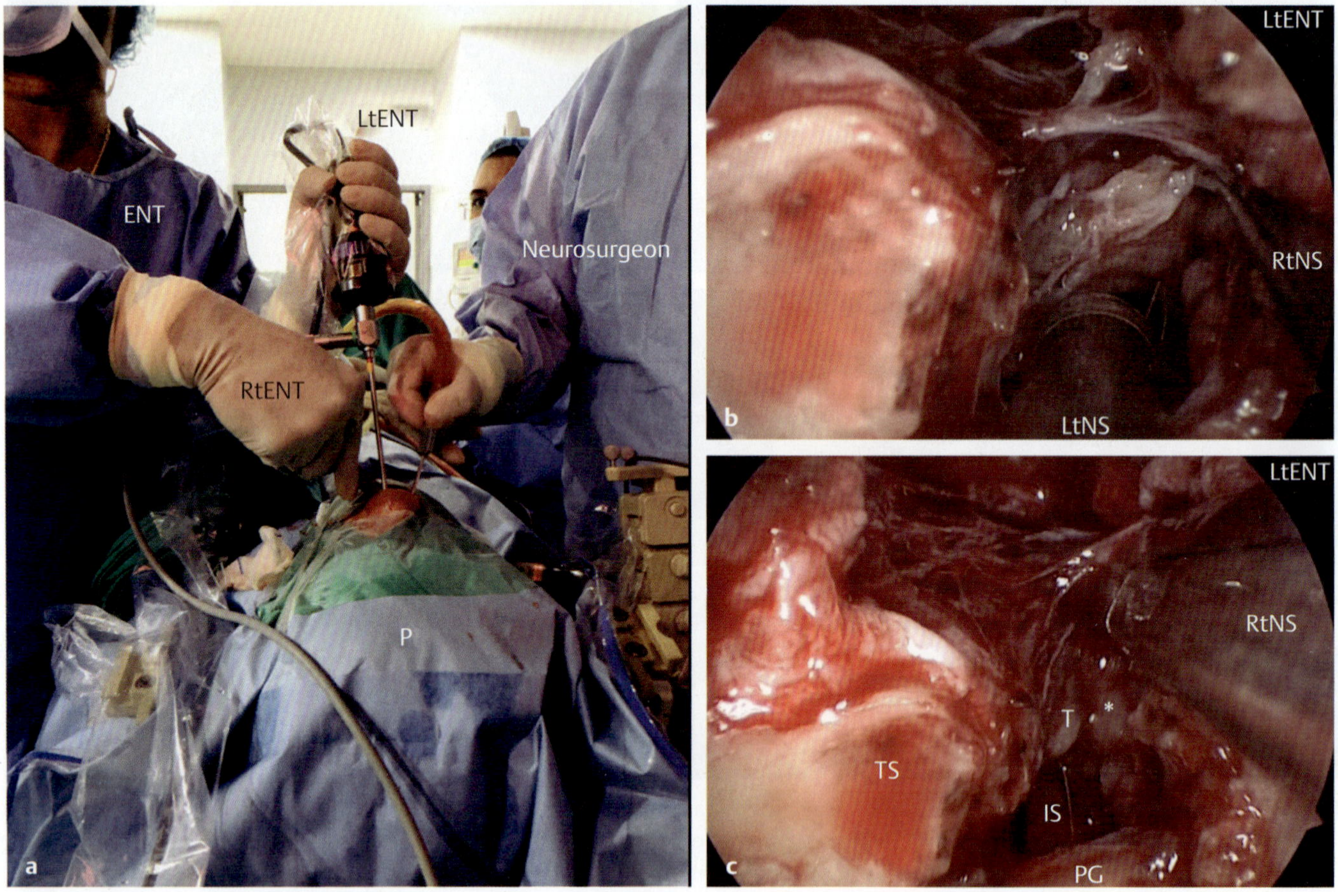

Fig. 1.43 Institutional experience in ergonomical aspects for the two-surgeon, three- and four-hand binostril technique. **(a)** The ENT surgeon (ENT) must position his or her left hand and arm (LtENT), the light and the camera cable ergonomically and comfortably to provide a tangential parallel working trajectory. The ENT surgeon can assist with his free right hand (RtENT) using a grasping instrument and by this present the dissection plane. The neurosurgeon is then able to ergonomically perform microsurgical maneuvers with this working trajectory with one or both hands (bimanual dissection). **(b)** Two-surgeon, three-hand procedure: The ENT surgeon only stabilizes the endoscope with his or her left hand and arm (LtENT). The NS performs a bimanual microsurgical dissection using a microdissector in his or her right hand (RtNS) and a suction device in his or her left hand (LtNS). **(c)** While holding and stabilizing the endoscope with his or her left hand (LtENT), the ENT surgeon can assist with his or her free right hand (RtENT) using a grasping instrument and by this present the dissection plane (*) in more complex maneuvers.

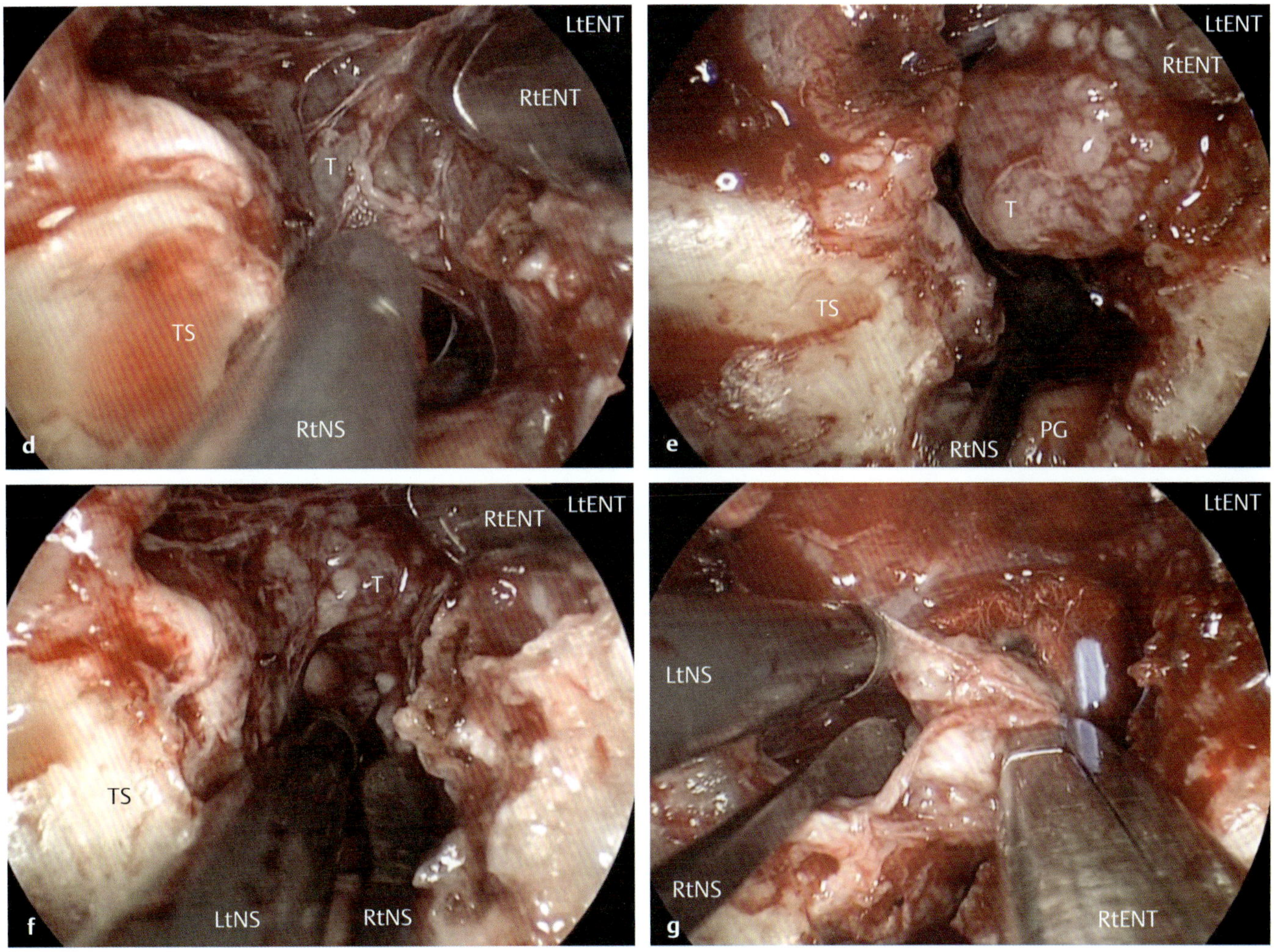

Fig. 1.43 (*Continued*) **(d)** Two-surgeon, three-hand procedure: While the ENT-surgeon holds the endoscope in his or her left hand (LtENT), he or she applies slight traction with a grasping instrument in his or her right hand (RtENT) to present the resection plane. The neurosurgeon can use an aspirator to debulk tumor tissue (RtNS). **(e)** Two-surgeon, three-hand procedure: While the ENT surgeon holds the endoscope in his or her left hand (LtENT), he or she applies slight traction with a grasping instrument in his or her right hand (RtENT) to present the dissection plane. The neurosurgeon can use a microdissector to dissect tumor away from critical neurovascular structures (RtNS). **(f, g)** Two-surgeon, four-hand procedure: While the ENT surgeon holds the endoscope in his or her left hand (LtENT), he or she applies slight traction with a grasping instrument in his or her right hand (RtENT) to present the dissection plane. The neurosurgeon can use a microdissector in his or her right hand (RtNS) and a suction device in his or her left hand (LtNS)] to bimanually dissect tumor away from critical neurovascular structures.

- The mucoperichondrial flap is raised off the septum with a Freer elevator posteriorly until the sphenoid ostia and posterior choana are visible (**Fig. 1.48b**).
- After dislocation of the bony cartilaginous junction, the exposed bony septum is fractured to the contralateral side and removed in a piecemeal fashion, freeing it from the overlying contralateral septal mucoperichondrium (**Fig. 1.49a–c**).
- Superiorly, the flap may be taken until about 0.5 to 1 cm below the skull base to preserve the olfactory function. Inferiorly, the flap can be taken as far as half the nasal floor if a large skull base defect is expected (Hadad–Bassagasteguy flap) (**Fig. 1.50a, b**).
- The sphenoid rostrum is fully exposed by dissecting the septal mucosa at the sphenovomerine junctions laterally. Both sphenoid ostia have to be visible and the

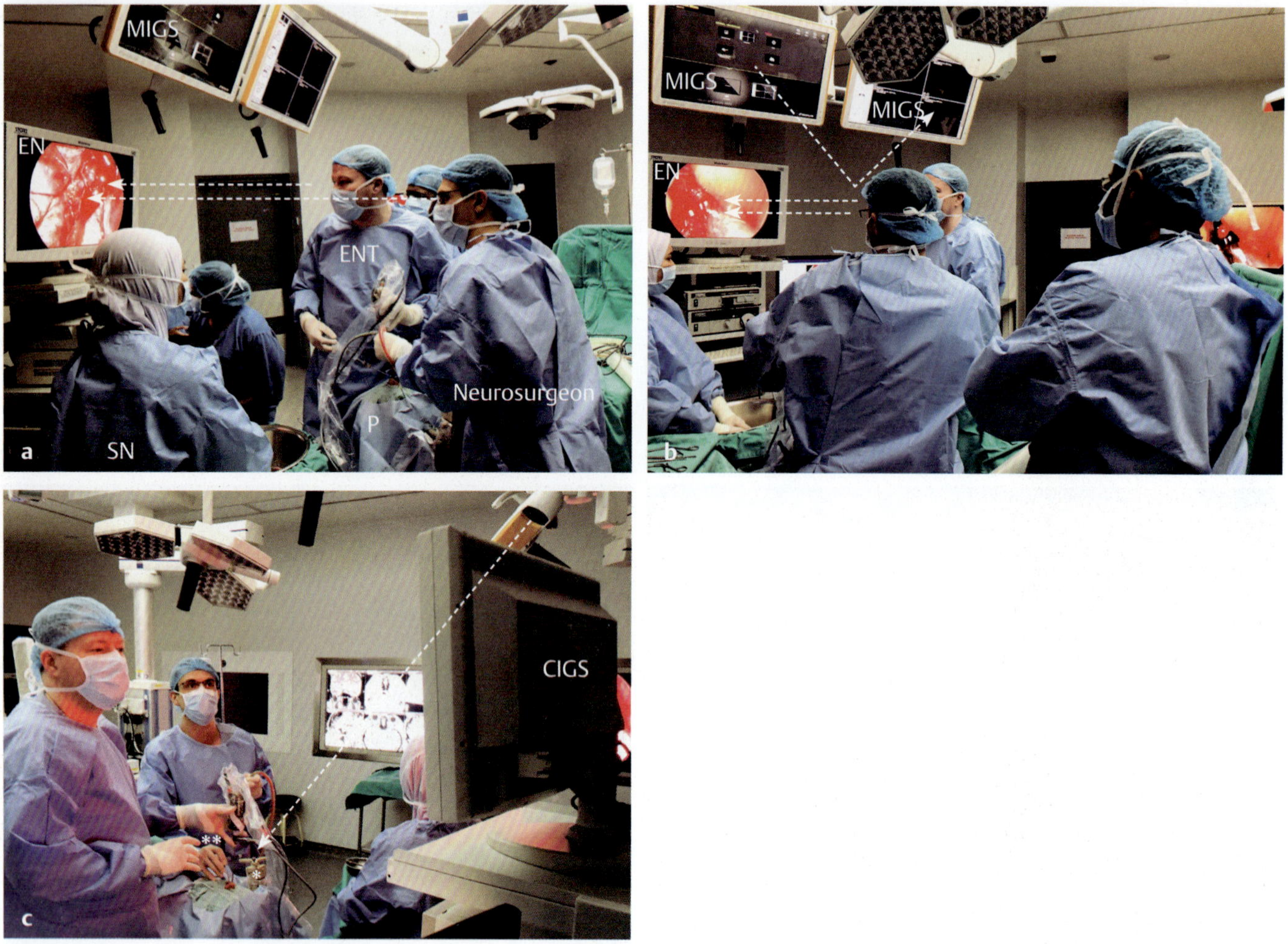

Fig. 1.44 Institutional experience in the operating room setup showing the positions of the ENT surgeon (ENT), neurosurgeon, monitor for the endoscope (EM), monitor for image-guided surgery (MIGS), infrared camera for image-guided surgery (CIGS) reference points for image-guided surgery (*), pointing instrument for image-guided surgery (**), and scrub nurse around the operating table and the patient head (P). **(a)** The EM is positioned at a physiological height in front of the surgeons (*white arrow*) to avoid nonergonomical posture during longer and more complex procedures. **(b)** The MIGS is positioned superior to the EM to allow a fluent workflow when using image-guided surgery during endonasal endoscopic surgeries (*white arrows*). **(c)** The position of the CIGS, the reference-points (*), and the pointing instrument (**) for image-guided surgery need to be arranged accordingly to allow a fluent workflow when using image-guided surgery during endonasal endoscopic surgeries (*white arrows*). The ENT surgeon has to control the endoscope, the light and the camera cable to avoid interruption of the infrared signal (*white arrow*) between the reference points (*), the pointing instrument (**), and the CIGS for image-guided surgery during endonasal endoscopic surgery.

anatomical midline has to be in view when a primary surgery is performed (**Fig. 1.51a, b**).

- The sphenoid ostia are widened using a Kerrison punch (**sphenoidotomy**), and the anterior wall of sphenoid sinus is removed in total or by piecemeal to give a wide exposure of the sphenoid cavity and the anterior, middle, and inferior midline skull base (planum sphenoidale, tuberculum sphenoidale, sella turcica, clivus, and paraclival ICAs) (**Fig. 1.52a, b**).
- Main and accessory intersinus septae in the sphenoid cavity have to be removed carefully, paying particular attention on septations inserting laterally along the paraclival or cavernous ICA or the opticocarotid recess (**Fig. 1.53**).

Endoscopic Endonasal Double Nostril Transseptal Transsphenoidal Approach

Using both narices for the surgical resection of sellar lesions allows a broader range of maneuvers for the two-surgeon four-hand technique as well as more flexibility for the ENT surgeon in terms of positioning of the endoscope. A **double nostril technique** may as well be utilized in patients with a narrow nostril with expected limited exposure. This approach can be used for microadenomas depending on unilaterality of the lesion, larger adenomas with relevant suprasellar extension or tumor cysts, and recurrent cases.

As a variation to the single nostril transseptal transsphenoidal approach, the bilateral removal of the superoposterior nasoseptal mucoperiosteum using a microdebrider/shaver allows an opening of the posterior septum (**Fig. 1.54a–e**). This allows both nostrils to be used for instrumentation.

Endonasal Endoscopic Revision Surgery for Recurrent Sellar Lesions

Transsphenoidal reoperations remain a challenging procedure because of scar tissue, loss of anatomical landmarks, and more invasive biological behavior of the recurrent lesions in

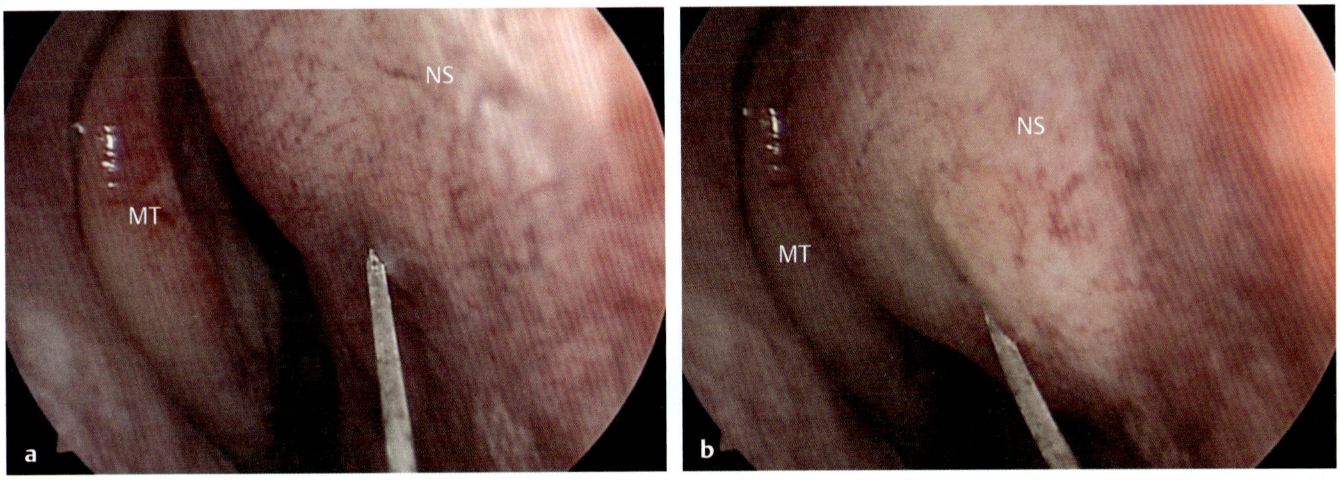

Fig. 1.45 Endoscopic endonasal mononostril transseptal transsphenoidal approach. **(a, b)** Mucosal infiltration of the osteocartilaginous junction.

Table 1.11c Predrape checklist for intraoperative MRI

No.	Details	Yes ✓	No ×	Comment
1	Patient position—no pressure points			
2	Insert fully assembled top coil			
3	Check MRI bore gauge			
4	Ensure that anesthetist/nurse has no metallic objects on person			
5	Ensure that no metallic objects on the operating table are present, and especially below the canvas and the warming blankets			
6	Note if any attached clamps and restraints are present that will need to be removed upon transfer for iMRI			
7	Anesthetist has to ensure tubs and monitoring cables are compatible with MRI: • Disconnect arterial line and keep only one drip			
8	Seat belt for transfer fastened			

Abbreviation: iMRI, intraoperative magnetic resonance imaging.

Note: This checklist has to be carried out prior to draping and is in the surgeon's responsibility. This checklist is also applicable for a preoperative MRI with the patient anesthetized and intubated (University Malaya Medical Centre, intraoperative MRI checklist, Centre for Image Guided and Minimally Invasive Therapy 1 [CIGMIT 1]).

Table 1.11d Patient transfer for intraoperative MRI checklist

No.	Details	Yes ✓	No ×	Comment
1	Inform radiographer with suitable timing			
2	The surgeon has to remove all metallic devices (clips, retractors, forceps)			
3	The surgeon has to manage wound exposure suitably			
4	The scrub nurse has to remove: • All cables • All devices (drills, forceps, suckers) • All quivers			
5	Remove diathermy pad			
6	The anesthetist has to ensure tubes and cables are ready for transfer: • Disconnect arterial and CVP lines • Check the patient is hemodynamically stable before transfer			
7	The anesthetist and the anesthetist's assistant are ferromagnetic free			
8	The O2 trolley, O2 cylinder, regulator, self-inflating bag, drip stand, and connectors are in good function, with enough pressure (cylinder) and MRI compatible			
9	The infusion machine is closed and no ferromagnetic objects are present on the surface or the drawer			
10	The table is at MRI height			
11	Remove sterile IGS array			
12	Cover with suitable drape (note top will become unsterile)			
13	Put on top-coil fully assembled			
14	Cut collection bag and cover with plastic shower cap			
15	Expose coil connectors			
16	Docking complete			
17	Walk about and release brake (surgeon)			
18	Transfer of patient supervised by surgeon			
19	Ensure the drape are not stuck			

Abbreviation: IGS, image-guided surgery.

Note: This checklist is carried out prior to the transfer of the patient from the operating room into the intraoperative MRI room. This checklist is for the responsible anesthetist, assistant anesthetist, surgeon, and scrub nurse only (University Malaya Medical Centre, intraoperative MRI checklist, Centre for Image Guided and Minimally Invasive Therapy 1 [CIGMIT 1]).

Table 1.11e Intraoperative MR room checklist

No.	Details	Yes ✓	No ×	Comment
	Anesthetist			
1	IPPV ventilation instituted			
2	MRI compatible SpO2 ECG and NIBP complete			
3	IV line and drug perfusion running well			
4	Handover to radiographer			

Abbreviations: ECG, electrocardiography; IIPV, intermittent positive pressure ventilation; IV, intravenous; NIBP, noninvasive blood pressure.

Note: This checklist is carried in the intraoperative MRI room. This checklist is for the responsible anesthetist, assistant anesthetist, and the radiographer only (University Malaya Medical Centre, intraoperative MRI checklist, Centre for Image Guided and Minimally Invasive Therapy 1 [CIGMIT 1]).

Table 1.11f Transfer back into operating room checklist

No.	Details	Yes ✓	No ×	Comment
	Anesthetist			
1	Reconnect all lines, circuits in a neat fashion in event of retransfer			
	Surgeon			
2	Remove drapes making sure no tears at the side rail of the head clamp			
3	Redrape top portion and reattach navigation array			

Note: This checklist is carried in the intraoperative MRI room. This checklist is for the responsible anesthetist and assistant anesthetist only (University Malaya Medical Centre, intraoperative MRI checklist, Centre for Image Guided and Minimally Invasive Therapy 1 [CIGMIT 1]).

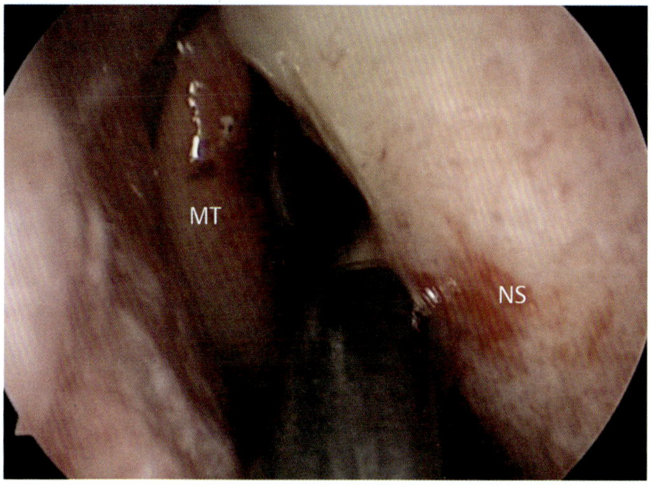

Fig. 1.46 Cauterization of the site of incision along the nasal septum (NS) on the level of the middle turbinate (MT).

certain cases.[272] Therefore, it is imperative to have information on pre- and postoperative endocrine status, pre- and postoperative visual field tests. Information on the approach, flap reconstruction, anatomical variations encountered, and postoperative complications are relevant; hence, the operative notes of the previous surgery should be consulted.[273] Radiological imaging (pre- and postoperative T1-weighted gadolinium-enhanced MRI sequences) will provide additional information on the previous surgical procedure: tumor size, tumor extension such as suprasellar and cavernous sinus invasion, and the extent of tumor resection.[273,274]

When performing an endonasal endoscopic approach for a recurrent sellar lesion, adhesions between the nasal septum and the turbinates need to be released if present. If a large posterior septal opening has already been done previously, the entry into the sphenoid sinus is easier and relatively safe. However, it must also be determined if a posterior septal flap was used to reconstruct the sella which is then cauterized and elevated off the bone. Using a suction, debris that may have collected within sphenoid sinus cavity has to be removed carefully. Dehiscent critical neurovascular structures have to be considered, and even this simple step has to be done carefully. Mucosal growth over the anterior aspect of sphenoid may reduce the view of the surgical field and removal might be necessary. Equally important is the size of posterior septectomy that may need to be enlarged anteriorly. This can be done easily with backbiting forceps. Bony regeneration over the sellar and adjacent bone has been seen to occur and affect the sellar exposure in revision surgery. In most cases, this requires drilling or piecemeal removal with a Kerrisons's punch to expose the dural covering of the pituitary gland. Intraoperative IGS is often helpful to identify fixed critical structures that serve as a landmark (pituitary fossa, planum sphenoidale, clivus) and also the position of ICAs. If available, iMRI is employed to look for residual tumor. Literature on morbidity and mortality of recurrent pituitary surgery is rare. A study by Jahangiri et al. retrospectively determined the morbidity associated with repeat versus initial transsphenoidal surgery in 1,015 consecutive operations of 916 patients (108 transsphenoidal reoperations with 907 primary surgeries). The incidence of postoperative diabetes insipidus, postoperative CSF leaks, and a longer duration of hospitalization was found to be more likely in patients undergoing repeat transsphenoidal surgery.[272]

Osteodural Phase (Zonal Dissection)

The osteodural exposure can be tailored according to the anatomical configuration of the lesion. With the aid of IGS, a zonal dissection of the skull base to sufficiently expose the lesion is possible. For normal-sized sellar lesions, a transsellar approach usually allows for a sufficient exposure of the sella turcica to safely remove these lesions:

- The exposure is defined by the cavernous internal carotid eminences laterally, the planum sphenoidale and tuberculum sellae superiorly, and the clivus inferiorly. The sphenoidal mucosa covering the sellar bone is meticulously cauterized, elevated off, and removed. The bony dehiscence over ICAs is sometimes

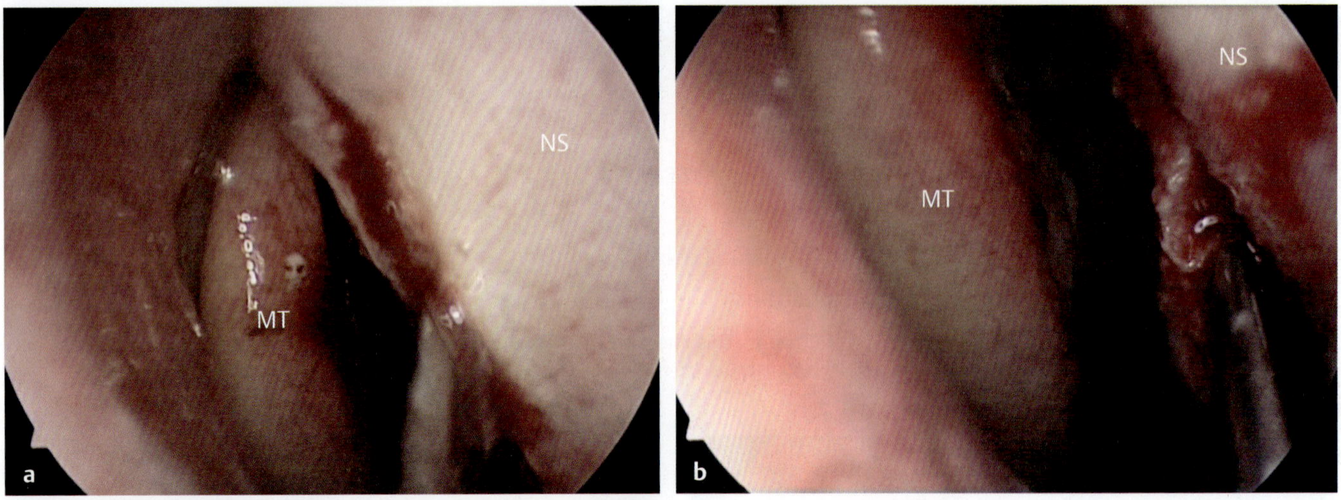

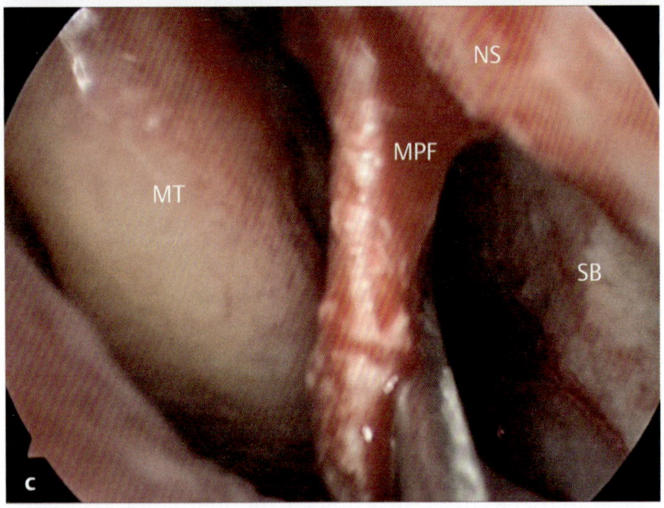

Fig. 1.47 Elevation of the mucoperichondrial flap (MPF). **(a)** Vertical sharp incision with a 15-mm blade. **(b)** Mucoperichondrial dissection using a Freer elevator. **(c)** The MPF is elevated posteriorly and the septal bone (SB) is exposed.

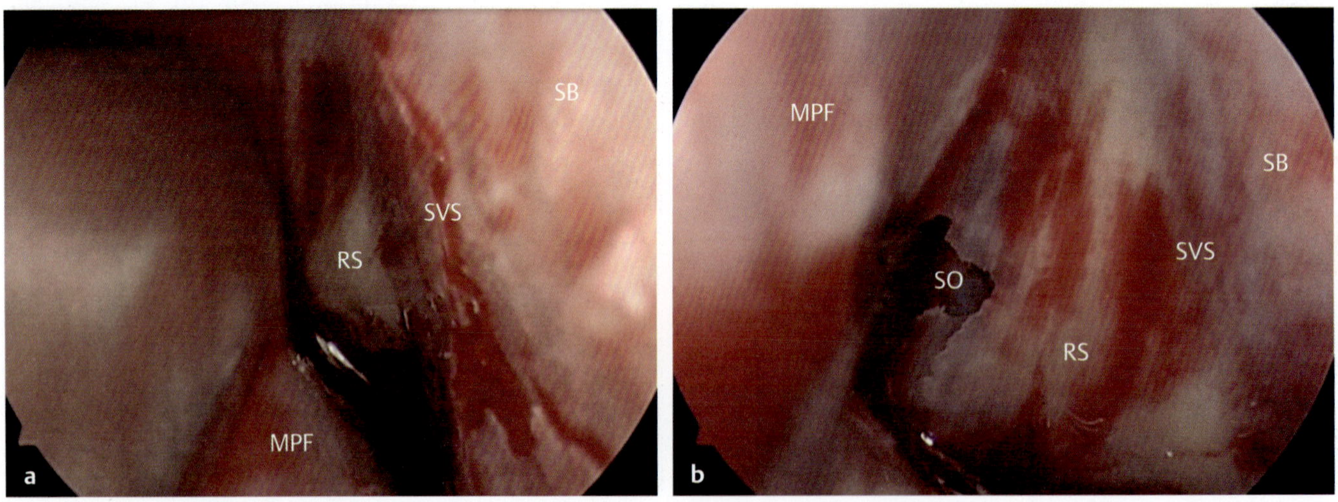

Fig. 1.48 **(a)** The mucoperichondrial flap (MFP) elevation is extended along the septal bone (SB) to the sphenovomerine suture (SVS) and the rostrum sphenoidale (RS) is located ipsilaterally. **(b)** The MPF is raised off the bony septum (BS) with a Freer elevator posteriorly until the RS and the sphenoid ostium (SO) are visible.

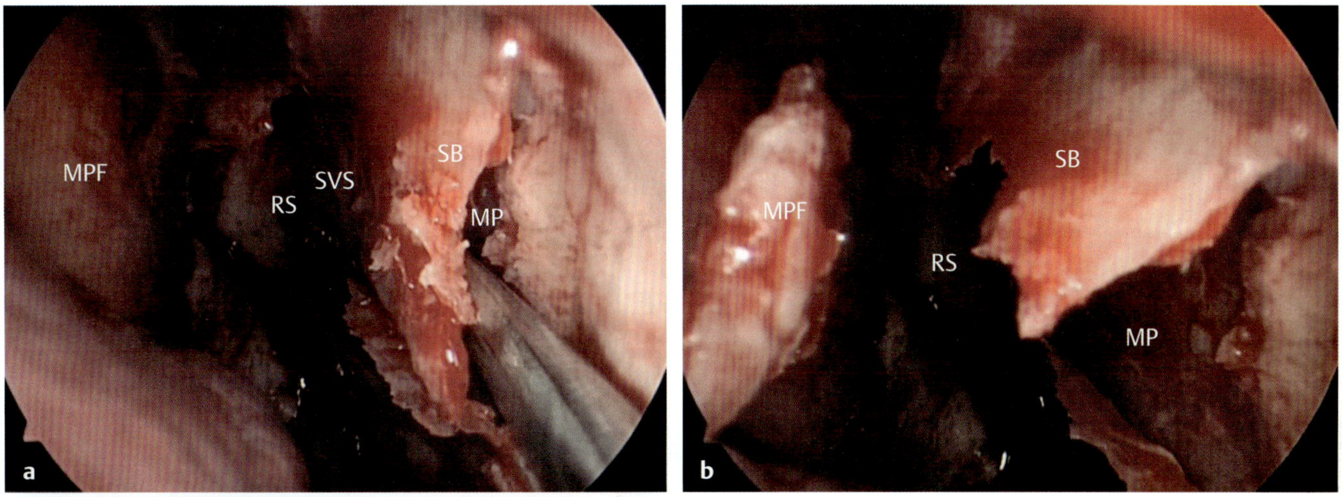

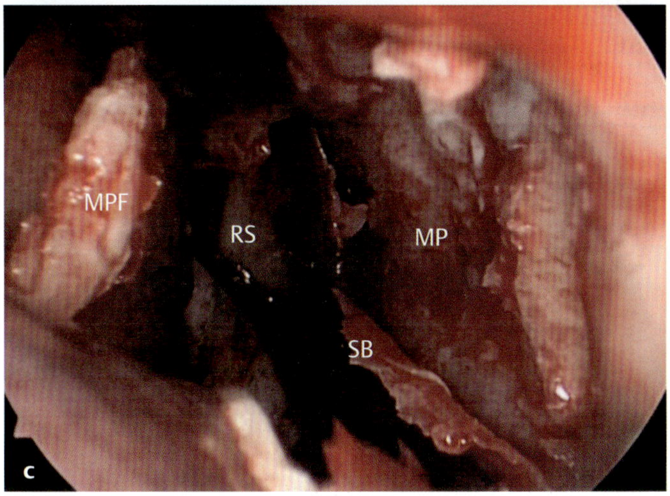

Fig. 1.49 **(a, b)** The exposed bony septum (BS) is fractured through at the osteocartilaginous junction to the contralateral side and **(c)** removed in a piecemeal fashion.

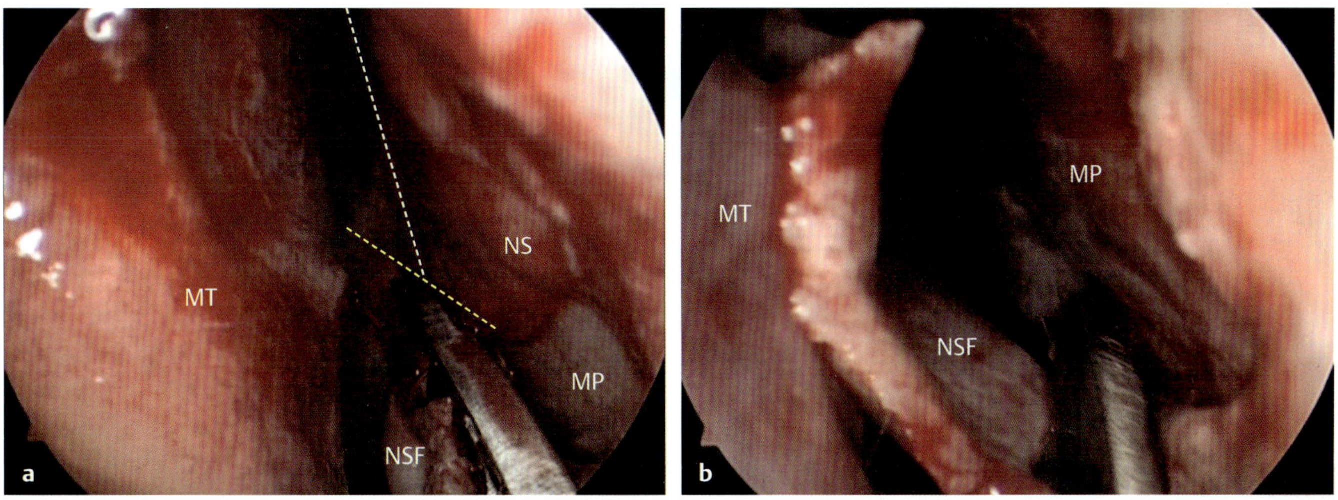

Fig. 1.50 **(a)** The superior cut (*yellow line*) for the nasoseptal flap (NSF) may be taken until about 0.5 to 1 cm below the skull base (*white line*) to preserve the olfactory function. **(b)** The inferior cut for the NSF can be taken as far as half the nasal floor if a large skull base defect is expected (Hadad–Bassagasteguy flap).

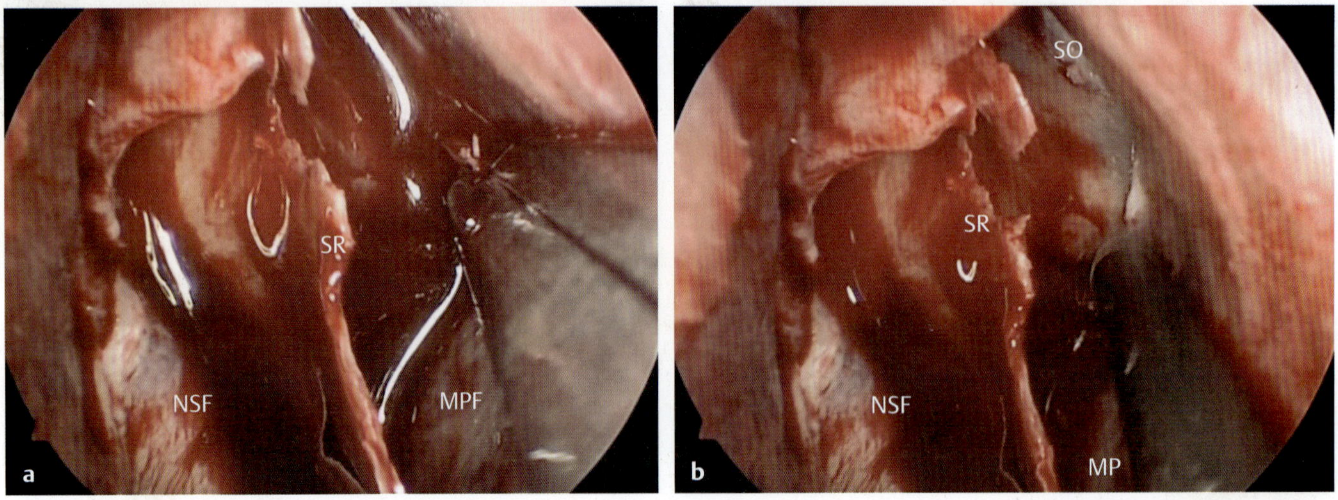

Fig. 1.51 **(a)** The sphenoid rostrum (SR) is fully exposed by dissecting the septal mucosa laterally. **(b)** Identification of the sphenoid ostium.

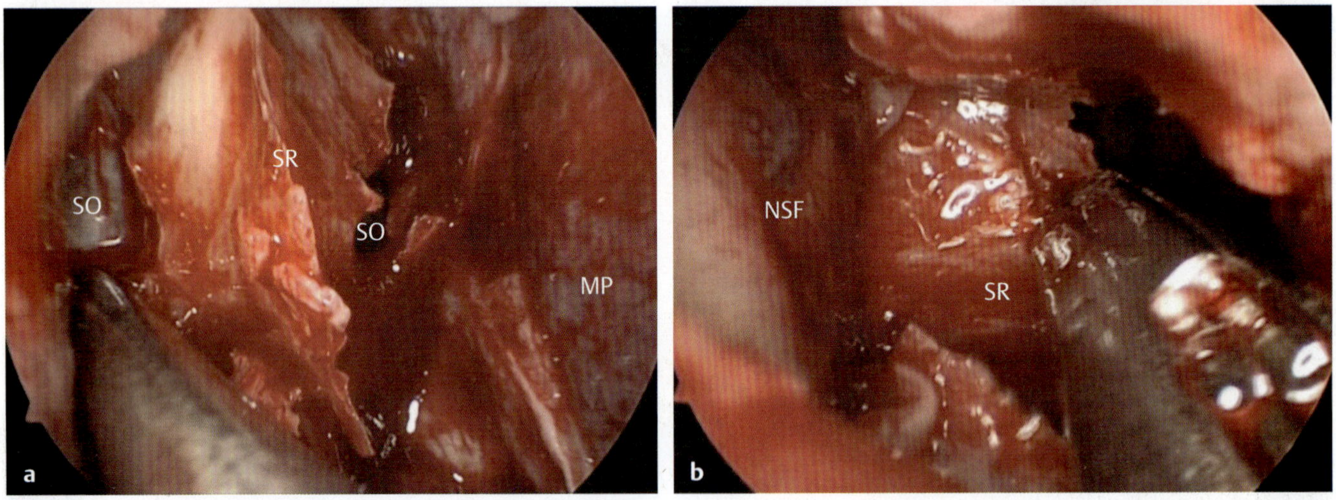

Fig. 1.52 **(a)** Sphenoidotomy: The sphenoid ostia (SO) are widened using a Kerrison punch. **(b)** The anterior wall of the sphenoid sinus (sphenoid rostrum [SR) is removed in total or by piecemeal.

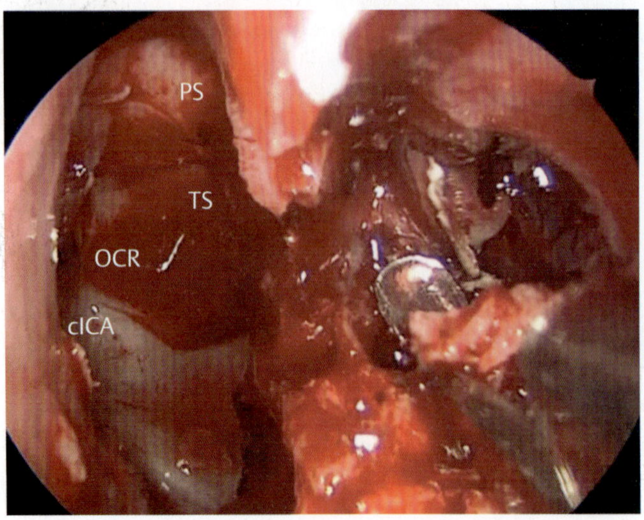

Fig. 1.53 Removal of a main intersinus septum of the sphenoid cavity.

encountered, and tearing of the mucosa should be done carefully after in-depth studies of the radiological imaging studies (**Fig. 1.55a, b**).

- If the bone overlying the sella turcica is thick and a controlled fracturing with a suction device or a dissector in the midline is not possible, the use of a high-speed drill is recommended to thin out the bone. In larger tumor eroding and remodeling the sella turcica, the bone is usually thin enough to be flicked off with either a right-angled probe or a Freer elevator exposing the corresponding dura (**Fig. 1.56a**).
- A right-angled probe is used to carefully lift away the sellar dura from the bone covering the sella turcica before proceeding with a wide bony removal. The lateral limit of bony removal is the cavernous sinus, inferiorly the sellar floor, and superiorly the intercavernous sinus (**Fig. 1.56b**).

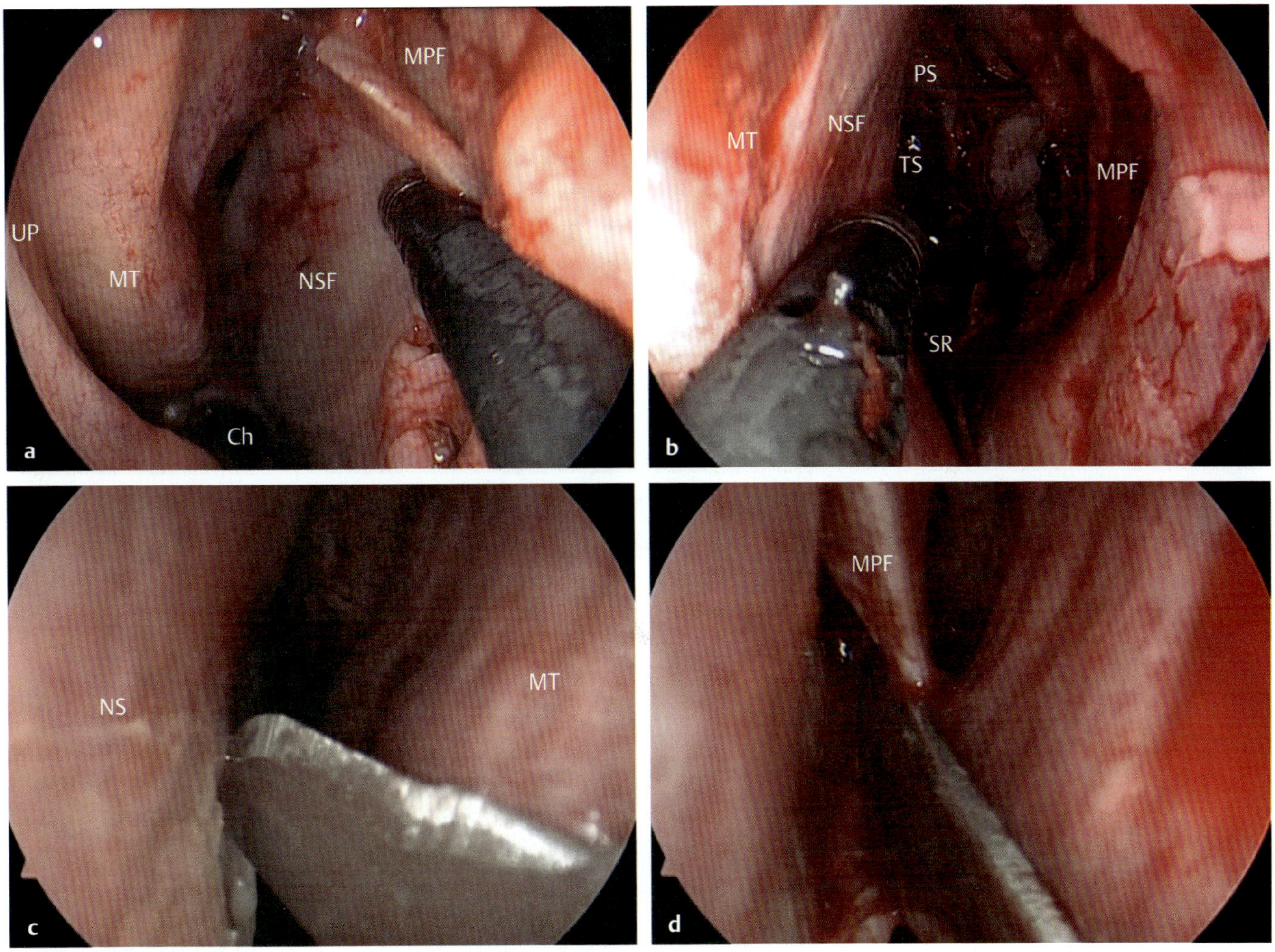

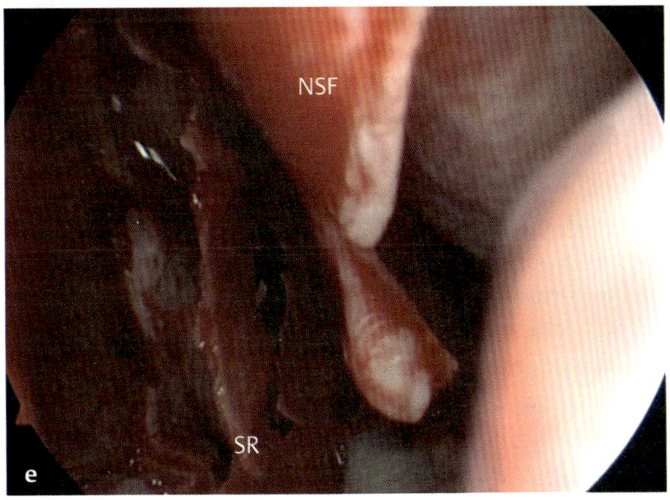

Fig. 1.54 Endoscopic endonasal double nostril transseptal transsphenoidal approach. **(a)** The medialized ipsilateral nasoseptal flap (NSF) is demonstrated after the mononostril transseptal transsphenoidal approach. The contralateral mucoperichondrial flap (MPF) can be elevated contralaterally along the way. **(b)** When the NSF is lateralized, the MPF is visible. **(c)** Sharp incision of the contralateral nasal mucosa in the contralateral nostril on the level of the middle turbinate (MT). **(d)** Elevation of the MPF. **(e)** The NSF can be created as described in **Fig. 1.50**. The binostril access is granted by identifying the midline structures from the contralateral nostril as they were identified using the ipsilateral nostril during the initial approach.

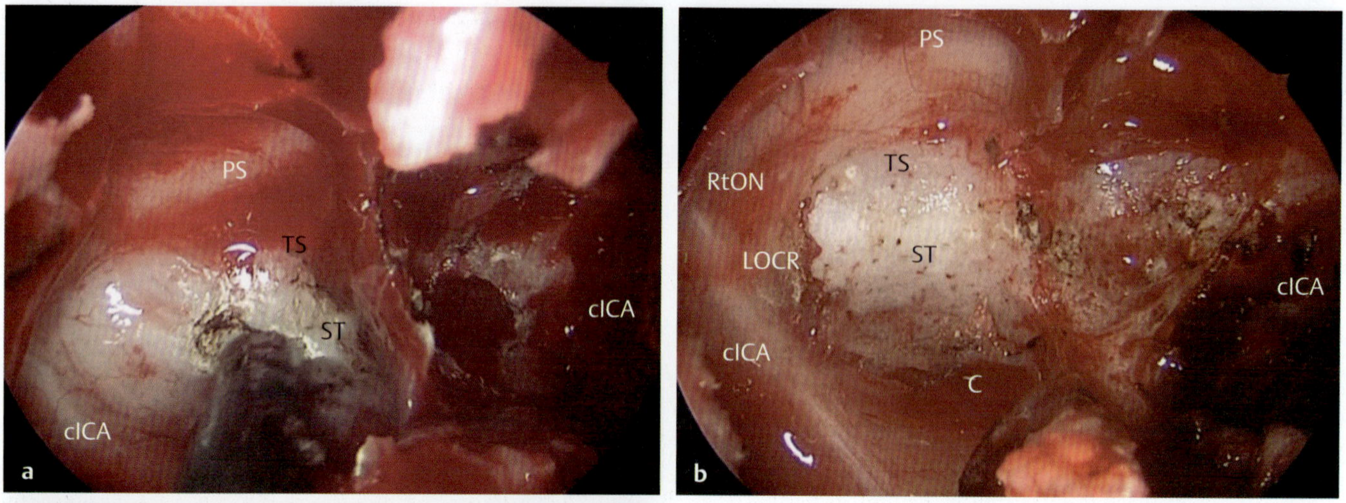

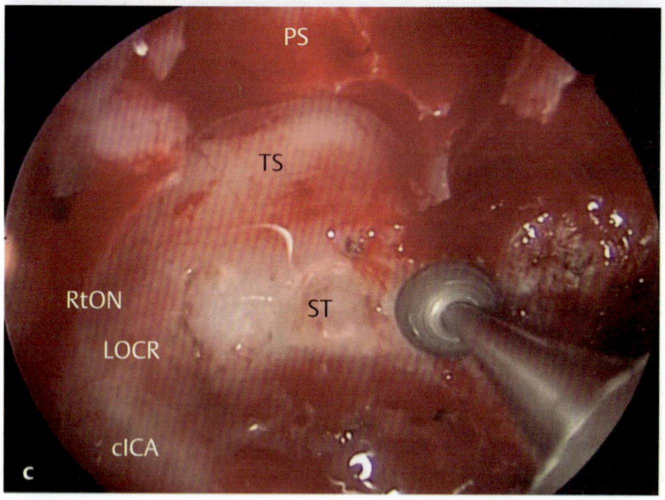

Fig. 1.55 Osteodural phase of the transsellar approach (zonal dissection) **(a)** The mucosa covering the sellar bone is cauterized and elevated off. **(b)** The exposure is defined by the cavernous internal carotid eminences (cICA) laterally, the planum sphenoidale (PS) and tuberculum sellae (TS) superiorly, and the clivus (C) inferiorly. **(c)** A high-speed drill can be used to thin out the bone covering the sella turcica (ST).

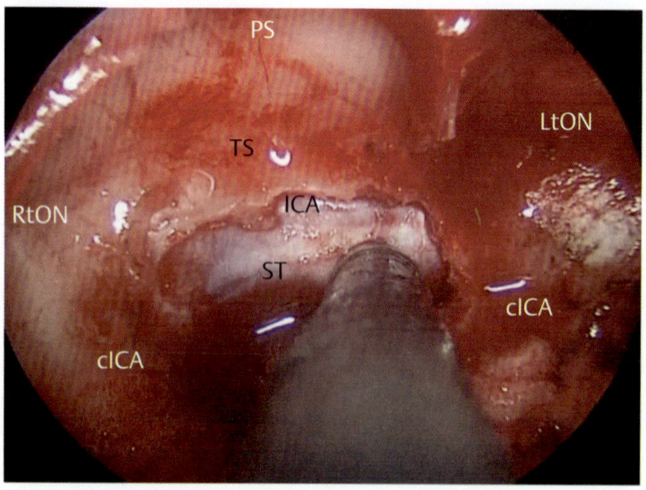

Fig. 1.56 Osteodural phase of the transsellar approach (zonal dissection). The transsellar approach can be completed using a Kerrison's punch. The lateral limit of the bony removal is the cavernous sinus with the carotid eminences [cICA], the sellar floor inferiorly, and the intercavernous sinus (ICS) and the tuberculum sellae (TS) superiorly.

Extended Endoscopic Endonasal Transseptal Transsphenoidal Approach

The extension of the sellar opening using a transtuberculum and transplanum extension can be part of the tailored approach concept. These extensions depend on the surgical route, the size and the firmness of the pituitary adenoma. In general, these approaches are advocated for the extracapsular dissection using the pituitary pseudocapsule in the suprasellar compartment.[275,276] Schwartz et al. did point out the difficulties, when a downward slope of the planum and cribriform plate is present, particularly with a 0-degree scope. They hence advocate the removal of the posterior ethmoid sinuses, and the use of a 30-degree scope to facilitate this approach.[128]

Intradural Phase (Tumor Resection)

Pituitary macroadenomas are the most frequent lesions encountered when performing endonasal endoscopic surgery. A systematic approach in resecting these lesions leads to a higher routine for the surgeon and therefore better results in terms of extent of resection.

Neurosurgical Considerations for Intradural Resection of Pituitary Macroadenomas

- The dura is cauterized at the site of incision. Often cruciate incision is made over the dural covering of the pituitary, but occasionally it is also tailored to the content and site of the cystic component. Incision is made lower in a case of superolateral cystic component to prevent early descend of the diaphragm which can obscure the surgical field (**Fig. 1.57**).
- A sample of tumor is removed for histopathological examination (**Fig. 1.58**).
- The rest of the tumor removal is performed using suction, dissectors, and also ring curettes.
- Tumor removal should be performed systemically starting with the inferior central tumor compartment and then continued laterally. This minimizes the risk of leaving tumor behind and prevents early descend of diaphragm and thus obscuring the surgeon's view.
- Inferior tumor debulking should be started in the midline along the sellar floor (central pillar) and then extended to the lateral on each side (lateral pillars) (**Fig. 1.59a, b**).
- Superior tumor debulking should be started posterior to avoid diaphragmal dura to bulge into the field and block the surgeon's view (**Fig. 1.60**).
- The anterior superior part should be approached as a last step. The likelihood for CSF leaks is higher while resecting these tumor parts near the planum sphenoidale (**Fig. 1.61**).
- The dural incision can be extended in any direction if residual tumor is suspected.
- When extending the dural opening laterally, the cavernous sinus and the carotid arteries have to be considered.
- When extending the dural opening superiorly, the intercavernous sinus has to be considered.
- If the anterior superior tumor aspects cannot be released, removal of the tuberculum sellae and even part of the planum sphenoidale might be necessary to reach the apex of the tumor and use extracapsular dissection from the neurovascular structures.
- To assure a complete removal of the pituitary adenoma, particular attention should be paid to corners and clefts between the cavernous sinus and diaphragma sellae. In most instances the dome of diaphragm descends symmetrically once tumor removal is adequate. Inspection is done using the suction to hold up the diaphragma sellae (**Fig. 1.62**).
- If there is an asymmetry in the diaphragmal bulge, residual tumor or strings might be hidden in the apical aspects of the resection cavity.

Neurosurgical Considerations for Intradural Resection of Functioning Microadenomas

In the case of a pituitary microadenoma, the laterality and the localization in the anterior posterior aspect are relevant.[218,277] Especially, very lateral microadenomas might not automatically be amenable for a single-nostril approach, as angulation of the endoscope and bimanual dissection might be limited. Usually, a unilateral opening of the sella and inspection of the pituitary gland are performed.[233] Pituitary gland dissection in cases where a microadenoma location is less clear is sometimes necessary. If the lesion is identified, resection using microdissectors and suction is performed. Minimal manipulation of the healthy pituitary gland tissue should be the goal while reaching radical resection of the functioning microadenoma.

Neurosurgical Consideration for the Management of Rathke's Cleft Cysts

Whether symptomatic Rathke's cleft cysts need aggressive resection or not remains controversial. A full evacuation of the cyst contents and liberal opening of the cyst wall have been advocated in the early years.[52] In general, small incidental cysts can be followed up with interval imaging to survey presence or absence of progression.[44,45] Patients who present with visual or endocrine symptoms need a surgical treatment. There is likewise uncertainty in patients who present with headache. One study elucidated resolution or improvement of headaches in 52 and 39% of patients with Rathke's cleft cyst, respectively.[69] The patient should be informed about the possibility of treatment failure with surgery, as headaches are a very unspecific symptom.

A surgical resection has impact on visual function as well as endocrinological status. However, an aggressive approach has repeatedly been shown to increase the risk of postoperative electrolyte disturbances and endocrinopathies.[127,174,278] The majority of patients with symptomatic Rathke's cleft cysts will experience a certain degree of improvement or resolution of visual field disturbances.[127,174] However, in terms of endocrine dysfunction data are less reliable, with one series demonstrating 10% new anterior pituitary deficiencies postoperatively and 27% of patients with improvement when preoperative dysfunction was present.[174] A large series of 87 patients with symptomatic Rathke's cleft cysts was stratified

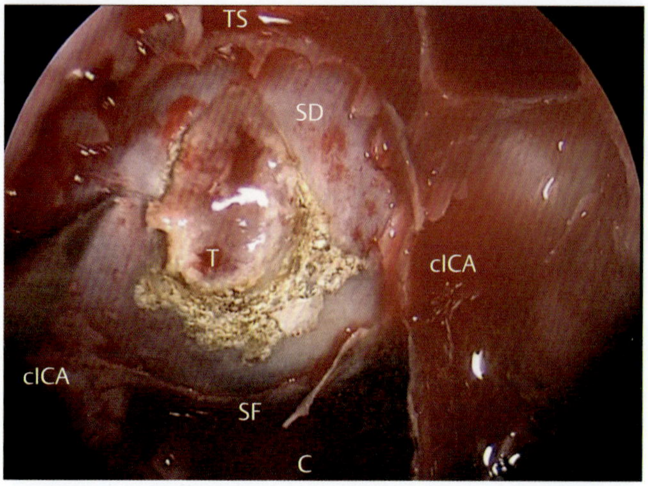

Fig. 1.57 Intradural resection of a pituitary macroadenoma. Cauterization and incision of the sellar dura (SD). Typical adenoma tissue (T) is visible.

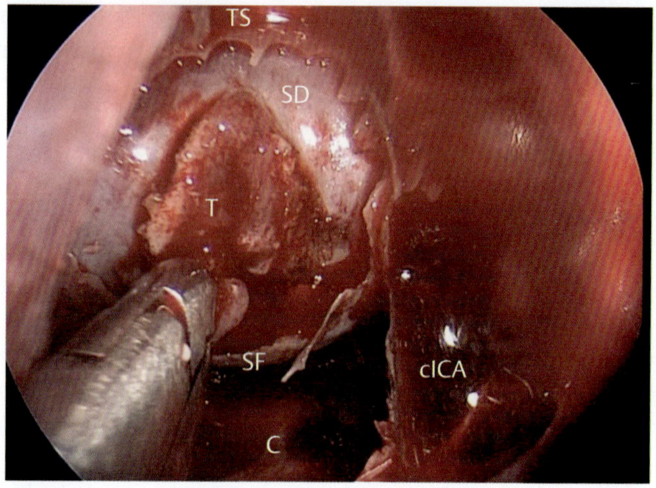

Fig. 1.58 A sample of the tumor is removed for histopathological examination.

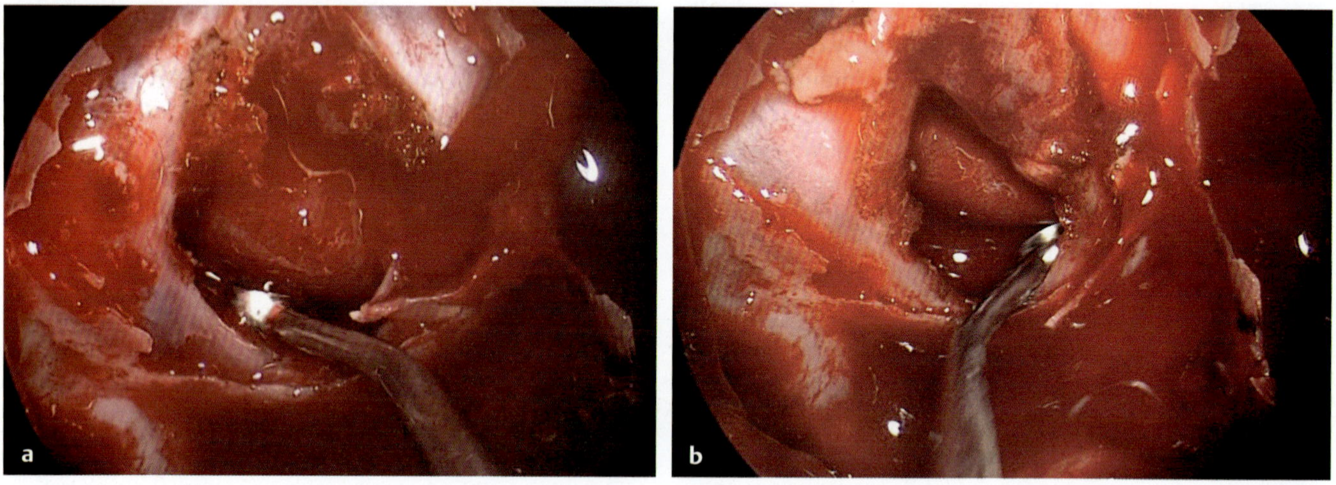

Fig. 1.59 Intradural resection of a pituitary macroadenoma. **(a)** Inferior tumor debulking along the midline sellar floor (central pillar). **(b)** Inferior tumor debulking along the lateral aspects of the medial cavernous sinus wall (lateral pillars).

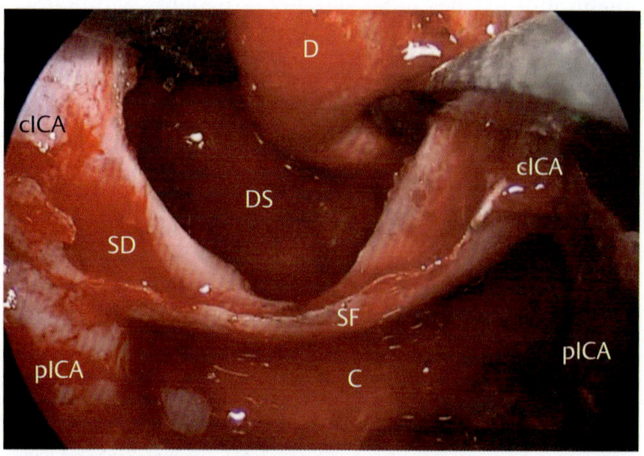

Fig. 1.60 Superior posterior tumor debulking to avoid diaphragm dura bulging into the field. The anterior superior part should be approached as a last step.

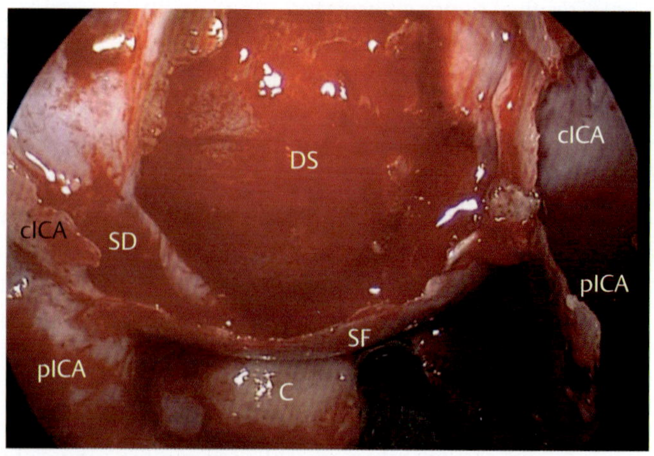

Fig. 1.61 In most instances the dome of diaphragm descends symmetrically once tumor removal is adequate.

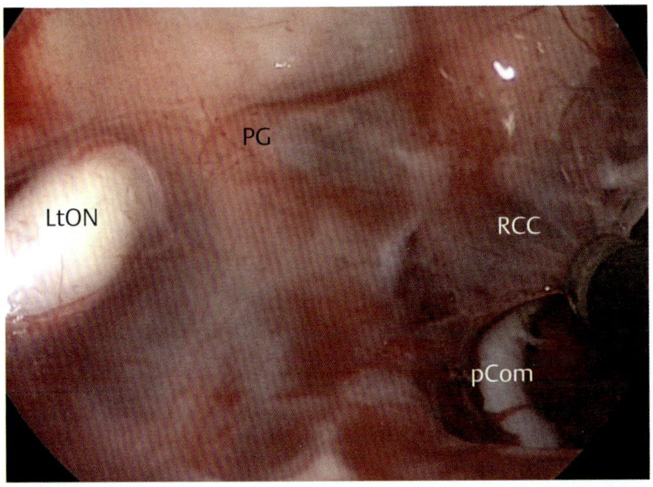

Fig. 1.62 Intraoperative view of a Rathke's cleft cyst (RCC) involving the left optic nerve (LtON), compressing the pituitary gland (PG) and the posterior communicating artery (pCom).

by Fan et al. in a transsphenoidal subtotal (n = 49), transcranial subtotal (n = 23), and a transcranial total (n = 15) resection group. Grade of resection was classified in a complete versus a subtotal resection of the cyst wall. Eventually, 8 and 9% in the subtotal and 47% in the complete resected group had postoperative complications, respectively. CSF leakage was present in 3% (exclusively in the endonasal group), new hypopituitarism in 9%, and postoperative diabetes insipidus in 6%. Complete resected cysts had the highest rate of postoperative hypopituitarism, while supraorbital keyhole surgery seemed to be superior when compared to classic open approaches. The Kaplan-Meier 3-year recurrence-free rates were 84, 87, and 86%, respectively.[278] Lower recurrence rates can be expected for Rathke's cleft cysts and arachnoid cysts after treatment as compared to craniopharyngioma. One study found cyst size to be a significant predictor of recurrence rate for Rathke's cleft cysts.[44]

Our institutional experience consists of an individualized approach depending on the cyst's anatomical location (intra- or suprasellar). As an aggressive resection is generally associated with complications without impacting the recurrence rate,[174, 278,279] we perform an endonasal endoscopic approach for the evacuation and conservative resection of the cyst wall for intrasellar lesions (inferior compartment), leaving the cyst wall along all vital structures and the pituitary gland if a very distinct plane is not evident (**Fig. 1.62**). Suprasellar lesions might be amenable for a more aggressive resection depending on their relationship to the infundibular stalk (superior compartment) and additional intrasellar extension, either via an endonasal endoscopic approach or a transcranial approach.

Neurosurgical Consideration for the Management of Intrasellar Arachnoid Cysts

Indication for the surgical treatment of intrasellar arachnoid cysts is in accordance to Rathke's cleft cysts causing locoregional mass effect symptoms. Size, location, and suprasellar extent dictate the surgical approach, respectively. Intra- and parasellar arachnoid cysts are amenable for an endonasal endoscopic transsphenoidal approach with cyst biopsy and fenestration. Transcranial open or endoscopic approaches for cyst fenestration or intracystic fluid diversion placement are necessary when the main part of the cyst is extrasellar and causing a global mass effect (**Fig. 1.35 e and f**).

Management of Intraoperative Bleeding

The management of intraoperative hemorrhage during skull base surgery is essential. Common tools used include diathermy or electrocautery, vessel clips, hemostatic agents, bone wax, and hot saline irrigation. In case of diffuse "oozing" from sinonasal mucosa or pathological tissue, hot saline irrigation (40°C) and slight head elevation (30 degrees) are effective in most cases. As a main principle, the endonasal endoscopic exposure should allow sufficient space for instrumentation in order to deal with intraoperative bleeding, especially in high-flow venous or arterial bleeding. Sources of intraoperative bleeding during endonasal endoscopic skull base surgery arise from the posterior septal branch of the sphenopalatine artery, endonasal or sphenoidal mucosa, the anterior or posterior ethmoidal artery, exposed bone, dural veins, the cavernous sinus, or very rarely from the ICA. Mucosal bleeding can usually be arrested with monopolar or bipolar cauterization. Bleeding from exposed bone may occasionally require bone wax if cautery is insufficient to control the ooze. Bleeding from dural veins and cavernous sinus can often be controlled with use of Surgicel (Fibrillar Absorbable matrix sealant agent, Baxter) (**Fig. 1.63**). In our institution, hemostasis is achieved using Taming Sari, a device designed by Waran et al., that allows for the delivery of a hemostatic agent accurately over the site of hemorrhage while simultaneously maintaining compression and suction.[264,265] This is particularly useful in endoscopic surgery through a long narrow tunnel, where the device is also able to prevent the hemostatic agent from being washed away by brisk bleeding.[264,265] The system has been used successfully in endoscopic skull base surgery and endoscopic surgery within the parenchyma of the brain using tube systems.[265] In a retrospective study by Brand et al. on endonasal endoscopic surgeries, the Taming Sari device allowed controlled application of small amounts of hemostatic agents (0.5–1 mL) to the site of bleeding. The controlled application hence reduced

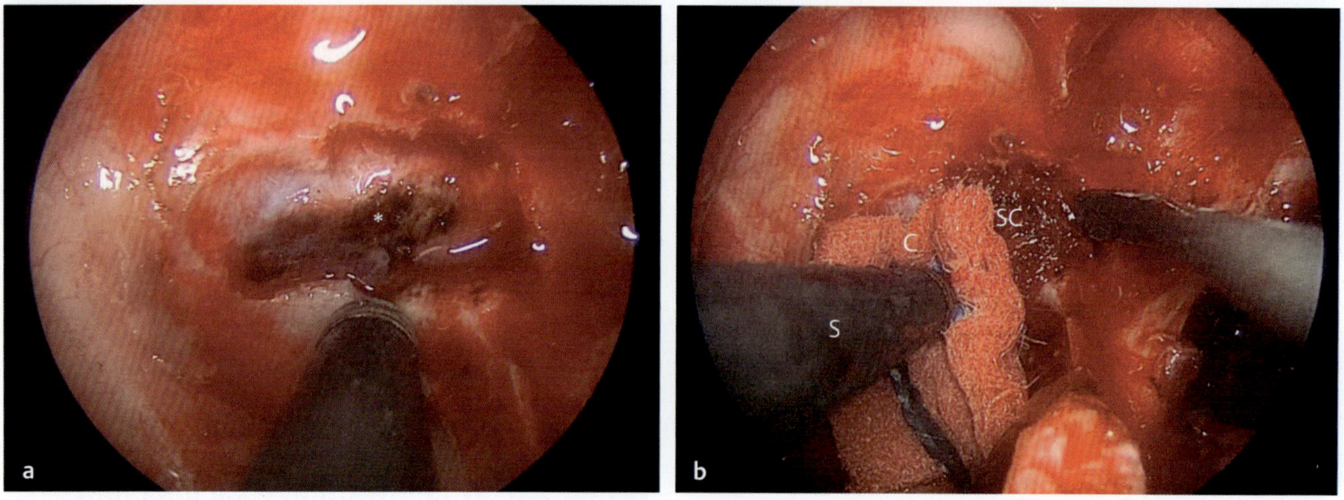

Fig. 1.63 (a, b) Bleeding from dural veins can often be controlled by cauterization (*) or with the use of Surgicel (SC) (Fibrillar Absorbable Hemostat, Johnson & Johnson) in combination with a cottonoid (C) and a suction device (S).

the amount required within an individual procedure (5–10 applications per 5-mL ampule of FloSeal) and increased the visibility during its application (**Fig. 1.64**).[264]

Internal Carotid Artery Injuries

Intraoperative injury to the ICA during endonasal endoscopic surgery for skull base lesions has been described as a rare but disastrous complication with an incidence of 0.2 to 1%, associated with high rates of morbidity and mortality.[187,280,281] Traumatic injury to the ICA during endonasal endoscopic surgery may cause sudden and massive intraoperative bleeding eventually leading to hypotension and hemodynamic shock with potential death within minutes.[282] Emergency local repair with large suctions, lens cleansing devices, crushed rectus abdominal muscle graft and multiple cottonoids, or a Teflon mesh and methyl methacrylate to form an external artificial wall over the laceration, and consecutive nasal packing, have been described.[187,280–282] If the hemodynamic situation of the patient after bleeding control is stable, a conventional angiography should be performed. This is based on the fact that even when hemostasis and a local repair is successfully implemented during endonasal endoscopic surgery, ICA pseudoaneurysms or a carotid cavernous fistula may be formed.[281,282–284] Endovascular treatment with parent vessel occlusion or stent graft placement has emerged to be the major therapeutic option for this complication[187,280–284] (**Fig. 1.65**).

Skull Base Defect Closure

The expansions of endoscopic endonasal approaches for the resection of benign or malignant skull base tumors have led to improved techniques for reconstructing large skull base defects. As the last step of the endonasal endoscopic approach, a watertight closure of the generated skull base defect is essential. This step is of crucial importance and several risk factors for intraoperative and postoperative CSF leakage have been described in the literature.[285] CSF leakage can occur during or after the tumor removal, during the exploration of cavernous sinus and diaphragmatic recesses particularly seen in revision surgery, and with suprasellar extension of a macroadenoma.[286] A meticulous technique and sufficient time should be invested to achieve an adequate closure.[287–290]

Management without Cerebrospinal Fluid Leakage

If there is no evident CSF leakage, sellar reconstruction is not required to complete the surgery.[287] In our institution, the cavity is usually packed with Surgicel (Fibrillar Absorbable Hemostat, Johnson & Johnson) and Gelfoam supported by the remaining floor of the sphenoid cavity, covered by an artificial dural or fibrin sealant. The mucoperiosteal flap of the septum is brought back into position, and a nasal packing with resorbable material is placed in both nostrils, bringing the middle turbinates back into position. If a nonresorbable nasal packing is used, it is usually left in situ for at about 5 days.

Management of Small Intraoperative Cerebrospinal Fluid Leakage

In the case of a small intraoperative CSF leak, a small piece of abdominal fat at the arachnoid break point followed by a bigger piece of fat is used to cover the defect. Optimally, the

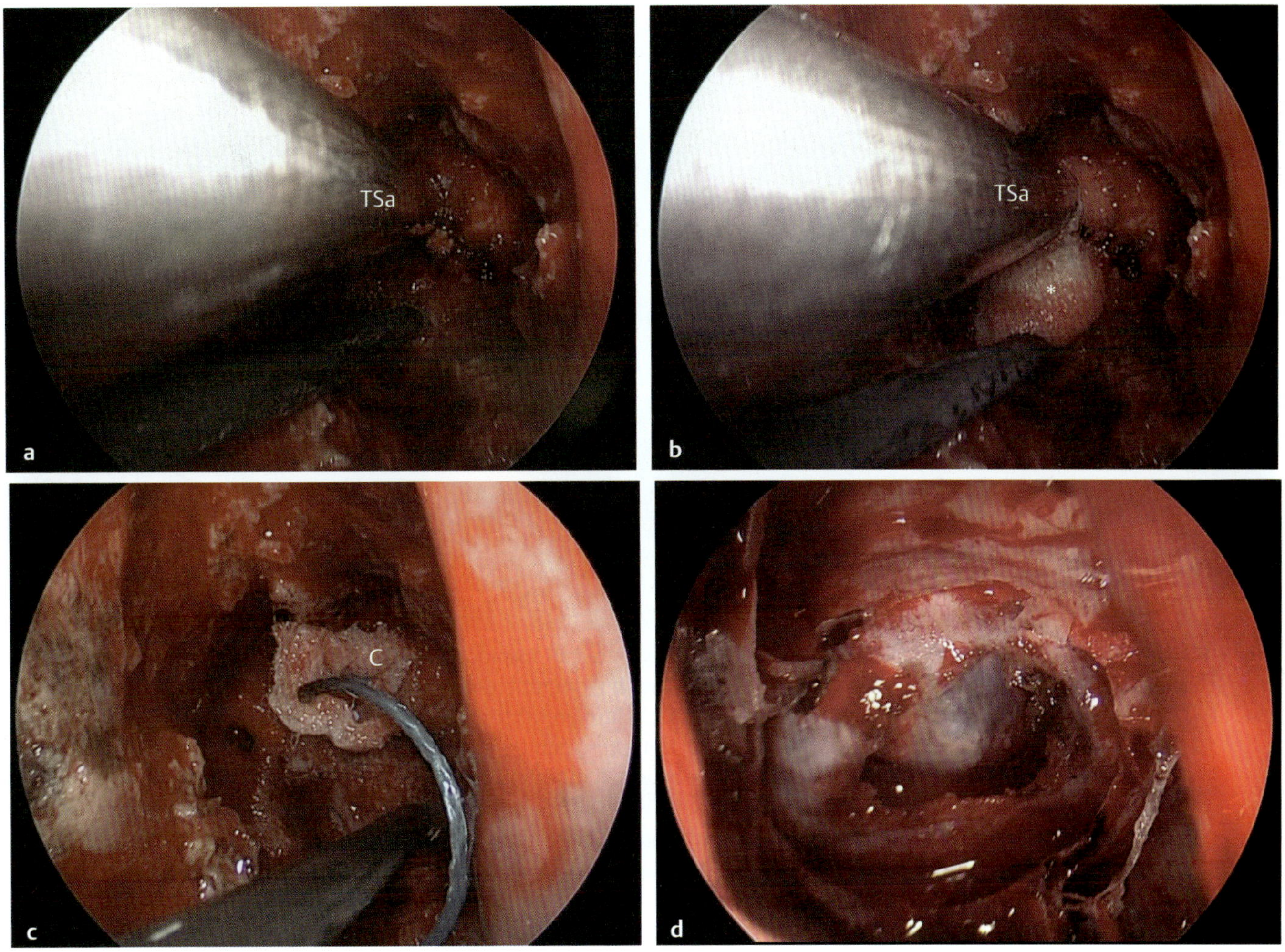

Fig. 1.64 **(a)** The Taming Sari (TSa) device has been designed by Vicknes Waran. **(b)** This device allows the delivery of hemostatic agents (*) accurately over the site of hemorrhage. **(c)** The device allows simultaneously maintaining compression with a cottonoid (C) and suction. **(d)** Controlled situs after the use of Taming Sari.

fat graft covers the dural edges intradurally. The construct is covered with an artificial dural sealant and Surgicel (Fibrillar Absorbable Hemostat, Johnson & Johnson). The nasoseptal flap is brought back into position and a nasal packing is applied (**Fig. 1.66**).

Autologous Abdominal Fat Graft

The use of an autologous abdominal free fat graft is a traditional surgical method for the repair of anterior skull base defects. A typical site of harvesting this graft is the periumbilical area, and the abdominal fat graft remains a safe and easily accessible material to repair CSF leaks.[291] In a small retrospective study by Lam et al., 25 out of 27 (93%) patients undergoing an endoscopic repair of a skull base defect with an abdominal free fat graft demonstrated successful repair of preoperative or intraoperative CSF leakage. Only two patients developed a recurrent CSF leakage using this technique, occurring in about 1 week after the primary closure with a secondary closure rate of 96%.[291] Local complications described in the literature are seroma and hematoma formation at the abdominal donor sites.

For most of the cases with no or small intraoperative CSF leakage, the postoperative control shows excellent healing with sufficient epithelialization of the operative site using this strategy (**Fig. 1.67**).

Management of Large Skull Base Defects with Cerebrospinal Fluid Leakage

The issue of the most appropriate repair of skull base defects remains unresolved and several strategies have been recommended and described in the literature.[291–295] When addressing larger lesions with the endonasal endoscopic approach,

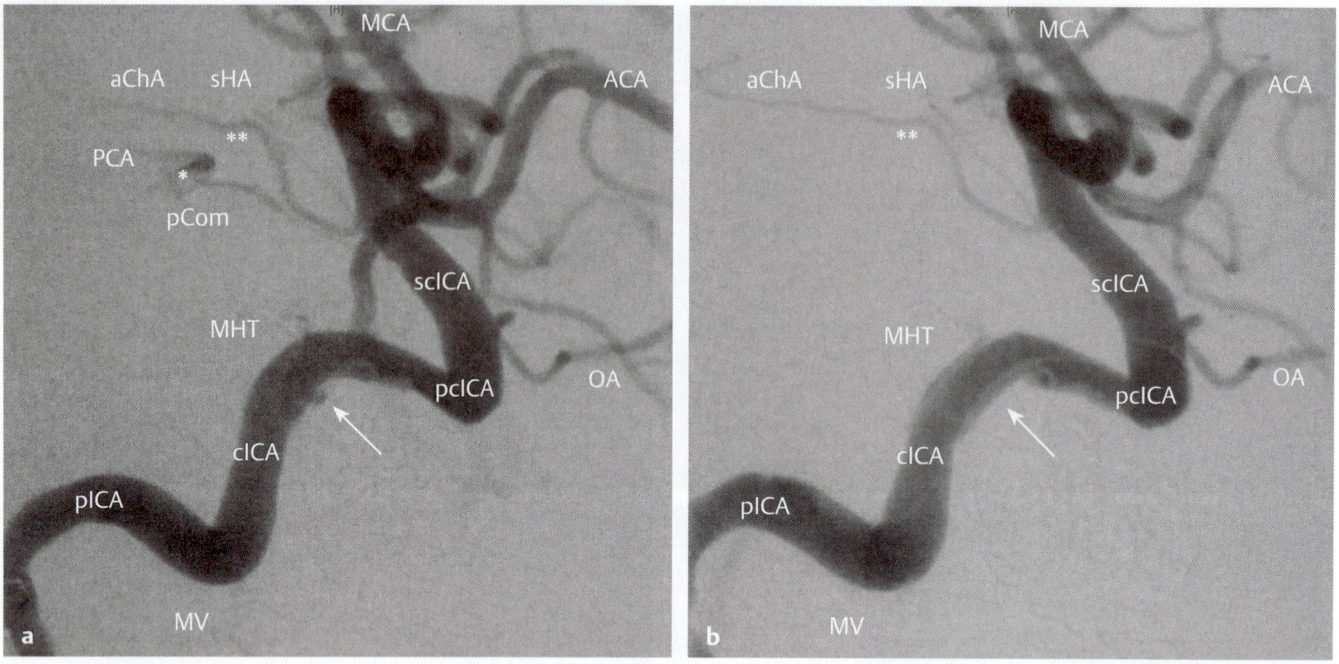

Fig. 1.65 **(a)** Lateral digital subtraction arteriogram performed after an intraoperative internal carotid artery injury with the formation of a pseudoaneurysm (*white arrow*). The arteriogram demonstrates the standard configuration most commonly seen. The mandibulovidian artery (MV), inferolateral trunk (not visible), and the meningohypophyseal trunk (MHT) are sometimes visible. The proximal dural ring can be assumed to be just proximal to the origin of the ophthalmic artery (OA) that runs anteriorly. The posterior communicating artery (pCom) with its posterior course and "flash-filling" (*) of the posterior cerebral artery (PCA) is visible. The junction is identifiable by the change in vessel caliber and the appearance of laminar mixing with unopacified blood from the basilar artery (*). The anterior choroidal artery (aChA) arises slightly more distal heading posteriorly and has a distinct "plexal point" (**). Finally, the superior hypophyseal artery (sHA) and the carotid bifurcation with the middle (MCA) and anterior (ACA) cerebral arteries are visible. **(b)** The pseudoaneurysm (*white arrow*) is not visible after the endovascular placement of a "Willis covered stent graft." Alternatively, parent artery occlusion of the internal carotid artery is a possible treatment option for this rare but serious complication.

complex reconstruction of the surgically created defects might be necessary.[66] An increasing diversity of tissues and grafts is available to reach a watertight defect closure.[296]

Larger dural skull base defects are usually filled with autologous grafts, either abdominal fat or fascia lata.[291–293] It is of great importance that these grafts cover the dural edges from intracranially to provide a watertight closure. The construct can be stabilized and held in position with an artificial dural sealant and Surgicel (Fibrillar Absorbable Hemostat, Johnson & Johnson).

Autologous Fascia Lata Graft

A multilayer technique using autologous FL is widely used and an accepted strategy for reconstruction of large skull base defects with CSF leakage.[126,293–295] The FL graft is usually harvested from the ipsilateral lateral thigh in the area of the iliotibial band using an approximately 3 to 5 cm longitudinal incision over the upper and middle one-third of the upper leg. The incision is carried down to the iliotibial band of the FL. A medial longitudinal incision in the fascia followed by a lateral longitudinal incision should be performed with care not to harm the underlying muscle tissue. A distal transverse incision allows to gently elevate off the fascia from the underlying muscle. The proximal transverse incision is made at the end. It is recommended to leave the surrounding fat tissue along the FL graft to optimize adherence along the bony borders and to allow a watertight closure of the skull base defect (**Fig. 1.68**).

For larger skull base defects with CSF leakage, it is also recommended to use previously harvested uni- or bilateral vascularized nasoseptal flaps. In the case of large skull base defects, a watertight closure is an absolute crucial step in managing the surgical resection of larger lesions. Postoperative CSF leakage has relevant impact on the outcome of these patients, when intracranial complications occur. The goal of harvesting pedicled nasoseptal flaps is to seal the skull base dura and separate the intracranial space

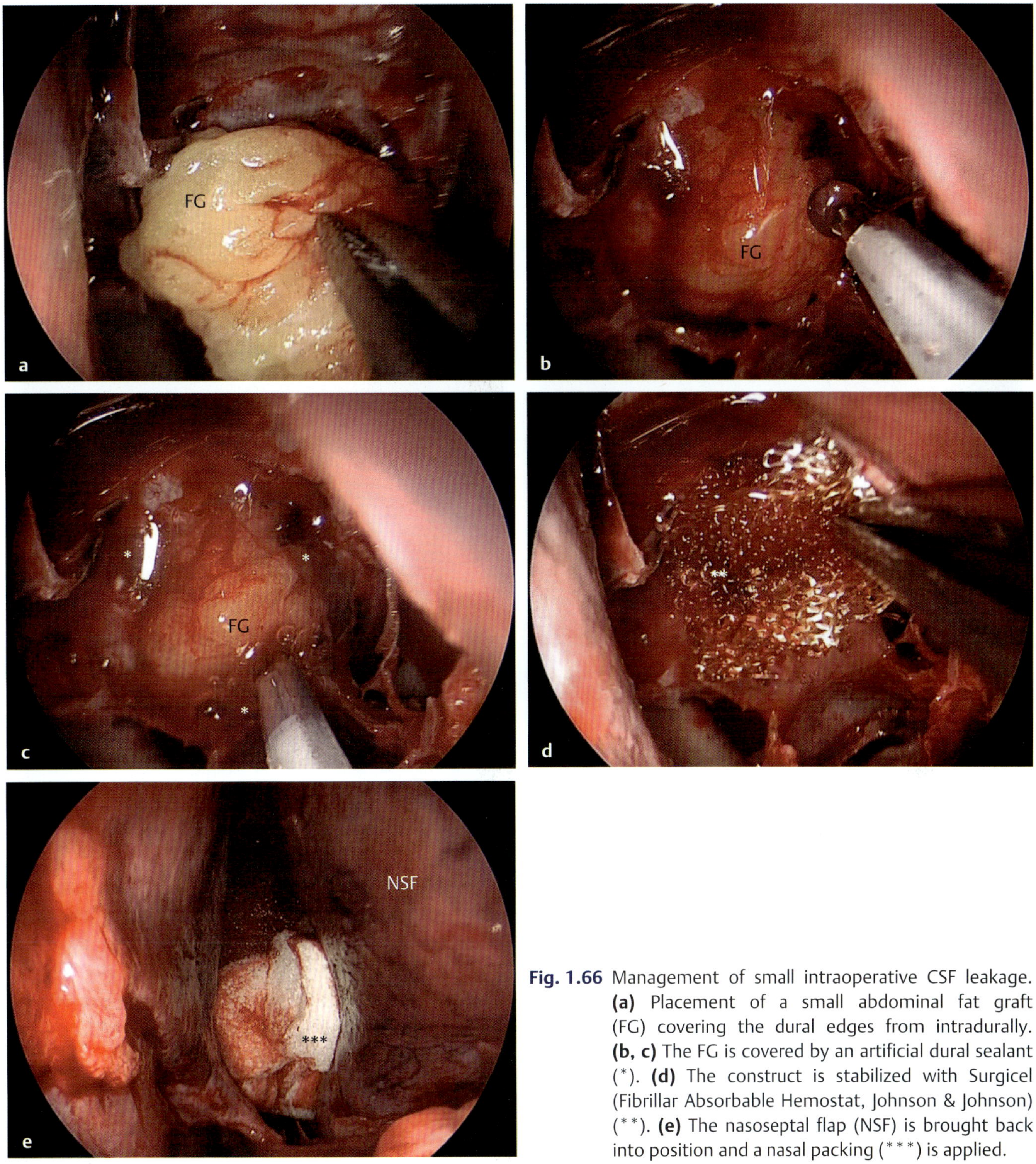

Fig. 1.66 Management of small intraoperative CSF leakage. **(a)** Placement of a small abdominal fat graft (FG) covering the dural edges from intradurally. **(b, c)** The FG is covered by an artificial dural sealant (*). **(d)** The construct is stabilized with Surgicel (Fibrillar Absorbable Hemostat, Johnson & Johnson) (**). **(e)** The nasoseptal flap (NSF) is brought back into position and a nasal packing (***) is applied.

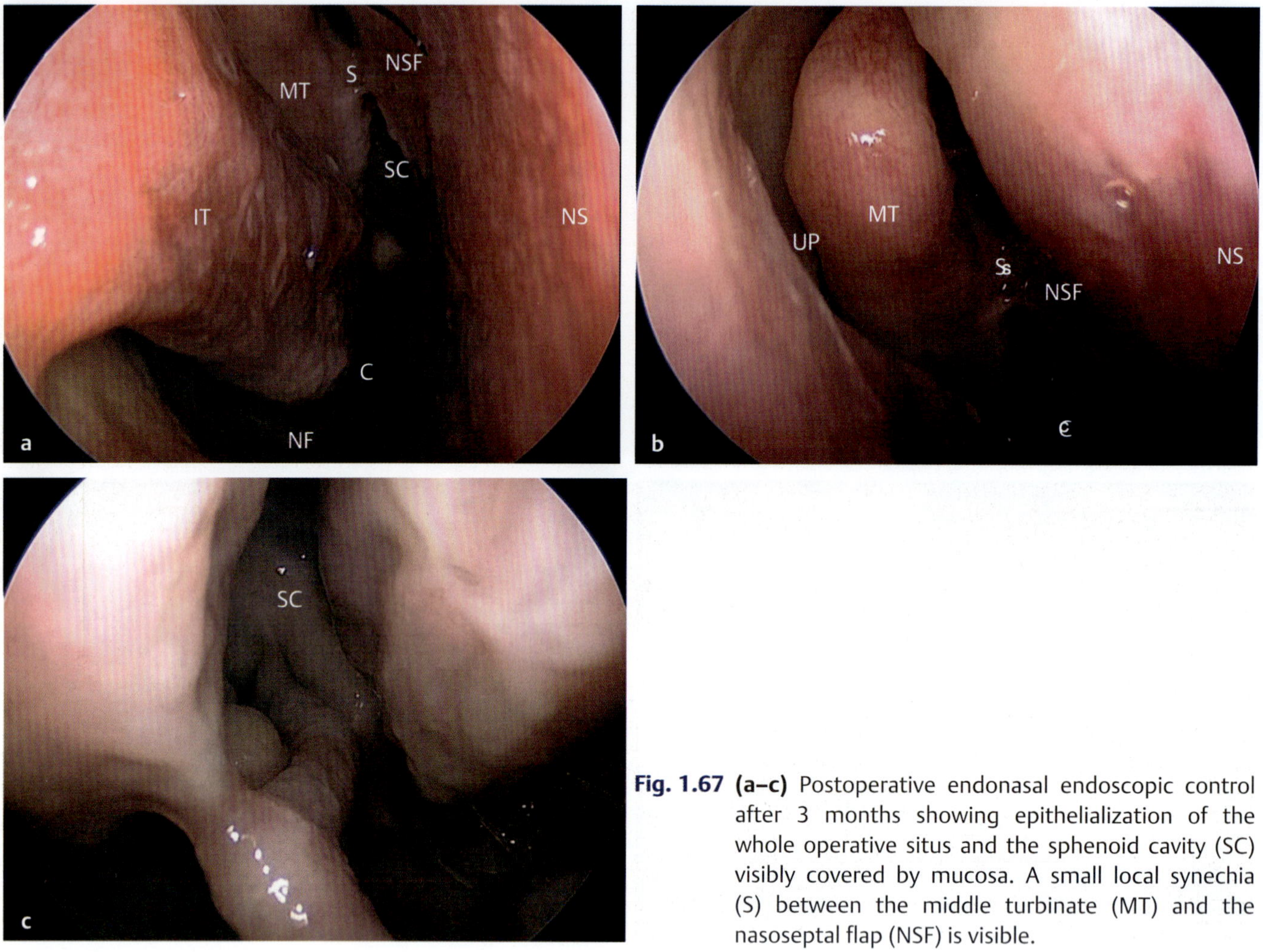

Fig. 1.67 **(a–c)** Postoperative endonasal endoscopic control after 3 months showing epithelialization of the whole operative situs and the sphenoid cavity (SC) visibly covered by mucosa. A small local synechia (S) between the middle turbinate (MT) and the nasoseptal flap (NSF) is visible.

from the sinonasal cavity.[297–299] Hadad et al. were the first to describe the use of a vascularized pedicled nasoseptal flap from the nasal septum mucoperiosteum and mucoperichondrium based on the nasoseptal artery arising from the sphenopalatine artery.[297] This technique has consecutively shown to significantly reduce the incidence of postoperative CSF leakage in endonasal endoscopic skull base surgery.[298–300] The viability of these vascularized nasoseptal flaps and a meticulous multilayer reconstruction contribute to faster and more complete healing with a lower incidence of CSF leaks, eventually being superior to free tissue grafts by promoting restoration of the local blood supply.[297–299,301,302] Since the introduction of the concept, various modifications in size, extent, and location of pedicled nasoseptal flaps have been developed and described in the literature (**Fig. 1.69**).[299] With increasing sizes of such defects, postoperative imaging and radiological follow-up remain challenging.[66,300,303,304] In the immediate postoperative period, a characteristic enhancing arc is usually seen, while free graft tissues present without enhancement and variable T2 hyperintensity. The construct will generally reduce in thickness over time and show enhancement. The intracranial fat packing generally undergoes resorption. Detection of the residual tumor remains challenging within this context.[66,300,303,304] The use of iMRI might be an interesting approach to assess residual tissue prior to complex skull base reconstruction.[66]

Postoperative Care

The nasal packs are usually removed within 24 to 48 hours. They may remain in situ for a longer time (72–120 hours) if a repair for CSF leakage was necessary. The patient is advised to avoid straining (no sneezing, coughing, straining during defecation). Endoscopic inspection and toileting are usually performed during the first week after the operation.

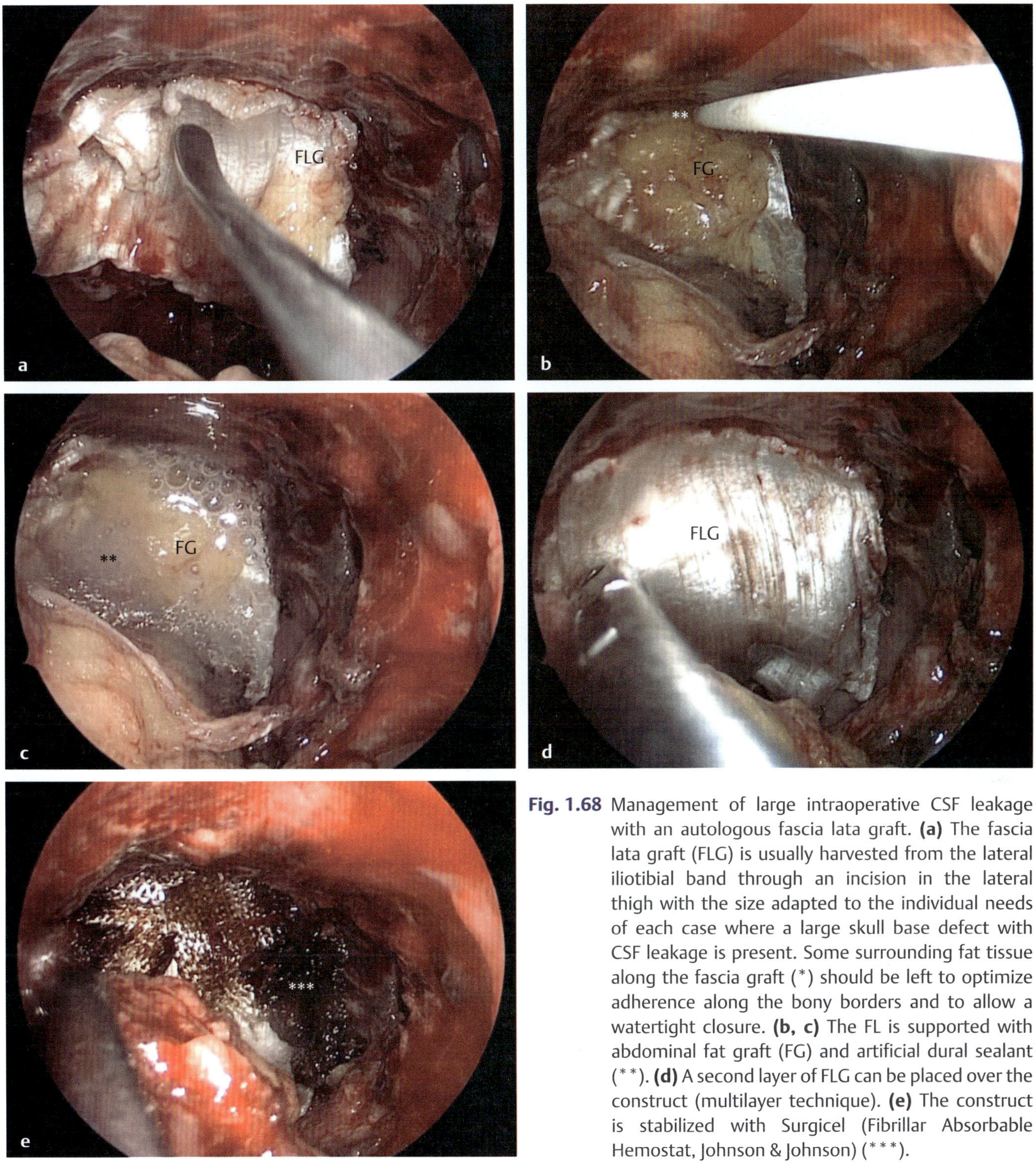

Fig. 1.68 Management of large intraoperative CSF leakage with an autologous fascia lata graft. **(a)** The fascia lata graft (FLG) is usually harvested from the lateral iliotibial band through an incision in the lateral thigh with the size adapted to the individual needs of each case where a large skull base defect with CSF leakage is present. Some surrounding fat tissue along the fascia graft (*) should be left to optimize adherence along the bony borders and to allow a watertight closure. **(b, c)** The FL is supported with abdominal fat graft (FG) and artificial dural sealant (**). **(d)** A second layer of FLG can be placed over the construct (multilayer technique). **(e)** The construct is stabilized with Surgicel (Fibrillar Absorbable Hemostat, Johnson & Johnson) (***).

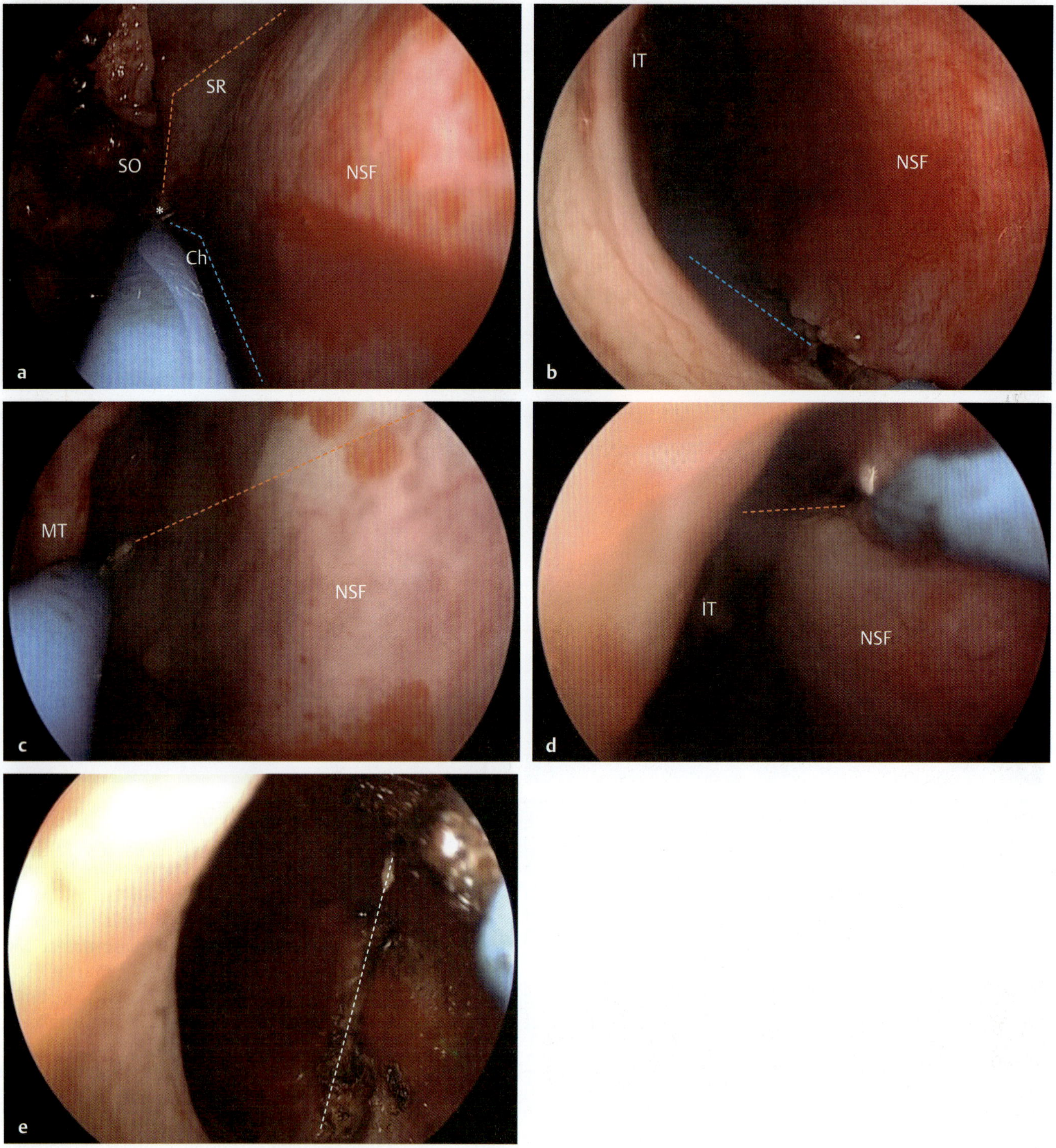

Fig. 1.69 Management of large intraoperative CSF leakage with a pedicled nasoseptal flap (Hadad–Bassagasteguy flap). **(a)** The nasoseptal flap (NSF) incisions at the right posterior nasal cavity are the initial steps.[297,298] The inferior incision (*blue line*) starts above the level of the choana (Ch) following the maxillary crest. The superior incision (*orange line*) extends laterally to cross the sphenoid rostrum (SR) at the level of the sphenoid ostium (SO) 1 to 2 cm inferior to the olfactory cleft. An angled Colorado-tipped Bovie cautery is used (*). **(b)** The inferior posterior incision (*blue line*) is carried down onto the septum above the maxillary crest and brought forward. This incision can be carried onto the nasal floor to create a larger flap.[299] **(c, d)** The superior incision (*orange line*) is carried forward onto the nasal septum (NS) until it crosses the anterior edge of the inferior turbinate (IT) at a level approximately 1 to 2 cm below and parallel to the most superior aspect of the septum avoiding the olfactory epithelium. **(e)** Anteriorly, the incision is carried downward in a vertical orientation (*white line*) to create a connection with the inferior aspect of the flap.

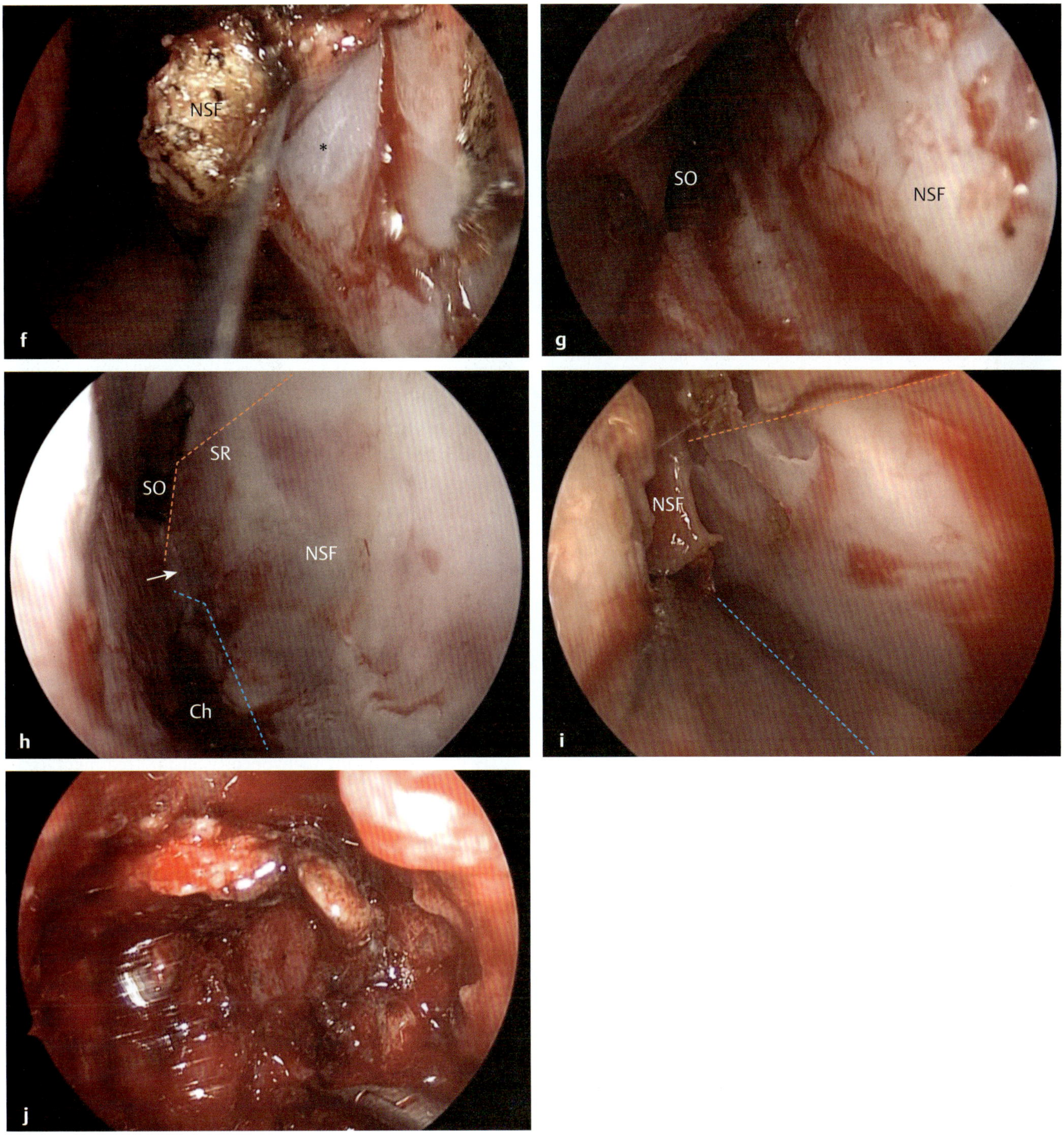

Fig. 1.69 *(Continued)* **(f–h)** The flap incision can be completed using the sharp edge of a Cottle or Freer elevator. The NSF is then elevated following a subperichondrial and subperiosteal plane (*) using an elevating instrument, back to the anterior face of the sphenoid sinus between where the posterior inferior (*blue line*) and superior (*orange line*) incisions have been made, preserving the pedicle of the septal branch of the sphenopalatine artery (*white arrow*). **(i)** Once fully elevated, the NSF is tucked into the sphenoethmoidal recess or the nasopharynx until it is needed for closure. A large middle antrostomy and exposure of the terminal internal maxillary artery might only be necessary if the flap will be stored in the maxilla when approaching clival and paraclival areas.[298] **(j)** For skull base defect closure, after placement of an abdominal free fat graft and supporting material, the NSF has to be placed along the nasal septum in order to avoid any rotation or twisting that might occur during temporary storage. The NSF is placed over the defect primarily covering the skull base defect. The mucosal surface has to face the nasal cavity, not the intracranial defect, to avoid the development of intracranial mucoceles. The NSF should cover the bony edges of the defect to assure appropriate healing.

Nonsurgical Treatment Modalities

Nonsurgical treatment modalities of pituitary adenomas include medical management and radiotherapy.

Medical Management

Prolactinoma

Prolactinomas are the only pituitary adenomas for which medical therapy is the first-line therapy, even in cases of mass effect with a stable neurological condition. Because of the physiological inhibitory stimulus of dopamine on lactotroph cells, dopamine agonists such as cabergoline and bromocriptine are the medical treatment of choice for prolactinoma. Cabergoline has a more favorable side effect profile and is also more efficient in women with hyperprolactinemic amenorrhea than bromocriptine, and should therefore be considered as the first-line medical therapy.[305] Surgery for prolactinoma is usually reserved for adenomas that are resistant to medical therapy, patients who do not tolerate medical therapy or for large invasive tumors with mass effect and neurological deterioration.[306]

Somatotroph, Thyrotroph, Corticotroph, Gonadotroph, and Hormone-Inactive Adenomas

Surgical therapy is classically the first-line therapy for somatotroph, thyrotroph, corticotroph, gonadotroph, and hormone-inactive macroadenomas as medical management is typically ineffective for those tumors. In patients with acromegaly and contraindications for surgical intervention or failed surgery, somatostatin analogs (e.g., octreotide) can be used as medical therapy. Somatostatin analogs act as potent suppressor of growth hormone secretion and potentially lead to tumor shrinkage. Octreotide can also be used in TSH-secreting adenomas as somatostatin receptors are also expressed on normal and neoplastic thyrotroph cells. In patients with Cushing's disease, ketoconazole (an antifungal agent that blocks adrenal steroid synthesis) can be used. Gonadotropin-secreting tumors may respond to long-acting gonadotropin-releasing hormone (GnRH) agonists (by downregulating receptors) or GnRH antagonists, but tumor size reduction is modest. In hormonally inactive macroadenomas, dopamine agonists and somatostatin analogs have been tried with only mild reduction in tumor size in 10 to 20% of the patients.[307]

Radiation Therapy

Radiation therapy is generally not a first-line treatment modality for pituitary adenomas.[308] The goal of radiation therapy with residual/recurrent nonfunctioning pituitary adenomas is tumor growth control. In functioning adenomas, it is tumor growth control and biochemical control, which require higher radiation doses. Radiation therapy can be delivered in multiple fractions (fractionated radiation therapy, requiring 25–30 treatments) or in a single large dose (stereotactic radiosurgery). Fractionated radiation therapy should be used for adenomas that are larger than 3 cm and/or close to the optic pathway. For adenomas that are smaller than 3 cm and at least 3 to 5 mm away from the optic apparatus, stereotactic radiosurgery should be offered. Either form of radiation controls adenoma size in at least 90% of patients at 5 to 10 years.[309-312] Radiation therapy may also reduce hormonal hypersecretion, but the effect is variable and slow. Complete biochemical normalization occurs approximately in 50% of patients after 10 years.[313-317] The risk for hypopituitarism after radiation therapy is about 80% after 10 years, whereas the risk for optic pathway damage and other long-term side effects are low.[312,318,319] Pharmacological treatment to reduce hormonal secretion should be discontinued 1 month prior and 1 month after radiation therapy. Because of the long-term risk of hypopituitarism after radiation therapy, lifelong surveillance is warranted.

Medical Management of Hypopituitarism

ACTH Deficiency

ACTH deficiency leads to hypocortisolism. Treatment consists in the administration of hydrocortisone in an amount and timing that mimics the physiological pattern of cortisol secretion. Hydrocortisone doses of 15 to 25 mg/d are recommended (with the largest dose administered in the morning).[320,321] Patients should be instructed that higher doses are needed in times of illness, surgery, procedures, and other stressful situations. Unlike replacement of other pituitary-dependent hormones, there is no laboratory test to objectively access the adequacy of cortisol replacement. An inadequate dose may result in persistence of hypocortisolism symptoms, whereas an excessive dose can lead to symptoms of cortisol excess.

TSH Deficiency

TSH deficiency results in thyroxine (T4) deficiency and is treated with T4 hormone (levothyroxine). It is very important to evaluate and treat hypocortisolism before levothyroxine is administered. In a patient with simultaneous hypothyroidism and hypocortisolism, treatment of hypothyroidism alone may increase the clearance of the little cortisol that is produced, thereby exacerbating cortisol deficiency. Measurement of serum TSH cannot be used as a marker of the adequacy of T4 replacement. An initial T4 dose of 1.6 µg/

kg/d is recommended and should be adjusted in order to reach a serum-free T4 concentration in the upper half of the reference range.[322]

LH and FSH Deficiency

In men who are not interested in fertility, testosterone replacement is indicated in the case of secondary hypogonadism. Adequacy of hormone replacement should be monitored by measuring serum testosterone, not LH. In men who wish to become fertile, a treatment with gonadotropins (in the case of pituitary dysfunction) or GnRH (in the case of hypothalamic insufficiency) can be offered. In women who are not interested in fertility, hormone replacement therapy with estrogen–progestin is administered. In women who wish to become fertile, ovulation induction can be offered. Women with hypothalamic dysfunction are candidates for either gonadotropin or pulsatile GnRH therapy, while those with pituitary disease are candidates only for gonadotropin therapy.

Growth Hormone Deficiency

Routine treatment with recombinant human GH is not recommended in patients with adult-onset GH deficiency, because the weak clinical benefits do not warrant the high cost of daily injections. In children with GH deficiency, replacement therapy is mandatory to ensure normal growth.

Prolactin Deficiency

Prolactin deficiency leads to the inability to lactate after delivery. There currently is no available treatment.

ADH Deficiency

ADH deficiency leads to central diabetes insipidus. Desmopressin (an ADH analog) is the therapy of choice for almost all patients. Desmopressin can be administered intranasally, orally, subcutaneously, or intravenously. The intranasal application form should be used initially as not all patients respond to oral therapy. The initial intranasal dose is 5 µg and can be increased depending on the response of nocturia. The usual daily maintenance dose is 5 to 20 µg (administered once or twice a day). After 24 hours of initiation of the desmopressin therapy, the serum sodium concentration should be checked as desmopressin can lead to water retention and hyponatremia. In mild diabetes insipidus, a low-solute (low sodium and low protein) diet may be sufficient to control polyuria and nocturia.[323]

Management of Complications

In transsphenoidal pituitary surgery, there is a strong relationship between the outcome and the caseload of the hospital and the experience of the surgeon. Experienced surgeons in high-volume centers have greater success in removing the adenoma completely and a lower incidence of complications.[324] The risks of transsphenoidal pituitary surgery include hormonal deficiencies, damage to sellar, parasellar, and suprasellar structures as well as general surgical risks. Kassam et al. retrospectively reviewed a cohort of 800 individuals, comprising 399 male (49.9%) and 401 female (50.1%) patients operated via an endonasal endoscopic approach, mainly for pituitary adenoma (39.1%) and meningioma (11.8%). The most common reported complications besides CSF leakage were transient neurological deficits (2.5%), permanent neurological deficits (1.8%), intracranial infections (1.6%), systemic complications (2.1%), and death (0.9%). The 30-days mortality rate within the perioperative period was 7 out of 800 (0.9%), 6 of which eventually died from systemic illnesses and 1 from an infectious complication. The authors conclude, that the endonasal endoscopic approach has an acceptable rate of complications in the hands of a skilled team of neurosurgeons and otorhinolaryngologists in selected patients presenting with a myriad of skull base pathologies.[231]

Endocrine Management and Complications

Pituitary function should be assessed before and after surgery. Perioperatively, a glucocorticoid stress prophylaxis is administered (except in the case of Morbus Cushing).

Anterior Pituitary Deficiencies

Anterior pituitary deficiencies may become apparent postoperatively and are believed to be secondary to excessive use of the tumor aspirator in the sellar cavity, inappropriate manipulation, resection of the normal pituitary gland adjacent to the adenoma, and the use of bipolar cauterization in the sellar cavity after tumor removal. The rate of postoperative anterior pituitary insufficiency was reported to be approximately 20%.[325]

Posterior Pituitary Deficiencies

After pituitary surgery, fluid intake and output, serum sodium, and urine osmolality should be measured at least once a day for a few days to monitor a potential diabetes insipidus, followed by the syndrome of inappropriate secretion of ADH, followed again by diabetes insipidus, which may be transient or permanent. Diabetes insipidus is caused by a dysfunction of vasopressin-producing neurons secondary to surgical trauma and thermal injury by cauterization or a dysfunction of the posterior pituitary gland. The risk of developing postoperative diabetes insipidus is approximately 18%.[325] Recovery is reported to occur within 6 months.[286]

The management of hormone deficiencies and hypopituitarism has been discussed earlier.

Cerebrospinal Fluid Leakage

The most common complication after endoscopic skull base surgery is CSF leakage. The introduction of vascular pedicled flaps significantly decreased the rate to an incidence of approximately 4%.[231] If a CSF leak is suspected, the fluid should be analyzed for beta-transferrin. The first step in the management of rhinoliquorrhea is to place a lumbar drain to to higher the chance of spontaneous healing. If this procedure remains unsuccessful after a few days, reoperation and reconstruction of the skull base defect should be performed. Failure to stop the leak increases the risk of meningitis.

Rhinological Complications

As described earlier, the removal of endonasal bone and bony coverage of the base of skull and mucosa is necessary to allow access for a binostril, four-handed surgical approach. This results in the disruption of the sinonasal tracts with the loss of normal nasal epithelium, ciliary and potentially the olfactory function. The loss of ciliary function is associated with nasal crusting.[217] Nasal crusting, causing patient discomfort, malodor, and inflammation, occurs in more than 95% of patients 1 month postoperatively and can be treated with saline irrigations and regular endoscopic debridement. About 50% of patients were found to be free of nasal crusting after 3 months.[235] Other postoperative sinonasal complications include the formation of nasal synechia, alar sill burn, hyposthesia in the areas innervated by the maxillary, palatal, or incisor nerve, taste disturbances, and serous otitis media.[236] Most of the patients regained their full nasal function 6 months postoperatively with an adequate rhinological postoperative care.[235,326] Postoperative hyposmia can occur after excessive coagulation of the superior turbinate and superior part of the middle turbinate or if turbinectomies are performed.[327–329]

Postoperative Tumor Residual and Recurrence

Complete resection of pituitary adenoma (any type and size) after transsphenoidal surgery can be achieved in 64 to 69% of the cases.[252] There is no significant difference in the extent of resection when comparing endoscopic with microscopic transsphenoidal techniques.[252] Negative prognostic factors for complete tumor resection are Knosp's grades 3 and 4, tumor diameter greater than 40 mm, and nodular extension.[15,23]

The recurrence incidence is about 12% with most adenoma recurring 4 to 8 years after surgery.[325] For tumors demonstrating significant regrowth or symptoms following initial resection, reoperation should be considered. After reoperation, radiation therapy can be discussed in the case of residual tumor or in the case of regrowth after the second surgery (see the section Nonsurgical treatment modalities of pituitary adenomas).

Tips and Pearls

- Hormone-active and hormone-inactive pituitary micro- and macroadenomas are the most frequent lesions encountered within the sellar region.
- The WHO morphofunctional as opposed to the DNA methylation-based classification does have similarities and discrepancies in the case of pituitary adenomas.
- To date, there is no neuropathological procedure to make solid statements about the aggressiveness of a pituitary adenoma.
- Nonadenomatous physiological causes for pituitary enlargement are pregnancy, primary hypothyroidism, and primary hypogonadism.
- The most frequent benign nonadenomatous lesions of the sellar and parasellar region are craniopharyngioma, meningioma, and Rathke's cleft cysts.
- The most frequent malignant lesions of the sellar and parasellar region are germ cell tumors, chordoma, primary CNS lymphoma, and metastases from breast and lung cancer.
- In-depth anatomical knowledge and repeated practice on cadavers are of paramount importance when surgically treating pathologies of the sellar region.
- MRI is mandatory for the diagnostic evaluation of sellar masses.
- Preoperative and postoperative evaluation of hypothalamic–pituitary function, hormonal hypersecretion and deficiencies allow an adequate perioperative monitoring of patients undergoing transsphenoidal surgery for hormone-inactive as well as hormone-active pituitary adenoma (level of evidence 1B).
- The preoperative assessment of the patiens' radiological images in terms of anatomical variants and tumor extension is invaluable during surgery.
- Image-guided surgery is important and should be used. However, it should only be seen as an adjunct to

the surgeon's anatomical knowledge and landmarks of the base of skull.

- Airway management of patients with hormone-active lesions (e.g., acromegalic patients) undergoing transsphenoidal surgery bears a potential risk for a higher perioperative morbidity during anesthesia.
- The risk of serious complications, including visual loss, intraoperative hemorrhage, carotid artery injuries, and postoperative meningitis is low and does not differ between the endonasal endoscopic and the microscopic technique.
- Extent of resection and endocrinological and visual outcomes are similar when comparing the endonasal endoscopic and the microscopic technique. Experienced surgeons familiar with either of both techniques have higher resection rate with less complications (level of evidence 1B).
- While approaching the sellar region with the endonasal endoscopic approach, the sphenoid rostrum should be preserved as a solid midline structure in its inferior aspect to maintain the anatomical orientation.
- Never use intersinus sphenoid septations as landmarks to keep the midline during endonasal endoscopic skull base surgery.
- Always expose the lateral opticocarotid recesses bilaterally, the tuberculum sellae and the planum sphenoidale superiorly, and the clival recess inferiorly.
- Use the four "blues" as dural landmarks: the cavernous sinuses laterally and the intercavernous sinuses superiorly and inferiorly, eventually even the venous plexus of the clivus inferiorly.
- Always preserve the posterior septal artery as a branch of the sphenopalatine artery, if a vascularized nasoseptal flap is required to repair larger skull base defects with CSF leakage.
- It is recommended to drill the bony covering of the skull base and flick the bony pieces rather than breaking or tearing the bony coverage of the sella.
- The resection of pituitary adenoma should be performed in a standardized way with initial debulking of the central inferior and bilateral lateral inferior pillars before approaching the superior compartments.
- The posterior superior compartment should be debulked first to avoid the diaphragma sellae to obstruct the surgical field.
- While removing the anterior superior compartment, the risk for CSF leakage is higher.
- A transtuberculum approach and extracapsular dissection of a suprasellar extending pituitary adenoma might be necessary in certain cases.
- In the rare case of an ICA injury during endonasal endoscopic surgery, endovascular treatment of potential pseudoaneurysms with apparent vessel occlusion or graft stent placement is the mainstay of treatment.
- Autologous abdominal fat graft and heterologous graft material should be used for small CSF leakage intraoperatively (level of evidence 5).
- Large skull base defects with CSF leakage should be approached with either autologous fascia lata graft or uni- or bilateral pedicled vascularized nasoseptal flaps supported by heterologous graft materials (level of evidence 5).
- The first-line therapy for LH- and FSH-producing macroadenoma (gonadotroph adenoma) with radiological contact to the optic chiasm, radiological progression, or visual symptoms is transsphenoidal surgery (level of evidence 1B).
- The first-line therapy for PRL-producing adenoma (lactotroph adenoma or prolactinoma) should be a medical therapy with a dopamine agonist (e.g., cabergoline). Transsphenoidal surgery is indicated for large tumors with visual impairment not responding to medical therapy or with intolerable side effects (level of evidence 1B).
- The first-line therapy for GH-producing adenoma (somatotroph adenoma) is transsphenoidal surgery with the goal of either GTR (level of evidence 1B) or significant tumor mass reduction for adjuvant treatment (level of evidence 2C).
- The first-line therapy for ACTH-producing adenoma (corticotroph adenoma) is transsphenoidal surgery with the goal of GTR including early reexploration (level of evidence 1B) prior to adjuvant treatments including adrenalectomy and pharmacological and radiotherapeutic strategies.

Acknowledgments

This chapter was written based on funding from the Martin Allgöwer Foundation, Department of Surgery, University Hospital of Basel (Basel, Switzerland), the Gottfried and Julia Bangerter-Rhyner Foundation (Bern, Switzerland), the Ministry of Health of Malaysia Scholarship (Malaysia), and the Adelaide Ear-Nose-Throat Research Institute (Australia). The Department of Neurosurgery of the University Hospital of Basel (Basel, Switzerland) and the Departments of Neurosurgery and Otorhinolaryngology of the University of Malaya (Kuala Lumpur, Malaysia) supported the creation of this chapter.

References

1. Lopes MBS. The 2017 World Health Organization classification of tumors of the pituitary gland: a summary. Acta Neuropathol 2017;134(4):521–535
2. Louis DN, Perry A, Reifenberger G, et al. The 2016 world health organization classification of tumors of the central nervous system: a summary. Acta Neuropathol 2016;131(6): 803–820
3. Louis DN, Reifenberger G. WHO Classification of Tumours of the Central Nervous System. Lyon: IARC; 2016.
4. Capper D, Jones DTW, Sill M, et al. DNA methylation-based classification of central nervous system tumours. Nature 2018;555(7697):469–474
5. Euskirchen P, Bielle F, Labreche K, et al. Same-day genomic and epigenomic diagnosis of brain tumors using real-time nanopore sequencing. Acta Neuropathol 2017;134(5): 691–703
6. Farrell WE, Clayton RN. Molecular pathogenesis of pituitary tumors. Front Neuroendocrinol 2000;21(3):174–198
7. Melmed S. Mechanisms for pituitary tumorigenesis: the plastic pituitary. J Clin Invest 2003;112(11):1603–1618
8. Scheithauer BW, Gaffey TA, Lloyd RV, et al. Pathobiology of pituitary adenomas and carcinomas. Neurosurgery 2006; 59(2):341–353, discussion 341–353
9. Dudley KJ, Revill K, Clayton RN, Farrell WE. Pituitary tumours: all silent on the epigenetics front. J Mol Endocrinol 2009;42(6):461–468
10. Lania A, Mantovani G, Spada A. Molecular Pathogenesis of Pituitary Adenomas. Totowa, NJ: Humana Press; 2008.
11. Burrow GN, Wortzman G, Rewcastle NB, Holgate RC, Kovacs K. Microadenomas of the pituitary and abnormal sellar tomograms in an unselected autopsy series. N Engl J Med 1981;304(3):156–158
12. Scoazec JY, Couvelard A; Réseau TENpath. [Classification of pancreatic neuroendocrine tumours: changes made in the 2017 WHO classification of tumours of endocrine organs and perspectives for the future]. Ann Pathol 2017;37(6): 444–456
13. Fernandez A, Karavitaki N, Wass JA. Prevalence of pituitary adenomas: a community-based, cross-sectional study in Banbury (Oxfordshire, UK). Clin Endocrinol (Oxf) 2010; 72(3):377–382
14. Raappana A, Koivukangas J, Ebeling T, Pirilä T. Incidence of pituitary adenomas in Northern Finland in 1992-2007. J Clin Endocrinol Metab 2010;95(9):4268–4275
15. Knosp E, Steiner E, Kitz K, Matula C. Pituitary adenomas with invasion of the cavernous sinus space: a magnetic resonance imaging classification compared with surgical findings. Neurosurgery 1993;33(4):610–617, discussion 617–618
16. Mete O, Lopes MB. Overview of the 2017 who classification of pituitary tumors. Endocr Pathol 2017;28(3):228–243
17. Sarkar S, Philip VJ, Cherukuri SK, Chacko AG, Chacko G. Implications of the World Health Organization definition of atypia on surgically treated functional and non-functional pituitary adenomas. Acta Neurochir (Wien) 2017;159(11): 2179–2186
18. Amar AP, Hinton DR, Krieger MD, Weiss MH. Invasive pituitary adenomas: significance of proliferation parameters. Pituitary 1999;2(2):117–122
19. Honegger J, Prettin C, Feuerhake F, Petrick M, Schulte-Mönting J, Reincke M. Expression of Ki-67 antigen in non-functioning pituitary adenomas: correlation with growth velocity and invasiveness. J Neurosurg 2003;99(4):674–679
20. Mastronardi L, Guiducci A, Spera C, Puzzilli F, Liberati F, Maira G. Ki-67 labelling index and invasiveness among anterior pituitary adenomas: analysis of 103 cases using the MIB-1 monoclonal antibody. J Clin Pathol 1999;52(2):107–111
21. Sarkar S, Chacko AG, Chacko G. Clinicopathological correlates of extrasellar growth patterns in pituitary adenomas. J Clin Neurosci 2015;22(7):1173–1177
22. Wilson CB. A decade of pituitary microsurgery. The Herbert Olivecrona lecture. J Neurosurg 1984;61(5):814–833
23. Mooney MA, Sarris CE, Zhou JJ, et al; TRANSSPHER Study Group. Proposal and validation of a simple grading scale (transspher grade) for predicting gross total resection of nonfunctioning pituitary macroadenomas after trans-sphenoidal surgery. Oper Neurosurg (Hagerstown) 2019; 17(5):460–469
24. Di Ieva A, Rotondo F, Syro LV, Cusimano MD, Kovacs K. Aggressive pituitary adenomas—diagnosis and emerging treatments. Nat Rev Endocrinol 2014;10(7):423–435
25. Saeger W, Honegger J, Theodoropoulou M, et al. Clinical impact of the current who classification of pituitary adenomas. Endocr Pathol 2016;27(2):104–114
26. Martins AN, Hayes GJ, Kempe LG. Invasive pituitary adenomas. J Neurosurg 1965;22:268–276
27. Mete O, Ezzat S, Asa SL. Biomarkers of aggressive pituitary adenomas. J Mol Endocrinol 2012;49(2):R69–R78
28. Dai C, Feng M, Liu X, et al. Refractory pituitary adenoma: a novel classification for pituitary tumors. Oncotarget 2016;7(50):83657–83668
29. Raverot G, Jouanneau E, Trouillas J. Management of endocrine disease: clinicopathological classification and molecular markers of pituitary tumours for personalized therapeutic strategies. Eur J Endocrinol 2014;170(4):R121–R132
30. Delellis RL, Lloyd RV, Heitz PU, Eng C. Pathology and Genetics of Tumors of Endocrine Organs. Lyon: IARC; 2004.
31. Scheithauer BW, Kovacs KT, Laws ER Jr, Randall RV. Pathology of invasive pituitary tumors with special reference to functional classification. J Neurosurg 1986;65(6):733–744

32. Pernicone PJ, Scheithauer BW, Sebo TJ, et al. Pituitary carcinoma: a clinicopathologic study of 15 cases. Cancer 1997;79(4):804–812
33. Gejman R, Tessa Hedley-Whyte E. Pathology of Pituitary Adenomas. Totowa, NJ: Humana Press; 2008.
34. Shimono T, Hatabu H, Kasagi K, et al. Rapid progression of pituitary hyperplasia in humans with primary hypothyroidism: demonstration with MR imaging. Radiology 1999;213(2):383–388
35. Alkhani AM, Cusimano M, Kovacs K, Bilbao JM, Horvath E, Singer W. Cytology of pituitary thyrotroph hyperplasia in protracted primary hypothyroidism. Pituitary 1999;1(3-4): 291–295
36. Scheithauer BW, Moschopulos M, Kovacs K, Jhaveri BS, Percek T, Lloyd RV. The pituitary in klinefelter syndrome. Endocr Pathol 2005;16(2):133–138
37. Ezzat S, Asa SL, Stefaneanu L, et al. Somatotroph hyperplasia without pituitary adenoma associated with a long standing growth hormone-releasing hormone-producing bronchial carcinoid. J Clin Endocrinol Metab 1994;78(3):555–560
38. Salbenblatt JA, Bender BG, Puck MH, Robinson A, Faiman C, Winter JS. Pituitary-gonadal function in Klinefelter syndrome before and during puberty. Pediatr Res 1985; 19(1):82–86
39. Lee L, Saran F, Hargrave D, Bódi I, Bassi S, Hortobágyi T. Germinoma with synchronous lesions in the pineal and suprasellar regions. Childs Nerv Syst 2006;22(12):1513–1518
40. Castle-Kirszbaum M, Goldschlager T, Ho B, Wang YY, King J. Twelve cases of pituitary metastasis: a case series and review of the literature. Pituitary 2018;21(5):463–473
41. Sogani J, Yang W, Lavi E, Zimmerman RD, Gupta A. Sellar collision tumor involving metastatic lung cancer and pituitary adenoma: radiologic-pathologic correlation and review of the literature. Clin Imaging 2014;38(3):318–321
42. Harrison MJ, Morgello S, Post KD. Epithelial cystic lesions of the sellar and parasellar region: a continuum of ectodermal derivatives? J Neurosurg 1994;80(6):1018–1025
43. Iqbal J, Kanaan I, Al Homsi M. Non-neoplastic cystic lesions of the sellar region presentation, diagnosis and management of eight cases and review of the literature. Acta Neurochir (Wien) 1999;141(4):389–397, discussion 397–398
44. Shin JL, Asa SL, Woodhouse LJ, Smyth HS, Ezzat S. Cystic lesions of the pituitary: clinicopathological features distinguishing craniopharyngioma, Rathke's cleft cyst, and arachnoid cyst. J Clin Endocrinol Metab 1999;84(11):3972–3982
45. Zada G, Lin N, Ojerholm E, Ramkissoon S, Laws ER. Craniopharyngioma and other cystic epithelial lesions of the sellar region: a review of clinical, imaging, and histopathological relationships. Neurosurg Focus 2010;28(4):E4
46. Snyder BJ, Naidich TP, Post KD. Cystic Lesions of the Sella. Totowa, NJ: Humana Press; 2008.
47. Park M, Lee SK, Choi J, et al. Differentiation between cystic pituitary adenomas and Rathke cleft cysts: a diagnostic model using MRI. AJNR Am J Neuroradiol 2015;36(10): 1866–1873
48. Choi SH, Kwon BJ, Na DG, Kim JH, Han MH, Chang KH. Pituitary adenoma, craniopharyngioma, and Rathke cleft cyst involving both intrasellar and suprasellar regions: differentiation using MRI. Clin Radiol 2007;62(5):453–462
49. Goyal A, Singh AK, Gupta V, Singh D, Tatke M, Kumar S. Suprasellar cystic meningioma: unusual presentation and review of the literature. J Clin Neurosci 2002;9(6):702–704
50. Kulah A, Ilçayto R, Fiskeci C. Cystic meningiomas. Acta Neurochir (Wien) 1991;111(3-4):108–113
51. Burger P, Scheithauer BW, Vogel F. Surgical Pathology of the Nervous System and Its Coverings. 4th ed. Baltimore, MD: Churchill Livingstone; 2003
52. Fager CA, Carter H. Intrasellar epithelial cysts. J Neurosurg 1966;24(1):77–81
53. Teramoto A, Hirakawa K, Sanno N, Osamura Y. Incidental pituitary lesions in 1,000 unselected autopsy specimens. Radiology 1994;193(1):161–164
54. Pierre-Kahn A, Capelle L, Brauner R, et al. Presentation and management of suprasellar arachnoid cysts. Review of 20 cases. J Neurosurg 1990;73(3):355–359
55. Sani S, Smith A, Leppla DC, Ilangovan S, Glick R. Epidermoid cyst of the sphenoid sinus with extension into the sella turcica presenting as pituitary apoplexy: case report. Surg Neurol 2005;63(4):394–397, discussion 397
56. Bahgat M, Bahgat Y, Bahgat A. Sphenoid sinus mucocele. BMJ Case Rep 2012;2012
57. Li E, Howard MA, Vining EM, Becker RD, Silbert J, Lesser RL. Visual prognosis in compressive optic neuropathy secondary to sphenoid sinus mucocele: a systematic review. Orbit 2018;37(4):280–286
58. Friedman A, Batra PS, Fakhri S, Citardi MJ, Lanza DC. Isolated sphenoid sinus disease: etiology and management. Otolaryngol Head Neck Surg 2005;133(4):544–550
59. Kösling S, Hintner M, Brandt S, Schulz T, Bloching M. Mucoceles of the sphenoid sinus. Eur J Radiol 2004;51(1):1–5
60. Sethi DS. Isolated sphenoid lesions: diagnosis and management. Otolaryngol Head Neck Surg 1999;120(5):730–736
61. Soon SR, Lim CM, Singh H, Sethi DS. Sphenoid sinus mucocele: 10 cases and literature review. J Laryngol Otol 2010; 124(1): 44–47
62. Tang IP, Chai CK, Kumar G, Prepageran N, Waran V. Intrasellar pituitary mucocele: diagnostic dilemma. Br J Neurosurg 2014;28(3):390–392
63. Abla AA, Maroon JC, Wilberger JE Jr, Kennerdell JS, Deeb ZL. Intrasellar mucocele simulating pituitary adenoma: case report. Neurosurgery 1986;18(2):197–199

64. Koutourousiou M, Kontogeorgos G, Wesseling P, Grotenhuis AJ, Seretis A. Collision sellar lesions: experience with eight cases and review of the literature. Pituitary 2010;13(1): 8–17

65. Furtado SV, Venkatesh PK, Ghosal N, Hegde AS. Coexisting intracranial tumors with pituitary adenomas: genetic association or coincidence? J Cancer Res Ther 2010;6(2): 221–223

66. Roethlisberger M, Jayapalan RR, Hostettler IC, et al. Evolving strategies for resection of sellar/parasellar synchronous tumors via endoscopic endonasal approach—a technical case report and systematic review of the literature. World Neurosurg 2020;133:381–391.e2

67. Syed S, Karambizi DI, Baker A, Groh DM, Toms SA. A comparative report on intracranial tumor-to-tumor metastasis and collision tumors. World Neurosurg 2018;116: 454–463.e2

68. Ogando-Rivas E, Alalade AF, Boatey J, Schwartz TH. Double pituitary adenomas are most commonly associated with GH- and ACTH-secreting tumors: systematic review of the literature. Pituitary 2017;20(6):702–708

69. Cannavò S, Curtò L, Fazio R, et al. Coexistence of growth hormone-secreting pituitary adenoma and intracranial meningioma: a case report and review of the literature. J Endocrinol Invest 1993;16(9):703–708

70. Zhao Y, Zhang H, Lian W, et al. Collision tumors composed of meningioma and growth hormone-secreting pituitary adenoma in the sellar region: case reports and a literature review. Medicine (Baltimore) 2017;96(50):e9139

71. Amirjamshidi A, Mortazavi SA, Shirani M, Saeedinia S, Hanif H. Coexisting pituitary adenoma and suprasellar meningioma-a coincidence or causation effect: report of two cases and review of the literature. J Surg Case Rep 2017;2017(5):rjx039

72. Lim KZ, Goldschlager T, Chandra RV, Hall J, Uren B, Pullar M. Co-occurrence of pituitary adenoma with suprasellar and olfactory groove meningiomas. Basic Clin Neurosci 2016; 7(4):361–365

73. Mahvash M, Igressa A, Pechlivanis I, Weber F, Charalampaki P. Endoscopic endonasal transsphenoidal approach for resection of a coexistent pituitary macroadenoma and a tuberculum sellae meningioma. Asian J Neurosurg 2014; 9(4):236

74. Prevedello DM, Thomas A, Gardner P, Snyderman CH, Carrau RL, Kassam AB. Endoscopic endonasal resection of a synchronous pituitary adenoma and a tuberculum sellae meningioma: technical case report. Neurosurgery 2007;60(4, Suppl 2):E401, discussion E401

75. Yamada K, Hatayama T, Ohta M, Sakoda K, Uozumi T. Coincidental pituitary adenoma and parasellar meningioma: case report. Neurosurgery 1986;19(2):267–270

76. Yoshida A, Sen C, Asa SL, Rosenblum MK. Composite pituitary adenoma and craniopharyngioma?: an unusual sellar neoplasm with divergent differentiation. Am J Surg Pathol 2008;32(11):1736–1741

77. Jin G, Hao S, Xie J, Mi R, Liu F. Collision tumors of the sella: coexistence of pituitary adenoma and craniopharyngioma in the sellar region. World J Surg Oncol 2013;11:178

78. Tanriover N, Aydin O, Kucukyuruk B, et al. Endoscopic approach to a collision tumor of growth hormone-secreting adenoma and gangliocytoma in the pituitary gland. J Craniofac Surg 2014;25(4):1277–1279

79. Valdes CJ, Tewfik MA, Guiot MC, Di Maio S. Synchronous esthesioneuroblastoma and growth-hormone-secreting pituitary macroadenoma: combined open and endoscopic management. J Neurol Surg Rep 2014;75(2):e194–e199

80. Miyagi N, Doi R, Kuramoto T, et al. Double pituitary adenomas associated with persistent trigeminal artery: a rare case report and the review of literature. Neurosurg Rev 2018;41(1):341–345

81. Yoshida K, Fukaya R, Fukuchi M, Hiraga Y, Ichimura S, Fuji K. Incidental ethmoidal dural arteriovenous fistula coexisting with a pituitary adenoma exacerbating post-transsphenoidal epistaxis. Br J Neurosurg 2019;33(6): 681–683

82. Black PM, Carroll R, Glowacka D, Riley K, Dashner K. Platelet-derived growth factor expression and stimulation in human meningiomas. J Neurosurg 1994;81(3):388–393

83. Partington MD, Davis DH. Radiation-induced meningioma after treatment for pituitary adenoma: case report and literature review. Neurosurgery 1990;26(2):329–331

84. Gadgil N, Thomas JG, Takashima M, Yoshor D. Endoscopic resection of tuberculum sellae meningiomas. J Neurol Surg B Skull Base 2013;74(4):201–210

85. Chowdhury FH, Haque MR, Goel AH, Kawsar KA. Endoscopic endonasal extended transsphenoidal removal of tuberculum sellae meningioma (TSM): an experience of six cases. Br J Neurosurg 2012;26(5):692–699

86. Vates GE, Berger MS, Wilson CB. Diagnosis and management of pituitary abscess: a review of twenty-four cases. J Neurosurg 2001;95(2):233–241

87. Solari D, Chiaramonte C, Di Somma A, et al. Endoscopic anatomy of the skull base explored through the nose. World Neurosurg 2014;82(6, Suppl):S164–S170

88. Solari D, Villa A, De Angelis M, Esposito F, Cavallo LM, Cappabianca P. Anatomy and surgery of the endoscopic endonasal approach to the skull base. Transl Med UniSa 2012;2:36–46

89. Orlandi RR, Lanza DC, Bolger WE, Clerico DM, Kennedy DW. The forgotten turbinate: the role of the superior turbinate in endoscopic sinus surgery. Am J Rhinol 1999;13(4):251–259

90. Millar DA, Orlandi RR. The sphenoid sinus natural ostium is consistently medial to the superior turbinate. Am J Rhinol 2006;20(2):180–181

91. Hidir Y, Battal B, Durmaz A, Karaman B, Tosun F. Optimum height from the roof of the choana for seeking the sphenoid ostium. J Craniofac Surg 2011;22(3):1077–1079

92. Kim HU, Kim SS, Kang SS, Chung IH, Lee JG, Yoon JH. Surgical anatomy of the natural ostium of the sphenoid sinus. Laryngoscope 2001;111(9):1599–1602

93. Eweiss AZ, Ibrahim AA, Khalil HS. The safe gate to the posterior paranasal sinuses: reassessing the role of the superior turbinate. Eur Arch Otorhinolaryngol 2012;269(5): 1451–1456

94. Halawi AM, Simon PE, Lidder AK, Chandra RK. The relationship of the natural sphenoid ostium to the skull base. Laryngoscope 2015;125(1):75–79

95. Cappabianca P, Cavallo LM, de Divitiis E. Endoscopic endonasal transsphenoidal surgery. Neurosurgery 2004; 55(4):933–940, discussion 940–941

96. Campero A, Martins C, Yasuda A, Rhoton AL Jr. Microsurgical anatomy of the diaphragma sellae and its role in directing the pattern of growth of pituitary adenomas. Neurosurgery 2008;62(3):717–723, discussion 717–723

97. Inoue K, Seker A, Osawa S, Alencastro LF, Matsushima T, Rhoton AL Jr. Microsurgical and endoscopic anatomy of the supratentorial arachnoidal membranes and cisterns. Neurosurgery 2009;65(4):644–664, discussion 665

98. Truong HQ, Borghei-Razavi H, Najera E, et al. Bilateral coagulation of inferior hypophyseal artery and pituitary transposition during endoscopic endonasal interdural posterior clinoidectomy: do they affect pituitary function? J Neurosurg 2018;131(1):141–146

99. Fernandez-Miranda JC, Zwagerman NT, Abhinav K, et al. Cavernous sinus compartments from the endoscopic endonasal approach: anatomical considerations and surgical relevance to adenoma surgery. J Neurosurg 2018; 129(2):430–441

100. Cohen-Cohen S, Gardner PA, Alves-Belo JT, et al. The medial wall of the cavernous sinus. Part 2: selective medial wall resection in 50 pituitary adenoma patients. J Neurosurg 2018;131(1):131–140

101. Truong HQ, Lieber S, Najera E, Alves-Belo JT, Gardner PA, Fernandez-Miranda JC. The medial wall of the cavernous sinus. Part 1: surgical anatomy, ligaments, and surgical technique for its mobilization and/or resection. J Neurosurg 2018;131(1):122–130

102. Labib MA, Prevedello DM, Carrau R, et al. A road map to the internal carotid artery in expanded endoscopic endonasal approaches to the ventral cranial base. Neurosurgery 2014;10(Suppl 3):448–471, discussion 471

103. Kassam AB, Gardner P, Snyderman C, Mintz A, Carrau R. Expanded endonasal approach: fully endoscopic, completely transnasal approach to the middle third of the clivus, petrous bone, middle cranial fossa, and infratemporal fossa. Neurosurg Focus 2005;19(1):E6

104. Kassam AB, Vescan AD, Carrau RL, et al. Expanded endonasal approach: vidian canal as a landmark to the petrous internal carotid artery. J Neurosurg 2008;108(1):177–183

105. Vescan AD, Snyderman CH, Carrau RL, et al. Vidian canal: analysis and relationship to the internal carotid artery. Laryngoscope 2007;117(8):1338–1342

106. Barges-Coll J, Fernandez-Miranda JC, Prevedello DM, et al. Avoiding injury to the abducens nerve during expanded endonasal endoscopic surgery: anatomic and clinical case studies. Neurosurgery 2010;67(1):144–154, discussion 154

107. Osawa S, Rhoton AL Jr, Seker A, Shimizu S, Fujii K, Kassam AB. Microsurgical and endoscopic anatomy of the vidian canal. Neurosurgery 2009;64(5, Suppl 2):385–411, discussion 411–412

108. Curragh DS, Valentine R, Selva D. Optic strut terminology. Ophthal Plast Reconstr Surg 2019;35(4):407–408

109. Souza AD, Ankolekar VH, Nayak N, Hosapatna M, Souza AS. Morphometric study of anterior clinoid process and optic strut and the ossification of carotico-clinoid ligament with their clinical importance. J Clin Diagn Res 2016;10(4): AC05–AC07

110. Cavallo LM, de Divitiis O, Aydin S, et al. Extended endoscopic endonasal transsphenoidal approach to the suprasellar area: anatomic considerations—part 1. Neurosurgery 2007;61 (3, Suppl):24–33, discussion 33–34

111. de Divitiis E, Cavallo LM, Cappabianca P, Esposito F. Extended endoscopic endonasal transsphenoidal approach for the removal of suprasellar tumors: part 2. Neurosurgery 2007; 60(1):46–58, discussion 58–59

112. Ouaknine GE, Hardy J. Microsurgical anatomy of the pituitary gland and the sellar region. 1. The pituitary gland. Am Surg 1987;53(5):285–290

113. Ouaknine GE, Hardy J. Microsurgical anatomy of the pituitary gland and the sellar region. 2. The bony structures. Am Surg 1987;53(5):291–297

114. Melmed S. The Pituitary. 3rd ed. San Diego, CA: Elsevier; 2011.

115. Melmed S. Pituitary medicine from discovery to patient-focused outcomes. J Clin Endocrinol Metab 2016;101(3): 769–777

116. Bao Y, Pan J, Qi ST, Lu YT, Peng JX. Origin of craniopharyngiomas: implications for growth pattern, clinical characteristics, and outcomes of tumor recurrence. J Neurosurg 2016;125(1):24–32

117. Fahlbusch R, Honegger J, Paulus W, Huk W, Buchfelder M. Surgical treatment of craniopharyngiomas: experience with 168 patients. J Neurosurg 1999;90(2):237–250

118. Honegger J, Buchfelder M, Fahlbusch R, Däubler B, Dörr HG. Transsphenoidal microsurgery for craniopharyngioma. Surg Neurol 1992;37(3):189–196

119. Cappabianca P, Cavallo LM, Esposito I, Barakat M, Esposito F. Bone removal with a new ultrasonic bone curette during endoscopic endonasal approach to the sellar-suprasellar area: technical note. Neurosurgery 2010;66(suppl_1):ons-E118

120. de Divitiis E, Cappabianca P, Cavallo LM. Endoscopic transsphenoidal approach: adaptability of the procedure to different sellar lesions. Neurosurgery 2002;51(3):699–705, discussion 705–707

121. Couldwell WT. Transsphenoidal and transcranial surgery for pituitary adenomas. J Neurooncol 2004;69(1-3):237–256

122. Couldwell WT, Weiss MH, Rabb C, Liu JK, Apfelbaum RI, Fukushima T. Variations on the standard transsphenoidal approach to the sellar region, with emphasis on the extended approaches and parasellar approaches: surgical experience in 105 cases. Neurosurgery 2004;55(3):539–547, discussion 547–550

123. Liu JK, Christiano LD, Patel SK, Eloy JA. Surgical nuances for removal of retrochiasmatic craniopharyngioma via the endoscopic endonasal extended transsphenoidal transplanum transtuberculum approach. Neurosurg Focus 2011;30(4):E14

124. Liu JK, Christiano LD, Patel SK, Tubbs RS, Eloy JA. Surgical nuances for removal of tuberculum sellae meningiomas with optic canal involvement using the endoscopic endonasal extended transsphenoidal transplanum transtuberculum approach. Neurosurg Focus 2011;30(5):E2

125. Liu JK, Eloy JA. Endoscopic endonasal transplanum transtuberculum approach for resection of retrochiasmatic craniopharyngioma. J Neurosurg 2012;32(Suppl):E2

126. Mangussi-Gomes J, Vellutini EA, Truong HQ, Pahl FH, Stamm AC. Endoscopic endonasal transplanum transtuberculum approach for the resection of a large suprasellar craniopharyngioma. J Neurol Surg B Skull Base 2018;79(Suppl 3):S249–S250

127. Aho CJ, Liu C, Zelman V, Couldwell WT, Weiss MH. Surgical outcomes in 118 patients with Rathke cleft cysts. J Neurosurg 2005;102(2):189–193

128. Schwartz TH, Anand VK. The endoscopic endonasal transsphenoidal approach to the suprasellar cistern. Clin Neurosurg 2007;54:226–235

129. Abuzayed B, Tanriover N, Akar Z, Eraslan BS, Gazioglu N. Extended endoscopic endonasal approach to the suprasellar parachiasmatic cisterns: anatomic study. Childs Nerv Syst 2010;26(9):1161–1170

130. Puchades-Orts A, Nombela-Gomez M, Ortuño-Pacheco G. Variation in form of circle of Willis: some anatomical and embryological considerations. Anat Rec 1976;185(1):119–123

131. Riggs HE, Rupp C. Variation in form of circle of Willis. The relation of the variations to collateral circulation: anatomic analysis. Arch Neurol 1963;8:8–14

132. Perlmutter D, Rhoton AL Jr. Microsurgical anatomy of the distal anterior cerebral artery. J Neurosurg 1978;49(2):204–228

133. Perlmutter D, Rhoton AL Jr. Microsurgical anatomy of anterior cerebral anterior communicating recurrent artery complex. Surg Forum 1976;27(62):464–465

134. Dias DA, Castro FL, Yared JH, Lucas Júnior A, Ferreira Filho LA, Ferreira NF. Liliequist membrane: radiological evaluation, clinical and therapeutic implications. Radiol Bras 2014;47(3):182–185

135. Froelich SC, Abdel Aziz KM, Cohen PD, van Loveren HR, Keller JT. Microsurgical and endoscopic anatomy of Liliequist's membrane: a complex and variable structure of the basal cisterns. Neurosurgery 2008;63(1, Suppl 1):ONS1–ONS8, discussion ONS8–ONS9

136. Fushimi Y, Miki Y, Ueba T, et al. Liliequist membrane: three-dimensional constructive interference in steady state MR imaging. Radiology 2003;229(2):360–365, discussion 365

137. Wilson CB. Surgical management of pituitary tumors. J Clin Endocrinol Metab 1997;82(8):2381–2385

138. Ezzat S, Asa SL, Couldwell WT, et al. The prevalence of pituitary adenomas: a systematic review. Cancer 2004;101(3):613–619

139. Snyder PJ. Gonadotroph adenomas. Curr Ther Endocrinol Metab 1997;6:56–58

140. Snyder PJ. Extensive personal experience: gonadotroph adenomas. J Clin Endocrinol Metab 1995;80(4):1059–1061

141. Melmed S, Casanueva FF, Hoffman AR, et al; Endocrine Society. Diagnosis and treatment of hyperprolactinemia: an Endocrine Society clinical practice guideline. J Clin Endocrinol Metab 2011;96(2):273–288

142. Ciccarelli A, Daly AF, Beckers A. The epidemiology of prolactinomas. Pituitary 2005;8(1):3–6

143. Vroonen L, Daly AF, Beckers A. Epidemiology and management challenges in prolactinomas. Neuroendocrinology 2019;109(1):20–27

144. Guignat L, Bertherat J. The diagnosis of Cushing's syndrome: an Endocrine Society Clinical Practice Guideline: commentary from a European perspective. Eur J Endocrinol 2010;163(1):9–13

145. Katznelson L, Laws ER Jr, Melmed S, et al; Endocrine Society. Acromegaly: an endocrine society clinical practice guideline. J Clin Endocrinol Metab 2014;99(11):3933–3951

146. Bertholon-Grégoire M, Trouillas J, Guigard MP, Loras B, Tourniaire J. Mono- and plurihormonal thyrotropic pituitary adenomas: pathological, hormonal and clinical studies in 12 patients. Eur J Endocrinol 1999;140(6):519–527

147. Smallridge RC. Thyrotropin-secreting pituitary tumors. Endocrinol Metab Clin North Am 1987;16(3):765–792

148. Smallridge RC, Smith CE. Hyperthyroidism due to thyrotropin-secreting pituitary tumors. Diagnostic and therapeutic considerations. Arch Intern Med 1983;143(3):503–507

149. Beck-Peccoz P, Lania A, Beckers A, Chatterjee K, Wemeau JL. 2013 European thyroid association guidelines for the diagnosis and treatment of thyrotropin-secreting pituitary tumors. Eur Thyroid J 2013;2(2):76–82

150. Beck-Peccoz P, Persani L, Asteria C, et al. Thyrotropin-secreting pituitary tumors in hyper- and hypothyroidism. Acta Med Austriaca 1996;23(1-2):41–46

151. Bassetti M, Spada A, Arosio M, Vallar L, Brina M, Giannattasio G. Morphological studies on mixed growth hormone (GH)- and prolactin (PRL)-secreting human pituitary adenomas. Coexistence of GH and PRL in the same secretory granule. J Clin Endocrinol Metab 1986;62(6):1093–1100

152. Russel SJ, Klahr-Miller K. Pituitary Apoplexy. Totowa, NJ:Humana Press; 2008.

153. Bonicki W, Kasperlik-Załuska A, Koszewski W, Zgliczyński W, Wisławski J. Pituitary apoplexy: endocrine, surgical and oncological emergency. Incidence, clinical course and treatment with reference to 799 cases of pituitary adenomas. Acta Neurochir (Wien) 1993;120(3-4):118–122

154. Bills DC, Meyer FB, Laws ER Jr, et al. A retrospective analysis of pituitary apoplexy. Neurosurgery 1993;33(4):602–608, discussion 608–609

155. Liu JK, Couldwell WT. Pituitary apoplexy in the magnetic resonance imaging era: clinical significance of sphenoid sinus mucosal thickening. J Neurosurg 2006;104(6):892–898

156. Randeva HS, Schoebel J, Byrne J, Esiri M, Adams CB, Wass JA. Classical pituitary apoplexy: clinical features, management and outcome. Clin Endocrinol (Oxf) 1999;51(2):181–188

157. Wakai S, Fukushima T, Teramoto A, Sano K. Pituitary apoplexy: its incidence and clinical significance. J Neurosurg 1981;55(2):187–193

158. Müller-Jensen A, Lüdecke D. Clinical aspects of spontaneous necrosis of pituitary tumors (pituitary apoplexy). J Neurol 1981;224(4):267–271

159. Brougham M, Heusner AP, Adams RD. Acute degenerative changes in adenomas of the pituitary body—with special reference to pituitary apoplexy. J Neurosurg 1950;7(5): 421–439

160. Rovit RL, Fein JM. Pituitary apoplexy: a review and reappraisal. J Neurosurg 1972;37(3):280–288

161. Patronas NJ, Liu CY. State of art imaging of the pituitary tumors. J Neurooncol 2014;117(3):395–405

162. Dubuisson AS, Beckers A, Stevenaert A. Classical pituitary tumour apoplexy: clinical features, management and outcomes in a series of 24 patients. Clin Neurol Neurosurg 2007;109(1):63–70

163. Nielsen EH, Lindholm J, Bjerre P, et al. Frequent occurrence of pituitary apoplexy in patients with non-functioning pituitary adenoma. Clin Endocrinol (Oxf) 2006;64(3): 319–322

164. Arita K, Tominaga A, Sugiyama K, et al. Natural course of incidentally found nonfunctioning pituitary adenoma, with special reference to pituitary apoplexy during follow-up examination. J Neurosurg 2006;104(6):884–891

165. Ayuk J, McGregor EJ, Mitchell RD, Gittoes NJ. Acute management of pituitary apoplexy—surgery or conservative management? Clin Endocrinol (Oxf) 2004;61(6):747–752

166. Sibal L, Ball SG, Connolly V, et al. Pituitary apoplexy: a review of clinical presentation, management and outcome in 45 cases. Pituitary 2004;7(3):157–163

167. Gruber A, Clayton J, Kumar S, Robertson I, Howlett TA, Mansell P. Pituitary apoplexy: retrospective review of 30 patients—is surgical intervention always necessary? Br J Neurosurg 2006;20(6):379–385

168. Karavitaki N, Wass JA. Craniopharyngiomas. Endocrinol Metab Clin North Am 2008;37(1):173–193, ix–x

169. Karavitaki N, Brufani C, Warner JT, et al. Craniopharyngiomas in children and adults: systematic analysis of 121 cases with long-term follow-up. Clin Endocrinol (Oxf) 2005;62(4): 397–409

170. Laws ER. Craniopharyngiomas in children and young adults. Prog Exp Tumor Res 1987;30:335–340

171. Karavitaki N. Hypopituitarism oddities: craniopharyngiomas. Horm Res 2007;68(Suppl 5):151–153

172. Isono M, Kamida T, Kobayashi H, Shimomura T, Matsuyama J. Clinical features of symptomatic Rathke's cleft cyst. Clin Neurol Neurosurg 2001;103(2):96–100

173. Raper DM, Besser M. Clinical features, management and recurrence of symptomatic Rathke's cleft cyst. J Clin Neurosci 2009;16(3):385–389

174. Benveniste RJ, King WA, Walsh J, Lee JS, Naidich TP, Post KD. Surgery for Rathke cleft cysts: technical considerations and outcomes. J Neurosurg 2004;101(4):577–584

175. el-Mahdy W, Powell M. Transsphenoidal management of 28 symptomatic Rathke's cleft cysts, with special reference to visual and hormonal recovery. Neurosurgery 1998;42(1): 7–16, discussion 16–17

176. Wiebracht ND, Zimmer LA. Complex anatomy of the sphenoid sinus: a radiographic study and literature review. J Neurol Surg B Skull Base 2014;75(6):378–382

177. Zada G, Agarwalla PK, Mukundan S Jr, Dunn I, Golby AJ, Laws ER Jr. The neurosurgical anatomy of the sphenoid sinus and sellar floor in endoscopic transsphenoidal surgery. J Neurosurg 2011;114(5):1319–1330

178. Fujii K, Chambers SM, Rhoton AL Jr. Neurovascular relationships of the sphenoid sinus. A microsurgical study. J Neurosurg 1979;50(1):31–39

179. Rhoton AL Jr. The sellar region. Neurosurgery 2002;51 (4, Suppl):S335–S374

180. Renn WH, Rhoton AL Jr. Microsurgical anatomy of the sellar region. J Neurosurg 1975;43(3):288–298

181. Hamberger CA, Hammer G, Marcusson G. Experiences in transantrosphenoidal hypophysectomy. Trans Pac Coast Otoophthalmol Soc Annu Meet 1961;42:273–286

182. Hamid O, El Fiky L, Hassan O, Kotb A, El Fiky S. Anatomic variations of the sphenoid sinus and their impact on trans-sphenoid pituitary surgery. Skull Base 2008;18(1):9–15

183. Inoue T, Rhoton AL Jr, Theele D, Barry ME. Surgical approaches to the cavernous sinus: a microsurgical study. Neurosurgery 1990;26(6):903–932

184. DeLano MC, Fun FY, Zinreich SJ. Relationship of the optic nerve to the posterior paranasal sinuses: a CT anatomic study. AJNR Am J Neuroradiol 1996;17(4):669–675

185. Kazkayasi M, Karadeniz Y, Arikan OK. Anatomic variations of the sphenoid sinus on computed tomography. Rhinology 2005;43(2):109–114

186. Turkdogan FT, Turkdogan KA, Dogan M, Atalar MH. Assessment of sphenoid sinus related anatomic variations with computed tomography. Pan Afr Med J 2017;27:109

187. Raymond J, Hardy J, Czepko R, Roy D. Arterial injuries in transsphenoidal surgery for pituitary adenoma; the role of angiography and endovascular treatment. AJNR Am J Neuroradiol 1997;18(4):655–665

188. Lysack JT, Schaefer PW. Imaging of the pituitary gland, sella, and parasellar region. Totowa, NJ:Humana Press; 2008.

189. Chaudhary V, Bano S. Imaging of the pituitary: recent advances. Indian J Endocrinol Metab 2011;15(Suppl 3): S216–S223

190. Bonneville JF, Bonneville F, Cattin F. Magnetic resonance imaging of pituitary adenomas. Eur Radiol 2005;15(3): 543–548

191. Bartynski WS, Lin L. Dynamic and conventional spin-echo MR of pituitary microlesions. AJNR Am J Neuroradiol 1997;18(5):965–972

192. Hainc N, Stippich C, Reinhardt J, et al. Golden-angle radial sparse parallel (GRASP) MRI in clinical routine detection of pituitary microadenomas: first experience and feasibility. Magn Reson Imaging 2019;60:38–43

193. Donovan JL, Nesbit GM. Distinction of masses involving the sella and suprasellar space: specificity of imaging features. AJR Am J Roentgenol 1996;167(3):597–603

194. Scotti G, Yu CY, Dillon WP, et al. MR imaging of cavernous sinus involvement by pituitary adenomas. AJR Am J Roentgenol 1988;151(4):799–806

195. Vieira JO Jr, Cukiert A, Liberman B. Evaluation of magnetic resonance imaging criteria for cavernous sinus invasion in patients with pituitary adenomas: logistic regression analysis and correlation with surgical findings. Surg Neurol 2006;65(2):130–135, discussion 135

196. Cottier JP, Destrieux C, Brunereau L, et al. Cavernous sinus invasion by pituitary adenoma: MR imaging. Radiology 2000;215(2):463–469

197. Dhandapani S, Singh H, Negm HM, Cohen S, Anand VK, Schwartz TH. Cavernous sinus invasion in pituitary adenomas: systematic review and pooled data meta-analysis of radiologic criteria and comparison of endoscopic and microscopic surgery. World Neurosurg 2016;96:36–46

198. Sumida M, Migita K, Tominaga A, Iida K, Kurisu K. Concomitant pituitary adenoma and Rathke's cleft cyst. Neuroradiology 2001;43(9):755–759

199. Kleinschmidt-DeMasters BK, Lillehei KO, Stears JC. The pathologic, surgical, and MR spectrum of Rathke cleft cysts. Surg Neurol 1995;44(1):19–26, discussion 26–27

200. Sartoretti-Schefer S, Wichmann W, Aguzzi A, Valavanis A. MR differentiation of adamantinous and squamous-papillary craniopharyngiomas. AJNR Am J Neuroradiol 1997;18(1):77–87

201. Osborn AG, Preece MT. Intracranial cysts: radiologic-pathologic correlation and imaging approach. Radiology 2006;239(3):650–664

202. Heier LA, Zimmerman RD, Amster JL, Gandy SE, Deck MD. Magnetic resonance imaging of arachnoid cysts. Clin Imaging 1989;13(4):281–291

203. Tsuruda JS, Chew WM, Moseley ME, Norman D. Diffusion-weighted MR imaging of the brain: value of differentiating between extraaxial cysts and epidermoid tumors. AJR Am J Roentgenol 1990;155(5):1059–1065, discussion 1066–1068

204. Gore RM, Weinberg PE, Kim KS, Ramsey RG. Sphenoid sinus mucoceles presenting as intracranial masses on computed tomography. Surg Neurol 1980;13(5):375–379

205. Abele TA, Yetkin ZF, Raisanen JM, Mickey BE, Mendelsohn DB. Non-pituitary origin sellar tumours mimicking pituitary macroadenomas. Clin Radiol 2012;67(8):821–827

206. Rennert J, Doerfler A. Imaging of sellar and parasellar lesions. Clin Neurol Neurosurg 2007;109(2):111–124

207. Pisaneschi M, Kapoor G. Imaging the sella and parasellar region. Neuroimaging Clin N Am 2005;15(1):203–219

208 Doglietto F, Prevedello DM, Jane JA Jr, Han J, Laws ER Jr. Brief history of endoscopic transsphenoidal surgery—from Philipp Bozzini to the First World Congress of Endoscopic Skull Base Surgery. Neurosurg Focus 2005;19(6): E3.

209. Gao Y, Zhong C, Wang Y, et al. Endoscopic versus microscopic transsphenoidal pituitary adenoma surgery: a meta-analysis. World J Surg Oncol 2014;12:94

210. de Divitiis E, Laws ER, Giani U, Iuliano SL, de Divitiis O, Apuzzo ML. The current status of endoscopy in transsphenoidal surgery: an international survey. World Neurosurg 2015;83(4):447–454

211. Zhang M, Singh H, Almodovar-Mercado GJ, Anand VK, Schwartz TH. Required reading: the most impactful articles in endoscopic endonasal skull base surgery. World Neurosurg 2016;92:499–512.e2

212. Waran V, Tang IP, Karuppiah R, et al. A new modified speculum guided single nostril technique for endoscopic transnasal transsphenoidal surgery: an analysis of nasal complications. Br J Neurosurg 2013;27(6):742–746

213. Wen G, Tang C, Zhong C, et al. Mononostril versus binostril endoscopic transsphenoidal approach for pituitary adenomas: a systematic review and meta-analysis. PLoS One 2016;11(4):e0153397

214. Conrad J, Ayyad A, Wüster C, et al. Binostril versus mononostril approaches in endoscopic transsphenoidal pituitary surgery: clinical evaluation and cadaver study. J Neurosurg 2016;125(2):334–345

215 Little AS, Kelly DF, White WL, et al; TRANSSPHER Study Group. Results of a prospective multicenter controlled study comparing surgical outcomes of microscopic versus fully endoscopic transsphenoidal surgery for nonfunctioning pituitary adenomas: the Transsphenoidal Extent of Resection (TRANSSPHER) Study. J Neurosurg 2019;1–11

216 Bastos RV, Silva CM, Tagliarini JV, et al. Endoscopic versus microscopic transsphenoidal surgery in the treatment of pituitary tumors: systematic review and meta-analysis of randomized and nonrandomized controlled trials. Arch Endocrinol Metab 2016;60(5):411–419

217 Kasemsiri P, Carrau RL, Ditzel Filho LF, et al. Advantages and limitations of endoscopic endonasal approaches to the skull base. World Neurosurg 2014;82(6 Suppl):S12–S21

218 Buchfelder M, Schlaffer S. Surgical treatment of pituitary tumours. Best Pract Res Clin Endocrinol Metab 2009; 23(5):677–692

219. Abou-Jaoude PM, Zeitouni AG, Soualmi L, Leblanc R. Multimodal multidisciplinary surgical approach for the treatment of pituitary tumours. J Otolaryngol 2007;36(6): 322–326

220. Gaillard S. The transition from microscopic to endoscopic transsphenoidal surgery in high-caseload neurosurgical centers: the experience of Foch Hospital. World Neurosurg 2014;82(6, Suppl):S116–S120

221. Laws ER Jr, Barkhoudarian G. The transition from microscopic to endoscopic transsphenoidal surgery: the experience at Brigham and Women's Hospital. World Neurosurg 2014;82(6, Suppl):S152–S154

222. Semple P. The transition from microscopic to endoscopic transsphenoidal surgery in high case load neurosurgical centers: the Groote Schuur Hospital experience. World Neurosurg 2014;82(6, Suppl):S162–S163

223. Karppinen A, Kivipelto L, Vehkavaara S, et al. Transition from microscopic to endoscopic transsphenoidal surgery for nonfunctional pituitary adenomas. World Neurosurg 2015;84(1):48–57

224. Little AS, Kelly DF, Milligan J, et al. Comparison of sinonasal quality of life and health status in patients undergoing microscopic and endoscopic transsphenoidal surgery for pituitary lesions: a prospective cohort study. J Neurosurg 2015;123(3):799–807

225. Chi F, Wang Y, Lin Y, Ge J, Qiu Y, Guo L. A learning curve of endoscopic transsphenoidal surgery for pituitary adenoma. J Craniofac Surg 2013;24(6):2064–2067

226. Ding H, Gu Y, Zhang X, et al. Learning curve for the endoscopic endonasal approach for suprasellar craniopharyngiomas. J Clin Neurosci 2017;42:209–216

227. Kshettry VR, Do H, Elshazly K, et al. The learning curve in endoscopic endonasal resection of craniopharyngiomas. Neurosurg Focus 2016;41(6):E9

228. Lofrese G, Vigo V, Rigante M, et al. Learning curve of endoscopic pituitary surgery: Experience of a neurosurgery/ENT collaboration. J Clin Neurosci 2018;47:299–303

229. Castelnuovo P, Pistochini A, Locatelli D. Different surgical approaches to the sellar region: focusing on the "two nostrils four hands technique". Rhinology 2006;44(1):2–7

230. Cavallo LM, Dal Fabbro M, Jalalod'din H, et al. Endoscopic endonasal transsphenoidal surgery. Before scrubbing in: tips and tricks. Surg Neurol 2007;67(4):342–347

231 Kassam AB, Prevedello DM, Carrau RL, et al. Endoscopic endonasal skull base surgery: analysis of complications in the authors' initial 800 patients. J Neurosurg 2011;114(6): 1544–1568

232. Cheng RX, Tian HL, Gao WW, Li ZQ. A comparison between endoscopic trans-sphenoidal surgery and traditional trans-sphenoidal microsurgery for functioning pituitary adenomas. J Int Med Res 2011;39(5):1985–1993

233. D'Haens J, Van Rompaey K, Stadnik T, Haentjens P, Poppe K, Velkeniers B. Fully endoscopic transsphenoidal surgery

for functioning pituitary adenomas: a retrospective comparison with traditional transsphenoidal microsurgery in the same institution. Surg Neurol 2009;72(4):336–340

234. Higgins TS, Courtemanche C, Karakla D, et al. Analysis of transnasal endoscopic versus transseptal microscopic approach for excision of pituitary tumors. Am J Rhinol 2008;22(6):649–652

235. O'Malley BW Jr, Grady MS, Gabel BC, et al. Comparison of endoscopic and microscopic removal of pituitary adenomas: single-surgeon experience and the learning curve. Neurosurg Focus 2008;25(6):E10

236. Choe JH, Lee KS, Jeun SS, Cho JH, Hong YK. Endocrine outcome of endoscopic endonasal transsphenoidal surgery in functioning pituitary adenomas. J Korean Neurosurg Soc 2008;44(3):151–155

237. Casler JD, Doolittle AM, Mair EA. Endoscopic surgery of the anterior skull base. Laryngoscope 2005;115(1):16–24

238. Atkinson JL, Young WF Jr, Meyer FB, et al. Sublabial transseptal vs transnasal combined endoscopic microsurgery in patients with Cushing disease and MRI-depicted microadenomas. Mayo Clin Proc 2008;83(5):550–553

239. Sheehan MT, Atkinson JL, Kasperbauer JL, Erickson BJ, Nippoldt TB. Preliminary comparison of the endoscopic transnasal vs the sublabial transseptal approach for clinically nonfunctioning pituitary macroadenomas. Mayo Clin Proc 1999;74(7):661–670

240. White DR, Sonnenburg RE, Ewend MG, Senior BA. Safety of minimally invasive pituitary surgery (MIPS) compared with a traditional approach. Laryngoscope 2004;114(11):1945–1948

241. Razak AA, Horridge M, Connolly DJ, et al. Comparison of endoscopic and microscopic trans-sphenoidal pituitary surgery: early results in a single centre. Br J Neurosurg 2013;27(1):40–43

242. Messerer M, De Battista JC, Raverot G, et al. Evidence of improved surgical outcome following endoscopy for nonfunctioning pituitary adenoma removal. Neurosurg Focus 2011;30(4):E11

243. Cappabianca P, Alfieri A, Colao A, Ferone D, Lombardi G, de Divitiis E. Endoscopic endonasal transsphenoidal approach: an additional reason in support of surgery in the management of pituitary lesions. Skull Base Surg 1999;9(2):109–117

244. Koren I, Hadar T, Rappaport ZH, Yaniv E. Endoscopic transnasal transsphenoidal microsurgery versus the sublabial approach for the treatment of pituitary tumors: endonasal complications. Laryngoscope 1999;109(11):1838–1840

245. Duz B, Harman F, Secer HI, Bolu E, Gonul E. Transsphenoidal approaches to the pituitary: a progression in experience in a single centre. Acta Neurochir (Wien) 2008;150(11):1133–1138, discussion 1138–1139

246. Neal JG, Patel SJ, Kulbersh JS, Osguthorpe JD, Schlosser RJ. Comparison of techniques for transsphenoidal pituitary surgery. Am J Rhinol 2007;21(2):203–206

247. Li A, Liu W, Cao P, Zheng Y, Bu Z, Zhou T. Endoscopic versus microscopic transsphenoidal surgery in the treatment of pituitary adenoma: A systematic review and meta-analysis. World Neurosurg 2017;101:236–246

248. Li K, Zhang J, Wang XS, Ye X, Zhao YL. A systematic review of effects and complications after transsphenoidal pituitary surgery: endoscopic versus microscopic approach. Minim Invasive Ther Allied Technol 2019;1–9

249. Goudakos JK, Markou KD, Georgalas C. Endoscopic versus microscopic trans-sphenoidal pituitary surgery: A systematic review and meta-analysis. Clin Otolaryngol 2011;36:212–220

250. Rotenberg B, Tam S, Ryu WH, Duggal N. Microscopic versus endoscopic pituitary surgery: a systematic review. Laryngoscope 2010;120(7):1292–1297

251. Strychowsky J, Nayan S, Reddy K, Farrokhyar F, Sommer D. Purely endoscopic transsphenoidal surgery versus traditional microsurgery for resection of pituitary adenomas: systematic review. J Otolaryngol Head Neck Surg 2011;40(2):175–185

252. Ammirati M, Wei L, Ciric I. Short-term outcome of endoscopic versus microscopic pituitary adenoma surgery: a systematic review and meta-analysis. J Neurol Neurosurg Psychiatry 2013;84(8):843–849

253. Dehdashti AR, Ganna A, Witterick I, Gentili F. Expanded endoscopic endonasal approach for anterior cranial base and suprasellar lesions: indications and limitations. Neurosurgery 2009;64(4):677–687, discussion 687–689

254. Bourdelot A, Coste J, Hazebroucq V, et al. Clinical, hormonal and magnetic resonance imaging (MRI) predictors of transsphenoidal surgery outcome in acromegaly. Eur J Endocrinol 2004;150(6):763–771

255. van Bunderen CC, van Varsseveld NC, Baayen JC, et al. Predictors of endoscopic transsphenoidal surgery outcome in acromegaly: patient and tumor characteristics evaluated by magnetic resonance imaging. Pituitary 2013;16(2):158–167

256. Pal'a A, Knoll A, Brand C, et al. The value of intraoperative magnetic resonance imaging in endoscopic and microsurgical transsphenoidal pituitary adenoma resection. World Neurosurg 2017;102:144–150

257. Neumann AM Jr, Pasquale-Niebles K, Bhuta T, Sillers MJ. Image-guided transnasal endoscopic surgery of the paranasal sinuses and anterior skull base. Am J Rhinol 1999;13(6):449–454

258. Hajdari S, Kellner G, Meyer A, Rosahl S, Gerlach R. Endoscopic endonasal surgery for removal of pituitary adenomas: a surgical case series of treatment results using different 2- and 3-dimensional visualization systems. World Neurosurg 2018;119:e80–e86

259. Schmitt H, Buchfelder M, Radespiel-Tröger M, Fahlbusch R. Difficult intubation in acromegalic patients: incidence and predictability. Anesthesiology 2000;93(1):110–114

260. Ahmed-Nusrath A. Anaesthesia for head and neck cancer surgery. BJA Educ 2017;17:383–389

261. Jellish WS, Murdoch J, Leonetti JP. Perioperative management of complex skull base surgery: the anesthesiologist's point of view. Neurosurg Focus 2002;12(5):e5

262. Stienen MN, Fierstra J, Pangalu A, Regli L, Bozinov O. The zurich checklist for safety in the intraoperative magnetic resonance imaging suite: technical note. Oper Neurosurg (Hagerstown) 2019;16(6):756–765

263. Cappabianca P, Cavallo LM, Esposito F, de Divitiis E. Endoscopic endonasal transsphenoidal surgery: procedure, endoscopic equipment and instrumentation. Childs Nerv Syst 2004;20(11-12):796–801

264. Brand Y, Narayanan V, Prepageran N, Waran V. A cost-effective delivery system for floseal during endoscopic and microscopic brain surgery. World Neurosurg 2016;90: 492–495

265. Waran V, Sek K, Bahuri NF, Narayanan P, Chandran H. A haemostatic agent delivery system for endoscopic neurosurgical procedures. Minim Invasive Neurosurg 2011; 54(5-6):279–281

266. Zaidi HA, De Los Reyes K, Barkhoudarian G, et al. The utility of high-resolution intraoperative MRI in endoscopic transsphenoidal surgery for pituitary macroadenomas: early experience in the Advanced Multimodality Image Guided Operating suite. Neurosurg Focus 2016;40(3):E18

267. Coburger J, König R, Seitz K, Bäzner U, Wirtz CR, Hlavac M. Determining the utility of intraoperative magnetic resonance imaging for transsphenoidal surgery: a retrospective study. J Neurosurg 2014;120(2):346–356

268. Serra C, Burkhardt JK, Esposito G, et al. Pituitary surgery and volumetric assessment of extent of resection: a paradigm shift in the use of intraoperative magnetic resonance imaging. Neurosurg Focus 2016;40(3):E17

269. Li J, Cong Z, Ji X, et al. Application of intraoperative magnetic resonance imaging in large invasive pituitary adenoma surgery. Asian J Surg 2015;38(3):168–173

270. Bayer S, Maier A, Ostermeier M, Fahrig R. Intraoperative imaging modalities and compensation for brain shift in tumor resection surgery. Int J Biomed Imaging 2017;2017: 6028645

271. Zaidi HA, Chowdhry SA, Wilson DA, Spetzler RF. The dilemma of early postoperative magnetic resonance imaging: when efficiency compromises accuracy: case report. Neurosurgery 2014;74(3):E335–E340, discussion E340

272. Jahangiri A, Wagner J, Han SW, et al. Morbidity of repeat transsphenoidal surgery assessed in more than 1000 operations. J Neurosurg 2014;121(1):67–74

273. Chang EF, Sughrue ME, Zada G, Wilson CB, Blevins LS Jr, Kunwar S. Long term outcome following repeat transsphenoidal surgery for recurrent endocrine-inactive pituitary adenomas. Pituitary 2010;13(3):223–229

274. Schuss P, Hadjiathanasiou A, Klingmüller D, Güresir Á, Vatter H, Güresir E. Transsphenoidal pituitary surgery: comparison of two sellar reconstruction techniques and their effect on postoperative cerebrospinal fluid leakage. Neurosurg Rev 2018;41(4):1053–1058

275. Chamoun R, Takashima M, Yoshor D. Endoscopic extracapsular dissection for resection of pituitary macroadenomas: technical note. J Neurol Surg A Cent Eur Neurosurg 2014; 75(1):48–52

276. Prevedello DM, Ebner FH, de Lara D, Ditzel Filho L, Otto BA, Carrau RL. Extracapsular dissection technique with the cotton swab for pituitary adenomas through an endoscopic endonasal approach—how I do it. Acta Neurochir (Wien) 2013;155(9):1629–1632

277. Jane JA Jr, Laws ER Jr. Surgical treatment of pituitary adenomas. In: Feingold KR, Anawalt B, Boyce A, eds. Endotext. South Dartmouth, MA; 2000.

278. Fan J, Peng Y, Qi S, Zhang XA, Qiu B, Pan J. Individualized surgical strategies for Rathke cleft cyst based on cyst location. J Neurosurg 2013;119(6):1437–1446

279. Kim JE, Kim JH, Kim OL, et al. Surgical treatment of symptomatic Rathke cleft cysts: clinical features and results with special attention to recurrence. J Neurosurg 2004; 100(1):33–40

280. Chin OY, Ghosh R, Fang CH, Baredes S, Liu JK, Eloy JA. Internal carotid artery injury in endoscopic endonasal surgery: a systematic review. Laryngoscope 2016;126(3):582–590

281. Fukushima T, Maroon JC. Repair of carotid artery perforations during transsphenoidal surgery. Surg Neurol 1998;50(2): 174–177

282. Zhang Y, Tian Z, Li C, et al. A modified endovascular treatment protocol for iatrogenic internal carotid artery injuries following endoscopic endonasal surgery. J Neurosurg 2019;1–8

283. Cobb MI, Nimjee S, Gonzalez LF, Jang DW, Zomorodi A. Direct repair of iatrogenic internal carotid artery injury during endoscopic endonasal approach surgery with temporary endovascular balloon-assisted occlusion: technical case

report. Neurosurgery 2015;11(Suppl 3):E483–E486, discussion E486–E487

284. Duek I, Sviri GE, Amit M, Gil Z. Endoscopic endonasal repair of internal carotid artery injury during endoscopic endonasal surgery. J Neurol Surg Rep 2017;78(4):e125–e128

285. Patel PN, Stafford AM, Patrinely JR, et al. Risk factors for intraoperative and postoperative cerebrospinal fluid leaks in endoscopic transsphenoidal sellar surgery. Otolaryngol Head Neck Surg 2018;158(5):952–960

286. Berker M, Hazer DB, Yücel T, et al. Complications of endoscopic surgery of the pituitary adenomas: analysis of 570 patients and review of the literature. Pituitary 2012;15(3): 288–300

287. Conger A, Zhao F, Wang X, et al. Evolution of the graded repair of CSF leaks and skull base defects in endonasal endoscopic tumor surgery: trends in repair failure and meningitis rates in 509 patients. J Neurosurg 2018;130(3): 861–875

288. Esposito F, Dusick JR, Fatemi N, Kelly DF. Graded repair of cranial base defects and cerebrospinal fluid leaks in transsphenoidal surgery. Oper Neurosurg (Hagerstown) 2007;60(4, Suppl 2):295–303, discussion 303–304

289. Park JH, Choi JH, Kim YI, Kim SW, Hong YK. Modified graded repair of cerebrospinal fluid leaks in endoscopic endonasal transsphenoidal surgery. J Korean Neurosurg Soc 2015;58(1):36–42

290. Zhang C, Ding X, Lu Y, Hu L, Hu G. Cerebrospinal fluid rhinorrhoea following transsphenoidal surgery for pituitary adenoma: experience in a Chinese centre. Acta Otorhinolaryngol Ital 2017;37(4):303–307

291. Lam K, Luong AU, Yao WC, Citardi MJ. Use of autologous fat grafts for the endoscopic reconstruction of skull base defects: indications, outcomes, and complications. Am J Rhinol Allergy 2018;32(4):310–317

292. Fiorindi A, Gioffrè G, Boaro A, et al. Banked fascia lata in sellar dura reconstruction after endoscopic transsphenoidal skull base surgery. J Neurol Surg B Skull Base 2015;76(4): 303–309

293. Gök A, Erkutlu I, Alptekin M, Kanlikama M. Three-layer reconstruction with fascia lata and vascularized pericranium for anterior skull base defects. Acta Neurochir (Wien) 2004;146(1):53–56, discussion 56–57

294. Locatelli D, Pozzi F, Agresta G, Padovan S, Karligkiotis A, Castelnuovo P. Extended endoscopic endonasal approach for suprasellar craniopharyngioma. J Neurol Surg B Skull Base 2018;79(2):S196–S198

295. Zada G, Fredrickson VL, Wrobel BB. Extended endoscopic endonasal approach for resection of tuberculum sellae meningioma. Neurosurg Focus 2017;43(VideoSuppl2):V2

296. Sigler AC, D'Anza B, Lobo BC, Woodard TD, Recinos PF, Sindwani R. Endoscopic skull base reconstruction: an evolution of materials and methods. Otolaryngol Clin North Am 2017;50(3):643–653

297. Hadad G, Bassagasteguy L, Carrau RL, et al. A novel reconstructive technique after endoscopic expanded endonasal approaches: vascular pedicle nasoseptal flap. Laryngoscope 2006;116(10):1882–1886

298. Kassam AB, Thomas A, Carrau RL, et al. Endoscopic reconstruction of the cranial base using a pedicled nasoseptal flap. Neurosurgery 2008;63(1, Suppl 1):ONS44–ONS52, discussion ONS52–ONS53

299. Moon JH, Kim EH, Kim SH. Various modifications of a vascularized nasoseptal flap for repair of extensive skull base dural defects. J Neurosurg 2019;1–9

300. Kang MD, Escott E, Thomas AJ, et al. The MR imaging appearance of the vascular pedicle nasoseptal flap. AJNR Am J Neuroradiol 2009;30(4):781–786

301. Thorp BD, Sreenath SB, Ebert CS, Zanation AM. Endoscopic skull base reconstruction: a review and clinical case series of 152 vascularized flaps used for surgical skull base defects in the setting of intraoperative cerebrospinal fluid leak. Neurosurg Focus 2014;37(4):E4

302. Prevedello DM, Barges-Coll J, Fernandez-Miranda JC, et al. Middle turbinate flap for skull base reconstruction: cadaveric feasibility study. Laryngoscope 2009;119(11):2094–2098

303. Learned KO, Adappa ND, Loevner LA, Palmer JN, Newman JG, Lee JY. MR imaging evaluation of endoscopic cranial base reconstruction with pedicled nasoseptal flap following endoscopic endonasal skull base surgery. Eur J Radiol 2013;82(3):544–551

304. Learned KOM, Maralani PJ, Malloy K, Loevner LA. Skull base reconstruction: demystifying postoperative imaging evaluation. Neurographics 2015;5(2):56–63

305. Webster J, Piscitelli G, Polli A, Ferrari CI, Ismail I, Scanlon MF; Cabergoline Comparative Study Group. A comparison of cabergoline and bromocriptine in the treatment of hyperprolactinemic amenorrhea. N Engl J Med 1994;331(14): 904–909

306. Andereggen L, Frey J, Andres RH, et al. Long-term follow-up of primary medical versus surgical treatment of prolactinomas in men: effects on hyperprolactinemia, hypogonadism, and bone health. World Neurosurg 2017;97:595–602

307. Greenman Y. Management of endocrine disease: present and future perspectives for medical therapy of nonfunctioning pituitary adenomas. Eur J Endocrinol 2017;177(3): R113–R124

308. Loeffler JS, Shih HA. Radiation therapy in the management of pituitary adenomas. J Clin Endocrinol Metab 2011;96(7): 1992–2003

309. Sheehan JP, Kondziolka D, Flickinger J, Lunsford LD. Radiosurgery for residual or recurrent nonfunctioning pituitary adenoma. J Neurosurg 2002;97(5, Suppl):408–414

310. Sheehan JP, Pouratian N, Steiner L, Laws ER, Vance ML. Gamma Knife surgery for pituitary adenomas: factors related to radiological and endocrine outcomes. J Neurosurg 2011;114(2):303–309

311. Liscák R, Vladyka V, Marek J, Simonová G, Vymazal J. Gamma knife radiosurgery for endocrine-inactive pituitary adenomas. Acta Neurochir (Wien) 2007;149(10):999–1006, discussion 1006

312. Erridge SC, Conkey DS, Stockton D, et al. Radiotherapy for pituitary adenomas: long-term efficacy and toxicity. Radiother Oncol 2009;93(3):597–601

313. Ding D, Mehta GU, Patibandla MR, et al. Stereotactic radiosurgery for acromegaly: an international multicenter retrospective cohort study. Neurosurgery 2019;84(3): 717–725

314. Pai FY, Chen CJ, Wang WH, et al. Low-dose gamma knife radiosurgery for acromegaly. Neurosurgery 2019;85(1): E20–E30

315. Mehta GU, Ding D, Patibandla MR, et al. Stereotactic radiosurgery for cushing disease: Results of an international, multicenter study. J Clin Endocrinol Metab 2017; 102(11):4284–4291

316. Moore JM, Sala E, Amorin A, et al. Cyberknife radiosurgery in the multimodal management of patients with Cushing disease. World Neurosurg 2018;112:e425–e430

317. Shrivastava A, Mohammed N, Xu Z, et al. Outcomes after gamma knife stereotactic radiosurgery in pediatric patients with cushing disease or acromegaly: a multi-institutional study. World Neurosurg 2019;125:e1104–e1113

318. van den Bergh AC, van den Berg G, Schoorl MA, et al. Immediate postoperative radiotherapy in residual nonfunctioning pituitary adenoma: beneficial effect on local control without additional negative impact on pituitary function and life expectancy. Int J Radiat Oncol Biol Phys 2007;67(3):863–869

319. Minniti G, Osti M, Jaffrain-Rea ML, Esposito V, Cantore G, Maurizi Enrici R. Long-term follow-up results of postoperative radiation therapy for Cushing's disease. J Neurooncol 2007;84(1):79–84

320. Arafah BM. Medical management of hypopituitarism in patients with pituitary adenomas. Pituitary 2002;5(2): 109–117

321. Grossman AB. Clinical Review#: the diagnosis and management of central hypoadrenalism. J Clin Endocrinol Metab 2010;95(11):4855–4863

322. Jonklaas J, Bianco AC, Bauer AJ, et al; American Thyroid Association Task Force on Thyroid Hormone Replacement. Guidelines for the treatment of hypothyroidism: prepared by the American Thyroid Association Task Force on thyroid hormone replacement. Thyroid 2014;24(12):1670–1751

323. Oiso Y, Robertson GL, Nørgaard JP, Juul KV. Clinical review: treatment of neurohypophyseal diabetes insipidus. J Clin Endocrinol Metab 2013;98(10):3958–3967

324. Barker FG II, Klibanski A, Swearingen B. Transsphenoidal surgery for pituitary tumors in the United States, 1996–2000: mortality, morbidity, and the effects of hospital and surgeon volume. J Clin Endocrinol Metab 2003;88(10): 4709–4719

325. Ciric I, Ragin A, Baumgartner C, Pierce D. Complications of transsphenoidal surgery: results of a national survey, review of the literature, and personal experience. Neurosurgery 1997;40(2):225–236, discussion 236–237

326. de Almeida JR, et al. Defining the nasopalatine line: the limit for endonasal surgery of the spine. Laryngoscope 2009; 119(2):239-244

327. Yahia-Cherif M, Delpierre I, Hassid S, De Witte O. Bony regeneration of the sella after transsphenoidal pituitary surgery. World Neurosurg 2016;88:497–502

328. Guthikonda B, Nourbakhsh A, Notarianni C, Vannemreddy P, Nanda A. Middle turbinectomy for exposure in endoscopic endonasal transsphenoidal surgery: when is it necessary? Laryngoscope 2010;120(12):2360–2366

329. Nyquist GG, Anand VK, Brown S, Singh A, Tabaee A, Schwartz TH. Middle turbinate preservation in endoscopic transsphenoidal surgery of the anterior skull base. Skull Base 2010;20(5):343–347

330. Micko AS, Wöhrer A, Wolfsberger S, Knosp E. Invasion of the cavernous sinus space in pituitary adenomas: endoscopic verification and its correlation with an MRI-based classification. J Neurosurg 2015;122(4):803–811

Chapter 2

Endoscopic Transnasal Approach for Pituitary Tumors

Narayan Jayashankar, Rajan Shah, and Suresh Sankhla

Introduction

Pituitary tumors are most commonly benign but can be slow growing or aggressive. They are either nonfunctional where there is no disturbance of various hormonal levels, or can be functional where the hormonal levels are deranged. In functional tumors especially, it is important to achieve gross total tumor excision. They are also classified as microadenomas (<10 mm in diameter) and macroadenomas (>10 mm in diameter).

Endoscopic transnasal approach to the sella offers the distinct advantage of distal illumination as also wide distal view as compared to microscope. It enhances capability to look into various corners of the sellar cavity especially the sellar–suprasellar areas as also the medial cavernous sinus to determine complete removal of tumor. With the technical improvements in the approach, the endoscopic approach is now widely considered the standard for excision of pituitary tumors.[1,2,3,4]

Indications

1. Nonfunctioning pituitary adenomas most commonly causing some visual disturbances. **Fig. 2.1** depicts MRI of a subject with pituitary macroadenoma.
2. Micro- or macroadenomas causing Cushing's disease.[5]
3. Micro- or macroadenomas causing acromegaly.
4. Rarely, in failed medical management of prolactinomas. It must be noted that medical therapy is the first line of treatment for prolactinomas.

Surgical Steps

1. The nasal cavity is decongested on both sides using dilute adrenaline-soaked patties. A view of the right nasal cavity is seen (**Fig. 2.2a, b**).
2. The middle turbinate is bipolarized and cut close to its anterior attachment to the skull base leaving a small tail behind for future identification of the axilla of the middle turbinate (**Fig. 2.3** and **Fig. 2.4**). Note that the scissor blades are horizontal and after cutting the middle turbinate anterior attachment, the turbinate is gently pushed inferiorly toward its posterior attachment. Cutting the anterior attachment of the turbinate flush with the skull base may cause undesirable cerebrospinal fluid (CSF) leak. The scissor blades are vertical when cutting the posterior attachment of the middle turbinate close to the lateral nasal wall (**Fig. 2.5**). The sump of middle turbinate at the posterior end is bipolarized close to its attachment to the lateral nasal wall (**Fig. 2.6**). Care is taken not to bipolarize the area of the sphenopalatine artery so as to preserve the arterial

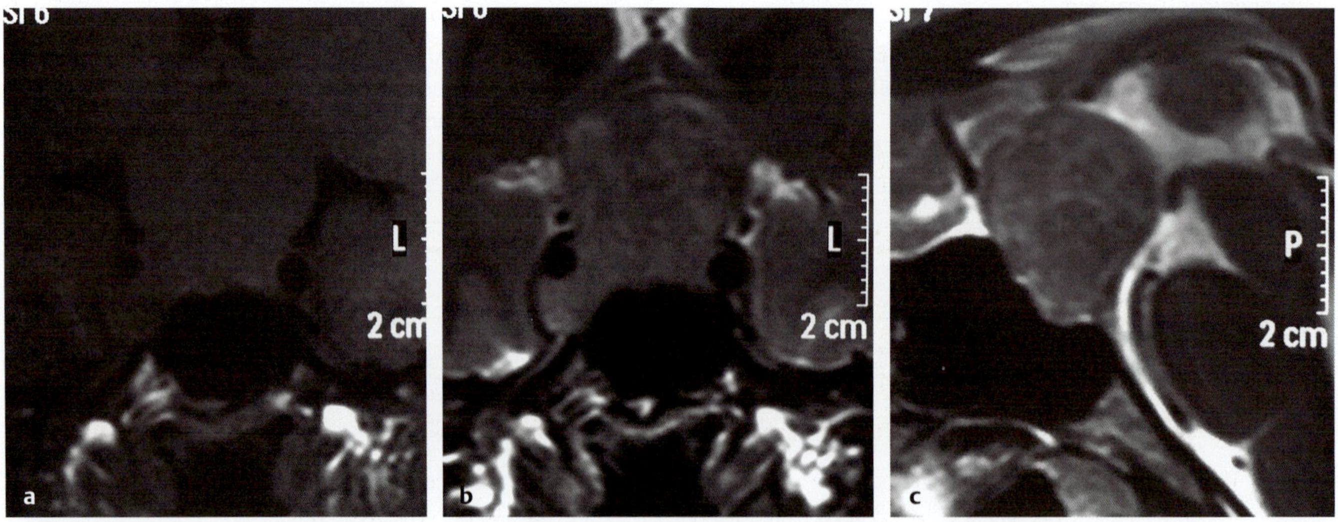

Fig. 2.1 MRI scans depicting the pituitary tumor. **(a)** T1W coronal. **(b)** T2W coronal. **(c)** T2W sagittal.

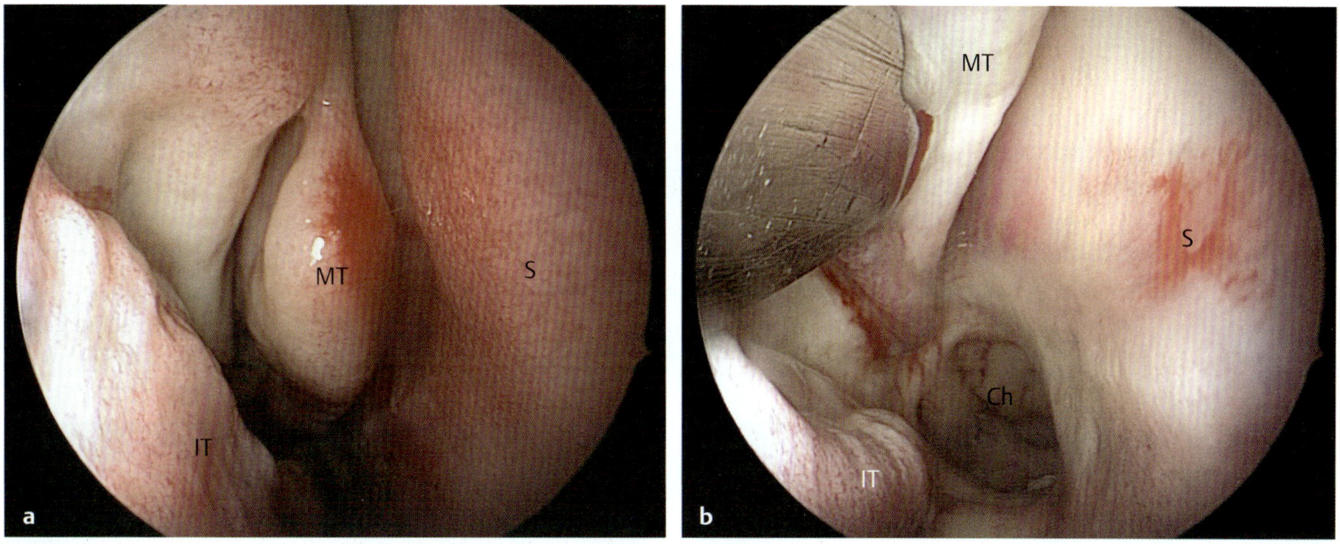

Fig. 2.2 **(a)** Right nasal cavity; **(b)** Posterior end of nasal cavity.

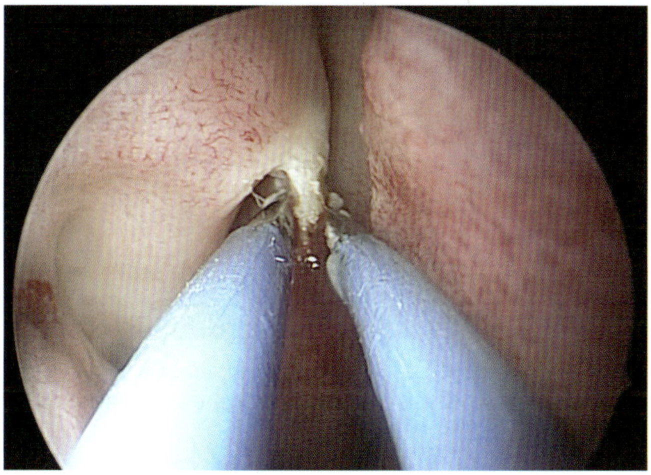

Fig. 2.3 Right middle turbinate is bipolarized close to axilla of the turbinate.

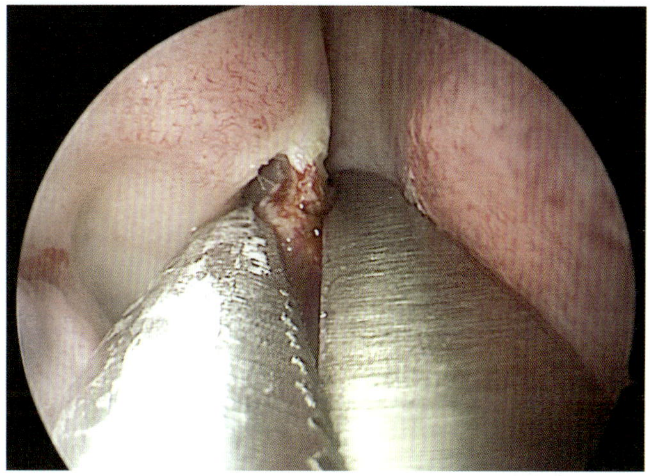

Fig. 2.4 Note that the scissors is horizontal when excising the middle turbinate close to the axilla.

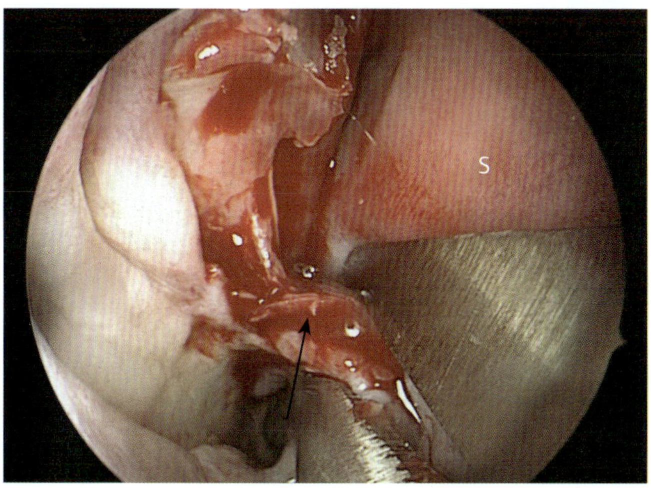

Fig. 2.5 The posterior attachment of the middle turbinate to the lateral nasal wall (*black arrow*) is seen which is cut with the scissor blades vertical.

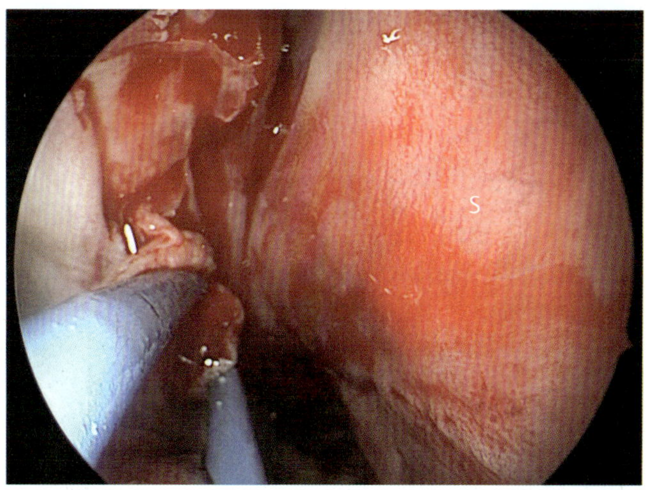

Fig. 2.6 The posterior sump of the middle turbinate is bipolarized to prevent bleeding.

supply to the Hadad-Bassagasteguy flap which is to be used for reconstruction. The middle turbinate is then removed.

3. A complete ethmoidectomy is performed on the right side, the posterior limit being the fovea ethmoidalis and the lateral limit being the lamina papyracea (**Fig. 2.7**). Care is taken to preoperatively identify an Onodi cell on computed tomography (CT) scan, if any, as the optic nerve in these cases may lie along the posterolateral wall of the Onodi cell rather than the sphenoid sinus.
4. The sphenoid ostium is identified. The inferior half of the superior turbinate that covers the sphenoid ostium is excised by bipolarizing it and then using a microdebrider (**Fig. 2.8**). The sphenoid ostium is identified just above the sphenoethmoid recess adjacent to the septum (**Fig. 2.9**). The sphenoid ostium is widened laterally using a Kerrison punch. It is safe to start from the sphenoid ostium and clear the bony overhangs toward the posterior ethmoids especially in cases where an Onodi cell exists (**Fig. 2.10**). In these cases, coming from posterior ethmoids to sphenoid may

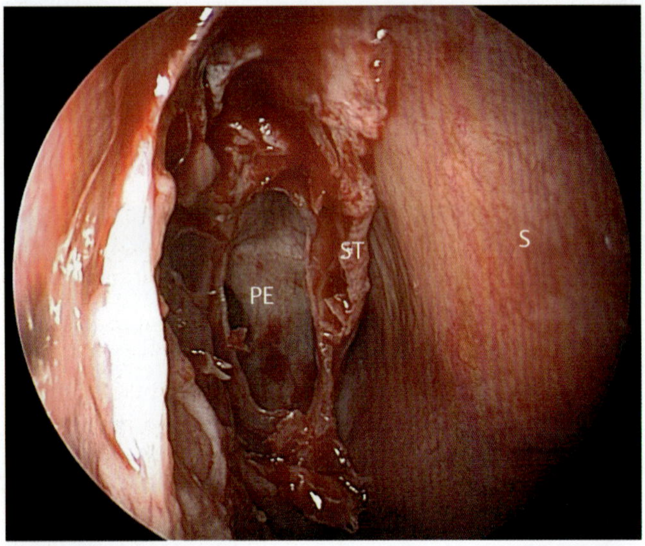

Fig. 2.7 Ethmoidectomy has been performed on the right side. A part of fovea ethmoidalis is seen. The superior turbinate is seen.

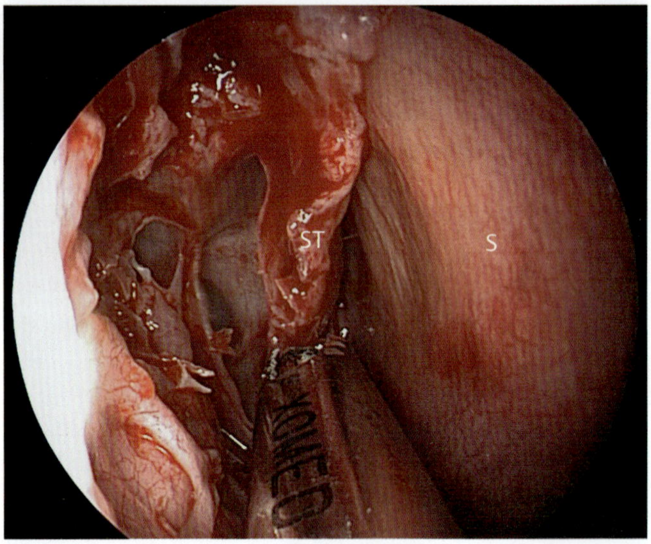

Fig. 2.8 The inferior half of the superior turbinate covering the sphenoid ostium is bipolarized and shaved off.

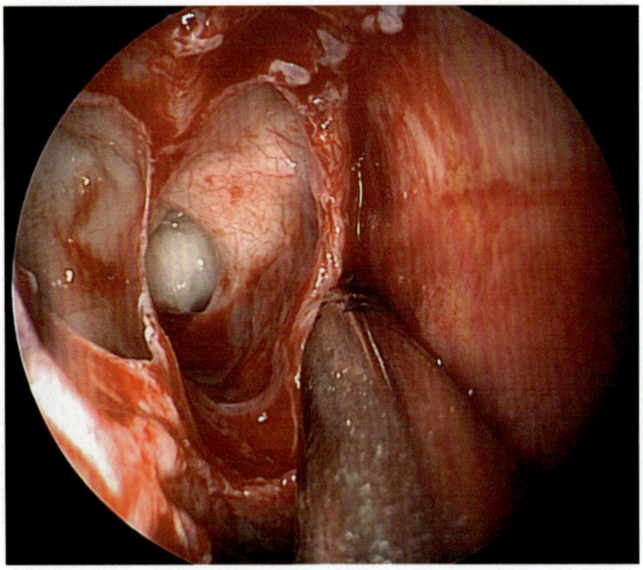

Fig. 2.9 The right sphenoid ostium is entered above the sphenoethmoidal recess, The Onodi cell with optic canal is seen.

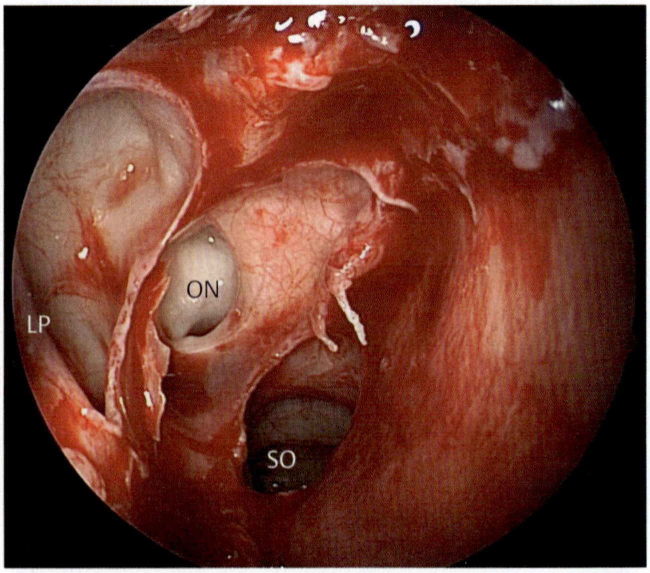

Fig. 2.10 The sphenoid sinus, Onodi cell, and lamina papyracea are seen. Note how the optic canal is present in the Onodi cell lateral wall.

risk injury to the optic nerve, especially so if the optic nerve is dehiscent.

5. Although many surgeons preserve the middle turbinate on the right side, removal of the middle turbinate and the ethmoids on the right side gives an unhindered view of the lateral sphenoid wall with the endoscope placed more proximally with additional improved space for instrument manipulation. This is the based on the concept of creating one and half cavity on the right side. The endoscope is placed in the extra space procured which gives a wide roomy cavity for instrument manipulation on the same side especially so when the surgery proceeds toward the right cavernous sinus area.
6. The Hadad-Bassagasteguy flap is harvested only when CSF leak is anticipated. Authors harvest the flap on the right side. A horizontal incision is taken at the inferior end of the sphenoid sinus ostium. A second incision is taken at the upper end of the posterior choanae. This incision is extended horizontally onto the inferior end of nasal septum. The anterior limit of this incision is at the mucocutaneous junction on the septum. The incision taken at the inferior end of sphenoid ostium is continued forward on to the septum about 1 cm below the level of the cribriform plate till we cross the anterior genu of the middle turbinate; it is then arched superiorly and a horizontal incision is continued forward at the upper end of septum till the mucocutaneous junction. A vertical incision at the mucocutaneous junction joins the upper and lower horizontal incisions over the nasal septum. The vascularized pedicled flap is then harvested retaining its vascularity from the sphenopalatine artery. In case a wider flap is required, the mucoperiosteum of the nasal floor is additionally included in the flap. The flap is tucked away in the nasopharynx for reconstruction, till the surgical procedure is complete.
7. In most cases, however, a rescue Hadad-Bassagasteguy flap is preserved for harvesting, in case needed. In this case, it is necessary to preserve the pedicle of the nasoseptal flap that runs in the sphenoethmoid recess before widening the sphenoid ostium inferiorly. In case of CSF leak, the rescue flap incisions are extended anteriorly as described in the earlier point and the Haddad Bassagasteguy flap is harvested.
8. The sphenoid ostia are now widened bilaterally along its inferior wall to the maximum permissible limit using a Kerrison punch. Next, the posterior third of the bony septum is resected (**Fig. 2.11**). The perpendicular plates of ethmoid and vomer are resected and preserved in saline for reconstruction. The rostrum of the sphenoid is then clearly seen. The mucoperiosteal flap on the opposite side (left side) is lifted off the rostrum so as to preserve the opposite vascular pedicle in case additional flap is required (**Fig. 2.12**). Once the palatovaginal canals are identified on both sides, the rostrum is drilled down to the level of the floor of the sphenoid, from one palatovaginal canal to the other. Alternatively, it is taken down with chisel and hammer by making controlled cuts on both sides as

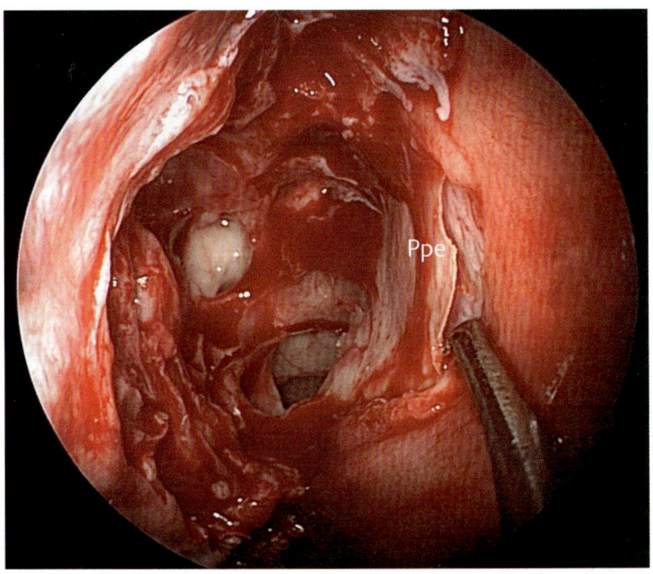

Fig. 2.11 A posterior septectomy is performed. The perpendicular plate of ethmoid and the vomer are removed. Ppe, perpendicular plate of ethmoid (posterior end of septum).

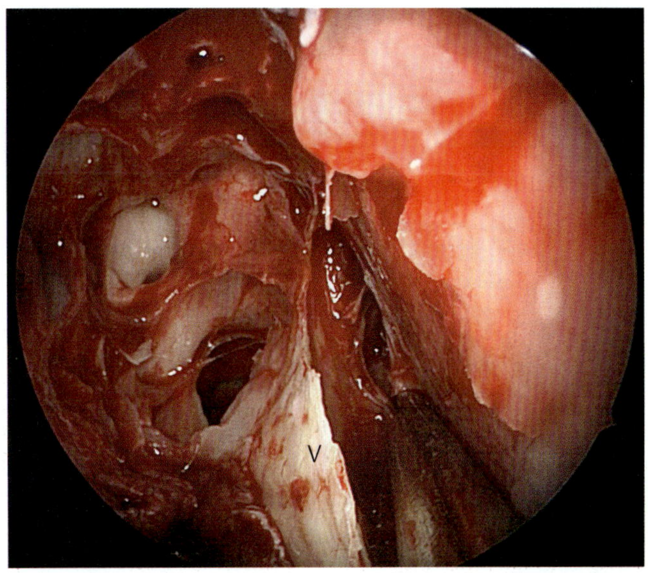

Fig. 2.12 The mucoperiosteal flap on both sides of the rostrum of sphenoid are separated to identify the palatovaginal and vidian canals. V, vomer.

also inferiorly (**Fig. 2.13**). The rostrum of sphenoid is then removed (**Fig. 2.14**).

9. The bony overhangs on all sides are then drilled off. Inferiorly, we should have an unhindered view of the upper clivus and sphenoid floor with no overhangs (**Fig. 2.15**). This additionally helps for Hadad-Bassagasteguy flap replacement at the end of the procedure. Superiorly, removal of any bony overhangs offers a nice view of the tuberculum as also the planum right up to the location of the posterior ethmoid arteries on both sides. Laterally, on both sides, we expose the area lateral to the paraclival carotids. In case a lateral sinus is present in sphenoid, the lateral sinus is exposed completely. It may be necessary in these cases to drill the pterygoid base as required. The posterior wall of Onodi cell, in case present, is also removed (**Fig. 2.16**) to convert the Onodi and sphenoid sinus into a single smooth cavity.

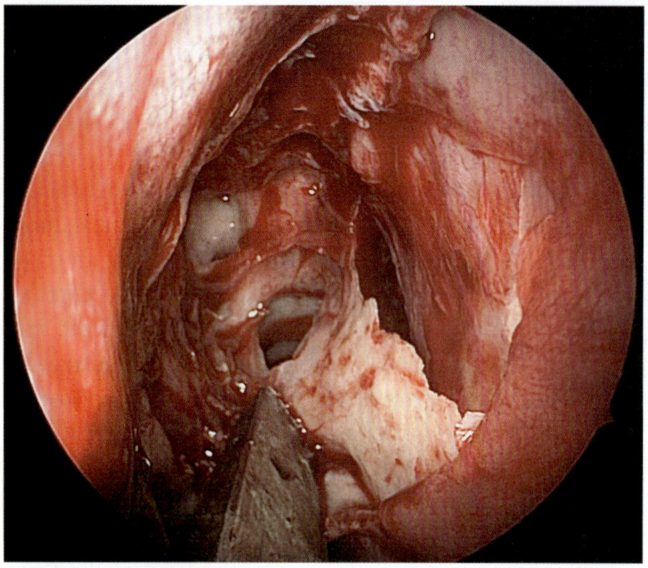

Fig. 2.13 A chisel and hammer is used to create cuts in the plane of palatovaginal canals to excise the rostrum of sphenoid.

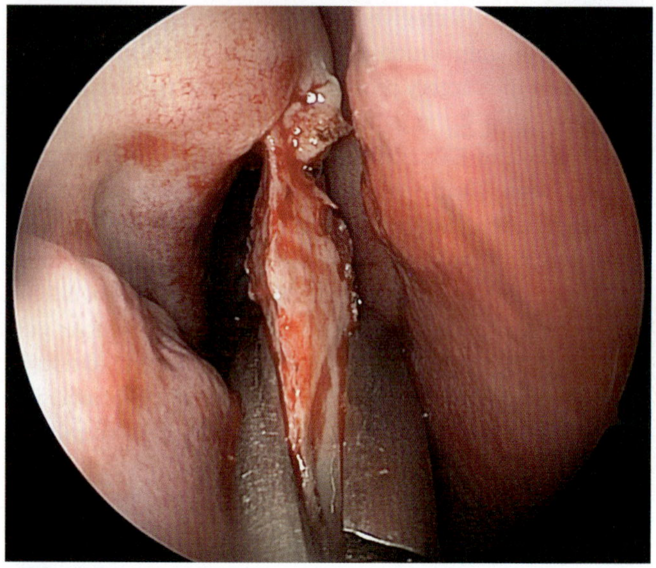

Fig. 2.14 The sphenoid rostrum is excised.

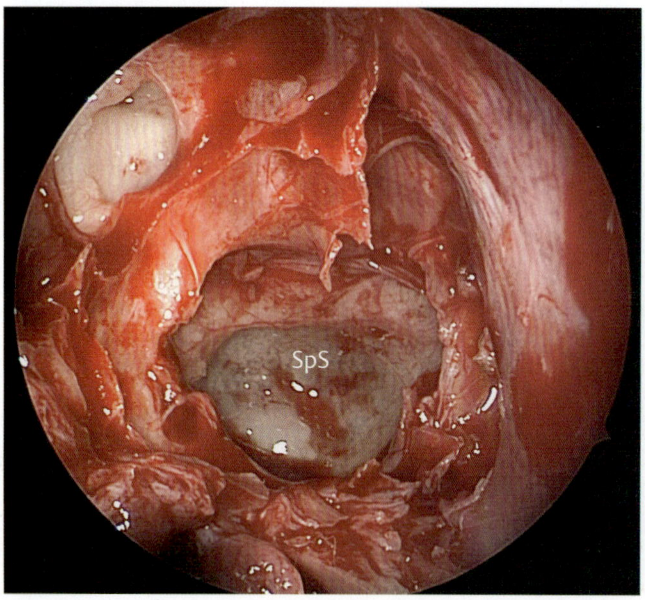

Fig. 2.15 The floor of the sphenoid is exposed. Any bony overhangs are drilled off to expose the floor of sphenoid as also the lateral sinus. SpS, sphenoid sinus.

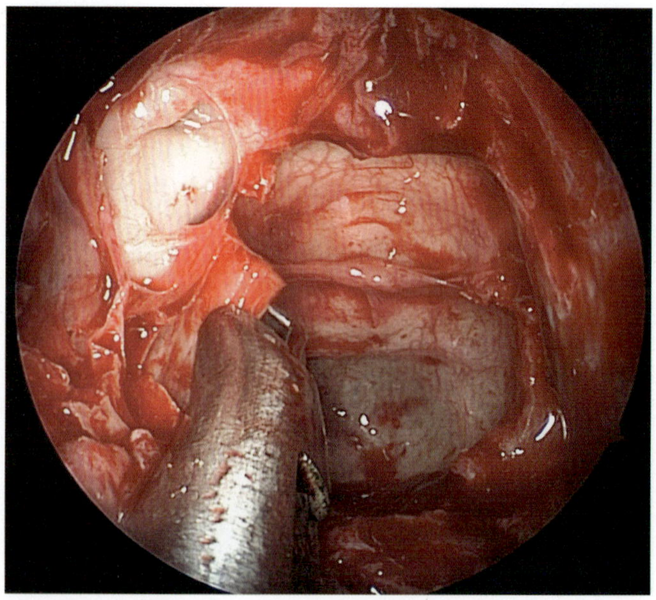

Fig. 2.16 The posterior wall of the Onodi cell is taken off.

10. The sphenoid sinus mucosa is stripped off. All bony sphenoid septations are drilled off with a coarse diamond burr (**Fig. 2.17**). If the sellar bone is thick at places, it is drilled down to make it uniformly eggshell thin. Depending on the pathology and the extent of the lesion, it may be necessary to also thin the bone over the cavernous and clinoidal carotids.

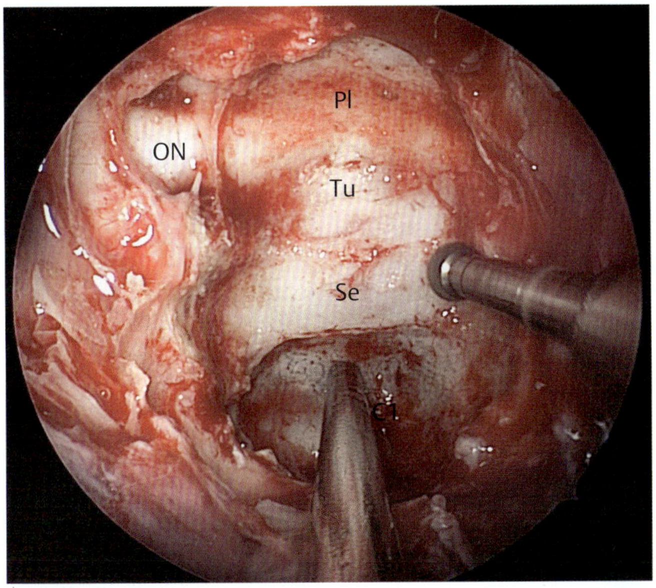

Fig. 2.17 All sphenoid septations, bony overhangs, and thick bone over the medial opticocarotid recess are drilled off.

11. The eggshell thin bone over the sella is fractured (**Fig. 2.18**) and the remaining shells of bone are lifted off using a Kerrison punch. It should be noted that the Kerrison punch is not used to bite, but the jaw is kept open, the anterior jaw of the Kerrison punch is put in between sellar dura and overlying thin bone, and then, the eggshell bone is gently lifted off the underlying dura (**Fig. 2.19**). The bone of the sellar floor is also taken off. It is very important to remove the bone completely over the medial opticocarotid recess on both sides. The extent of bone removal is the bluish hue of the cavernous sinuses laterally, the superior intercavernous sinus superiorly, and the inferior intercavernous sinus inferiorly.
12. In case of lesions extending to the medial cavernous sinus, the bone is taken off the ipsilateral cavernous and clinoidal carotid. Removal of this bone helps to gently retract the carotid artery laterally to gain access to the medial cavernous sinus.
13. The sellar dura is incised in a + shape (**Fig. 2.20**). It is important to incise the dura to the maximum permissible limits so that the sellar cavity can be inspected better. The dural edges are reflected to expose the pituitary tumor (**Fig. 2.21**). Bleeding from dural edges, if any, can be controlled with bipolar cauterization.
14. Biopsy is taken from the tumor before clearance of the tumor. As tumor removal progresses, a part of diaphragm is visible and identified (**Fig. 2.22**). It is important to clear the lateral gutters of tumor before

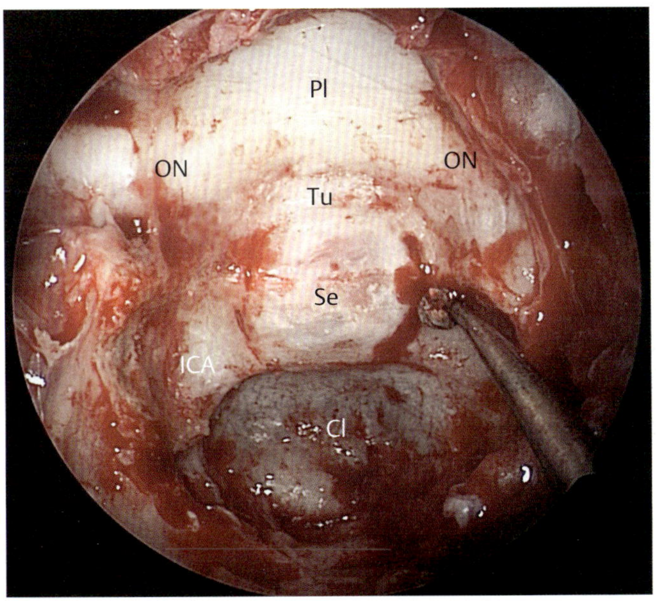

Fig. 2.18 Gentle fracture is created on both sides of the sella. Cl, clivus; ICA, internal carotid artery (paraclival segment); ON, optic nerve; Pl, planum; Se, sella; Tu, tuberculum sellae.

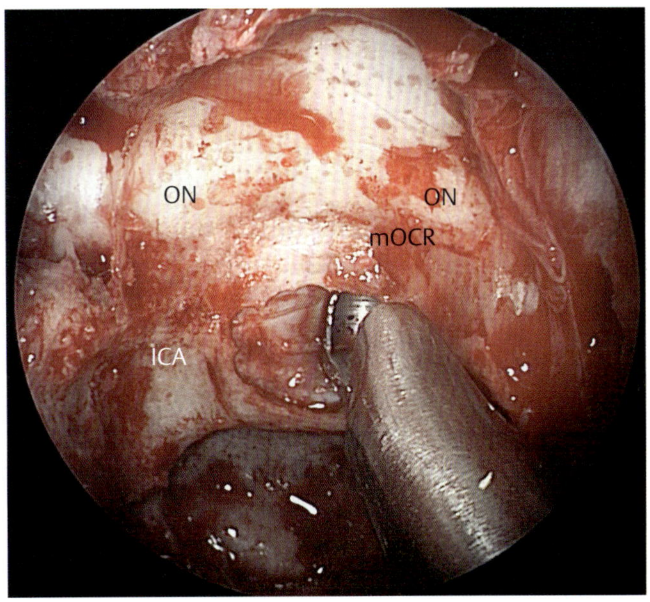

Fig. 2.19 The edges are taken off with a Kerrison punch to widen the bony opening to the maximum desired. ICA, internal carotid artery; mOCR, medial opticocarotid recess; ON, optic nerve.

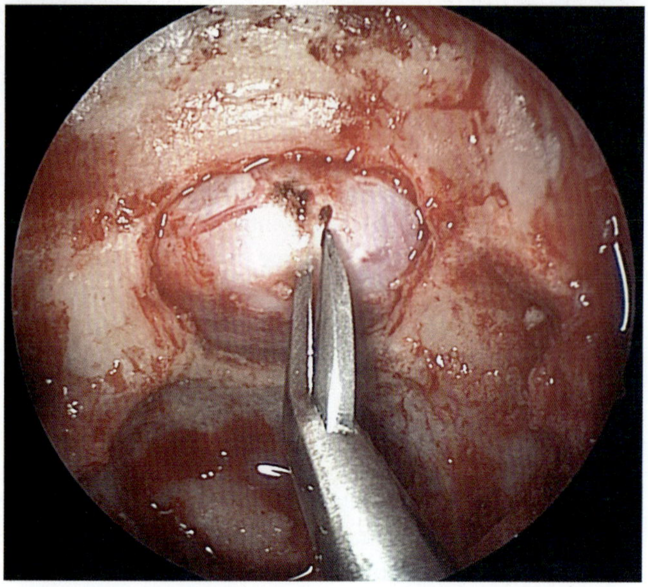

Fig. 2.20 Dura over the sella is incised.

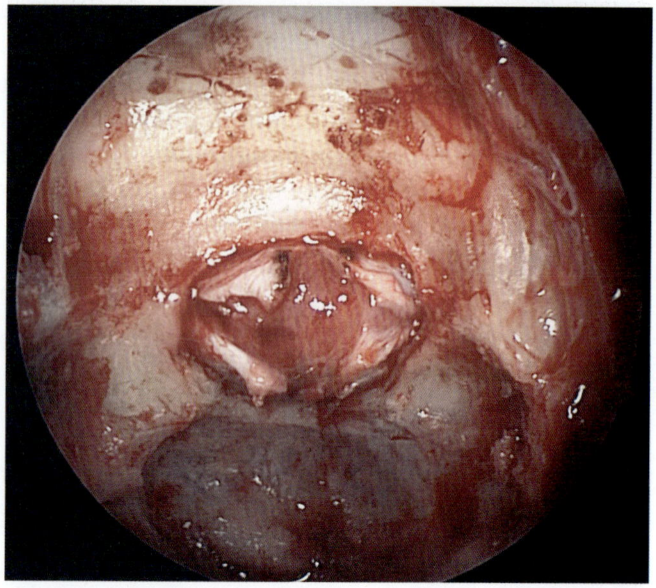

Fig. 2.21 The pituitary adenoma is seen on incising and reflecting the dural flaps.

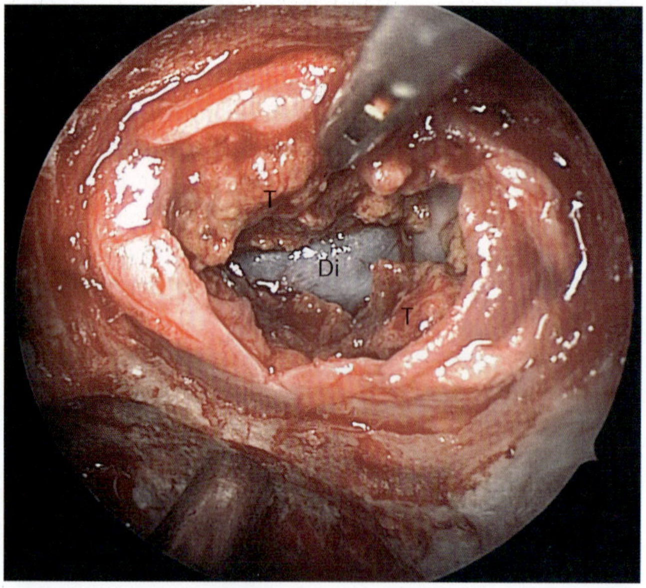

Fig. 2.22 Pituitary adenoma is partially debulked. The diaphragm is seen posteriorly.

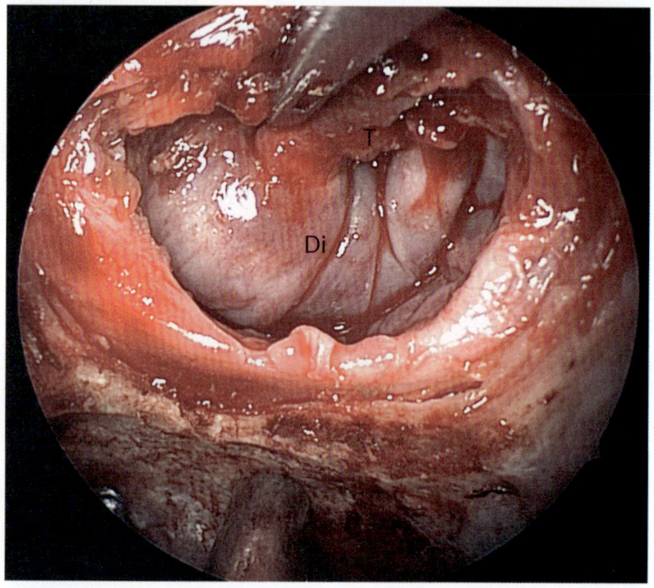

Fig. 2.23 The diaphragm is seen more prominently falling into the sella when tumor is removed.

completely excising the superior part to prevent diaphragm from prolapsing and obscuring the field. On removal of tumor, the diaphragm prolapses into the sellar cavity (**Fig. 2.23**). A cotton patty is used to lift the diaphragm and once again look into the lateral gutters for complete clearance of the tumor (**Fig. 2.24**). Herein lies the biggest advantage of the endoscope to look into the sellar cavity and confirm clearance of the tumor. The pituitary gland location relative to the tumor is identified on the preoperative scans, and inadvertent injury to the gland is avoided during surgery.

15. Hemostasis is confirmed.
16. In case there is no CSF leak, we use a small piece of vomer to seal the anterior face of sella (**Fig. 2.25**).
17. In case of CSF leakage, fat is packed into the sellar cavity (**Fig. 2.26**) and a Hadad-Bassagasteguy pedicled nasoseptal flap is used to cover the whole area (**Fig. 2.27**). Tissue glue is used at the periphery of the flap. Care is taken that the pedicled flap rests on bone

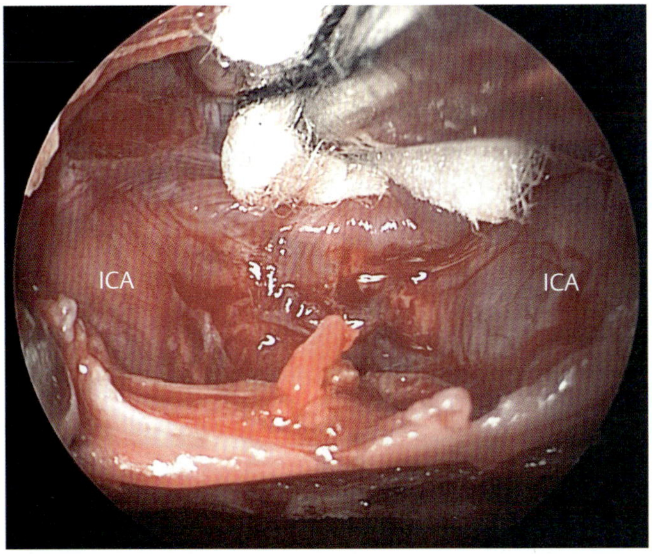

Fig. 2.24 A cotton patty is used to retract the diaphragm gently and look into the lateral gutters of the sella. ICA, internal carotid artery.

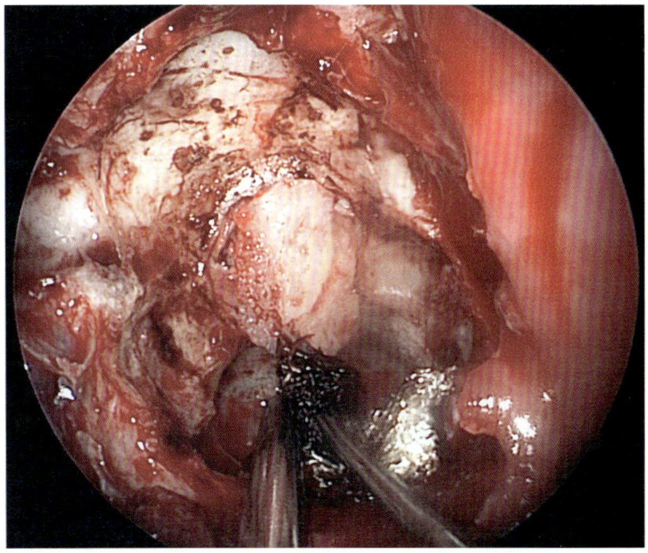

Fig. 2.25 A piece of vomer is used to close the anterior face of sella.

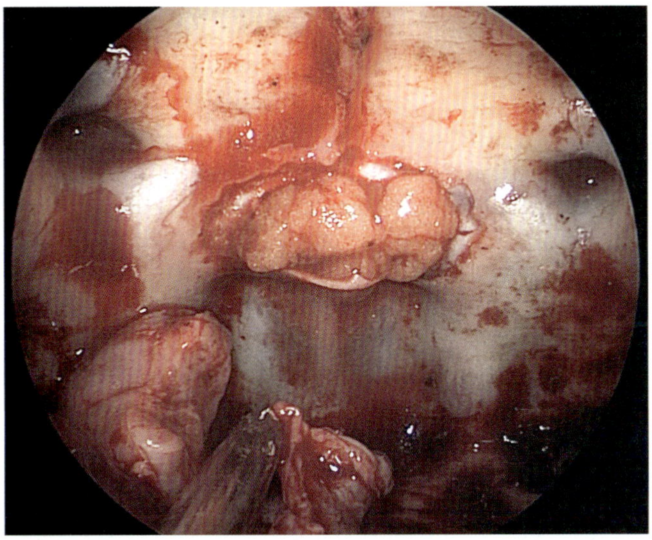

Fig. 2.26 Fat used to seal the sellar cavity in case of CSF leak.

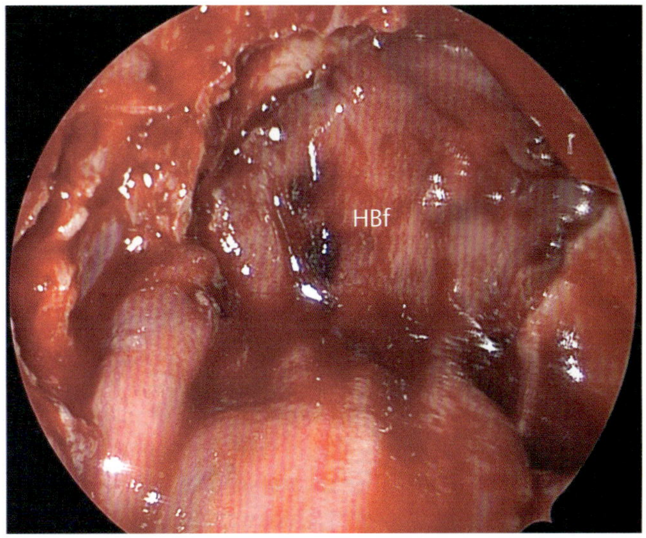

Fig. 2.27 Pedicled nasoseptal flap is used to cover the operative site.

all around, and there should not be any material interposed between the flap and bone.

18. In cases where a Hadad-Bassagasteguy flap has been harvested, we harvest a reverse flap to cover the donor site of septum. Details of reverse flap are described in Chapter 36.
19. We do not routinely use lumbar drains.

Extensions of the Approach

1. In pituitary adenomas with a large suprasellar extension/giant pituitary adenomas, fibrous tumors or dumbbell-shaped tumors, the extended approach, endoscopic transsellar transtubercular approach, is used.[6,7,8,9,10,11] This allows the tumor neck to free up allowing subsequent descent of the tumor into the sellar cavity as excision proceeds.
2. In pituitary adenomas with a large frontal extension, the bone over the tuberculum as also the planum is drilled off to gain access to the superior pole of the tumor.
3. This approach is useful to clear pituitary adenomas from medial cavernous sinus[12,13,14,15] (**Fig. 2.28a, b**). However, access to the lateral cavernous sinus is

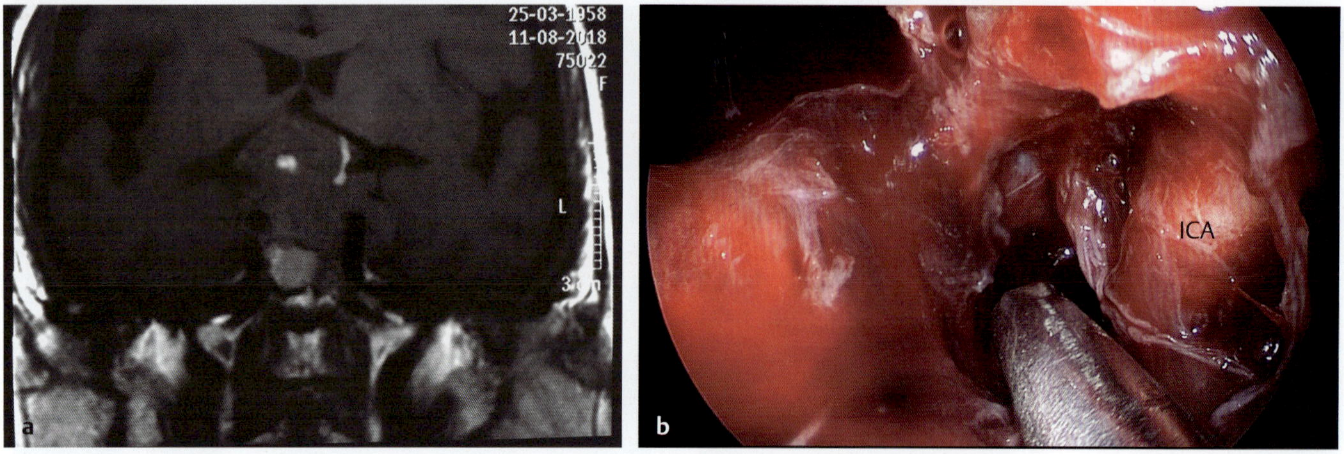

Fig. 2.28 **(a)** Preoperative MRI showing tumor extension into the left cavernous sinus. **(b)** The tumor has been cleared from medial cavernous sinus, both, anterior and posterior to the left internal carotid artery

obtained by doing a transpterygoid approach.[16] We avoid surgery on the lateral cavernous sinus in nonfunctional tumors.

Tips and Pearls

- It is essential to plan reconstruction preoperatively. Pedicle of Hadad-Bassagasteguy nasoseptal flap is preserved carefully in all cases.
- It is advisable to always have a maximal approach for even small tumors, that is, maximal exposure for four-hand technique, maximal widening of sphenoid cavity to visualize area lateral to the internal carotid artery (ICA) on both sides, good visualization of planum and sphenoid floor. There should be a wide opening of the sellar bone to visualize cavernous blue laterally, superior and inferior intercavernous sinuses, respectively. Similarly, dural opening should be wide, that is, up to bony sellar opening so that visualization into sellar cavity is not hampered.
- Although we prefer intracapsular removal of tumor, it is also feasible to perform extracapsular excision of tumor in experienced hands. Care is to be taken not to injure the pituitary gland.
- Use of intraoperative navigation and intraoperative MRI are very useful to ensure complete tumor excision (especially so in functional tumors). Similarly, intraoperative Doppler is extremely useful to locate the position of IC•

4. Preservation of olfaction and prevention of crusting (by preserving mucosa) help improve the postoperative quality of life scores.

References

1. Jho HD, Carrau RL. Endoscopic endonasal transsphenoidal surgery: experience with 50 patients. J Neurosurg 1997; 87:44–51
2. Cappabianca P, Cavallo LM, Colao A, et al. Endoscopic endonasal transsphenoidal approach: outcome analysis of 100 consecutive procedures. Minim Invasive Neurosurg 2002;45: 193–200
3. Schwartz TH, Anand VK. The endoscopic, endonasal transsphenoidal approach to the sella. In: Anand VK, Schwartz TH, eds. Practical Endoscopic Skull Base Surgery. San Diego, CA: Plural Publishing; 2007:89–104
4. Cappabianca P, Cavallo LM, de Divitiis O, Solari D, Esposito F, Colao A. Endoscopic pituitary surgery. Pituitary 2008;11(4): 385–390
5. Dehdashti AR, Gentili F. Current state of the art in the diagnosis and surgical treatment of Cushing disease: early experience with a purely endoscopic endonasal technique. Neurosurg Focus 2007;23:E9
6. Elshazly K, Kshetry VR, Farrell CJ, Nyquist G, Rosen M, Evans JJ. Clinical outcomes after endoscopic endonasal resection of giant pituitary adenomas. World Neurosurg 2018;114: 447–456
7. Yano S, Hide T, Shinojima N. Efficacy and complications of endoscopic skull base surgery for giant pituitary adenomas. World Neurosurg 2017;99:533–542
8. Cappabianca P, Cavallo LM, de Divitiis O, de Angelis M, Chiaramonte C, Solari D. Endoscopic endonasal extended approaches for the management of large pituitary adenomas. Neurosurg Clin N Am 2015;26(3):323–331

9. Koutourousiou M, Gardner PA, Fernandez-Miranda JC, Paluzzi A, Wang EW, Snyderman CH. Endoscopic endonasal surgery for giant pituitary adenomas: advantages and limitations. J Neurosurg 2013;118(3):621–631

10. Sankhla SK, Jayashankar N, Khan GM. Surgical management of selected pituitary macroadenomas using extended endoscopic endonasal transsphenoidal approach: early experience. Neurol India 2013;61(2):122–130

11. Komotar RJ, Starke RM, Raper DM, Anand VK, Schwartz TH. Endoscopic endonasal compared with microscopic transsphenoidal and open transcranial resection of giant pituitary adenomas. Pituitary 2012;15(2):150–159

12. Knosp E, Kitz K, Steiner E, Matula C. Pituitary adenomas with parasellar invasion. Acta Neurochir Suppl (Wien). 1991;53: 65–71

13. Ceylan S, Koc K, Anik I. Endoscopic endonasal transsphenoidal approach for pituitary adenomas invading the cavernous sinus. J Neurosurg 2010;112(1):99–107

14. Micko AS, Wöhrer A, Wolfsberger S, Knosp E. Invasion of the cavernous sinus space in pituitary adenomas: endoscopic verification and its correlation with an MRI-based classification. J Neurosurg 2015;122(4):803–811

15. Paluzzi A, Fernandez-Miranda JC, Tonya Stefko S, Challinor S, Snyderman CH, Gardner PA. Endoscopic endonasal approach for pituitary adenomas: a series of 555 patients. Pituitary 2014;17(4):307–319

16. Hardesty DA, Montaser AS, Carrau RL, Prevedello DM. Limits of endoscopic endonasal transpterygoid approach to cavernous sinus and Meckel's cave. J Neurosurg Sci 2018;62(3):332–338

Chapter 3 Endoscopic Endonasal Surgeries for Pituitary Macroadenoma

Case 3A

Single Nostril Endoscopic Transseptal Transsphenoidal Approach for a Pituitary Macroadenoma

Adzreil Bakri, Michel Roethlisberger, Prepageran Narayanan, and Vicknes Waran

History

A 35-year-old lady presented with a 6-month history of headache and a 2-week history of blurry vision. Ophthalmological examination revealed bitemporal hemianopia with normal visual acuity. A magnetic resonance imaging (MRI) of the brain revealed a pituitary macroadenoma measuring 20 × 19 mm (**Fig. 3A.1**). A *single nostril endoscopic transseptal transsphenoidal excision* of the tumor was planned with intraoperative MRI (iMRI) for the extent of resection control.

Surgical Steps

1. *Single nostril approach:* Local anesthetics and adrenaline (1:10000 units) are infiltrated into the septum (**Fig. 3A.2**).
2. The septum is then incised with a size 15 blade on one side, and the mucoperichondrial flap is raised posteriorly until the choana is reached (**Fig. 3A.3**).
3. Through the same septal incision, the cartilaginous septum is incised, and a mucoperichondrial flap is raised on the opposite side (**Fig. 3A.4**).
4. The cartilaginous and bony septum are removed until the sphenoid keel is exposed.
5. Suction monopolar cautery is used to remove any residual mucosa covering bilateral sphenoid ostia.
6. The bilateral sphenoid ostia are widened inferomedially in a V shape with a Kerrison punch, and once the bony removal is sufficient, the sphenoid keel is then removed with a pituitary rongeur forceps (**Fig. 3A.5**).
7. After removal of the sphenoid keel, any residual mucosa or bony septations is removed to make the bilateral sphenoid sinus a single common cavity. Attention must be given to critical neurovascular structures underlying a thin bone coverage or even dehiscence of the structures when cauterizing the sphenoid mucosa. Care must be taken when removing sphenoid septae. When these structures are cracked rather than drilled or punched, the risk for indirect damage of neurovascular structures is higher (**Fig. 3A.6**).
8. *Transsellar approach:* Prior to the removal of the bone overlying the sella, the exact location of the tumor has to be confirmed using image-guided surgery (IGS). Laterality, planum sphenoidale and the floor of the sella are important landmarks. Besides IGS, the midline can be estimated using landmarks such as the bilateral opticocarotid recesses, the paraclival carotid arteries, and the floor of the remaining sphenoid keel. Anatomical variations and asymmetries have to be considered when assessing the midline without neuronavigation.
9. The bone overlying this area is then thinned out with a drill or curette. Alternatively, a small opening into the sella using a small chisel is possible. Generally, drilling and punching is performed from medial to lateral to avoid injury of the carotid siphons of the cavernous sinuses bilaterally (**Fig. 3A.7**).
10. Once a window is made, a right-angle dissector can be inserted to separate the bone and the underlying dura (**Fig. 3A.8**).
11. This bony opening is then widened adequately in the shape of a rectangle using a Kerrison punch (**Fig. 3A.9**).
12. After adequate exposure, a cruciate incision is made on the dura with a size 15 blade (**Fig. 3A.10**, **Fig. 3A.11**, and **Fig. 3A.12**).
13. Using suction and a blunt ring curette, the tumor is debulked along the sellar floor with curettage (central pillar) to the back side of the sella (clival bone). The resection is then widened to the lateral pillars (left and right sides) with gentle suction and curetting along the cavernous sinus wall. The cavernous carotid artery might be palpable.

14. In invasive cases, the cavernous sinus wall can be missing. This has to be appreciated when assessing preoperative imaging.
15. When the lower pillars of the tumor are removed, the apical parts of the tumor are resected, and these are gently dissected from the normal pituitary gland tissue and the diaphragma sellae (**Fig. 3A.13**).
16. The diaphragma sellae prolapses into the resection cavity. The appearance of the symmetric "frog bladder" is a sign of complete removal. The normal gland can be appreciated and preserved (**Fig. 3A.14**).
17. The extent of resection is then controlled using iMRI (**Fig. 3A.15**).
18. The small skull base defect is closed with Surgicel (oxidized cellulose polymer), and the sphenoid sinus is filled with Gelfoam (absorbable gelatin sponge; **Fig. 3A.16**).
19. Both septal flaps are approximated in the midline, and the septal incision is covered with Nasopore (synthetic biodegradable foam) while making sure that adequate airway along the nasal floor is provided (**Fig. 3A.17**).

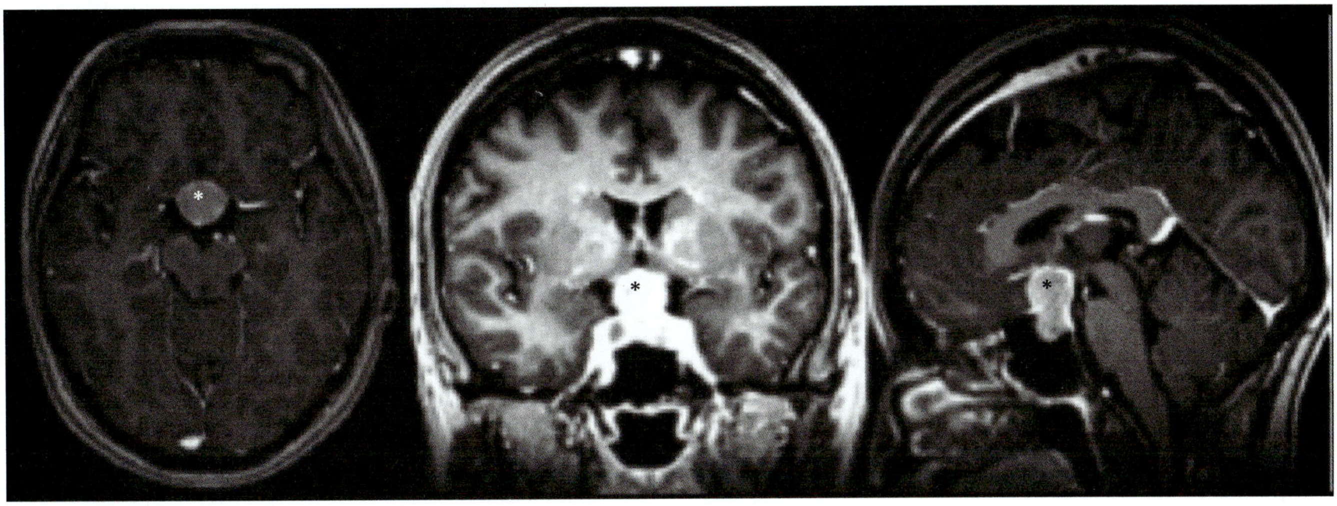

Fig. 3A.1 Preoperative T1-weighted gadolinium contrast-enhanced MRI sections demonstrating a 20 × 19 × 18 mm isointense intrasellar mass (*) with moderate homogenous enhancement along with areas of signal shortening, suggestive for microhemorrhage or necrosis. The pituitary gland is present with slightly more enhancement and is displaced posterosuperiorly. There is compression of the optic chiasm and both optic nerves. Left: Axial section. Middle: Coronal section. Right: Sagittal section.

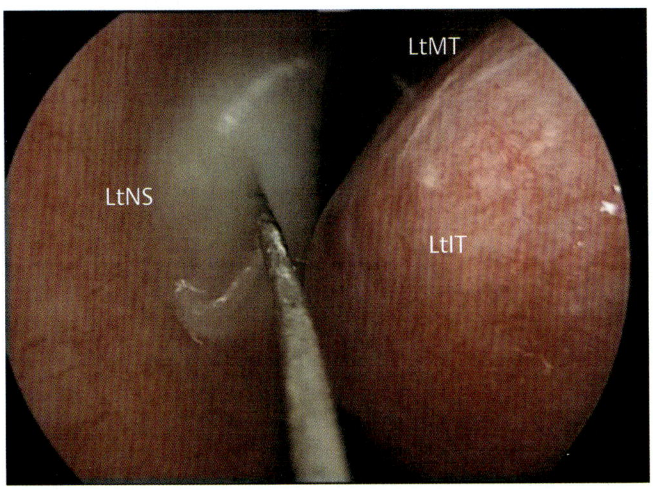

Fig. 3A.2 Local anesthesia infiltration into the nasal septum of the left nasal cavity.

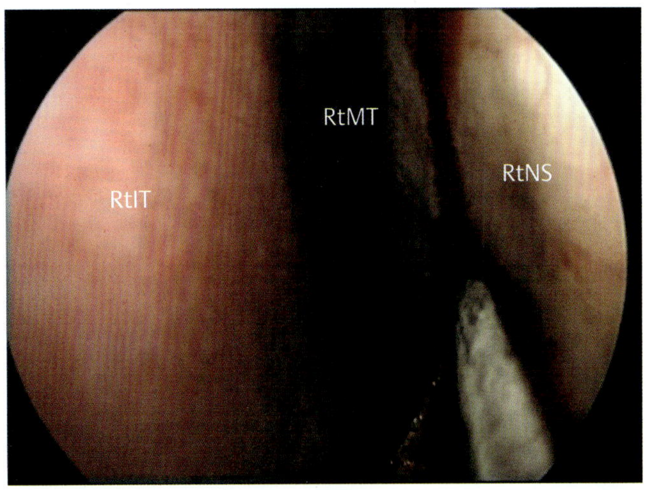

Fig. 3A.3 Incision on the nasal septum of the right nasal cavity opposite to the anterior part of the middle turbinate.

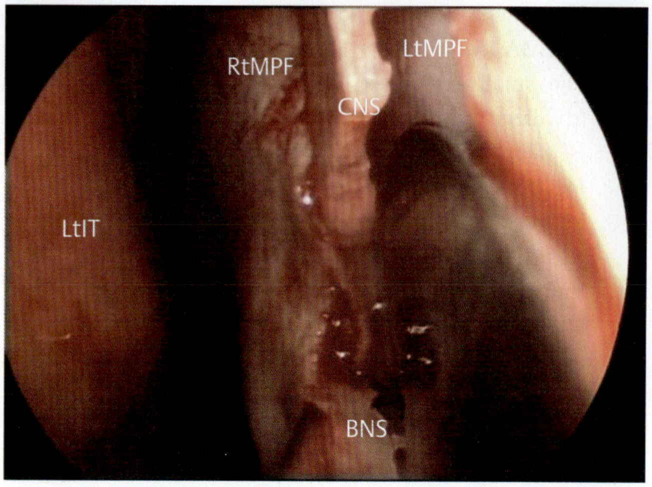

Fig. 3A.4 Raising of bilateral mucoperichondrial flaps and removal of the cartilaginous and bony septum.

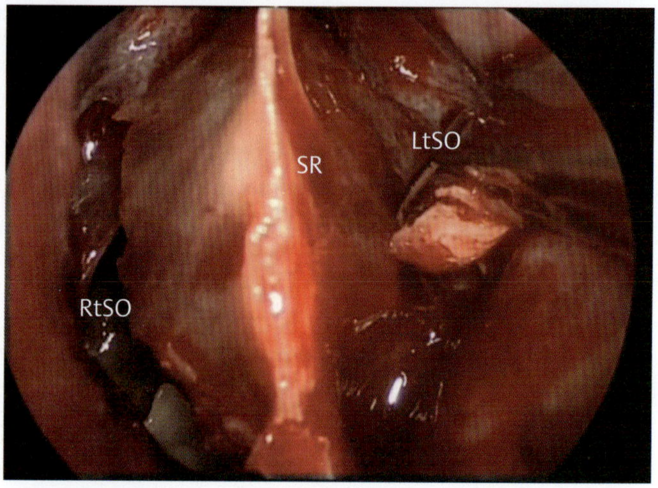

Fig. 3A.5 Exposure and removal of the sphenoid rostrum (SR).

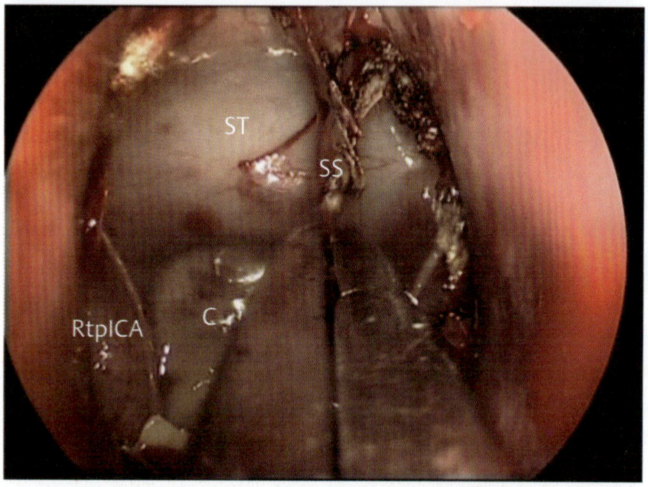

Fig. 3A.6 Removal of residual mucosa and bony septations creating a single large sphenoid cavity.

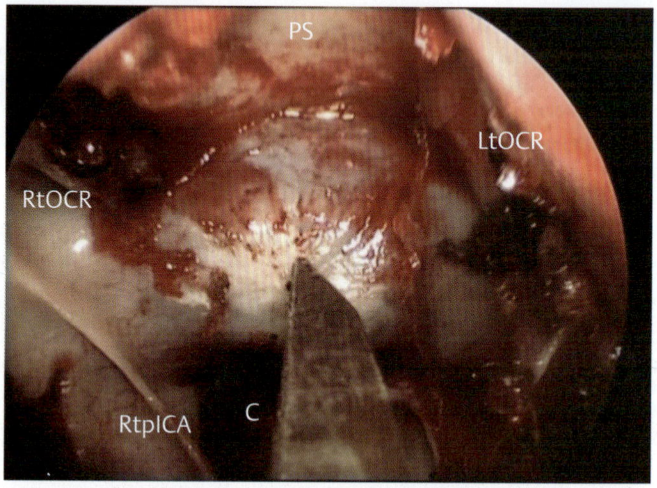

Fig. 3A.7 Transsellar approach: The bone overlying the sella is gently chiseled to create a small opening.

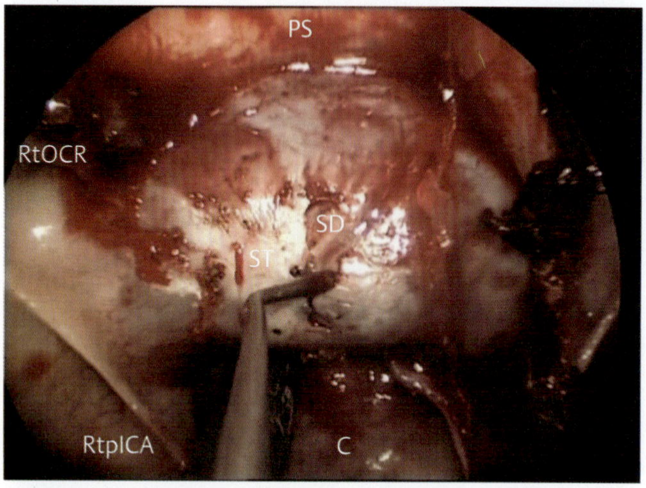

Fig. 3A.8 A right-angle dissector is insinuated between the bone and the underlying dura.

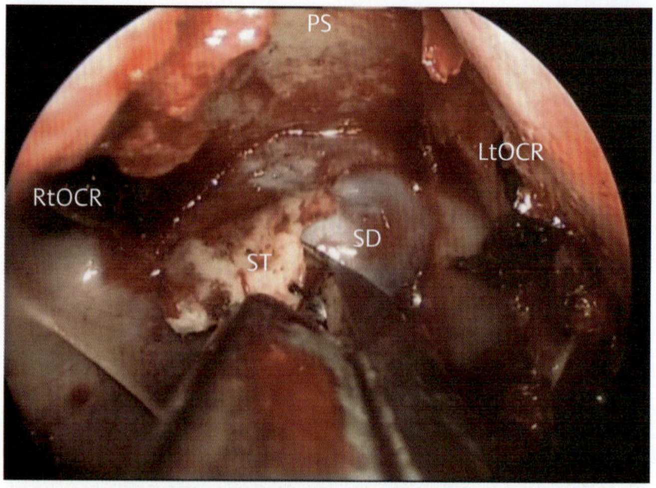

Fig. 3A.9 The bony opening is widened using a Kerrison punch.

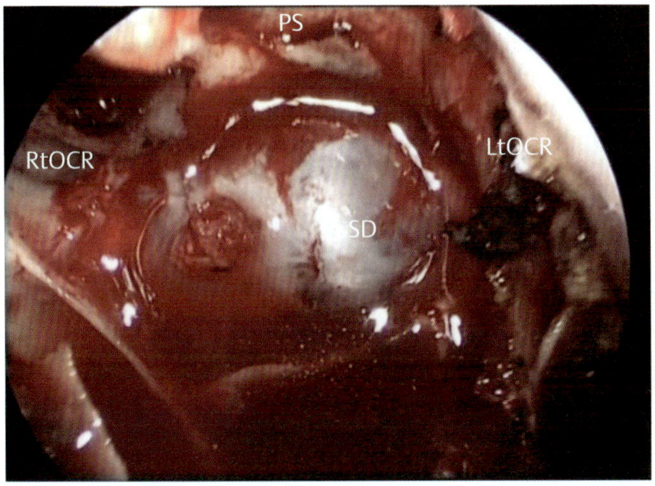

Fig. 3A.10 Transsellar approach: adequate bony removal for the exposure of tumor.

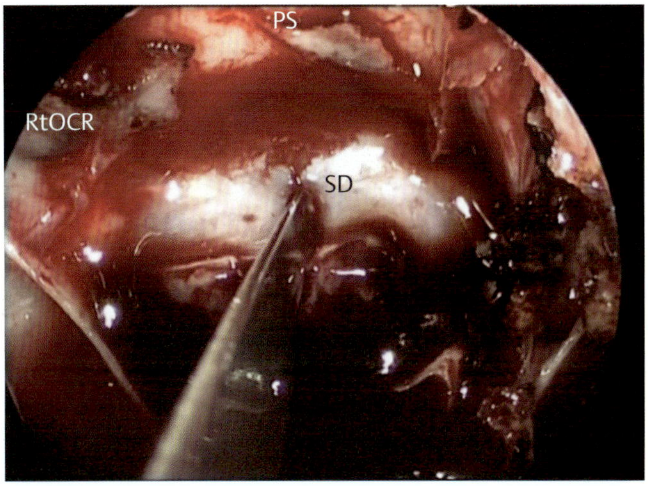

Fig. 3A.11 Cruciate incision of the sellar dura.

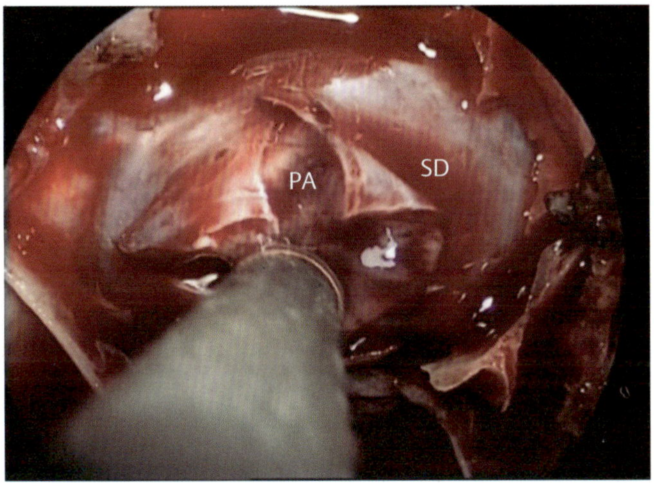

Fig. 3A.12 Blunt dissection and removal of the tumor using suction.

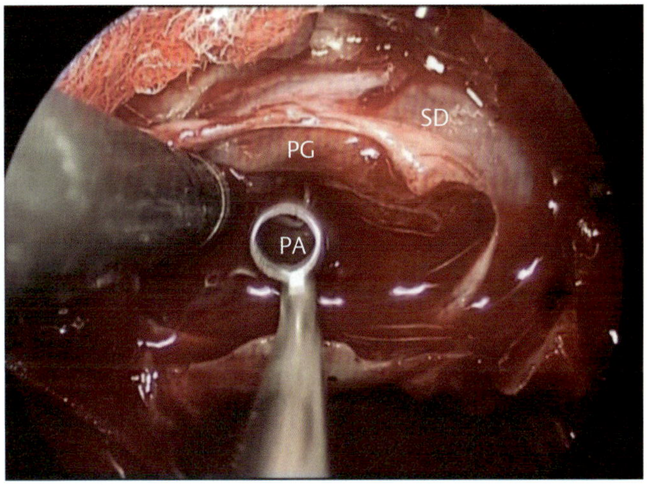

Fig. 3A.13 Removal of the tumor using a blunt ring curette.

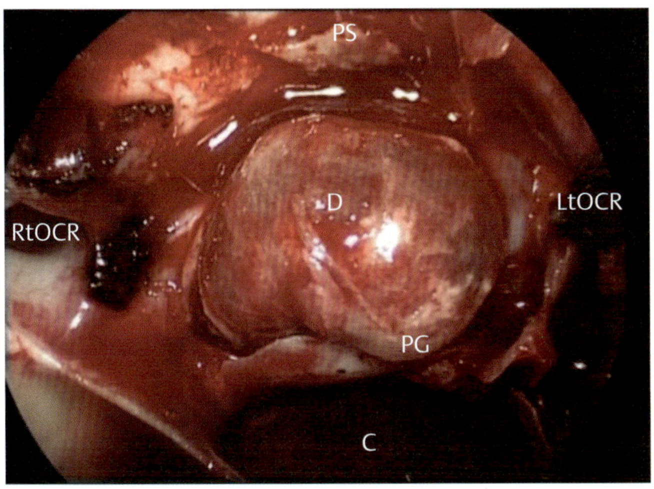

Fig. 3A.14 Final view of the prolapsed diaphragma sellae after complete tumor removal.

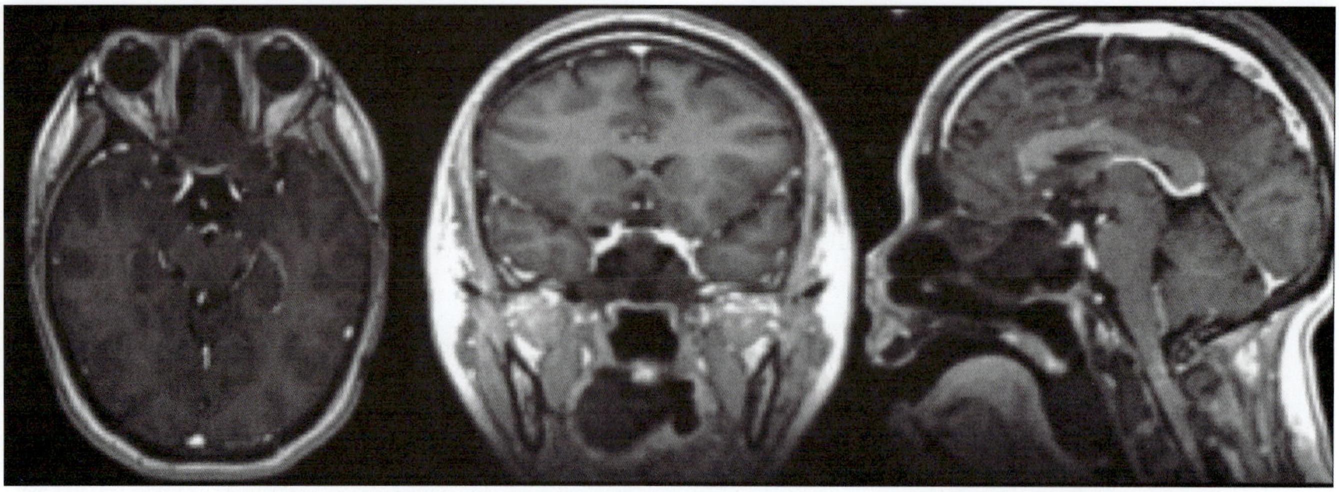

Fig. 3A.15 Intraoperative MRI for resection control demonstrating complete removal of the lesion without residual tumor.

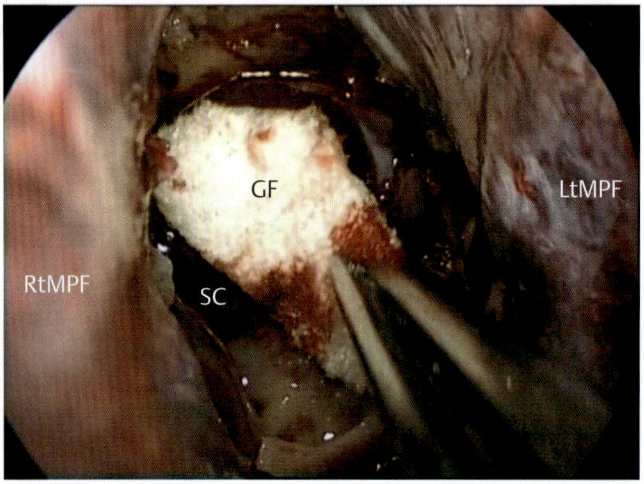

Fig. 3A.16 Skullbase defect closure: the sphenoid cavity is packed with layers of Gelfoam (gelatin sponge).

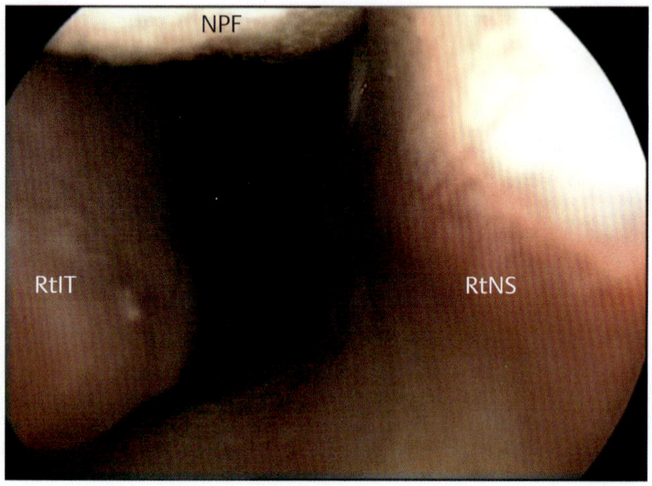

Fig. 3A.17 Closure of septal incision and nasal packing with a synthetic biodegradable foam providing adequate nasal airway along the floor of the nose.

Case 3B

Extended Endoscopic Transseptal Transsphenoidal Transplanum (Single Nostril) Excision of a Pituitary Macroadenoma

Kong Yew Liew, Michel Roethlisberger, Adzreil Bakri, Saif Al-Zahid, Prepageran Narayanan, and Vicknes Waran

History

A 46-year-old man was referred with a prolonged history of fatigue and reduced libido. An endocrinological work-up revealed low blood testosterone values. Accordingly, bitemporal hemianopia was documented using a Goldman perimetry. Neurocranial imaging confirmed a pituitary macroadenoma with compression of the optic chiasm and dislocation of the pituitary gland and infundibular stalk.

To account for the superior extension of the lesion, an endonasal endoscopic mononostril approach with expansion of the sellar opening to the planum sphenoidale was planned.

Surgical Steps

1. Local anesthesia is infiltrated into the septum to raise the mucoperichondrial flaps bilaterally in preparation for the creation of the pedicled nasoseptal flaps.
2. An incision is made with a no. 15 blade anterior to the middle turbinate down to the cartilaginous septum.
3. The nasoseptal flap is then raised off the septum with a Freer elevator posteriorly until the sphenoid ostia and posterior choana are visible. Superiorly, the flap may be taken until about 0.5 to 1 cm below the skull base to preserve the olfactory function. Inferiorly, the flap can be taken as far as half the nasal floor if a large skull base defect is expected.
4. The nasoseptal flap is then freed with a microscissors superiorly and inferiorly aiming for the sphenoid ostia and posterior choana, respectively.
5. The pedicled flap can then be stored in the nasopharynx until reconstruction is required.
6. The exposed cartilaginous septum is fractured through to the contralateral side and removed by piecemeal, all the while freeing it from the overlying contralateral septal mucoperichondrium.
7. This is continued until the sphenoid keel is exposed with the sphenoid ostia visible bilaterally.
8. At this point, the contralateral nasoseptal flap can be created in the same manner as in steps 6 and 7.
9. Once the sphenoid keel is fully exposed, the ostia are widened inferomedially using a Kerrison punch in a V shape toward the midline.
10. Using the Kerrison punch, the ostia are then widened medially toward the midline, and the keel is removed with a pituitary rongeur forceps.
11. Remnant sphenoid keel and sphenoid sinus septations are then removed to allow an unobstructed view.
12. The posterior wall of the sphenoid sinus is demucosalized with a monopolar cautery tipped aspirator. This allows for drilling of the sella and tuberculum and prevents oozing from mucosal edges. Care has to be taken laterally as there may be dehiscence of the optic nerve or carotid artery, which should be identified by inspection of the sphenoid sinus prior to commencement.
13. Transsellar approach: Drilling is then commenced with a diamond burr to thin the bone overlying the sella and tuberculum (**Fig. 3B.1**). An aspirator is kept within the nasal cavity to allow clearance of bone dust and smoke for an unobstructed view.
14. Once the bone has been sufficiently thinned, a right-angle dissector can be insinuated between the bone and the dura, and the bone is flaked off.
15. After enough bone has been removed, the exposure can be completed with a Kerrison punch. The use of a Kerrison punch allows for a better control during bone removal. The exposure should be extended laterally until the cavernous sinuses are visible. The superior and inferior extents of the exposure are dictated by the size of the lesion and can be confirmed with IGS (**Fig. 3B.2**).
16. Transtuberculum and trans-planum approach: expansions of the exposure by removing the bone covering the tuberculum sellae and the planum sphenoidale. (**Fig. 3B.3**).
17. The dura of the planum sphenoidale is then incised horizontally (**Fig. 3B.4**).
18. The underlying tissue is freed with a right-angle dissector.
19. A second horizontal incision is then made over the sella turcica to expand the access. The two incisions are joined vertically (**Fig. 3B.5**).
20. The overlying dura is freed from underlying tissue, and the two horizontal incisions are joined with a vertical incision, that is brought to the border of the anterior intercavernous sinus.

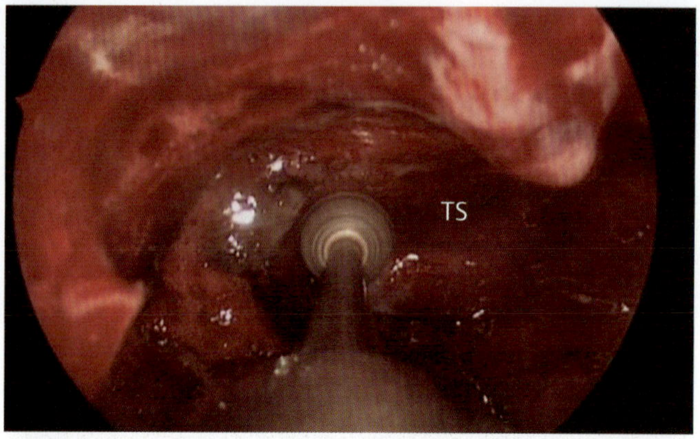

Fig. 3B.1 Transtuberculum approach: Drilling and thinning of the tuberculum sellae prior to bone removal.

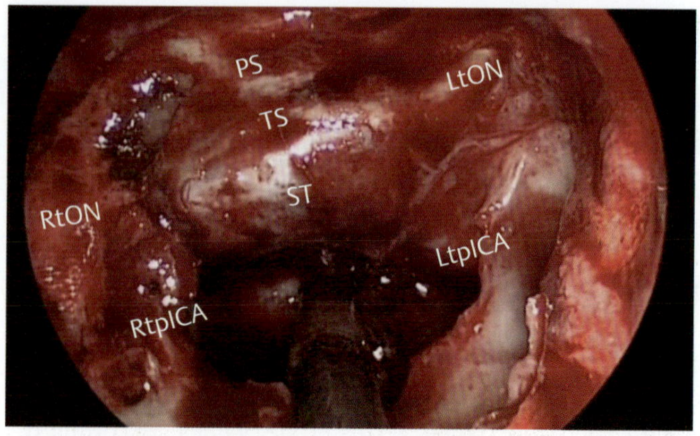

Fig. 3B.2 Panoramic view of the exposed dura of the sella turcica (ST), tuberculum sellae (TS), and planum sphenoidale (PS) after removal of the bony coverage.

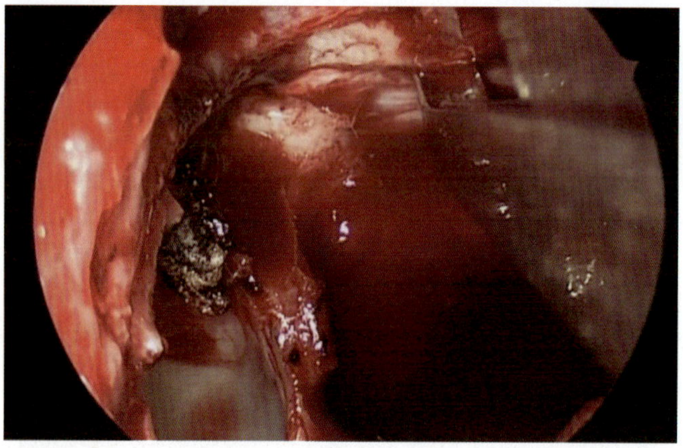

Fig. 3B.3 Transplanum approach: Bone removal from the planum sphenoidale using a Kerrison punch insinuated between the bone and the dura.

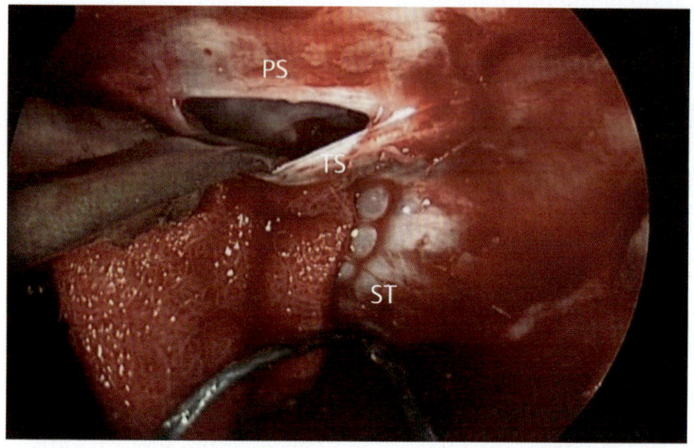

Fig. 3B.4 Horizontal dural incision between the planum sphenoidale (PS) and tuberculum sellae (TS).

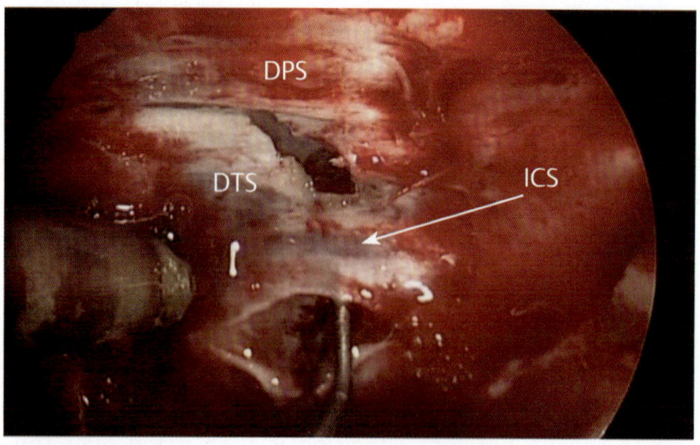

Fig. 3B.5 After a second horizontal incision over the sella turcica, a right-angle dissector is used to free the overlying dura prior to the vertical incision. The translucent dura shows the dissector just inferior to the anterior intercavernous sinus (ICS). Tumour tissue is noted through the inferior horizontal incision. The vertical incision is brought posteriorly to the ICS.

21. The anterior intercavernous sinus is freed from the underlying tissue, grasped with bipolar cautery and cauterized along its length (**Fig. 3B.6**).
22. The anterior intercavernous sinus can then be divided sharply using microscissors (**Fig. 3B.7**).
23. Initial excision of the central tumor compartment allows for a better visualization of the lateral compartments and facilitates central collapse. Thus, the lateral aspects of the tumor are easier to remove (**Fig. 3B.8**).
24. Once the central component has been debulked, the lateral and inferior edges are debulked with a ring curette in a similar fashion.
25. As the tumor collapses inward, the lateral and superior compartments are debulked until the tumor capsule is reached. Following the tumor capsule, an arachnoid plane can be identified and slightly peeled laterally with a dissector.
26. With the central, inferior, and lateral parts of the tumor removed, the superior component is addressed.

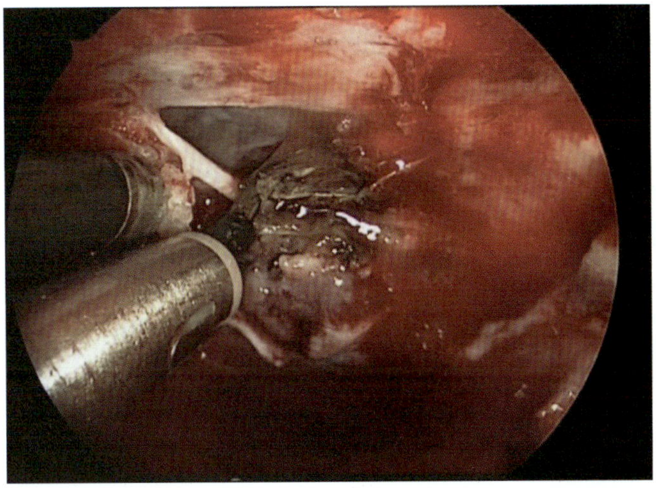

Fig. 3B.6 Bipolar cautery of the anterior intercavernous sinus.

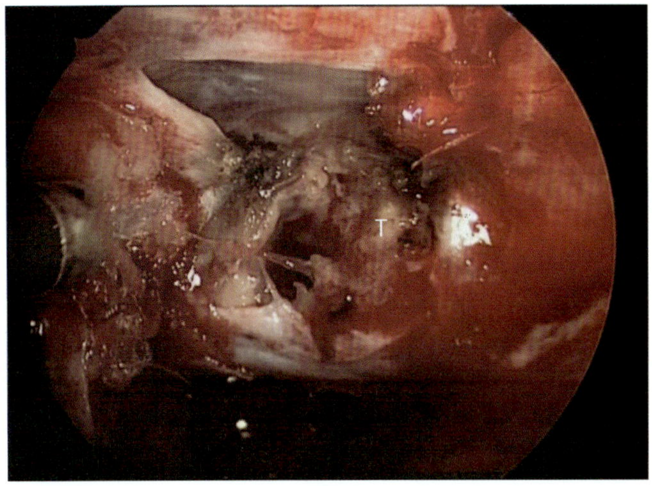

Fig. 3B.7 The tumor (T) is exposed after sharp division of the anterior intercavernous sinus.

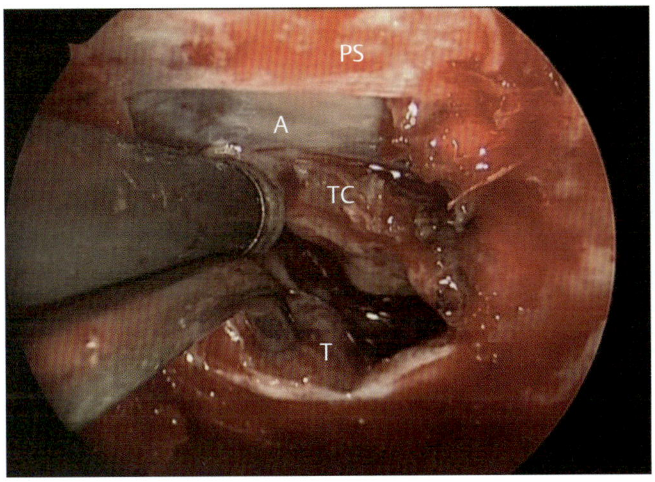

Fig. 3B.8 A ring curette delivering tumor (T) from the right side of the cavity to the central zone.

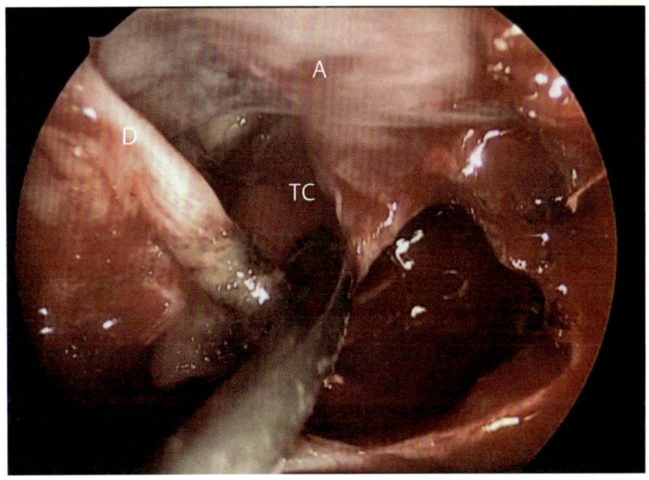

Fig. 3B.9 The superior tumor capsule (TC) is dissected off the arachnoid plane (A) with caution to not inadvertently harm an overlying arterial vessel.

The arachnoid mater is retracted superiorly to visualize the superior compartment, which is then dissected gradually and brought inferiorly into the central zone with a combination of aspiration and blunt dissection (**Fig. 3B.9**).

27. Tumor debulking is then carried superiorly to deliver the tumor centrally with a combination of ring curette and aspiration (**Fig. 3B.10**).
28. Meticulous hemostasis is achieved with neuropatties and absorbable hemostats. The cavity is then inspected for remnant tumor.
29. The defect is reconstructed with an abdominal fat graft. The graft is placed intracranially to ensure a watertight seal without causing compression to the underlying physiological structures (**Fig. 3B.11**).
30. The repair is then reinforced with an absorbable followed by a synthetic dural sealant. A pedicled nasoseptal flap may be used to further strengthen the repair at this step if desired.
31. The construct is again covered with an absorbable hemostat, and absorbable gelatin sponges are packed within the sphenoid cavity to complete the repair.
32. An intraoperative magnetic resonance imaging (MRI) is performed to confirm tumor clearance prior to reconstruction and closure (**Fig. 3B.12**).

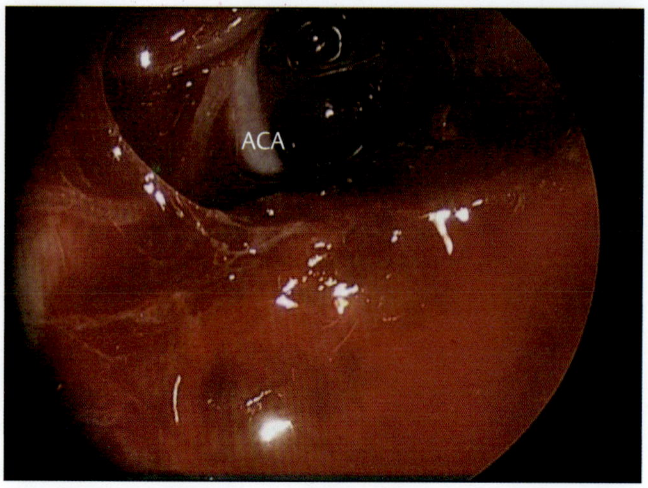

Fig. 3B.10 Superior margin clearance with a view of the right anterior cerebral artery (ACA).

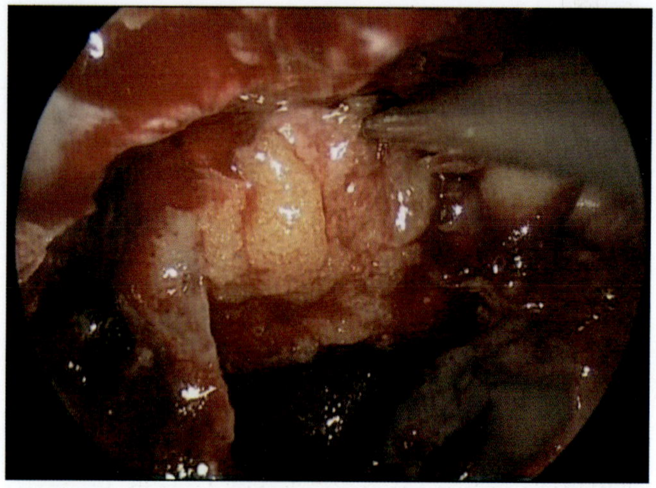

Fig. 3B.11 Abdominal fat graft being tucked under the edges of the skullbase defect to achieve a watertight closure.

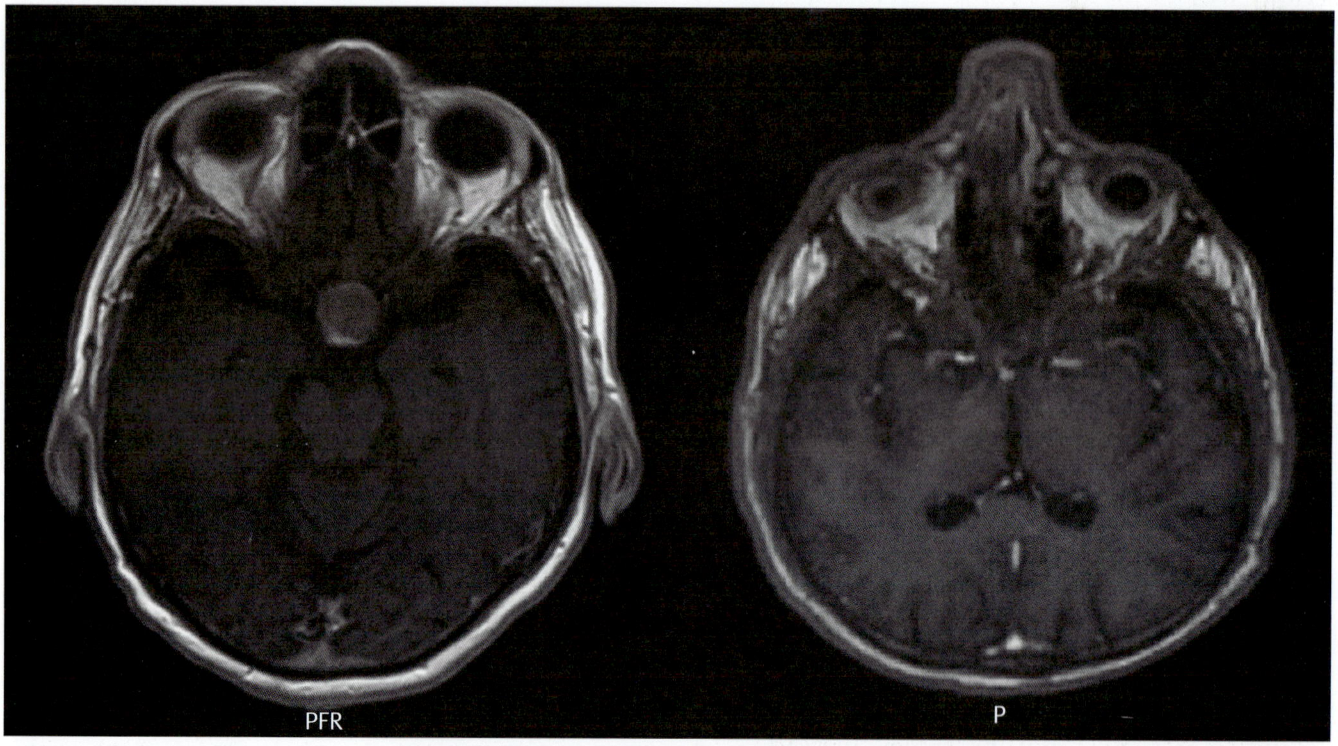

Fig. 3B.12 A comparison between the preoperative axial MRI (*left*) and the intraoperative postcontrast T1-weighted axial MRI (*right*) showing complete removal of the tumor.

Case 3C

Endoscopic Transseptal Transsphenoidal Excision of a Pituitary Macroadenoma with Left Anterior Cerebral Artery Involvement

Michel Roethlisberger, Kong Yew Liew, Adzreil Bakri, Prepageran Narayanan, and Vicknes Waran

History

A 76-year-old man with a known history of hypertension, diabetes mellitus, and chronic airway obstruction disease underwent resection of a urinary bladder carcinoma with adjuvant chemotherapy 7 years ago. He also has documented blindness of the right eye for 5 years and a cataract in the left eye. He presented with hoarseness of his voice for 3 months. Clinical examination revealed a right vocal cord palsy. As part of an investigation for the vocal cord palsy, a neurocranial magnetic resonance imaging (MRI) was performed, and, incidentally, an extensive pituitary mass was seen on the scan with extensive suprasellar component and lateral extension above and beyond the plane of the internal carotid artery on the right side (**Fig. 3C.1a–c**). Endocrinological blood investigations confirmed reduced levels of gonadotropins, thyroid hormones, and cortisol.

Surgical Steps

1. A **binostril transnasal transseptal transsphenoidal approach** is performed as previously described (refer to **Chapter 1**), and the sphenoid cavity is exposed.
2. The posterior wall of the sphenoid sinus is then demucosalized with a monopolar-cautery–tipped aspirator. This allows for the drilling of the sella turcica and tuberculum sellae and prevents oozing from the mucosal edges. Care has to be taken laterally as there may be dehiscence of the optic nerve or the carotid arteries. These landmarks have to be identified prior to commencement of the osteo-dural exposure.
3. **Transsellar and transtuberculum approach:** The bone overlying the sella turcica and the tuberculum sellae is then thinned out using a diamond high speed drill. An aspirator is kept within the nasal cavity to clear bone dust and smoke to allow for an unobstructed view.
4. Once the bone has been sufficiently thinned out, a right-angle dissector can be insinuated between the bone and the dura, and the bone is flaked off.
5. After enough bone has been removed, the osteodural exposure can be completed with a Kerrison punch. This allows for better control while removing the bone covering the skullbase. The anterior and posterior as well as lateral limitations of the exposure are dictated by the size of the lesion and can be confirmed using IGS. (**Fig. 3C.2**).
6. The sellar dura is opened horizontally over the capsule of the lesion and then extended superiorly with microscissors after freeing the underlying tissue using a right-angle dissector (**Fig. 3C.3**).
7. A ring curette is then used to debulk the lesion in a zonal manner, focusing on the central inferior compartment first, followed by the right and left inferior lateral compartments (lateral pillars), along the dura of the cavernous sinus. The loose tumor is cleared with an aspirator.
8. The additional space gained within the inferior resection cavity will allow for the lesion to be pushed downward and delivered inferiorly, away from the neurovascular structures (**Fig. 3C.4**).
9. To expose the superior compartment of the lesion along its entire length, the dura of the planum sphenoidale close to the tuberculum sellae is incised horizontally with a microblade in a further step (**Fig. 3C.5**).
10. The dura is freed from the underlying tissue with a right-angle dissector (**Fig. 3C.6**).
11. The dura is then incised vertically with microscissors in a T-shaped manner (**Fig. 3C.7**).
12. The anterior intercavernous sinus is defined and dissected with a right-angle dissector, controlled with bipolar cautery, and divided using microscissors to expose the entire lesion (**Fig. 3C.8**).
13. The debulking of the superior tumor compartment is continued with aspirators clearing the tumor, going from inferior to superior. Parts of the lesion that are slightly more lateral can be aspirated with an olive-tipped 'J' aspirator (**Fig. 3C.9**).
14. Due to the extended transplanum and transtuberculum approach, the superior component of the pituitary adenoma can be dissected in an extracapsular manner along the arachnoid plane. It can be removed after defining the neurovascular structures (**Fig. 3C.10**, **Fig. 3C.11**, **Fig. 3C.12**, and **Fig. 3C.13**).
15. The tumor extending superior and lateral is removed with an olive-tipped 'J' aspirator (**Fig. 3C.14** and **Fig. 3C.15**).
16. An intraoperative MRI (iMRI) is performed, which demonstrates a small piece of remnant tumor far

lateral on the right side between the anterior cerebral artery and the supraclinoidal internal carotid artery. This remnant tumor was inaccessible and could not be removed in a re-explorative step after the iMRI (**Fig. 3C.16**).

17. A decision is made to stop the surgery at this point as attempts to access and remove the remnant tumor may present an unnecessary risk for the patient.
18. Meticulous hemostasis is performed.
19. The defect is plugged with an abdominal fat graft. The edges are tucked intradurally to create a watertight seal. Care is taken not to pack too much fat tightly into the cavity (**Fig. 3C.17**).
20. The construct is sealed with a synthetic dural sealant and layered with absorbable hemostat.
21. The nasoseptal flap is then rotated over the defect to complete the repair. The construct is reinforced with gelatin sponges to keep the flap in position. No other nasal packing is required (**Fig. 3C.18**).

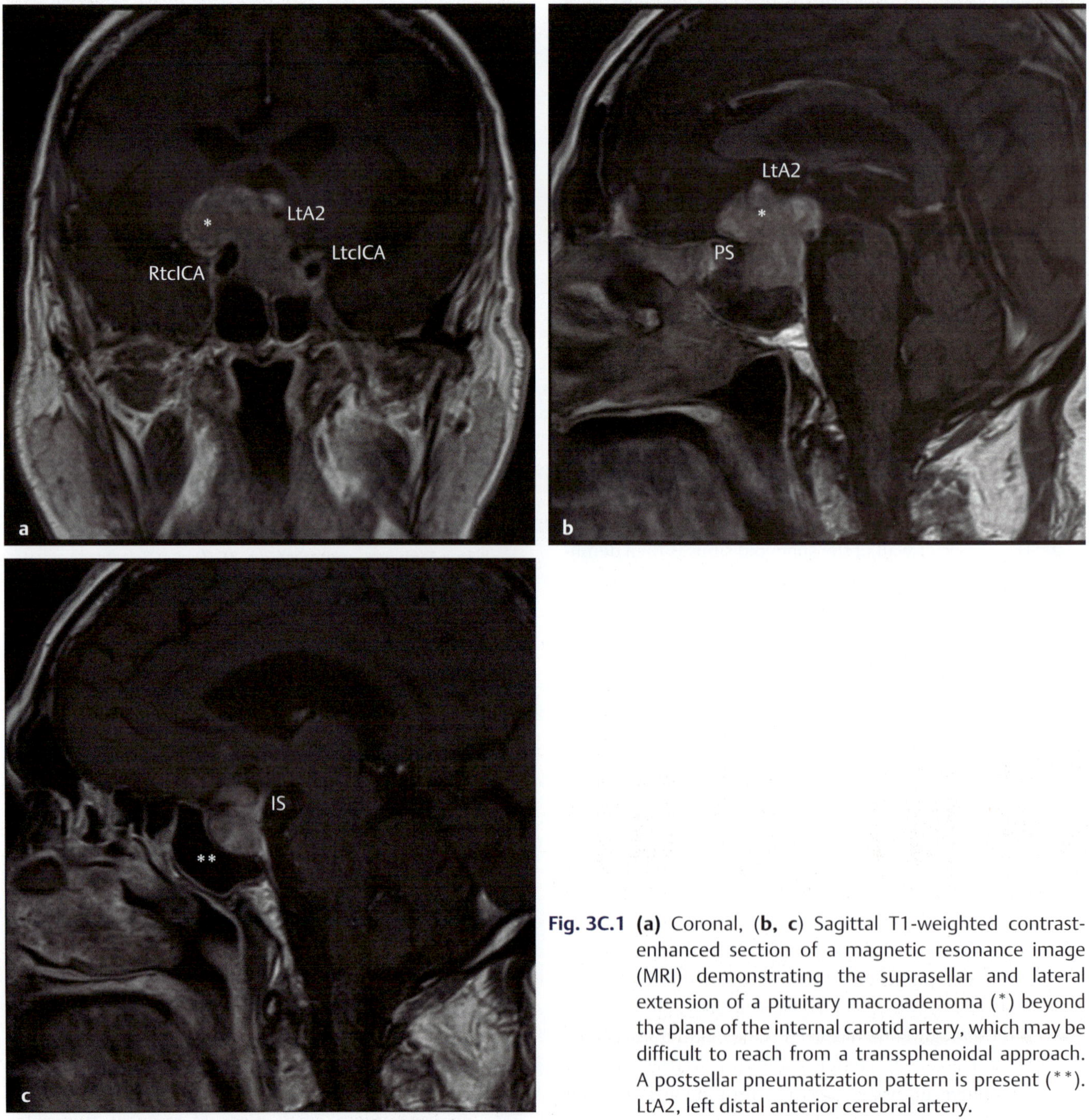

Fig. 3C.1 **(a)** Coronal, (**b, c**) Sagittal T1-weighted contrast-enhanced section of a magnetic resonance image (MRI) demonstrating the suprasellar and lateral extension of a pituitary macroadenoma (*) beyond the plane of the internal carotid artery, which may be difficult to reach from a transsphenoidal approach. A postsellar pneumatization pattern is present (**). LtA2, left distal anterior cerebral artery.

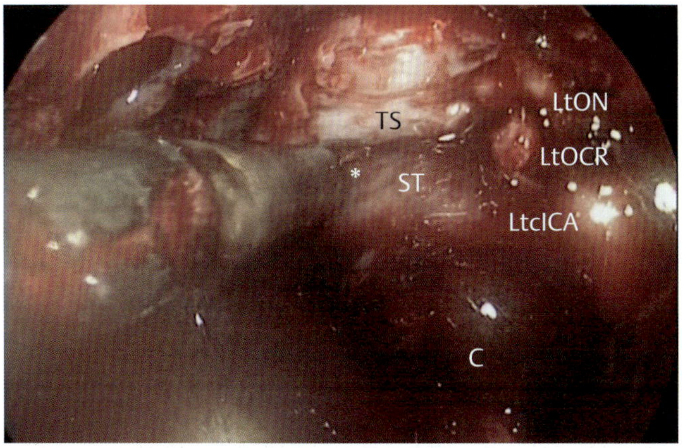

Fig. 3C.2 Endonasal endoscopic view after osteodural exposure using a transsellar, transtubercular, and transplanum approach. Part of the tumor (*) can be seen to the left and inferior to the aspirator. Superior to the aspirator, the dura of the tuberculum and planum is visible between the bony edges.

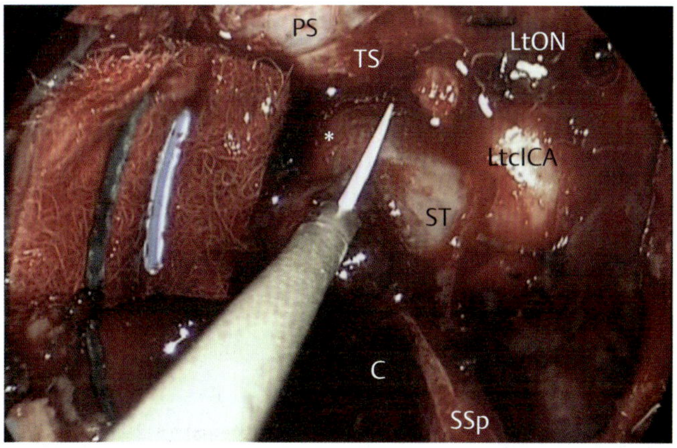

Fig. 3C.3 The incision is extended vertically and superiorly using microscissors. Tumor (*).

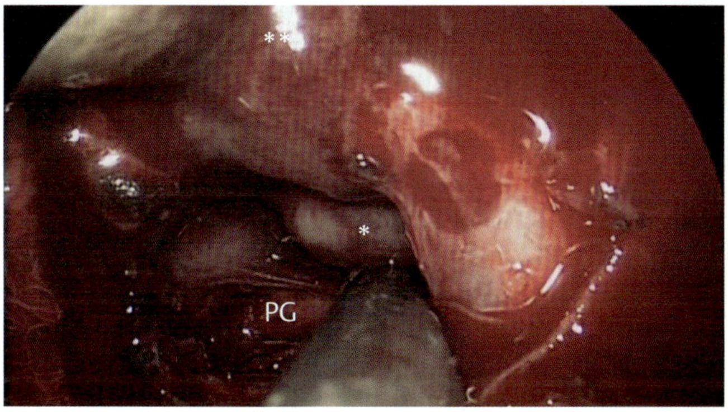

Fig 3C.4 The inferior compartment of the tumor is debulked using a bimanual technique. To the left, suction is used to hold up the superior tumor compartment (**) to prevent tumor collapse and an obscured view, whereas to the right, another aspirator is used to debulk the inferior compartment of the tumor (*) posteriorly.

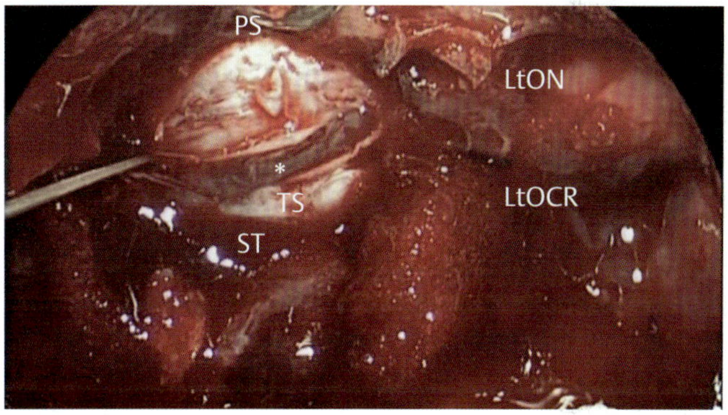

Fig 3C.5 Horizontal incision of the dura over the planum sphenoidale (PS). The tumor (*) is visible under the incision.

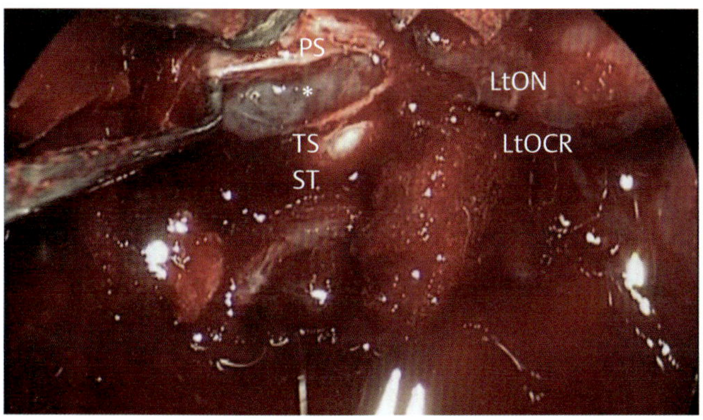

Fig. 3C.6 A right-angle dissector is being used to free the underlying tissue away from the dura. The tumor (*) is visible under the incision.

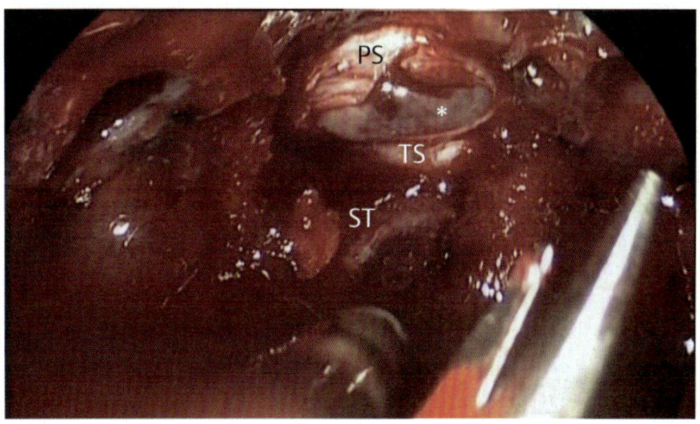

Fig. 3C.7 Vertical incision over the planum sphenoidale (PS) with microscissors. The tumor (*) is visible under the incision.

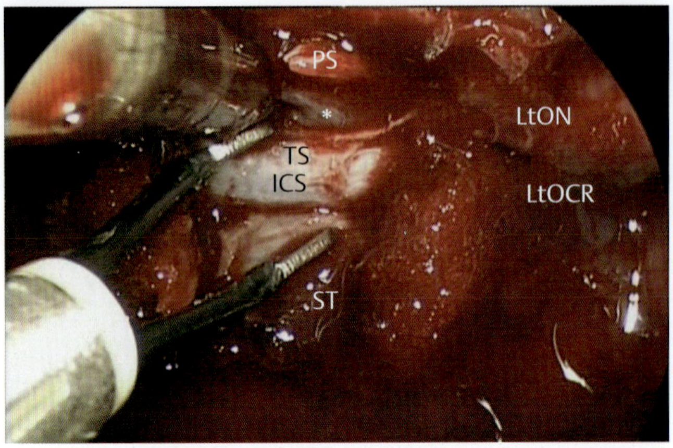

Fig. 3C.8 The intercavernous sinus (ICS) is cauterized and divided using microscissors. The tumor (*) is visible under the incision.

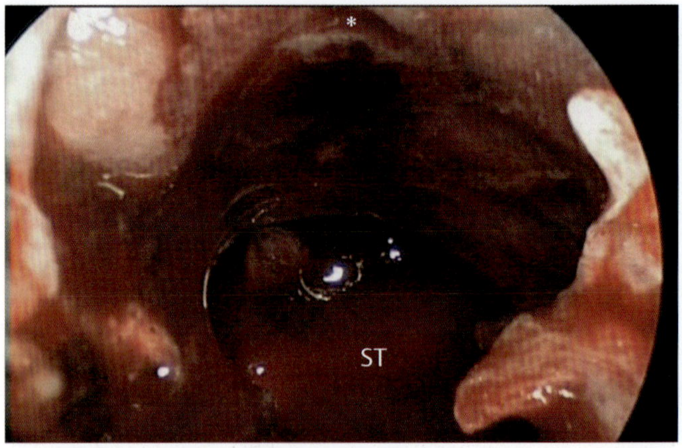

Fig. 3C.9 Resection cavity after clearance of the central component of the tumor. The superior tumor compartment is visible (*).

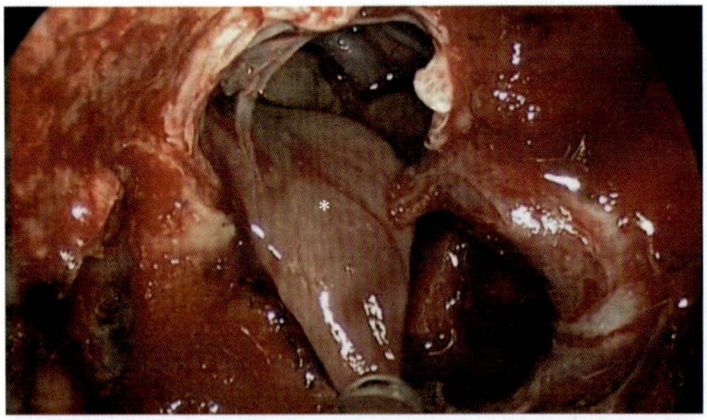

Fig. 3C.10 After interior debulking of the superior tumor compartment, the tumor capsule (*) is dissected along the arachnoid layer.

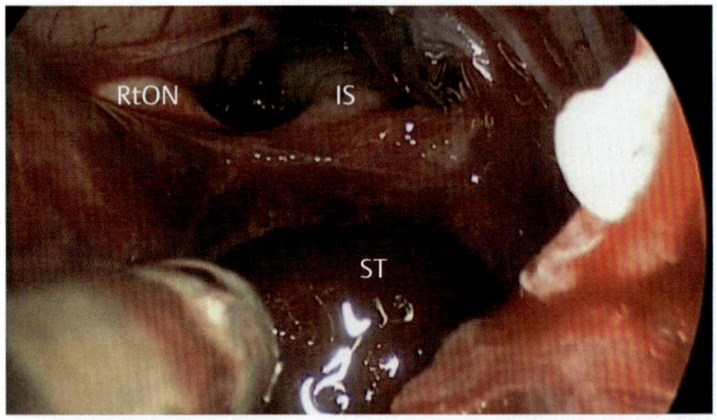

Fig. 3C.11 Remnant tumor being peeled away from the brain-tumor interface divided by an arachnoid plane using a microdissector.

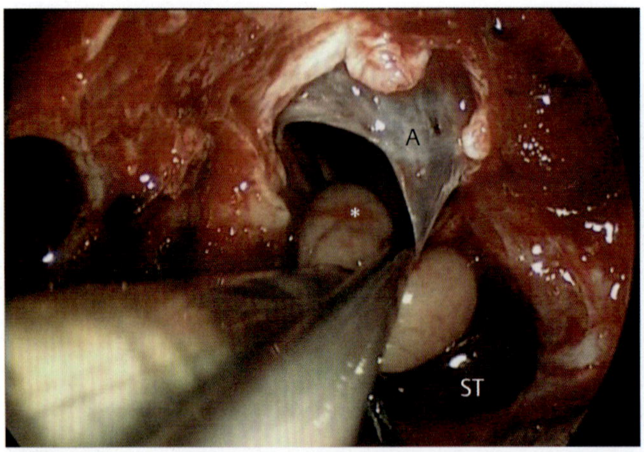

Fig. 3C.12 The remnant tumor of the superior compartment (*) is removed from the arachnoid layer (A).

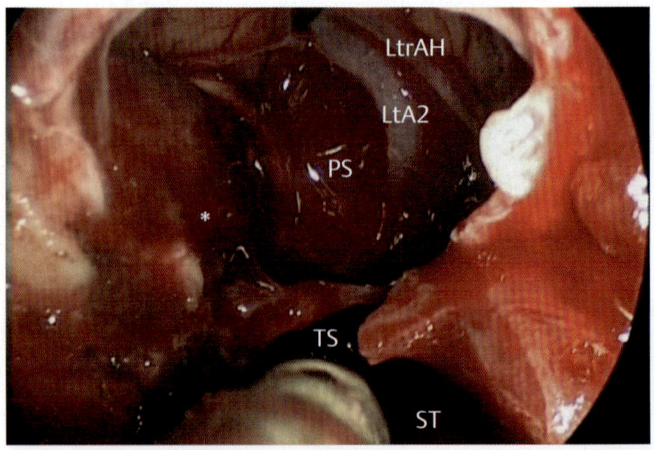

Fig. 3C.13 The medial superior tumor compartment is removed, whereas the superior lateral extending portion is still visible (*).

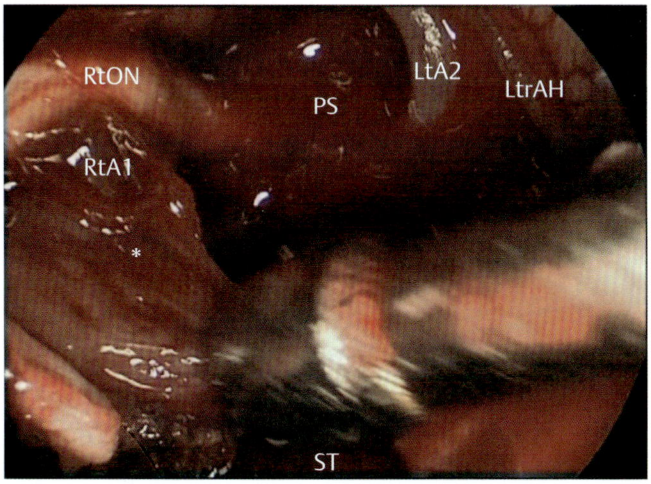

Fig. 3C.14 The superior lateral extending tumor remnant (*) is removed using the maxillary 'J' aspirator. The right anterior cerebral artery (RtA1) is visible superior to the tumor.

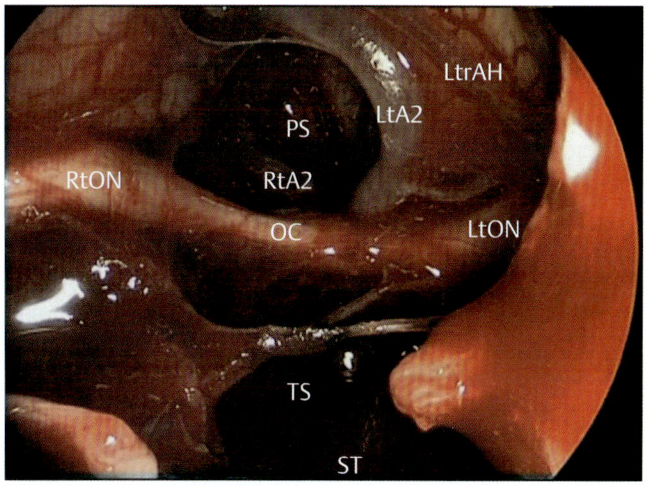

Fig. 3C.15 Final view of the resection cavity.

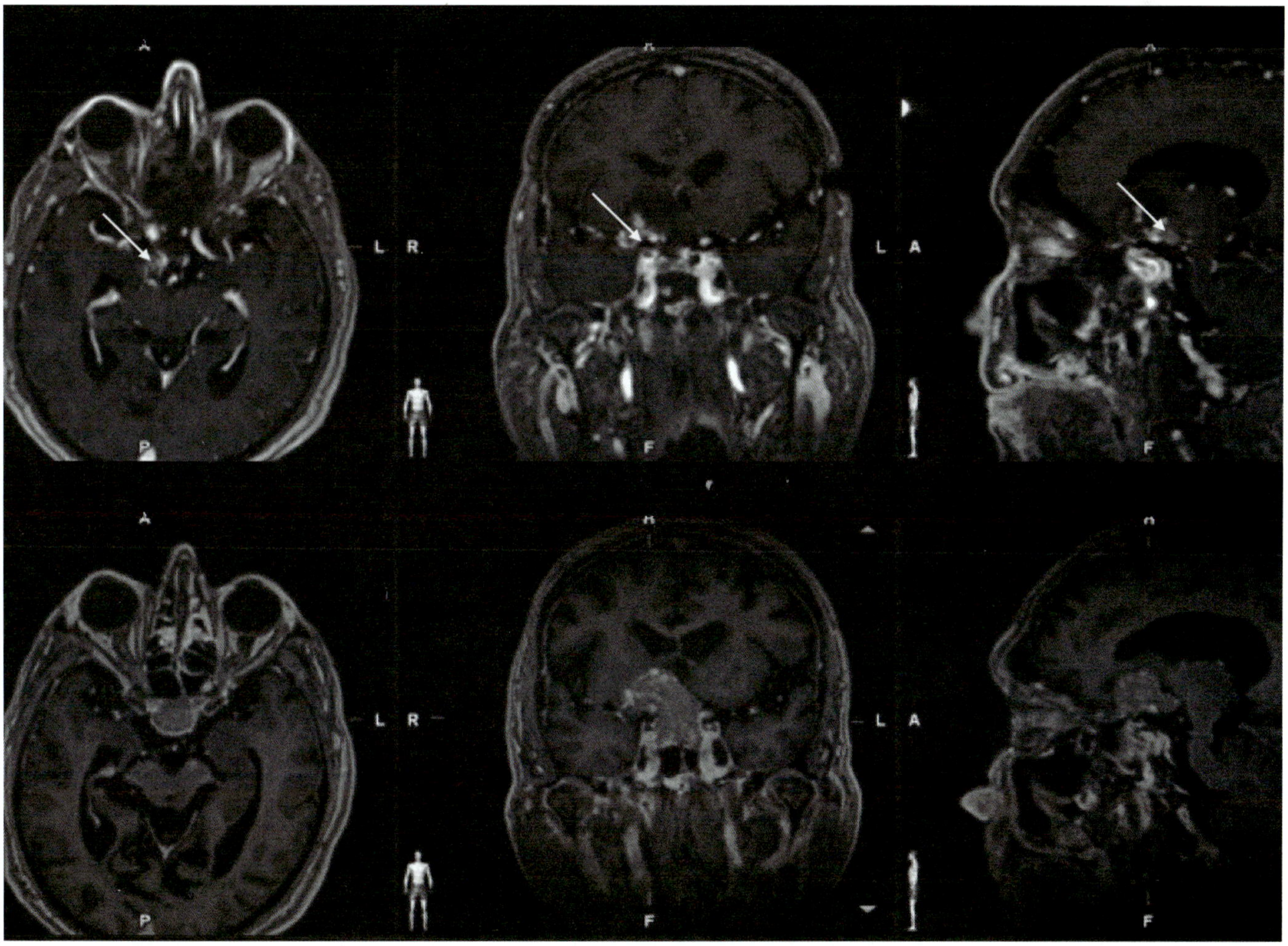

Fig. 3C.16 Axial, coronal, and sagittal T1-weighted contrast-enhanced intraoperative (upper row) and preoperative (lower row) MRI sections. Complete excision of the lesion is achieved except for a small cuff, which is seen as the hyperintense area on the intraoperative coronal cut between the anterior cerebral artery and the internal carotid artery (*white arrow*).

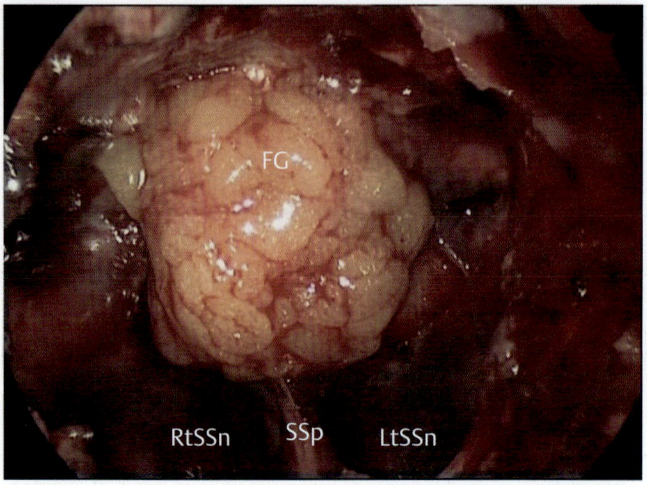

Fig. 3C.17 Autologous abdominal fat graft (FG) for skull base defect reconstruction.

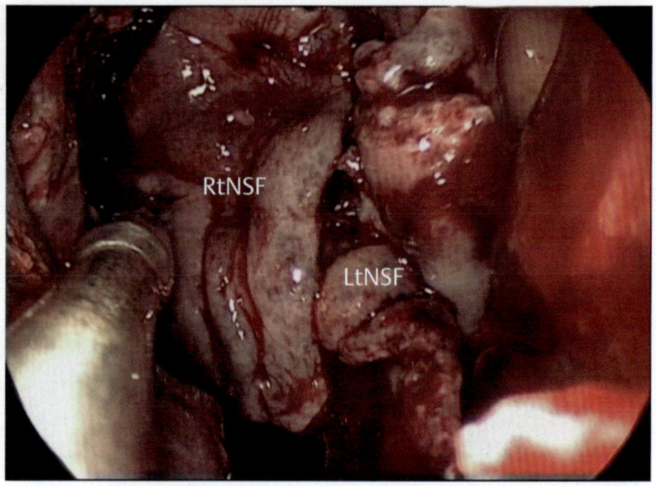

Fig. 3C.18 The right (RtNSF) and left nasoseptal flap (LtNSF) are placed over the construct to complete the repair.

Case 3D

Binostril Endoscopic Transseptal Transsphenoidal Intra- and Extracapsular Excision of a Pituitary Macroadenoma

Michel Roethlisberger, Yves Brand, and Luigi Mariani

History

A 70-year-old patient was admitted to an external hospital with progressive confusion and decreased consciousness. Emergency workup revealed acute hyponatremia with serum sodium values of 114 mmol/L and urinary sodium values of 84 mmol/L. A Syndrome of inappropriate antidiuretic hormone secretion (SIADH) was suspected, and the patient was admitted to the medical ward and treated with fluid intake restriction. Serum values normalized during the same hospitalization. Patient history revealed a prolonged history of hyponatremia with regular intake of bouillon prescribed by his or her physician. Endocrinological workup did not reveal any chemical or clinical hormonal abnormalities. Ophthalmological examination demonstrated a left superotemporal visual field defect without impairment of the visual acuity.

Neurocranial imaging was performed confirming a 22 × 22 × 23 mm intra- and suprasellar lesion with cranial extension and compression of the optic chiasm without lateral cavernous sinus invasion (**Fig. 3D.1a–c**).

Surgical Steps

1. A *binostril transseptal transsphenoidal approach* is performed as described in Chapter 1.
2. The dissection is continued until the sphenoid keel is exposed with the sphenoid ostia visible bilaterally.
3. Once the sphenoid keel is fully exposed, the ostia are widened inferomedially using a Kerrison punch in a V shape toward the midline (**Fig. 3D.2**).
4. The keel is removed with a pituitary rongeur forceps.
5. The remaining superior parts of the sphenoid rostrum and sphenoid sinus septations are then removed to allow an unobstructed view (**Fig. 3D.3**).
6. The mucosa covering the posterior ethmoidal cells is removed to allow an unobstructed view (**Fig. 3D.4** and **Fig. 3D.5**).
7. The posterior wall of the sphenoid sinus is then demucosalized, and the landmarks of the skull base are identified (**Fig. 3D.6**).
8. *Transsellar approach:* Opening of the sella is started with a diamond burr in the midline, reducing the thickness of the overlying septal insertion (**Fig. 3D.7**).

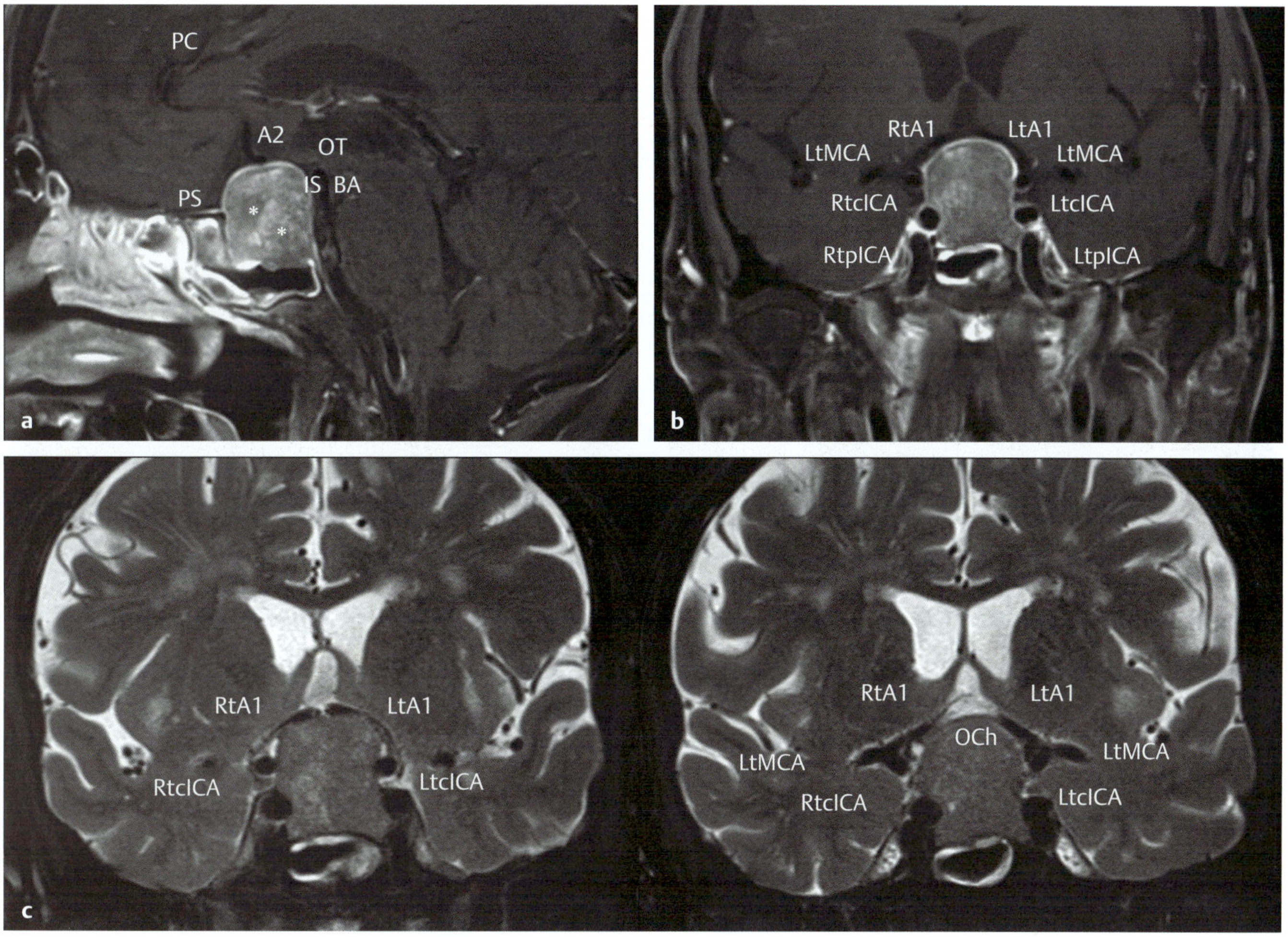

Fig. 3D.1 **(a)** Sagittal and **(b)** coronal T1-weighted gadolinium contrast-enhanced MRI section; **(c)** coronal T2-weighed MRI sections. A large isointense intra- and suprasellar lesion with moderate homogenous enhancement along with areas of signal shortening (*) suggestive for microhemorrhage or necrosis is seen. The infundibular stalk (IS) and the pituitary gland are compressed by the tumor. The cranial extension of the lesion leads to cranial displacement of the optic chiasm (OCh) and the left (LtA1) and right proximal anterior cerebral arteries (RtA1).

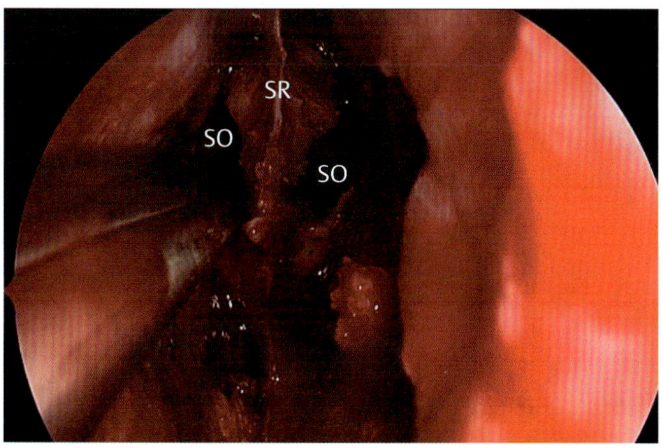

Fig. 3D.2 Exposed sphenoid rostrum (SR) using a binostril posterior transseptal approach. V-shaped opening of the sphenoid ostia (SO) using a Kerrison punch.

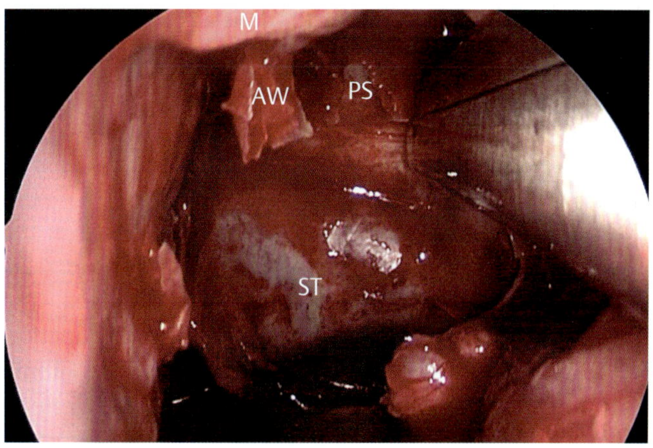

Fig. 3D.3 Parts of the anterior wall (AW) are still visible. Removal of the remaining sphenoid AW bone and mucosa (M) along the skull base. The sella turcica (ST) and the planum sphenoidale (PS) are visible within the sphenoid cavity.

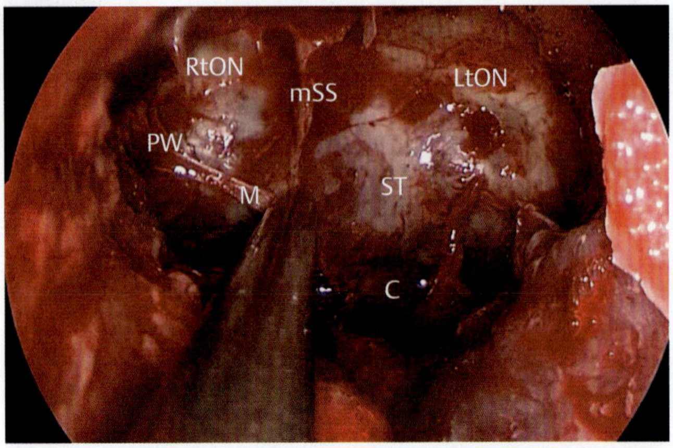

Fig. 3D.4 Removal of sphenoid mucosa (M) and a sphenoid main dividing septum (mSS) along the posterior wall (PW) of the sphenoid sinus and identification of the landmarks including the left (LtON) and right optic nerve (RtON), sella turcica (ST), and the clivus (C).

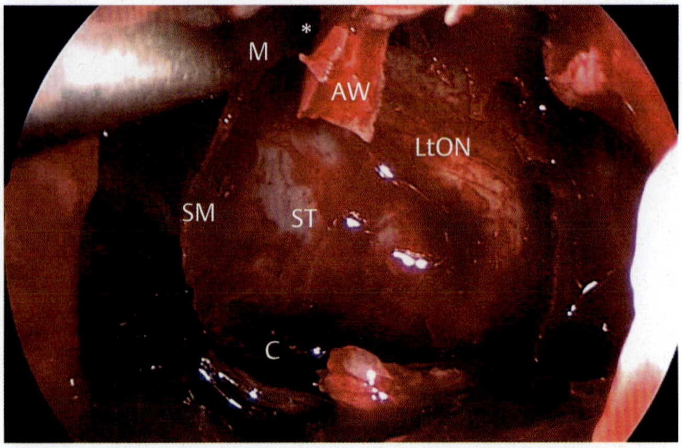

Fig. 3D.5 Removal of the anterior sphenoid wall (PW), ethmoidal cells (*), and mucosa (M).

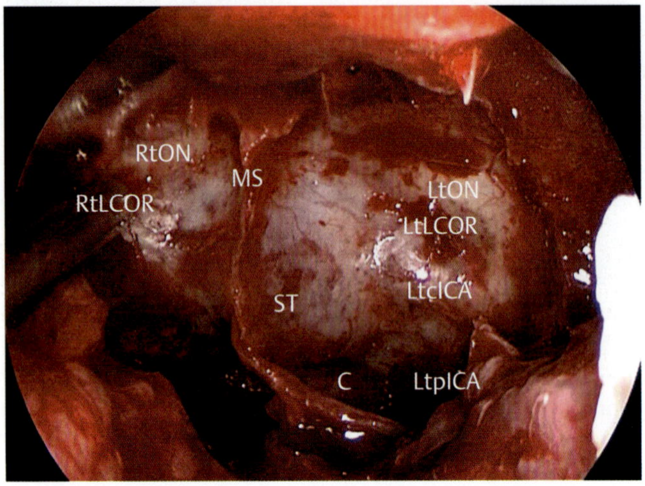

Fig. 3D.6 The left (LtLOCR) and the right lateral optico-carotid recess (RtLOCR) are identified and confirmed using image-guided surgery.

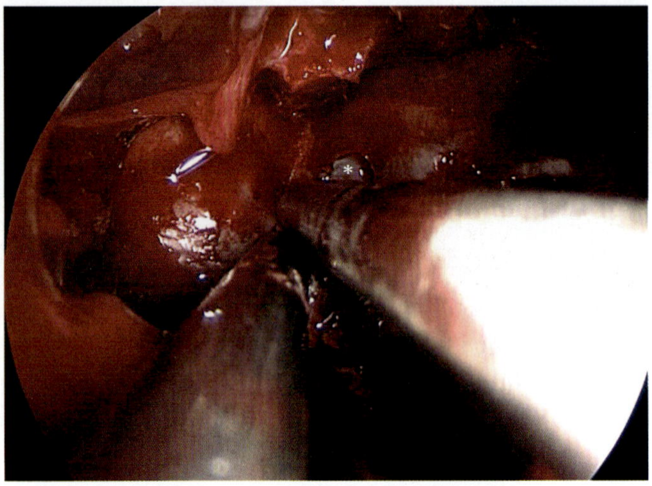

Fig. 3D.7 Widening of the sellar opening after defining a plane between the sellar bone and dura (*) using a Kerrison punch.

9. Once the bone has been sufficiently thinned out, a right-angle dissector can be insinuated between the bone and the dura and with the use of a Kerrison punch, the sellar opening can be completed. The anatomical landmarks of the sella turcica (superior: intercavernous sinus and planum sphenoidale, lateral: cavernous sinus, inferior: sellar floor) have to be in clear view, and orientation can be supported by image-guided surgery.
10. A cruciate incision of the sellar dura allows exposure of the pituitary gland bulging into the surgical field. No normal tumor tissue is visible (**Fig. 3D.8**).
11. To widen the access, a plane between the sellar dura and the flattened bulging pituitary gland is defined and the dura is pushed laterally (**Fig. 3D.9**).
12. The pituitary gland is incised and divided medially to allow access to the posteriorly located lesion (**Fig. 3D.10**).
13. A 90-degree ring curette is then used to debulk the lesion in a zonal manner, focusing on the central inferior zone first (**Fig. 3D.11** and **Fig. 3D.12**).
14. Tumor specimen should be retained for histological examination using pituitary forceps (**Fig. 3D.13**).

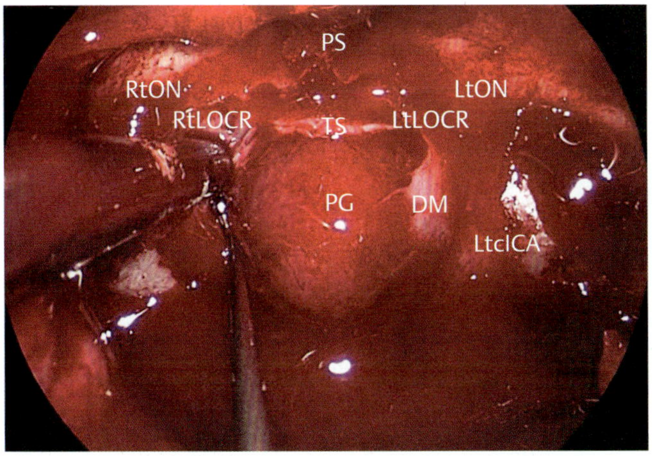

Fig. 3D.8 Defining a plane between the bulging pituitary gland (PG) anterior to the tumor and the dura mater (DM) to lateralize the dural opening.

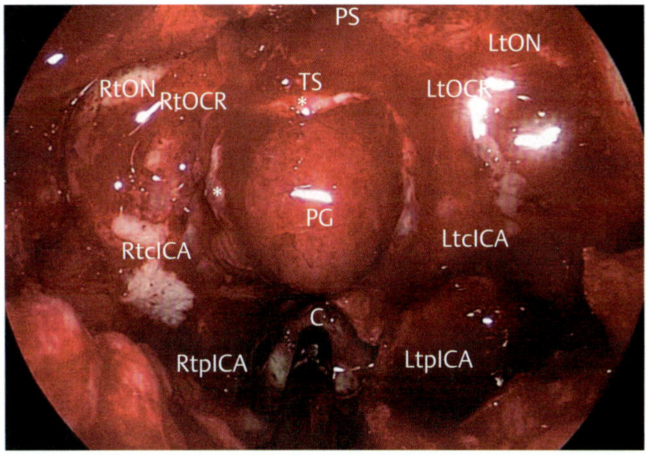

Fig. 3D.9 The dural flaps (*) can then be folded laterally to provide unobstructed view.

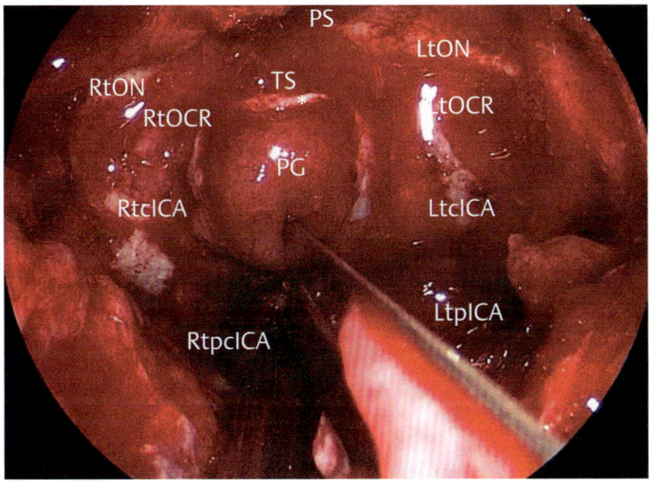

Fig. 3D.10 Midline sharp incision of the pituitary gland (PG) to release the tumor.

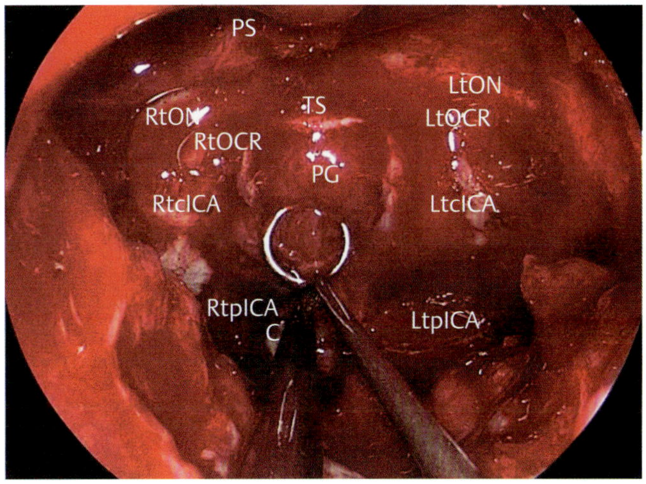

Fig. 3D.11 Initial midline inferior debulking using a 90-degree curette.

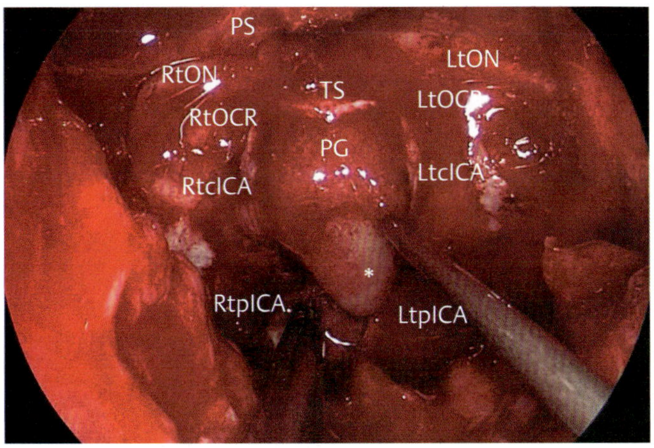

Fig. 3D.12 Liquid whitish tumor mass (*) evacuates under pressure.

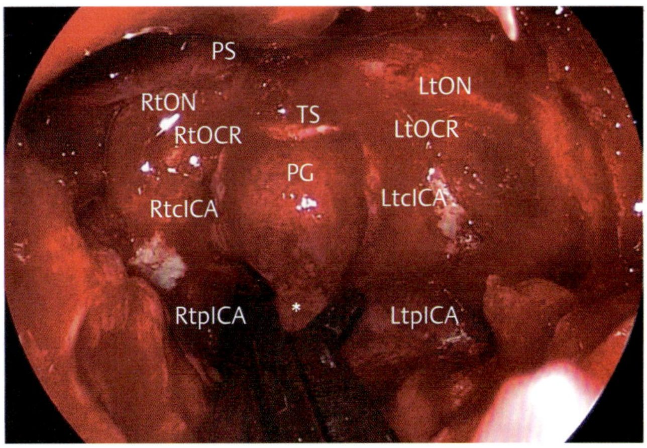

Fig. 3D.13 Asservation of tumor tissue (*).

15. Inferior central tumor debulking along the sellar floor to the dorsum sellae (formed by the anterior clival wall) is continued bimanually with a 90-degree ring curette and suction. Consecutively, the same maneuver is done bilaterally inferior within the tumor capsule (**Fig. 3D.14** and **Fig. 3D.15**).
16. The anterior superior compartment is debulked, and solid tumor components are removed from the tumor pseudocapsule (**Fig. 3D.16**).
17. Extracapsular dissection is performed superiorly to find the plane between the tumor and the diaphragma sellae, and to identify the thinned-out pituitary gland (**Fig. 3D.17**).
18. The extracapsular dissection is widened laterally to have a broad dissection plane along the diaphragma sellae (**Fig. 3D.18**).
19. The dissection plane between the pseudocapsule and the diaphragma sellae is continued posteriorly (**Fig. 3D.19**).
20. Microdissectors can be used to perform a bimanual dissection (**Fig. 3D.20**).
21. After circumferential dissection of the capsule and clearance of potential adherences, resection of the tumor capsule is possible (**Fig. 3D.21**).
22. Solid tumor components can be encapsulated within smaller chambers that open during dissection along this plane (**Fig. 3D.22** and **Fig. 3D.23**).
23. The normal pituitary gland is flattened out along the diaphragma sellae and can be identified while removing the superoposterior tumor compartment consisting of solid–liquid and capsular tumor components (**Fig. 3D.24**).

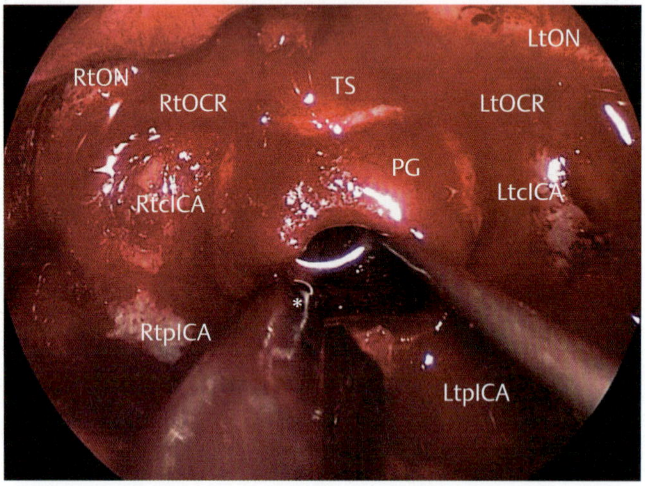

Fig. 3D.14 Zonal tumor (*) debulking posterior to the pituitary gland (PG).

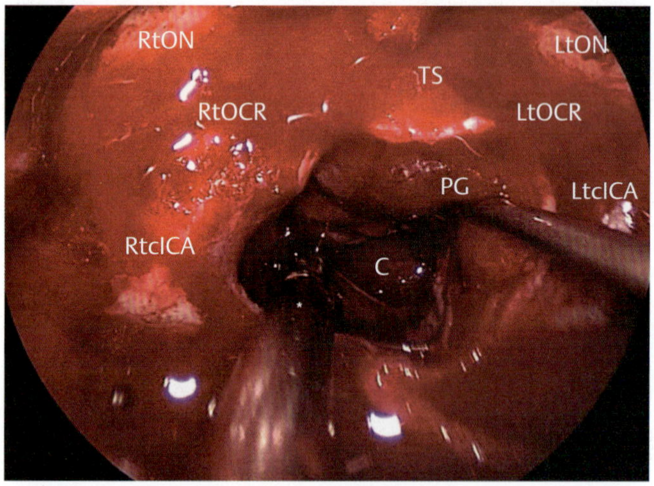

Fig. 3D.15 Bimanual dissection and identification of the clival (C) dura (posterior limitation).

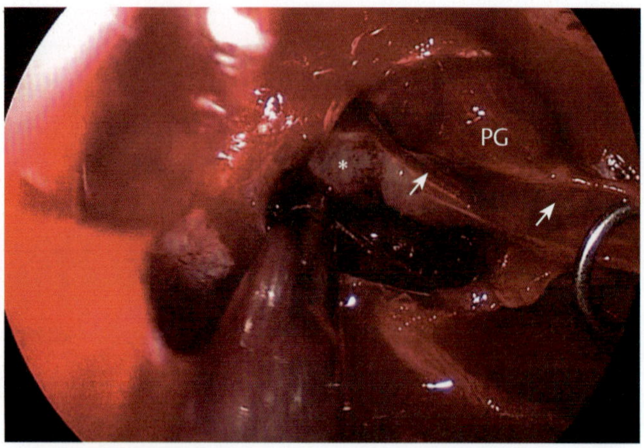

Fig. 3D.16 Debulking of the superior compartment of the tumor (*) and identification of the pseudocapsule (*arrows*).

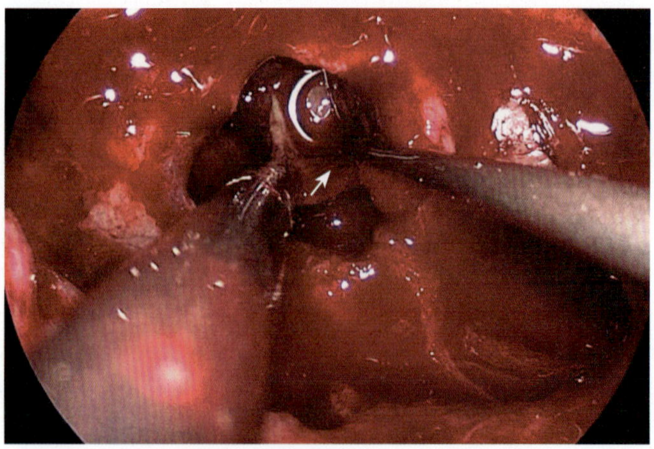

Fig. 3D.17 Bimanual extracapsular dissection. Tumor pseudocapsule (*arrow*).

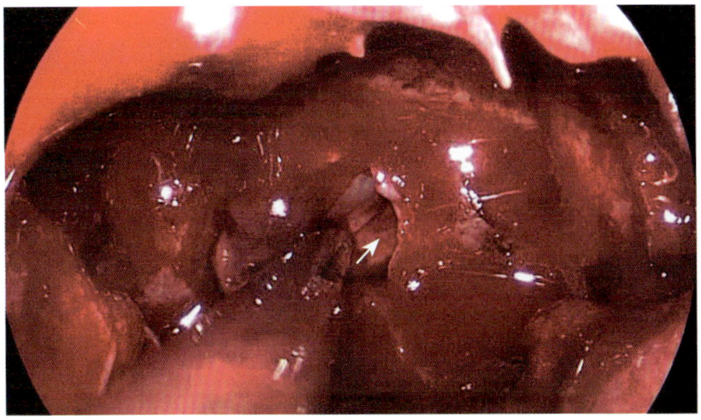

Fig. 3D.18 Lateral extracapsular dissection. Tumor pseudocapsule (*arrow*).

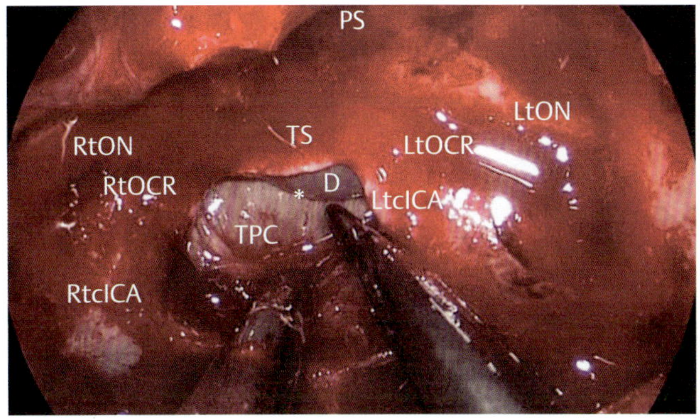

Fig. 3D.19 A plane (*) between the tumor pseudocapsule (TPC) and the diaphragma sellae (D) is identified.

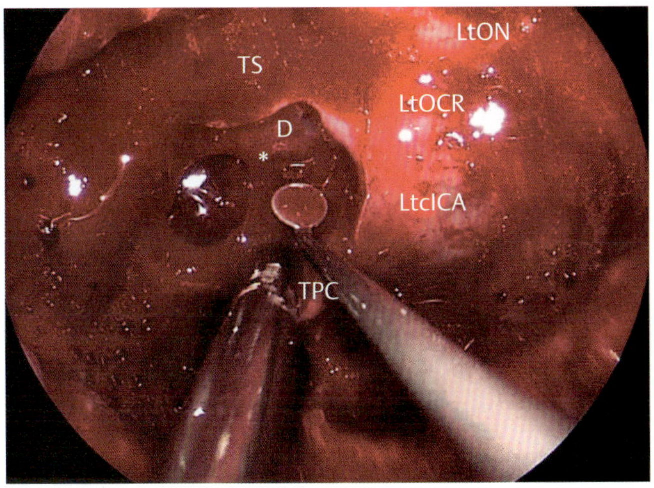

Fig. 3D.20 The use of a microdissector for the dissection along the defined plane (*).

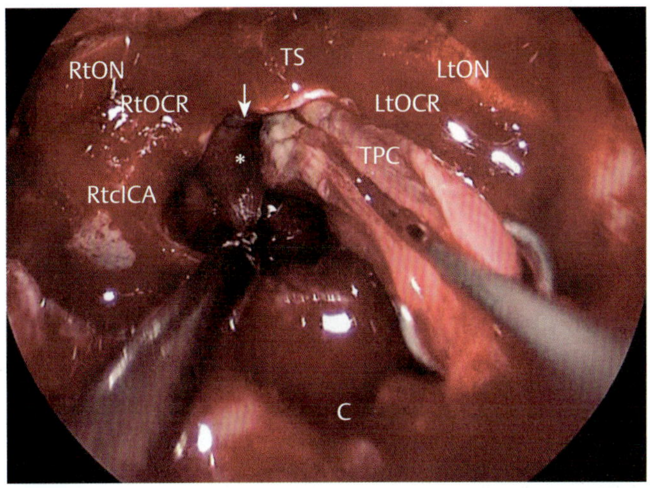

Fig. 3D.21 Removal of tumor pseudocapsule (TPC) from the diaphragma sellae *(white arrow)* along the dissection plane (*).

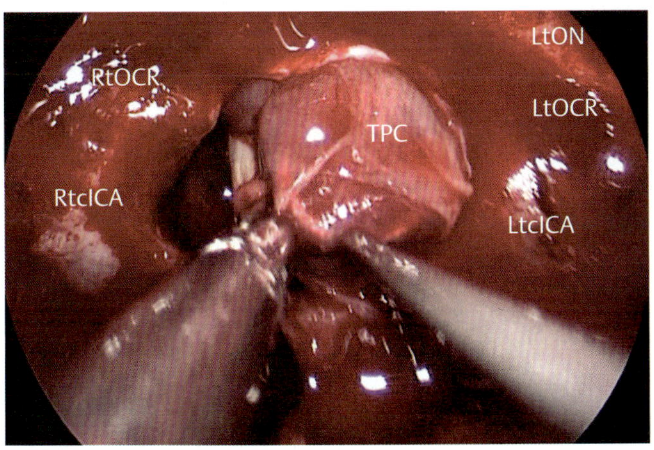

Fig. 3D.22 Removal of solid tumor and tumor pseudocapsule (TPC) from superior anterior to superior posterior.

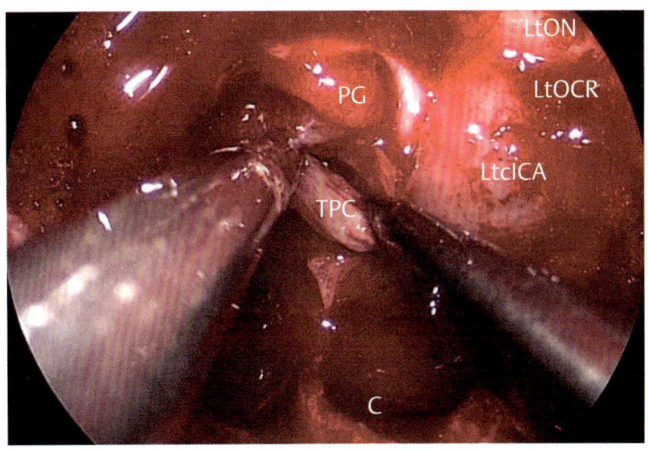

Fig. 3D.23 Removal of solid tumor and tumor pseudocapsule (TPC) from superior anterior to superior posterior. The anteriorly located pituitary gland (PG) has retracted superiorly and is flattened along the diaphragma sellae.

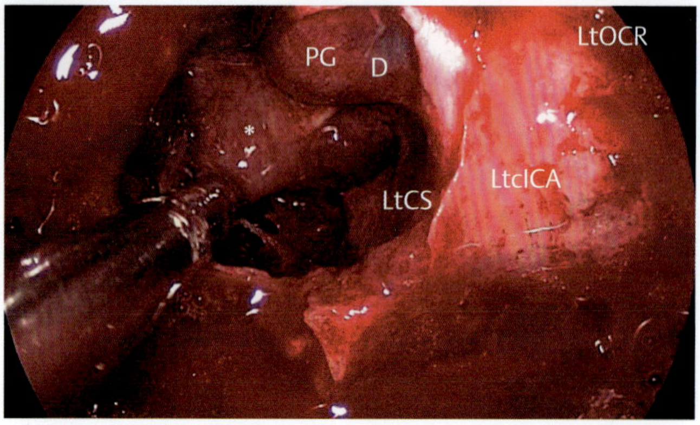

Fig. 3D.24 Removal of solid tumor (*) superior posteriorly. The pituitary gland (PG) is flattened along the diaphragma sellae (D).

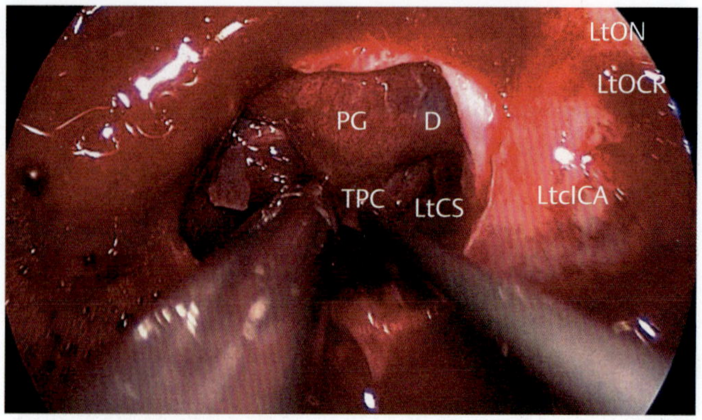

Fig. 3D.25 Removal of the remaining tumor pseudocapsule (TPC) in the most posterior aspect along the clival dura. The pituitary gland (PG) is flattened along the diaphragma sellae (D).

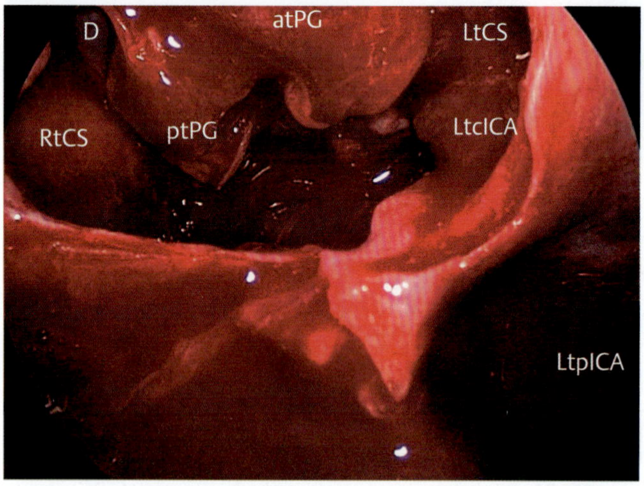

Fig. 3D.26 Final view showing the medial wall of the left cavernous sinus (LtCS), the flattened anterior (atPG) and posterior pituitary gland (ptPG) along the diaphragma sellae (D).

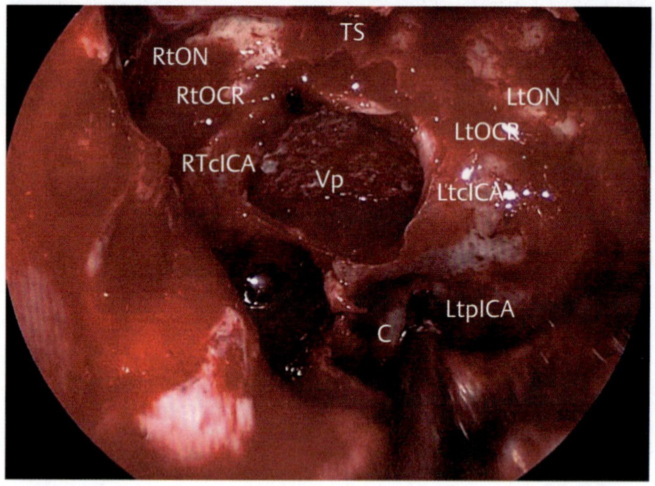

Fig. 3D.27 Sellar reconstruction with a Vicryl patch (Vp).

24. The inferoposterior and the superoposterior dissection planes are connected and the remaining tumor capsule is removed (**Fig. 3D.25**).
25. The resection cavity is inspected, and the medial cavernous sinus walls are cleared from residual tumor tissue. The flattened anterior lobe of the pituitary gland, the posterior pituitary gland, and the flattened pituitary stalk can be visualized (**Fig. 3D.26**).
26. The diaphragma sellae can be supported with a fitting Vicryl patch to prevent downward herniation of the chiasma opticum (**Fig. 3D.27**).
27. The skull base defect is closed with an abdominal fat graft, an artificial dural replace, and a dural sealant.
28. The sphenoid cavity is filled with Surgifoam, and the nasoseptal flaps are brought back in position. The middle turbinates are brought back into position and stabilized with resorbable nasal packs with slight compression of both nasoseptal flaps.
29. A postoperative magnetic resonance imaging (MRI) 6 weeks after the surgery confirms complete resection of the macroadenoma with decompression of the chiasma opticum (**Fig. 3D.28**).

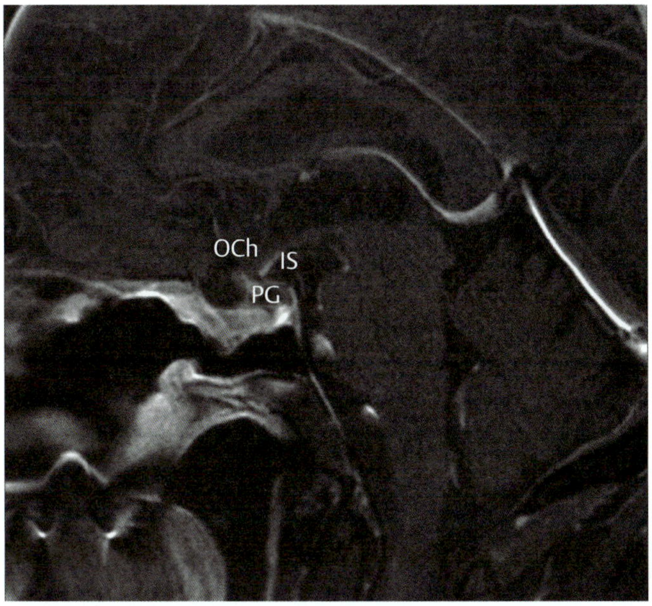

Fig. 3D.28 Six-week postoperative sagittal T1-weighted gadolinium contrast-enhanced MRI section demonstrating removal of the pituitary macroadenoma with the infundibular stalk (IS) and the pituitary gland (PG) visible together with decompression of the optic chiasm (OCh).

Case 3E

Endoscopic Transseptal Transsphenoidal (Binostril) Resection of a Suprasellar Pituitary Adenoma

Michel Roethlisberger, Yves Brand, and Luigi Mariani

History

A 67-year-old patient with a history of an atypical frontal lobe hemorrhage and transcranial excision of an arteriovenous malformation 5 years ago presents for regular clinical and radiological follow-up. An incidental suprasellar mass was identified in the neuroimaging studies and underwent regular follow-up. The patient suffers from a residual sensorimotor palsy of the right side. Initially, the lesion was 7 × 9 mm in progressive growth (9 × 13 × 23 mm) over the years with new compression of the optic chiasm (**Fig. 3E.1a–d**). Endocrinological and ophthalmological examinations did not show any pathological findings. The patient agreed after 2 years of hesitation to undergo *endoscopic endonasal transsphenoidal resection* of the lesion for histological analysis and decompression of the optic chiasm.

Surgical Steps

1. A *binostril transnasal transseptal transsphenoidal approach* is performed as described previously (**Chapter 1**).
2. The mucosa covering the posterior ethmoid cells is removed to allow an unobstructed view (**Fig. 3E.2**).
3. The posterior wall of the sphenoid sinus is demucosalized and the landmarks of the skull base are identified (**Fig. 3E.3** and **Fig. 3E.4**).
4. *Transsellar approach*: Opening of the sella is started in the midline using a high-speed diamond burr and the opening widened with the aid of a Kerrison punch (**Fig. 3E.5** and **Fig. 3E.6**).
5. The bone covering the sellar dura is removed along the sellar floor (**Fig. 3E.7**).
6. *Transtuberculum approach*: The bone of the tuberculum sellae covering the anterior intercavernous sinus is removed after meticulous separation of the dura from the bone and hemostasis (**Fig. 3E.8** and **Fig. 3E.9**).
7. The dura of the sella turcica is opened in the midline using a 15-mm knife (**Fig. 3E.10**).
8. The lesion is identifiable superior to the pituitary gland. A plane can be defined between the gland and the tumorous lesion. An initial central medial debulking with asservation of tumor tissue is performed (**Fig. 3E.11**).

9. The pituitary gland is located inferiorly within the sella turcica, while the suprasellar portion extends along the infundibular stalk. Hence, the dissection plane is followed in a superior direction without traction or pressure on the pituitary gland (**Fig. 3E.12** and **Fig. 3E.13**).
10. The suprasellar adenoma is further removed systematically using curettes, starting from the right superior (**Fig. 3E.14** and **Fig. 3E.15**) to the left superior (**Fig. 3E.16** and **Fig. 3E.17**) compartment.
11. After clearing the superior lateral pillars, the midline compartment along the tubercular dura is cleaned using curettes (**Fig. 3E.18**).
12. The resection cavity is inspected and filled with resorbable hemostatic material (**Fig. 3E.19** and **Fig. 3E.20**).
13. The skull base defect is covered using a Vicryl patch and sealed with an artificial dural sealant (**Fig. 3E.21** and **Fig. 3E.22**).
14. The nasoseptal flaps and the middle turbinates are brought back into position.
15. A 3 months' postoperative magnetic resonance imaging (MRI) revealed no residual tumor with decompression of the optic chiasm (**Fig. 3E.23a, b**).
16. Histological workup confirmed the histology of a typical pituitary macroadenoma.

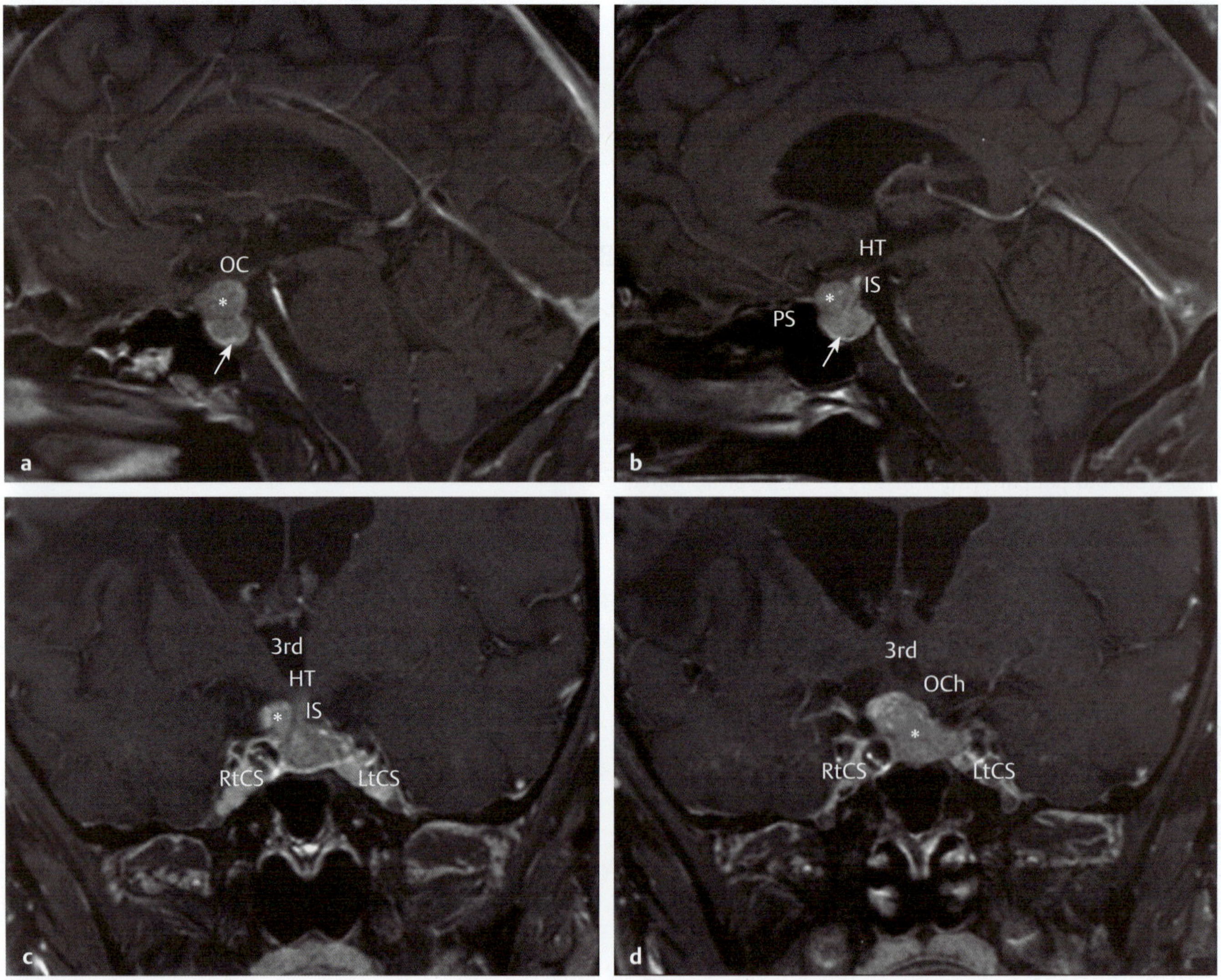

Fig. 3E.1 **(a, b)** Sagittal, and **(c, d)** coronal T1-weighted gadolinium-enhanced MRI sequences demonstrating an intra- and suprasellar hyperintense enhancing lesion (*) superior to the pituitary gland (*arrow*) and anterior to the infundibular stalk (IS) with extension superior to the planum sphenoidale (PS) level on the right side. There is compression of the optic chiasm (OCh). 3rd, third ventricle; HT, hypothalamus; LtCS, left cavernous sinus; RtCS, right cavernous sinus.

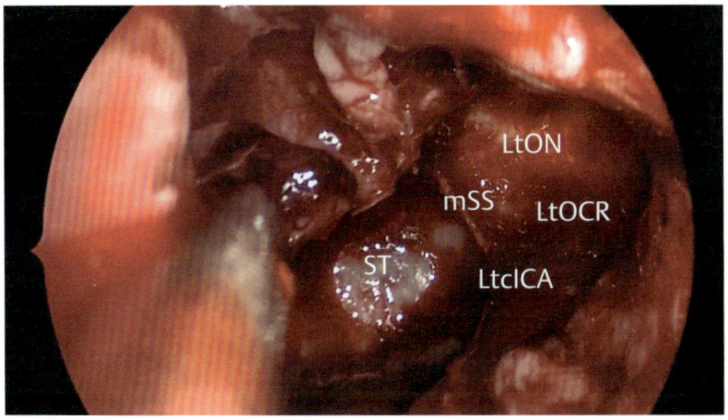

Fig. 3E.2 Removal of the anterior sphenoidal wall and mucosa of the posterior ethmoid cells. A dividing sphenoid main septum (mSS) is inserting along left cavernous internal carotid artery (LtcICA).

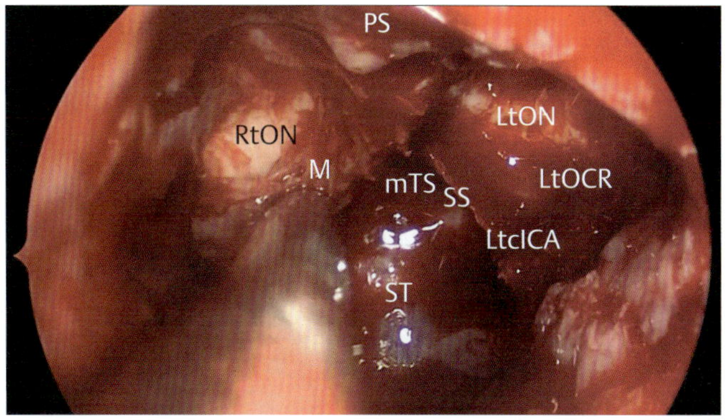

Fig. 3E.3 Removal of the mucosa (M) covering the posterior sphenoidal wall.

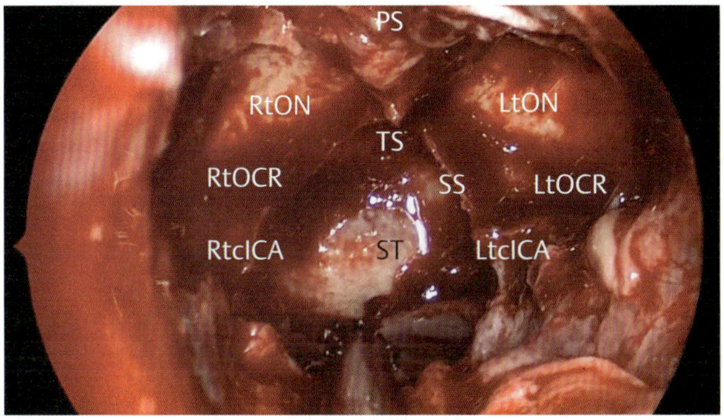

Fig. 3E.4 Overview of the landmark structures of the skull base after demucosalization of the posterior sphenoid sinus wall.

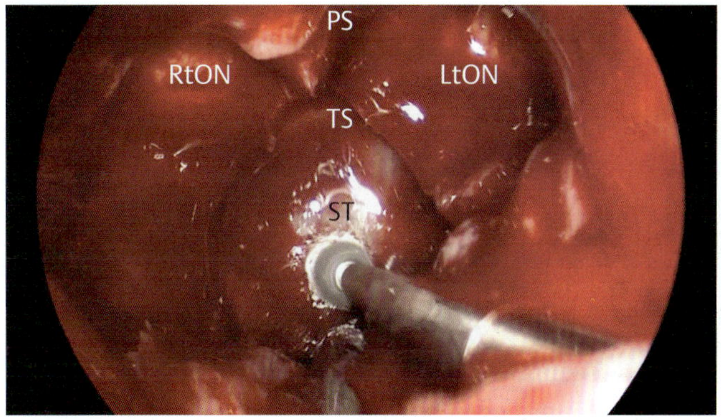

Fig. 3E.5 Transsellar approach: Midline opening of the sella turcica (ST) with a high-speed diamond burr.

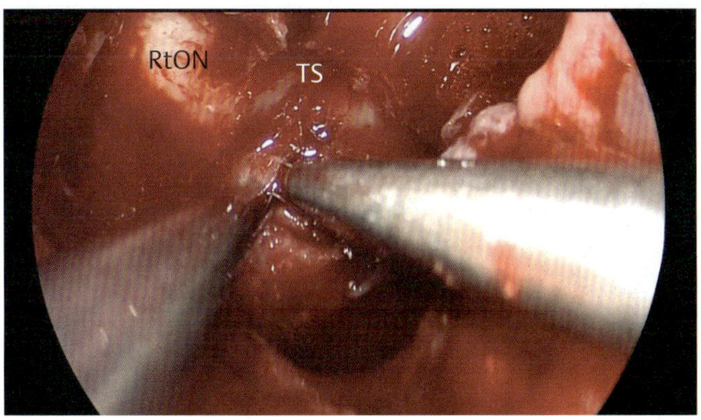

Fig. 3E.6 Transsellar approach: Removal of the bone covering the sella turcica with a Kerrison punch.

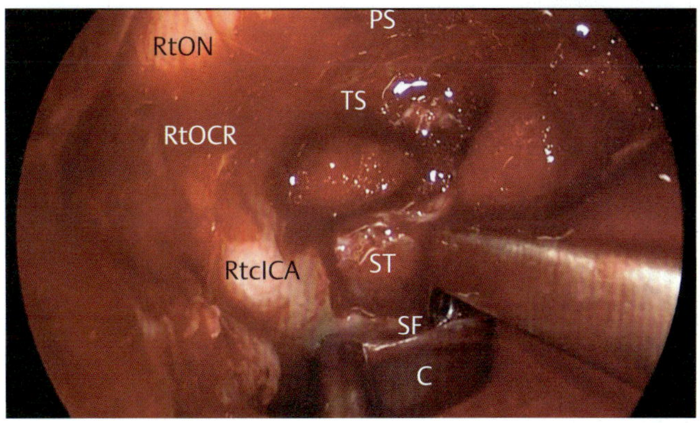

Fig. 3E.7 Transsellar approach: Inferior extension along the sellar floor.

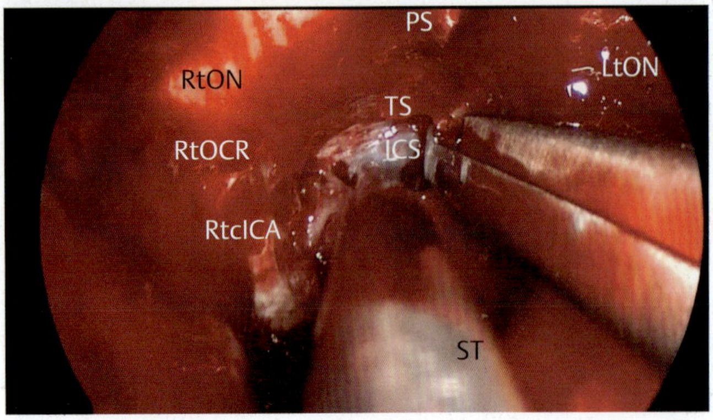

Fig. 3E.8 Transtuberculum approach: The bone covering the anterior intercavernous sinus (ICS) is removed.

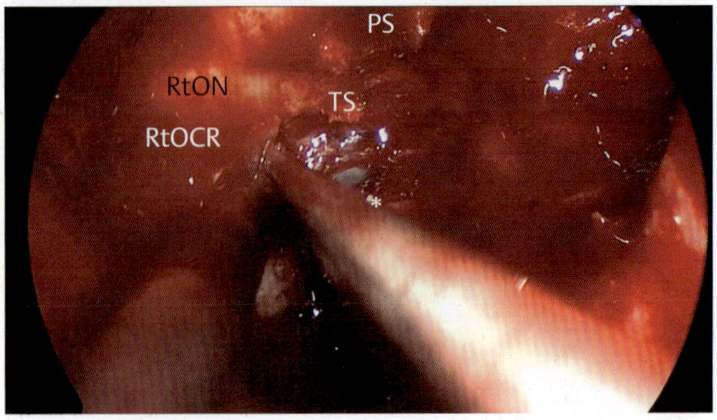

Fig. 3E.9 Transtuberculum approach: Removal of the bone covering the more lateral aspects of the anterior intercavernous sinus (*).

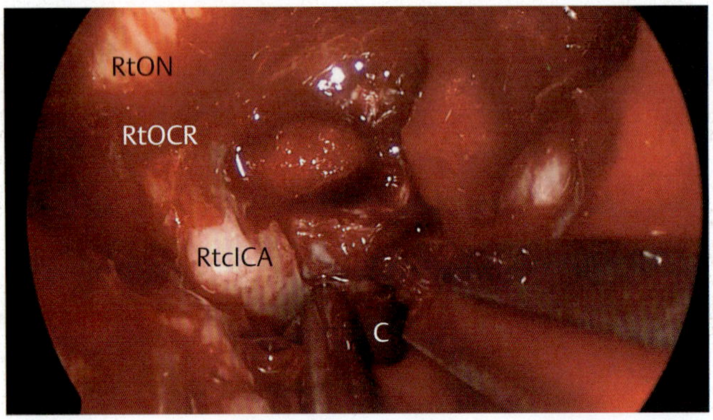

Fig. 3E.10 Sharp opening of the sellar dura strictly following the midline.

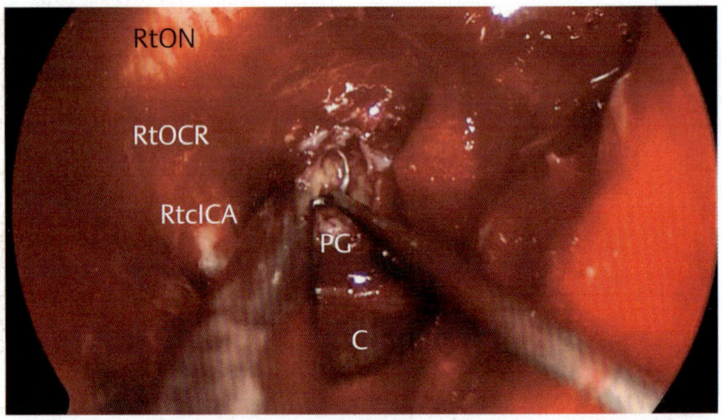

Fig. 3E.11 Central medial debulking of the lesion located superiorly to the normal pituitary gland (PG).

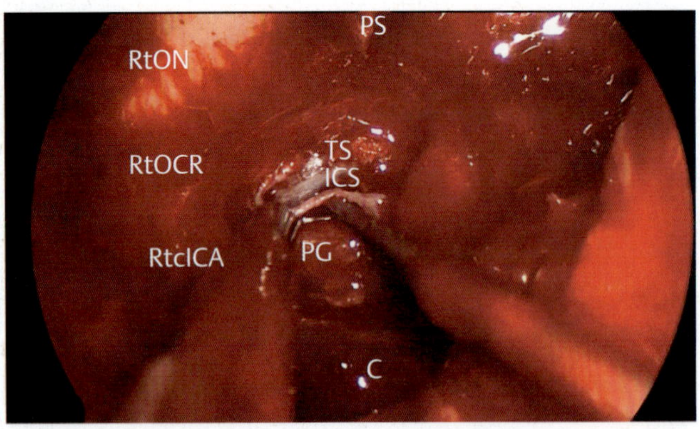

Fig. 3E.12 Elevation of the dura and the anterior intercavernous sinus (ICS).

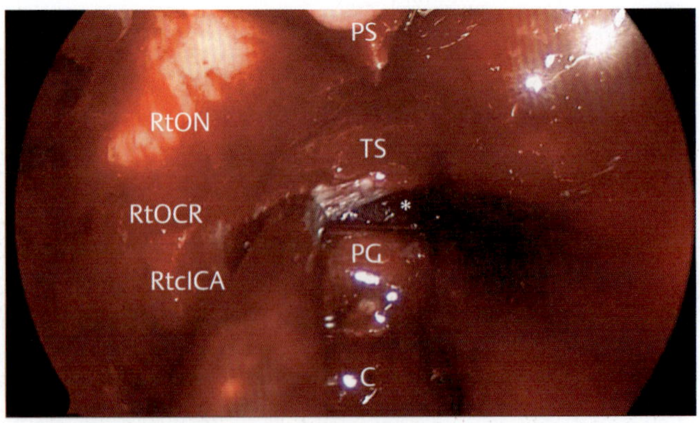

Fig. 3E.13 Definition of a dissection plane (*) between the lesion and the pituitary gland (PG).

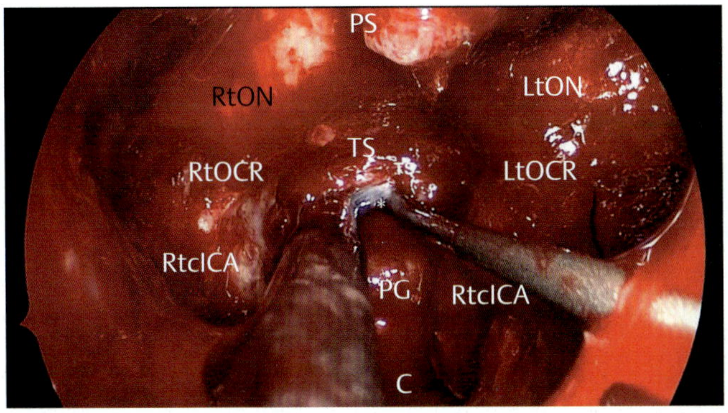

Fig. 3E.14 Insertion of a curette to reach the superior compartment of the tumor right anterior to the infundibular stalk with the elevation of the anterior intercavernous sinus (*).

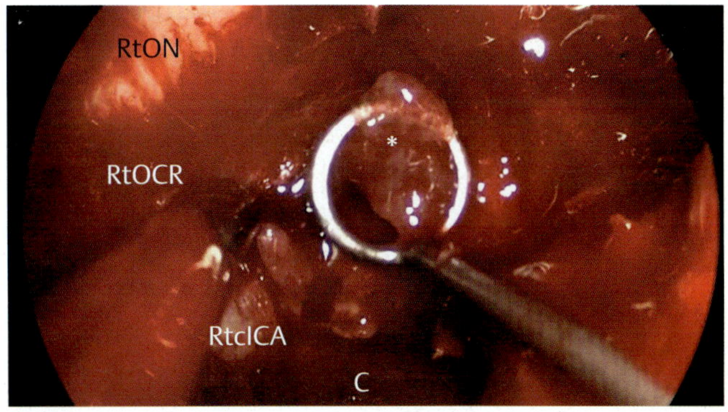

Fig. 3E.15 The left lateral pillar of the tumor (*) can be removed.

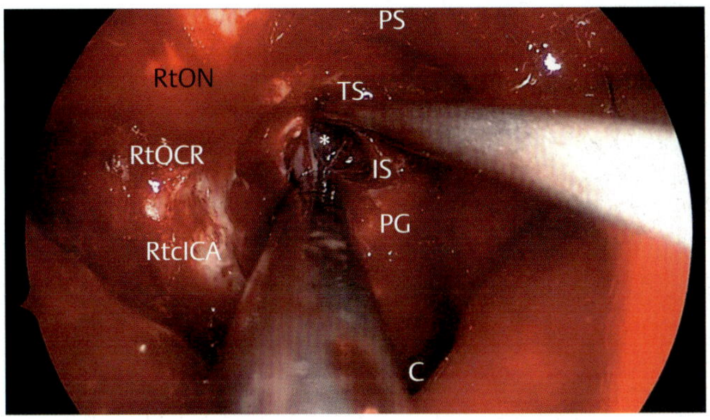

Fig. 3E.16 The tumor resection cavity (*) superior to the pituitary gland (PG) and right anterior to the infundibular stalk (IS) is further dissected posteriorly and toward the midline.

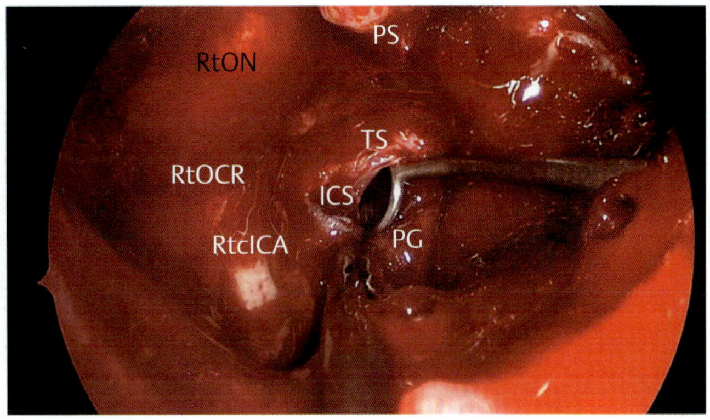

Fig. 3E.17 The right lateral tumor compartment is removed using a 45-degree curette.

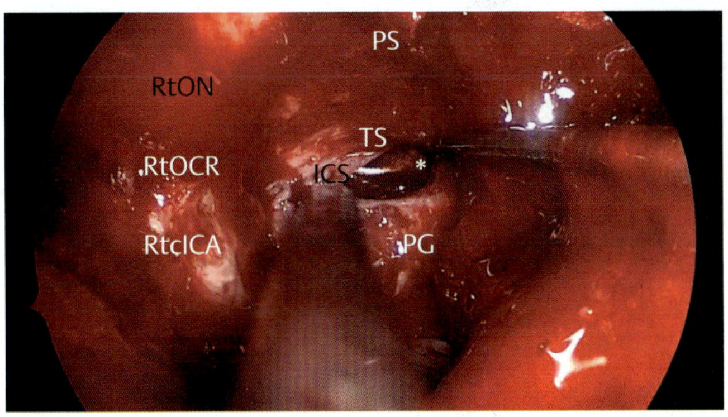

Fig. 3E.18 The suprasellar tumor compartment (*) is removed using a 90-degree curette.

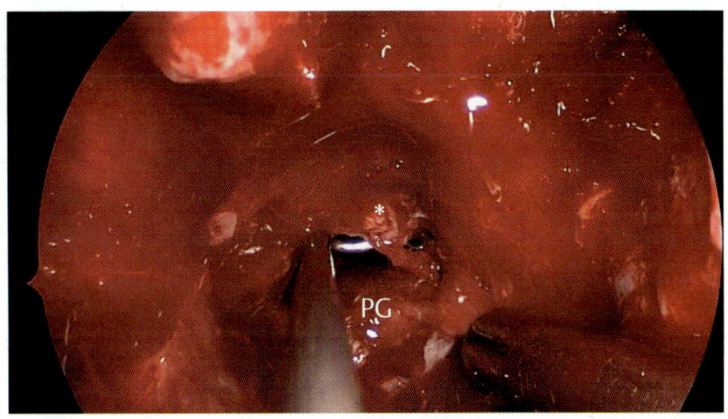

Fig. 3E.19 Suprasellar tumor remnants (*) removed along the dura covering the tuberculum sellae using a 90-degree curette.

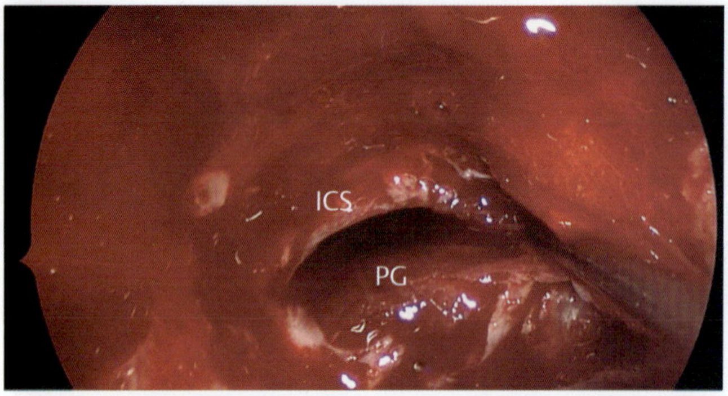

Fig. 3E.20 Inspection of the tumor resection cavity located superior to the pituitary gland (PG).

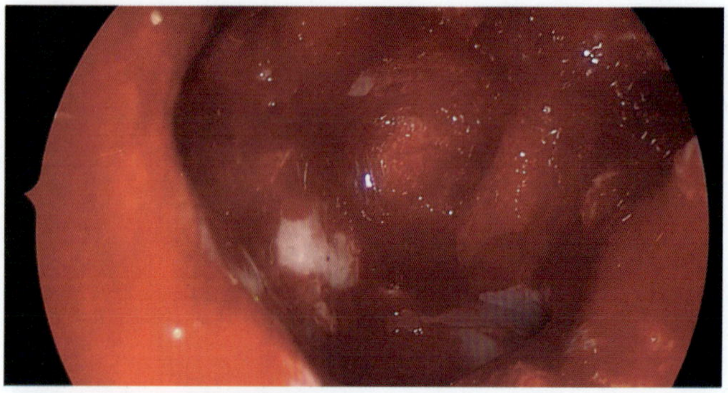

Fig. 3E.21 The resection cavity is filled with resorbable hemostatic agents.

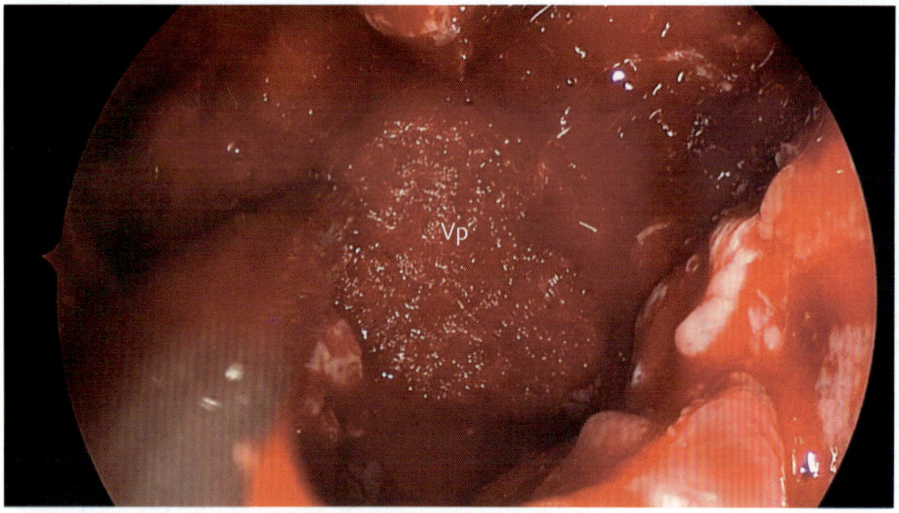

Fig. 3E.22 A Vicryl patch (Vp) is used to cover the sellar defect.

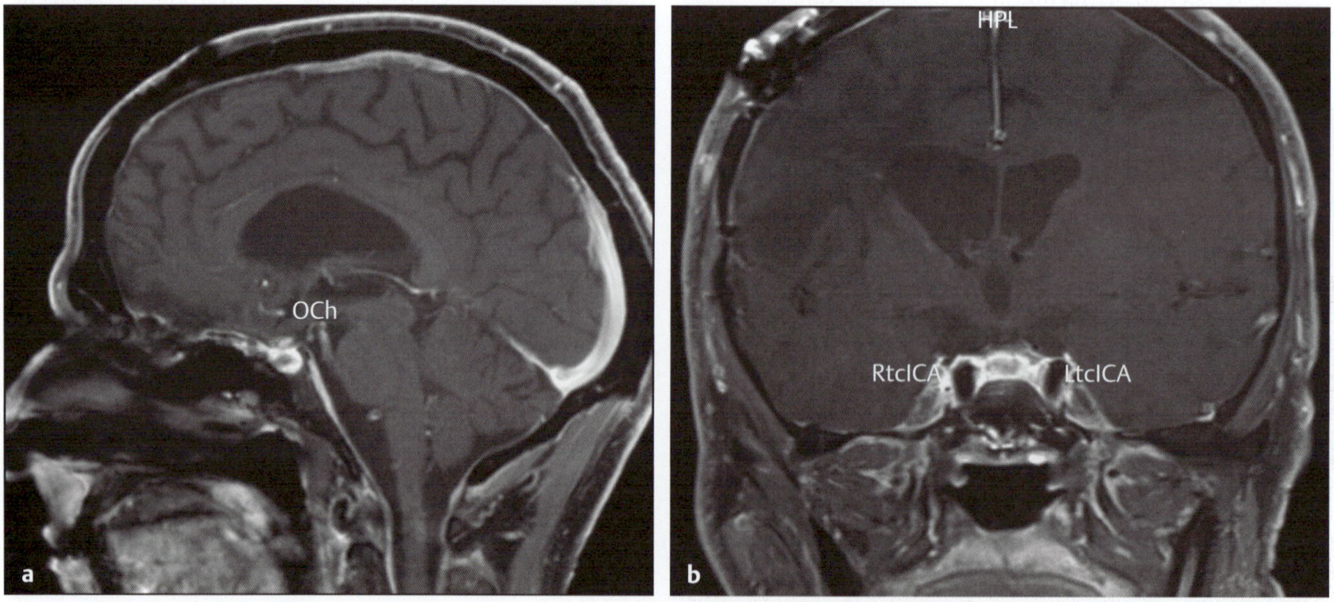

Fig. 3E.23 **(a)** Sagittal and **(b)** coronal T1-weighted gadolinium-enhanced MRI sequences demonstrating the resected pituitary adenoma with the pituitary gland and the infundibular stalk (*arrow*) in their physiological position together with the decompressed optic chiasm (OCh).

Case 3F

Single Nostril Endoscopic Transseptal Transsphenoidal Excision of a Pituitary Macroadenoma with an Anteriorly Located Pituitary Gland

Revadi Govindaraju, Michel Roethlisberger, Saif Al-Zahid, Prepageran Narayanan, and Vicknes Waran

History

A 57-year-old woman with underlying hypertension was investigated for persistent hyponatremia. A pituitary macroadenoma was found as an incidental finding on magnetic resonance imaging (MRI) scan. Investigations of the hypothalamic-pituitary-adrenal axis hormones and other endocrine investigations were normal. Her vision was normal, and there was no evidence of optic nerve or chiasma compression (**Fig. 3F.1**). MRI findings showed a tumor wedged between an anteriorly located adenohypophysis and posteriorly placed posterior pituitary gland (**Fig. 3F.2a, b**). She underwent *endoscopic transseptal transsphenoidal excision* of the tumor. However, the hyponatremia remained unchanged postoperatively.

Surgical Steps

1. A *single nostril transseptal transsphenoidal approach* is performed as described in Chapter 1.
2. Once a wide opening of the anterior wall of the sphenoid sinus is obtained, the bony septations within the sphenoid sinus are evaluated (**Fig. 3F.3**). The mucosal edges are cauterized using a monopolar suction diathermy to minimize bleeding (**Fig. 3F.4**), and the septations toward the sella are removed (**Fig. 3F.5**).
3. *Transsellar approach:* In the present case, where the bony wall is thick, a burr/drill or alternatively, a chisel is used to perform osteotomy (**Fig. 3F.6**). Once there is sufficient opening, an angled probe and/or dissector can be insinuated between the bone and the dura to elevate the dura away from the bone (**Fig. 3F.7** and **Fig. 3F.8**).
4. The bone is removed in piecemeals with a Kerrison punch (**Fig. 3F.9**). An angled probe is used to dissect the dura away from the bony edges prior removal. This avoids the dura from being caught in the punch/rongeur and torn during bony removal (**Fig. 3F.9**).
5. Dural opening is performed inferiorly to avoid injury of the anterosuperiorly located normal pituitary gland (**Fig. 3F.10**). Specimen is retained for pathology as the tumor protrudes out of the cavity (**Fig. 3F.11**).
6. The dural opening is further extended vertically and inferolaterally after freeing it from the underlying tissue using an angled probe (**Fig. 3F.12, Fig. 3F.13, Fig. 3F.14**, and **Fig. 3F.15**).
7. Tumor removal is performed in a systematic fashion, with more specimen obtained for biopsy as required. The tumor is removed using micro-dissectors, suction, and ring curettes (**Fig. 3F.16** and **Fig. 3F.17)**.
8. Meticulous tumor removal and an appropriate placement of the incision will ensure that the pituitary gland is preserved at the end of the surgery. (**Fig. 3F.18**).
9. Intraoperative MRI is a useful tool to evaluate residual tumor, together with serial postoperative imaging for comparison (**Fig. 3F.19**).

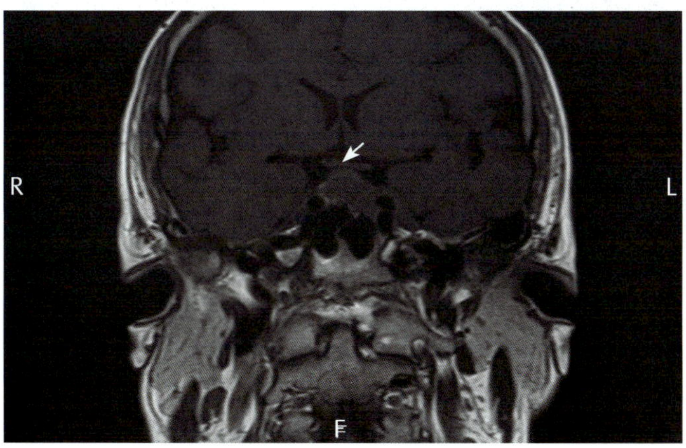

Fig. 3F.1 A non-contrast T1-weighted MRI scan in the coronal plane shows the pituitary macroadenoma affecting the optic chiasm (*arrow*) without compressive effect.

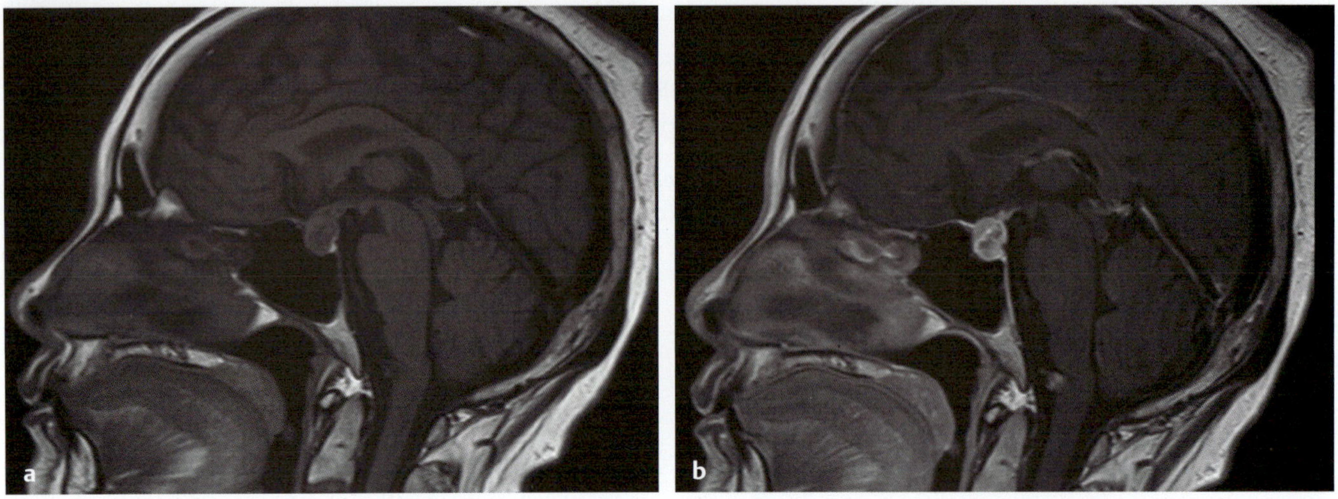

Fig. 3F.2 Sagittal views of the T1-weighted MRI scan **(a)** pre- and **(b)** postcontrast administration a pituitary adenoma between an anteriorly located adenohypophysis and posteriorly displaced posterior pituitary gland. The tumor is hypointense in the noncontrasted image and is not enhancing postcontrast.

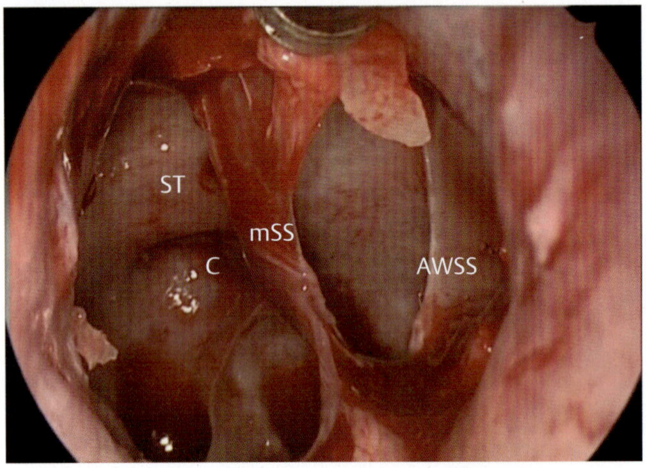

Fig. 3F.3 A midline bony main septum within the sphenoid sinus is seen inserting into the sellar region.

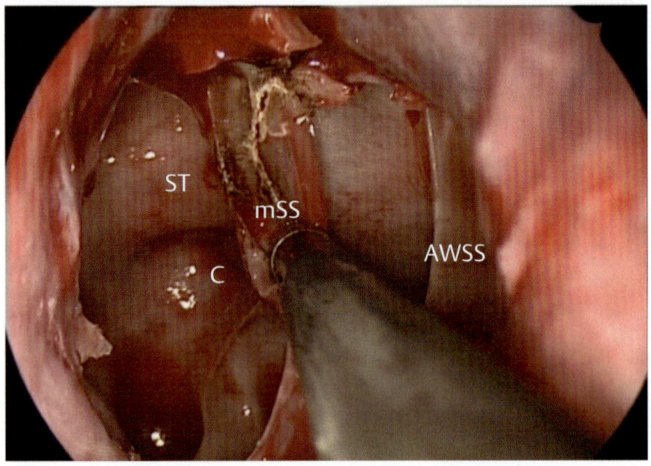

Fig. 3F.4 Mucosal edges of the bony septations are cauterized with a monopolar suction diathermy.

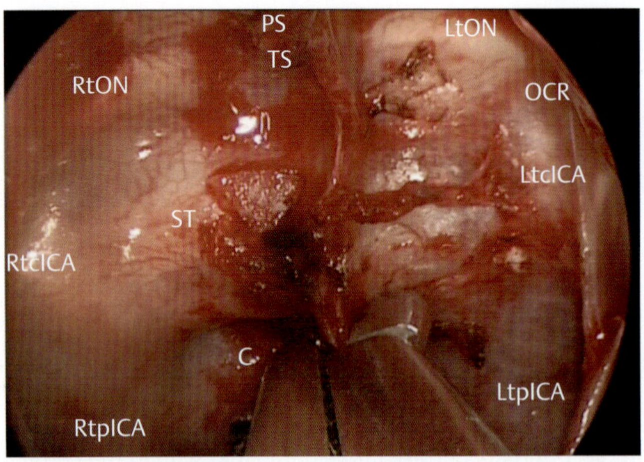

Fig. 3F.5 Removal of the bony septation at the sellar region using a Blakesley forceps.

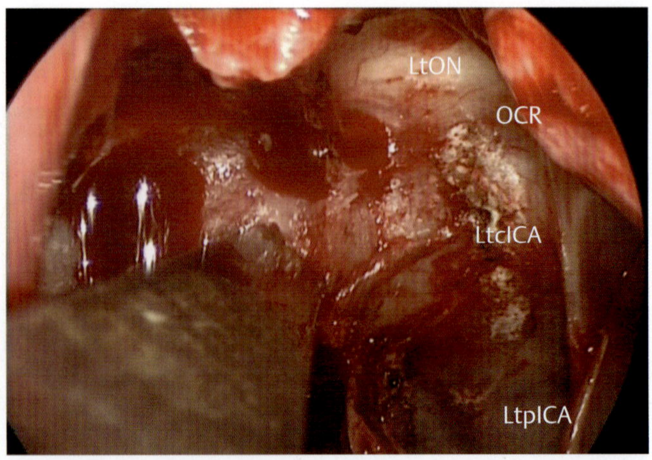

Fig. 3F.6 An osteotomy is performed using a 4-mm chisel to create the transsellar approach.

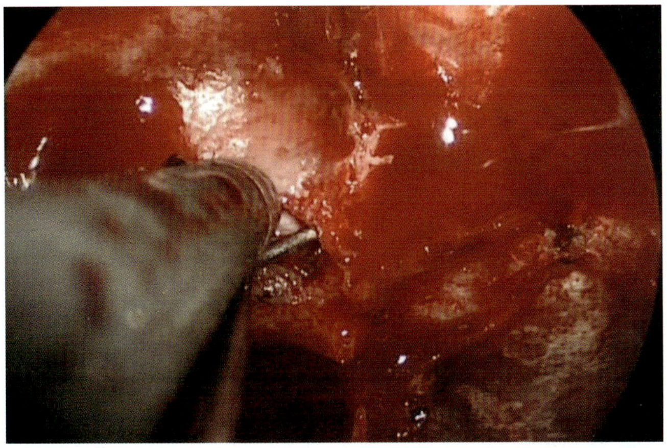

Fig. 3F.7 Transsellar approach: An angled probe is slid through the small opening to elevate the dura off the bony shelf prior to removal of the anterior wall of the sella.

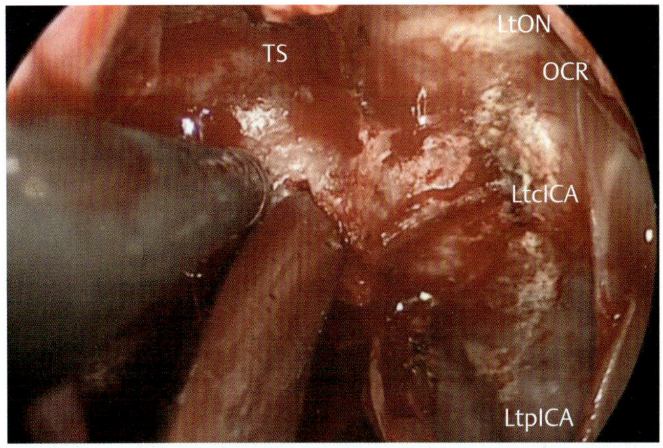

Fig. 3F.8 Transsellar approach: when the bony exposure in the anterior wall of sella is adequate, a dissector is introduced into the opening to carefully elevate the dura away from the bone.

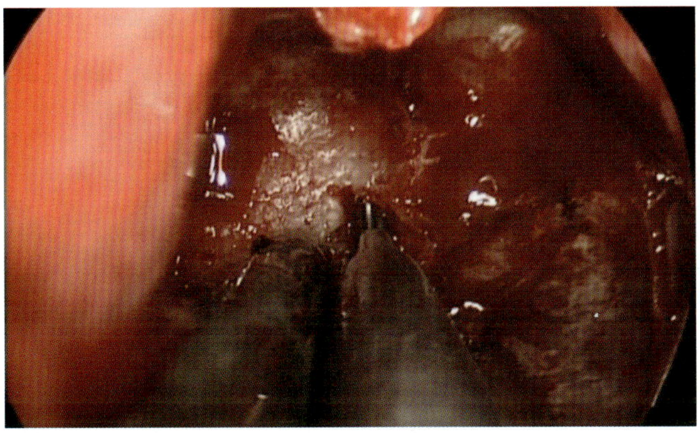

Fig. 3F.9 Transsellar approach: a rongeur or Kerrison's punch is used to enlarge the opening of the sella turcica in a stepwise manner, removing the bone in piecemeals.

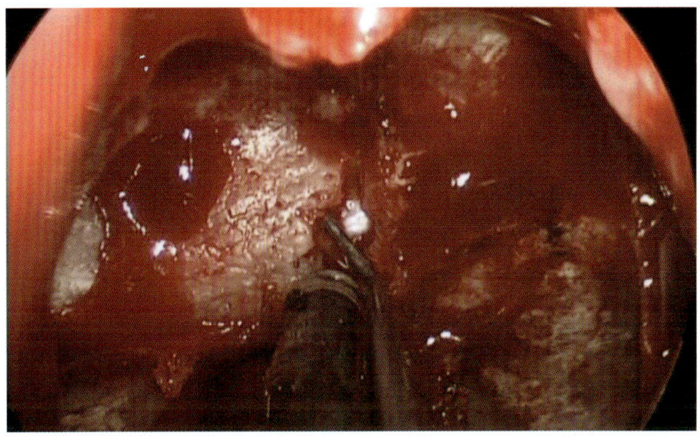

Fig. 3F.10 Transsellar approach: as the opening is enlarged, probes are continuously used in between to ensure that the dura is dissected away from the bone.

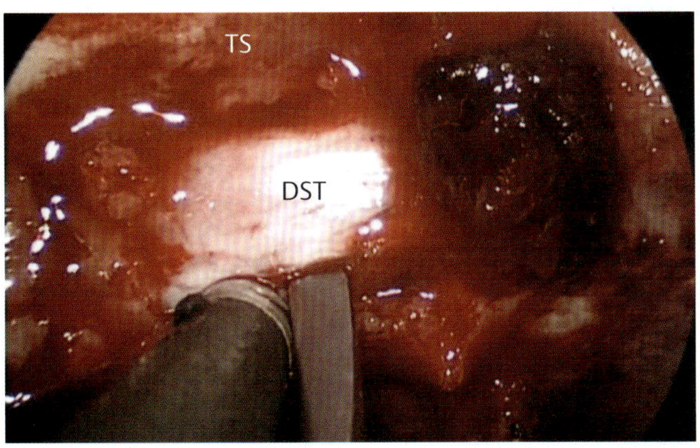

Fig. 3F.11 An incision is made in the inferior aspect of the sella turcica dura (DST) to avoid incising through the normal gland located more anterosuperiorly.

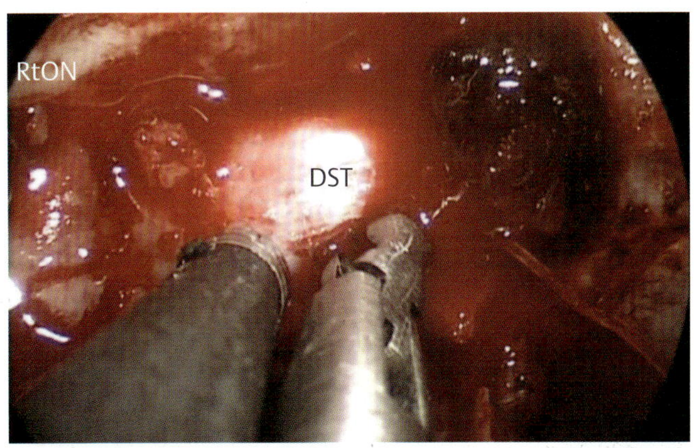

Fig. 3F.12 A biopsy is obtained from the tumor protruding out of the cavity.

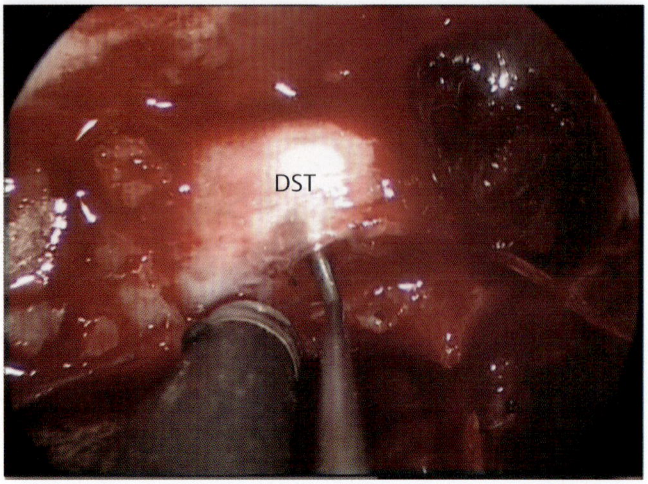

Fig. 3F.13 An angled probe is used to free the dura from the underlying tumor and normal pituitary gland.

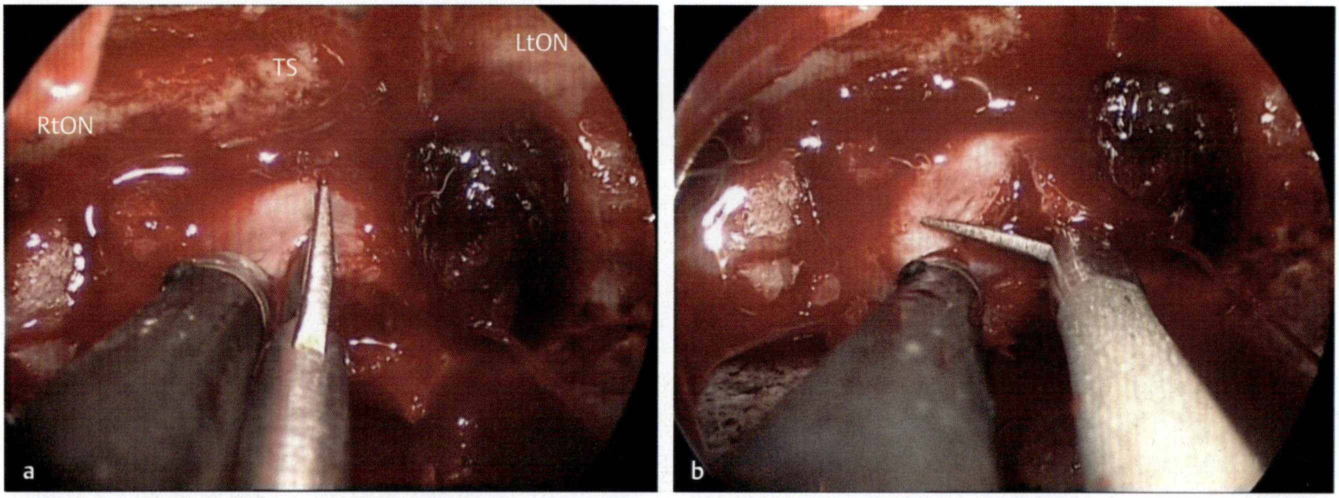

Fig. 3F.14 A microscissor is used to cut open the dura carefully without damaging the normal gland located anterosuperiorly, vertically along the **(a)** midline and continuing **(b)** inferolaterally.

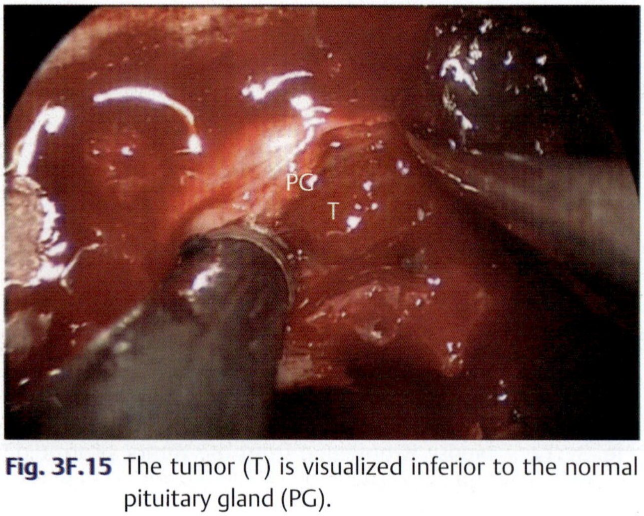

Fig. 3F.15 The tumor (T) is visualized inferior to the normal pituitary gland (PG).

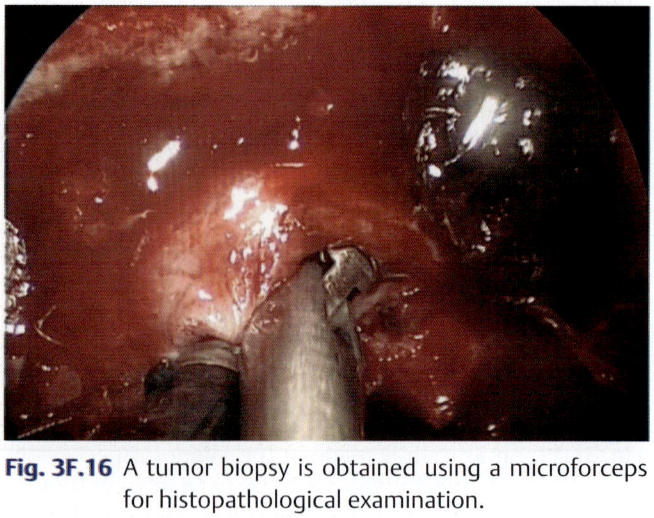

Fig. 3F.16 A tumor biopsy is obtained using a microforceps for histopathological examination.

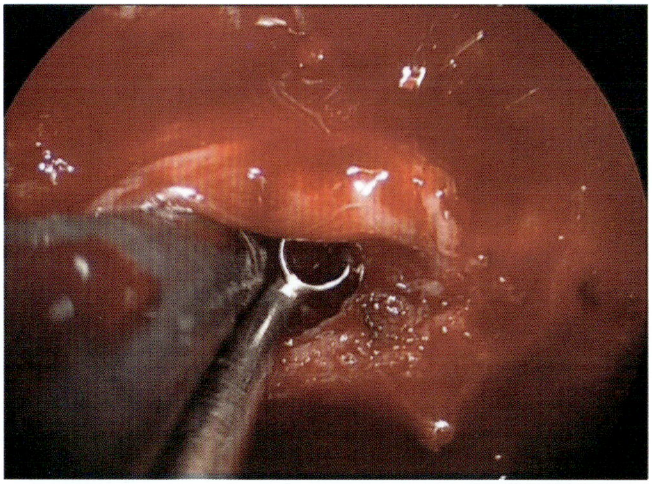

Fig. 3F.17 The tumor is carefully removed from the medial wall of the cavernous sinus with a ring curette.

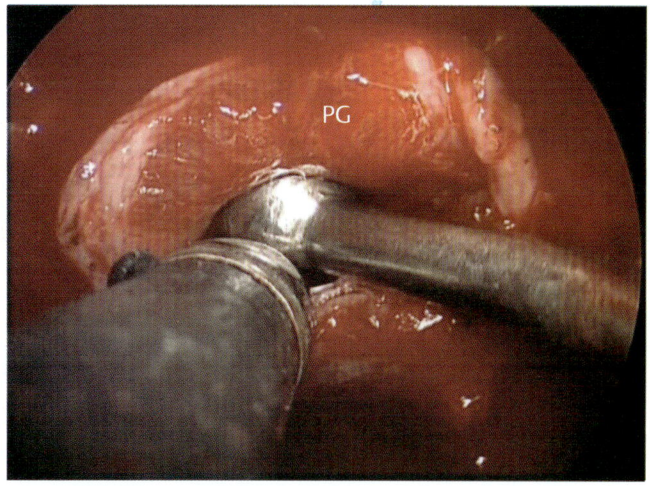

Fig. 3F.18 The normal pituitary gland (PG) is preserved at the end of the surgery.

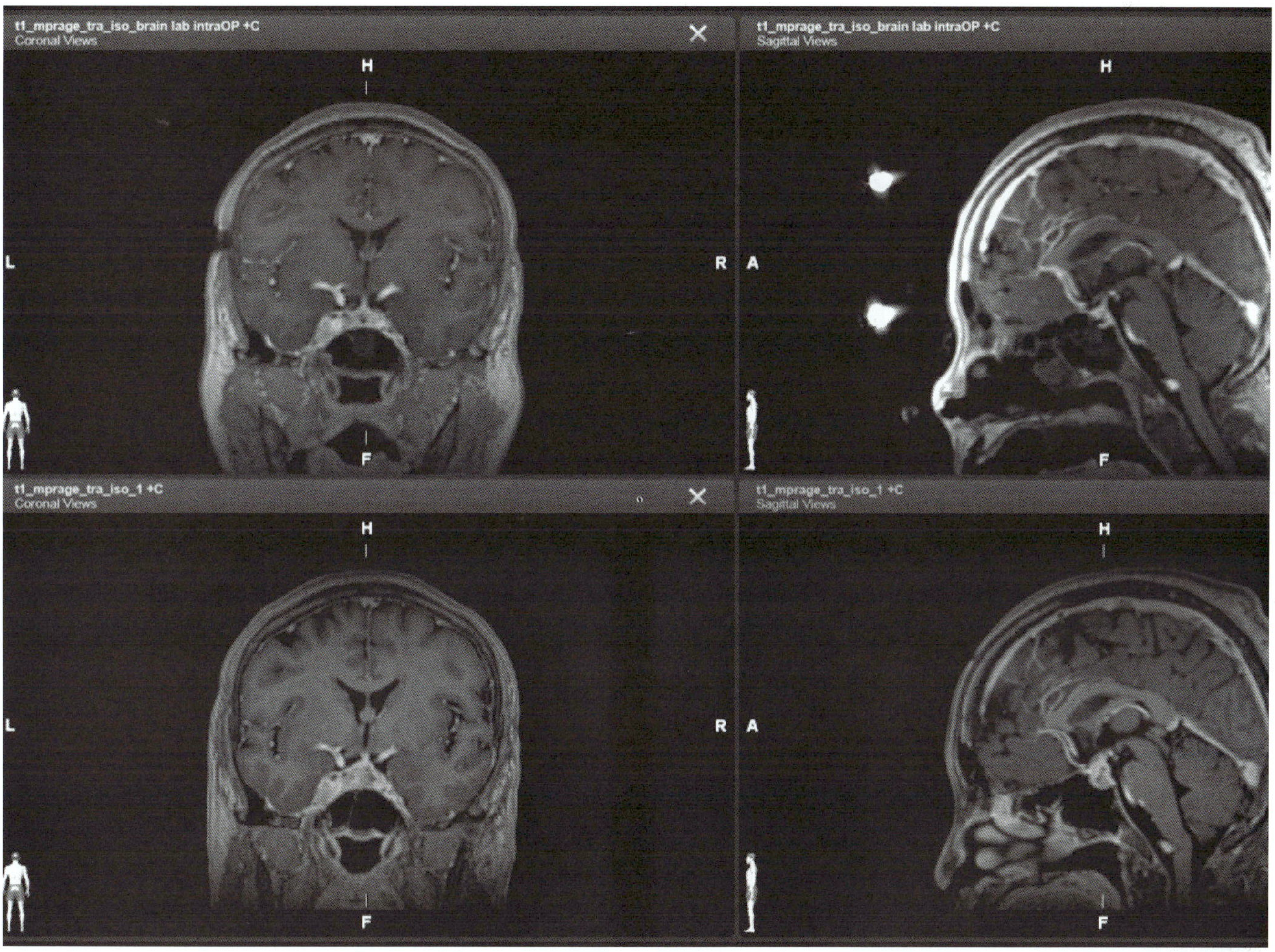

Fig. 3F.19 Intraoperative images of the T1-weighted postcontrast MRI scan on the upper panel synchronized with preoperative scans in the lower panel for direct comparison.

Case 3G

Endoscopic Transseptal Transsphenoidal (Single Nostril) Resection of a Pituitary Macroadenoma Complicated with a Postoperative Cerebrospinal Fluid Leak

Adzreil Bakri, Michel Roethlisberger, Prepageran Narayanan, and Vicknes Waran

History

A 53-year-old gentleman presented with a 2-month history of blurry vision and mild persistent headache. Ophthalmological examination revealed a bitemporal hemianopia with normal visual acuity. A magnetic resonance imaging (MRI) of the brain revealed a pituitary macroadenoma (**Fig. 3G.1**). A *single nostril endoscopic transseptal transsphenoidal excision* of the tumor was planned.

Surgical Steps

1. An endoscopic *single nostril transseptal transsphenoidal approach* is performed as previously described (Chapter 1).
2. Prior to the removal of the bone overlying the sella, the exact location of the tumor is confirmed using image-guided surgery (IGS).
3. The bone overlying the sella is thinned out using a high-speed drill. A small opening into the sella could also be made with a small chisel (**Fig. 3G.2** and **Fig. 3G.3**). In the present case, the bone is thinned by the tumor, and it cracks easily with gentle pressure. Care must be taken so that drilling or curetting is performed medially to avoid injury to the carotid siphons of the cavernous sinuses bilaterally.
4. Once a window is made, a right-angle dissector can be inserted to separate the bone and the underlying dura (**Fig. 3G.4**). This bony opening is then widened adequately in the shape of a rectangle using a Kerrison

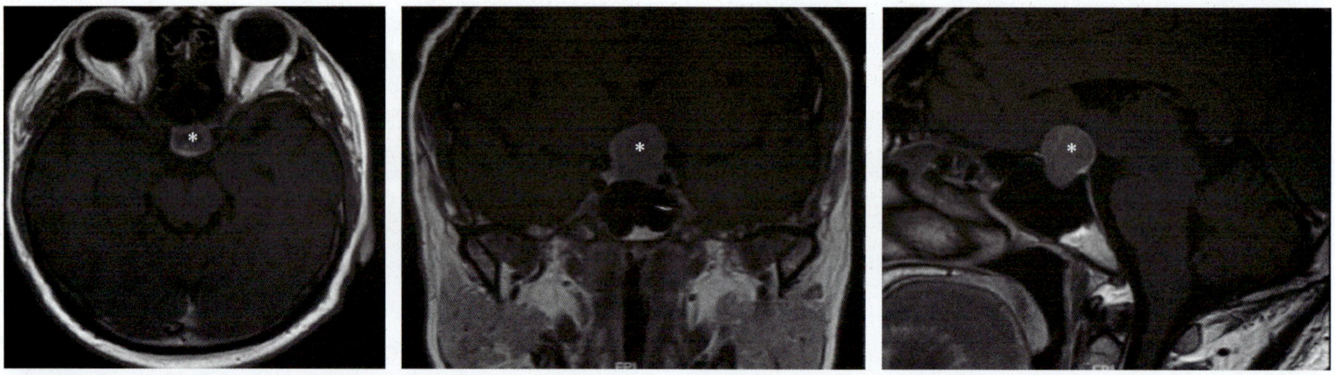

Fig. 3G.1 Preoperative T1-weighted noncontrasted MRI showing a pituitary macroadenoma (*).

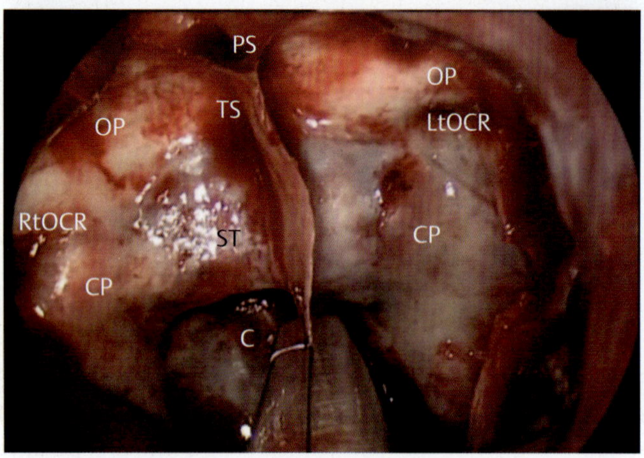

Fig. 3G.2 Removal of residual mucosa and bony septations creating a single large sphenoid cavity.

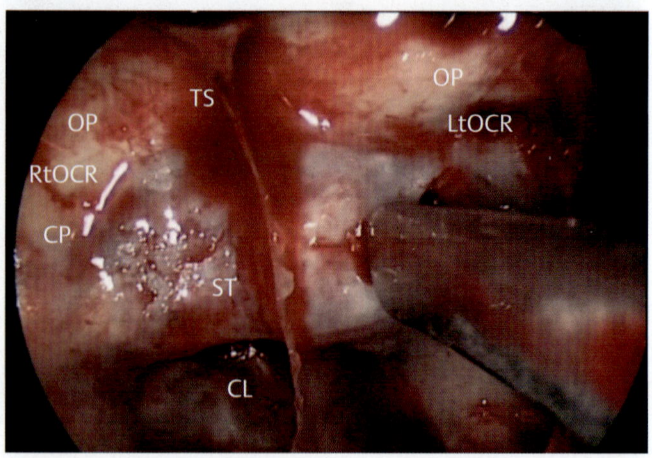

Fig. 3G.3 The bone overlying the sella is gently chiseled to create a small opening or window.

punch, making sure that the dura is always separated from the bone before each bite (**Fig. 3G.5**).

5. After adequate exposure (**Fig. 3G.6**), a horizontal and vertical incision in the shape of a cruciate is made on the dura with a size 15 blade (**Fig. 3G.7**).
6. The tumor is exposed, and a biopsy is taken for histopathological examination (**Fig. 3G.8**). The tumor is then gently dissected away from the normal pituitary gland tissue with suction and blunt ring curette (**Fig. 3G.9** and **Fig. 3G.10**).
7. In this case, the tumor is adherent anterosuperiorly in the sella, the incision is extended, and parts of the adherent tumor are removed using microscissors (**Fig. 3G.11** and **Fig. 3G.12**).
8. After the complete removal of the tumor is confirmed by intraoperative MRI (**Fig. 3G.13**), a large dural defect is noted posterior to the sella which is leaking cerebrospinal fluid (CSF; **Fig. 3G.14**). This defect is repaired in layers with fat graft harvested from the abdomen, Surgicel (oxidized cellulose polymer), and tissue glue (**Fig. 3G.15**, **Fig. 3G.16**, and **Fig. 3G.17**).
9. The sphenoid cavity is then packed with Gelfoam (gelatin sponge) (**Fig. 3G.18**).
10. The septal incision is approximated and the nasal cavity is packed loosely with Nasopore (synthetic biodegradable foam) while making sure that adequate airway along the nasal floor is provided (**Fig. 3G.19**).

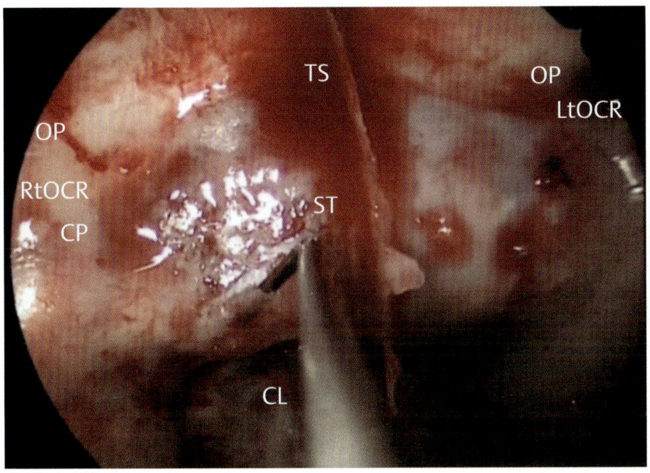

Fig. 3G.4 A right-angle dissector is insinuated between the bone of the sella turcica and the underlying dura.

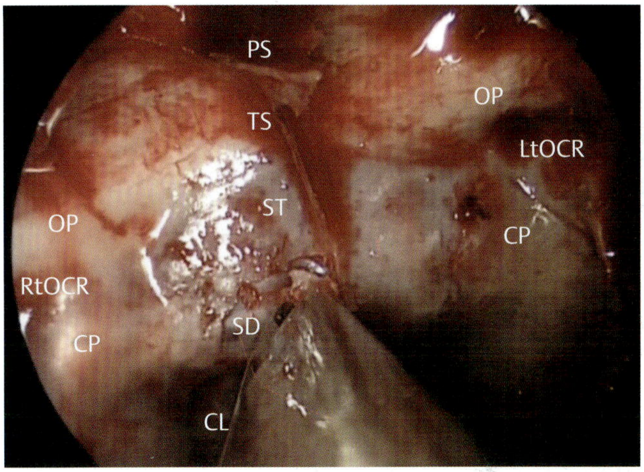

Fig. 3G.5 The bony opening is widened using a Kerrison punch.

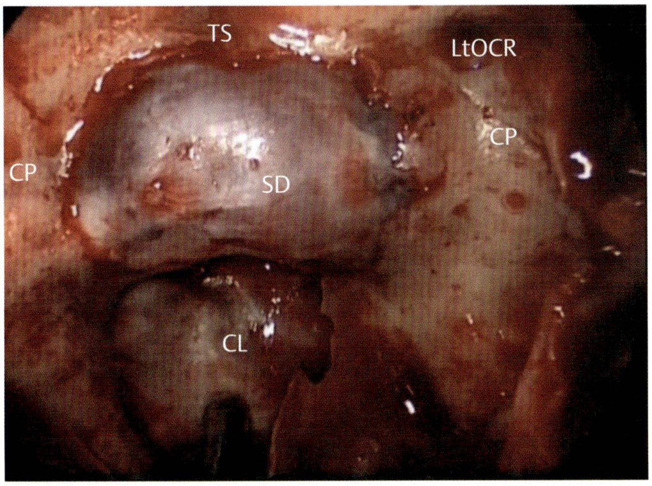

Fig. 3G.6 An adequate bony opening with exposure of the tumor.

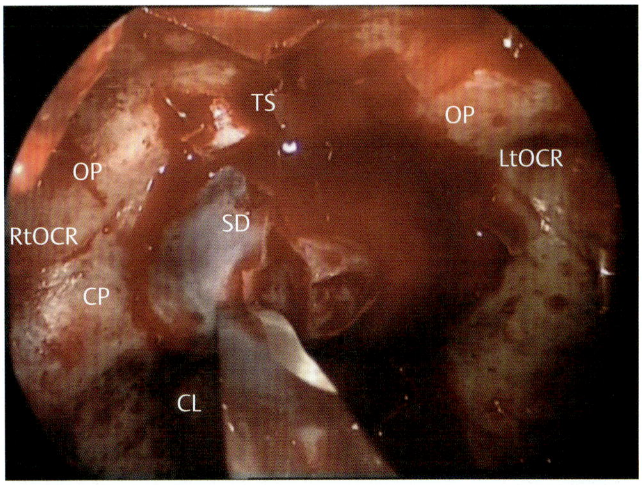

Fig. 3G.7 Cruciate incision of the dura.

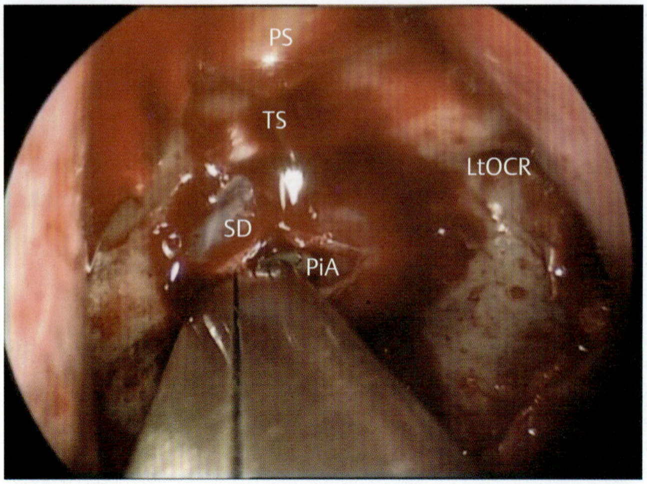

Fig. 3G.8 A biopsy is taken from the pituitary adenoma (PiA).

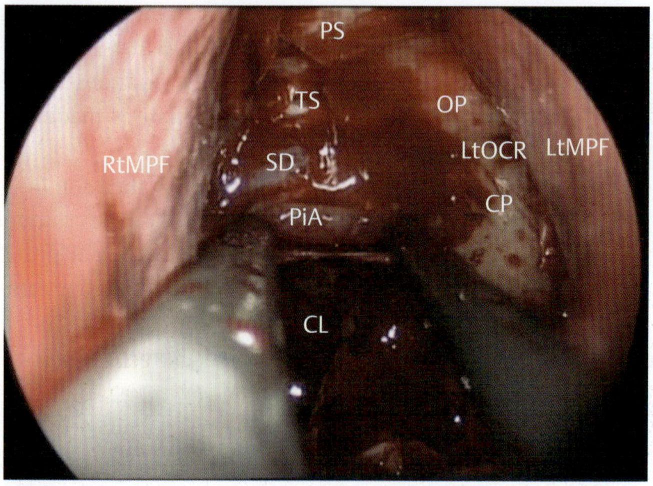

Fig. 3G.9 Blunt dissection and removal of the pituitary adenoma (PiA) using the dual suction method.

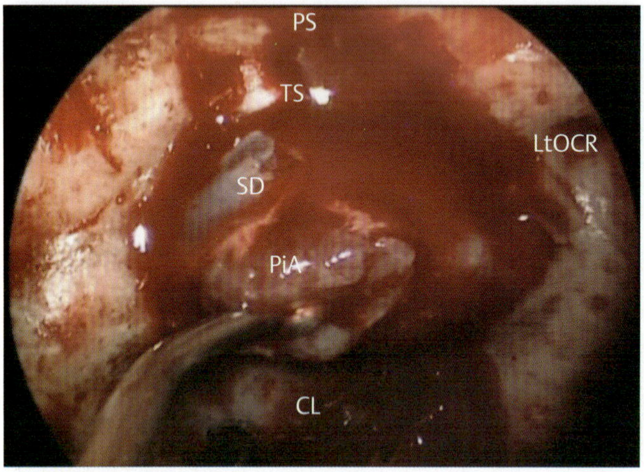

Fig. 3G.10 Pituitary adenoma (PiA) removal using a blunt ring curette.

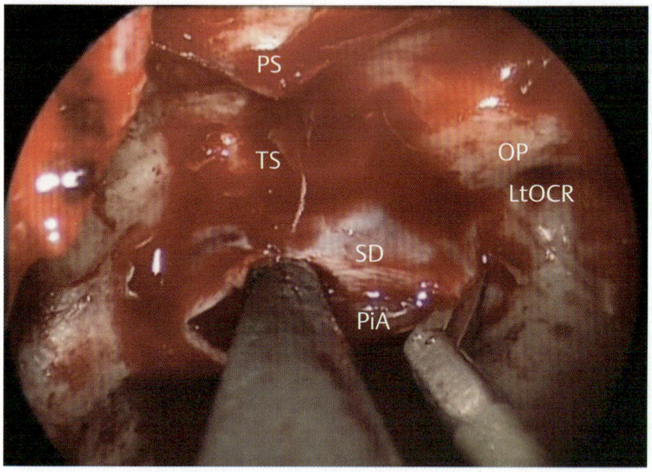

Fig. 3G.11 The dural incision is extended as the pituitary adenoma (PiA) is adherent anterosuperiorly.

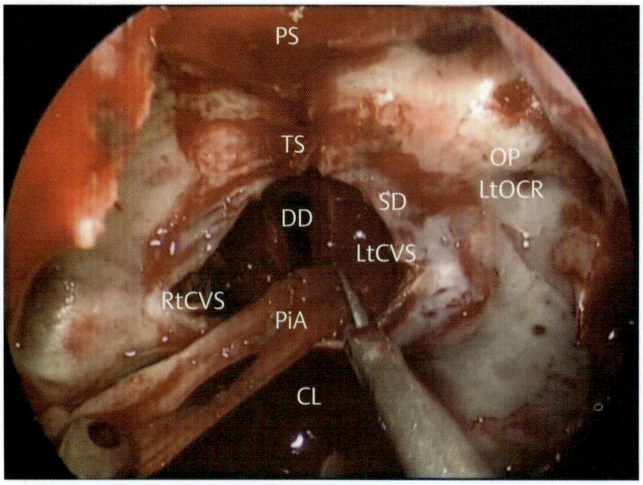

Fig. 3G.12 Excision of adherent pituitary adenoma capsule (PiA) with microscissors.

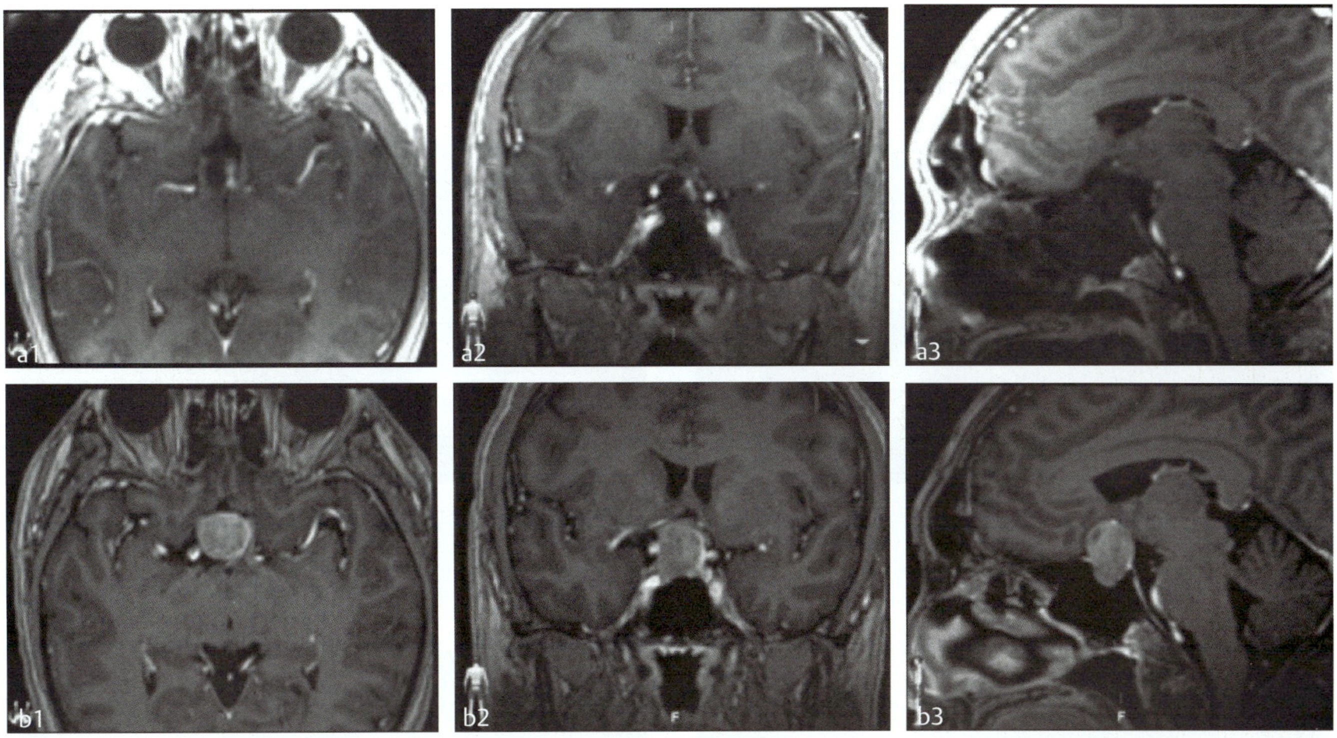

Fig. 3G.13 **(a1)** Axial; **(a2)** coronal; **(a3)** sagittal intraoperative T1-weighted contrast-enhanced MRI section confirming complete resection of the pituitary macroadenoma, as compared to the preoperative **(b1)** axial; **(b2)** coronal; **(b3)** sagittal T1-weighted contrast-enhanced MRI sections.

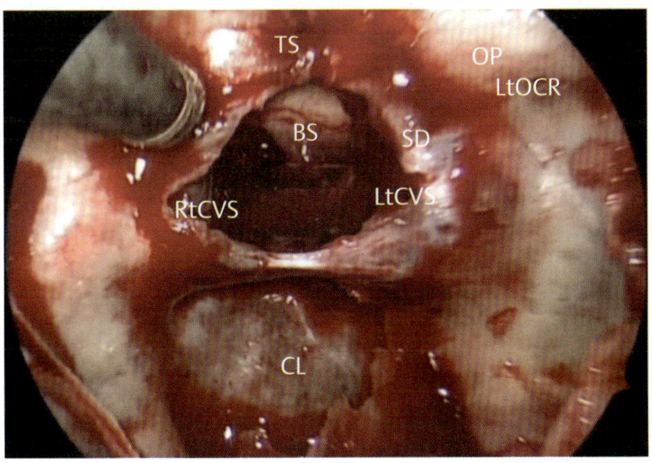

Fig. 3G.14 A dural defect with a posteriorly located intermediate-flow cerebrospinal fluid leak is identified.

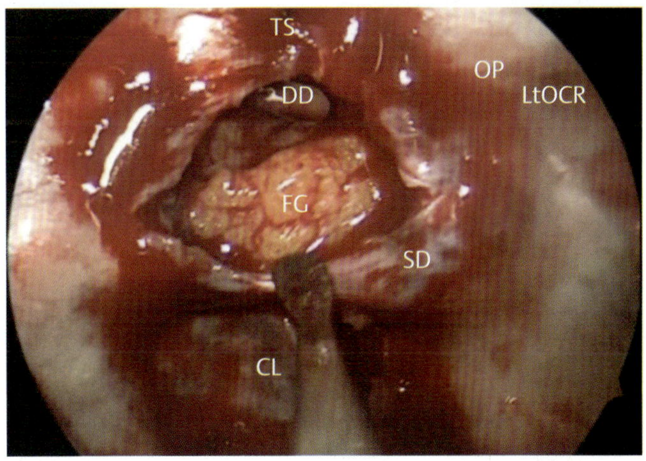

Fig. 3G.15 The dural defect is repaired with an abdominal fat graft (FG).

Repair of an Iatrogenic Intraoperative Cerebrospinal Fluid Leak

Case Continuation

The patient developed CSF-leakage on the second postoperative day after severe bouts of coughing and retching. He was brought to the operation theatre for the repair of the CSF leak.

Surgical Steps

1. The patient is placed in a supine position under general anesthesia with the head slightly extended.
2. The nose is decongested with nasal packing as per the usual methods of the institution.
3. The nasal cavity is inspected for the potential leakage site. The septal incision is reopened, and the previous

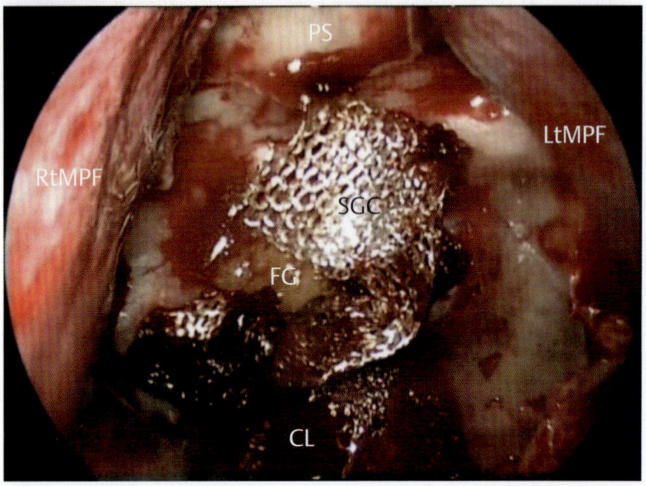

Fig. 3G.16 Surgicel (SGC) is layered over the abdominal fat graft (FG).

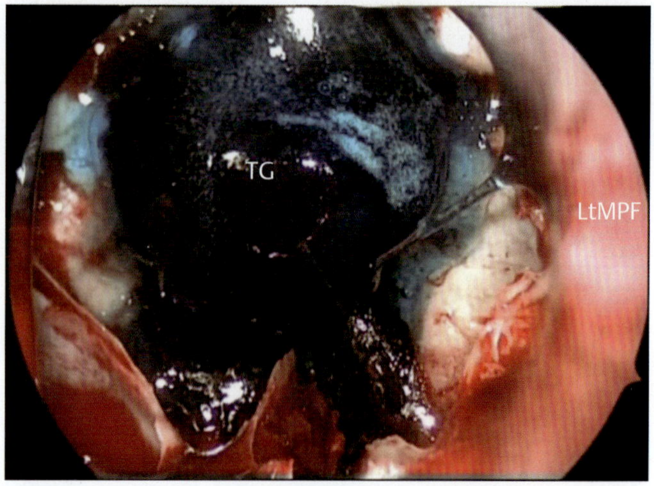

Fig. 3G.17 Tissue glue (TG) is deposited over the fat graft.

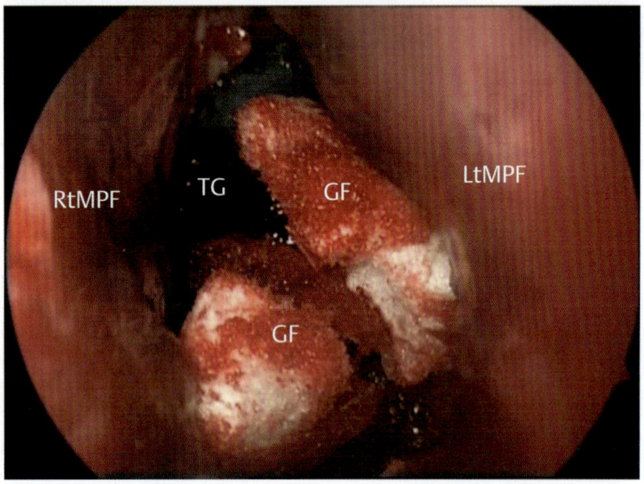

Fig. 3G.18 The sphenoid cavity is packed with Gelfoam (GF).

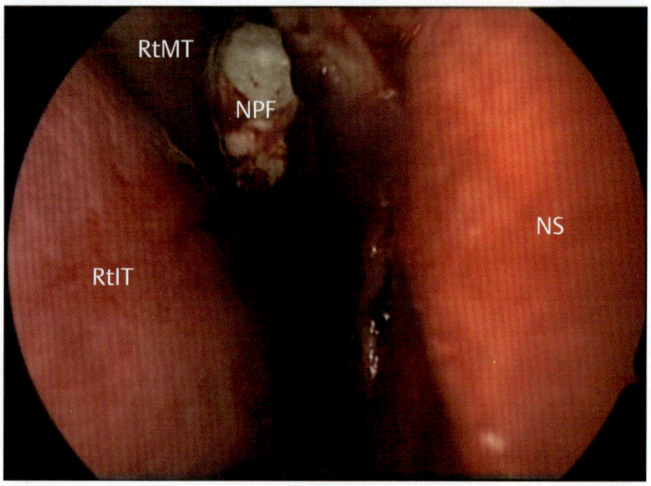

Fig. 3G.19 Closure of the septal incision and loose nasal packing with Nasopore (NPF).

layers of repair are gently removed layer-by-layer (**Fig. 3G.20** and **Fig. 3G.21**).

4. Once all the previous layers of repair are removed, the actual leakage site is clearly identified and assessed (**Fig. 3G.22**).
5. The defect is repaired using an abdominal fat graft (underlay method), and the sella is packed with another fat graft (**Fig. 3G.23**). A Valsalva maneuver is performed to assess the patency of the first layer of repair (**Fig. 3G.24**). If there is no sign of CSF leakage through the repair, the fat graft is reinforced using tissue glue (**Fig. 3G.25**).
6. A second layer of fat is applied and reinforced with Surgicel and tissue glue (**Fig. 3G.26** and **Fig. 3G.27**).
7. The sphenoid cavity is packed with Surgicel and Gelfoam (**Fig. 3G.28**).
8. The septal incision is reapproximated, and the nasal cavity is packed loosely with Nasopore allowing adequate nasal airway passage along the floor of the nose (**Fig. 3G.29**).

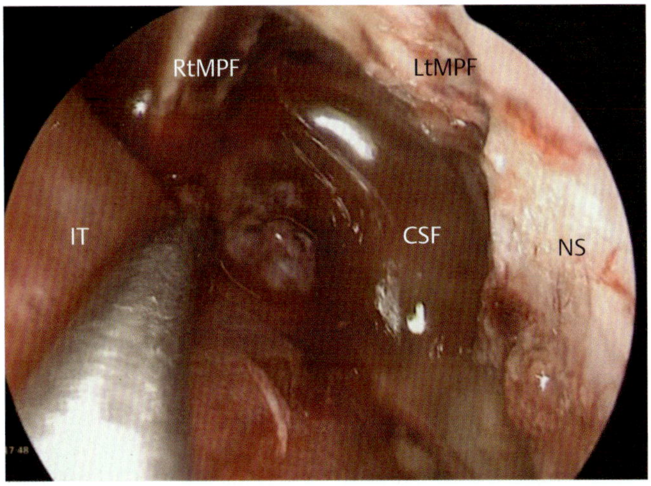

Fig. 3G.20 The septal incision in the right nasal cavity is reopened exposing cerebrospinal fluid (CSF).

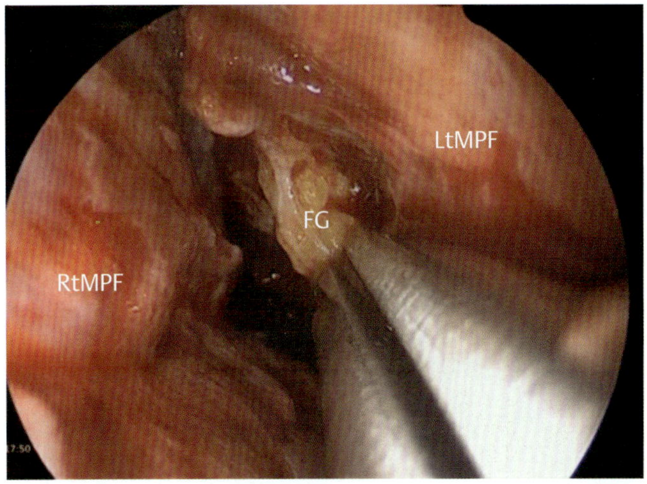

Fig. 3G.21 Gentle removal of previous repair material in layers.

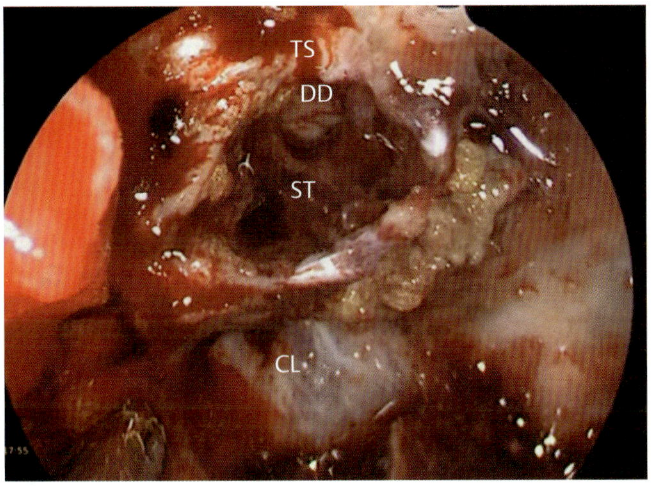

Fig. 3G.22 The leakage site is noted to be similar to the initial dural defect of the first operation.

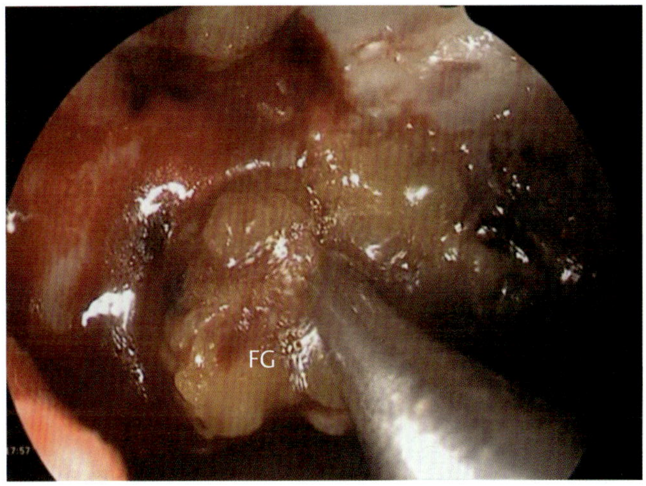

Fig. 3G.23 Repair of the defect with an abdominal fat graft (FG).

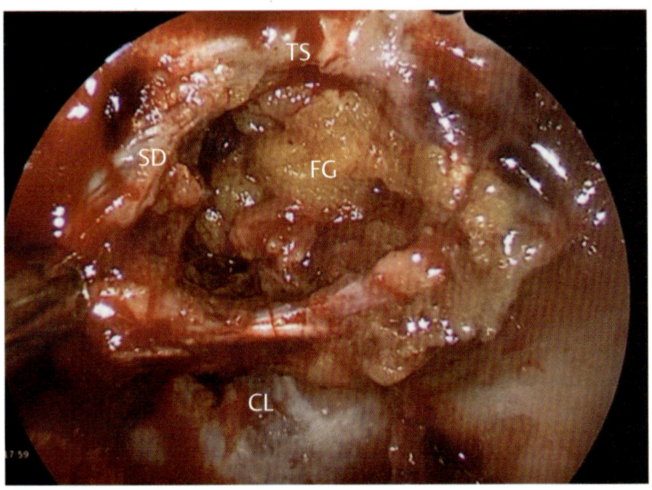

Fig. 3G.24 The sella is packed with fat (FG), and Valsalva maneuver is performed to check any further CSF leak.

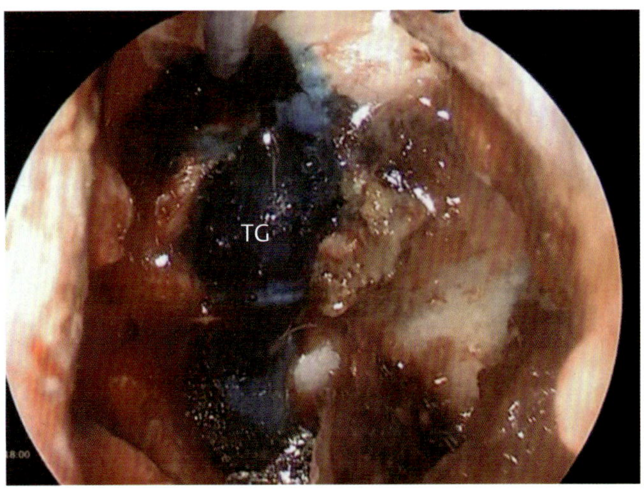

Fig. 3G.25 Tissue glue (TG) is applied over the fat graft.

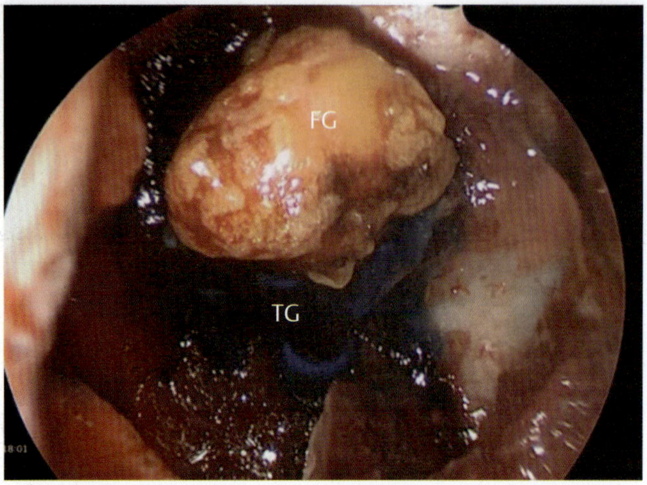

Fig. 3G.26 A second layer of fat (FG) is applied.

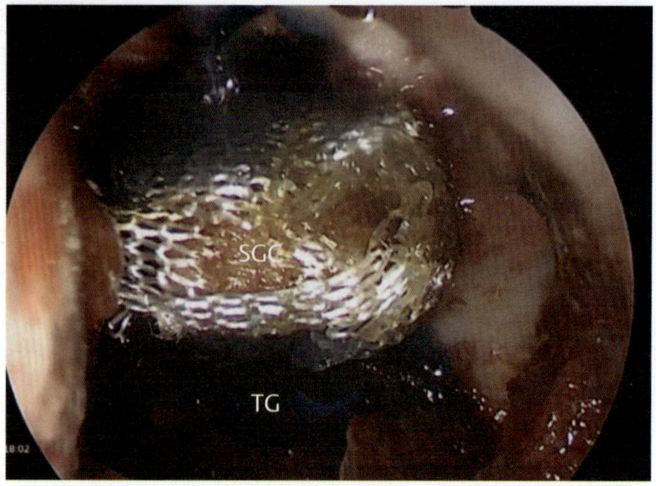

Fig. 3G.27 This second layer of repair is reinforced with Surgicel (SGC) and tissue glue (TG).

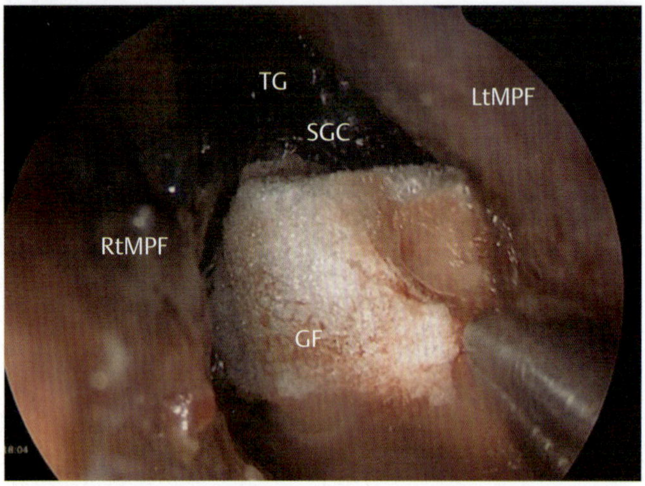

Fig. 3G.28 Packing of the sphenoid cavity with Surgicel (SGC) and Gelfoam (GF).

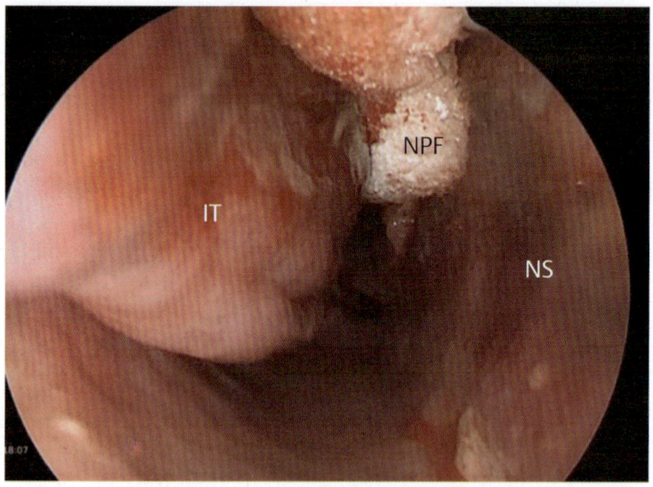

Fig. 3G.29 Approximation of the septal incision and loose nasal packing with Nasopore (NPF).

Case 3H

Endonasal Endoscopic Mononostril Transsphenoidal Approach for a Macroadenoma with Detected Residual in Intraoperative MRI

Michel Roethlisberger, Warren O. Bennett, Prepageran Narayanan, and Vicknes Waran

History

This is a case of a 71-year-old lady who presented with a large nonsecretory pituitary macroadenoma. This was causing the visual disturbance. The magnetic resonance imaging (MRI) shows a macroadenoma with suprasellar extension and a cystic component within (**Fig. 3H.1**). It was felt that this case would be suitable for a mononostril transsphenoidal approach rather than the more common binostril approach, meaning less nasal cavity trauma and disturbance. We highlight the importance of the intraoperative MRI (iMRI) so making sure all tumor is removed.

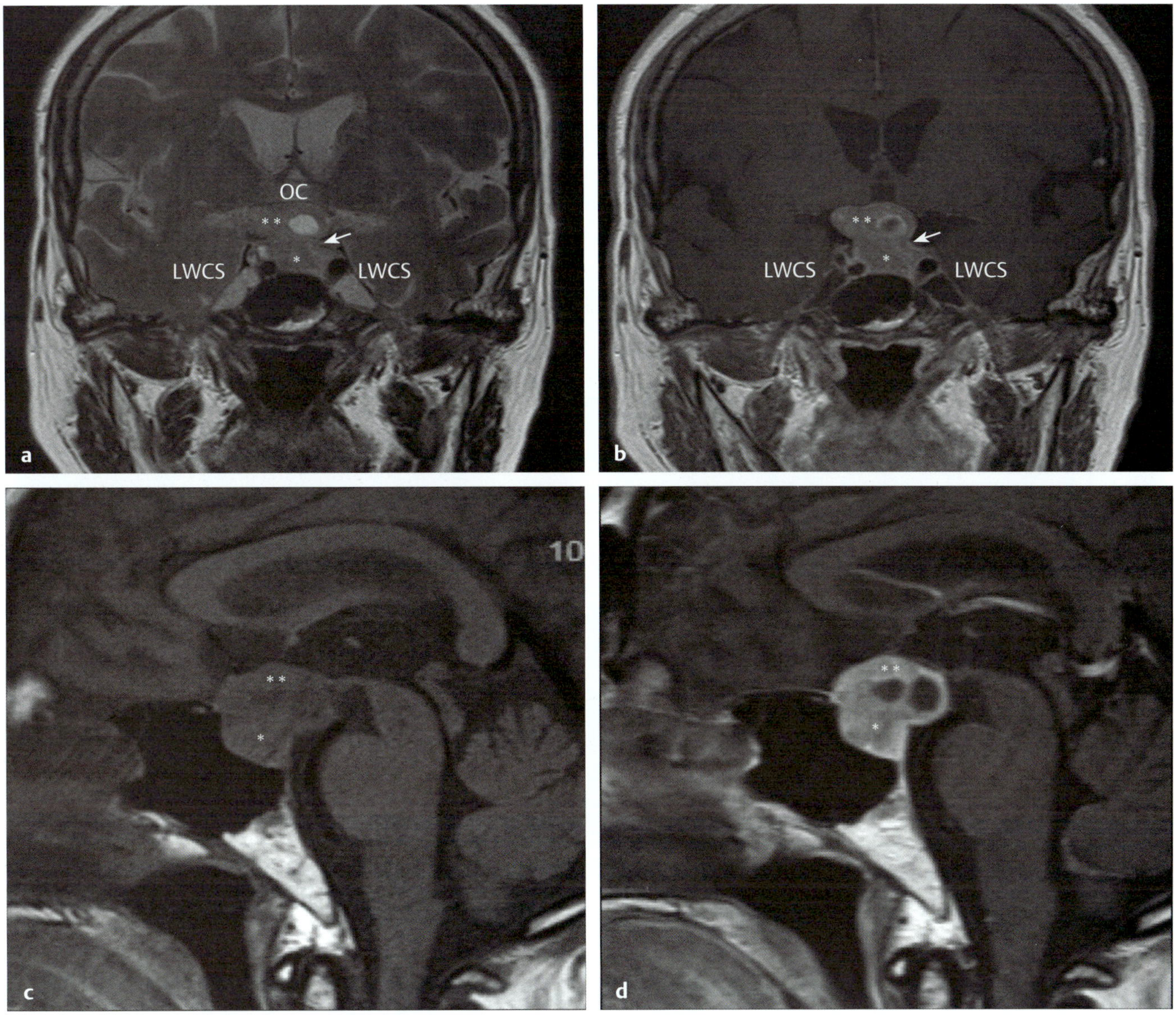

Fig. 3H.1 **(a)** Coronal T2-weighted and **(b)** coronal T1-weighted gadolinium contrast-enhanced, **(c)** sagittal T1-weighted noncontrast-enhanced and **(d)** sagittal T1-weighted gadolinium contrast-enhanced MRI section showing a pituitary tumor with intra- (*), suprasellar (**) extension and a dumbbell-like shape (*white arrow*).

Surgical Steps

1. A *mononostril transseptal transsphenoidal approach* is performed as previously described.
2. The exposed cartilaginous and bony septum can then be removed in a piecemeal fashion (**Fig. 3H.2**).
3. The mucosal flaps are further elevated to expose the anterior face of the sphenoid and both ostia of the sphenoid sinus. The flap should be elevated as far lateral as possible to the lateral wall of the nasal cavity. If elevated in the correct plane, both flaps will maintain their blood supply from the posterior branch of the sphenopalatine artery and can be used for reconstruction if required. With the mononostril approach, the elevated mucosal flaps can be brought back to the midline to give a membranous nasal septum.
4. The rostrum sphenoidale or keel can then be taken down. This can be done with many different instruments or a combination of instruments, including downward Kerrison's punch, pituitary rongeur forceps, or a drill (**Fig. 3H.3**).
5. The sphenoid ostium can now be widened using a downward Kerrison punch. This should be done in an inferior and medial direction to avoid damaging important structures.

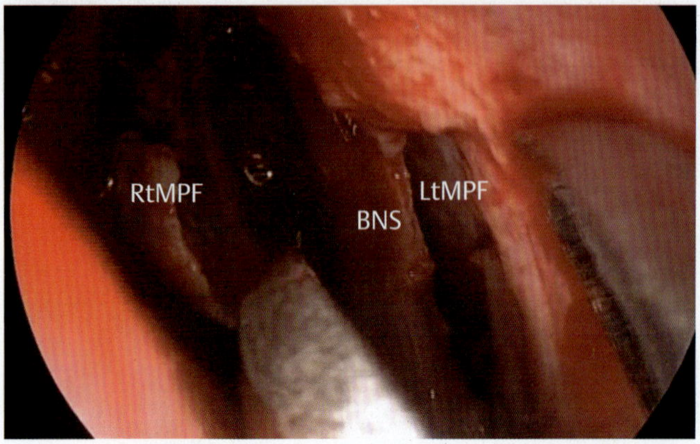

Fig. 3H.2 The mononostril approach requires the removal of the nasal septum to allow midline access and also means that the contralateral septal mucosa may be elevated but not interrupted. This allows less nasal trauma postoperatively.

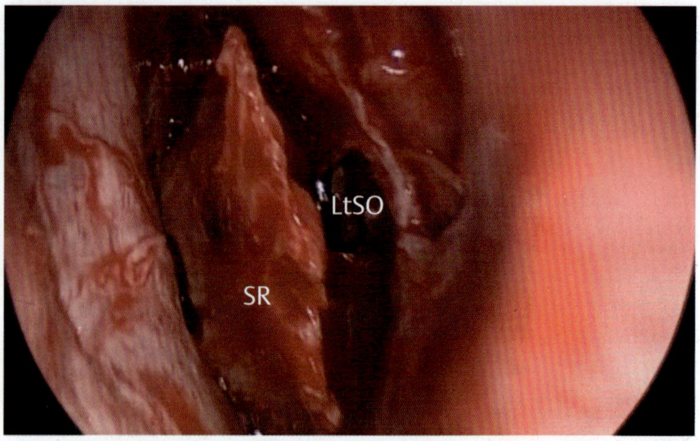

Fig. 3H.3 The sphenoid rostrum (SR) has been exposed with both sphenoid ostia visible. The rostrum must be removed and the ostia widened for sufficient access for the pituitary surgery.

6. The amount of bone to be removed has to be enough to allow an unobstructed view of the sella and the parasellar critical structures (optic nerve, internal carotid artery [ICA], midclivus, and planum sphenoidale) and to allow adequate access for instruments. This often requires removing bone to the level of the floor of the sphenoid.
7. Sphenoid septations can be carefully removed with either a drill or pituitary rongeur forceps. This allows small controlled bites of bone to be removed, instead of uncontrolled fractures which may result in ICA injury or CSF-leakage.
8. A suction monopolar is then used to cauterize and remove the mucosa over the posterior wall of the sphenoid sinus.
9. The extension of the lesion can be defined using intraoperative IGS.
10. In most cases of pituitary macroadenoma, the bone over the sella is thin as in this case. Therefore, a gentle fracture in the midline will allow a right-angle dissector to be insinuated between the bone and the dura, and the bone is flaked off (**Fig. 3H.4**).
11. The osteodural exposure is continued with removal of the lateral limit next to the parasellar ICA and inferiorly the floor of the sella.
12. The dural opening is done with a knife, and the extension is done with microscissors after freeing the underlying tissue using a right-angle dissector.
13. Bleeding at this stage can occur from the intercavernous venous sinus. This can be dealt with using hemostats such as Surgicel (Ethicon US, LLC) or Floseal (Baxter Healthcare Corporation) (**Fig. 3H.5**).
14. The tumor is then debulked using a ring curette. This must be done in controlled and orderly manner (**Fig. 3H.5**).
15. The inferior aspect of the tumor is usually removed first from the floor of the pituitary fossa and then the lateral inferior aspects can be cleared. Debulking is continued with the aim to clear the inferior margin of the tumor before proceeding superiorly.
16. If it is not done in this order, the diaphragm will fall into the surgical view covering the inferior posterior aspect of the tumor (**Fig. 3H.6, Fig. 3H.7, Fig. 3H.8,** and **Fig. 3H.9**).
17. A piece of the tumor must always be sent for histology.
18. With the inferior and central components of the tumor removed, the remnant superior component can be delivered centrally and removed until the diaphragm prolapses into the pituitary fossa (**Fig. 3H.10**).
19. The extent of resection is matched with IGS and the pituitary fossa temporarily packed with cottonoids prior to the iMRI control (**Fig. 3H.11**, and **Fig. 3H.12a**).
20. Intraoperative gadolinium contrast-enhanced MRI was performed at this stage. The intraoperative noncontrast- and contrast-enhanced images reveal residual tumor in the right suprasellar region (**Fig. 3H.12b–d**).
21. The surgery was recommenced. Further tumor was found superior and was hidden within folds of the diaphragm. This was successfully removed (**Fig. 3H.13, Fig. 3H.14, Fig. 3H.15, Fig. 3H.16, Fig. 3H.17,** and **Fig. 3H.18**).
22. Thorough hemostasis is then performed to make sure there will not be a residual hematoma.

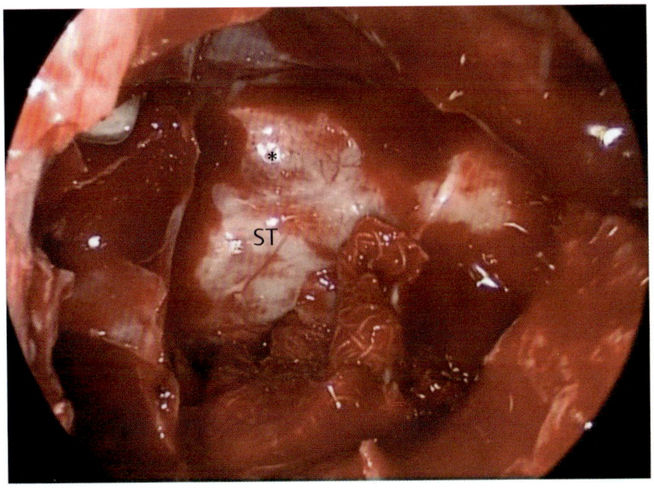

Fig. 3H.4 The bone covering the sella turcica (ST) is thinned (*) over the anterior wall of the pituitary fossa.

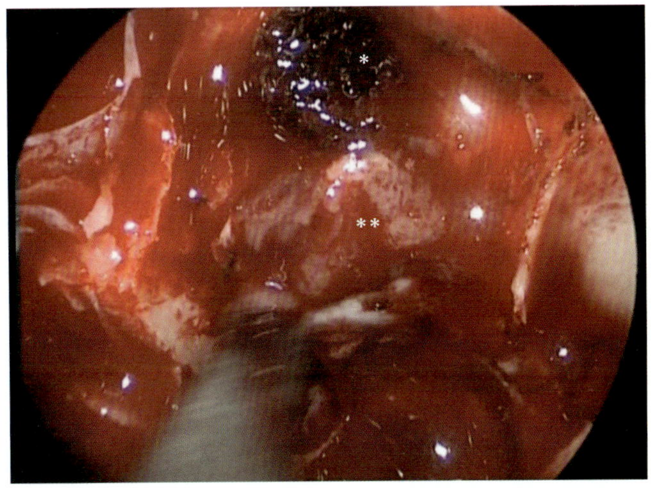

Fig. 3H.5 After the opening of the sellar dura, bleeding from the intercavernous sinus can be managed with hemostatic agents (*). A ring curette is carefully used to remove the central pillar (**) of the pituitary adenoma along the sellar floor.

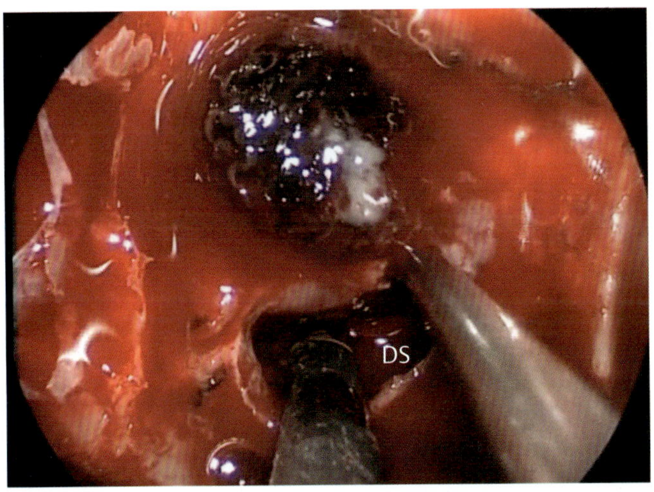

Fig. 3H.6 The dorsum sellae (DS) is reached, and the lateral pillars of the pituitary adenoma are removed using a suction device. The superior aspects of the tumor are still visible (*).

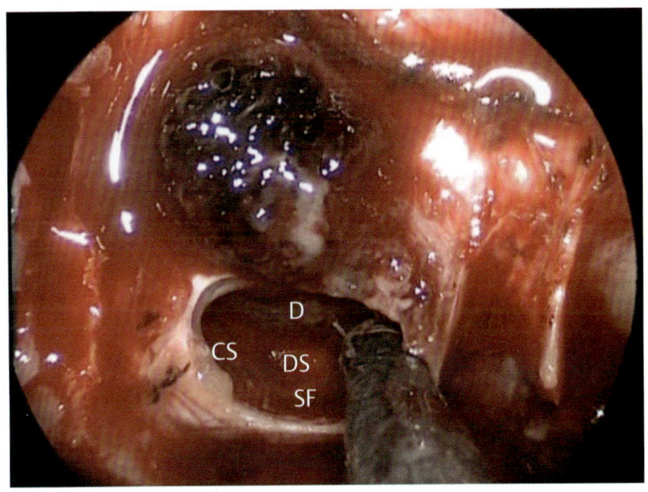

Fig. 3H.7 While following a systematic resection of the pituitary adenoma, the dorsum sellae (DS), the sellar floor (SF), the medial wall of the cavernous sinus (CS), and the diaphragma sellae (D) are identifiable.

23. Abdominal fat is harvested from around the umbilicus. This can be done by an assistant during the surgery and stored in saline. The defect in the anterior wall of the pituitary fossa is plugged with the fat and the edges are tucked into edges of the fossa to create a watertight seal (**Fig. 3H.19**).
24. This is then sealed with a synthetic dural sealant and layered with absorbable hemostat.
25. The elevated nasoseptal flaps are then placed back into the midline, and absorbable nasal dressings can be placed in the nasal cavity to keep these in place.
26. A postoperative radiological follow-up reveals complete tumor removal with resolving visual deficits and normal pituitary function (**Fig. 3H.20**).

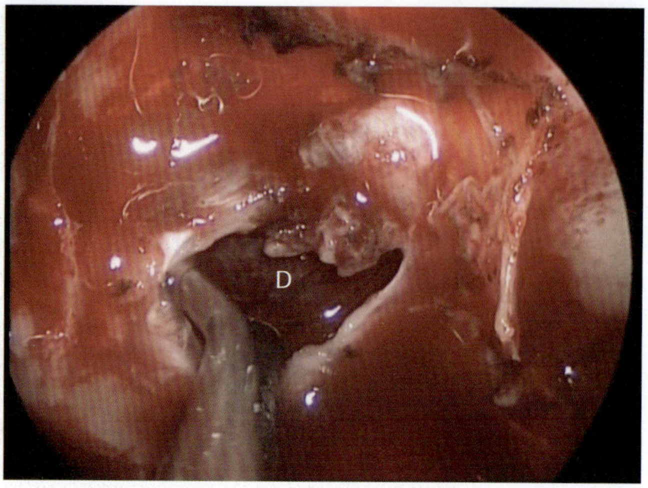

Fig. 3H.8 The lateral aspects along the medial wall of the cavernous sinus are cleaned from tumor using an angled ring curette.

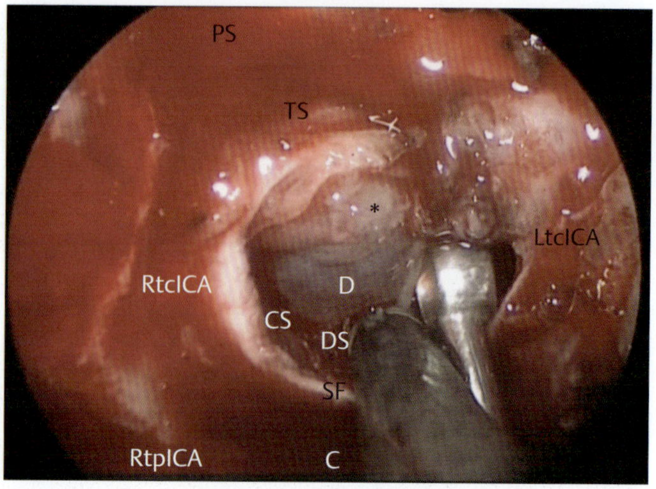

Fig. 3H.9 The lateral and anterosuperior aspects along the prolapsing diaphragm sellae (D) are cleaned from the residual tumor (*) using an angled ring curette.

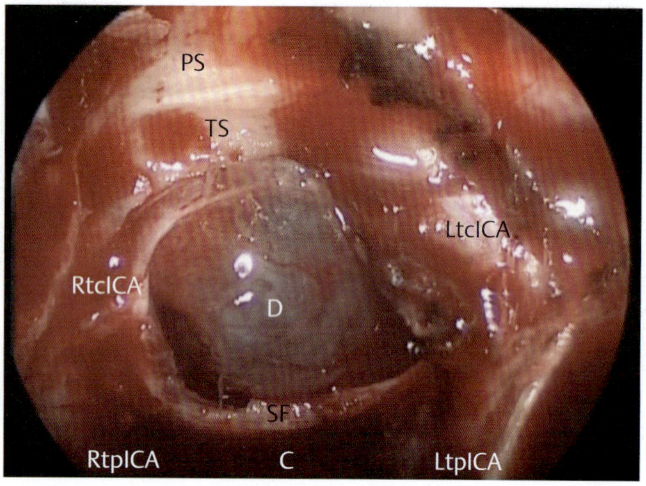

Fig. 3H.10 Final inspection shows a symmetrically prolapsed diaphragm sellae (D) giving the impression of complete tumor removal.

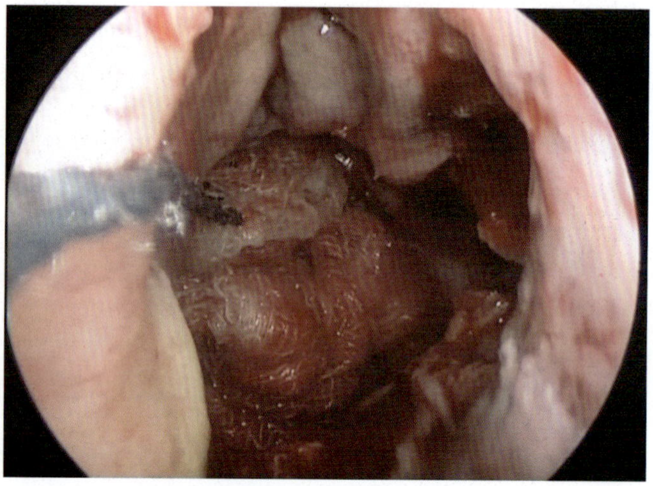

Fig. 3H.11 Temporary packing with cottonoids prior to intraoperative MRI for the extent of resection control.

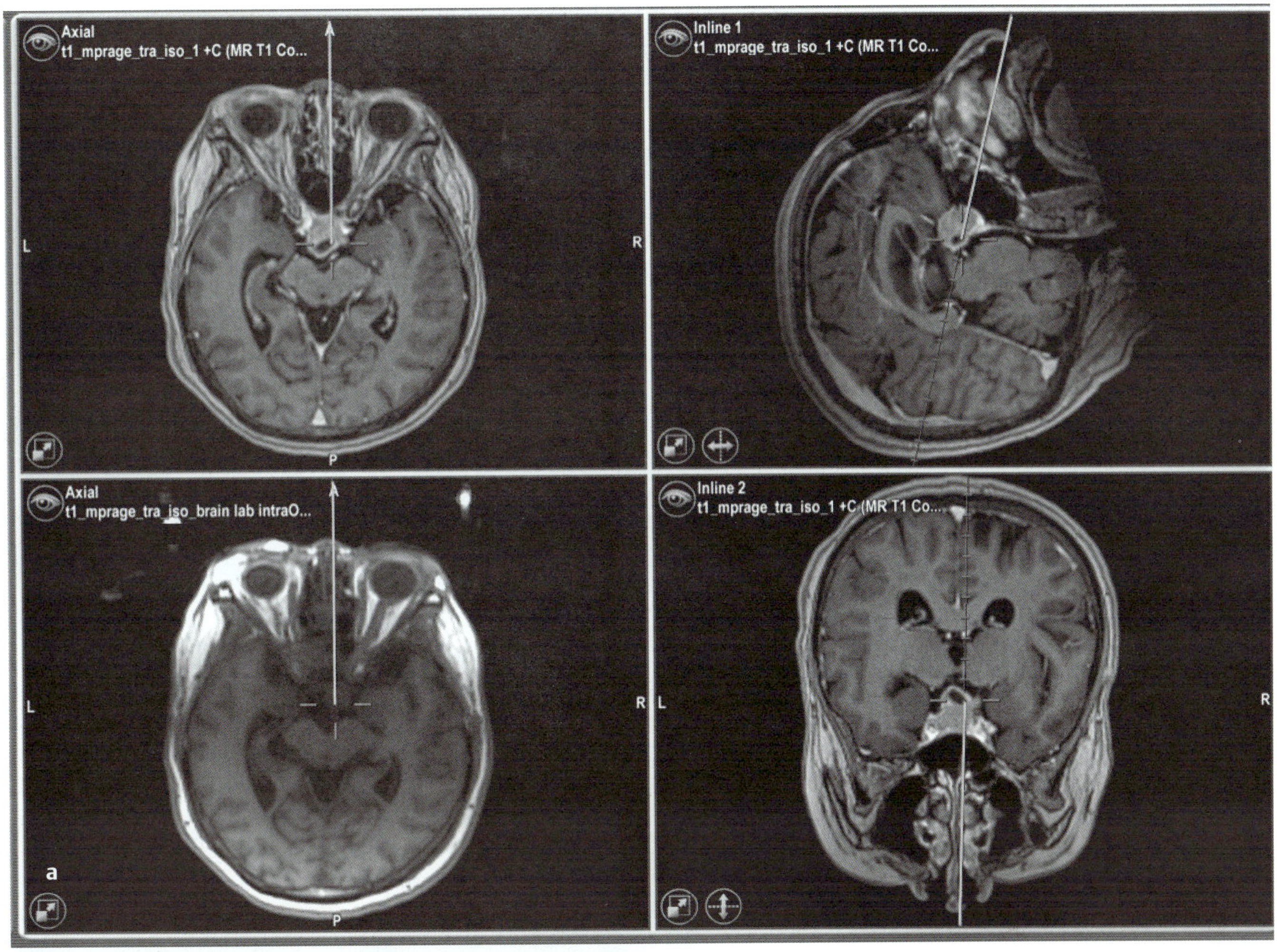

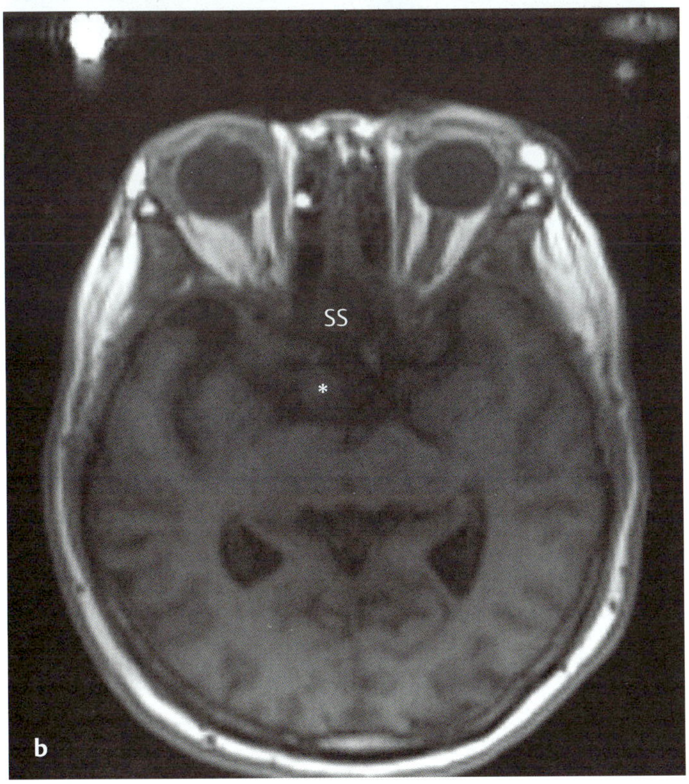

Fig. 3H.12 **(a)** Intraoperative image-guided surgery confirms the pointer-tip located at the posterior resection borders of the pituitary adenoma. **(b)** Intraoperative T1-weighted noncontrast-enhanced axial. *(Continued)*

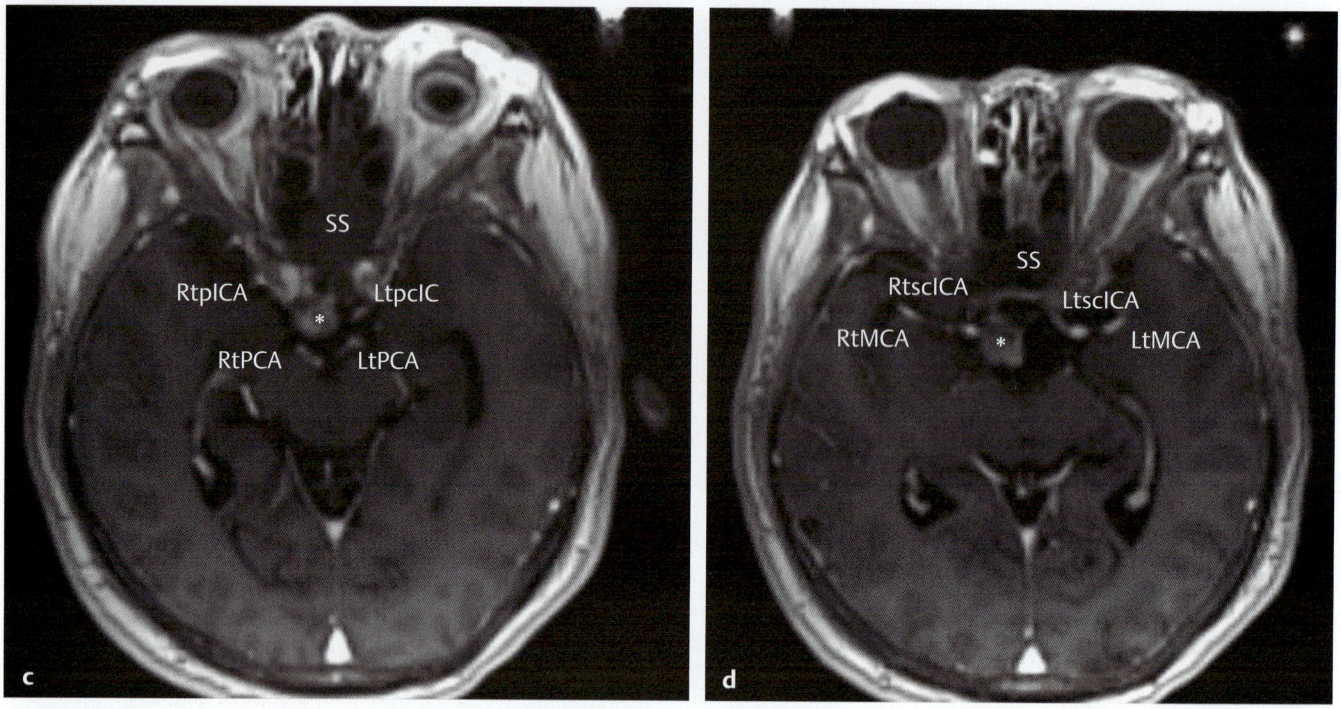

Fig. 3H.12 *(Continued)* **(c, d)** Intraoperative T1-weighted gadolinium contrast-enhanced axial MRI sections demonstrating residual right-sided suprasellar tumor tissue (*).

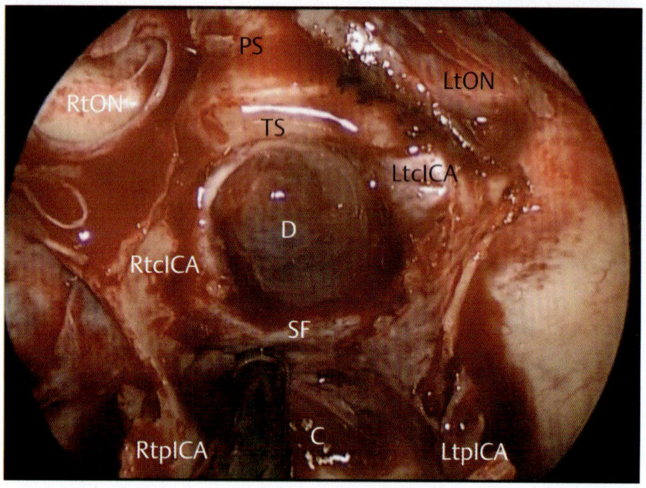

Fig. 3H.13 Reinspection of the operative situs shows no obvious residual tumor with the prolapsing diaphragma sellae (D) in the field.

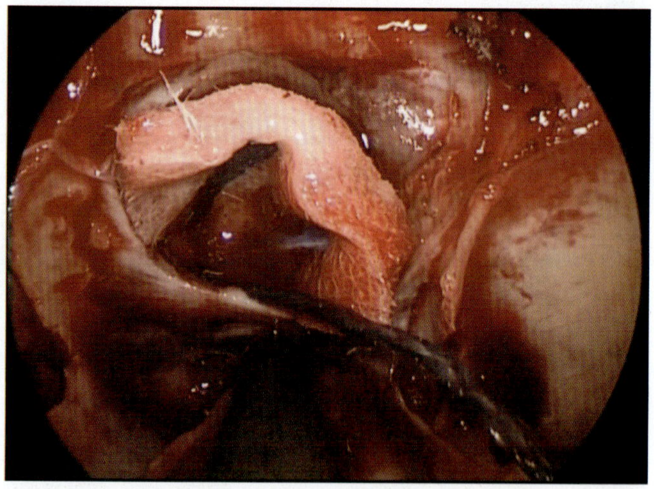

Fig. 3H.14 Small cottonoids are helpful to manipulate the prolapsing diaphragm sellae to systematically inspect the sella for residual tumor within the diaphragmal folds.

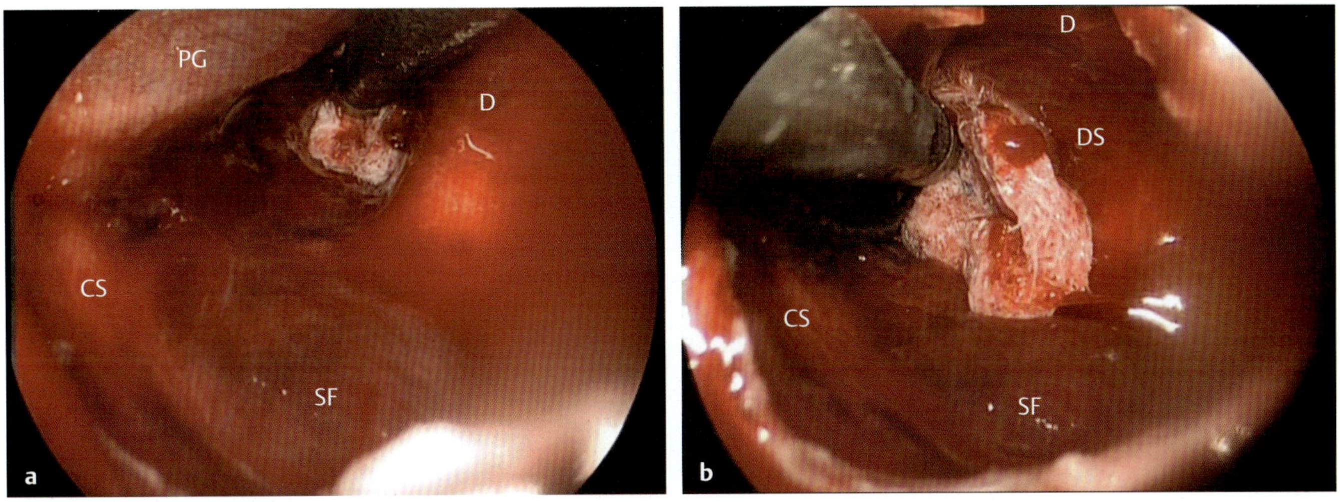

Fig. 3H.15 **(a, b)** Posterosuperior elevation of the diaphragm sellae using a cottonoid allows for further exploration the diaphragmal folds.

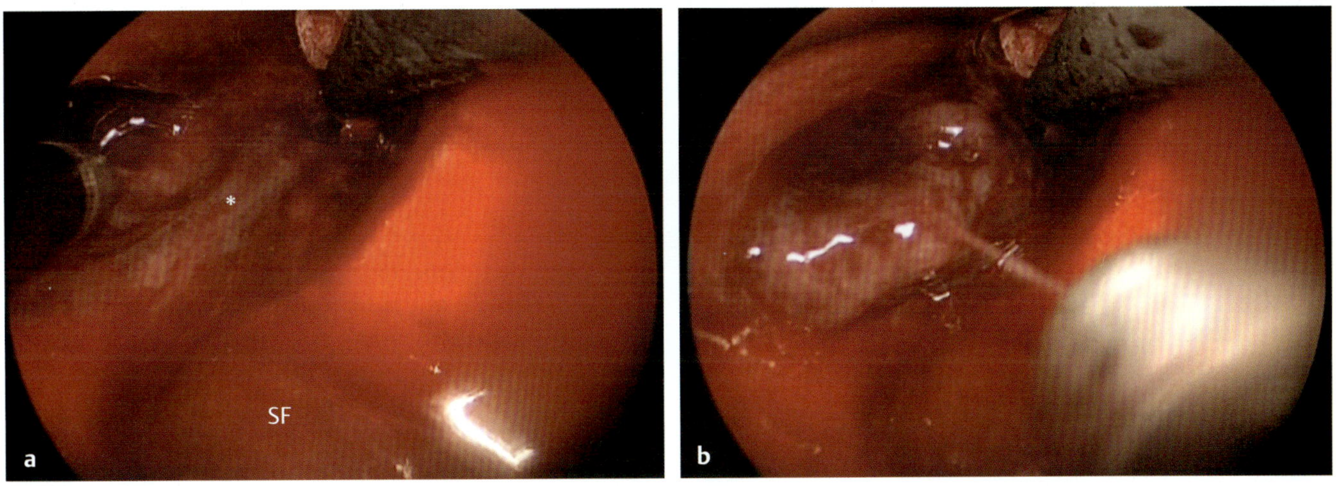

Fig. 3H.16 **(a, b)** Residual tumor (*) is identified and can be removed using two suction devices and the cottonoid in place displacing the prolapsing diaphragm sellae superiorly.

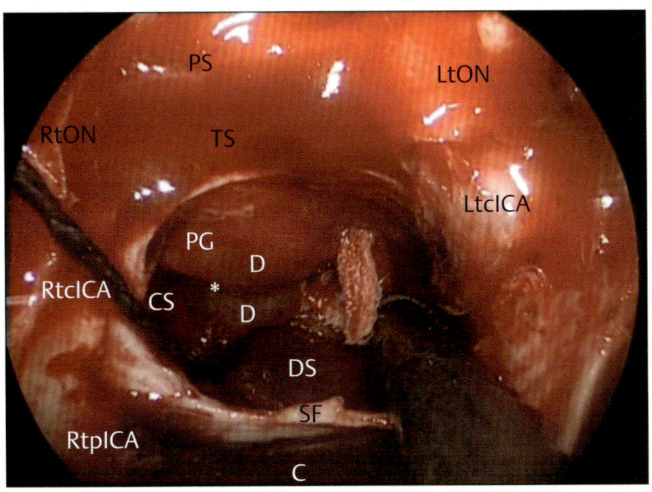

Fig. 3H.17 The diaphragm sellae (D) does not prolapse symmetrically indicating that residual tumor might still be stuck within the dura fold (*).

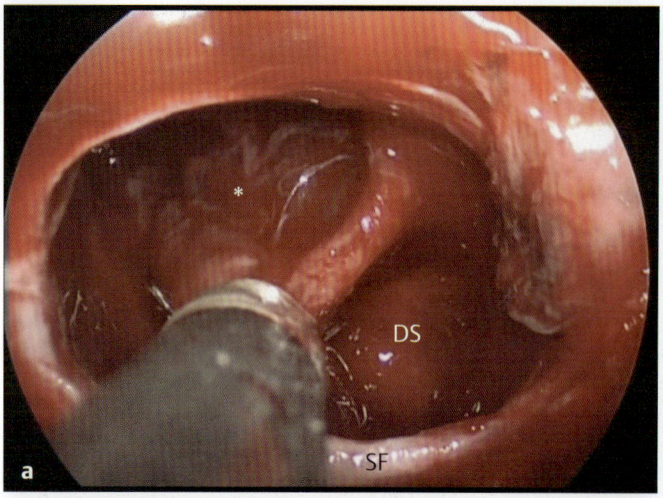

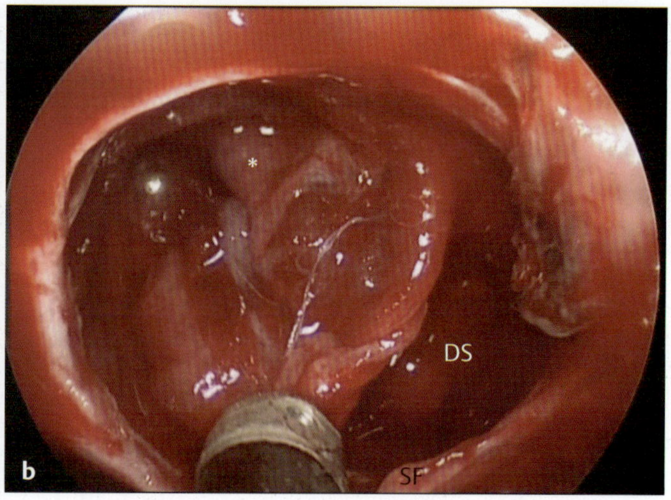

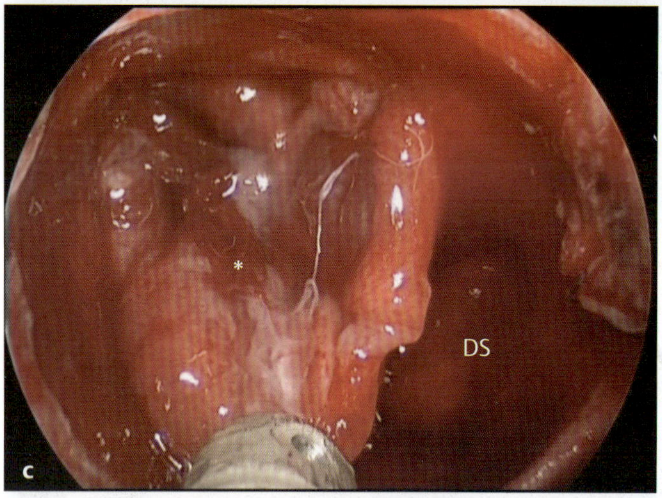

Fig. 3H.18 **(a–c)** Further dissection within the dural fold reveals the rest of the suprasellar tumor (*) which can be removed using two suction devices.

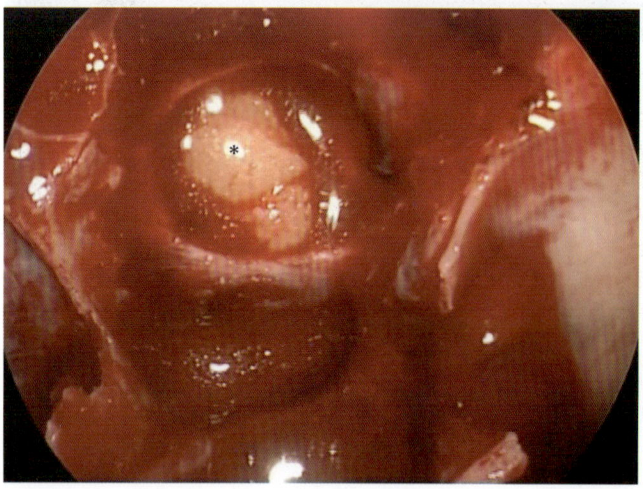

Fig. 3H.19 The closure with the abdominal fat graft (*). Note that it is tucked under the bony edges to allow a watertight seal.

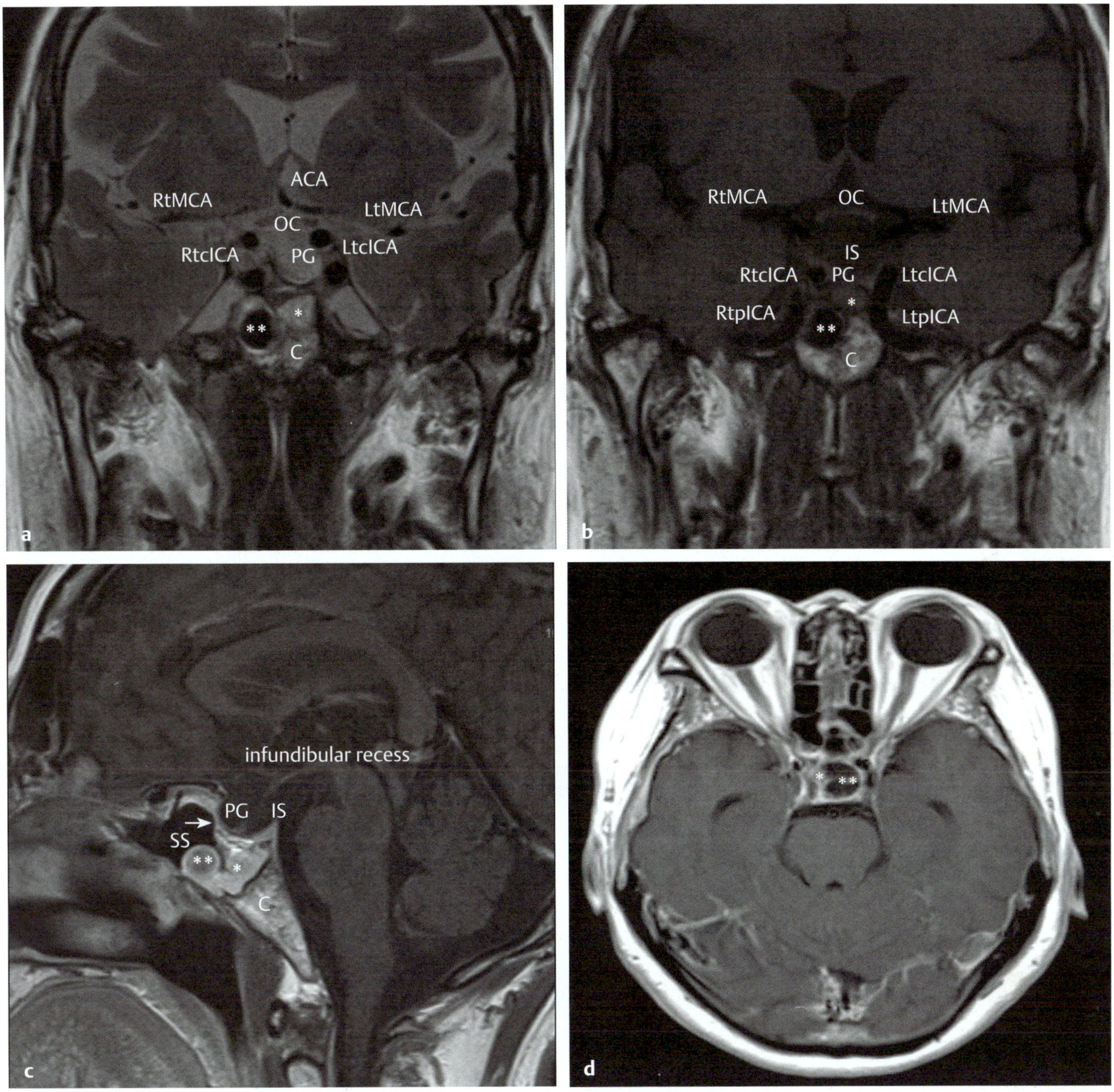

Fig. 3H.20 Three months' postoperative radiological follow-up. **(a)** Coronal T2-weighted, **(b)** coronal noncontrast-enhanced T1-weighted, **(c)** sagittal and **(d)** axial gadolinium-enhanced T1-weighted MRI sections showing complete tumor removal with the infundibular stalk (IS) deviated to the right side and the flattened but identifiable pituitary gland (PG) within the pituitary fossa. Postoperative changes (*) within the sphenoid sinus (SS), postoperative scaring over the sella turcica (*white arrow*), and a small postoperative sphenoidal mucocele (**) are identifiable.

Case 3I

Resection of a Giant Pituitary Macroadenoma Complicated by Intraoperative Hemorrhage

Asiya Kamber Zaidi, Michel Roethlisberger, Prepageran Narayanan, and Vicknes Waran

History

A 39-year-old man was admitted with 7-month history of headache and 6-month history of progressive blurring of vision initially in the right eye followed by the left eye. He had a history of renal transplant done 28 years ago and has been on long-term steroids (currently 10 mg OD and cyclosporine). He also developed hypertension secondary to renal transplantation and was on antihypertensives since the last 10 years. On neuro-ophthalmological examination, the vision was reduced to only light perception in the right eye and only hand motion at the superonasal quadrant in the left eye. The relative afferent pupillary defect (RAPD) could not be assessed, but both pupils were sluggish (right eye—4 mm, left eye—5 mm). Bilateral steroid-induced posterior subcapsular cataract with bilateral pale disc was observed.

Magnetic resonance imaging (MRI) of the brain revealed a sellar mass measuring 3.6 (Wt) × 4.2 (Ht) × 2.9 cm (Ap) isointense on axial T1-weighted imaging (T1W1) with hypointense focal areas suggestive of old hemorrhage/necrosis (**Fig. 3I.1a**). On axial T2-weighted imaging (T2W1) the sellar mass seems to obliterate the entire sphenoid sinus cavity with protrusion through the anterior wall of the sinus on the right side (**Fig. 3I.1b**). Superiorly, on coronal T1- and T2-weighted imaging, the mass extends upward into the suprasellar cistern with abutment of the hypothalamus, compressing the brain tissue, the optic chiasm, and the third ventricle. Laterally, it infiltrates the cavernous sinuses bilaterally with encasement of the carotid arteries on both sides. Inferiorly, the mass erodes the floor of the widened sella extending into the sphenoid sinus (**Fig. 3I.2**).

A binostril endoscopic transsphenoidal excision of the tumor was planned with intraoperative MRI (iMRI), which provides an objective basis for real-time judgement of completeness of resection.

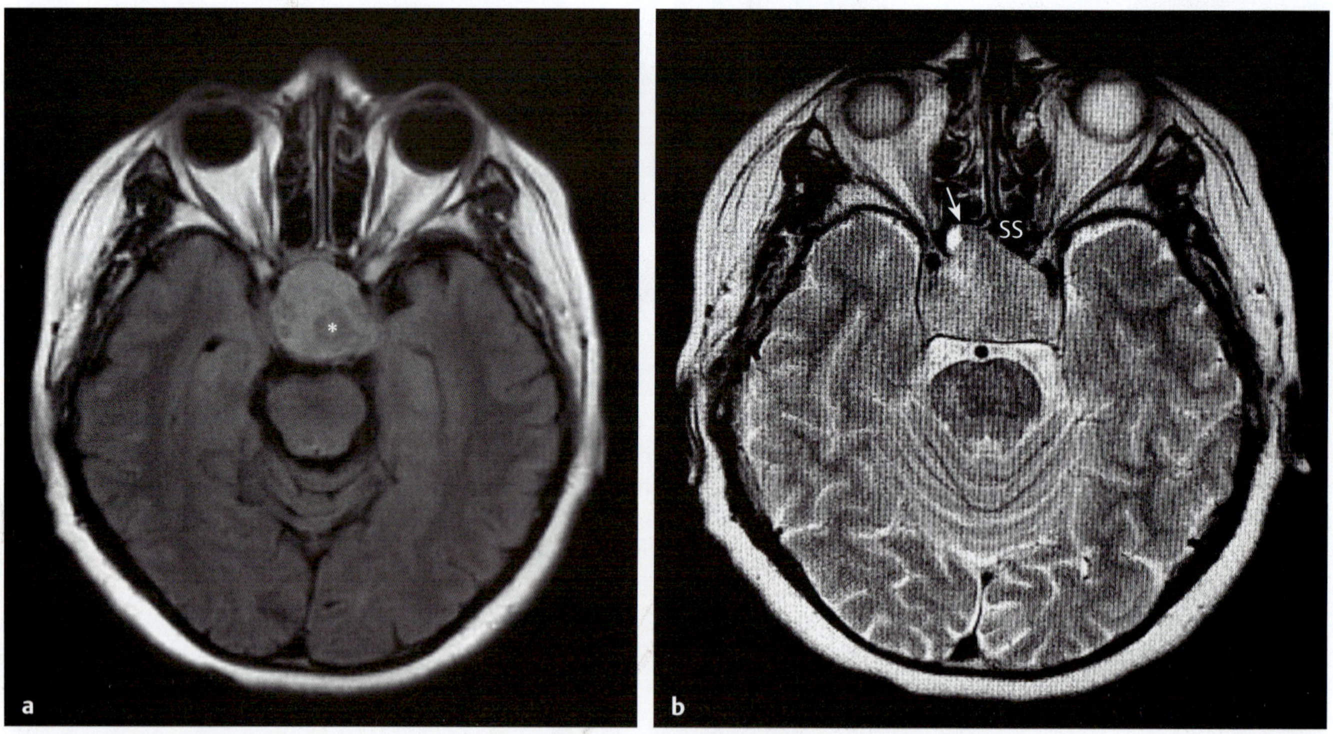

Fig. 3I.1 **(a)** Preoperative axial T1-weighted MRI section showing a well-defined isointense intrasellar lesion with areas of focal hypointensity (*) suggestive for necrosis. There is compression of the optic chiasm and both optic nerves. **(b)** Axial T2-weighted MRI demonstrating the lesion obliterating the sphenoid sinus (SS) cavity and parts of the tumor protruding through the anterior wall (*white arrow*).

Surgical Steps

1. The patient is placed under general anesthesia in supine position and the head fixed slightly retroflexed within a NORAS frame for iMRI.
2. Registration for IGS (Brainlab, Munich, Germany) was done.
3. *Nasal stage*: Nasal endoscopy is performed for initial assessment of bilateral nasal cavities to evaluate the ease of access to the sphenoid sinus. Selective packing using two to three ribbon gauze soaked in xylocaine and adrenaline 1:1,000 units is performed between the middle turbinate and the septum (sphenoethmoidal recess) and left in situ for a few minutes, to decongest the nasal mucosa and also to widen the nasal corridor for easy instrumentation.
4. Infiltration is done with local anesthetic and adrenaline 1:1,000 units into the nasal septum.
5. A pedicled nasoseptal flap is fashioned. The superior incision for the flap may be taken just beneath the sphenoid ostium and then carried forward along the septum until about 0.5 to 1 cm below and parallel to the skull base to preserve the olfactory function. Inferiorly the flap can be taken as far as half the nasal floor if a large skull base defect is expected (Hadad–Bassagasteguy flap).
6. The flap is then raised off the septum in a subperichondrial and subperiosteal plane using a Freer elevator until the sphenoid ostia and posterior choana are visible bilaterally.
7. *Sphenoid stage*: The dissection is continued until the sphenoid keel is visualized and the sphenoid ostia are identified bilaterally (posteroinferior to the attachment of superior turbinate) (**Fig. 31.3**).
8. The mucosa over the rostrum of sphenoid sinus and around the ostium is cauterized to provide a relatively bloodless surgical field. This prevents frequent soiling of the endoscope which hampers visualization. This is an important step during the surgery.
9. Once the sphenoid keel is fully exposed, a bite of the bone is taken inferomedially using a Kerrison punch in a V shape on the left side toward the midline to achieve a wide anterior sphenoidotomy.
10. *Tumor exposure*: In this case, asymmetrical septation of the sphenoid sinus is present and the tumor is visualized extruding between the two limbs of the Y-shaped septa (**Fig. 31.4**).
11. The sellar bone is thinned out, and the dura mater is identified beneath the tumor in the midline (**Fig. 31.5**).
12. A right-angled dissector is insinuated between the tumor and the dura mater such that the entire crescentic superior aspect of the tumor attached to the thinned out sellar bone along with a part of sphenoid septa was flaked off. The remnant sphenoid keel and sphenoid sinus septations are also removed to allow an unobstructed view.
13. *Sellar stage*: The dura is incised, and the soft grayish red suctionable tumor with "*marrow-like consistency*" comes into view.

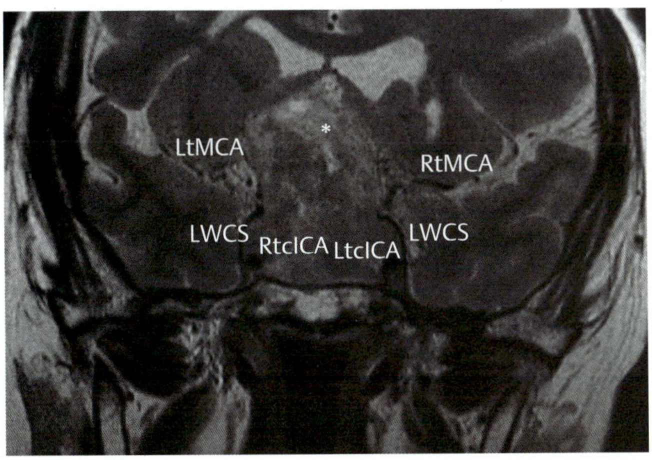

Fig. 31.2 Preoperative coronal T2-weighted MRI image demonstrating the suprasellar extension of the lesion (*), bulging into the floor of the third ventricle with mass effect compressing the optic chiasm. The mass extends bilaterally into the cavernous sinus with encasement and narrowing of the left (LtcICA) and right (RtcICA) cavernous ICA.

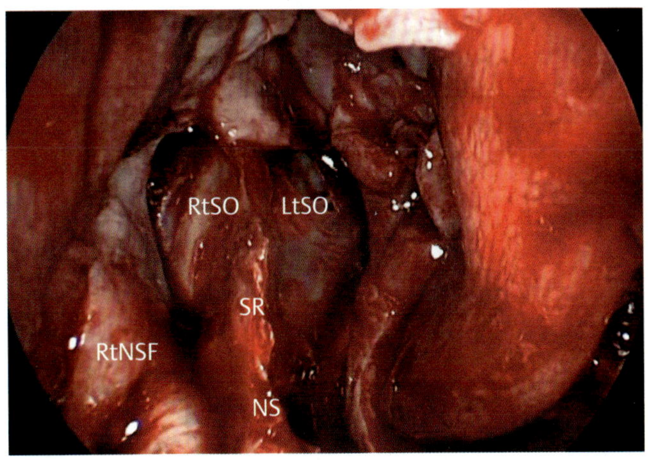

Fig. 31.3 Sphenoid stage. Endonasal endoscopic exposure of sphenoid rostrum (SR) and bilateral sphenoid ostia.

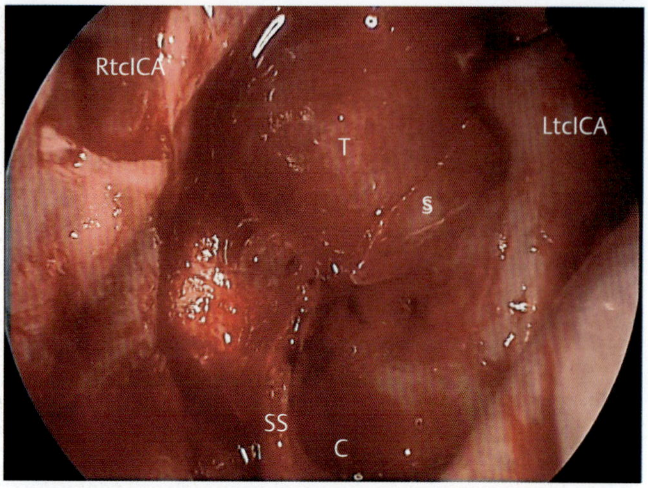

Fig. 31.4 After removal of the sphenoid rostrum, the tumor (T) protruding out through the thinned out sellar wall (S) can be visualized.

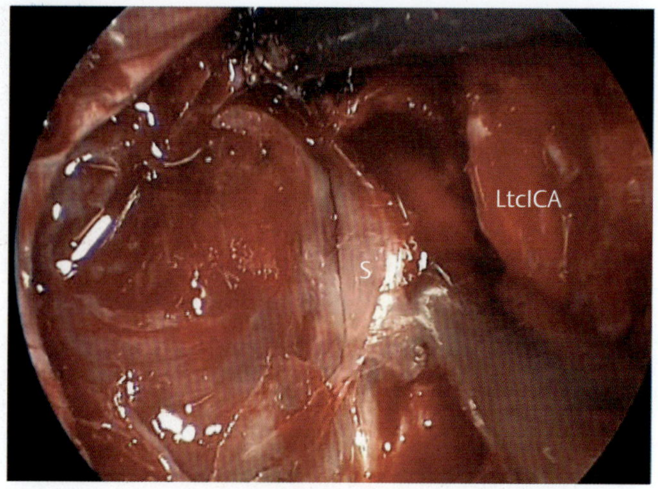

Fig. 31.5 The thinned sellar bone (S) is removed.

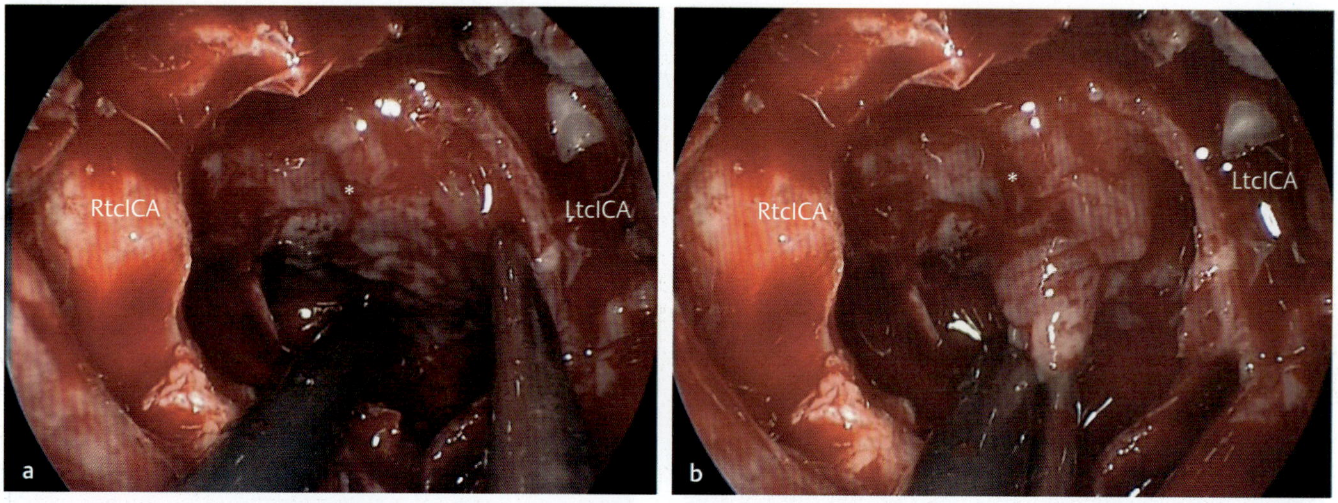

Fig. 31.6 **(a, b)** The suprasellar part of the lesion (*) is resected after removal of the inferior central and bilateral inferior tumor compartments using a blunt curette and suction.

14. A blunt ring curette and a suction are then used to debulk the tumor sequentially in zones, focusing on the inferior zone first, then both the right and left inferior zones (**Fig. 31.6a, b**). Biopsy is taken for histopathological examination.
15. Extracapsular sharp dissection with gradual traction and countertraction with a suction device and a blunt currette is performed. Care is taken during the lateral curettage because of the proximity of the cavernous sinus and carotids.
16. Debulking is continued with the aim to clear the inferior margin of the tumor before proceeding superiorly. The additional space gained within the cavity allows for the suprasellar component to be delivered inferiorly and suctioned out away from the suprasellar structures.
17. The posterior part of the tumor is addressed and the posterior aspect of the dura is identified.
18. The diaphragma sellae then prolapses into the resection cavity. A symmetric "frog bladder" appearance is a sign for complete removal (**Fig. 31.7a, b**).

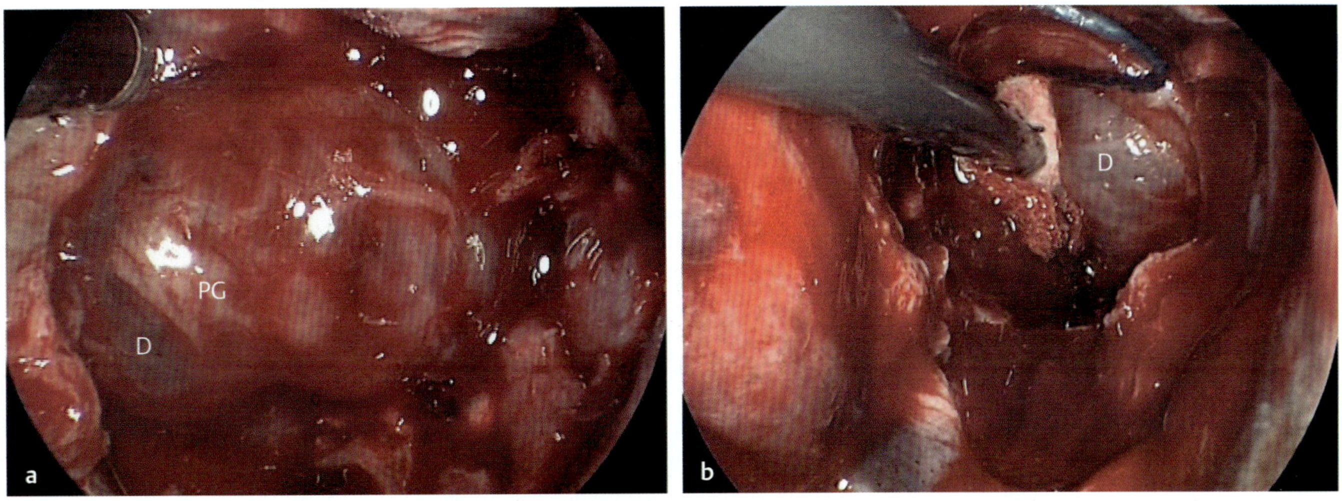

Fig. 31.7 **(a, b)** After resection of the suprasellar tumor compartment, the diaphragma sellae (D) prolapses into the pituitary fossa. The normal pituitary gland (PG) tissue can be appreciated along the surface of the diaphragma sellae. With the aid of a cottonoid, the pituitary fossa can be inspected for remnant tumor while pushing the prolapsing diaphragma away.

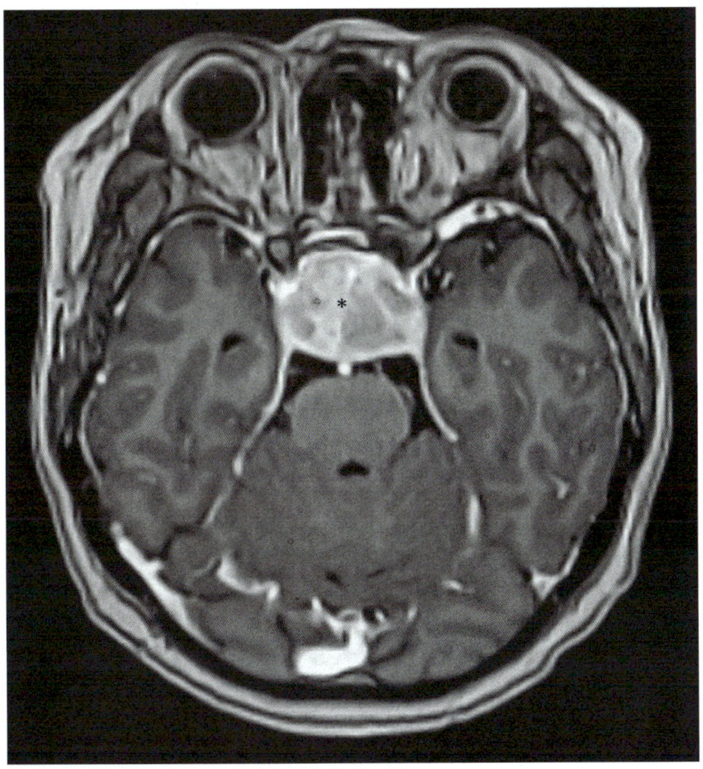

Fig. 31.8 Intraoperative gadolinium contrast-enhanced axial MRI section showing evidence of an acute hemorrhage within the pituitary fossa that most likely developed immediately after tumor removal.

19. Intraoperative contrast-enhanced MRI is performed showing a hematoma that had developed within the cavity and a near-total resection of the large supra-/parasellar and sellar lesion (**Fig. 31.8**).
20. To arrest the hemorrhage, meticulous hemostasis is performed using Surgicel (oxidized cellulose polymer), Floseal (gelatin and thrombin component mixture) delivered accurately at the site of hemorrhage through the hemostatic agent delivery system *Taming sari* (**Fig. 31.9a, b**). No further resection of the small residual tumor is attempted.
21. The defect was plugged with abdominal fat harvested at the beginning of the surgery and the edges of the fat are tucked underneath to create a watertight seal. Care is taken not to pack too much fat tightly into the cavity.
22. The area is sealed with a synthetic dural sealant and layered with absorbable hemostat.
23. The nasoseptal flap is then teased out and rotated over the defect to complete the repair and reinforced with gelatin sponges to keep the flaps in position (**Fig. 31.10**).
24. The septal incision is covered with Nasopore (synthetic biodegradable foam) while making sure to provide adequate airway along the nasal floor.

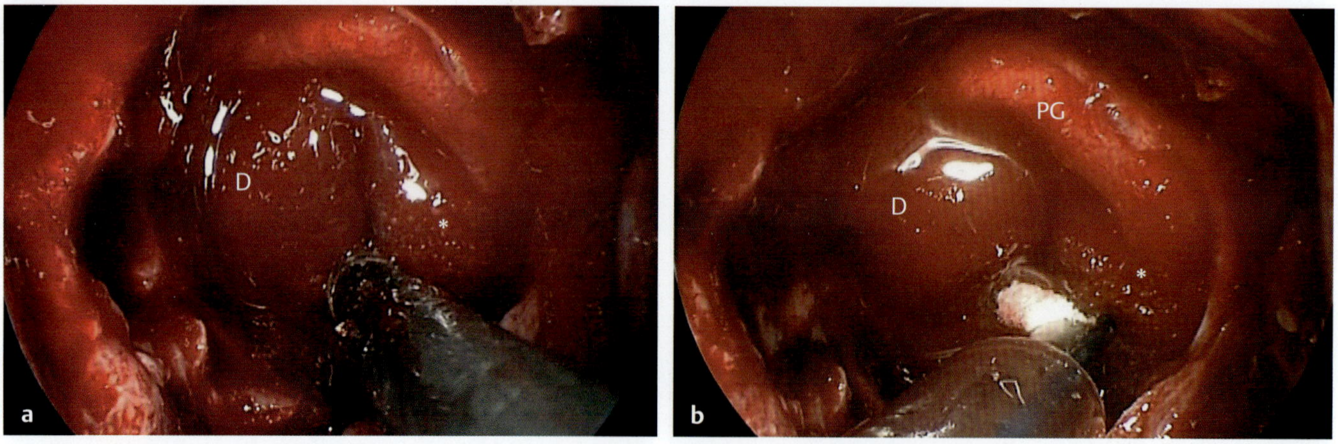

Fig. 3I.9 (a, b) The acute hematoma is removed immediately after diagnosis until the diaphragma (D) is visualized again. Hemostasis is achieved using Floseal (*), a gelatin and thrombin component mixture, delivered accurately at the site of hemorrhage at the suprasellar cistern area through the hemostatic agent delivery system *Taming sari* (TS). The residual pituitary gland (PG) is identified and preserved.

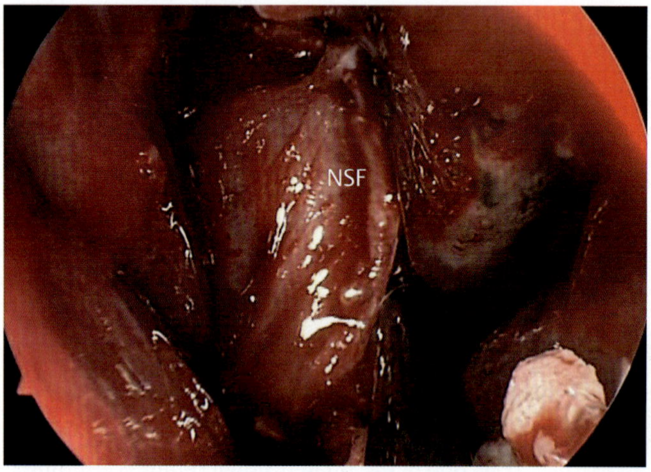

Fig. 3I.10 The nasoseptal flap (NSF) is teased out from the nasopharynx and rotated over the defect to complete the repair.

There was a minor cerebrospinal fluid leakage on the third postoperative day which resolved spontaneously. After a month postoperatively, nasal endoscopy revealed nasal mucosa in the healing stage. Only occasional headaches were reported, and the visual acuity improved with hand motion (HM) in both eyes.

A 3 months postoperative MRI was performed. Sagittal T1-weighted image shows iatrogenic hyperintense lipid (fat used as graft for reconstruction) in the sphenoid sinus with a rim of hypointensity which is most likely hemosiderin. During the degradation of hemoglobin, methemoglobin becomes oxidized to hemosiderin causing hypointensity on both T1- and T2-weighted images (**Fig. 3I.11a–c**). The optic chiasm is decompressed.

Histopathological examination confirmed the diagnosis of pituitary macroadenoma.

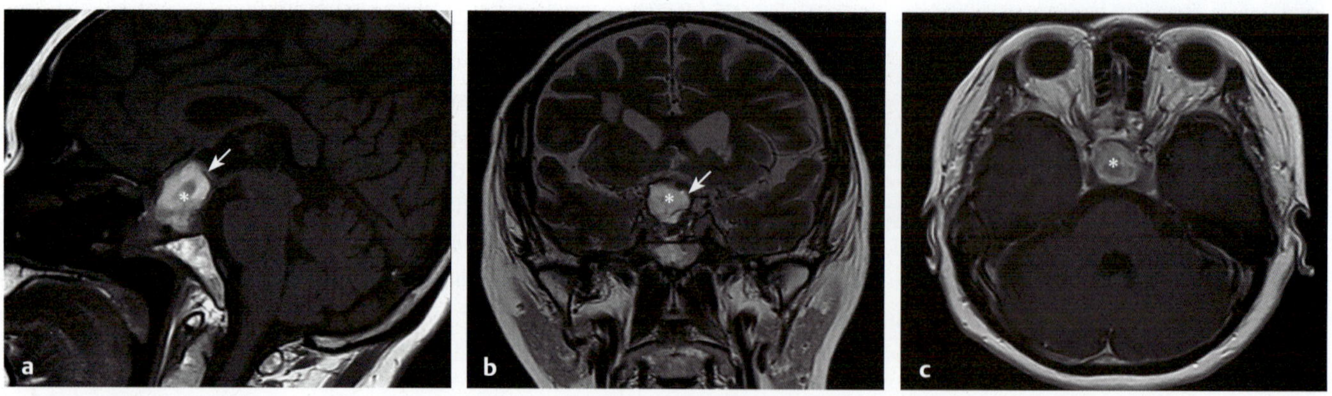

Fig. 3I.11 Postoperative changes after transnasal transsphenoidal binostril endoscopic surgery for resection of nonfunctioning pituitary macroadenoma. **(a)** Sagittal T1-weighted MRI section. **(b)** Coronal T2-weighted MR image. **(c)** Axial T1-weighted MRI section obtained 1 month after surgery shows heterogenous opacification (*) representing fat graft/blood products with a rim of hypointensity (*white arrow*) suggestive of hemosiderin.

Chapter 4 Endoscopic Endonasal Revision Surgery for Pituitary Adenoma

Case 4A

Endoscopic Endonasal Transsphenoidal Revision Surgery for a Recurrent Pituitary Adenoma

Liew Yew Toong, Michel Roethlisberger, Saif Al-Zahid, Prepageran Narayanan, and Vicknes Waran

History

A 55-year-old gentleman, who had transsphenoidal hypophysectomy 5 years ago, presented with gradual bitemporal hemianopia with vertex headache for the last 6 months. Surgery was done previously in a nearby hospital, and recent magnetic resonance imaging (MRI) showed a recurrent pituitary macroadenoma. Clinical findings and biochemical tests revealed a nonfunctioning pituitary tumor.

Surgical Steps

1. Endoscopic evaluation noted a posterior septectomy and wide sphenoidotomy from previous surgeries with fibrotic bands at 3, 6, and 9 o'clock position toward the sella (**Fig. 4A.1**).
2. The fibrotic bands are divided with monopolar suction diathermy (**Fig. 4A.2**).
3. An angled probe is used to open up the adhesions at the sellar floor and look for the bony edges, which act as a surgical landmark (**Fig. 4A.3**). The sellar floor is widened with a Kerrison punch to ease the process of tumor removal (**Fig. 4A.4**).
4. The scar tissue covering the pituitary is opened with a cruciate incision (**Fig. 4A.5**).
5. The intrasellar tumor is removed using a suction device, an angled ball probe, ring curettes, and ultrasonic aspiration. The dissection planes are identified where possible. In revision cases, fibrous bands and scars can separate the recurrent tumor (**Fig. 4A.6**).
6. During dissection, an arachnoid membrane tear with profuse cerebrospinal fluid (CSF) leakage is identified. The torn membrane is temporarily occluded with patties to improve the surgical field so as not to disturb the tumor removal (**Fig. 4A.7**).
7. After complete removal of the tumor, the defect is reconstructed with an abdominal fat graft. The edges are tucked in just enough to ensure a watertight seal taking care not to cause compression to underlying structures by overpacking with fat (**Fig. 4A.8**).
8. This is then covered with synthetic dural sealant or tissue glue (**Fig. 4A.9**).
9. Intraoperative MRI shows residual tumor (**Fig. 4A.10**), and further clearance is performed using image-guided surgery (IGS). (**Fig. 4A.11**).

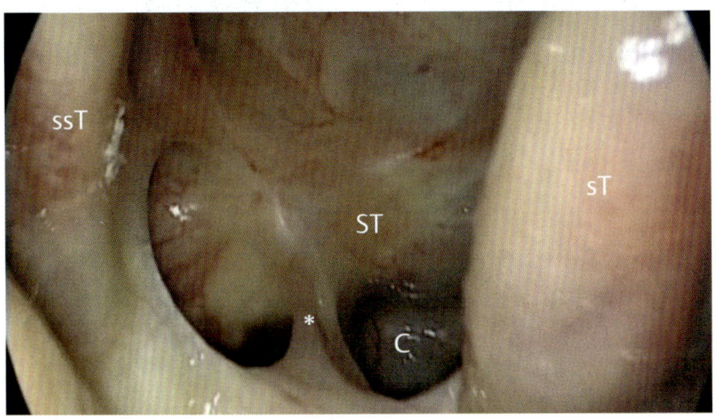

Fig. 4A.1 Fibrotic bands (*) at 3, 6, and 9 o'clock positions are seen through a wide sphenoidotomy from a previous surgery.

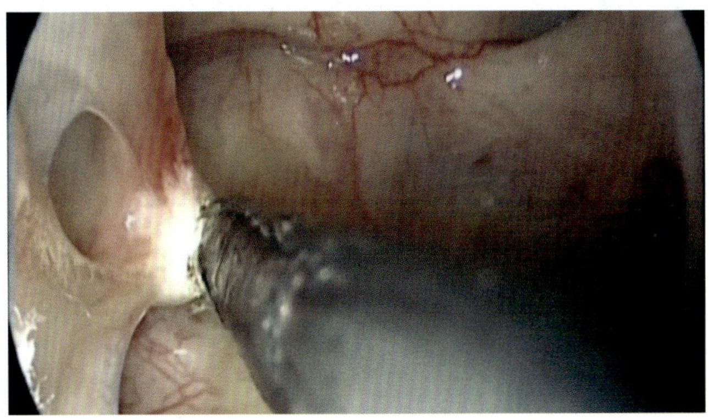

Fig. 4A.2 A suction monopolar diathermy is used to divide the adhesion bands.

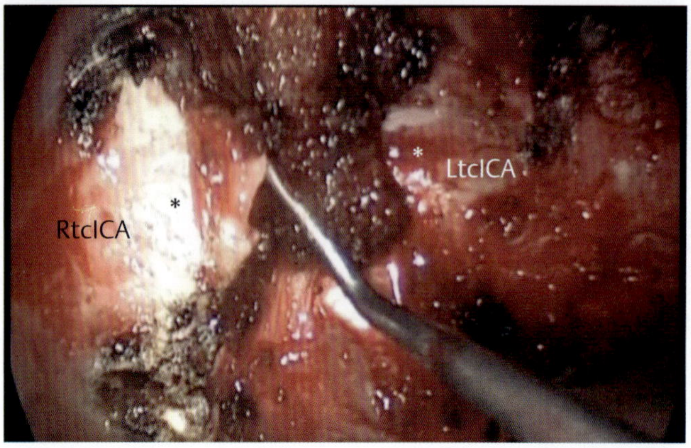

Fig. 4A.3 The bony edges (*) are acting as a surgical landmark.

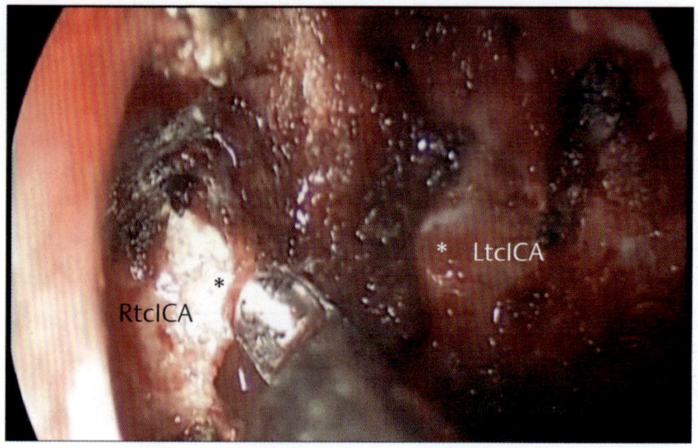

Fig. 4A.4 The transsellar opening is widened on both sides using a Kerrison punch by removing the bony edges (*).

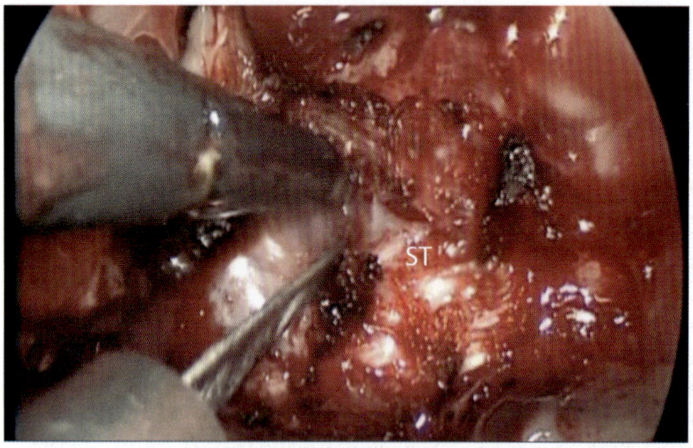

Fig. 4A.5 Sharp opening of the scar tissue covering the sella turcica (ST).

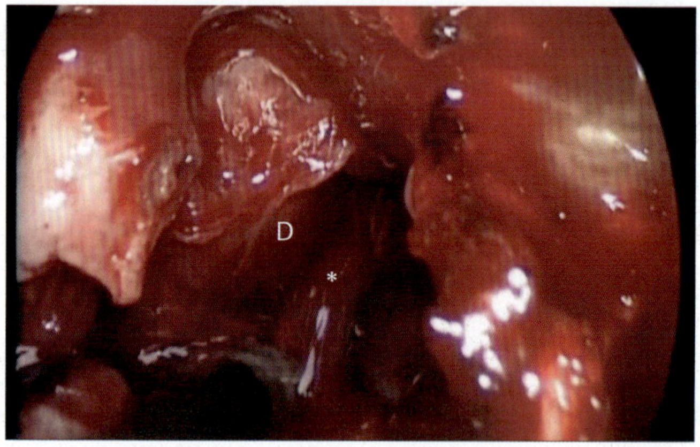

Fig. 4A.6 Tumor (*) removal and identification of the diaphragma sellae (D).

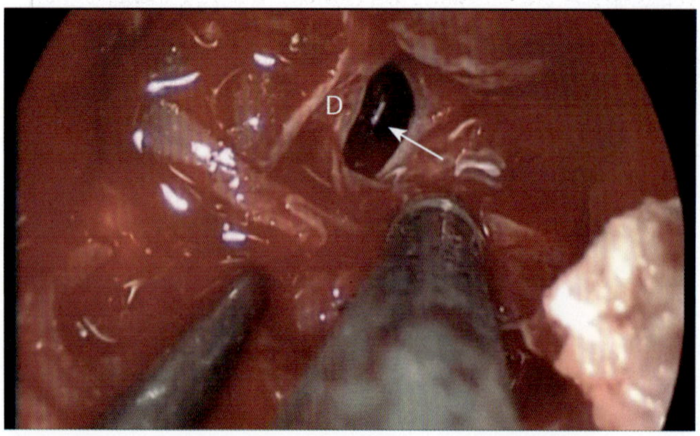

Fig. 4A.7 A intermediate flow CSF leak is encountered through a tear (*white arrow*) at the site of the diaphragma sellae (D) during dissection of the tumor (*).

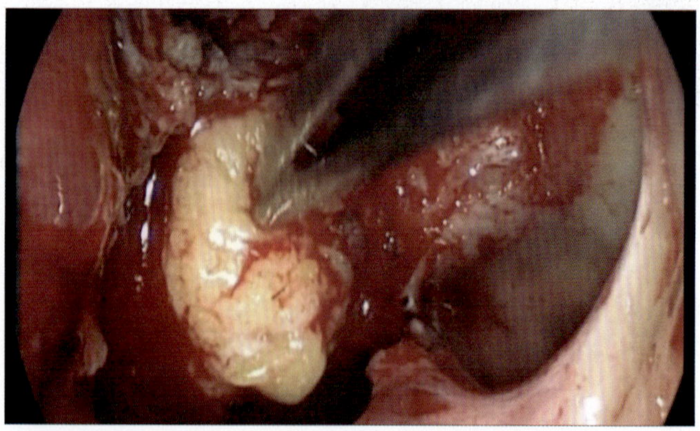

Fig. 4A.8 An abdominal fat graft is used to seal the leak.

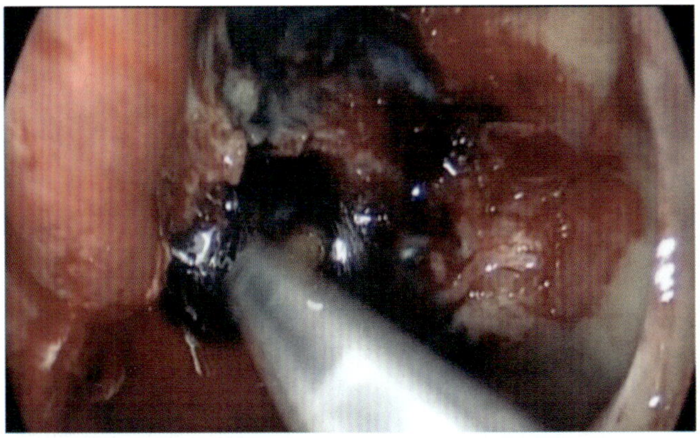

Fig. 4A.9 An artificial dural sealant is applied over the construct at the end of procedure.

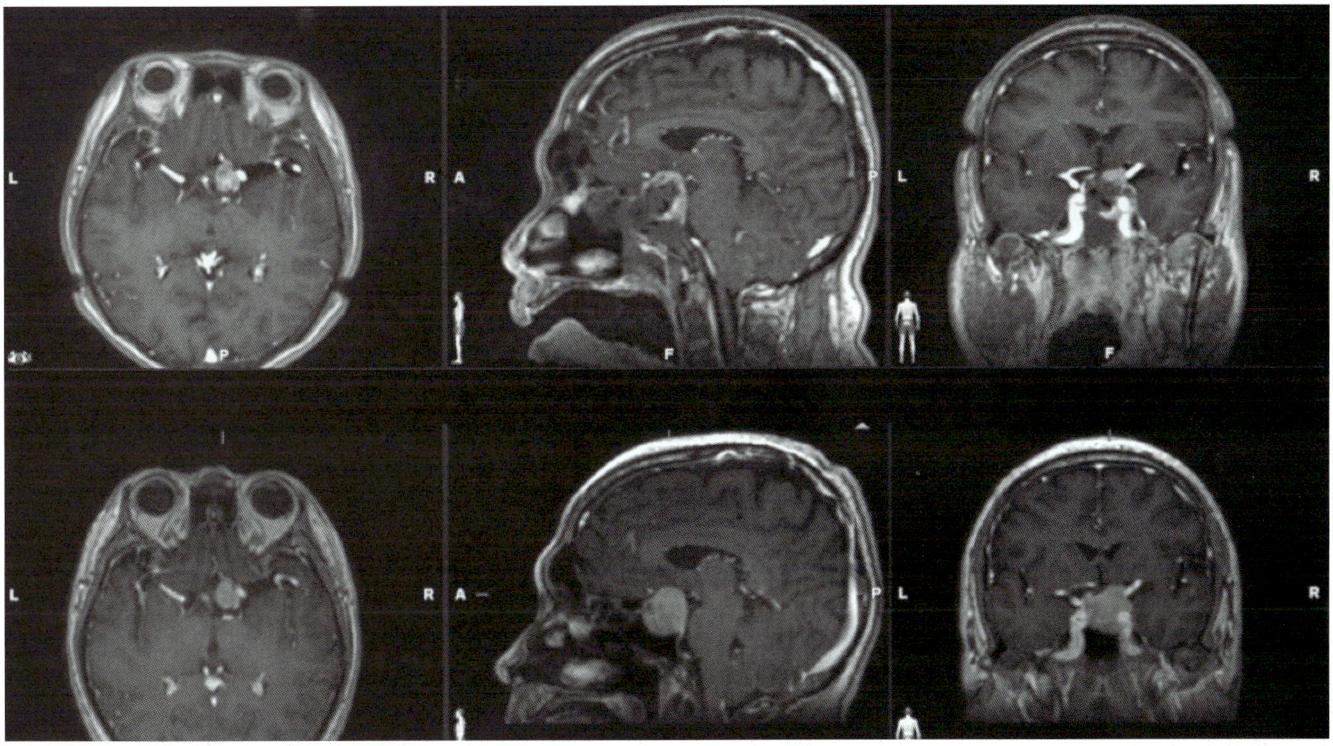

Fig. 4A.10 T1-weighted MRI with contrast at upper row demonstrating residual tumor at the right upper corner; the lower row is the preoperative MRI scan.

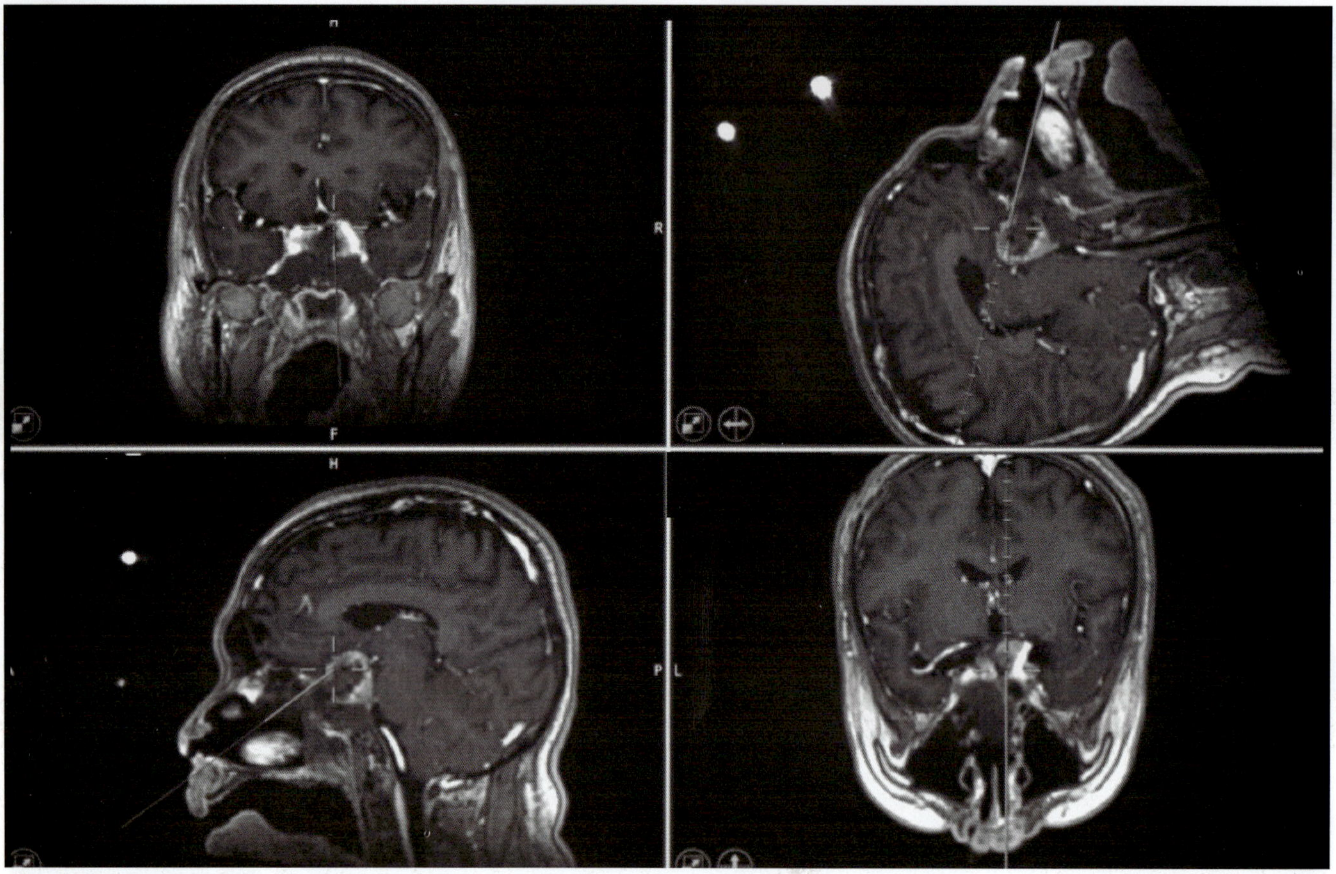

Fig. 4A.11 Verification of the residual tumor using image-guided surgery.

Case 4B

Endoscopic Endonasal Transsphenoidal Resection of a Transcranially Preoperated Recurrent Pituitary Adenoma

Michel Roethlisberger, Warren O. Bennett, Saif Al-Zahid, Prepageran Narayanan, and Vicknes Waran

History

A 69-year-old female patient underwent transcranial surgery for a giant pituitary adenoma more than a decade ago in an external hospital. She suffered from documented blindness of her right eye ever since. The patient receives substitution of the thyrotropin and the gonadotropin axis. The functional level is good, and the patient is able to perform daily activities independently. Since three months, the patient notes a slowly progressive loss of vision on the left side. The ophthalmological assessment revealed a new left temporal visual defect. Neurocranial imaging revealed a recurrent pituitary macroadenoma with compression of the optic chiasm and the left optic nerve (**Fig. 4B.1a–d**).

Therefore, an **endonasal endoscopic transsphenoidal resection** of the recurrent lesion was recommended.

Surgical Steps

1. A **binostril posterior transseptal transsphenoidal approach** is performed as previously described.
2. In the present case, a main sphenoid intersinus septum and an accessory horizontal sphenoid septum (shelf) are present and can be appreciated in the preoperative imaging (**Fig. 4B.2a–d**).
3. Once the sphenoid keel is fully exposed, the ostia are widened inferomedially using a Kerrison punch in a V shape manner toward the midline.

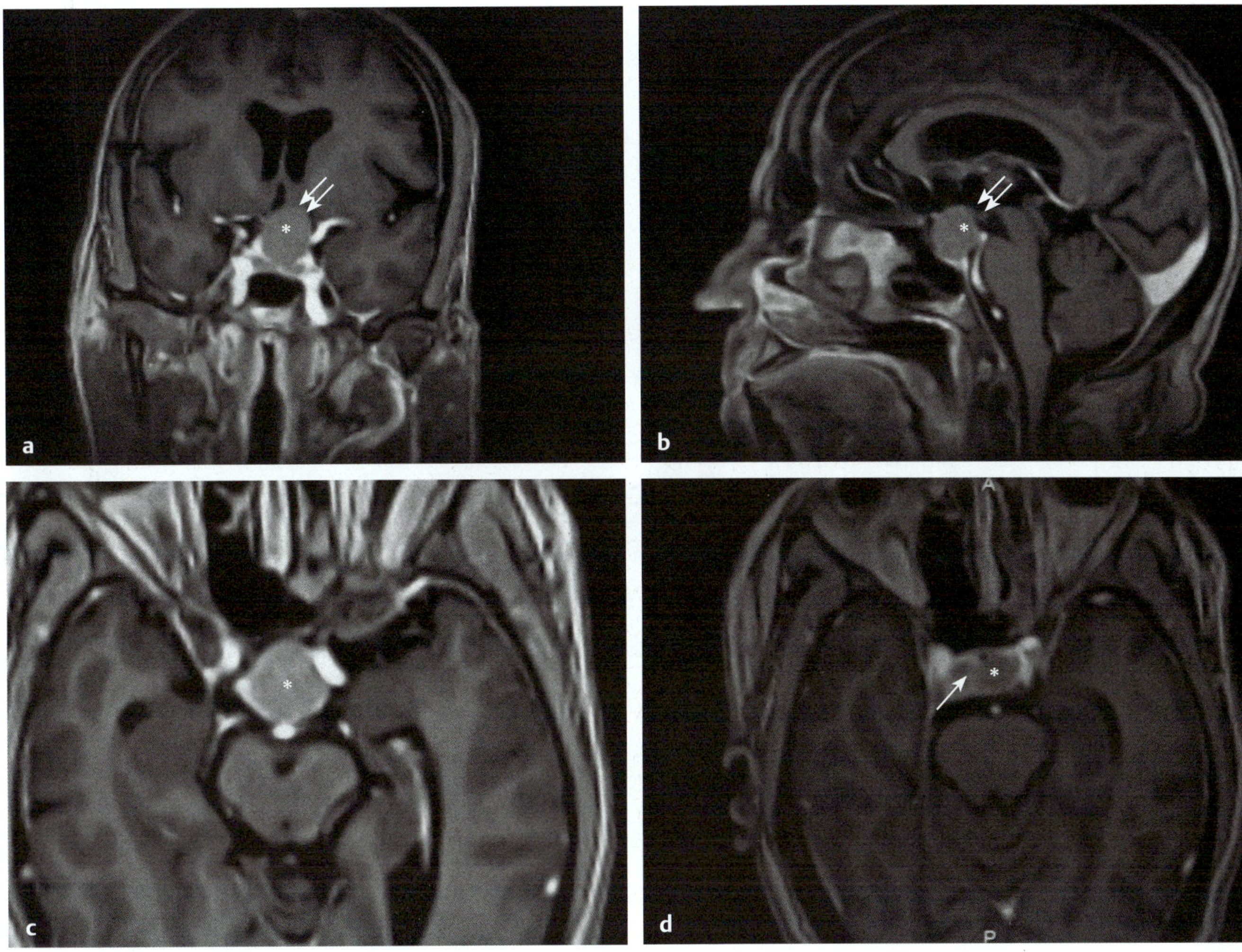

Fig. 4B.1 **(a)** Coronal, **(b)** sagittal, **(c, d)** axial, T1-weighted gadolinium contrast-enhanced section. An isointense intrasellar mass with moderate homogenous enhancement (*) is seen. An enhancing ring posterior to the mass is noted, most likely being the posterior pituitary gland. The lesion is divided by enhancing strings most probably reflecting scar tissue from the first transcranial operation (*arrow*). The optic chiasm and the left optic nerve are displaced and compressed by the lesion (*double arrow*). No cavernous sinus invasion is present.

4. The keel is removed with pituitary rongeur forceps.
5. The main intersinus septum is divided anteriorly imitating an additional rostrum sphenoidale. The remaining superior parts of the intersinus septum skew the surgeons view when entering the sphenoid cavity (**Fig. 4B.3** and **Fig. 4B.4**).
6. The sphenoid main divider inserts at the right paraclinoid carotid skewing the symmetry of the sphenoid cavity. It has to be removed meticulously to allow insight into the sphenoid cavity and the base of skull (**Fig. 4B.5**).
7. The suspected sphenoid shelf is identified, imitating the planum sphenoidale (**Fig. 4B.6**). Meticulous removal allows insight into the superior sphenoid cavity and the actual planum sphenoidale (**Fig. 4B.7**).
8. The mucosa covering the posterior ethmoid and posterior ethmoid cells can be removed to allow an unobstructed view.
9. As the main sphenoid sinus septum is inserting into the paraclinoid carotid of the left side, fracturing or cracking the septum away from the skull base is not recommended (**Fig. 4B.8**).
10. The main sphenoid sinus septum is removed in piecemeal fashion or with a high-speed diamond burr (**Fig. 4B.9**).

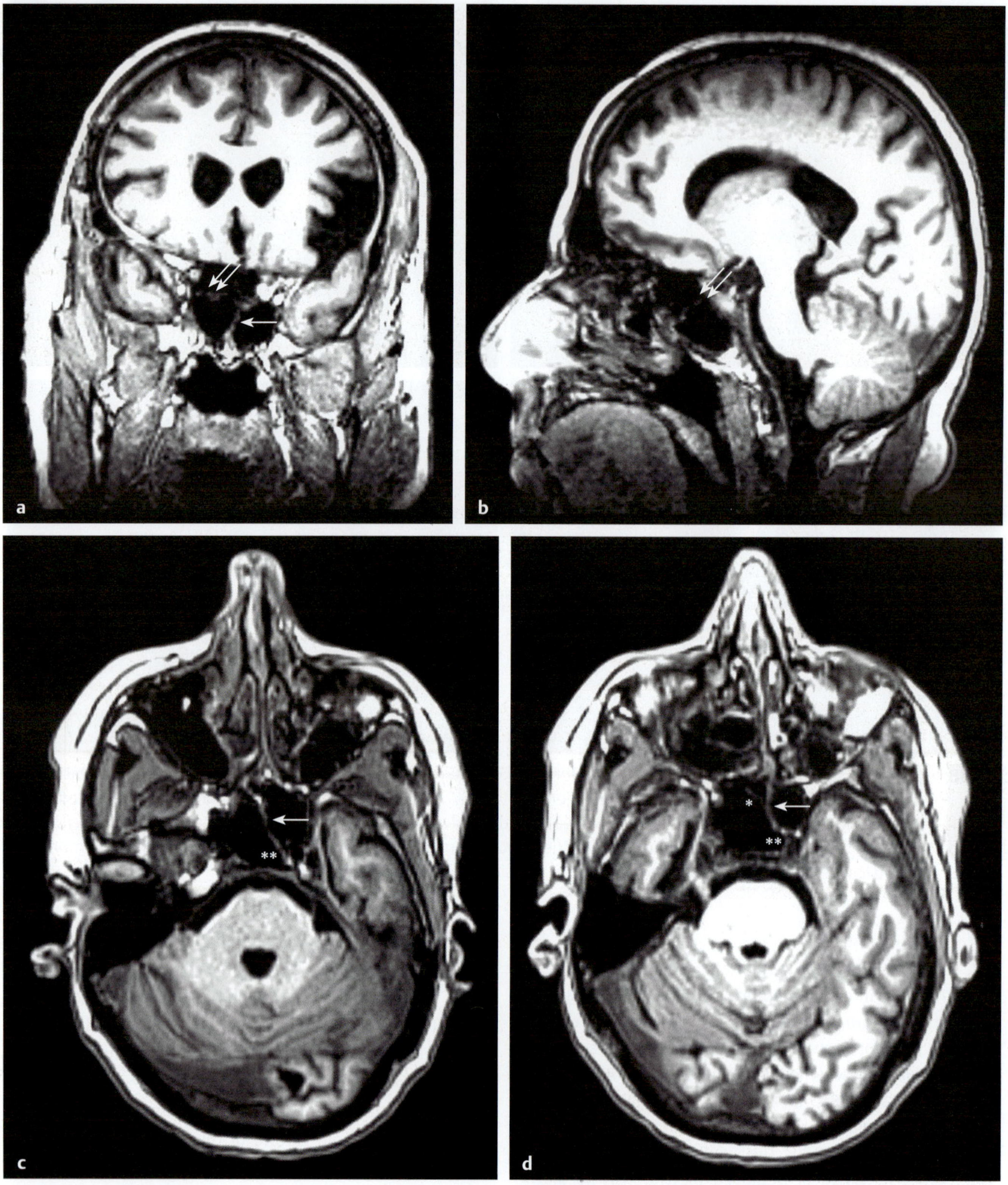

Fig. 4B.2 **(a)** Coronal, **(b)** sagittal, **(c, d)** axial, T1-weighted gadolinium contrast-enhanced MRI sections. A main vertical sphenoid intersinus septum (divider) (*arrow*) and an accessory horizontal sphenoid septum (shelf) (*double arrow*) are present. The dividing main septum is Y shaped anteriorly (*) and is inserting in the bony coverage over the left paraclival and cavernous internal carotid artery (**).

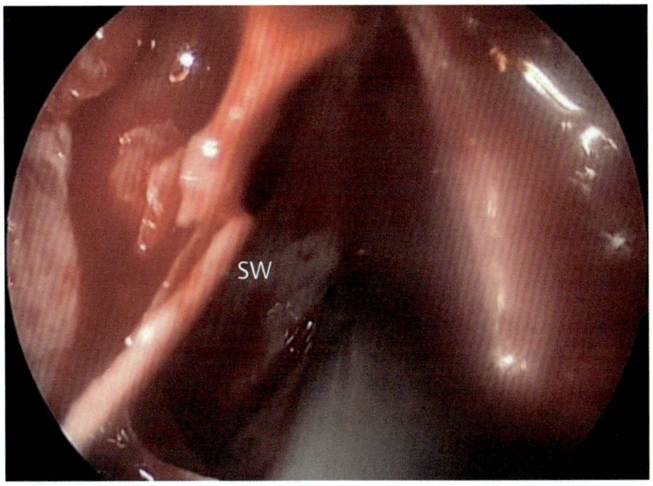

Fig. 4B.3 An Y-shaped main sphenoid septation, a divider with two wings oriented in the coronal plane, forms a sphenoid wall (SW) obstructing the view into the sphenoid cavity. This configuration imitates the sphenoid rostrum.

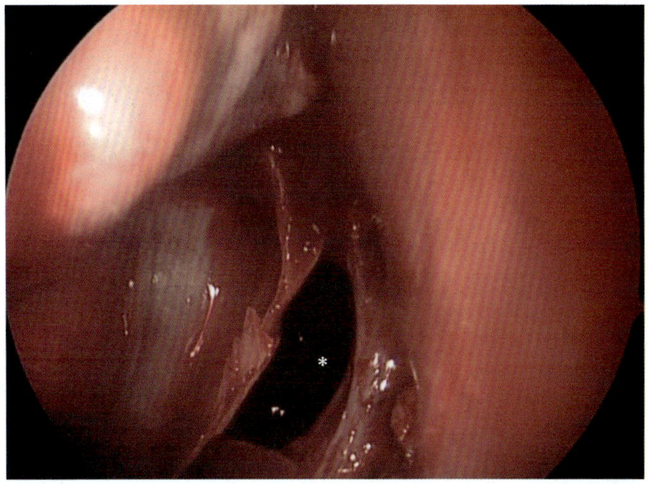

Fig. 4B.4 The left wing of the Y-shaped sphenoid wall is removed (*) without identification of relevant skull base landmarks.

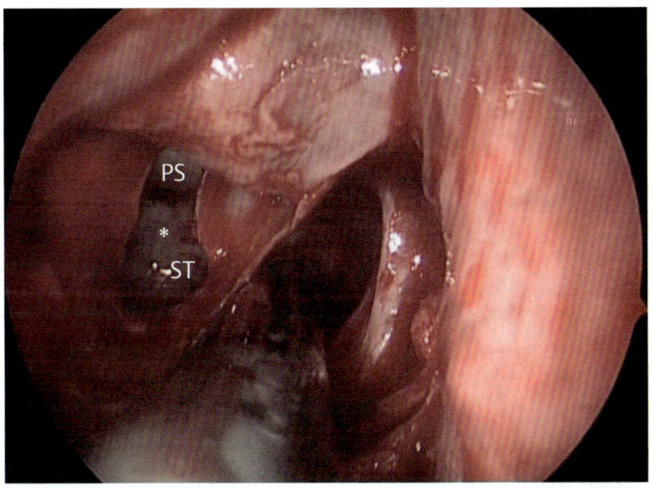

Fig. 4B.5 The right wing of the Y-shaped sphenoid wall is removed (*). The planum sphenoidale (PS) and the sella turcica (ST) are visible.

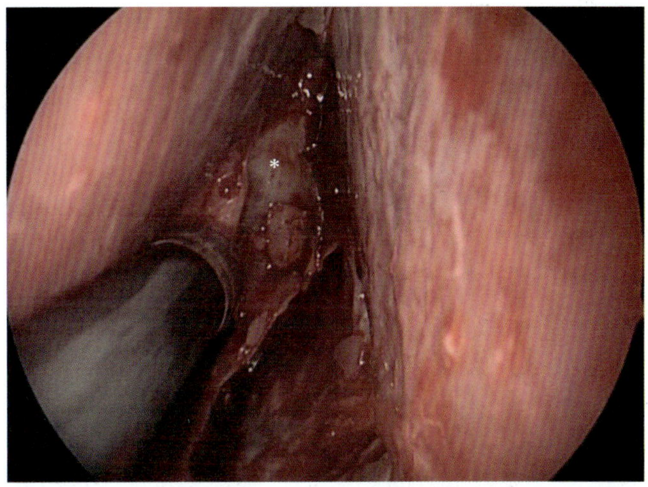

Fig. 4B.6 A horizontally oriented sphenoid septation (shelf) is identified (*). This configuration can imitate the sella turcica or the planum sphenoidale.

11. The identified landmarks of the skull base and the midline are identified using image-guided surgery (**Fig. 4B.10**).
12. **Transsellar approach:** The mucosa covering the sella turcica is cauterized and removed from medial to lateral (**Fig. 4B.11** and **Fig. 4B.12**). Care has to be taken when a dehiscent cavernous carotid artery or optic nerves are present.
13. Opening of the sella is started in the midline (**Fig. 4B.13**).
14. With the use of the Kerrison punch, the sellar opening is completed. The anatomical landmarks of the sella turcica (superior intercavernous sinus and planum sphenoidale, lateral cavernous sinus, inferior sellar floor) have to be in clear view (**Fig. 4B.14**).
15. A cruciate incision of the sellar dura allows exposure of the scared pituitary gland and tumor tissue (**Fig. 4B.15** and **Fig. 4B.16**).
16. A 90-degree ring curette and a suction using bimanual technique is then used to debulk the lesion in a zonal

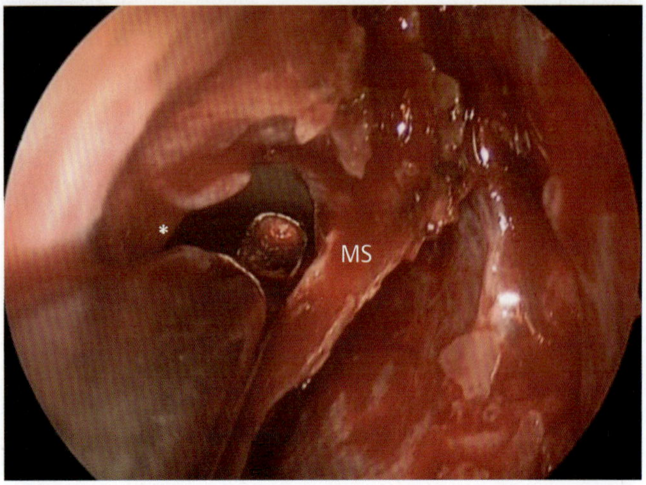

Fig. 4B.7 Removal of the sphenoid shelf (*) using a Kerrison punch.

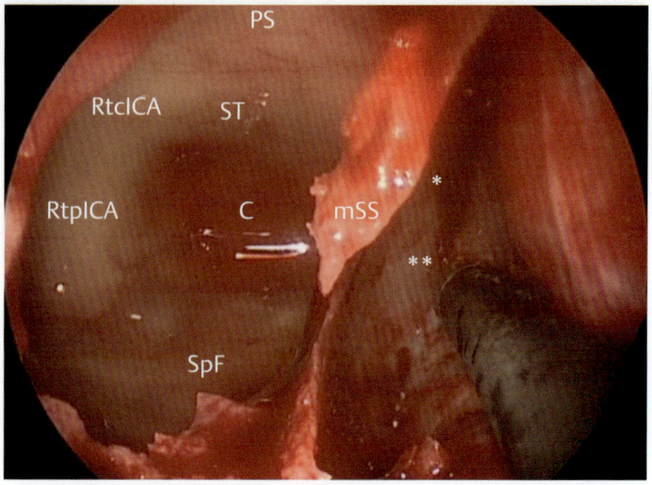

Fig. 4B.8 The dividing sphenoid main septum (mSS) is inserting into the bony coverage over the left paraclinoid (*) and cavernous internal carotid artery (**).

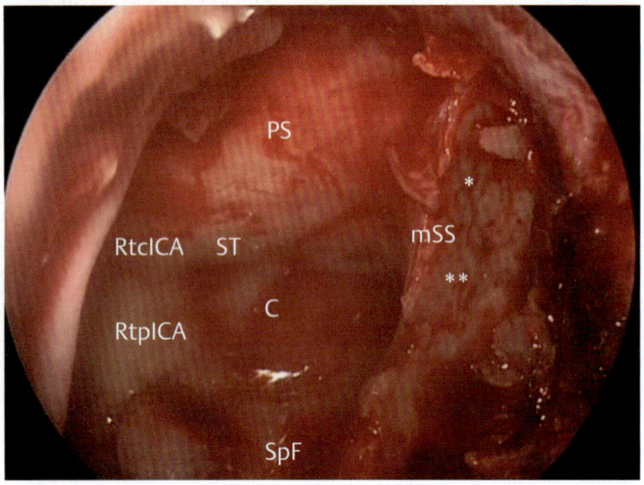

Fig. 4B.9 The dividing sphenoid main septum (MS) has been meticulously removed by piecemeal without cracking. The insertion site along the bony coverage over the left paraclinoid (*) and cavernous internal carotid artery (**) is visible.

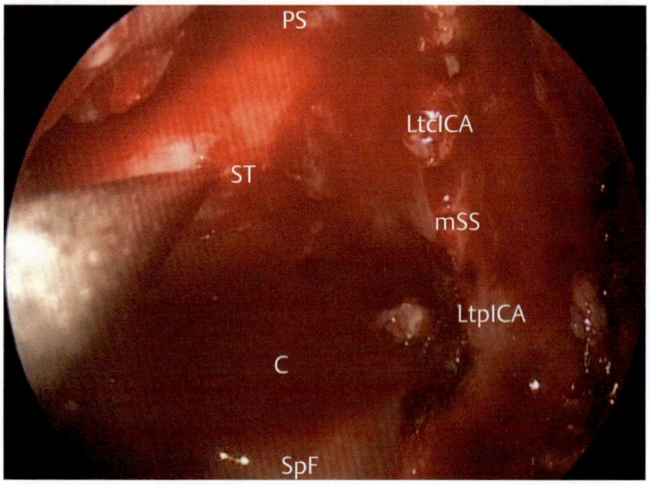

Fig. 4B.10 The midline is verified using image-guided surgery.

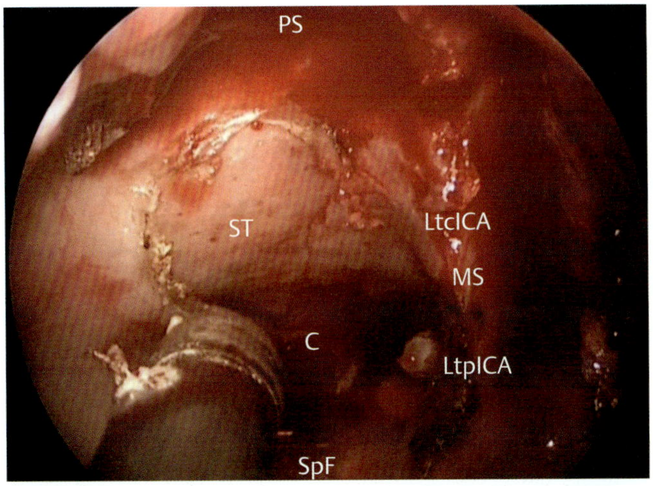

Fig. 4B.11 The mucosa covering the sella turcica (ST) is cauterized using a monopolar suction. Care has to be taken with dehiscent structures like the internal carotid arteries or optic nerves.

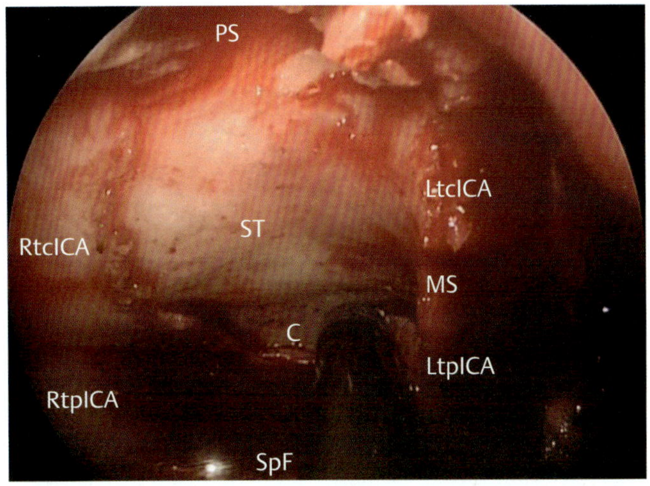

Fig. 4B.12 The clivus (C) is exposed and visualized.

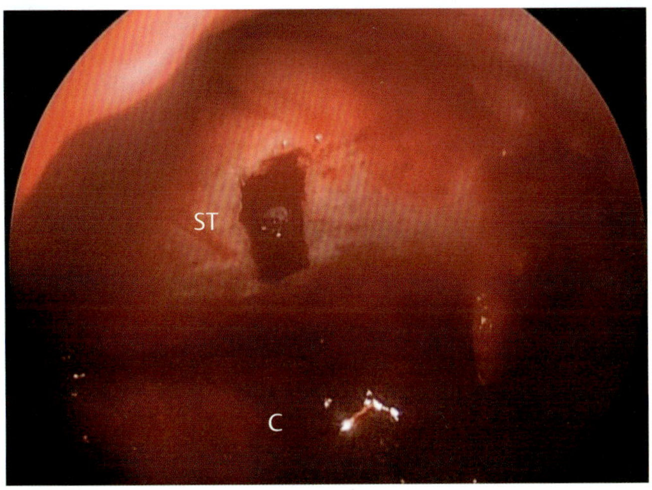

Fig. 4B.13 The sella turcica (ST) is opened using a Jizzle.

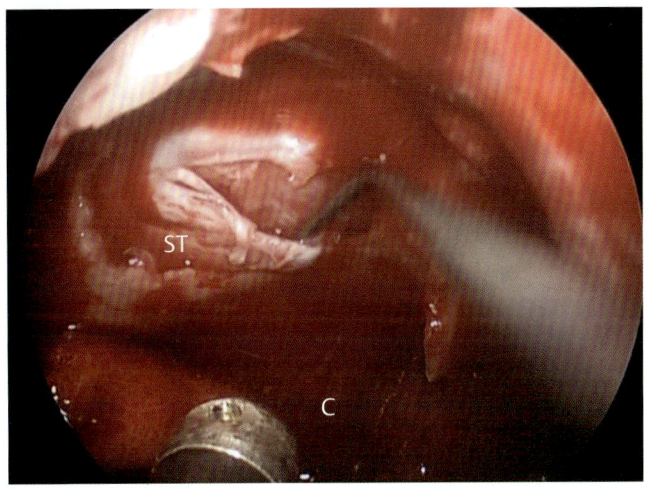

Fig. 4B.14 The dura of the sella turcica (ST) is opened with a horizontal cut and a plane between the dura and the scared pituitary tissue is defined using a blunt dissector.

manner, focusing on the central inferior zone first (**Fig. 4B.17**).

17. Resection is continued until the sellar floor and the posterior wall of the sella turcica are identified (**Fig. 4B.18**). Scar tissue and septations might compartmentalize the tumor in preoperated cases, and division of the latter might be necessary to further debulk the tumor. In previously transcranially operated cases, detailed assessment of the preoperative imaging is necessary and identification of bone covering the posterior sella has to be identified. Otherwise, this maneuver has to be done very carefully to not harm the more posterior structures including the basilar artery in the prepontine cistern and its perforators to the pons cerebri.
18. Then, the anterior superior compartment is debulked and tumor components are removed from thickened scar tissue and the tumor pseudocapsule (**Fig. 4B.19, Fig. 4B.20, Fig. 4B.21**).
19. The posterior margin of the resection cavity is the clival dura covering the posterior wall of the sella turcica and the Liliequist membrane dividing the space

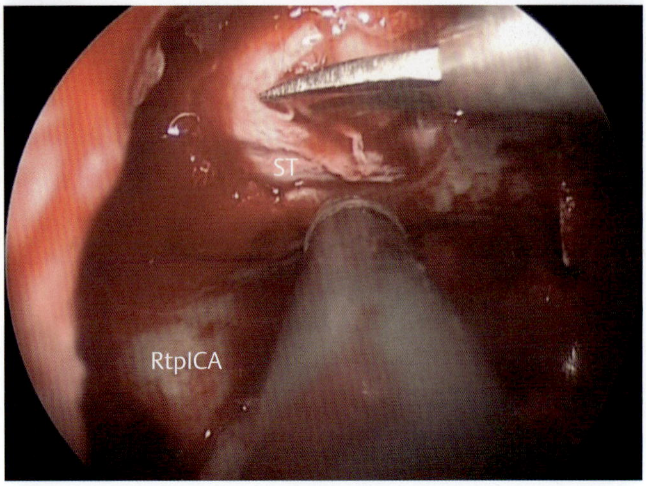

Fig. 4B.15 The sellar opening is widened laterally on both sides.

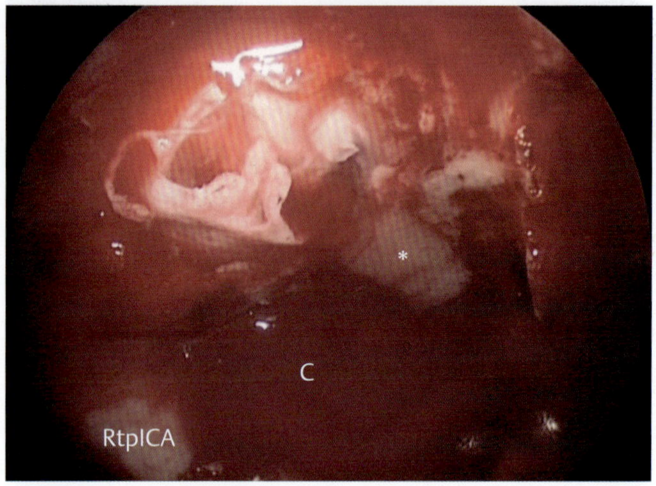

Fig. 4B.16 Whitish liquid tumor tissue (*) spontaneously evacuates.

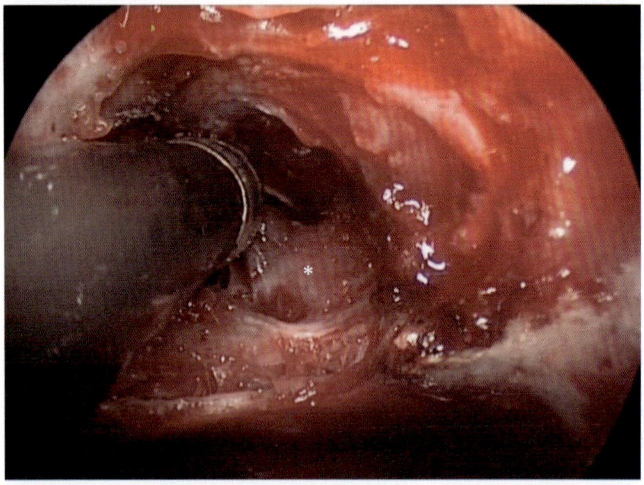

Fig. 4B.17 Central tumor debulking. The intrasellar scar tissue consists of various fibrous strands (*).

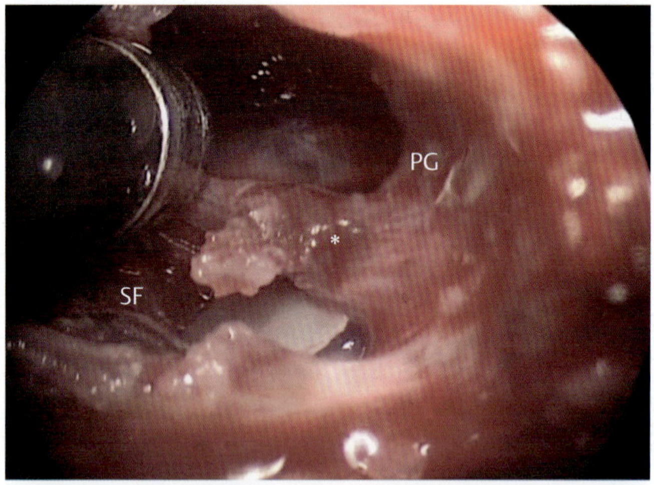

Fig. 4B.18 The intrasellar scar tissue forms fibrous strands (*).

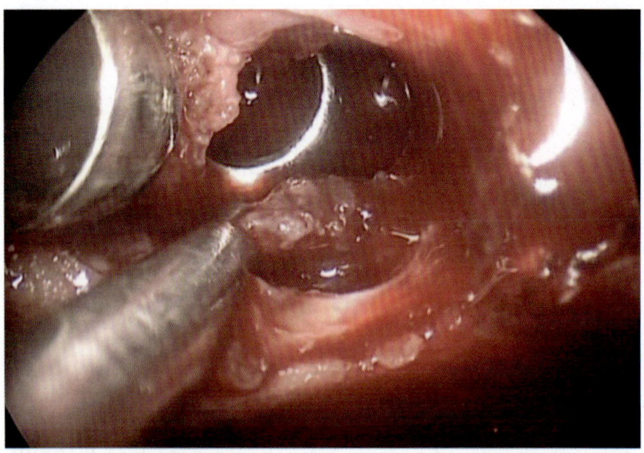

Fig. 4B.19 Debulking of the anterior superior tumor compartment.

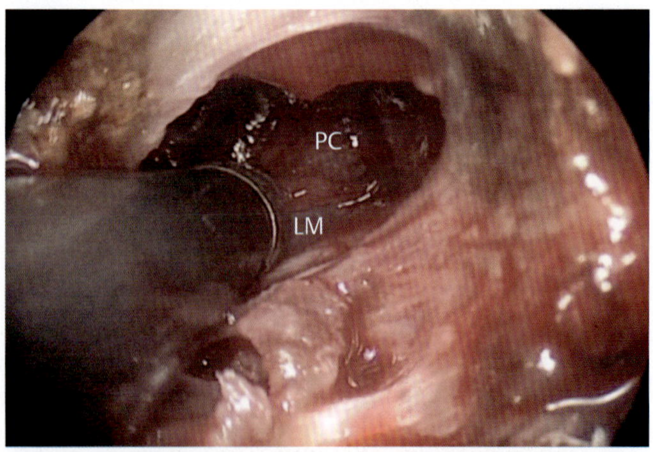

Fig. 4B.20 Identification of a thickened pseudocapsule from the posterior sellar wall and the Liliequist membrane (LM).

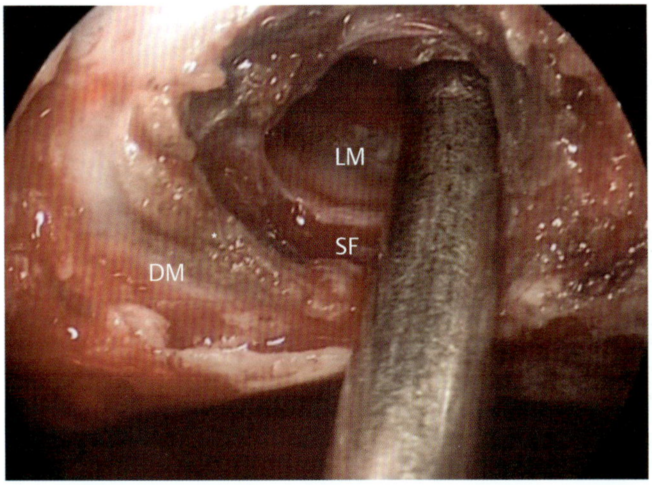

Fig. 4B.21 Debulking of the posterior superior tumor compartment.

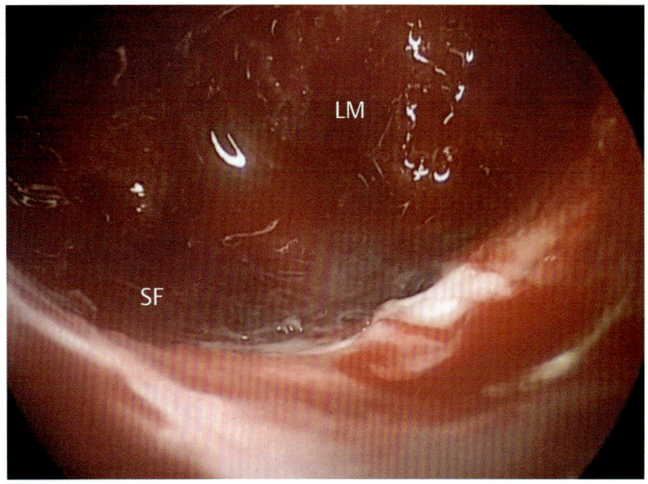

Fig. 4B.22 Resection cavity after tumor removal.

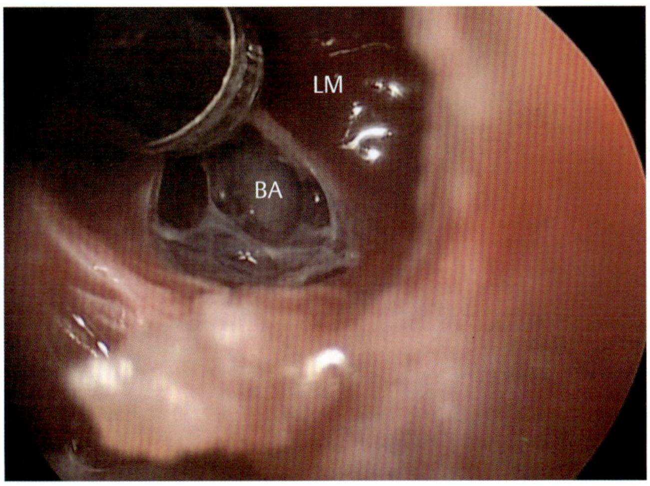

Fig. 4B.23 Opening of the thickened Liliequist's membrane (LM) reveals the basilar artery (BA).

between the suprasellar and the prepontine cistern (**Fig. 4B.22** and **Fig. 4B.23**).

20. In preoperated recurrent pituitary adenoma cases, the use of intraoperative magnetic resonance imaging (iMRI) is very helpful after initial tumor removal to assess the extent of resection. In the present case, the assumed resection of the recurrent pituitary macroadenoma was incomplete in the suprasellar compartment, which was confirmed by intraoperative MRI (iMRI) (**Fig. 4B.24**).
21. To reach the suprasellar remaining tumor, a superior expansion of the transsellar osteodural exposure is necessary (**Fig. 4B.25**).
22. **Transtuberculum approach:** After removal of the bone covering the midline tuberculum sellae, the dural opening is extended superiorly. The anterior intercavernous sinus has to be identified, cauterized, and transected when performing this extension (**Fig. 4B.26** and **Fig. 4B.27**).
23. Solid tumor components can be encapsulated within smaller chambers along the suprasellar compartment, allowing the identification of the thickened and scared diaphragma sellae, the optic nerve, and the optic chiasm (**Fig. 4B.28, Fig. 4B.29, Fig. 4B 30, and Fig. 4B.31**).
24. The skull base defect is closed with an abdominal fat graft and an artificial dural sealant (**Fig. 4B.32**).
25. The sphenoid cavity is filled with Surgifoam, and the nasoseptal flaps are brought back in position.
26. The middle turbinates are brought back into position and stabilized with resorbable nasal packs with slight compression.

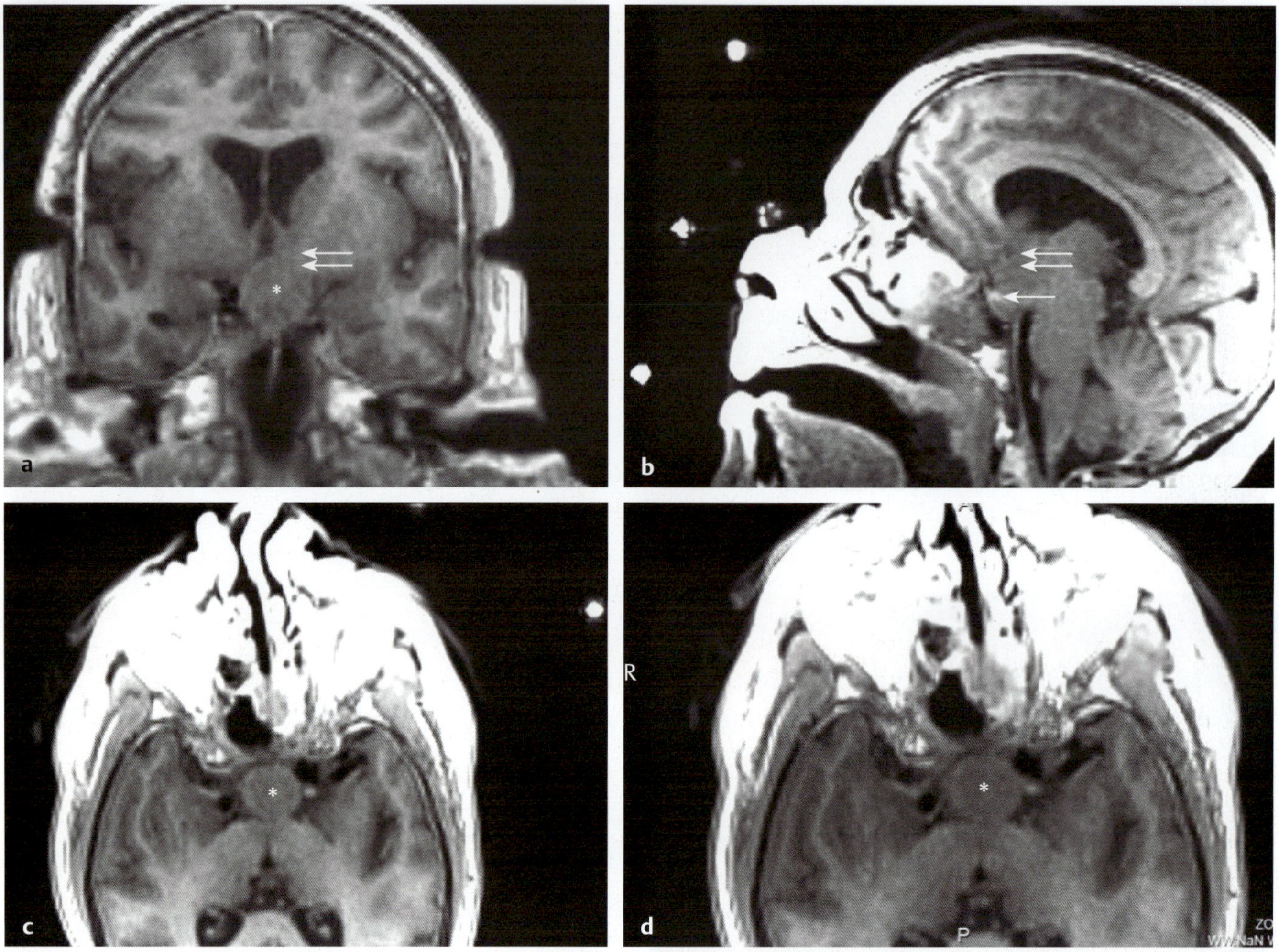

Fig. 4B.24 **(a)** Coronal, **(b)** sagittal, **(c, d)** axial, T1-weighted section of the intraoperative MRI. The intraoperative imaging demonstrated sufficient tumor removal of the intrasellar compartment with remaining suprasellar extension of the recurrent pituitary adenoma (*), divided by a thick scar layer (*arrow*). Compression of the optic chiasm (*double arrow*) and left optic nerve (*double arrow*) is still present.

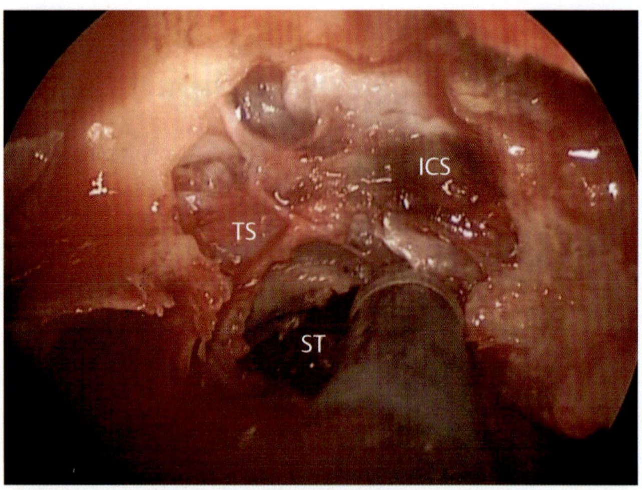

Fig. 4B.25 Superior extension of the bone covering the sella turcica (ST), the tuberculum sellae (TS), and the anterior intercavernous sinus (ICS).

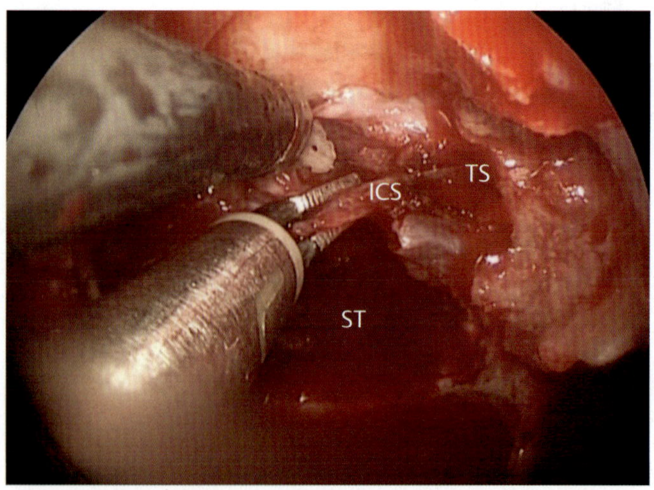

Fig. 4B.26 Cauterization of the anterior intercavernous sinus (ICS).

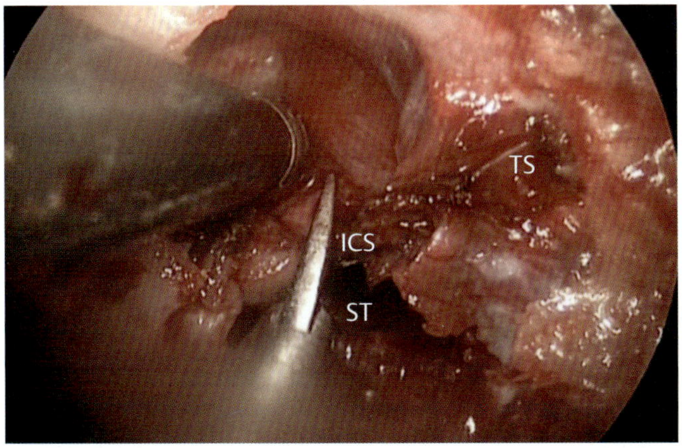

Fig. 4B.27 Cutting of the anterior intercavernous sinus (ICS).

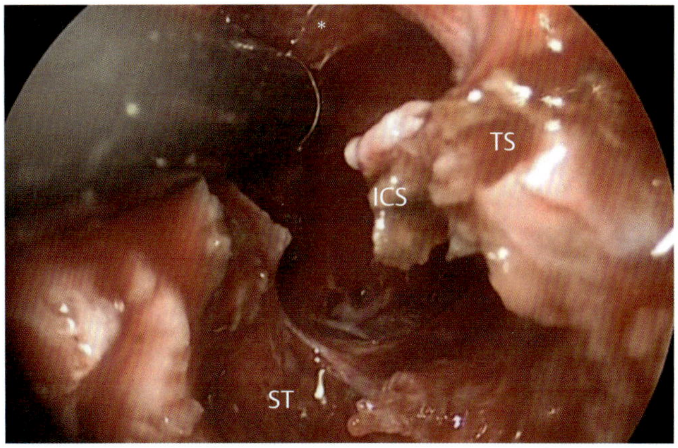

Fig. 4B.28 Resection of the suprasellar residual tumor compartment (*) after transection of the intercavernous sinus (IICS).

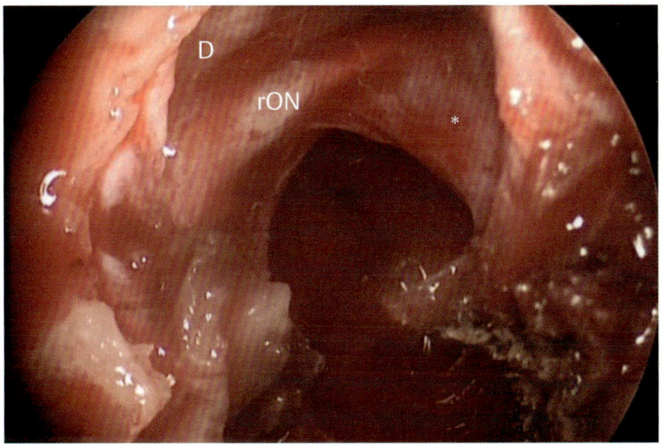

Fig. 4B.29 The thickened and scared diaphragma sellae (D) and the right optic nerve (rON) are visible after removal of the suprasellar tumor compartment. Tumor tissue (*) is still present within a left suprasellar compartment.

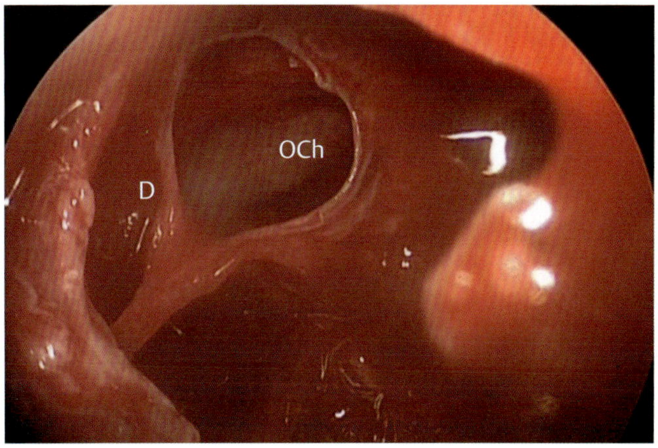

Fig. 4B.30 The left suprasellar tumor remnant has been removed and the thickened and scared diaphragma sellae (D) has been opened. The optic chiasm is identified.

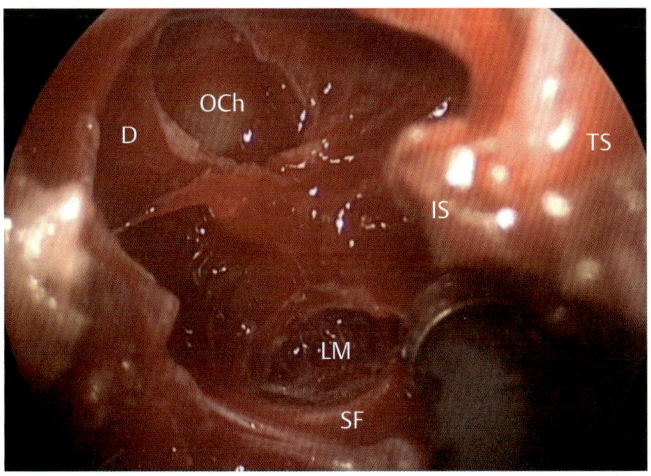

Fig. 4B.31 Resection cavity after intra- and suprasellar tumor removal.

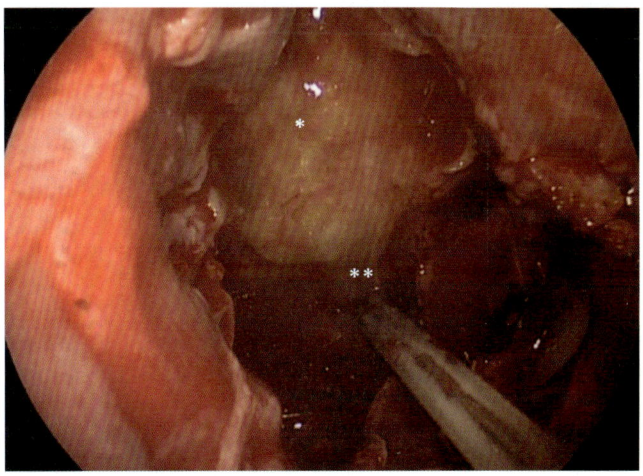

Fig. 4B.32 Repair of the skull base defect using abdominal fat graft (*) an artificial dural sealant (**).

Chapter 5 Endoscopic Endonasal Surgery for Functioning Pituitary Adenoma

Case 5A

Single Nostril Endoscopic Transseptal Transsphenoidal Excision of an ACTH-Producing Microadenoma

Adzreil Bakri, Michel Roethlisberger, Prepageran Narayanan, and Vicknes Waran

History

A 35-year-old lady with Cushing's disease presented with a 1-year history of weight gain, headache, anxiety, and hypertension. Her urine, blood cortisol, and adrenocorticotrophic hormone (ACTH) levels were elevated. A magnetic resonance imaging (MRI) of the brain revealed a pituitary microadenoma measuring approximately 5 × 5 mm (**Fig. 5A.1**).

A single nostril endoscopic transseptal transsphenoidal excision of the tumor was planned. This approach was chosen due to the small size of the tumor.

Surgical Steps

1. The patient is placed under general anesthesia in the supine position with her head slightly extended and fixed within a NORAS® (NORAS MRI Products, Germany)-frame for intraoperative MRI (iMRI). Registration for neuronavigation (Brainlab, Munich, Germany) is performed.
2. Local anesthesia is infiltrated into both sides of the septum to raise the mucoperichondrium away from the bony septum (**Fig. 5A.2**).
3. The septum is then incised with a size-15 blade on one side, and the mucoperichondrial flap is raised posteriorly toward the choana (**Fig. 5A.3**).
4. Through the same septal incision, the cartilaginous septum is incised, and a mucoperichondrial flap is raised on the opposite side (**Fig. 5A.4**).
5. The cartilaginous and bony septum is removed until the sphenoid rostrum is exposed (**Fig. 5A.5**).
6. Suction monopolar cautery is used to remove any residual mucosa covering the sphenoid ostiae bilaterally.

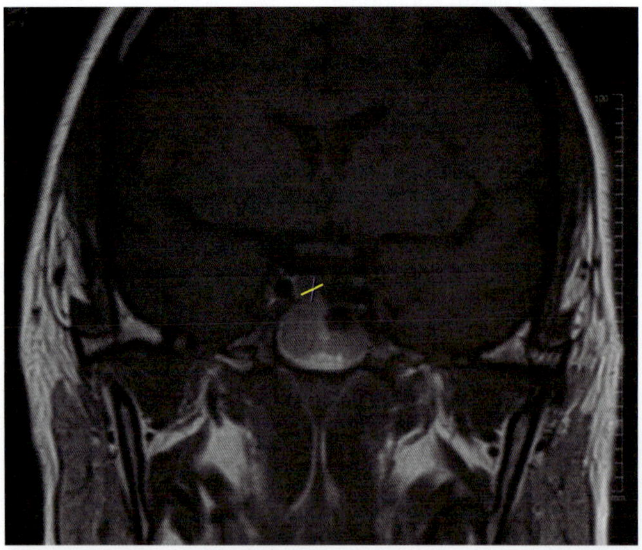

Fig. 5A.1 A T1-weighted MRI showing a 4.7 mm *(yellow line)* x 4.5 mm *(blue line)* tumor at the right side of the pituitary gland.

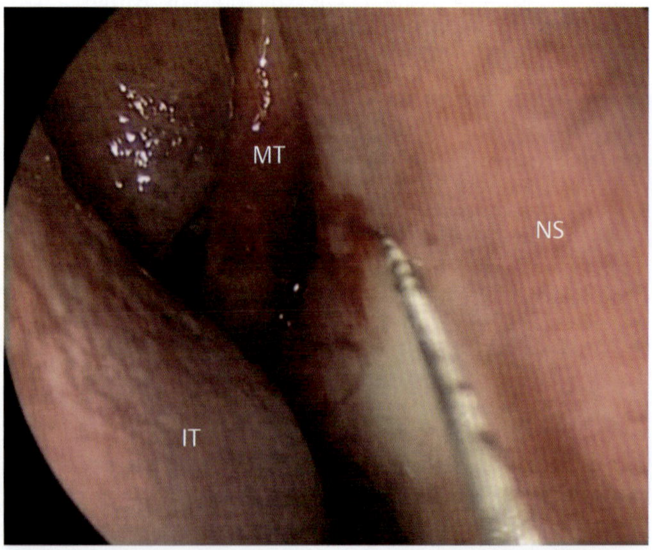

Fig. 5A.2 View of the right nasal cavity. Local anesthesia infiltration into the nasal septum (NS).

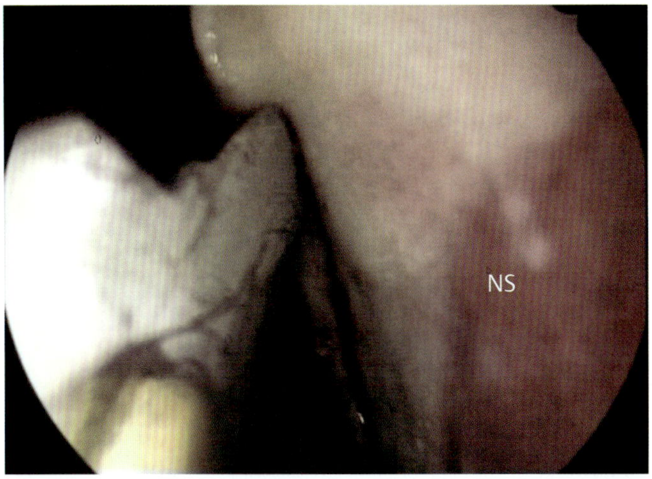

Fig. 5A.3 View of the right nasal cavity. Incision on the nasal septum (NS) opposite to the anterior part of the middle turbinate.

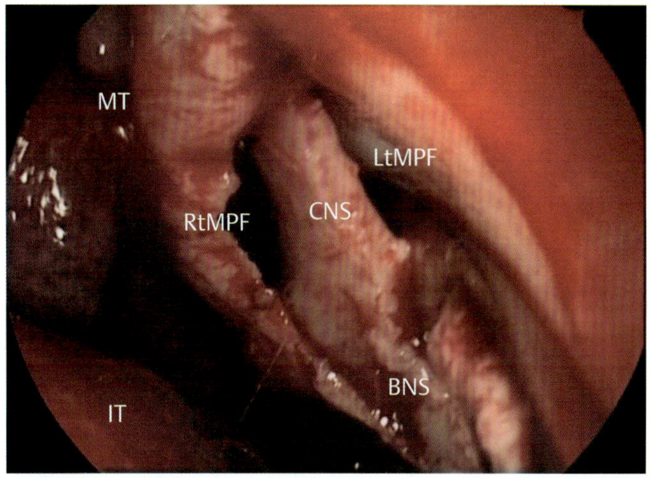

Fig. 5A.4 View from the right nasal cavity. Raising of bilateral mucoperichondrial flaps and removal of the cartilaginous and bony septum.

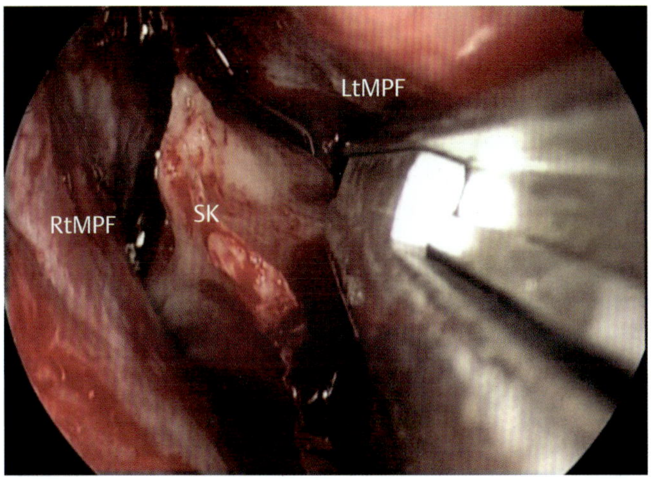

Fig. 5A.5 Exposure and removal of the sphenoid keel (SK).

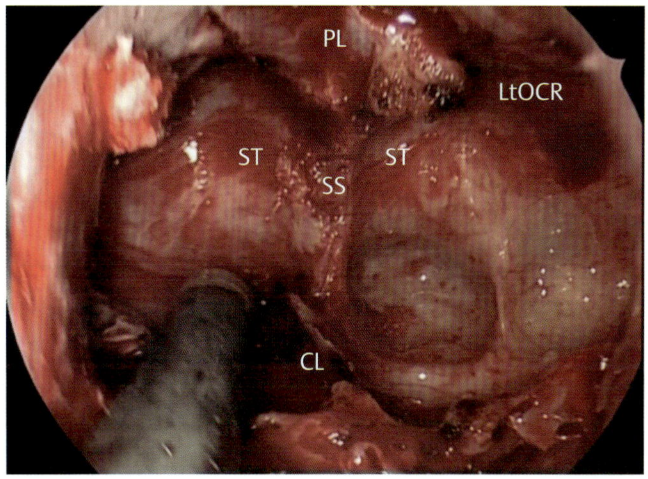

Fig. 5A.6 Removal of residual mucosa and bony septations creating a single large sphenoid cavity.

7. The bilateral sphenoid ostiae are widened inferomedially in a V-shaped manner with a Kerrison's punch, and once the bony removal is sufficient, the sphenoid keel is removed with pituitary rongeur forceps.
8. After the removal of the sphenoid keel, any residual mucosa or bony septations are carefully removed to make the bilateral sphenoid sinus a single common cavity (**Fig. 5A.6**).
9. Prior to the removal of the bone overlying the sella, the exact location of the tumor is confirmed using image-guided surgery (IGS).
10. The bone overlying this area is then thinned out with a drill or a curette. Drilling and curetting maneuvers should be performed medially to avoid injury to the carotid siphons of the cavernous sinuses bilaterally (**Fig. 5A.7**).
11. Once the bone is thin enough, a right-angle dissector can be inserted to separate the bone and the underlying dura (**Fig. 5A.8**). This bony opening is then widened adequately in the shape of a rectangle using a Kerrison's punch, making sure that the dura is always separated from the bone (**Fig. 5A.9** and **Fig. 5A.10**).
12. After adequate exposure, a horizontal and vertical incision in the shape of a cruciate is made on the dura with a size-15 blade (**Fig. 5A.11** and **Fig. 5A.12**).

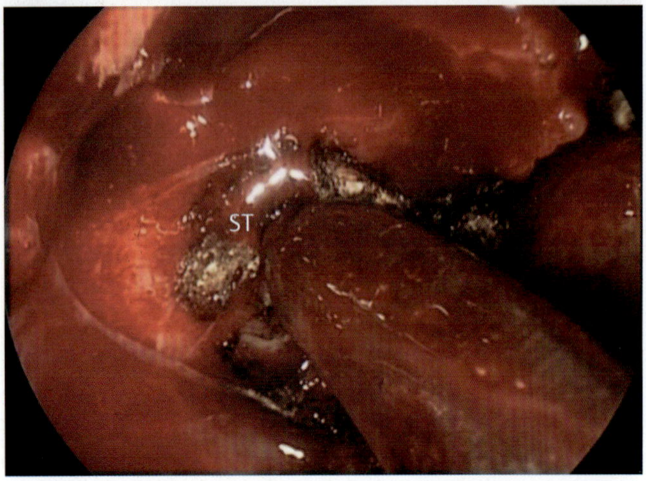

Fig. 5A.7 Bone overlying the tumor is thinned out with a curette.

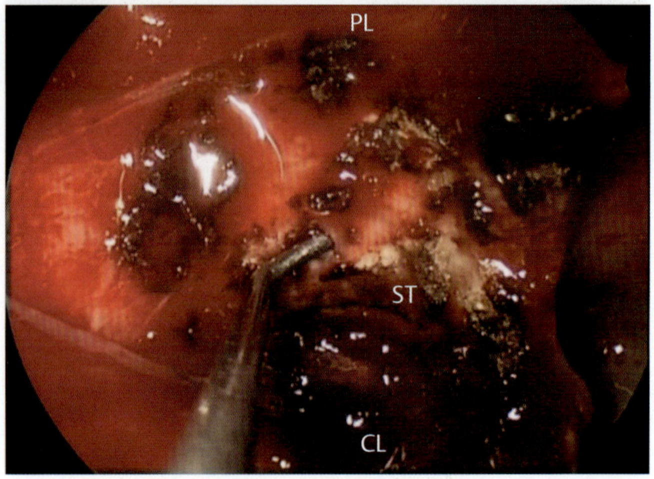

Fig. 5A.8 A right-angle dissector is insinuated between the bone and the underlying dura.

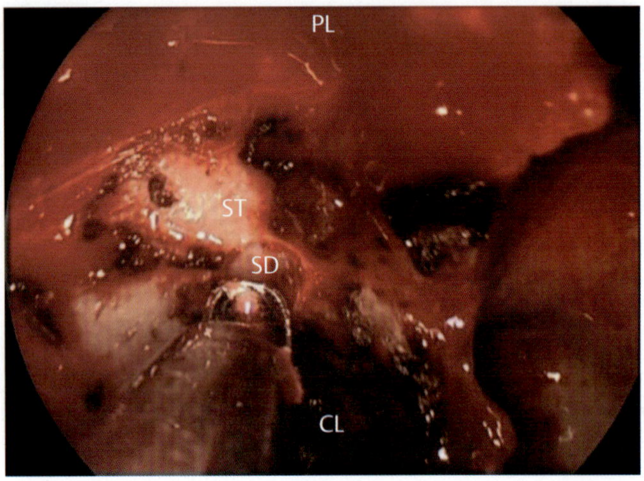

Fig. 5A.9 The bony opening is widened using a Kerrison's punch.

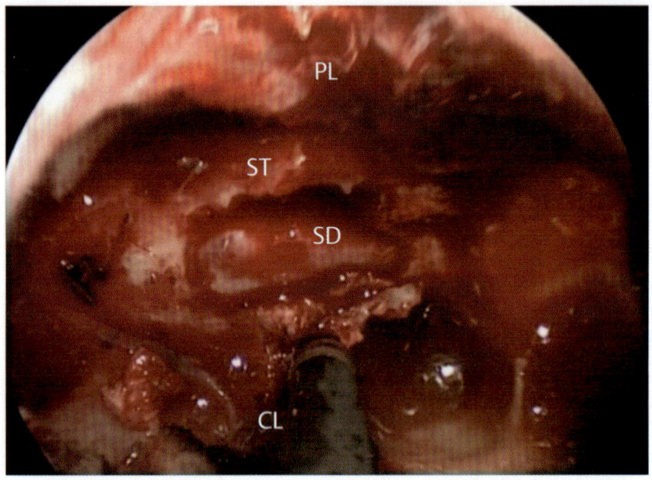

Fig. 5A.10 An adequate bony opening is made in the shape of a rectangle.

13. The tumor is exposed and gently dissected away from the normal pituitary gland tissue with a blunt ring curette (**Fig. 5A.13** and **Fig. 5A.14**).
14. Once the tumor removal is complete, the small defect is closed with oxidized cellulose polymer (Surgicel, Ethicon, USA), and the sphenoid sinus is filled with absorbable gelatin sponges (Gelfoam, Pfizer, USA) (**Fig. 5A.15** and **Fig. 5A.16**).
15. Both septal flaps are approximated in the midline, and the septal incision is covered with synthetic biodegradable foams (Nasopore, Stryker, USA) while making sure to provide an adequate airway along the nasal floor (**Fig. 5A.17**).

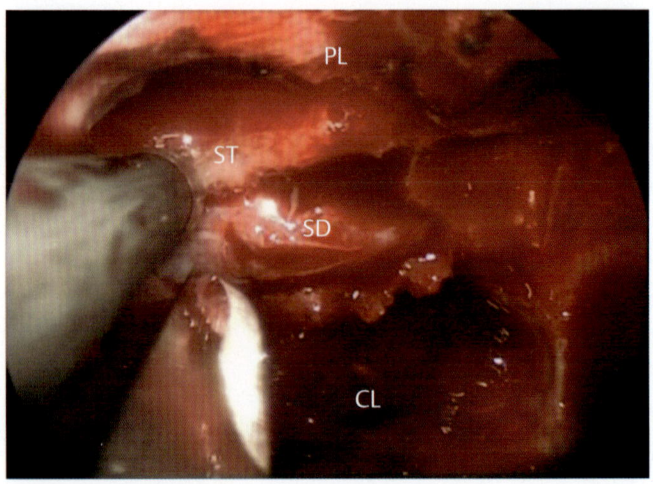

Fig. 5A.11 Cruciate incision on the dura.

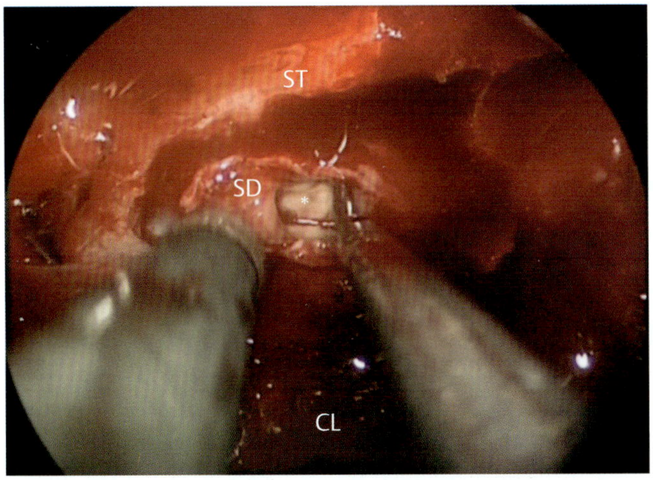

Fig. 5A.12 Vertical incision of the sellar dura using micro scissors. The tumor has been depicted by *.

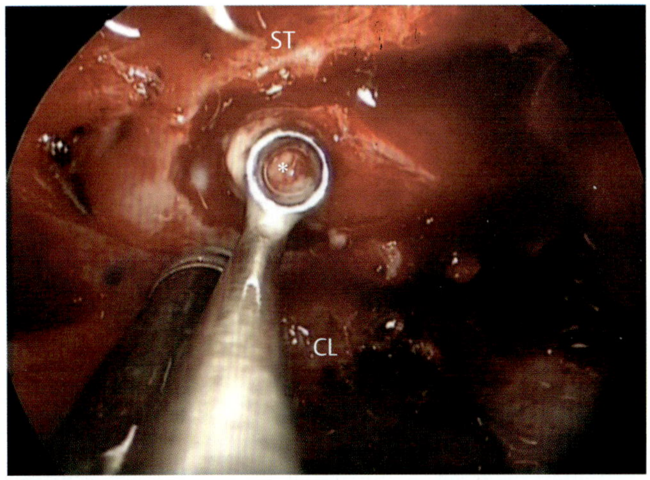

Fig. 5A.13 Tumor (*) removal using a blunt ring curette.

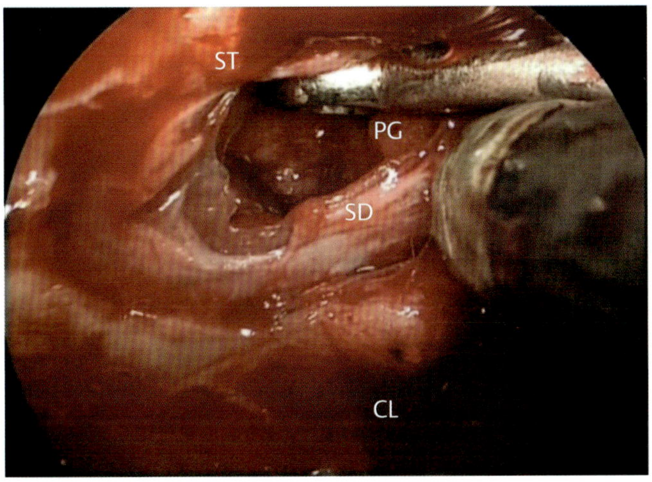

Fig. 5A.14 Final view after complete tumor removal.

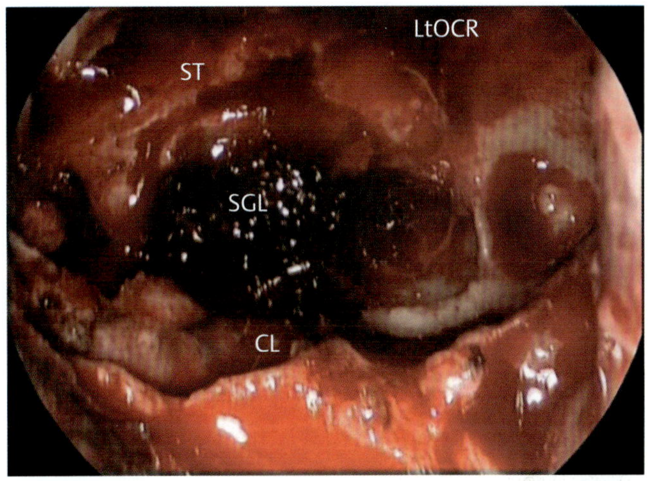

Fig. 5A.15 Defect closed using Surgicel (SGL ; Ethicon, USA).

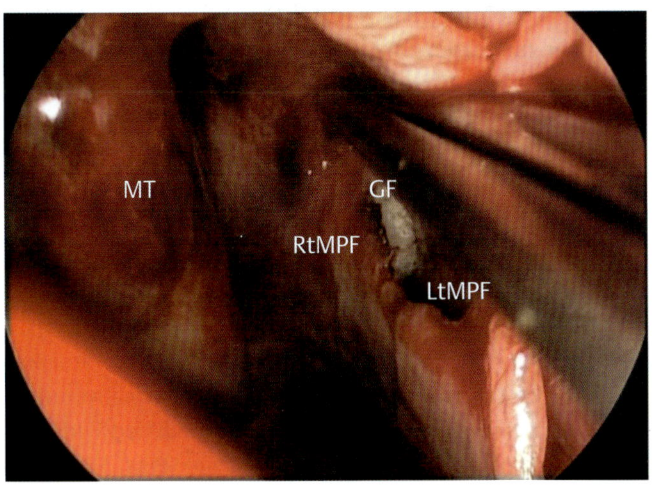

Fig. 5A.16 View from the right nasal cavity. Packing of the sphenoid cavity with Gelfoam (GF; Pfizer, USA) and midline reapproximation of the septal flaps.

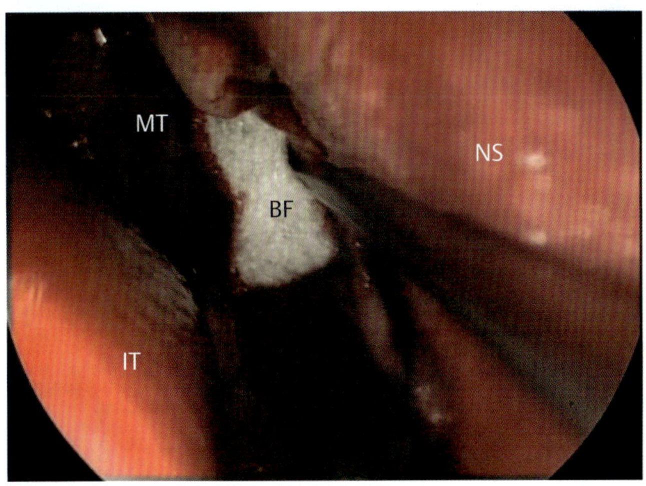

Fig. 5A.17 View of the right nasal cavity. Closure of the septal incision and nasal packing with synthetic biodegradable foams (BF) providing adequate nasal airway along the floor of the nose.

Case 5B

Binostril Endoscopic Transseptal Transsphenoidal Excision of an ACTH-Producing Pituitary Microadenoma

Michel Roethlisberger, Prepageran Narayanan, and Vicknes Waran

History

A 27-year-old lady presented with an 8-month history of weight gain, hypertension, and a progressive rounded face (**Fig. 5B.1**) with pink or purple stretch marks on the skin in the abdominal region (striae). Decreased glucose tolerance was detected. A further workup revealed elevated urine, blood cortisol, and adrenocorticotrophic hormone (ACTH) levels. Consecutive neuroimaging demonstrated the presence of a pituitary microadenoma in the right basal pituitary hemisphere measuring approximately 3 × 4 mm (**Fig. 5B.2**).

A double nostril endoscopic transseptal transsphenoidal excision of the tumor was planned.

On the third postoperative day, morning (7–9 am) serum cortisol levels were 91 mmol/L (145–691 mmol/L), while the other hormonal axis remained within a normal range.

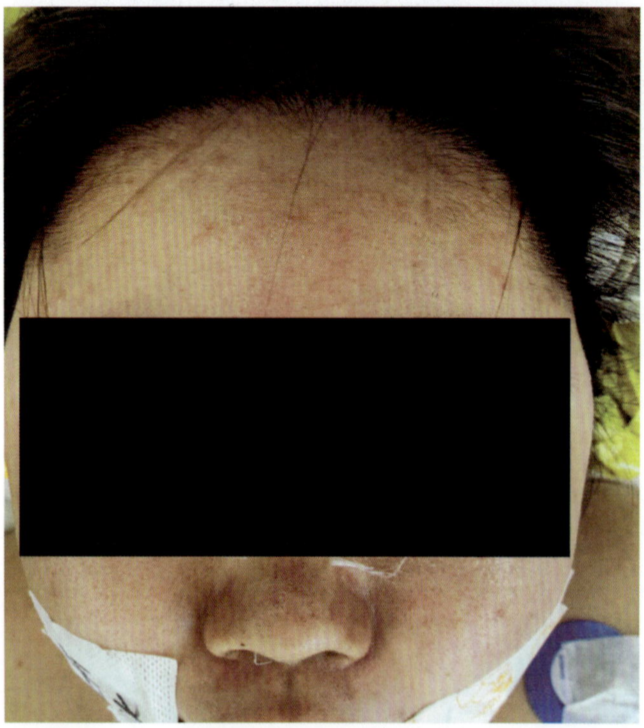

Fig. 5B.1 One of the hallmark signs of Cushing's syndrome is the rounded face, facial acne, and hyperpigmentation around the nose with signs of easy bruising.

Surgical Steps

1. A *transnasal transseptal transsphenoidal binostril approach* is performed as described in Chapter 1.
2. The sphenoid cavity is exposed, and the anatomical landmarks of the skull base are inspected and verified using image-guided surgery (**Figs. 5B.3** and **Fig. 5B.4**).
3. Remaining bone and mucosa of the anterior sphenoidal wall and posterior ethmoidal cells are removed (**Fig. 5B.5**).
4. Sphenoid septae are removed using punches or a high-speed drill (**Fig. 5B.6**).
5. The sella turcica is opened using a Kerrison Punch (**Fig. 5B.7**).
6. The osteodural exposure is placed on the right-lateral side, where the microadenoma is suspected. The exposition of the dura covering the right cavernous internal carotid artery is relevant to have sufficient laterality when approaching the microadenoma (**Figs. 5B.8** and **Fig. 5B.9**).
7. The dura of the sella turcica is opened over the right lateral aspect, where the microadenoma is suspected (**Fig. 5B.10**).
8. The ACTH-producing microadenoma is clearly distinguishable from the healthy right pituitary gland lobe, as it is located in the right-lateral anterior inferior aspect of the gland (**Fig. 5B.11**).
9. The microadenoma is dissected from the healthy pituitary gland tissue using a micro dissector. The plane is followed in a circumferential way (**Fig. 5B.12a–d**).
10. The microadenoma can be isolated up to the point where it protrudes out of the dissection cavity. It can then be removed using a pituitary rongeur (**Fig. 5B.13**).
11. The tumor cavity is systematically cleaned using curettes and flushing of sterile saline (**Fig. 5B.14**).
12. Widening of the tumor cavity, its inspection and visualization is necessary to identify even the smallest tumor tissues that may remain. The normal pituitary gland should be preserved and manipulated with care when inspecting the resection cavity (**Figs. 5B.15** and **Fig. 5B.16**).
13. Closure with Surgifoam and the nasoseptal flap without any graft is possible, when no leakage of cerebrospinal fluid (CSF) is identified.

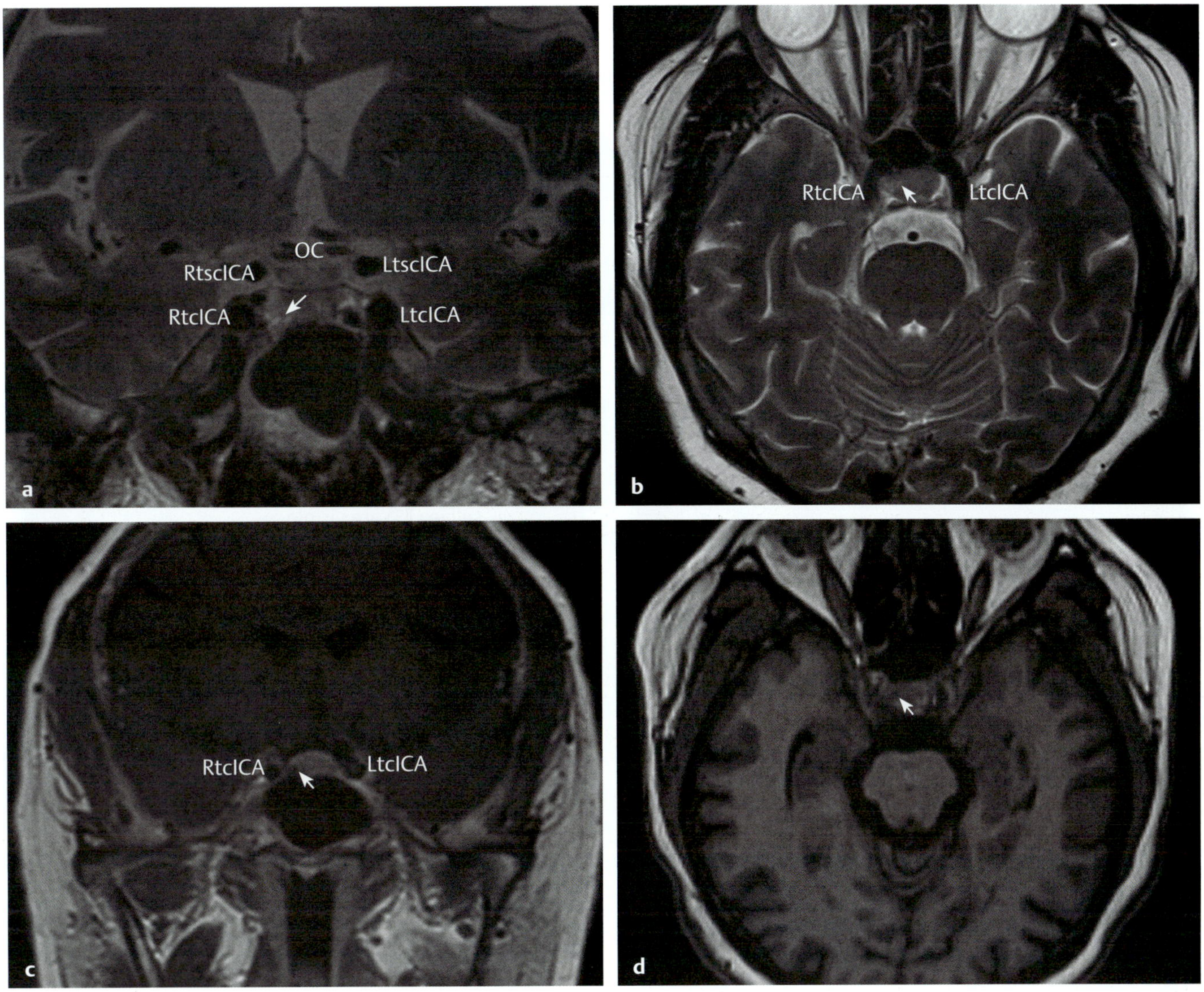

Fig. 5B.2 **(a)** Coronal; and **(b)** Axial; T2-weighted MRI sequences demonstrating a hyperintense lesion within the right pituitary gland lobe (arrow) next to the right cavernous internal carotid artery (RtcICA). **(c)** T1 contrast-enhanced dynamic sequence demonstrating hypoenhancement compared to the more enhancing pituitary gland in the right-lateral anterior inferior aspect next to the right cavernous internal carotid artery (RtcICA), suggestive of a microadenoma. **(d)** axial T1-weighted contrast-enhanced MRI section showing hypoenhancement within the right pituitary gland lobe, suggestive of a microadenoma.

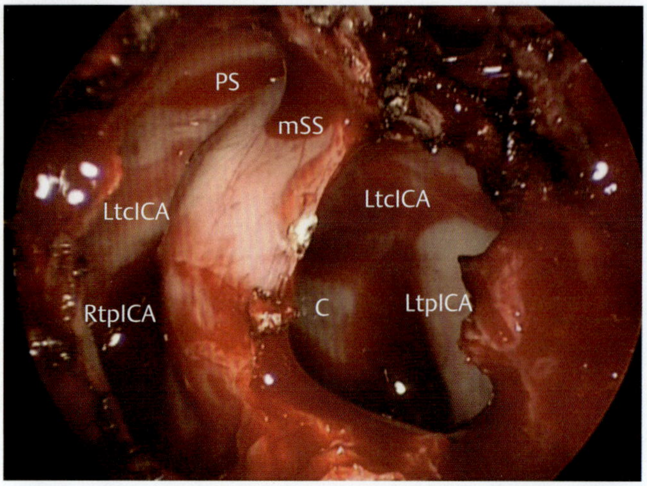

Fig. 5B.3 A main dividing septum (mSS) obstructs the view of the sella turcica within the sphenoid cavity.

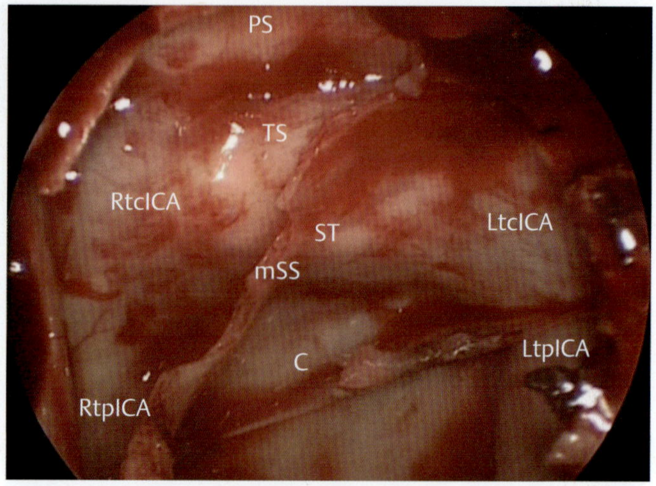

Fig. 5B.4 After the removal of the main dividing septum (mSS), the sella turcica (ST) and the tuberculum sellae (TS) are visible.

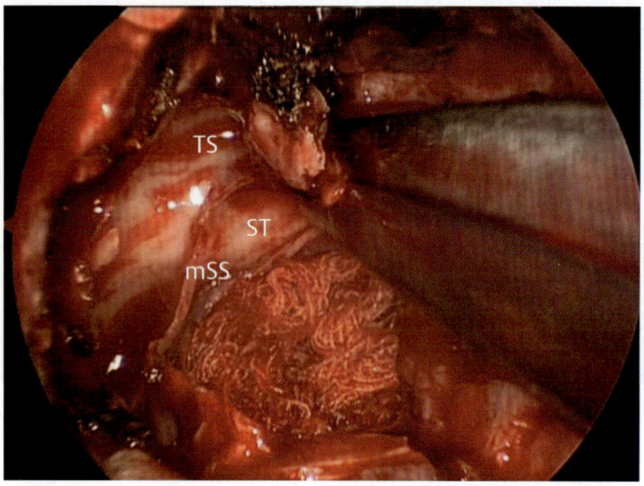

Fig. 5B.5 Removal of the remaining anterior sphenoid wall and mucosa of the posterior ethmoidal cells.

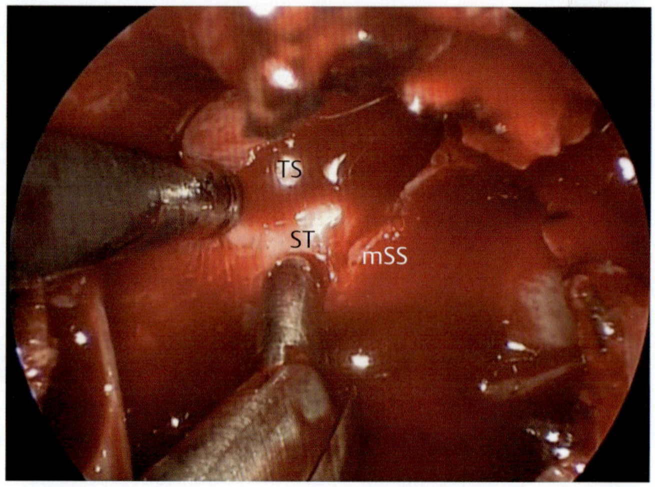

Fig. 5B.6 Piecemeal removal of the main dividing septum (SS).

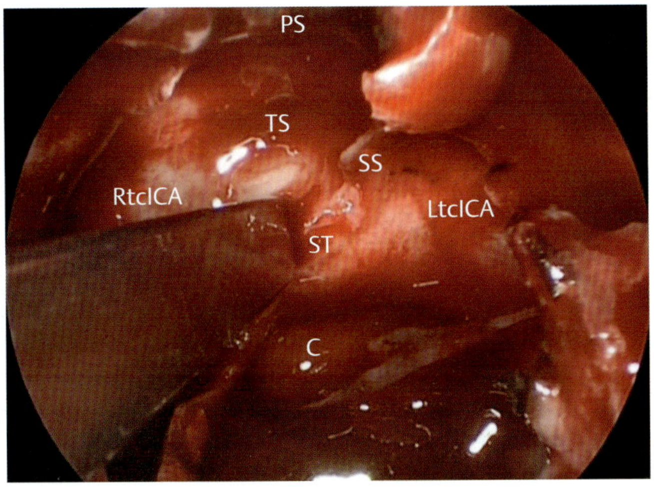

Fig. 5B.7 Opening of the sella turcica (TS).

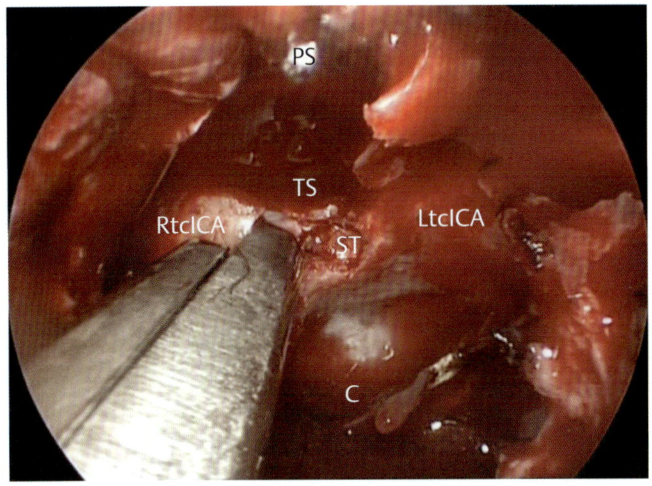

Fig. 5B.8 Opening of the sella turcica (ST) toward the right lateral using a Kerrison punch. The lateral limitation is visualization of the right cavernous internal carotid artery (RtcICA) to fully expose the microadenoma.

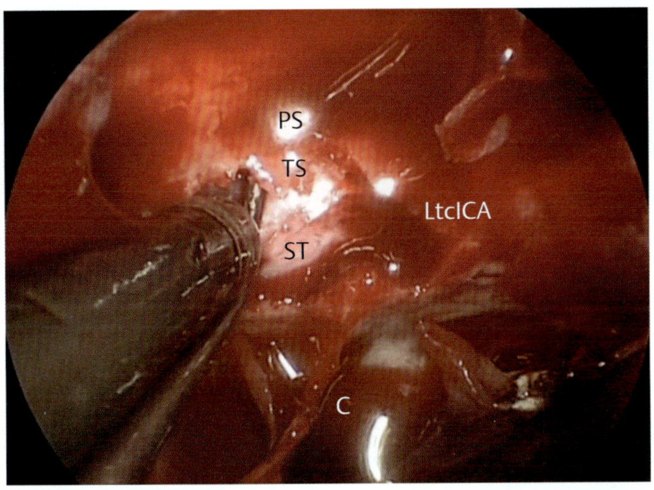

Fig. 5B.9 Opening of the sella turcica (ST) in a superior direction. The superior limitation is the anterior intercavernous sinus.

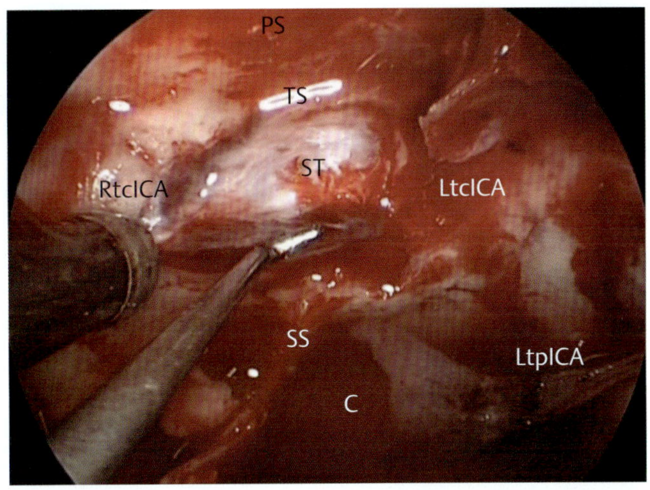

Fig. 5B.10 Opening of the sellar dura has to be performed carefully to not harm the normal pituitary gland or the integrity of the microadenoma before inspection of the surface is possible.

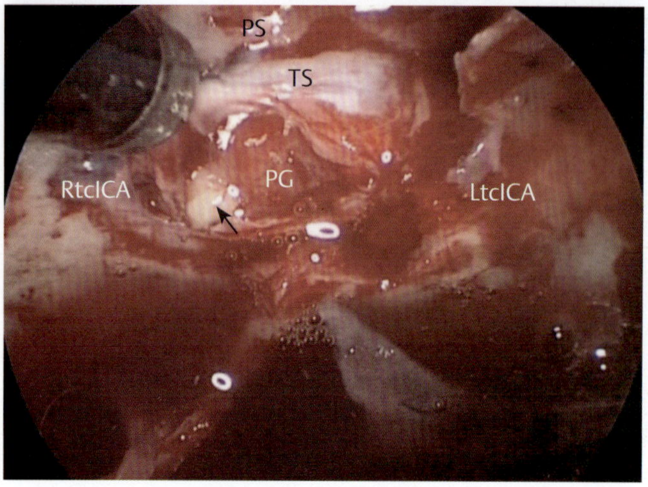

Fig. 5B.11 Inspection of the right anterior pituitary gland (PG) surface. The microadenoma is spontaneously visible in this case, as it is located within the lateral anterior inferior aspect of the sella turcica next to the right cavernous internal carotid artery (RtcICA).

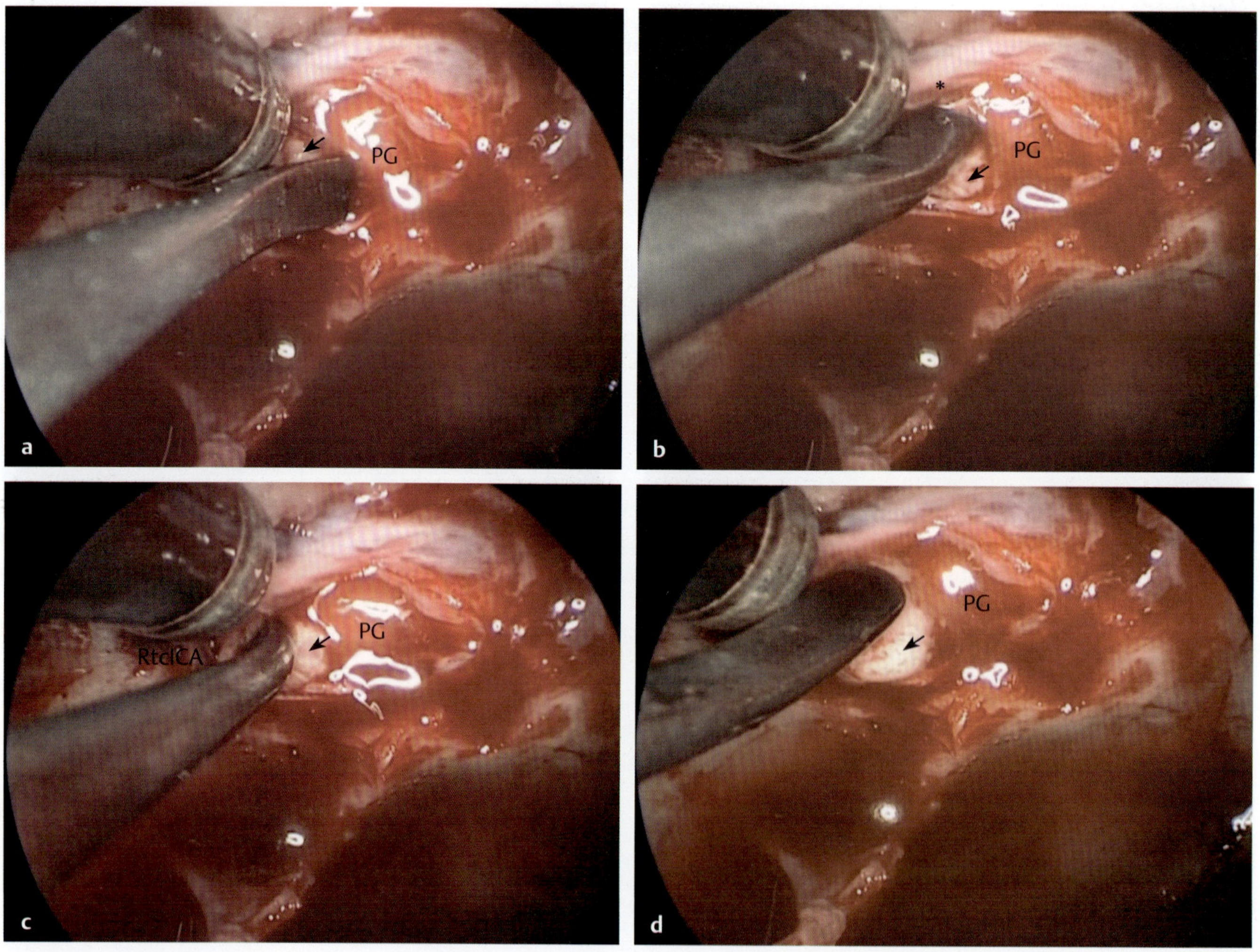

Fig. 5B.12 **(a–d)** Circumferential dissection of the plane (*) between the microadenoma (*arrow*) and the normal right pituitary gland (PG) lobe.

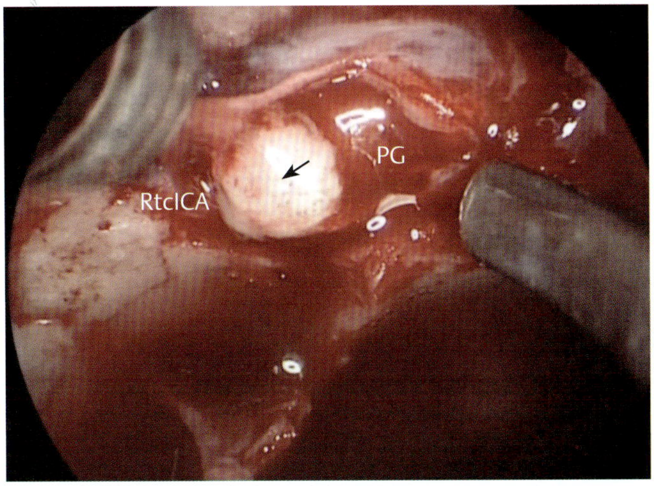

Fig. 5B.13 Circumferentially dissected and defined planes between the microadenoma (*arrow*) and the normal right pituitary gland (PG) lobe.

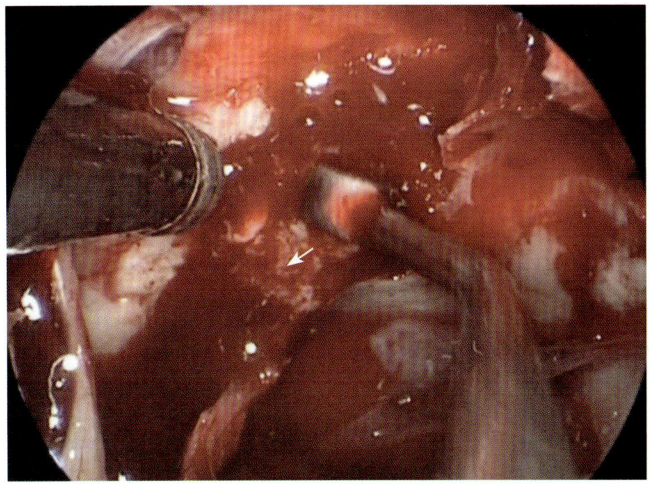

Fig. 5B.14 After the removal of the microadenoma, liquid tumor components are resected with the use of a curette.

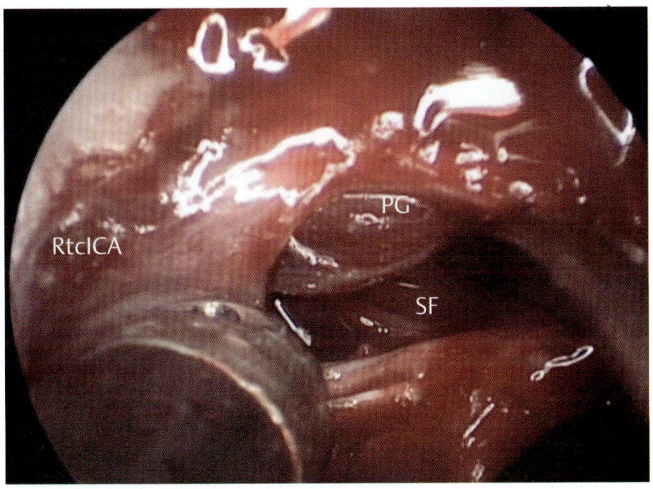

Fig. 5B.15 Meticulous inspection of the resection cavity after flushing with sterile saline.

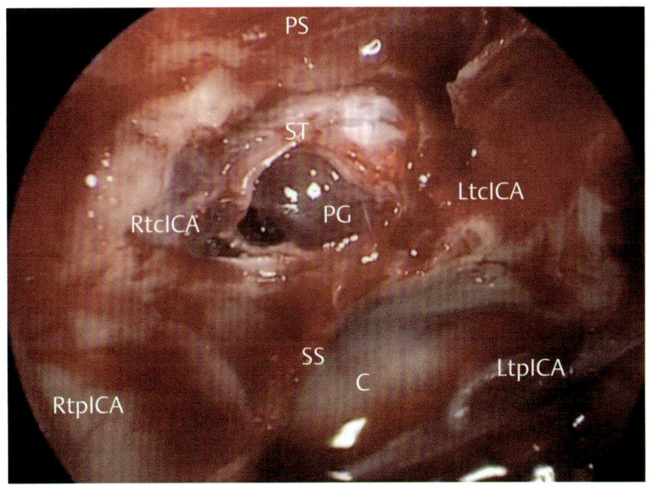

Fig. 5B.16 Inspection of the postoperative situs after tumor resection.

Case 5C

Mononostril Endonasal Endoscopic Resection of a Growth Hormone–Producing Pituitary Microadenoma

Michel Roethlisberger, Prepageran Narayanan, and Vicknes Waran

History

A 35-year-old male patient was assessed for acromegaly with slowly progressive onset of classical clinical symptoms including abnormal growth of his distal extremities. The patient noticed swelling of his hands and feet about 2 years ago. The associated bone changes consecutively altered the patient's facial appearance (**Fig. 5C.1**). Chemical endocrinological assessment confirmed acromegaly with elevated insulin-like growth factor 1 (IGF-1) and growth hormone (GH) levels.

Neuroimaging confirmed an intrasellar left dominant isointense lesion anterior-inferior to the pituitary gland with less enhancement when compared to the gland itself. The lesion erodes into the sphenoid cavity along a midline sphenoid septum. This finding is highly suspicious for an GH-producing pituitary macroadenoma (**Fig. 5C.2a–c**).

An *endonasal endoscopic transsphenoidal resection* of the lesion was recommended. Postoperative IGF-1 and GH levels dropped significantly after the operative resection.

Surgical Steps

1. A *mononostril transnasal transseptal transsphenoidal approach* is performed as in Case 5A.
2. The sphenoid main septum is removed meticulously. Parts of the tumorous lesion evacuate spontaneously as the sphenoid septum is removed.
3. The *transsellar zonal opening of the skull base* is completed.
4. The lesion appears to be whitish and semiliquid with crumbly tumor components.
5. Resection of the adenoma is started in the anterior central aspect along the sellar floor (**Fig. 5C.3**).
6. The left lateral pillar is then removed using curettes and suction (**Fig. 5C.4** and **Fig. 5C.5**).
7. The same maneuver is then performed for the right lateral pillar (**Fig. 5C.6**).
8. The resection is continued for the more superior lateral aspects between the pituitary gland and the left cavernous sinus wall (**Fig. 5C.7**).
9. Following the tumor tissue that is well distinguishable from the normal pituitary gland, the resection is continued superiorly posteriorly following the left cavernous sinus wall between the diaphragma sellae and the pituitary gland (**Fig. 5C.8**).

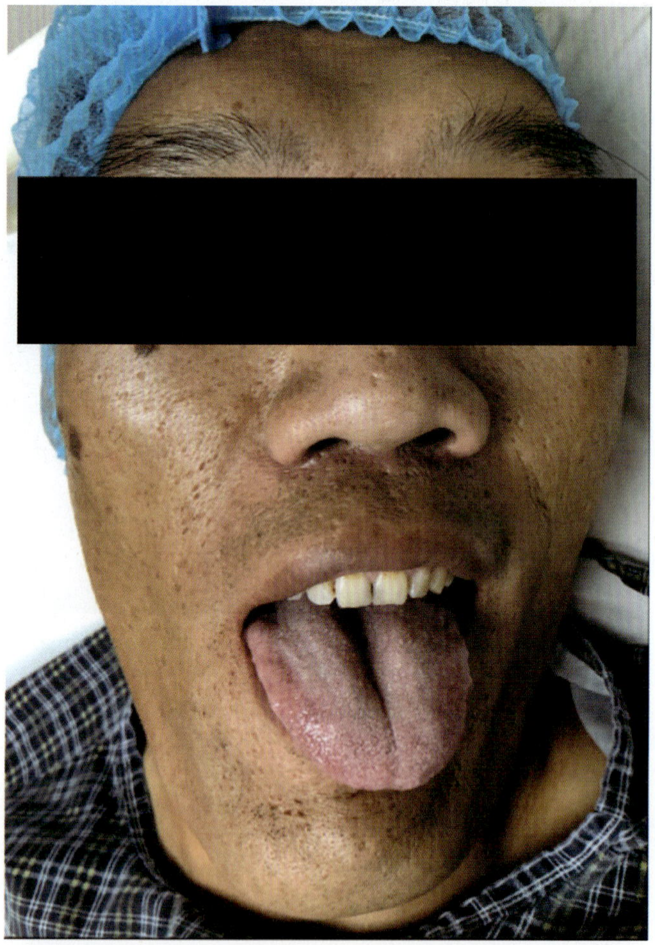

Fig. 5C.1 Typical facial changes in adult acromegaly with protrusion of the brows and the lower jaw, enlarged nasal bone, and discrete macroglossia.

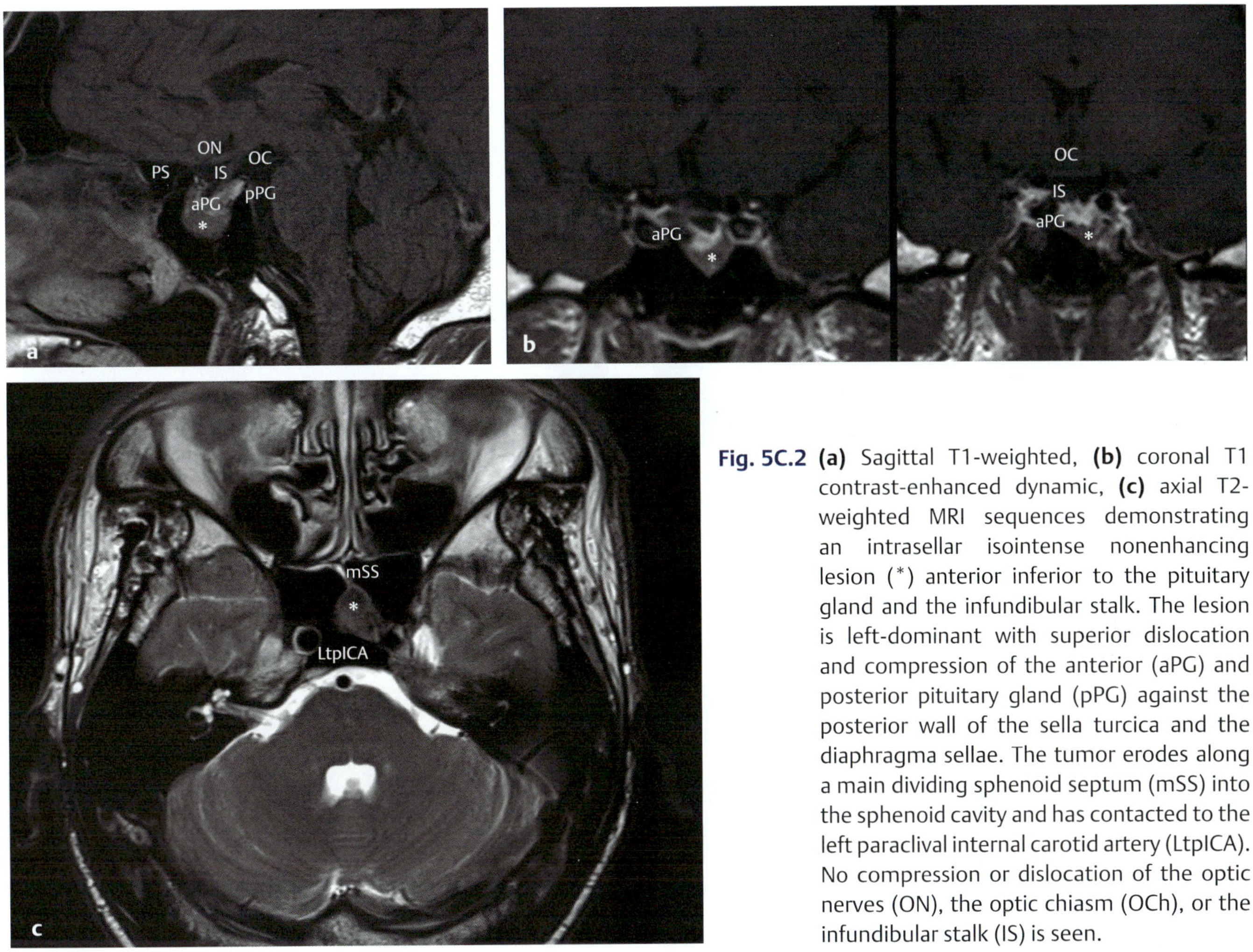

Fig. 5C.2 **(a)** Sagittal T1-weighted, **(b)** coronal T1 contrast-enhanced dynamic, **(c)** axial T2-weighted MRI sequences demonstrating an intrasellar isointense nonenhancing lesion (*) anterior inferior to the pituitary gland and the infundibular stalk. The lesion is left-dominant with superior dislocation and compression of the anterior (aPG) and posterior pituitary gland (pPG) against the posterior wall of the sella turcica and the diaphragma sellae. The tumor erodes along a main dividing sphenoid septum (mSS) into the sphenoid cavity and has contacted to the left paraclival internal carotid artery (LtpICA). No compression or dislocation of the optic nerves (ON), the optic chiasm (OCh), or the infundibular stalk (IS) is seen.

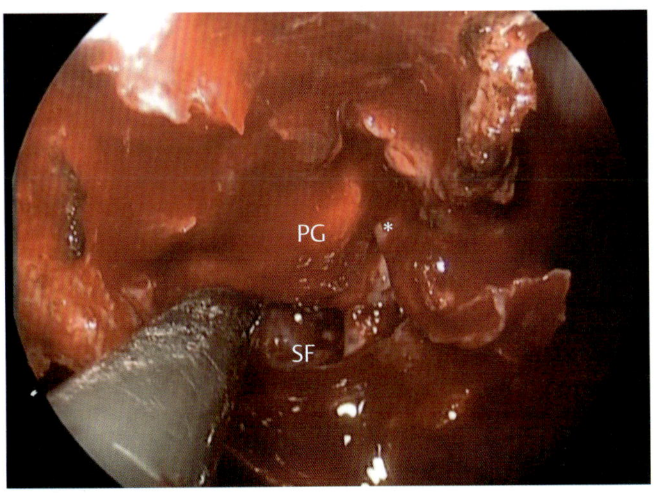

Fig. 5C.3 Resection of the anterior central aspect of the GH-producing adenoma along the sellar floor (SF) with preservation of the normal pituitary gland (PG). Next to the left lateral aspect of the tumor cavity, the left tumor pillar (*) is visible. The tumor tissue is well distinguishable from the normal pituitary gland.

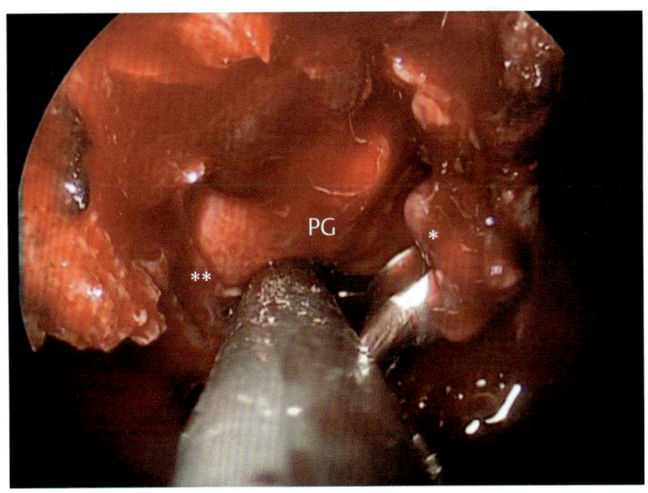

Fig. 5C.4 Removal of the left lateral inferior pillar (*) of the macroadenoma using a curette. The right lateral pillar (**) is still visible.

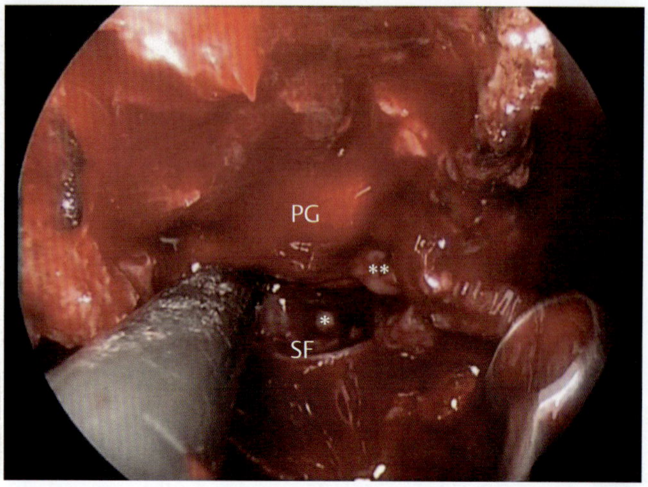

Fig. 5C.5 Removal of the left lateral inferior pillar (*) of the macroadenoma using a curette. Tumor remnants along the sellar floor (SF) are still visible. More superior aspects of the left lateral pillar are not resected yet (**).

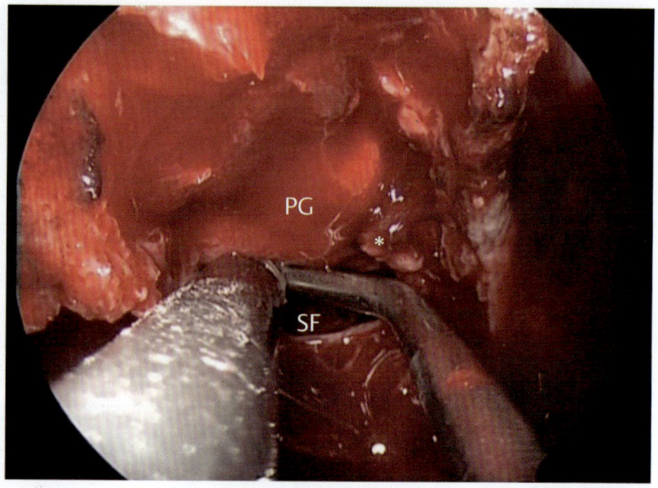

Fig. 5C.6 Removal of the right lateral inferior pillar of the macroadenoma using a curette. More superior aspects of the left lateral pillar are not resected yet (*).

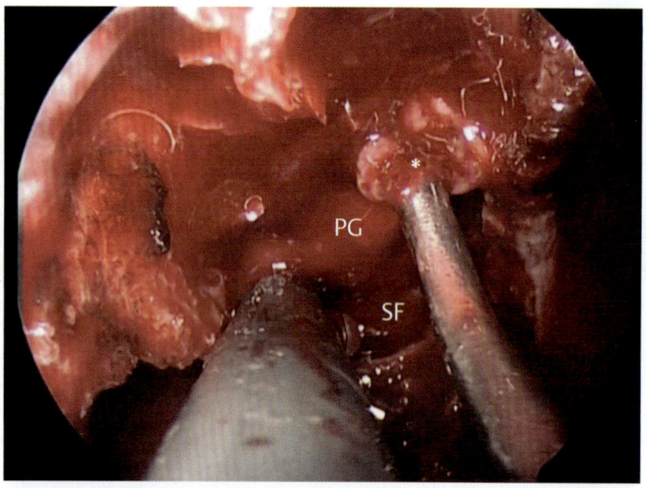

Fig. 5C.7 Removal of the superior aspect of the left lateral pillar (*).

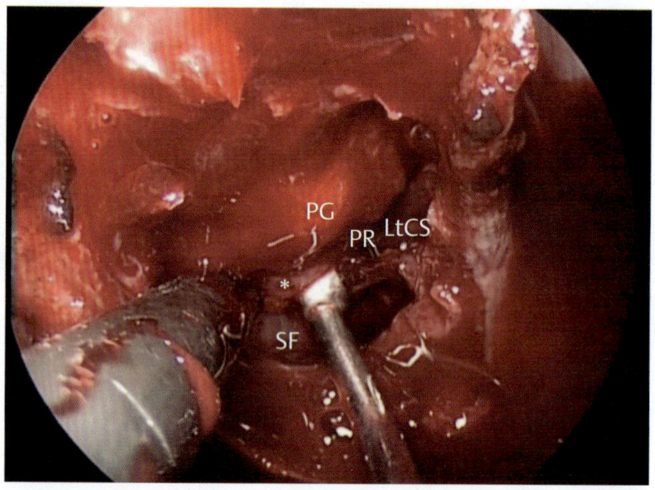

Fig. 5C.8 Removal of the superior posterior aspect of the tumor (*) along the left cavernous sinus (LtCS) wall and the posterior wall of the sella turcica, forming the posterior recess (PR).

10. The surfaces of the anatomical structures have to be visualized, and tumor remnants along the resection cavity have to be identified and removed meticulously in hormone-producing adenomas (**Fig. 5C.9**).
11. The same maneuver as described in step 9 has to be performed anteriorly to the pituitary gland between the anterior diaphragmal dura and the dura of the anterior recess using curettes. The risk for causing a cerebrospinal fluid (CSF) leak is higher in this region (**Fig. 5C.10** and **Fig. 5C.11**).
12. The surfaces of the defined anatomical structures have to be inspected for remnant adenoma circumferentially and in a systematic way around the pituitary gland (**Fig. 5C.12, Fig. 5C.13,** and **Fig. 5C.14**).

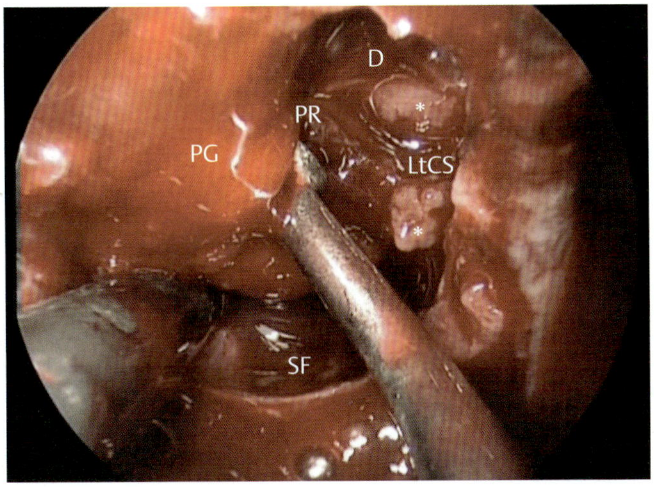

Fig. 5C.9 Careful dislocation of the pituitary gland (PG) reveals the dural surfaces of the sellar floor (SF), the left cavernous sinus (LtCS), and the diaphragma sellae (D). Several tumor remnants (*) are identifiable and are removed using suction and curettes.

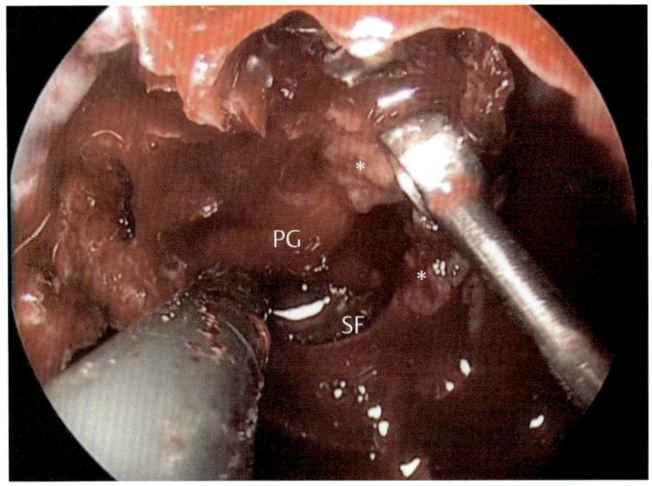

Fig. 5C.10 Continuation along the anterior superior aspect of the adenoma (*) between the pituitary gland (PG) and the anterior sellar dura forming the anterior recess.

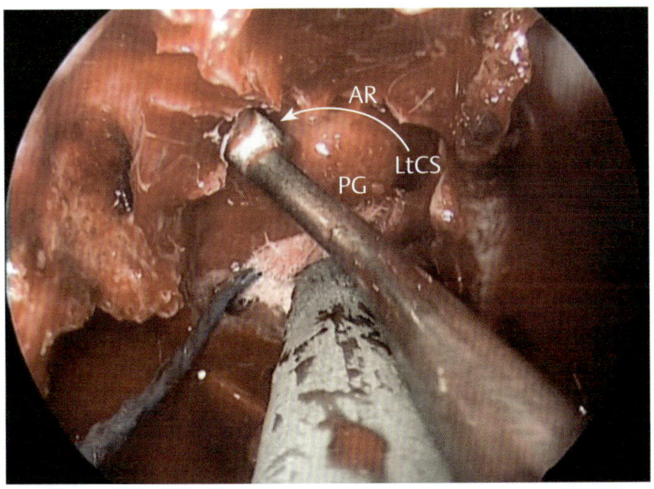

Fig. 5C.11 The curette follows (*arrow*) along the anterior superior aspect of the adenoma (*) between the pituitary gland (PG) and the anterior sellar dura forming the anterior recess (AR).

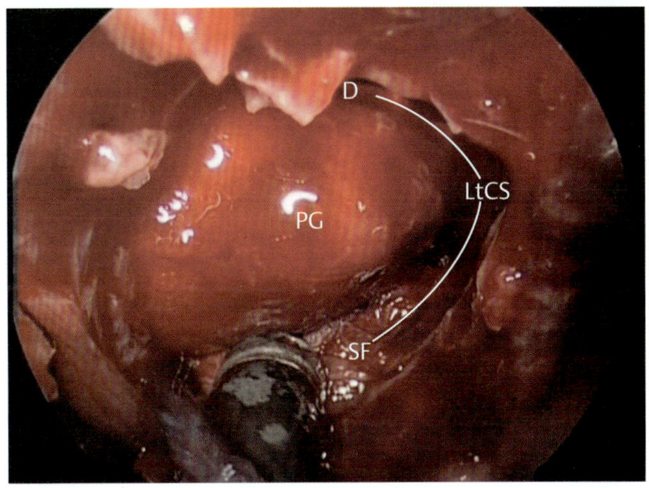

Fig. 5C.12 Inspection of the resection cavity: The lesion was left-dominant surrounding the pituitary gland (PG). Hence, the sellar floor (SF), the left medial cavernous sinus wall (LtCS), and the diaphragma sellae (D) as well as the anterior and posterior recess are visible and free of tumor.

13. The resection cavity is filled with an absorbable hemostatic agent (**Fig. 5C.15**).
14. The sphenoid cavity is filled with resorbable hemostatic sponge material. (**Fig. 5C.16**).
15. The nasoseptal flap is brought back into position, and the middle turbinate is medialized and stabilized with a resorbable nasal packing (**Fig. 5C.17**).

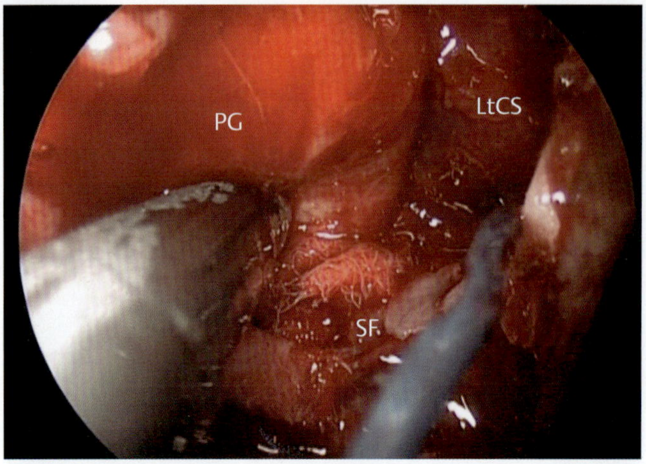

Fig. 5C.13 Inspection of the resection cavity: The sellar floor (SF) and the left medial cavernous sinus wall (LtCS) are free of tumor.

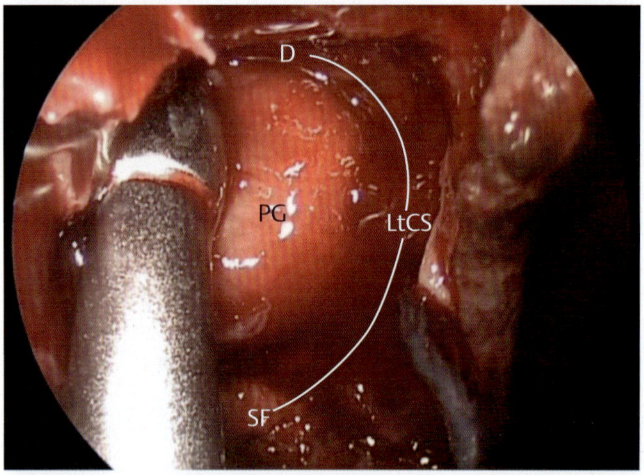

Fig. 5C.14 Inspection of the resection cavity: The sellar floor (SF), the left cavernous sinus wall (LtCS), and the anterior and posterior recess between the pituitary gland (PG) and the diaphragma sellae (D) are free of tumor.

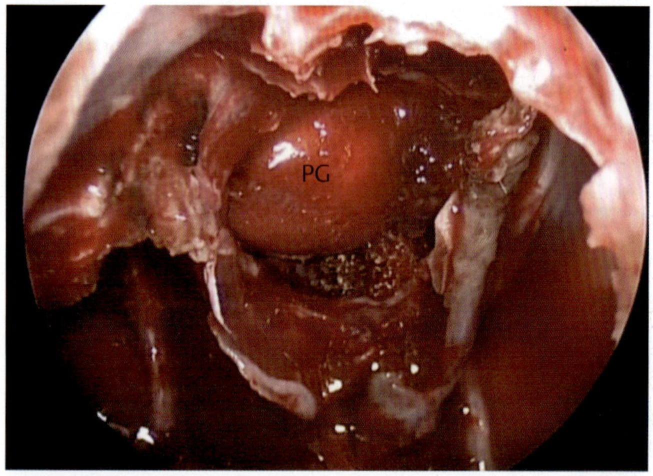

Fig. 5C.15 The resection cavity is filled with a resorbable hemostatic agent. PG, pituitary gland.

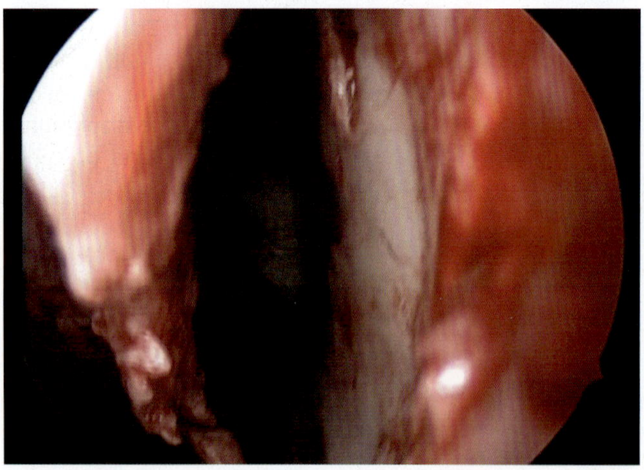

Fig. 5C.16 The sphenoid cavity is filled with resorbable hemostatic sponge material.

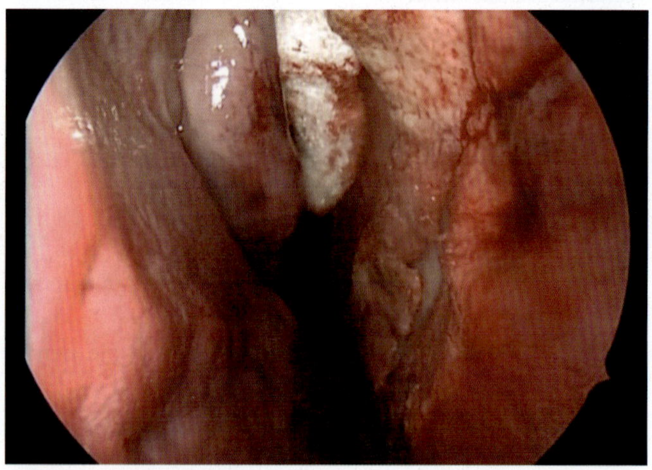

Fig. 5C.17 The nasoseptal flap is held in place with resorbable nasal packing that brings the middle turbinate back into the physiological position.

Case 5D

Endonasal Endoscopic Binostril Excision of a Growth Hormone–Producing Extrasellar Macroadenoma Involving the Sphenoid Sinus and the Clival Region

Michel Roethlisberger and Luigi Mariani

History

A 70-year-old female patient was diagnosed with a growth hormone (GH)-producing macroadenoma during the endocrinological evaluation of a dysthyreosis in 2013. The lesion was predominantly located in the clivus with involvement of the paraclival area and the sphenoid bone, without infiltration of the sella turcica or the suprasellar region (**Fig. 5D.1a–i**). The patient refused surgical and radiotherapeutical options and was treated with different somatostatin analogues and dopaminergic medication, even in combination because of cosecretion of prolactin. Pituitary function remained intact,

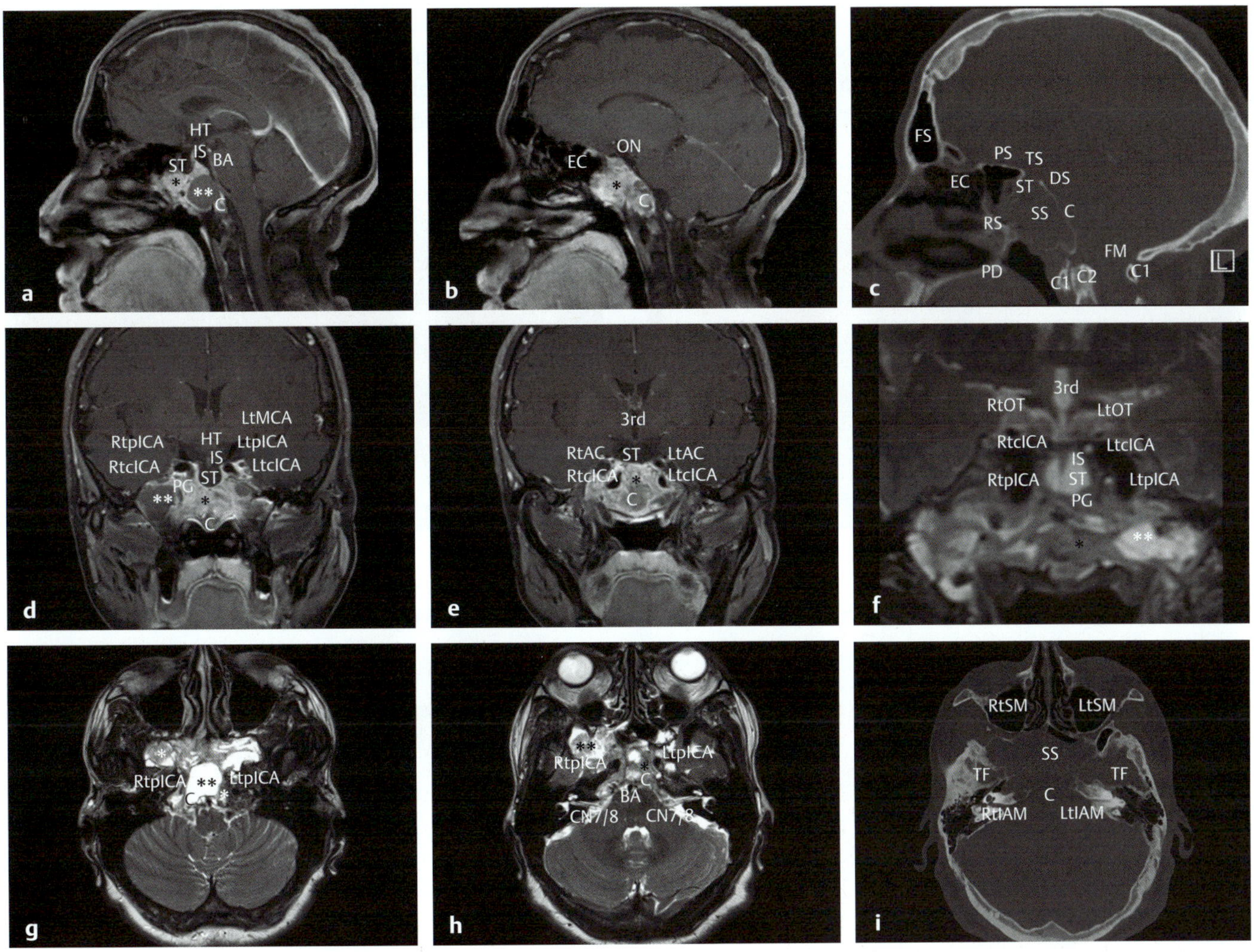

Fig. 5D.1 (a,b) Sagittal T1-weighted gadolinium contrast-enhanced MRI, **(c)** bone-weighted computed tomography, **(d,e)** coronal T1-weighted gadolinium contrast-enhanced MRI, **(f)** coronal, **(g,h)** axial T2-weighted MRI, and **(i)** bone-weighted computed tomography sequences demonstrating an T2-hyperintense and T1-hyperintense solid (*) and cystic (**) lesion of the clivus (65 × 46 × 25 mm) extending into the sphenoid bone and sinus (SS) as well as the right anterior clinoid process (RtAC) and bilateral pterygoid processes. Infiltration of the cavernous sinus with encasement of the right (RtcICA) and left (LtcICA) cavernous internal carotid arteries, predominantly on the right side is present. The sella turcica (ST) is not infiltrated. The infundibular stalk (IS) as well as the pituitary gland (PG) can appreciated within the "empty sella–like" configured ST. Bony erosion of the ST, the SS, and the clivus (C) is present with thinned-out bone and remodeling.

and no visual disturbances were noted. However, a chemical control of the disease was not achieved with this conservative approach and the lesion did not demonstrate any radiological changes over time. Consecutively, the patient developed classic systemic sequelae of acromegaly including diabetes mellitus (HbA_1C 6.4%), arterial hypertonia, bronchopathy with obstructive sleep apnea syndrome (OSAS), dilated cardiomyopathy with a worsening ejection fraction of 40 to 50% in consecutive echocardiographic examinations, and bilateral gonarthrosis. Additionally, a colonoscopy revealed intestinal polyposis. Six years after the initial diagnosis, the patient finally accepted the recommended surgical treatment to achieve a significant reduction in the volume of the GH-producing lesion for a better chemical control of the disease. Hence, an endonasal endoscopic transsphenoidal subtotal resection of the lesion was performed.

Surgical Steps

1. A binostril transseptal transsphenoidal approach is performed as described in Chapter 1.
2. The dissection is continued until the sphenoid rostrum is exposed with the sphenoid ostia visible bilaterally (**Fig. 5D.1** and **Fig. 5D.2**).
3. Once the sphenoid rostrum is fully exposed, the sphenoid ostiae are widened inferomedially using a Kerrison punch in a V shape toward the midline (**Fig. 5D.3** and **Fig. 5D.4**).
4. The keel is removed with a pituitary Rongeur forceps (**Fig. 5D.5**).
5. The remaining superior parts of the sphenoid rostrum are removed, and the intrasphenoidal extension of the lesion involving the sphenoid bone and sinus, the clivus as well as the right anterior clinoid process can be visualized (**Fig. 5D.6**).

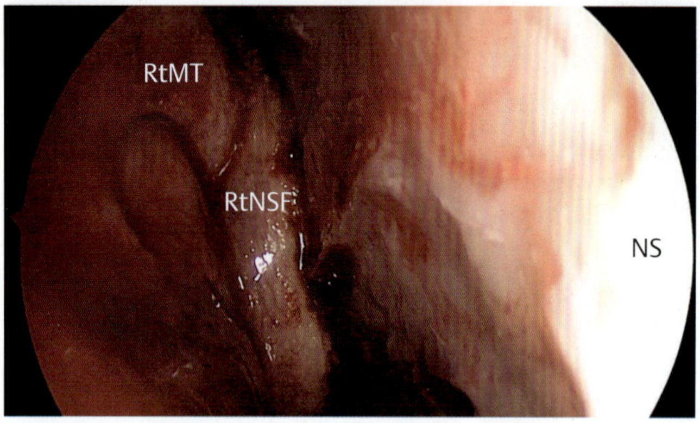

Fig. 5D.2 Mucoperichondrial dissection along the nasal septum (NS) with elevation of a right-sided vascularized nasoseptal flap (RtNSF).

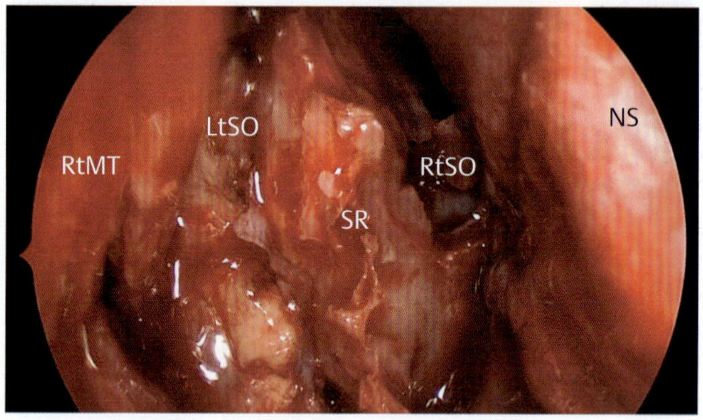

Fig. 5D.3 Exposed sphenoid rostrum (SR) using a binostril posterior transseptal approach with the left (LtSO) and the right (RtSO) sphenoid ostia visible.

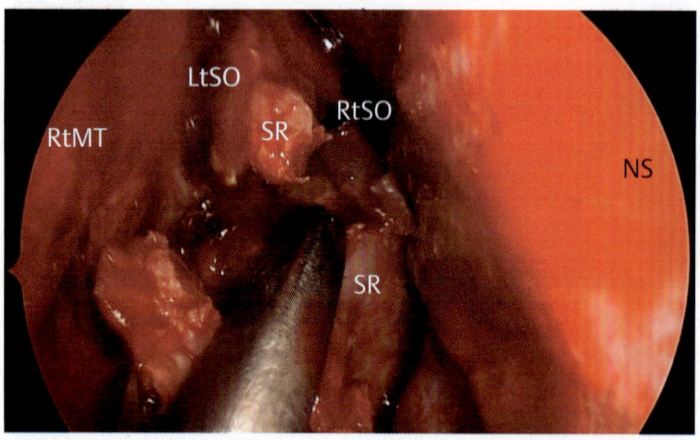

Fig. 5D.4 V-shaped opening of the left (LtSO) and right (RtSO) sphenoid ostia toward the midline defined by the exposed sphenoid rostrum (SR) using a Kerrison punch. The tumor mass within the sphenoid cavity is visible (*).

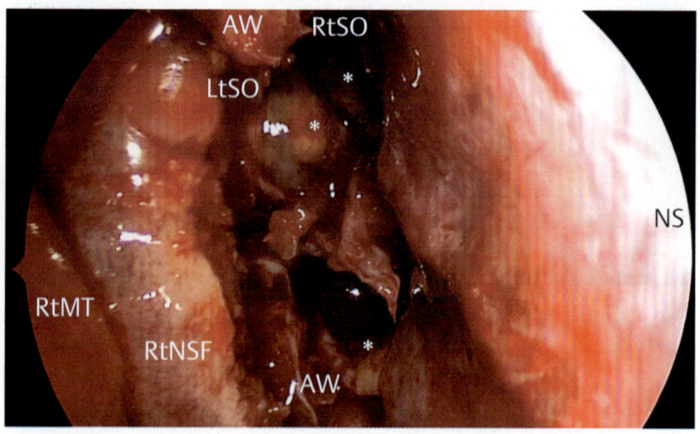

Fig. 5D.5 Parts of the anterior wall (AW) of the sphenoid rostrum (SR) with the left (LtSO) and right (RtSO) sphenoid ostia are still present. The tumor mass within the sphenoid cavity is visible (*).

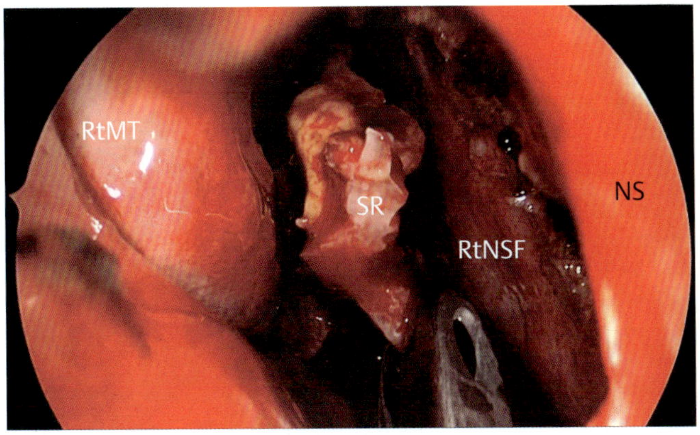

Fig. 5D.6 Removal of the remaining sphenoid rostrum (SR) bone with tumor mass within the sphenoid cavity (*).

6. The same systematic approach to resect the lesion within the sphenoid sinus is used as described for intrasellar lesions, starting with tissue sampling (**Fig. 5D.7**) and debulking of the central parts using curettes and suction devices along the sphenoid floor (**Fig. 5D.8**). This allows to identify the posterior midline clivus as posterior border (**Fig. 5D.9a**) and avoids injury of the dehiscent paraclival internal carotid arteries, which are embedded within the right dominant extensive tumor mass.
7. The lateral extensions of the lesion are defined by the lateral recesses of the sphenoid cavity. These can be used as anatomical landmarks while removing the tumor masses (**Fig. 5D.9b** and **Fig. 5D.10a–c**).

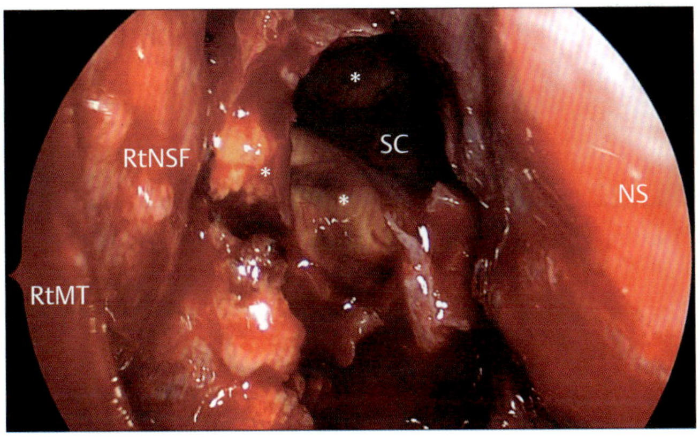

Fig. 5D.7 The tumor mass (*) with the typical yellowish and grayish appearance is visible within the sphenoid cavity (SC).

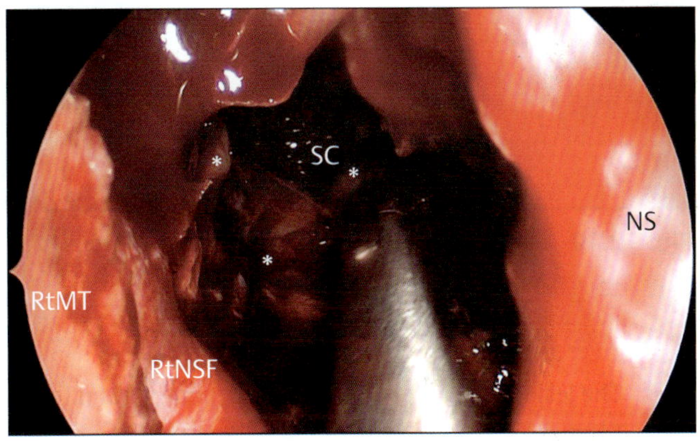

Fig. 5D.8 Asservation and removal of tumor mass (*) within the sphenoid cavity (SC) for histological work-up.

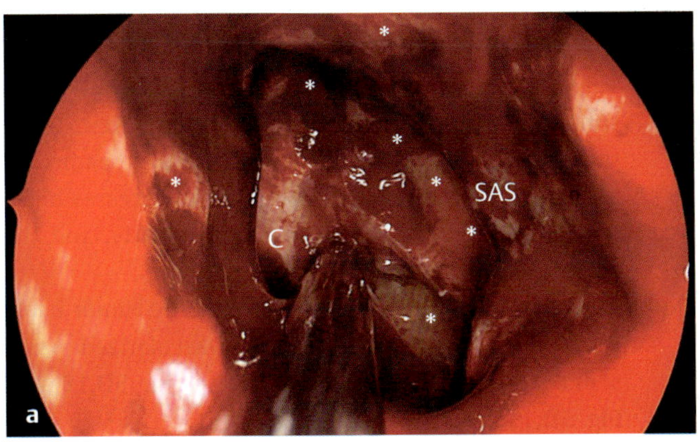

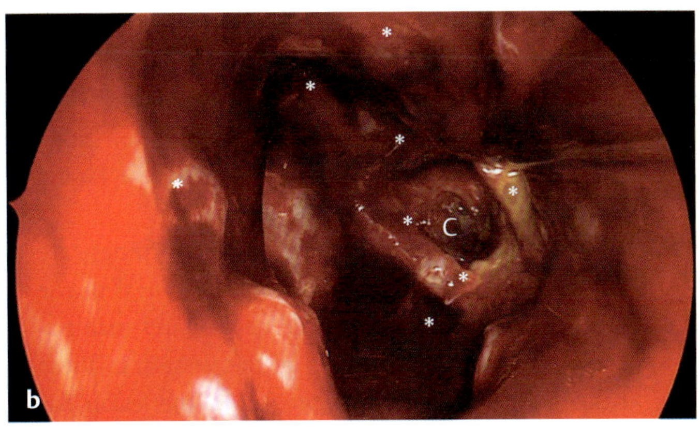

Fig. 5D.9 **(a,b)** The central main tumor mass (*) within the sphenoid cavity (SC) is removed using curettes and suction devices. The lateral, superior, and inferior extensions of the tumor (*) can be appreciated with the midline approach. Posteriorly, the bony clivus (C) is reached defining the posterior tumor border, and a right-sided partial accessory sphenoid septum (SAS) near the left paraclival internal carotid artery is identified.

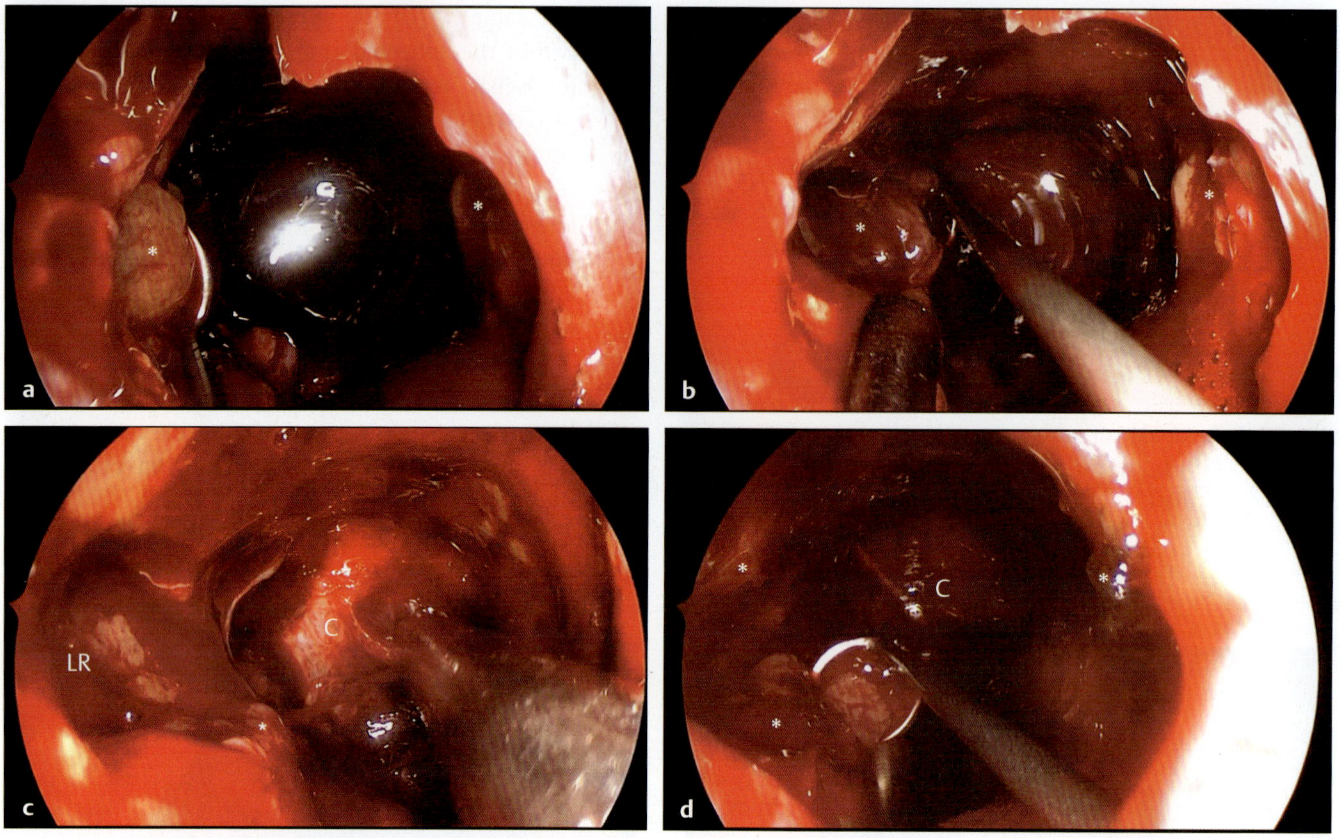

Fig. 5D.10 (a–d) The lateral extension of the tumorous masses (*) within the sphenoid cavity and the lateral recesses (LR) are evacuated using curettes.

8. The lesion has liquid and fleshy components and forms fibrous strands that potentially are attached to the dehiscent paraclival internal carotid arteries. These need to be manipulated and dissected carefully, and uncontrolled tearing should be avoided (**Fig. 5D.10d**).
9. If an incomplete accessory sphenoid septum obstructs the view to the lateral aspect of the sphenoid posterior wall and the clivus, careful removal is necessary using a high-speed drill and Kerrison's punches. This maneuver is necessary to expose tumorous extension along the paraclival internal carotid artery and the lateral recess (**Fig. 5D.11a–c** and **Fig. 5D.12a, b**).
10. When the paraclival internal carotid arteries are embedded within the tumor, careful removal of the surrounding pathological tissue necessitates manipulation and careful dislocation of the vessels. In these cases, no bony coverage is present as the lesion has eroded the whole clival and paraclival region (**Fig. 5D.12c**, **Fig. 5D.13**, and **Fig. 5D.14a–c**).
11. The same accounts for the clival bone, forming the posterior wall of the sphenoid sinus that is thinned out and eroded by the tumor. Careful removal of tumor along the clival bone and dura is possible to clean the tumor resection cavity (**Fig. 5D.15**).
12. Venous oozing of the clival bone and plexus has to be expected and managed accordingly prior to skull base defect closure (**Fig. 5D.16**).
13. The resection cavity inferior to the sella within the sphenoid sinus is defined by the sella turcica with the flattened pituitary gland superiorly, the paraclival internal carotid arteries and the lateral recesses bilaterally, the clival bone and dura posteriorly, and the sphenoid floor inferiorly (**Fig. 5D.17**).
14. The large skull base defect, caused by the tumor itself, is covered using the right-sided vascularized nasoseptal (Hadad–Bassagasteguy) flap (**Fig. 5D.18** and **Fig. 5D.19a, b**).
15. The construct is stabilized using artificial dural sealant and hemostyptic material (**Fig. 5D.20a–c**).

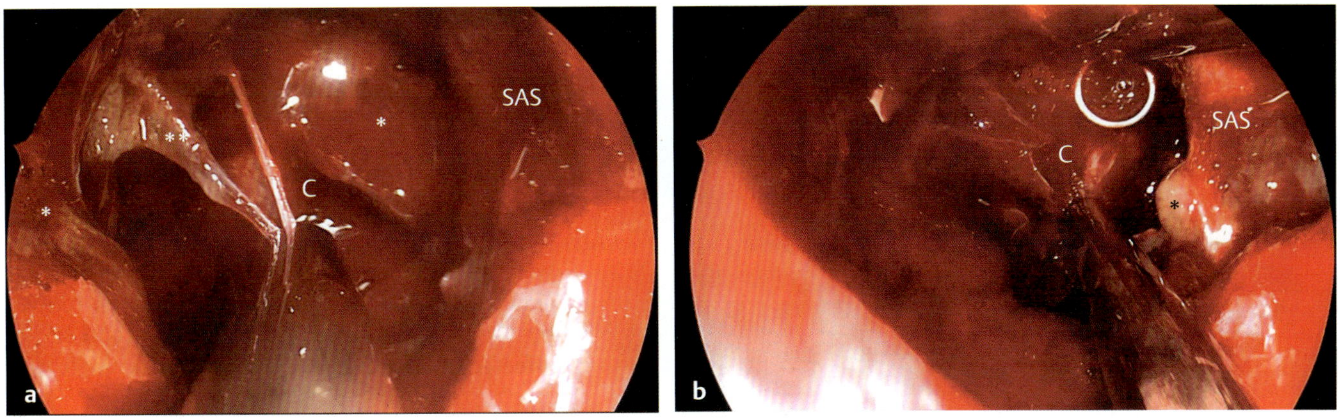

Fig. 5D.11 **(a,b)** The extensive tumor mass (*) is semiliquid and can be removed with curettes and suction devices. Fibrous strands (**) are found within the tumor mass, and uncontrolled traction should be avoided. The paraclival internal carotid arteries are embedded within the loose tumor mass and are not covered by bone. This can be anticipated in the presurgical radiological assessment (**Fig. 5D.1a–i**).

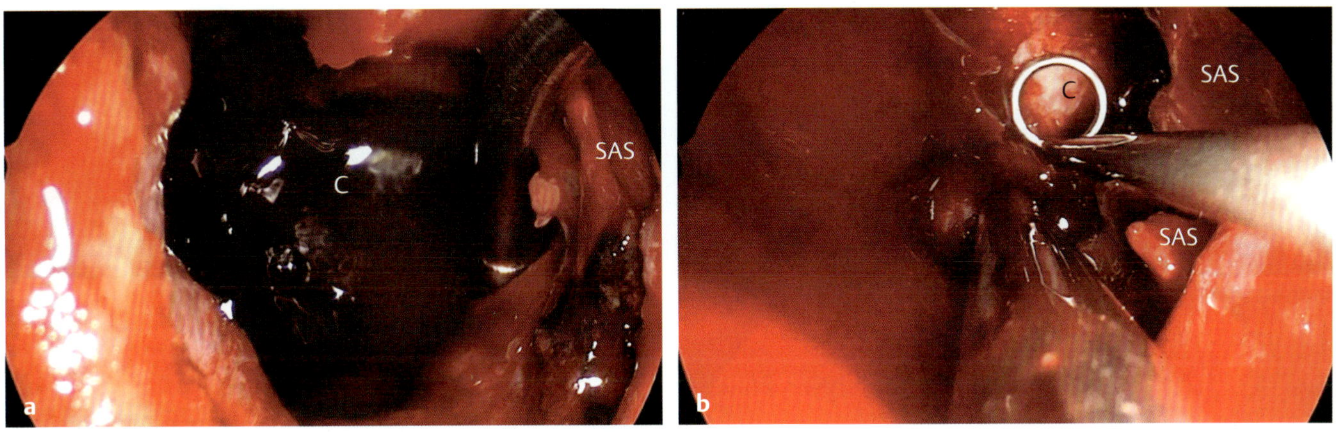

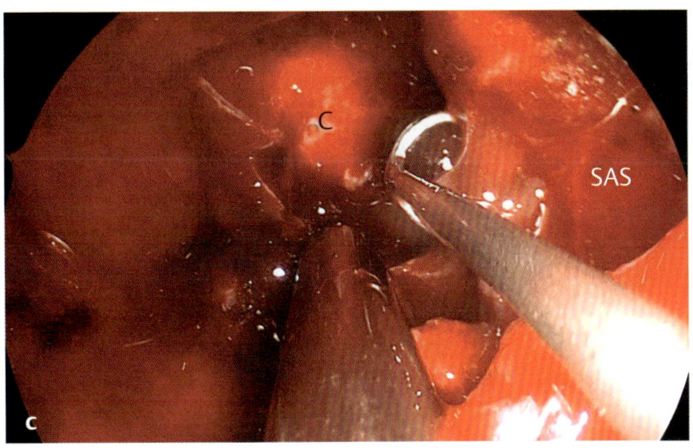

Fig. 5D.12 **(a–c)** To reach suspected tumor mass posterior to the left-sided accessory sphenoid septum (SAS), a maxillary suction device is used after partial drilling and removal of the latter. The septum and tumor mass are in close relationship with the left paraclival carotid artery.

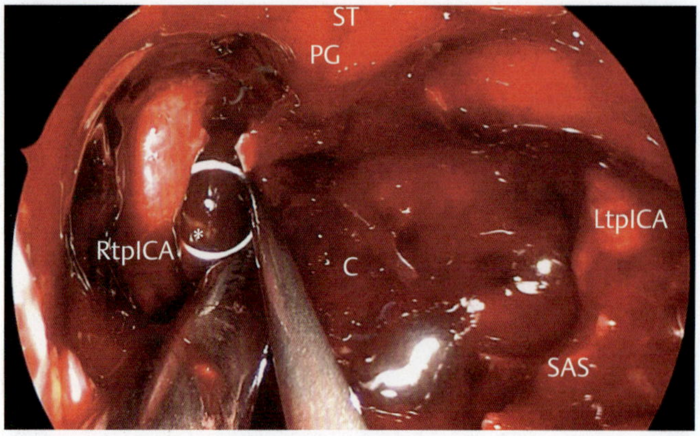

Fig. 5D.13 The extensive tumor mass (*) has been removed with curettes and suction devices within the sphenoid cavity and lateral recesses as well as the posterior aspect along the clivus (C). The left-sided accessory sphenoid septum (SAS) has been removed partially to remove tumor in the posterolateral compartment. The left (LtpICA) and right (RtpICA) paraclival internal carotid arteries are dehiscent and were embedded by tumor mass. The sella turcica (ST) is visible without bony coverage and is formed by the flattened pituitary gland (PG) and is not affected or infiltrated by tumor.

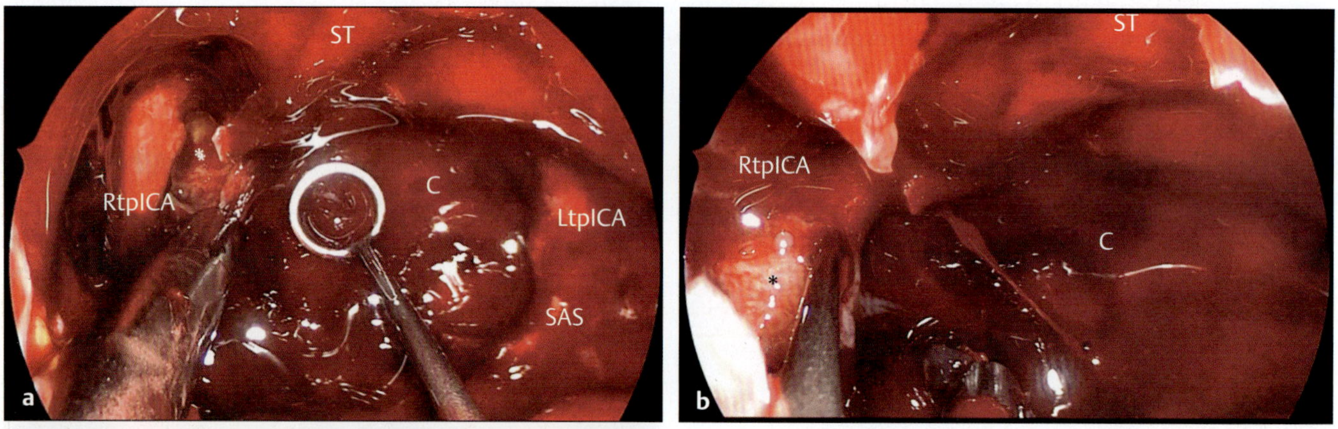

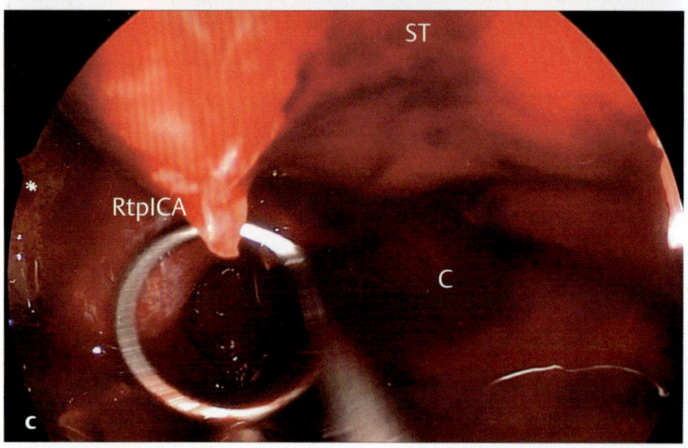

Fig. 5D.14 **(a–c)** Bimanual dissection technique to reach suspected tumor mass (*) posterior to the right paraclival internal carotid artery (RtpICA). A curette and a suction device are used; the vessel is handled carefully. Left paraclival internal carotid artery (LtpICA), sella turcica (ST), pituitary gland (PG), left sided accessory sphenoid septum (SAS).

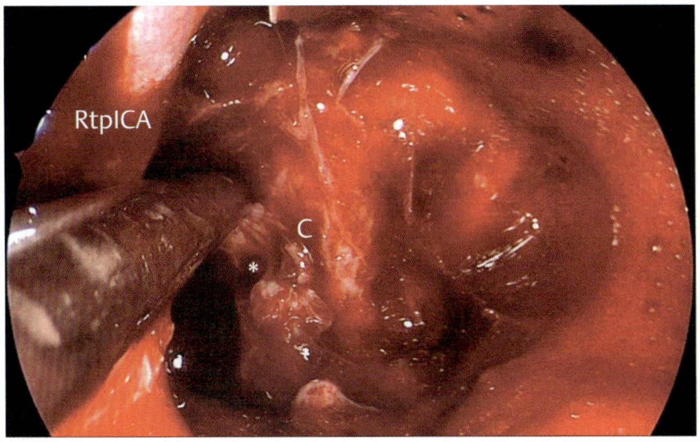

Fig. 5D.15 Tumor remnants (*) along the posterior border of the sphenoid sinus and involving the clivus (C) and the sphenoid floor is carefully removed.

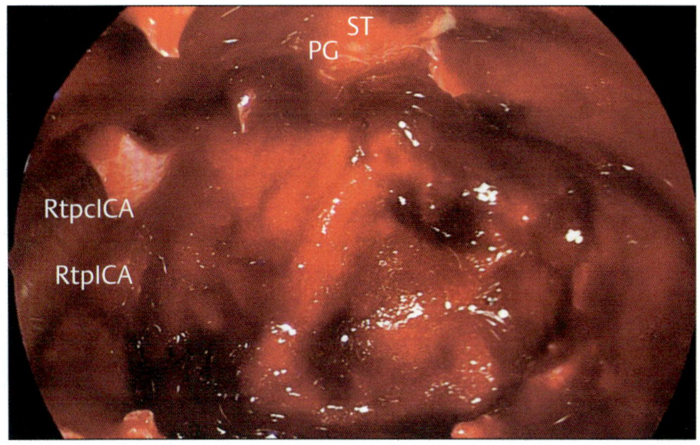

Fig. 5D.16 The eroded clival bone and plexus cause profuse venous oozing that is managed using hemostyptic material.

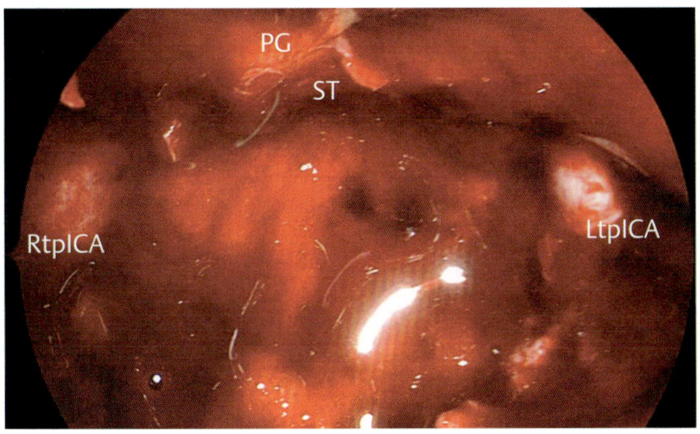

Fig. 5D.17 Final view of the resection cavity with dehiscent left (LtpICA) and right (RtpICA) paraclival internal carotid arteries, the eroded sella turcica (ST) without bony coverage, and the flattened pituitary gland (PG).

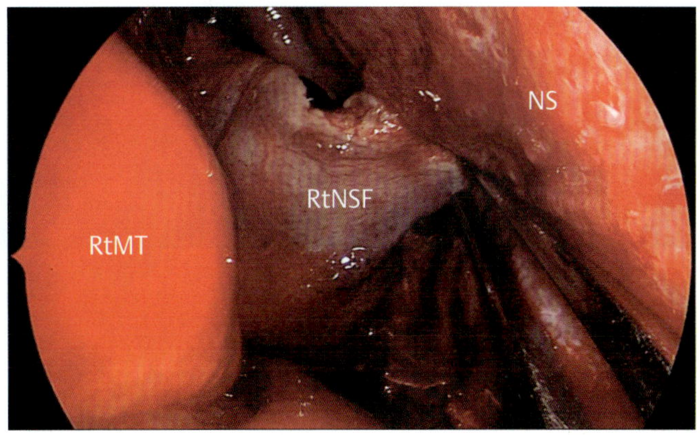

Fig. 5D.18 The right-sided nasoseptal flap (RtNSF) is harvested from the sphenoethmoidal recess, where it was stored during the tumor removal.

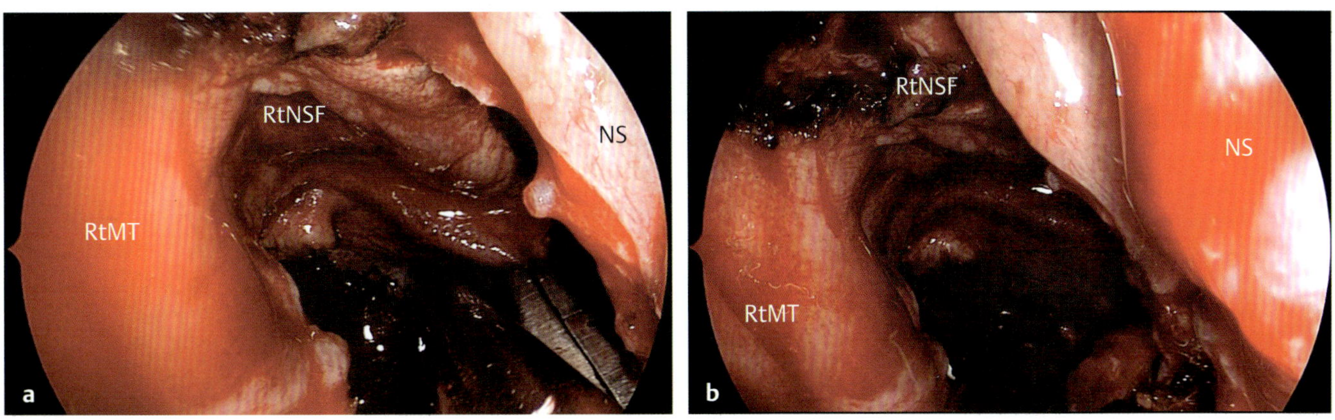

Fig. 5D.19 **(a, b)** The right-sided nasoseptal flap (RtNSF) is placed over the large skull base defect. It is crucial to place the flap without torsion along the pedicle to avoid flap necrosis. Liberation of all adherences allows better manipulation and placement of the flap.

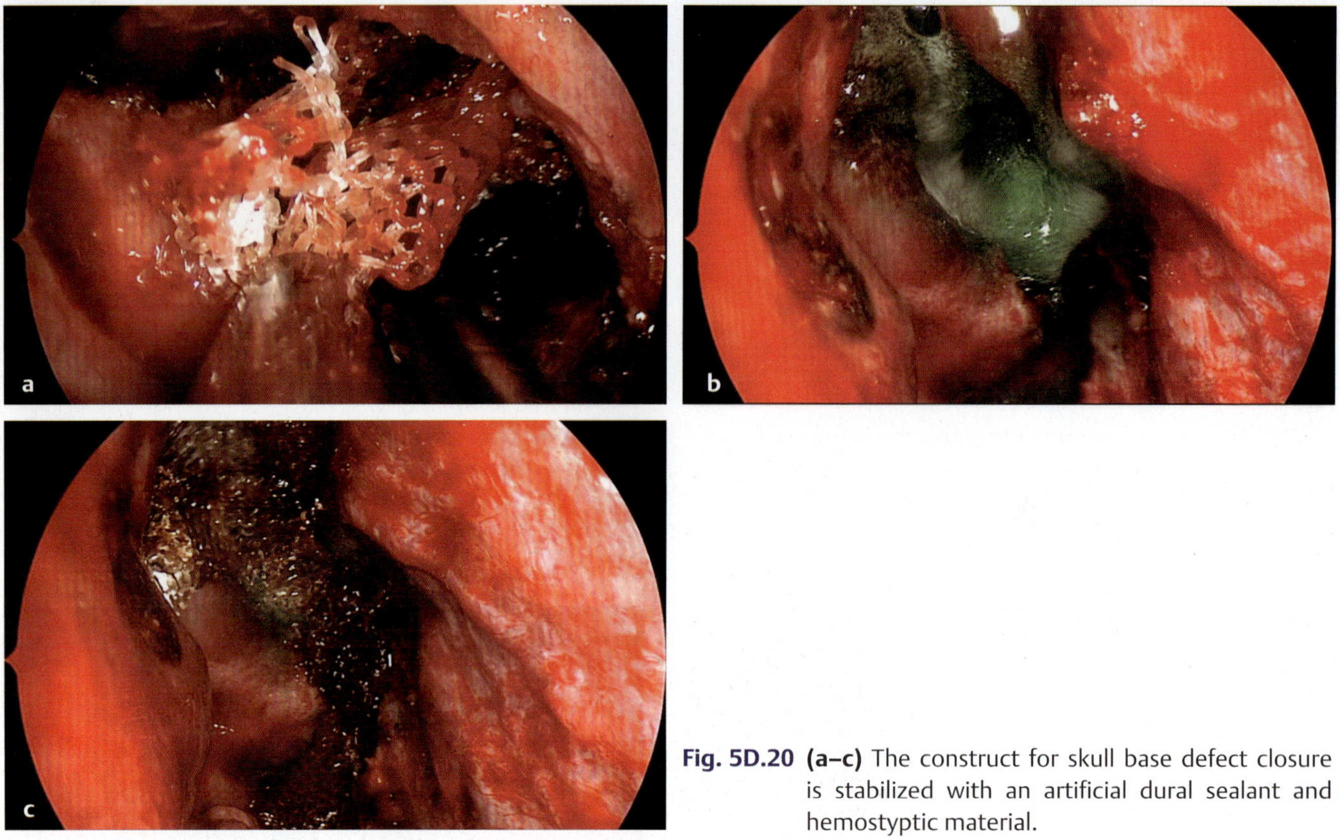

Fig. 5D.20 **(a–c)** The construct for skull base defect closure is stabilized with an artificial dural sealant and hemostyptic material.

Chapter 6 Endoscopic Endonasal Surgery for Cystic Lesions of the Sella

Case 6A

Endoscopic Endonasal Excision of a Rathke Cleft Cyst

Michel Roethlisberger, Kong Yew Liew, Saif Al-Zahid, Adzreil Bakri, Prepageran Narayanan, and Vicknes Waran

History

A 70-year-old male with underlying hypertension presented himself with aggravating blurring of vision, diplopia, dizziness, and headache. Clinical examination revealed ptosis of the right eyelid. Neurocranial magnetic resonance imaging (MRI) revealed a right-sided T1-weighted (T1W) hyperintense and T2W isointense suprasellar mass of approximately 1 cm (**Fig. 6A.1**). An endoscopic transnasal transseptal excision was planned.

Surgical Steps

1. Local anesthesia is infiltrated into the posterior septum to raise the mucoperichondrium away from the bony septum (**Fig. 6A.2**).
2. The septum is then incised with a size 15 blade, and the mucoperichondrial flap is raised posteriorly to the level of the choana (**Fig. 6A.3**).
3. The nasoseptal flap is then developed by incising the superior mucoperichondrial flap with a microscissor, angling the direction toward the sphenoid ostia. About 1 cm of mucosa is preserved superiorly to the flap to maintain olfactory function (**Fig. 6A.4**).
4. The flap can then be freed from the floor of the nasal cavity in a similar fashion, following the floor perpendicularly. To fully free the naso-septal flap, the elevation is followed posteriorly to the choana. The flap can then be stored in the nasopharynx for later use during the skull base reconstruction phase.
5. The contralateral nasoseptal flap can be incised anteriorly and superiorly to develop a rescue flap, which can be freed completely for use should the need arise.
6. The bony and cartilaginous septum is removed to expose the sphenoid rostrum (**Fig. 6A.5**). Suction monopolar cautery can be used to clear any overlying residual mucosa to properly visualize the sphenoid ostia bilaterally.

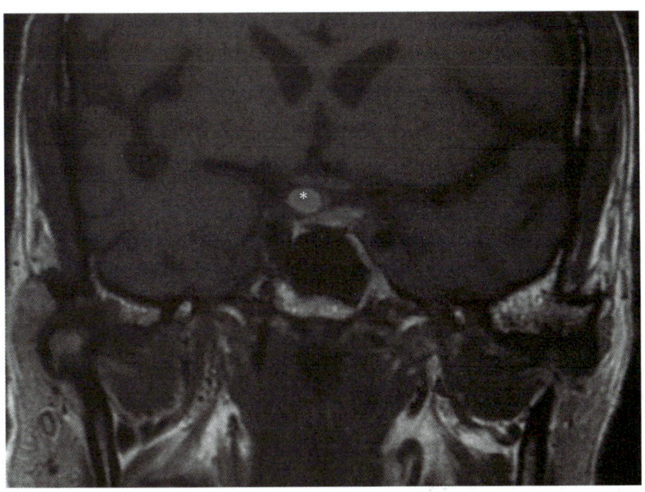

Fig. 6A.1 T1-weighted coronal MRI section revealing a right suprasellar hyperintense lesion (*) measuring approximately 1 cm in size.

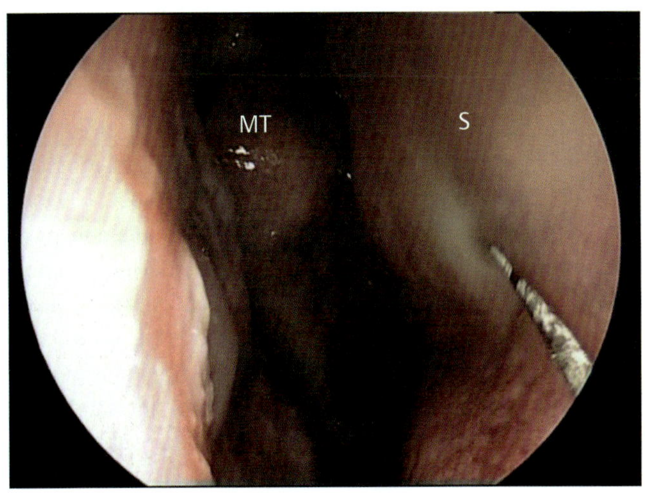

Fig. 6A.2 Local anesthesia being injected into the nasal septum with blanching of the mucosa.

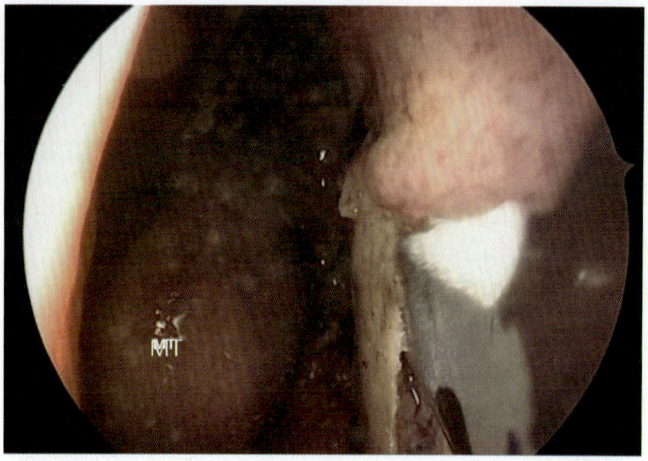

Fig. 6A.3 Anterior incision over the septum to develop the mucoperichondrial flap.

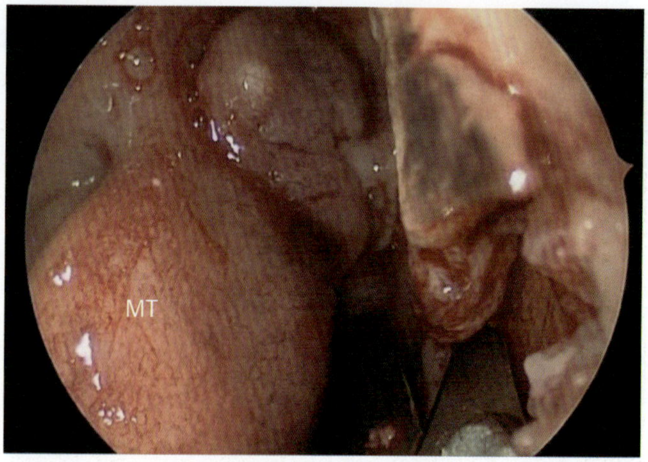

Fig. 6A.4 The superior incision over the nasal septum with microscissors, taken below the axilla of the middle turbinate (MT).

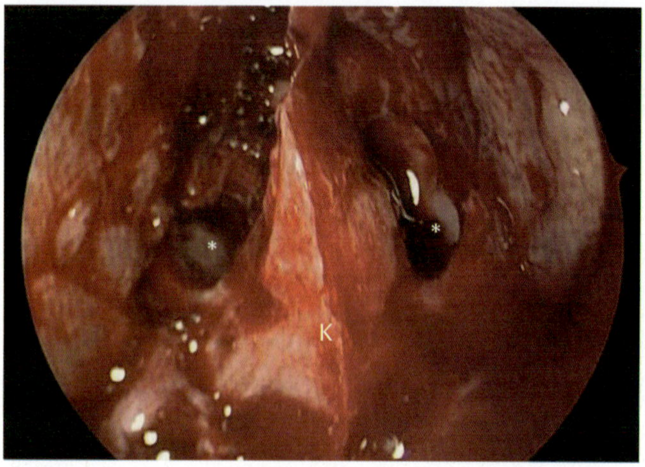

Fig. 6A.5 Exposure of the sphenoid keel (K) with the ostia visible (*) bilaterally.

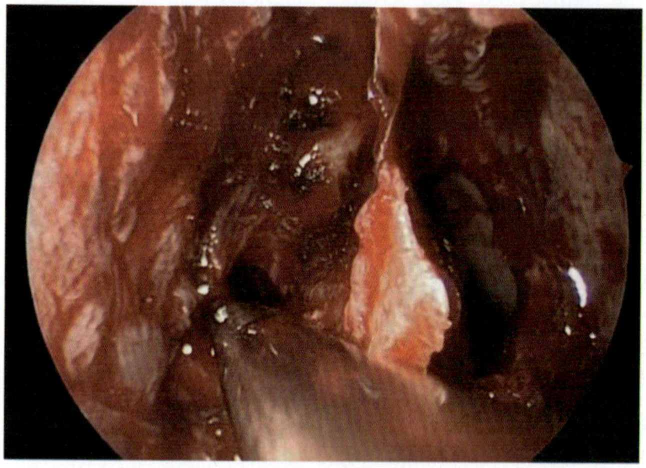

Fig. 6A.6 A Kerrison punch engaged in the right sphenoid ostia.

7. The sphenoid ostia are then widened inferiorly toward the midline in a V shape with bone rongeurs, such as a Kerrison punch (**Fig. 6A.6**).
8. After sufficient bone removal, the keel is removed with a twisting motion using a pituitary rongeur forceps (**Fig. 6A.7**).
9. After removal of the sphenoid keel, all sphenoid septations are removed to minimize visual obstruction within the sphenoid cavity and the relevant neurovascular landmarks of the base of skull (**Fig. 6A.8**).
10. The sphenoid sinus mucosa may be stripped or cauterized to expose the bare bone to allow for safe high-speed drilling during the osteo-dural exposure.
11. The osteo-dural exposure is performed using a high-speed diamond burr to thin the bone overlying the sella (trans-sellar approach) and tuberculum sellae

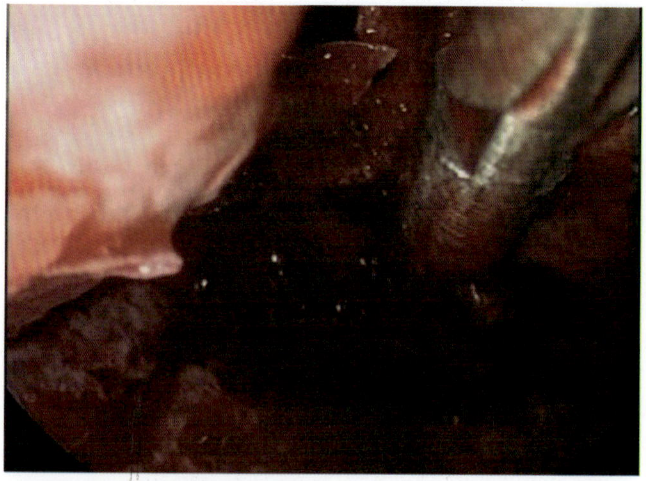

Fig. 6A.7 The sphenoid keel grasped with a pituitary rongeur forceps for removal.

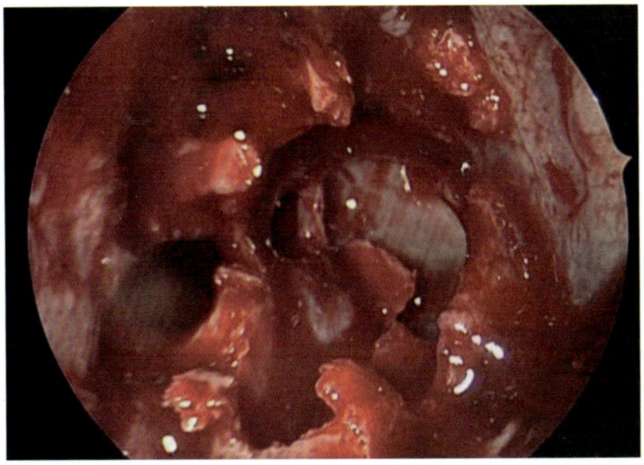

Fig. 6A.8 View of the sphenoid cavity after removal of the keel.

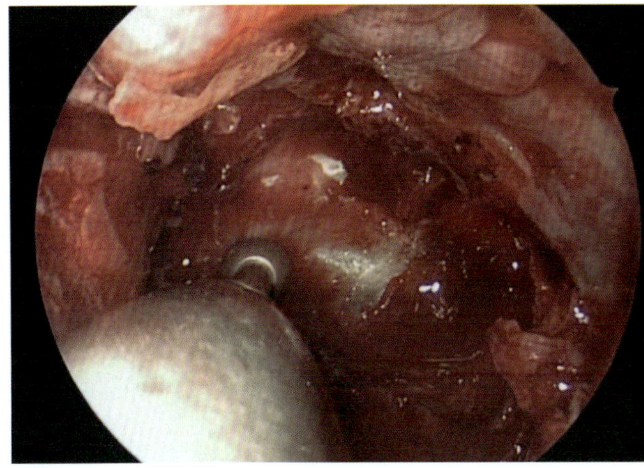

Fig. 6A.9 Trans-sellar approach: The underlying anterior intercavernous sinus is visible.

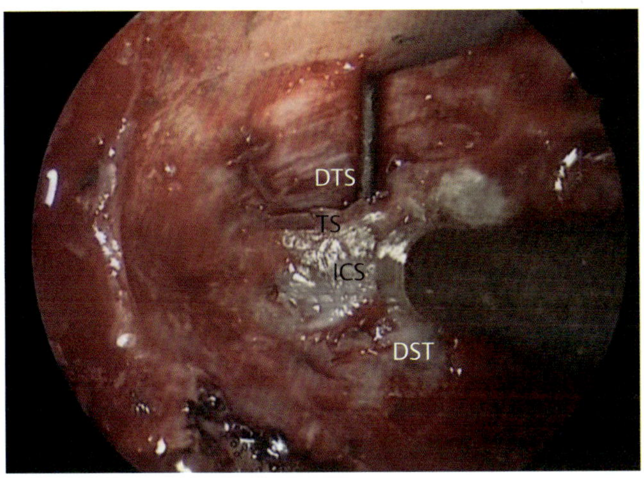

Fig. 6A.10 A right-angle dissector is used to free the dura from the underlying bone. Note the dura is already exposed under the majority of the dissector.

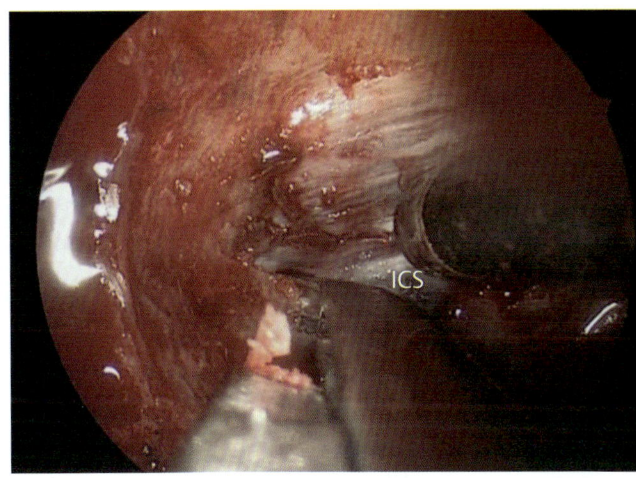

Fig. 6A.11 A Kerrison punch engaged to remove bone from the dura overlying the anterior intercavernous sinus (ICS).

(trans-tuberculum approach). Care should be taken to maintain a midline orientation to avoid the risk of damaging the carotid siphons or cavernous sinuses bilaterally. Localization should be confirmed with image-guided surgery at regular intervals. The anterior intercavernous sinus may also be encountered as the drilling proceeds deeper (**Fig. 6A.9**).

12. Once the bone has been sufficiently thinned, a right-angle dissector can be insinuated between the bone and the dura, and the bone flaked off to expose the dura of the tuberculum sellae, sella turcica, and the anterior intercavernous sinus (**Fig. 6A.10**).
13. Access to the dura can then be widened carefully with a Kerrison punch, making sure to free the underlying dura before removal of the bone. Dural exposure should be taken laterally until the bluish cavernous sinus is identifiable, and superiorly and inferiorly as much as is required for removal of the lesion, which can be confirmed on image-guided surgery (**Fig. 6A.11** and **Fig. 6A.12**).
14. The dura is incised in a transverse fashion, and is joined with a vertical incision superiorly. (**Fig. 6A.13**). The overlying arachnoid membrane should be visible at this stage (**Fig. 6A.14**).

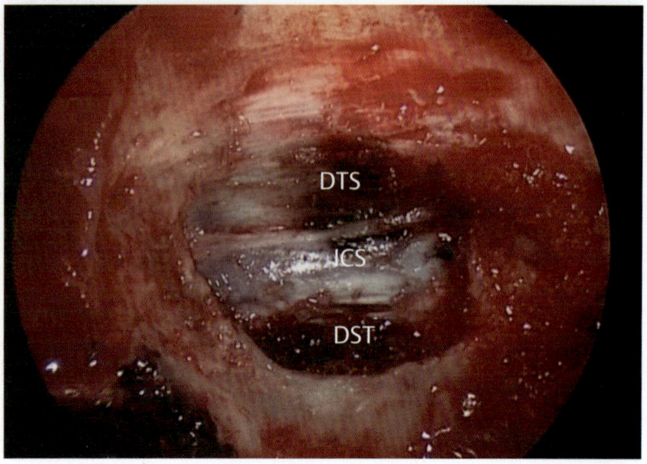

Fig. 6A.12 Final osteo-dural exposure: the anterior intercavernous sinus (ICS), dura of the sella turcica (DST), and tuberculum sellae (DTS) are exposed.

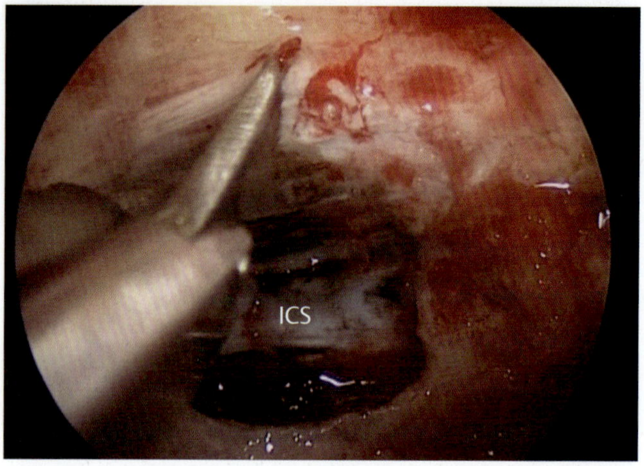

Fig. 6A.13 Dural incision anterior and superior to the anterior intercavernous sinus (ICS).

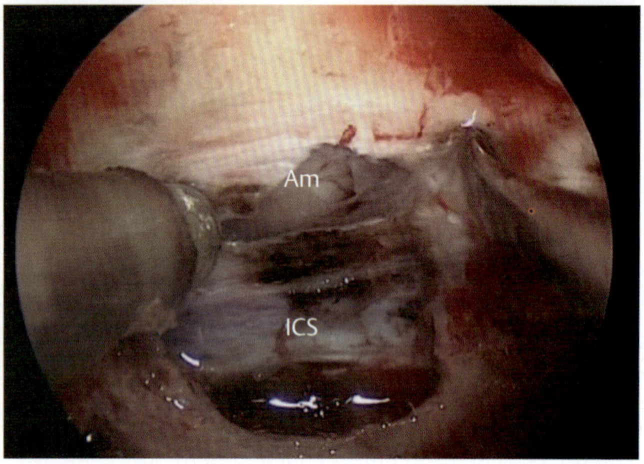

Fig. 6A.14 Exposure of the arachnoid membrane (Am). ICS, anterior intercavernous sinus.

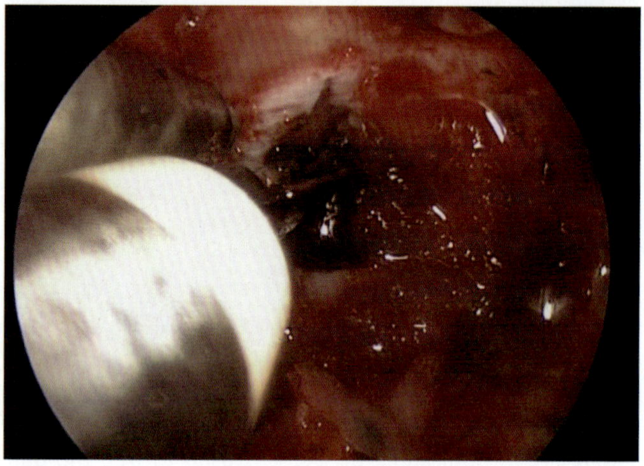

Fig. 6A.15 The anterior intercavernous sinus grasped with bipolar cautery prior to cauterization. Both the right and left sides should be cauterized.

15. The anterior intercavernous sinus is cauterized on both sides with a bipolar cautery and then divided (**Fig. 6A.15**). Troublesome bleeding from this site can usually be stopped with direct application of an absorbable hemostat such as Surgicel and compression for a few minutes.
16. The arachnoid membrane is opened between the pituitary gland and the optic chiasm (**Fig. 6A.16**), and the suprasellar region is visualized where the cyst can be seen to the right of the pituitary stalk (**Fig. 6A.17**).
17. The arachnoid membrane can be dissected away laterally to provide further access and visualization (**Fig. 6A.18**).
18. The lesion is gently dissected away from the pituitary stalk, and a biopsy is asserved for histological

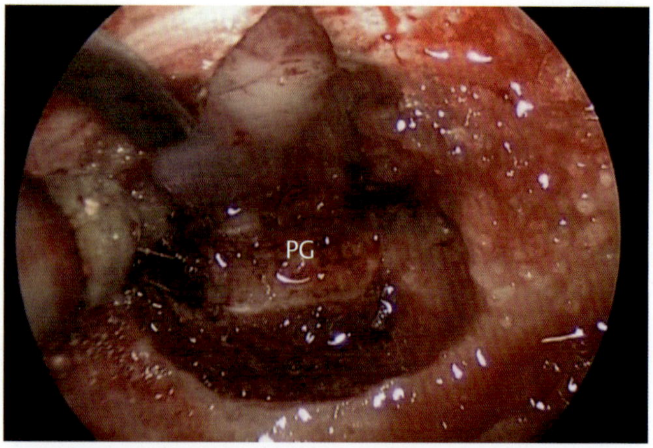

Fig. 6A.16 View after division of the anterior intercavernous sinus. The pituitary gland (PG) is visible.

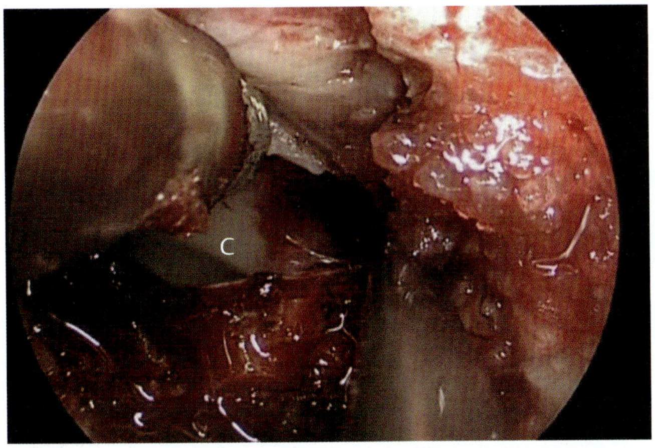

Fig. 6A.17 The arachnoid membrane being opened laterally, with the cyst (C) in view.

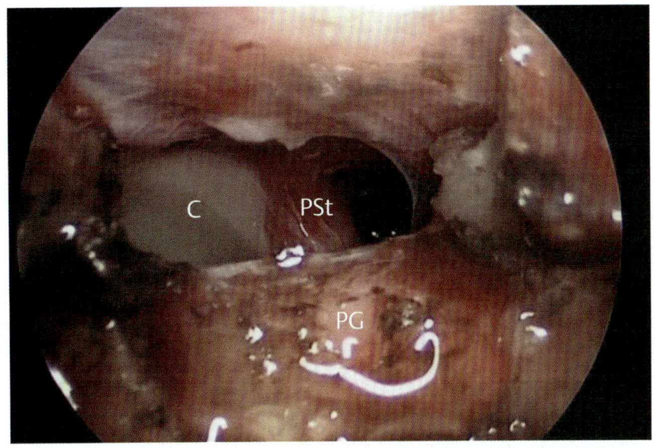

Fig. 6A.18 View of the suprasellar region. The pituitary gland (PG) can be seen inferior to the opening and the pituitary stalk (PSt) directly in the center of the view. The cyst (C) is seen on the right of the pituitary stalk.

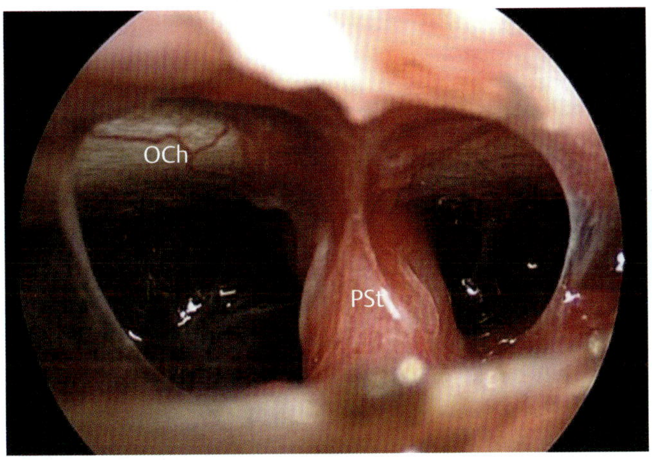

Fig. 6A.19 Endonasal endoscopic view of the supra-sellar region after resection: The pituitary stalk (PSt) remains in its physiological position with the optic chiasm (OCh) superiorly.

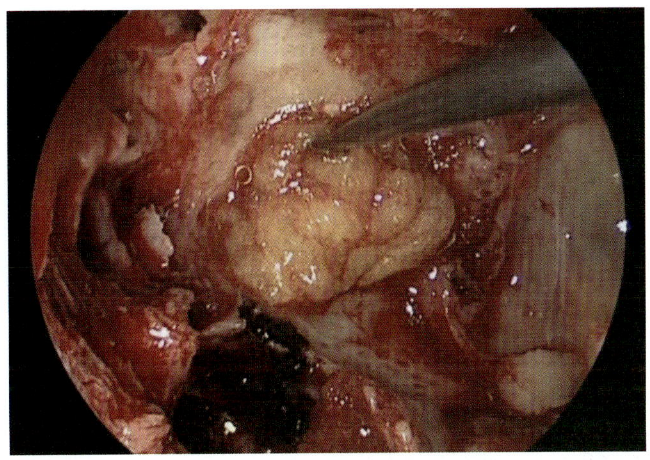

Fig. 6A.20 Bony sphenoid defect being plugged with fat.

examination. The lesion is then completely removed with a combination of dissection and aspiration (**Fig. 6A.19**).

19. The defect is reconstructed with an abdominal fat graft. The edges are tucked intradurally to ensure a watertight seal but not tightly enough to cause compression to underlying structures (**Fig. 6A.20**).
20. The construct is covered with a synthetic dural sealant or tissue glue. The nasoseptal flap is placed over the construct to reinforce the repair (**Fig. 6A.21**).
21. A postoperative MRI is performed which confirms complete resection of the lesion **(Fig. 6A.22** and **Fig. 6A.23**).

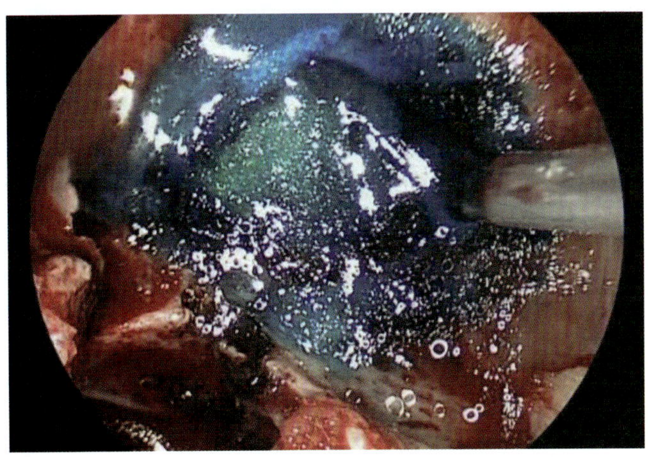

Fig. 6A.21 Synthetic dural sealant applied to reinforce the repair prior to the nasoseptal flap placement.

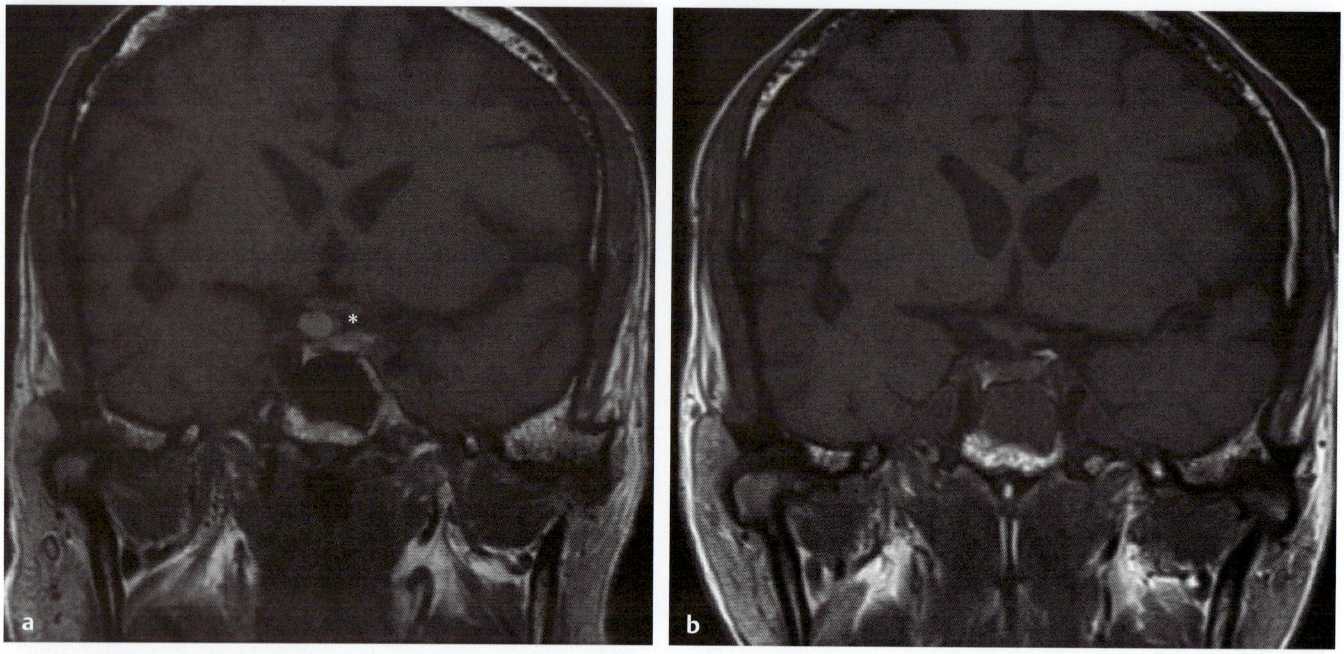

Fig. 6A.22 Comparison between the preoperative T1-weighted coronal MRI section **(a)**, showing the lesion (*) just to the right and above the pituitary stalk and gland, respectively, and the postoperative T1-weighted coronal MRI section **(b)** demonstrating complete resection of the supra-sellar lesion.

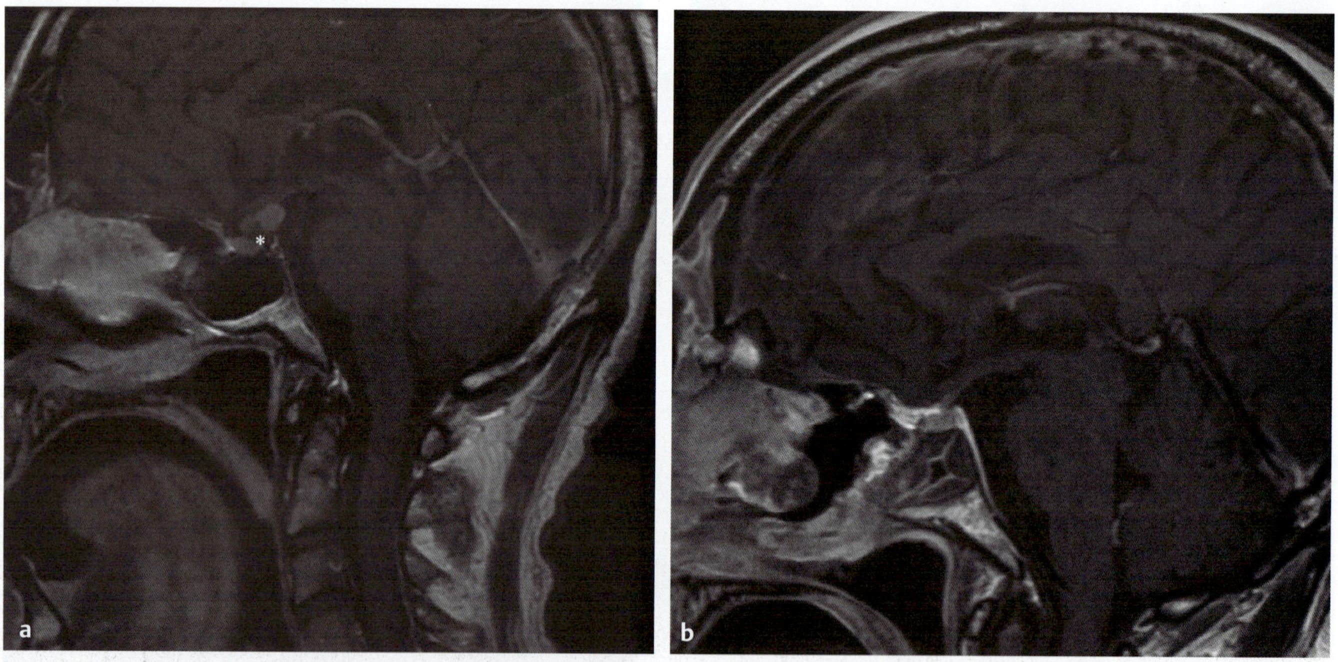

Fig. 6A.23 Comparison between the T1-weighted preoperative sagittal MRI **(a)** and the postoperative sagittal MRI **(b)** showing complete resection of the supra-sellar lesion.

Case 6B

Single Nostril Endoscopic Transseptal Transsphenoidal Excision of an Intrasellar Pituitary Mucocele

Adzreil Bakri, Prepageran Narayanan, Vicknes Waran, and Michel Roethlisberger

History

A 55-year-old Chinese gentleman presented with a history of sublabial transseptal pituitary surgery 15 years ago. On follow-up magnetic resonance imaging (MRI), there was an incidental finding of a nonenhancing lesion in the sella (**Fig. 6B.1**) with low signal intensity on T1-weighted images and high intensity on T2-weighted images measuring 1.8 cm × 1 cm × 0.9 cm. The patient is otherwise well with no symptoms. Based on the MRI findings, a slowly recurring pituitary adenoma could not be excluded, although the imaging was suggestive for a mucocele. The patient was amenable for an "endonasal endoscopic transsphenoidal resection" of the lesion for exclusion of a recurrent disease. Intraoperatively and based on histology, an intrasellar mucocele was confirmed.

Surgical Steps

1. Local anesthesia is infiltrated into both sides of the septum to raise the septal mucoperichondrium (**Fig. 6B.2**).
2. **Single nostril transseptal transsphenoidal approach:** After bipolar diathermy, the septum is incised unilaterally with a no. 15 blade opposite to the anterior aspect of the middle turbinate. The mucoperichondrial flap is raised in a posterior direction until the choana is reached. (**Fig. 6B.3**). Since this is a revision case, the septal cartilage and bone are absent and gentle care is taken when removing adhesions and raising the flaps to prevent flap tearing or perforation (**Fig. 6B.4**).

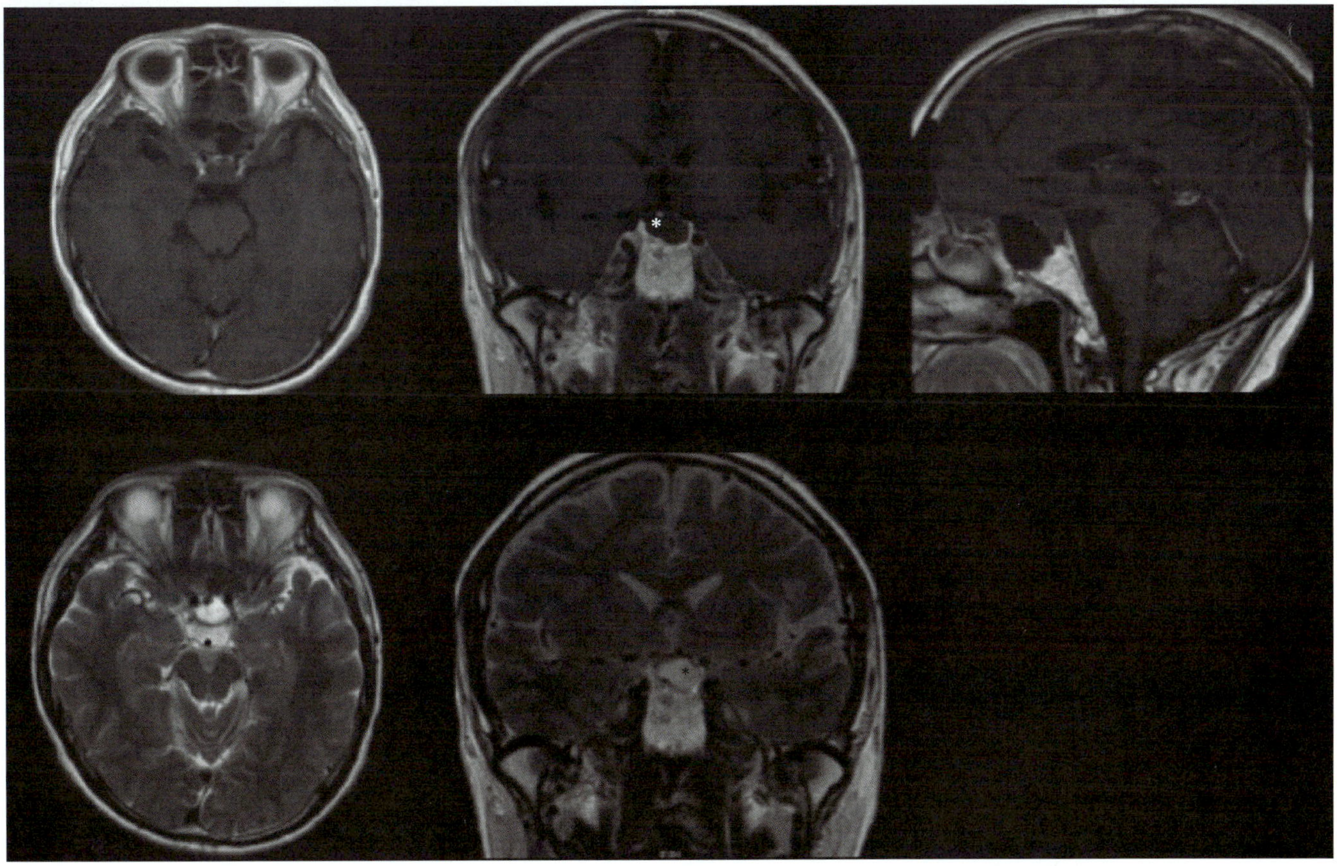

Fig. 6B.1 Preoperative axial, coronal and sagittal T1-(first row) and axial and coronal T2-weighted (second row) MRI sections demonstrating a sellar and supra-sellar cystic lesion (*).

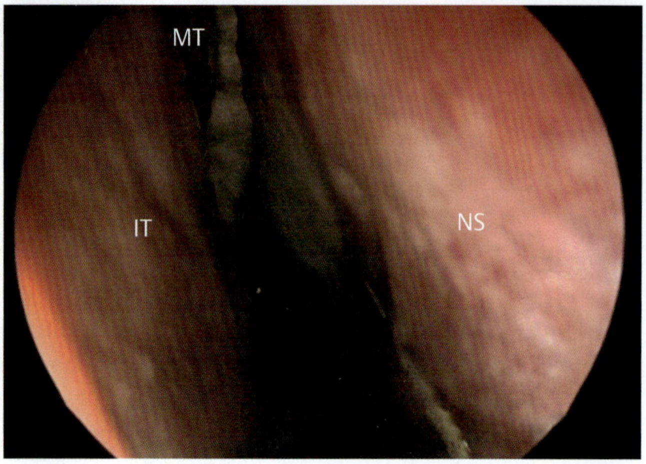

Fig. 6B.2 Local anesthesia of the right nasal septum mucosa.

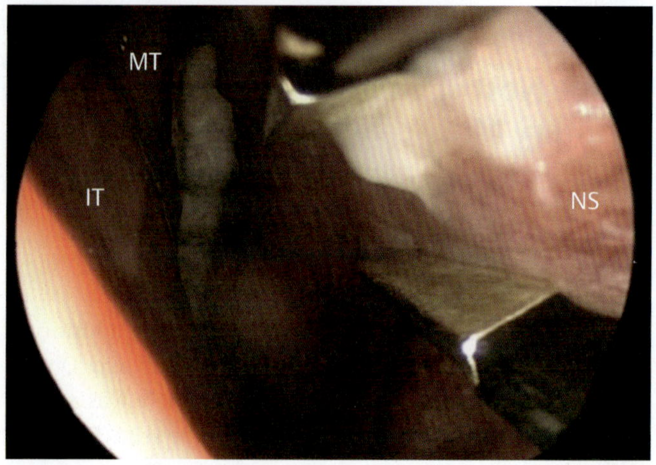

Fig. 6B.3 Bipolar diathermy prior to the incision of the right nasal septum mucosa opposite to the anterior part of the middle turbinate.

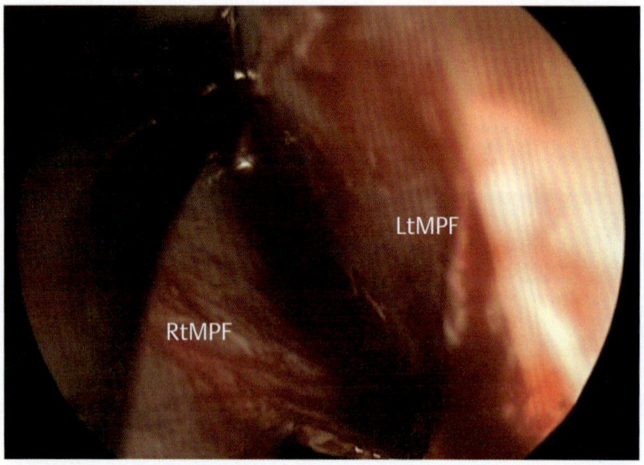

Fig. 6B.4 Raising of bilateral mucoperichondrial flaps: Note that the septal bone and cartilage are absent because of the previous surgery, and care is taken to remove adhesions and prevent flap tearing or perforation

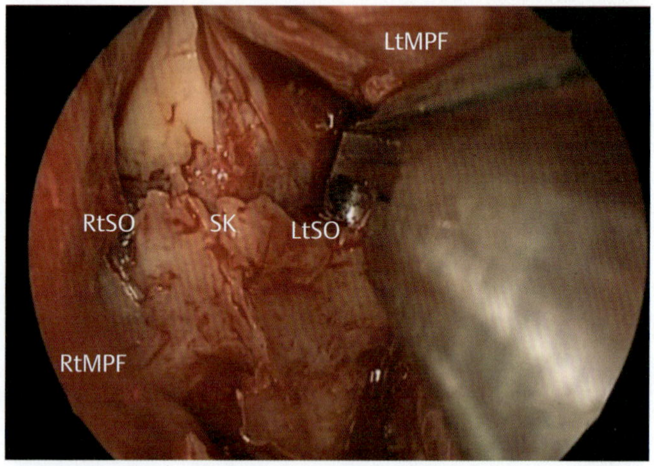

Fig. 6B.5 Exposure and removal of the sphenoid keel. Note adhesions and residual bone at the superior half of the keel with the inferior half still intact.

3. The sphenoid keel is exposed and any residual mucosa or adhesions are cauterized using a monopolar diathermy.
4. The sphenoid ostia are identified bilaterally and widened inferomedially in a V-shaped manner using a Kerrison punch, and once the bony removal is sufficient, the sphenoid keel is then removed with a pituitary rongeur forceps (**Fig. 6B.5**).
5. After removal of the sphenoid keel, any residual mucosa or bony septations are removed to make the bilateral sphenoid sinus a single common cavity (**Fig. 6B.6**).
6. Prior to the removal of bone overlying the sella, the exact location of the mucocele is confirmed with neuronavigation (**Fig. 6B.7**).
7. A small bony opening into the sella is made with a chisel (**Fig. 6B.8**). Care must be taken when removing bone laterally to avoid injury to the carotid siphon of the cavernous sinuses bilaterally.

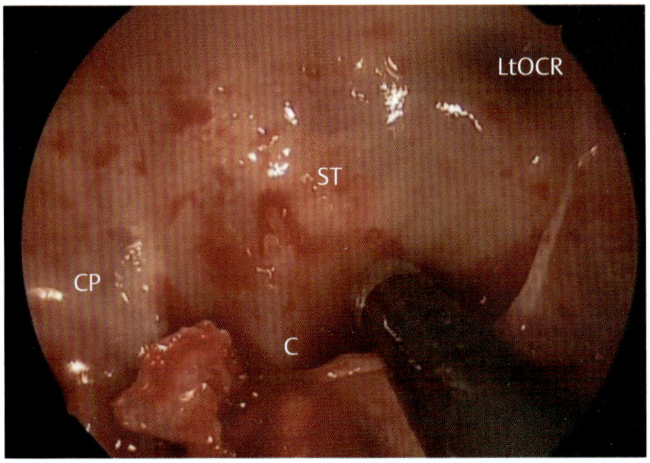

Fig. 6B.6 Removal of residual mucosa and bony septations creating a single large sphenoid cavity.

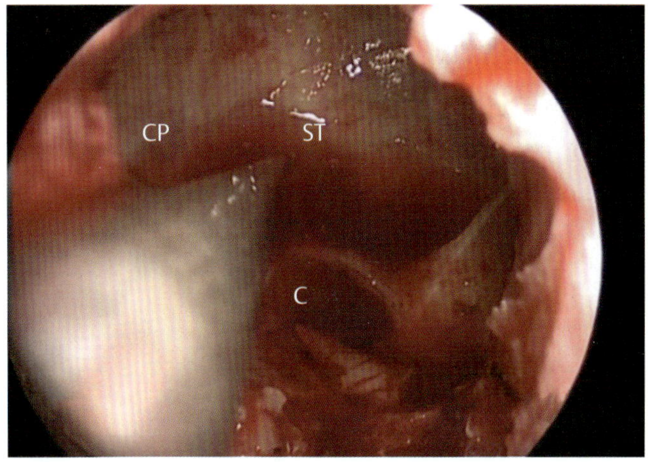

Fig. 6B.7 Neuronavigation probe over the sella turcica to determine the exact location of the mucocele.

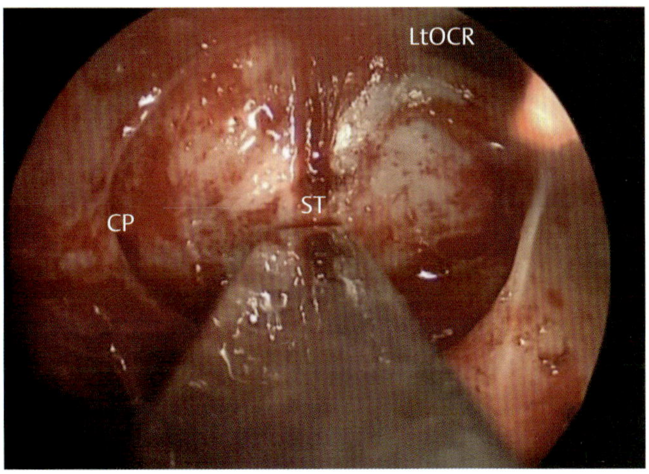

Fig. 6B.8 The bone overlying the sella turcica is gently chiseled to create a small opening or window. Carotid prominence can be seen.

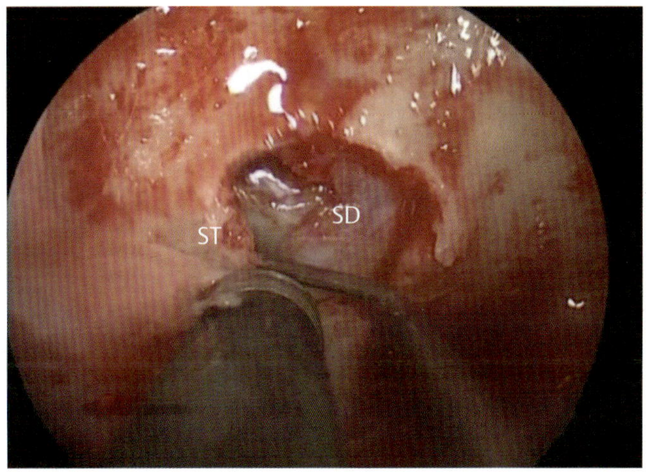

Fig. 6B.9 A right-angle dissector is inserted to separate bone and underlying dura.

8. A right-angle dissector is inserted to separate bone from the underlying dura. The bony opening is widened adequately using a Kerrison punch, making sure that the dura is always separated from the bone before each bite (**Fig. 6B.9** and **Fig. 6B.10**).
9. After adequate exposure, a cruciate incision is made on the dura with a no. 15 blade (**Fig. 6B.11**).
10. The incised dura is then elevated off the wall of the mucocele with an elevator (**Fig. 6B.12**).
11. Once adequate exposure of the mucocele is performed, an incision is made on the mucocele itself with a no. 15 blade (**Fig. 6B.13**).
12. The mucocele is drained and its wall is then marsupialized (**Fig. 6B.14** and **Fig. 6B.15**).
13. Once the mucocele is removed, its cavity is left open and oxidized cellulose polymers (Surgicel) and absorbable gelatin sponges (Gelfoam) are applied within the sphenoid cavity (**Fig. 6B.16**).
14. Both septal flaps are approximated in the midline, and the septal incision is covered with Gelfoam and synthetic biodegradable foams (Nasopore) while making sure to provide an adequate airway along the nasal floor (**Fig. 6B.17**).

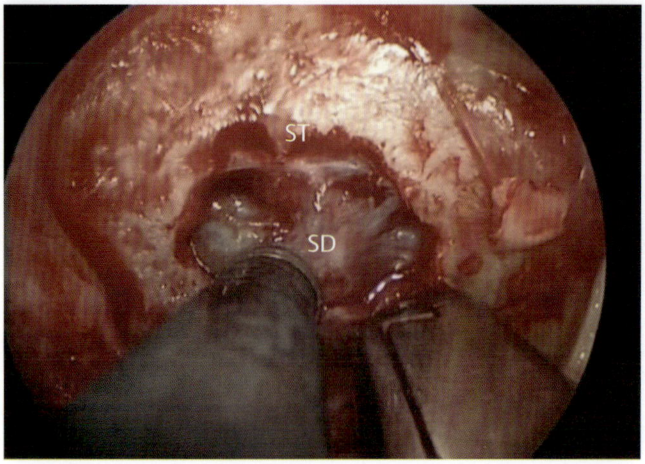

Fig. 6B.10 The bony opening is widened using a Kerrison punch. SD, sellar dura; ST, sella turcica.

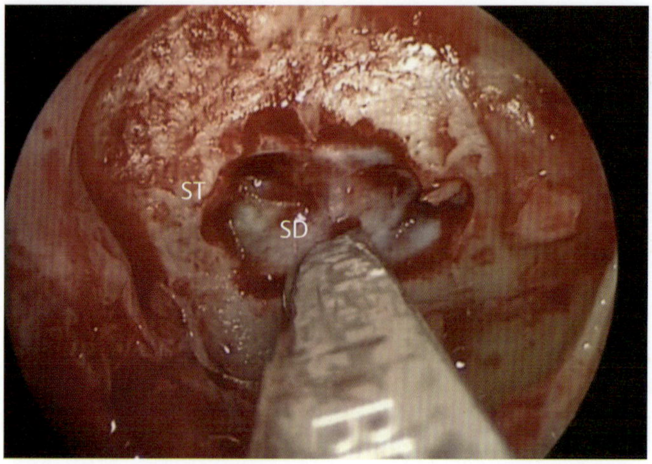

Fig. 6B.11 Cruciate incision on the dura.

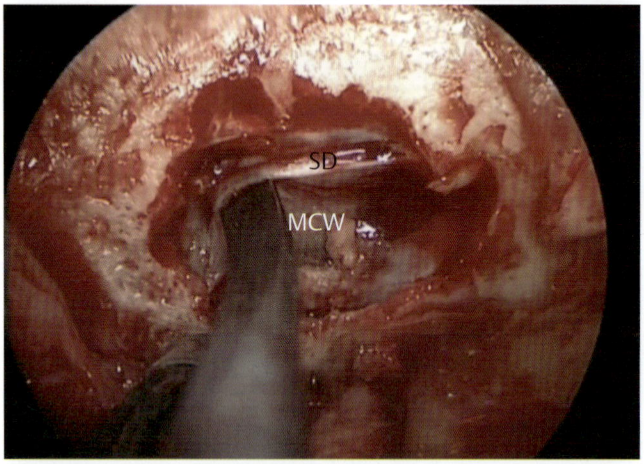

Fig. 6B.12 Elevation of dura from the mucocele wall (MCW).

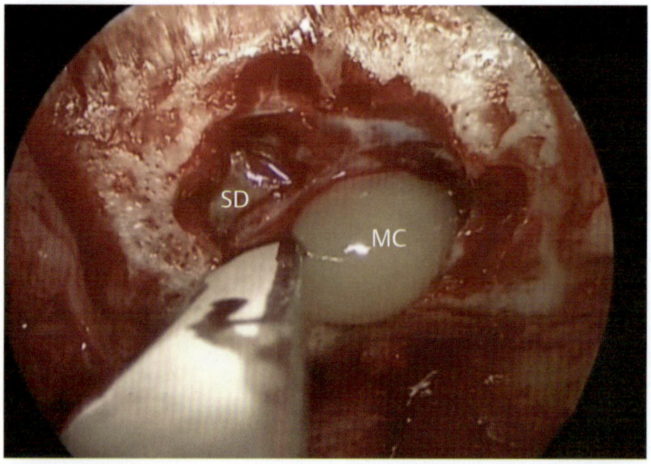

Fig. 6B.13 Incision on the mucocele (MC) with a no. 15 blade.

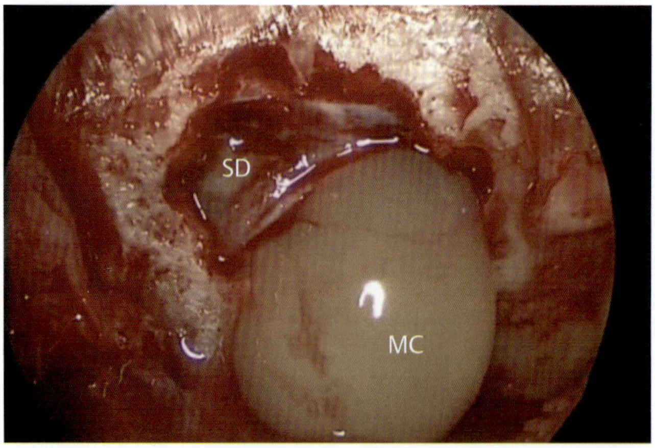

Fig. 6B.14 The mucocele (MC) is drained and samples are sent for histological examination, microbial culture and antibiotic sensitivity testing.

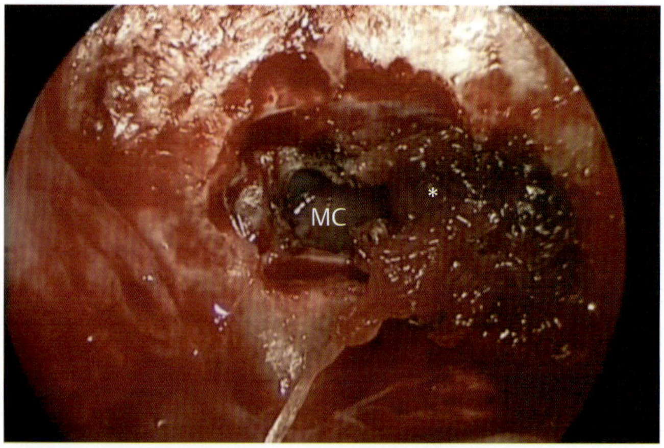

Fig. 6B.15 Final view after removal of the mucocele. Note a Surgicel patch over the left surgical field which was used to stop bleeding from the left cavernous sinus (*).

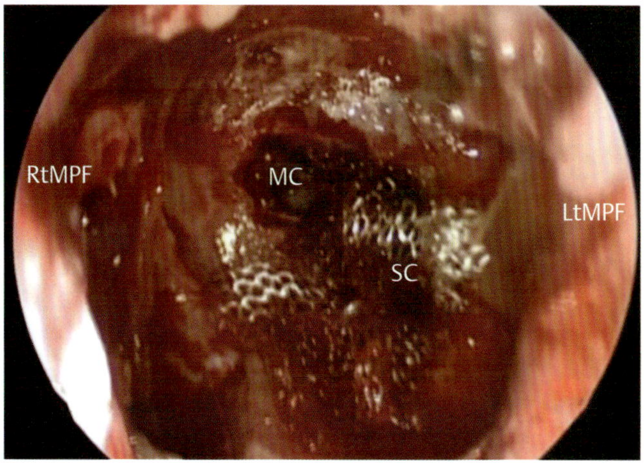

Fig. 6B.16 Surgicel (SC) and Gelfoam are applied surrounding the defect (MC) but not occluding it in the sphenoid cavity.

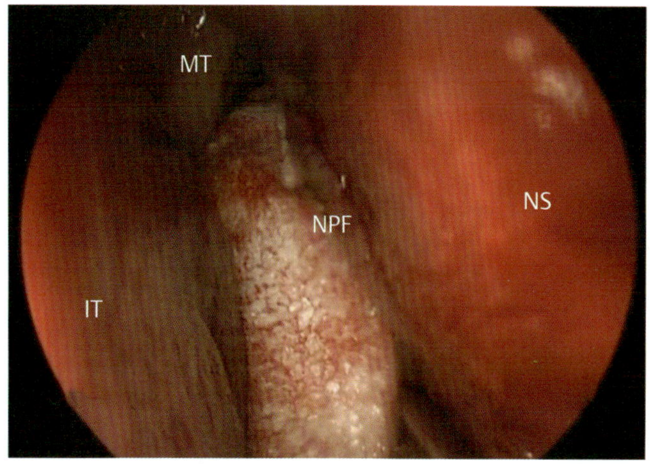

Fig. 6B.17 Closure of the septal incision and nasal packing with Gelfoam and Nasopore (NPF) providing adequate nasal airway along the floor of the nose.

Section II

Supra-sellar Region

Chapter 7 Craniopharyngioma

Michel Roethlisberger, Raphael Guzman, Jonathan Rychen, Adam Jadczak, Yves Brand, Kein Seong Mun, Jürgen Hench, Luigi Mariani, Prepageran Narayanan, and Vicknes Waran

Introduction

Craniopharyngiomas account for approximately 2 to 5% of all central nervous system tumors.[1] They present as solid or mixed solid-cystic benign primary brain tumors of the sellar and suprasellar region.[2] However, craniopharyngiomas do not display a benign behavior, although they are classified as World Health Organization (WHO) grade I tumors. Their tendency for recurrence and the inherent risk of consecutive reoperations have led to the concept of radical surgical resection, when these tumors are treated.[3] However, gross total resection (GTR) is not feasible in many cases, as these lesions, in contrast to pituitary adenomas, are adhesive to crucial adjacent neurovascular structures, namely the optic chiasm, the hypothalamus, and cerebral arterial vessels. Hence, craniopharyngiomas are one of the most challenging central nervous system neoplasms. Questions concerning the management have caused a lot of controversy in the past decades. With approximately half of these tumors presenting during childhood and adolescence and a half after the age of 20 years, and with newly available treatment modalities, including endonasal endoscopic techniques, subtotal resection (STR), and adjuvant radiotherapies, even more questions arise concerning optimal treatment strategies. The growing field of endonasal endoscopic procedures reveals new insights for the understanding of the origin, growth patterns, and anatomical relationship of this tumor entitiy.[2,4]

The natural course of the disease and/or consecutive treatments, in the pediatric as well as the adult population, has a significant impact on the quality of life (QOL) of these patients. Besides endocrine deficiencies, one of the most serious complications is hypothalamic obesity (hypothalamic syndrome), which can be clinically apparent before and/or after treatment, and needs to be addressed by an interdisciplinary approach.[5–9]

Pathological Considerations

Craniopharyngiomas appear as solid or partially cystic tumors originating along the vestiges of the stomodeal diverticulum. They are encountered most commonly in the region of the infundibular stalk, but may arise along a line from the nasopharynx to the diencephalon where epithelial tissue forms the pharyngohypophyseal duct during embryological development. The squamous epithelium commonly persists after involution of this so-called Rathke's cleft. Mutations in the respective precursor cells can lead to the formation of this neoplasm and ultimately culminate in tumorous growth.[10]

Craniopharyngiomas are slow-growing, histologically benign lesions with well-defined borders (**Fig. 7.1**).[11] However, they are locally aggressive and often present adherence to adjacent neurovascular structures, including the optic nerves, blood vessels, pituitary gland, and hypothalamus.[12,13]

Histologically, as well as on the base of their mutational spectrum and consecutive alterations of their methylome, two distinct types of craniopharyngioma are currently distinguished.[14] These types, in fact representing rather different neoplasms, also show characteristic age distributions with the adamantinomatous craniopharyngioma having a bimodal age distribution, peaking in the first and sixth decades of life, while papillary craniopharyngioma is much less common and peaks in the sixth decade.[10,11,15,16]

Both entities, taken together, account for 1 to 5% of all intracranial tumors and 6 to 13% of pediatric brain tumors, with a prevalence of 1 to 3 per 100,000 and an estimated incidence of 0.13 to 2 per 100,000 individuals.[15–17]

Adamantinomatous Craniopharyngioma

This tumor type, derived from squamous embryonic rests, is histologically characterized by a distinctively keratinizing squamous epithelium, termed "wet keratin." It is the most common variant in childhood. Mutations of the beta-catenin (*CTNNB1*) gene with WNT-pathway upregulation are characteristic for this tumor subentity.[11,18–21] Adamantinomatous craniopharyngiomas are composed of nests and cords of squamoid epithelium with a peripheral palisade of columnar cells (**Fig. 7.2**). The solid parts of the tumor are hard because of frequent calcifications (**Fig. 7.3** and **Fig. 7.4**).[10,12] The cystic components frequently contain a "machine oil" fluid composed of desquamated squamous epithelium which has a high protein concentration, sometimes being mixed with cholesterol crystals[10,22] (**Fig. 7.5**).

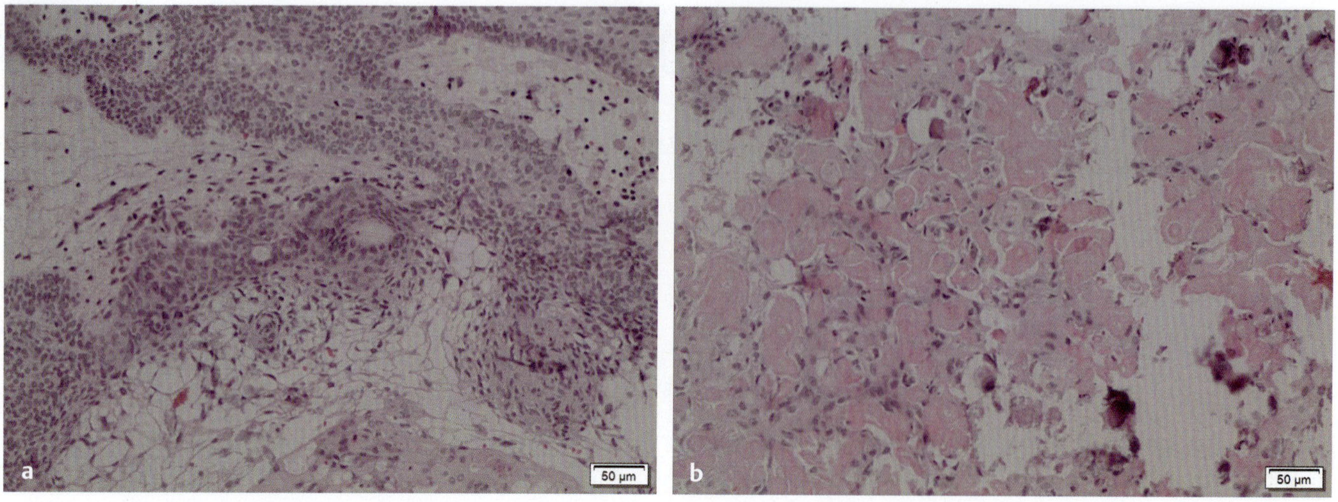

Fig. 7.1 Histomorphological features of a cystic intra- and suprasellar craniopharyngioma (WHO grade 1). The tumor is composed of solid sheets of neoplastic cells with vague palisading at the periphery. Looser areas (stellate reticulum) of neoplastic cells are seen at the center focally. Wet keratin and dystrophic calcification are also evident. **(a)** The tumor is composed of squamous epithelia with loose reticulum pattern and peripheral nuclear palisading in areas (hematoxylin and eosin, original magnification ×100). **(b)** Other areas show clumps of wet keratin and calcification (hematoxylin and eosin, original magnification ×100). The correlating radiological and intraoperative features of the same case are demonstrated in Chapter 1 (**Fig. 1.33**), and Case 9A, Chapter 9.

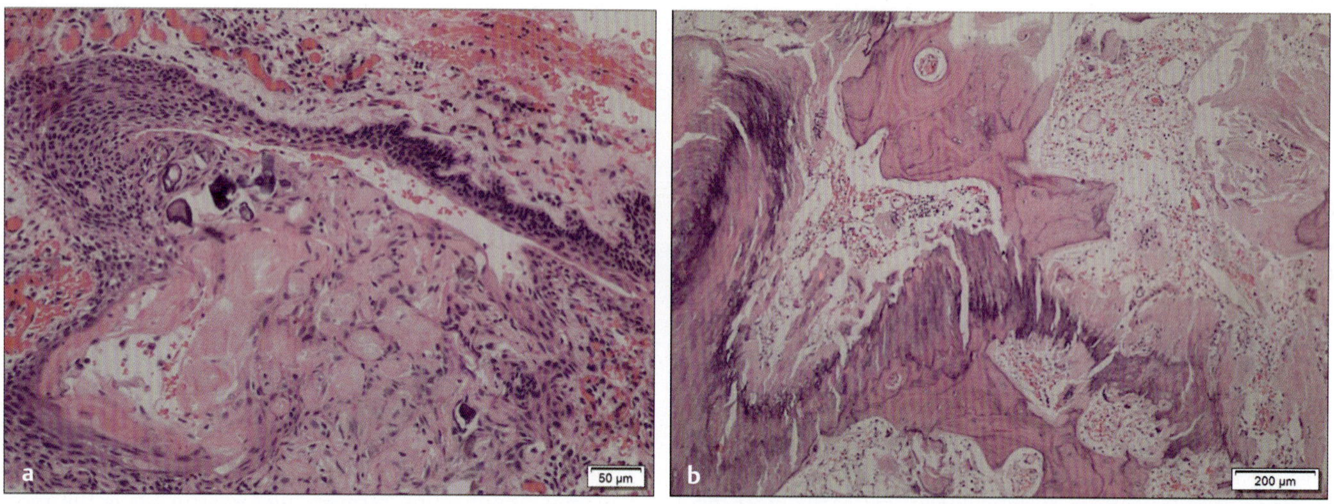

Fig. 7.2 Histomorphological features of an adamantinomatous craniopharyngioma (WHO grade I). Multiple deeper levels show fragments of ossified bony trabeculae admixed with some nonviable bone. One fragment of vascularized stroma tissue is lined by well-differentiated squamous epithelium with focal peripheral basal palisading. Multiple clusters of wet keratin can be seen. No definite stellate reticulum is identified. Areas of tumor necrosis and calcifications can be seen. The histological sections show clumps of partly calcified and ossified pinkish anucleate keratin admixed along with many fragments of squamous epithelium. The squamous cells are polygonal with a regular vesicular nucleus and peripheral nuclear palisading. In several fragments the central portion of the squamous epithelium exhibits a loose stellate reticulum pattern. Scattered inflammatory cells are noted. Adjacent neural tissue shows gliosis. Foreign body multinucleated giant cell reaction is also evident. No evidence of malignancy can be seen. **(a)** The tumor is congested with connective tissue surrounded by sheets of well-differentiated squamous epithelium with focal peripheral basal palisading and multiple clusters of wet keratin as well as calcifications (hematoxylin and eosin, original magnification ×100). **(b)** Tracts of ossified bony trabeculae are also seen (hematoxylin and eosin, original magnification ×40).

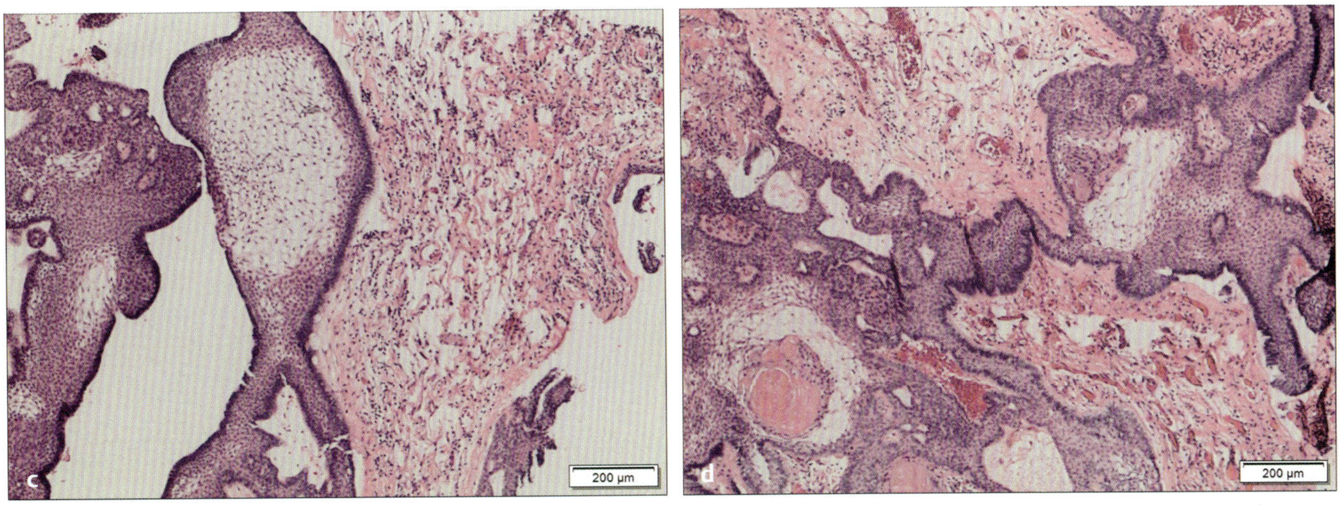

Fig. 7.2 *(Continued)* **(c)** The tumor is made up of fragments of squamous epithelium admixed with clumps of anucleate keratin. The squamous cells are polygonal with a regular vesicular nucleus and peripheral nuclear palisading. The central portion of the squamous epithelium exhibits a loose stellate reticulum pattern (hematoxylin and eosin, original magnification ×40). **(d)** The squamous epithelium shows peripheral nuclear palisading, with a central loose stellate reticulum pattern (hematoxylin and eosin, original magnification ×40). The correlating radiological and intraoperative features of the same case are demonstrated in **Fig. 7.9** (see also Case 9B, Chapter 9).

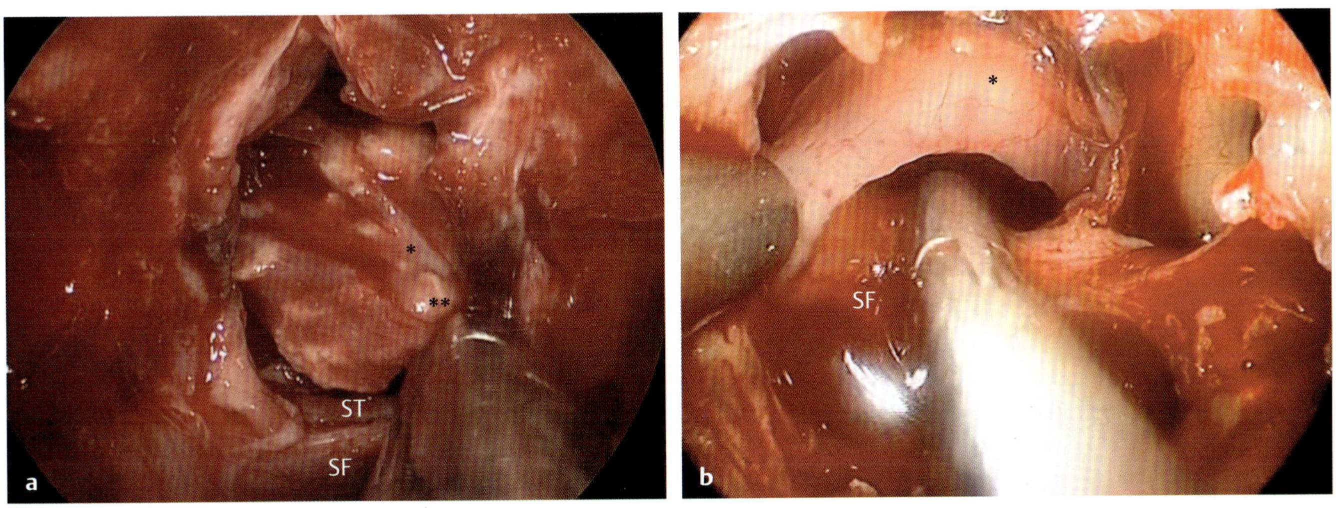

Fig. 7.3 **(a, b)** The solid parts of the tumor are vascularized, have a fleshy firm consistency (*) and frequently express calcifications (**).

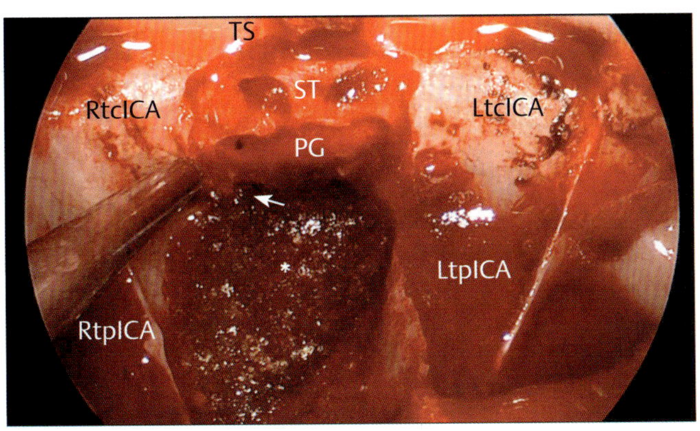

Fig. 7.4 The cystic components of craniopharyngioma frequently contain a "machine oil" fluid (*white arrow*), sometimes being mixed with cholesterol crystals (*).

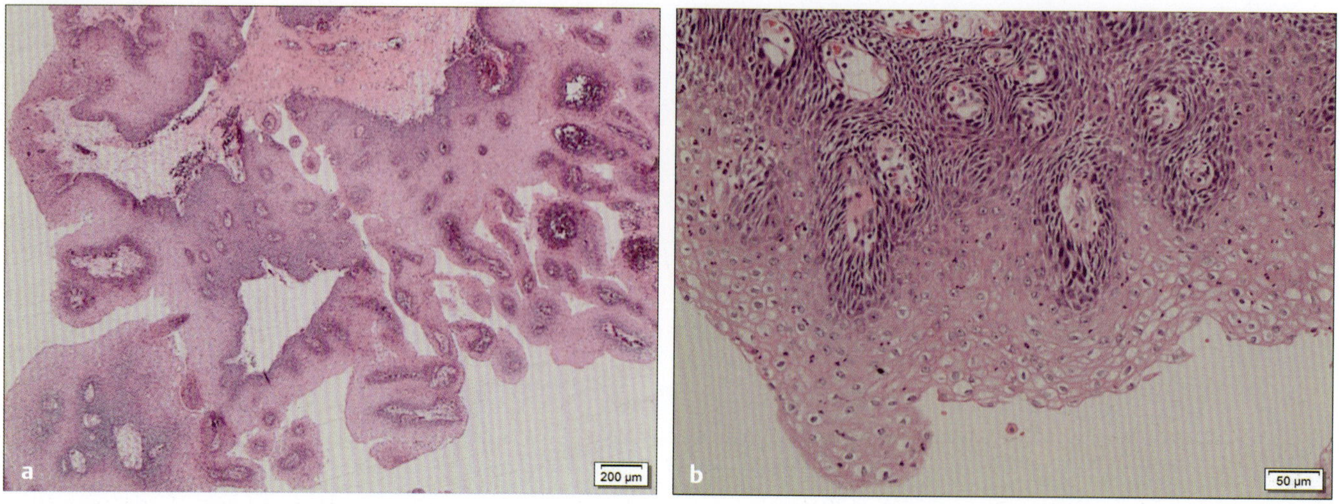

Fig. 7.5 Histomorphological features of a papillary craniopharyngioma (WHO grade I). The histological sections show sheets of differentiated stratified nonkeratinizing squamous epithelium surrounding broad crude papillary structures. No keratohyalin granules, mucocytes, or columnar epithelial cells are seen. No wet keratin or squamous whorls are present. The loose connective fibrovascular tissue is patchily infiltrated by neutrophils and lymphocytes with occasional foamy histiocytes. No evidence of malignancy can be detected. **(a)** The tumor is made up of papillary structures composed of fibrovascular cores covered by layers of nonkeratinizing stratified squamous epithelium (hematoxylin and eosin, original magnification ×20). **(b)** The squamous epithelium shows normal maturation (hematoxylin and eosin, original magnification ×100). The correlating radiological features of the same case are demonstrated in **Fig. 7.14 (a, b)**.

Papillary Craniopharyngioma

This tumor type shows a papillary histoarchitecture with fibrovascular cores covered by nonkeratinizing squamous epithelium.[11] It imitates the oropharyngeal mucosa and is reported to be the common type in adults.[10] Mutations in the *BRAF p.V600E* gene are typical of this tumor subentity.[18,19] Papillary craniopharyngiomas rarely exhibit calcification. The cystic parts are typically yellow and viscous (**Fig. 7.6**).[10,12]

Anatomical Considerations

The anatomical origin, growth pattern, and final extension of the craniopharyngioma have an impact on the surgical approach. Several proposed classifications tried to cluster the lesions to predict resectability, visual and endocrine outcome, and to assist in the surgical approach selection.[24–28] Transcranial observations revealed the anatomical origin of the tumor in relation to the optic chiasm. The diaphragma sellae does determine the growth pattern of these lesions.[24–28] Especially, surgical features and adhesion patterns reportedly seem to depend on these specific relationships.[4,26]

Anatomy-based classification: Yaşargil et al. described six types of craniopharyngiomas using an anatomy-based classification concept:[29]

- Purely intrasellar—infradiaphragmatic.
- Intra- and suprasellar, infra- and supradiaphragmatic.
- Supradiaphragmatic, parachiasmatic, extraventricular.
- Intra- and extraventricular.
- Paraventricular in relation to the third ventricle.
- Purely intraventricular.

Relationship to the optic chiasm: Relative to the optic chiasm, craniopharyngiomas were classified by Wang et al. to be located:[26]

- Prechiasmatic.
- Subchiasmatic.
- Retrochiasmatic.

Relationship to the third ventricle: Steno et al. anatomically classified craniopharyngioma relative to the third ventricle:[30]

- Intraventricular.
- Extraventricular.
- Below the ventricle.

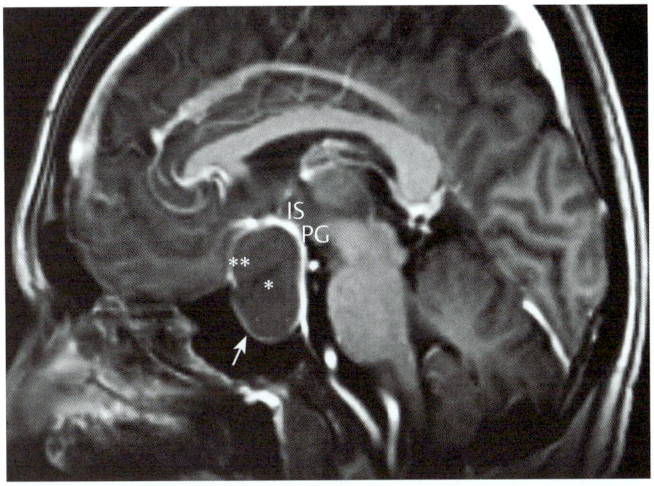

Fig. 7.6 Adult adamantinomatous preinfundibular (type I) craniopharyngioma.[23] Sagittal T1 contrast-enhanced MRI section demonstrating a cystic intra- and suprasellar lesion (*) with typical ring enhancement of the cyst wall (**). The lesion displaces the pituitary gland (PG) and the infundibular stalk (IS) posteriorly. Remodeling of the sella turcica can be appreciated (*white arrow*).

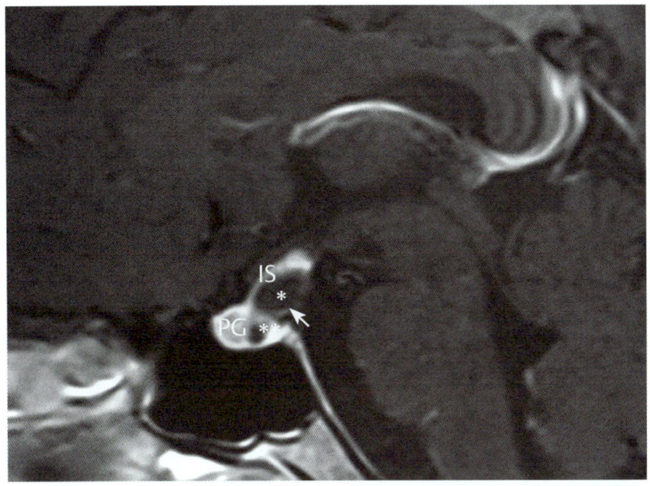

Fig. 7.7 Adult adamantinomatous transinfundibular (type II) craniopharyngioma with extension into the infundibular stalk.[23] This patient initially presented with galactorrhea and elevated prolactin due to the stalk effect. The craniopharyngioma cyst (*) shows peripheral ring enhancement of the cyst wall (*white arrow*) and extends into the infundibular stalk (IS) with anterior displacement and stretching of the latter. A solid tumor part (**) can be appreciated in the intrasellar compartment posteriorly to the normal pituitary gland (PG).

Relationship to the diaphragma sellae: In another publication, Wang et al. classified the tumor's location and growth pattern in relation to the diaphragma sellae:[25]

- Sellar (infradiaphragmatic).
- Suprasellar (supradiaphragmatic).
- Sellar and suprasellar (infra- and supradiaphragmatic).

Suprasellar extension and relationship to the infundibular stalk: In the era of endoscopic surgeries, Kassam et al. established a classification scheme based on the suprasellar extension and the relationship between the infundibular stalk and the craniopharyngioma (**Fig. 7.6**, **Fig. 7.7**, **Fig. 7.8**, **Fig. 7.9** and **Fig. 7.10**):[23]

- *Type I:* Preinfundibular.
- *Type II:* Transinfundibular (with extension into the infundibular stalk).
- *Type III:* Retroinfundibular (extending behind the pituitary gland and infundibular stalk).
  - *Type IIIa:* Extending into the third ventricle.
  - *Type IIIb:* Extending into the interpeduncular cistern.
- *Type IV:* Isolated to the third ventricle and/or optic recess.

Several authors consecutively confirmed the findings associated with this classification reporting favorable results after endoscopic endonasal approach (EEA).[4,31–35]

Transinfundibular craniopharyngioma (Type II): Most of the transinfundibular craniopharyngiomas originate from the infundibulum–tuber cinereum and grow within and along the long axis of the infundibulum.[2]

Predictive value of anatomy-based classification: The concept of anatomy-based classifications relates to surgical outcomes, such as the possible extent of tumor resection and postoperative sequelae. A prominent example is endocrinological dysfunction of the pituitary gland, which is found to be more prevalent in subdiaphragmatic craniopharyngiomas, while hypothalamic dysfunction has been associated with craniopharyngiomas invading the third ventricle.[36,37] In a recent study by Dho et al., tumor invasion into the center of the pituitary stalk affected the postoperative outcomes most significantly, and had strong predictive power for worse postoperative endocrinological outcome.[4] Tang et al. demonstrated that the pituitary stalk could only be preserved in 20.6% of cases when compared to nontransinfundibular craniopharyngioma (80.3%).[2]

More recently, the hypothalamic involvement of craniopharyngiomas has been considered to be relevant for the functional outcome of especially the pediatric population.

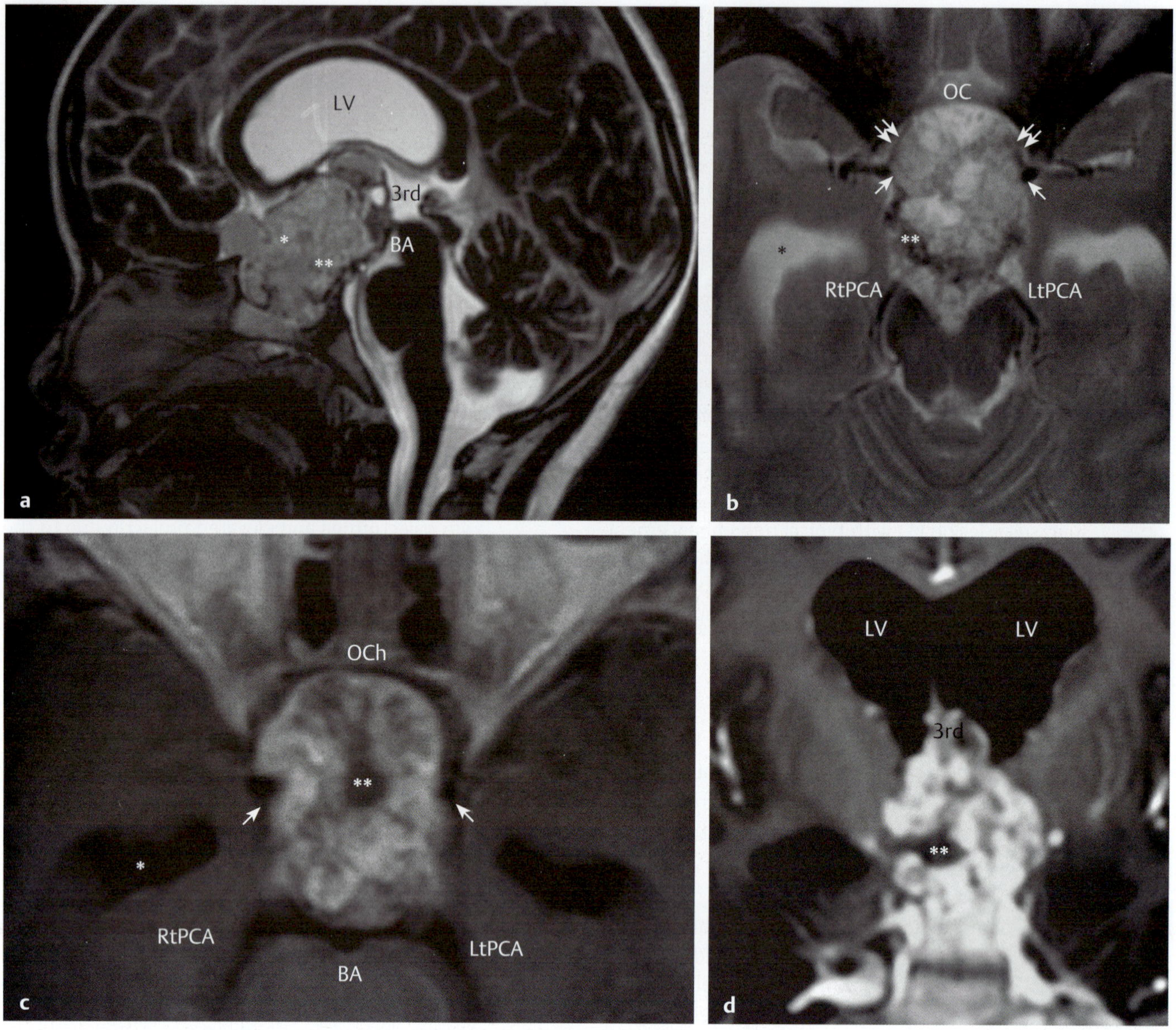

Fig. 7.8 Pediatric adamantinomatous retroinfundibular (type IIIa) craniopharyngioma extending into the third ventricle.[23] **(a)** T2-weighted sagittal MRI section showing a hyperintense mainly solid intra- and suprasellar mass (*) involving the third ventricle (3rd) and causing obstructive hydrocephalus with widened lateral ventricles (LV). Hypointense signals are suggestive for calcifications (**). **(b)** T2-weighted axial MRI section and **(c)** fluid-attenuated inversion recovery (FLAIR)-weighted axial MRI section demonstrating a hyperintense mainly solid suprasellar mass causing obstructive hydrocephalus (*). Hypointense signals are suggestive for calcifications (**). The optic chiasm (OCh) is prefixed and displaced anteriorly. The tumor seems to be adherent to the internal carotid artery bifurcations (*arrow*) and anterior cerebral arteries (*double arrow*). No cortical cuff is distinguishable. **(d)** T1-weighted gadolinium contrast-enhanced coronal MRI section showing a hyperintense contrast-enhancing mainly solid suprasellar mass extending into the third ventricle (3rd) with consecutive widening the lateral ventricles (LV) because of obstructive hydrocephalus. Hypointense nonenhancing areas are present and are suggestive for calcifications (**).

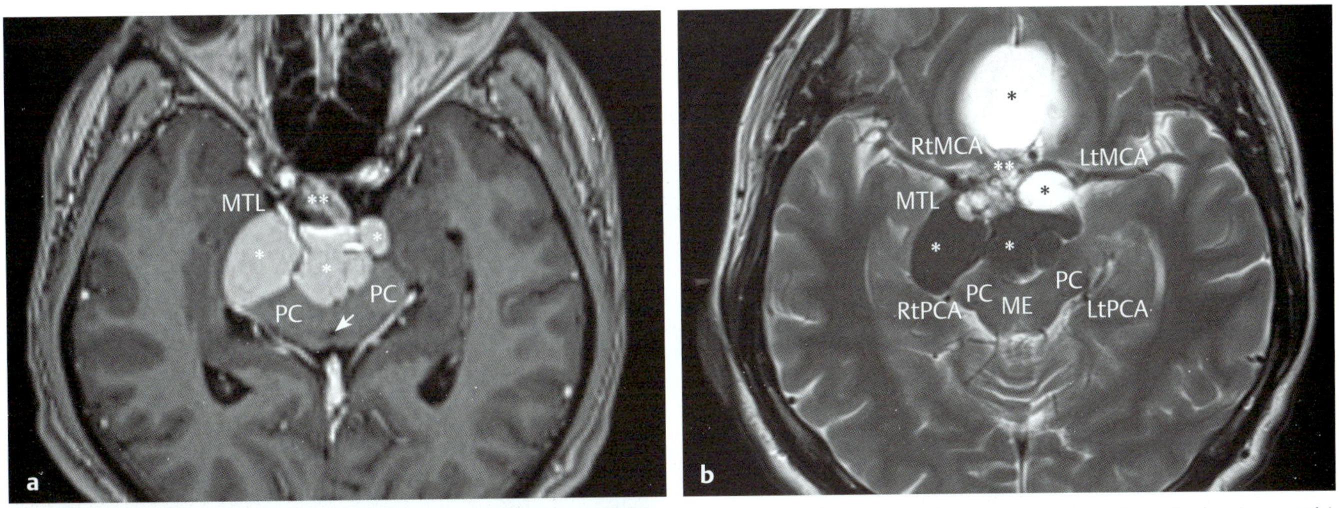

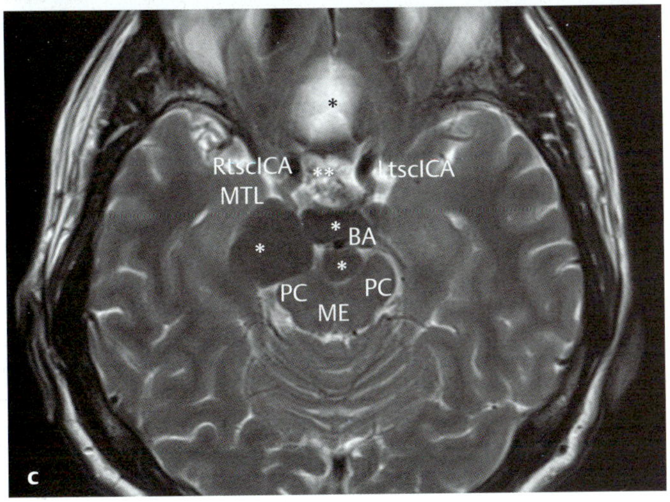

Fig. 7.9 Adult adamantinomatous retroinfundibular (type IIIb) craniopharyngioma extending into the interpeduncular cistern.[23] **(a)** T1-weighted gadolinium contrast-enhanced axial MRI section showing a multicystic (*) and solid (**) tumor extending into the interpeduncular cistern with compression and spreading of both cerebral pedunculi (CP) and mesial temporal lobe (MTL) of the right side. The cerebral aqueduct (*white arrow*) is patent. **(b, c)** T2-weighted axial MRI section demonstrating a multicystic (*) and solid (**) tumor extending into the interpeduncular cistern with compression and spreading of both (CP and MTL of the right side. The tumor cysts express variable intensity (hyperintense and hypointense) reflecting the variable content of desquamated squamous epithelium, which has a high protein concentration.

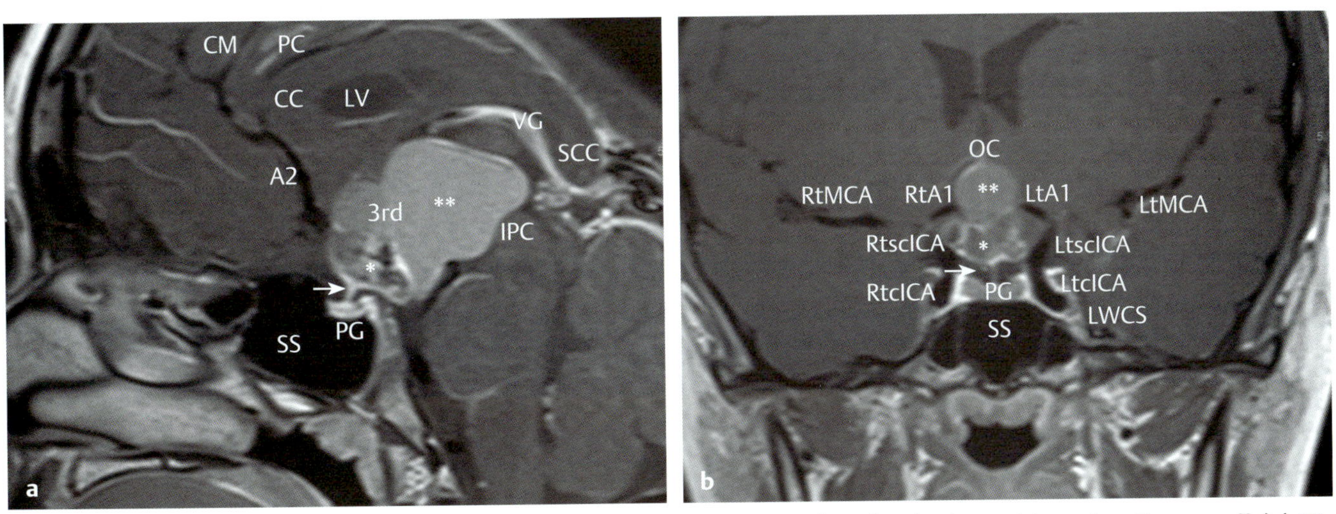

Fig. 7.10 Pediatric adamantinomatous (type IV) craniopharyngioma isolated to the third ventricle and optic recess.[23] **(a)** T1-weighted gadolinium contrast-enhanced sagittal MRI section demonstrating a large cystic (*) and solid (**) tumor located superiorly to the pituitary gland (PG) and the infundibular stalk (*arrow*) expanding the third ventricle (3rd) and the interpeduncular cistern (IPC). **(b)** Fluid-attenuated inversion recovery (FLAIR)-weighted coronal MRI section. *(Continued)*

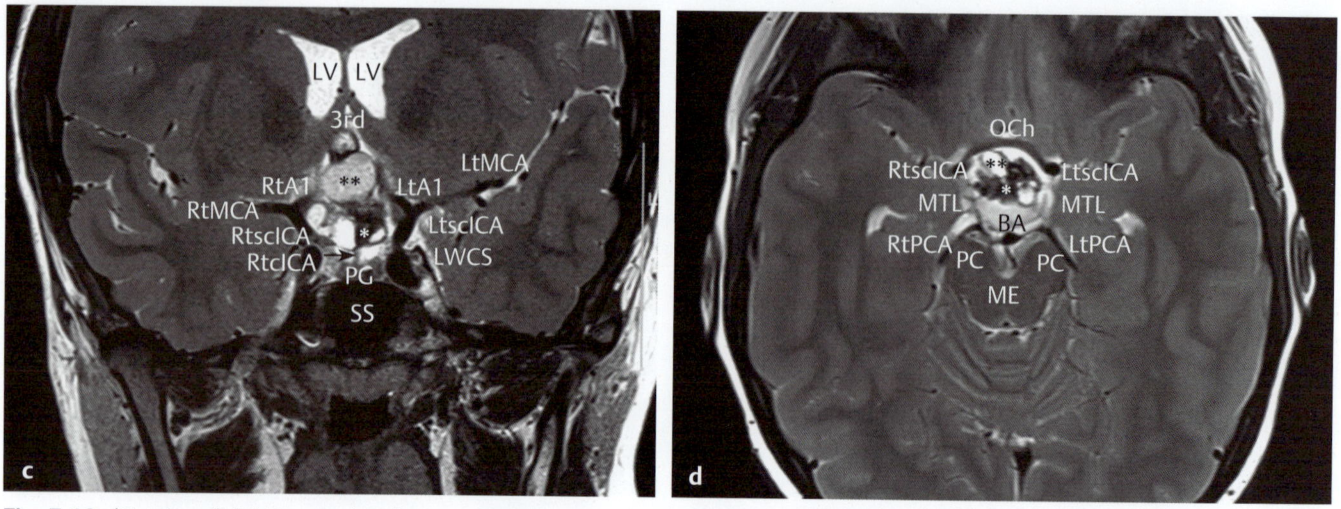

Fig. 7.10 *(Continued)* **(c)** T2-weighted coronal MRI section demonstrating a cystic (*) and solid (**) tumor located superiorly to the pituitary gland (PG) and the infundibular stalk (*white arrow*) with superior dislocation and compression of the optic chiasm (OCh). **(d)** T2-weighted axial MRI section demonstrating a cystic (*) and solid (**) tumor located in the optic recess with anterior dislocation and compression of the prefixed optic chiasm.

Puget et al. therefore correlated craniopharyngiomas according to the hypothalamic involvement in the preoperative magnetic resonance imaging (MRI) as compared to postoperative hypothalamic damage reflected by the body mass index (BMI):[38]

- *Grade 0:* No hypothalamic involvement, no hypothalamic damage.
- *Grade 1:* Hypothalamus displaced by the tumor, minimal hypothalamic damage.
- *Grade 2:* Hypothalamic involvement, severe hypothalamic damage.

Clinical Features

The clinical features arise from a direct impact on locoregional anatomical structures. Symptoms are caused by compression of the adjacent hypothalamic–pituitary axis, optic pathways, thalamus, and frontal lobes. Craniopharyngiomas are slow growing, and diagnosis is often established 1 to 2 years after the onset of symptoms.[39,40]

The clinical features of craniopharyngioma include visual disturbances (45%) and endocrine deficiencies, the latter being more frequent in children. Cognitive deterioration and personality changes have been found in half of the patients. Symptoms of intracranial hypertension can be present in larger lesions (70%) and are associated with obstructive hydrocephalus.[13]

Endocrine abnormalities are present in 80 to 90% of patients but rarely are the chief complaint.[41] Growth hormone (GH) deficiency is the most common endocrinopathy observed in the pediatric craniopharyngioma population and is found in 75% of such patients.[42] Growth retardation has been reported in up to 30% of cases. With suprasellar extension and hypothalamic involvement, hyperphagia (26%), a BMI more than 1.15 higher than the standard deviation, and diencephalic syndrome (4.5%) are described.[38] Precocious puberty on the other hand is relatively rare.[43] The most common presenting sign in the adult patient is gonadotrophin deficiency and, in an adolescent, delayed puberty, both because of disruptions in the secretion of luteinizing hormone (LH) and follicle-stimulating hormone (FSH).[44] Hypothyroidism and adrenocorticotropic hormone (ACTH) dysfunction might occur in as initial endocrinopathy at the time of diagnosis with craniopharyngioma.[12,41,45,46] Disturbances of the neurohypophysis, namely diabetes insipidus, are found in 9 to 38% of patients at the time of presentation.[12,13]

Tumor growth into the frontal lobe can cause dementia, apathy, abulia, or psychomotor slowing. Tumor growth into the temporal lobe can cause seizures and amnesia.[47,48]

Radiological Features

Craniopharyngiomas may appear as solid or solid–cystic and are located anatomically sellar, suprasellar, and/or parasellar in their extent.[29] Craniopharyngiomas can be either retro- or prechiasmatic and occasionally wholly intrasellar.[17]

Radiologically, the two types of craniopharyngiomas are often distinguishable. Adamantinomatous craniopharyngiomas are more often cystic masses in children, while papillary craniopharyngiomas are rather solid masses in adults. The extent and the imaging criteria differ with the tumor type and the age of the patient.[49,50] In children, craniopharyngiomas appear as calcified, solid, and/or cystic enhancing lesions, and the majority of them involve the suprasellar space.[12,51] However, cystic intrasellar appearance is possible. In general, the cyst rim of craniopharyngioma enhances in MRI and CT.[12]

Radiographic Features in Computed Tomography

In general, computed tomography (CT) is the modality of choice for the detection of calcifications, and some authors suggest a strong correlation of calcification and type of the craniopharyngioma (**Fig. 7.11**).[50]

Calcifications are evident in more than 90% of pediatric and more than 70% of adult craniopharyngioma.[10,52] In the adamantinous type, there is mostly a hypodense cystic and an isodense solid component. Either the solid (mostly nodular pattern) or the cystic (mostly rim-like enhancement) component usually enhances. In the papillary type, the solid component is mostly isodense, the enhancement is less vivid, and calcifications are rarely seen.

Radiographic Features in Magnetic Resonance Imaging

In MRI, the appearance and signal behavior show some variation regarding tumor type and cyst content.[53,54] In T1-weighted sequences, the cystic elements can be of high to intermediate to low intensity, depending on the content of the cyst.[10,12,52] The solid elements are usually iso- or hypointense. In T2-weigted sequences, the intracystic signal can be variable but mostly hyperintense. The solid component appears often heterogenous.[22,52] Calcifications can correlate with hypointensity on T2-weighted images.[12,55]

The cystic elements of adamantinomatous craniopharyngioma are of high intensity on T1-weighted and high or mixed intensity on T2-weighted images.[10,12,52] Cysts of the solid–cystic papillary subtype are of low intensity on T1-weighted and high intensity on T2-weighted images (**Fig. 7.12**, **Fig. 7.13** and **Fig. 7.14**).

The solid parts of the craniopharyngioma heterogeneously enhance after contrast enhancement,[22,52] the cyst wall enhances vividly in T1 contrast-enhanced images.[10,12,52]

Fluid-attenuated inversion recovery (FLAIR) and diffusion-weighted imaging (DWI) are usually of no further use for the classification of the lesion but can be useful for the imaging of "surrounding structures."[10]

Contrast-free or contrast-enhanced MR angiography (e.g., time-of-flight [TOF] angiography) can be used to visualize displacement and/or encasement of adjacent arterial vessels. With MR spectroscopy, a broad lipid spectrum has been descriped.[56]

Surgical Considerations

Because of their geographical location, the surgical treatment of craniopharyngiomas has been a part of controversial discussion over the past decades. The selection of the optimal surgical route for maximal exposure to achieve complete tumor resection with minimal postoperative morbidity is of great importance and is mainly based on the knowledge of the surgical anatomy. Endonasal endoscopic techniques are widely used for craniopharyngioma nowadays. Several groups around the world have reported their institutional experiences and outcomes using this technique.

Gross Total Resection for Craniopharyngiomas

In the past decades, achieving GTR was generally considered to be difficult for craniopharyngioma, because of a higher likelihood of perioperative complications. Within the available body of literature, rates have been reported to range from 28.6 to 91.1%.[2,4,32,34,35,57] A retrospective series by Apra et al. on 22 adult craniopharyngioma patients revealed that no patient with GTR experienced tumor recurrence or was in need of any adjuvant treatment after a median period of approximately 4 years.[58]

Subtotal Resection for Craniopharyngiomas

Adjunctive treatment options including intracystic therapies, reactive agents (bleomycin, interferon [INF] alpha), and radiotherapy after STR have been investigated.[3,12,36,59,60] Certain studies have compared the rate of disease control for STR followed by adjuvant radiotherapy and GTR. A similar disease control rate, with fewer complications, has been found when not aggressively resecting these tumors.[61–63] Reported long-term complications after adjuvant radiotherapy, especially in the pediatric population, are cognitive dysfunction, hypopituitarism, and secondary tumors. These have to be considered in association with this treatment modality.[64] A retrospective series on 22 adult craniopharyngioma patients reported that out of 8 patients with STR, 4 (50%) showed tumor growth needing adjuvant radiotherapy.[58]

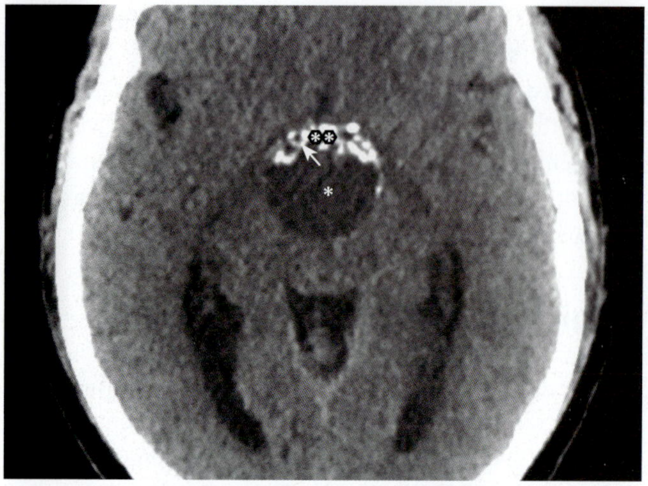

Fig. 7.11 Axial noncontrast-enhanced CT section demonstrating a cystic (*) and solid (**) tumor of the suprasellar region with calcification (*white arrow*). Lee et al. found that a T1 bright signal intensity and calcification on CT scans favor the adamantinomatous type over the papillary type of craniopharyngioma in the pediatric population.[50]

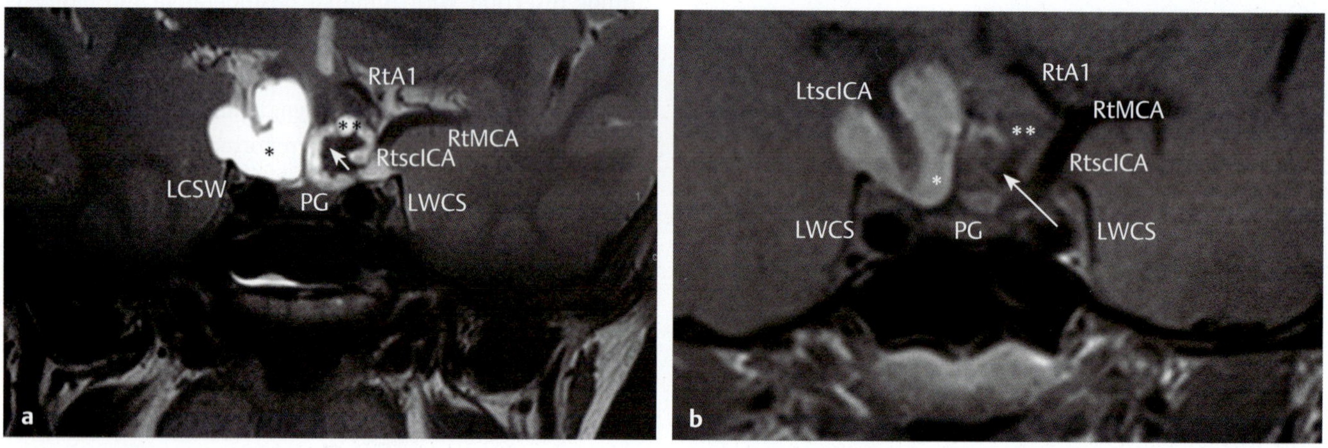

Fig. 7.12 **(a)** T2-weighted and **(b)** fluid-attenuated inversion recovery (FLAIR)-weighted coronal MRI section demonstrating characteristics of the cystic (*) and the solid (**) parts of a pediatric adamantinomatous type IV craniopharyngioma. The intracystic signal is hyperintense. The solid component appears heterogeneous. Calcifications can correlate with hypointensity (*white arrows*).

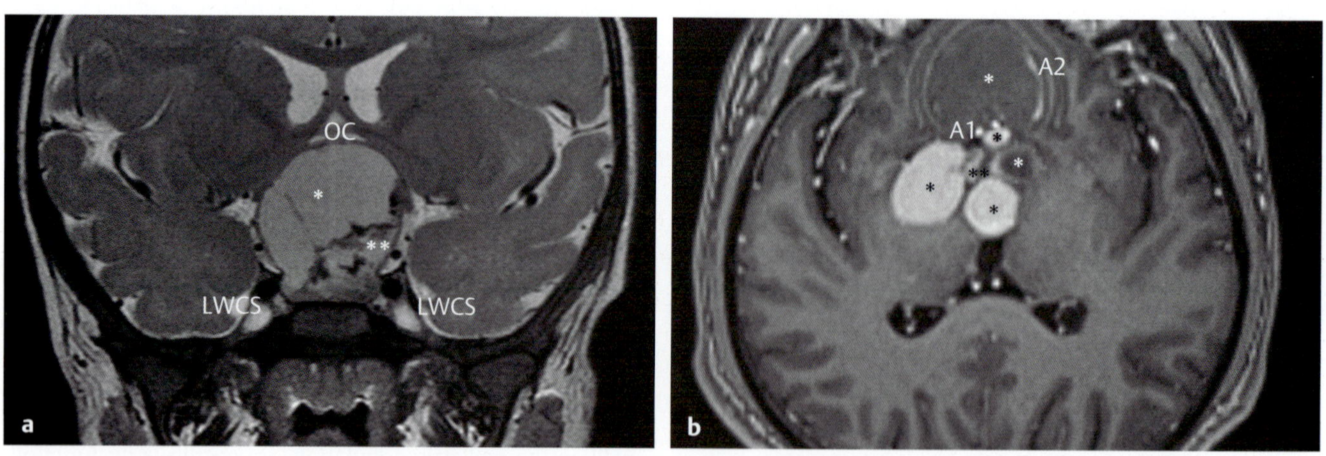

Fig. 7.13 **(a)** T2-weighted coronal and **(b)** T1-weighted contrast-enhanced axial MRI section demonstrating characteristics of the cystic (*) and the solid (**) parts of an adult adamantinomatous type IIIa/b craniopharyngioma. On T2-weighted images, the cyst content (*) is of high or mixed intensity. The solid parts (**) usually present themselves as iso- or hypointense. In T1-weighted contrast-enhanced sequences, the cystic elements (*) can be of high to intermediate to low intensity, reflecting the variable content of desquamated squamous epithelium with high protein concentration, while the solid parts (**) heterogeneously enhance after contrast enhancement.

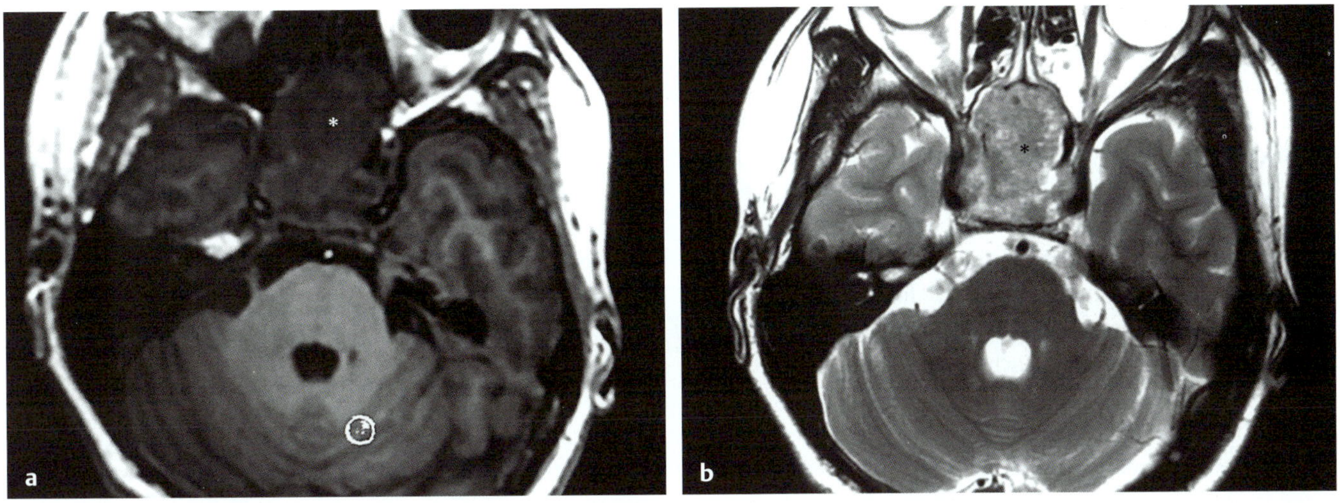

Fig. 7.14 **(a)** T1-weighted and **(b)** T2-weighted axial MRI section demonstrating characteristics of a large papillary craniopharyngioma in an adult patient extending into the sphenoid cavity. The solid elements of the papillary craniopharyngioma (*) are usually iso- or hypointense.

Special Considerations in Pediatric Craniopharyngioma

As previously described, childhood onset is different regarding histology and anatomy when compared to adult craniopharyngioma. The adamantinomatous type arises primarily in children.[19,58] The benign nature of these tumors implies that a total surgical excision leads to sufficient control and cure. Historically seen, the outcome on craniopharyngioma surgery was focused on vision, while endocrinological deficits were considered to be inevitable and normal.[9,48,65,66] Several series of surgically resected craniopharyngioma in the pediatric population demonstrate the burden and difficulties when treating such lesions. Yaşargil et al., for example, reported a 20% morbidity rate, while 60% of patients remained in good clinical condition.[29] Laws et al. reported successful results in 81%.[67] Mark et al. described a mortality rate of 12%, with a hypothalamic dysfunction rate of 40%, and visual deterioration in 19% in the pediatric population.[68] More recently, Sainte-Rose et al. reported GTR in 50%, STR in 36%, and partial resection in 14% of 66 consecutively treated pediatric craniopharyngiomas. One-third of patients with GTR did show recurrence and half of the studied population with residual tumor progressed within 7 years.[69]

In a meta-analysis by Clark et al. on 531 pediatric patients with craniopharyngioma, GTR was significantly associated with an increased rate of new endocrine dysfunction, panhypopituitarism, and new neurological deficits when compared with biopsy procedures. The latter was not found to be increased when following a STR strategy. GTR was associated with increased rates of diabetes insipidus when compared with STR and adjuvant radiotherapy. The latter was associated with increased rates of panhypopituitarism but otherwise similar rates of morbidities.[47]

In the past decades, concerns in terms of hypothalamic injury have been raised and were increasingly accounted as an unacceptable complication associated with the intention of GTR in the pediatric population. In an attempt to compare a cohort with GTR and a cohort with the goal of improved QOL and reduced morbidity, Thompson et al. focused on morbidity, mortality, and tumor recurrence in childhood craniopharyngioma. The authors concluded that they were able to improve the quality of outcome without compromising tumor recurrence based on a scoring grade for vision, cognition, motor function, hypothalamic dysfunction, and endocrine disturbances.[70] Experts in the field, such as Puget et al. hence advocate the preservation of function to be the more important therapeutic goal than just pure "cure of the disease," and thus recommend a less aggressive resection with adjuvant multimodal therapeutic options.[38,66]

In an intent to predict hypothalamic injury by surgical resection of craniopharyngiomas, Puget et al. correlated hypothalamic involvement in the preoperative MRI with postoperative morbidity to hypothalamic dysfunction in a retro- and prospective study of 103 patients with 66 eligible children.[38,66] As important findings, the preoperative radiological grade of hypothalamic involvement, the clinically assessed hypothalamic function, and the surgeon's operative experience showed a significant association with poor outcome. The same grading for hypothalamic involvement was used in a prospective cohort of 22 children with pediatric craniopharyngioma, where approximately 80%

were subtotally resected lesions or complete resection with avoidance of tumor dissection along the hypothalamic wall. Adjuvant radiotherapy was used in cases with indented residual lesions. With this strategy, the authors were able to avoid postoperative hyperphagia, morbid obesity, or behavioral dysfunction in all 22 children.[38] A large multicenter prospective study by Müller et al. confirmed the degree of hypothalamic involvement in the preoperative imaging as the only independent predictor for morbid obesity.[71] Nevertheless, the paradigm recommended was mainly based on transcranial approaches such as the transcallosal–transventricular, frontopterional, and subfrontal (uni- or bilateral) approaches.[38,66] With the development of extended EEA, a better hypothalamic exposure through a different surgical canal is possible, and new data have to confirm if this paradigm still remains feasible within the pediatric population.[58]

Puget et al. conclude that strategies to treat pediatric craniopharyngioma should be adapted to the degree of hypothalamic involvement, as previously described, to reduce postoperative morbidity in terms of morbid obesity. They recommend GTR to be feasible only for craniopharyngioma without hypothalamic involvement (type 0). If hypothalamic compression is present (type 1), the outcome of GTR will be influenced by the surgeon's experience. With hypothalamic involvement (type 2), STR with local adjuvant radiotherapy is recommended as appropriate management in childhood craniopharyngioma.[66]

Special Considerations in Adult Craniopharyngioma

In the adult population, the papillary craniopharyngiomas are found almost exclusively, more frequently located in the suprasellar and retrochiasmatic area.[19,58] Recommendations for tailored treatment strategies in adult patients with craniopharyngioma are based on less extensive data in the literature when compared with the pediatric population.[9,58,72] Thus, GTR or STR followed by watch and wait or adjuvant therapies has to be discussed on an individual basis considering topoanatomical and clinical factors, such as intra- or suprasellar extension and hypothalamic involvement. In parallel to the pediatric population, the benign biology of these tumors leads to a rather good long-term survival, but morbidities are relevant for the individual outcome and need regular follow-up and interdisciplinary management.[9,58,72] The most frequently reported morbidities in adults are long-term pituitary deficiencies, diabetes insipidus, and hypothalamic obesity.[73] Analogous to the pediatric population, a large study performed by Van Gompel et al. in 296 adult patients with craniopharyngioma demonstrated a good correlation of the degree of preoperative hypothalamic involvement and postoperative weight gain.[74] However, the concept of STR in adult patients has been controversial, as remnant tumor poses a risk of therapeutic failure when not responsive to radiotherapy. Some experts argue that treatment outcomes in pediatric studies might not be applicable to the adult population, as consequences of hypothalamic involvement and a potential worsening of preoperative morbid obesity might be different in children and adults.[58,75]

If GTR is a reasonable strategy in adult patients with hypothalamic involvement was studied in a small retrospective study by Apra et al. on 22 patients with craniopharyngioma operated via EEA. Fourteen out of these 22 patients (64%) underwent endonasal endoscopic GTR. Visual improvement occurred in 12 (63%) patients with 20 (91%) needing postoperative hormone replacement. Diabetes insipidus was present in 13 (65%) patients. No difference in weight gain was reported in the GTR when compared to the STR group.[58] According to the authors, this finding indicates that GTR of craniopharyngiomas in the adult population might not worsen a preoperative hypothalamic syndrome, even if the lesion invades the third ventricle.[58] They conclude that hypothalamic damage in adults may be caused by the tumor itself, as these findings are in contrast with findings in children operated by cranial approaches.[58] The same authors further conclude that the surgeon's experience is key in deciding when to stop the dissection, but achieving GTR whenever possible avoids tumor progression and radiotherapy.[58]

Potential Advantages of the Endonasal Endoscopic Approach

Tailoring the EEA using both nares for the surgical resection of craniopharyngioma allows a broader range of maneuvers. The binostril approach provides more flexibility for the ENT surgeon in terms of positioning of the endoscope and allows a two-surgeon four-hand technique.[76,77]

The extended endoscopic transnasal transsphenoidal approach provides direct midline access to lesions that extend along the anterior cranial base (planum sphenoidale), the chiasmatic region, the retrochiasmatic space, as well as the prepontine region. Thus, using the transplanum and transtuberculum approaches superiorly, and the transclival approach inferiorly may widen the standard transsphenoidal approach to deal with more extensive craniopharyngioma types.[78–80]

Endonasal endoscopic techniques provide an in-line access with superior visualization and illumination of the lesion and the relevant neurovascular structures like the optical chiasm, hypothalamus, and infundibular stalk.[23,32,33,35,81–88]

The possibility for the neurosurgeon to bimanually dissect using microsurgical instruments is of particular importance when addressing lesions like craniopharyngiomas that, when compared to pituitary adenoma, tend to adhere and be in close relationship with critical neurovascular structures and potential extension into the third ventricle.[89,90] Dho et al. describe the microdissection and preservation of the superior hypophyseal artery under direct surgical view being a possible explanation of the high rate of visual improvement besides direct decompression of the optic chiasm.[4] Other studies have reported better results in terms of hypothalamic dysfunction when using EEA,[66,91,92] mainly based on infradiaphragmatic lesions.[66,93] Difficulties when comparing surgical morbidities between transnasal endoscopic and transcranial approaches are the high influence of tumor location and heterogeneity, the extent of resection, and associated adjuvant treatment strategies that influence the relevant outcome parameters.[66]

However, studies comparing transcranial versus EEA revealed a trend toward better visual outcome for extended EEA.[23,94] A published series by Dho et al. described a GTR rate of 91.1% (62 of 68 patients) with an acceptable morbidity using EEA. There were no significant differences between the groups when using any of the classification systems.[4] A study by Madsen et al. did show similar, if not better, the extent of resection rates when using EEA. The authors further found significantly less incidence of postoperative weight gain with a fewer extent of ischemic injury, especially hypothalamic injury, when compared to transcranial open approaches.[66,95] GTR has the advantage of a low recurrence rate and thus no need for adjuvant therapy, such as radiotherapy. Several studies revealed that approximately 75 to 85% of patients who had visual impairment before surgery experienced significant improvement postoperatively.[31,34,35] Dho et al. reported a better visualization of the optic nerve and tumor with EEA when compared to transcranial approaches in cases where the tumor arose from the pituitary stalk. Tumor invasion into the center of the pituitary stalk affected the postoperative endocrine outcomes most significantly.[4]

Potential Disadvantages of the Endonasal Endoscopic Approach

The endoscopic endonasal transsphenoidal approach has limitations for suprasellar and high-riding lesions as well as lateral extension over the limitation of the clinoidal carotid artery. The relationship of the pituitary stalk and the tumor has to be taken into account when treating craniopharyngiomas with this approach.[4,90,96,97]

Preoperative Considerations

Every patient should get an endocrine diagnostic work-up since most patients have at least partial hypopituitarism. Hormone deficiencies should be replaced (Chapter 1). A detailed neuroopthalmological examination including visual acuity and visual field testing is also necessary.

The treatment and management of patients with craniopharyngioma is interdisciplinary. In larger institutions, the preoperative work-up of these patients involves endocrinologists, ophthalmologists, neurosurgeons, ENT surgeons, and neuroradiologists. Usually, patients are evaluated by multidisciplinary consensus at regularly held tumor boards. Adult patients with a severe preoperative hypothalamic syndrome and morbid obesity with relevant comorbidities potentially represent a contraindication for surgery because of the high risk of neurological and general complications.[58]

Endocrinological Assessment

Hypothalamic–pituitary hormonal function: Serum prolactin, total or free T4, thyroid-stimulating hormone (TSH), LH and FSH, free testosterone, estrogen and progesterone, morning cortisol 24-hour urinary-free cortisol, insulin-like growth factor.

Ophthalmological Assessment

Visual acuity and visual field using Goldman's perimetry as well as optometry in cases of double vision.

Neurological Assessment

Focal neurological deficits, neuropsychological changes in a large lesion with extrasellar extension with hypothalamic or frontal or temporal lobe involvement.

Rhinological Assessment

Endoscopic examination of the nose to rule out signs of infection, synechiae, or congenital anomalies.

Radiological Investigations

High-resolution (HR) MRI brain with image-guided surgery (IGS) protocol, HRCT scan of the paranasal sinuses if indicated.

Preoperative Radiological Considerations

The surgeon should systematically assess available imaging. This is of special importance when selecting surgical modalities and variations of the available approaches and tailoring the surgical corridor to reach the region of interest:

- *Nasal anatomy*: Signs of upper airway infection, septal deviations, signs of trauma.
- *Sphenoid anatomy*: Three-dimensional orientation (shelf, divider, wall) and insertion site (cavernous or paraclinoid internal carotid artery [ICA], opticocarotid recess, or optic nerves) of the sphenoid septations, mucosa, pneumatization pattern (sellar, presellar, or postsellar type), and bone thickness.
- *Cavernous carotid artery*: Space between carotid siphon (intercarotid distance), probable dehiscence, bulging into the sphenoid cavity.
- *Lesion*: Purely intrasellar, suprasellar, purely in the third ventricle or involving the third ventricle. Solid–cystic, extension of cysts, involvement of anterior skull base (frontal lobe) or clivus (prepontine cistern) region.
- *Neurovascular structures:*
  - ➢ *Main intracranial vessels involved*: Anterior cerebral artery (ACA) and branches, chiasmatic perforators, basilar artery and posterior cerebral artery (PCA), brainstem perforators.
  - ➢ *Relationship to the optic chiasm*:[26] Prechiasmatic, subchiasmatic, retrochiasmatic.
  - ➢ *Relationship to the third ventricle*:[30] Intraventricular, extraventricular, below the ventricle.
  - ➢ *Relationship to the diaphragma sellae*:[25] Sellar (infradiaphragmatic), suprasellar (supradiaphragmatic), sellar and suprasellar (infra- and supradiaphragmatic).
  - ➢ *Suprasellar extension and relationship to the infundibular stalk*:[23] Preinfundibular, transinfundibular (with extension into the stalk), retroinfundibular (extending behind the pituitary gland and stalk), extending into the third ventricle, extending into the interpeduncular cistern, or isolated to the third ventricle and/or optic recess.
  - ➢ *Relationship to the hypothalamus*: There are signs of hypothalamic displacement by the tumor or hypothalamic involvement.[38]
- *Recurrent case*: The presence or absence of endonasal structures has to be anticipated from preoperative imaging or endoscopy. Scars and adhesions can be present. The pituitary gland and infundibular stalk might not be identifiable in revision cases. Mucosal flaps over the surgical site or fat graft from the previous surgery. Branches of the ACA might have migrated near the sella and tumor residual because of scarring (sagittal plane T1 contrast-enhanced).

Selection of the Surgical Approach

Depending on the anatomical classification and relationship to critical neurovascular structures,[1,23,24,98–100] different surgical approaches are recommended and extensively described in the literature.[2–4,36] As previously discussed, the surgical treatment of craniopharyngioma remains challenging given the risk of recurrence and hypothalamic dysfunction following an aggressive GTR.[38,91,101] The extent of the lesion is used to determine the feasibility of a transsphenoidal resection. Entirely or mainly intrasellar craniopharyngioma and smaller lesions that were even unsuspected at the time of transsphenoidal surgery for a sellar mass were hence common indications for a surgical approach “from below.” Further on, the transsphenoidal approach was advocated when cyst drainage, biopsy, or a STR are the primary treatment concept.[12]

The selected approach is depending on the lesion’s anatomical extension and the surgeon’s preference. Classical transcranial approaches include the pterional–transsylvian for minimally superior extending lesions, or if extension into the interpeduncular cistern is present. In these cases, a wider splitting of the sylvian fissure is recommended. Some authors advocate taking the frontal bone opening more medial than usual to improve the visualization from a frontal and a temporal direction in the case of a suspected craniopharyngioma.[12,102] The bifrontal interhemispheric or transcortical approach has been described for lesions extending to the dorsal frontal lobe. The pterional or subfrontal transcallosal as well as the frontobasal interhemispheric approach have been described for suprasellar–parachiasmatic lesions.[12,91] The parasagittal transcallosal approaches are known to yield good results for lesions extending into the third ventricle.[29] More recently, minimally invasive keyhole approaches like the supraorbital eyebrow craniotomy have been proposed to remove these tumors depending on their extension.[29,103–105]

Retrochiasmatic craniopharyngiomas are challenging subset of tumors with a deep location and intimate proximity to critical neurovascular structures. Transcranial corridors are described as transbasal subfrontal, bifrontal interhemispheric, pterional, orbitopterional, supraorbital, or orbitozygomatic approaches.[90] The well-described conventional operative corridors through the interoptic and opticocarotid cisterns have their limitations in terms of the infra- and retrochiasmatic regions.[90,106,107] The translamina terminalis exposure has further been described to reach tumors in the retrochiasmatic region with anteriorly displaced or prefixed chiasm. Again, the limitation is the impaired visualization of the undersurface of the optic chiasm and optic nerves.[90,106,108] The posterior petrosal approach allows an upward trajectory with direct visualization of the hypothalamus and the infundibular stalk. Prolonged temporal lobe retraction and potential injury to the vein of Labbé, especially on the left side, contribute to relevant morbidity when using this approach.[90]

The transnasal transsphenoidal route provides a direct midline approach to the suprasellar region without any brain retraction.[109,110] Mainly infradiaphragmatic craniopharyngiomas with an enlarged sella have been operated using this approach. With the availability of extended EEA and the transplanum and transtuberculum approaches, more extensive lesions and retrochiasmatic tumors have been resected using this technique.[3,4]

In our institution, suprasellar lesions in the upper part or intraventricular lesions without intrasellar involvement are preferably operated via a transcranial route. If an endonasal endoscopic route is considered, the lesion should preferably involve the intrasellar or the lower suprasellar compartment. This provides a surgical corridor for the surgeon while resecting the tumor. Several topoanatomical and structural tumor characteristics might guide the surgeon's decision in the approach selection and surgical strategy:

- *Intrasellar extension*: Predominantly, intrasellar craniopharyngioma are the preferred indication in our institution. They provide optimal lesions for an endonasal endoscopic resection if they appear cystic and soft in the preoperative imaging. The relation to the infundibular stalk and the pituitary gland is of great importance when selecting this approach.[2,4]
- *Suprasellar extension*: The endonasal endoscopic resection of craniopharyngiomas extending into the suprasellar space can be considered if the tumor extends in the lower aspect of the suprasellar compartment. In this case, the relation to the infundibular stalk and the normal pituitary gland as well the absence of intervening vessels and the position of the optic chiasm have to be considered.[96]
- *Intratumoral calcification*: If the majority of the lesion is heavily calcified and located in the inferior compartments, removal through the endonasal route can be very difficult and crucial anatomical structures might not be identifiable. Ultrasonic aspiration is not possible in these cases.
- *Hypothalamic compression or involvement*: When cystic or solid components of a craniopharyngioma compress or involve the hypothalamic wall in preoperative MRI, postoperative hypothalamic injury is more likely. This might guide the surgeon's decision for GTR or STR in adult and especially in the pediatric population.[38,58,66]

When to prefer a transcranial approach for craniopharyngioma: The evidence of the transsphenoidal resection of craniopharyngioma, especially with the endoscopic technique, still remains somewhat equivocal, and transcranial approaches are well known and extensively described:[1,29,65,91,106,108]

- Suprasellar posterior to the infundibulum (pterional–transsylvian).
- Suprasellar–parachiasmatic (pterional or subfrontal, transcallosal, translamina terminalis).
- Retrochiasmatic (transpetrosal, transpetrosal–transtentorial).
- Dorsal frontal lobe (bifrontal interhemispheric or transcortical).
- Mainly in the third ventricle (transcallosal).

Presurgical Phase

Anesthesia, patient positioning, equipment, and ergonomical aspects for the endonasal endoscopic techniques have been described in Chapter 1.

Nasal Phase (Tailored Approach)

Endoscopic endonasal double nostril transseptal transsphenoidal approach

If a craniopharyngioma is suspected, a binostril approach is preferred in our institution, as two-surgeon four-hand maneuvers and bimanual microsurgical dissection are more likely to be necessary as compared to pituitary adenoma.

Osteodural Phase (Zonal Dissection)

The osteodural exposure can be tailored according to the anatomical configuration of the lesion. With the aid of IGS, a zonal dissection of the skull base to sufficiently expose the lesion is possible.

Extended Endoscopic Endonasal Transseptal Transsphenoidal Approach

As previously described, a common extension of the transsphenoidal transsellar approach consists of transtuberculum and transplanum as well as transclival expansions depending on the extension of the solid and cystic components of the craniopharyngioma (MRI sagittal plane).

Intradural Phase (Tumor resection)

Craniopharyngiomas are challenging lesions to resect microsurgically due to their geographical location, close proximity to important neurovascular structures, and adherences to the surrounding tissues (**Fig. 7.15** and **Fig. 7.16**). In our institution, certain nuances in terms of instrumental armamentarium are relevant when resecting craniopharyngiomas through an EEA:

- *Long slim ultrasonic aspirator*: Ultrasonic aspirators with high suction and low power modality are a useful tool to remove solid tumor components, dealing with remaining cystic parts, and reducing tumor mass along critical neurovascular structures in a controlled fashion. Calcifications can interfere with the ability to aspirate the solid tumor components.
- *Two-surgeon four-hand technique*: The two-surgeon four-hand technique allows the neurosurgeon to perform bimanual microsurgical dissection with either one suction and a microdissector or with two suctions. The ENT surgeon supports the dissection with gentle traction or elevation of tumor parts with a grasping instrument, while the neurosurgeon dissects the plane of capsule or solid tumor components from the neurovascular structures.
- *Sudden brain shift*: In larger lesions, the decompression of tumor cysts might cause a shift of the neurovascular structures and solid tumor components, and the intraoperative findings might potentially dyscorrelate with the presurgical radiological assessment.

Neurosurgical Considerations for Intradural Resection of Craniopharyngiomas

- The initial step of dissection defines a plane between the pituitary gland and tumor tissue. The pituitary gland can be mobilized back or sideways. Downward pressure is possible but might cause indirect tear of the infundibular stalk.
- The main dissection starts from the anterior aspect of the tumor continuing sideways and backward toward both ICAs.
- Further dissection is then performed following the tumor from the pituitary tumor junction with continuation forward toward both ICAs.

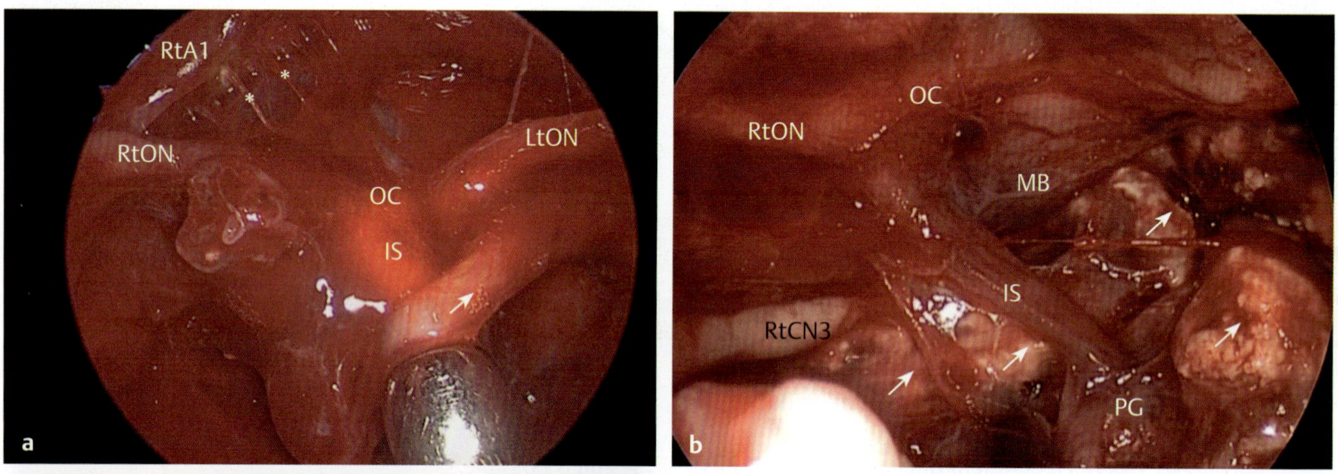

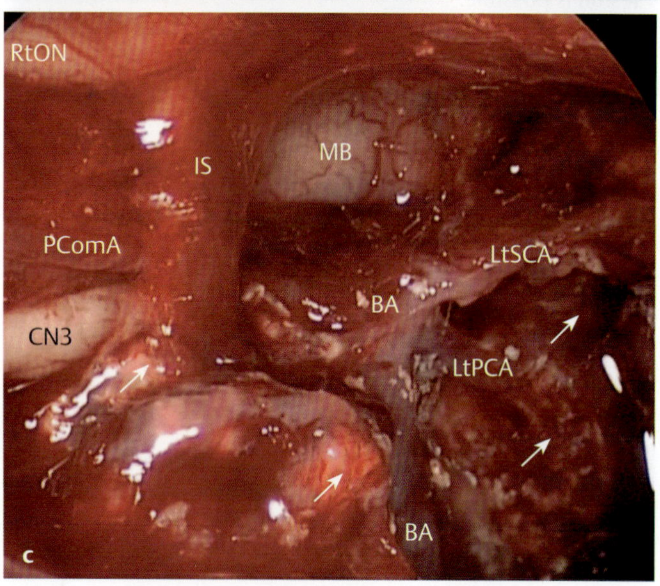

Fig. 7.15 Geographical location of craniopharyngiomas in the chiasmatic (suprasellar) region. **(a–c)** Endonasal endoscopic view of the chiasmatic (suprasellar) region during surgical resection of a pediatric adamantinomatous craniopharyngioma. The visualization of the relevant neurovascular structures involved by the tumor (*white arrows*) demonstrates the geographical location and the potential short-term and long-term morbidities associated with this disease. Surgical complications include hyponatremia because of diabetes insipidus caused by lesions of the infundibular stalk (IS) or the hypothalamus, visual impairment by lesioning the optic apparatus, long-term endocrine dysfunction with partial or panhypopituitarism by lesioning or resecting the pituitary gland (PG), cranial nerve dysfunction, and neurocognitive deficits. Vascular injuries and strokes are rare. Perforating arteries (*).

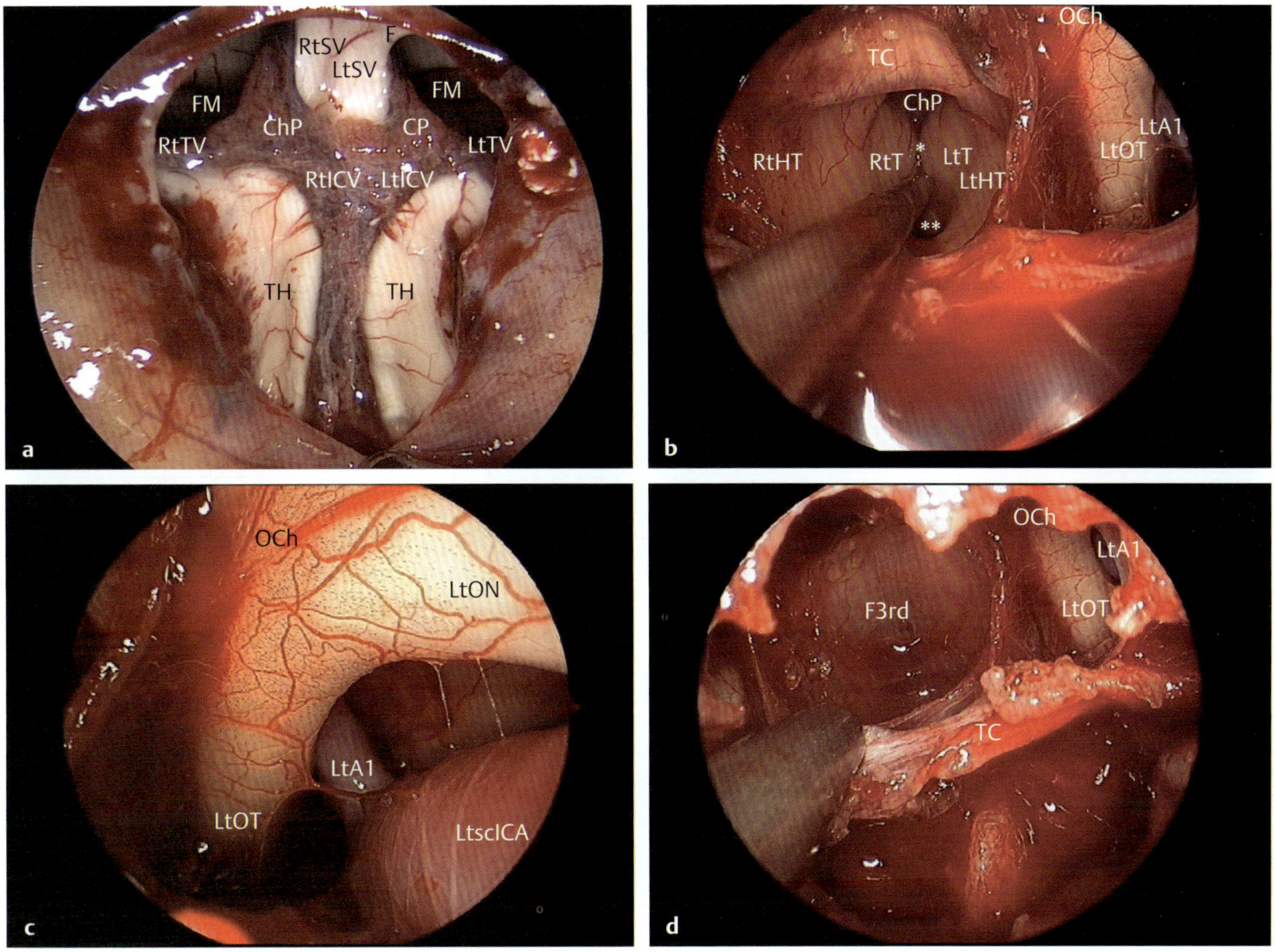

Fig. 7.16 Geographical location of craniopharyngiomas in the third ventricular region. **(a)** The anterior part of the third ventricle: The interventricular foramina of Monro (FM) are visible leading to the lateral ventricles, defined by the thalamus (TH) inferiorly and the fornix (F) superiorly. The choroid plexus (ChP) of the third ventricle is visible. The right (RtTV) and left (LtTV) thalamic vein are joining the right (RtSV) and left (LtSV) septal vein to form the right (RtICV) and left (LtICV) internal cerebral vein. **(b)** Endonasal endoscopic view of the third ventricle during surgical resection of a retrochiasmatic pediatric adamantinomatous craniopharyngioma demonstrating the posterior aspect of the third ventricle. The tumor capsule (TC) is still in situ. The left (LtHT) and right (RtHT) medial hypothalamic walls, the medial aspects of the left (LtT) and right (RtT) thalamus, the interthalamic connection (*) with the choroid plexus (ChP) of the third ventricle passing superior posterior to the latter are visible. The posterior recess of the third ventricle (**) leads to the cerebral aqueduct, posterior commissure, pineal recess, and habenular commissure. Laterally, the left optic tract (LtOT), the optic chiasm (OCh), and the left precommunicating anterior cerebral artery (LtA1) are visible. **(c)** Endonasal endoscopic projection lateral to the third ventricle toward the left side. The LtOT, the OC, and the left optic nerve (LtON) are visualized, together with the LtA1 arising from the left supraclinoid internal carotid artery (LtscICA). **(d)** After removal of the tumor capsule (TC), the floor of the third ventricle (F3rd) is visible. The LtOT, the OC, and the LtON are visualized, together with the LtA1.

Skull Base Defect Closure

The last step of the EEA is a watertight closure of the generated skull base defect. In craniopharyngioma and especially when resecting them with an extended zonal dissection of the skull base, adequate closure techniques are of crucial importance. Several techniques of a graded defect closure and postoperative care have been described in Chapter 1.

Craniopharyngioma Recurrence

Even though being benign, craniopharyngiomas generally have a recurrence rate of approximately 10 to 15% over time.

A study by Klimo et al. reported a tumor recurrence rate of 18% within a median time to recurrence of 4.2 years.[111] The most significant factor associated with recurrence is the extent of resection, while histopathological subtype and brain invasion are less relevant in totally resected tumors.[4,101] One study found cyst size to be a significant predictor of recurrence rate for craniopharyngoma.[112] The management of recurrent or residual craniopharyngiomas remains controversial. Generally, reoperation or radiation provides common retreatment options. Radiation therapy is effective to control solid tumors as compared to associated cysts.[111,113,114]

Several studies on reoperation in recurrent craniopharyngioma report a higher risk of complications and lower extents of resection, leading to a preference in radiation therapy in these cases.[63,114–116] The extent of resection in recurrent cases seems to impact the preoperative tumor volume and prior radiation therapy.[115] A study by Cavallo et al. on 22 recurrent craniopharyngioma cases reoperated via an extended EEA reported total removal in 9 patients (40.9%) and near-total removal (defined as >95% resection rate) in 8 patients (36.4%). Subtotal removal (>70%) was achieved in 4 patients (18.2%), and less than 50% was possible in only 1 case (4.5%).[117]

In the case of recurrence after STR and radiotherapy, surgery remains the therapy of choice. Respectively, surgery is reported to be difficult in this situation because of the severe adhesions.[4,25,115]

Neurosurgical Considerations for Intradural Resection of Recurrent Craniopharyngioma

In case of a recurrent craniopharyngioma, an adequate exposure is mandatory to manage sufficient extent of resection while visualizing all relevant neurovascular structures and potential cerebrospinal fluid (CSF) leaks.

Nasal Phase (Tailored Approach)

- Lateralization of the middle turbinates.
- Wide sphenoidotomy and posterior ethmoidectomy or definition of the remaining bony borders in the case of reoperation (rostrum sphenoidale, posterior ethmoid, cribriform plate).
- Raise of a previously placed nasoseptal flap with meticulous identification and dissection along the maintained bony structures. The use of IGS is very helpful in these cases. Adhesions, scaring, and dehiscence of neurovascular structure have to be considered. The vascular pedicle of the previously used nasoseptal flap has to be maintained, if replacement of the same flap is considered.
- Raise of a new ipsilateral (if not used previously) or contralateral vascularized nasoseptal flap for subsequent reconstruction.

Osteodural Exposure (Zonal Dissection)

- Transsella, transtuberculum, and transplanum sphenoidale defined by IGS.
- Lateral opticocarotid recesses as landmarks and medial opticocarotid recesses as lateral limitation of the osteodural exposure.
- Cauterization and dissection of the anterior intercavernous sinus.

Intradural Phase (Tumor Resection)

- Sufficient internal debulking of solid tumor parts.
- Meticulous separation of tumor parts from adjacent neurovascular structures using sharp microdissection.
- Preservation of the pituitary gland, the infundibular stalk, and superior hypophyseal arteries, resection in cases where GTR is the goal of the operation.
- With suprasellar extension, the roof of the third ventricle and identification of the foramina of Monro are important anatomical landmarks.

In a prospective study by Dhandapani et al. on 22 recurrent craniopharyngioma patients operated by an EEA, similar extent of resection, visual outcome, and improvement in QOL were found without a significant increase in complications when compared to a control group with first operations.[115] The authors conclude that reoperations are a safe option for patients with recurrent craniopharyngiomas and may even be preferable when GTR can be achieved, in comparison to radiation only.[115] A more recent study by Dho et al. on the other hand found lower rates of GTR in the group with recurrence when compared to primary resected tumors, with a lower rate of visual improvement and a higher rate of postoperative infections in recurrent cases.[4]

Nonsurgical Treatment Modalities

Although GTR should be the goal when surgically treating craniopharyngioma, the consequences of traction in an effort to aggressively strip the capsule away from crucial neurovascular structures might cause a high rate of morbidity with a significantly worse outcome. Hence, the recommendation is to leave adherent tumor to the optic apparatus, the pituitary stalk, and especially the walls of the hypothalamus. Another strategy consists of staged operations with initial endonasal resection and transcranial completion.

Symptomatic Treatment of Craniopharyngioma Cysts

Obstructive hydrocephalus or tumor cyst might lead to a rapid onset of raised intracranial pressure or visual loss. In these cases, an initial minimally invasive decompression with transventricular endoscopic marsupialization and intracystic catheters is indicated. Puget et al. reported emergency cyst drainage using an Ommaya reservoir placement (30 out of 66) or endoscopic fenestrations (3 out of 66) in 55% of the included children, prior to surgical resection (**Fig. 7.17**).[38]

If a tumor cyst cannot be completely resected and causes symptoms because of compression of visual or hypothalamic structures or obstruction of the third ventricle, transventricular endoscopic marsupialization may be an additional treatment option. Percutaneous aspiration of cyst contents has also been used to alleviate symptoms (**Fig. 7.18**).[118,119] An alternative is to place a subcutaneous reservoir system for intermittent aspiration of cyst content.[120] Purely cystic tumors may be managed with the placement of a catheter to allow repeated aspiration alone.

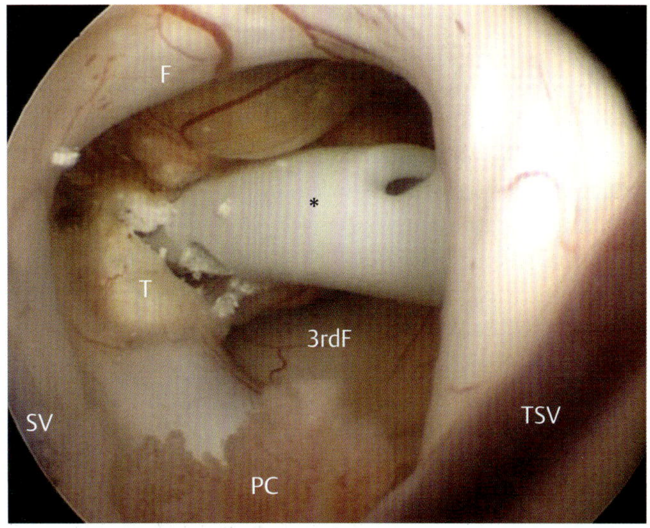

Fig. 7.17 Right-sided ventriculoscopy visualizing the third ventricle and a previously placed intracystic catheter (*) to relieve intracystic pressure in a patient with obstructive hydrocephalus. The ventriculoscopy was indicated after the recurrence of a tumor cyst causing a new cranial nerve deficit.

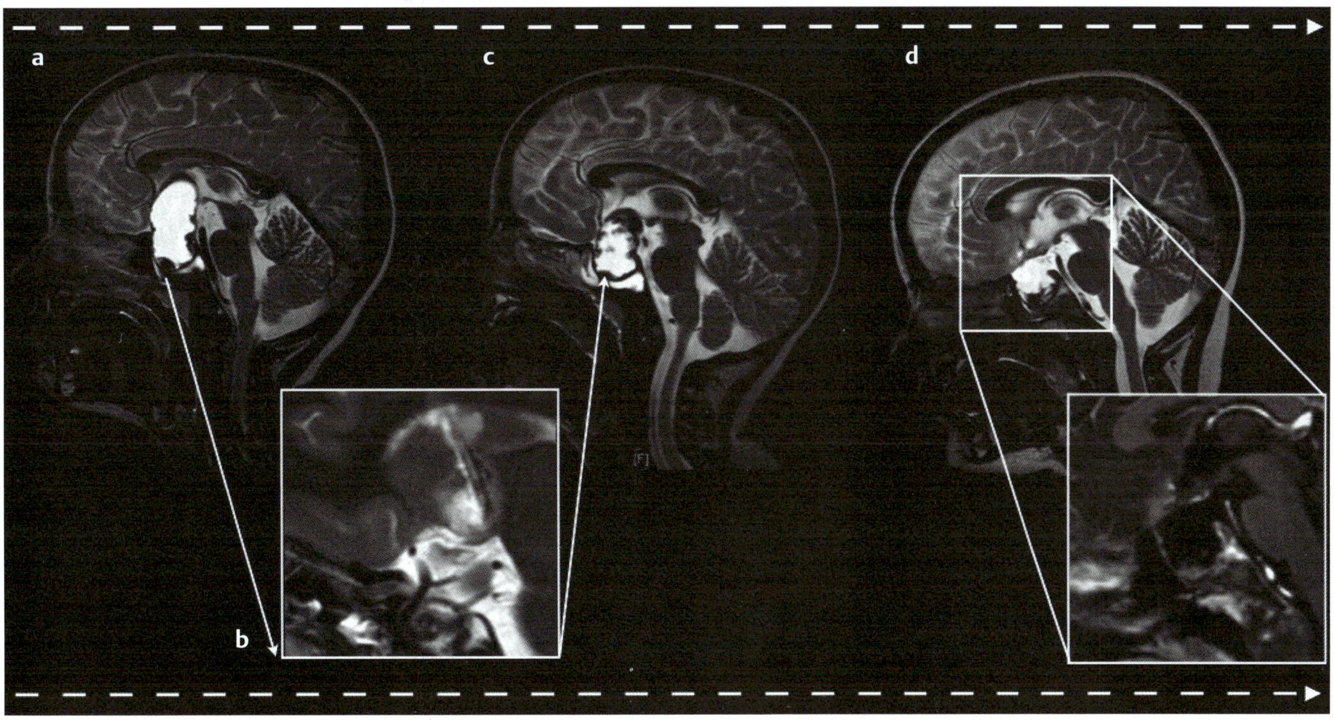

Fig. 7.18 Multimodal management of a pediatric adamantinomatous type IIIa craniopharyngioma. **(a)** T2-weighted sagittal MRI section demonstrating a solid–cystic sellar tumor with a large suprasellar cystic component (2.1 x 4.8 cm) at the time-point of presentation. **(b)** Initial insertion of an intracystic catheter with Ommaya's reservoir. **(c)** T2-weighted sagittal MRI section demonstrating the collapsed cystic component being smaller in size (1.8 x 3.5 cm). **(d)** Four months after the initial treatment, the tumor was subtotally resected using a transcranial approach. The tumor residual demonstrates the limitation of the transcranial resection with residual solid tumor along the floor of the sella turcica.

Intracavitary irradiation via stereotactically applied radioisotopes (yttrium-90 and phosphorus-32) is another possible treatment option for the management of symptomatic cysts.[121–126] As an alternative to intracavitary irradiation, intracavitary chemotherapy has been used. A study with the application of intracystic bleomycin in 100 patients reported a 94% response rate with a duration of less than a year in 47% of the treated individuals.[127–130] Intracystic INF-alpha, theoretically activating apoptosis, was used in 21 children, of which 11 (52%) demonstrated a complete and 7 (33%) a partial response. Resection was reported to be easier after INF-alpha treatment.[131–133] However, because of the low evidence of these therapy options, they do not reach enough strength to be recommended.[66]

If a nontraumatic resection of the tumor from the hypothalamic walls is less likely to be possible, symptomatic treatment of tumor cysts with minimally invasive procedures, STR, and radiosurgical treatment are established options.[38,58,66]

External Beam and Conformal Radiotherapy

Radiation therapy is recommended for the treatment of patients with the residual tumor or tumor recurrence.[134,135] Adjuvant radiation therapy after STR significantly reduces the risk of local recurrence.[136,137] Radiotherapy potentially provides long-term tumor control for childhood-onset craniopharyngioma, more recently reaching approximately 80% disease control at 10 years and favorable functional outcome in 42 to 86%.[64,66,138,139]

Radiation therapy can be delivered in multiple fractions (fractionated radiation therapy, requires 25–30 treatments) or in a single large dose (stereotactic radiosurgery). Merchant et al. reported a 36-month median follow-up of 28 children treated with conformal radiation therapy (54–55.8 Gy) with a 3-year progression-free survival of 90.3%.[139] Pemberton et al. treated 87 patients (28 children) with external beam radiation therapy (42 Gy) and reported a 10- and 20-year survival of 86 and 76% with a corresponding 10- and 20-year progression-free survival of 78 and 66%, respectively.[140] Thus, conformal radiation therapy can be considered as the most appropriate radiation technique with additionally documented reduced neurocognitive dysfunction when compared to conventional external beam radiotherapy.[64,66,134,135,139,141] In an adult series of 116 patients with craniopharyngioma resected using an extended EEA by Park et al., the overall tumor recurrence rate was 15.5%, with a median interval of 14.5 months. The patients who underwent a near-total resection or STR followed by adjuvant radiotherapy had a similar median recurrence-free survival rate compared with those who underwent GTR (26.5 vs. 20 months).[142]

For each technique, care must be taken to keep the dose within the tolerance of the optic nerves, chiasm, and tracts. It is important that irradiation is targeted to a mostly solid lesion with cystic components aspirated or resected prior to irradiation. Documented long-term sequelae of irradiation are visual deterioration, hypothalamic–pituitary dysfunction, cerebrovascular diseases including moyamoya syndrome (up to 21%), secondary tumor genesis (1.9% at 10 years), cavernous malformation, and cognitive decline.[66,139,143]

Proton Beam Therapy

Newer studies reported less documented neurocognitive disorders and less late effects on the optic pathways and hypothalamus with proton beam therapy (**Fig. 7.19**).[66,144–146] Fitzek et al. reported long-term results of combined proton and photon irradiation for craniopharyngioma with an actuarial 10-year survival rate of 72% and an actuarial 5- and 10-year local control rate of 93 and 85%, respectively. A preliminary report by Luu et al. on fractionated proton radiation treatment reported local control in 14 of 15 patients, while 12 out of 15 patients survived.[66,144–146]

Molecular Targeted Therapy

Adamantinomatous craniopharyngiomas are mostly driven by activation of the WNT signaling pathway and the majority harbor activating mutations in *CTNNB1*. By contrast, papillary craniopharyngiomas commonly carry mutations in the *BRAF* oncogene, a potential target for molecular therapy with *BRAF* inhibitors like murafenib and dabrafenib in the near future.[147–149]

Management of Complications

Childhood- and adult-onset initial hypothalamic tumor involvement predicts the lifelong effect on the clinical course. Hence, craniopharyngioma constitutes a chronic disease requiring constant monitoring to provide optimal QOL.[9]

Short-term surgical complications are hydrocephalus, meningitis (3%), CSF leakage (5–10%), hyponatremia, seizures, visual impairment, ICA injuries (<1%), and stroke (<1%). Long-term complications of treatment for craniopharyngiomas include mostly endocrine, neurological, and visual complications.[150] Hence, follow-up monitoring of endocrine deficiencies along with osteodensitometry, visual fields and optometry, early weight control programs, and a multidisciplinary care concept are very relevant when managing these adult patients with totally or subtotally resected craniopharyngioma.[73]

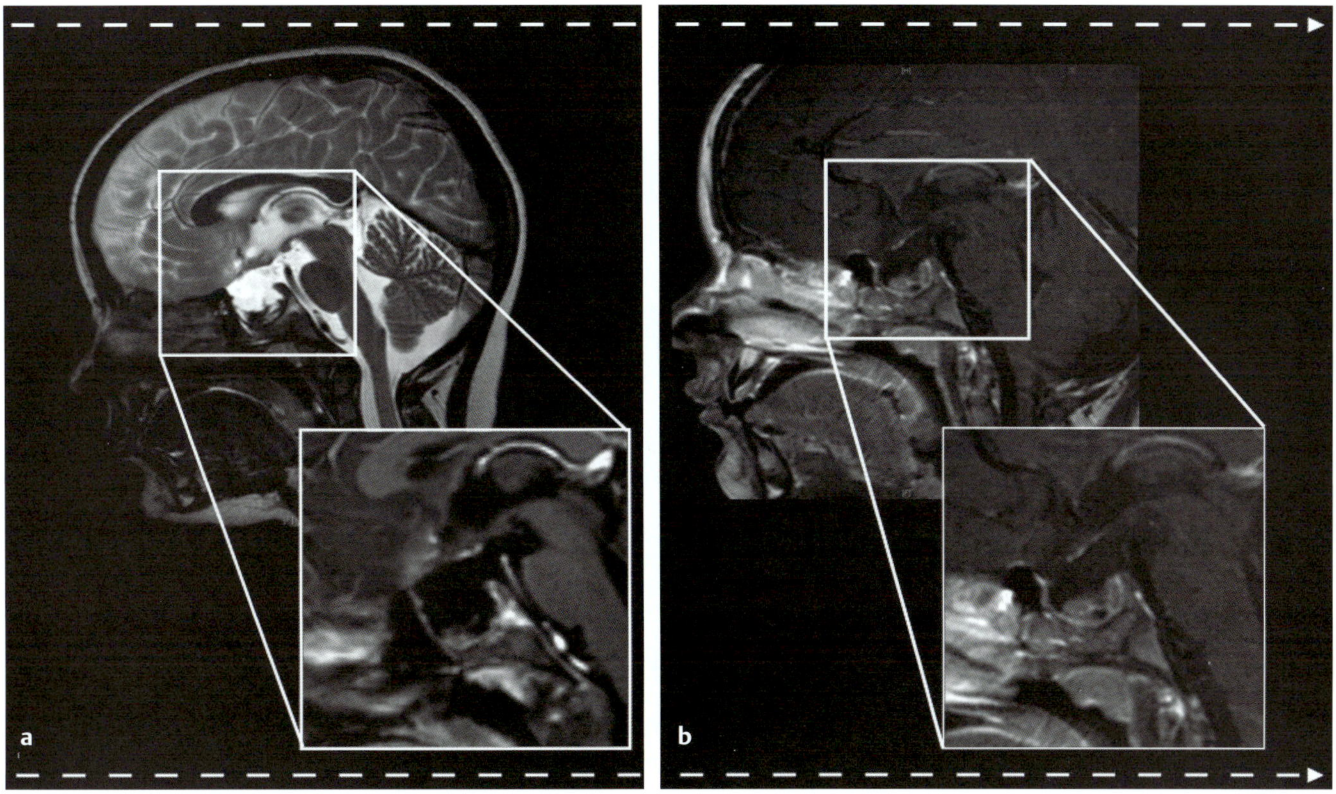

Fig. 7.19 T2- and T1-weighted contrast-enhanced sagittal MRI sections during the postoperative course of a multimodally treated pediatric adamantinomatous type IIIa craniopharyngioma. **(a)** Tumor residual along the sellar floor 4 months after subtotal resection using a transcranial approach. **(b)** A 12-month postoperative control reveals the regrowth of the residual tumor. The patient was referred for proton beam therapy to radiate the residual tumor.

Anterior Pituitary Deficiency

Anterior pituitary lobe dysfunction may become apparent postoperatively and is believed to be secondary to excessive use of the tumor aspirator in the sellar cavity, inappropriate manipulation and resection of the normal pituitary gland adjacent to the adenoma, and use of bipolar cauterization in the sellar cavity after the tumor removal. Hypothyroidism and ACTH deficiency can occur in children with craniopharyngioma following surgical resection with or without concomitant radiation therapy and is more frequently detected during posttreatment assessments.[12,41,45,46] Hence, appropriate postoperative screening, detection, and replacement is necessary, and an appropriate stress dosing should be used as needed.[12]

Posterior Pituitary Gland Disturbances

The incidence of disturbances of the neurohypophysis is much higher postoperatively. Some authors have correlated early postoperative deaths in pediatric craniopharyngioma patients with severe electrolyte disturbances.[41,42,44,45] Diabetes insipidus can occur due to temporary dysfunction of vasopressin-producing neurons secondary to surgical trauma and thermal injury of cautery or a dysfunction of posterior pituitary gland; however, recovery is reported to occur within 6 months. It is imperative to screen electrolytes, fluid intake, and urinary output as well as serum and urine osmolarity in the postoperative period and aggressively manage a potential diabetes insipidus with DDAVP.[12]

Postoperative diabetes insipidus is considered as a potential marker for the development of hypothalamic obesity.[73] Andereggen et al. followed up 32 adult patients with craniopharyngioma within a median follow-up of 10 years. During this period, hypothalamic obesity increased over time while long-term pituitary deficiencies remained high. On the other side, they found that postoperative diabetes insipidus, and not hypothalamic involvement, was an independent predictor for hypothalamic obesity.[73] Endocrinopathies, including diabetes insipidus, showed the worst prognosis after surgery.[112]

Pathological Bone Density in Osteodensitometry

Andereggen et al. followed up 32 adult patients with craniopharyngioma within a median follow-up of 10 years. In two-thirds of patients, osteodensitometry was performed and confirmed pathological bone density in half of them at last available follow-up.[73]

Hypothalamic Dysfunction after Gross Total Resection

Complications due to hypothalamic dysfunction are present in 65 to 80% of children with GTR. It causes disabling obesity (55%) because of hyperphagia, the autonomous nervous system dysregulation, disorders of temperature regulation, sleep disorders, or diabetes insipidus. Long-term complications of obesity include metabolic syndrome, type 2 diabetes mellitus, and fatty liver disease.[151–153] Notably, this complication and its sequelae significantly influence the QOL.[48] Treatment options for patients suffering from hypothalamic syndrome remain limited. Data on bariatric surgery suggest this therapy option to be the most tolerable and effective in weight reduction for severely obese adult patients.[9,154]

Neurological and Neuropsychological Outcome

Common neurological complications after surgery for craniopharyngiomas include visual disturbances, cranial nerve deficits, neurocognitive deficits (e.g., short-term memory deficits, limited concentration span), and behavioral problems, in particular, in patients with hypothalamic involvement.

- *Visual complications:* Most patients have ophthalmological deficits prior to surgery. These deficits may be exacerbated after surgery and/or radiation therapy. In a retrospective study by Giese et al. on 71 transcranially resected patients, visual acuity was significantly improved in 23 (32%), and remained stable in 32 (45%) patients.[155]
- *Neurocognitive deficits:* Patients frequently complain about neuropsychological deficits including fatigue, avolition, memory, and concentration.[48,113,156] In a retrospective study by Apra et al. on 22 adult patients with craniopharyngioma undergoing surgery with EEA, the cognitive status was stable or improved in all patients except for one.[58] A study by Giese et al. reported 27 out of 36 (75%) prospectively assessed transcranially resected craniopharyngioma patients with neuropsychological deviations in at least one test item, particularly attentiveness, cognitive speed, and short-term memory.[155]
- *Quality of life:* QOL is significantly affected in patients with craniopharyngioma, when morbid obesity is present.[48] The study by Giese et al. on 36 prospectively assessed transcranially resected craniopharyngioma patients reported affection in the mental score in 19.4% and one-third in the physical score. The risk factors affecting the QOL were a tumor volume larger than 9 cm^3, involvement of the third ventricle or the brainstem, and resection using a bifrontal translamina terminalis or left-sided approach. If endonasal endoscopic techniques contribute to less impairment by using a different corridor, or if the disease itself has this postoperative burden, remains to be shown in larger studies comparing outcomes in transcranial and endoscopic techniques.[155]

Further Long-term Complications

A variety of vascular abnormalities (temporal cavernomas, moyamoya syndrome, aneurysms, decrease in vessel caliber) can follow radiation therapy of pediatric craniopharyngioma.[143] Patients may also be at increased risk for ischemic attack or stroke after multimodal treatment.[152,157] Long-term follow-up have shown an association of radiation therapy with the secondary development of meningioma and malignant glial tumors.[157,158]

Overall Survival

Overall survival and QOL are impaired when hypothalamic involvement is present. In a large study with 216 patients (HIT-Endo trial), the 20-year overall survival was lower in patients with hypothalamic involvement compared to patients without hypothalamic involvement.[159]

Pearls and Points

- Craniopharyngiomas do not display a benign behavior, although they are classified as WHO grade I tumors.
- Total resection must remain the goal for those craniopharyngiomas that do not involve hypothalamic structures.
- More recently, the hypothalamic involvement of craniopharyngiomas has been considered to be relevant for the functional outcome of especially the pediatric population.
- For many children with craniopharyngiomas, the cost of resection is hypothalamic dysfunction and a poor QOL.

- The current treatment of craniopharyngiomas is evolving into one of a multimodal approach in which the aim is disease control and improved preservation of QOL.
- Patient with incomplete resected craniopharyngioma should preferably receive radiation therapy rather than observation with salvage radiation therapy in case of recurrent disease (level of evidence 1B).
- There is increasing advocacy among experts for limited resection followed by radiotherapy especially in the pediatric population.
- Whether outcome data based on pediatric craniopharyngioma with transcranial resection can be applied on either adult patients or the endonasal endoscopic surgery remains controversial and further data have to clarify this.
- Resection of craniopharyngiomas is frequently associated with postoperative neuropsychological deficits, long-term pituitary dysfunction, and an impaired QOL.

Acknowledgments

This chapter was written based on funding from the Martin Allgöwer Foundation, Department of Surgery, University Hospital of Basel (Basel, Switzerland) and the Gottfried and Julia Bangerter-Rhyner Foundation (Bern, Switzerland). The Departments of Neurosurgery of the University Hospital of Basel (Basel, Switzerland) and the Departments of Neurosurgery and Oto-Rhino-Lanryngology of the University of Malaya (Kuala Lumpur, Malaysia) supported the creation of this chapter.

References

1. Hoffman HJ. Surgical management of craniopharyngioma. Pediatr Neurosurg 1994;21(Suppl 1):44–49
2. Tang B, Xie S, Huang G, et al. Clinical features and operative technique of transinfundibular craniopharyngioma. J Neurosurg 2019;:1–10
3. Fernandez-Miranda JC, Gardner PA, Snyderman CH, et al. Craniopharyngioma: a pathologic, clinical, and surgical review. Head Neck 2012;34(7):1036–1044
4. Dho YS, Kim YH, Se YB, et al. Endoscopic endonasal approach for craniopharyngioma: the importance of the relationship between pituitary stalk and tumor. J Neurosurg 2018;129(3): 611–619
5. Elfers CT, Roth CL. Effects of methylphenidate on weight gain and food intake in hypothalamic obesity. Front Endocrinol (Lausanne) 2011;2:78
6. Lustig RH. Hypothalamic obesity after craniopharyngioma: mechanisms, diagnosis, and treatment. Front Endocrinol (Lausanne) 2011;2:60
7. Roth CL. Hypothalamic obesity in craniopharyngioma patients: disturbed energy homeostasis related to extent of hypothalamic damage and its implication for obesity intervention. J Clin Med 2015;4(9):1774–1797
8. Roth CL. Hypothalamic obesity in patients with craniopharyngioma: profound changes of several weight regulatory circuits. Front Endocrinol (Lausanne) 2011;2:49
9. Müller HL. Craniopharyngioma—a childhood and adult disease with challenging characteristics. Front Endocrinol (Lausanne) 2012;3:80
10. Zada G, Lin N, Ojerholm E, Ramkissoon S, Laws ER. Craniopharyngioma and other cystic epithelial lesions of the sellar region: a review of clinical, imaging, and histopathological relationships. Neurosurg Focus 2010;28(4):E4
11. Louis DP, Reifenberger G. WHO Classification of Tumours of the Central Nervous System. IARC; 2016
12. Snyder BJ, Naidich TP, Post KD. Cystic Lesions of the Sella. Totowa, NJ:Humana Press; 2008
13. Bao Y, Pan J, Qi ST, Lu YT, Peng JX. Origin of craniopharyngiomas: implications for growth pattern, clinical characteristics, and outcomes of tumor recurrence. J Neurosurg 2016;125(1):24–32
14. Capper D, Jones DTW, Sill M, et al. DNA methylation-based classification of central nervous system tumours. Nature 2018;555(7697):469–474
15. Bunin GR, Surawicz TS, Witman PA, Preston-Martin S, Davis F, Bruner JM. The descriptive epidemiology of craniopharyngioma. Neurosurg Focus 1997;3(6):e1
16. Bunin GR, Surawicz TS, Witman PA, Preston-Martin S, Davis F, Bruner JM. The descriptive epidemiology of craniopharyngioma. J Neurosurg 1998;89(4):547–551
17. Gejman R, Tessa Hedley-Whyte E. Pathology of Pituitary Adenomas. Totowa, NJ:Humana Press; 2008
18. Müller HL, Merchant TE, Puget S, Martinez-Barbera JP. New outlook on the diagnosis, treatment and follow-up of childhood-onset craniopharyngioma. Nat Rev Endocrinol 2017;13(5): 299–312
19. Hölsken A, Sill M, Merkle J, et al. Adamantinomatous and papillary craniopharyngiomas are characterized by distinct epigenomic as well as mutational and transcriptomic profiles. Acta Neuropathol Commun 2016;4:20
20. Feng Y, Ni M, Wang YG, Zhong LY. Comparison of neuroendocrine dysfunction in patients with adamantinomatous and papillary craniopharyngiomas. Exp Ther Med 2019;17(1):51–56
21. Malgulwar PB, Nambirajan A, Pathak P, et al. Study of β-catenin and BRAF alterations in adamantinomatous and papillary craniopharyngiomas: mutation analysis with immunohistochemical correlation in 54 cases. J Neurooncol 2017; 133(3):487–495

22. Choi SH, Kwon BJ, Na DG, Kim JH, Han MH, Chang KH. Pituitary adenoma, craniopharyngioma, and Rathke cleft cyst involving both intrasellar and suprasellar regions: differentiation using MRI. Clin Radiol 2007;62(5):453–462

23. Kassam AB, Gardner PA, Snyderman CH, Carrau RL, Mintz AH, Prevedello DM. Expanded endonasal approach, a fully endoscopic transnasal approach for the resection of midline suprasellar craniopharyngiomas: a new classification based on the infundibulum. J Neurosurg 2008;108(4):715–728

24. Pascual JM, Carrasco R, Prieto R, Gonzalez-Llanos F, Alvarez F, Roda JM. Craniopharyngioma classification. J Neurosurg 2008; 109(6):1180–1182, author reply 1182–1183

25. Wang KC, Hong SH, Kim SK, Cho BK. Origin of craniopharyngiomas: implication on the growth pattern. Childs Nervous System 2005;21:628–634

26. Wang KC, Kim SK, Choe G, Chi JG, Cho BK. Growth patterns of craniopharyngioma in children: role of the diaphragm sellae and its surgical implication. Surg Neurol 2002;57(1):25–33

27. Tang B, Xie SH, Xiao LM, et al. A novel endoscopic classification for craniopharyngioma based on its origin. Sci Rep 2018;8(1): 10215

28. Zhou L, You C. Craniopharyngioma classification. J Neurosurg 2009;111(1):197–199, author reply 199

29. Yaşargil MG, Curcic M, Kis M, Siegenthaler G, Teddy PJ, Roth P. Total removal of craniopharyngiomas. Approaches and long-term results in 144 patients. J Neurosurg 1990;73(1):3–11

30. Steno J, Malácek M, Bízik I. Tumor-third ventricular relationships in supradiaphragmatic craniopharyngiomas: correlation of morphological, magnetic resonance imaging, and operative findings. Neurosurgery 2004;54(5):1051–1058, discussion 1058–1060

31. Campbell PG, McGettigan B, Luginbuhl A, Yadla S, Rosen M, Evans JJ. Endocrinological and ophthalmological consequences of an initial endonasal endoscopic approach for resection of craniopharyngiomas. Neurosurg Focus 2010; 28(4):E8

32. Cavallo LM, Frank G, Cappabianca P, et al. The endoscopic endonasal approach for the management of craniopharyngiomas: a series of 103 patients. J Neurosurg 2014; 121(1):100–113

33. Frank G, Pasquini E, Doglietto F, et al. The endoscopic extended transsphenoidal approach for craniopharyngiomas. Neurosurgery 2006;59(1, Suppl 1):ONS75–ONS83, discussion ONS75–ONS83

34. Koutourousiou M, Gardner PA, Fernandez-Miranda JC, Tyler-Kabara EC, Wang EW, Snyderman CH. Endoscopic endonasal surgery for craniopharyngiomas: surgical outcome in 64 patients. J Neurosurg 2013;119(5):1194–1207

35. Leng LZ, Greenfield JP, Souweidane MM, Anand VK, Schwartz TH. Endoscopic, endonasal resection of craniopharyngiomas: analysis of outcome including extent of resection, cerebrospinal fluid leak, return to preoperative productivity, and body mass index. Neurosurgery 2012;70(1):110–123, discussion 123–124

36. Mortini P, Losa M, Pozzobon G, et al. Neurosurgical treatment of craniopharyngioma in adults and children: early and long-term results in a large case series. J Neurosurg 2011;114(5): 1350–1359

37. Qi S, Pan J, Lu Y, et al. The impact of the site of origin and rate of tumour growth on clinical outcome in children with craniopharyngiomas. Clin Endocrinol (Oxf) 2012;76(1): 103–110

38. Puget S, Garnett M, Wray A, et al. Pediatric craniopharyngiomas: classification and treatment according to the degree of hypothalamic involvement. J Neurosurg 2007;106(1, Suppl):3–12

39. Garnett MR, Puget S, Grill J, Sainte-Rose C. Craniopharyngioma. Orphanet J Rare Dis 2007;2:18

40. Duff J, Meyer FB, Ilstrup DM, Laws ER Jr, Schleck CD, Scheithauer BW. Long-term outcomes for surgically resected craniopharyngiomas. Neurosurgery 2000;46(2):291–302, discussion 302–305

41. Sklar CA. Craniopharyngioma: endocrine abnormalities at presentation. Pediatr Neurosurg 1994;21(Suppl 1):18–20

42. Halac I, Zimmerman D. Endocrine manifestations of craniopharyngioma. Childs Nervous System 2005;21: 640–648

43. Banna M, Hoare RD, Stanley P, Till K. Craniopharyngioma in children. J Pediatr 1973;83(5):781–785

44. Paja M, Lucas T, García-Uría J, Salamé F, Barceló B, Estrada J. Hypothalamicpituitary dysfunction in patients with craniopharyngioma. Clin Endocrinol (Oxf) 1995;42(5):467–473

45. Sklar CA. Craniopharyngioma: endocrine sequelae of treatment. Pediatr Neurosurg 1994;21(Suppl 1):120–123

46. de Vries L, Lazar L, Phillip M. Craniopharyngioma: presentation and endocrine sequelae in 36 children. J Pediatr Endocrinol Metab 2003;16(5):703–710

47. Clark AJ, Cage TA, Aranda D, Parsa AT, Auguste KI, Gupta N. Treatment-related morbidity and the management of pediatric craniopharyngioma: a systematic review. J Neurosurg Pediatr 2012;10(4):293–301

48. Cohen M, Guger S, Hamilton J. Long-term sequelae of pediatric craniopharyngioma—literature review and 20 years of experience. Front Endocrinol (Lausanne) 2011;2:81

49. Mollá E, Martí-Bonmatí L, Revert A, et al. Craniopharyngiomas: identification of different semiological patterns with MRI. Eur Radiol 2002;12(7):1829–1836

50. Lee IH, Zan E, Bell WR, Burger PC, Sung H, Yousem DM. Craniopharyngiomas: radiological differentiation of two types. J Korean Neurosurg Soc 2016;59(5):466–470

51. Curran JG, O'Connor E. Imaging of craniopharyngioma. Childs Nervous System 2005;21:635–639
52. Sartoretti-Schefer S, Wichmann W, Aguzzi A, Valavanis A. MR differentiation of adamantinous and squamous-papillary craniopharyngiomas. AJNR Am J Neuroradiol 1997;18(1):77–87
53. Pusey E, Kortman KE, Flannigan BD, Tsuruda J, Bradley WG. MR of craniopharyngiomas: tumor delineation and characterization. AJR Am J Roentgenol 1987;149(2):383–388
54. Freeman MP, Kessler RM, Allen JH, Price AC. Craniopharyngioma: CT and MR imaging in nine cases. J Comput Assist Tomogr 1987;11(5):810–814
55. Hald JK, Eldevik OP, Skalpe IO. Craniopharyngioma identification by CT and MR imaging at 1.5 T. Acta Radiol 1995;36(2): 142–147
56. Sener RN. Proton MR spectroscopy of craniopharyngiomas. Comput Med Imaging Graph 2001;25(5):417–422
57. Jane JA Jr, Kiehna E, Payne SC, Early SV, Laws ER Jr. Early outcomes of endoscopic transsphenoidal surgery for adult craniopharyngiomas. Neurosurg Focus 2010;28(4):E9
58. Apra C, Enachescu C, Lapras V, Raverot G, Jouanneau E. Is gross total resection reasonable in adults with craniopharyngiomas with hypothalamic involvement? World Neurosurg 2019;129:e803–e811
59. Müller HL. Consequences of craniopharyngioma surgery in children. J Clin Endocrinol Metab 2011;96(7):1981–1991
60. Sughrue ME, Yang I, Kane AJ, et al. Endocrinologic, neurologic, and visual morbidity after treatment for craniopharyngioma. J Neurooncol 2011;101(3):463–476
61. Veeravagu A, Lee M, Jiang B, Chang SD. The role of radiosurgery in the treatment of craniopharyngiomas. Neurosurg Focus 2010;28(4):E11
62. Winkfield KM, Tsai HK, Yao X, et al. Long-term clinical outcomes following treatment of childhood craniopharyngioma. Pediatr Blood Cancer 2011;56(7):1120–1126
63. Yang I, Sughrue ME, Rutkowski MJ, et al. Craniopharyngioma: a comparison of tumor control with various treatment strategies. Neurosurg Focus 2010;28(4):E5
64. Kiehna EN, Merchant TE. Radiation therapy for pediatric craniopharyngioma. Neurosurg Focus 2010;28(4):E10
65. Hoffman HJ, De Silva M, Humphreys RP, Drake JM, Smith ML, Blaser SI. Aggressive surgical management of craniopharyngiomas in children. J Neurosurg 1992;76(1): 47–52
66. Puget S. Treatment strategies in childhood craniopharyngioma. Front Endocrinol (Lausanne) 2012;3:64
67. Laws ER Jr. Transsphenoidal removal of craniopharyngioma. Pediatr Neurosurg 1994;21(Suppl 1):57–63
68. Mark RJ, Lutge WR, Shimizu KT, Tran LM, Selch MT, Parker RG. Craniopharyngioma: treatment in the CT and MR imaging era. Radiology 1995;197(1):195–198
69. Sainte-Rose C, Puget S, Wray A, et al. Craniopharyngioma: the pendulum of surgical management. Childs Nerv Syst 2005; 21(8-9):691–695
70. Thompson D, Phipps K, Hayward R. Craniopharyngioma in childhood: our evidence-based approach to management. Childs Nerv Syst 2005;21(8-9):660–668
71. Müller HL, Gebhardt U, Teske C, et al.; Study Committee of KRANIOPHARYNGEOM 2000. Post-operative hypothalamic lesions and obesity in childhood craniopharyngioma: results of the multinational prospective trial KRANIOPHARYNGEOM 2000 after 3-year follow-up. Eur J Endocrinol 2011;165(1): 17–24
72. Zoicas F, Schöfl C. Craniopharyngioma in adults. Front Endocrinol (Lausanne) 2012;3:46
73. Andereggen L, Hess B, Andres R, et al. A ten-year follow-up study of treatment outcome of craniopharyngiomas. Swiss Med Wkly 2018;148:w14521
74. Van Gompel JJ, Nippoldt TB, Higgins DM, Meyer FB. Magnetic resonance imaging-graded hypothalamic compression in surgically treated adult craniopharyngiomas determining postoperative obesity. Neurosurg Focus 2010;28(4):E3
75. Forbes JA, Ordóñez-Rubiano EG, Tomasiewicz HC, et al. Endonasal endoscopic transsphenoidal resection of intrinsic third ventricular craniopharyngioma: surgical results. J Neurosurg 2018;:1–11
76. Gao Y, Zhong C, Wang Y, et al. Endoscopic versus microscopic transsphenoidal pituitary adenoma surgery: a meta-analysis. World J Surg Oncol 2014;12:94
77. Little AS, Kelly DF, Milligan J, et al. Comparison of sinonasal quality of life and health status in patients undergoing microscopic and endoscopic transsphenoidal surgery for pituitary lesions: a prospective cohort study. J Neurosurg 2015;123(3):799–807
78. Abou-Al-Shaar H, Blitz AM, Rodriguez FJ, Ishii M, Gallia GL. Expanded endonasal endoscopic approach for resection of an infrasellar craniopharyngioma. World Neurosurg 2016;95: 618.e7–618.e12
79. Locatelli D, Pozzi F, Agresta G, Padovan S, Karligkiotis A, Castelnuovo P. Extended endoscopic endonasal approach for suprasellar craniopharyngioma. J Neurol Surg B Skull Base 2018;79(2):S196–S198
80. Messerer M, Maduri R, Daniel RT. Extended endoscopic endonasal approach for craniopharyngioma removal. J Neurol Surg B Skull Base 2018;79(2):S199–S200
81. Cappabianca P, Cavallo LM, Esposito F, De Divitiis O, Messina A, De Divitiis E. Extended endoscopic endonasal approach to

the midline skull base: the evolving role of transsphenoidal surgery. Adv Tech Stand Neurosurg 2008;33:151–199

82. Cavallo LM, de Divitiis O, Aydin S, et al. Extended endoscopic endonasal transsphenoidal approach to the suprasellar area: anatomic considerations—part 1. Neurosurgery 2007;61(3, Suppl):24–33, discussion 33–34

83. Cavallo LM, Messina A, Cappabianca P, et al. Endoscopic endonasal surgery of the midline skull base: anatomical study and clinical considerations. Neurosurg Focus 2005; 19(1):E2

84. Cavallo LM, Solari D, Esposito F, Cappabianca P. The endoscopic endonasal approach for the management of craniopharyngiomas involving the third ventricle. Neurosurg Rev 2013;36(1):27–37, discussion 38

85. de Divitiis E, Cappabianca P, Cavallo LM, Esposito F, de Divitiis O, Messina A. Extended endoscopic transsphenoidal approach for extrasellar craniopharyngiomas. Neurosurgery 2007;61(5, Suppl 2):219–227, discussion 228

86. de Divitiis E, Cavallo LM, Cappabianca P, Esposito F. Extended endoscopic endonasal transsphenoidal approach for the removal of suprasellar tumors: part 2. Neurosurgery 2007; 60(1):46–58, discussion 58–59

87. Gardner PA, Kassam AB, Snyderman CH, et al. Outcomes following endoscopic, expanded endonasal resection of suprasellar craniopharyngiomas: a case series. J Neurosurg 2008;109(1): 6–16

88. Komotar RJ, Starke RM, Raper DM, Anand VK, Schwartz TH. Endoscopic endonasal compared with microscopic transsphenoidal and open transcranial resection of giant pituitary adenomas. Pituitary 2012;15(2):150–159

89. de Divitiis E, Cappabianca P, Cavallo LM. Endoscopic transsphenoidal approach: adaptability of the procedure to different sellar lesions. Neurosurgery 2002;51(3):699–705, discussion 705–707

90. Liu JK, Christiano LD, Patel SK, Eloy JA. Surgical nuances for removal of retrochiasmatic craniopharyngioma via the endoscopic endonasal extended transsphenoidal transplanum transtuberculum approach. Neurosurg Focus 2011;30(4):E14

91. Fahlbusch R, Honegger J, Paulus W, Huk W, Buchfelder M. Surgical treatment of craniopharyngiomas: experience with 168 patients. J Neurosurg 1999;90(2):237–250

92. Zona G, Spaziante R. Management of cystic craniopharyngiomas in childhood by a transsphenoidal approach. J Pediatr Endo-crinol Metab 2006;19(Suppl 1):381–388

93. Jane JA Jr, Prevedello DM, Alden TD, Laws ER Jr. The transsphenoidal resection of pediatric craniopharyngiomas: a case series. J Neurosurg Pediatr 2010;5(1):49–60

94. Wannemuehler TJ, Rubel KE, Hendricks BK, et al. Outcomes in transcranial microsurgery versus extended endoscopic endonasal approach for primary resection of adult craniopharyngiomas. Neurosurg Focus 2016;41(6):E6

95. Madsen PJ, Buch VP, Douglas JE, et al. Endoscopic endonasal resection versus open surgery for pediatric craniopharyngioma: comparison of outcomes and complications. J Neurosurg Pediatr 2019;:1–10

96. Liu JK, Eloy JA. Endoscopic endonasal transplanum transtuberculum approach for resection of retrochiasmatic craniopharyngioma. J Neurosurg 2012;32(Suppl):E2

97. Todeschini AB, Montaser AS, Shahein M, et al. Endoscopic endonasal approach to a suprasellar craniopharyngioma. J Neurol Surg B Skull Base 2018;79(Suppl 3):S237–S238

98. Castro-Dufourny I, Carrasco R, Prieto R, Barrios L, Pascual JM. The infundibulotuberal syndrome caused by craniopharyngiomas: clinicopathological evidence from an historical French cohort (1705–1973). Pituitary 2015; 18(5):642–657

99. Pascual JM, Prieto R, Carrasco R. Infundibulotuberal or not strictly intraventricular craniopharyngioma: evidence for a major topographical category. Acta Neurochir (Wien) 2011;153(12):2403–2425, discussion 2426

100. Qi S, Lu Y, Pan J, Zhang X, Long H, Fan J. Anatomic relations of the arachnoidea around the pituitary stalk: relevance for surgical removal of craniopharyngiomas. Acta Neurochir (Wien) 2011;153(4):785–796

101. Weiner HL, Wisoff JH, Rosenberg ME, et al. Craniopharyngiomas: a clinicopathological analysis of factors predictive of recurrence and functional outcome. Neurosurgery 1994;35(6):1001–1010, discussion 1010–1011

102. Scott RM. Craniopharyngioma: a personal (Boston) experience. Childs Nerv Syst 2005;21(8-9):773–777

103. Couldwell WT, Weiss MH, Rabb C, Liu JK, Apfelbaum RI, Fukushima T. Variations on the standard transsphenoidal approach to the sellar region, with emphasis on the extended approaches and parasellar approaches: surgical experience in 105 cases. Neurosurgery 2004;55(3):539–547, discussion 547–550

104. Buchfelder M, Schlaffer SM, Lin F, Kleindienst A. Surgery for craniopharyngioma. Pituitary 2013;16(1):18–25

105. Gu Y, Zhang X, Hu F, et al. Suprachiasmatic translamina terminalis corridor used in endoscopic endonasal approach for resecting third ventricular craniopharyngioma. J Neurosurg 2015;122(5):1166–1172

106. Al-Mefty O, Ayoubi S, Kadri PA. The petrosal approach for the total removal of giant retrochiasmatic craniopharyngiomas in children. J Neurosurg 2007;106(2, Suppl):87–92

107. Van Effenterre R, Boch AL. Craniopharyngioma in adults and children: a study of 122 surgical cases. J Neurosurg 2002; 97(1):3–11

108. Hakuba A, Nishimura S, Inoue Y. Transpetrosal-transtentorial approach and its application in the therapy of retrochiasmatic craniopharyngiomas. Surg Neurol 1985;24(4):405–415

109. Dehdashti AR, Ganna A, Witterick I, Gentili F. Expanded endoscopic endonasal approach for anterior cranial base and suprasellar lesions: indications and limitations. Neurosurgery 2009;64(4):677–687, discussion 687–689

110. Dusick JR, Esposito F, Kelly DF, et al. The extended direct endonasal transsphenoidal approach for nonadenomatous suprasellar tumors. J Neurosurg 2005;102(5):832–841

111. Klimo P Jr, Venable GT, Boop FA, Merchant TE. Recurrent craniopharyngioma after conformal radiation in children and the burden of treatment. J Neurosurg Pediatr 2015; 15(5):499–505

112. Shin JL, Asa SL, Woodhouse LJ, Smyth HS, Ezzat S. Cystic lesions of the pituitary: clinicopathological features distinguishing craniopharyngioma, Rathke's cleft cyst, and arachnoid cyst. J Clin Endocrinol Metab 1999;84(11): 3972–3982

113. Karavitaki N, Wass JA. Craniopharyngiomas. Endocrinol Metab Clin North Am 2008;37(1):173–193, ix–x

114. Šteňo J, Bízik I, Šteňo A, Matejčík V. Recurrent craniopharyngiomas in children and adults: long-term recurrence rate and management. Acta Neurochir (Wien) 2014;156(1):113–122, discussion 122

115. Dhandapani S, Singh H, Negm HM, et al. Endonasal endoscopic reoperation for residual or recurrent craniopharyngiomas. J Neurosurg 2017;126(2):418–430

116. Rajan B, Ashley S, Gorman C, et al. Craniopharyngioma—a long-term results following limited surgery and radiotherapy. Radiother Oncol 1993;26(1):1–10

117. Cavallo LM, Prevedello DM, Solari D, et al. Extended endoscopic endonasal transsphenoidal approach for residual or recurrent craniopharyngiomas. J Neurosurg 2009;111(3):578–589

118. Ignelzi RJ, Squire LR. Recovery from anterograde and retrograde amnesia after percutaneous drainage of a cystic craniopharyngioma. J Neurol Neurosurg Psychiatry 1976;39(12):1231–1235

119. McMurry FG, Hardy RW Jr, Dohn DF, Sadar E, Gardner WJ. Long term results in the management of craniopharyngiomas. Neurosurgery 1977;1(3):238–241

120. Gutin PH, Klemme WM, Lagger RL, MacKay AR, Pitts LH, Hosobuchi Y. Management of the unresectable cystic craniopharyngioma by aspiration through an Ommaya reservoir drainage system. J Neurosurg 1980;52(1):36–40

121. Barriger RB, Chang A, Lo SS, et al. Phosphorus-32 therapy for cystic craniopharyngiomas. Radiother Oncol 2011;98(2):207–212

122. Huk WJ, Mahlstedt J. Intracystic radiotherapy (90Y) of craniopharyngiomas: CT-guided stereotaxic implantation of indwelling drainage system. AJNR Am J Neuroradiol 1983;4(3):803–806

123. Julow J, Lányi F, Hajda M, et al. The radiotherapy of cystic craniopharyngioma with intracystic installation of 90Y silicate col-loid. Acta Neurochir (Wien) 1985;74(3-4): 94–99

124. Pollock BE, Lunsford LD, Kondziolka D, Levine G, Flickinger JC. Phosphorus-32 intracavitary irradiation of cystic craniopharyngiomas: current technique and long-term results. Int J Radiat Oncol Biol Phys 1995;33(2):437–446

125. Van den Berge JH, Blaauw G, Breeman WA, Rahmy A, Wijngaarde R. Intracavitary brachytherapy of cystic craniopharyngiomas. J Neurosurg 1992;77(4):545–550

126. Voges J, Sturm V, Lehrke R, Treuer H, Gauss C, Berthold F. Cystic craniopharyngioma: long-term results after intracavitary irradiation with stereotactically applied colloidal beta-emitting radioactive sources. Neurosurgery 1997;40(2):263–269, discussion 269–270

127. Liu W, Fang Y, Cai B, Xu J, You C, Zhang H. Intracystic bleomycin for cystic craniopharyngiomas in children (abridged republication of cochrane systematic review). Neurosurgery 2012;71(5):909–915

128. Steinbok P, Hukin J. Intracystic treatments for craniopharyngioma. Neurosurg Focus 2010;28(4):E13

129. Zhang S, Fang Y, Cai BW, Xu JG, You C. Intracystic bleomycin for cystic craniopharyngiomas in children. Cochrane Database Syst Rev 2016;7:CD008890

130. Zheng J, Fang Y, Cai BW, et al. Intracystic bleomycin for cystic craniopharyngiomas in children. Cochrane Database Syst Rev 2014;(9):CD008890

131. Cavalheiro S, Dastoli PA, Silva NS, Toledo S, Lederman H, da Silva MC. Use of interferon alpha in intratumoral chemotherapy for cystic craniopharyngioma. Childs Nerv Syst 2005;21(8-9):719–724

132. Cavalheiro S, Di Rocco C, Valenzuela S, et al. Craniopharyngiomas: intratumoral chemotherapy with interferon-alpha: a multicenter preliminary study with 60 cases. Neurosurg Focus 2010;28(4):E12

133. Kilday JP, Caldarelli M, Massimi L, et al. Intracystic interferon-alpha in pediatric craniopharyngioma patients: an international multicenter assessment on behalf of SIOPE and ISPN. Neuro Oncol 2017;19(10):1398–1407

134. Minniti G, Esposito V, Amichetti M, Enrici RM. The role of fractionated radiotherapy and radiosurgery in the

management of patients with craniopharyngioma. Neurosurg Rev 2009;32(2):125–132, discussion 132

135. Minniti G, Saran F, Traish D, et al. Fractionated stereotactic conformal radiotherapy following conservative surgery in the control of craniopharyngiomas. Radiother Oncol 2007; 82(1):90–95

136. Lin LL, El Naqa I, Leonard JR, et al. Long-term outcome in children treated for craniopharyngioma with and without radiotherapy. J Neurosurg Pediatr 2008;1(2):126–130

137. Stripp DC, Maity A, Janss AJ, et al. Surgery with or without radiation therapy in the management of craniopharyngiomas in children and young adults. Int J Radiat Oncol Biol Phys 2004;58(3):714–720

138. Habrand JL, Saran F, Alapetite C, Noel G, El Boustany R, Grill J. Radiation therapy in the management of craniopharyngioma: current concepts and future developments. J Pediatr Endocrinol Metab 2006;19(Suppl 1):389–394

139. Merchant TE. Craniopharyngioma radiotherapy: endocrine and cognitive effects. J Pediatr Endocrinol Metab 2006; 19(Suppl 1):439–446

140. Pemberton LS, Dougal M, Magee B, Gattamaneni HR. Experience of external beam radiotherapy given adjuvantly or at relapse following surgery for craniopharyngioma. Radiother Oncol 2005;77(1):99–104

141. Scarzello G, Buzzaccarini MS, Perilongo G, et al. Acute and late morbidity after limited resection and focal radiation therapy in craniopharyngiomas. J Pediatr Endocrinol Metab 2006;19(Suppl 1):399–405

142. Park HR, Kshettry VR, Farrell CJ, et al. Clinical outcome after extended endoscopic endonasal resection of craniopharyngiomas: two-institution experience. World Neurosurg 2017;103:465–474

143. Liu AK, Bagrosky B, Fenton LZ, et al. Vascular abnormalities in pediatric craniopharyngioma patients treated with radiation therapy. Pediatr Blood Cancer 2009;52(2):227–230

144. Baumert BG, Norton IA, Lomax AJ, Davis JB. Dose conformation of intensity-modulated stereotactic photon beams, proton beams, and intensity-modulated proton beams for intracranial lesions. Int J Radiat Oncol Biol Phys 2004;60(4):1314–1324

145. Fitzek MM, Linggood RM, Adams J, Munzenrider JE. Combined proton and photon irradiation for craniopharyngioma: long-term results of the early cohort of patients treated at Harvard Cyclotron Laboratory and Massachusetts General Hospital. Int J Radiat Oncol Biol Phys 2006;64(5):1348–1354

146. Luu QT, Loredo LN, Archambeau JO, Yonemoto LT, Slater JM, Slater JD. Fractionated proton radiation treatment for pediatric craniopharyngioma: preliminary report. Cancer J 2006;12(2):155–159

147. Brastianos PK, Taylor-Weiner A, Manley PE, et al. Exome sequencing identifies BRAF mutations in papillary craniopharyngiomas. Nat Genet 2014;46(2):161–165

148. Buslei R, Nolde M, Hofmann B, et al. Common mutations of beta-catenin in adamantinomatous craniopharyngiomas but not in other tumours originating from the sellar region. Acta Neuropathol 2005;109(6):589–597

149. Sekine S, Shibata T, Kokubu A, et al. Craniopharyngiomas of adamantinomatous type harbor beta-catenin gene mutations. Am J Pathol 2002;161(6):1997–2001

150. Berker M, Hazer DB, Yücel T, et al. Complications of endoscopic surgery of the pituitary adenomas: analysis of 570 patients and review of the literature. Pituitary 2012;15(3):288–300

151. Hoffmann A, Bootsveld K, Gebhardt U, Daubenbüchel AM, Sterkenburg AS, Müller HL. Nonalcoholic fatty liver disease and fatigue in long-term survivors of childhood-onset craniopharyngioma. Eur J Endocrinol 2015;173(3): 389–397

152. Olsson DS, Andersson E, Bryngelsson IL, Nilsson AG, Johannsson G. Excess mortality and morbidity in patients with craniopharyngioma, especially in patients with childhood onset: a population-based study in Sweden. J Clin Endocrinol Metab 2015;100(2):467–474

153. Wijnen M, Olsson DS, van den Heuvel-Eibrink MM, et al. Excess morbidity and mortality in patients with craniopharyngioma: a hospital-based retrospective cohort study. Eur J Endocrinol 2018;178(1):93–102

154. Bingham NC, Rose SR, Inge TH. Bariatric surgery in hypothalamic obesity. Front Endocrinol (Lausanne) 2012; 3:23

155. Giese H, Haenig B, Haenig A, Unterberg A, Zweckberger K. Neurological and neuropsychological outcome after resection of craniopharyngiomas. J Neurosurg 2019;:1–10

156. Memmesheimer RM, Lange K, Dölle M, Heger S, Mueller I. Psychological well-being and independent living of young adults with childhood-onset craniopharyngioma. Dev Med Child Neurol 2017;59(8):829–836

157. Lo AC, Howard AF, Nichol A, et al. Long-term outcomes and complications in patients with craniopharyngioma: the British Columbia Cancer Agency experience. Int J Radiat Oncol Biol Phys 2014;88(5):1011–1018

158. Enchev Y, Ferdinandov D, Kounin G, Encheva E, Bussarsky V. Radiation-induced gliomas following radiotherapy for craniopharyngiomas: a case report and review of the literature. Clin Neurol Neurosurg 2009;111(7):591–596

159. Sterkenburg AS, Hoffmann A, Gebhardt U, Warmuth-Metz M, Daubenbüchel AM, Müller HL. Survival, hypothalamic obesity, and neuropsychological/psychosocial status after childhood-onset craniopharyngioma: newly reported long-term outcomes. Neuro Oncol 2015;17(7):1029–1038

Chapter 8

Endoscopic Endonasal Transsphenoidal Transplanum Transtuberculum Approach

Suresh Sankhla and Narayan Jayashankar

Introduction

The transtuberculum transplanum approach is an extension of the endoscopic endonasal transsphenoidal transsellar approach that was developed to remove lesions located in the suprasellar region, above or under the diaphragma sellae. The extra bone removal obtained at the anterior skull base provides a direct corridor to the midline suprasellar region and has the advantage of offering an unhindered view of the sellar, infra- and supradiaphragmatic, infra- and suprachiasmatic, anterior third ventricular, hypothalamic regions, and interpeduncular fossa.

Indications

- Pre-infundibular, transinfundibular, and retroinfundibular craniopharyngiomas.
- Rathke's cleft cysts.
- Tuberculum sellae or planum meningiomas.
- Giant pituitary macroadenomas with suprasellar extension.
- Suprasellar arachnoid cysts.
- Selected hypothalamic gliomas.

Surgical Steps

1. On the right nostril of the subject, the middle turbinate is bipolarized and cut close to its anterior attachment to the skull base leaving a small tail behind for future identification of the axilla of the middle turbinate (**Fig. 8.1**). Similarly, it is bipolarized at its posterior end close to its attachment to the lateral nasal wall and cut (**Fig. 8.2**). Care is taken not to bipolarize the area of the sphenopalatine artery to preserve the arterial supply to the Hadad-Bassagasteguy flap which is to be used for reconstruction. The middle turbinate is then excised. An ethmoidectomy is performed (**Fig. 8.3**), and the lamina papyracea is identified laterally (**Fig. 8.4**). Although many surgeons preserve the middle turbinate and anterior ethmoids on the right side, removal of the same gives an unhindered view of the lateral sphenoid wall with the endoscope placed

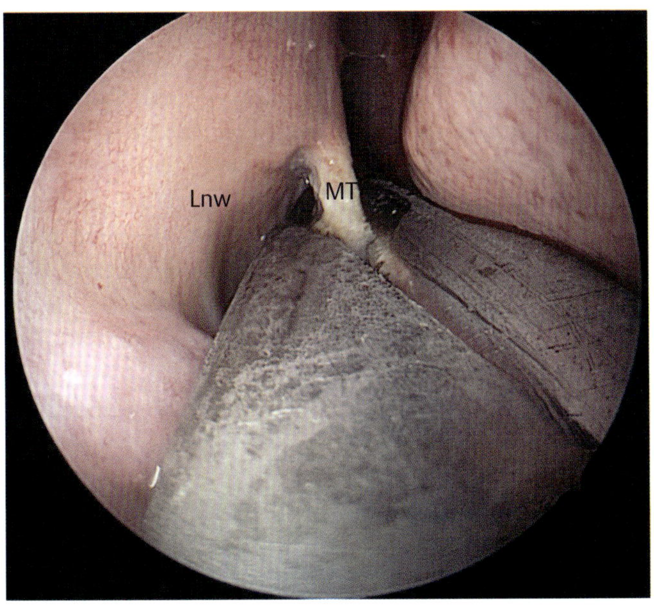

Fig. 8.1 Right middle turbinate attachment to skull base is bipolarized and cut a little away from the axilla.

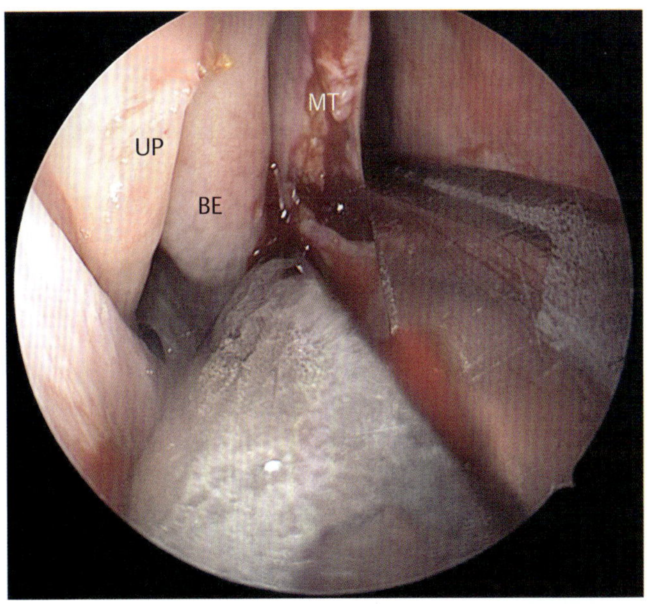

Fig. 8.2 The attachment of the posterior end of the middle turbinate to the lateral nasal wall is also bipolarized and cut a little away from the lateral nasal wall.

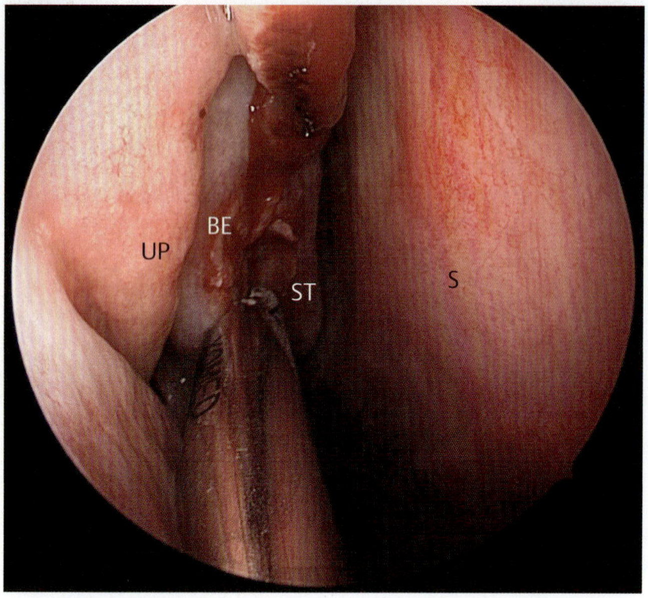

Fig. 8.3 A complete ethmoidectomy is performed on the right side.

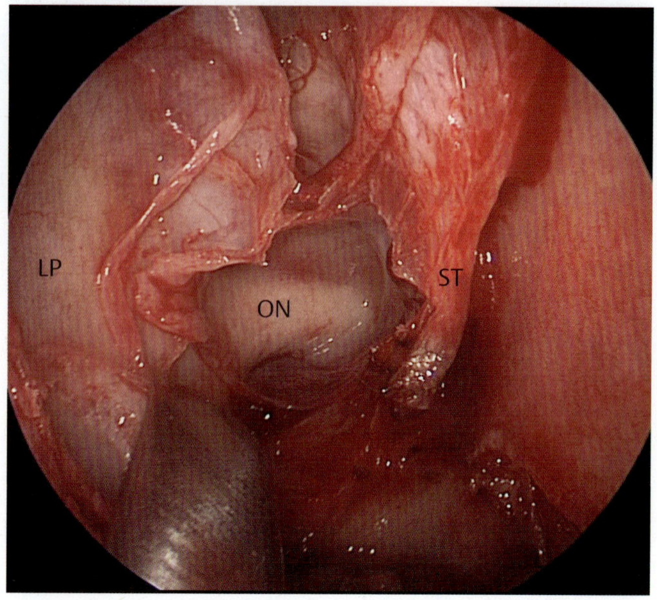

Fig. 8.4 The lamina papyracea is seen and also the optic nerve is seen from the orbital apex traversing in an Onodi cell.

more proximally with additional improved space for instrument manipulation. This is based on the concept of creating one and a half cavity on the right side. The endoscope is placed in the extra space procured which gives a wide roomy cavity for instrument manipulation on the same side, especially so when the surgery proceeds toward the right medial cavernous sinus area. The inferior half of the superior turbinate is excised and sphenoid ostia is uncovered.

2. The Hadad-Bassagasteguy flap is then harvested on the right side. A horizontal incision is taken at the inferior end of the sphenoid sinus ostium. A second incision is taken at the upper end of the posterior choanae. This incision is extended horizontally onto the inferior end of the nasal septum. The anterior limit of this incision is at the mucocutaneous junction on the septum. The incision taken at the inferior end of sphenoid ostium is continued forward onto the septum about 1 cm below the level of the cribriform plate till we cross the axilla of the middle turbinate; it is then arched superiorly and a horizontal incision is continued forward at the upper end of septum till the mucocutaneous junction. A vertical incision at the mucocutaneous junction joins the upper and lower horizontal incisions over the nasal septum. The vascularized pedicled flap is then harvested retaining its vascularity from the nasoseptal branch of the posterior septal artery, which is a branch of the sphenopalatine artery. In case a wider flap is required, the mucoperiosteum of the nasal floor is additionally included in the flap. The flap is tucked away in the nasopharynx for reconstruction, till the surgical procedure is complete (**Fig. 8.5**).
3. The sphenoid ostia are widened bilaterally to the maximum permissible limit using a Kerrison punch (**Fig. 8.6**). Next, the posterior third of the bony septum is resected (**Fig. 8.7**). A piece of vomer is preserved in saline for reconstruction. The rostrum of the sphenoid is then clearly seen. The mucoperiosteal flap on the opposite side (left side) is lifted off the rostrum so as to preserve the opposite vascular pedicle in case an additional flap is required. Once palatovaginal canals are identified on both sides, the rostrum is drilled down to the level of the floor of the sphenoid, from one palatovaginal canal to the other. Alternatively, it is taken down with chisel and hammer by making controlled cuts on both sides and also inferiorly (**Fig. 8.8**).
4. The bony overhangs on all sides are then drilled off. Inferiorly, one should have an unhindered view of the upper clivus and sphenoid floor with no overhangs. This additionally helps in Hadad-Bassagasteguy flap replacement at the end of the procedure. Superiorly, removal of any bony overhangs offers a nice view of the tuberculum as also the planum right up to the location of the posterior ethmoid arteries on both sides (**Fig. 8.9**). Laterally, on both sides, the area lateral to the paraclival carotids is exposed. In cases where

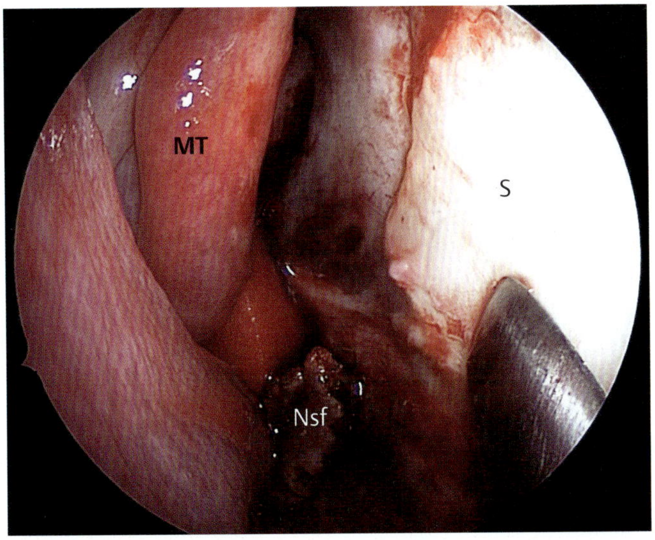

Fig. 8.5 Hadad-Bassagasteguy nasoseptal flap harvested and tucked away in the nasopharynx.

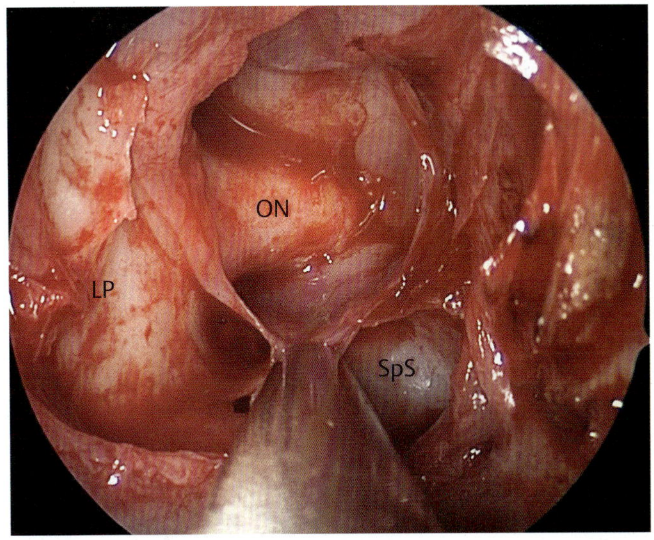

Fig. 8.6 Sphenoid ostia is widened.

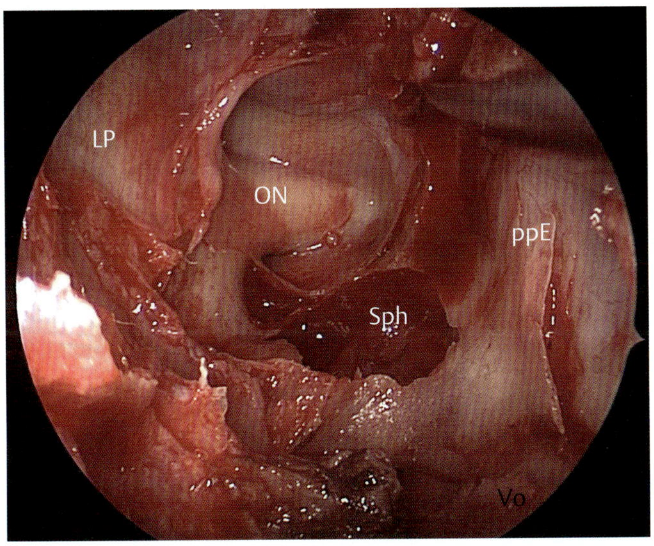

Fig. 8.7 Posterior third of bony septum including the vomer and the perpendicular plate of ethmoid is excised.

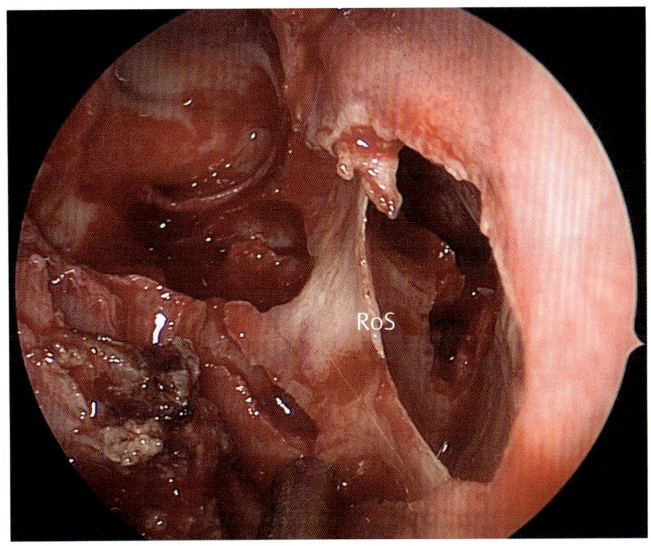

Fig. 8.8 Excision of the rostrum of sphenoid.

a lateral sinus of sphenoid exists, it must be exposed completely. It may be necessary in these cases to drill the pterygoid base as required.

5. All bony sphenoid septations are drilled off with a coarse diamond burr. It is important to identify the normal anatomical landmarks in the sphenoid sinus such as the optic and carotid protuberances, and the medial and lateral opticocarotid recesses before drilling of the bone is commenced.

The neuronavigation should be used to identify or confirm the position of the normal bony structures at the base of skull. The medial opticocarotid recess is a crucial structure as it represents pneumatization of the middle clinoid process and indicates the lateral aspect of the tuberculum sellae. The bone over the tubercular strut and both medial opticocarotid recesses are thinned down with a diamond drill and then removed gently with a blunt hook. This maneuver unroofs the medial aspect of the optic canals and facilitates exposure of the optic nerves and paraclinoid carotid arteries in the opticocarotid cistern. Extreme care should be exercised to avoid thermal injury to the optic nerves by using copious saline irrigation during bone drilling.

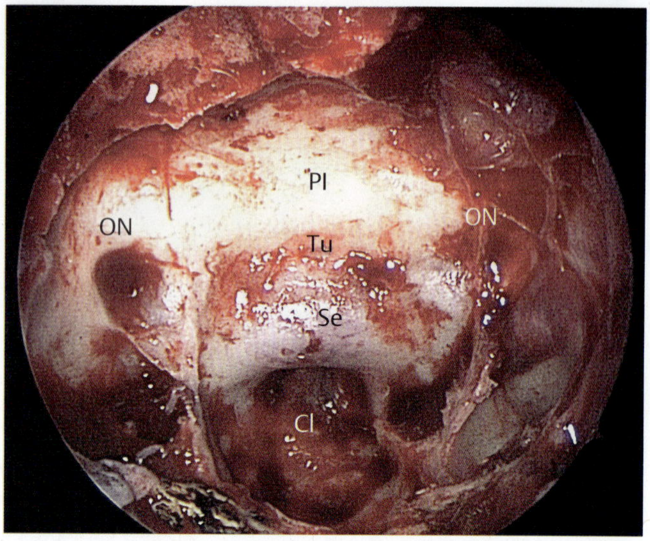

Fig. 8.9 Complete exposure of floor of sphenoid sinus inferiorly to planum superiorly and lateral wall of sphenoid on both sides is obtained.

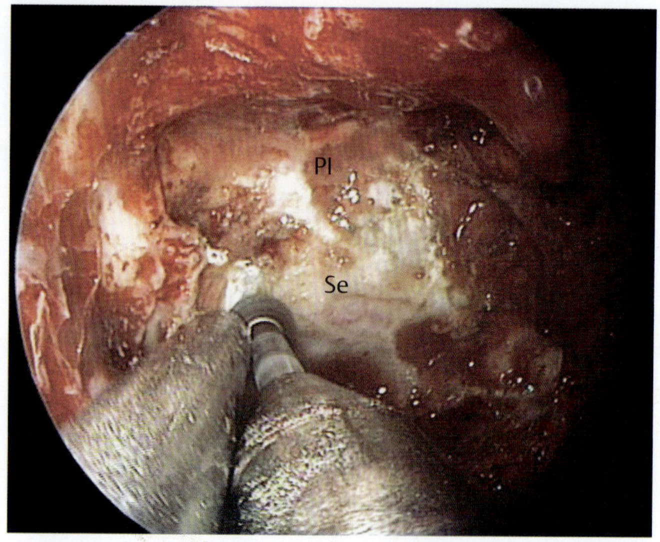

Fig. 8.10 Drilling the sella, tuberculum, and planum.

6. The normal bone of the sellar floor and posterior planum sphenoidale is drilled down carefully to make it eggshell thin (**Fig. 8.10**).

   Depending on the pathology and the extent of the lesion, it may also be necessary to thin the bone over the cavernous and clinoidal carotids. The eggshell thin bone over the sella is fractured and the remaining shells of bone are lifted off using a Kerrison punch. It should be noted that the Kerrison punch is not used to bite, but the jaw is kept open and the eggshell bone is gently lifted off the underlying dura (**Fig. 8.11**). The remnant bone over the superior intercavernous sinus, if any, is then dissected off the sinus using a blunt hook or Freer elevator. Punching the bone in this area leads to bleeding from the superior intercavernous sinus or an inadvertent tear of the dura.

   The optimal exposure usually includes bone removal of sella, from one optic protuberance to the other, and from the carotid artery on one side to the carotid on the other side in the lateral extent (**Fig. 8.12**).

   When tumor is extending laterally, the bone over the internal carotid artery (ICA) is removed gently in the same way as described above. The use of Doppler at this stage is extremely important. It not only helps identifying the location of the ICA and its dural course but also adds safety to the bone removal and dural opening. Bone removal inferiorly should include the entire floor of the sella so that it is flush with the upper clivus. Superiorly, it should include exposure of the superior intercavernous sinus and the dura of the tuberculum and planum up to the posterior ethmoid arteries. A precise bone removal can be determined by using neuronavigation during surgery.
7. The dura is opened using bimanual microsurgical techniques through both nostrils. The 0-degree scope is used for the most part of the dissection in a free-hand dynamic fashion to provide the depth perception. It is introduced through the right nostril and is placed in the superior part of the exposure (11 o'clock position), leaving adequate space in the cavity for manipulation of the surgical instruments, suction cannula, and irrigation. The site of dural incision can be variable and depends on the type and location of the intradural lesion. Generally, two parallel horizontal dural incisions are made above and below the superior intercavernous sinus and are extended superiorly and inferiorly after sectioning the cauterized dural venous sinus in the midline (**Fig. 8.13a–d**).

   In case of a large sellar tumor like a pituitary giant macroadenoma, the dura is opened in the sellar region initially and is extended superiorly as per the need. Conversely, in cases of supradiaphragmatic tumors with no sellar extension, like the tuberculum sellae meningiomas and craniopharyngiomas, the dural opening is made above the superior intercavernous sinus and the incision is extended inferiorly, only if necessary (**Fig. 8.14**). In tuberculum sellae meningiomas, the superior intercavernous sinus is often compressed by the tumor and is difficult to identify. The dural opening can sometimes be difficult because of the bleeding from the tumor attachment to the dura. It is, therefore, advisable to make the first dural incision

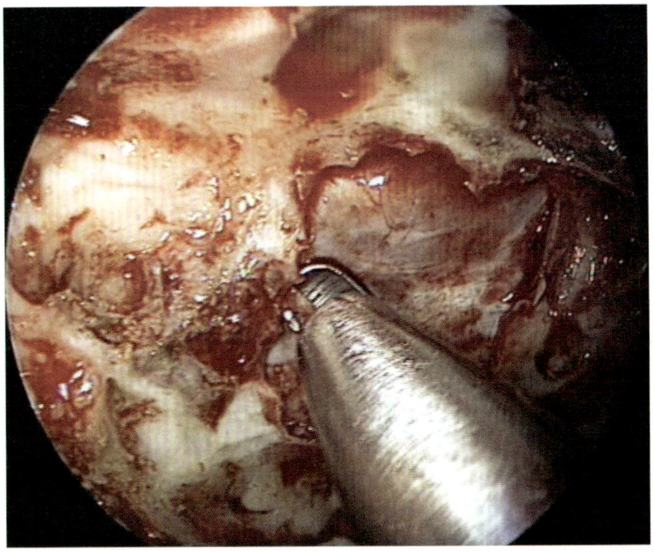

Fig. 8.11 Bone over the dura should be thinned down using a burr and eggshell bone lifted off using a Kerrison punch.

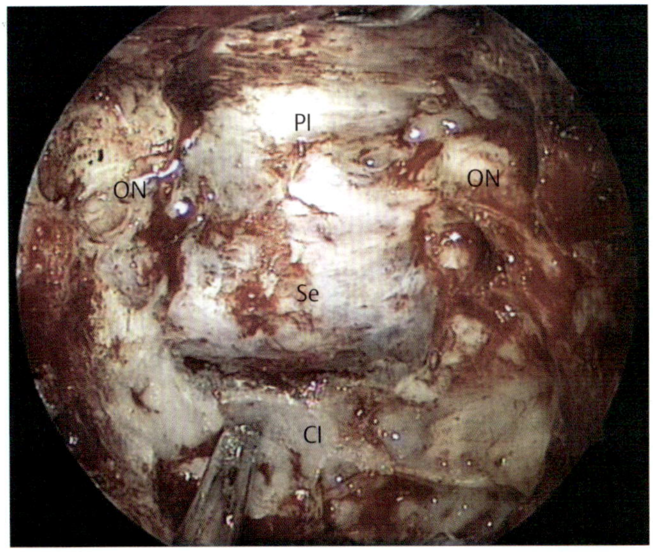

Fig. 8.12 Dura exposed from the floor of the sella inferiorly till planum superiorly and till carotids on both sides.

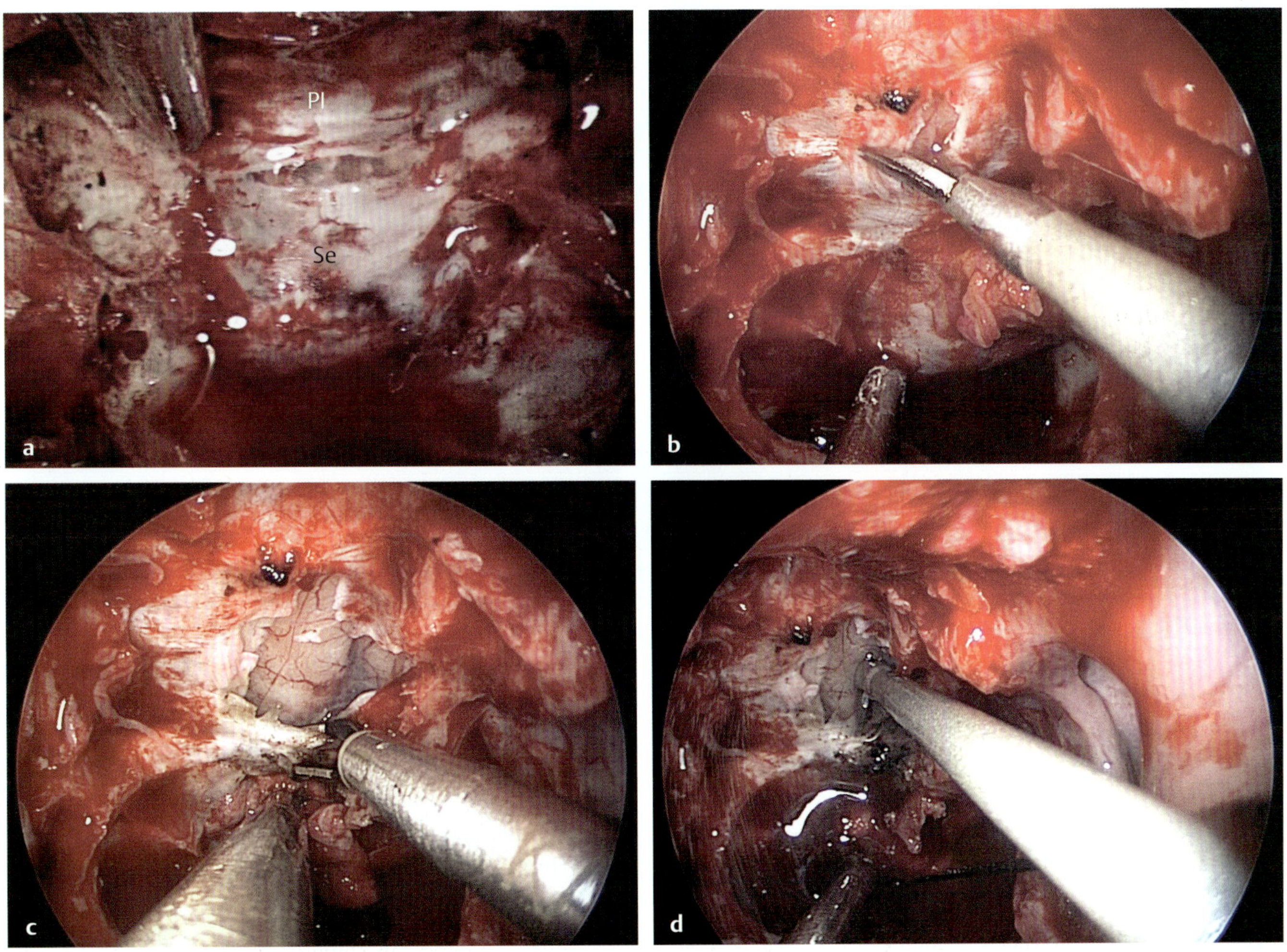

Fig. 8.13 **(a)** Horizontal dural incision just inferior to the superior intercavernous sinus. **(b)** Horizontal dural incision just superior to the superior intercavernous sinus. **(c)** Bipolarizing the superior intercavernous sinus. **(d)** Cutting the bipolarized superior intercavernous sinus to convert the sellar and suprasellar space into a single cavity.

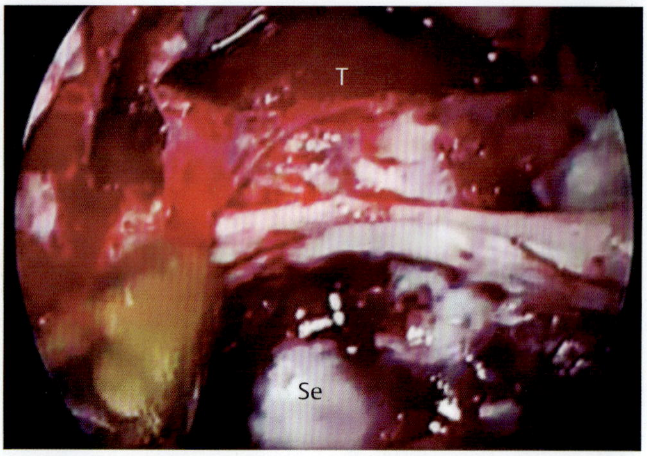

Fig. 8.14 First dural incision in suprasellar space in a case of tuberculum sellae meningioma.

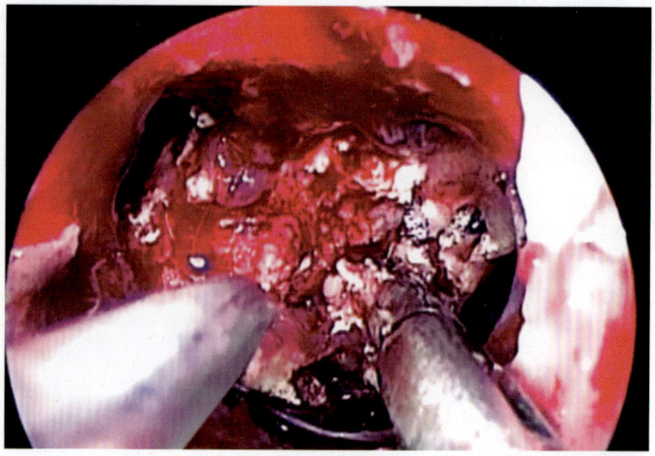

Fig. 8.15 Tumor debulking in a case of craniopharyngioma.

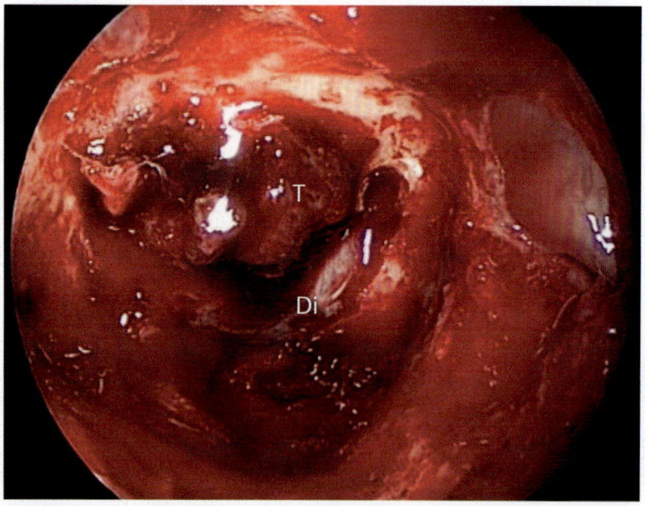

Fig. 8.16 The pituitary tumor is cleared from the floor of the sella and lateral gutters first.

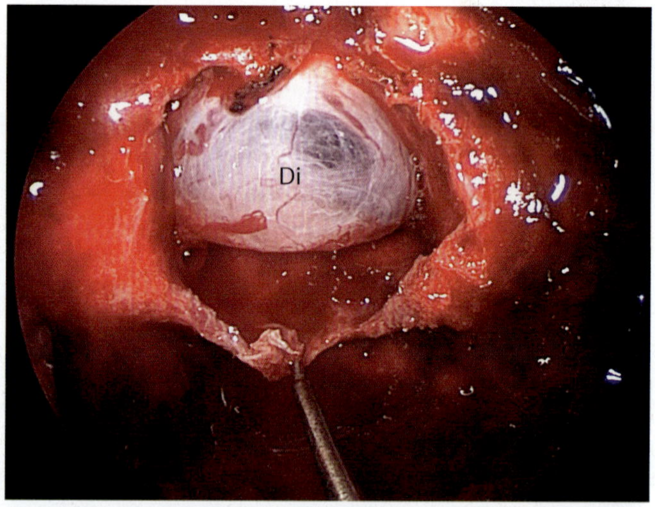

Fig. 8.17 Diaphragm prolapsing into the sellar cavity could impede complete clearance of the tumor.

above the tumor in the suprasellar dura and to continue subsequent dural opening under direct intradural visualization of the tumor margins.

8. It is important to maximize tumor decompression before attempting mobilization of the tumor capsule from the arachnoid over the optic nerves and chiasm, blood vessels, and the pituitary stalk (**Fig. 8.15**). It relieves the pressure from the optic chiasm and nerves, and provides enough room to mobilize the tumor capsule with no or minimal traction on the neurovascular structures. The tumor debulking is usually carried out in the same way as it is done in microsurgical tumor removal procedures. A soft pituitary adenoma can be removed easily with bimanual suction and tumor-holding forceps, whereas firm meningiomas and calcified craniopharyngiomas may require sharp cutting and piecemeal removal. Ultrasonic aspirator has been found to be a very useful tool for tumor decompression. Draining the tumor cyst (craniopharyngiomas and Rathke's cleft cysts) is a very effective method of internal decompression.
9. In cases of the soft pituitary macroadenomas, the internal decompression should be performed uniformly and systematically in all directions, beginning from the inferior and lateral parts. This maneuver allows the suprasellar tumor to fall slowly and spontaneously into the cavity because of gravity (**Fig. 8.16**).

A rapid and asymmetrical tumor removal leads to prolapse of the diaphragma sellae into the tumor cavity which may obscure visualization of the residual tumor (**Fig. 8.17**).

Care must be taken during Rathke's cyst surgery to avoid sudden and complete cyst drainage which can make the dissection of its thin wall extremely difficult. In the case of a meningioma, it is preferable to begin internal decompression from the most anterior part of the tumor, primarily because it is clearly visible to the surgeon and is least likely to involve critical neurovascular structures. Beginning tumor removal from the front also ensures that adequate bone removal has been obtained at the planum. Additional tumor removal should be performed intermittently whenever the tumor bulk is found to obstruct mobilization of the capsule. Once the anterior capsule has been mobilized adequately, it becomes easier to visualize optic chiasm and anterior cerebral arteries.

Tuberculum Sellae Meningioma

Magnetic resonance imaging (MRI) scans of a case of tuberculum sellae meningioma are shown in **Fig. 8.18a–d.** The initial steps of surgery (**Fig. 8.19** and **Fig. 8.20**) are same as described above. The tumor is gradually cleared keeping the arachnoid intact where possible (**Fig. 8.21** and **Fig. 8.22**).

It is safer to begin extracapsular dissection from the superior pole of the tumor where the capsule–arachnoid plane is easier to find once the tumor debulking has made the capsule lax and redundant. As tuberculum sellae meningiomas tend to displace the chiasm posteriorly, the first structures encountered at this point are the A2 branches and recurrent artery of Heubner covered by an arachnoid layer (**Fig. 8.23**). A sharp or careful blunt dissection is used to displace the arachnoid away from the capsule until chiasm is visualized (**Fig. 8.24**). Utmost care must be taken to avoid any manipulation of the chiasm during dissection. A plane of cleavage is developed between the tumor capsule and the arachnoid anterior to the chiasm by inserting gentle traction on the capsule with the help of a suction cannula or tumor-holding forceps. The A1 segments of the anterior cerebral artery (ACA) and the anterior communicating artery are usually in vision at this stage.

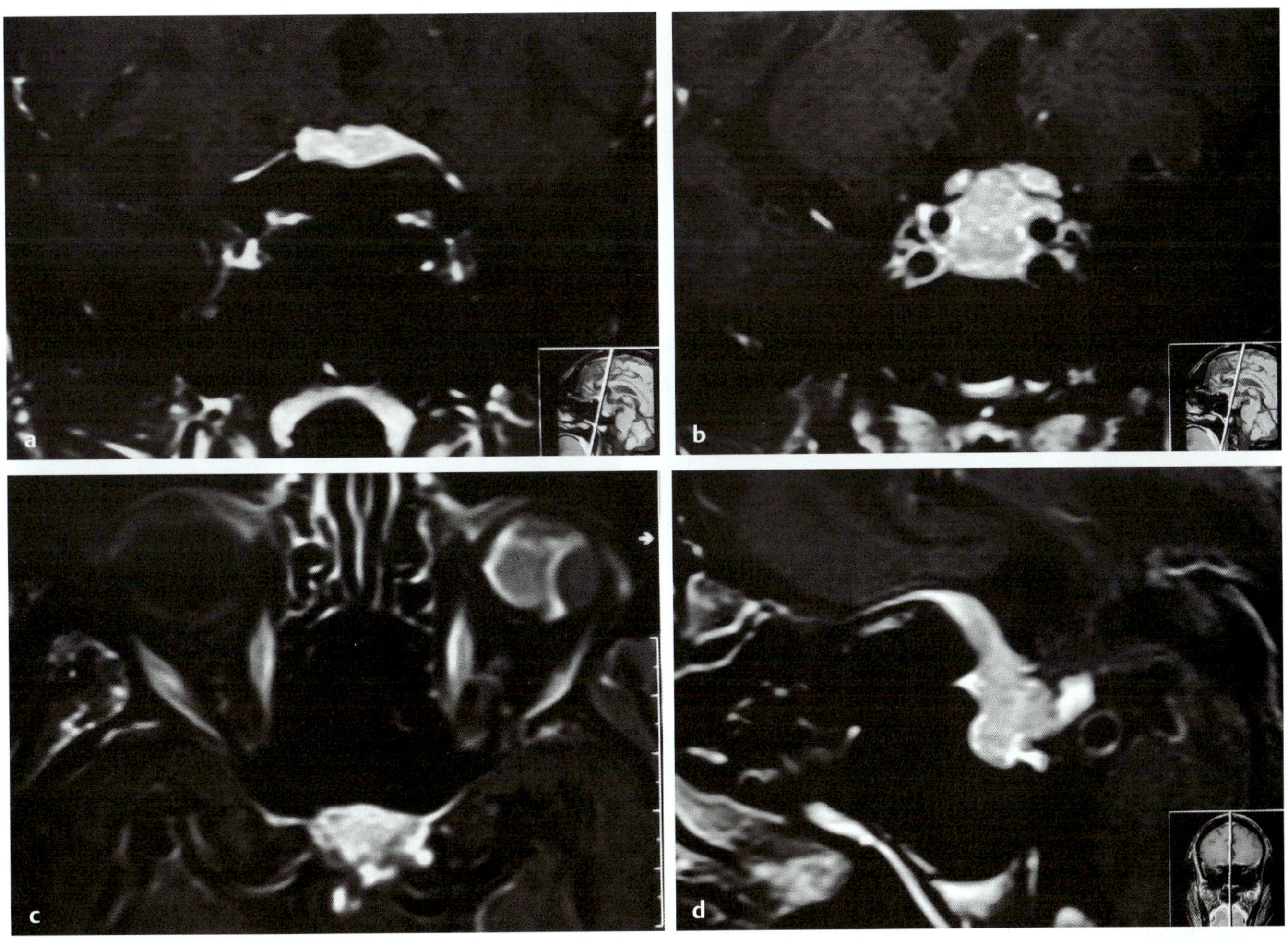

Fig. 8.18 (a–d) Coronal, axial, and sagittal scans showing the extent of the meningioma.

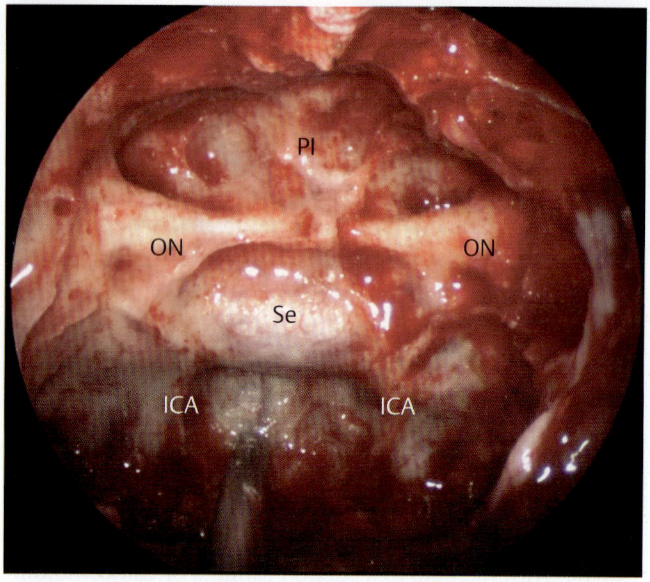

Fig. 8.19 Wide exposure from the floor of sphenoid to planum and lateral wall of sphenoid sinus on both sides with the drilling of sphenoid septations is desired as explained above.

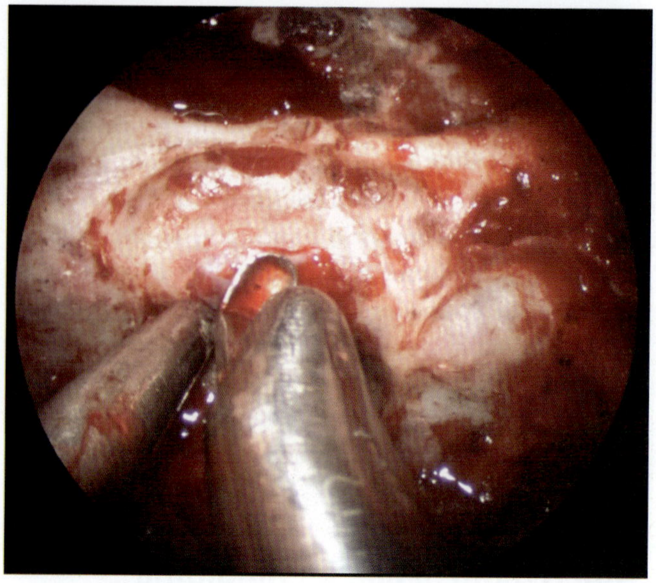

Fig. 8.20 Bone over the sella, planum, and tuberculum is taken off.

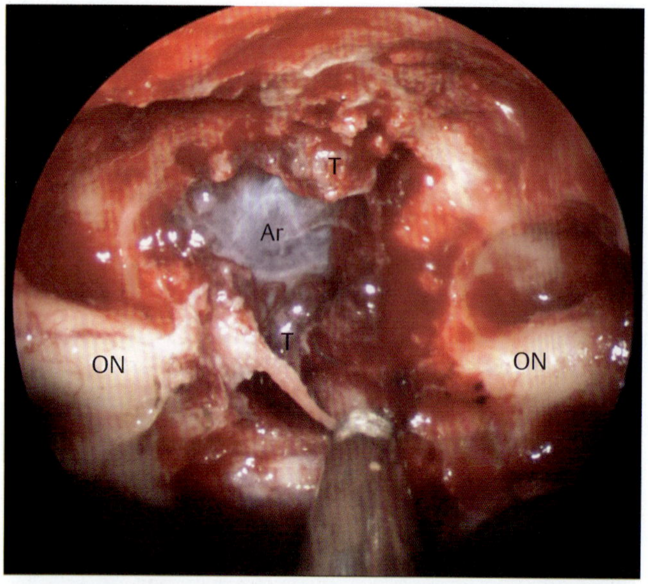

Fig. 8.21 Tumor is exposed. An area of arachnoid is seen after tumor clearance from that area.

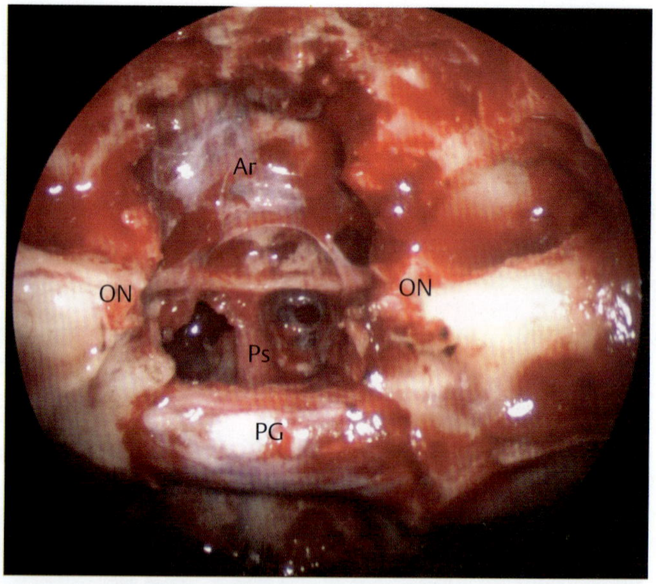

Fig. 8.22 Structures are seen after the excision of meningioma. Arachnoid preservation is seen.

Mobilization of the posterior capsule is critical because it is in close approximation with the perforating arteries supplying the optic chiasm and the pituitary stalk. Injury to any neurovascular structures in this region may lead to devastating visual or endocrinological complications. Using the same technique posteriorly and inferiorly, the capsule is elevated to separate mamillary bodies, displaced pituitary stalk and distorted gland, and diaphragma sellae, a step which may expose bifurcation of the basilar artery in interpeduncular fossa. Meningiomas at this location are frequently attached to the diaphragm, which should be resected if involved, along with the tumor extending into the sella. Care must be exercised during dissection at the inferior pole to avoid injury to the superior hypophyseal artery or its branches.

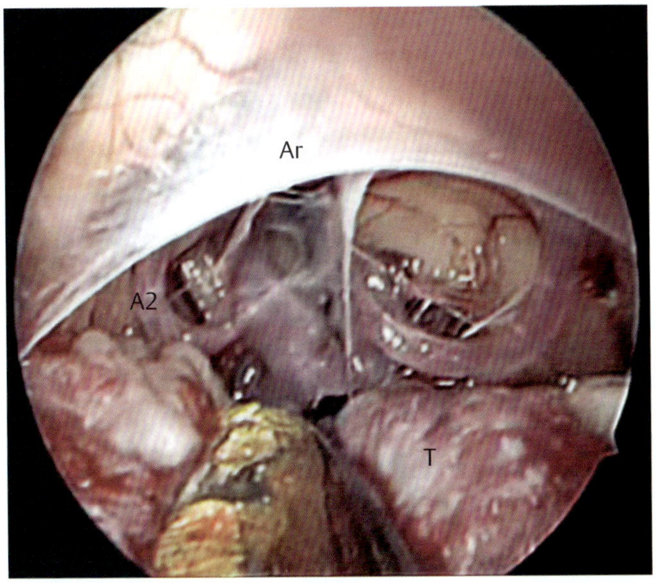

Fig. 8.23 A2 segments of anterior cerebral arteries are seen in another case.

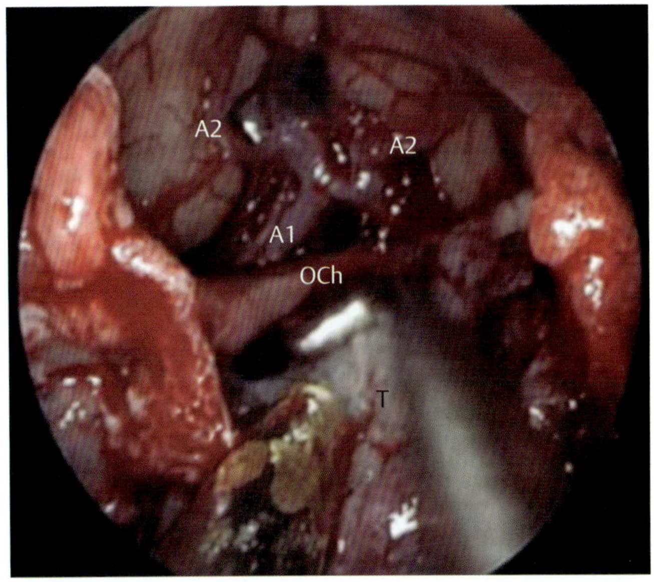

Fig. 8.24 Meningioma is separated from the optic chiasm.

Tumors extending into the optic canals require proper evaluation of the preoperative imaging and surgical planning. When the intracanalicular tumor is clearly visible on the MRI, drilling of the medial bony walls and roof should be performed at the beginning of the procedure along with the removal of the tumor. This maneuver untethers the optic nerves at the tight optic canals and minimizes traction on the nerves and chiasm during the subsequent part of the tumor dissection. The optic canal drilling can also be done in the latter part of the surgery when an unanticipated tumor extension is observed during surgery. Partial opening of the optic canals is done frequently to inspect the canals for the presence of any tumor tissue or thickened ligaments. There may be no need to open the canals if there is no suspicion about the presence of the tumor on the preoperative MRI, clinical evaluation, or intraoperative observation.

Craniopharyngioma

Because of the unique features of tumors like craniopharyngiomas, the surgical strategy of their removal requires some special techniques and considerations. First, these tumors are mostly found in the vicinity of the pituitary stalk and have a tendency to grow under the optic chiasm, which is usually displaced superiorly and posteriorly. Second, the presence of dense calcification in the tumor mass causes technical difficulties during its removal from the adherent optic nerves and chiasm, ICAs, pituitary stalk, and hypothalamus.

Attention is paid to identify the pituitary gland and stalk as early as possible during tumor decompression, and extreme care must be exercised to preserve it throughout the procedure (**Fig. 8.25**).

Although the tumor–stalk relationship can be variable in each case (preinfundibular, transinfundibular, or retroinfundibular), it is generally possible to localize the stalk position on the preoperative MRI. During surgery, the stalk is first identified at its junction with the pituitary gland, and then careful sharp dissection is performed to separate it gently from the tumor along with its accompanying vascular channels. However, it is not always possible to identify the stalk within the tumor mass or preserve it during surgery, even with a meticulous dissection, particularly in cases with large or transinfundibular (type II) tumors. The chunks of calcification adherent to the stalk often make its dissection from the tumor further difficult and hazardous. The surgical options in these situations may remain between complete tumor removal with sacrificing the stalk and resultant hormone replacement therapy for lifelong and an incomplete tumor removal with anatomical preservation of the stalk and a higher risk of tumor recurrence in the future.

Once the tumor (**Fig. 8.26**) has adequately been decompressed, extracapsular dissection is begun carefully using the bimanual microdissection technique. Constant saline irrigation during tumor dissection by the surgical colleague is very helpful. It removes blood, calcification, and debris, and keeps the operative field clear and tidy. The tumor capsule is often adherent to the undersurface of the optic nerves and

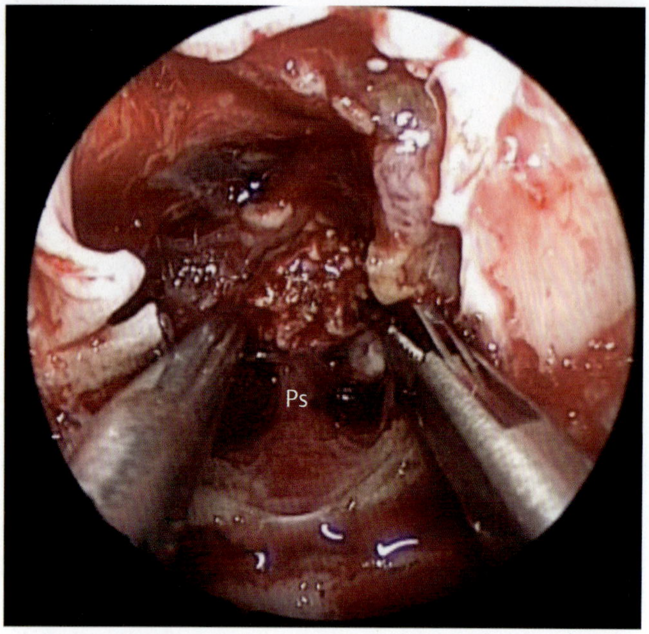

Fig. 8.25 Excision of craniopharyngioma is in progress. Pituitary stalk is seen.

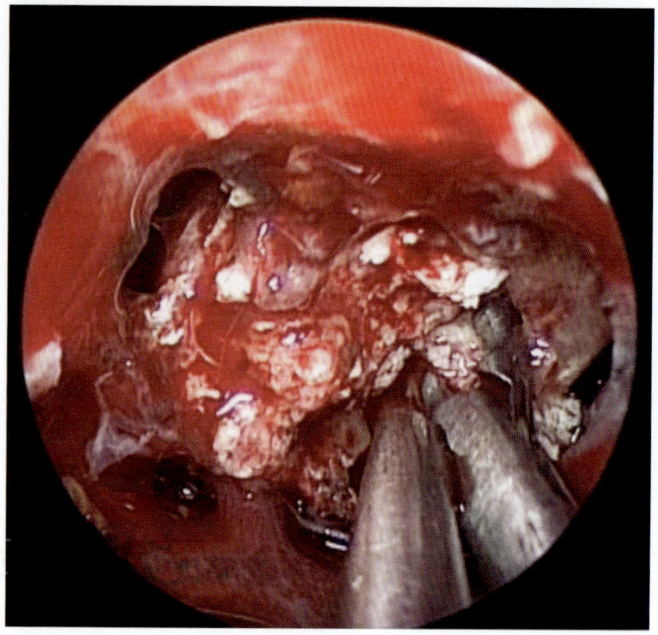

Fig. 8.26 Tumor debulking is in progress.

chiasm, and hypothalamus. It is, however, important to identify the double-layered arachnoid of the suprasellar cistern and to differentiate the tumor arachnoid from the cisternal arachnoid. The key to safe dissection is to find a plane of cleavage between the tumor capsule and tumor arachnoid, and not the cisternal arachnoid. As the tumor capsule is separated away on one side, the oculomotor nerve, superior cerebellar artery, and the bifurcation of the basilar artery come into view (**Fig. 8.27**). All efforts are made to preserve the hypophyseal arteries and the small perforating vessels supplying the undersurface of the chiasm and optic nerves. The anterior cerebral artery complex is located superior to the optic chiasm and is therefore protected from the plane of dissection. The extracapsular dissection is often facilitated by exerting gentle countertraction on the mobilized tumor capsule by holding it firmly with tumor-holding forceps and rolling it over toward the debulked tumor cavity. Care must be taken to avoid premature amputation of the capsule because it may result in the loss of the correct plane. Capsular dissection in the region of the hypothalamus and anterior third ventricle requires angular vision upward which can be obtained using a 30-degree scope from below. An angled scope is also useful to inspect the third ventricular cavity, if it is opened, for residual tumor or cyst, or blood clots. The Liliequist membrane is generally intact in most cases and acts as a protective layer for the basilar artery and its branches. At this stage, the abducent nerves can also be visualized traversing the lateral part of the interpeduncular fossa. Once the tumor capsule has been dissected from these vital structures, the remaining tumor can be dissected and delivered easily from the anterior third ventricular region (**Fig. 8.28**).

Pituitary Macroadenomas with Suprasellar Extension

Pituitary macroadenomas with large suprasellar extension require careful study of the preoperative MRI and computed tomography (CT) and meticulous surgical planning. Tumors with low signal intensities on T2-weighted images and homogenous appearance (**Fig. 8.29a, b**) are likely to be fibrous in consistency.

Generally, soft tumors (**Fig. 8.30**) can be removed easily from the endosellar route using standard tumor removal techniques with suction and curettage. With progressive internal decompression of the tumor from below, the soft tumor tissue tends to fall in the sellar cavity until a normal diaphragm becomes visible at the roof. Occasionally, techniques like the Valsalva maneuver are required to facilitate tumor descent into the empty sellar cavity. However, the old

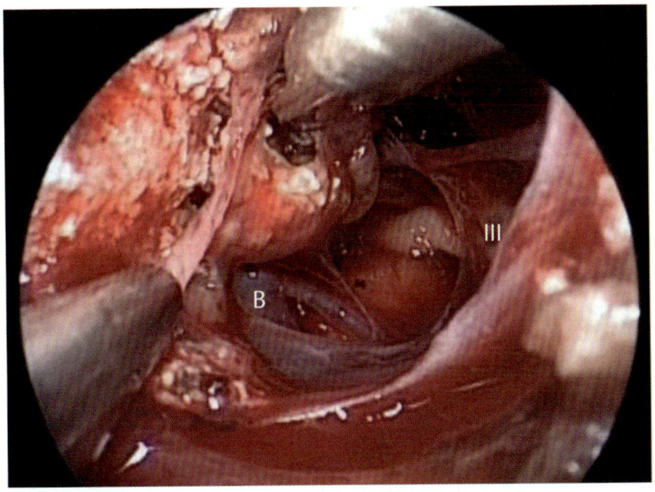

Fig. 8.27 Tumor is gently dissected off from structures deeper to it like basilar artery and III nerve.

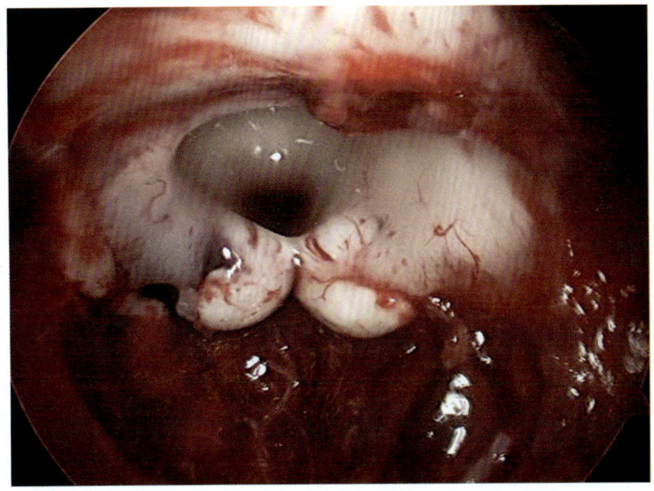

Fig. 8.28 Mammillary bodies and third ventricle are seen after tumor excision.

methods, like air inflation into the arachnoid space through a lumbar catheter, are rarely necessary and not advocated routinely. The tumors with a large globular extension into the suprasellar space often pose difficulty in descending down because of the narrow space at the roof of the sella turcica. Enlarging the space by removing the bone of the tuberculum sella and posterior planum helps the soft tumor mass to fall spontaneously into the cavity or become visible for dissection. It also allows unobstructed and free manipulation of the instruments in different angles during tumor removal.

The conventional maneuvers of tumor removal are often ineffective when the adenoma is firm or fibrous. In that case, the bimanual microsurgical techniques with piecemeal tumor removal become necessary. The same strategy is adapted for the removal of pituitary adenomas that are either dumbbell shaped or are located in the suprasellar region primarily. Surgery is begun with intracapsular removal or internal decompression of the tumor, and once the tumor has been debulked adequately, the suprasellar part of the tumor is approached and mobilized by dissecting the arachnoid layer away from the tumor. An intermittent gentle push to the capsule from above helps in the descent of the suprasellar portion of the tumor down into the sellar cavity from where it can be removed easily. The same procedure of extracapsular dissection and intracapsular tumor removal is repeated until complete removal has been achieved from the sellar and suprasellar regions. Angled scopes (30 or 45 degrees) are used in the end to ensure total tumor removal and hemostasis.

Closure and Skull Base Reconstruction

The closure is of critical importance in preventing postoperative cerebrospinal fluid (CSF) leak and meningitis. The authors use a piece of fat to plug the dural defect (**Fig. 8.31**) taking care that the fat does not prolapse into the intracranial space. An overlay graft of fascia lata is used over the defect. The vomer, which was preserved during the initial steps of the procedure, is reshaped to an adequate size to match the bony defect (**Fig. 8.32**). The edges of this bone graft are hinged to the edges of the bony defect over the fascia lata so that it forms a firm and fixed bony closure similar to a gasket seal. The vascularized nasoseptal flap is then rotated superiorly to cover the operative area (**Fig. 8.33**). Care is taken to ensure that the edges of the nasoseptal flap are in contact with bone all around. A thin layer of Tisseel (Baxter Healthcare Corp.) fibrin glue is spread over the nasoseptal flap, followed by gentamicin-soaked Gelfoam pledgets to buttress the flap repair. A Merocel (Medtronic Xomed) nasal pack is then placed in the nasal cavity to bolster the Gelfoam layer and is left in place for approximately 3 days. The authors use postoperative lumbar drainage for 2 days.

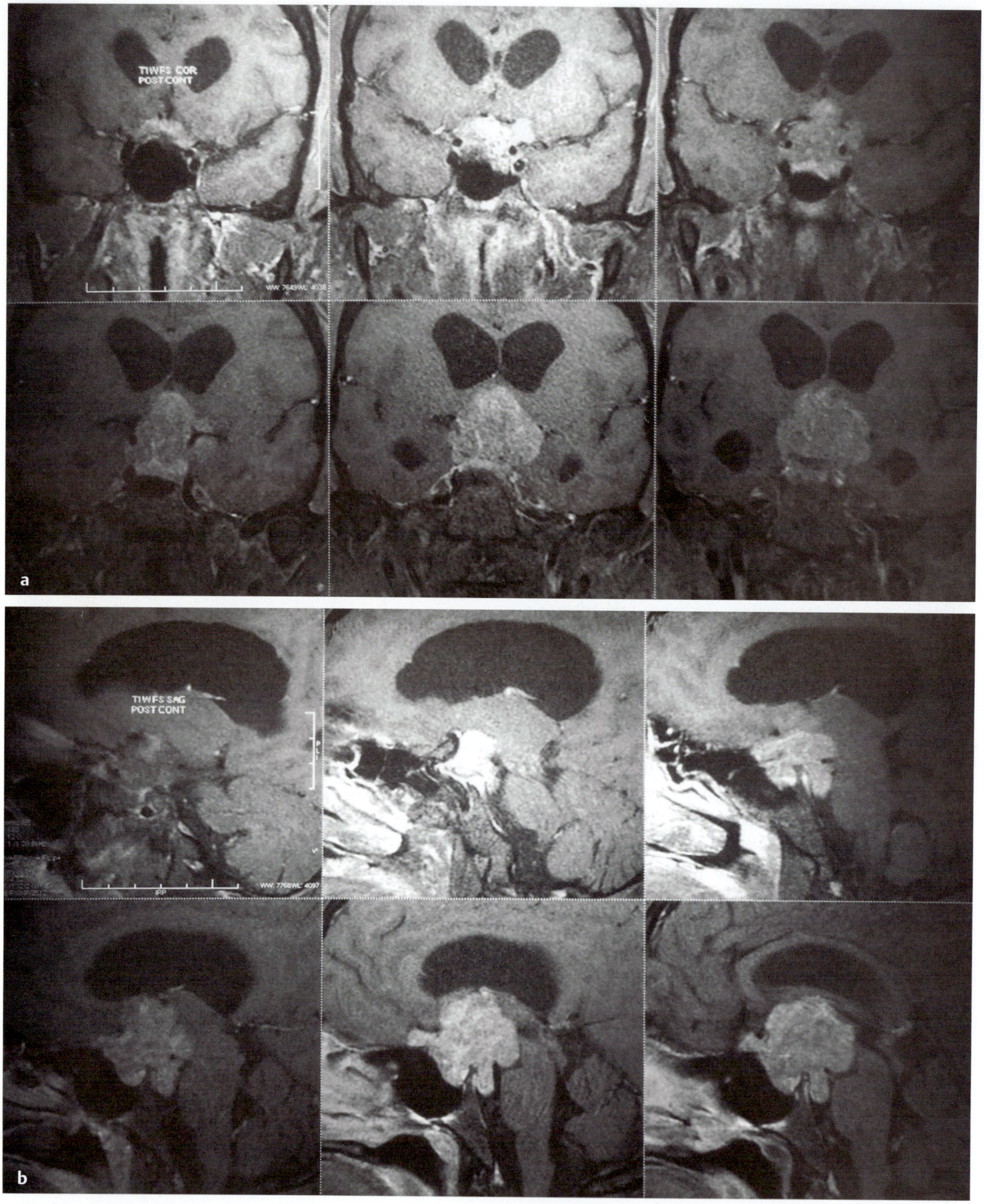

Fig. 8.29 (a, b) A homogenous appearance of the pituitary tumor suggests that the tumor could be fibrous in consistency.

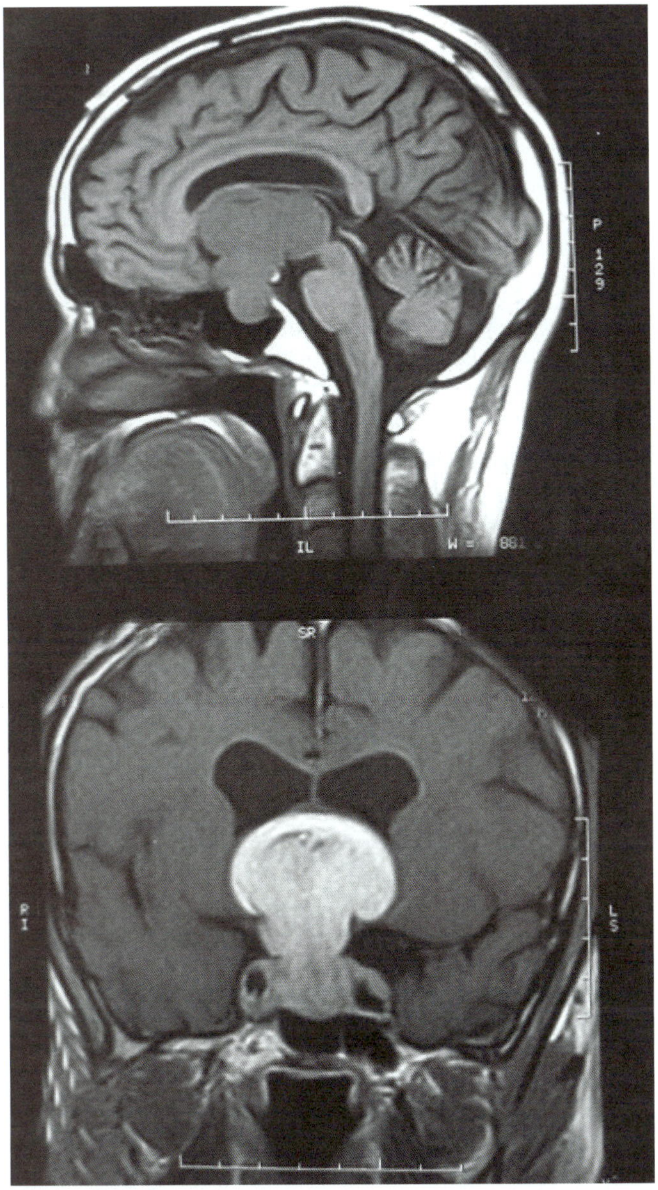

Fig. 8.30 Coronal and sagittal postcontrast MR scans showing a pituitary macroadenoma with a large suprasellar extension. The mosaic appearance with hyperintense dots suggest that the tumor has a soft consistency.

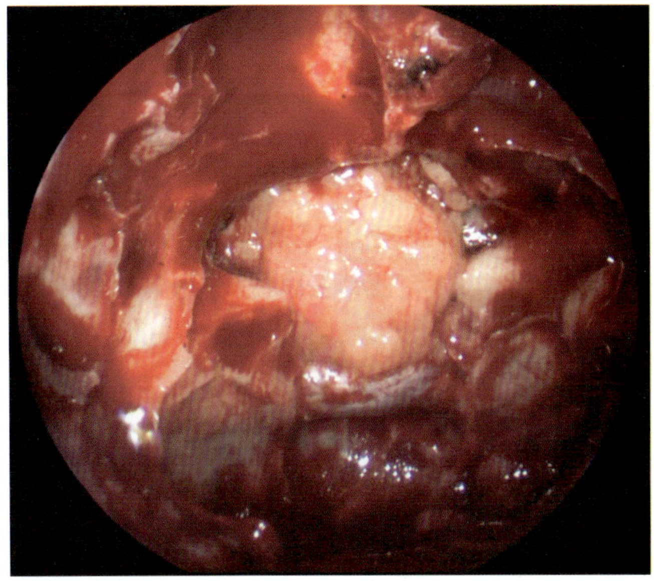

Fig. 8.31 Fat is used to plug the dural defect.

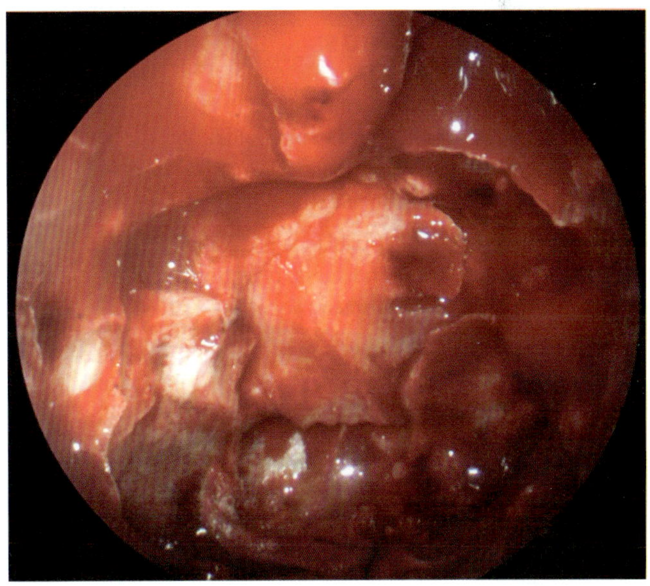

Fig. 8.32 A piece of the vomer is snugly fitted in the bony defect.

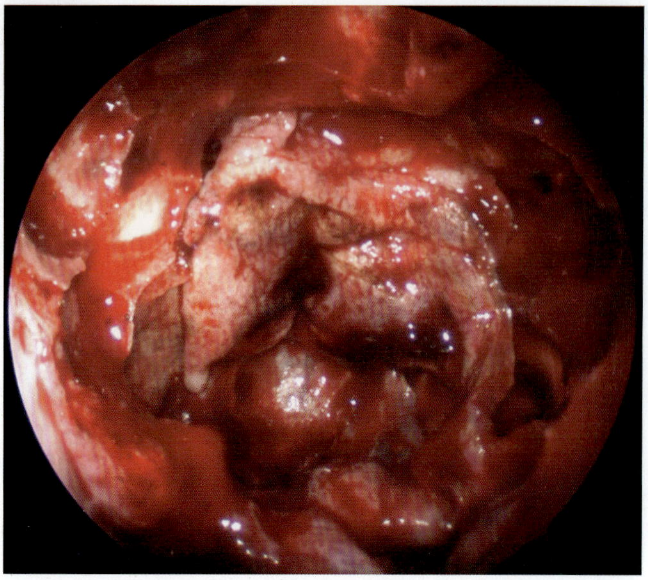

Fig. 8.33 A Hadad-Bassagasteguy pedicled nasoseptal flap is used to cover the operated area.

Suggested Readings

de Divitiis E, Cavallo LM, Cappabianca P, Esposito F. Extended endoscopic endonasal transsphenoidal approach for the removal of suprasellar tumors: part 2. Neurosurgery 2007; 60(1):46–58; discussion 58–59

de Divitiis E, Esposito F, Cappabianca P, Cavallo LM, de Divitiis O, Esposito I. Endoscopic transnasal resection of anterior cranial fossa meningiomas. Neurosurg Focus 2008; 25(6):E8

Ditzel Filho LF, Prevedello DM, Jamshidi AO, et al. Endoscopic endonasal approach for removal of tuberculum sellae meningiomas. Neurosurg Clin N Am 2015;26(3):349–361

Kassam A, Snyderman CH, Mintz A, Gardner P, Carrau RL. Expanded endonasal approach: the rostrocaudal axis. Part I. Crista galli to the sella turcica. Neurosurg Focus 2005;19(1):E3

Khan OH, Anand VK, Schwartz TH. Endoscopic endonasal resection of skull base meningiomas: the significance of a "cortical cuff" and brain edema compared with careful case selection and surgical experience in predicting morbidity and extent of resection. Neurosurg Focus 2014; 37(4):E7

Koutourousiou M, Fernandez-Miranda JC, Stefko ST, Wang EW, Snyderman CH, Gardner PA. Endoscopic endonasal surgery for suprasellar meningiomas: experience with 75 patients. J Neurosurg 2014;120(6):1326–1339

Koutourousiou M, Fernandez-Miranda JC, Wang EW, Snyderman CH, Gardner PA. The limits of transsellar/transtuberculum surgery for craniopharyngioma. J Neurosurg Sci 2018;62(3): 301–309

Liu JK, Christiano LD, Patel SK, Tubbs RS, Eloy JA. Surgical nuances for removal of tuberculum sellae meningiomas with optic canal involvement using the endoscopic endonasal extended transsphenoidal transplanum transtuberculum approach. Neurosurg Focus 2011;30(5):E2

Sankhla SK, Jayashankar N, Khan GM. Endoscopic endonasal transplanum transtuberculum approach for retrochiasmatic craniopharyngiomas: operative nuances. Neurol India 2015;63(3):405–413

Solari D, Morace R, Cavallo LM, et al. The endoscopic endonasal approach for the management of craniopharyngiomas. J Neurosurg Sci 2016;60(4):454–462

Turel MK, Tsermoulas G, Reddy D, Andrade-Barazarte H, Zadeh G, Gentili F. Endonasal endoscopic transsphenoidal excision of tuberculum sellae meningiomas: a systematic review. J Neurosurg Sci 2016;60(4):463–475

Zacharia BE, Amine M, Anand V, Schwartz TH. Endoscopic endonasal management of craniopharyngioma. Otolaryngol Clin North Am 2016;49(1):201–212

Zoli M, Guaraldi F, Pasquini E, Frank G, Mazzatenta D. The endoscopic endonasal management of anterior skull base meningiomas. J Neurol Surg B Skull Base 2018; 79(Suppl 4):S300–S310

Chapter 9 Endoscopic Endonasal Surgeries for Craniopharyngioma

Case 9A

Endonasal Transnasal Transseptal Transsphenoidal Excision of a Solitary Cystic Craniopharyngioma

Michel Roethlisberger, Prepageran Narayanan, and Vicknes Waran

History

A 34-year-old male presents with a slowly progressive bitemporal hemianopia. Clinically, no signs for an endocrinopathy or excessive hormone production are present. Laboratory workup did show partial hypopituitarism with depressed thyrotropin and gonadotropin axes with an otherwise normal function of the pituitary gland.

Contrast-enhanced magnetic resonance imaging (MRI) revealed a cystic intra- and suprasellar mass with an enhancement of the cyst wall and compression of the optic chiasm and optic nerve (**Fig. 9A.1a–d**).

An **endoscopic transnasal transsphenoidal resection** of the lesion was recommended.

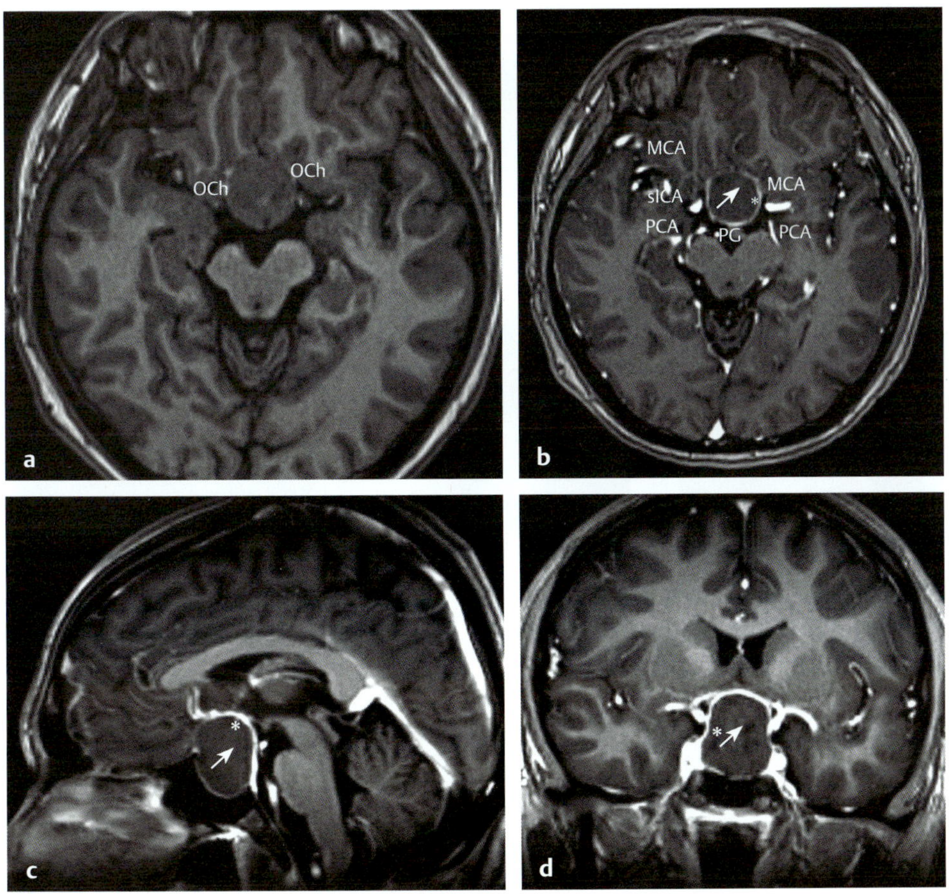

Fig. 9A.1 **(a)** Axial T1-weighted, **(b)** axial, **(c)** sagittal, **(d)** coronal T1-weighted gadolinium contrast-enhanced MRI section. A T1-isointense homogenous lesion (*arrow*) in the non-enhancing sequences being slightly hypointense in contrast sequences is present. The lesion is intra- and suprasellar with a prominent rim enhancement (*). The optic chiasm (OCh) is elevated and compressed. The normal pituitary gland (PG) and the infundibular stalk are difficult to distinguish within the enhancing rim.

Surgical Steps

1. A **binostril transnasal transseptal transsphenoidal approach** with harvesting of bilateral pedicled nasoseptal flaps is performed as previously described (Chapter 1).
2. The sphenoid cavity is exposed, and the common anatomical landmarks of the skull base are identified (**Fig. 9A.2**).
3. The sphenoid septae are removed by piecemeal resection. Care has to be taken while removing the septae that are close to the relevant neurovascular structures. In toto removal with cracking is not recommended, while piecemeal removal within a controlled range is possible (**Fig. 9A.3**).
4. While thinning out the insertion site of the sphenoid septae, the sellar dura can be identified at one point, and a dissection plane between the bone covering the sella turcica and the sellar dura can be defined (**Fig. 9A.4**).
5. The sellar opening is completed using a Kerrison punch and should reach the cavernous internal carotid arteries, the sellar floor, and the anterior intercavernous sinus (**Figs. 9A.5**, **9A.6**, and **9A.7**).
6. The sellar dura is then opened along the midline using a cruciate incision (**Figs. 9A.8** and **9A.9**).
7. The underlying tumor capsule is then separated and dissected away from the sellar dura (**Fig. 9A.10**).
8. The tumor capsule can then be opened in a controlled manner, and a brown oily thick fluid is evacuated into the sphenoid cavity. Crystalline shining components can be appreciated consisting of cholesterol crystals (**Fig. 9A.11**).
9. Tumor capsule, fleshy tumor components, and calcifications are removed using grasping instruments, curettes, and suction (**Figs. 9A.12** and **9A.13**).
10. After resection of the antero-medial and -lateral portions, the sellar opening is extended superiorly to address the suprasellar part and the diaphragma sellae (**Fig. 9A.14**).
11. The solid tumor components can then be dissected away from the diaphragma sellae along an anatomical dissection plane (**Figs. 9A.15**, **9A.16**, and **9A.17**).

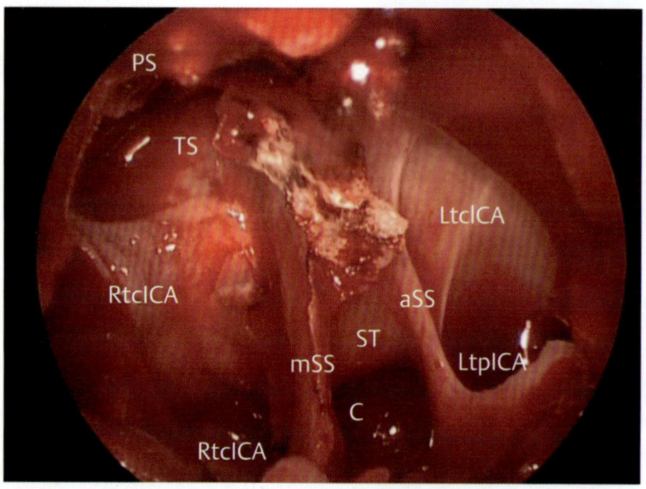

Fig. 9A.2 Exposure of the sphenoid cavity via a binostril transseptal transsphenoidal approach. The common landmarks of the skull base are skewed and covered by a main dividing septum (mSS) and an accessory dividing septum (aSS) inserting along the medial aspect of the left cavernous internal carotid artery (LtcICA).

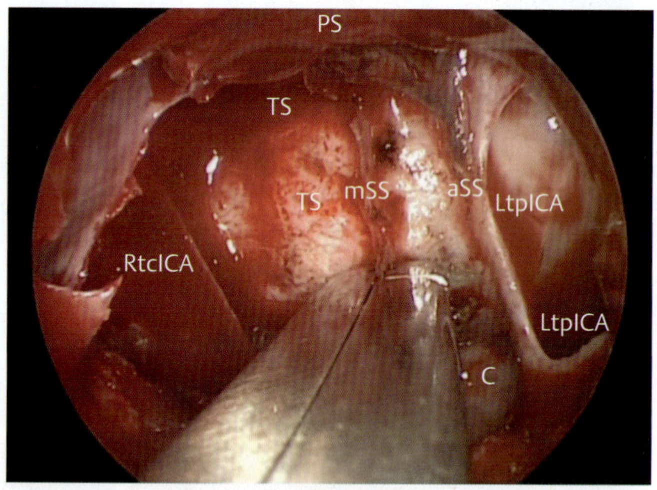

Fig. 9A.3 Piecemeal removal of the main dividing septum (mSS).

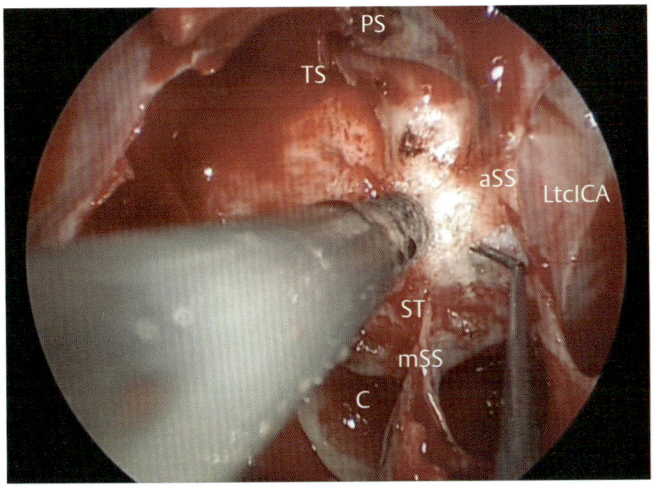

Fig. 9A.4 Defining the plane between the bone covering the sellar dura using a blunt hooked instrument.

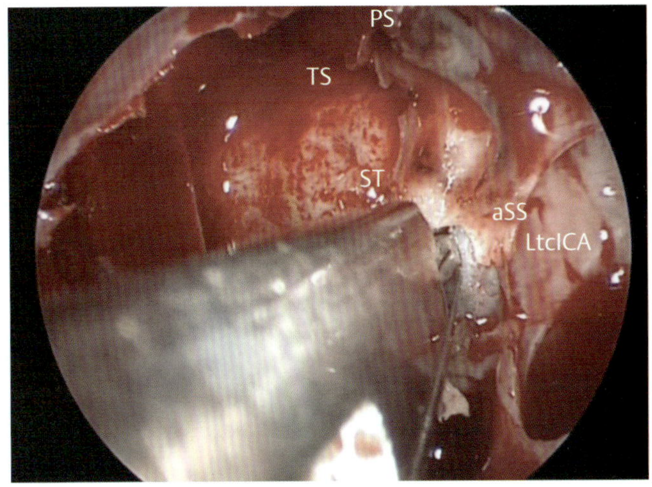

Fig. 9A.5 Opening the sella turcica using a Kerrison punch.

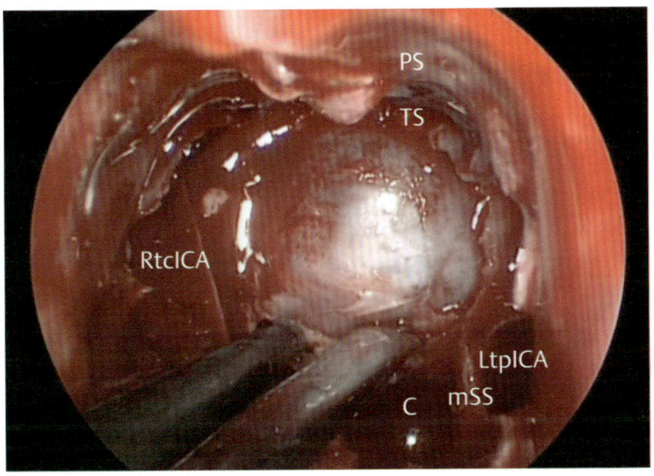

Fig. 9A.6 Transsellar approach and opening. The sellar floor is identified using a dissector.

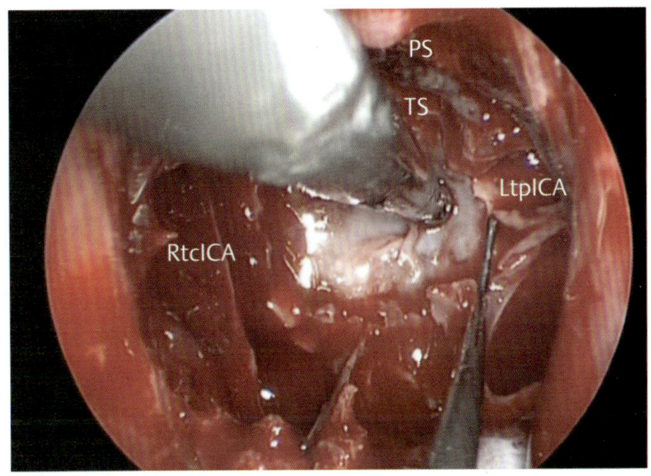

Fig. 9A.7 Transsellar approach and opening. Definition of the lateral sellar dura and left cavernous internal carotid artery (LtcICA) using a blunt hooked instrument.

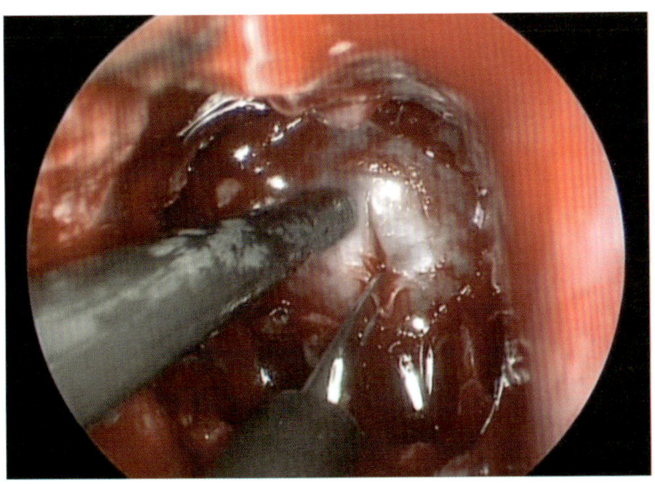

Fig. 9A.8 Sharp vertical opening of the sellar dura with a 15-mm blade.

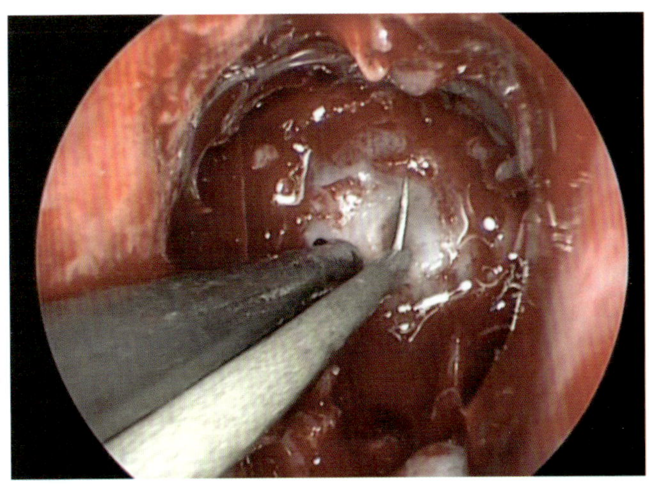

Fig. 9A.9 Sharp vertical opening of the sellar dura with microscissors.

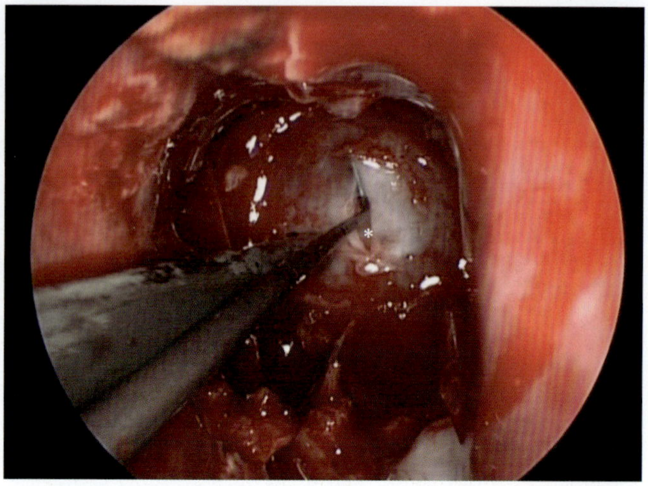

Fig. 9A.10 Definition of a plane between the tumor capsule and the sellar dura using a blunt hooked instrument prior to evacuation of the tumor cyst (*).

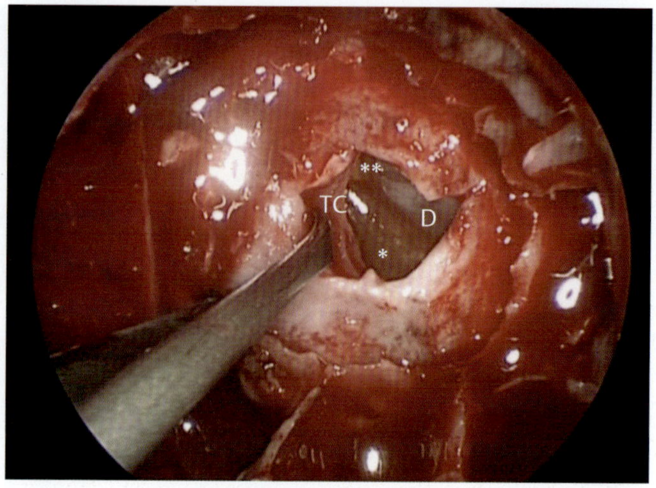

Fig. 9A.11 After opening of the tumor capsule (TC) and evacuation of brownish oily liquid with cholesterol crystals (*), smaller solid tumor components and calcifications (**) are identified superiorly in contact with the diaphragma sellae (D).

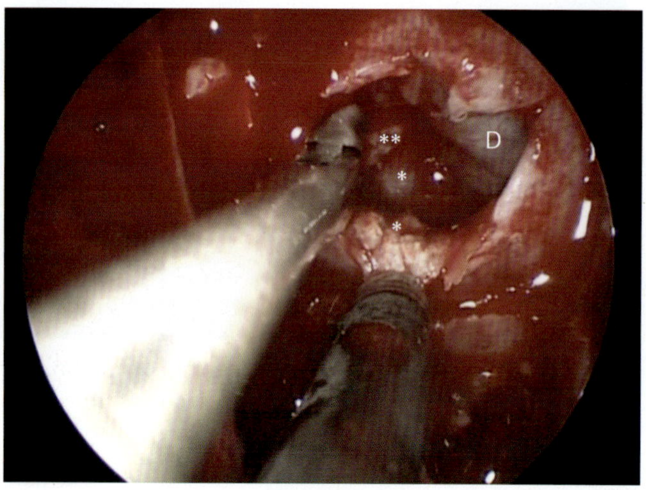

Fig. 9A.12 Solid (*) and calcified (**) tumor components are removed using grasping instruments and suction. The diaphragma sellae (D) is used as anatomical landmark, and it has to be protected from accidental laceration or tearing while removing pieces of the tumorous lesion.

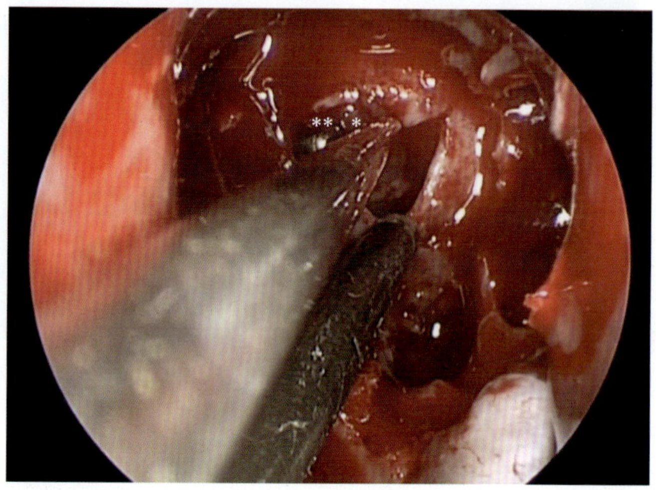

Fig. 9A.13 Solid (*) and calcified (**) tumor components are removed using a 45-degree curette.

12. The resection is continued posteriorly along the diaphragma sellae, and the posterior tumor compartments are resected (**Figs. 9A.18** and **9A.19**).
13. The prolapsing diaphragma sellae is held in place using a neuropatty and a suction to minimize laceration and manipulation of the diaphragmal dura (**Fig. 9A.20**).
14. The posterior inferior solid and calcified tumor components can then be removed until the clival dura is identified (**Figs. 9A.21** and **9A.22**).
15. After complete tumor removal and hemostasis, the diaphragma sellae prolapses symmetrically into the sphenoid cavity (**Figs. 9A.23** and **9A.24**).

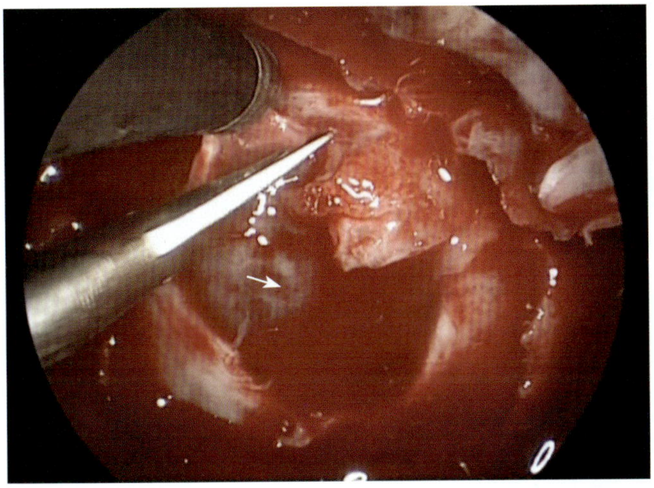

Fig. 9A.14 The solid tumor component (*arrow*) is located superiorly and is exposed by widening the dural opening.

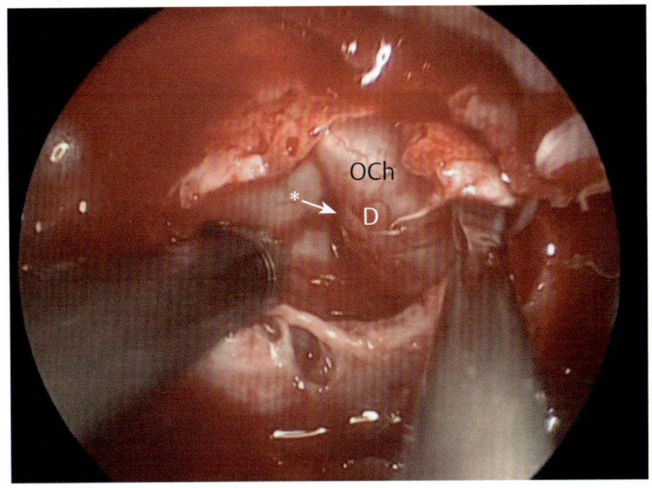

Fig. 9A.15 The solid tumor component (*) is resected following the anatomical dissection plane (*arrow*) between the tumor and the diaphragma sellae (D) posteriorly. The flattened and compressed optic chiasm (OCh) is visible.

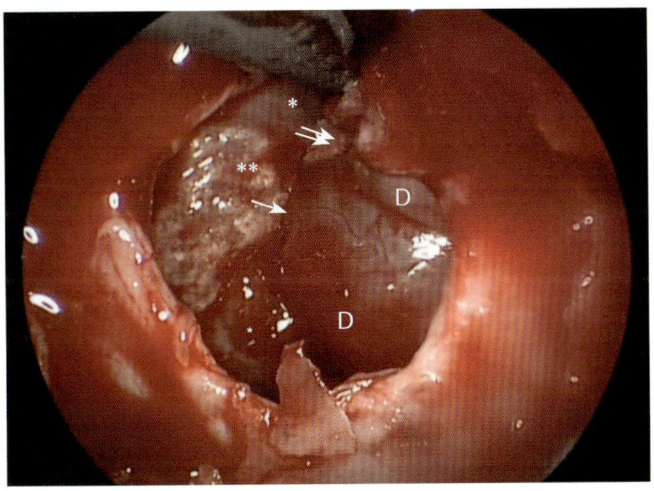

Fig. 9A.16 The solid (*) and calcified (**) tumor components are resected following the anatomical dissection plane (*arrow*) between the tumor and the diaphragma sellae (D) posteriorly. The diaphragma sellae is protected and pushed superiorly using a neuropatty and suction (*double arrow*).

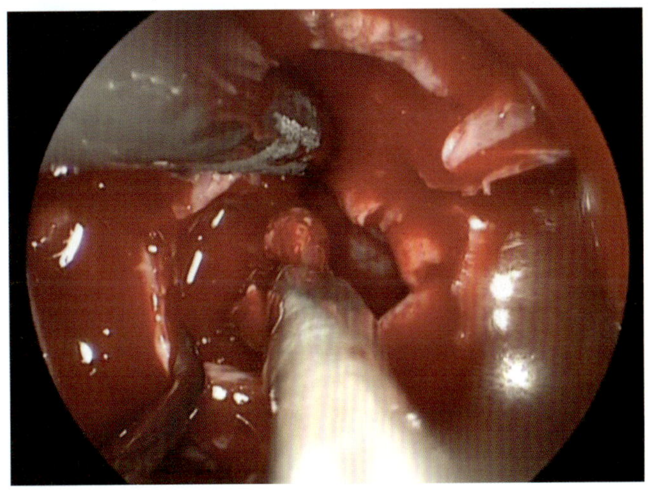

Fig. 9A.17 Removal of the solid calcified tumor components using a grasping instrument.

16. Reconstruction of the skull base defect is started with an intrasellar abdominal fat graft plug (**Fig. 9A.25**).
17. The construct is supported with Surgicel and an artificial dural sealant (**Figs. 9A.26**, **9A.27**, and **9A.28**).
18. The pedicled nasoseptal flaps are brought into place and are supported with Surgifoam and a resorbable endonasal packing (**Figs. 9A.29** and **9A.30**).

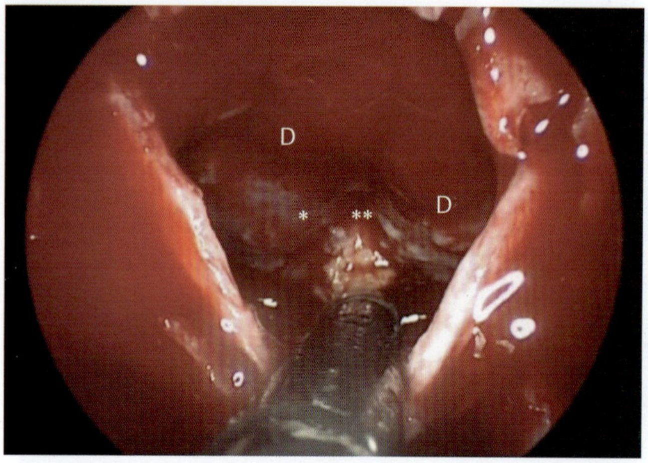

Fig. 9A.18 Superior posterior solid (*) and (**) calcified tumor components along the diaphragma sellae (D) cause irregularities and folds that indicate remnants of the tumor.

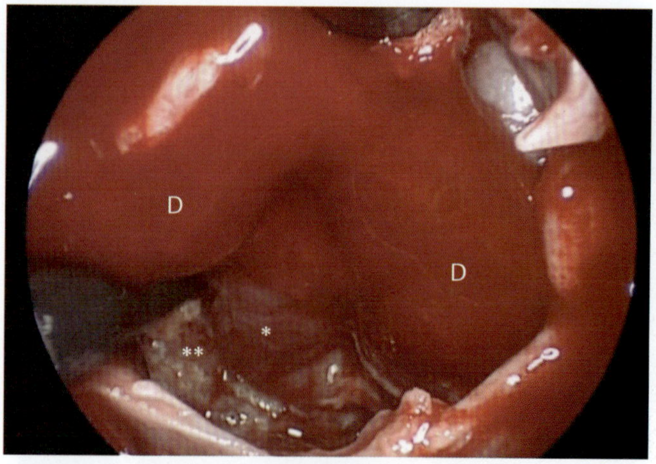

Fig. 9A.19 Posterior solid (*) and (**) calcified tumor components along the diaphragma sellae (D) cause irregularities and folds that indicate remnants of the tumor.

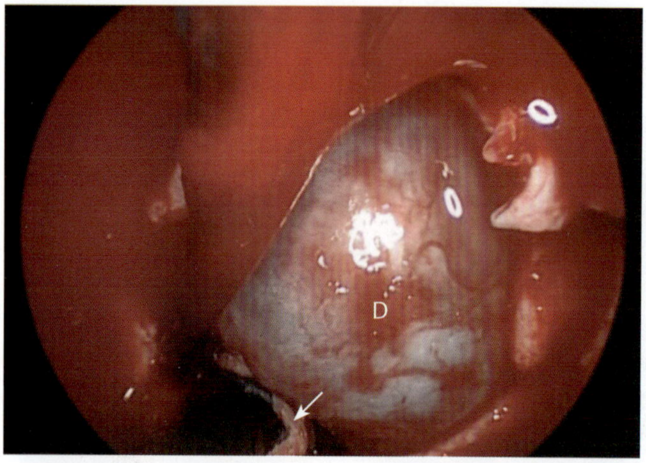

Fig. 9A.20 To reach the most posterior aspect of the solid tumor component, the prolapsing diaphragma sellae (D) is elevated and protected using a neuropatty (*arrow*) and a suction device.

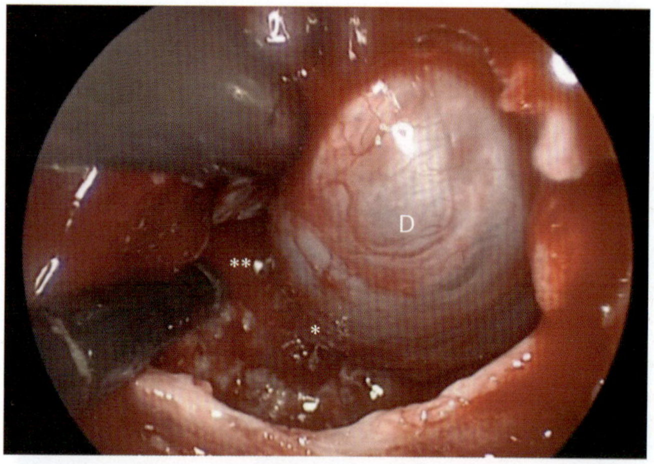

Fig. 9A.21 The posterior solid (*) and calcified (**) tumor components are removed.

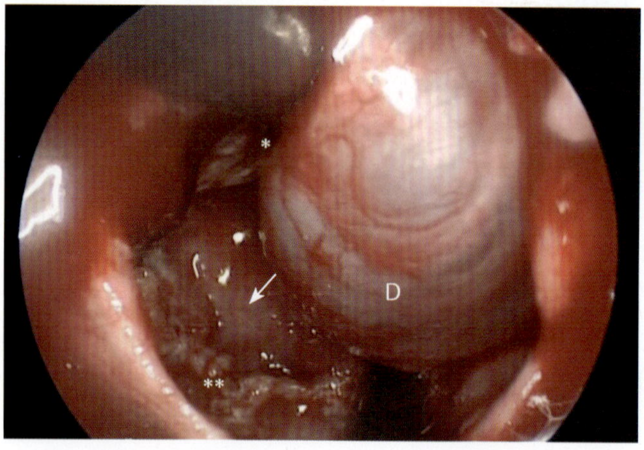

Fig. 9A.22 The resection of the most posterior solid (*) and calcified (**) tumor components is continued until the clival dura is identified (*arrow*).

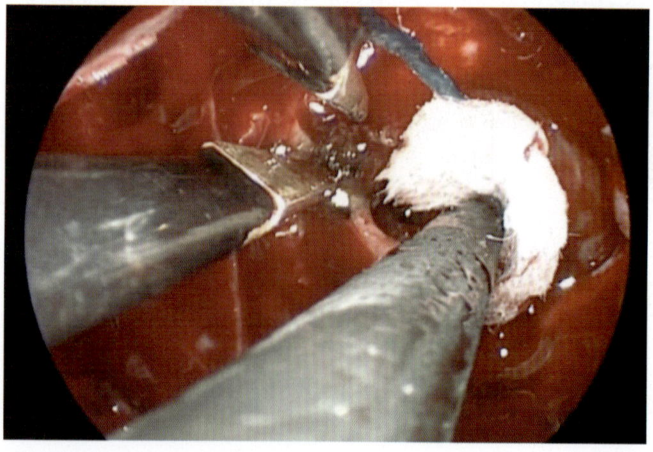

Fig. 9A.23 Hemostasis of the sellar dura after complete resection and inspection of the sella.

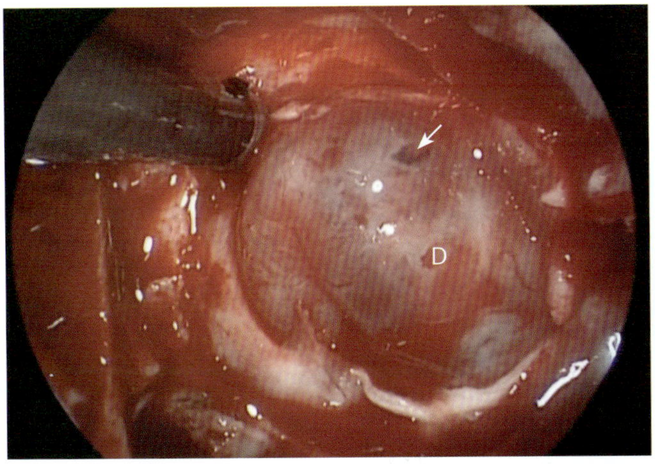

Fig. 9A.24 Symmetrical prolapse of the diaphragma sellae (D) indicates a complete resection of the lesion. A laceration of the diaphragmal dura (*arrow*) is identified with relevant CSF-leakage.

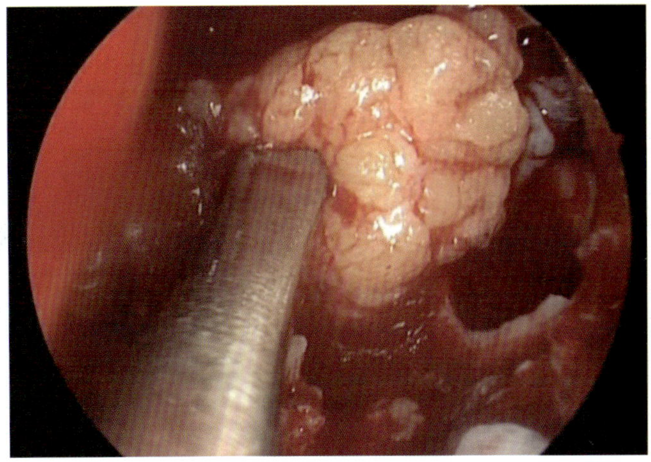

Fig. 9A.25 Placement of an intrasellar abdominal fat graft. The edges of the fat plug have to be placed intradurally and cover the whole sella.

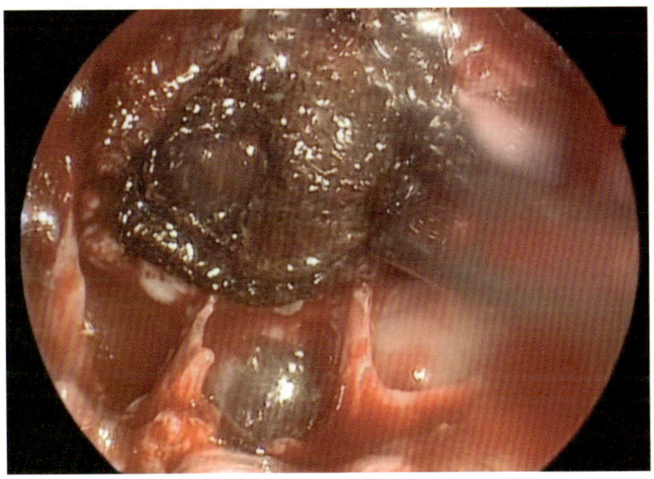

Fig. 9A.26 The abdominal fat graft is stabilized using Surgicel.

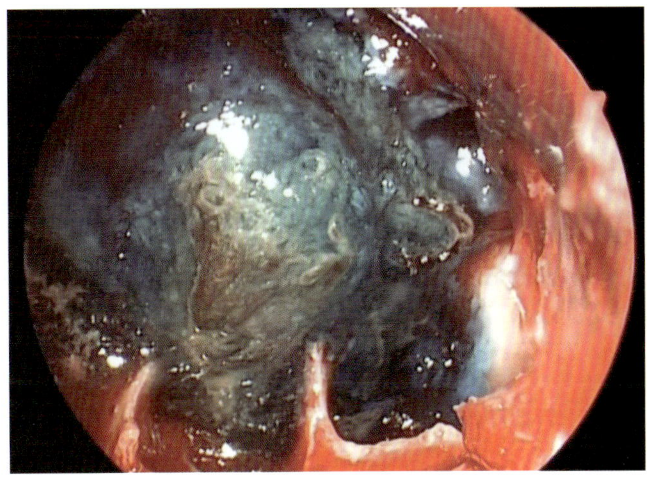

Fig. 9A.27 The construct is stabilized using an artificial dural sealant.

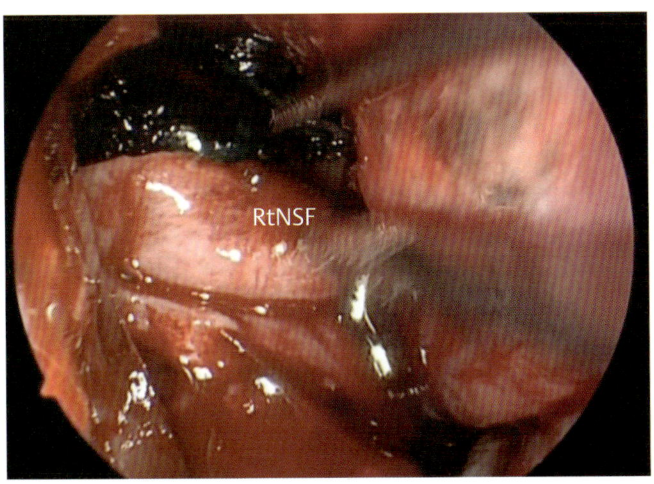

Fig. 9A.28 The right nasoseptal flap (RtNSF) is brought into the field and placed over the construct.

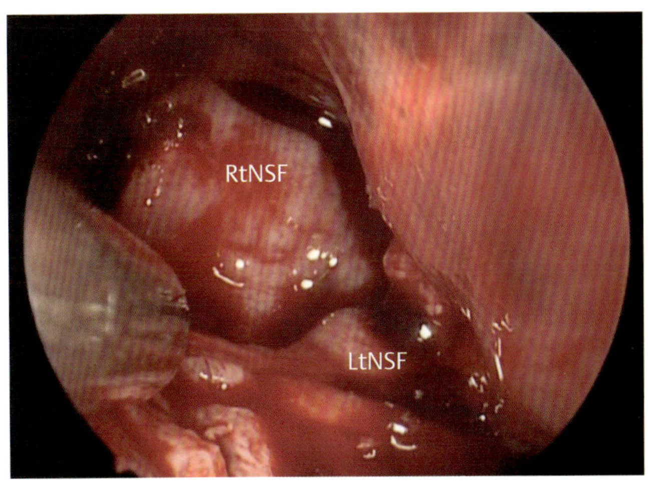

Fig. 9A.29 The left nasoseptal flap (LtNSF) is brought into the field and placed over the construct.

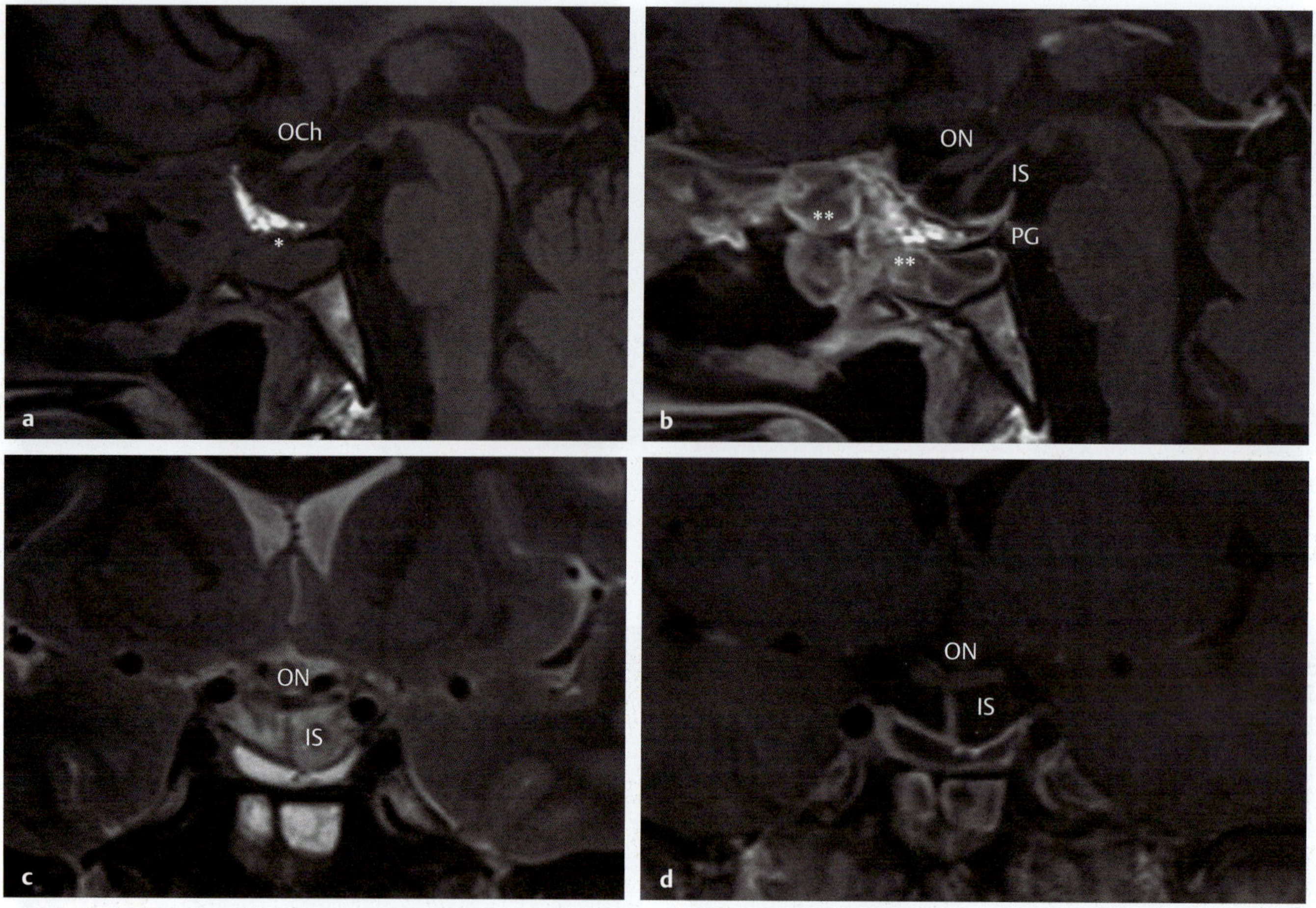

Fig. 9A.30 **(a)** Sagittal T1-weighted, **(b)** Sagittal T1-weighted contrast-enhanced, **(c)** Coronal T2-weighted, **(d)** Coronal T1-weighted MRI sequences demonstrating postoperative changes with resorption of the abdominal fat graft (*) and vital enhancement of the pedicled nasoseptal flaps (**). The optic chiasm (OCh) and the optic nerves (ON) are decompressed, and the infundibular stalk (IS) and pituitary gland (PG) are back in a physiological position.

Case 9B

A Tailored Extended Endonasal Endoscopic Approach for a Large Multicystic-Solid Craniopharyngioma

Michel Roethlisberger, Prepageran Narayanan, and Vicknes Waran

History

A 48-year-old man presented with progressive bilateral loss of vision and discrete personality changes with loss of memory noted by his family. Endocrinological examination revealed an insufficiency of the hypothalamic-pituitary-adrenal axis. Further diagnostic workup with neurocranial imaging revealed a large sellar/parasellar lesion with cystic components extending over the planum sphenoidale, an intra- and suprasellar solid component. A second cyst was present extending to the clival region with compression of the midbrain area and the cerebral peduncles (**Fig. 9B.1a–d**).

Due to the extension along the skull base as well as the solid intrasellar and paraclival component, a **binostril extended endoscopic tailored approach** was selected to treat this patient's lesion.

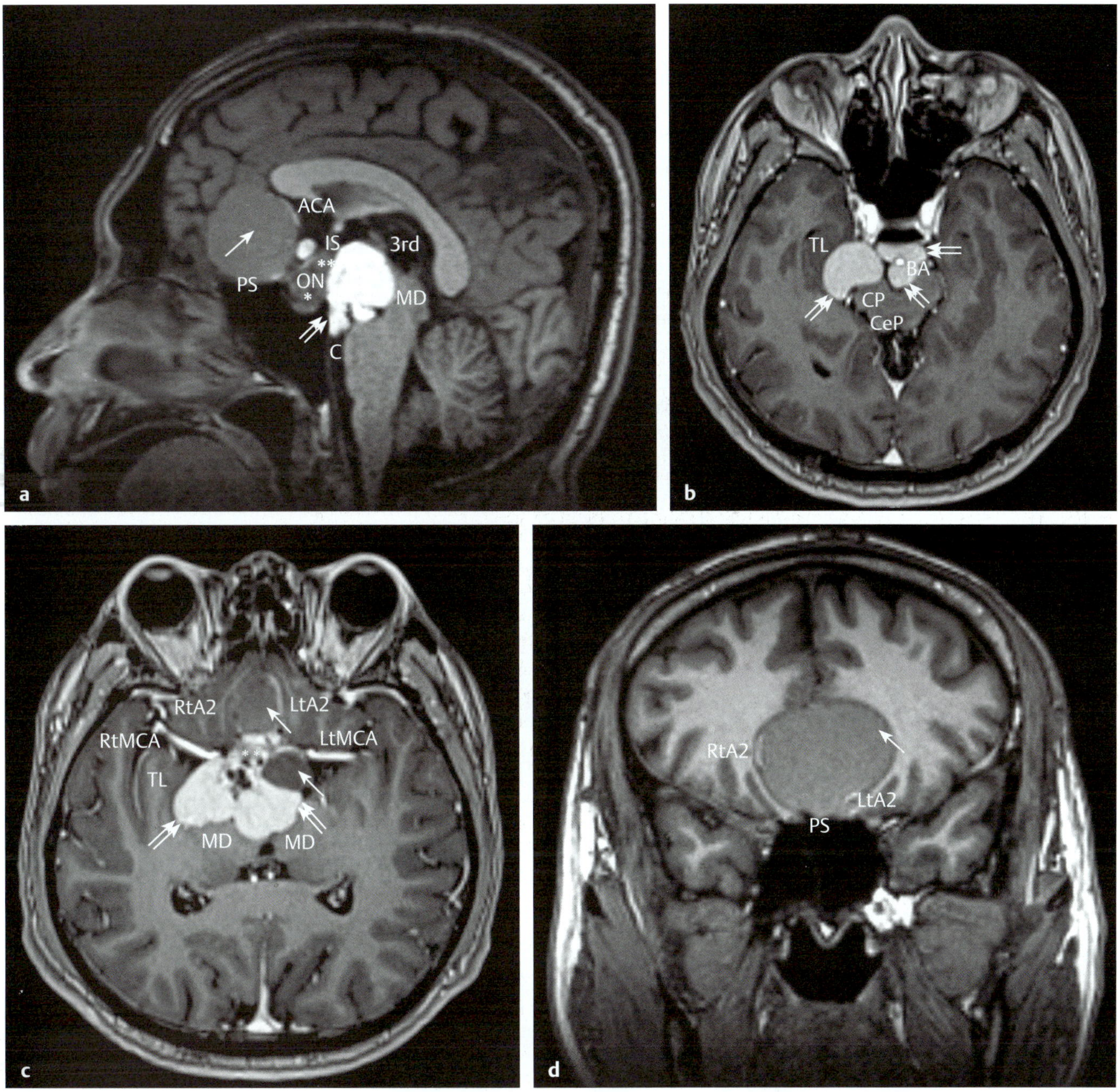

Fig. 9B.1 **(a)** Sagittal, **(b, c)** axial, and **(d)** coronal T1-weighted gadolinium contrast-enhanced sections showing a large sellar/ parasellar lesion with a cystic component (*arrow*) extending over the planum sphenoidale (PS) with a second cyst (*double arrows*) extending to the prepontine cistern and clival area (C) with compression of the midbrain, the cerebral peduncles (CP) and the right mesial temporal lobe (TL). Encasement of the basilar artery (BA) by the posterior cyst is seen. The anterior cyst demonstrates a brain isointense signal while the posterior cyst is hyperintense indicating high proteinaceous content. The cysts are divided by an intra- (*) and suprasellar (**) solid component without extension into the 3rd ventricle. There is dislocation the optic nerves (ON), the infundibular stalk (IS), as well as the anterior cerebral arteries (ACA).

Surgical Steps

1. Local anesthesia is infiltrated into the septum to raise the mucoperichondrial flaps bilaterally in preparation for the creation of bilateral pedicled nasoseptal flaps.
2. An incision is made with a size-15 blade anteriorly to the middle turbinate down to the cartilaginous septum with more anterior extension than in a standard situation (**Fig. 9B.2**).
3. The pedicled nasoseptal flap is then raised off the septum with a Freer elevator from anterior to posterior (**Fig. 9B.3**).
4. The exposed cartilaginous septum is fractured through to the contralateral side and removed in a piecemeal manner, all the while freeing it from the overlying contralateral septal mucoperichondrium (**Fig. 9B.4**).
5. The elevation of septal mucoperichondrium is continued posteriorly until the sphenoid ostia and the posterior choana are visible (**Fig. 9B.5**).
6. Superiorly, the flap may be taken until about 0.5 to 1 cm below the skull base to preserve the olfactory function. Inferiorly, the flap can be taken as far as half the nasal floor if a large skull base defect is expected (Hadad-Bassagasteguy flap) (**Fig. 9B.6**).
7. The nasoseptal flap is then freed superiorly and inferiorly using microscissors aiming for the sphenoid ostia and posterior choana, respectively (**Fig. 9B.7**).
8. The pedicled flap can then be stored in the nasopharynx until it is required for reconstruction (**Fig. 9B.8**).
9. This is continued until the sphenoid rostrum is exposed with the sphenoid ostia visible bilaterally.
10. At this point, the contralateral nasoseptal flap can be created in the same manner as described in steps 5 and 6.
11. Once the sphenoid rostrum is fully exposed, the ostia are widened inferomedially using a Kerrison punch in a V-shape fashion toward the midline (**Fig. 9B.9**).
12. Using the Kerrison punch, the ostia are then widened medially toward the midline, and the sphenoid rostrum is removed using a pituitary rongeur forceps.
13. The remnant sphenoid rostrum and the sphenoid sinus septations are then removed to allow an unobstructed view (**Fig. 9B.10**).
14. The posterior wall of the sphenoid sinus is then demucosalized with a monopolar cautery-tipped aspirator. This allows an overview of the sphenoid cavity and the crucial neurovascular landmarks of the bony skull base. Care is taken laterally as there may be dehiscence of the optic nerve or carotid artery, which should be identified by inspection of the sphenoid sinus prior to commencement.
15. A tailored extended approach for this lesion is appropriate, involving the anterior extending cyst, the solid intrasellar part, as well as the posteriorly extending paraclival tumor cyst.
16. Drilling is commenced at the bone covering the planum sphenoidale using a high-speed diamond burr (Medtronic, Minneapolis, USA) and extended to the tuberculum and the sella turcica. An aspirator is kept within the nasal cavity to allow bone dust and smoke that is formed to be cleared to allow for an unobstructed view (**Fig. 9B.11**).
17. Both posterior ethmoidal arteries are identified.

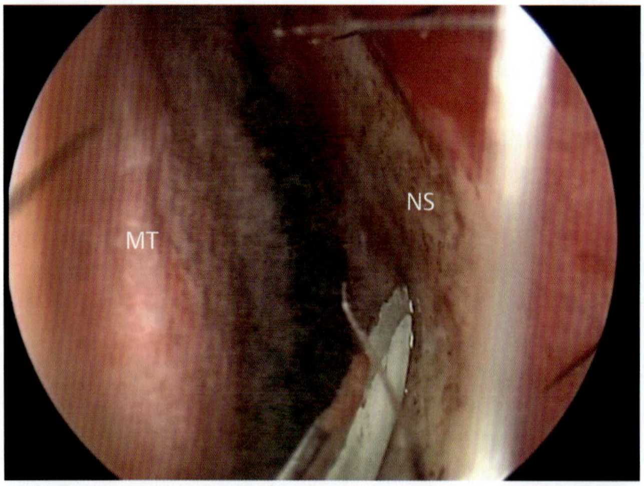

Fig. 9B.2 Mucosal incision anterior to the middle turbinate (MT) down to the cartilaginous nasal septum (NS).

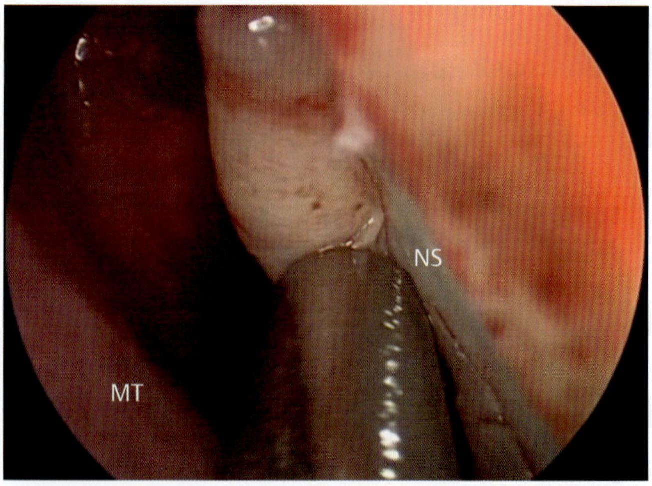

Fig. 9B.3 Elevation of the mucoperichondrium from the nasal septum (NS).

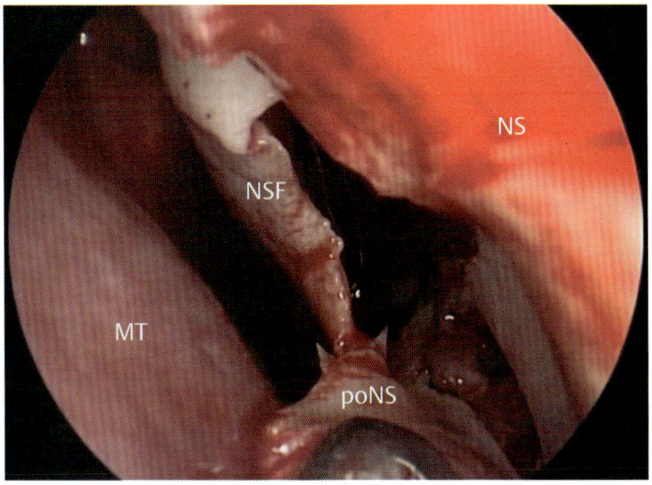

Fig. 9B.4 Piecemeal removal of the posterior septal bone (poNS).

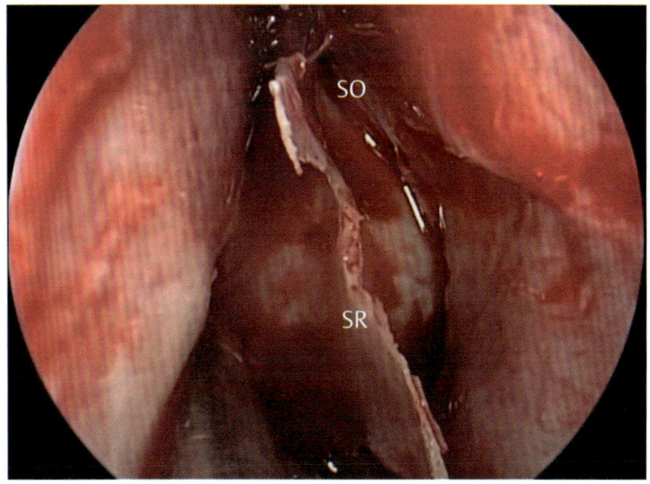

Fig. 9B.5 Exposure of the sphenoid rostrum (SR) and bilateral sphenoid ostia (SO).

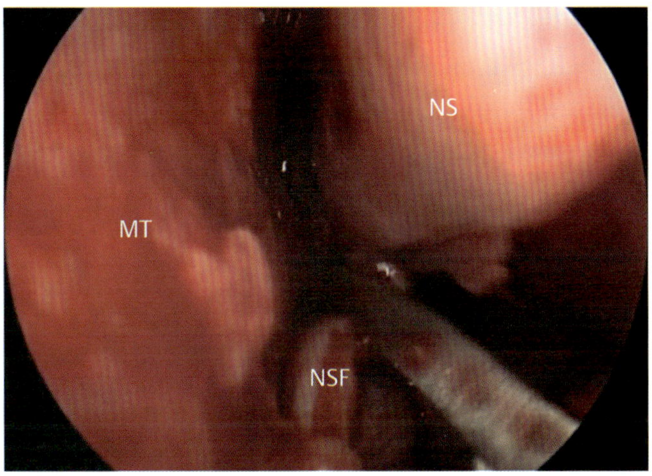

Fig. 9B.6 Cutting of the superior margin of the pedicled nasoseptal flap (NSF) 0.5 to 1 cm below the skull base to preserve the olfactory function.

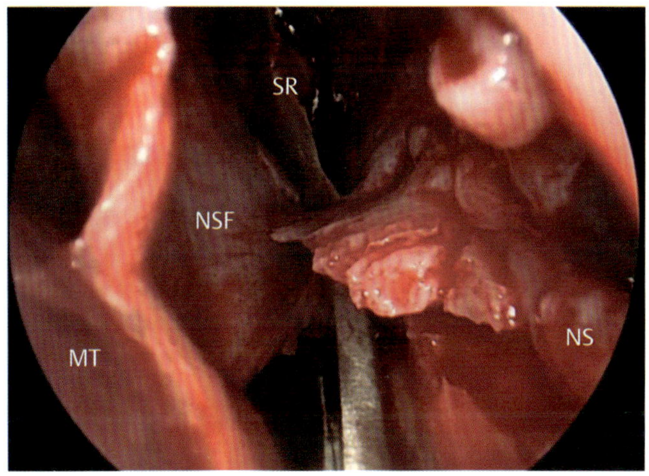

Fig. 9B.7 Inferior margin of the pedicled nasoseptal flap (NSF).

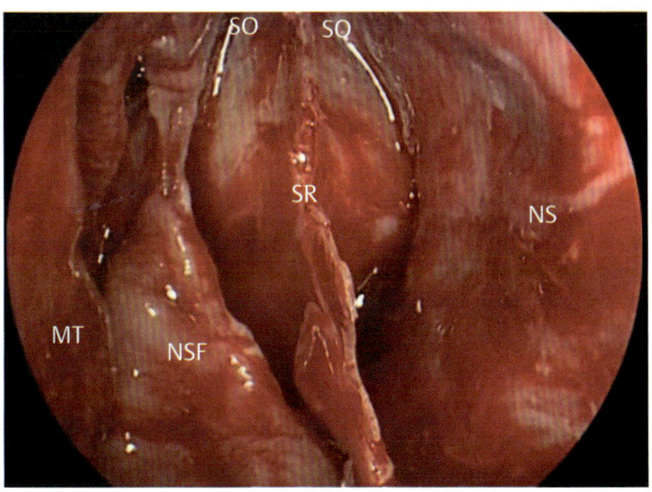

Fig. 9B.8 The nasoseptal flap (NSF) can be stored in the sphenoethmoid recess.

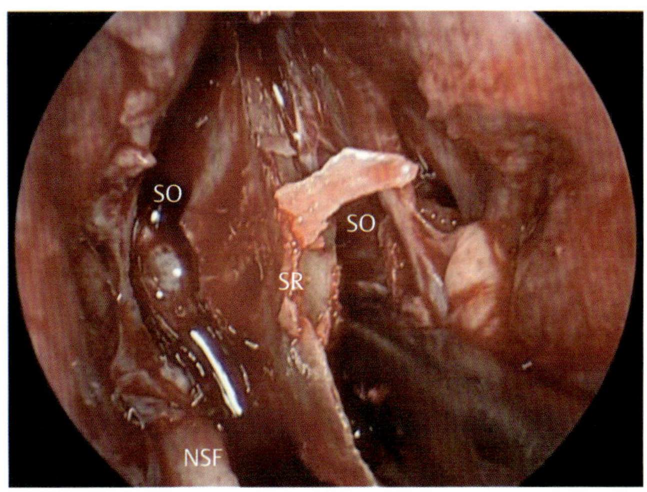

Fig. 9B.9 V-shaped opening of the sphenoid ostium using a Kerrison punch and bilateral connection.

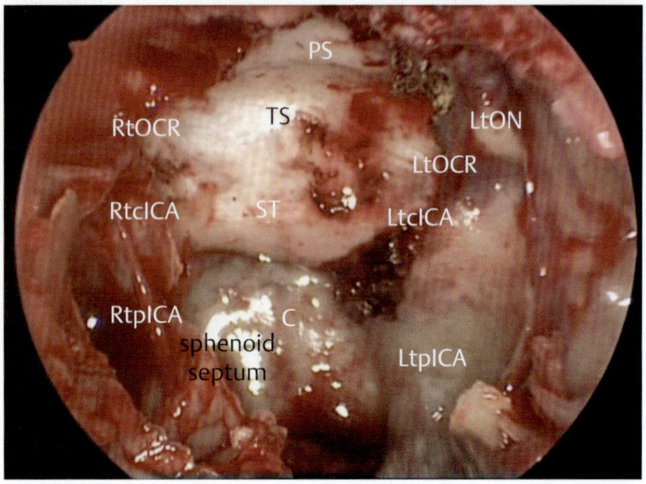

Fig. 9B.10 Exposure of the sphenoid cavity. A right-sided sphenoid septum is inserting at the right cavernous internal carotid artery (RtcICA) and paraclival internal carotid artery (RtpICA). The planum sphenoidale (PS), the tuberculum sellae (TS), and the sella turcica (ST) are visible.

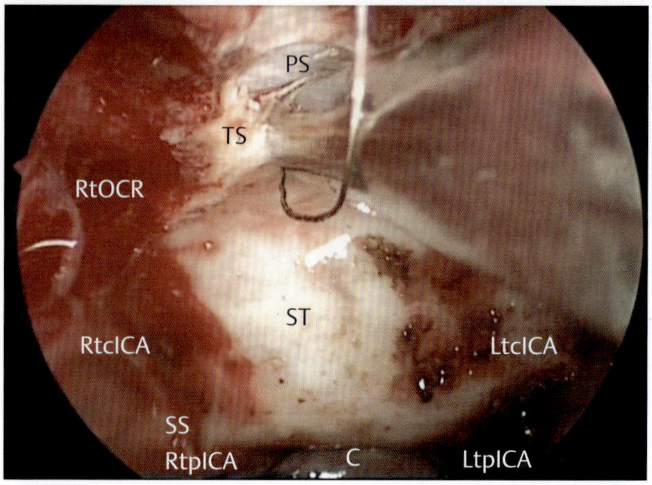

Fig. 9B.11 Drilling of the planum sphenoidale (PS) and blunt removal of bone.

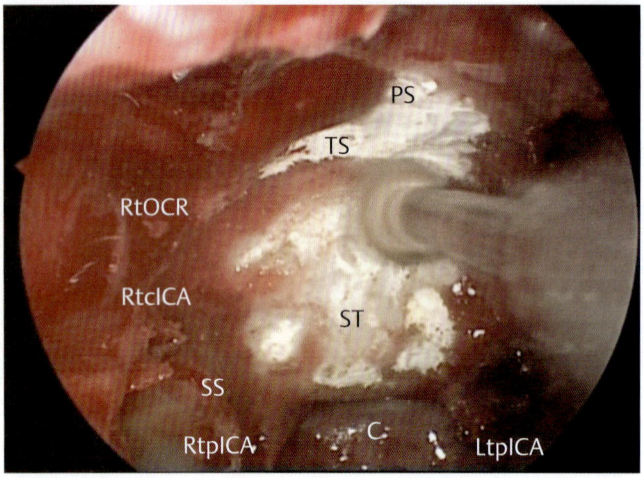

Fig. 9B.12 Drilling of the sella turcica (ST) and the tuberculum sellae (TS).

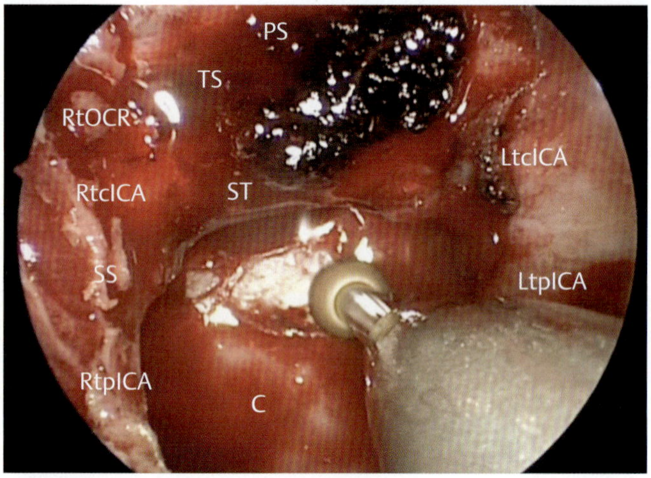

Fig. 9B.13 Drilling of the clival bone (C) between both paraclinoidal arteries.

18. Once the bone has been sufficiently thinned out, a right-angle dissector can be insinuated between the bone and the dura, and the bone is flaked off.
19. The osteodural exposure is continued with the removal of the tuberculum sellae and the bone covering the sella turcica (**Fig. 9B.12**).
20. After enough bone has been removed, the exposure can be completed with a Kerrison punch. The use of a Kerrison punch allows for better control during bone removal.
21. To reach the inferior tumor cyst, the clivus is drilled and thinned out as an inferior extension of the sellar opening. Hemostasis and bone wax should be ready to use due to venous hemorrhage of the clival bone (**Fig. 9B.13**).
22. Finally, the remaining bone covering the lateral aspects of the tuberculum sellae that covers the optic nerves are removed (**Fig. 9B.14**). This allows a tailored exposure of the complete lesion (**Fig. 9B.15**).
23. The dural opening is started at the sella turcica using microscissors after freeing the underlying tissue with a right-angle dissector.
24. Meticulous coagulation and division of the anterior intercavernous sinus are necessary to connect the planum sphenoidale with the sellar region. For this maneuver, the dural structure is freed with a

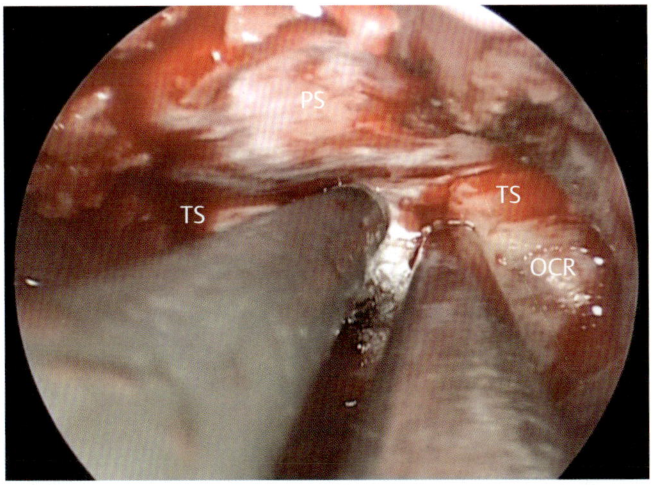

Fig. 9B.14 Connection of the anterior and sellar osteodural exposure and lateral removal of bone covering both optic nerves.

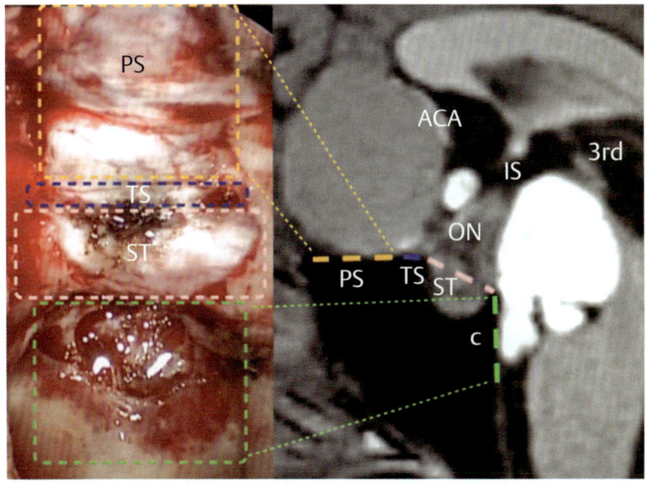

Fig. 9B.15 Tailored approach to the skull base with osteodural exposure of the planum sphenoidale (*orange square*), tuberculum sellae and intercavernous sinus (*blue square*), sella turcica (rose square), and clivus (*green square*) according to the anterior (*orange line*), tubercular (*blue line*), sellar (*rose line*), and paraclival (*green line*) extension of the craniopharyngioma.

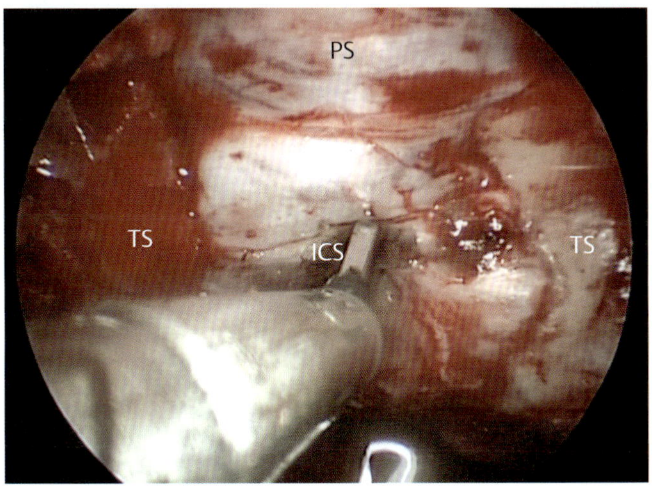

Fig. 9B.16 Cauterization and splitting of the intercavernous sinus (ICS).

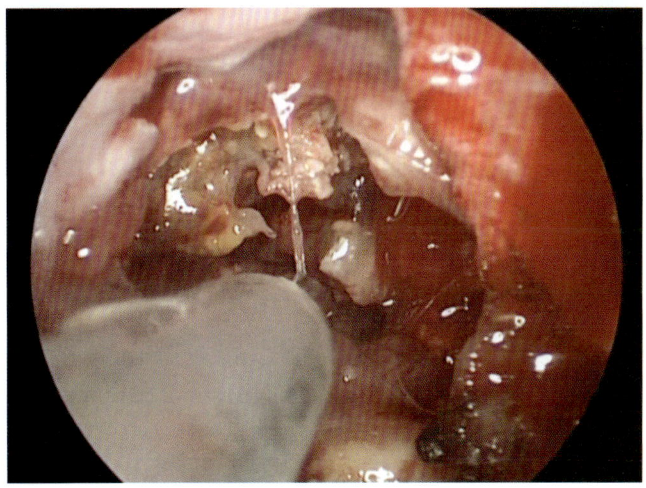

Fig. 9B.17 Blunt dissection and ultrasonic aspiration of the intra- and suprasellar solid tumor component.

right-angle dissector, controlled with bipolar cautery, and divided using microscissors to expose the entire lesion (**Fig. 9B.16**).

25. The solid tumor part within the sella is removed using blunt dissection, suction, and ultrasonic aspiration (**Fig. 9B.17**). Following the tumorous structures as well as calcified components, dissections planes can be identified. The infundibular stalk as well as the pituitary gland can be identified (**Fig. 9B.18**).
26. While blunt dissection and aspiration are continued posteriorly, the posterior tumor cyst, that is high in protein content, opens up and a greenish cyst component is identified (**Fig. 9B.19**).
27. As a next step, the dural opening is continued along the planum sphenoidale with microscissors after freeing the underlying tissue using a right-angle dissector. Hereby, the anterior tumor cyst wall is identified and preserved while completing the anterior opening under neuronavigational control (**Fig. 9B.20**).
28. The anterior cyst collapses after opening and can be removed extracapsularly from the brain surface due to an intact arachnoid plane. The anterior vessels

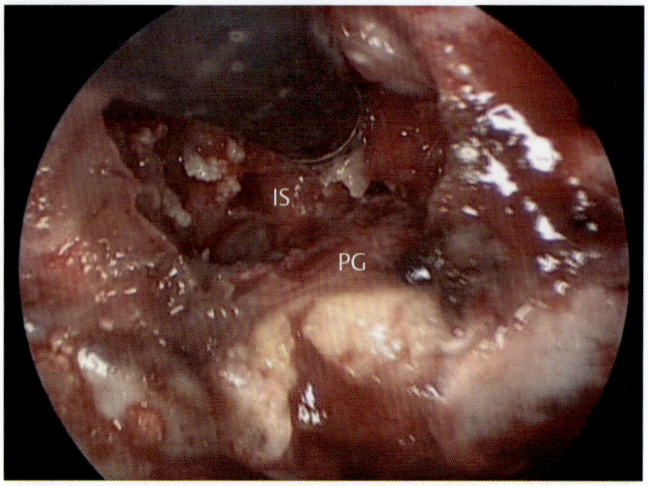

Fig. 9B.18 Identification of the infundibular stalk (IS) and the anterior pituitary gland (PG).

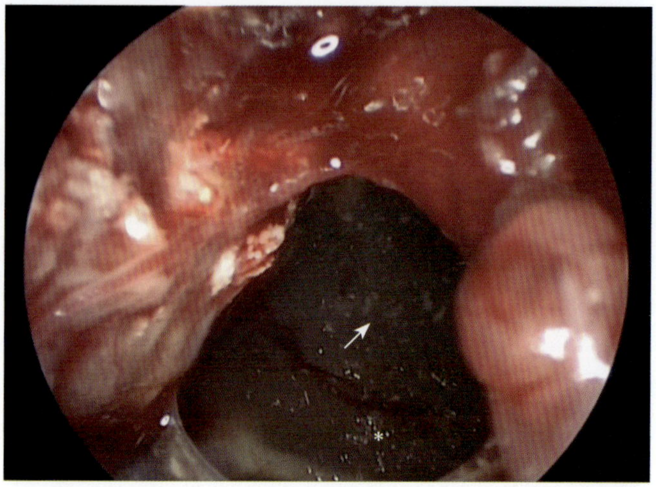

Fig. 9B.19 Opening of the posterior tumor cyst (*arrow*), which is rich in protein and presents with cholesterol crystals (*) and greenish mucoid fluid.

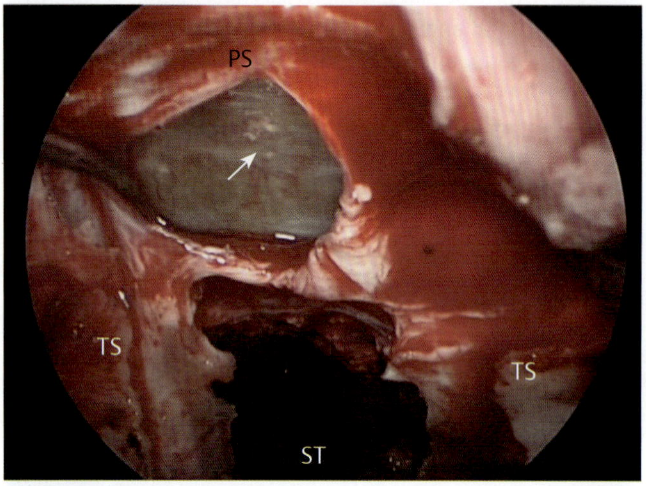

Fig. 9B.20 Opening of the dura covering the planum sphenoidale (PS) and identification of a dissection plane between the dura and the anterior tumor cyst (*arrow*).

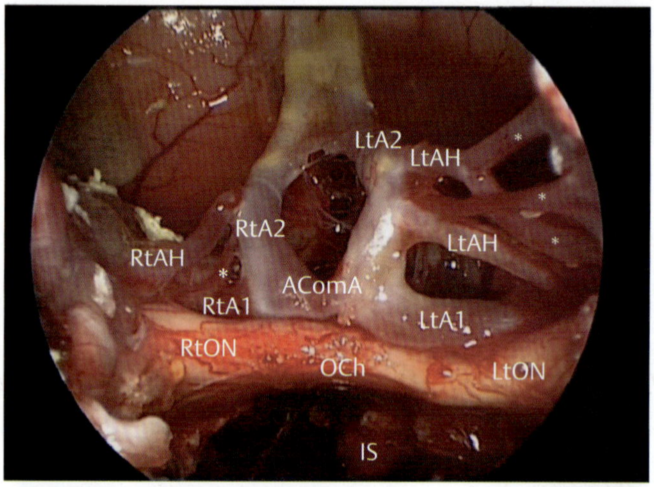

Fig. 9B.21 Resection cavity after removal of the anterior tumor cyst from anterior to posterior. The right distal anterior cerebral artery (RtA2) and left distal anterior cerebral artery (LtA2), the right recurrent arteries of Heubner (RtAH) and left recurrent arteries of Heubner (LtAH) with a duplicated anatomical variant on the left side, perforating arteries (*), the anterior communicating artery (AComA) as well as the right proximal anterior cerebral arteries (RtA1) and left proximal anterior cerebral arteries (LtA1) are visible. In close anatomical relation, the optic chiasm (OCh) and the right optic nerves (RtON) and left optic nerves (LtON) as well as the infundibular stalk (IS) are visible.

including the frontopolar branches, distal anterior cerebral artery (ACA, A2), the recurrent artery of Heubner, the anterior communicating artery (AComA), as well as the proximal anterior cerebral arteries (ACA, A1) have to be identified and preserved. In close anatomical relation are the optic chiasm and the optic nerves (**Fig. 9B.21**).

29. While dissecting posteriorly, the resection cavity of the anterior tumor cyst connects with the resection cavity of the solid intra- and suprasellar tumor component,

the mesencephalon and the mamillary bodies, as well as small perforating arteries can be identified and have to be preserved (**Figs. 9B.22** and **9B.23**).

30. An intraoperative contrast-enhanced MRI was performed showing complete resection of the large supra/parasellar and sellar lesion (**Fig. 9B.24 a–d**).
31. Meticulous hemostasis is then performed.
32. The defect is then plugged with fat taken from the abdomen, and the edges of the fat are tucked underneath to create a watertight seal. Care is taken not to pack too much fat tightly into the cavity (**Fig. 9B.25**).
33. This is then sealed with a synthetic dural sealant and layered with an absorbable hemostat.
34. The bilateral nasoseptal flaps are then rotated over the defect to complete the repair and reinforced with gelatin sponges to keep the flaps in position. No other nasal packing is required (**Fig. 9B.26**).

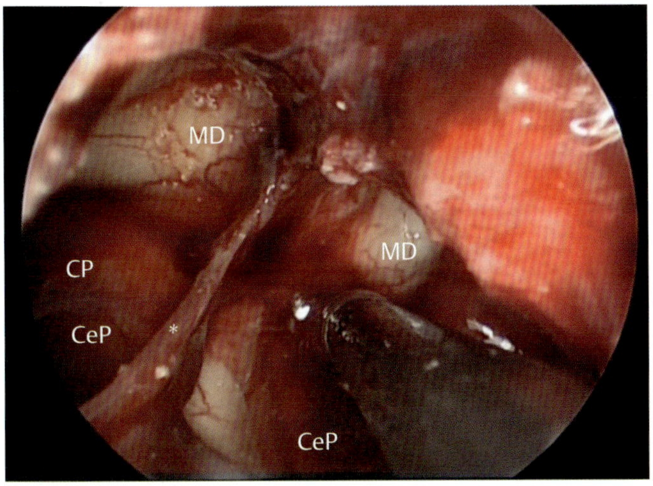

Fig. 9B.22 The cerebral peduncles (CeP), the mamillary bodies (MB), and midbrain perforators (*) are visible after resection of the anterior tumor cyst and the suprasellar solid tumor component.

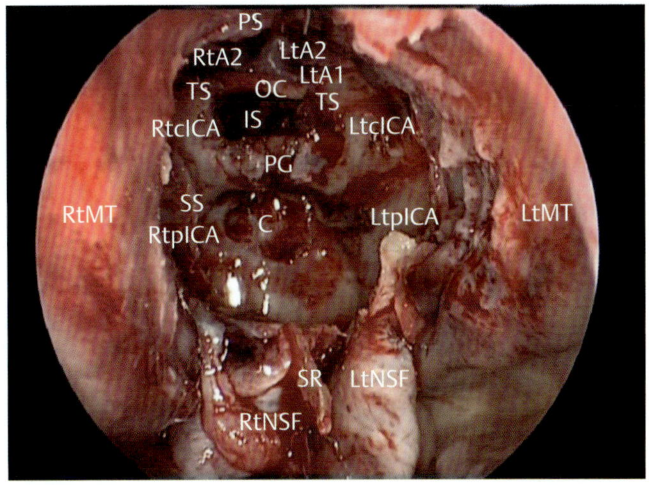

Fig. 9B.23 Full view of the resection cavity with the right (RtNSF) and left pedicled nasoseptal flaps (LtNSF) in the field.

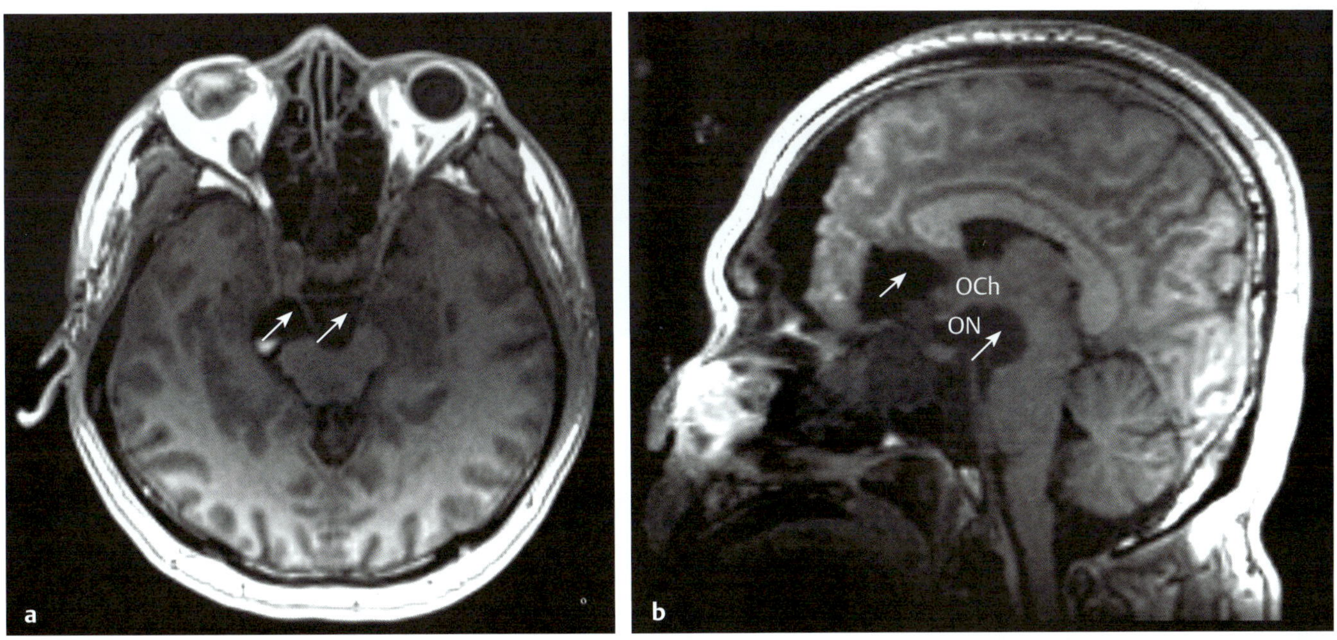

Fig. 9B.24 **(a)** Axial and **(b)** coronal intraoperative T1-weighted MRI section demonstrating complete resection of the tumorous lesion (*arrows*). The optic chiasm (OCh) and the optic nerves (ON) are decompressed. There is no evidence of an acute hemorrhage. *(Continued)*

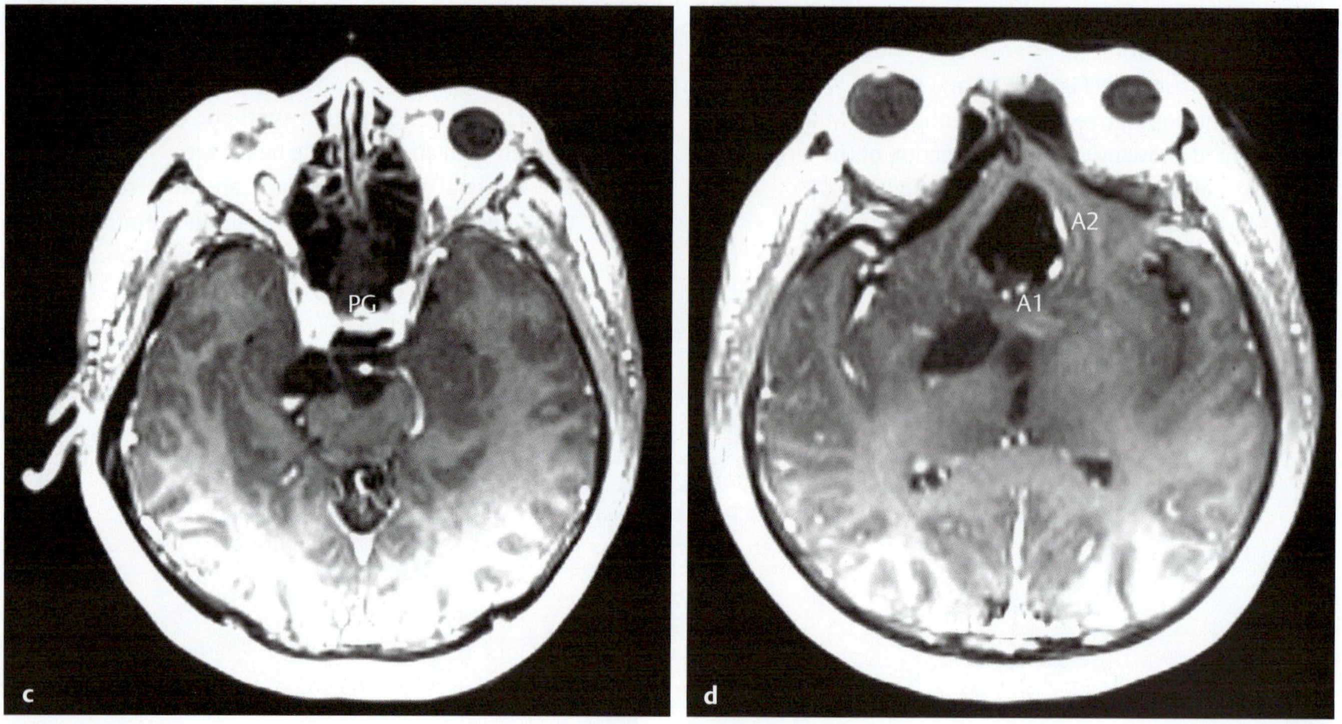

Fig. 9B.24 *(Continued)* **(c, d)** Axial intraoperative T1-weighted contrast-enhanced MRI section demonstrating the enhancing posterior pituitary gland (PG). The pre- (A1) and postcommunicating segments (A2) of the anterior cerebral arteries are perfused and clearly visible.

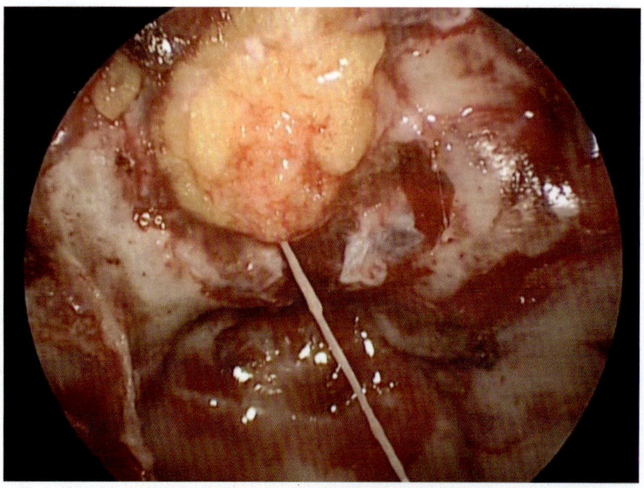

Fig. 9B.25 Closure of the large dural skull base defect using an abdominal fat graft.

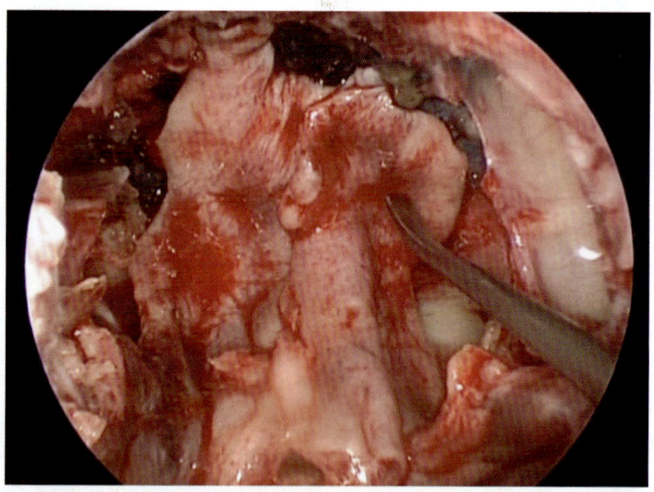

Fig. 9B.26 Coverage of the fat graft with an artificial dural sealant and bilateral pedicled nasoseptal flaps with contact to the surrounding bony margin.

Case 9C

A Tailored Extended Endoscopic Transseptal Transsphenoidal Excision of a Solid-Cystic Craniopharyngioma Extending to the Third Ventricle

Michel Roethlisberger, Kong Yew Liew, Saif Al-Zahid, Prepageran Narayanan, and Vicknes Waran

History

A 55-year-old female patient with a history of underlying hypertension presented with slowly progressive memory impairment, urinary incontinence, headaches, and an unsteady gait. A neurocranial MRI revealed a large suprasellar a partly cystic partly solid lesion with the involvement of the intrasellar compartment and extending to the third ventricle with compression of the hypothalamic walls and consecutive obstructive hydrocephalus.

Surgical Steps

1. A **binostril endoscopic transseptal transsphenoidal approach** is performed as previously described (**Chapter 1**).
2. The posterior wall of the sphenoid sinus is then demucosalized with a monopolar cautery-tipped aspirator. This allows for drilling of the sella and tuberculum and to prevent oozing from the mucosal edges (**Fig. 9C.1**).
3. Drilling is then commenced with a diamond burr to thin the bone overlying the sella and tuberculum. An aspirator is kept within the nasal cavity to allow bone dust and smoke that is formed to be cleared to give an unobstructed view (**Fig. 9C.2**).
4. Once the bone has been sufficiently thinned out, a right-angle dissector can be insinuated between the bone and the dura, and the bone can be removed (**Fig. 9C.3**).
5. The osteodural exposure is completed with a Kerrison punch. The use of a Kerrison punch allows for better control when removing bone. The superior and inferior extent of the exposure is dictated by the size of the lesion and can be confirmed through image guided surgery (IGS).
6. The sellar dura is opened in a horizontal manner. The underlying tissue is separated superiorly and inferiorly from the incision, and the dura is then cut superiorly using microscissors (**Fig. 9C.4**).
7. The dura of the planum sphenoidale close to the tuberculum sellae is incised horizontally. With this maneuver, the anterior intercavernous sinus, which is located between the two horizontal incisions, is freed and cauterized with a bipolar cautery and divided with microscissors consecutively (**Fig. 9C.5**).
8. The excision is then started at the central component of the lesion with a combination of an aspirator, dissection and ultrasonic aspiration. As the central component is debulked, the weight of the surrounding soft tissue will cause the tumor edges to collapse into the

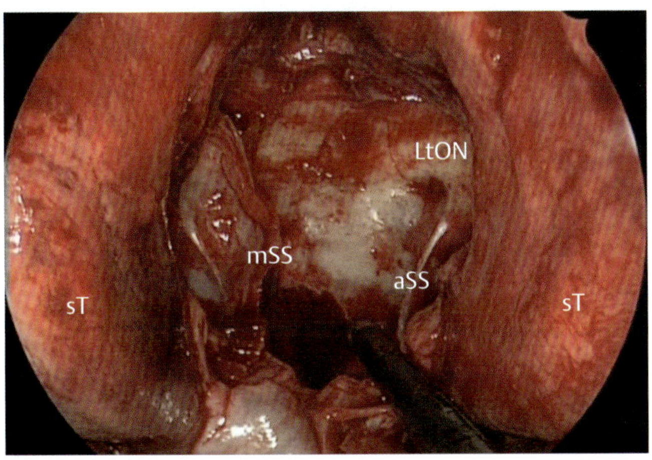

Fig. 9C.1 The view of the sphenoid sinus after removal of the sphenoid rostrum. The superior turbinates (sT) are visible bilaterally and the pedicle of the right nasoseptal flap can be seen opposite to the aspirator.

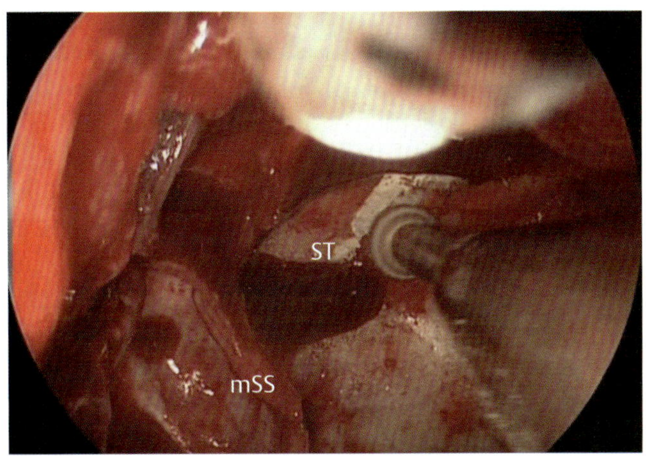

Fig. 9C.2 Transplanum approach. The aspirator is visible superiorly keeping the smoke and dust out of view.

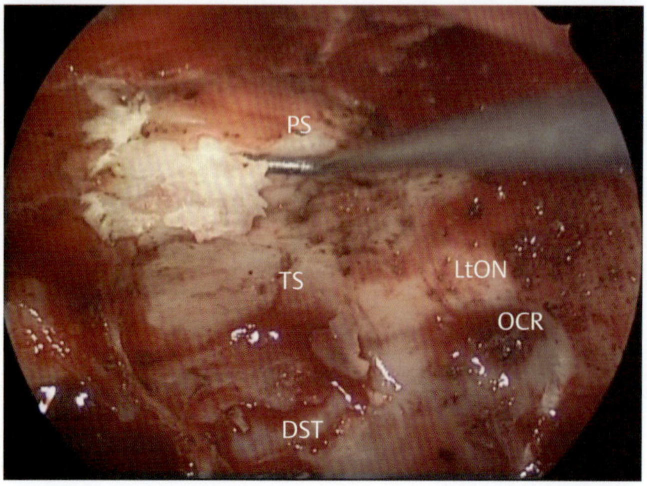

Fig. 9C.3 Transplanum and transtuberculum approach. The bone between the planum sphenoidale (PS) and tuberculum sellae (TS) is removed using a right-angle dissector. The sella turcica dura (DST) is already exposed.

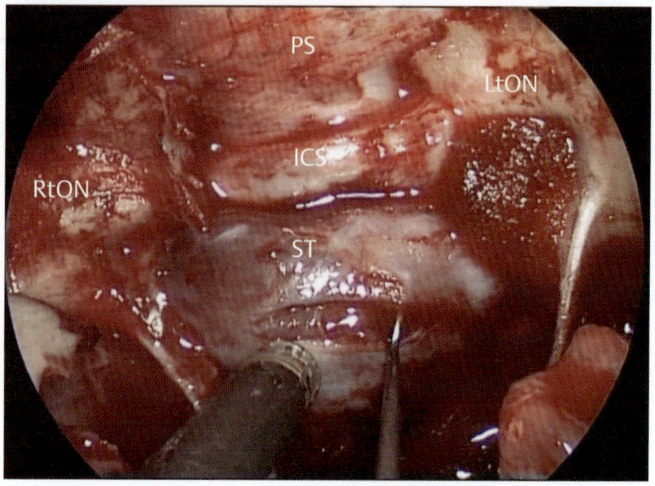

Fig. 9C.4 Transplanum and transtuberculum osteodural exposure. The intercavernous sinus (ICS) is seen between the dura of the sella turcica (ST) and planum sphenoidale (PS). A right-angle dissector is used to free the dura overlying the lesion superior to the incision.

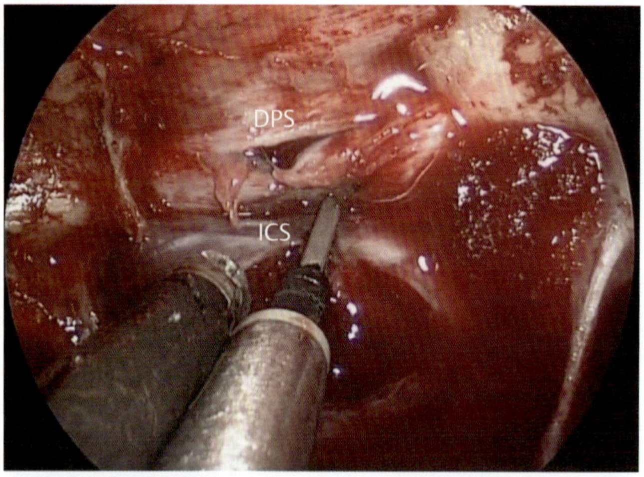

Fig. 9C.5 The anterior intercavernous sinus (ICS) is cauterized with bipolar cautery.

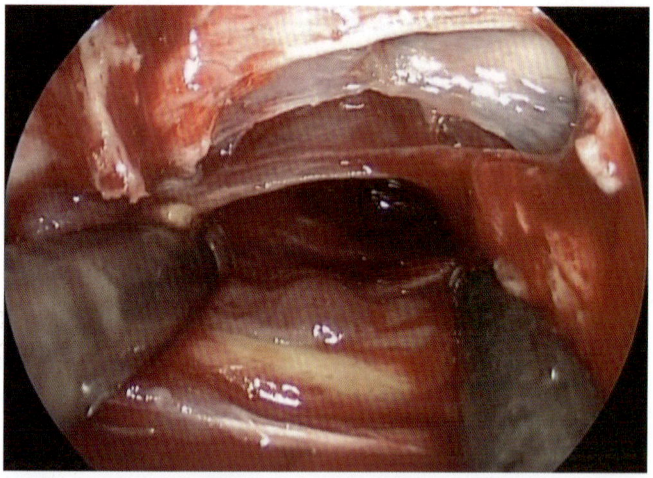

Fig. 9C.6 Debulking of the central tumor mass. The superior edge can be seen gradually falling into the surgical field.

central zone. This allows the periphery of the lesion and the edges to be delivered through a smaller opening rather than having to expand the exposure along the skull base (**Fig. 9C.6**).

9. The central debulking should be continued as far as it is visualized safely. Positioning should be confirmed through IGS regularly, and the surgical dissection should not continue if the depth cannot be seen.
10. The superior edge is then delivered into view. This step should be performed gently to not put too much traction on the optic chiasm superiorly. The tumor is then freed from the optic chiasm, and the superior component is delivered centrally into view (**Figs. 9C.7** and **Fig. 9C.8**).
11. The lateral aspects of the tumor are dissected circumferentially and collapsed into the central cavity (**Fig. 9C.9**).
12. As the tumor is delivered centrally, it may be debulked further to allow for an easier extracapsular dissection. However, the capsule should be maintained to keep the correct dissection plane (**Fig. 9C.10**).
13. After complete excision, the cavity is examined for any remnants of the tumor (**Fig. 9C.11**).

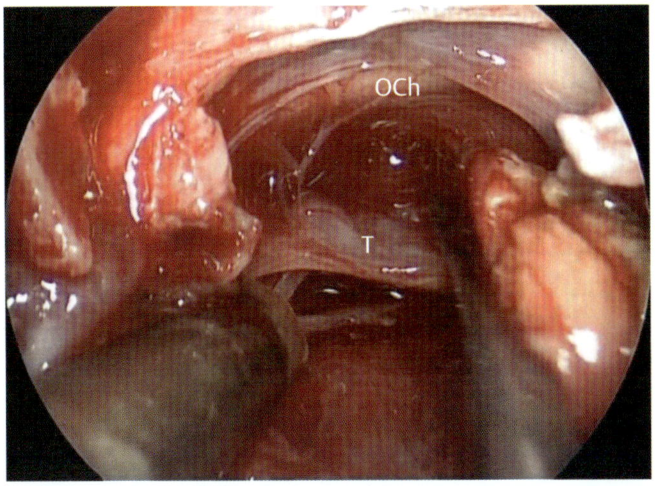

Fig. 9C.7 The superior tumor edge (T) is delivered centrally. The optic chiasm (OCh) is visible superiorly.

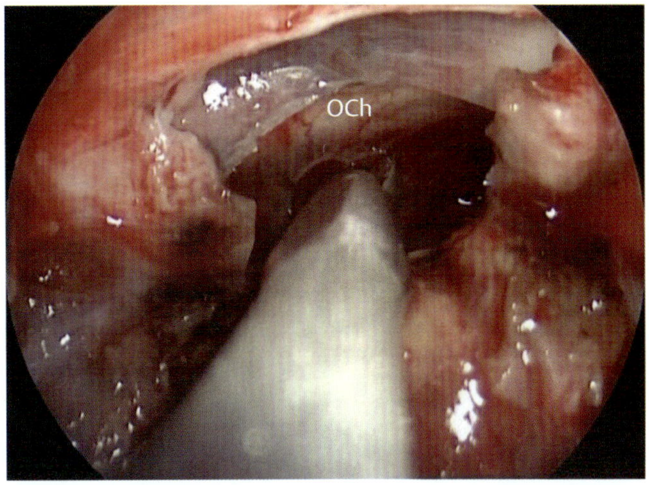

Fig. 9C.8 Tumor attachments to the optic chiasm (OCh) are cut with microscissors.

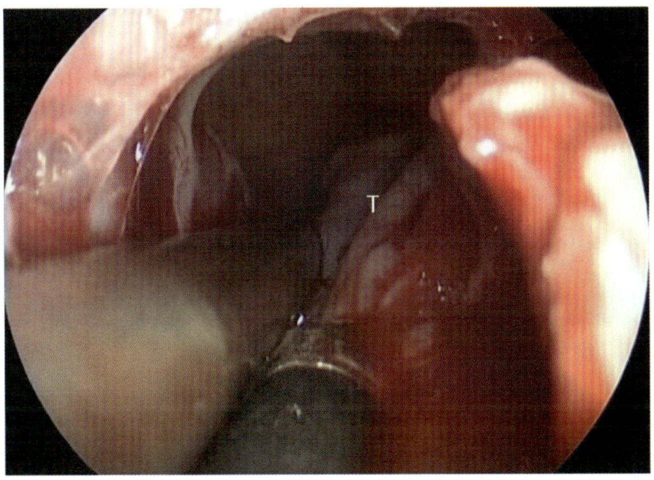

Fig. 9C.9 The superior edge of the tumor (T) is brought into the central zone after freeing it from the optic chiasm. The posterior limit of the tumor has been reached as normal tissue can be seen deep posteriorly.

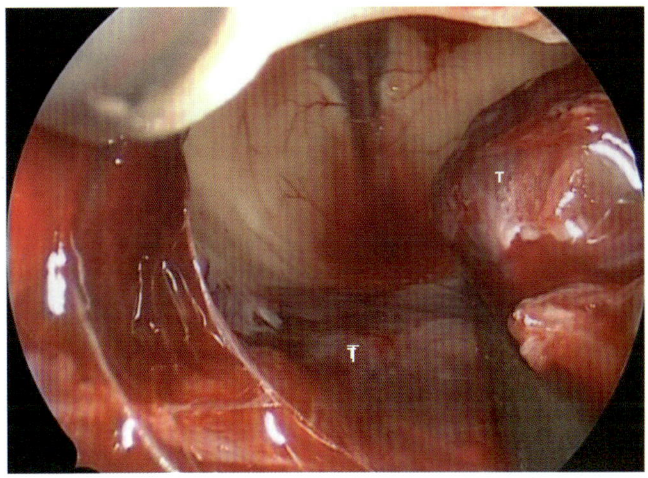

Fig. 9C.10 View after the superior and right tumor (T) edges have been mobilized. The inferior component of the tumor is still attached and is visible inferiorly. The third ventricle can be seen posteriorly.

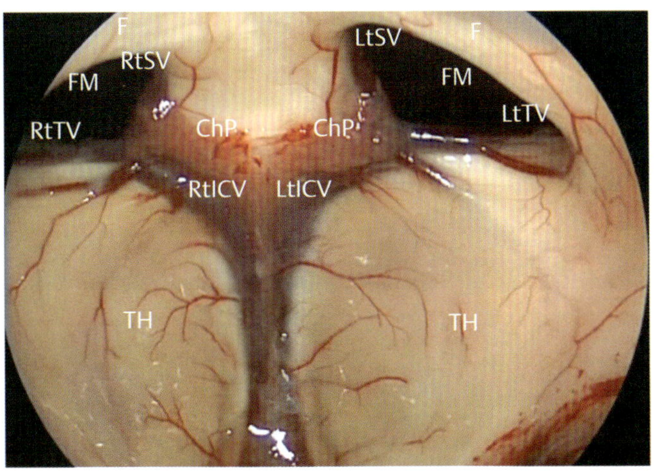

Fig. 9C.11 Endonasal endoscopic view into the third ventricle with no remnant tumor identified. The interventricular foramina of Monro (FM) are visible leading to the lateral ventricles, defined by the thalamus (TH) inferiorly and the fornix (F) superiorly. The choroid plexus (ChP) of the third ventricle is visible. The right thalamic vein (RtTV) and the left thalamic vein (LtTV) are joining the right septal vein (RtSV) and the left septal vein (LtSV) to form the right internal cerebral vein (RtICV) and left internal cerebral vein (LtICV).

14. Meticulous hemostasis is achieved with neuropatties and absorbable hemostat as needed.
15. The dural defect is then plugged using an abdominal fat graft. The edges are tucked under the defect for a watertight closure (**Fig. 9C.12**).
16. A layer of absorbable hemostat is placed over the fat plug, and a synthetic dural sealant is applied over the construct.
17. The repair can be reinforced with a further layer of fat, absorbable hemostat and dural sealant as needed.
18. Finally, the pedicled nasoseptal flaps are rotated over the repair as a final layer.
19. The nasoseptal flaps are then held in place with absorbable gelatin sponges. No nasal packing is required (**Fig. 9C.13**).
20. An intraoperative magnetic resonance imaging (iMRI) was performed to confirm the complete resection of the tumor (**Fig. 9C.14**).

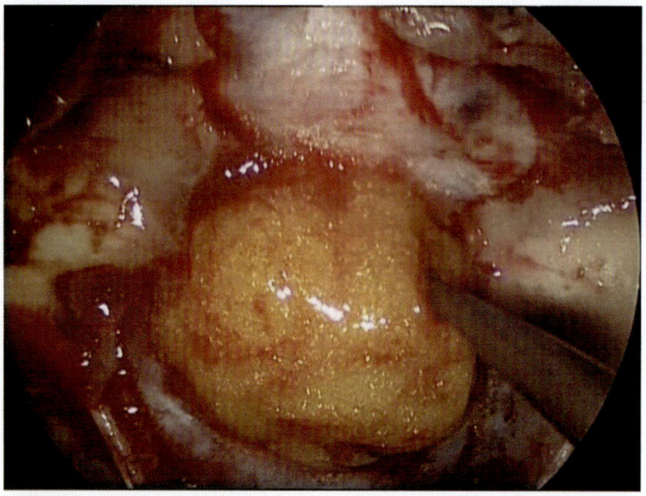

Fig. 9C.12 Fat plug being tucked under the defect edges.

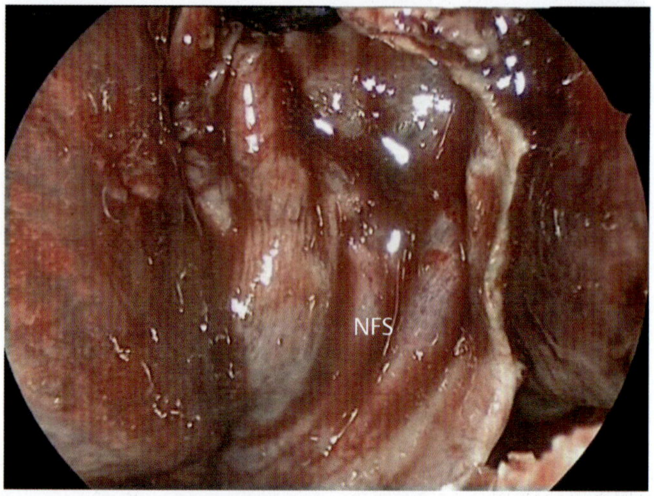

Fig. 9C.13 Final view after nasoseptal flap (NSF) reconstruction.

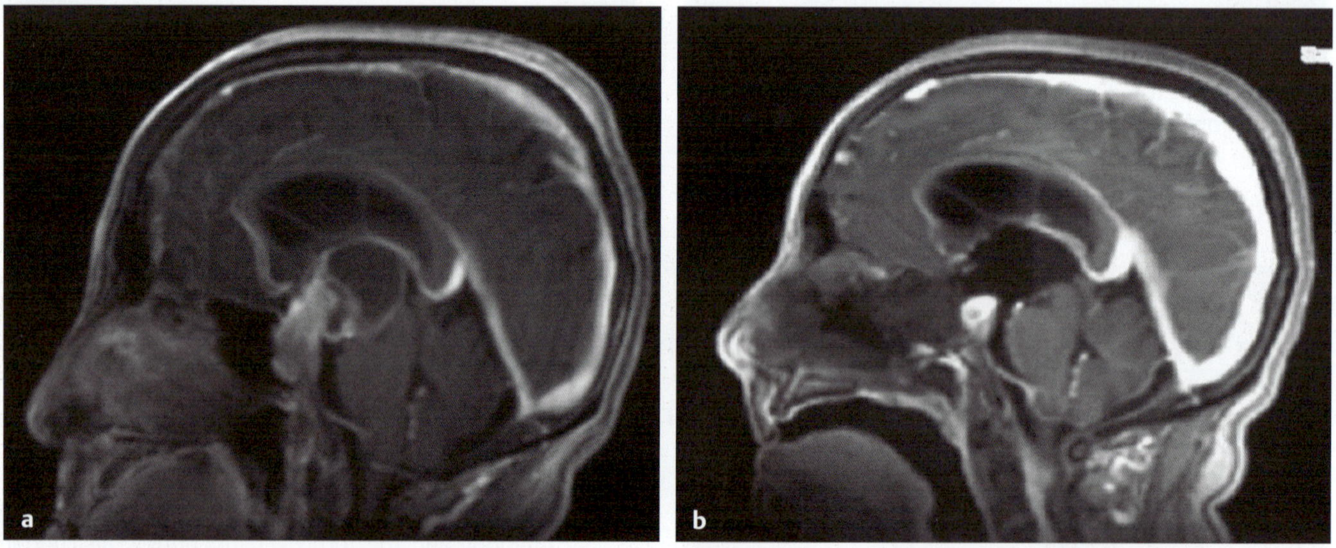

Fig. 9C.14 Comparison between the preoperative **(a)** and intraoperative **(b)** sagittal T1-weighted MRI with contrast which shows the complete resection of the tumor.

Case 9D

Endoscopic Transseptal Transsphenoidal Debulking of an Adult Solid-Cystic Adamantinomatous Craniopharyngioma with Hypothalamic Invasion

Michel Roethlisberger, Yves Brand, and Raphael Guzman

History

A 34-year-old male presented in the emergency department with progressive headaches, dizziness, nausea, and vomiting. His wife noted progressive neuropsychological changes with loss of short-term memory, distraction, and personality changes. The patient has gained weight over the last years and had a BMI-score of approximately 30. Initial neurocranial imaging with CT confirmed a large solid-cystic sellar and parasellar lesion with cystic extension into the third ventricle and consecutive obstructive hydrocephalus (**Figs. 9D.1** and **9D.2**). On the day of admission, the patient developed progressive signs of elevated intracranial pressure. An emergency ventriculoscopy with fenestration of the tumor cyst and implantation of an intra-cystic catheter with a connected subcutaneous Rickham reservoir was performed (**Fig. 9D.3**). The reservoir would be available for emergency puncture in case a recurrent deterioration would occur. Neurocranial imaging with MRI was performed the next day after the patient was stable. The suprasellar solid-cystic lesion with correct placement of the intra-cystic catheter was confirmed with regression of the obstructive hydrocephalus and a collapsed cystic tumor component. In the adult population, the impact of hypothalamic invasion remains less clear as compared to pediatric craniopharyngioma, especially, when gross-total resection is the goal. The present case would correlate with a pediatric PUGET Grade 2 (**Figs. 9D.4**, **9D.5**, and **9D.6**), and major hypothalamic worsening is less likely when an aggressive surgical resection is used. However, it remains an intraoperative and individual decision when to

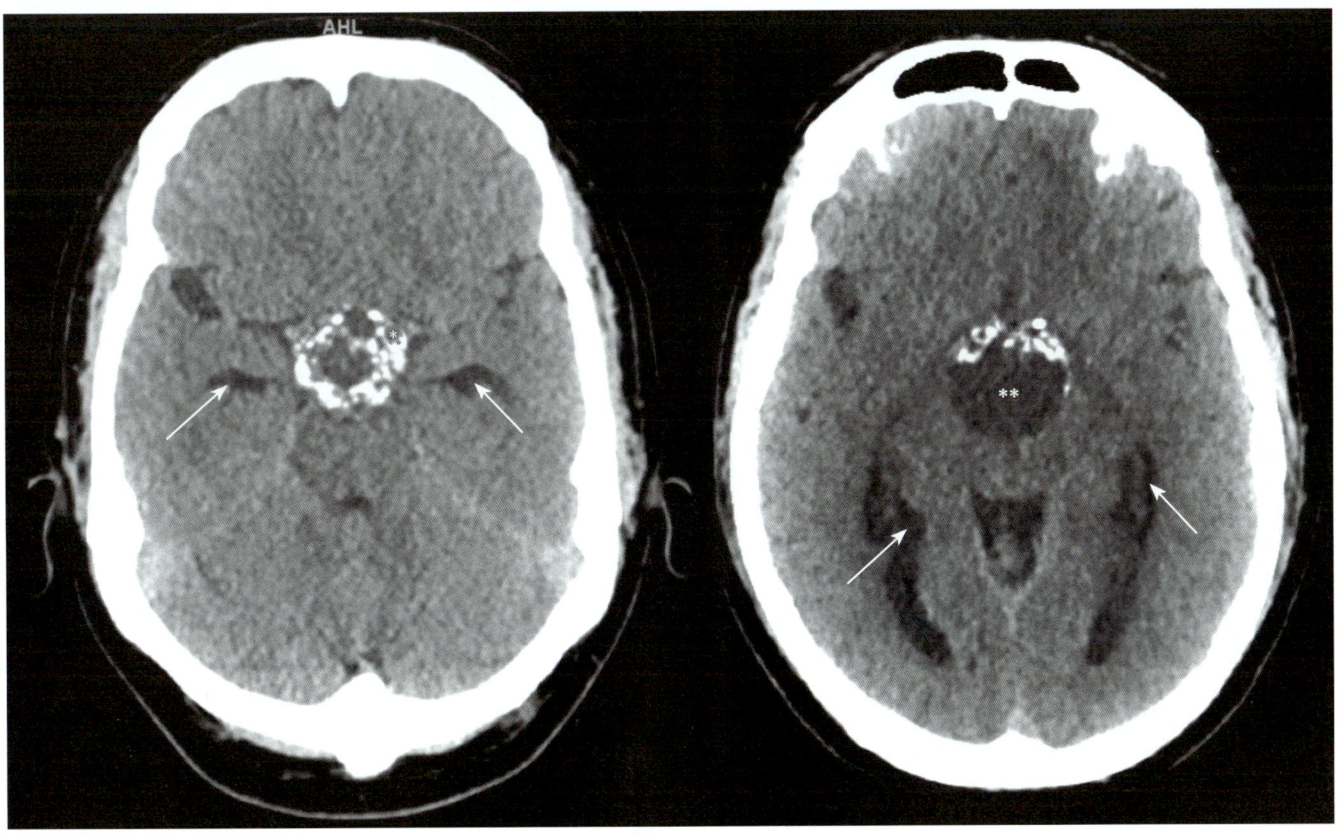

Fig. 9D.1 Axial non-contrast-enhanced CT section at presentation demonstrating a suprasellar lesion with solid calcified components (*) and a cystic component (**) causing obstructive hydrocephalus (*arrows*). The finding is highly suggestive of a craniopharyngioma.

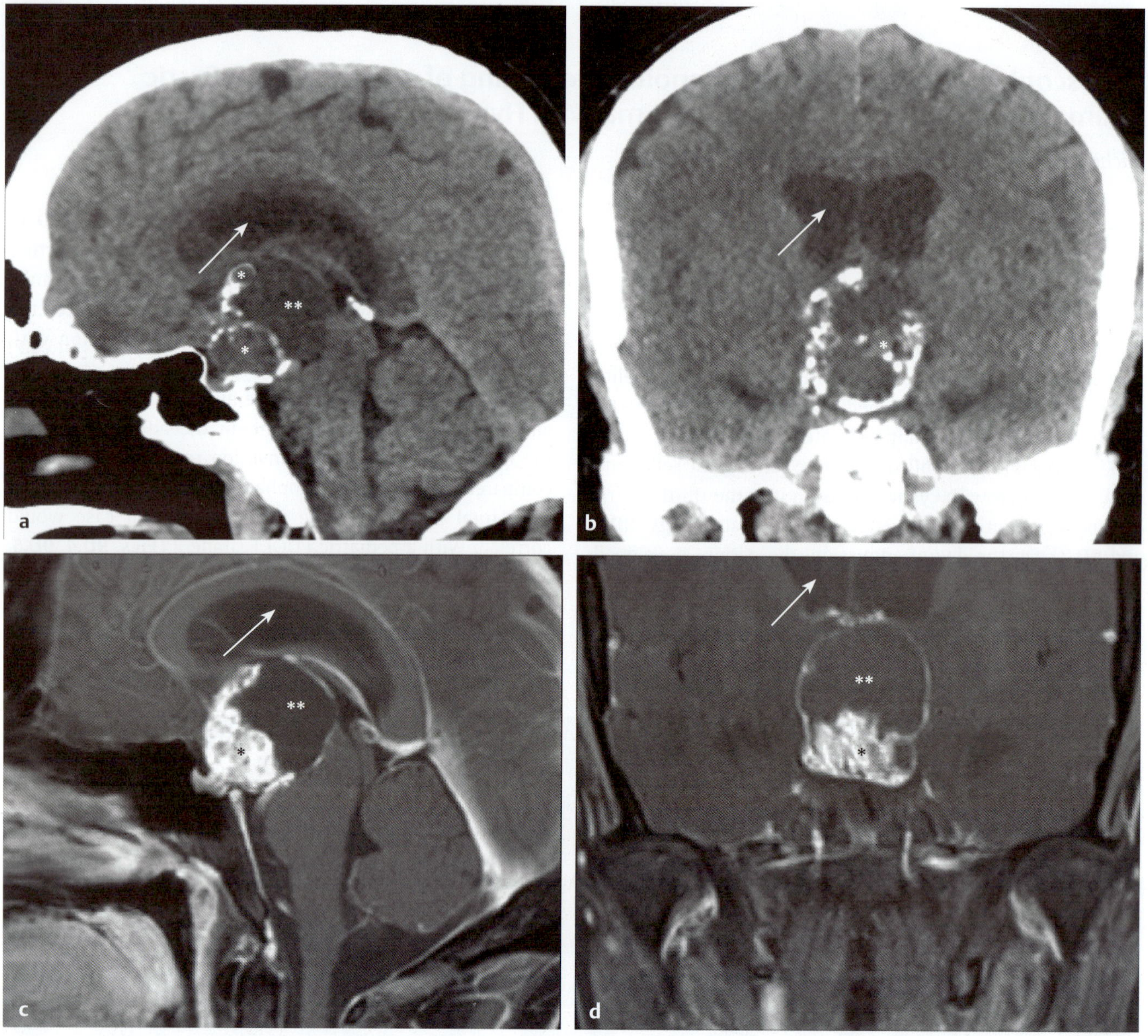

Fig. 9D.2 **(a)** Sagittal, **(b)** coronal; non-contrast-enhanced CT section, **(c)** sagittal, **(d)** coronal; T1-weighted gadolinium contrast-enhanced MRI sections at presentation demonstrating a suprasellar lesion with solid calcified components (*) and a cystic component (**) causing an obstructive hydrocephalus (*arrows*). The finding is highly suggestive of a craniopharyngioma.

stop the dissection between the tumor capsule and the hypothalamic walls.

In the following days, endocrinological evaluation revealed no abnormalities, while an ophthalmological workup documented a bitemporal hemianopsia.

The decision for an endonasal endoscopic approach was based on the concept of removing the solid part located mainly in the sellar region, and an attempt was made to resect the tumor capsule. Intraoperatively, the tumor capsule was very adherent to the hypothalamic structures on both sides, and the decision for a subtotal resection was made. The patient recovered from the mass effect symptoms but developed postoperative diabetes insipidus and panhypopituitarism.

A couple of weeks later, the patient presented with a new onset diplopia, and a small recurrent tumor cyst was found compressing the right oculomotor nerve in its cisternal segment. Hence, a transventricular endoscopic fenestration of the cyst was necessary.

After this procedure, the patient received proton-beam therapy with 54/1.8 Gy (RBE) to treat the remaining lesion. There was neither tumor progression nor the new onset of

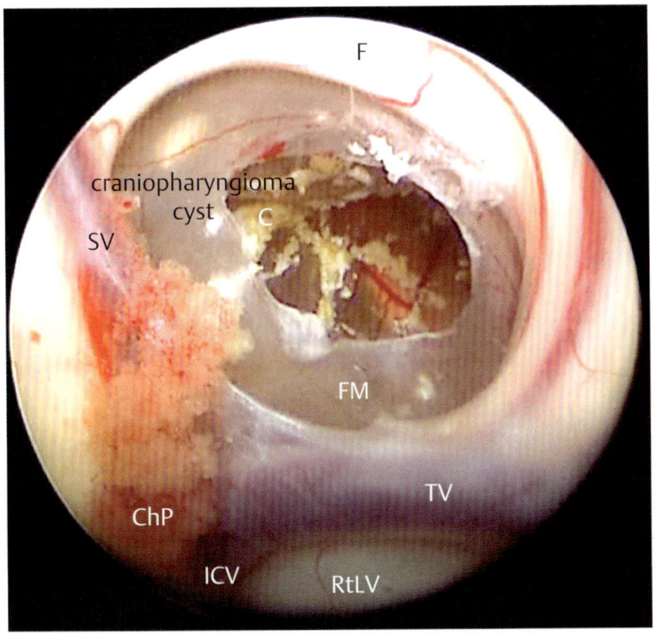

Fig. 9D.3 Neuroendoscopy of the right lateral ventricle (RtLV) with the foramen of Monro (FM) insight. The fornix (F) and the confluence of the thalamic (TV) and the septal vein (SV) forming the internal cerebral vein (ICV) can be appreciated, covered by the choroid plexus (ChP). The craniopharyngioma cyst was fenestrated to release intracystic pressure. Calcifications (C) within the cyst can be appreciated.

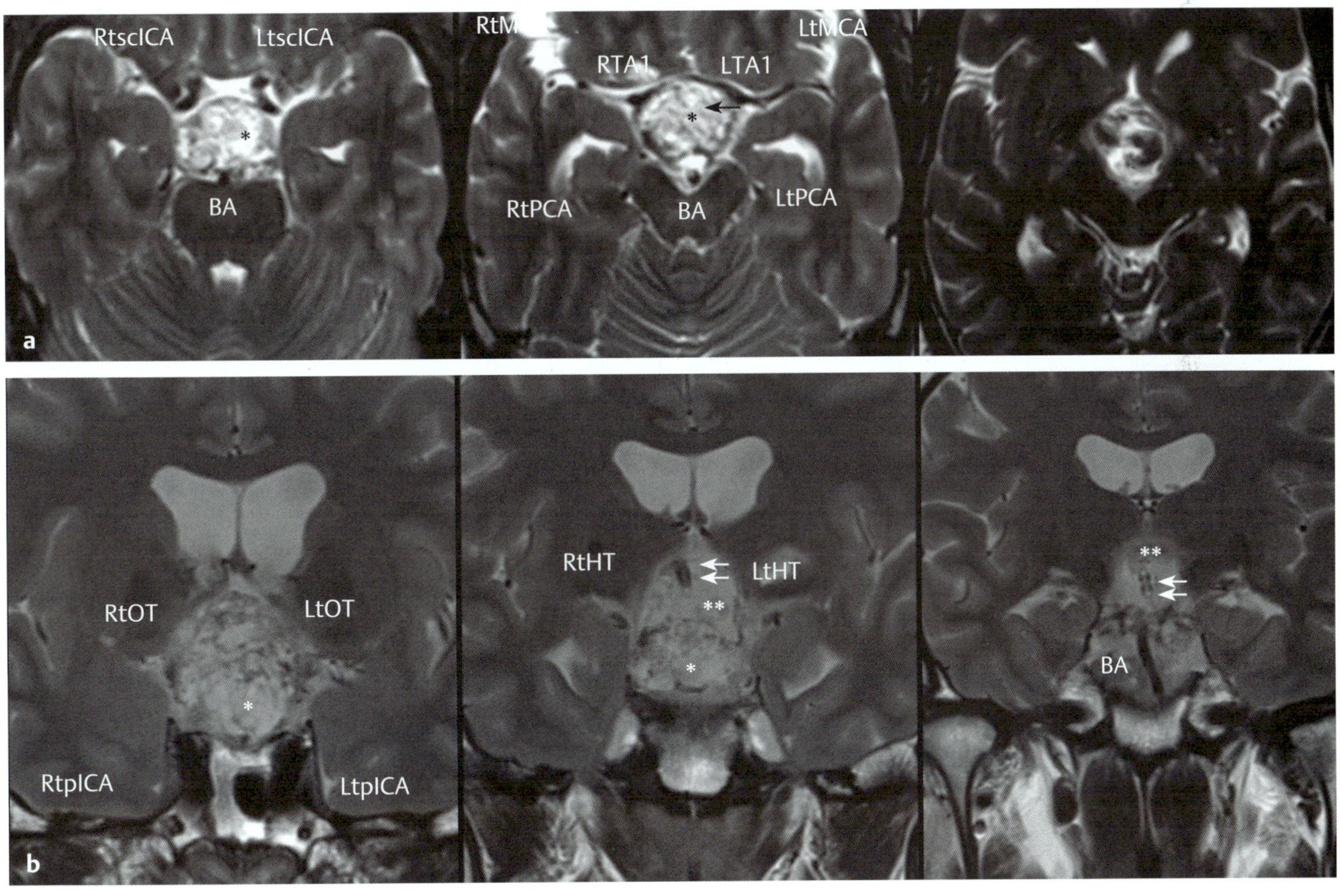

Fig. 9D.4 **(a)** Axial, **(b)** coronal T2-weighted MRI sections after right frontal ventriculoscopy and insertion of a right frontal intracystic catheter for immediate resolution of the obstructive hydrocephalus. The suprasellar hyperintense solid tumor component (*) shows hypointense signals suggestive for calcifications (*arrow*). Due to the cranial extension, the arteries of the circle of Willis are spread by the lesion. The right intracystic catheter (*double arrows*) is placed within the cystic component of the tumor (**). No cleft between the right medial hypothalamic wall (RtHT) and the left medial hypothalamic walls (LtHT) can be identified.

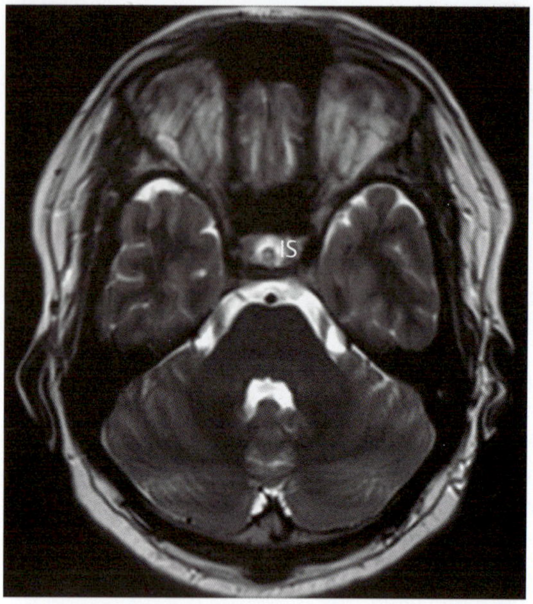

Fig. 9D.5 Axial T2-weighted MRI-section demonstrating the infundibular stalk (IS) and a cerebrospinal fluid cleft between the pituitary gland and the tumor.

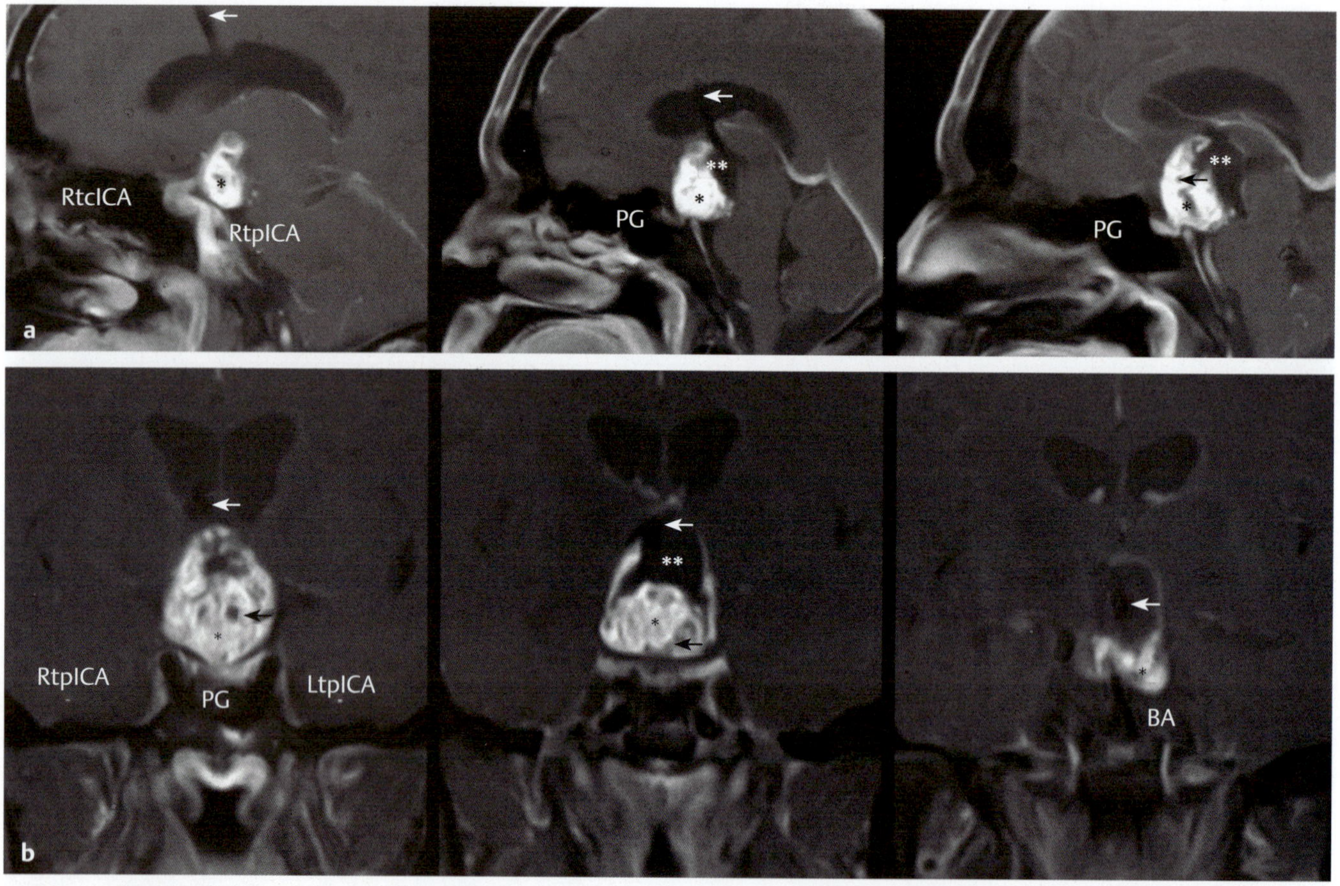

Fig. 9D.6 **(a)** Sagittal, **(b)** coronal T1-weighted gadolinium contrast-enhanced MRI sections after right frontal ventriculoscopy and insertion of a right frontal intracystic catheter for immediate resolution of the obstructive hydrocephalus. The suprasellar hyperintense solid tumor component (*) shows signal shortening, suggestive of calcifications (*arrow*). Due to the cranial extension, the arteries of the circle of Willis are spread by the lesion. The right intracystic catheter (*double arrow*) is placed within the cystic component of the tumor (**). The tumor cyst is hyperintense and enhances with expansion into the prepontine cistern and the third ventricle. The pituitary gland (PG) can be identified as inferior to the lesion within the sella turcica.

symptoms, as the adjuvant treatment and the hemianopsia and diplopia gradually resolved. Although the infundibular stalk (IS) was identified and preserved, the patient subsequently developed hypopituitarism and also suffered from diabetes insipidus.

Surgical Steps

1. A **binostril posterior transseptal transsphenoidal approach** with a posterior septectomy and sphenoidotomy is performed as described in Chapter 1.
2. The posterior wall of the sphenoid sinus is demucosalized, and the landmarks of the skull base are identified (**Fig. 9D.7**).
3. The opening of the sella is started with a diamond burr in the midline, reducing the thickness of the overlying septal insertion (**Fig. 9D.8**).
4. Once the bone has been sufficiently thinned out, a right-angle dissector can be insinuated between the bone and the dura. With the use of a Kerrison punch, the sellar opening can then be widened (**Fig. 9D.9**).
5. A right-angle hook can be used to separate the bone from the dura laterally covering the cavernous carotid artery (**Fig. 9D.10**).
6. The anatomical landmarks of the sella turcica have to be in clear view. Superior: intercavernous sinus and planum sphenoidale, lateral: cavernous sinus, inferior: sellar floor; the orientation can be supported by image guided surgery (**Fig. 9D.11**).
7. A cruciate incision of the sellar dura can be done with a sickle knife in the midline (**Fig. 9D.12**). A 15-mm knife allows for the opening of the laterally extending dura in a controlled manner (**Fig. 9D.13**).
8. To expand the dural opening of the sella superiorly, the anterior intercavernous sinus has to be cauterized and divided. The adenohypophysis and the diaphragma sellae are identified. No normal tumor tissue is visible, as the lesion is located superior posterior to the pituitary gland (**Fig. 9D.14**).

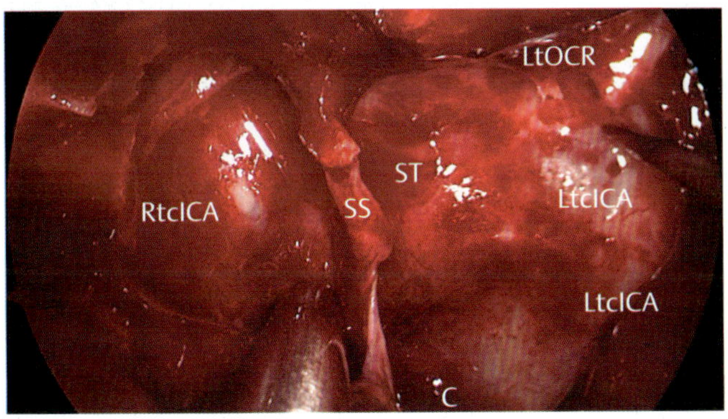

Fig. 9D.7 Verification of the visualized landmarks of the skull base with image guided surgery.

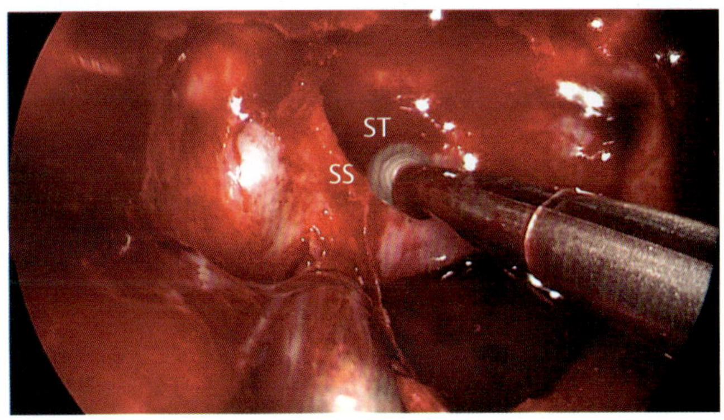

Fig. 9D.8 Reduction of bone thickness at the insertion of the sphenoid main septum using a high-speed diamond burr.

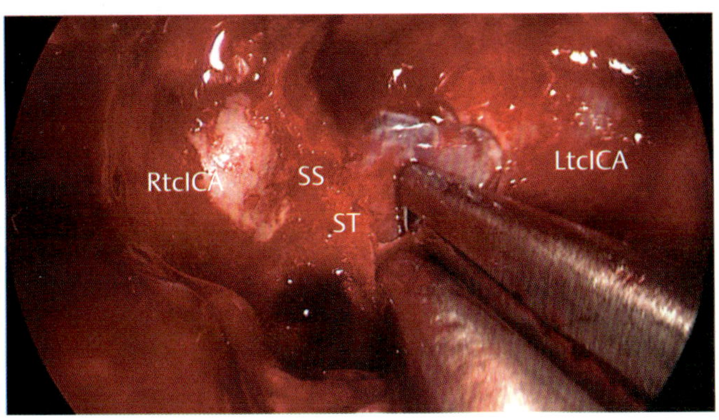

Fig. 9D.9 Osteodural exposure of the sella turcica (ST) with the aid of a Kerrison punch.

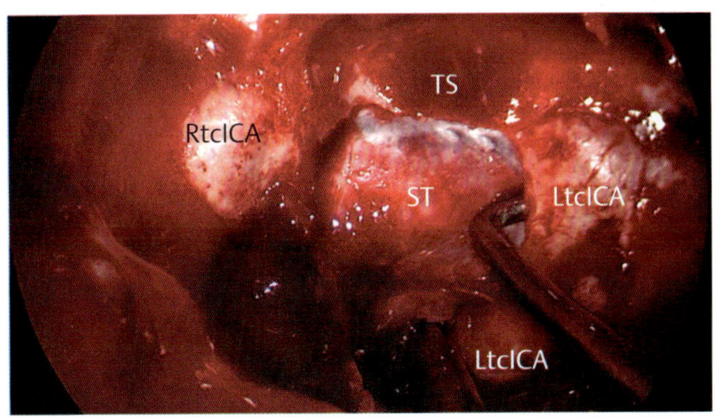

Fig. 9D.10 Lateral osteodural exposure: dissection of the dura from the bone covering the left cavernous internal carotid artery (LtcICA) with a blunt hooked instrument.

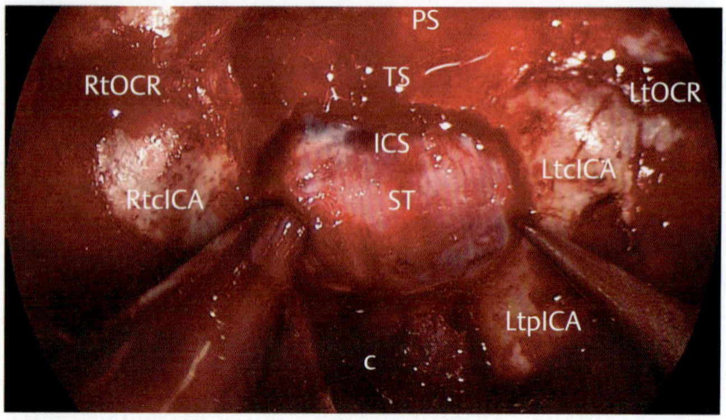

Fig. 9D.11 Verification of the laterality with image guided surgery.

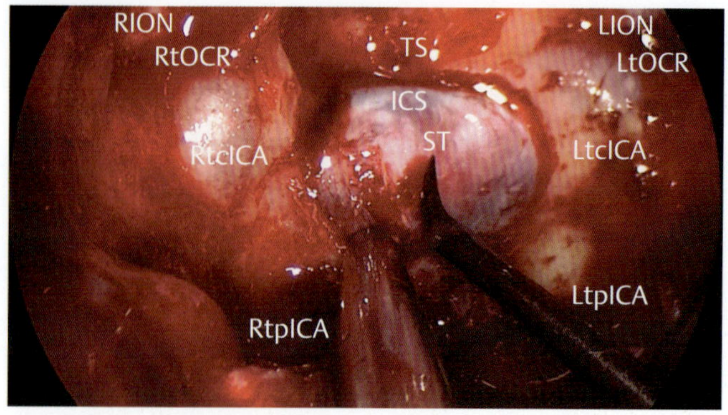

Fig. 9D.12 Midline dural opening using a sickle knife.

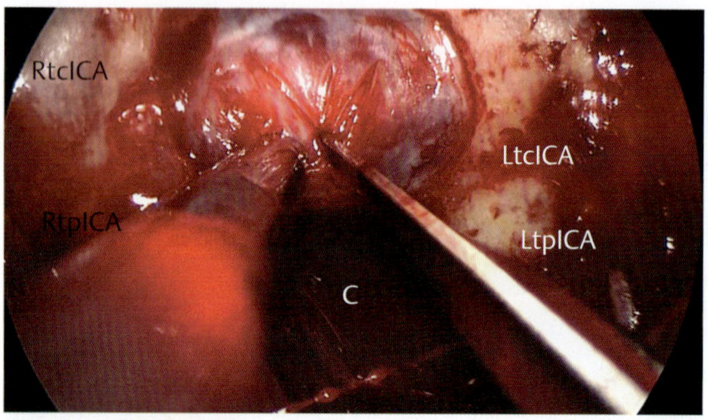

Fig. 9D.13 Cruciate incision using a 15 mm scalpel.

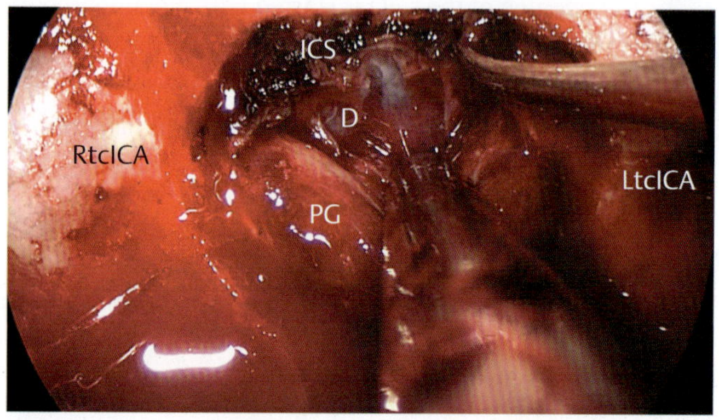

Fig. 9D.14 Cauterization and division of the intercavernous sinus (ICS). The anterior pituitary gland (PG) is visible as well as the diaphgrama sellae (D).

9. The IS passes through the diaphragma sellae and should be identified superiorly to the pituitary gland. The diaphragmal dura can be thickened due to the tumoral process, and the stalk can be dislocated to one side (**Fig. 9D.15**).
10. After identification of the pituitary stalk, the diaphragma sellae has to be opened to gain access to the suprasellar space. The IS and the pituitary gland (PG) can be pushed slightly laterally, but the risk of postoperative dysfunction is higher due to indirect traction of the stalk (**Fig. 9D.16**).
11. After the opening of the diaphragmal dura, the tumor capsule should be identified in the suprasellar space. Cauterization and sharp incision might be necessary (**Fig. 9D.17**).
12. Tumor specimen is retained for histological examination using pituitary forceps (**Fig. 9D.18**).
13. Bimanual anterior central tumor debulking along the sellar floor is commenced using with a 90° ring curette and suction. Consecutively, the same maneuver is done bilaterally within the tumor capsule (**Figs. 9D.19** and **9D.20**).
14. Further debulking of the solid tumor component should be done in a zonal manner. The solid component extends posteriorly with an adjacent tumor cyst and has a superior solid compartment (**Figs. 9D.21** and **9D.22**).
15. The intraventricular intracystic catheter is used as a depth reference when resecting the posterior tumor compartment, and it indicates the location of the tumor cyst in the third ventricle (**Figs. 9D.23** and **9D.24**).
16. The superior solid tumor components can be resected with bimanual curettes and suction or dissection and mobilization using blunt hooked instruments (**Fig. 9D.25**). These maneuvers have to be continued until all solid tumor components are removed and the tumor capsule is visible.

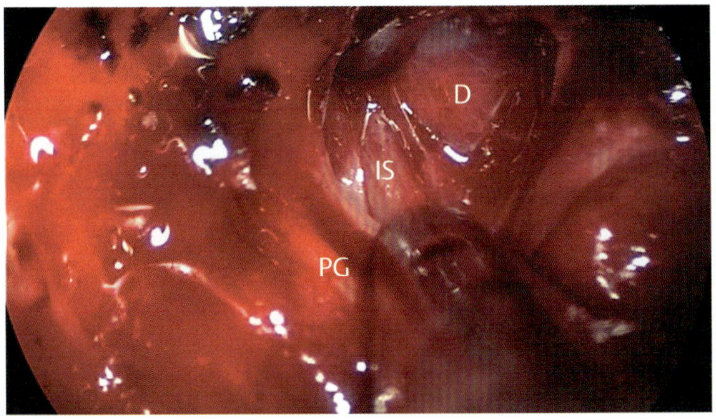

Fig. 9D.15 The infundibular stalk (IS) can be visualized at its entrance into the dura of the diaphragma sellae (D).

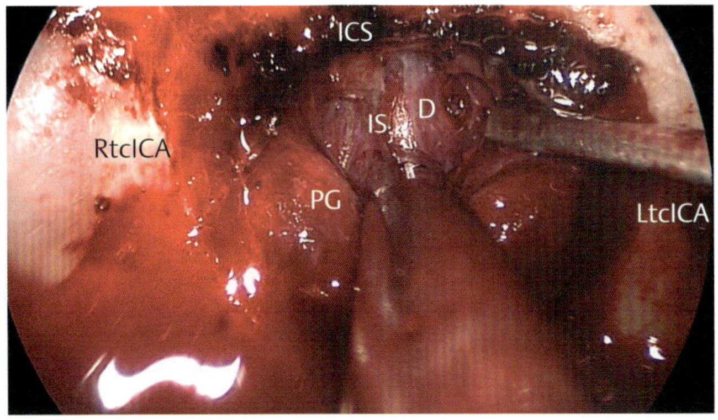

Fig. 9D.16 The dura of the diaphragma sellae (D) is incised with a diamond knife lateral to the infundibular stalk (IS) and the supradiaphragmal space is exposed.

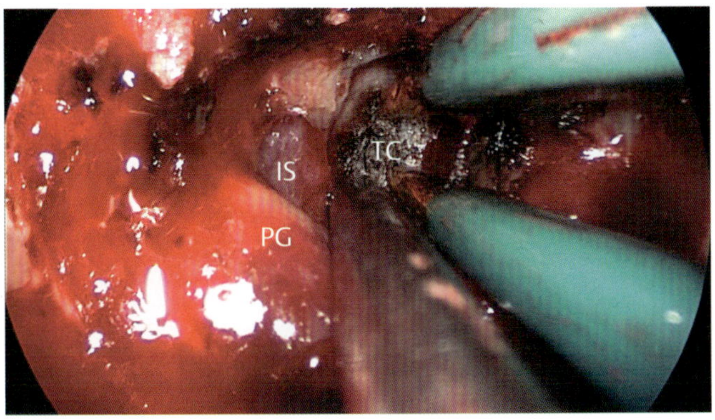

Fig. 9D.17 Cauterization of tumor capsule (TC).

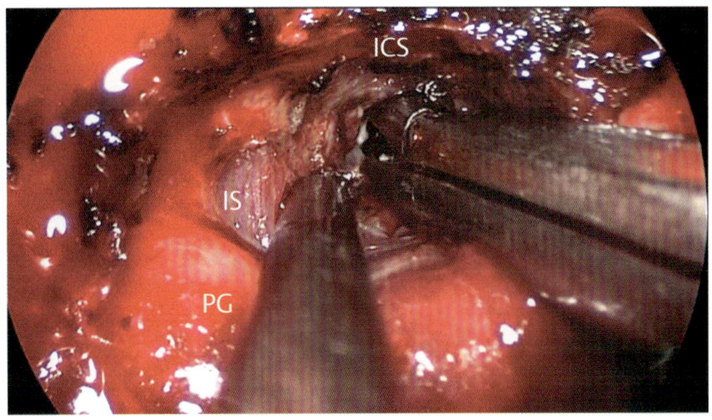

Fig. 9D.18 Tumor specimen is retained for histological examination.

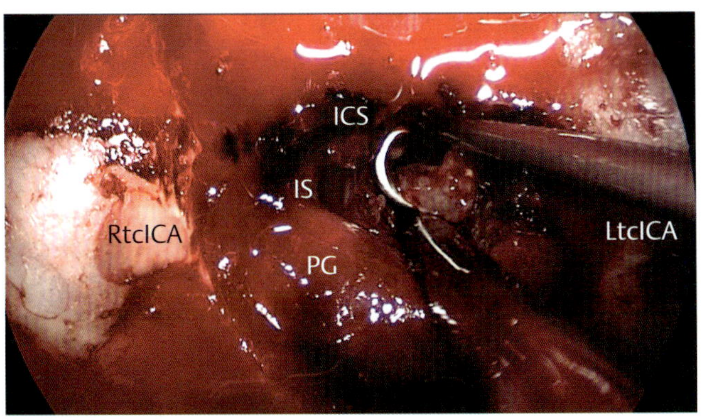

Fig. 9D.19 90-degree curettes are used to debulk the anterior solid tumor compartment.

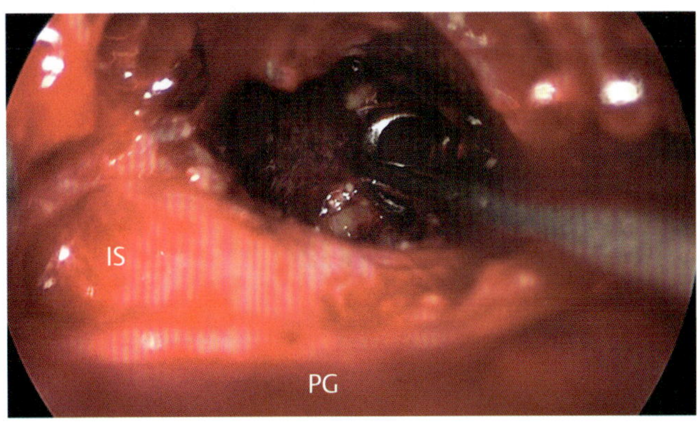

Fig. 9D.20 Intratumoral debulking along the left-sided solid tumor capsule.

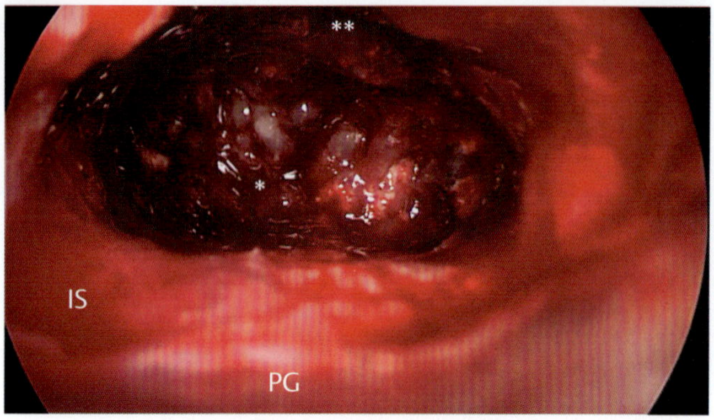

Fig. 9D.21 The posterior (*) and the superior (**) compartments of the solid tumor are visible in relation to the pituitary gland (PG) and the infundibular stalk (IS).

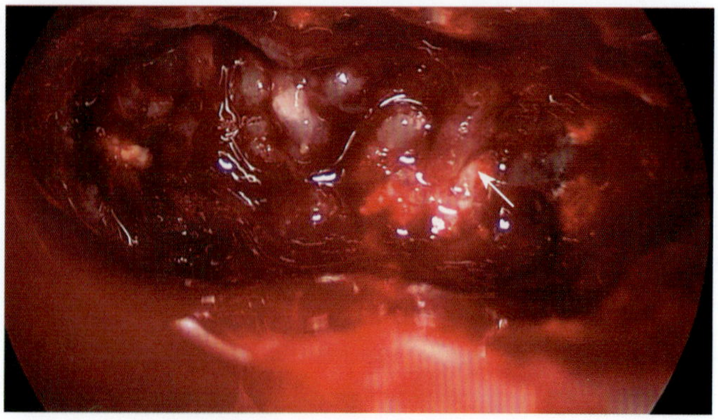

Fig. 9D.22 Heterogenous appearance of the solid tumor of the posterior compartment. Calcifications are visible (*arrow*).

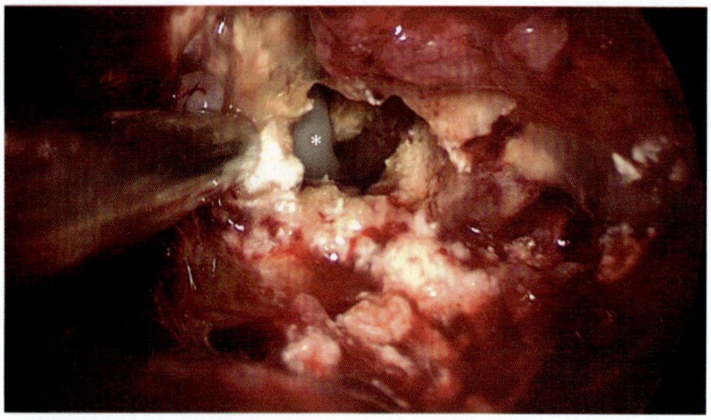

Fig. 9D.23 Resection of the posterior compartment leads to the intraventricular intracystic catheter (*).

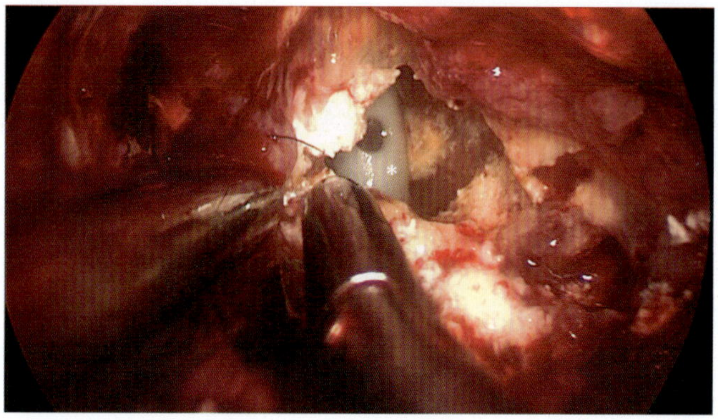

Fig. 9D.24 The posterior solid tumor compartments are removed around the catheter (*).

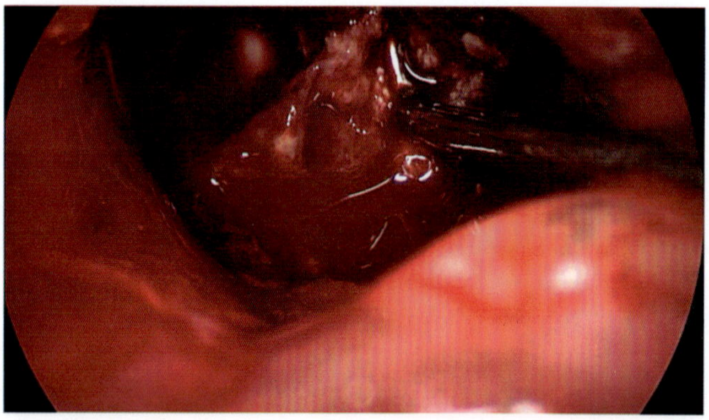

Fig. 9D.25 The superior tumor compartment is resected with the aid of curettes and blunt hooked instruments.

17. An extracapsular dissection plane can then be defined between the tumor capsule and the adjacent hypothalamic structures using a blunt dissecting instrument and low suction. A broad dissection plane should be defined (**Fig. 9D.26**).
18. The tumor capsule can be mobilized using grasping instruments and high-power suction. Attachments and a thick tumor capsule increase the chance of traumatizing and injuring the hypothalamic wall and might cause postoperative hypothalamic dysfunction, although this is less likely in adults as compared to pediatric cases (**Figs. 9D.27, 9D.28**, and **9D.29**).
19. Removal of the solid components is completed as far as possible. The adherent tumor capsule is left behind along the hypothalamic structures (**Fig. 9D.30**).

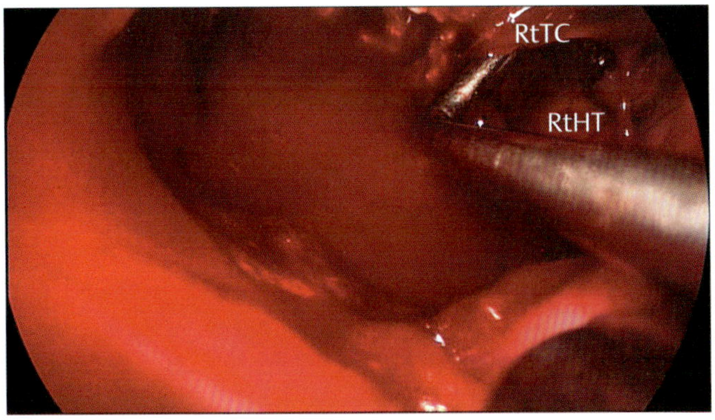

Fig. 9D.26 The right lateral tumor capsule (RtTC) is dissected along the right hypothalamic wall (RtHT) until strong attachments are encountered.

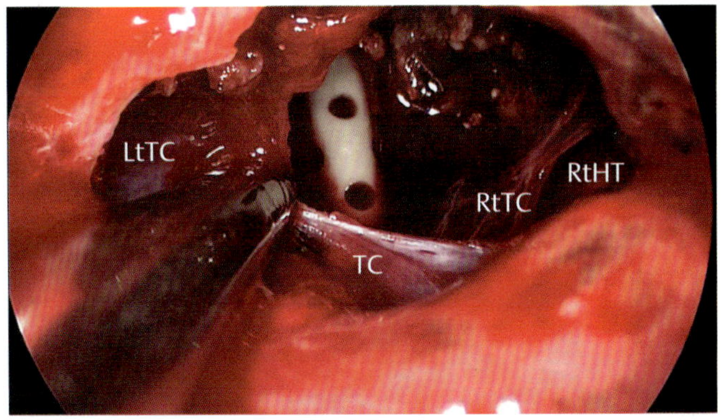

Fig. 9D.27 The left lateral tumor capsule (LtTC) is then dissected and brought into the surgical field.

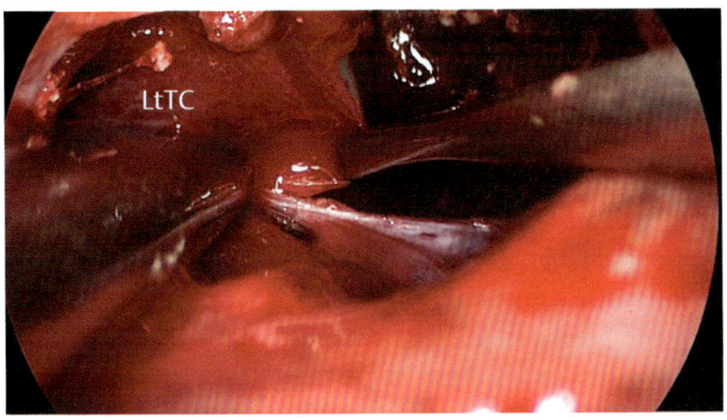

Fig. 9D.28 Several attempts are made to mobilize the left lateral tumor capsule (LtTC).

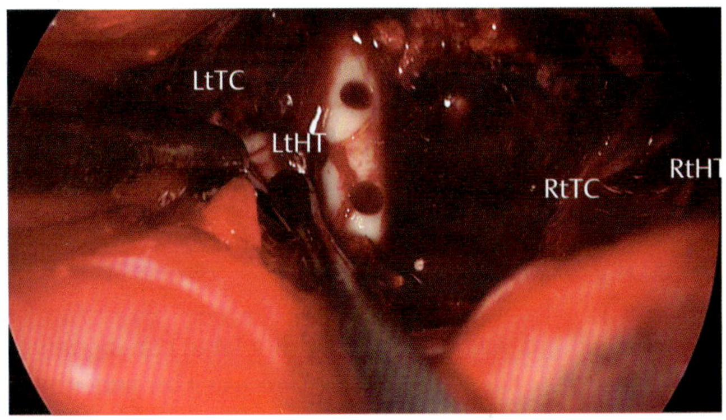

Fig. 9D.29 The left lateral tumor capsule (LtTC) is adherent to the left hypothalamic wall (LtHT) and cannot be removed.

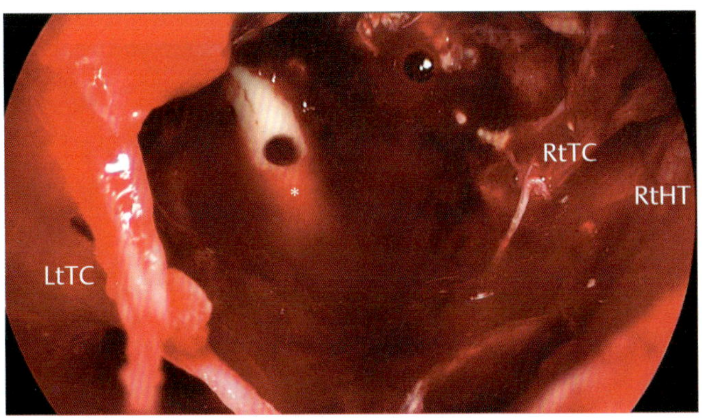

Fig. 9D.30 Final view of the debulked craniopharyngioma.

20. The skull base defect is reconstructed using a vicryl patch, an artificial dura replacement (TachoSil, Takeda Pharma Vertrieb GmbH&Co., Germany), and an artificial dural sealant (Adherus, HyperBranch Medical Technology, Inc., Stryker, Durham, North Carolina, USA) (**Fig. 9D.31**).
21. The nasoseptal flaps are placed over the cartilaginous septum, and the middle turbinates are brought back into position and covered with a lateral and a medial resorbable nasal pack on each side.
22. A 6-week postoperative MRI demonstrates a subtotal resection of the tumor cyst with near-total resection of the solid tumor components and the correct placement of an intracystic catheter (**Fig. 9D.32**).

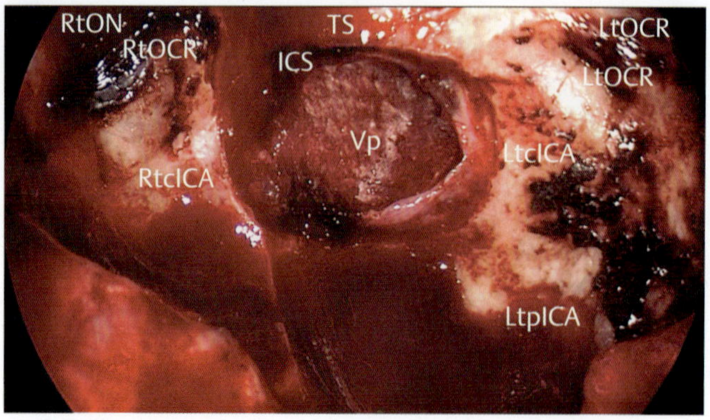

Fig. 9D.31 Sellar reconstruction using a vicryl patch (Vp).

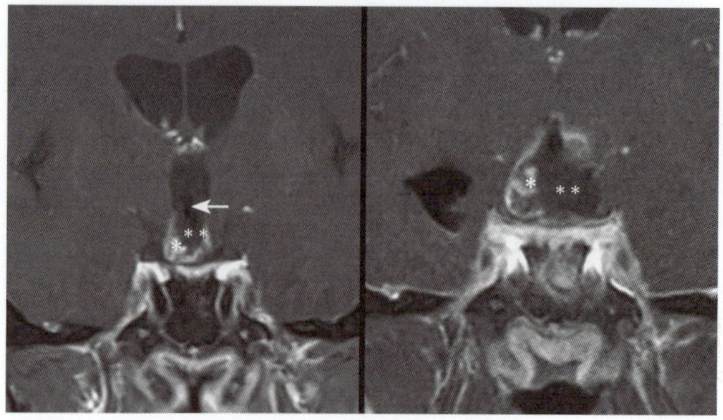

Fig. 9D.32 Coronal T1-weighted gadolinium contrast-enhanced sections demonstrating the subtotal removal of the adherent tumor cyst (*) while the majority of the solid component (**) is resected. The intracystic catheter is still in place (*arrow*).

Case 9E

A Tailored Extended Endoscopic Approach for a Pediatric Craniopharyngioma

Michel Roethlisberger, Wong HT, Sien Hui Tan, Saif Al-Zahid, Prepageran Narayanan, and Vicknes Waran

History

A 6-year-old girl was diagnosed with a large craniopharyngomia and underwent surgical exision using an endoscopic transsellar and transplanum approach. The girl was born uneventfully until 2 months ago where she presented with a left eye squint and worsening headache. She was underweight at 14 kg. Ophthalmological assessment revealed a reduced visual acuity with 6/12 in the right eye and 6/45 in the left eye, with the presence of papilledema in the left eye.

Neurocranial imaging revealed a predominantly cystic lesion with a maximal diameter of 5 cm with extension into the prechiasmatic and retrochiasmatic region, and the left middle cranial fossa. There is evidence of compression of the midbrain, pons and cerebellum, with obstructive hydrocephalus. (**Fig. 9E.1a–c**).

The authors used a two surgeon, dual nostril, four-handed technique to endoscopically excise the tumor through a transplanum and transsellar approach.

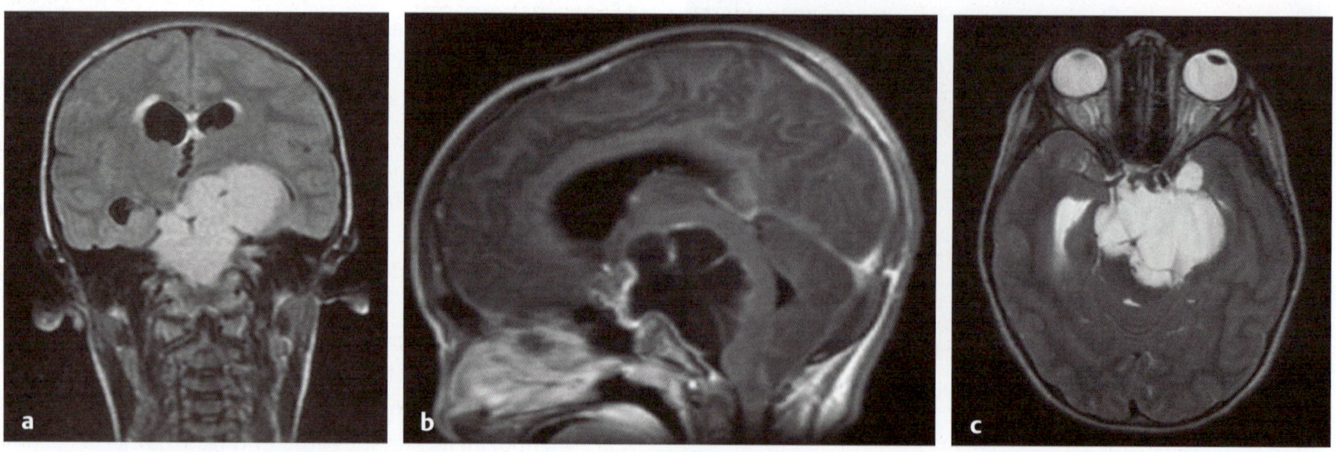

Fig. 9E.1 **(a)** Coronal fluid-attenuated inversion recovery (FLAIR), **(b)** sagittal T1-weighted contrast-enhanced, and **(c)** axial T2-weighted MRI sections demonstrating the extension of the cystic tumorous lesion with compression of the adjacent neurovascular structures.

Surgical Steps

1. A **dual nostril, four-handed technique with a right-sided nasoseptal flap** is performed as described in Chapter 1.
2. Trans-tuberculum and trans-planum approach: After identification of the critical neurovascular landmarks of the skull base (**Fig. 9E.2**), the planum sphenoidale is thinned out using a high-speed drill (**Figs. 9E.3** and **9E.4**).
3. Transsellar approach: The bone over the sellar region is removed. A right-angle dissector is used to separate the bone from the dura.
4. Intradural phase: An H-shaped vertical horizontal incision is made at the sellar dura (**Fig. 9E.5**).
5. After the dural opening, the solid and cystic components of the tumor can be identified. Cystic fluid can be collected and retained for histopathological examination (**Fig. 9E.6**).
6. The tumorous lesion has soft and cystic as well as hard and calcified components. (**Fig. 9E.7**).
7. The tumor is dissected away from the superior and lateral attachment. An ultrasonic aspirator (Cavitron Ultrasonic Surgical Aspirator) is used to debulk the calcified parts (**Fig. 9E.8**).

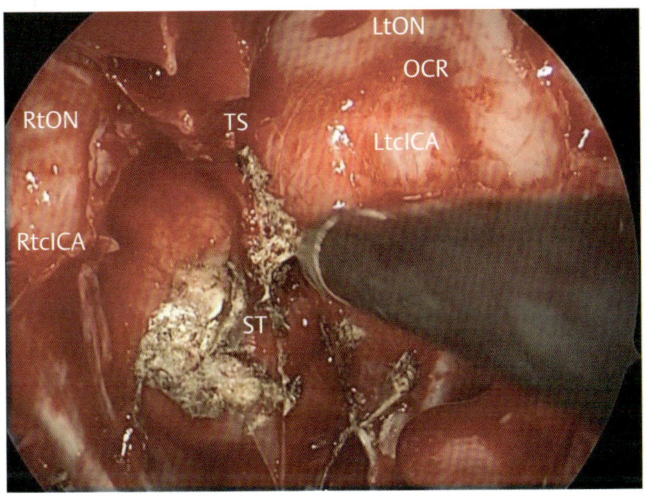

Fig. 9E.2 Cauterization of sphenoid sinus mucosa after identification of the critical neurovascular structures.

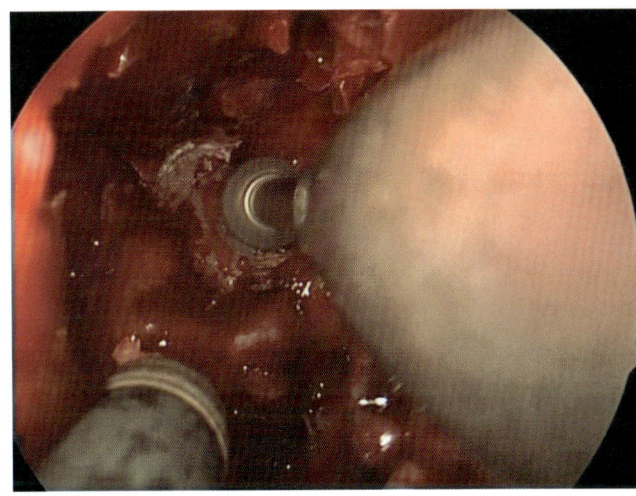

Fig. 9E.3 Drilling of the planum sphenoidale using a high-speed drill.

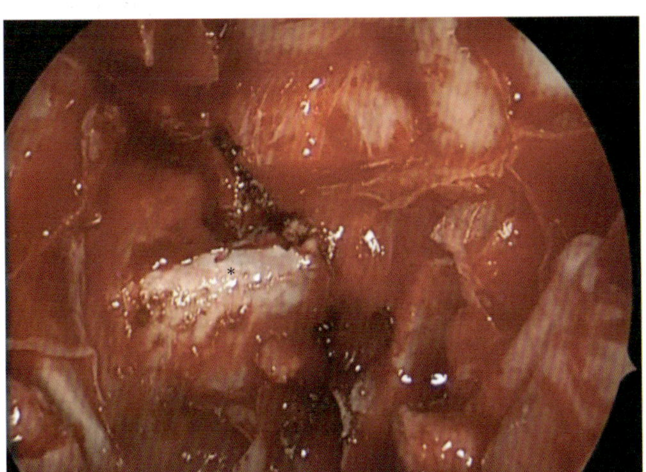

Fig. 9E.4 Partially thinned out sella turcica (*).

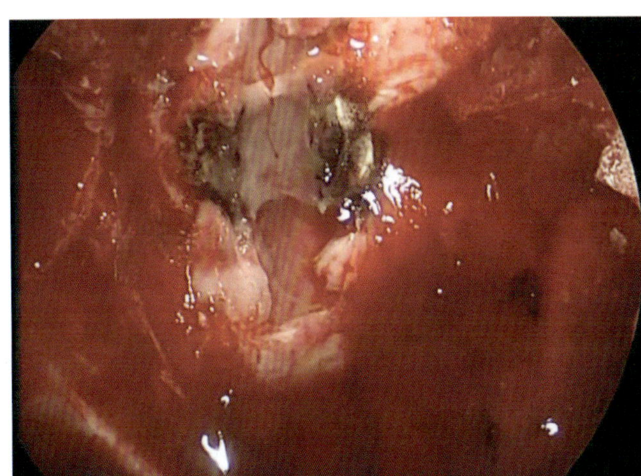

Fig. 9E.5 An H-shaped vertical horizontal incision of the sellar dura with a knife and curved scissors.

8. The thinned out tumor mass is elevated superiorly to allow for a dissection plane along the inferior aspect of the lesion (**Fig. 9E.9**).
9. While resecting the tumor posteriorly, the posterior communicating arteries, the basilar artery and its perforating branches are at risk for accidental injury. The residual tumor is hidden underneath the posterior cerebral arteries and the superior cerebellar arteries (**Fig. 9E.10**).
10. Once the tumor has been dissected off the right posterior cerebral artery and the right superior cerebellar artery, the oculomotor nerve, coursing between these two arteries, is at risk of accidental injury and has to be identified (**Fig. 9E.11a–c**).
11. Intraoperative magnetic resonance imaging (MRI) confirmed tumor clearance and a sufficient decompression of the brainstem prior to the reconstruction of the skull base defect (**Fig. 9E.12**).
12. A DuraGen patch (Integra Lifesciences Service, France) is used to close the defect using an underlay technique. The edges of the patch are tucked below the bony edges (**Fig. 9E.13**).
13. A dural sealant is applied over the DuraGen patch followed by a second layer of DuraGen. An abdominal fat graft is applied over the second layer of DuraGen. The right nasoseptal flap is then placed over the construct. A dural sealant is then applied over the reconstruction (**Fig. 9E.14**).

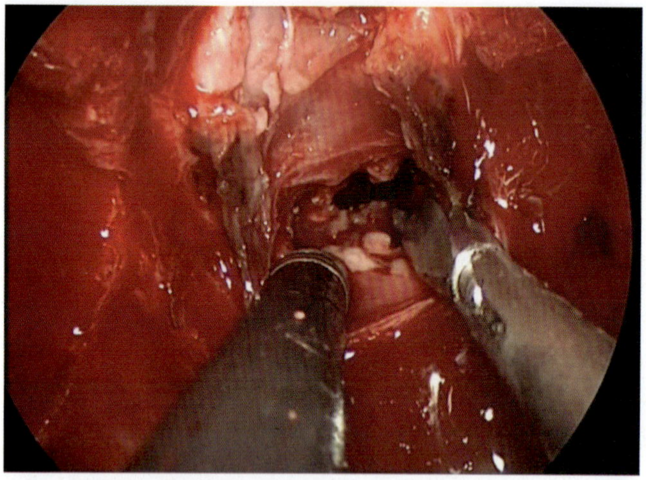

Fig. 9E.6 Endonasal endoscopic view of the solid tumor components after the evacuation of the tumor cyst.

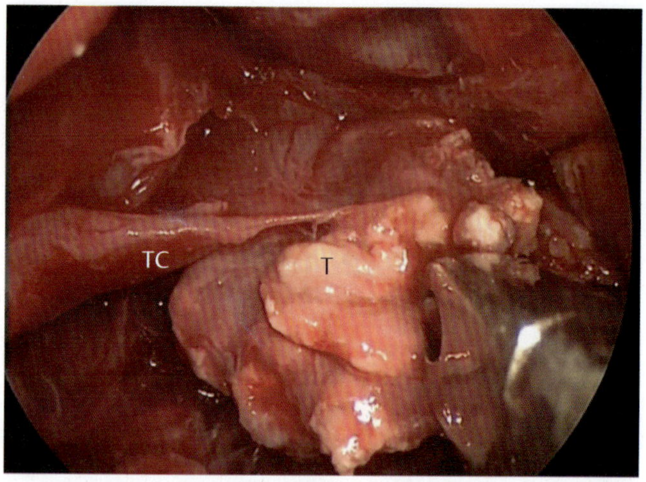

Fig. 9E.7 The calcified components of the tumor (T) are removed to decompress the adherent tumor capsule (TC).

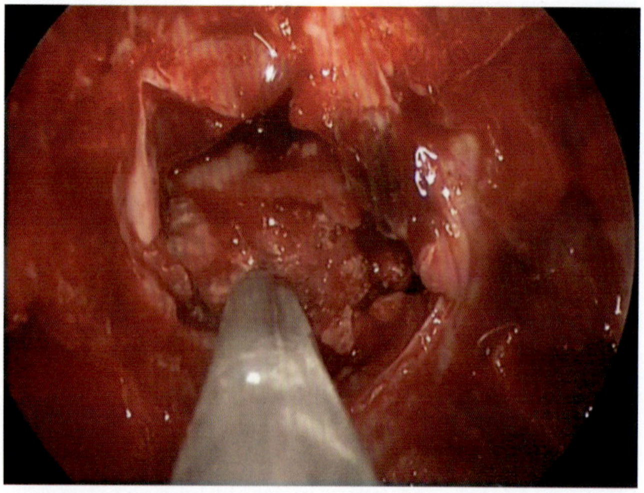

Fig. 9E.8 Debulking of the calcified tumor components using an ultrasonic aspirator.

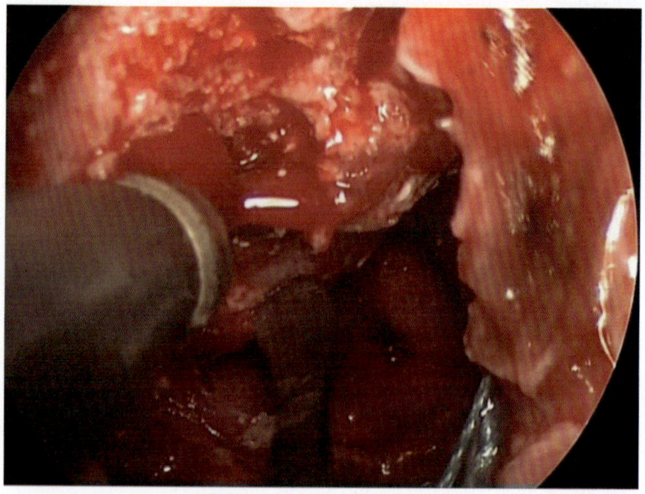

Fig. 9E.9 The remaining tumor is elevated superiorly to create a dissection plane along the inferior tumor aspect.

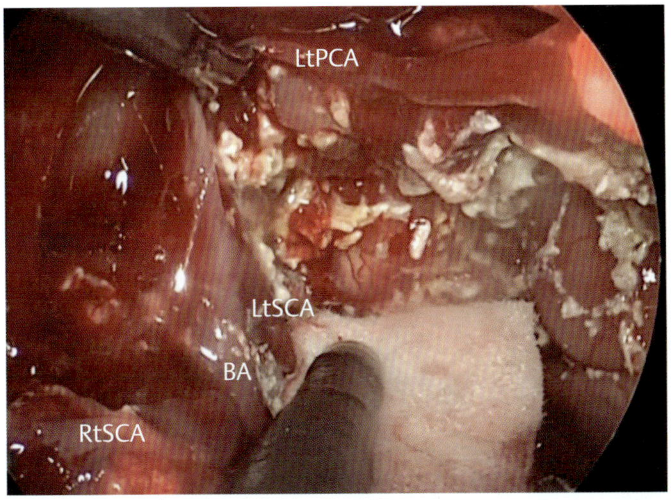

Fig. 9E.10 The basilar artery (BA) and its perforating branches are identified. The left posterior cerebral artery (LtPCA) is lifted up to clear the tumor (T) underneath.

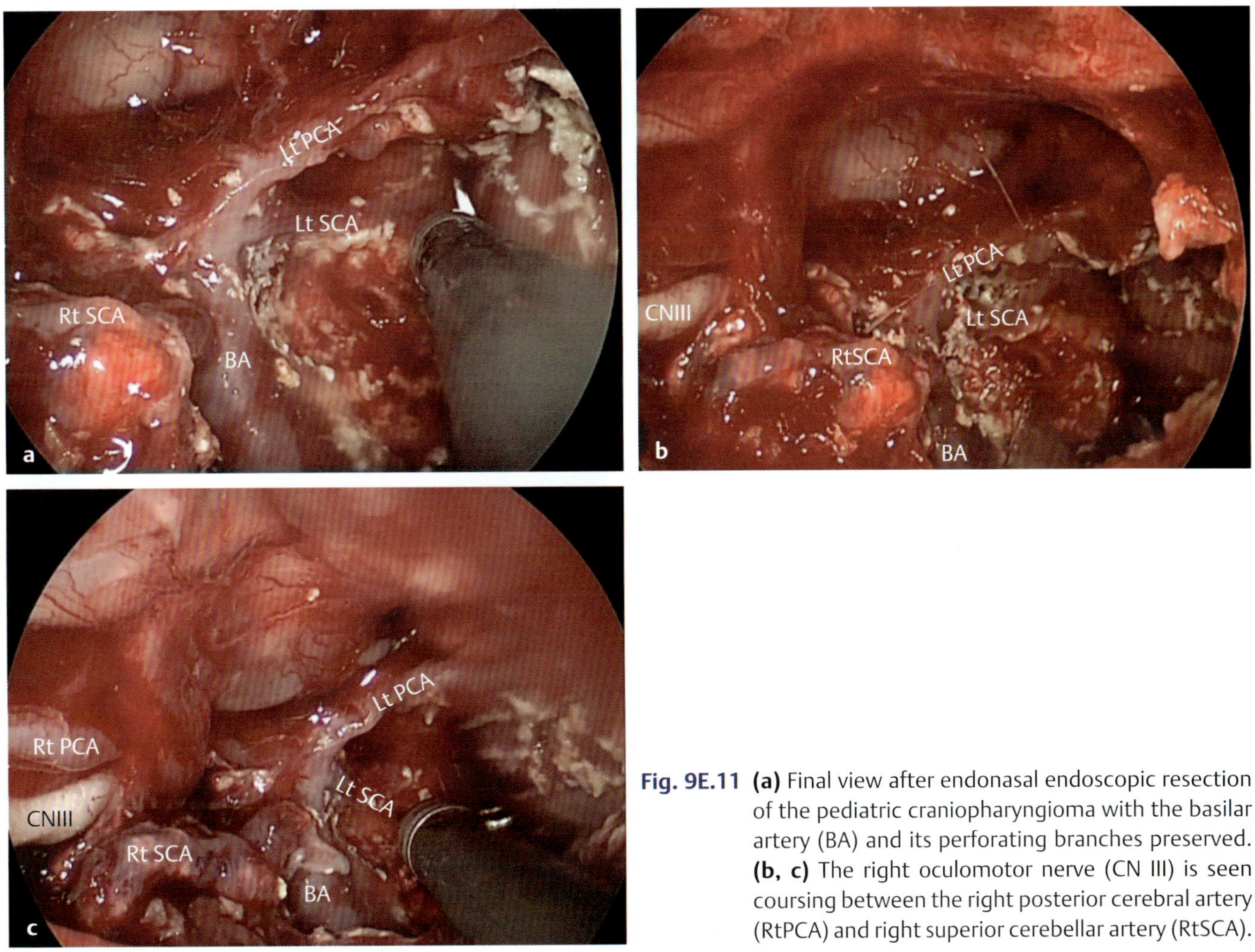

Fig. 9E.11 **(a)** Final view after endonasal endoscopic resection of the pediatric craniopharyngioma with the basilar artery (BA) and its perforating branches preserved. **(b, c)** The right oculomotor nerve (CN III) is seen coursing between the right posterior cerebral artery (RtPCA) and right superior cerebellar artery (RtSCA).

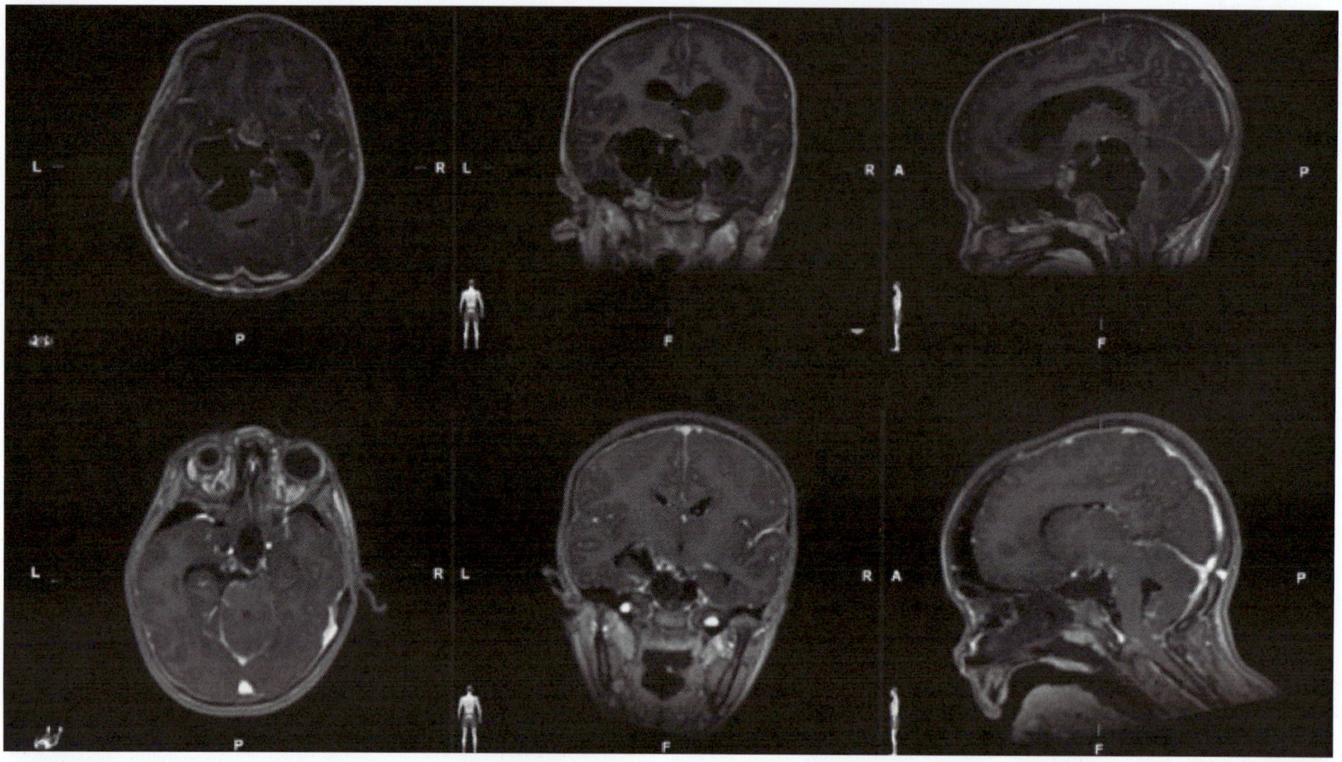

Fig. 9E.12 Intraoperative MRI control: The superior row demonstrates axial, coronal and sagittal sections preoperatively compared to the inferior row after resection of the pediatric craniopharyngioma.

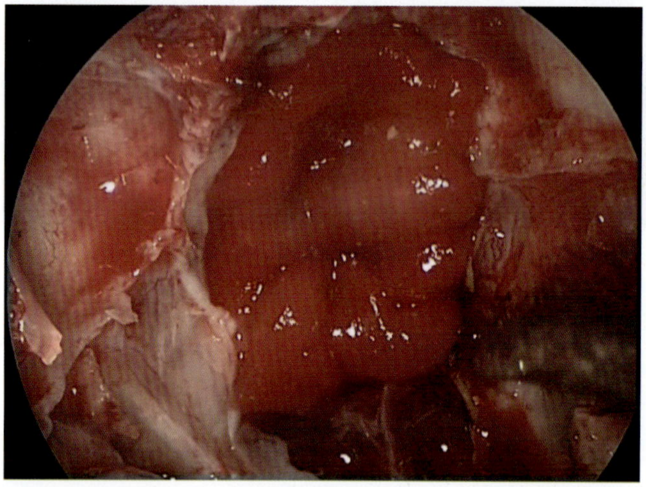

Fig. 9E.13 DuraGen (Integra Lifesciences Service, France) is used to reconstruct the skull base defect and is applied using an underlay technique.

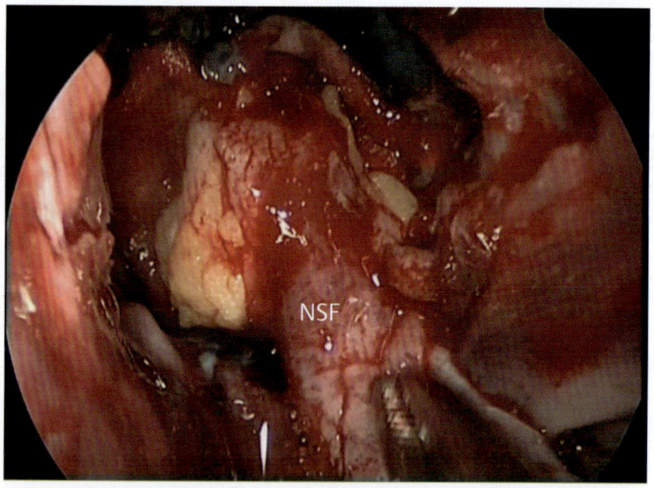

Fig. 9E.14 An abdominal fat graft and a nasoseptal flap (NSF) are applied over the multilayered DuraGen. A final layer of dural sealant is used to stabilize the construct.

Chapter 10 Microsurgical Approach for Suprasellar Lesions

Rajan Shah, Prashik Waghmare, and Sudhendoo Babhulkar

Case 10

Frontotemporal Approach for Sellar and Suprasellar Lesions

Introduction

Skull base approaches are designed to provide better exposure to the normal and abnormal structures in the skull base. Owing to the sheer location, manipulation of these regions is a herculean task for the skull base surgeons during any surgical interventions. Through this chapter, we would like to discuss an extended transcranial skull base approach which gives us better maneuverability compared to conventional cranial approaches. The most significant advantage of this technique is the prevention of retraction and manipulation injuries to the intracranial structures which occur during convention approaches.

An understanding of the complex microanatomy is key in preserving the critical structures involved in each approach. The frontotemporal approach with variations of orbitozygomatic extension is one of the most commonly used skull base approaches. It is helpful in the treatment of both vascular and neoplastic pathologies involving the anterior and middle cranial fossa, orbit, orbital apex and cavernous sinus, paraclinoid and parasellar regions, and with better expertise, even the basilar apex.

Surgical Anatomical Considerations

Neurosurgeons over the past several decades, starting with Sir Walter Dandy, Sir Krause, to the father of modern neurosurgery, Prof. Yasargil, to name a few, have mastered the fronto-temporal approach for skull base diseases. This approach is also known as the fronto-pterional approach.

Pterion is an H-shaped area identified by the union of four bones namely frontal, parietal, temporal, and sphenoidal.[1] Landmark to identify the pterion is 4 cm above the zygoma and 3.5 cm behind the frontozygomatic arch. The skin incision should be fashioned in such a way as to get maximum exposure of pterion. The soft tissue covering this area comprises five layers: skin, subcutaneous tissue, galea aponeurotica, loose connective tissue, and pericranium.

Yasargil referred to the sphenoid wing as "the key landmark" in the approach to the circle of Willis.[2] Drilling the sphenoid bone as far down as the superior orbital fissure, the orbital roof projections, and, occasionally, a part of the orbital ridge and the roof should be performed to reach to the base. This preferably should be done extradurally. Curvilinear dural flap is opened to center Sylvian fissure in its center. Yasargil emphasized the importance of opening Sylvian fissure for relaxing the frontal and temporal lobes of the brain (**Fig. 10.1**).

Anatomically, the Sylvian fissure carries middle cerebral artery (MCA) and its perforators. Dissection will lead the operating surgeon to the internal carotid artery (ICA). The arachnoid is dissected to open the Sylvian fissure, which also helps drain the cerebrospinal fluid (CSF) to reduce the need for retraction of the frontal and temporal lobes. The opening of the fissure could be done from inside out or lateral to medial. It is important to preserve the veins during this step and prevent possibilities of a venous infarct. Also, in the event of an inadvertent breach of the venous structure, it would be prudent to avoid self-retraining retraction on the cerebral lobes (**Fig. 10.2**).

The lamina terminalis cistern is located in the anterior incisural space, above the optic chiasm and delimitated superiorly by the rostrum of the corpus callosum, posteriorly by the lamina terminalis, and laterally by the portions of the medial surfaces of the frontal lobes.[3]

The optic chiasm is a quadrilateral X-shaped structure, situated at the bottom of the brain, immediately below the hypothalamus. It is possible to describe three anatomical variations in the relationship between the optic chiasm and the sella turcica: the so-called normal fixed variant, overlies the diaphragma sellae; the prefixed variant, located above the tuberculum sellae; and the postfixed variant, situated superior to the dorsum sellae.[4]

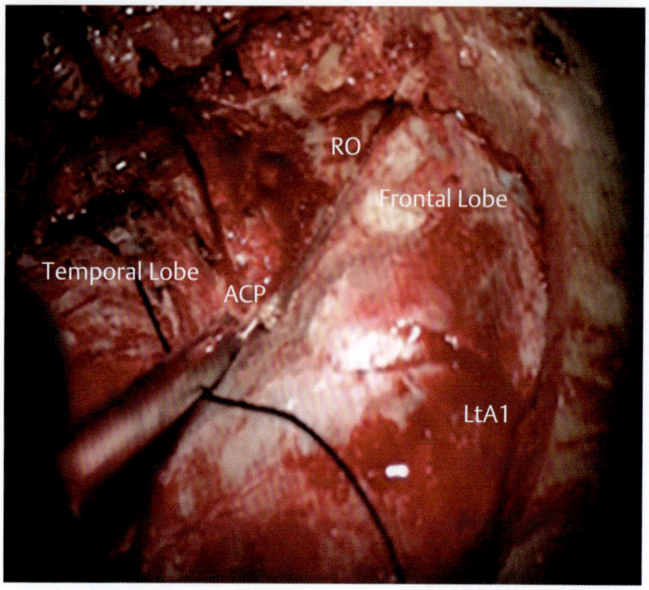

Fig. 10.1 Microscopic image showing the anatomical location of the anterior clinoid process (ACP) after extradural drilling of sphenoid wing and spine of sphenoid bone, the roof of the orbit (RO), and frontal and temporal lobes after craniotomy.

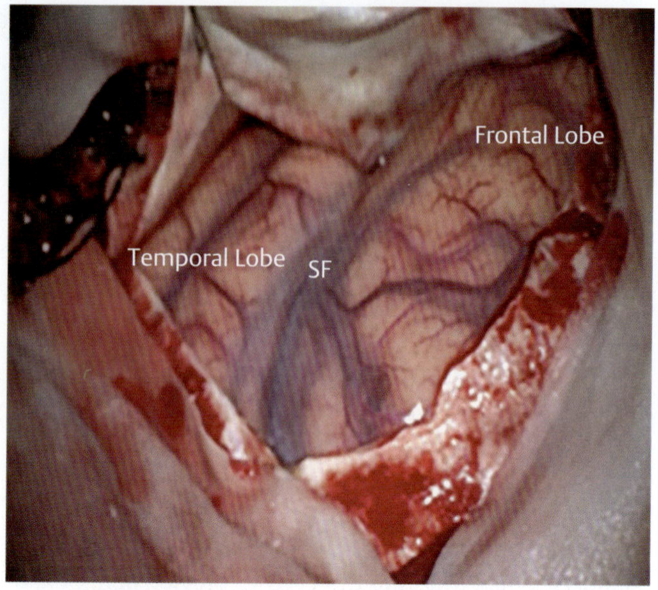

Fig. 10.2 Microscopic image showing frontal and temporal lobes with the sylvian fissure (SF) after the opening of dura.

Indications

Transsphenoidal approach is the most commonly used method for the sellar lesion. However, few indications of fronto-temporal approach used for sellar-suprasellar lesions are enumerated below:

- Large suprasellar component.
- Parasellar tumor.
- Lesion involving the cavernous sinus.
- Active sinus infection.
- Kissing carotid arteries.
- Previously failed transsphenoidal surgeries.

Surgical Steps

The patient is placed supine with a soft gelatin roll under the ipsilateral shoulder to reduce neck torsion and to improve venous drainage. The operating table is adjusted so that the trunk and head are elevated about 20 degrees for additional improvement of cerebral venous outflow. Once secured to a Mayfield three-point headrest, taking care that the pins are kept far away from the planned incision site, the head is extended backward over the neck about 10 to 15 degrees so that the malar eminence remains the highest point in the operative field; this maneuver allows the frontal and temporal lobes to fall by gravity away from the bony basal structures for better surgical access with minimal need for retraction.[5] Finally, the head is rotated 15 to 60 degrees to the contralateral side, and the degree of rotation is dictated by the location and extension of the targeted lesion.

The skin incision is started below the posterior root of the zygomatic arch, 1 cm anterior to the tragus, continued superiorly along the line of the posterior third of the temporal muscle, and then frontally curved toward the opposite superior temporal line, in a bicoronal fashion remaining whenever possible at least 1 cm behind the hairline. The position of this incision preserves the main trunk of the superficial temporal artery.[6]

The scalp flap is dissected, with sharp and blunt dissection, from the galea and from the outer layer of the fascia temporalis superficialis in two layers. The frontotemporal branch of the facial nerve is left intact, mobilized inferiorly between the two layers of the fascia temporalis superficialis. The temporalis muscle is then dissected from the temporal line inferiorly to its attachment near the zygoma.

The craniotomy is then performed.[7] A keyhole burr hole is placed over the frontosphenoidal suture 1 cm behind the frontozygomatic suture. Two accessory holes are made: one in the lowest exposed squamous temporal bone just superior to the posterior root of the zygomatic arch, and the other at the level of the temporoparietal suture inferior to the temporal line (**Fig. 10.3**).

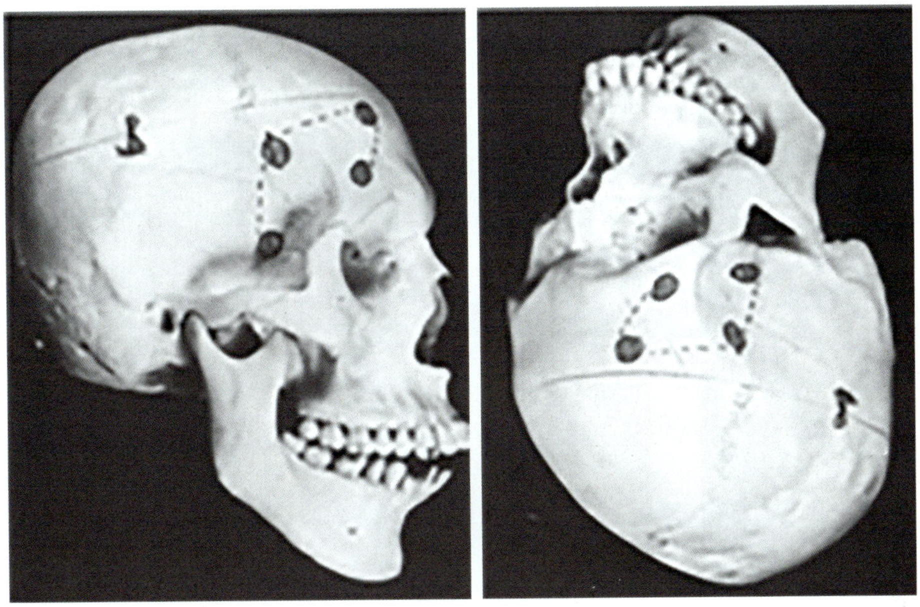

Fig. 10.3 Image showing anatomical landmark for craniotomy.

Extradural Dissection

Drilling of the superior orbital rim is optional as one of the variations for this approach. However, the sphenoid wing and spine of sphenoid bone are drilled extradurally with a diamond burr to create working space. The sphenoid bone is drilled as far as the falciform ligament lateral to the superior orbital fissure.

At this point, the basal frontal and medial temporal dura is completely exposed, separated from the periorbita by a bony bridge formed superiorly by the roof of the optic canal and the anterior clinoid process and laterally by the most posterior residual of the lateral orbital wall. The anterior clinoid process is drilled, together with the optic strut, using small diamond-tipped burrs to expose the subclinoid portion of the ICA (**Fig. 10.4**).

These maneuvers are performed in most cases because they allow better mobilization of the ICA and optic nerve after the dural opening, which facilitates the surgical treatment of lesions extensively involving the anterior and middle cranial base or expanding into the parasellar region and/or the interpeduncular cistern.

The dura mater is widely opened in a standard fashion. The Sylvian fissure is widely opened as a rule and further space may be gained by opening the dura propria of the optic nerve and incising the dural ring encircling the ICA at its intradural entrance. Intradural mobilization of the optic nerve and ICA allows the surgical corridor located between these structures (interopticocarotid cistern) and the corridor between the ICA siphon and the third cranial nerve (laterocarotid cistern) to be enlarged. The third cranial nerve may be further mobilized by sectioning the insertion of the dura at the tentorial notch lateral to the nerve. This maneuver may enlarge the working space lateral to the ICA (moving laterally the third cranial nerve) and also may create a surgical corridor lateral to the nerve (if it is retracted medially; **Fig. 10.5**).[5]

Conclusion

This approach is best to deal with the cavernous sinus and parasellar pathologies especially lateral to the ICA and the third, fourth, fifth, and sixth cranial nerves in the lateral wall of the cavernous sinus.

With the advances in the anesthesia and knowledge of the microanatomy of the skull base especially the CSF cisterns, it is possible to reach the cavernous sinus with almost no retraction trauma to the brain by letting out CSF at every stage of dissection. This has significantly reduced the postoperative morbidity, making this approach for the lesions not clearly amenable to transnasal endoscopic procedures.

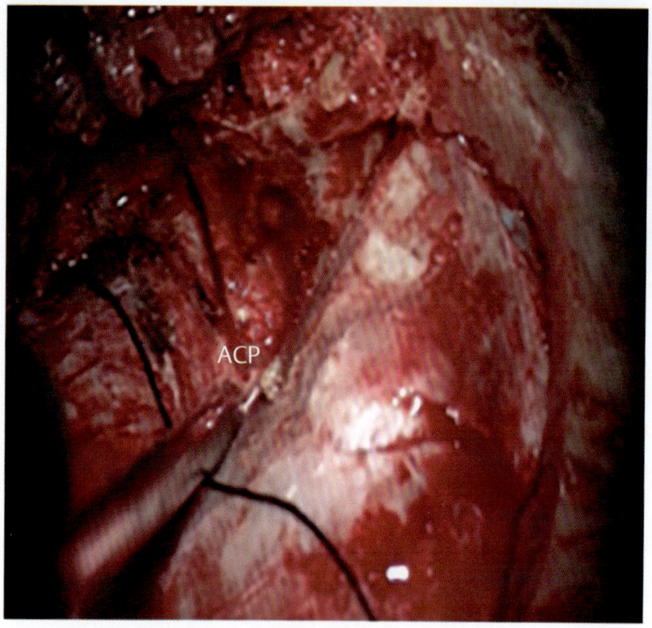

Fig. 10.4 Microscopic image showing exposed anterior clinoid process after extradural drilling of sphenoid ridge.

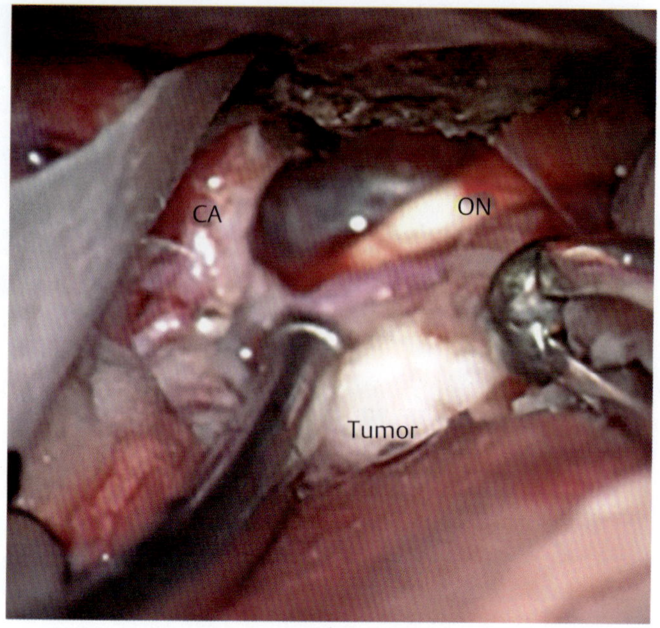

Fig. 10.5 image showing the parasellar tumor in proximity with optic nerve (ON) and carotid artery (CA) after Sylvian fissure dissection.

References

1. McMinn RM. Last's Anatomy Regional and Applied. 9th ed. Edinburgh: Churchill Livingstone; 1994:645
2. Yasargil MG, Antic J, Laciga R, Jain KK, Hodosh RM, Smith RD. Microsurgical pterional approach to aneurysms of the basilar bifurcation. Surg Neurol 1976;6(2):83–91
3. Yamamoto I, Rhoton AL Jr, Peace DA. Microsurgery of the third ventricle: part I. Microsurgical anatomy. Neurosurgery 1981;8(3):334–356
4. Renn WH, Rhoton AL Jr. Microsurgical anatomy of the sellar region. J Neurosurg 1975;43(3):288–298
5. Galzio RJ, Tschabitscher M, Ricci A. Orbitozygomatic approach. Cranial, Craniofacial and Skull Base Surgery. Milano: Springer; 2010:61–86
6. Yaşargil MG, Reichman MV, Kubik S. Preservation of the frontotemporal branch of the facial nerve using the interfascial temporalis flap for pterional craniotomy. Technical article. J Neurosurg 1987;67(3):463–466
7. Aziz KM, Froelich SC, Cohen PL, Sanan A, Keller JT, van Loveren HR. The one-piece orbitozygomatic approach: the MacCarty burr hole and the inferior orbital fissure as keys to technique and application. Acta Neurochir (Wien) 2002;144(1):15–24

Chapter 11

Sellar, Parasellar, and Suprasellar Meningioma

Michel Roethlisberger, Dominik Cordier, Jürgen Hench, Adam Jadczak, Yves Brand, Luigi Mariani, Prepageran Narayanan, and Vicknes Waran

Introduction

Although benign skull base lesions, meningiomas of the sellar, parasellar, and suprasellar region represent a unique set of surgically challenging tumors, given their three-dimensional relationship with the optic apparatus, vascular structures, the pituitary stalk, and the pituitary gland. These challenges are encountered within the context of a surgical goal that provides long-term tumor control, preservation or improvement of visual function, and minimal morbidity. Advancements in skull base surgery with improvements in traditional and minimally invasive transcranial (TCA) and endonasal endoscopic approaches (EEA) have hence enlarged the surgical strategies available.

Pathological Considerations

Histological and Molecular Features

Because of the fact that meningiomas are common intracranial neoplasms presenting with a wide spectrum of clinical and biological behavior, experts have sought to resolve this by the introduction of histology-based classification systems. To date, 15 morphological meningioma variants are listed in the World Health Organization (WHO) classification.[1] These have been attributed to one of three WHO grades (I–III) each, and this system bears substantial gray zones between these grades. In recent years, methylome analysis,[2,3] and subsequent whole-genome sequencing efforts have finally resolved these discrepancies.[4] Six distinct types of meningioma have been identified,[2] each of which shows rather consistent clinical behavior[2] and also shares genetic aberrations in terms of the specifically deregulated pathways, enabling future targeted therapies (**Table 11.1**).[3] At the same time, the molecular analyses highlighted the high error rate of histological classification with respect to biological behavior and clinical outcome. In fact, the six molecular meningioma types exhibit a type-specific prognosis, which led to their nomenclature: The "benign-1, -2, and -3" types have a prognosis slightly more favorable than the average WHO grade I tumor, the "intermediate-A and -B" types are more aggressive than WHO grade II tumors, and the "malignant" meningiomas are even more progressive than anaplastic meningioma (WHO grade III). As shown for brain tumors in general,[2] the misclassification rate of meningiomas based on histology is higher than 10%.[3] Since meningiomas are typically large tumors and are so far best characterized of all brain tumors on a molecular level, it is almost imperative to the neurosurgeon and neuropathologist to preserve DNA in the best possible state from such specimens to subject it to methylome analysis. Histological features to allow for grading in accordance with the WHO should be reported, but recurrence risk and aggressiveness should be commented on after completion of molecular stratification only. Immunohistochemical analysis can be reduced to determining the proliferation fraction (Ki-67/MIB-1 labeling). Concerning the many morphological variants, it has now been demonstrated that they are not well suited to predict biological behavior despite being the mainstay of diagnostics according to the WHO. It is highly likely that this will be changed in the upcoming WHO classifications.

Anatomical Considerations

Meningiomas arising in the anterior skull base are the most common primary tumors in this region (20%).[5,6] When including meningiomas of the sphenoid wing, they even account for 40% of all primary anterior skull base tumors (**Fig. 11.1**).[5,6] These, usually benign and slow-growing lesions are surrounded by multiple arachnoidal layers that separate the tumor from the physiological neurovascular structures of the base of skull.

Olfactory Groove Meningioma

Meningiomas arising from the cribriform plate of the ethmoid bone involving anatomical structures from the crista galli to the planum sphenoidale are frequently encountered and account for approximately one-fifth of all intracranial meningiomas.[5,7,8] When these lesions extend posteriorly, they involve the pituitary fossa and the orbital roofs.[9,10]

Table 11.1 Methylation classes of meningioma

Methylation class	Description
Benign-1	Usually harbors deletions of 22q and *NF2* mutations. Other chromosomal aberrations or mutations are rare. Histology mostly resembles the fibroblastic or transitional subtype. Risk of recurrence after complete resection is low.
Benign-2	These have usually flat copy number profiles and are enriched for cases with TRAF7 mutations in combination with mutations of *AKT1* or *KLF4*, and for *SMO* mutations. Cases with meningothelial (particularly enriched for *AKT1/TRAF7* mutations) or secretory (*KLF4* mutation) histology mostly fall into this methylation class. Risk of recurrence after complete resection is low. If present, *AKT1E17K* mutations offer a target for treatment in cases in which complete resection is not feasible.
Benign-3	These often show chromosomal gains, particularly including chromosome 5. About half of these cases also have 22q deletions and *NF2* mutations. The histological variants of metaplastic, microcytic, and angiomatous meningioma are enriched in this methylation class. Risk of recurrence after complete resection is low.
Intermediate A/B	Intermediate A/B meningiomas have frequently deletion of 22q and mutations of *NF2*, but in addition often deletions of 1p, 10, and 14. A subset can also present with *CDKN2A/B* deletion. TERT promoter mutations can occur but are rare in this methylation class. A large share shows increased mitotic count, but some cases may by histologically inconspicuous. Risk of recurrence is about 50% within 48 months.
Malignant	They show usually highly perturbed copy number profiles, including deletions of 22q, 1p, 10, 14, and *CDKN2A/B*. However, focal deletions of *BAP1* with otherwise flat copy number profiles have also been observed. Most cases have *NF2* mutations, some in addition have mutations of the TERT promoter. The risk of recurrence is higher than for the average of cases histologically diagnosed as grade III meningioma with approximately 75% recurrence rate at 24 months.

Note: The methylation profile of a given tumor typically falls into one of these six methylation classes. Note that the A/B nomenclature is separate of any other A/B nomenclature in meningioma. This classification is likely to supersede the grading philosophy currently proposed by the WHO.
Source: Adapted from www.molecularneuropathology.org.

Planum Sphenoidale and Tuberculum Sellae Meningioma

Meningiomas arising from the planum sphenoidale, tuberculum sellae, and the diaphragma sellae represent 5 to 10% of all intracranial meningiomas.[11–13] These subtypes differ in terms of anatomical origin, dural involvement, vascular blood supply, and their relationship to neurovascular structures (**Fig. 11.1** and **Fig. 11.2**).[12–14]

- *Planum sphenoidale meningioma*: These meningiomas are the second most common suprasellar meningioma. They are the most anteriorly located meningiomas of this subgroup.[7,9,15,16]
- *Tuberculum sellae meningioma (type A)*: Tuberculum sellae meningioma primarily arise from the dura covering the tuberculum sellae and chiasmatic sulcus and can involve the dura of the limbus sphenoidalis anteriorly and/or diaphragma sellae posteriorly (**Fig. 11.3**).[17,18] They represent the most common type of tuberculum sellae meningioma.[9]
- *Combined tubercular and diaphragma sellae (type B) or diaphragma sellae meningioma (type C)*: These tumors arise from the diaphragma sellae and often demonstrate significant tumor extension into the sella turcica. The pituitary stalk can be adherent along the posterior aspect of the capsule but is generally easy to locate because of its vascular and fleshy appearance.[18] True diaphragma sellae meningiomas are rare.[13,19]

Topoanatomical Relationships

- *High-lying tuberculum sellae meningioma*: When a pneumosinus sphenoidalis dilatans of more than 5 mm is present, the tumor lies high in relation to the frontobasal line.[20] In preoperative magnetic resonance imaging (MRI) of surgically treated tuberculum sellae meningioma, 24% were classified as high-lying tumors.[20]
- *Low-lying tuberculum sellae meningioma*: Tumor extension into the pituitary fossa more than 5 mm below the tuberculum sellae.[20] In preoperative MRI of surgically treated tuberculum sellae meningioma, 71% were classified as low-lying, and 5% as nonspecific tumors.[20]

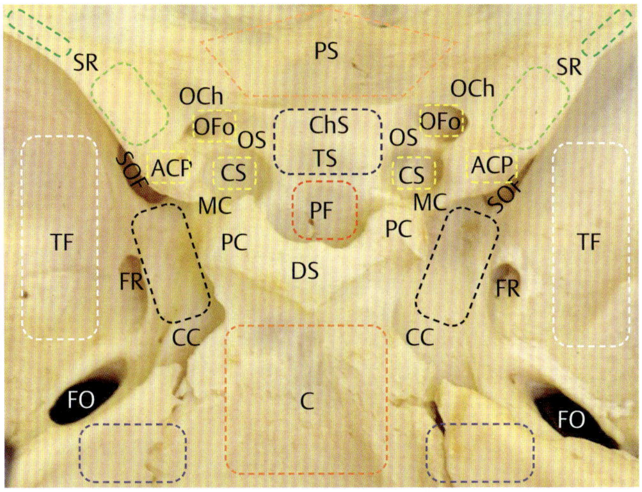

Fig. 11.1 Superior oblique view of the skull base to demonstrate the topoanatomical relationship of anterior skull base meningiomas in a dry bone specimen. The pituitary fossa (PF) lies in the body of the sphenoid bone, bounded anteriorly by the tuberculum sellae (TS) and posteriorly by the dorsum sellae (DS). The planum sphenoidale (PS) is the bony continuation anterior to the TS. Between these two structures is a shallow groove, the chiasmatic sulcus (ChS). The optic chiasm lies posterior and superior to the sulcus, the optic foramina (OFo) with the optic nerves are lateral to the ChS. The limbus sphenoidalis is a ridge of bone at the anterior aspect of the ChS. Lateral sphenoidal wing (pterional) meningioma (*dark green squares*), middle sphenoidal wing meningioma (*light green squares*), clinoidal meningioma (*yellow squares*), planum sphenoidale meningioma (*orange square*), tuberculum sellae meningioma (*blue square*), intrasellar meningioma (*red square*), cavernous sinus meningioma (*black squares*), middle temporal fossa meningioma (*white squares*), clival meningioma (*rose square*), petroclival meningioma (*violet squares*).

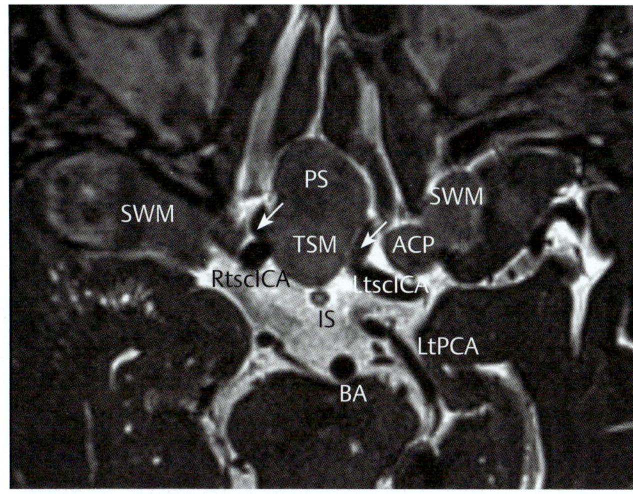

Fig. 11.2 T1-weighted noncontrast-enhanced axial MRI section of a patient with meningiomatosis cerebri demonstrating a concomitant lateral sphenoid wing meningioma (SWM), a tuberculum sellae meningioma (TSM) extending into the planum sphenoidale (PS) and a meningioma of the anterior clinoid process (ACP). There is a postfixed optic chiasm and hence close proximity to the left and right optic nerve (*white arrow*). The infundibular stalk (IS) lies posterior to the lesion.

- *Relationships to neural structures*: With consecutive growth over time, tuberculum sellae meningiomas displace the optic nerves laterally and the chiasm posterosuperiorly. In extensive lesions, the optic nerve may even be lateral to the carotid arteries. The relationship of the optic chiasm in relation to the tuberculum sellae meningioma is characteristic and differentiates them from planum sphenoidale and olfactory groove meningiomas. An important feature of tuberculum sellae meningioma is the tendency to extend into the optic canals and into the pituitary fossa with dislocation of the infundibular stalk and consecutive contact with the pituitary gland (**Fig. 11.3a–i**).[18]

Neurovascular Relationships

The posterior ethmoidal arteries and the meningeal branches of the cavernous internal carotid artery (ICA) usually provide the blood supply of tuberculum sellae meningiomas and consecutively from the anterior communicating and anterior cerebral arteries in later stages.[18] The superior hypophyseal arteries are displaced laterally.[18] The basilar artery and posterior circulation branches are usually protected by the membrane of Liliequist as an arachnoidal barrier[18] (**Fig. 11.4**). Larger tuberculum sellae meningiomas displace or even encase the intradural ICA laterally and the anterior H-complex superiorly. The postcommunicating segments of the anterior cerebral arteries are usually separated from the superior–posterior apex of the tuberculum sellae meningioma by arachnoid layers of the interhemispheric fissure (**Fig. 11.5** and **Fig. 11.6**).[18]

Clinoidal Meningioma

Pure clinoidal meningiomas arise from the meninges of the anterior clinoid process and hence inhere specific characteristics related to their anatomical origin. Three types are described in the literature (**Fig. 11.1**).[5,21–24]

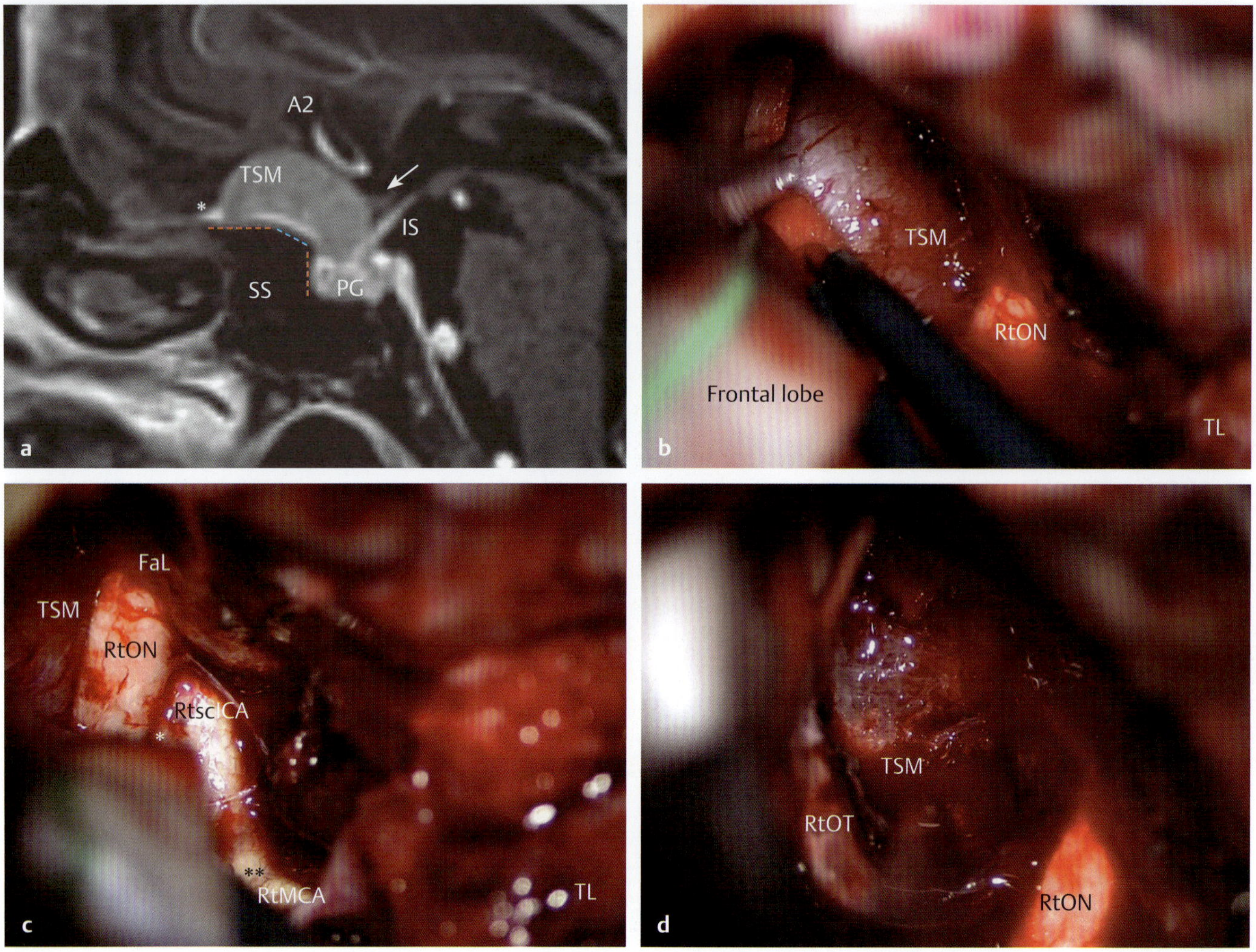

Fig. 11.3 Topoanatomical relationship of a tuberculum sellae meningioma extending toward the planum sphenoidale. **(a)** T1-weighted noncontrast-enhanced sagittal MRI section of a patient with meningiomatosis cerebri demonstrating a tuberculum sellae meningioma (TSM) extending anteriorly over the planum sphenoidale (*orange line*) with a typical dural tail (*). Posteriorly, the meningioma grows from the tuberculum sellae (*blue line*) over the limbus sphenoidale toward the pituitary fossa (*red line*) and develops a close contact with the pituitary gland (PG) and the infundibular stalk (IS). The optic chiasm (*white arrow*) is postfixed. The apex of the lesion is in proximity with the distal anterior cerebral artery (A2). **(b)** Exposure of the tuberculum sellae meningioma (TSM) extending toward the planum sphenoidale through a right pterional craniotomy. Using the subfrontal approach, the suprachiasmatic cistern has been opened, and cerebrospinal fluid has been released to relax the surgical field. The cisternal arachnoid membrane has been dissected, and the lateral aspect of the tumor is exposed after gentle retraction of the frontal lobe. The right optic nerve (RtON) is dislocated and compressed laterally by the tumor. **(c)** Topoanatomical relations of the tuberculum sellae meningioma (TSM) after microsurgical splitting of the right sylvian fissure. The right optic nerve (RtON) is dislocated and compressed laterally, entering the optic canal covered by the falciform ligament (FaL). Laterally, the opticocarotid window (*) and the right supraclinoid internal carotid artery (RtscICA) with the carotid bifurcation (**) are exposed. **(d)** The tuberculum sellae meningioma (TSM) is debulked between the right olfactory tract (RtOT) and the right optic nerve (RtON).

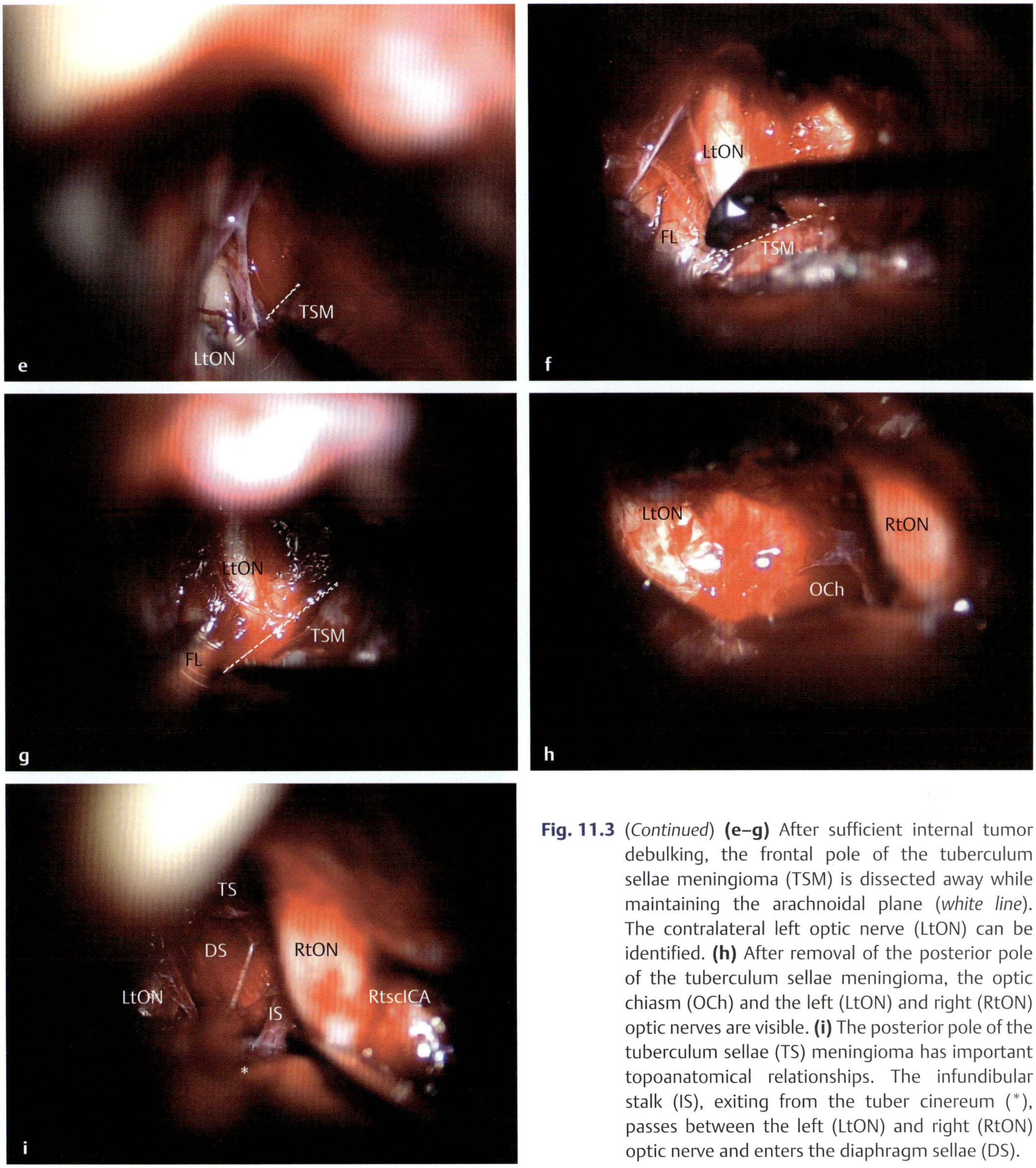

Fig. 11.3 (*Continued*) **(e–g)** After sufficient internal tumor debulking, the frontal pole of the tuberculum sellae meningioma (TSM) is dissected away while maintaining the arachnoidal plane (*white line*). The contralateral left optic nerve (LtON) can be identified. **(h)** After removal of the posterior pole of the tuberculum sellae meningioma, the optic chiasm (OCh) and the left (LtON) and right (RtON) optic nerves are visible. **(i)** The posterior pole of the tuberculum sellae (TS) meningioma has important topoanatomical relationships. The infundibular stalk (IS), exiting from the tuber cinereum (*), passes between the left (LtON) and right (RtON) optic nerve and enters the diaphragm sellae (DS).

- *Type I:* Originate from the subclinoid dura medial to the anterior clinoid process in the carotid sulcus near the ICA.
- *Type II:* Located superolateral to the anterior clinoid process. They are separated from the ICA and the optic nerve by arachnoidal membrane layers of the carotid cistern.
- *Type III*: Originate from the optic foramen and can extend into the optic canal.

Clinical Considerations

Clinical signs and symptoms of anterior (olfactory groove and planum sphenoidale) and central skull base (tuberculum sellae and clinoidal) meningiomas depend of the exact topo-anatomical location, growth pattern, and size of the lesion.

Nonspecific symptoms involve headache and vertigo, even occurring in asymptomatic meningiomas. Migraine, nonspecific headaches, and vertigo are common neurological signs leading to neurocranial MRI revealing incidental findings of smaller meningiomas of the base of skull.

Trigeminal nerve dysfunctions are suggestive for cavernous sinus involvement. Orthoptic disturbances including diplopia, oculomotor and abducent dysfunction, are possible when meningiomas involve the cavernous sinus, or in purely intracavernous meningiomas (**Fig. 11.7**). Orthoptic disturbances can be present when meningiomas involve the orbital fissures or the orbit apex or conus. Exophthalmos is more a sign of spheno-orbital meningiomas, but can be found with cavernous sinus involvement as well.[5,18]

Focal neurological deficits include aphasia, hemiparesis, behavioral changes, psychiatric symptoms, mental deterioration, short-term memory loss, somnolence and seizures, and usually correlate with large lesions compressing the surrounding frontal or temporal lobes with perifocal edema.[5,25–28]

- *Olfactory groove meningioma:* Slow and often subclinical loss of olfaction (anosmia), cacosmia and behavioral or mental changes, personality changes, and "frontal lobe syndrome" because of compression of the frontal lobes, frequently with extensive "vasogenic edema" in radiological work-up.[25–30] Long-term headache is a possible symptom.[5,6,31] If they involve the tuberculum sellae and the pituitary fossa, visual and endocrinological disturbances are possible.
- *Planum sphenoidale meningioma:* Even though they are slow-growing benign tumors, significant morbidity may result from compression of the oculomotor nerve, anterior visual pathways, or trigeminal nerve.[32] Tumor expansion may lead to visual disturbances (inferior or

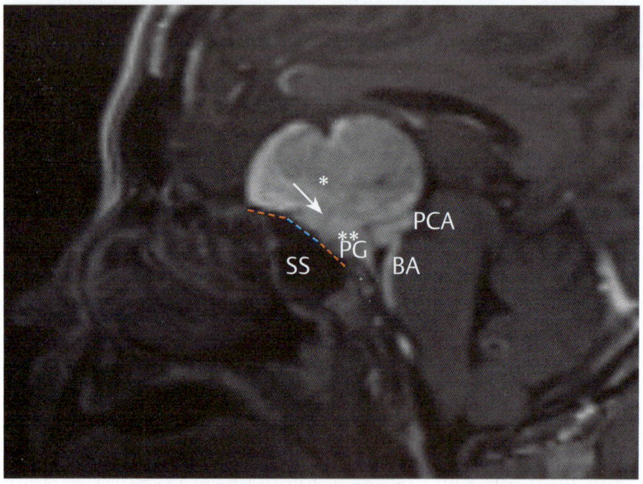

Fig. 11.4 T1-weighted gadolinium contrast-enhanced sagittal MRI section showing the suprasellar mass extending from the tuberculum sellae (*blue line*) to the planum sphenoidale (*orange line*). A typical sunburst pattern (*white arrow*) is suggestive that the meningioma is emerging from the tuberculum sellae with the blood supply arising from this region. Hypointense nonenhancing areas are present and are suggestive for calcifications (*). The pituitary gland (PG) is separated by a hypointense arachnoid cleft (**) from the lesion. Sella turcica (*green line*).

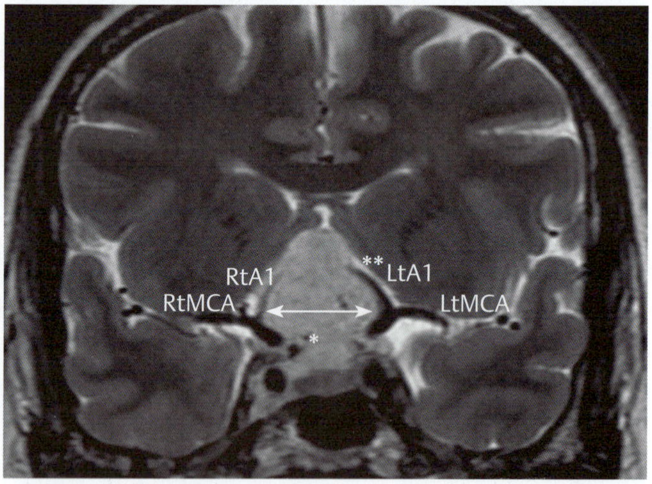

Fig. 11.5 T2-weighted coronal MRI section showing a T2-isointense extra-axial solid mass emerging from the tuberculum sellae. The apex of the lesion is in close contact with the precommunicating segments of the left (LtA1) and right (RtA1) anterior cerebral arteries and spreads the carotid bifurcations apart bilaterally (*white arrow*). Hypointense signals are suggestive for calcifications (*). A cortical cuff sign can be appreciated, suggestive for a good brain–tumor interface during endonasal endoscopic resection of the lesion (**).

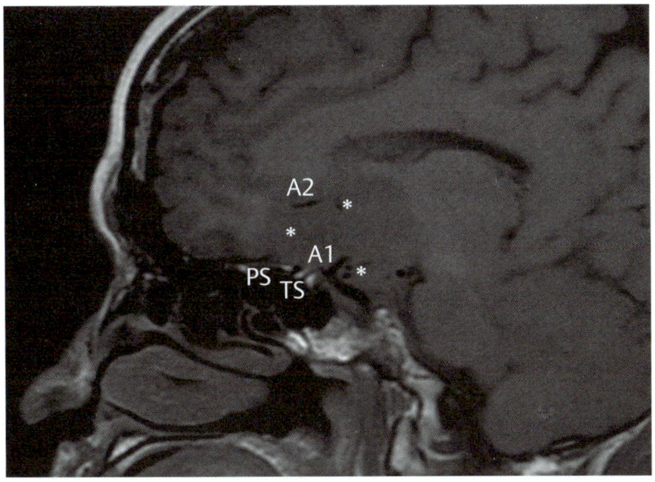

Fig. 11.6 T1-weighted noncontrast-enhanced sagittal MRI section showing an iso- to hypointense suprasellar mass extending from the tuberculum sellae (TS) to the planum sphenoidale (PS). Hypointense nonenhancing areas are present and are suggestive for calcifications (*).

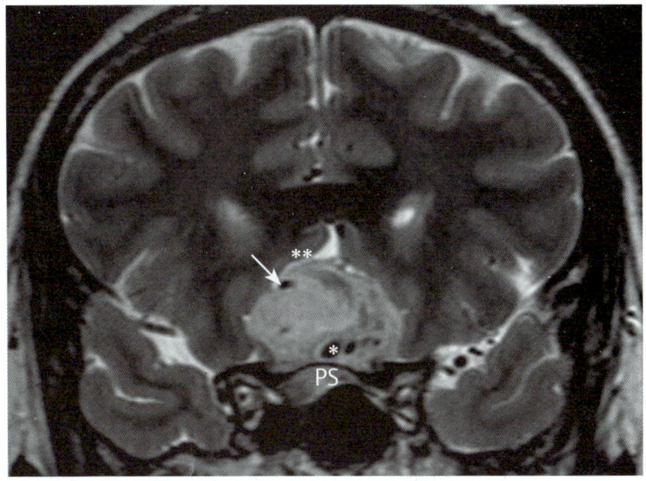

Fig. 11.7 T2-weighted coronal MRI section showing a T2-isointense extra-axial solid mass extending along the planum sphenoidale (PS). The apex is in contact with the postcommunicating segment of the anterior cerebral arteries (*arrow*). Hypointense signals are suggestive for calcifications (*). A cortical cuff sign can be appreciated, suggestive for a good brain–tumor interface during endonasal endoscopic resection of the lesion (**).

bitemporal visual field defect), visual loss, and endocrinological disturbances.[33]

- *Tuberculum sellae meningioma:* Typically present with slowly progressive visual symptoms, including visual loss (98%), depending on the grade of involvement of the optic chiasm, optic nerve atrophy (78%), and inferior or bitemporal visual field deficits.[6,16,18,34,35] The long-term compression of the optic apparatus leads to thinning and demyelination with consecutive impairment of vision.[16] A higher grade of compression and involvement along the tumor and inside of the optic canals leads to a higher risk of surgical injury intraoperatively.[18,36] A classic clinical finding that has been described in the literature for approximately two-thirds of tuberculum sellae meningiomas is a unilateral temporal field defect with a contralateral quadrantanopia.[18,37–39] More laterally growing tuberculum sellae meningioma with asymmetric invasion of the optic canals can cause a relative afferent pupillary defect with a unilateral optic atrophy.[5] Other symptoms include hemiparesis (15%) and anosmia (11%).[18,37–39] Endocrinological dysfunction is possible when the infundibular stalk and the pituitary fossa are involved.
- *Clinoidal meningiomas:* Blindness, optic nerve atrophy, and visual field deficits are common symptoms. Type III clinoidal meningiomas can present very early because of invasion of the optic canal and hence ophthalmological disturbances.[5,21–24]

Radiological Features

Suprasellar meningiomas can be classified as planum sphenoidale, tuberculum sellae, combined tubercular and diaphragmatic, or diaphragmatic.[12] These radiological variants differ in terms of origin, dural involvement, vascular blood supply, and topoanatomical relationships.

Generally, the intensity and homogeneity of enhancement, the visualization of a dural attachment, and the dural "tail" in MRI may provide a strong suggestion that the patient has a meningioma (**Fig. 11.3**).[40] Meningiomas are known to calcify in 15 to 20% of cases (**Fig. 11.7**). Hence, the addition of computed tomography (CT) may reveal hyperostosis or calcifications.[41,42] MRI with fat suppression is helpful for detecting intraorbital involvement of a skull base meningioma. MRI angiography reveals the topoanatomical relationship of a meningioma with the internal carotid and anterior cerebral arteries. Parasellar involvement into the cavernous sinus (**Fig. 11.8**), orbit apex, or ethmoidal and sphenoidal involvement is possible. If cystic components are present, meningiomas might be difficult to differentiate from craniopharyngiomas.[43] Further on, typical features of each tumor entity might not necessarily be present in the case of a synchronous tumorous lesion.[44,45]

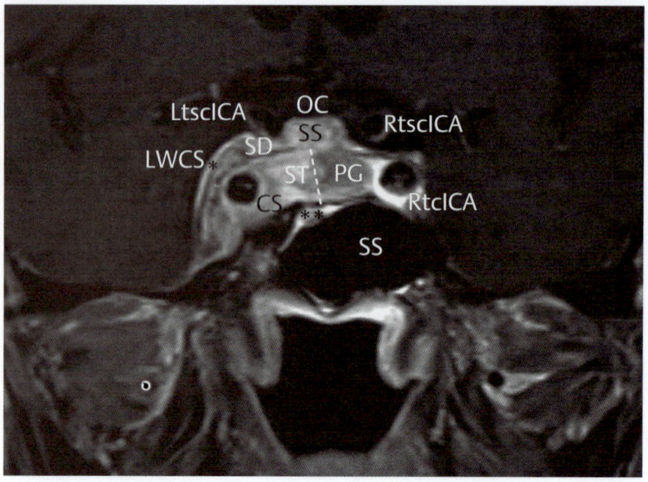

Fig. 11.8 Intra-, para-, and suprasellar meningioma with cavernous sinus involvement. T1-weighted gadolinium contrast-enhanced coronal MRI section demonstrating a meningioma extending into the sella turcica (ST), left cavernous sinus (CS), suprasellar region (SS), supradiaphragmal (SD) region, along the lateral wall (*) of the cavernous sinus (LWCS) and en plaque along the roof (**) of the sphenoid sinus (SS). The pituitary gland (PG) can be distinguished from the intrasellar portion of the meningioma (*white line*).

Olfactory Groove Meningioma

These tumors displace the optic chiasm inferiorly while extending posteriorly. Invasion of the ethmoidal cells is present in approximately one-fifth of cases, and bony erosion of the base of skull is possible.[25,27,30] The olfactory nerves are displaced laterally and compressed, encased, or invaded in larger lesions.[25,27,30]

Planum Sphenoidale Meningioma

These tumors have the most anterior site of origin and predominant area of dural involvement. Hence, a posterior and inferior displacement of the optic nerves, the optic chiasm, and the anterior cerebral arteries complex is encountered when assessing these lesions.[11,12,15]

Tuberculum Sellae Meningioma

This subgroup combines meningioma involving the dura covering the limbus sphenoidale, chiasmatic sulcus, and tuberculum sellae (**Fig. 11.1, Fig. 11.2, Fig. 11.3,** and **Fig. 11.4**].[6,16,46] Meningioma in this anatomical region lead to a displacement of the optic nerves superolaterally, the optic chiasm posteriorly, and the anterior cerebral H-complex superiorly (**Fig. 11.5** and **Fig. 11.6**).[6,46] These lesions may extend into both optic canals. This specific feature might have a higher prevalence intraoperatively than anticipated when assessing these lesions preoperatively.[18,47]

- *Tuberculum sellae meningioma (type A):* This meningioma subgroup demonstrates a significant elongation of the tuberculum–sellar floor interval and planum–tuberculum interval (**Fig. 11.3** and **Fig. 11.4**).[12]
- *Combined tubercular and diaphragmal meningioma (type B):* This meningioma subgroup demonstrates a relative elongation of both the tuberculum–sellar floor interval and planum–tuberculum interval.[12]
- *Diaphragma sellae meningioma (type C):* This meningioma subgroup can be differentiated from type A meningiomas radiologically when an elongation of neither the tuberculum–sellar floor interval nor the planum–tuberculum interval is present.[12,19]

Surgical Considerations

Incidentally discovered meningiomas in the sella can be observed if they are small, and there is no encroachment of the optic apparatus, neurological deficit, or endocrine dysfunction. Cases of purely intrasellar meningiomas have long since been considered amenable for a transsphenoidal operation. In some cases, pathological examination reveals the diagnosis of a meningioma after resection.

In the modern era of endonasal endoscopic surgeries, indications to resect suprasellar meningiomas have been set to a broader extent.[16,48–51] Extending the zonal dissection of the skull base beyond the sellar opening has been extensively described in the literature.[52–57] Possible extensions that can be applied when addressing larger lesions of the skull base include transcribriform, transplanum, transtuberculum, and transclivus extensions.[58,59] These extensions depend on the surgical route dictated by the size and firmness of the treated lesion.[60,61] In the past decades, suprasellar meningiomas have been more and more amenable for pure endoscopic endonasal resection. The proximity to critical surrounding neurovascular structures remains a challenging feature of these tumors.[11] Many groups around the world report the extension of the classic midline corridor to the tuberculum sellae and planum sphenoidale.[18,31] However, transcranial approaches (TCAs) have repeatedly been shown to be an equivocal, safe, and efficient way to treat suprasellar meningiomas.[62–66] The correct indication and assessment of factors that predict unsuccessful or incomplete resection of skull base meningioma prior to surgery are of great importance.[20,67] Thus, TCAs remain a well described option and have to be considered when resection of these lesions is necessary.[63–66]

The surgical route for suprasellar meningioma is either through a superior transcranial route or an inferior transnasal route.[38,62,68–70] Advantages and disadvantages of the EEA for suprasellar meningiomas remain somewhat equivocal in terms of complications and extent of resection.[12,16,38,71–73]

Planum Sphenoidale Meningioma

These meningiomas usually do not extend below the level of the planum spheniodale.[20,62,74,75] This important feature allows a surgical approach by a subfrontal or pterional transcranial route. The more inferior the point of the anatomical origin and predominant dural involvement toward the tuberculum and diaphragma sellae, the more angulation and inferior dissection is necessary. Hence, more brain retraction with potentially higher surgical access morbidity is necessary.[13,76] This might be even more accentuated, when an elongation of the tuberculum sellae is present.[13,76] In the modern era of extended endonasal endoscopic surgery, this region has been more and more accessible for lesions extending below the planum level.[20,62,74,75]

Tuberculum Sellae Meningiomas

- *Type A meningiomas (tubercular origin)*: This anatomical subgroup of meningioma requires a supradiaphragmatic dissection and exposure. Type A meningiomas are associated with an elongation of the tuberculum–sellar floor interval and planum–tuberculum interval.[12,13,76] This specific feature and the consecutive expansion of the sella turcica have been reported to facilitate the EEA for these tumors.[12,76]
- *Type B (combined diaphragmal and tubercular) and type C (exclusive diaphragmal origin)*: These anatomical subgroups require a combined infra- and supradiaphragmatic dissection an exposure for a radical surgical resection.[12]

Potential Advantages of the Endonasal Endoscopic Approach

Several reviews comparing the TCA and EEA for tuberculum sellae meningiomas did not demonstrate superiority of one of both surgical techniques in regard of mortality and extent of resection.

1. *Approach-related morbidity and mortality:* Mortality rates were recently reported to be similar in EEA compared to TCA.[72]
2. *Visual outcome:* One of the most frequently stated advantages of the endonasal route for suprasellar (planum sphenoidale and tuberculum sellae) meningioma is an improved visual outcome and lower rates of visual deterioration compared to modern craniotomy studies.[51,65,66,71,74]

In a retrospective comparison study by Song et al., 44 patients with tuberculum sellae meningiomas receiving EEA and 40 patients with tuberculum sellae meningiomas receiving TCA in two institutions between 2004 and 2015 were analyzed.[66] Visual improvement (partial or full recovery) was found in 98% of patients. About 24% transcranially treated patients did experience visual deterioration after surgery. EEA and younger age (< 55 years) were found to be independent predictors for a favorable visual outcome.[66]

A study performed by Kong et al. retrospectively reviewed 84 patients with a tuberculum sellae meningioma treated by EEA against 94 patients treated by TCA. One hundred and forty out of 157 patients with preoperative visual disturbance had improved or stable vision postoperatively, while 17 (9.6%) patients experienced postoperative visual deterioration. Preoperative optic canal involvement was an independent predictor for worse visual outcome in patients treated via a TCA when compared to the EEA group.[20] The topoanatomical height of the tumors, for example, high-lying or low-lying tumors, did not influence the visual outcome.[20]

A possible explanation for these findings is a lower rate of manipulation of the optic chiasm and the optic nerves because tumor debulking is the first step in this procedure when compared to TCA.[51,65,66,71,74]

Potential Disadvantages of the Endonasal Endoscopic Approach

In general, a lower complication rate is associated with less extensive tumor removal.[16,38,71–73]

- Approach-related morbidity and mortality:
  - *Postoperative cerebrospinal fluid (CSF) leakage:* The anterior extension of the meningioma might need opening of the planum sphenoidale up to the most anterior aspect of the lesion. An extension passing over the cribriform plate results in a large bone opening and might carry a higher risk for postoperative CSF leakage.[31,65,74,77,78]
  - *Vascular injury:* Vascular injury was found to be higher using EEA compared to TCA.[65] The absence of vascular encasement and identification of a cortical cuff as predictor for vascular injury during endonasal endoscopic surgery for suprasellar meningiomas, however, has been challenged in the literature during the past years. Intended remnants can be left behind if dissection seems too dangerous to cause vascular injury.[74,79] An adequate internal decompression of the tumor before starting the extracapsular dissection is recommended.[20,62,74,75]

- ➢ *Brain edema:* Concomitant brain edema caused by the meningioma itself was another factor reported to complicate EEA in meningioma,[65] and the correct selection of the approach to minimize brain retraction is even more important when taking surrounding tumor edema into account.
- ➢ *Mortality:* Recently, Muskens et al.[65] have reported similar mortality rates for EEA and TCA.

- *Extent of resection and relapse-free survival:* Compared to TCA, gross total resection (GTR) rates and relapse-free survival seem to be similar. The strength of each route is represented in the location of tumor recurrences, being mainly in the sella turcica when resected through a TCA, and lateral or superior of the clinoid process when resected via an EEA.[66] In the context of tuberculum sellae meningioma, a recent meta-analysis could not demonstrate superiority for GTR using TCA compared to EEA.[65] A meticulous case selection is mandatory, as the literature reveals multiple reasons for unsuccessful endonasal endoscopic removal of tuberculum sellae meningioma:
  - ➢ *High- versus low-lying tumors:* Whether the tumor was higher than 5 mm over the frontobasal line (pneumosinus sphenoidalis dilatans) or lower than 5 mm below the tuberculum sellae did not influence the extent of resection rates (GTR rates) neither in patients undergoing EEA nor in patients undergoing TCA for tuberculum sellae meningiomas.[20]
  - ➢ *Lateral extension:* Lateral extension of the meningioma itself or the dural tail and its ratio to the interfovea ethmoidalis distance might require extended removal of the bone overlying the medial opticocarotid recess or the medial orbital wall.[67,74] Lateral extension to the anterior clinoid or lateral to the ICA bifurcation might result in incomplete resection.[67,74]
  - ➢ *Internal carotid artery involvement:* Cavernous ICA involvement has been reported to be a risk factor for incomplete resection.[67]
  - ➢ *Optic canal involvement:* Precise identification of optic canal involvement is relevant when a GTR using an EEA is considered.[80] Invasion of the optic canal has been shown to require resection through a TCA to reach the lateral and in most of the cases even the medial portion of the canal.[74]

A retrospective review by Pamir et al. correlated the presence of asymmetric visual findings in the preoperative ophthalmological examinations with the intraoperative presence of optic canal invasion and recommended the intraoperative transcranial optic canal unroofing and exploration.[81]

A retrospective study performed by Kong et al. reviewed 84 patients with tuberculum sellae meningiomas treated by EEA against 94 patients treated by TCA. GTR was achieved in 145 patients (81.5%) and did not differ significantly between both groups, again demonstrating the nonsuperiority for GTR using the EEA when compared to TCA.[20]

Preoperative Considerations

Every patient should get an endocrine diagnostic work-up, since most patients have at least partial hypopituitarism. Hormone deficiencies should be replaced (Chapter 1.1, medical therapy of hypopituitarism). A detailed neuro-ophthalmologic examination including visual acuity and visual field testing is also necessary.

The treatment and management of patients with sellar and parasellar meningiomas is interdisciplinary. In larger institutions, the preoperative work-up of these patients involves endocrinologists, ophthalmologists, neurosurgeons, ENT surgeons, and neuroradiologists. Usually, patients are evaluated by multidisciplinary consensus at regularly held tumor boards.

Endocrinological Assessment

Hypothalamic–pituitary hormonal function: Serum prolactin, total or free T4, thyroid-stimulating hormone (TSH), luteinizing hormone (LH) and follicle-stimulating hormone (FSH), free testosterone, estrogen and progesterone, morning 24-hour urinary-free cortisol, insulin-like growth factor.

Ophthalmological Assessment

Visual acuity and visual field using Goldman's perimetry as well as optometry in cases of double vision.

Neurological Assessment

Focal neurological deficits, neuropsychological changes in large lesion with extrasellar extension with frontal or temporal lobe involvement.

Rhinological Assessment

Endoscopic examination of the nose to rule out signs of infection, synechiae, or congenital anomalies.

Radiological Investigations

High-resolution MRI brain with image-guided surgery (IGS) protocol, high-resolution CT (HRCT) scan of the paranasal sinuses if indicated.

Preoperative Radiological Considerations

The surgeon should systematically assess available imaging. This is of special importance when selecting surgical modalities and variations of the available approaches and tailoring the surgical corridor to reach the region of interest:

- *Nasal anatomy:* Signs of upper airway infection, septal deviations, signs of trauma.
- *Sphenoid anatomy:* Three-dimensional orientation (shelf, divider, wall) and insertion site (cavernous or paraclinoid ICA, opticocarotid recess, or optic nerves) of the sphenoid septations, mucosa, pneumatization pattern (sellar, presellar, or postsellar type) and bone thickness.
- *High-lying tumor:* When a pneumosinus sphenoidalis dilatans of more than 5 mm is present, the tumor lies high in relation to the frontobasal line.[20]
- *Low-lying tumor:* Tumor extension into the pituitary fossa more than 5 mm below the tuberculum sellae.[20]
- *Cavernous carotid artery:* Space between the carotid eminences (intercarotid distance), probable dehiscence, bulging into the sphenoid cavity.
- *Lesion:* Purely intrasellar or suprasellar and parasellar involvement. The sellar dimensions, elongation of the tuberculum sellae, and the relative position of the planum sphenoidale. Lateral extension to the carotid arteries or beyond the clinoid portion of the carotid artery. Cortical cuff sign (CSF clefts around the tumor). T2 hyperintensity: most likely soft tumor and therefore amenable for endoscopic resection.
- Neurovascular structures
  - ➢ *Relationship to the cerebral intracranial vessels:* Anterior circulation vessels including the anterior "H-complex" might be displaced or encased with these tumors (**Fig. 11.4, Fig. 11.5** and **Fig. 11.6**). Relevant intracranial vessels to be considered are the ICA bifurcations, the proximal precommunicating segment of the cerebral artery (A1), the anterior communicating artery (AComA) and the postcommunicating segment of the anterior cerebral arteries (A2), as well as the recurrent arteries of Heubner (bilateral) **Fig. 11.4, Fig. 11.5** and **Fig. 11.6**). Posterior extension usually displaces the basilar artery and its branches and the posterior cerebral artery (PCA) as well as midbrain and brainstem perforators without encasement because of protective arachnoid layers of the Liliequist membrane (**Fig. 11.4**).
  - ➢ *Relationship to the brainstem:* Relevant brainstem compression should be acknowledged (medial, from lateral to one side) (**Fig. 11.6**).
  - ➢ *Relationship to the optic chiasm, optic nerves, and pituitary stalk:* The position of the optic nerves (dislocation) and the optic chiasm (prefixed, normal, postfixed) with corresponding perforators are relevant, as well as the relationship of the tumor with the pituitary stalk (**Fig. 11.2, Fig. 11.3**).[82] Further, optic foramen and canal infiltration should be assessed on the preoperative MRI, as these findings significantly limit the success using an EEA. However, these features can be difficult to assess in larger tumors.
  - ➢ *Relationship to the parasellar region:* Orbital apex or conus involvement, cavernous sinus invasion or extension into the sphenoid cavity, and posterior ethmoidal cells are relevant.
- *Recurrent case:* Radiation therapy usually is a good option to treat residual or small recurrent meningioma. If surgery is necessary, presence or absence of endonasal structures, scars, and adhesions have to be considered. Mucosal flaps over surgical site or fat graft from the previous surgery have to be identified. Abdominal fat graft might have created cystic cavities and scarring intradurally. Branches of the anterior cerebral artery might have migrated near the planum sphenoidale, tuberculum sellae, or sella turcica because of scarring (assessable on sagittal T1 contrast enhanced MRI sections).

Selection of the Surgical Approach

When addressing anterior skull base meningiomas using an EEA, an adequate removal of the bone covering the skull base beneath the entire tumor is mandatory, as compared to pituitary adenoma surgery. The nasal approach and the zonal dissection of the skull base needs to follow the extent of the lesion (tailored approach). There are special considerations for the intradural resection and the closure of the dural skull base defect when treating these lesions endoscopically.

When to prefer a transcranial approach for meningiomas of the planum sphenoidale and tuberculum sellae

- *Relevant frontobasal extension:* Subfrontal interhemispheric, frontal, or frontotemporal (pterional) subfrontal or transsylvian approach.
- *Relevant suprasellar extension:* Orbitozygomatic extension of the frontotemporal approach, frontal parasagittal interhemispheric approaches.
- *Relevant infratentorial extension:* Retrosigmoid, presigmoid, or posterior or anterior transpetrosal approaches (described for petroclival and petrous apex meningioma), staged operation concept or combined supra- and infratentorial approaches with tentorial division (Chapter 10.3.2 presigmoid retrolabyrinthine approach and 10.3.3 retrosigmoid craniotomy).

- *Relevant lateral extension, medial sphenoid wing, and anterior clinoid process:* Frontotemporal (pterional) subfrontal or transsylvian approach, especially when beyond the paraclinoidal portion of the internal carotid or involvement of the sphenoid wing, anterior clinoid process, and lateral wall of the cavernous sinus.
- *T2-hypointense or calcifications:* Suggestive for a most likely hard or fibrous meningioma, not amenable for endoscopic resection.
- *Encasement of neurovascular structures:* High probability of postoperative complications. However, this has been challenged in the literature.

Presurgical Phase

Anesthesia, patient positioning, equipment, and ergonomical aspects for the endonasal endoscopic techniques have been described previously (Chapter 1).

Nasal Phase (Tailored Approach)

Endoscopic endonasal double nostril transseptal transsphenoidal approach: After decongestion of the nose with pure adrenaline 1:1,000 units and mucosal infiltration with local anesthetics and adrenaline 1:10,000 units, bilateral pedicled nasoseptal flaps (NSFs) are usually harvested in case of a tuberculum sellae or a planum sphenoidale meningioma. After posterior resection of the nasal septum and bilateral identification of the sphenoid ostia, the rostrum of the sphenoid is removed and the sphenoid sinus is exposed.[45]

Osteodural Phase (Zonal Dissection)

The osteodural exposure can be tailored according to the anatomical configuration of the lesion. With the aid of image-guided surgery, a zonal dissection of the skull base to sufficiently expose the lesion is possible.

Extended endoscopic endonasal transseptal transsphenoidal approach: Transtuberculum and transplanum approaches are necessary to treat these lesions using an EEA. The remaining bone might act as an abutment that potentially prevents the surgeon from adequately debulking and dissecting the capsule away from critical neurovascular structures (**Fig. 11.9**).[45,48]

1. Use bone wax and drill it into the bone when venous bleeding occurs in the bone.
2. Sufficient exposure below the meningioma is mandatory to "release" the tumor and facilitate extracapsular dissection.
3. Sufficient exposure anterior to the tumor is necessary to define the anterior extracapsular dissection plane (image-guided surgery).
4. Remove the medial orbital walls as well as the lateral aspects of the tuberculum sellae to gain a better osteodural exposure.
5. Remove the bone covering the sella turcica to be able to identify the posterior brain-tumor interface and push the pituitary gland backward.

Intradural Phase (Tumor Resection)

An adequate internal decompression of the tumor before starting the extracapsular dissection is recommended.[20,62,74,75] The latter is achieved with the use of sharp microsurgical instruments to successfully dissect surrounding blood vessels from the tumor capsule. If the dissection poses a high risk for vascular injury, intended remnants can be left behind.[74,79]

Neurosurgical Considerations for Intradural Resection of Meningiomas:

1. *Step 1:* Wide dural opening from the planum sphenoidale toward the anterior intercavernous sinus. This allows the tumor to fall down (**Fig. 11.10** and **Fig. 11.11**).
2. *Step 2:* Debulking of the tumor (ultrasonic aspirator) especially in the anterior aspects to facilitate the extracapsular dissection (**Fig. 11.10** and **Fig. 11.11**).

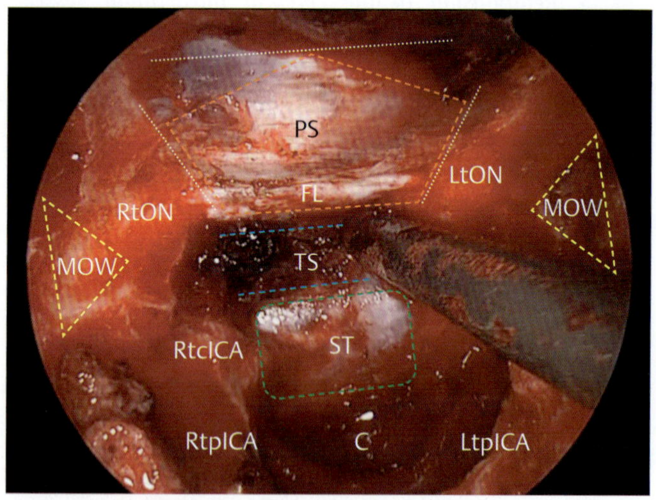

Fig. 11.9 Completed zonal dissection including a transplanum (*orange pentagon*), transtuberculum (*blue square*), and transsellar (*green square*) osteodural exposure for the resection of a tuberculum sellae meningioma. The medial orbital walls (MOW) have been removed to faciliate the lateral exposure (*yellow triangles*). Image-guided surgery is helpful to define the anterior and lateral extension of the removed bone of the base of skull (*white lines*).

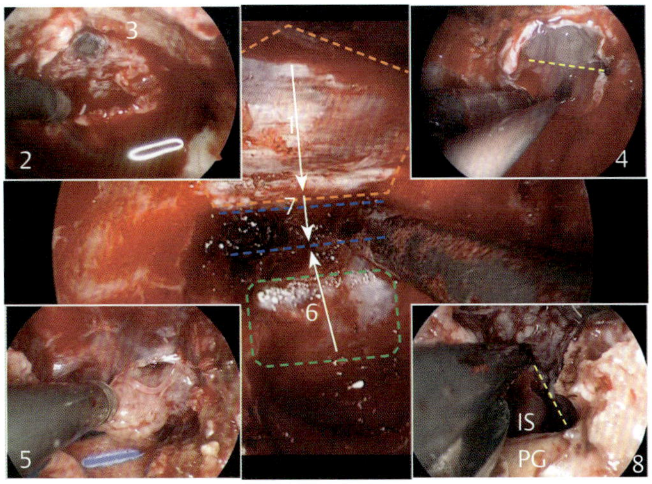

Fig. 11.10 Systematic approach for the resection of a tuberculum sellae meningioma after extended transplanum, transtuberculum, and transsellar osteodural exposure. Wide dural opening from the planum sphenoidale (*orange pentagon*) toward the tuberculum sellae (*blue square*) and the anterior intercavernous sinus (*step 1*). Tumor debulking in the anterior aspects is performed to facilitate the extracapsular dissection (*step 2*). Anterior extension of the dural opening to the brain–tumor interface (*step 3*). Bilateral extracapsular dissection along the brain–tumor interface (*yellow line*) using the arachnoid layer (*step 4*). Intratumoral debulking laterally and posteriorly (*step 5*). Dural opening from the sella turcica toward the tuberculum sellae with cauterization and dissection of the intercavernous sinus (*step 6*). Extension of the dural opening toward the sella turcica (*green square*) in a posterior direction (*step 7*). Definition of a dissection plane (*yellow line*) between the pituitary gland (PG), the infundibular stalk (IS), and the posterior tumor aspects (*step 8*). Final tumor removal is then performed in an anterior to posterior direction.

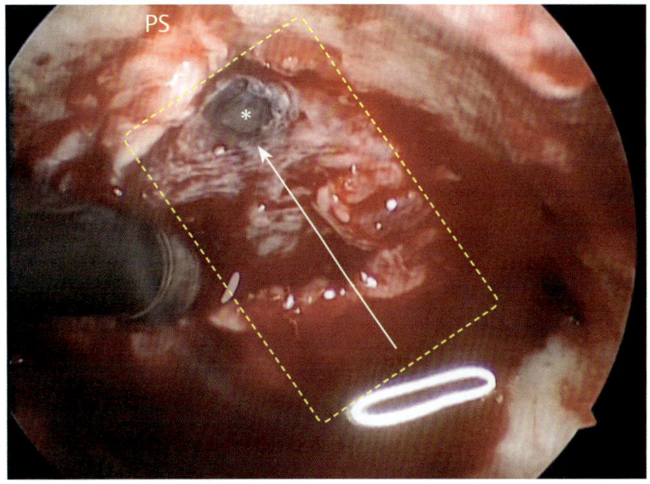

Fig. 11.11 Anterior extension of the dural opening (*white arrow*) to the brain–tumor interface (*) for the resection of a tuberculum sellae meningioma. Internal debulking of the tumor especially in the anterior aspects (*yellow square*) facilitates the extracapsular dissection. A sufficient osteodural exposure without bony abutments allows the lesion to fall down.

3. *Step 3:* Extension of the dural opening to the brain–tumor interface anteriorly (**Fig. 11.9** and **Fig. 11.10**).
4. *Step 4:* The extracapsular dissection is started sideways bilaterally. The arachnoid layer leads the surgeon to the relevant neurovascular structures. Cauterization of the arachnoid or the tumor capsule is not recommended to prevent the loss of the dissection plane. When performing the extracapsular dissection, the tumor surface is pushed away from the arachnoid membranes protecting the relevant neurovascular structures (**Fig. 11.10, Fig. 11.12**).
5. *Step 5:* Intratumoral debulking is continued laterally and posteriorly. The tumor capsule and arachnoid layer will fall into the center of the resection cavity (**Fig. 11.10, Fig. 11.13** and **Fig. 11.14**).
6. *Step 6:* Dural opening from the sella turcica toward the tuberculum sellae, cauterization and dissection of the intercavernous sinus (**Fig. 11.10**).
7. *Step 7:* Extension of the dural opening posteriorly over the sella brings the pituitary gland and infundibular stalk into view (**Fig. 11.10** and **Fig. 11.15**).
8. *Step 8:* A dissection plane between the pituitary gland and the posterior tumor aspects has to be identified. The dissection is then completed from an anterior to posterior direction bilaterally (**Fig. 11.10** and **Fig. 11.15**).

The vessels of the anterior H-complex including the pre- and postcommunicating segments of the anterior cerebral artery, the anterior communicating artery, and the recurrent arteries of Heubner usually are protected by arachnoidal layers from the interhemispheric fissure. Careful extracapsular dissection after adequate tumor debulking, gentle microsurgical and sharp dissection is mandatory to identify and preserve these vessels (**Fig. 11.16**).

Intraoperative Magnetic Resonance Imaging

The literature on intraoperative (iMRI) use in nonadenomatous sellar lesions is scant.[45,83] Recently, two publications addressed the use of iMRI in the setting of tuberculum sellae meningioma and synchronous tumors of the sella.

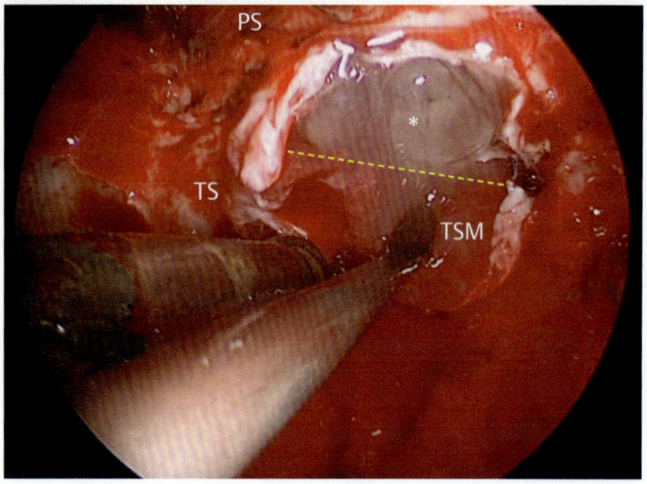

Fig. 11.12 Definition of the anterior brain–tumor interface (*yellow line*) using the arachnoid layer (*). Cauterization of the arachnoid layer or the tumor capsule is not recommended to maintain the dissection plane.

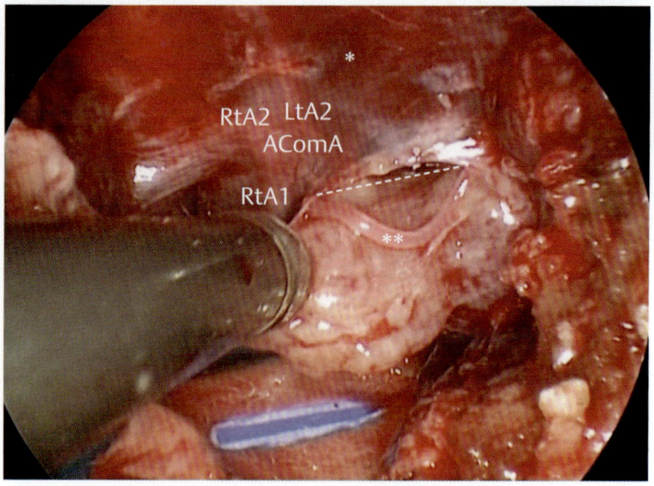

Fig. 11.13 Internal tumor debulking and piecemeal tumor removal in the case of a tuberculum sellae meningioma. The arachnoid layer (*) protects the relevant neurovascular structures. However, careful resection of tumor pieces with dissection of adhering arterial vessels (**) is necessary, when the lesion breaks through the arachnoid layer (*white line*). When performing the extracapsular dissection, the tumor surface is pushed away from the arachnoid membranes protecting the relevant neurovascular structures.

The retrospective study by Giordano et al. reported further tumor resection after the first iMRI scan in 40% of cases, with a substantial additional volume reduction in cavernous sinus lesions. No complications were found related to the use of iMRI scan.[83] Roethlisberger et al. reported that iMRI was useful in confirming complete resection of a meningioma in the setting of a synchronous tumor, while intended remnants of a pituitary adenoma were confirmed intraoperatively. The authors state that detection of residual tumor might be challenging in the postoperative period.[84–86] They conclude that there might be a potential advantage in using iMRI for the detection of residual disease in the context of large synchronous tumors, especially when a complex skull base defect reconstruction is necessary.[45]

Skull Base Defect Closure

The large dural defects caused by the transtuberculum, transplanum, and transcribriform approaches for the resection of anterior cranial fossa meningioma are usually closed using intradural and extradural autologous fat grafts and an artificial dural sealant system. This construct is sealed with an artificial dural sealant covered by vascularized nasoseptal flaps.[87–89] Contact to the surrounding bony edges is necessary for an adequate watertight closure and healing of the skull

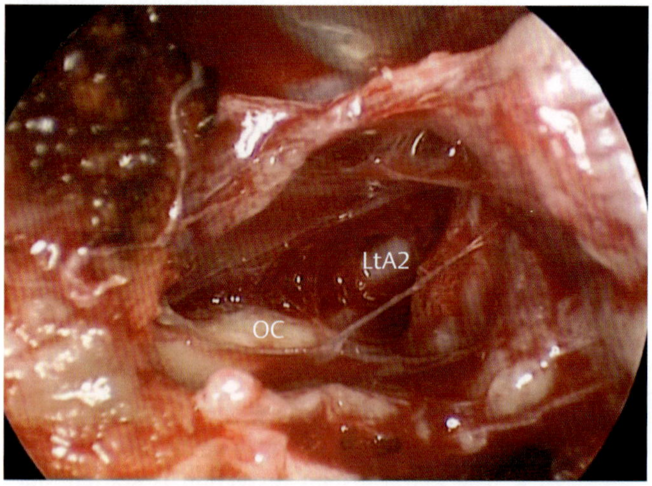

Fig. 11.14 When resecting the tubercular portion of tuberculum sellae meningiomas, the arachnoid layer (*) leads the surgeon to the relevant neurovascular structures.

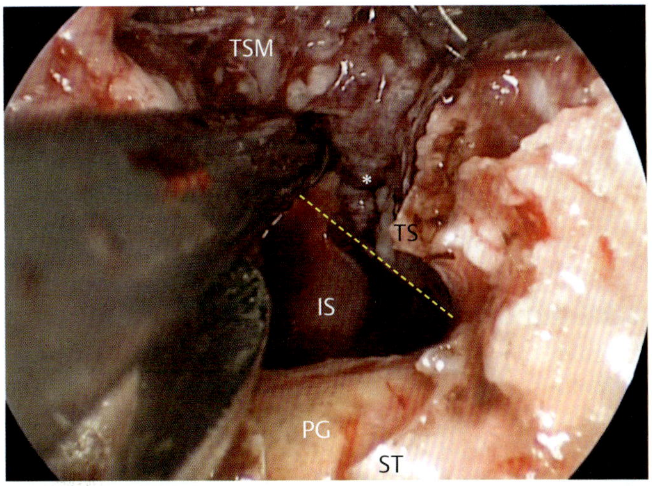

Fig. 11.15 Definition of the posterior dissection plane (*yellow line*) between the pituitary gland (PG), the infundibular stalk (IS), and the posterior tumor pole (*) in the case of a tuberculum sellae meningioma (TSM).

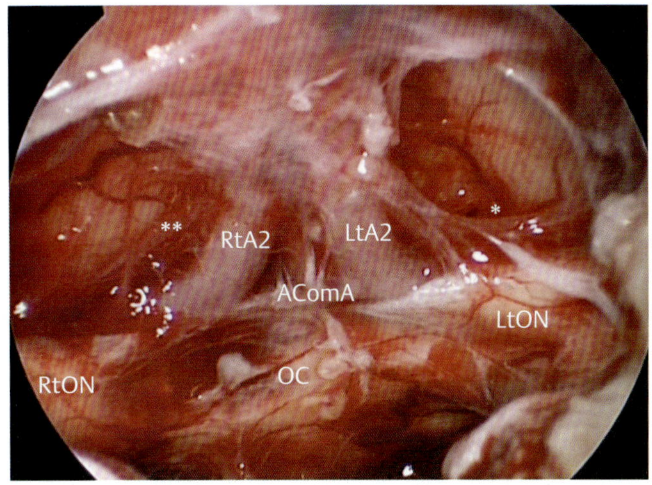

Fig. 11.16 Exposure of the chiasmatic cistern demonstrating the close relationship of a tuberculum sellae meningioma with the critical neurovascular structures. Frontopolar branches (*) and recurrent perforating branches (**) arising from the right postcommunicating segment of the anterior cerebral arteries.

base defect. Several techniques of graded defect closure and postoperative care have been described in Chapter 1.1, Skull base defect closure.

Postoperative Care

The nasal packs are usually removed within 24 to 48 hours. They may remain in situ for longer time (72–120 hours) if a CSF leak repair has been performed. The patient is advised to avoid straining (no sneezing, coughing, straining during defecation) if a concomitant intraoperative CSF leak repair was necessary. Endoscopic inspection and suction clearance are usually performed during the first week after the operation.

Nonsurgical Treatment of Perisellar Meningiomas

Despite all advances in the surgical therapy of meningiomas in the perisellar region, there is a subset of patients who cannot be treated satisfactorily by surgical means (**Fig. 11.17, Fig. 11.18, Fig. 11.19, Fig. 11.20, Fig. 11.21, Fig. 11.22, Fig. 11.23, Fig. 11.24, Fig. 11.25** and **Fig. 11.26**).

- One group in this subset are patients who have had multiple surgeries for recurrence. With every recurrence, the surgical option becomes more hazardous concerning injury of nerovascular structures and surgical morbidity, and carries less chance of success concerning the achievable extent of resection.
- Other tumors might be small, but they primarily infiltrate functionally critical structures resulting in an unfavorable surgical risk-to-benefit ratio.
- Patients, who are, because of severe medical comorbidity, high-risk candidates for surgery or who simply refuse surgical treatment, represent a third group.

For these complex cases without promising surgical options, the goal of treatment needs to be redefined. Shrinkage of the tumor volume or inhibition of further growth then becomes the main intention of treatment.

Oncological Treatment Modalities

In neuro-oncology, the additional standard options to surgery are oncological treatment and radiation therapy. Concerning oncological meningioma treatment, there are, disregarding salvage strategies such as bevacizumab or sunitinib, no promising standard options.[90,91]

Radiation Therapy Modalities

Radiation oncology offers opportunities for the postoperative treatment of atypical meningiomas, but the optimal moment for initiation of treatment is still subject of ongoing studies (e.g., EORTC 1308).[92] The irradiation of WHO grade I meningiomas might become reasonable in the situations previously mentioned in the first paragraph. From a technical point of view, "standard" radio-oncological treatment needs to be

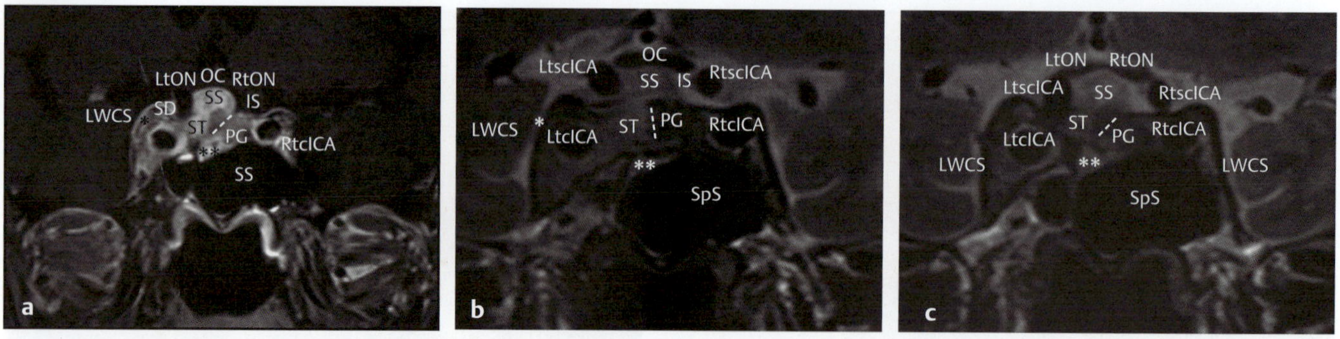

Fig. 11.17 Multimodal treatment of an intra-, para-, and suprasellar meningioma. A 68-year-old patient presented with sudden-onset diplopia and a third nerve palsy of the right side with ptosis and pupillary dysfunction. Endocrinological work-up revealed a slightly elevated prolactin, interpreted as "stalk effect" because of the deviation of the infundibular stalk (IS) to the left side. **(a)** T1-weighted gadolinium contrast-enhanced coronal MRI section. **(b, c)** T2-weighted coronal MRI sections demonstrating a meningioma extending into the sella turcica (ST), left cavernous sinus (LtCS), suprasellar region (SS), supradiaphragmal region (SD), along (*) the lateral wall of the cavernous sinus (LWCS) and en plaque along the roof (**) of the sphenoid sinus (SpS). The pituitary gland (PG) can be distinguished from the intrasellar portion of the meningioma (*white line*).

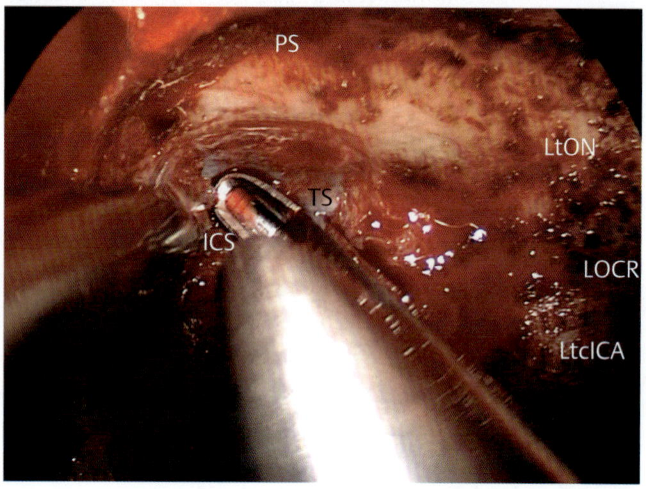

Fig. 11.18 Multimodal treatment of intra-, para-, and suprasellar meningioma. An endonasal endoscopic binostril transseptal transsphenoidal surgery is used to biopsy the lesion and confirm the diagnosis of a meningioma. A transsellar and transtuberculum sellae (TS) osteodural exposure is necessary to expose the suprasellar and supradiaphragmal aspects of the lesion.

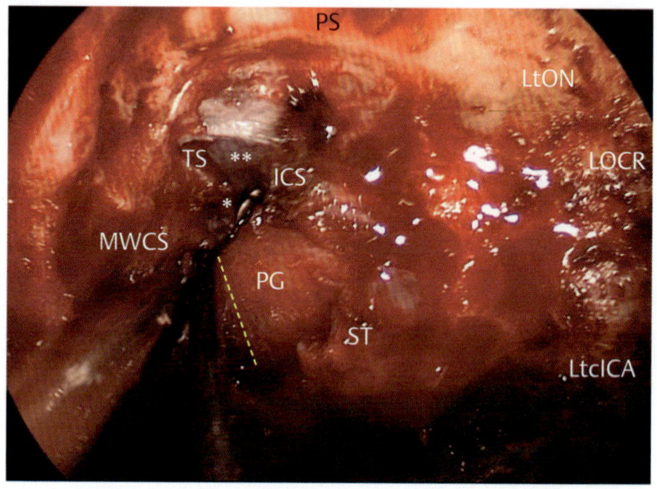

Fig. 11.19 After cauterization and transsection of the intercavernous sinus (ICS), the sellar and tubercular dura can be opened and the intrasellar (*) as well as the suprasellar (**) portion of the meningioma can be distinguished from the physiological structures of the pituitary fossa (*yellow line*). The continuation of the meningioma through the medial wall of the cavernous sinus (MWCS) is visible.

differentiated from radiosurgical treatment. Depending on WHO grade, size, and location of the meningioma, different fractionated or hypofractionated treatment protocols are available as "standard" treatment.[93] Radiosurgery using either a cobalt radiation source or a linear accelerator represents a valuable option especially in cases of small and localized perisellar meningiomas. A size larger than 2 cm in diameter (other authors: 3 cm), an irregular shape, or en plaque growth pattern of the meningioma might reduce the otherwise high success rates of radiosurgery with a usually acceptable risk profile (**Fig. 11.27a–c**).[94,95] A relevant feature of all radiotherapeutic options is the fact that there is only a limited possibility to repeat treatment in case of treatment failure or tumor recurrence.

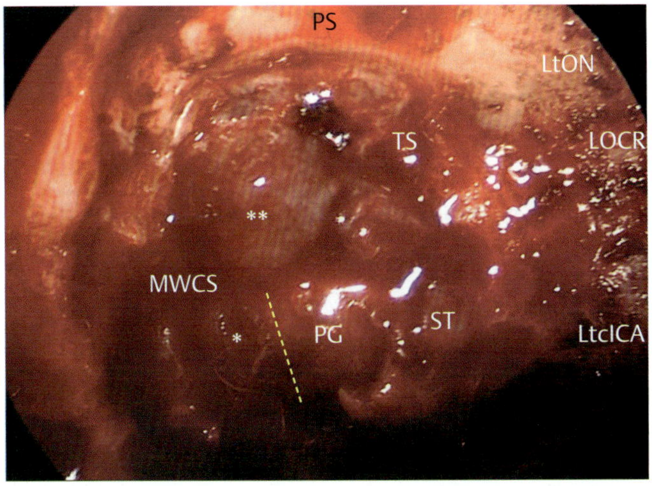

Fig. 11.20 While the intrasellar (*) portion of the meningioma is firmer in consistency, the suprasellar (**) portion of the meningioma evacuates after dissection with a curette and sufficient exposure given by the transtubercular approach. The pituitary gland (PG) can be distinguished from the intrasellar portion of the meningioma (*yellow line*). The continuation of the meningioma through the medial wall of the cavernous sinus (MWCS) is visible.

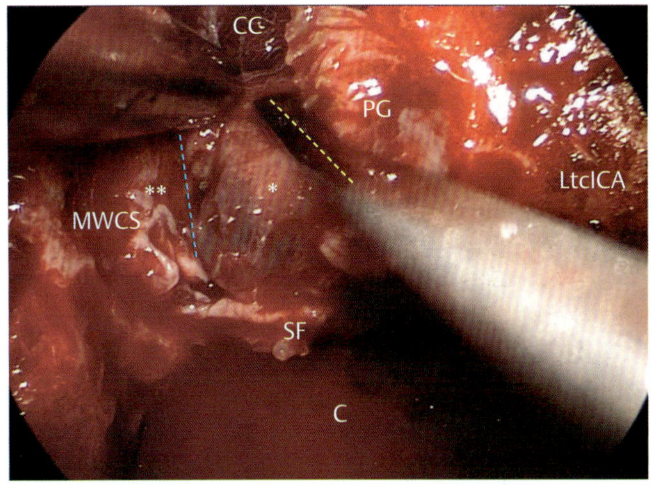

Fig. 11.21 After removal of the suprasellar portion of the meningioma, the arachnoid membranes of the chiasmatic cistern (CC) are visible. A dissection plane (*yellow line*) between the intrasellar portion of the meningioma (*) and the pituitary gland (PG) and a plane (*blue line*) toward the intracavernous portion of the meningioma (**) is defined.

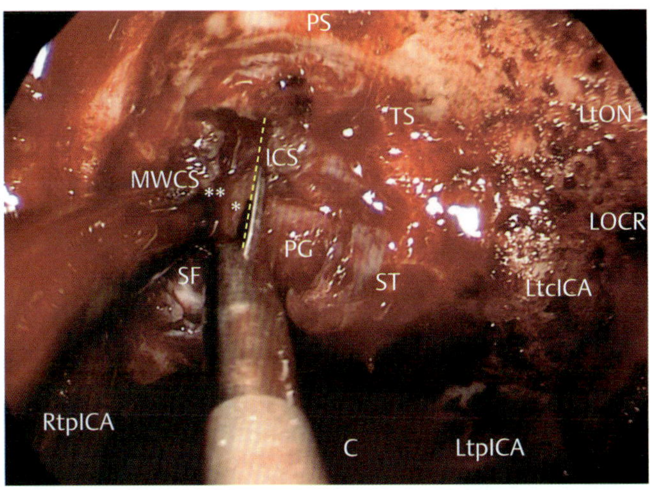

Fig. 11.22 Sharp dissection with a scissors (*yellow line*) between the intrasellar portion of the meningioma (*) and the pituitary gland (PG). The continuation of the meningioma through the medial wall of the cavernous sinus (MWCS) is visible (**).

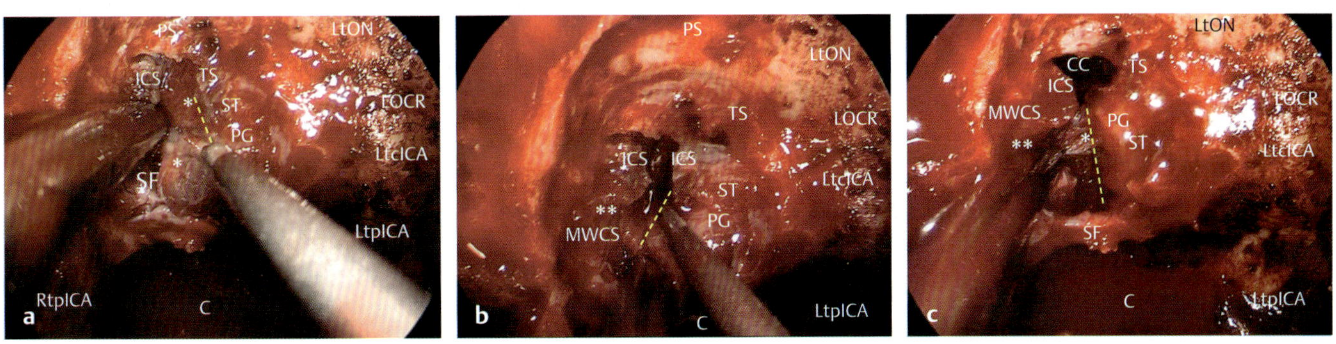

Fig. 11.23 **(a–c)** Removal of the intrasellar portion of the meningioma (*) after sharp dissection (*yellow line*) from the pituitary gland (PG). The continuation of the meningioma through the medial wall of the cavernous sinus (MWCS) is visible (**).

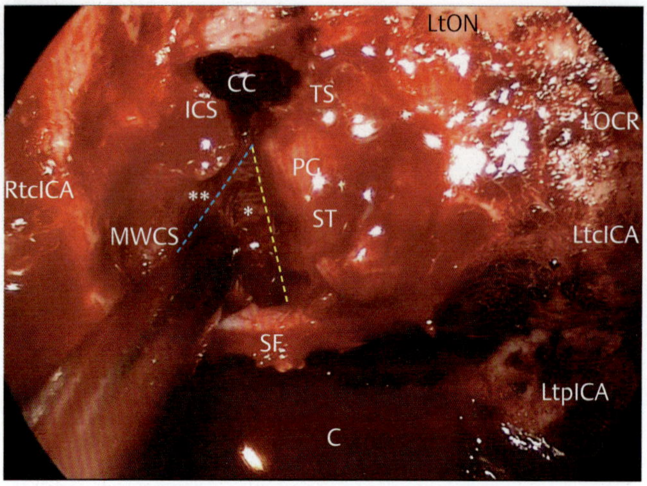

Fig. 11.24 Subtotal resection of the meningioma with artificial borders (*yellow line*) between the intrasellar portion of the meningioma (*) and the pituitary gland (PG) and a plane (*blue line*) toward the intracavernous portion of the meningioma (**).

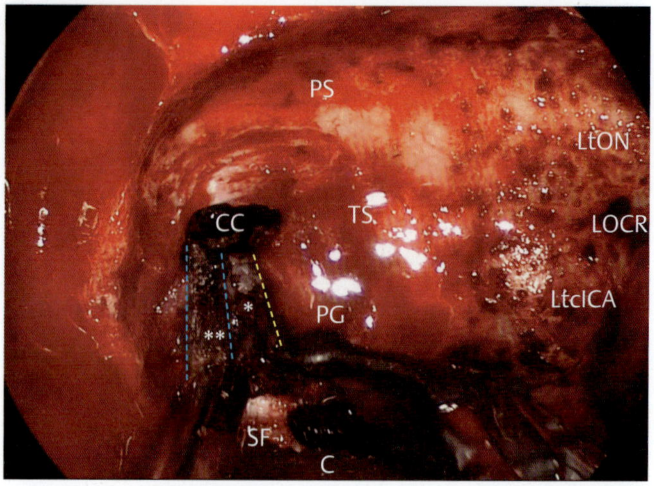

Fig. 11.25 Subtotal resection of the meningioma with artificial borders (*yellow line*) between the intrasellar portion of the meningioma (*) and the pituitary gland (PG) and a plane (*blue lines*) toward the intracavernous portion of the meningioma (**). The medial surface of the intracavernous portion of the meningioma (*blue lines*) is cauterized with an endoscopic diathermy to shrink the volume toward the sella turcica.

Treatment Modalities in Nuclear Medicine

A mentionable treatment alternative in case of surgical and radio-oncological treatment failure is the therapy with radiolabeled somatostatin analogues. About 70 to 100% of all meningiomas overexpress somatostatin receptors (SSTR), which can be targeted by the systemically applied and radionuclide-labeled SSTR agonist Y-90-DOTATOC. Before initiation of DOTATOC treatment, the expression of SSTR needs to be confirmed. DOTATOC treatment represents an option especially in complex configurations or recurrent meningiomas with proximity to critical vascular or neural structures or meningiomas with a diffuse growth pattern (**Fig. 11.28**). Main limitations of this modality are impaired renal function or sparse SSTR expression on the meningioma cells.[96]

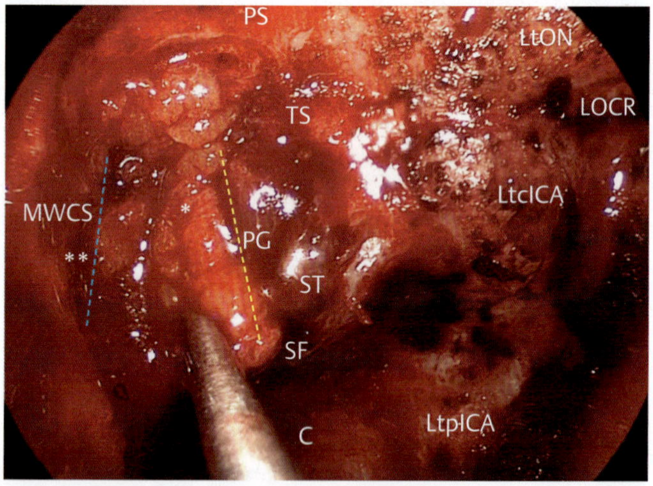

Fig. 11.26 The resection cavity between (*yellow line*) the intrasellar portion of the meningioma (*) and the pituitary gland (PG) and toward (*blue line*) the intracavernous portion of the meningioma (**) is filled with an abdominal fat graft (*). The graft acts as a protection for the pituitary gland when the cavernous portion of the meningioma is radiated postoperatively.

Tips and Pearls

- Make sure to preserve sufficient amounts of DNA for molecular risk stratification of meningiomas. This is best performed from native (intraoperative) cryosections, which are verified for high tumor cell content by microscopy and then used to extract DNA.
- No prospective randomized trial comparing transcranial versus endonasal endoscopic surgery for

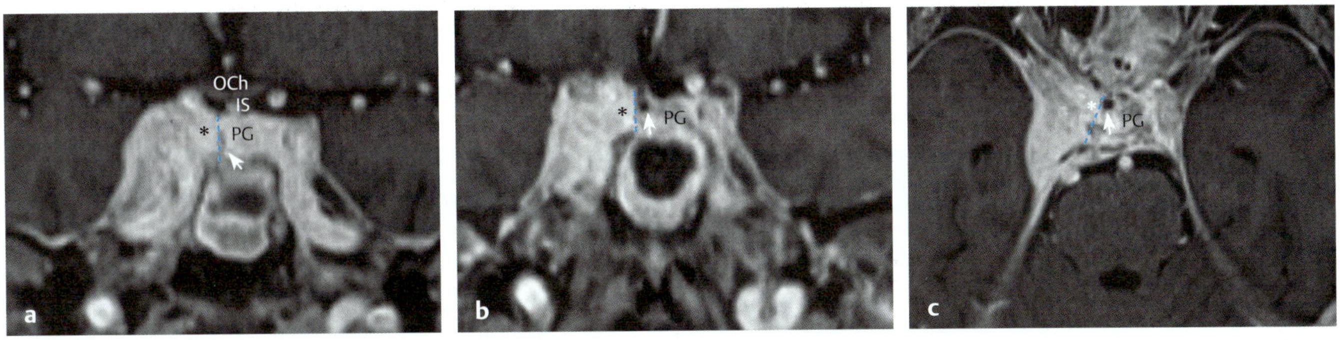

Fig. 11.27 **(a, b)** Multimodal treatment of intra-, para-, and suprasellar meningioma. After endonasal endoscopic resection of the intra- and suprasellar portion of the meningioma, the patient was treated with high-dose steroids for a couple of weeks to treat the oculomotor and abducens palsy. A couple of weeks after the surgery, the main intracavernous portion was treated with stereotactic dynamic intensity-modulated radiotherapy (IMRT) (volumetric modulated arc therapy [VMAT] stereotaxy) fractioned radiotherapy. **(c)** Three months postoperative T1-weighted gadolinium contrast-enhanced coronal, T1-weighted gadolinium contrast-enhanced axial MRI section demonstrating removal of the intrasellar and suprasellar portion of the meningioma with the abdominal fat graft (*white arrow*) between (*blue line*) the pituitary gland (PG) and the intracavernous portion of the meningioma (*). The optic chiasm (OCh) and the infundibular stalk have a physiological configuration. The patient's condition improved after the surgery with resolving oculomotor and abducens palsy and a nonremarkable visual field. High-dose steroids were consecutively reduced and finished under endocrinological surveillance for adrenal function.

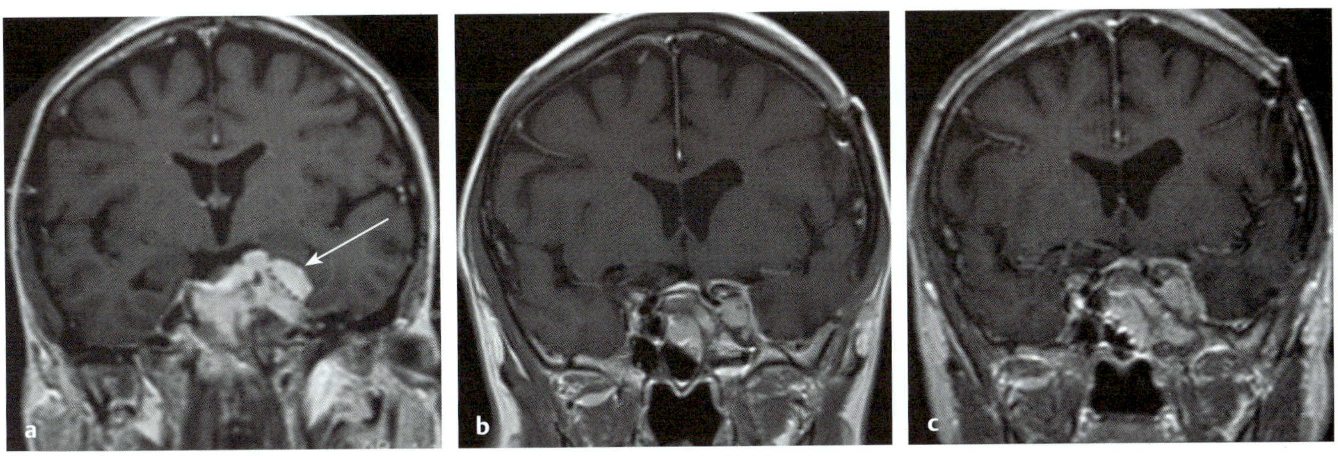

Fig. 11.28 Multimodal treatment of a WHO grade I cavernous/extracavernous meningioma. Following surgical decompression of the left optic nerve and chiasm, two therapeutic cycles of Y-90-DOTATOC were applied. **(a)** Coronal contrast-enhanced T1-weighted MRI section at initiation of a Y-90-DOTATOC therapy. **(b)** Coronal contrast-enhanced T1-weighted MRI section at 60 months after the Y-90-DOTATOC therapy. **(c)** Coronal contrast-enhanced T1-weighted MRI section 87 months after Y-90-DOTATOC treatment. Tumor localization (*white arrow*). (Reproduced with permission of Gerster-Gilliéron et al. 2015.[96])

suprasellar meningioma is available. Level of evidence 3 (observational studies) and 4 (expert opinions), and systematic reviews and meta-analysis based on these studies (not qualifying as Level 2 or more) are available with following recommendations:

- Endoscopic approaches can obtain an extent of resection equal to transcranial techniques, being potentially higher for giant midline located tumors.
- Endoscopic approaches are safer and more effective in alleviating symptoms from neurovascular compression including the visual outcome.
- Endoscopic approaches can be recommended over transcranial approaches in selected tuberculum sellae meningiomas (small soft midline lesions, without major vessel encasement, or parasellar extension) with respect to visual improvement with an acceptable complication rate.

  - ➢ Transcranial approaches still provide an effective and safe treatment strategy for tuberculum sellae meningiomas.
  - ➢ Transcranial approaches are favored for tumors extending to the middle or anterior fossa.
- Radiation therapy has an important role to play in controlling residual disease or recurrences.

Acknowledgments

This chapter was written based on funding from the Martin Allgöwer Foundation, Department of Surgery, University Hospital of Basel (Basel, Switzerland) and the Gottfried and Julia Bangerter-Rhyner Foundation (Bern, Switzerland). The Department of Neurosurgery of the University Hospital of Basel (Basel, Switzerland) and the Departments of Neurosurgery and Otorhinolaryngology of the University of Malaya (Kuala Lumpur, Malaysia) supported the creation of this chapter.

References

1. Louis DPA, Reifenberger G. WHO Classification of Tumours of the Central Nervous System. Lyon: IARC; 2016
2. Capper D, Jones DTW, Sill M, et al. DNA methylation-based classification of central nervous system tumours. Nature 2018;555(7697):469–474
3. Sahm F, Schrimpf D, Stichel D, et al. DNA methylation-based classification and grading system for meningioma: a multicentre, retrospective analysis. Lancet Oncol 2017; 18(5):682–694
4. Paramasivam N, Hübschmann D, Toprak UH, et al. Mutational patterns and regulatory networks in epigenetic subgroups of meningioma. Acta Neuropathol 2019;138(2):295–308
5. Di Ieva A, Lee JM, Cusimano M. Handbook of Skull Base Surgery. New York, NY: Thieme Medical Publishers; 2016
6. DeMonte F. Surgical treatment of anterior basal meningiomas. J Neurooncol 1996;29(3):239–248
7. Chan RC, Thompson GB. Morbidity, mortality, and quality of life following surgery for intracranial meningiomas. A retrospective study in 257 cases. J Neurosurg 1984;60(1):52–60
8. Solero CL, Giombini S, Morello G. Suprasellar and olfactory meningiomas. Report on a series of 153 personal cases. Acta Neurochir (Wien) 1983;67(3-4):181–194
9. Rubin G, Ben David U, Gornish M, Rappaport ZH. Meningiomas of the anterior cranial fossa floor. Review of 67 cases. Acta Neurochir (Wien) 1994;129(1-2):26–30
10. Spektor S, Valarezo J, Fliss DM, et al. Olfactory groove meningiomas from neurosurgical and ear, nose, and throat perspectives: approaches, techniques, and outcomes. Neurosurgery 2005;57(4, Suppl):268–280, discussion 268–280
11. Jallo GI, Benjamin V. Tuberculum sellae meningiomas: microsurgical anatomy and surgical technique. Neurosurgery 2002;51(6):1432–1439, discussion 1439–1440
12. Ajlan AM, Choudhri O, Hwang P, Harsh G. Meningiomas of the tuberculum and diaphragma sellae. J Neurol Surg B Skull Base 2015;76(1):74–79
13. Al-Mefty O, Holoubi A, Rifai A, Fox JL. Microsurgical removal of suprasellar meningiomas. Neurosurgery 1985;16(3): 364–372
14. de Divitiis E, Esposito F, Cappabianca P, Cavallo LM, de Divitiis O, Esposito I. Endoscopic transnasal resection of anterior cranial fossa meningiomas. Neurosurg Focus 2008;25(6):E8
15. Nanda A, Ambekar S, Javalkar V, Sharma M. Technical nuances in the management of tuberculum sellae and diaphragma sellae meningiomas. Neurosurg Focus 2013;35(6):E7
16. Hayhurst C, Teo C. Tuberculum sella meningioma. Otolaryngol Clin North Am 2011;44(4):953–963, viii–ix
17. Kulwin C, Schwartz TH, Cohen-Gadol AA. Endoscopic extended transsphenoidal resection of tuberculum sellae meningiomas: nuances of neurosurgical technique. Neurosurg Focus 2013;35(6):E6
18. Raza SM, Effendi ST, DeMonte F. Tuberculum sellae meningiomas: evolving surgical strategies. 2014. Curr Surg Rep 2014;2:73
19. Kinjo T, al-Mefty O, Ciric I. Diaphragma sellae meningiomas. Neurosurgery 1995;36(6):1082–1092
20. Kong DS, Hong CK, Hong SD, et al. Selection of endoscopic or transcranial surgery for tuberculum sellae meningiomas according to specific anatomical features: a retrospective multicenter analysis (KOSEN-002). J Neurosurg 2018; 130(3):838–847
21. Giammattei L, Starnoni D, Levivier M, Messerer M, Daniel RT. Surgery for clinoidal meningiomas: case series and meta-analysis of outcomes and complications. World Neurosurg 2019;129:e700–e717
22. Al-Mefty O. Clinoidal meningiomas. J Neurosurg 1990; 73(6):840–849
23. al-Mefty O, Ayoubi S. Clinoidal meningiomas. Acta Neurochir Suppl (Wien) 1991;53:92–97
24. Salas S, Gamble A, Dehdashti AR. Surgical nuances for resection of a large anterior clinoidal meningioma. Oper Neurosurg (Hagerstown) 2017;13(5):640
25. Adappa ND, Lee JY, Chiu AG, Palmer JN. Olfactory groove meningioma. Otolaryngol Clin North Am 2011;44(4):965–980, ix
26. Chiang GS, Goh LG. Olfactory groove and planum sphenoidale meningioma: Dementia masquerade. Can Fam Physician 2017;63(4):288–291

27. Pepper JP, Hecht SL, Gebarski SS, Lin EM, Sullivan SE, Marentette LJ. Olfactory groove meningioma: discussion of clinical presentation and surgical outcomes following excision via the subcranial approach. Laryngoscope 2011;121(11):2282–2289
28. Ravikanth R, Pinto DS, Mathew S. Olfactory groove meningioma masquerading as psychiatric disturbances. Indian J Psychiatry 2018;60(3):367–369
29. Ayad T, Khoueir P, Saliba I, Moumdjian R. Cacosmia secondary to an olfactory groove meningioma. J Otolaryngol 2007;36(4):E51–E53
30. Zhang J, Sai K, Zhu ZQ, et al. Prognostic factors for olfactory groove meningioma with nasal cavity extension. Oncotarget 2017;9(4):4607–4613
31. Lu VM, Goyal A, Rovin RA. Olfactory groove and tuberculum sellae meningioma resection by endoscopic endonasal approach versus transcranial approach: a systematic review and meta-analysis of comparative studies. Clin Neurol Neurosurg 2018;174:13–20
32. Lutwak N, Dill C, Wieczorek R. Planum sphenoidale meningioma leading to visual disturbance. BMJ Case Rep 2011;2011
33. Galal A, Faisal A, Al-Werdany M, El Shehaby A, Lotfy T, Moharram H. Determinants of postoperative visual recovery in suprasellar meningiomas. Acta Neurochir (Wien) 2010;152(1):69–77
34. Kwancharoen R, Blitz AM, Tavares F, Caturegli P, Gallia GL, Salvatori R. Clinical features of sellar and suprasellar meningiomas. Pituitary 2014;17(4):342–348
35. Leu CH, Hu TL, Shen CC, Wang YC. Tuberculum sellae meningiomas: clinical manifestation, radiologic diagnosis, surgery and visual outcome. Zhonghua Yi Xue Za Zhi (Taipei) 1998;61(1):1–7
36. Lee JH, Sade B, Park BJ. A surgical technique for the removal of clinoidal meningiomas. Neurosurgery 2006;59(1, Suppl 1): ONS108–ONS114, discussion ONS108–ONS114
37. Goel A, Muzumdar D, Desai KI. Tuberculum sellae meningioma: a report on management on the basis of a surgical experience with 70 patients. Neurosurgery 2002;51(6): 1358–1363, discussion 1363–1364
38. Nakamura M, Roser F, Struck M, Vorkapic P, Samii M. Tuberculum sellae meningiomas: clinical outcome considering different surgical approaches. Neurosurgery 2006; 59(5):1019–1028, discussion 1028–1029
39. Mahmoud M, Nader R, Al-Mefty O. Optic canal involvement in tuberculum sellae meningiomas: influence on approach, recurrence, and visual recovery. Neurosurgery 2010;67(3, Suppl Operative):ons108–ons118, discussion ons118–ons119
40. Bilder RM, Wu H, Bogerts B, et al. Absence of regional hemispheric volume asymmetries in first-episode schizophrenia. Am J Psychiatry 1994;151(10):1437–1447
41. Rennert J, Doerfler A. Imaging of sellar and parasellar lesions. Clin Neurol Neurosurg 2007;109(2):111–124
42. Pisaneschi M, Kapoor G. Imaging the sella and parasellar region. Neuroimaging Clin N Am 2005;15(1):203–219
43. Snyder BJ, Naidich TP, Post KD. Cystic lesions of the sella. Totowa, NJ:Humana Press; 2008
44. Abele TA, Yetkin ZF, Raisanen JM, Mickey BE, Mendelsohn DB. Non-pituitary origin sellar tumours mimicking pituitary macroadenomas. Clin Radiol 2012;67(8):821–827
45. Roethlisberger M, Jayapalan RR, Hostettler IC, et al. Evolving strategies for resection of sellar/parasellar synchronous tumors via endoscopic endonasal approach—a technical case report and systematic review of the literature. World Neurosurg 2020 Jan;133:381-391.e2. doi: 10.1016/j.wneu.2019.08.102.
46. Landeiro JA, Gonçalves MB, Guimarães RD, et al. Tuberculum sellae meningiomas: surgical considerations. Arq Neuropsiquiatr 2010;68(3):424–429
47. Margalit NS, Lesser JB, Moche J, Sen C. Meningiomas involving the optic nerve: technical aspects and outcomes for a series of 50 patients. Neurosurgery 2003;53(3):523–532, discussion 532–533
48. Hayhurst C, Sughrue ME, Gore PA, Bonney PA, Burks JD, Teo C. Results with expanded endonasal resection of skull base meningiomas technical nuances and approach selection based on an early experience. Turk Neurosurg 2016;26(5):662–670
49. Zwagerman NT, Zenonos G, Lieber S, et al. Endoscopic transnasal skull base surgery: pushing the boundaries. J Neurooncol 2016;130(2):319–330
50. Frank G, Pasquini E. Tuberculum sellae meningioma: the extended transsphenoidal approach—for the virtuoso only? World Neurosurg 2010;73(6):625–626
51. Koutourousiou M, Fernandez-Miranda JC, Stefko ST, Wang EW, Snyderman CH, Gardner PA. Endoscopic endonasal surgery for suprasellar meningiomas: experience with 75 patients. J Neurosurg 2014;120(6):1326–1339
52. Dehdashti AR, Ganna A, Witterick I, Gentili F. Expanded endoscopic endonasal approach for anterior cranial base and suprasellar lesions: indications and limitations. Neurosurgery 2009;64(4):677–687, discussion 687–689
53. de Divitiis E, Cavallo LM, Cappabianca P, Esposito F. Extended endoscopic endonasal transsphenoidal approach for the removal of suprasellar tumors: part 2. Neurosurgery 2007;60(1):46–58, discussion 58–59
54. de Divitiis E, Cappabianca P, Cavallo LM. Endoscopic transsphenoidal approach: adaptability of the procedure to different sellar lesions. Neurosurgery 2002;51(3):699–705, discussion 705–707
55. Lee SC, Senior BA. Endoscopic skull base surgery. Clin Exp Otorhinolaryngol 2008;1(2):53–62

56. Lobo B, Heng A, Barkhoudarian G, Griffiths CF, Kelly DF. The expanding role of the endonasal endoscopic approach in pituitary and skull base surgery: a 2014 perspective. Surg Neurol Int 2015;6:82

57. Paluzzi A, Gardner P, Fernandez-Miranda JC, Snyderman C. The expanding role of endoscopic skull base surgery. Br J Neurosurg 2012;26(5):649–661

58. Solari D, Chiaramonte C, Di Somma A, et al. Endoscopic anatomy of the skull base explored through the nose. World Neurosurg 2014;82(6, Suppl):S164–S170

59. Solari D, Villa A, De Angelis M, Esposito F, Cavallo LM, Cappabianca P. Anatomy and surgery of the endoscopic endonasal approach to the skull base. Transl Med UniSa 2012;2:36–46

60. Couldwell WT, Weiss MH, Rabb C, Liu JK, Apfelbaum RI, Fukushima T. Variations on the standard transsphenoidal approach to the sellar region, with emphasis on the extended approaches and parasellar approaches: surgical experience in 105 cases. Neurosurgery 2004;55(3):539–547, discussion 547–550

61. Couldwell WT. Transsphenoidal and transcranial surgery for pituitary adenomas. J Neurooncol 2004;69(1-3):237–256

62. Soni RS, Patel SK, Husain Q, Dahodwala MQ, Eloy JA, Liu JK. From above or below: the controversy and historical evolution of tuberculum sellae meningioma resection from open to endoscopic skull base approaches. J Clin Neurosci 2014;21(4):559–568

63. Bohman LE, Stein SC, Newman JG, et al. Endoscopic versus open resection of tuberculum sellae meningiomas: a decision analysis. ORL J Otorhinolaryngol Relat Spec 2012;74(5): 255–263

64. de Divitiis E, Esposito F, Cappabianca P, Cavallo LM, de Divitiis O. Tuberculum sellae meningiomas: high route or low route? A series of 51 consecutive cases. Neurosurgery 2008;62(3):556–563, discussion 556–563

65. Muskens IS, Briceno V, Ouwehand TL, et al. The endoscopic endonasal approach is not superior to the microscopic transcranial approach for anterior skull base meningiomas-a meta-analysis. Acta Neurochir (Wien) 2018;160(1):59–75

66. Song SW, Kim YH, Kim JW, et al. Outcomes after transcranial and endoscopic endonasal approach for tuberculum meningiomas-a retrospective comparison. World Neurosurg 2018;109:e434–e445

67. Mascarella MA, Tewfik MA, Aldosari M, Sirhan D, Zeitouni A, Di Maio S. A simple scoring system to predict the resectability of skull base meningiomas via an endoscopic endonasal approach. World Neurosurg 2016;91:582–591.e1

68. Fernandez-Miranda JC, Pinheiro-Nieto C, Gardner PA, Snyderman CH. Endoscopic endonasal approach for a tuberculum sellae meningioma. J Neurosurg 2012;32(Suppl):E8

69. Prosser JD, Vender JR, Alleyne CH, Solares CA. Expanded endoscopic endonasal approaches to skull base meningiomas. J Neurol Surg B Skull Base 2012;73(3):147–156

70. Chowdhury FH, Haque MR, Goel AH, Kawsar KA. Endoscopic endonasal extended transsphenoidal removal of tuberculum sellae meningioma (TSM): an experience of six cases. Br J Neurosurg 2012;26(5):692–699

71. Komotar RJ, Starke RM, Raper DM, Anand VK, Schwartz TH. Endoscopic endonasal versus open transcranial resection of anterior midline skull base meningiomas. World Neurosurg 2012;77(5-6):713–724

72. Clark AJ, Jahangiri A, Garcia RM, et al. Endoscopic surgery for tuberculum sellae meningiomas: a systematic review and meta-analysis. Neurosurg Rev 2013;36(3):349–359

73. Chokyu I, Goto T, Ishibashi K, Nagata T, Ohata K. Bilateral subfrontal approach for tuberculum sellae meningiomas in long-term postoperative visual outcome. J Neurosurg 2011;115(4):802–810

74. Ottenhausen M, Banu MA, Placantonakis DG, et al. Endoscopic endonasal resection of suprasellar meningiomas: the importance of case selection and experience in determining extent of resection, visual improvement, and complications. World Neurosurg 2014;82(3-4):442–449

75. Abuzayed B, Tanriover N, Akar Z, Eraslan BS, Gazioglu N. Extended endoscopic endonasal approach to the suprasellar parachiasmatic cisterns: anatomic study. Childs Nerv Syst 2010;26(9):1161–1170

76. Zada G, Agarwalla PK, Mukundan S Jr, Dunn I, Golby AJ, Laws ER Jr. The neurosurgical anatomy of the sphenoid sinus and sellar floor in endoscopic transsphenoidal surgery. J Neurosurg 2011;114(5):1319–1330

77. Khan OH, Krischek B, Holliman D, et al. Pure endoscopic expanded endonasal approach for olfactory groove and tuberculum sellae meningiomas. J Clin Neurosci 2014;21(6):927–933

78. Gadgil N, Thomas JG, Takashima M, Yoshor D. Endoscopic resection of tuberculum sellae meningiomas. J Neurol Surg B Skull Base 2013;74(4):201–210

79. Dhandapani S, Negm HM, Cohen S, Anand VK, Schwartz TH. Endonasal endoscopic transsphenoidal resection of tuberculum sella meningioma with anterior cerebral artery encasement. Cureus 2015;7(8):e311

80. Liu JK, Christiano LD, Patel SK, Tubbs RS, Eloy JA. Surgical nuances for removal of tuberculum sellae meningiomas with optic canal involvement using the endoscopic endonasal extended transsphenoidal transplanum transtuberculum approach. Neurosurg Focus 2011;30(5):E2

81. Pamir MN, Ozduman K, Belirgen M, Kilic T, Ozek MM. Outcome determinants of pterional surgery for tuberculum sellae meningiomas. Acta Neurochir (Wien) 2005;147(11): 1121–1130, discussion 1130

82. Gulsen S, Dinc AH, Unal M, Cantürk N, Altinors N. Characterization of the anatomic location of the pituitary stalk and its relationship to the dorsum sellae, tuberculum sellae and chiasmatic cistern. J Korean Neurosurg Soc 2010;47(3):169–173

83. Giordano M, Gallieni M, Metwali H, Fahlbusch R, Samii M, Samii A. Can intraoperative magnetic resonance imaging be helpful in the surgical resection of parasellar meningiomas? A case series. World Neurosurg 2019;132:e577–e584

84. Learned KO, Adappa ND, Loevner LA, Palmer JN, Newman JG, Lee JY. MR imaging evaluation of endoscopic cranial base reconstruction with pedicled nasoseptal flap following endoscopic endonasal skull base surgery. Eur J Radiol 2013;82(3):544–551

85. Learned KO, Maralani PJ, Malloy K, Loevner LA. Skull base reconstruction: demystifying postoperative imaging evaluation. Neurographics 2015;5(2):56–63

86. Kang MD, Escott E, Thomas AJ, et al. The MR imaging appearance of the vascular pedicle nasoseptal flap. AJNR Am J Neuroradiol 2009;30(4):781–786

87. Hadad G, Bassagasteguy L, Carrau RL, et al. A novel reconstructive technique after endoscopic expanded endonasal approaches: vascular pedicle nasoseptal flap. Laryngoscope 2006;116(10):1882–1886

88. Kassam AB, Thomas A, Carrau RL, et al. Endoscopic reconstruction of the cranial base using a pedicled nasoseptal flap. Neurosurgery 2008;63(1, Suppl 1):ONS44–ONS52, discussion ONS52–ONS53

89. Moon JH, Kim EH, Kim SH. Various modifications of a vascularized nasoseptal flap for repair of extensive skull base dural defects. J Neurosurg 2019:1–9

90. Nayak L, Iwamoto FM, Rudnick JD, et al. Atypical and anaplastic meningiomas treated with bevacizumab. J Neurooncol 2012;109(1):187–193

91. Rahman A. Sunitinib for atypical and anaplastic meningioma. Lancet Oncol 2014;15(10):e424

92. Jenkinson MD, Javadpour M, Haylock BJ, et al. The ROAM/EORTC-1308 trial: Radiation versus Observation following surgical resection of Atypical Meningioma: study protocol for a randomised controlled trial. Trials 2015;16:519

93. Nguyen EK, Nguyen TK, Boldt G, Louie AV, Bauman GS. Hypofractionated stereotactic radiotherapy for intracranial meningioma: a systematic review. Neurooncol Pract 2019;6(5):346–353

94. Akyoldas G, Hergunsel OB, Yilmaz M, Sengoz M, Peker S. Gamma knife radiosurgery for anterior clinoid process meningiomas: a series of 61 consecutive patients. World Neurosurg 2020;133:e529–e534

95. Graffeo CS, Link MJ, Stafford SL, Parney IF, Foote RL, Pollock BE. Risk of internal carotid artery stenosis or occlusion after single-fraction radiosurgery for benign parasellar tumors. J Neurosurg 2019:1–8

96. Gerster-Gilliéron K, Forrer F, Maecke H, Mueller-Brand J, Merlo A, Cordier D. 90Y-DOTATOC as a therapeutic option for complex recurrent or progressive meningiomas. J Nucl Med 2015;56(11):1748–1751

Chapter 12 Tailored Endonasal Endoscopic Approaches for Meningioma Involving the Planum Sphenoidale and Tuberculum Sellae

Case 12A

Extended Endoscopic Endonasal Transethmoidal Approach for a Midline Meningioma of the Planum Sphenoidale and Olfactory Groove

Michel Roethlisberger and Yves Brand

History

34-year-old male patient with a history of surgically resected cerebellar medulloblastoma and the whole brain radiation therapy in childhood. His clinical course was complicated with a malabsorptive hydrocephalus treated with a permanent CSF-diversion. In the past decades, the patient underwent multiple bilateral frontal and occipital revisions and re-implantations of his CSF-diversion device. The patient was followed up regularly with neurocranial imaging. There are no endocrinological, ophthalmological, or neurological complaints except for cognitive impairment due to his underlying disease.

A slowly growing enhancing lesion of the planum sphenoidale with the erosion of the skull base and extension into the sphenoid cavity and posterior ethmoidal cells has been observed (**Fig. 12A.1** and **12A.2**). The lesions demonstrated a constant growth rate. Therefore, a surgical resection for histological confirmation of a most likely post radiation meningioma of the skull base has been indicated.

Due to its favorable location with intranasal extension and with the history of multiple revisions of his CSF-diversion device, the resection via a **binostril transethmoidal transsphenoidal approach with image-guided surgery** was selected.

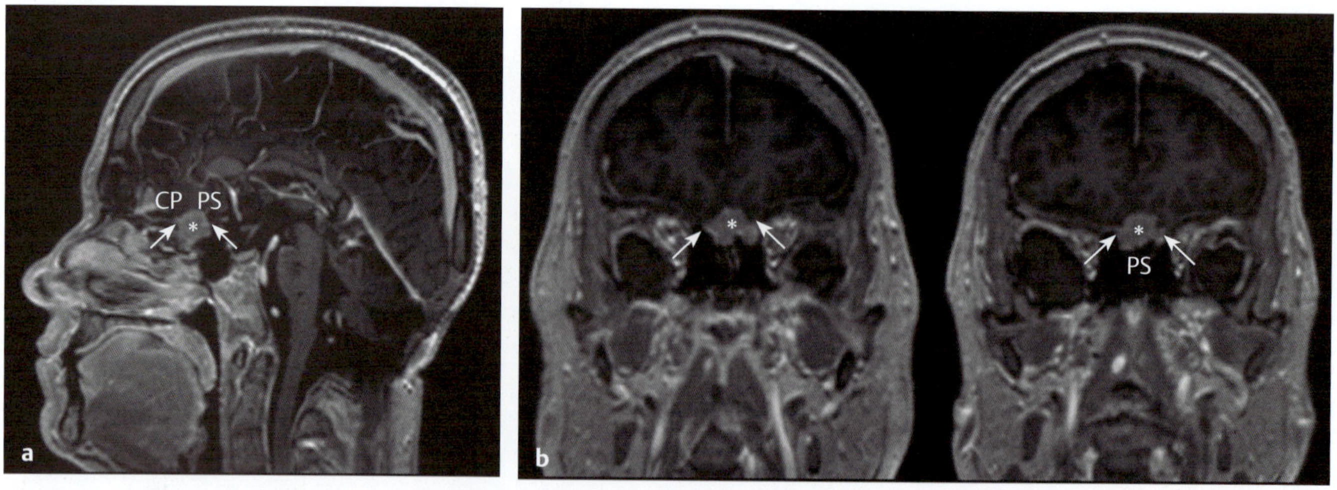

Fig. 12A.1 **(a)** Sagittal, **(b)** coronal T1-weighted gadolinium-enhanced MRI sections showing a dural based enhancing lesion (*) of the anterior skull base with erosion (*arrow*) of the ethmoidal bone and invasion of the anterior aspect of the planum sphenoidale (PS), the olfactory groove, and the cribriform plate (CP). There is no involvement of the medial orbit wall and discrete impacting of the inferior anterior lobe surface.

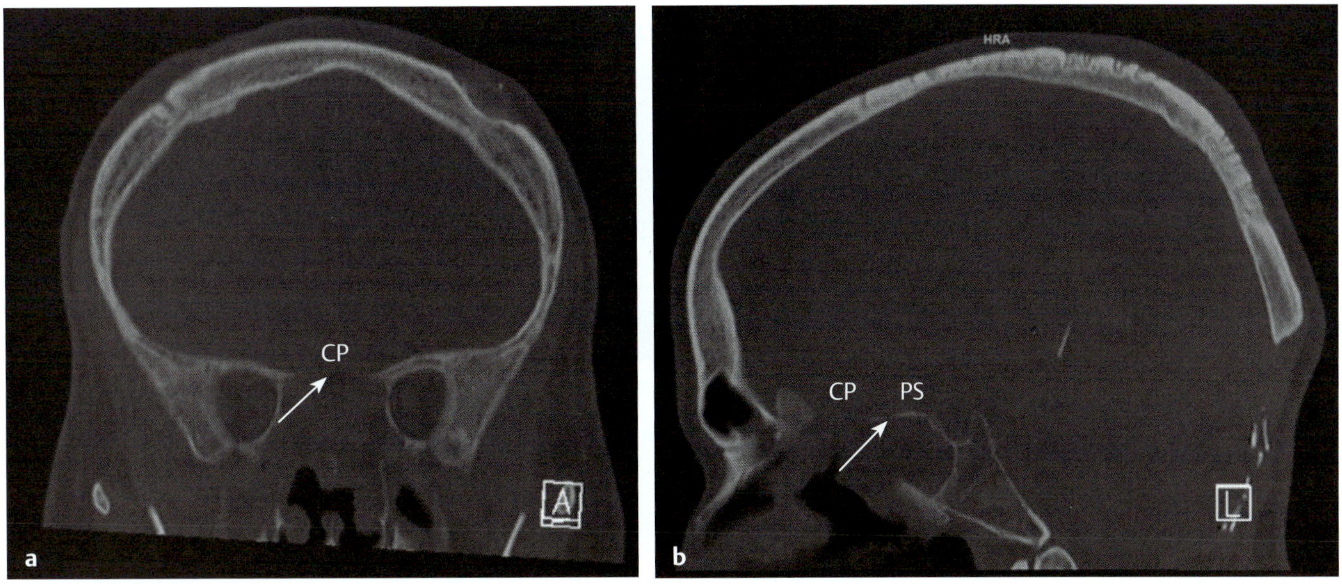

Fig. 12A.2 **(a)** Coronal, **(b)** sagittal non-enhanced CT sections (bone window) demonstrating the bony erosion (*arrow*) of the anterior aspect of the planum sphenoidale (PS), the olfactory groove, and the cribriform plate (CP). The reservoir and the catheter of the ventriculo peritoneal CSF-diversion device are visible. Postoperative changes after a suboccipital craniectomy and tumor resection are visible.

Surgical Steps

1. Nasal inspection and identification of the endonasal landmarks are of crucial importance when planning a transethmoidal approach to the sphenoid cavity.
2. Identification of the uncinate process and the ethmoidal bulla when medializing the middle turbinate show the access to the anterior and the posterior ethmoidal cells. This should be done on both sides if a bilateral approach is planned (**Fig. 12A.3**).
3. A vertical incision of the mucosa covering the lower third of the uncinate process allows entering the ethmoidal bulla, which is the most constant anterior ethmoidal air cell.
4. Step-wise removal of the lamellar bones following the anatomical sequence allows the surgeon to advance posteriorly and reach the posterior ethmoid cells. The trajectory can be controlled with the use of image-guided surgery. Laterally, the medial orbital wall, defined by the lamina papyracea, is the limitation. Superiorly, the frontal skull base is the limitation (**Fig. 12A.4**).
5. When passing the lamella of the middle turbinate and posterior ethmoidal air cells, the anterior wall of the sphenoid sinus and the spheno-ethmoidal recess come into view. The sphenoid ostium and the superior turbinate should be identified (**Fig. 12A.5**).
6. A sphenoidotomy with the widening of the sphenoid ostium allows to access the sphenoid cavity (**Fig. 12A.6**).
7. The septum is then incised with a size-15 blade on one side, and a mucoperichondrial flap is raised (**Fig. 12A.7**).
8. The posterior superior nasal septum removed.
9. The transethmoidal approach is then repeated on the contralateral side. The anterior superior wall of the sphenoid, including the superior aspect of the sphenoid keel, is removed (**Fig. 12A.8**).
10. By connecting the two approaches in the midline, the planum sphenoidale is exposed. Remaining posterior ethmoidal cells and mucosa are removed, and the intranasal portion of the meningioma is exposed (**Fig. 12A.9** and **12A.10**).
11. The locations and the margins are confirmed using image-guided surgery (IGS).
12. Osteodural exposure of the tumor is achieved by meticulously dissecting the bony edges from the fronto-basal dura around the tumor eroding the skull base (**Fig. 12A.11** and **12A.12**).

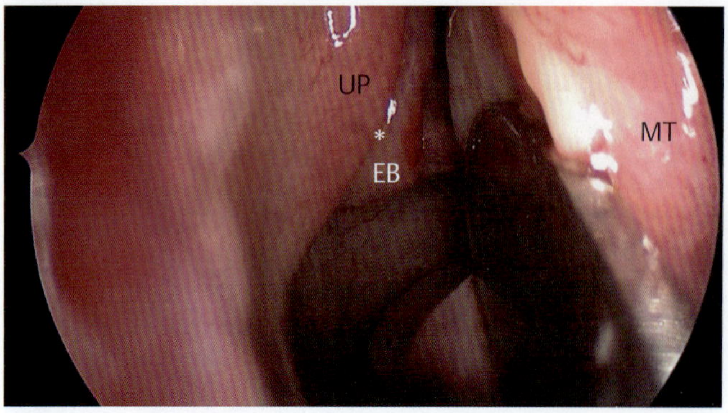

Fig. 12A.3 Endoscopic inspection of the right nostril. The middle turbinate (MT) is medialized using a Freer elevator. The uncinate process (UP), the hiatus semilunaris (*), and the ethmoidal bulla (EB) are identified.

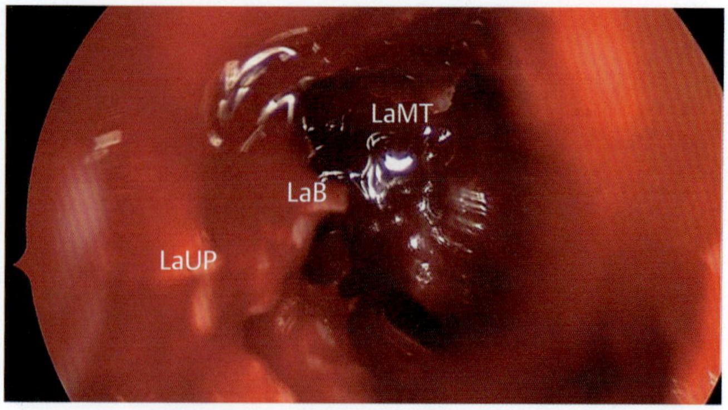

Fig. 12A.4 The lamella of the uncinate process (LaUP) and the lamella of the bulla (LaB) are removed. Lamella of the middle turbinate (LaMT).

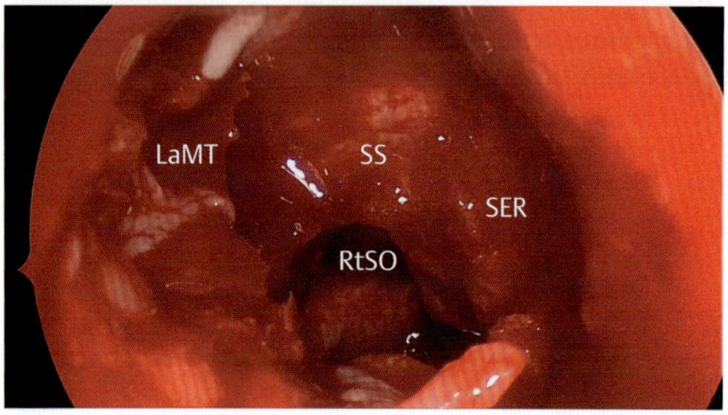

Fig. 12A.5 The middle part of the lamella of the middle turbinate (LaMT) and the posterior ethmoidal air cells are removed. The sphenoethmoid recess (SER) is visible with the anterior wall of the sphenoid sinus (SS) and the right sphenoid ostium (RtSO).

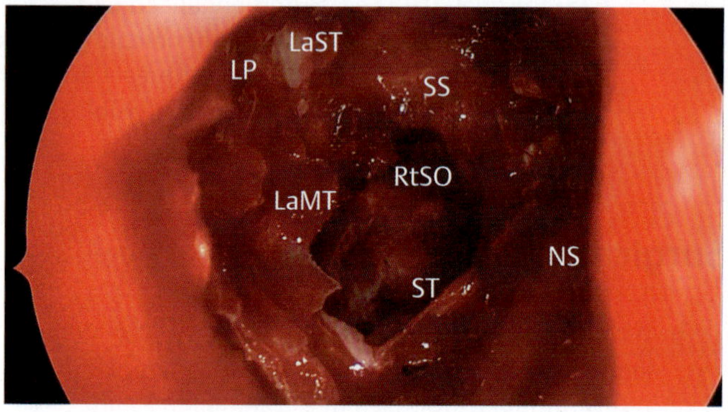

Fig. 12A.6 A sphenoidotomy of the right sphenoid ostium (RtSO) is performed.

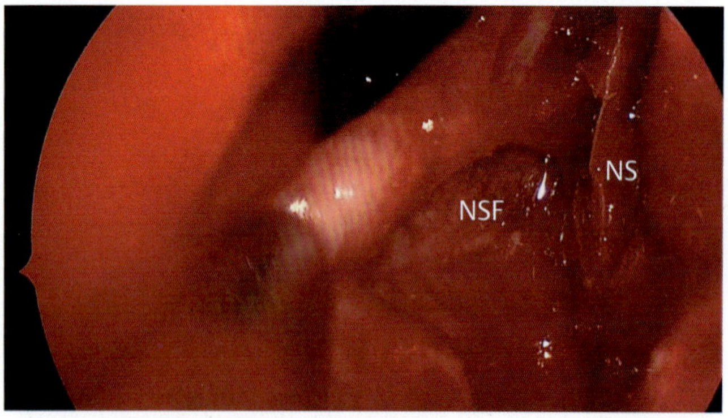

Fig. 12A.7 Harvesting of a right naso-septal flap (NSF) from the right nasal septum (NS).

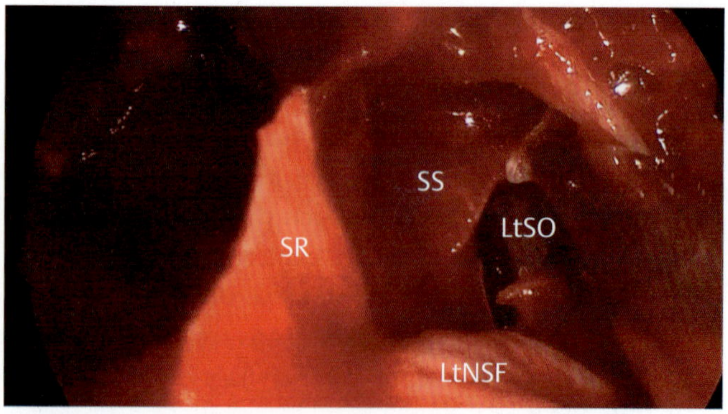

Fig. 12A.8 Left transethmoidal approach and exposition of the left sphenoid ostium (LtSO).

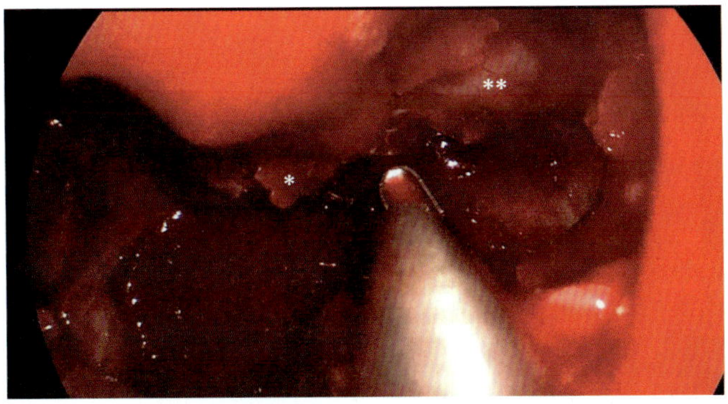

Fig. 12A.9 Removal of remaining ethmoidal air cells (*) posterior to the meningioma. The tumor erodes the skull base in the midline and the sinonasal portion can be visualized (**).

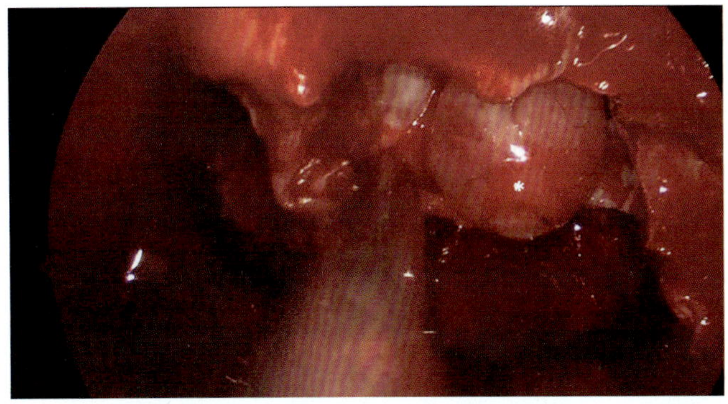

Fig. 12A.10 Further removal of the posterior ethmoidal cells expose the sinonasal portion (*) of the meningioma.

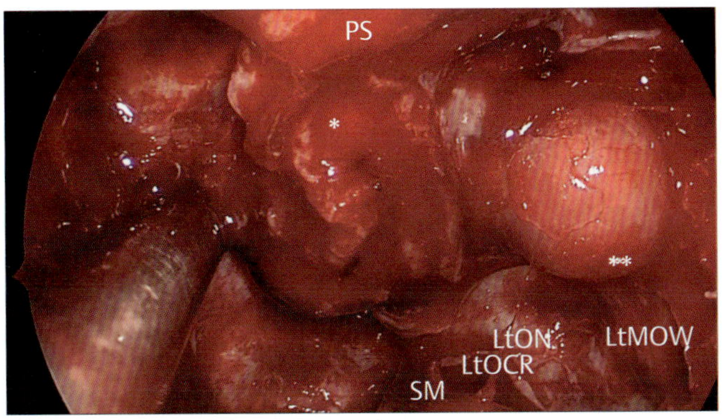

Fig. 12A.11 Overview after resection of the posterior ethmoidal cells. The tumor erodes the skull base in the midline (*). The sinonasal portion can be visualized (**).

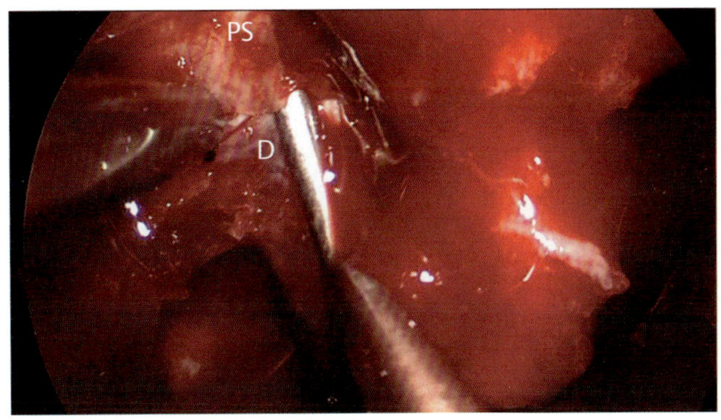

Fig. 12A.12 Dissection of the dural plane (D) around the meningioma using a blunt hooked instrument.

13. The posterior ethmoidal artery, a branch of the ophthalmic artery, passes through the fissure between the frontal bone and the lamina papyracea to enter the nasal cavity in the roof of the ethmoid bone. This vessel has to be identified and ligated when defining the planes around the tumor (**Fig. 12A.13**, **12A.14**, and **12A.15**).
14. After clearing of the tumor margins, debulking of the internal tumor is started using cauterization, piecemeal removal with forceps, and ultrasonic aspiration (**Fig. 12A.16**, **12A.17**, and **12A.18**).
15. The intracranial portion of the planum sphenoidale meningioma is then visible. In the first step, the brain tumor interface and an arachnoid have to be identified (**Fig. 12A.19a**).
16. A 90° ring curette and suction are useful with a bimanual technique to mobilize and remove the smaller intracranial portions (**Fig. 12A.19b**).
17. A tumor specimen should be preserved for histological examination.
18. Using a blunt hooked instrument, the plane between the dura and the arachnoid layer of the brain surface can be dissected carefully. Any resistance might be indicative of a small vessel.
19. With a 90° ring curette, the intracranial surface of the dura is cleaned and explored for any remaining tumor (**Fig. 12A.19c**).
20. The dural edges can be widened using a Kerrison punch. As there is a blind area of punching, this should be performed with care to not harm an intracranial vessel. By widening the opening, the dural involvement of the meningioma and a dural tail can be removed.
21. The dural edges can be punched and cauterized to further reduce remnant tumor cells (**Fig. 12A.20**).

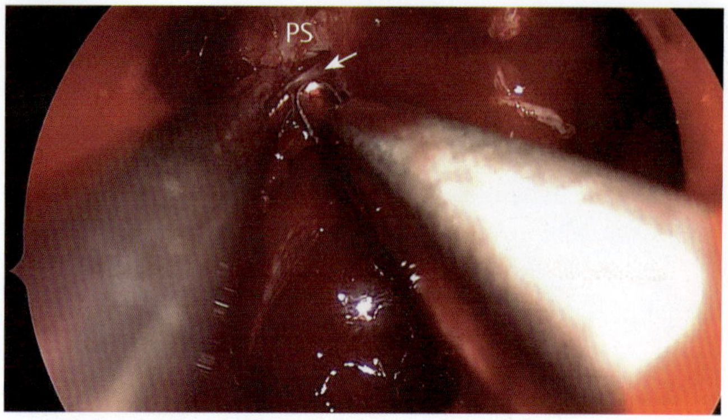

Fig. 12A.13 The posterior ethmoidal artery (*arrow*) is identified.

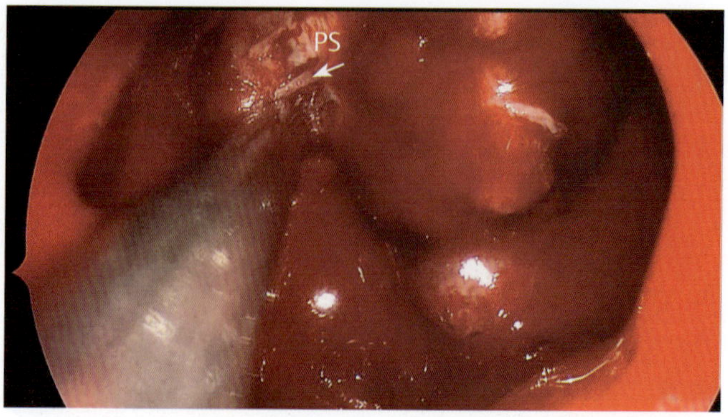

Fig. 12A.14 The bone covering the posterior ethmoidal artery (*arrow*) is removed using a Kerrison punch.

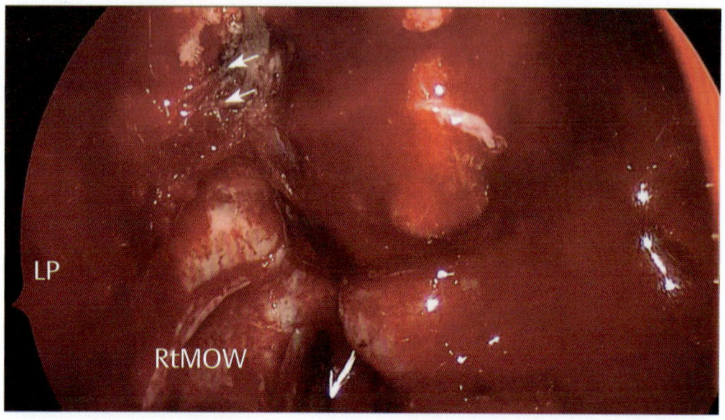

Fig. 12A.15 Sufficient exposure of the posterior ethmoidal artery (*arrows*) allows a controlled cauterization of the vessel and avoids retraction below the bony coverage.

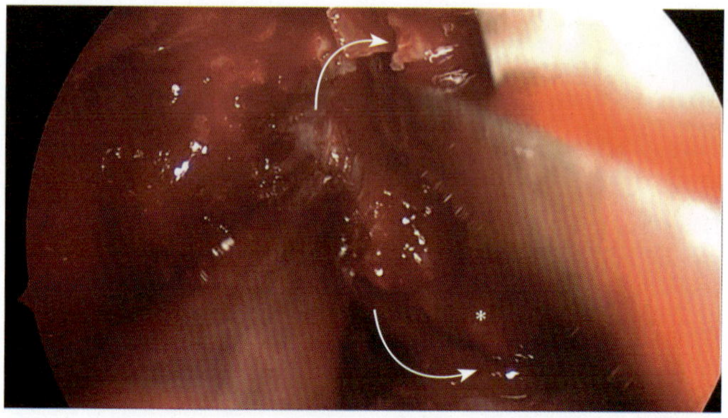

Fig. 12A.16 The osteodural exposure of the sinonasal portion of the meningioma (*) is continued circumferentially (*arrows*). This allows a downwards shift of the whole lesion into the nasal cavity.

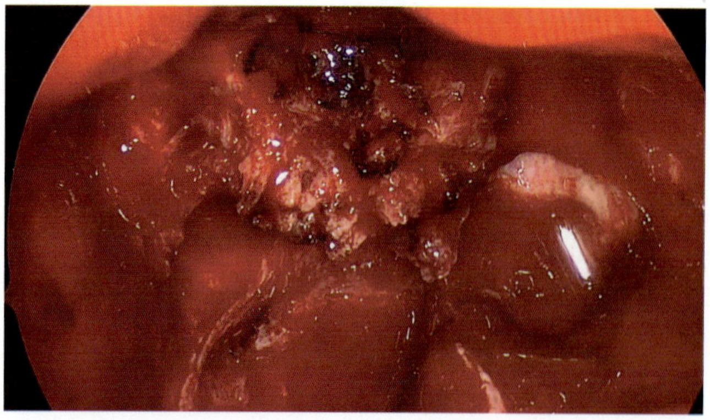

Fig. 12A.17 Cauterization of the tumor surface to shrink the lesion. This maneuver should be avoided in the brain-tumor interface, where the arachnoid plane is important.

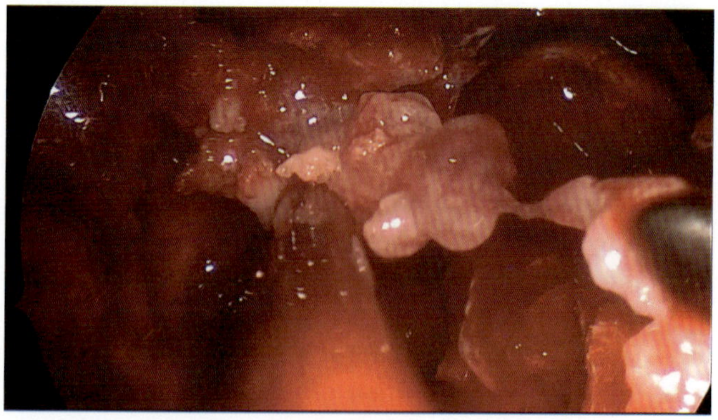

Fig. 12A.18 Piecemeal resection of the tumor.

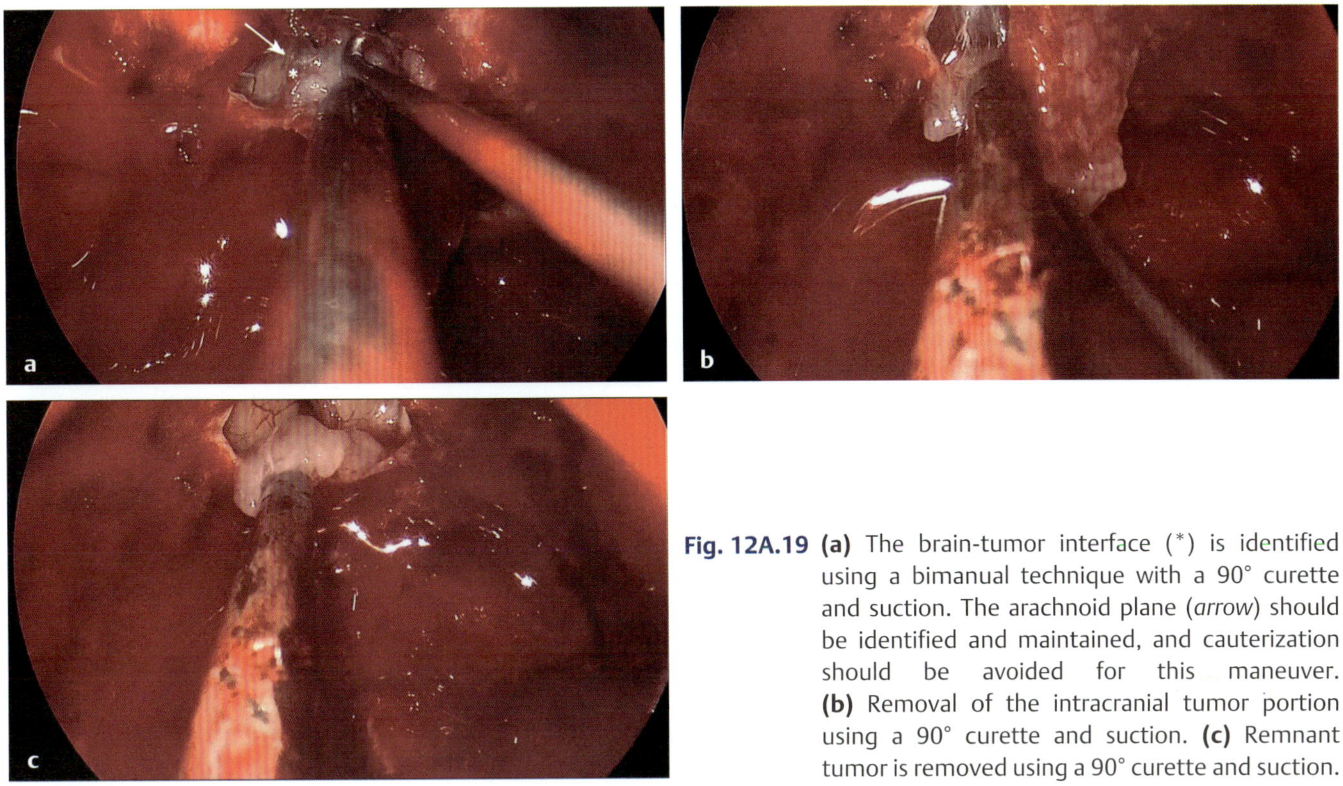

Fig. 12A.19 (a) The brain-tumor interface (*) is identified using a bimanual technique with a 90° curette and suction. The arachnoid plane (*arrow*) should be identified and maintained, and cauterization should be avoided for this maneuver. **(b)** Removal of the intracranial tumor portion using a 90° curette and suction. **(c)** Remnant tumor is removed using a 90° curette and suction.

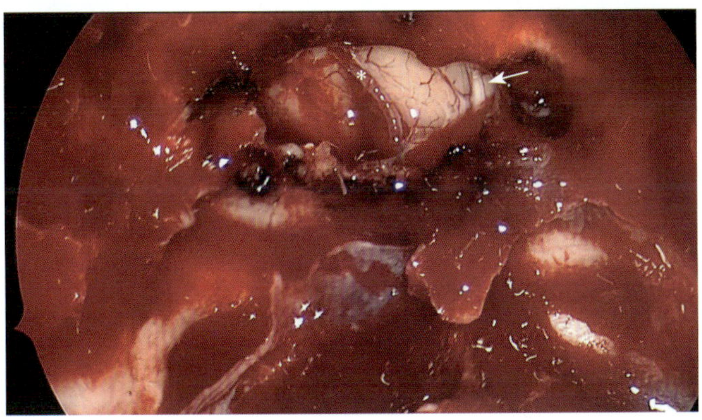

Fig. 12A.20 Circumferential excision and cauterization of the surrounding dura to reach a potential Simpson Grade 1 resection. A branch of the frontopolar artery (*) and the right olfactory tract (*arrow*) are visible.

22. Skull base dural defect closure is started with a tailored fascia lata inlay, harvested from the right thigh via a straight longitudinal cut (**Fig. 12A.21a–d**).
23. The inlay is supported with an extradural graft of subcutaneous fat (**Fig. 12A.22a** and **b**).
24. A first layer of artificial dural sealant and SURGICEL® Original Absorbable Hemostat (Ethicon, Johnson&Johnson, USA) hold the construct in place (**Fig. 12A.22c**).
25. A big piece of fascia lata harvested from the right thigh is then placed over the exposed anterior skull base and held in place with an artificial dural sealant (**Fig. 12A.23a** and **b**).
26. The remaining posterior ethmoidal cavity is filled with larger pieces of subcutaneous fat and SURGIFOAM® Absorbable Gelatin Sponge (Ethicon, Johnson&Johnson, USA) to further support the construct (**Fig. 12A.24**).
27. The nasoseptal flaps are brought back into position, and bilateral nasal packing with resorbable packs in the lateral and medial recess hold the middle turbinates in place (**Fig. 12A.25**).
28. A postoperative resection control after 6 weeks confirmed successful tumor removal, without clinical evidence of rhinoliquorrhea or new neurological symptoms (**Fig. 12A.26a** and **b**).

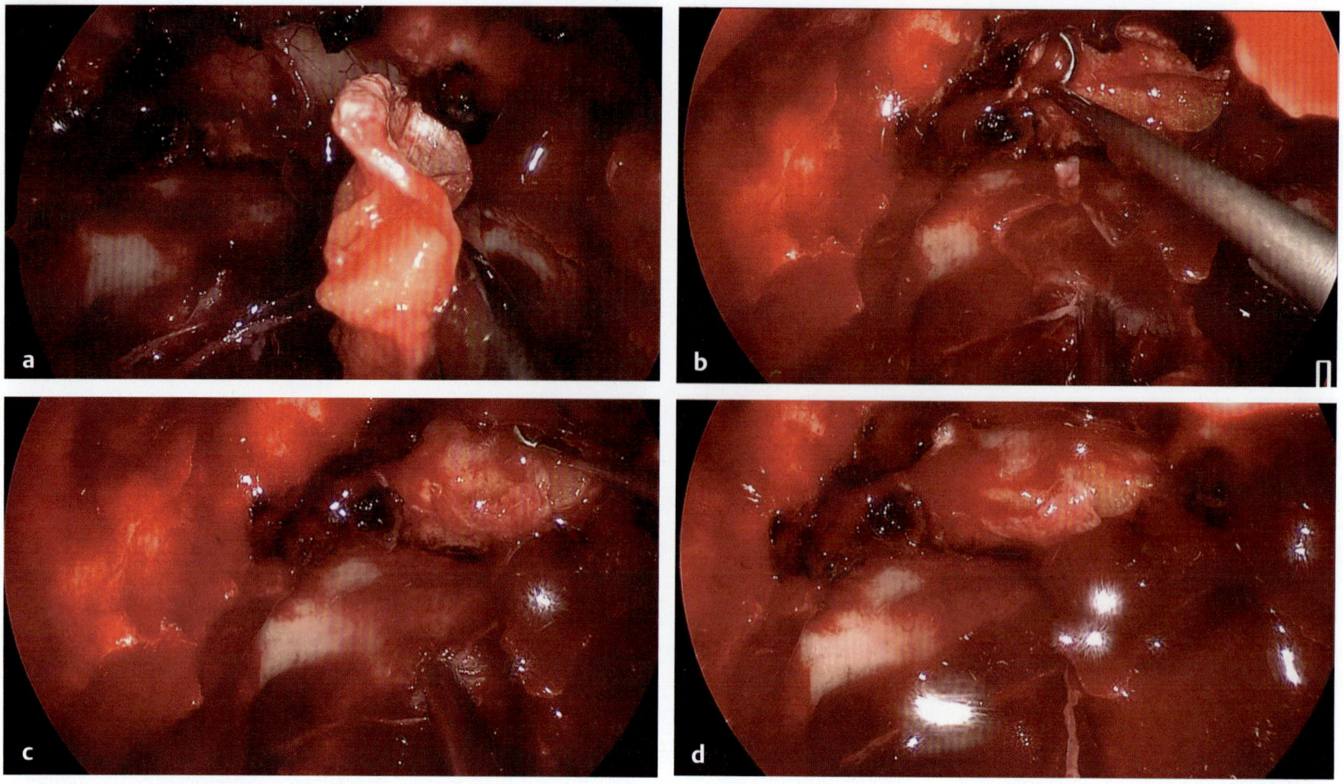

Fig. 12A.21 **(a)** Reconstruction of the dural skull base defect using a tailored fascia lata graft inlay. **(b, c)** A curette can be used to place the fascia lata graft intradurally. **(d)** The dural margins should be visible along the whole defect to ensure correct position of the inlay.

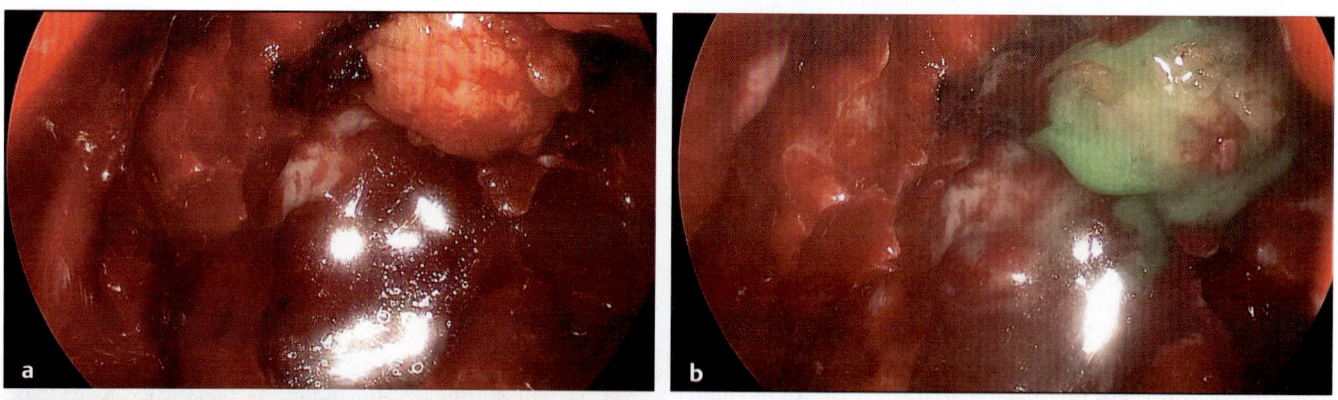

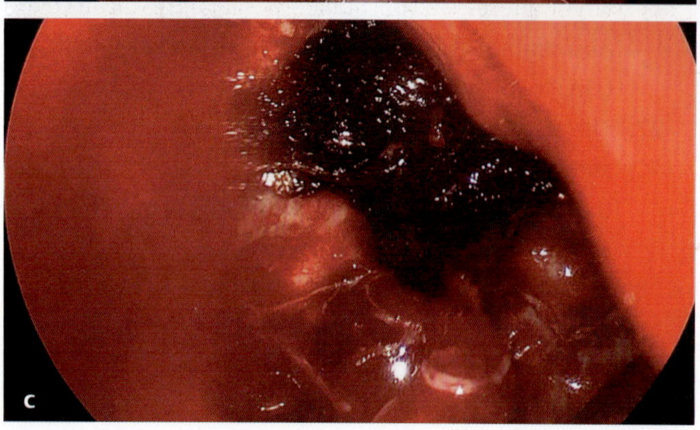

Fig. 12A.22 **(a)** A tailored subcutaneous fat graft from the thigh is used to support the fascia lata inlay as a first measure. **(b, c)** An artificial dural sealant and Surgicel© absorbable haemostat (Ethicon, Johnson & Johnson, USA) are used to support the first layer of the construct.

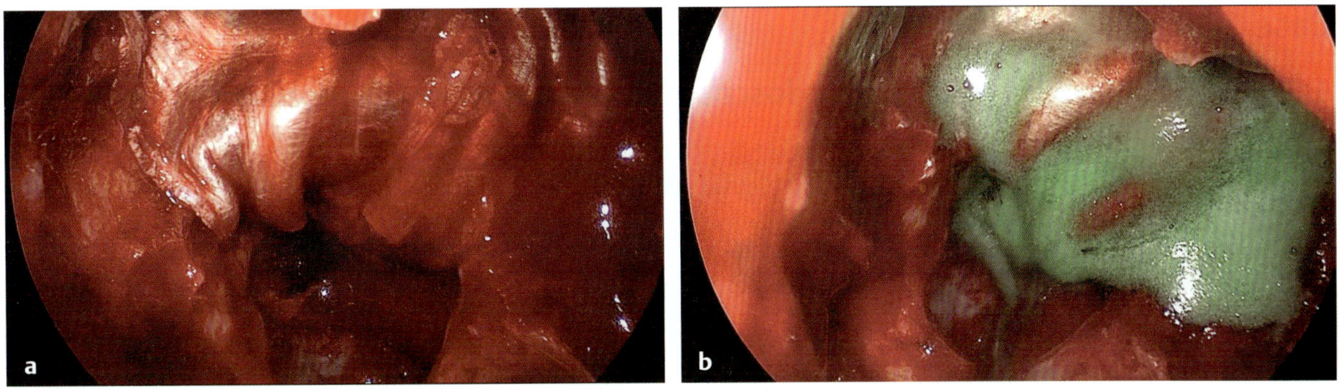

Fig. 12A.23 **(a, b)** A broad piece of fascia lata is placed along the whole aspect of the planum sphenoidale and sealed with an artificial dural sealant.

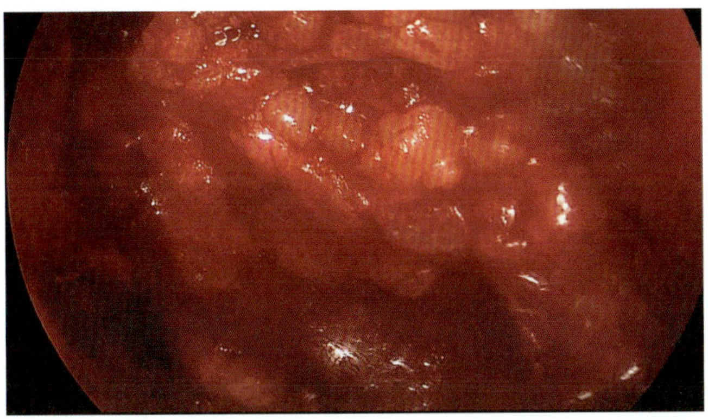

Fig. 12A.24 Larger pieces of a subcutaneous fat graft are used to support the fascia lata, which is stabilized with an artificial dural sealant and Surgicel© absorbable haemostat (Ethicon, Johnson & Johnson, USA).

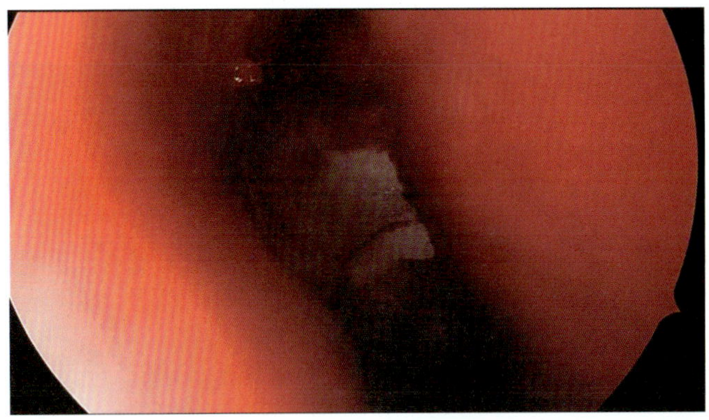

Fig. 12A.25 The construct is supported with Surgifoam© absorbable gelatine sponge (Ethicon, Johnson & Johnson, USA). The nasal mucosa is brought back into place and the nasal cavity packed with resorbable nasal packing.

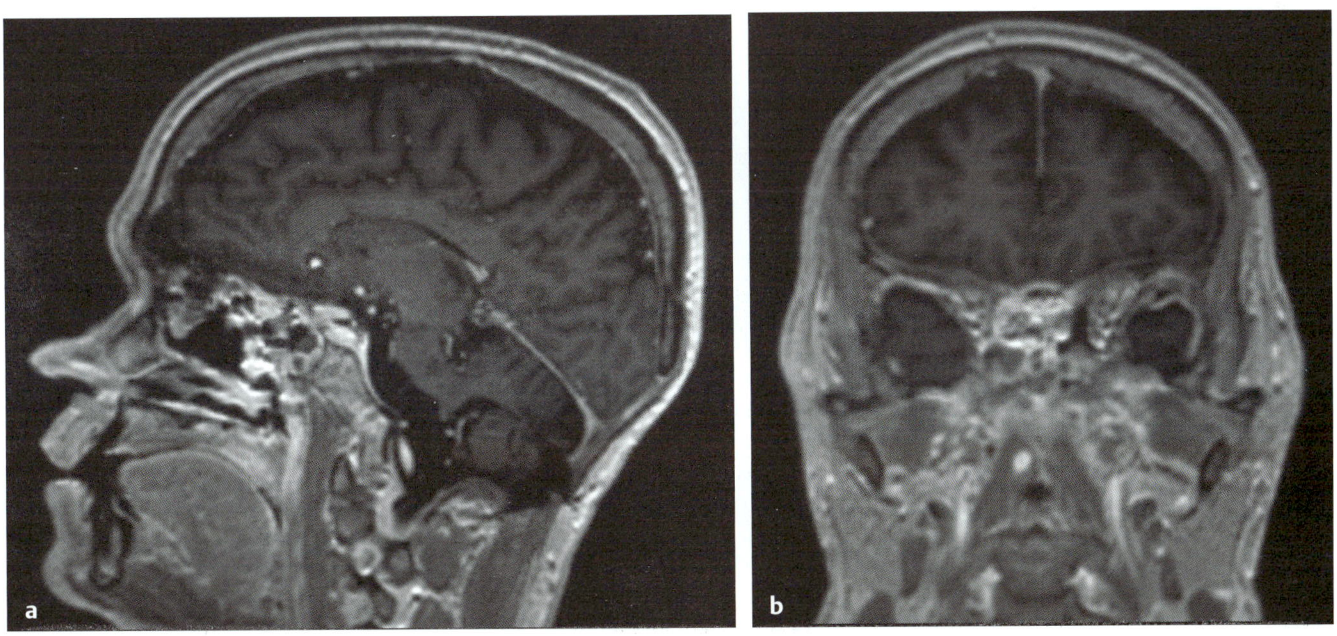

Fig. 12A.26 **(a)** Sagittal, **(b)** coronal postoperative T1-weighted gadolinium-enhanced MRI section after 6 weeks demonstrating complete resection of the planum sphenoidale and olfactory groove meningioma with postoperative changes of the abdominal fat and fascia lata graft.

Case 12B

A Tailored Extended Endonasal Endoscopic Approach for an Intrasellar Tuberculum Sellae Meningioma

Michel Roethlisberger, Prepageran Narayanan, and Vicknes Waran

History

A 46-year-old woman underwent transcranial resections of multiple intracranial meningiomas over the past decade. Clinical, ophthalmological, and endocrinological functions are within the normal range, and regular radiological follow-up is indicated because of her underlying diseases of meningiomatosis cerebri (**Fig. 12B.1a–f**). Over the last years, an enhancing lesion within the sella turcica demonstrated slow but steady growth, being suggestive for an intrasellar meningioma (**Fig. 12B.2**). Hence, an endonasal endoscopic transsphenoidal resection of the lesion was recommended.

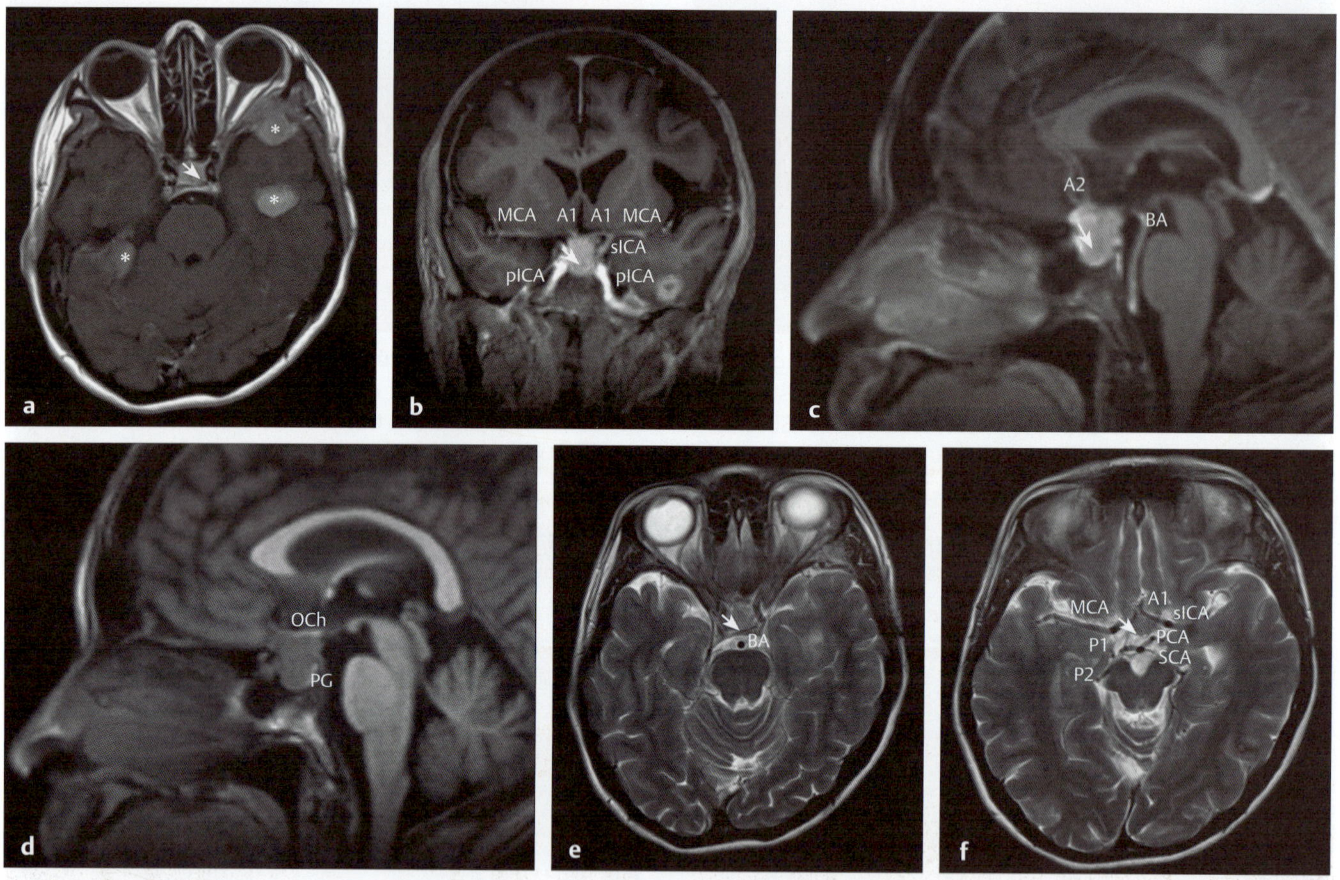

Fig. 12B.1 **(a)** Axial; **(b)** coronal; **(c)** sagittal T1-weighted gadolinium contrast-enhanced sections showing multiple dural-based contrast-enhancing lesions (*). One of these lesions (*arrow*) extending from the tuberculum sellae mainly into the sella turcica and partially into the suprasellar space. There is no vascular encasement. **(d)** Sagittal T1-weighted nonenhanced section demonstrating the isointensity of the lesion and the slightly more hyperintensive optic chiasm (OCh) as well as the posterior pituitary gland (PG) in relation to the tumor. **(e, f)** Axial T2-weighted sections showing isointensity of the lesion suggesting soft tumor consistency (*arrow*) without vascular encasement.

Surgical Steps

1. An endonasal endoscopic binostril transseptal transsphenoidal approach is performed as described in Chapter 1. The remaining anterior wall of the sphenoid cavity as well as the posterior ethmoidal cells and mucosa is removed using a debrider and Kerrison's punches (**Fig. 12B.3 and Fig. 12B.4**).
2. After the posterior ethmoidectomy and debriding of mucosal remnants along the posterior skull base, this approach provides a sufficient overview of the sphenoid cavity, the opticocarotid recesses, the planum sphenoidale, as well as the medial orbital apex walls (**Fig. 12B.5**).
3. These relevant landmarks can be verified using image-guided surgery (IGS).

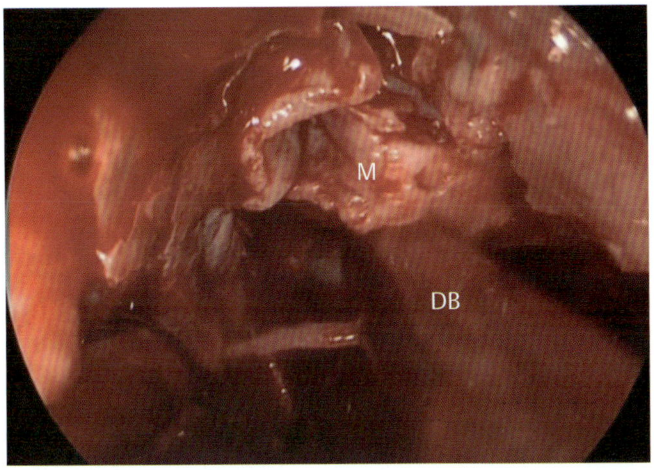

Fig. 12B.2 Removal of mucosa (M) covering the posterior ethmoidal cells with a debrider (DB).

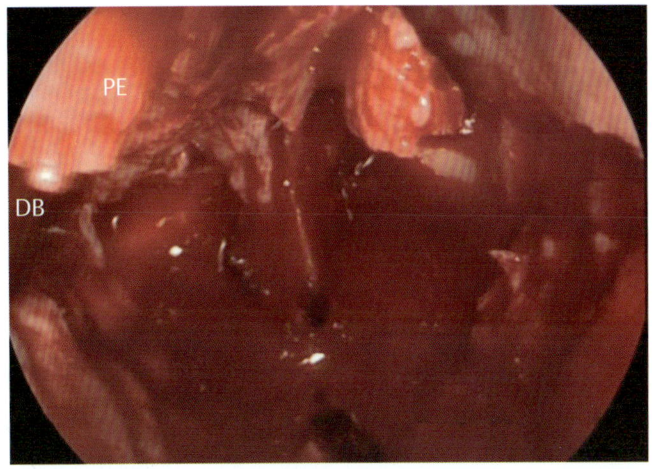

Fig. 12B.3 Removal of the posterior ethmoidal cells (PE) with a debrider (DB) to allow unobstructed view of the planum sphenoidale.

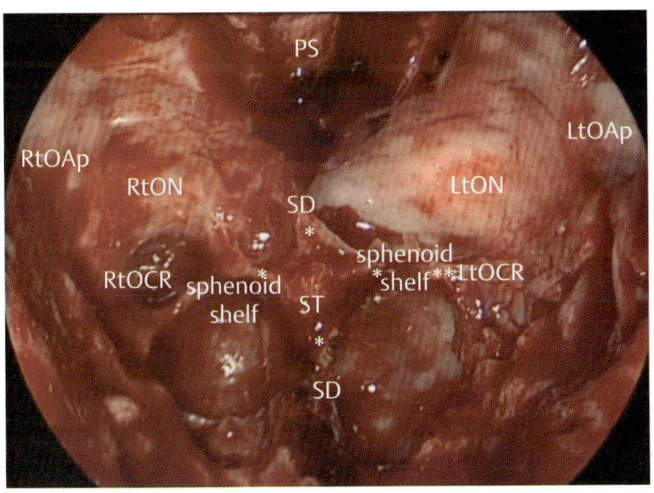

Fig. 12B.4 The sphenoid cavity is exposed. A complex sphenoid septation pattern is identified including a sphenoid main divider (SD) and a sphenoid shelf. The sella turcica (ST) is covered by the thick bony insertion site of the dividing septae (*). The left opticocarotid recess (LtOCR) is pneumatized while the right opticocarotid recess (RtOCR) is covered by the sphenoid shelf (**). The planum sphenoidale (PS), the left (LtOAp) and right medial orbital apex walls (RtOAp) are visible with the provided exposure.

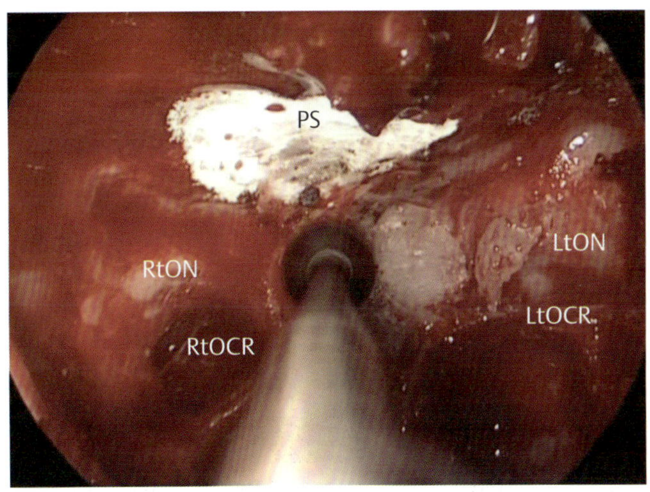

Fig. 12B.5 Transplanum approach: Thinning out the bony covering of the planum sphenoidale (PS) using a high-speed drill.

4. Drilling is commenced at the bone covering the planum sphenoidale using a high-speed diamond burr (Medtronic, Minneapolis, MN). An aspirator is kept within the nasal cavity to allow bone dust and smoke that are formed to be cleared to give an unobstructed view (**Fig. 12B.6**).
5. Once the bone has been sufficiently thinned out, a right angle dissector can be insinuated between the bone and the dura, and the osteodural exposure of the planum sphenoidale can be widened using Kerrison's punches (**Fig. 12B.7 and Fig. 12B.8**).
6. The bone thinning with a high-speed diamond burr is extended to the tuberculum sellae and the sella turcica (**Fig. 12B.9**). The osteodural exposure of the sella turcica is performed as described in Chapter 1.

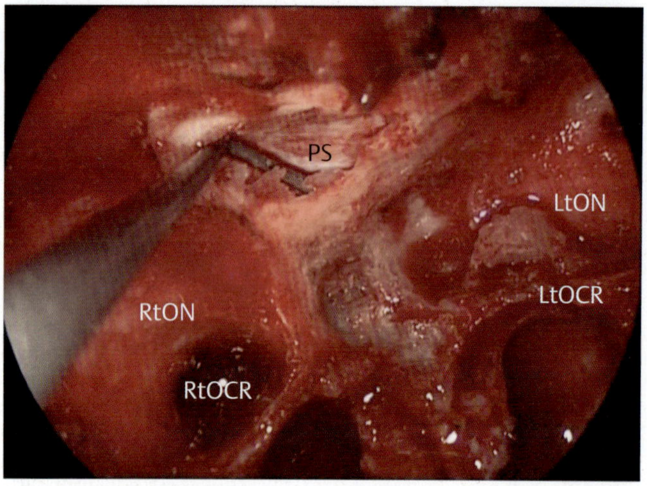

Fig. 12B.6 Transplanum approach: A blunt hooked instrument can be used to dissect the dura from the bony covering to avoid injury while using the Kerrison punch.

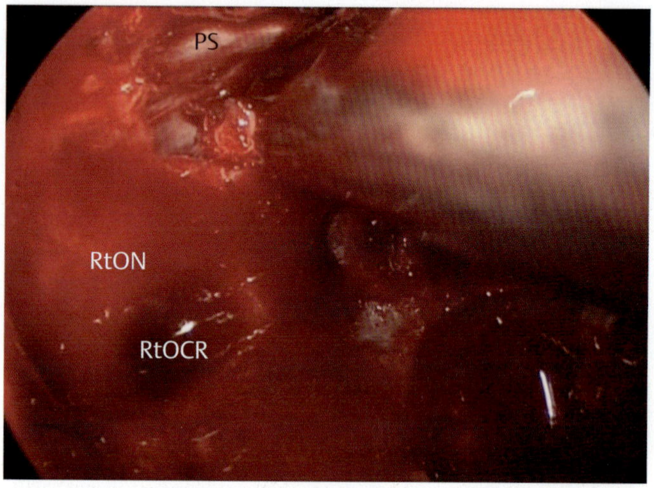

Fig. 12B.7 Transplanum approach: Extension of the osteodural exposure with a Kerrison punch.

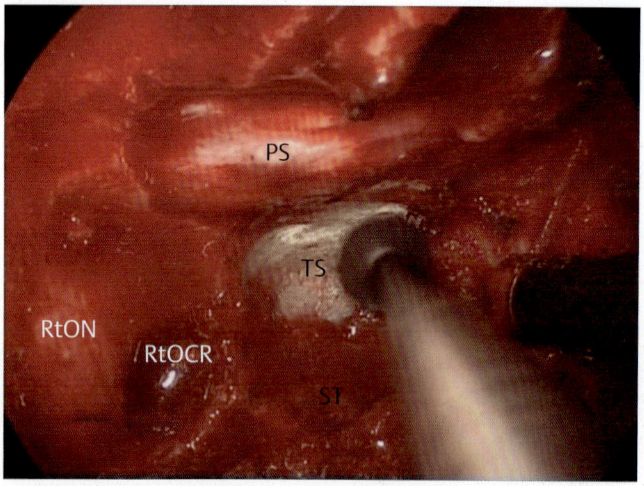

Fig. 12B.8 Transtuberculum approach: Thinning out the bony covering of the tuberculum sellae (TS) and the sella turcica (ST) with a high-speed drill.

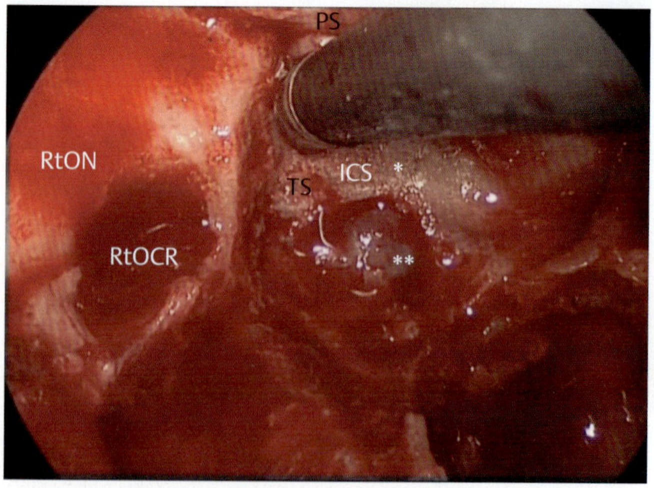

Fig. 12B.9 Bone bridge (*) of the tuberculum sellae (TS) covering the anterior intercavernous sinus (ICS). The meningioma has eroded parts of the sellar dura and is visible (**).

7. In cases with a thick bony coverage of the tubercular dura, a remaining bone bridge between the planum sphenoidale and the sella turcica (**Fig. 12B.10**) has to be removed piece by piece with a meticulous definition of the dural plane (**Fig. 12B.11**).
8. A wide dural osteodural exposure from the planum sphenoidale and the sella turcica toward the anterior intercavernous sinus should be seen before tumor resection is initiated (**Fig. 12B.12**). The lateral extension of the osteodural exposure has to be tailored for the size and location of the lesion. Meticulous definition of a plane between the covering bone and the dura should be emphasized (**Fig. 12B.13, Fig. 12B.14, Fig. 12B.15**). Verification of the laterality with IGS is useful (**Fig. 12B.16, 12B.17**).
9. The dural opening is started anteriorly to the brain–tumor interface in a T-shaped manner and is extended posteriorly to the sella turcica (**Fig. 12B.18, Fig. 12B.19, Fig. 12B.20**).

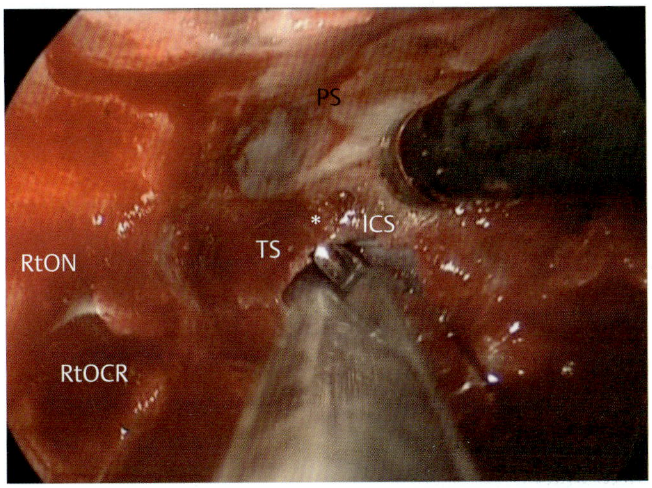

Fig. 12B.10 Removing the bone (*) of the tuberculum sellae (TS) covering the anterior intercavernous sinus (ICS).

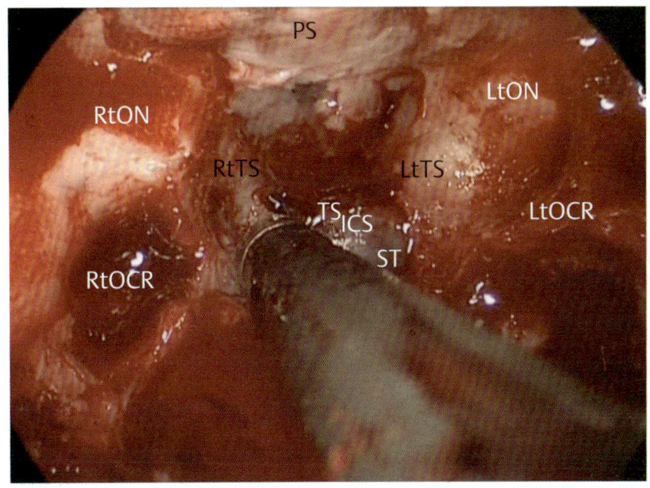

Fig. 12B.11 Midline osteodural exposure of the meningioma from the planum sphenoidale (PS), tuberculum sellae (TS), anterior intercavernous sinus (ICS) to the sella turcica (ST). The laterality of the bony exposure is not sufficient.

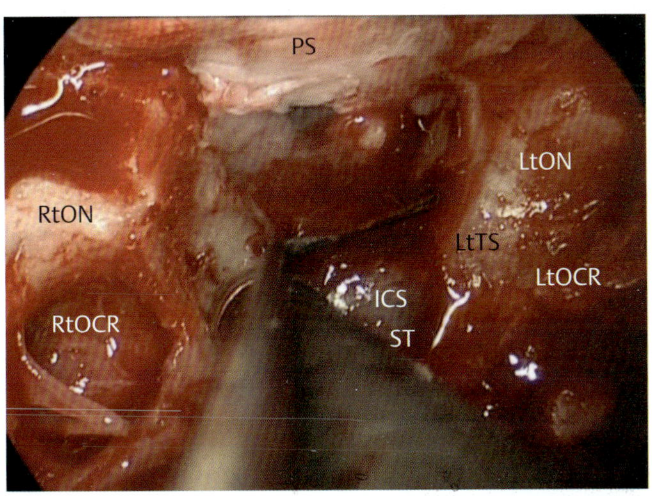

Fig. 12B.12 Definition of a plane between the left lateral dura and left lateral aspect of the tuberculum sellae (LtTS).

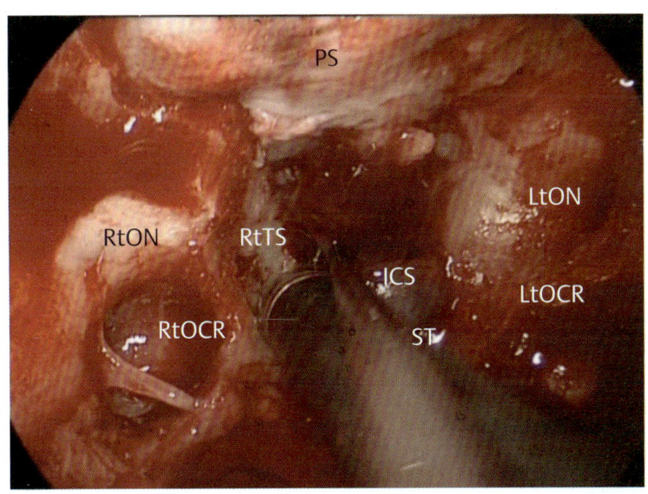

Fig. 12B.13 Definition of a plane between the right lateral dura and right lateral aspect of the tuberculum sellae (RtTS).

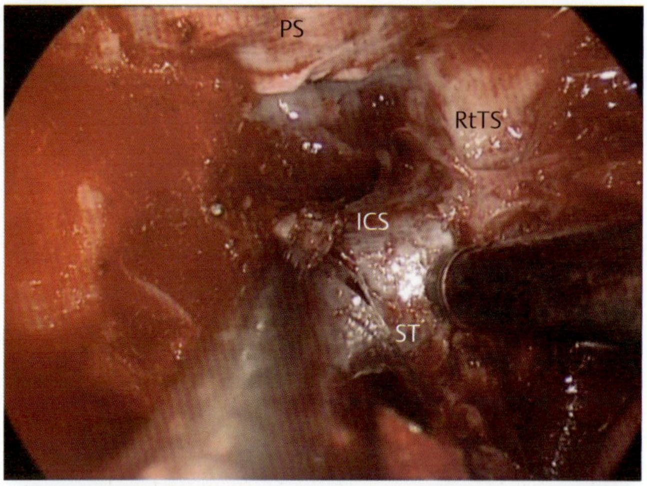

Fig. 12B.14 Transsellar approach: Removal of bone covering the right cavernous internal carotid artery (ICS).

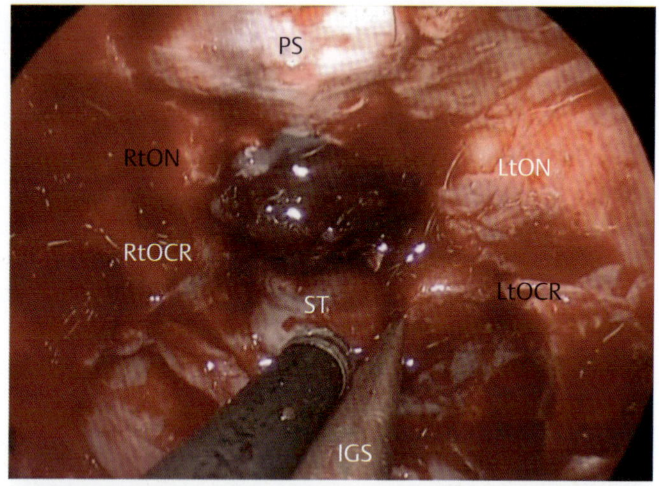

Fig. 12B.15 Confirming the left lateral osteodural exposure of the sella with image-guided surgery (IGS).

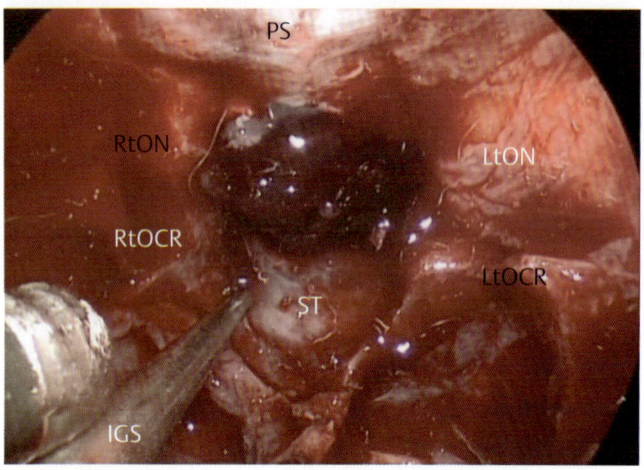

Fig. 12B.16 Confirming the right lateral osteodural exposure of the sella with image-guided surgery (IGS).

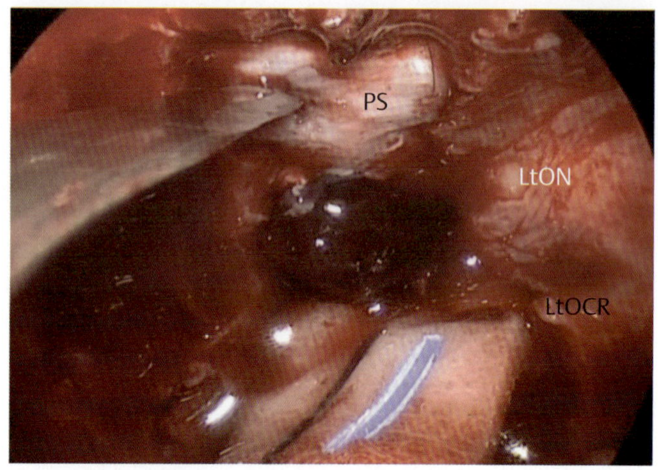

Fig. 12B.17 Anterior horizontal incision of the planum sphenoidale (PS) dura.

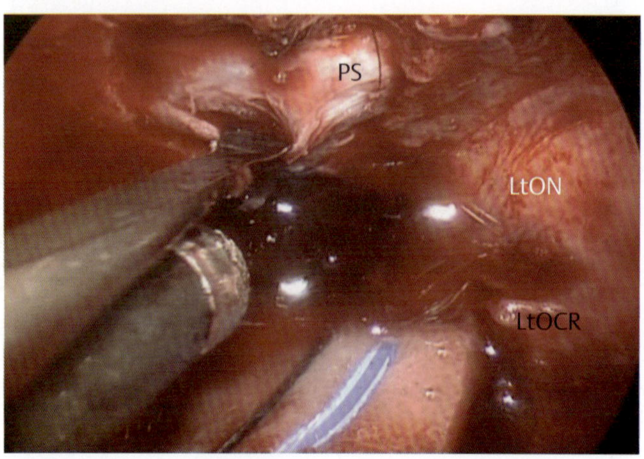

Fig. 12B.18 The dissection plane between the dura mater and the arachnoidal membrane is defined using a microdissector.

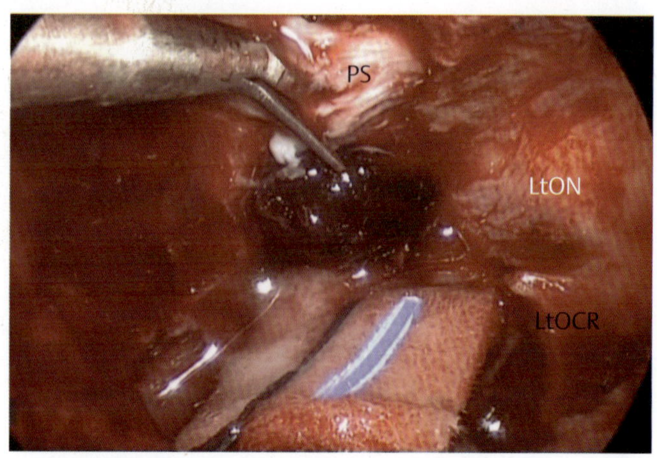

Fig. 12B.19 Vertical posterior dural incision along the planum sphenoidale (PS).

10. Meticulous coagulation and division of the anterior intercavernous sinus is necessary to connect the planum sphenoidale with the sellar region. For this maneuver, the dural structure is freed with a right angle dissector, controlled with bipolar cautery, and divided using a microscissors to expose the entire lesion (**Fig. 12B.21 and Fig. 12.22**).
11. The anterior brain–tumor interface is defined using the arachnoid plane between the brain surface and the tumor (**Fig. 12B.23 and 12B.24**). The tumor can then be debulked starting anteriorly and continuing sideways bilaterally (**Fig. 12B.25**).
12. When removing the tubercular portion of the meningioma, the optic chiasm, the optic nerves, and the postcommunicating segments of the anterior cerebral artery have to be identified and preserved.
13. To reach the sellar portion of the meningioma, opening of the dura covering the sella turcica is necessary (**Fig. 12B.26** and **Fig. 12B.27**).

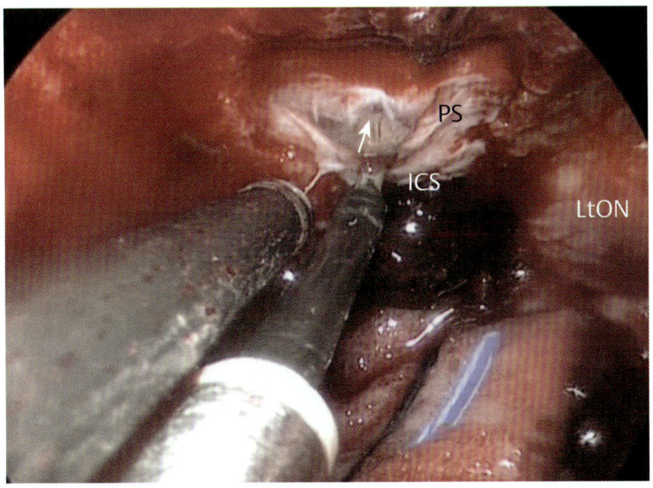

Fig. 12B.20 Cauterization of the anterior intercavernous sinus (ICS) using bipolar forceps. Arachnoid membrane (*white arrow*).

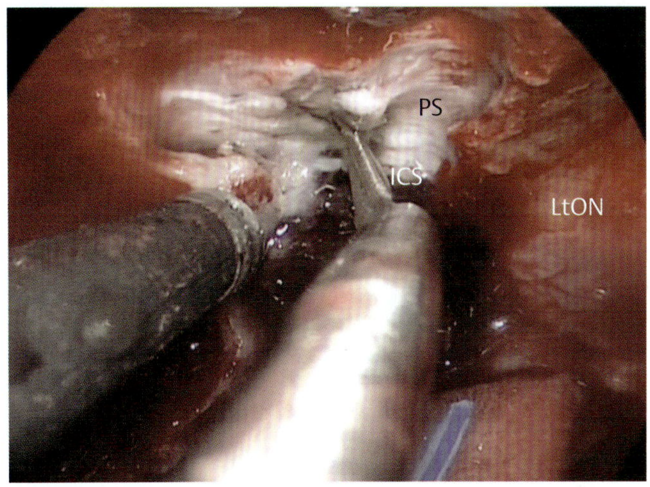

Fig. 12B.21 The vertical cut is continued posteriorly, and the anterior intercavernous sinus (ICS) is divided.

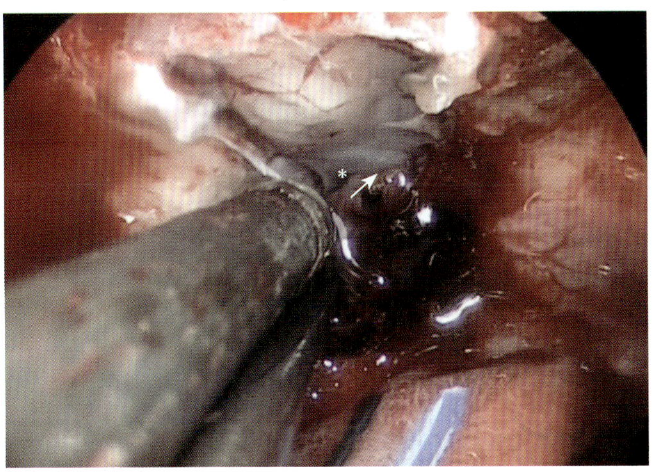

Fig. 12B.22 The superior tumor margin (*arrow*) and arachnoid plane (*) to the brain surface is defined using a microdissector.

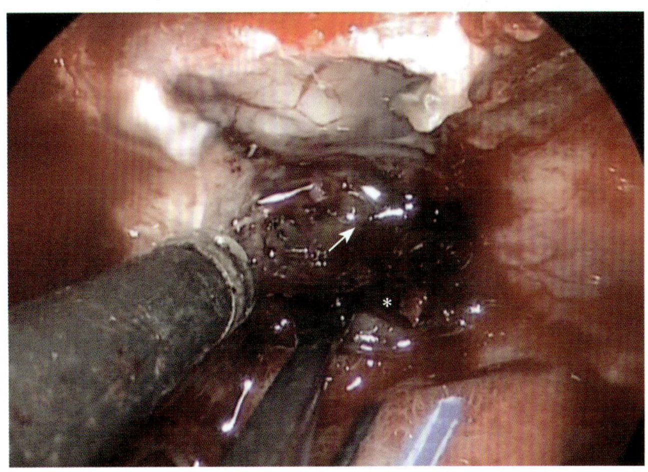

Fig. 12B.23 The tubercular portion of the tumor (*arrow*) and the plane (*) to the sella turcica (ST) are defined using a microdissector.

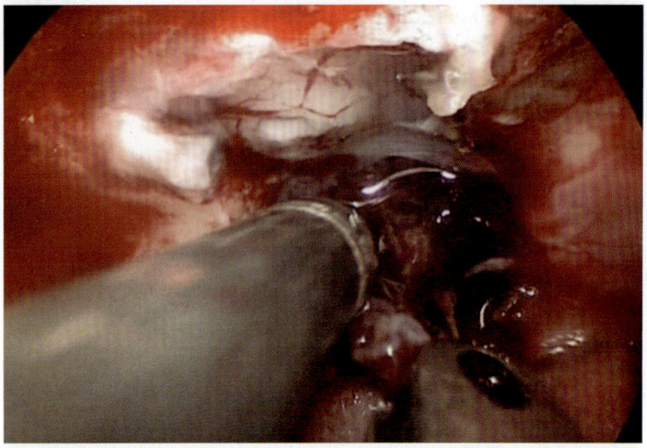

Fig. 12B.24 Bimanual removal of the tubercular tumor compartment with grasping instruments and suction.

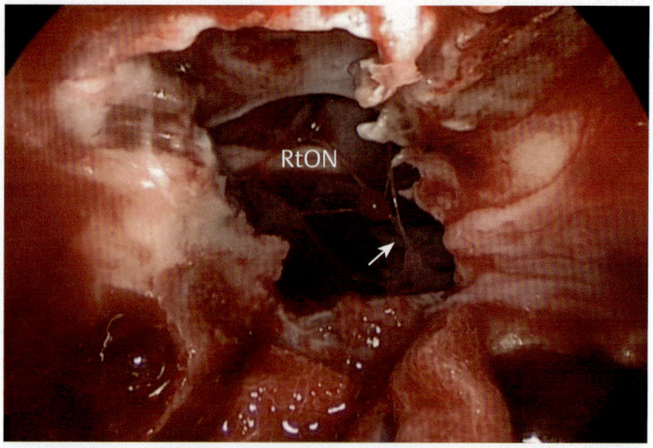

Fig. 12B.25 The right optic nerve (RtON) is visible after the removal of the superior tumor compartment. The intrasellar tumor compartment is visible (*arrow*).

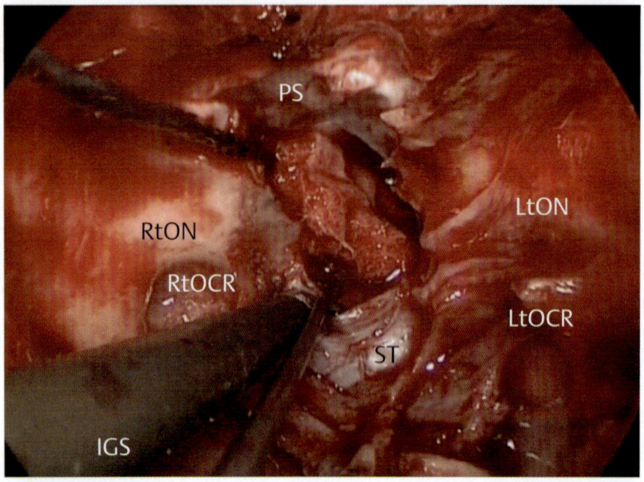

Fig. 12B.26 The plane between the sellar dura and the sellar tumor compartment is defined using a blunt hooked instrument.

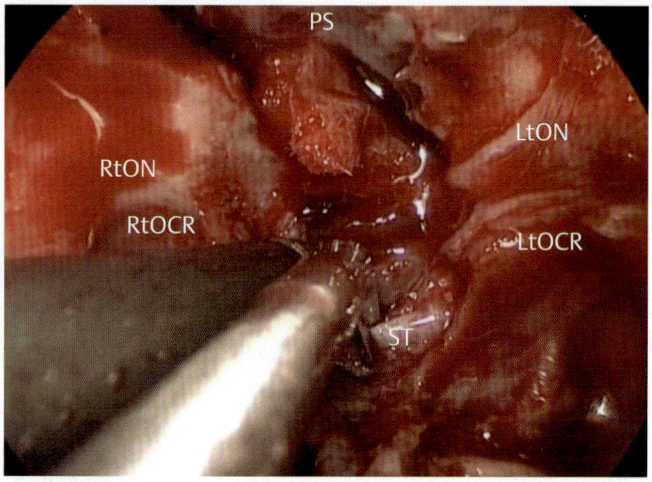

Fig. 12B.27 The vertical cut is continued inferiorly to open the sella turcica (ST).

14. The intrasellar inferior tumor margin is defined using the arachnoid plane when the tumor is suspected to arise from the tuberculum sellae. The tumor is cleared using a bimanual microsurgical dissection technique and suction (**Fig. 12B.28, Fig. 12B.29, Fig. 12B.30**).
15. When removing the sellar portion of the meningioma, the infundibular stalk and the pituitary gland have to be identified and preserved (**Fig 12B. 31** and **Fig. 12B.32**).
16. Intraoperative contrast-enhanced magnetic resonance imaging (MRI) is performed showing a complete resection of the mainly intrasellar located tuberculum sellae meningioma.
17. Meticulous hemostasis is then performed.
18. The defect is plugged with an abdominal fat graft, and the edges of the fat are brought intracranially to create a watertight seal (**Fig. 12B.33**).
19. This is then sealed with a synthetic dural sealant and layered with an absorbable hemostat (**Fig. 12B.34**).
20. The dural skull base defects are usually closed using vascularized pedicled nasoseptal flaps (Hadad's flaps). These are harvested during the approach and stored in the caudal nasal cavity. The flaps should cover the whole construct and have contact with the bony edges of the osteodural opening (**Fig. 12B.35**).

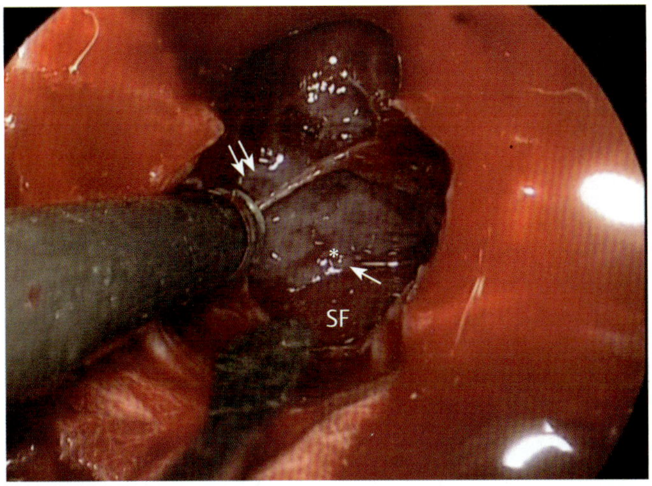

Fig. 12B.28 The inferior (*arrow*) and lateral (*double arrow*) margins of the sellar tumor compartment and the arachnoidal plane (*) to the sellar floor (SF) are defined using a microdissector.

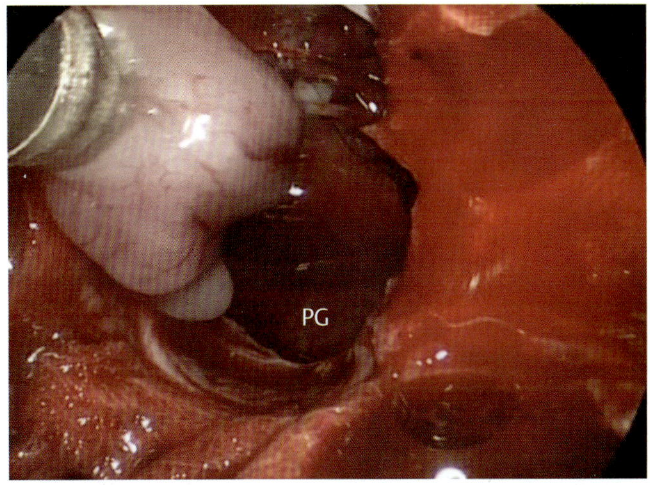

Fig. 12B.29 Removal of the intrasellar tumor compartment.

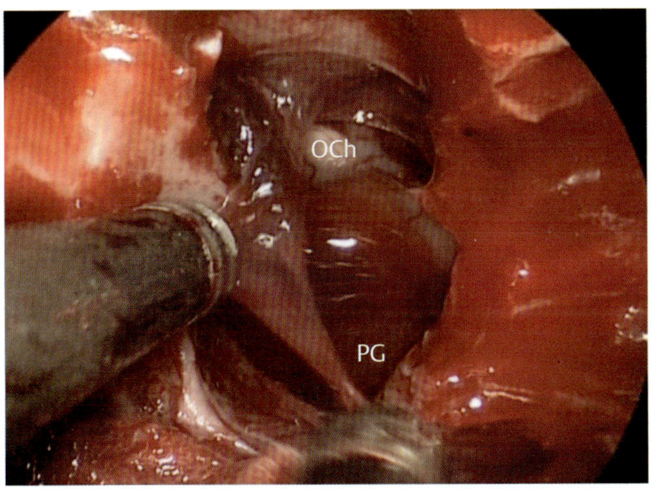

Fig. 12B.30 Remaining tumor and arachnoidal strands are removed using two suctions.

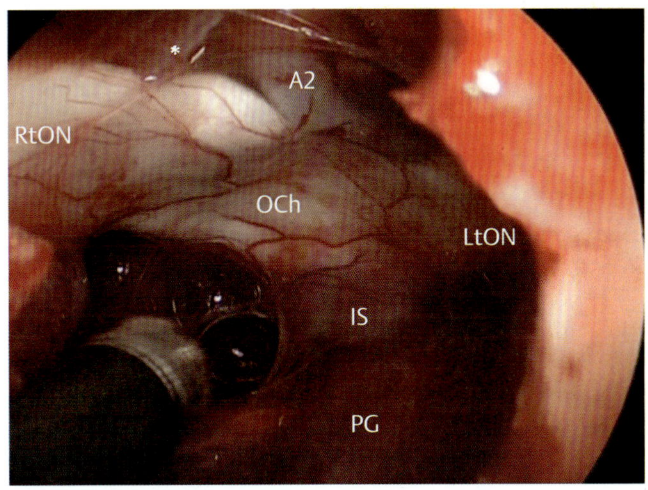

Fig. 12B.31 Endoscopic view of the suprasellar anatomy after tumor removal. The flattened optic chiasm (OCh) and left (LtON) and right optic nerves (RtON), the infundibular stalk (IS), and the pituitary gland (PG) are visible. Small perforators (*) arise from the distal anterior cerebral artery (A2) supplying the left optic nerve (LtON).

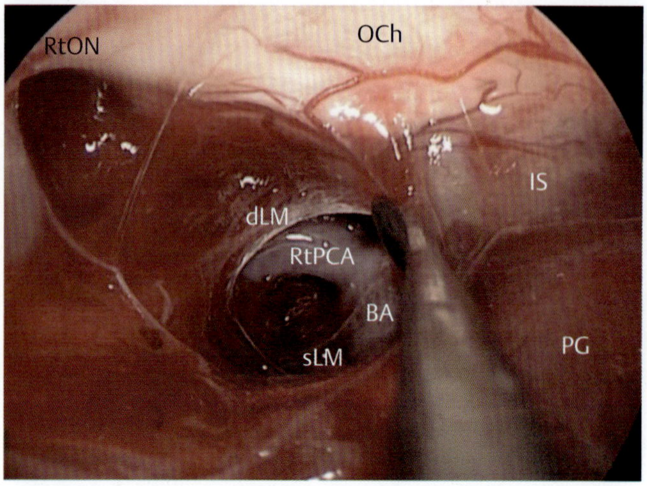

Fig. 12B.32 Dissection of the sellar (sLM) Liliequist membrane reveals an endoscopic view of the prepontine cistern with the tip of the basilar artery (BA) and the right posterior cerebral artery (RtPCA). The flattened optic chiasm (OCh), right optic nerve (RtON), the infundibular stalk (IS), and the pituitary gland (PG) are visible.

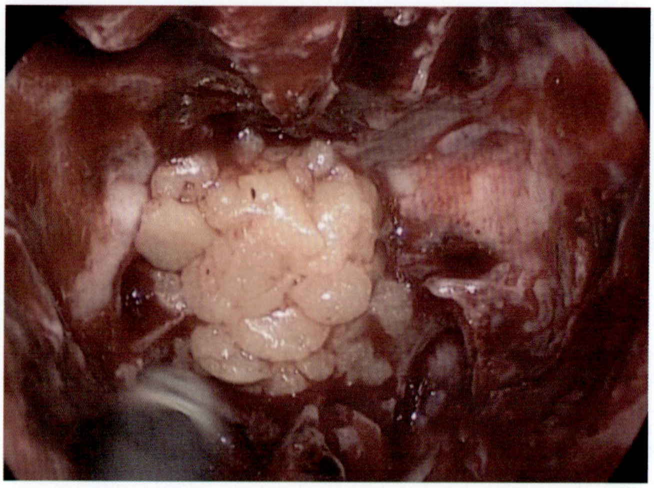

Fig. 12B.33 Placement of an abdominal fat graft in the tumor cavity.

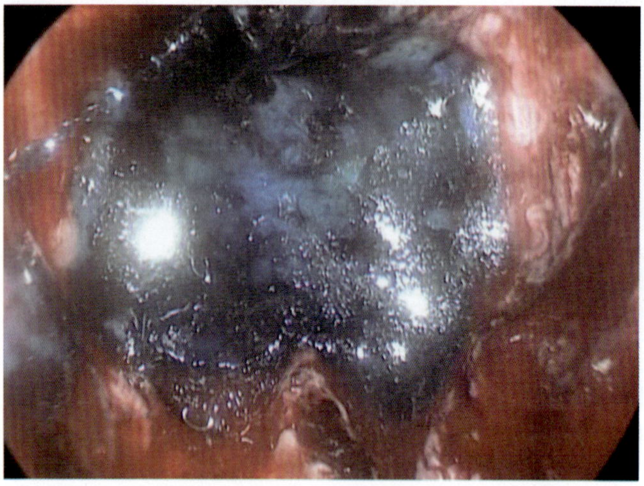

Fig. 12B.34 Application of an artificial dural sealant.

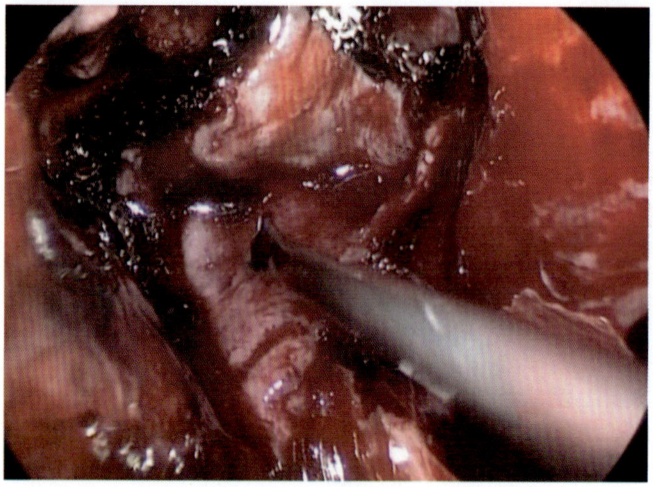

Fig. 12B.35 A harvested and stored pedicled nasoseptal flap is placed over the construct along the bony edges.

Case 12C

A Tailored Extended Endonasal Endoscopic Approach for a Medium-Sized Tuberculum Sellae Meningioma

Michel Roethlisberger, Prepageran Narayanan, and Vicknes Waran

History

A 43-year-old male patient was referred to the neurosurgical clinic with slowly progressing loss of visual acuity and documented unilateral temporal field defect with a contralateral quadrantanopsia. Otherwise, the patient was healthy. Endocrinological work-up did not reveal any dysfunction of the endocrine axis.

Contrast-enhanced magnetic resonance imaging (MRI) demonstrates a homogenous enhancing T1- and T2- isointense extra-axial solid mass on the tuberculum sella with the extension on the planum sphenoidale with lateral displacement of the intracranial carotid arteries and carotid bifurcations and in close relation with the anterior H-complex of the anterior cerebral artery (ACA). The infundibular stalk and the pituitary gland are posterior inferior to the lesions without significant compression (**Fig. 12C.1, Fig. 12C.2,** and **Fig. 12C.3**).

An elongated tuberculum sellae, the soft appearance of the tumor in the T2-weighted sequences, and absence of optic canal involvement made this tumor amenable for endonasal endoscopic resection. A binostril transsphenoidal transplanum transtuberculum approach with image-guided surgery was selected to gain adequate exposure of this tumor.

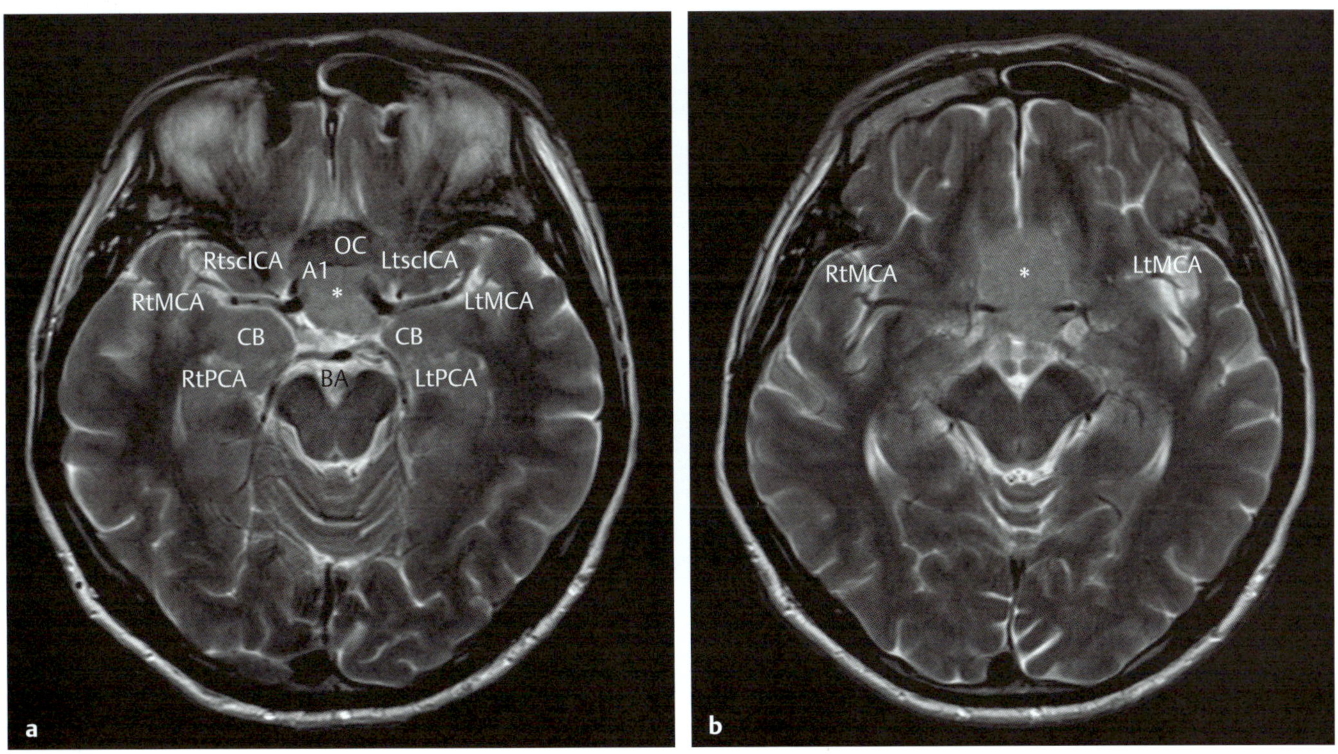

Fig. 12C.1 (a, b) Axial T2-weighted sections.

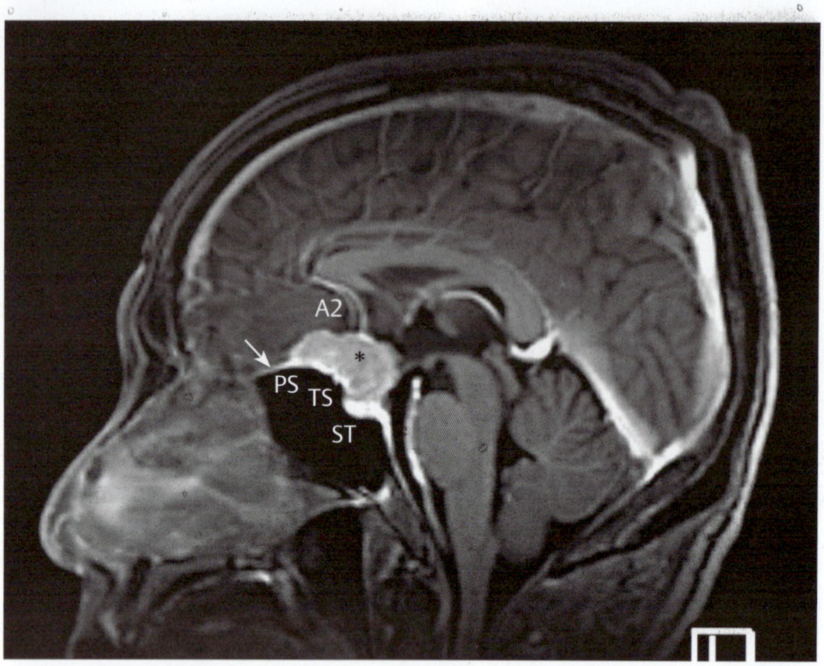

Fig. 12C.2 Sagittal T1-weighted gadolinium contrast-enhanced section.

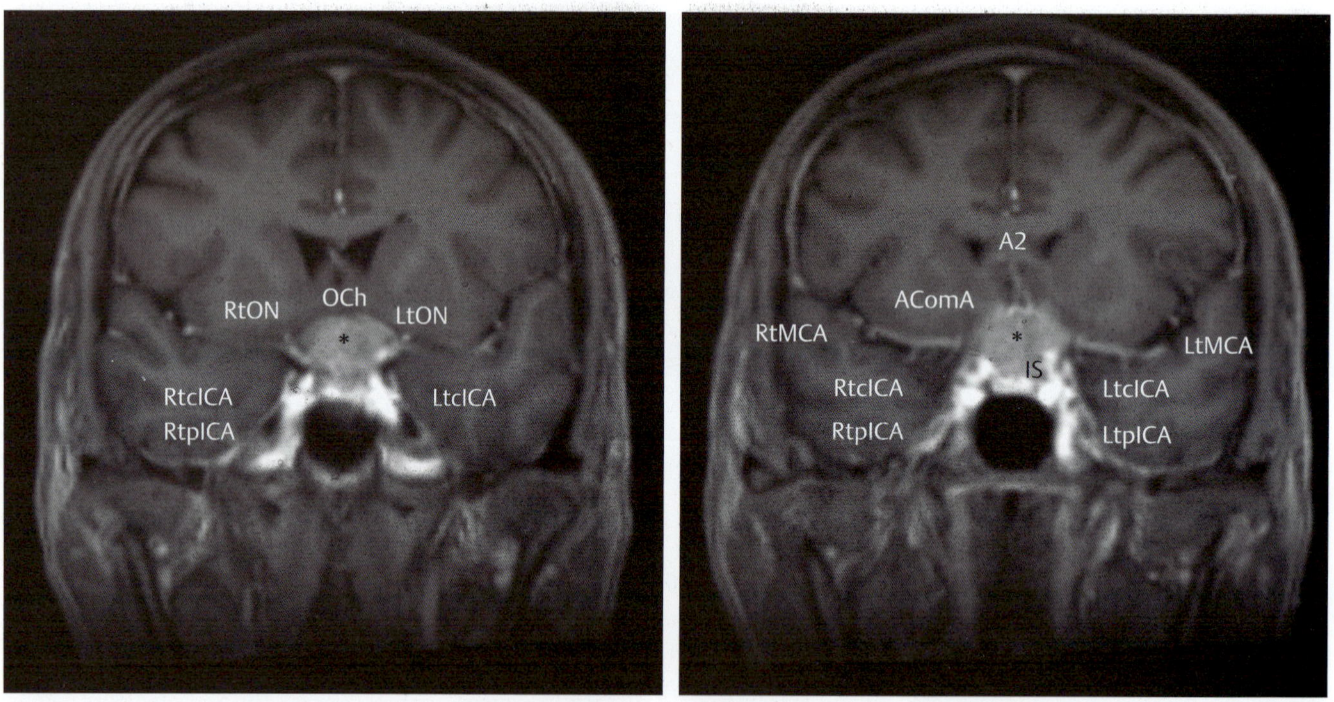

Fig. 12C.3 Coronal T1-weighted gadolinium contrast-enhanced section. **Fig. 12C.1**, **Fig. 12C.2**, and **Fig. 12C.3** show a homogenous enhancing T1- and T2-isointense extraaxial solid mass on the tuberculum sella and planum sphenoidale is present (*). A typical dural tail (*arrow*) extends anteriorly along the planum sphenoidale (PS). The posterior pole is in contanct with the anterior communicating artery (AComA) and the pre- (A1) and postcommunicating segments (A2) of the anterior cerebral arteries without signs of encasement. The pituitary gland (PG) presents with slightly more enhancement within the sella turcia (ST) and without significant dislocation. The infundibular stalk (IS) is displaced slightly posterior by the tumor mass. There is compression of the optic chiasm (OCh), and the right (RtON) and left optic nerves (LtON) are pushed superiorly and laterally. The right (RtscICA) and left supraclinoid internal carotid arteries (LtscICA) and the carotid bifurcations (CB) are pushed laterally by the tumor mass.

Surgical Steps

1. An incision is made with a no. 15 blade anterior to the middle turbinate down to the cartilaginous septum with more anterior extension than in standard cases (**Fig. 12C.4**).
2. The pedicled nasoseptal flap is then raised off the septum with a Freer elevator posteriorly until the sphenoid ostia and posterior choana are visible. Superiorly, the flap may be taken until about 0.5 to 1 cm below the skull base to preserve the olfactory function. Inferiorly, the flap can be taken as far as half the nasal floor if a large skull base defect is expected (Hadad-Bassagasteguy flap).
3. The nasoseptal flap is then freed with microscissors superiorly and inferiorly aiming for the sphenoid ostia and the posterior choana, respectively (**Fig. 12C.5** and **Fig. 12C.6**].
4. The exposed bony septum is fractured through to the contralateral side and removed by piecemeal, all the while freeing it from the overlying contralateral septal mucoperichondrium (**Fig. 12C.7**).
5. This is continued until the sphenoid keel is exposed with the sphenoid ostia visible bilaterally (**Fig. 12C.8**).

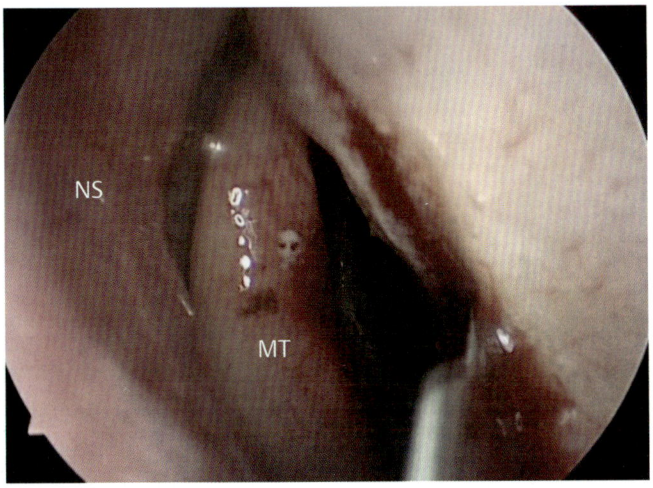

Fig. 12C.4 Vertical incision of the nasoseptal mucosa anterior to the middle turbinate down to the cartilaginous septum.

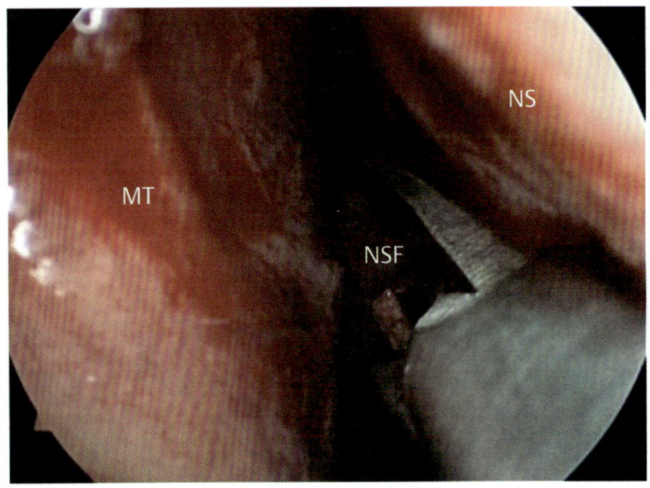

Fig. 12C.5 Superior horizontal cut for the pedicled nasoseptal flap (NSF) about 0.5 to 1 cm below the skull base.

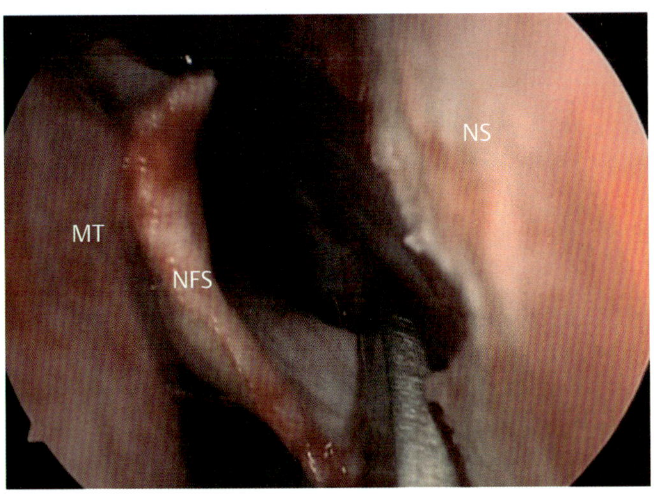

Fig. 12C.6 Inferior horizontal cut for the pedicled nasoseptal flap (NSF).

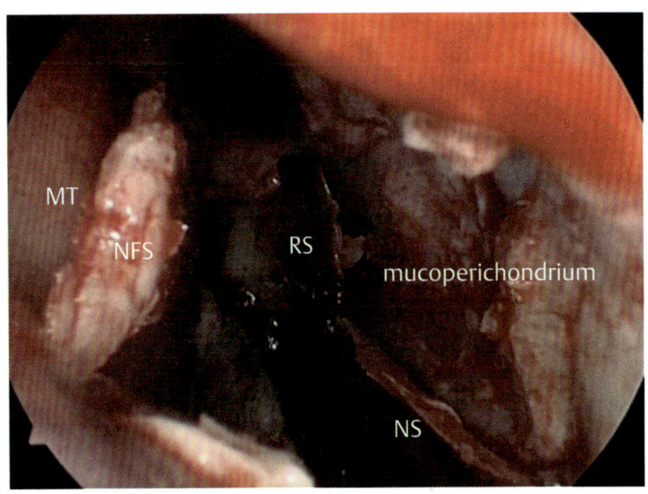

Fig. 12C.7 The posterior bony nasal septum (NS) has been removed and the contralateral mucoperichondrium is visible.

6. At this point, the contralateral nasoseptal flap can be created with the previously illustrated steps. Both pedicled nasoseptal flaps can be stored in the medial recess of the lower nasal cavity or the nasopharynx (**Fig. 12C.9**).
7. The sphenoid ostia are widened inferomedially using a Kerrison punch in a V-shaped manner toward the midline (**Fig. 12C.10**).
8. The sphenoid rostrum is removed with a pituitary rongeur forceps, either as one piece or in several pieces.
9. An unobstructed view of the sphenoid cavity and the planum sphenoidale is of special importance when a transplanum approach is planned. In this case, overhanging bony and mucosal tissues from either the posterior ethmoidal cells or the anterior wall of the sphenoid cavity have to be removed meticulously using a microdebrider (**Fig. 12C.11**).
10. The posterior wall of the sphenoid sinus is then demucosalized. This allows an overview of the sphenoid cavity and the neurovascular landmarks of the bony skull base (**Fig. 12C.12**). There may be dehiscence of the optic nerve or carotid artery, which should be identified by inspection of the sphenoid sinus and in depth knowledge of preoperative imaging.

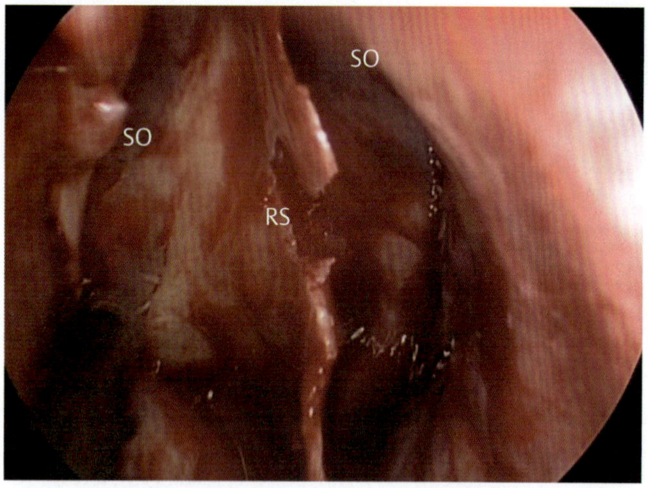

Fig. 12C.8 The rostrum sphenoidale (RS) is fully exposed with both sphenoid ostia (SO) in view.

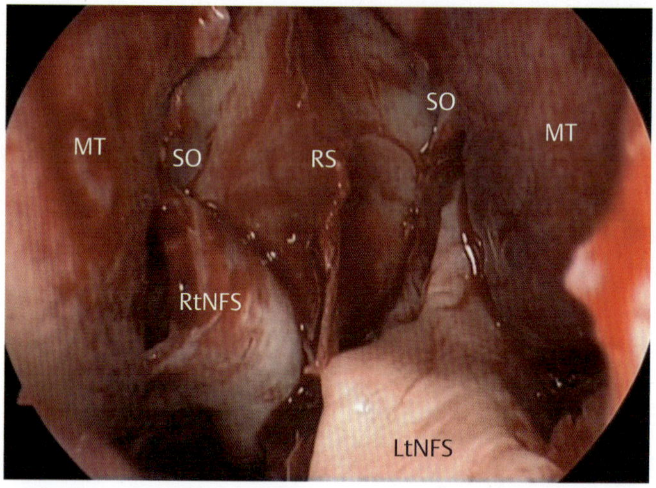

Fig. 12C.9 The right (RtNSF) and left nasoseptal flaps (LtNSF) are stored in the sphenoethmoidal recess.

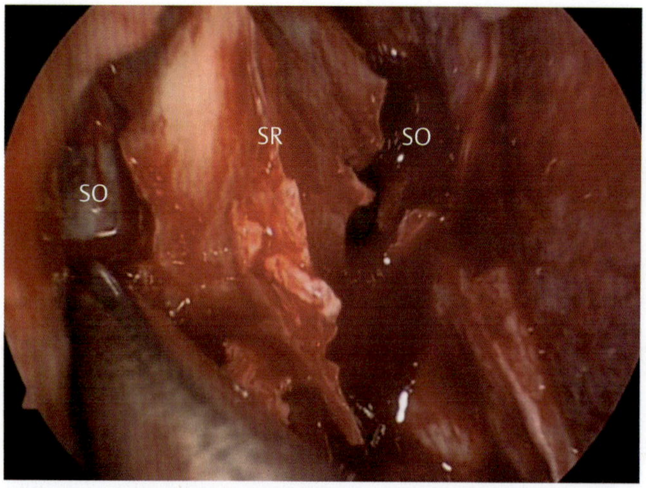

Fig. 12C.10 The sphenoid ostia (SO) are widened inferomedially using a Kerrison punch.

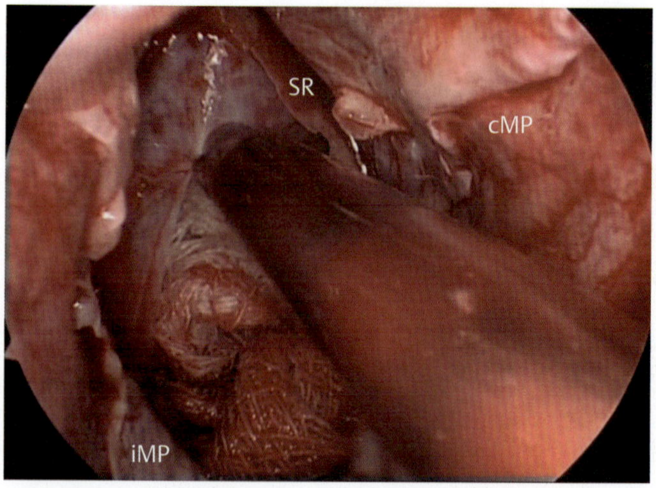

Fig. 12C.11 Mucosa (M) of the sphenoid cavity and bony remnants of the sphenoidal rostrum (SR) are removed using a microdebrider.

11. The planum sphenoidale has to be exposed sufficiently before the osteodural exposure of the meningioma is started (**Fig. 12C.13**).
12. The most anterior and lateral extension of the anterior lesion can be defined using image-guided surgery (IGS).
13. For the transplanum approach, the bony covering of the planum sphenoidale is thinned out using a high-speed diamond burr (**Fig. 12C.14**).
14. The thinned-out bone should be dissected away from the dura and a circumferential widening of the osteodural exposure can be continued. The use of Kerrison punches allows better control of the bone removal (**Fig. 12C.15** and **Fig. 12C.16a, b**).
15. In medium-to-large-sized meningiomas, sufficient osteodural exposure is mandatory to "release" the tumor. This will facilitate internal debulking of the anterior portion and facilitate extracapsular dissection of the anterior pole during the later stages. Hence, the wide opening of the planum sphenoidale is continued posteriorly toward the tuberculum sellae (**Fig. 12C.17a, b**).

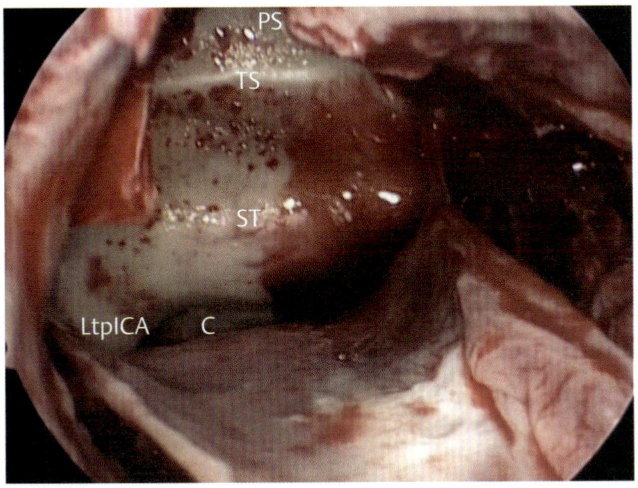

Fig. 12C.12 Demucolarization of the sphenoid cavity.

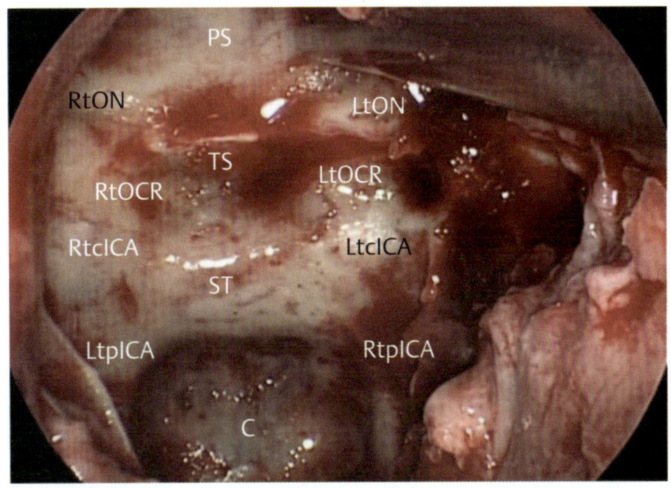

Fig. 12C.13 Identification of the planum sphenoidale (PS) and the neurovascular landmarks of the skull base: sella turcica (ST), tuberculum sellae (TS), left optic nerve (LtON), right optic nerve (RtON), left (LtcICA) and right cavernous internal carotid arteries (RtcICA); left (LtOCR) and right opticocarotid recess (RtOCR); left (LtpICA) and right paraclival internal carotid arteries (RtpICA).

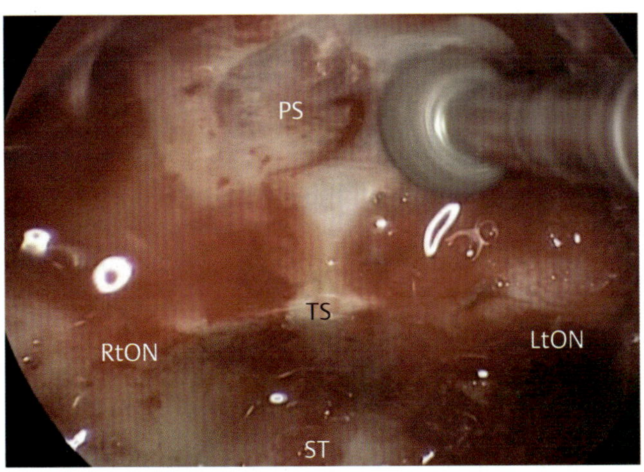

Fig. 12C.14 Transplanum approach. The bone covering the planum sphenoidale (PS) is removed using a high-speed diamond burr (Medtronic, Minneapolis, MN).

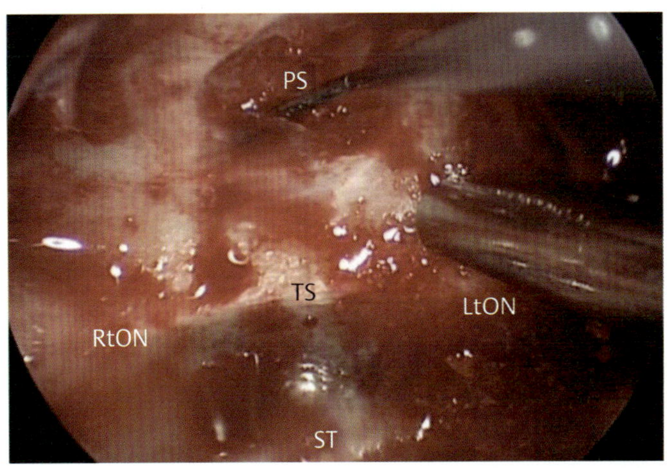

Fig. 12C.15 Transplanum approach. The thinned-out bone is dissected from the dura with a blunt hooked instrument and can be flicked off.

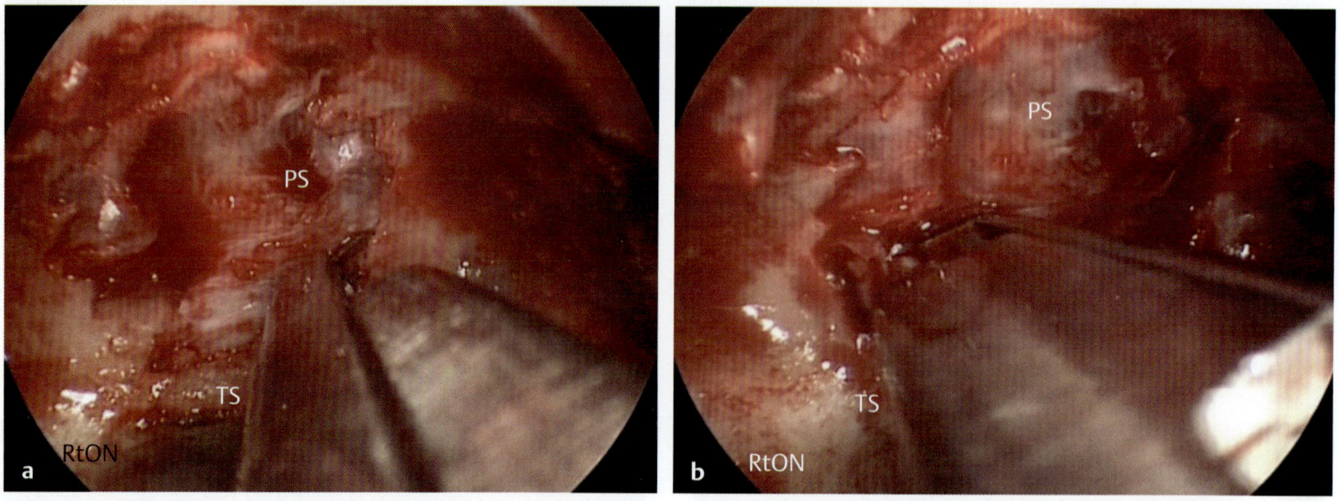

Fig. 12C.16 (a, b) Transplanum approach. The osteodural exposure is widened using a Kerrison punch. The laterality of left and right sides is verified with image-guided surgery.

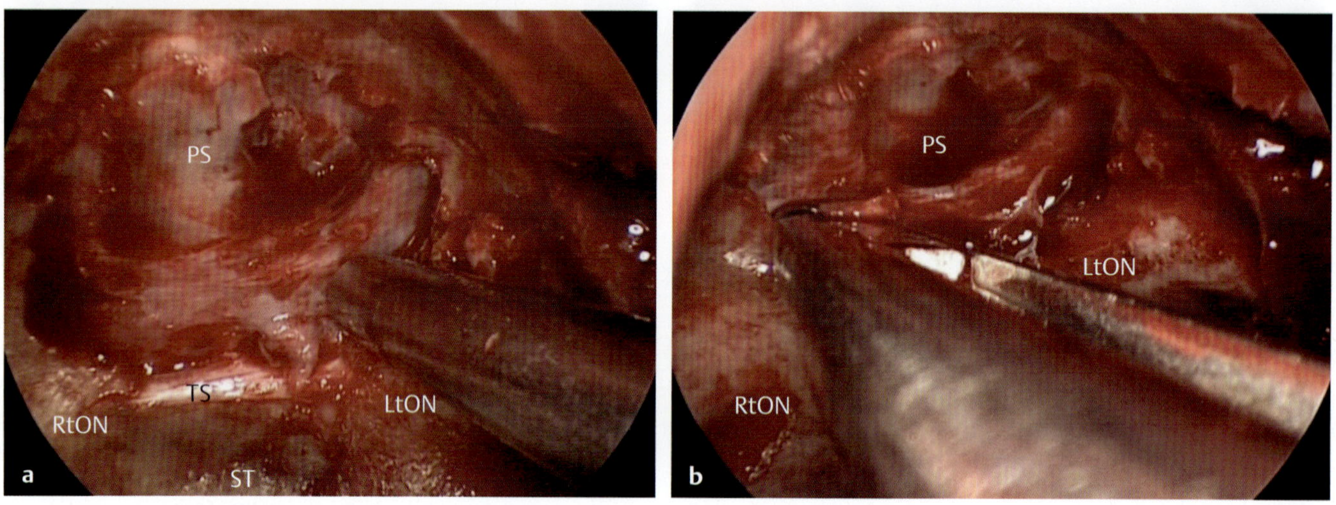

Fig. 12C.17 (a, b) Transplanum approach. The laterality of the osteodural exposure is continued posteriorly toward the tuberculum sellae (TS).

16. For the transsellar and transtuberculum approach, the bone of the tuberculum sellae and the bony coverage of the anterior intercavernous sinus are thinned out with a high-seed diamond burr. The drilling can be continued to the bone covering the sella turcica, when a relevant bone thickness is expected. This can be appreciated with the tip of suction or a dissecting instrument (**Fig. 12C.18**).
17. To facilitate the removal of the tuberculum sellae, the osteodural exposure of the sella turcica is done first. This allows to define a plane between the tubercular bone and the dura covering the intercavernous sinus (**Fig. 12C.19**).
18. The tubercular bone is removed by piecemeal using Kerrison's punches and continued to define the osteodural exposure cranially. If the tubercular bone has a relevant thickness, reduction with a high-speed diamond drill might be mandatory (**Fig. 12C.20**, **Fig. 12C.21**, and **Fig. 12C.22**).
19. When removing the bony covering of the anterior intercavernous sinus, venous bleeding has to be expected. Hemostatic agents precisely delivered to the point of bleeding with simultaneous pressure, and suction through a device tip (Taming Sari, V. Waran, Kuala Lumpur, Malaysia.) allows controlled management of the bleeding (**Fig. 12C.23** and **Fig. 12C.24**).

20. Removal of the lateral aspects of the tuberculum sellae allows for sufficient osteodural exposure and "release" of the meningioma in the posterior aspects. This will facilitate internal debulking of the posterior portion and extracapsular dissection along the brain–tumor interface in a later stage (**Fig. 12C.25**).
21. Using IGS, the anterior and lateral osteodural exposure has to be verified following the principle of a tailored approach with zonal dissection of the skull base. For a sufficient tumor release, a widening of the bony exposure might be necessary (**Fig. 12C.26, Fig. 12C.27,** and **Fig. 12C.28**).
22. Dural opening is started at the planum sphenoidale in a T-shaped manner. Using a dissecting instrument and microscissors, the most anterior extension of the tumor has to be identified and an arachnoid layer has to be visible. This might need an anterior extension of the dural opening (**Fig. 12C.29, Fig. 12C.30, Fig. 12C.31,** and **Fig. 12C.32**).
23. The dural opening is extended posteriorly to the tuberculum sellae and the anterior intercavernous sinus after freeing the underlying tissue using a right-angle dissector (**Fig. 12C.33**).

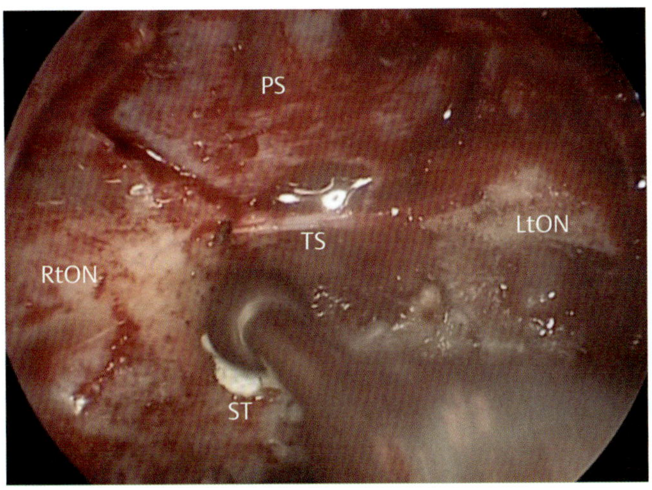

Fig. 12C.18 Transsellar approach. The bone over the sella turcica (ST) is thinned out using a high-speed diamond burr.

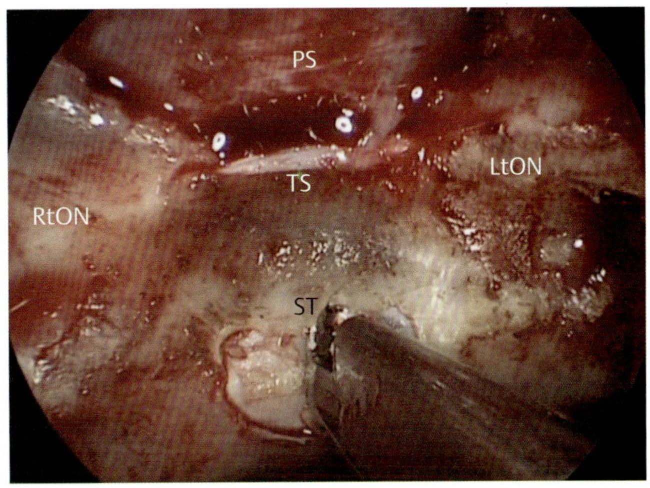

Fig. 12C.19 Transsellar approach. Osteodural exposure of the sella turcica (ST) with a Kerrison punch.

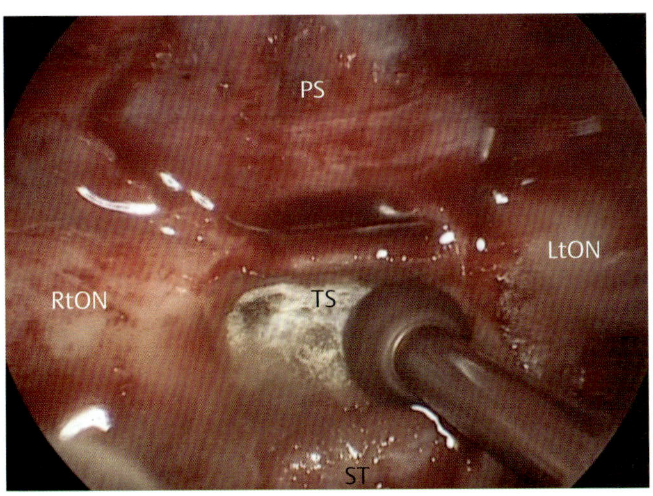

Fig. 12C.20 Transtuberculum approach. The bone over the sella turcica (ST) is thinned out using a high-speed diamond burr.

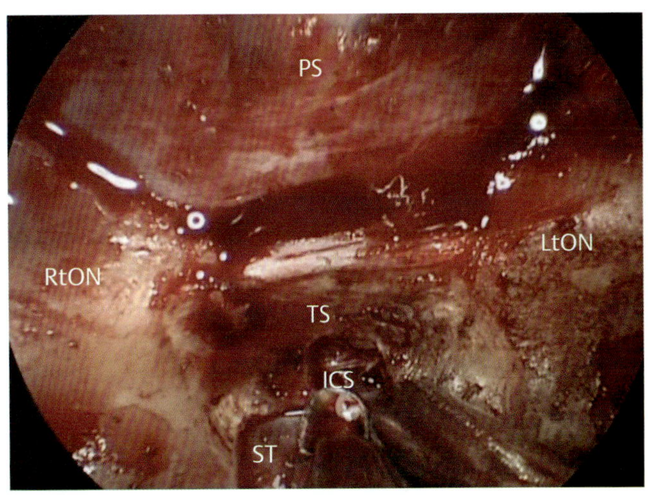

Fig. 12C.21 Transtuberculum approach. The thinned-out bone is removed from a caudal to cranial direction. Hemostatic agents should be ready to use, when venous bleeding from the anterior intercavernous sinus (ICS) occurs.

24. Initial internal tumor debulking using suction or an ultrasonic aspirator with high power and low suction is started in the anterior portion of the tumor. The initial debulking should not be too aggressive and the tumor capsule should not be breached.
25. The anterior extracapsular dissection is started from the most anterior point sideways bilaterally and continued posteriorly.
26. The dura of the sella turcica is then opened using a reversed T-shaped cut. Careful cranial continuation of the incision is necessary to not open the anterior intercavernous sinus (**Fig. 12C.34** and **Fig. 12C.35**).
27. This maneuver brings the pituitary gland and infundibular stalk into view, and definition of a posterior arachnoid dissection plane leading to the posterior brain–tumor interface is possible (**Fig. 12C.36**).
28. Meticulous coagulation and division of the anterior intercavernous sinus is necessary to connect the planum sphenoidale with the sellar region. For this maneuver, the dural structure is freed with a right angle dissector, controlled with bipolar cautery, and divided using a microscissors to expose the entire lesion (**Fig. 12C.37, Fig. 12C.38, Fig. 12C.39,** and **Fig. 12C.40**).

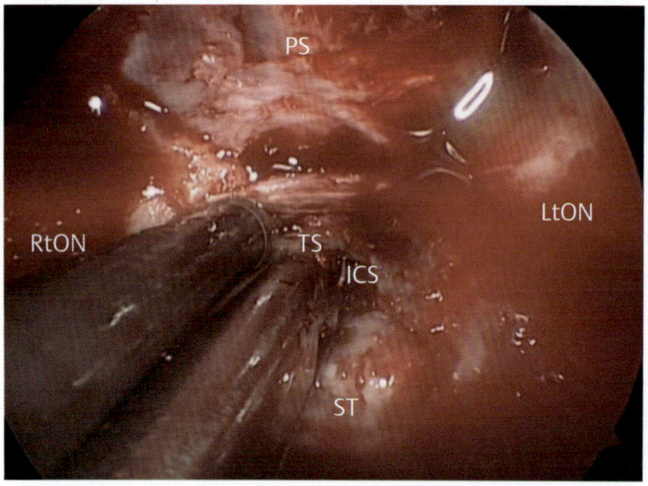

Fig. 12C.22 Transtuberculum approach. Removal of the bone bridge connects the transplanum and the transtuberculum osteodural exposure.

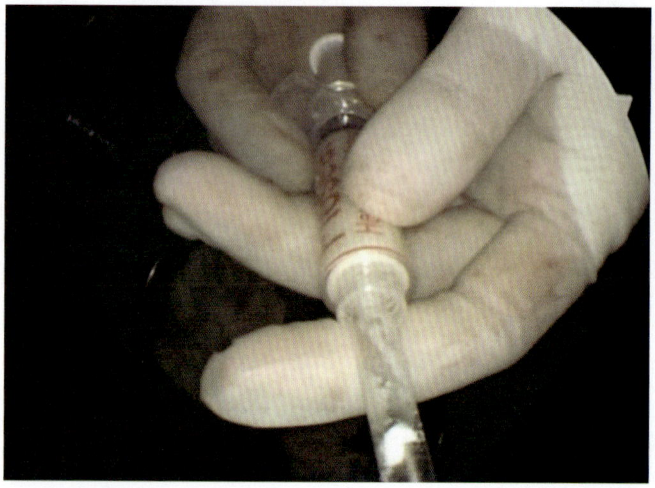

Fig. 12C.23 Hemostatic agents are filled into the applicator of the Taming Sari device (V. Waran, Kuala Lumpur, Malaysia). Hemostatic agents should be ready to use when venous bleeding from the anterior intercavernous sinus (ICS) occurs.

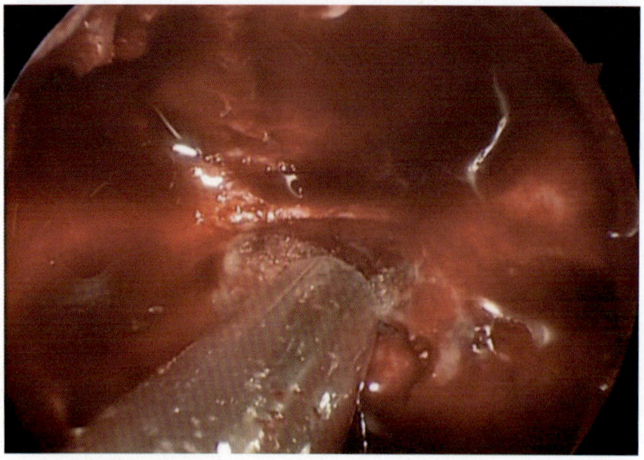

Fig. 12C.24 The tip of the applicator is brought precisely to the point of bleeding, and the hemostatic agent is delivered with light pressure through a cottonoid.

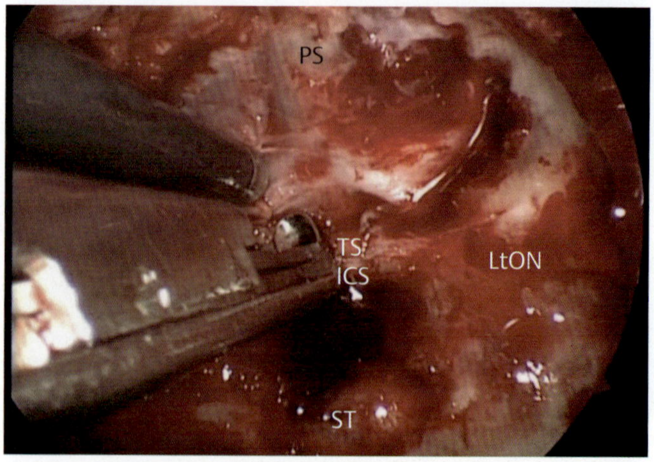

Fig. 12C.25 Removal of the right lateral tuberculum sellae (TS).

29. Interior debulking of the posterior and tubercular portion of the tumor is then continued using an ultrasonic aspirator and a suction device (**Fig. 12C.41**).
30. The extracapsular dissection using the arachnoid layer along the brain–tumor interface is continued bilaterally posteriorly. This might need a two-surgeon three-hand or two-surgeon four-hand technique to define a dissection plane and allowing bimanual microsurgical dissection by the neurosurgeon (**Fig. 12C.42** and **Fig. 12C.43**).
31. The arachnoid layer protects the arterial vessels from the tumor interface when strictly following the plane and no vascular encasement is seen in the preoperative imaging. Cauterization of the arachnoid or the tumor capsule is not recommended to not lose this dissection plane (**Fig. 12C.44**).
32. The lateral tumor aspects of the tubercular portion are in anatomical relation with the optic nerve and the clinoidal portion of the carotid artery. Removal of these parts needs microsurgical dissection, the use of an olive-tipped maxillary J-sucker and ultrasonic aspiration (**Fig. 12C.45, Fig. 12C.46, Fig. 12C.47,** and **Fig. 12C.48**).

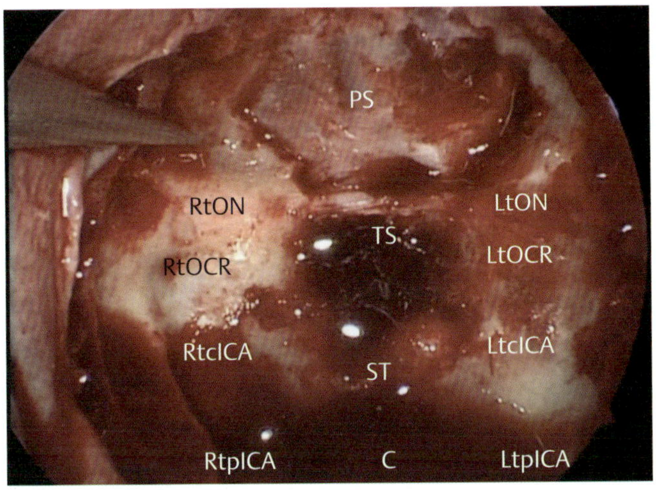

Fig. 12C.26 Verification of the osteodural exposure with image-guided surgery. The laterality of the transplanum and transtuberculum osteodural exposure has to be sufficient to "release" the meningioma.

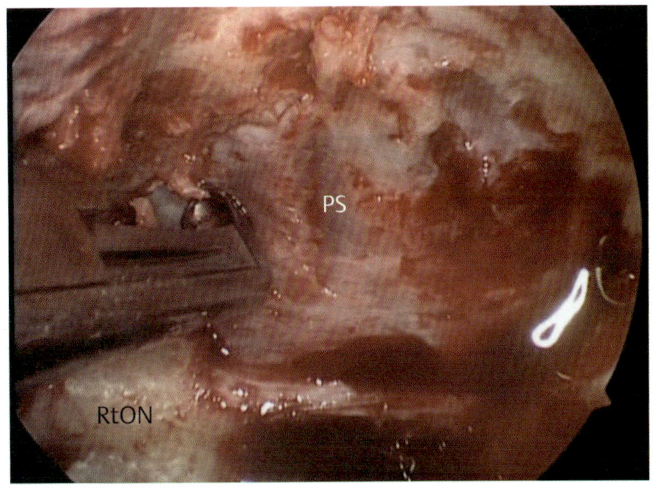

Fig. 12C.27 Right lateral extension of the transplanum osteodural exposure according to image guidance.

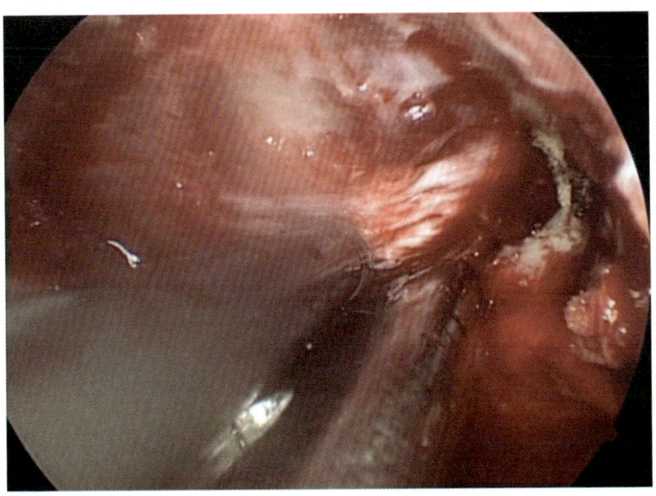

Fig. 12C.28 Left lateral extension of the transplanum osteodural exposure according to image guidance.

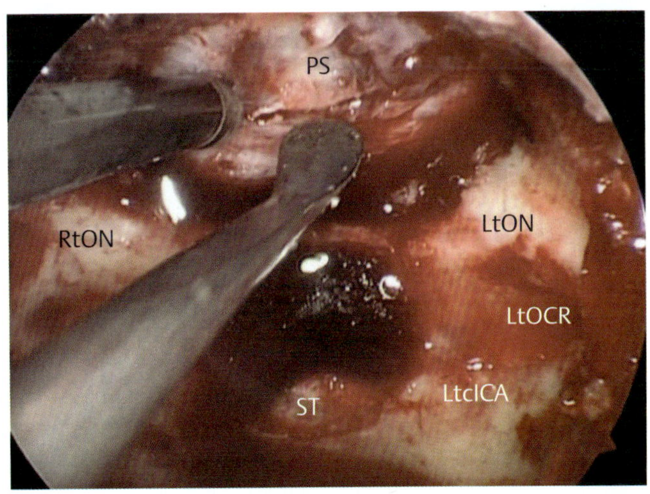

Fig. 12C.29 Dural opening is started at the most anterior extension of the tumor at the planum sphenoidale in a T-shaped manner.

33. The defined arachnoid layer between the pituitary gland and the infundibular stalk is used to define the posterior brain–tumor interface and remove the posterior pole of the tubercular and sellar portion (**Fig. 12C.49** and **Fig. 12C.50**).
34. Parts of the meningioma might breach the dural layer. These nodular remnants have to be dissected from the arachnoid membranes and removed microsurgically. As there is no protecting tissue layer, smaller or larger arterial vessels can be attached to these tumor parts. Hence, dissection has to be very careful with preservation of these vessels (**Fig. 12C.51, Fig. 12C.52, Fig. 12C.53,** and **Fig. 12C.54**).
35. The optic nerves, the optic chiasm, the pre- and post-communicating segments of both anterior cerebral arteries, the anterior communicating artery, and both recurrent arteries of Heubner have to be considered and preserved, when the superior aspect of the posterior portion is resected (**Fig. 12C.55** and **12C.56**).
36. The defect is plugged with an abdominal fat graft, and the edges of the fat are brought intracranially to create a watertight seal. Care is taken not to pack too much fat tightly into the cavity (**Fig. 12C.57**).

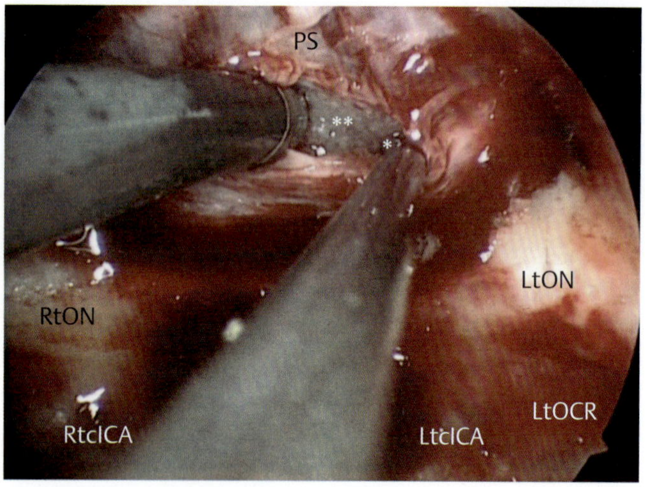

Fig. 12C.30 Definition of a plane (*) between the meningioma (**) and the dura of the planum sphenoidale (PS). An arachnoid plane is not visible.

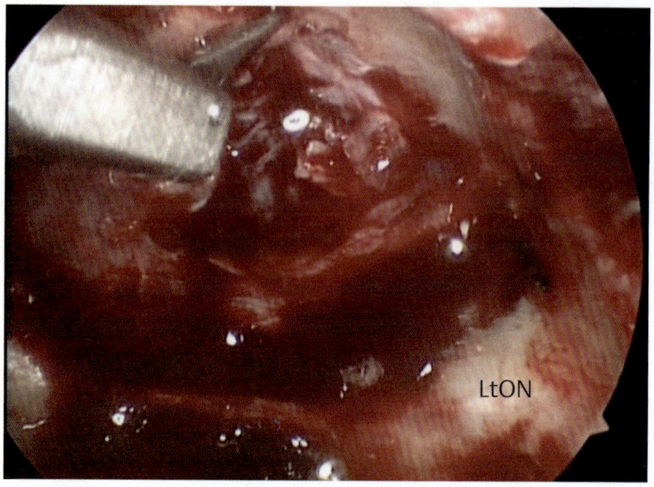

Fig. 12C.31 Dural opening is continued anteriorly to the most anterior extension of the tumor.

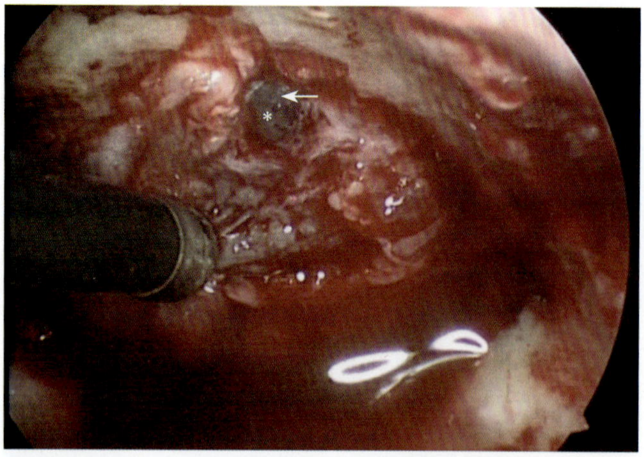

Fig. 12C.32 The most anterior extension of the tumor can be appreciated when the arachnoid dura (*arrow*) and the arachnoid space (*) are visible.

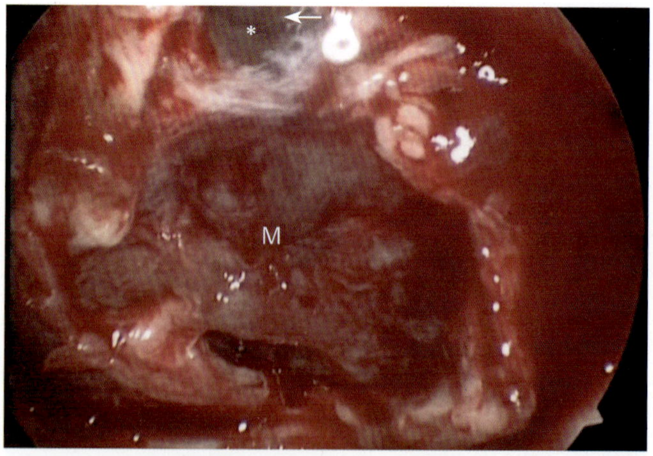

Fig. 12C.33 The dural opening is continued posteriorly along the midline (T shape) to expose the anterior portion of the meningioma (M). Posterior limitation is the dura next to the anterior intercavernous sinus. Arachnoid dura (*arrow*) and arachnoid space (*).

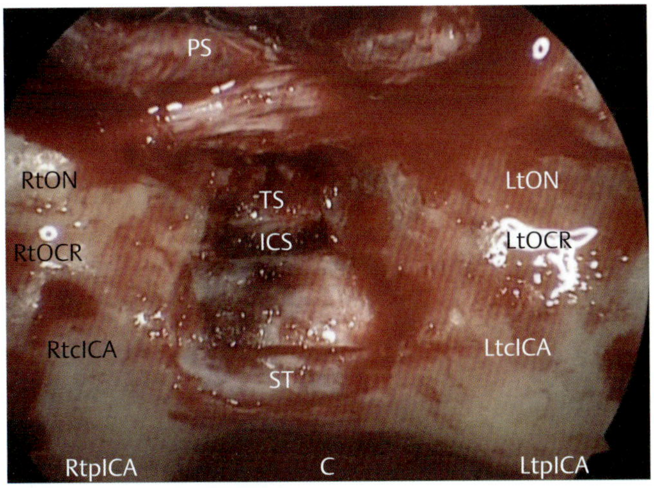

Fig. 12C.34 Horizontal incision of the dura covering the sella turcica (ST).

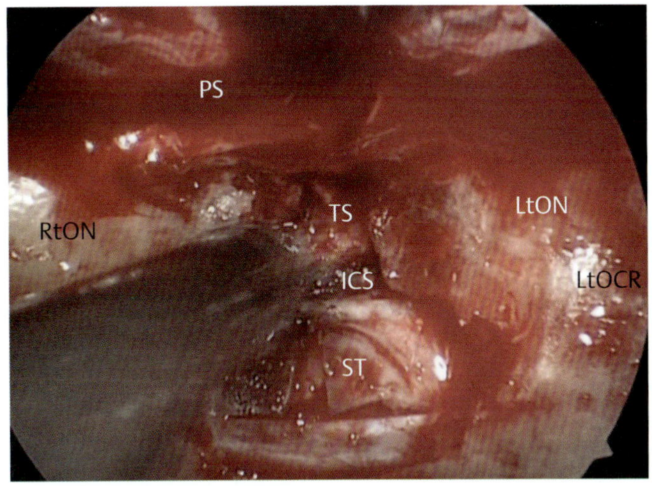

Fig. 12C.35 Vertical incision of the dura covering the sella turcica (reversed T shape). Superior limitation is the anterior intercavernous sinus (ICS).

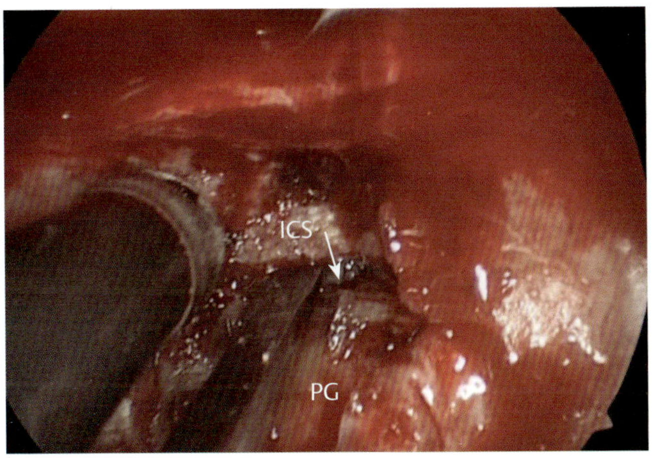

Fig. 12C.36 Definition of the brain–tumor interface (*arrow*) between the pituitary gland (PG) and the inferior anterior pole of the tuberculum sellae meningioma.

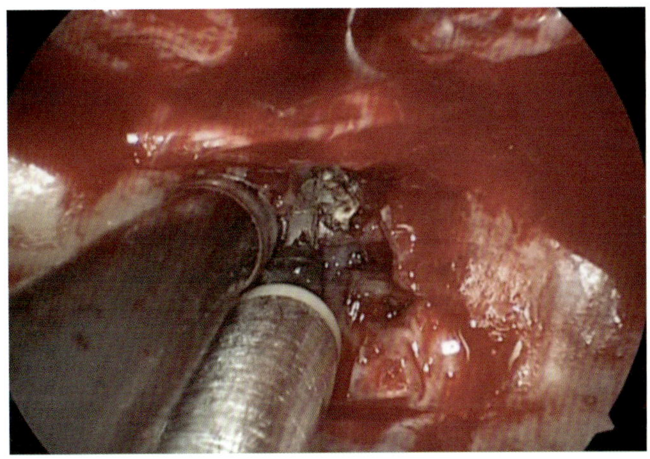

Fig. 12C.37 Cauterization of the anterior intercavernous sinus.

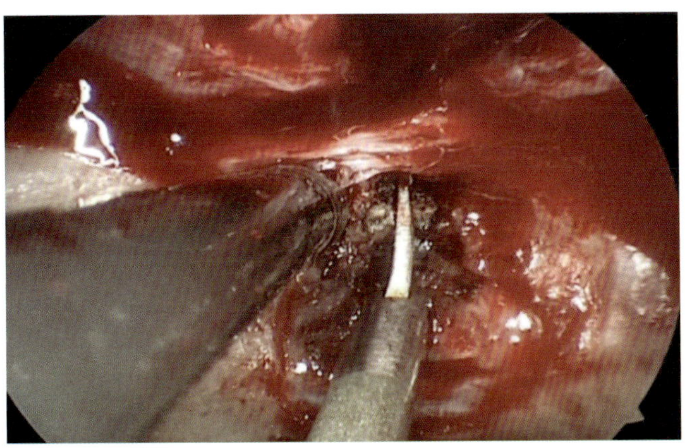

Fig. 12C.38 Division of the anterior intercavernous sinus.

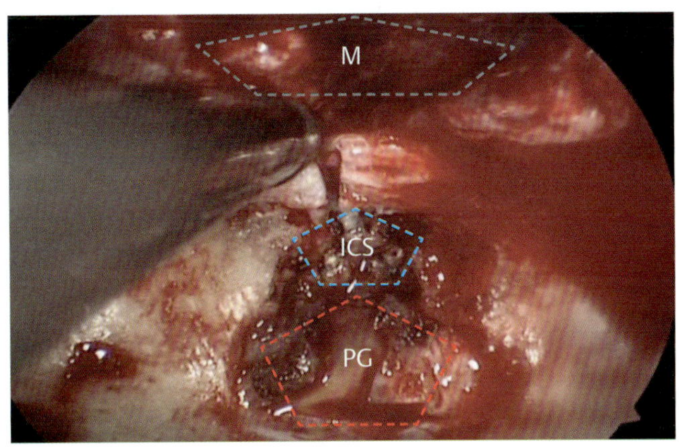

Fig. 12C.39 Connection of the dural opening between the transplanum (*gray pentagon*), transtuberculum (*blue pentagon*), and transsellar (*red pentagon*) approach.

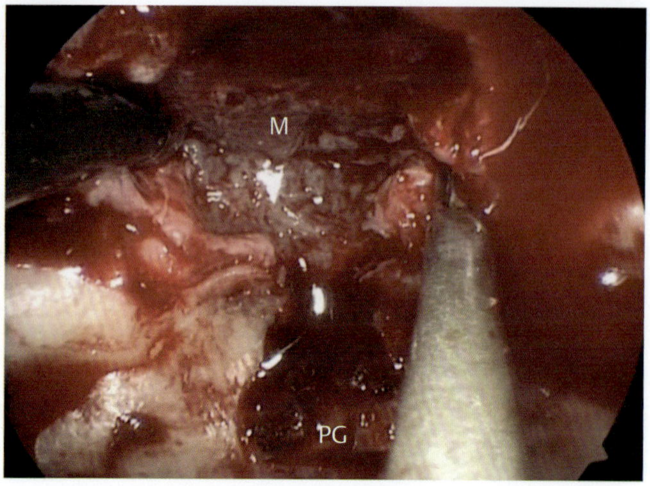

Fig. 12C.40 The wide osteodural opening "releases" the meningioma (M) prior to internal tumor debulking and facilitates extracapsular dissection.

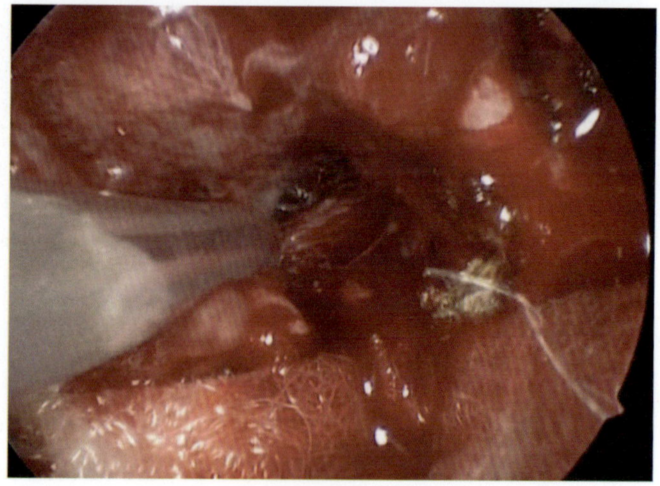

Fig. 12C.41 Internal tumor debulking using a long small ultrasonic aspirator.

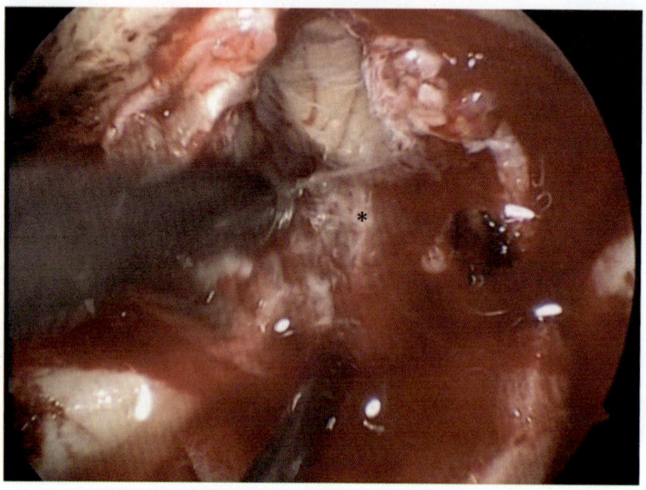

Fig. 12C.42 Extracapsular dissection along the brain–tumor interface from anterior to posterior and sideways bilaterally. The arachnoid layer (*) is used to continue the bimanual microdissection posteriorly.

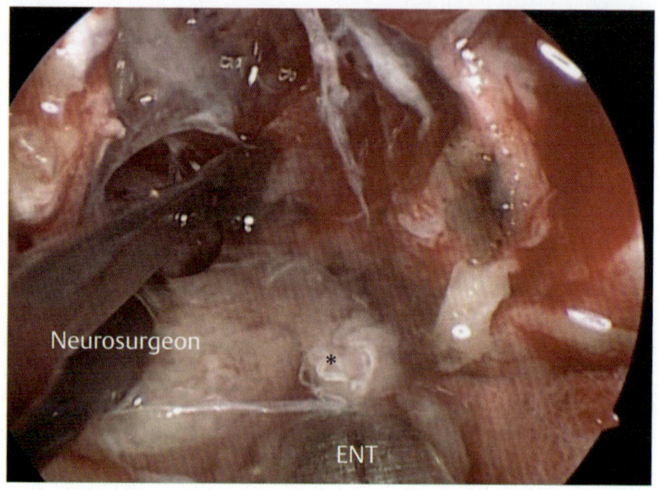

Fig. 12C.43 Extracapsular dissection of the brain–tumor interface along the superior aspect of the tubercular portion of the meningioma. The two-surgeon four-hand technique allows the ear, nose, and throat surgeon (ENT) to present the arachnoid dissection plane (*), while the neurosurgeon can perform a bimanual microdissection and tumor removal with a microdissector and suction.

37. This is sealed with a synthetic dural sealant and layered with an absorbable hemostat (**Fig. 12C.58**).
38. The bilateral vascularized nasoseptal flaps are rotated over the defect to complete the repair and are reinforced with gelatine sponges to keep the flaps in position. No other nasal packing is required (**Fig. 12C.59** and **12C.60**).

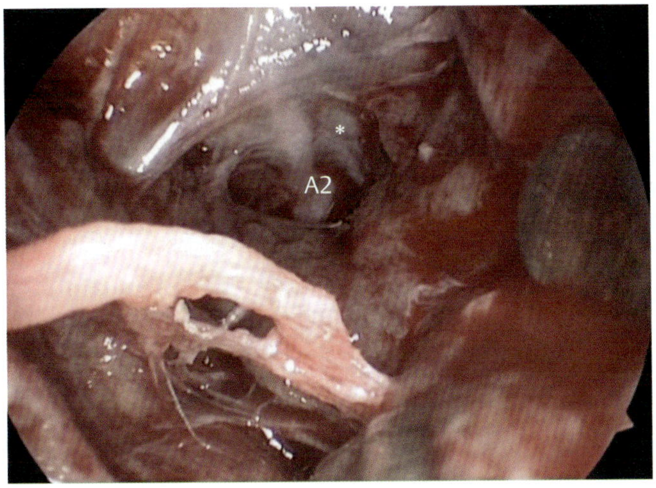

Fig. 12C.44 Extracapsular dissection of the brain–tumor interface and removal of the tubercular portion of the meningioma. The arachnoid dura (*) is intact and the distal anterior cerebral arteries (A2) come into view.

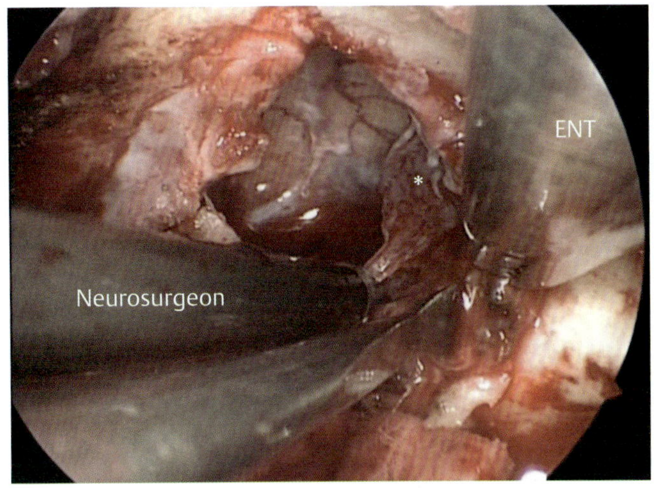

Fig. 12C.45 Removal of the left lateral tubercular portion of the meningioma (*). The two-surgeon four-hand technique allows the ear, nose, and throat surgeon (ENT) to present the arachnoid dissection plane (*), while the neurosurgeon can perform a bimanual dissector and tumor removal with a microdissector and suction.

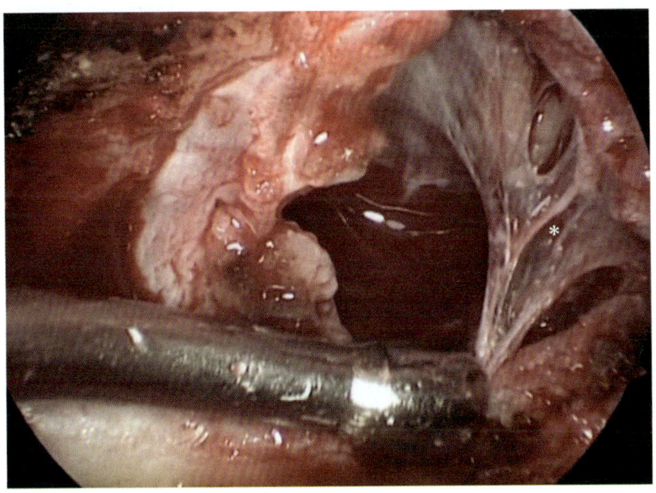

Fig. 12C.46 An olive-tipped maxillary suction is used to remove the left lateral tubercular portion of the meningioma (*).

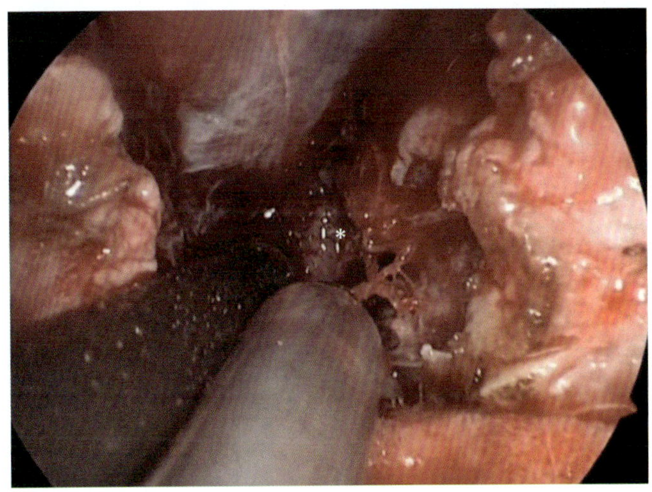

Fig. 12C.47 Bimanual ultrasonic aspiration and suction is used to remove the left lateral tubercular portion of the meningioma (*).

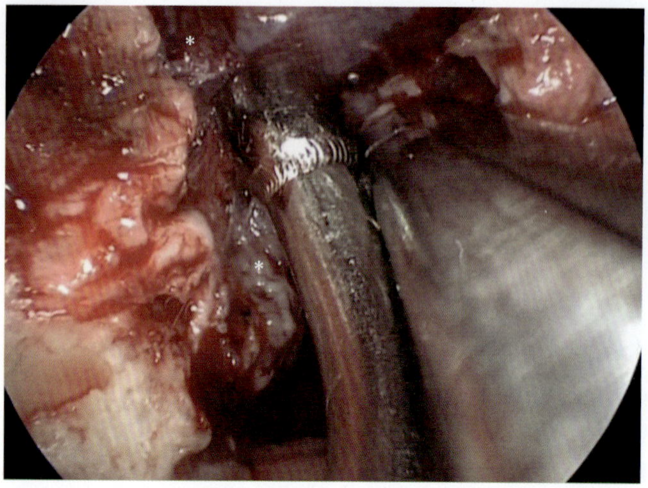

Fig. 12C.48 An olive-tipped maxillary suction is used to remove the right lateral tubercular portion of the meningioma (*).

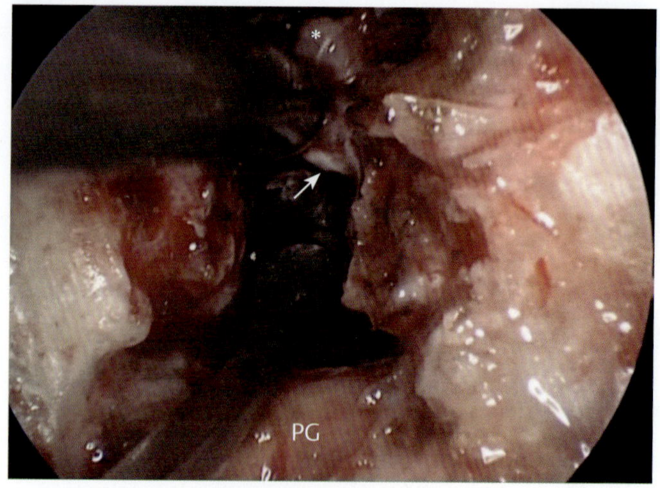

Fig. 12C.49 The posterior inferior tubercular portion is removed using the brain–tumor interface (*arrow*) between the meningioma (*) and the pituitary gland (PG).

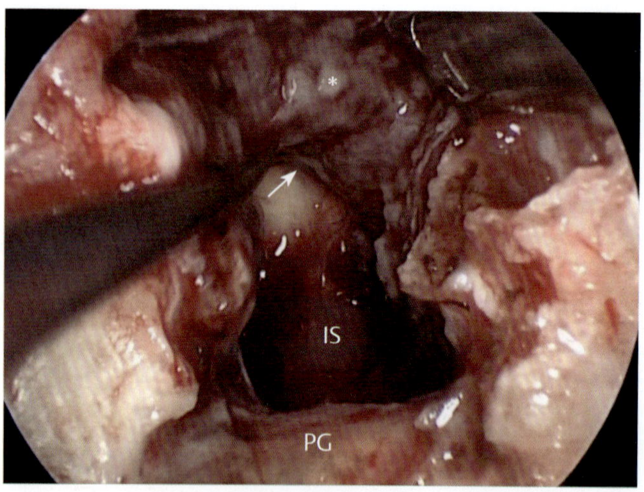

Fig. 12C.50 The posterior inferior tubercular portion is removed using the brain–tumor interface (*arrow*) between the meningioma (*), the pituitary gland (PG), and the infundibular stalk (IS).

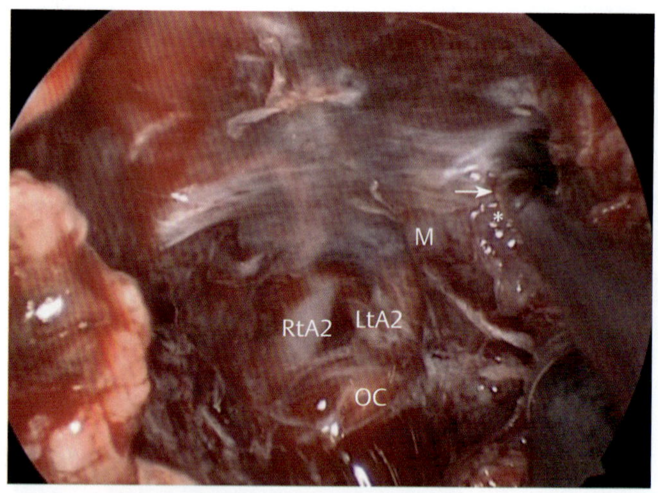

Fig. 12C.51 The tubercular portion of the meningioma (*) is removed following the brain–tumor interface (*arrow*) between the meningioma and the arachnoid plane covering the neurovascular structures of the suprasellar (chiasmatic) cistern. Meningioma remnants breaching the dural plane (M) are visible on both sides.

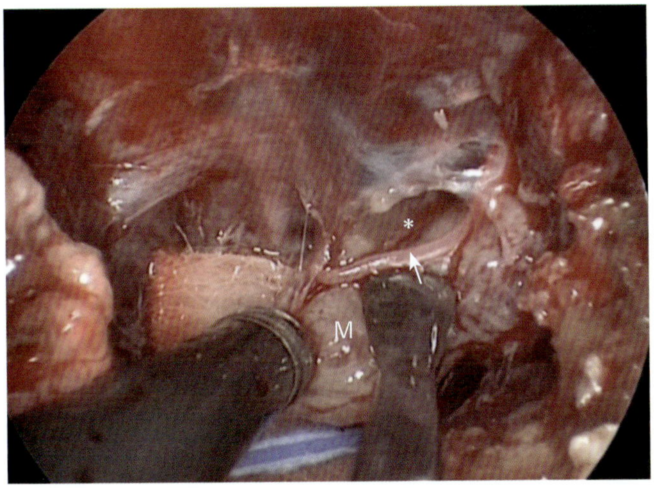

Fig. 12C.52 A left nodular extension of the meningioma (M) breaching through the arachnoid layer (*) is adherent to small arterial vessels (perforating artery, recurrent artery of Heubner) (*arrow*). Hence, careful and meticulous dissection and removal of these tumor parts is necessary.

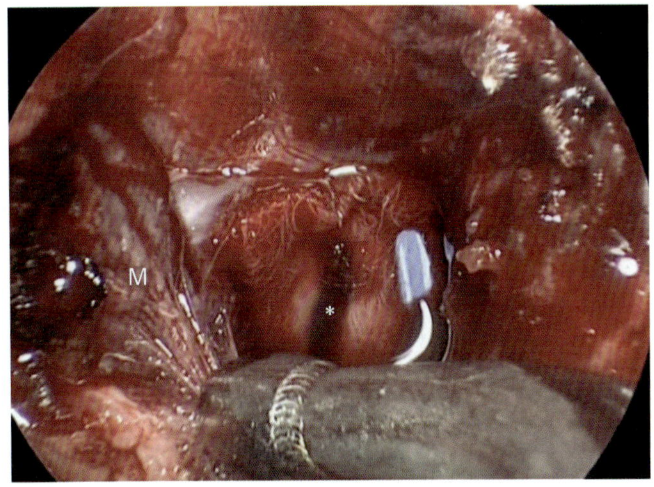

Fig. 12C.53 Removal of the right lateral tubercular portion of the meningioma (M) with an olive-tipped J-sucker. A cottonoid (*) has been placed to protect the neurovascular structures of the chiasmatic cistern.

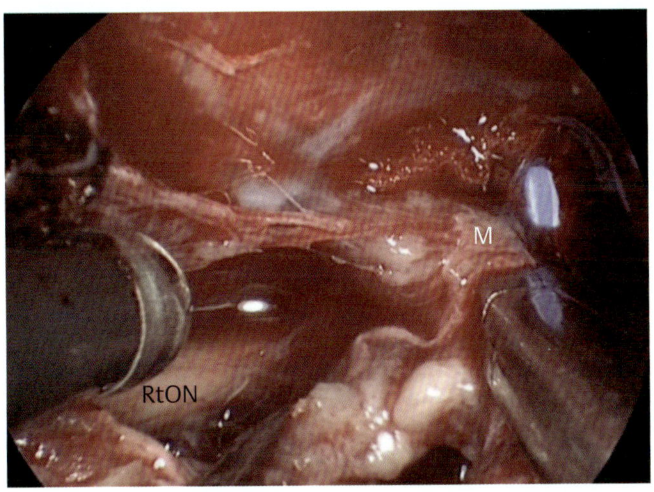

Fig. 12C.54 Removal of the left lateral tubercular portion of the meningioma (M) with the two-surgeon three-hand technique. The ENT surgeon presents the dissecting plane to the neurosurgeon by holding the tumor with a grasping instrument. The right optic nerve (RtON) is revealed.

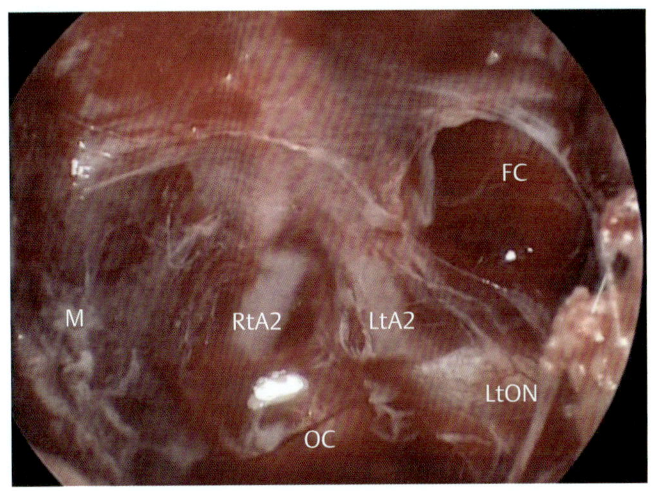

Fig. 12C.55 Removal of the right nodular extension reveals the left optic nerve (LtON).

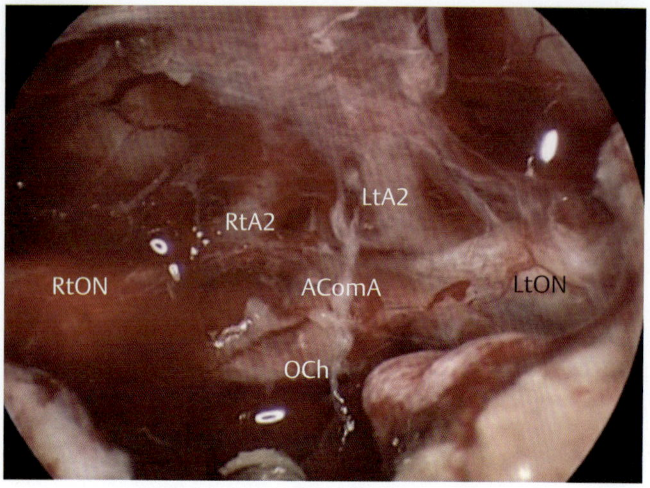

Fig. 12C.56 Inspection of the tumor resection cavity. Postcommunicating segments of the left anterior cerebral artery (LtA2), right distal anterior cerebral artery (RtA2), anterior communicating artery (AComA), left optic nerve (LtON), right optic nerve (RtON), optic chiasm (OCh).

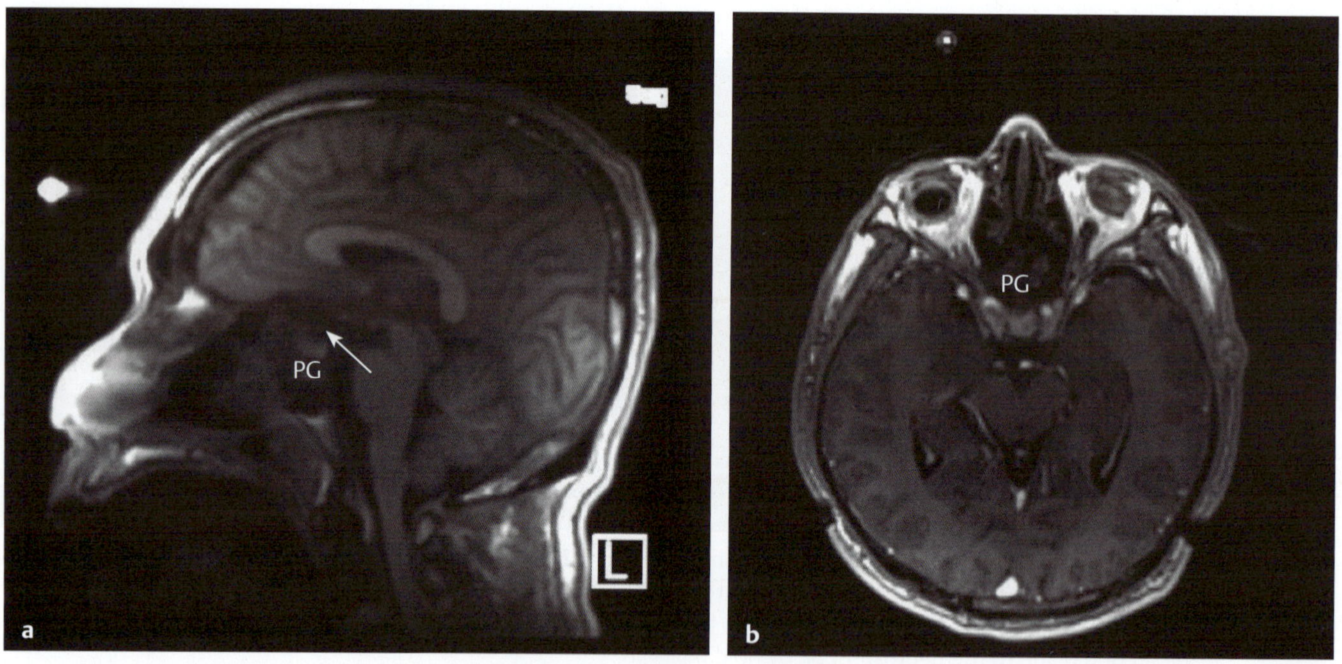

Fig. 12C.57 **(a)** Sagittal intraoperative T1–noncontrast-enhanced and **(b)** axial T1 contrast-enhanced MRI sections demonstrating complete resection of the meningioma with the pituitary gland (PG) and the infundibular stalk (*arrow*) in physiological position.

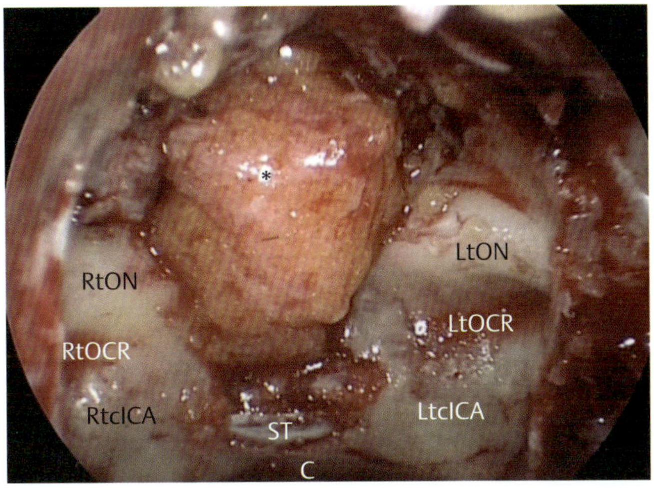

Fig. 12C.58 The anterior skull base defect is closed using intradural autologous abdominal fat graft (*). The construct is stabilized using Surgicel.

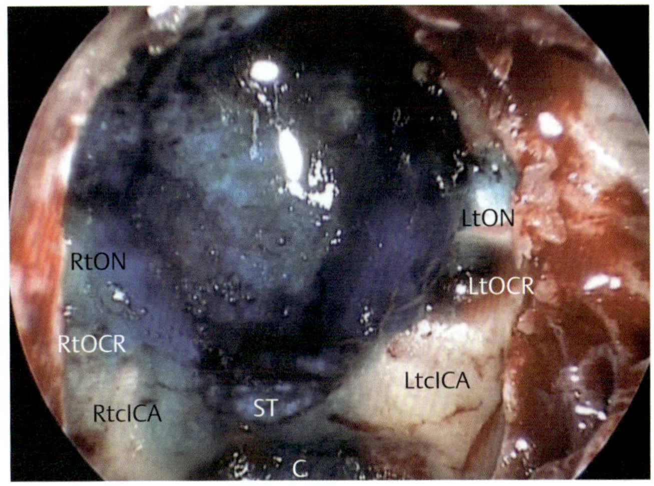

Fig. 12C.59 The whole skull base reconstruction is sealed with an artificial dural sealant system.

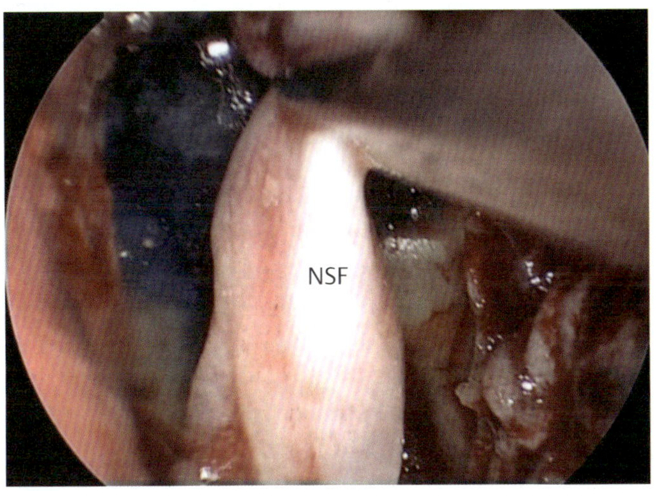

Fig. 12C.60 The harvested right- and left-sided pedicled nasoseptal flaps (NSF) are carefully placed over the construct.

Case 12D

A Tailored Endonasal Endoscopic Approach for a Large Tuberculum Sellae Meningioma

Michel Roethlisberger, Prepageran Narayanan, and Vicknes Waran

History

A 44-year-old man was assessed because of frontal headaches and a slowly progressive loss of vision. Ophthalmological examination revealed a right-sided unilateral temporal field defect. The endocrinological examination did not reveal any hormonal abnormalities.

Contrast-enhanced magnetic resonance imaging (MRI) confirmed a large homogeneously enhancing T1- and T2-isointense extra-axial suprasellar lesion involving the tuberculum sellae and the planum sphenoidale in close contact with the anterior cerebral artery complex. Dislocation of the chiasma opticum and the optic nerves was found to correlate with the ophthalmological symptoms (**Fig. 12D.1a–d**).

The lesion was considered amenable for a binostril endonasal endoscopic transsphenoidal resection using a transsphenoidal transplanum transtuberculum approach with image-guided surgery (IGS).

Surgical Steps

1. A binostril transsphenoidal approach with elevation of bilateral pedicled nasoseptal flaps is performed as previously described.
2. The planum sphenoidale has to be exposed sufficiently prior to starting the osteodural exposure of the meningioma.
3. The most anterior and lateral extension of the lesion can be defined using IGS.
4. For the transsellar and transtuberculum approach, the bone of the tuberculum sellae and the bony coverage of the anterior intercavernous sinus are thinned out with a high-seed diamond burr. The drilling can be continued to the bone covering the sella turcica, when a relevant bone thickness is expected (**Fig. 12D.2**).
5. The thinned-out bone should be dissected away from the dura, and a circumferential widening of the osteodural exposure can be continued (**Fig. 12D.3**).
6. For large tuberculum sellae meningiomas, a sufficient osteodural exposure is mandatory to "release" the tumor. This will facilitate internal debulking of the anterior portion and extracapsular dissection of the anterior pole in a later stage.
7. To facilitate the removal of the tuberculum sellae, the osteodural exposure of the sella turcica is done first. This allows to define a plane between the tubercular bone and the dura covering the intercavernous sinus (**Fig. 12D.4a**).
8. The tubercular bone is removed by piecemeal using Kerrison's punches and continuing to define a dural plane cranially. Removal of the lateral aspects of the tuberculum sellae allows a sufficient osteodural exposure and "release" of the meningioma in the posterior aspects. This will facilitate the internal debulking of the posterior portion and extracapsular dissection along the brain–tumor interface in a later stage (**Fig. 12D.4b** and **Fig. 12D.5**).
9. Using IGS, the anterior and lateral osteodural exposure has to be verified to assure a sufficient tumor release. The dural opening is started at the planum sphenoidale in a T-shaped manner (**Fig. 12D.6**).
10. Using a dissecting instrument and microscissors, the most anterior extension of the tumor has to be identified and an arachnoid layer has to be visible. This might need an anterior extension of the dural opening (**Fig. 12D.7**).
11. The dural opening is extended posteriorly to the tuberculum sellae and the anterior intercavernous sinus after freeing the underlying tissue using a right-angle dissector.
12. The dura of the sella turcica is then opened using a reversed T-shaped cut (**Fig. 12D.8a, b**).
13. Careful cranial continuation of the incision is necessary to not accidentally open the anterior intercavernous sinus (**Fig. 12D.9**).
14. Meticulous coagulation and division of the anterior intercavernous sinus is necessary to connect the planum sphenoidale with the sellar region. For this maneuver, the dural structure is freed with a right-angle dissector, controlled with bipolar cautery and divided using a microscissors (**Fig. 12D.10** and **Fig. 12D.11a, b**).

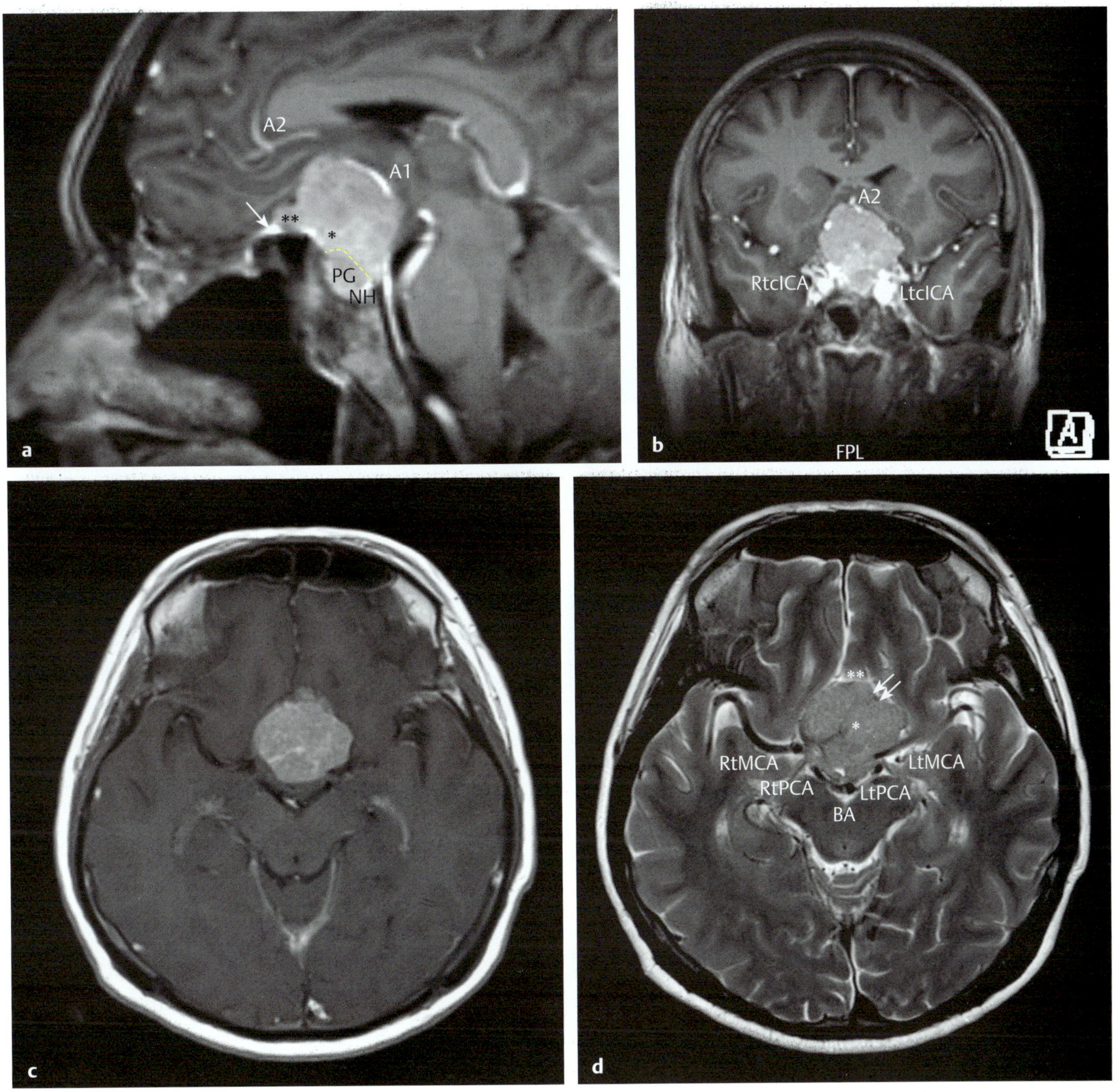

Fig. 12D.1 **(a)** Sagittal and **(b)** coronal T1-weighted gadolinium contrast-enhanced, **(c)** axial T2-weighted fluid-attenuated inversion recovery (FLAIR), **(d)** axial T2-weighted MRI section. A homogeneous, enhancing, and T2-isointense extra-axial solid mass on the tuberculum sellae (*) and planum sphenoidale (**) can be appreciated. A typical dural tail is present (*arrow*). The apex is in contact with the pre- (A1) and postcommunicating segments (A2) of the anterior cerebral arteries and dislocates the carotid bifurcations laterally on each side. A cortical cuff sign can be appreciated (*double arrow*). The pituitary gland (PG) can be differentiated from the lesion because of slightly less contrast enhancement (*yellow line*) and the typical bright spot of the neurohypophysis is visible (NH).

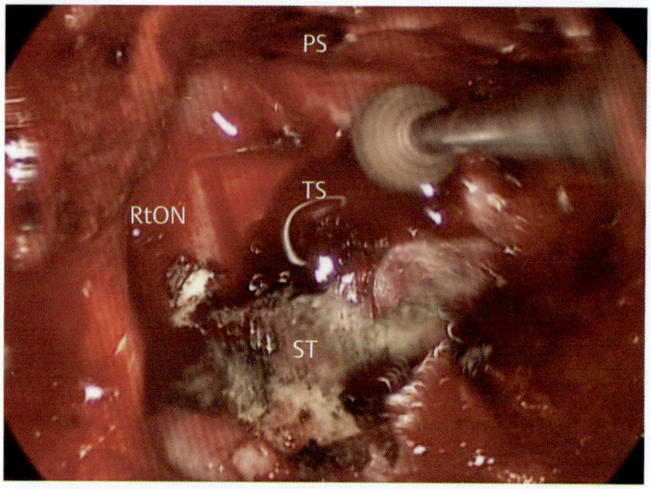

Fig. 12D.2 Transplanum transtuberculum approach. The bone covering the planum sphenoidale (PS) is removed using a high-speed diamond burr (Medtronic, MN).

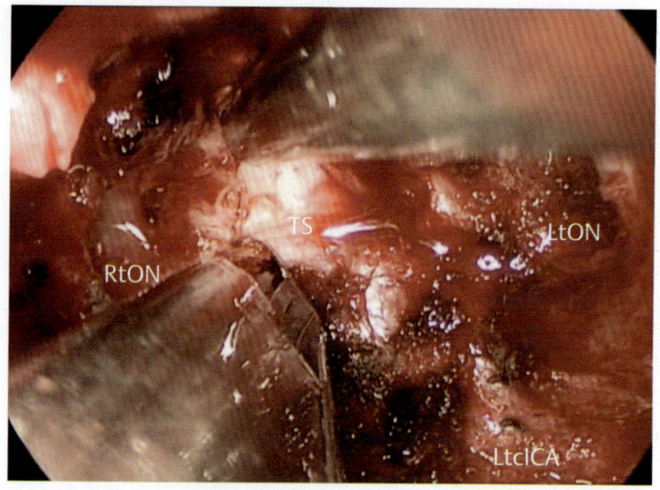

Fig. 12D.3 Transplanum approach. The osteodural exposure is widened using a Kerrison punch. The laterality of the left and right side is verified with IGS.

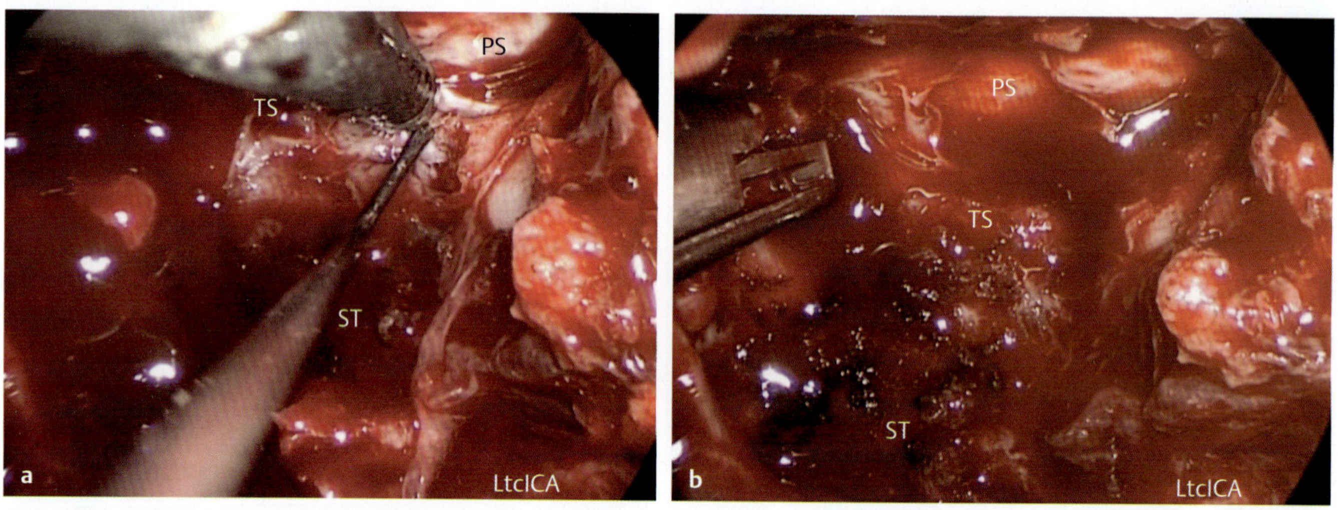

Fig. 12D.4 **(a, b)** Transplanum transtuberculum approach. The thinned-out bone is dissected from the dura with a blunt hooked instrument and can be flicked off.

15. The pituitary gland and infundibular stalk have to be identified, and the definition of a posterior arachnoid dissection plane leading to the posterior brain–tumor interface is mandatory (**Fig. 12D.12**).
16. The anterior extracapsular dissection is started from the most anterior point sideway bilaterally and continued posteriorly (**Fig. 12D.13** and **Fig. 12D.14**).
17. Initial internal tumor debulking using suction or an ultrasonic aspirator with high power and low suction is started in the anterior portion of the tumor (**Fig. 12D.15**).
18. The arachnoid layer protects the arterial vessels from the tumor interface when strictly following the plane, and no vascular encasement is seen in the preoperative imaging (**Fig. 12D.16**).
19. The lateral tumor aspects of the tubercular portion are in anatomical relation with the optic nerve and the clinoidal portion of the carotid artery. Removal of these parts needs microsurgical dissection, the use of an olive-tipped maxillary J-sucker, and ultrasonic aspiration (**Fig. 12D.17a**).

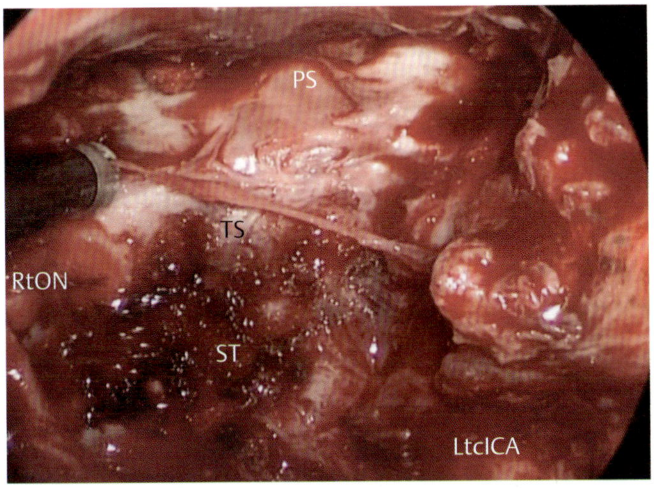

Fig. 12D.5 Verification of the osteodural exposure with IGS. The laterality of the transplanum transtuberculum osteodural exposure has to be sufficient to "release" the meningioma.

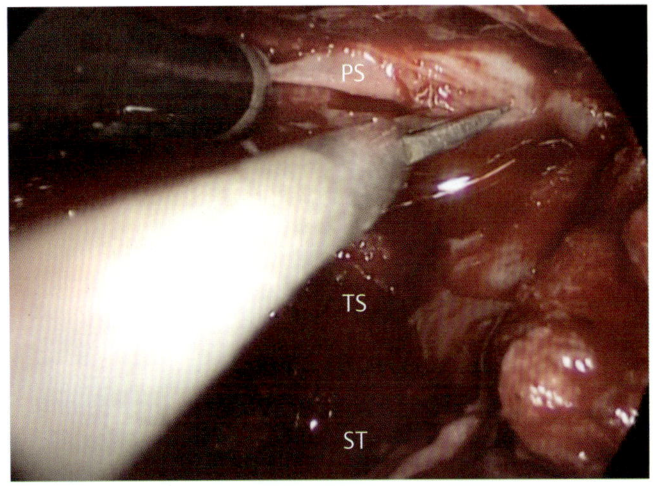

Fig. 12D.6 Dural opening is started at the most anterior extension of the tumor at the planum sphenoidale in a T-shaped manner.

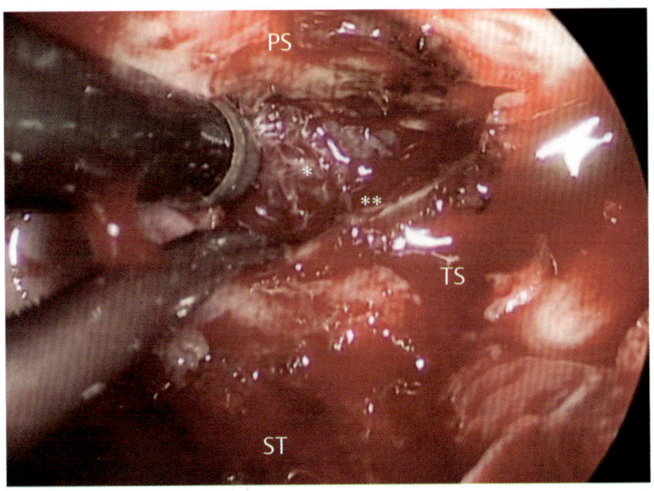

Fig. 12D.7 Definition of a plane (*) between the meningioma (**) and the dura of the planum sphenoidale (PS). An arachnoidal plane is not visible.

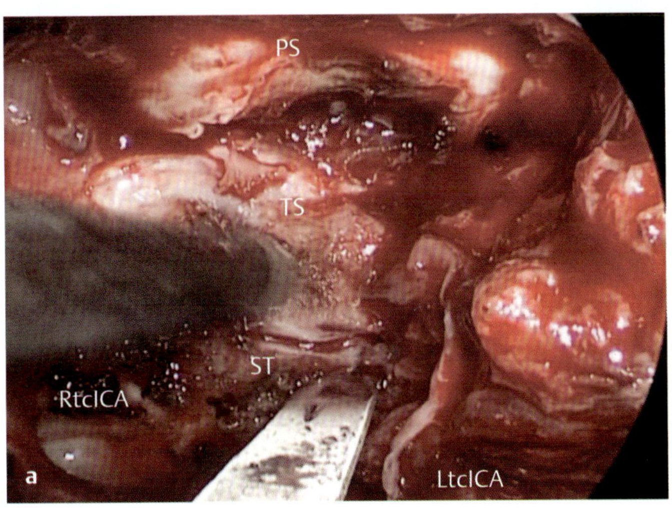

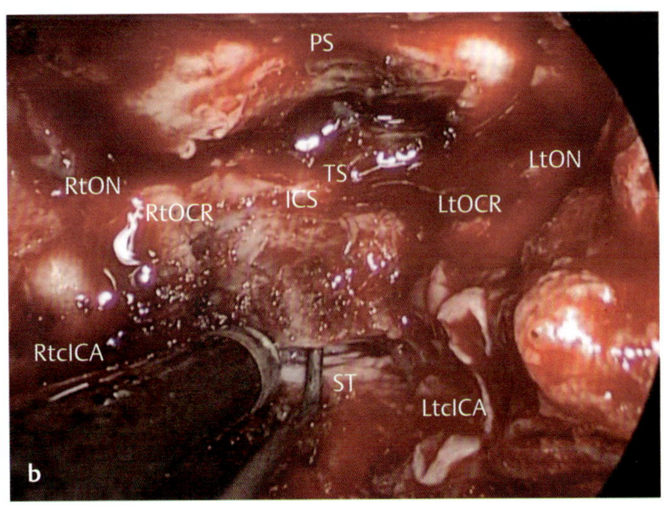

Fig. 12D.8 **(a, b)** Horizontal incision of the dura covering the sella turcica (ST).

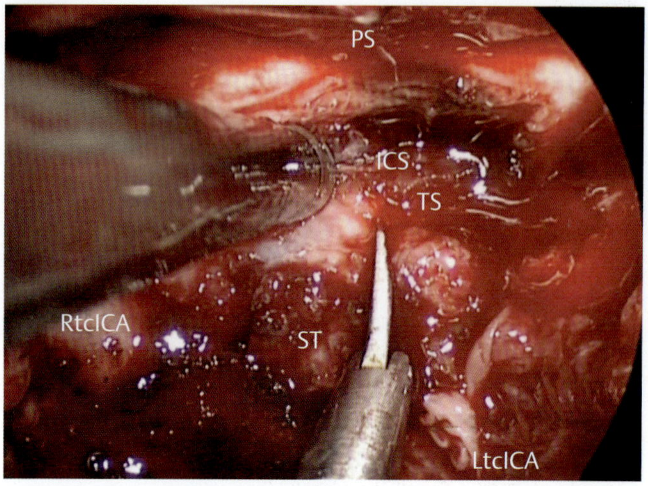

Fig. 12D.9 Vertical incision of the dura covering the sella turcica (reversed T-shape). Superior limitation is the anterior intercavernous sinus (ICS).

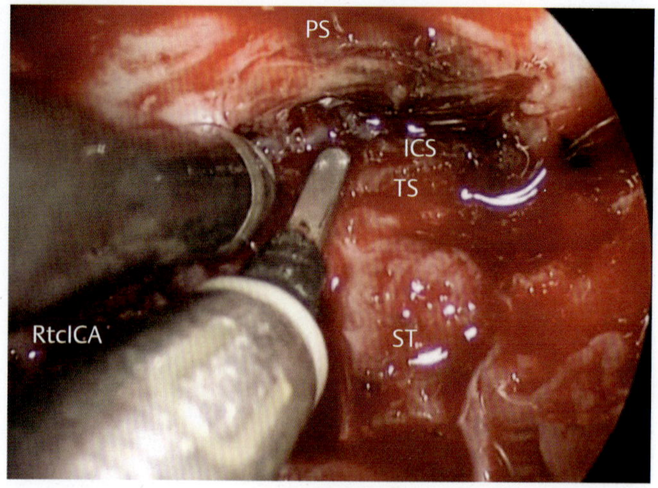

Fig. 12D.10 Cauterization of the anterior intercavernous sinus (ICS).

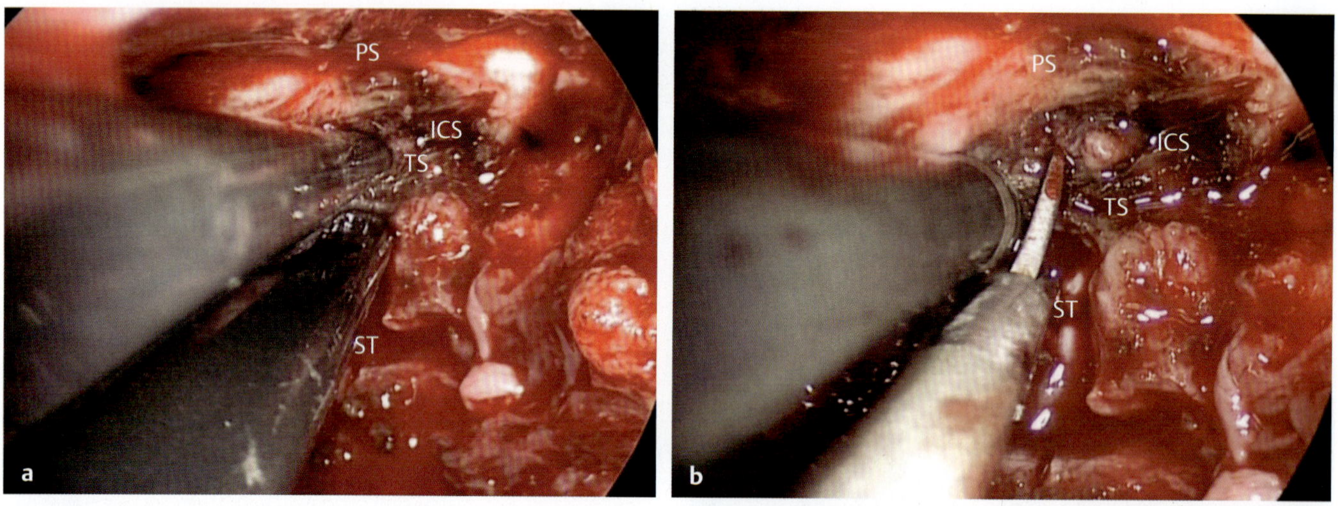

Fig. 12D.11 **(a, b)** Division of the anterior intercavernous sinus (ICS).

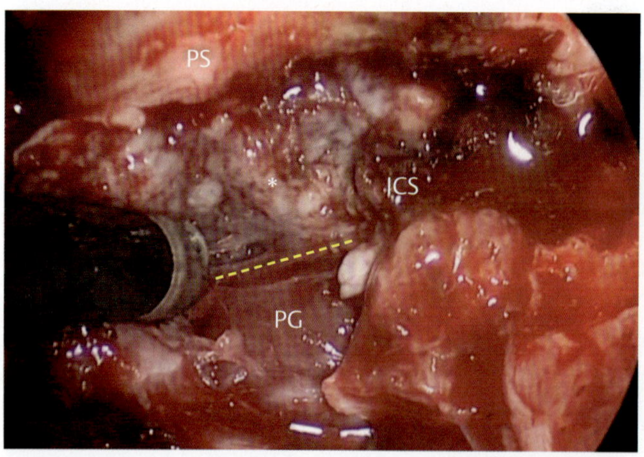

Fig. 12D.12 Definition of the brain–tumor interface (*yellow line*) between the pituitary gland (PG) and the inferior anterior pole of the tuberculum sellae meningioma (*).

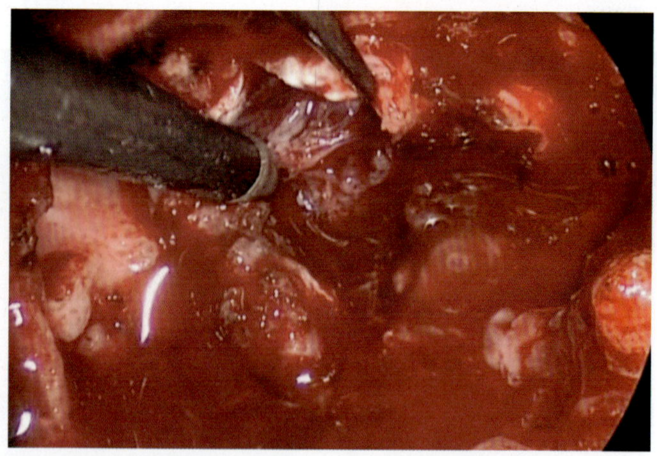

Fig. 12D.13 Initial internal tumor debulking.

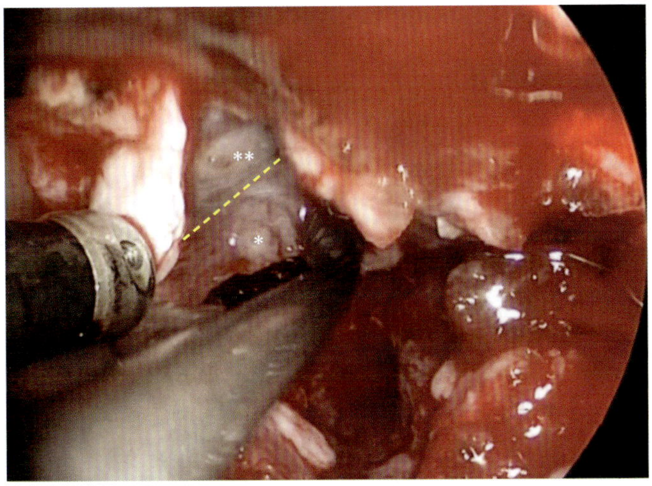

Fig. 12D.14 The initial internal tumor debulking facilitates the extracapsular dissection of the tumor capsule (*) and the arachnoidal plane (**) along the brain–tumor interface (*yellow line*) from anterior to posterior and sideways bilaterally. The arachnoid layer (**) is used to continue the bimanual microdissection posteriorly.

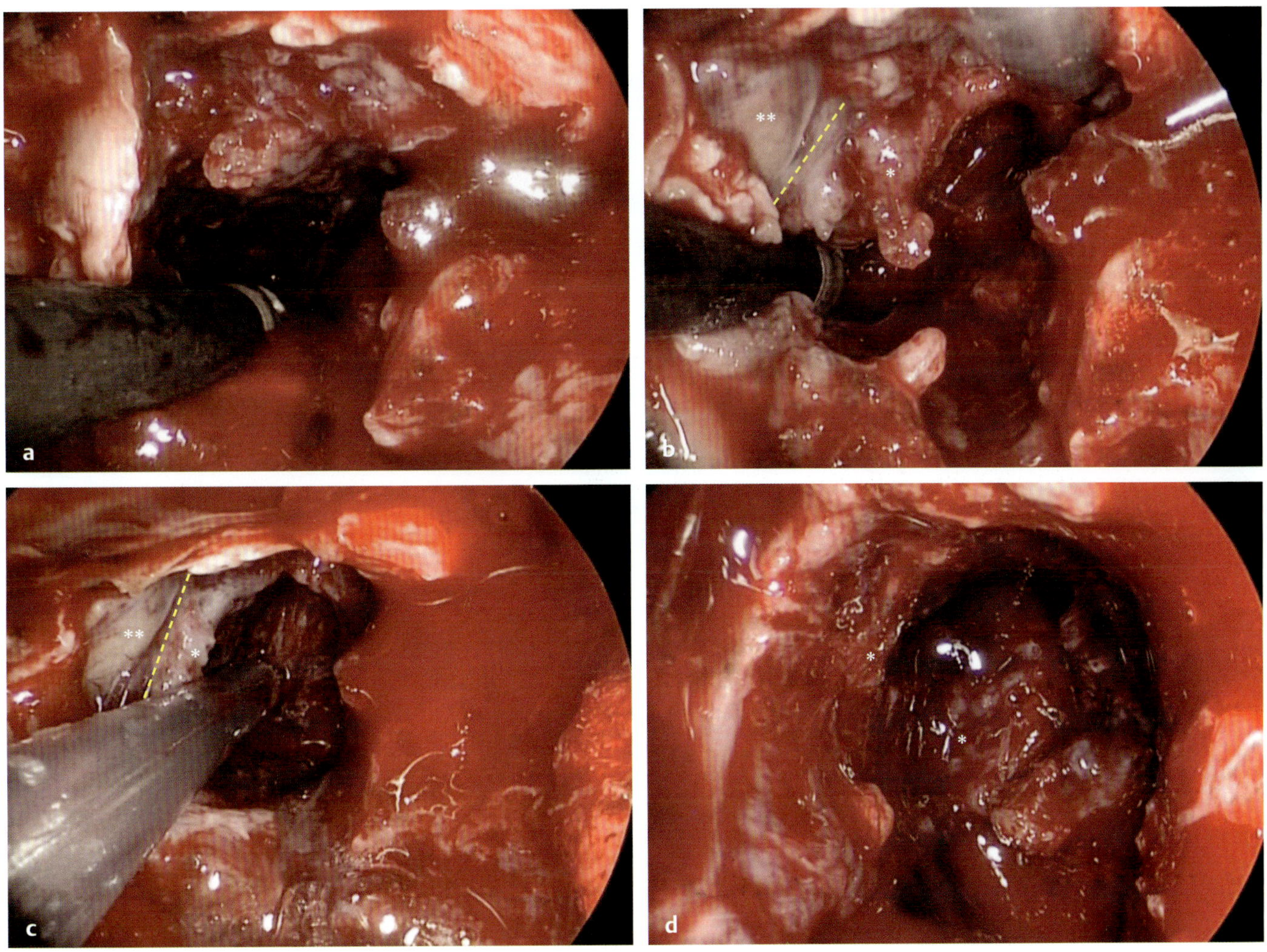

Fig. 12D.15 (a–d) Sufficient internal tumor debulking using a suction device or ultrasonic aspirator along the anteroposterior axis is necessary, when the extracapsular dissection of the tumor capsule (*) and the arachnoidal plane (**) along the brain–tumor interface (*yellow line*) is not easily possible because of a thick tumor shell diameter. Either a two-surgeon one-hand or two-surgeon three- or four-hand technique have to be used for these maneuvers.

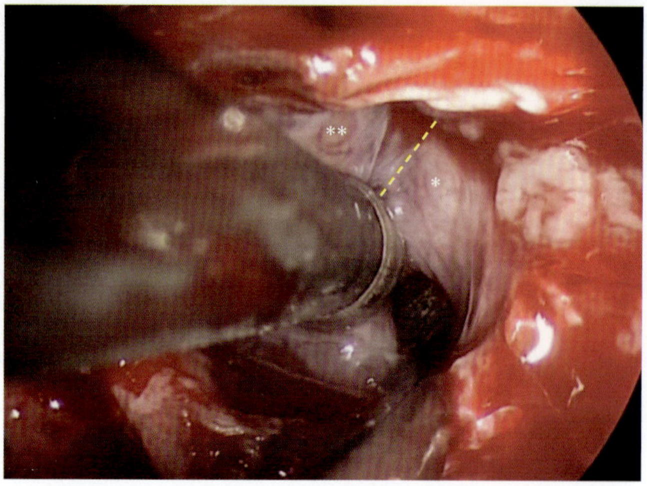

Fig. 12D.16 Extracapsular dissection of the tumor capsule (*) and the arachnoidal plane (**) along the brain–tumor interface (*yellow line*) in the posterior superior aspect of the tubercular portion of the meningioma.

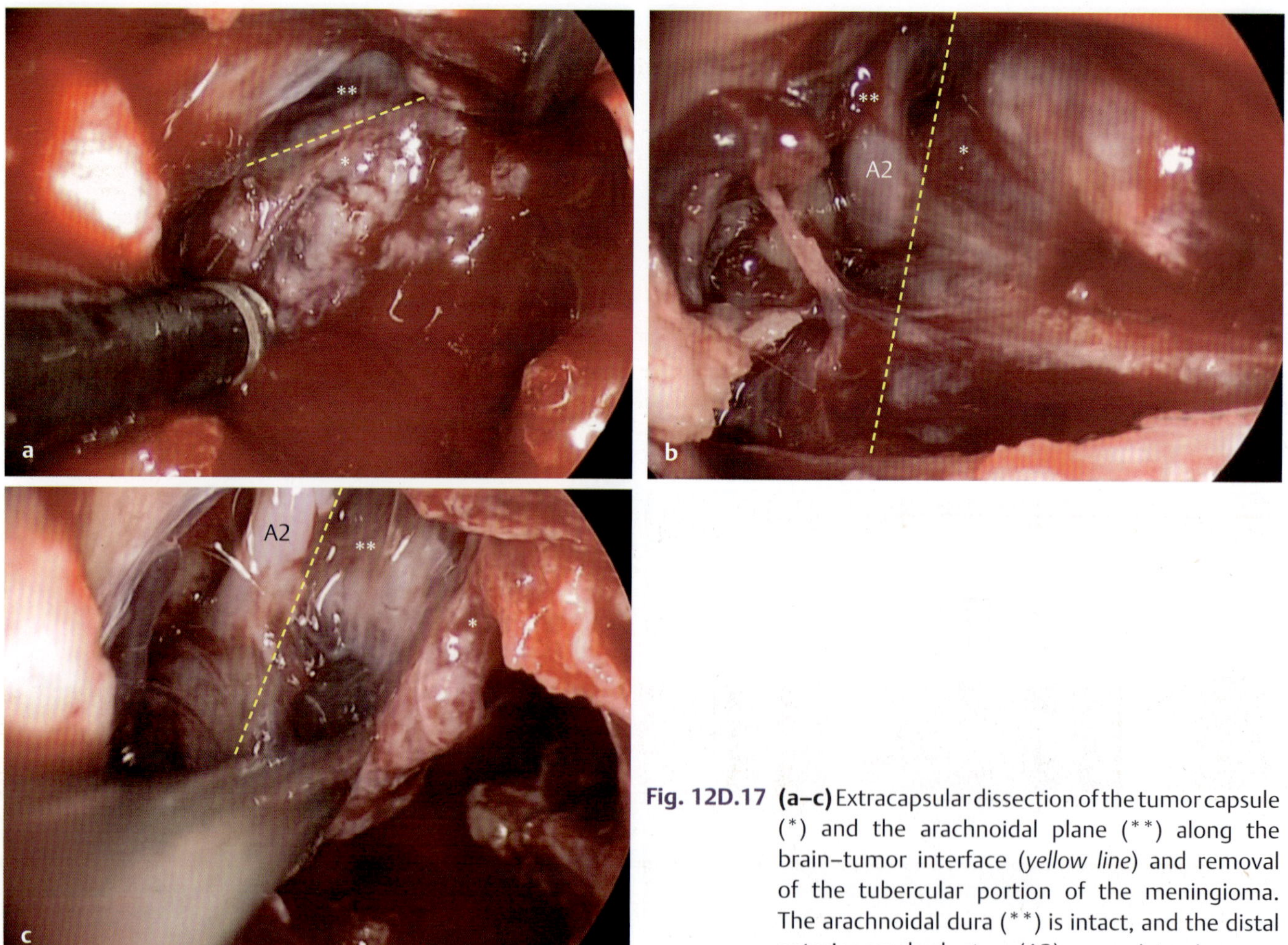

Fig. 12D.17 **(a–c)** Extracapsular dissection of the tumor capsule (*) and the arachnoidal plane (**) along the brain–tumor interface (*yellow line*) and removal of the tubercular portion of the meningioma. The arachnoidal dura (**) is intact, and the distal anterior cerebral artery (A2) comes into view.

20. The extracapsular dissection using the arachnoid layer along the brain–tumor interface is continued bilaterally posteriorly (**Fig. 12D.17b, c**).
21. Interior debulking of the posterior and tubercular portion of the tumor is continued using an ultrasonic aspirator and suction (**Fig. 12D.18**).
22. In larger meningiomas, smaller or larger arterial vessels can be attached to these tumor parts. Sharp dissection might be necessary to release stuck vessels from the tumor capsule. If adherence is too strong or there is a high risk for vascular injury, remnant tumor should be left behind (**Fig. 12D.19a–g**).
23. The anterior suprasellar tubercular portion of the meningioma is removed using the previously defined plane between the pituitary gland and the suprasellar portion, and the optic chiasm is identified (**Fig. 12D.20a, b**).

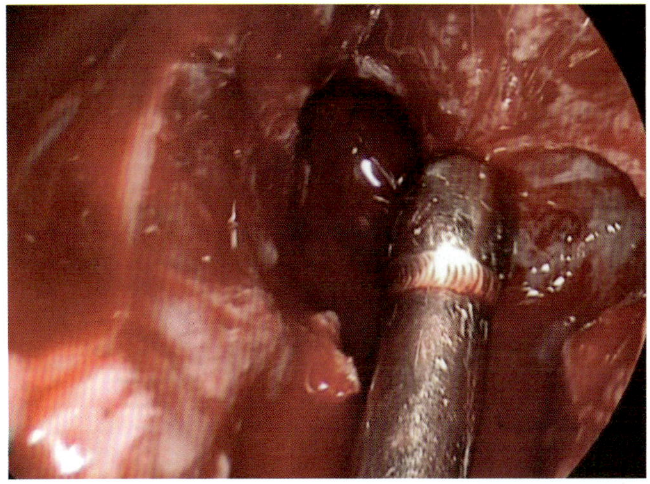

Fig. 12D.18 Removal of the superior aspect of the tubercular portion of the meningioma.

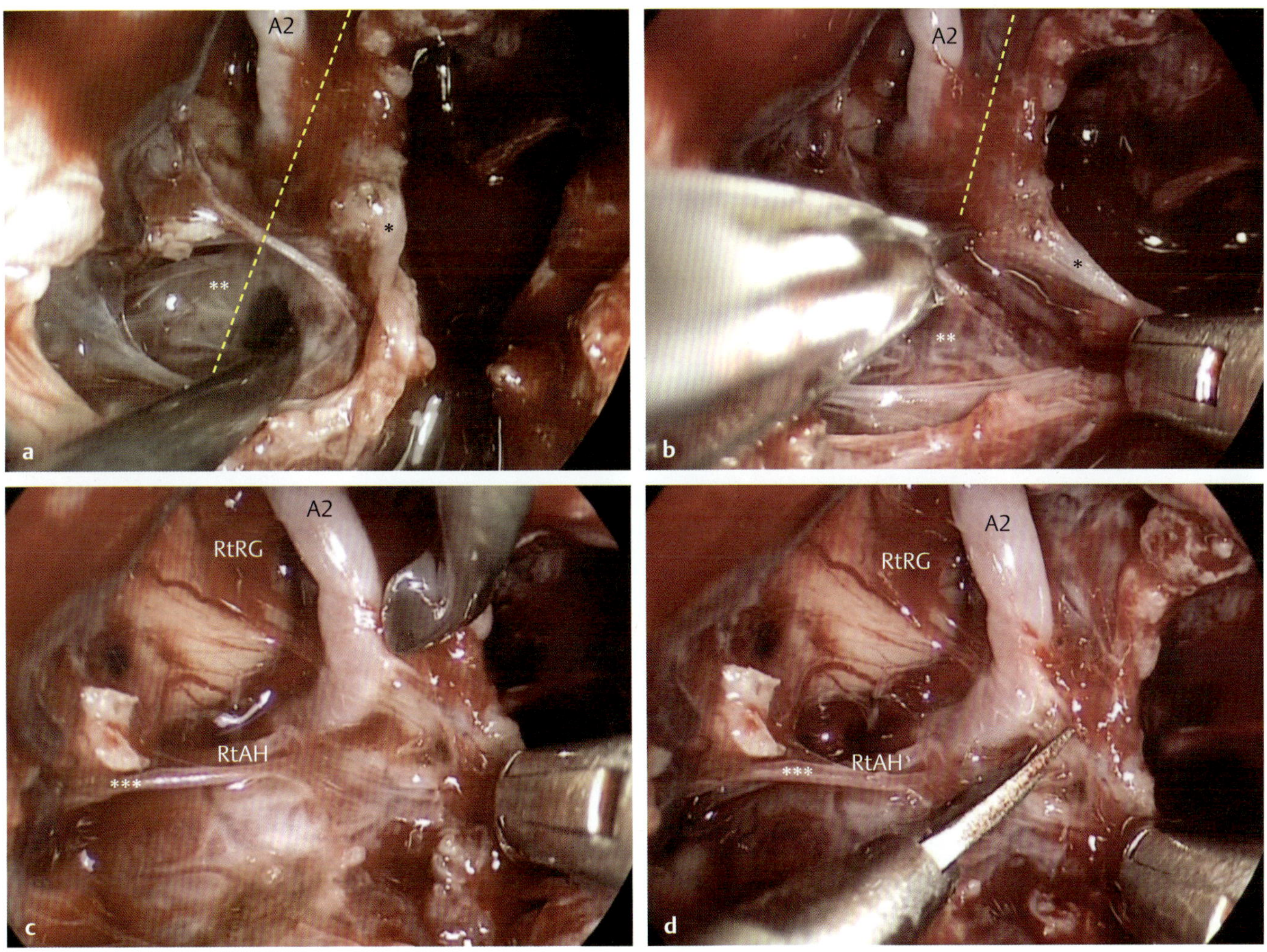

Fig. 12D.19 **(a–d)** Sharp extracapsular dissection of the tumor capsule (*) and the arachnoidal plane (**) along the brain–tumor interface (*yellow line*) while removing the tubercular superior apex of the meningioma. The tumor capsule (*) is adherent to the distal anterior cerebral artery (A2), and sharp dissection using microscissors is performed. Perforating artery (***). *(Continued)*

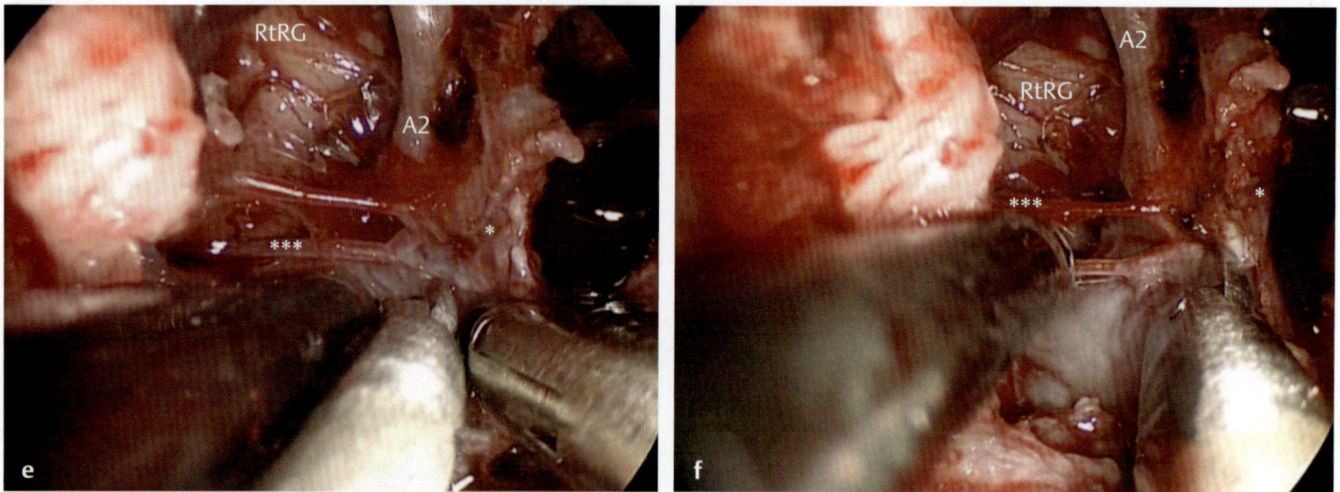

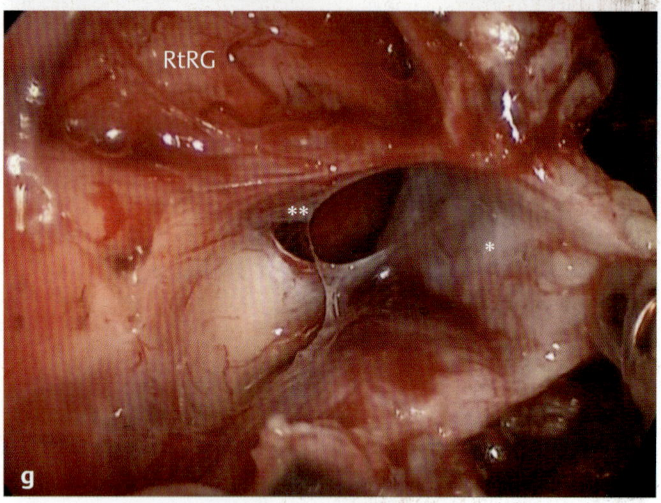

Fig. 12D.19 *(Continued)* **(e–g)** Sharp extracapsular dissection of the tumor capsule (*) and the arachnoidal plane (**) along the brain–tumor interface while removing the tubercular superior apex of the meningioma. The tumor capsule (*) is adherent to the distal anterior cerebral artery (A2), and sharp dissection using microscissors is performed. Perforating artery (***).

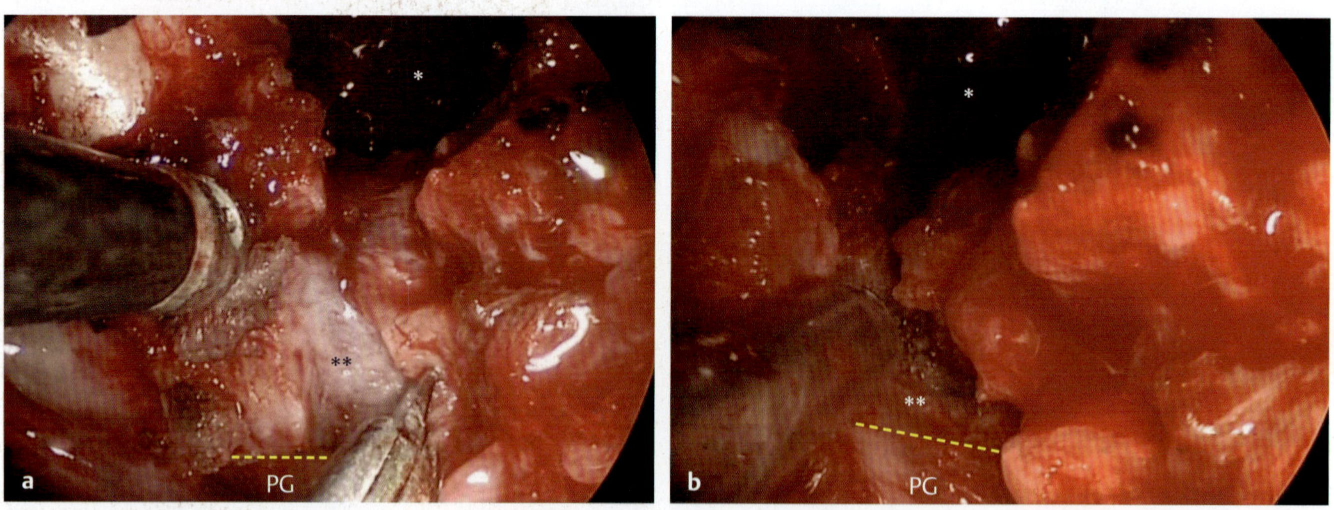

Fig. 12D.20 **(a, b)** After removal of the superior tubercular portion of the meningioma (*), the anterior suprasellar tubercular portion (**) is approached and debulked accordingly. The brain–tumor interface (*yellow line*) between the pituitary gland (PG) and the inferior anterior pole of the tuberculum sellae meningioma (**) is visible.

24. After sufficient internal debulking of the posterior and the tubercular portion of the tumor, the apex of the lesion can be carefully dissected along the arachnoidal plane and pushed downward into the surgical field (**Fig. 12D.21** and **Fig. 12D.22**).
25. Extracapsular dissection along the vessels of the anterior communicating complex has to be performed very carefully.
26. If the liberation of the vessels from the superolateral and apical tumor compartments is not possible, even when using sharp dissection, the intended remnant should left behind to not injure a main or perforating vessel (**Fig. 12D.23**, **Fig. 12D.24**, and **Fig. 12D.25**).
27. The defect is plugged with an abdominal fat graft, and the edges of the fat are brought intracranially to create a watertight seal. Care is taken not to pack too much fat tightly into the cavity (**Fig. 12D.26**).

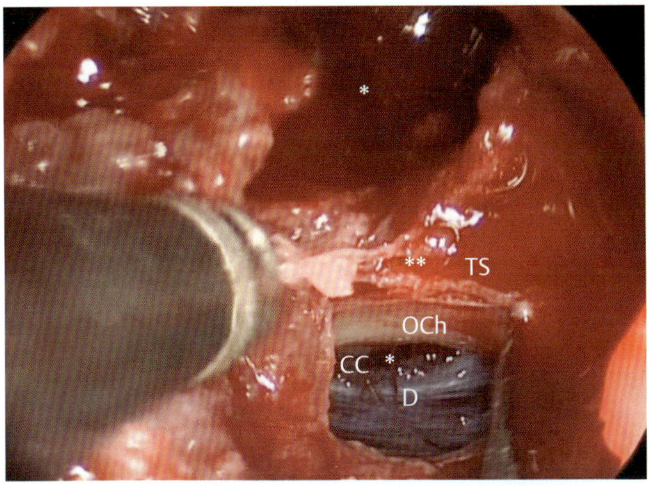

Fig. 12D.21 The optic chiasm (OCh) is identified after removal of the anterior suprasellar tubercular portion (**) of the meningioma, and the chiasmatic cistern (CC) with arteries perforating the optic chiasm (*) and the diaphragma sellae (D) are identified. Removed superior tubercular portion of the meningioma (*).

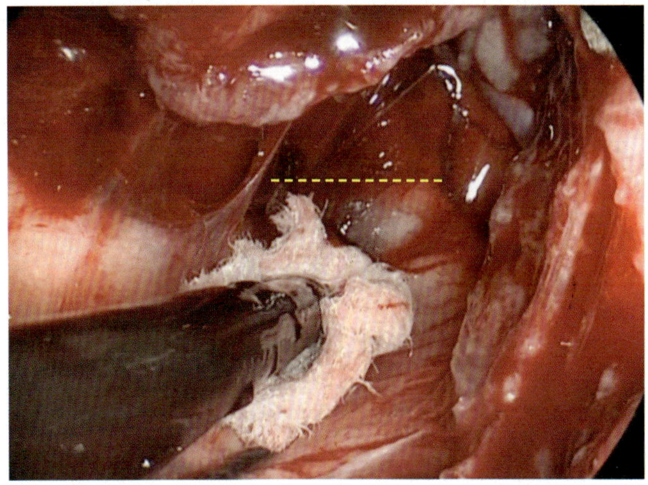

Fig. 12D.22 The posterior inferior tubercular portion is removed using the brain–tumor interface (*yellow line*).

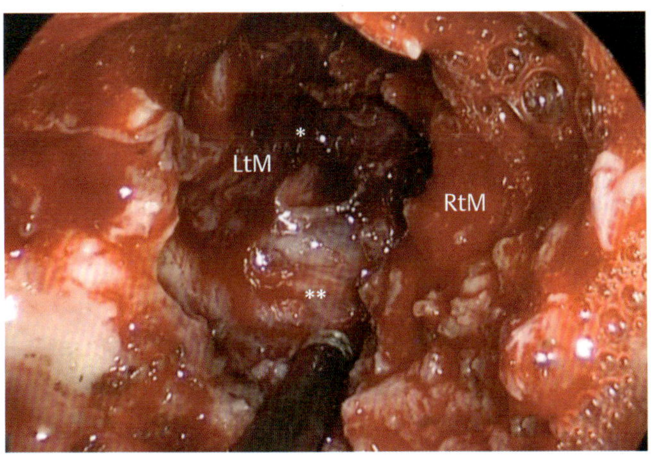

Fig. 12D.23 Tumor cavity after resection of the superior tubercular (*) and the anterior suprasellar tubercular portion (**) of the meningioma. The left (LtM) and right (RtM) lateral tubercular portions of the meningioma are still in situ. The pituitary gland is located below the suction device.

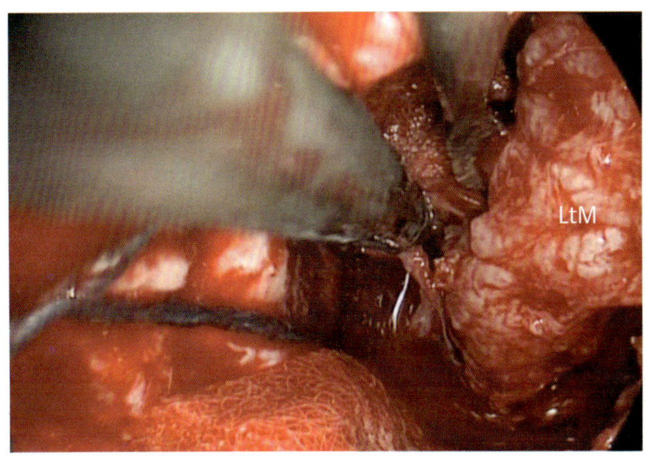

Fig. 12D.24 Removal of the left lateral tubercular portion of the meningioma (LtM) with the two-surgeon three-hand technique. The ENT surgeon presents the dissecting plane to the neurosurgeon by holding the tumor with a grasping instrument.

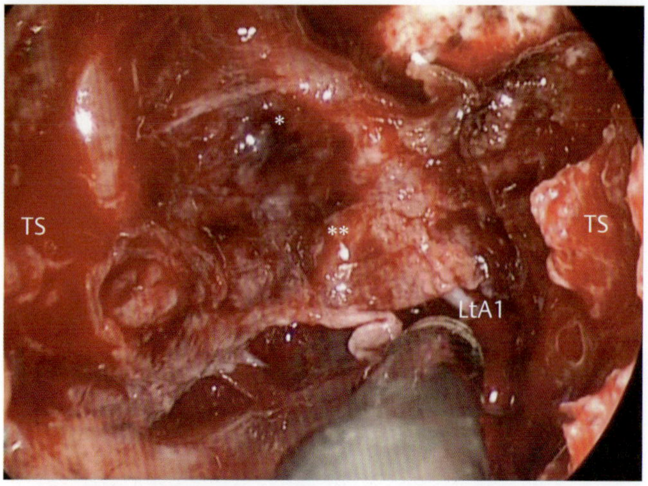

Fig. 12D.25 Inspection of the tumor resection cavity. The H-complex (*) is encased by the most cranial apex of the tuberculum sellae meningioma (**) and intended remnants are left to minimize the risk of vascular injury.

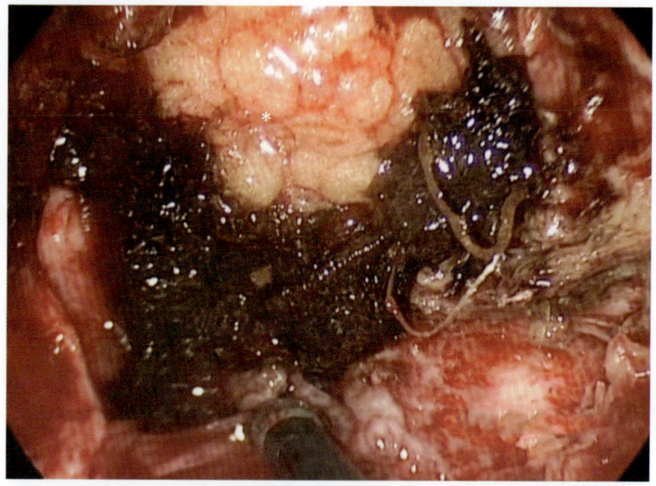

Fig. 12D.26 The anterior skull base defect is closed using intradural autologous abdominal fat graft (*). The construct is stabilized using Surgicel.

28. This is sealed with a synthetic dural sealant and layered with an absorbable hemostat (**Fig. 12D.27**).
29. The bilateral vascularized nasoseptal flaps are rotated over the defect to complete the repair and reinforced with gelatin sponges to keep the flaps in position. No other nasal packing is required.

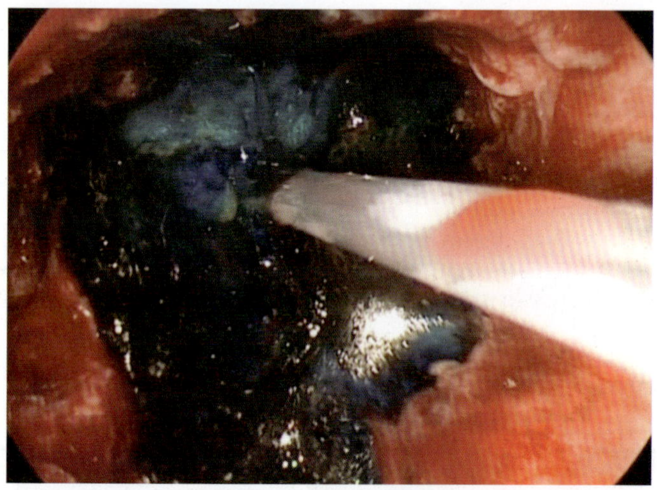

Fig. 12D.27 The whole skull base reconstruction is sealed with an artificial dural sealant system.

Case 12E

A Tailored Extended Endonasal Endoscopic Approach for a Large Synchronous Tumor of the Sellar and Parasellar Region

Michel Roethlisberger, Prepageran Narayanan, and Vicknes Waran

History

A 54-year-old female presented herself with progressive right dominant bilateral loss of vision, associated with occasional headaches and dizziness. Clinical visual examination revealed the ability to count fingers on the right eye while visual acuity was near normal on the left side. Visual field examination revealed severely depressed fields on all four quadrants on the right and temporal hemianopia on the left side. A fundoscopy revealed a right pale optic disc in contrast with a left pink optic disc with preservation of the cup-to-disc ratio. Clinical and laboratory work-up did not reveal any pathological signs.[1]

Neurocranial imaging with magnetic resonance imaging (MRI) revealed a sellar/suprasellar enhancing lesion (28 × 19 × 16 mm) suspicious for a pituitary macroadenoma. A colliding second extra-axial lesion (22 × 36 × 20 mm) expanding from the tuberculum sellae to the planum sphenoidale with encasement of the anterior communicating complex was found suspicious for a large meningioma (**Fig. 12E.1a–c**).[1]

The patient repeatedly refused transcranial resection of the lesion but agreed for an endoscopic resection. A transnasal transsphenoidal transplanum transtuberculum transsellar approach with removal of the medial orbital walls was recommended to assess this rare lesion.[1]

Postoperatively, the right temporal hemianopia recovered slowly with improvement of the visual field on the left side.[1]

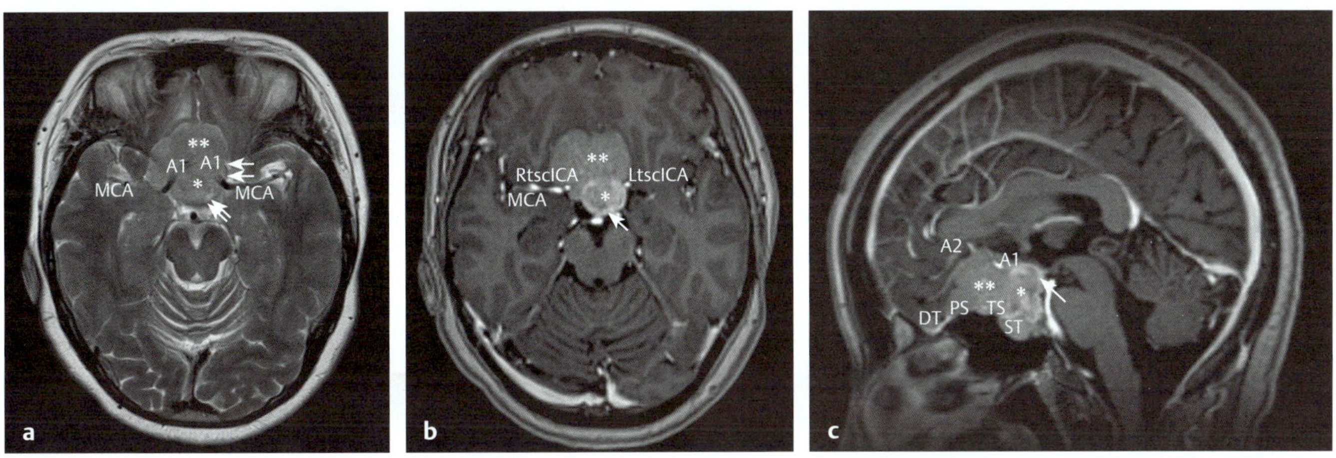

Fig. 12E.1 **(a)** Axial T2-weighted, **(b)** axial, and **(c)** sagittal T1-weighted gadolinium contrast-enhanced MRI sections. A biphasic lesion with an isointense mass in the sella turcica (ST) with moderate homogenous enhancement is seen (*). The pituitary gland presents with slightly higher enhancement and is displaced posteriorly along with the infundibular stalk (*arrow*). The optic chiasm is postfixed (*double arrow*), and both optic nerves are compressed and dislocated laterally. Cavernous sinus invasion is present on the right side (Knosp's grade 2). A second slightly less but still homogenous enhancing T1- and T2-isointense extra-axial lesion extending along the tuberculum sella (TS) and a dural tail (DT) extending to the planum sphenoidale (PS) is seen. The apex of this second lesion is extending more to the right side, with encasement of the pre- (A1) and postcommunicating segments (A2) of the anterior cerebral arteries.

Surgical Steps

1. The pedicled nasoseptal flap is raised off the septum with a Freer elevator posteriorly until the sphenoid ostia and posterior choana are visible (**Fig. 12E.2**).
2. The nasoseptal flap is freed with a microscissors superiorly and inferiorly aiming for the sphenoid ostia and posterior choana, respectively.
3. The exposed cartilaginous septum is fractured through to the contralateral side and removed by piecemeal, all the while freeing it from the overlying contralateral septal mucoperichondrium (**Fig. 12E.3**).
4. This is continued until the sphenoid rostrum is exposed with the sphenoid ostia visible bilaterally.
5. At this point, the contralateral nasoseptal flap can be created in the same manner as described in Case 12C.
6. Once the sphenoid keel is fully exposed, the ostia are widened inferomedially using a Kerrison punch in a V shape toward the midline (**Fig. 12E.4**).
7. The remnant sphenoid keel and sphenoid sinus septations are then removed to allow an unobstructed view. The pedicled flap can then be stored in the nasopharynx until reconstruction is necessary (**Fig. 12E.5**).
8. The posterior wall of the sphenoid sinus is demucosalized with a monopolar cautery-tipped aspirator.

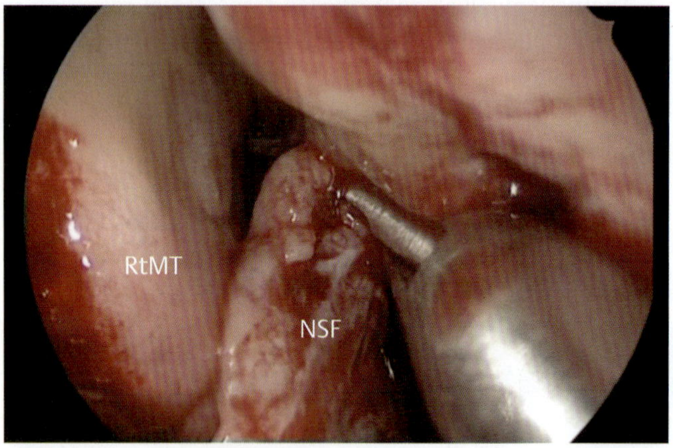

Fig. 12E.2 The superior margin of the pedicled nasoseptal flap (NSF)] is defined approximately 0.5 to 1 cm below the skull base to preserve the olfactory function. Inferiorly, the flap can be taken as far as half the nasal floor (Hadad-Bassagasteguy flap).

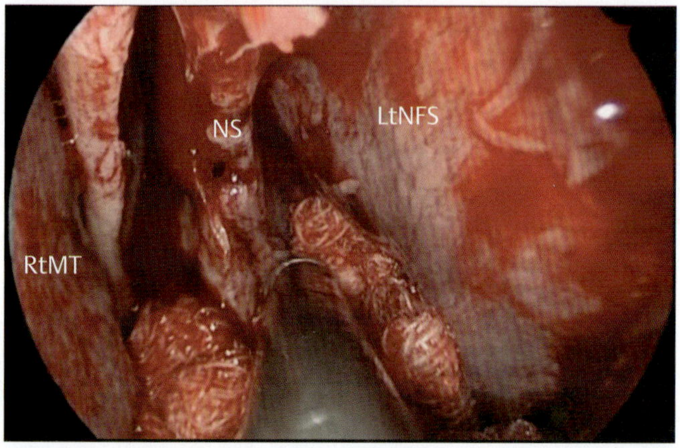

Fig. 12E.3 The posterior bony aspect of the nasal septum (NS), the vomer, has been removed, and exposition of the contralateral mucosa is used for the left contralateral nasoseptal flap (LtNFS).

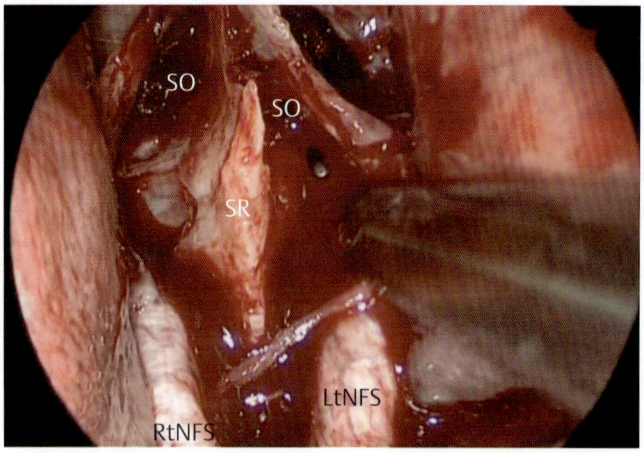

Fig. 12E.4 The sphenoid rostrum (SR) and both sphenoid ostia (SO) have been exposed. The left (LtNSF) and right nasoseptal flaps (RtNSF) have been stored in the sphenoethmoidal recess.

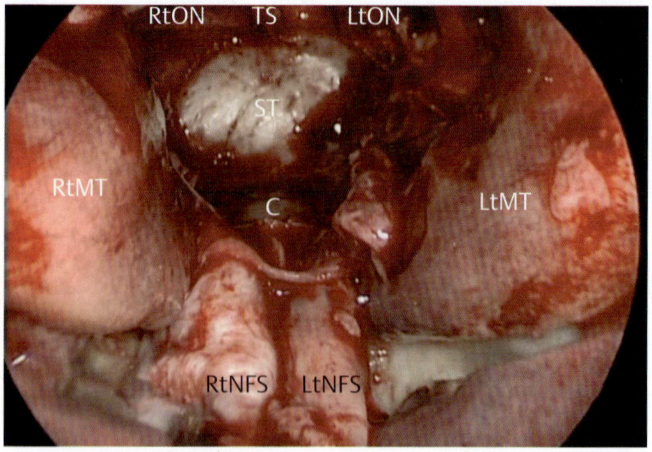

Fig. 12E.5 The sphenoid rostrum has been removed and the sphenoid cavity is exposed. The left (LtNSF) and right nasoseptal flaps (RtNSF) have been stored in the sphenoethmoidal recess and the right (RtMT) and left middle turbinates (LtMT) are preserved.

This allows an overview of the sphenoid cavity and the crucial neurovascular landmarks of the bony skull base (**Fig. 12E.6**).

9. The most anterior and lateral extension of the anterior lesion can be defined using intraoperative image-guided surgery (IGS).
10. In a first step, the bone covering the medial orbit is removed bilaterally (**Fig. 12E.7**).
11. Transplanum approach: Drilling is commenced at bone covering the planum sphenoidale using a high-speed diamond burr and extended to the tuberculum sellae and the sella turcica.

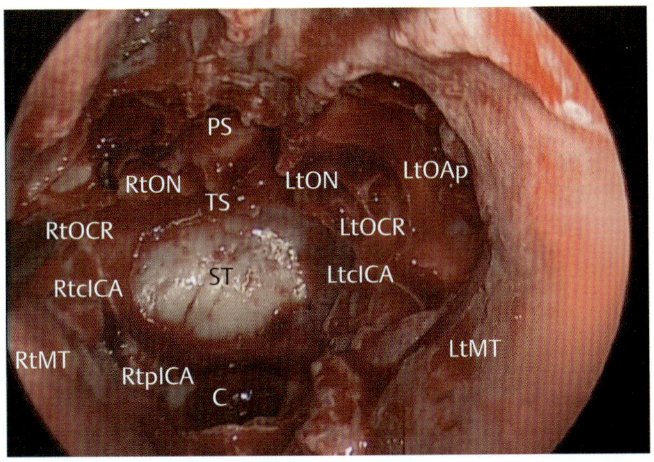

Fig. 12E.6 To allow an unobstructed view of the planum sphenoidale and the bilateral medial orbital walls, the anterior wall and posterior ethmoidal cells are removed and demucosalized.

12. Once the bone has been sufficiently thinned out, a right angle dissector can be insinuated between the bone and the dura, and the bone is flaked off (**Fig. 12E.8**).
13. Transtuberculum approach: The osteodural exposure is continued with removal of the tuberculum sellae as described in Cases 12B and 12C. (**Fig. 12E.9**).
14. Transsellar approach: The bone covering the sella turcica is thinned out using a high-speed drill and the bone is removed as described in Cases 12B and 12C. (**Fig. 12E.9**).
15. Dural opening is started at the most anterior extension of the tumor at the planum sphenoidale in a T-shaped manner and is extended posteriorly to the sella turcica with a microscissors after freeing the underlying tissue using a right angle dissector (**Fig. 12E.10**).
16. Interior debulking of the anterior lesion facilitates the stepwise resection of the capsule from the arachnoid layer of the brain surface (**Fig. 12E.11**).
17. When continuing the dissection more posteriorly, the tubercular portion of the meningioma reveals its close contact to the optic nerves and the H-complex of the anterior cerebral artery (**Fig. 12E.12**).
18. The apex of the meningioma shows encasement of the arterial vessels of the H-complex. Hence, microsurgical removal of tumor remnants is necessary (**Fig. 12E.13, Fig. 12E.14, Fig. 12E.15**).
19. The pre- and postcommunicating segments of both anterior cerebral arteries, the anterior communicating artery, and both recurrent arteries of Heubner have to be considered, identified, and preserved (**Fig. 12E.16**).

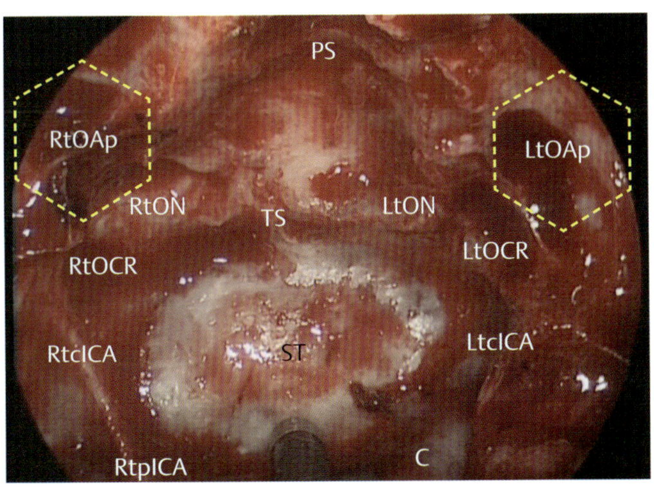

Fig. 12E.7 The right (RtOAp) and left medial orbital apex walls (LtOAp) (*yellow pentagon*) are removed bilaterally to account for the lateral expansion of the anterior lesion being suspicious for a tuberculum sellae meningioma.

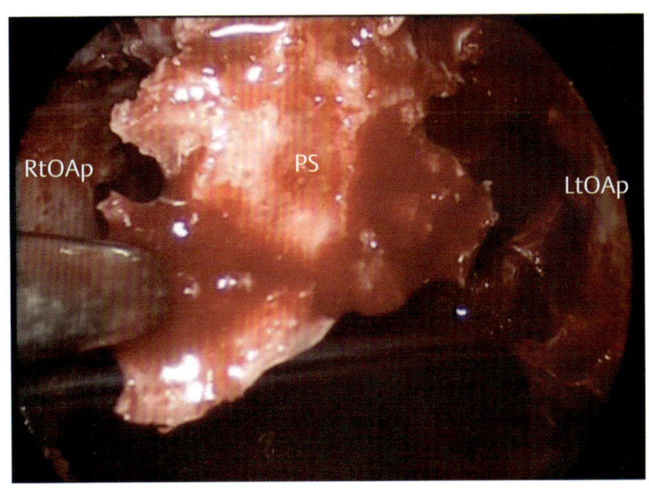

Fig. 12E.8 Transplanum approach: After thinning out the bone covering, the planum sphenoidale (PS), the bone can be flicked of. Right (RtOAp) and left medial orbital apex walls (LtOAp) with removed bony covering.

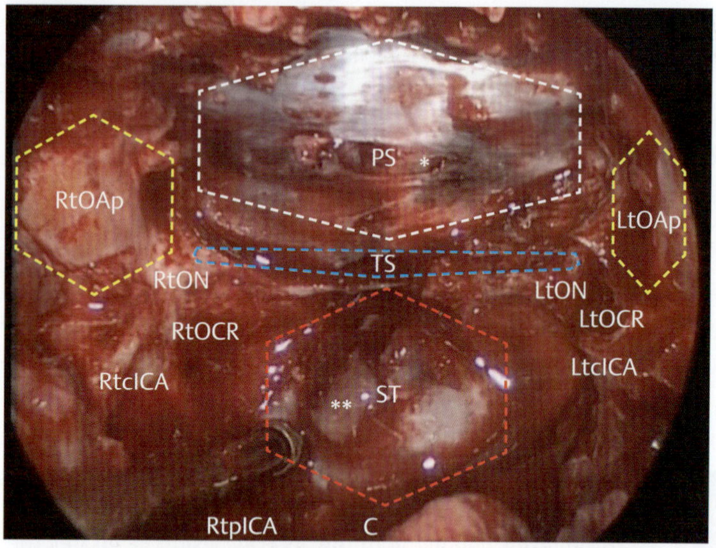

Fig. 12E.9 Tailored approach and zonal dissection of the skull base for the osteodural exposure of the synchronous tumor in the sellar/suprasellar and parasellar region. The transplanum approach (*gray pentagon*) is connected with the transtuberculum approach (*blue pentagon*) and the transsellar approach (*red pentagon*). The anterior lesion (*) and intra-/suprasellar lesion (**) can be addressed with this tailored approach to the skull base. The right and left medial orbits are visible after removal of the left and right medial orbital apex walls (LtOAp and RtOAp) (*yellow pentagon*) to account for the lateral extension of the anterior lesion.

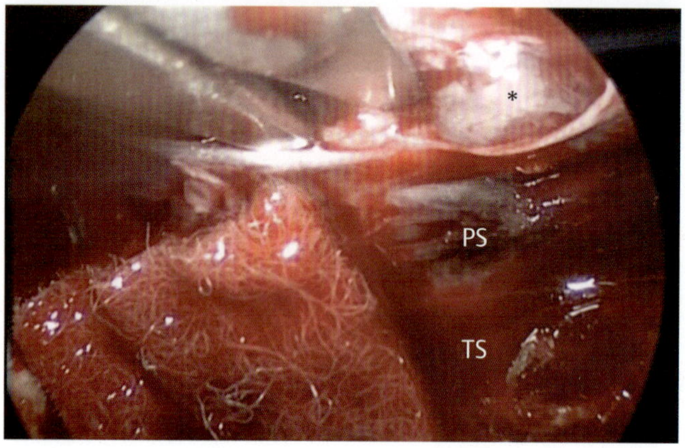

Fig. 12E.10 Anterior dural opening in a T-shaped manner to expose the most anterior planum sphenoidale (PS) portion of the meningioma (*).

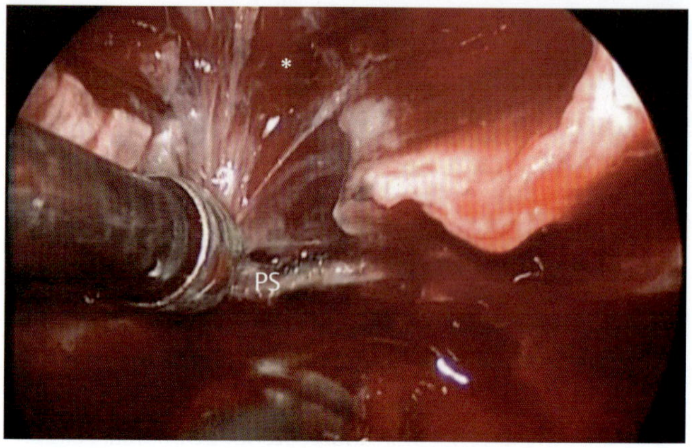

Fig. 12E.11 Internal debulking of the planum sphenoidale (PS) portion of the meningioma (*).

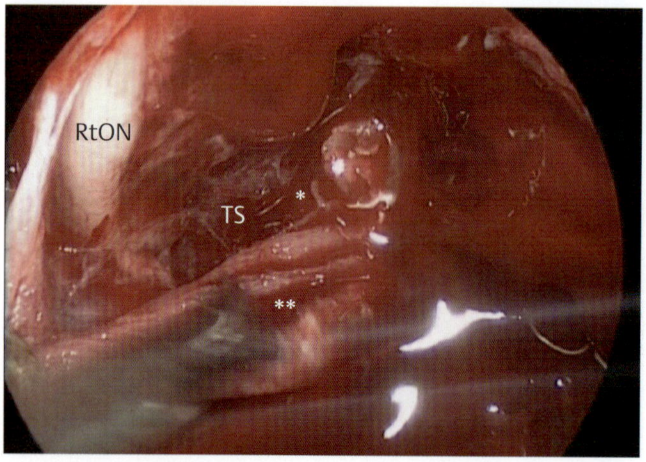

Fig. 12E.12 Resection of the tuberculum sellae (TS) portion of the meningioma (*). Fibrous strands can be removed within the tumor (**).

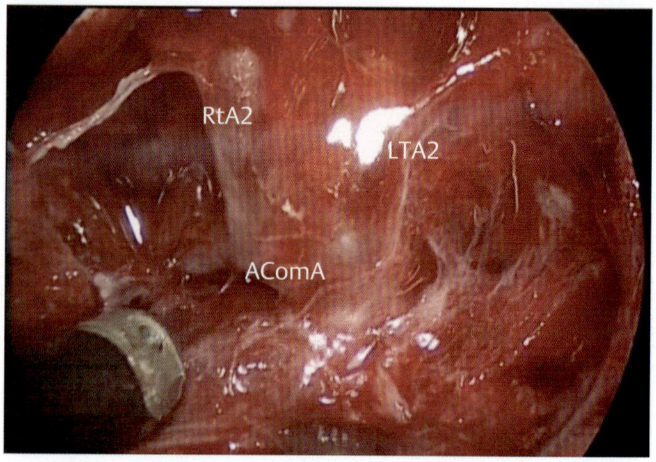

Fig. 12E.13 Microsurgical bimanual resection of the superior tubercular portion of the meningioma with encasement of the right (RtA2) and left (LtA2) distal anterior cerebral artery and the anterior communicating artery (AComA).

20. Meticulous coagulation and division of the anterior intercavernous sinus are necessary to connect the planum sphenoidale with the sellar region as described in Cases 12A, 12B, and 12C previously (**Fig. 12E.17**).
21. Opening of the dural covering the sella turcica reveals the typical aspect of a pituitary adenoma. A brighter more fibrous tissue belonging to the larger anterior parasellar lesion was distinguishable from softer and more deliquescent grayish tissue in the sellar/suprasellar lesion, identified as the contact zone between the two tumors (**Fig. 12E.18**).
22. Debulking is completed with aspirators, clearing the tumor from inferior to superior. Parts of the lesion that are slightly more lateral are aspirated with an olive-tipped J aspirator (**Fig. 12E.19**).
23. Intraoperative contrast-enhanced MRI is performed, demonstrating complete resection of the large supra-/parasellar and sellar lesion with suspected residual tumor along the right cavernous carotid artery (**Fig. 12E.20a, b**).
24. Meticulous hemostasis is performed.
25. The defect is plugged with fat taken from the abdomen, and the edges of the fat are tucked intradurally to create a watertight seal. Care is taken not to pack too much fat tightly into the cavity (**Fig. 12E.21**).
26. The construct is sealed with a synthetic dural sealant and layered with an absorbable hemostat.
27. The bilateral nasoseptal flaps are rotated over the defect to complete the repair and reinforced with gelatine sponges to keep the flaps in position. No other nasal packing is required (**Fig. 12E.22** and **12E.23**).

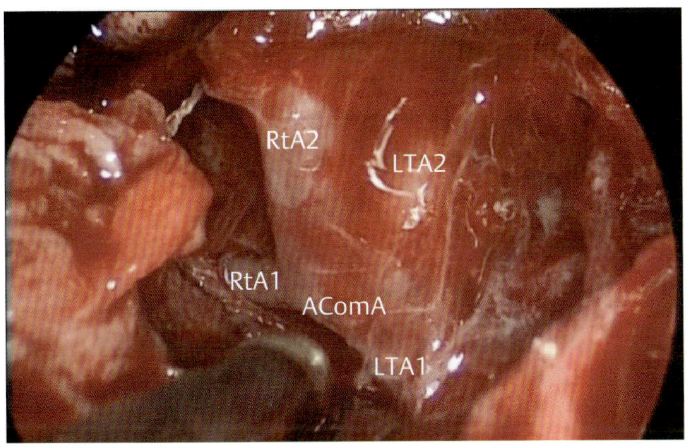

Fig. 12E.14 Microsurgical bimanual resection of the superior tubercular portion of the meningioma.

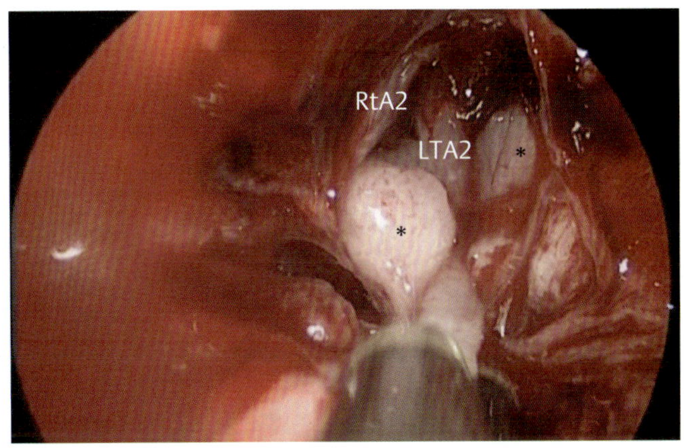

Fig. 12E.15 After bimanual microsurgical sharp dissection, the encasing superior part of the tubercular portion of the meningioma (*) can be mobilized and removed between the right (RtA2) and left distal anterior cerebral arteries (LtA2).

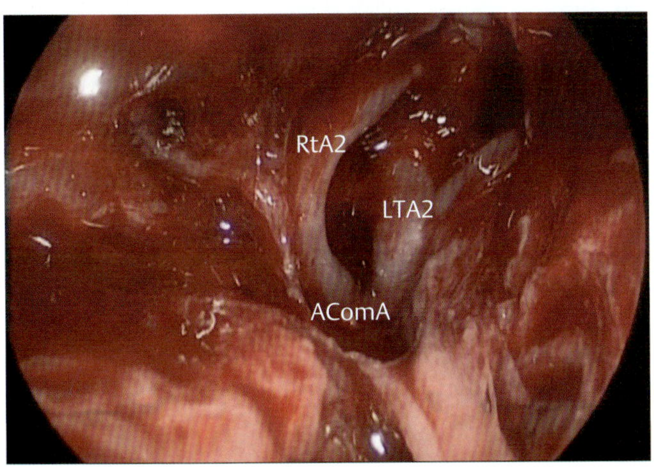

Fig. 12E.16 Suprasellar cistern after tumor resection including the encasing parts superiorly to the right (RtA2) and left distal anterior cerebral arteries (LtA2).

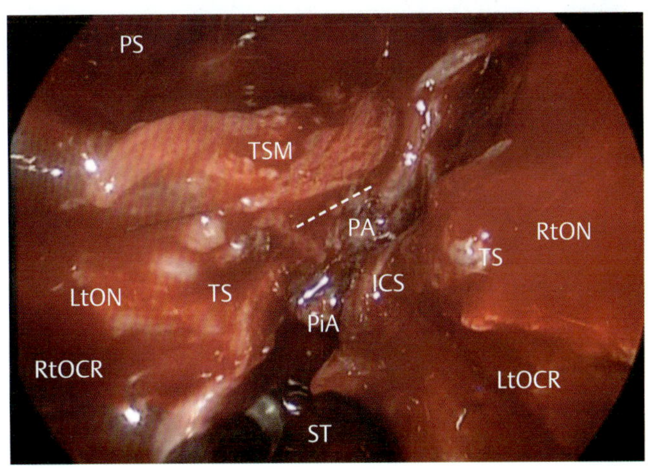

Fig. 12E.17 Contact zone (*white line*) between the tuberculum sellae meningioma (TSM) and the pituitary adenoma (PiA).

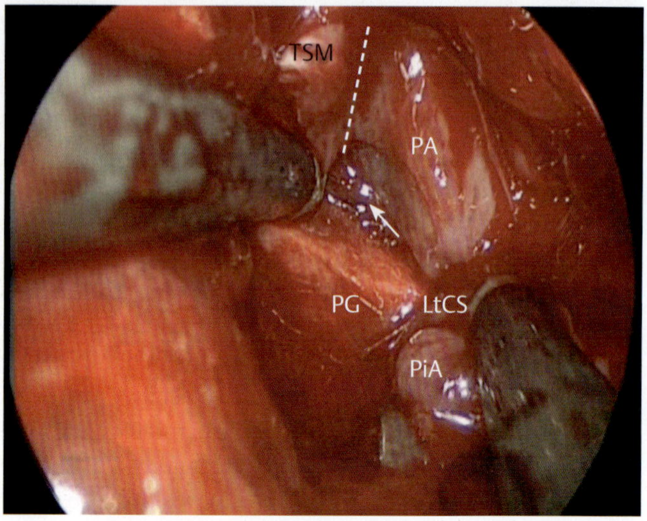

Fig. 12E.18 Two-surgeon four-hand technique. While the neurosurgeon uses two suckers, the ENT surgeon helps with a dissector to present a dissection plane. The collision zone (*white line*) between the tuberculum sellae meningioma (TSM) and the pituitary adenoma (PiA) is visible. The pituitary adenoma is partially removed and the posterior clival dura is visible (*arrow*).

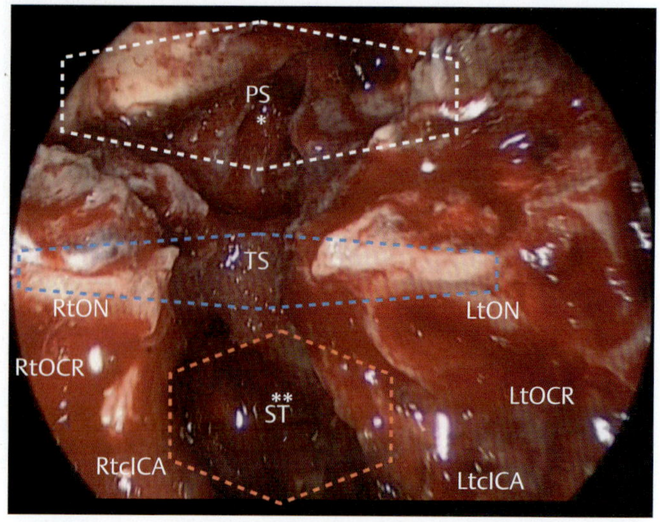

Fig. 12E.19 Resection cavity: The transplanum approach (*gray pentagon*) is connected with the transtuberculum approach (*blue pentagon*) and the transsellar approach (*red pentagon*). The anterior lesion (*) and the intra-/suprasellar lesion (**) can be addressed with this tailored approach to the base of skull.

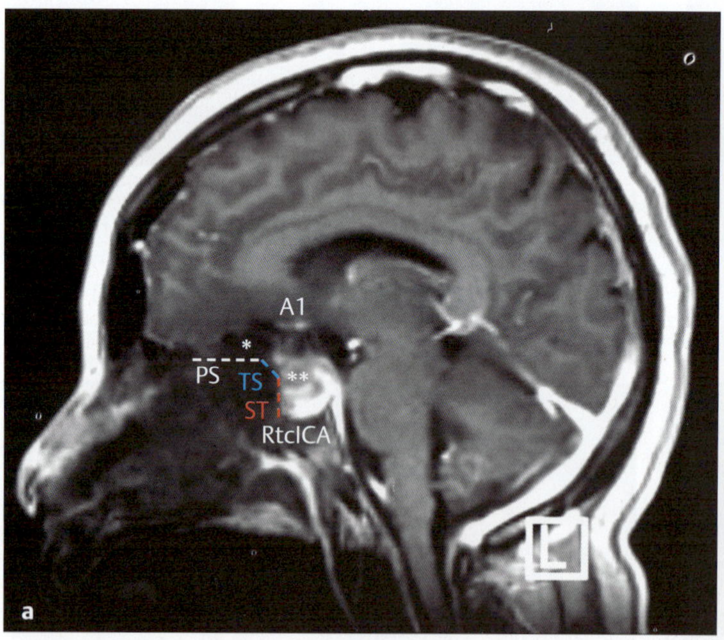

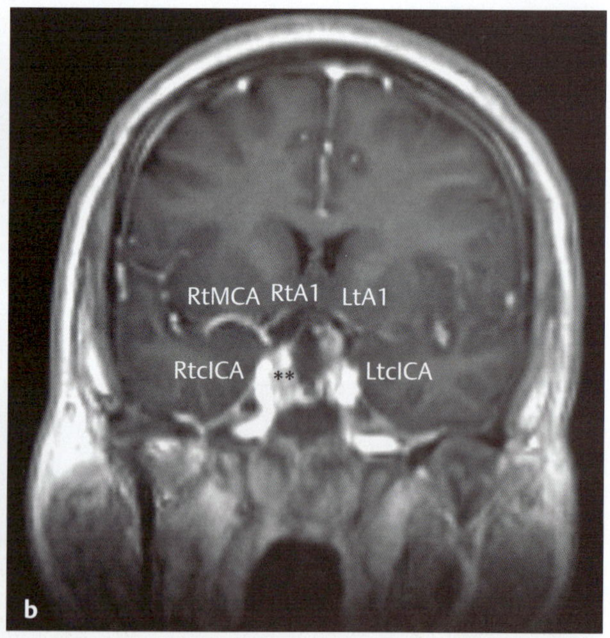

Fig. 12E.20 **(a)** Coronal, and **(b)** sagittal intraoperative T1-weighted gadolinium contrast-enhanced MRI sections. Complete resection of the large supra-/parasellar (*) and sellar lesion was achieved with the intended residual tumor (**) in close contact with the sixth cranial nerve and the right cavernous internal carotid artery (RtcICA). Planum sphenoidale (PS, *white line*), tuberculum sellae (TS, *blue line*), sella turcica (ST, *red line*).

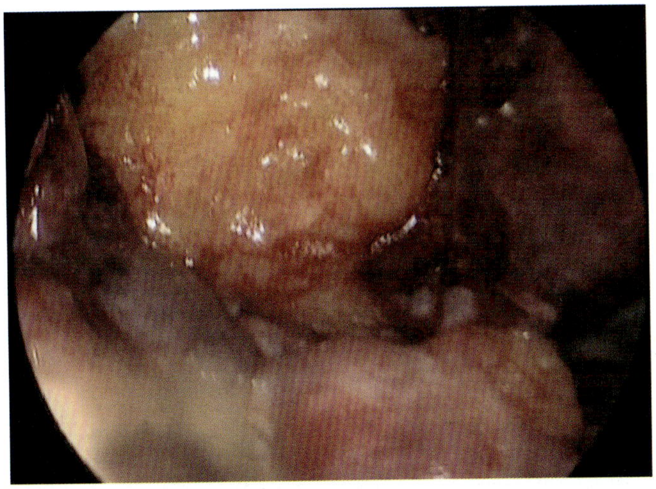

Fig. 12E.21 An abdominal fat graft is placed in each of the two resection cavities. The placement must be adequate and the dural edges must be visible to plug the fat intradurally. After fixation with resorbable hemostatic material and artificial dural sealant, a second fat layer is placed over the construct.

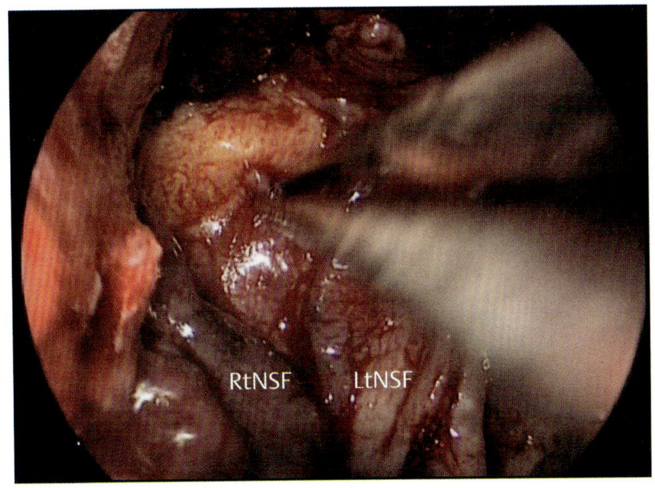

Fig. 12E.22 The right (RtNSF) and left nasoseptal flaps are rotated over the construct.

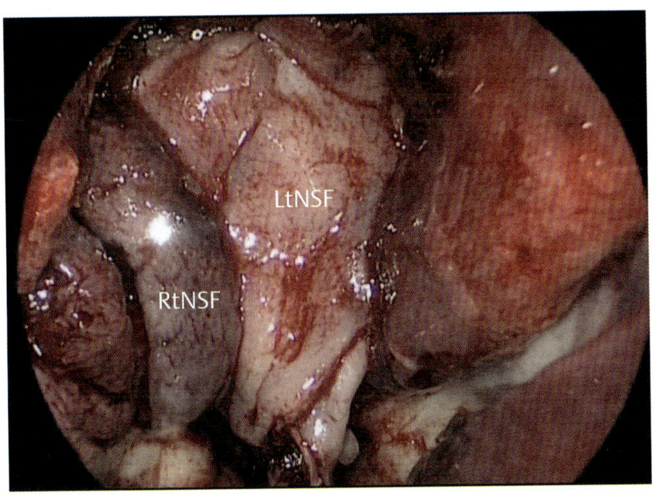

Fig. 12E.23 The edges of the nasoseptal flaps should have contact with the bony border of the skull base defect to assure adherence and epithelialization of the whole defect.

Chapter 13 Pterional Craniotomy and Resection of Tuberculum Sellae Meningioma

Amr Mohamed, Robert Iorga, and Sanjeeva Jeyaretna

History

A 43-year-old woman presented with a gradual worsening of left-sided vision. The visual acuity in the left eye was 6/60 and in the right eye was 6/12. The preoperative magnetic resonance imaging (MRI) is shown in **Fig. 13.1.**

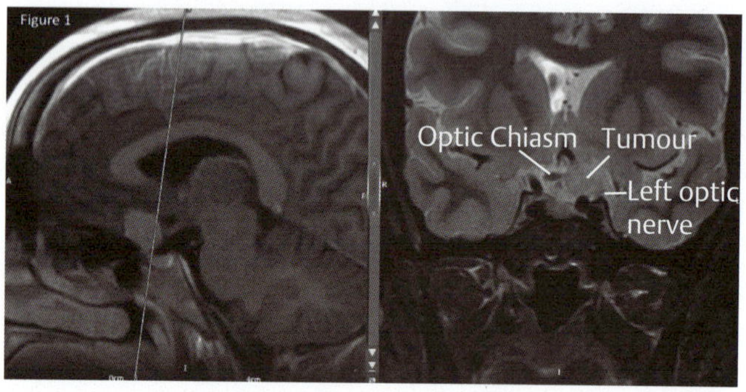

Fig. 13.1 Preoperative MRI scan. On the left, a sagittal T1 sequence with contrast and on the right a coronal image of a short tau inversion recovery (STIR) sequence showing the tuberculum sellae meningioma with compression and distortion of the left optic nerve.

Surgical Steps

1. The patient was positioned supine with a sandbag under the ipsilateral shoulder. The head is fixed in a Mayfield three-pin fixation system. The head position is raised above the level of the heart to improve venous drainage, turned 60 degrees to the contralateral side with lateral extension.
2. A curvilinear skin incision is performed from anterior to the tragus (< 1 cm to avoid injury to the temporal branch of the facial nerve) just above the upper border of the zygomatic arch (**Fig. 13.2a**), extending superiorly toward the superior temporal line and then turns anterior to cross the midline and ends on the contralateral side of the midline (**Fig. 13.2b**). (Right-sided incision is shown, all subsequent pictures demonstrate a left-sided operation). The temporalis fascia is not incised at this juncture, but the periosteum is cut in line with the incision. The superior temporal fascia fuses with the periosteum and both are dissected anteriorly with the skin flap to protect the temporal branch of the facial nerve (**Fig. 13.3**).
3. Interfascial dissection of the temporalis fascia: The dissection should continue anteriorly, exposing the

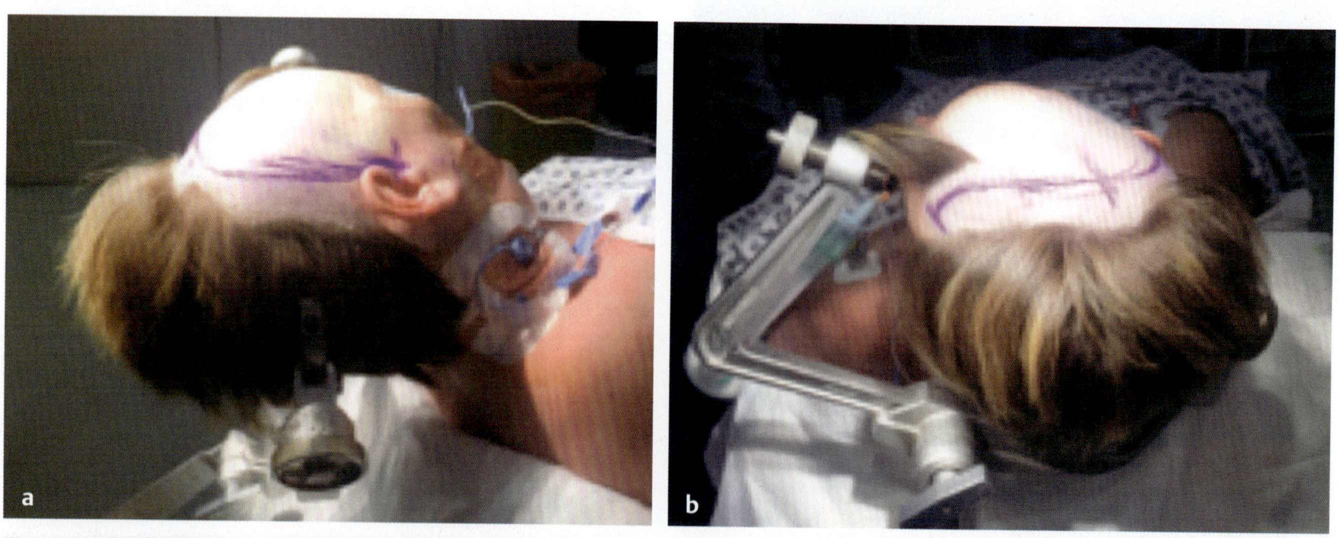

Fig. 13.2 (a, b) Patient positioning and skin incision (right-sided pterional craniotomy incision is shown).

zygomatic process of the frontal bone anteriorly (**Fig. 13.4** and **Fig. 13.5**).

4. The temporalis muscle is detached from the superior temporal line with monopolar cautery and then subperiosteally elevated from the squamous part of the temporal bone using a sharp periosteal elevator (e.g., Adson's periosteal elevator) to protect the deep nervous and vascular supply to the muscle (**Fig. 13.6**). The anterior attachment of the muscle on the sphenoid bone is dissected using monopolar coagulation because of the lack of a periosteal layer anteriorly because of the anastomosis of the deep temporal artery and middle meningeal artery.
5. The pterional craniotomy is performed next. The first burr hole is the keyhole, just posterior to the zygomatic process of the frontal bone and inferior to the superior temporal line. We drill across the sphenoid ridge using a 4-mm burr or a match head burr to create a trench. We complete the craniotomy by using a craniotome connecting the end of the trench to the keyhole then proceeding posteriorly till the edge of the wound and turn inferiorly to the middle fossa floor then anteriorly to the inferior end of the trench. After lifting the bone flap, we break through the remaining attachment of the sphenoid ridge (**Fig. 13.7**). This step is followed by drilling the lesser wing of sphenoid till reaching the lateral edge of the superior orbital fissure where the orbitomeningeal band is located. This is followed by dual incision and lifting it anteriorly.
6. Via a subfrontal approach, the tumor over the tuberculum sellae was exposed (**Fig. 13.8**).
7. Once we exposed the tumor, the arachnoid was dissected off the surface of the tumor to delineate its boundaries and early identification of the surrounding structures (**Fig. 13.9**). This step allowed to incise the tumor capsule safely to help us achieve central debulking of the tumor using the ultrasonic aspirator (e.g., CUSA, SONOPET, etc.) (**Fig. 13.10 and Fig. 13.11**).
8. After reducing the size of the meningioma to allow us to retract its edges, we managed to expose the left optic nerve and the left internal carotid artery (ICA) (**Fig. 13.12**). It is very important to remember the

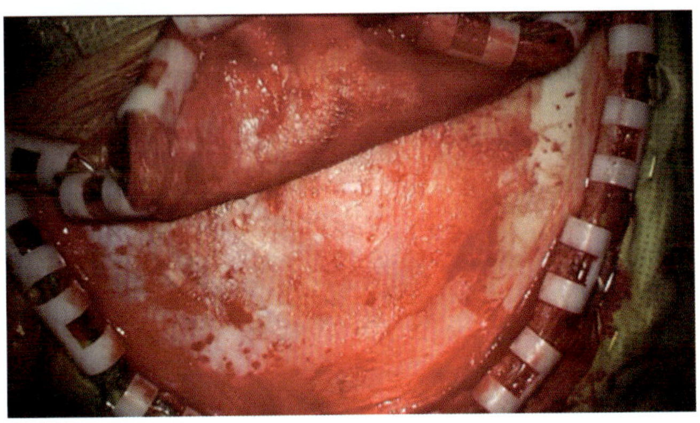

Fig. 13.3 The superior temporal fascia fuses with the periosteum, and both are dissected anteriorly with the skin flap to protect the temporal branch of the facial nerve.

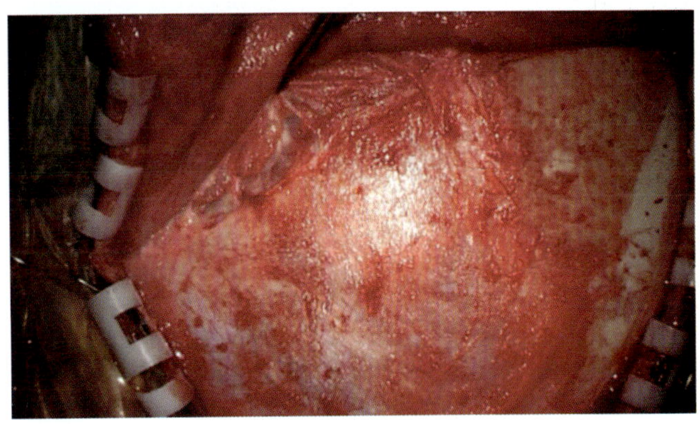

Fig. 13.4 An incision is made to separate the superficial and deep temporal fascia.

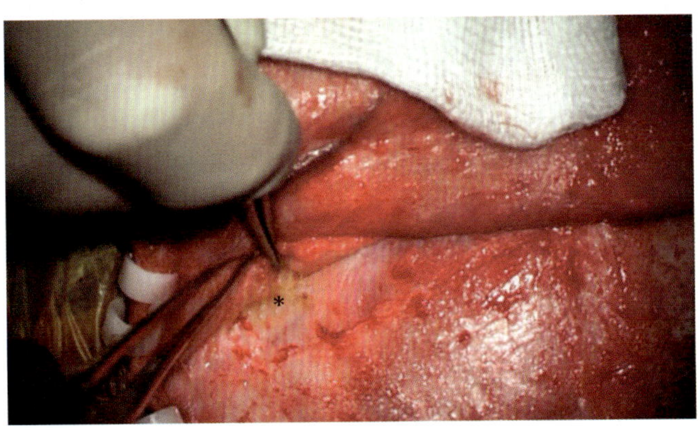

Fig. 13.5 This will expose the temporal fat pad (*).

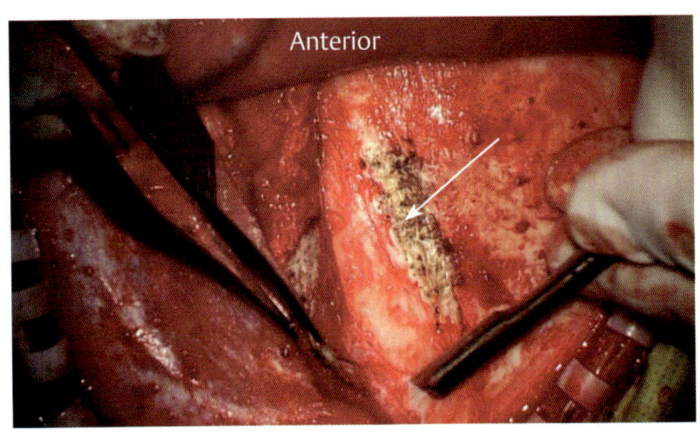

Fig. 13.6 Temporalis muscle dissection (*arrow*).

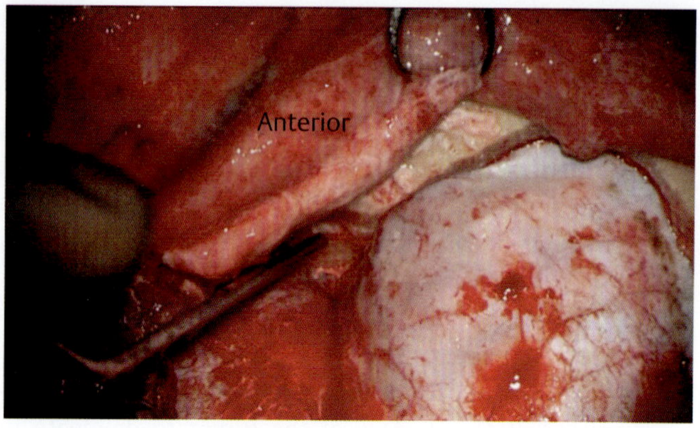

Fig. 13.7 Dura exposed after the elevation of the bone flap.

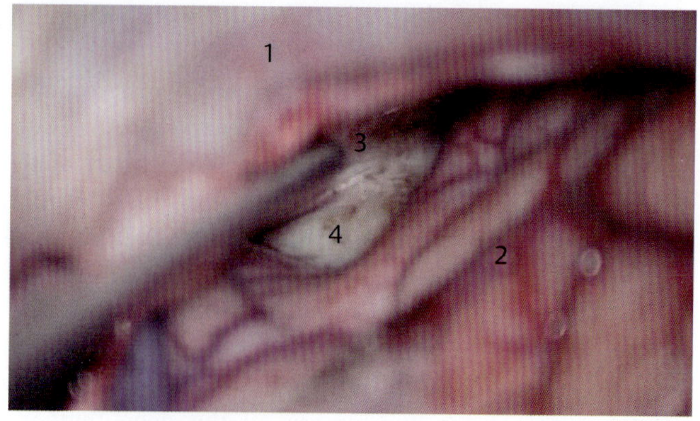

Fig. 13.8 Subfrontal approach and exposure of the tumor. A left-sided pterional craniotomy was performed. 1, the dura retracted anteriorly; 2, the orbital surface of the left frontal lobe; 3, the planum sphenoidale; 4, the meningioma on the tuberculum sellae.

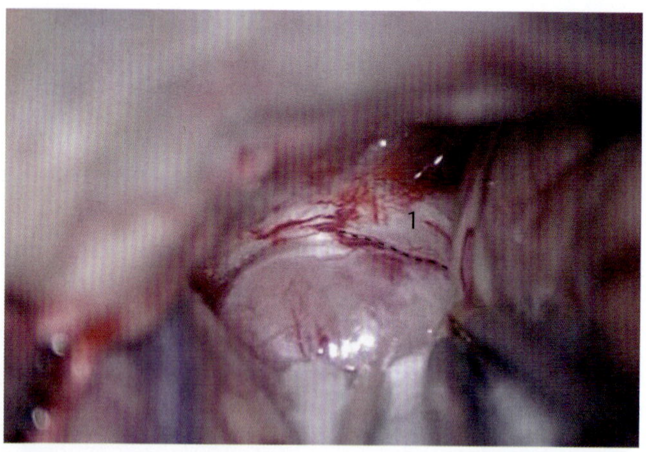

Fig. 13.9 The dissection of the arachnoid (1) of the tumor. The dotted line represents the arachnoid plane.

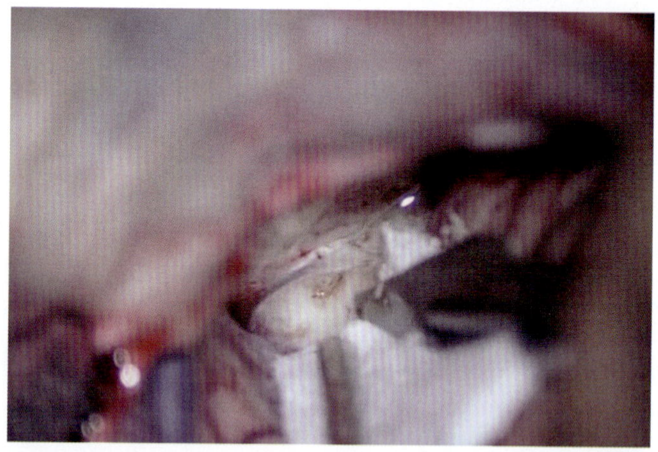

Fig. 13.10 Incision of the tumor capsule using a no. 11 blade.

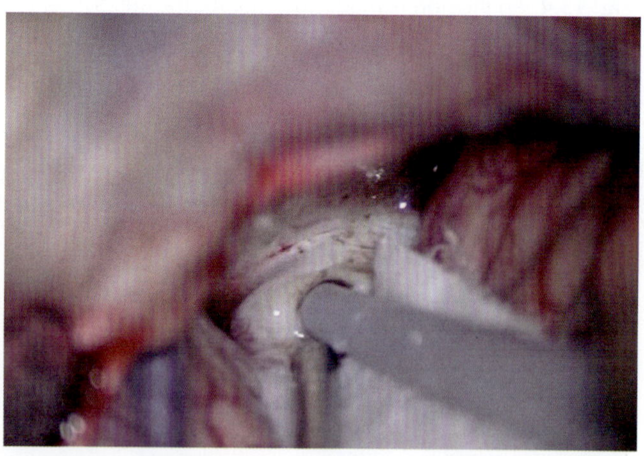

Fig. 13.11 Central debulking of the tumor using the ultrasonic aspirator using a SONOPET (Stryker) with a microtip.

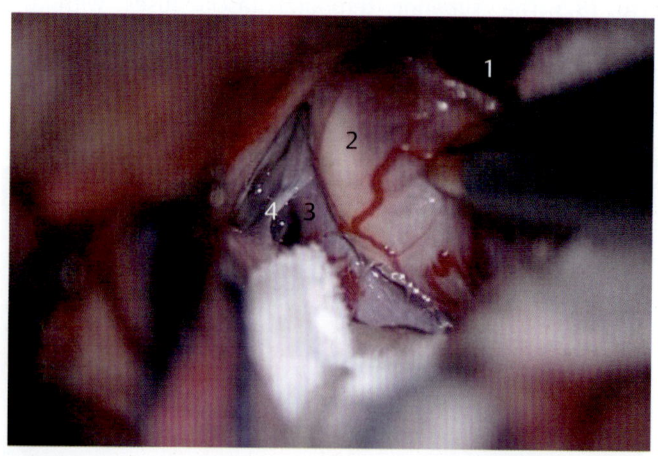

Fig. 13.12 Exposure of the left optic nerve by dissection of the arachnoid from over the meningioma. 1, the debulked tumor; 2, the left optic nerve; 3, the left ICA.

relationship of the optic nerve to the meningioma by careful reviewing of the preoperative MRI scan (**Fig. 13.1**). In our case, the left optic nerve was pushed inferiorly and laterally to the tumor.

9. Once the left optic nerve and the left ICA have been identified, further tumor debulking was carried out which led to the exposure of the right optic nerve dissection of the tumor (**Fig. 13.13**).
10. After resecting the meningioma, both optic nerves were visualized. Removal of the intracanalicular component of the meningioma in the left optic canal was achieved by the incision of the falciform ligament. A blunt hook was passed between the left optic nerve and the falciform ligament prior to dividing the falciform ligament (**Fig. 13.14**).
11. Deroofing of the left optic canal was done to achieve complete removal of the intracanalicular portion of the tumor. This was done by using a 1-mm up cutting Kerrison rongeur (**Fig. 13.15** and **Fig. 13.16**).

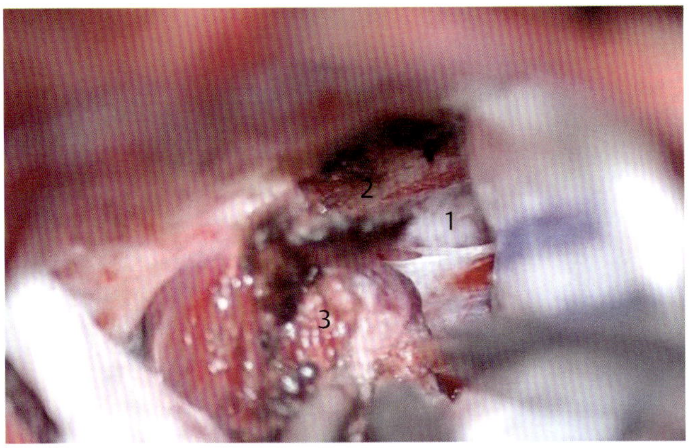

Fig. 13.13 Alternating between arachnoid dissection and central debulking of the meningioma. (1) the tuberculum sellae after debulking the majority of the meningioma; (2) the meningioma; (3) the left optic nerve.

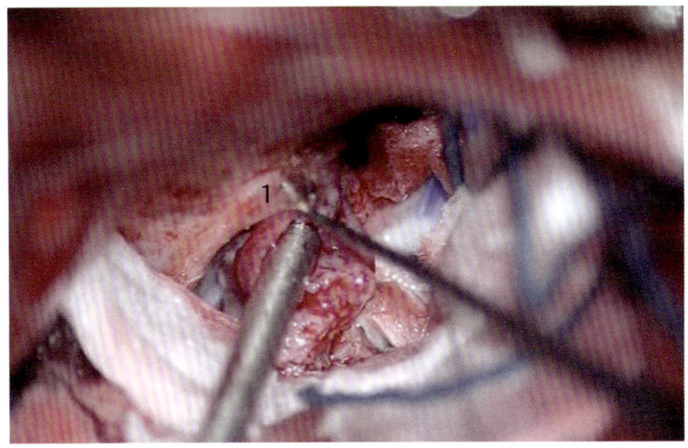

Fig. 13.14 Incision of the falciform ligament on the left to deliver the intracanalicular meningioma. , A blunt hook passed between the left optic nerve (1) and the falciform ligament prior to dividing the falciform ligament.

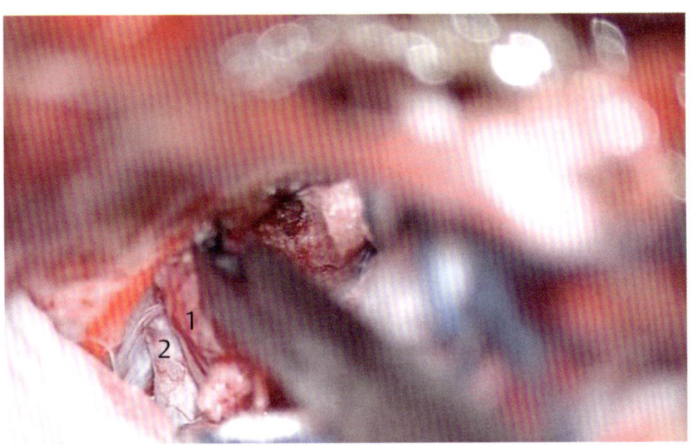

Fig. 13.15 Deroofing of the left optic canal using a 1-mm up cutting Kerrison rongeur to help deliver the intracanalicular meningioma. 1, the left optic nerve; 2, the left ICA.

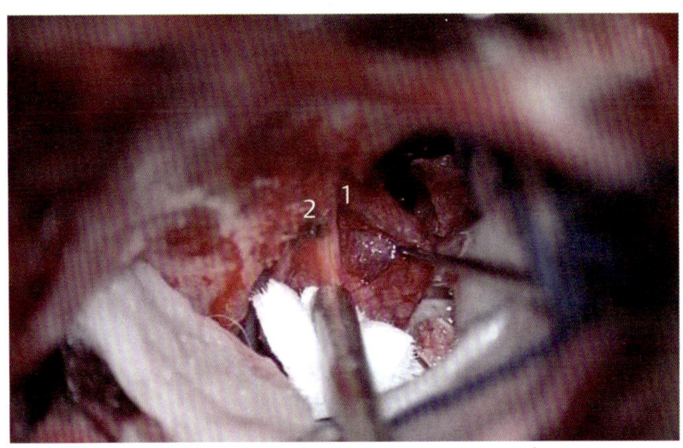

Fig. 13.16 Retrieval of the intracanalicular portion of the meningioma (1). 2, the left optic nerve.

12. The tumor capsule was adherent to the left optic nerve; hence, it was left to prevent damage to the optic nerve. **Fig. 13.17** demonstrates the final view under the microscope following the resection of the tumor.
13. After ensuring adequate hemostasis, watertight closure of the dura is done, followed by repositioning the bone flap and securing it with miniplates. The muscle and fascia are repositioned over the craniotomy and stitched to holes made in the skull over the superior temporal line. The subcutaneous and skin are closed in layers.
14. The postoperative MRI scan is seen in **Fig. 13.18**.

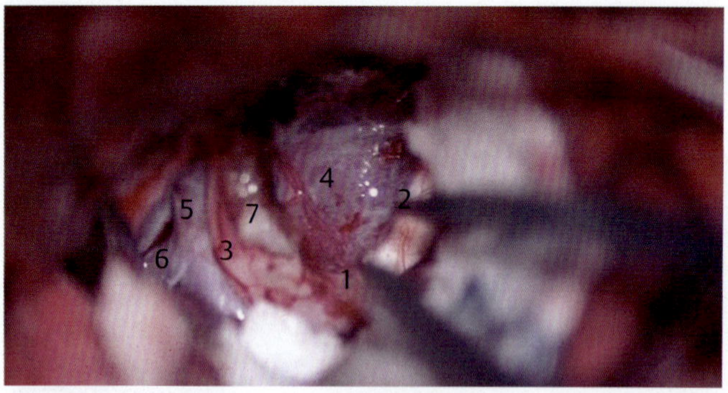

Fig. 13.17 The final picture following resection of the meningioma. 1, the optic chiasm; 2, the right optic nerve; 3, the left optic nerve; 4, the diaphragma sellae; 5, the left ICA; 6, the left posterior communicating artery; 7, residual meningioma capsule attached to the left optic nerve.

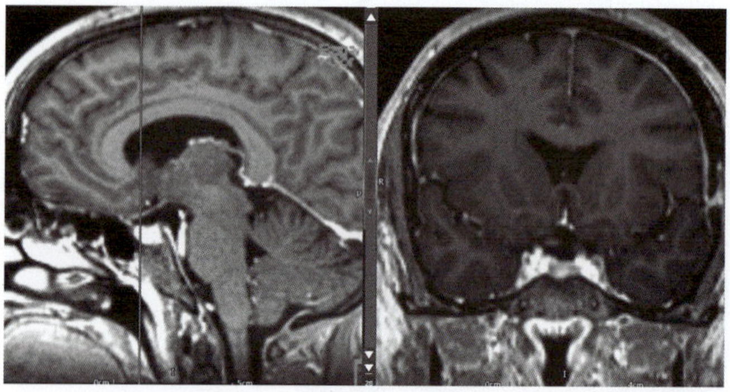

Fig. 13.18 T1 with contrast sequence, on the left a sagittal cut and on the right a coronal cut, revealing gross total resection of the tuberculum sellae meningioma.

Section III

Transcribriform Approach

Chapter 14 Endoscopic Resection of Sinonasal Tumors with Endonasal Craniectomy

Prathamesh S. Pai and Neelesh Tiwari

Introduction

Sinonasal tumors are uncommon tumors, and form less than 3% of all head and neck tumors. They are predominantly nonsquamous histology, subcranial and rarely metastasize to the neck nodes. Computed tomography (CT) scans and magnetic resonance imaging (MRI) can determine when the tumor has crossed the cribriform to involve the dura or brain. The systematic review of management of malignant sinonasal tumors over four decades suggests surgery with or without radiation to be the treatment of choice barring a few exceptions. Various surgical approaches have been described to manage sinonasal tumors. For subcranial diseases, transfacial approaches (medial maxillectomy, total maxillectomy) are adequate, while for intracranial extensions, craniofacial approach is suitable. Endoscopic surgery has over the past two decades proven to be safe oncologically with minimal morbidity.

Since Professor Messerklinger described "functional endoscopic sinus surgery," the transnasal access has been pursued with the microscope and later the endoscope for removal of sinonasal tumors. Professor Aldo Stamm and Professor Wolfgang Draf developed the microendoscopic transnasal route while the Pittsburgh group led by Professor Ricardo Carrau, Professor Carl Synderman, and Professor Amin Kassam described a modular "expanded endonasal approach" to access the entire ventral skull base. Their modular design simplified understanding of the complex skull base anatomy and paved the way for increased interest in endonasal tumor resection.

Transnasal Endoscopic Access

Experience in the transnasal access has come from working in confined spaces, controlling hemorrhage, and cerebrospinal fluid (CSF) leak management. Sinonasal tumors also lend themselves for endoscopic resection as they arise in the ethmoids, grow locally within the nasal cavity, and extend toward the eye, septum, cranium, and the palate. These tumors tend to hang into the nasal cavity rather than infiltrate the surrounding structures. A complete resection of these tumors is possible with margins similar to conventional techniques. The expanded endonasal approach is a methodical approach to the resection of the skull base in the coronal and sagittal plane. This approach while being minimally invasive is similar to conventional craniofacial resections. While en bloc resection was considered the gold standard in oncology, experiences from laryngeal, dermal, and other skull base tumor resections have proven that en bloc need not be sacrosanct for oncological safety. Another truism as far as sinonasal tumors is concerned is that these tumors seldom come out intact, and the posterior regions of these tumors are always removed piecemeal. En bloc resection involves extensive soft tissue and bone dissection but does not ensure wide margins as the limits are the orbits laterally and brain, carotid, and pituitary superiorly. Thus, a surgery wherein margins are structures to be resected clearly detailed, its execution via endonasal endoscopic resection would be as safe as conventional surgery. The only criterion to be adhered to is the surety that the tumor is resectable and is suitable for complete excision via conventional methods to ensure similar control rates.

Case Selection

The case selection for endoscopic approaches is critical.

- The anterior facial skeleton and nasolacrimal duct system should be free of disease.
- The palate and orbital contents should be free.
- The intracranial spread should be limited to paramedian region.
- The supraorbital extension should not cross the midpupillary line.

It is vital to evaluate the imaging in all the three planes, axial, coronal, and sagittal, as each plane provides information of disease spread vital for appropriate case selection.

Coronal plane provides information on the cribriform plate, the intracranial spread, the lamina papyracea, the midpupillary line, the maxillary sinus, and the palatal extent (**Fig. 14.1**).

Axial plane provides information on the anteroposterior length of the frontal sinus, the orbital apex, the nasolacrimal duct, the pterygopalatine fossa, and lateral sphenoid wall (**Fig. 14.2**).

Sagittal plane provides information on the anterior facial skeleton—the frontal bone, the maxilla, the nasal bones, as

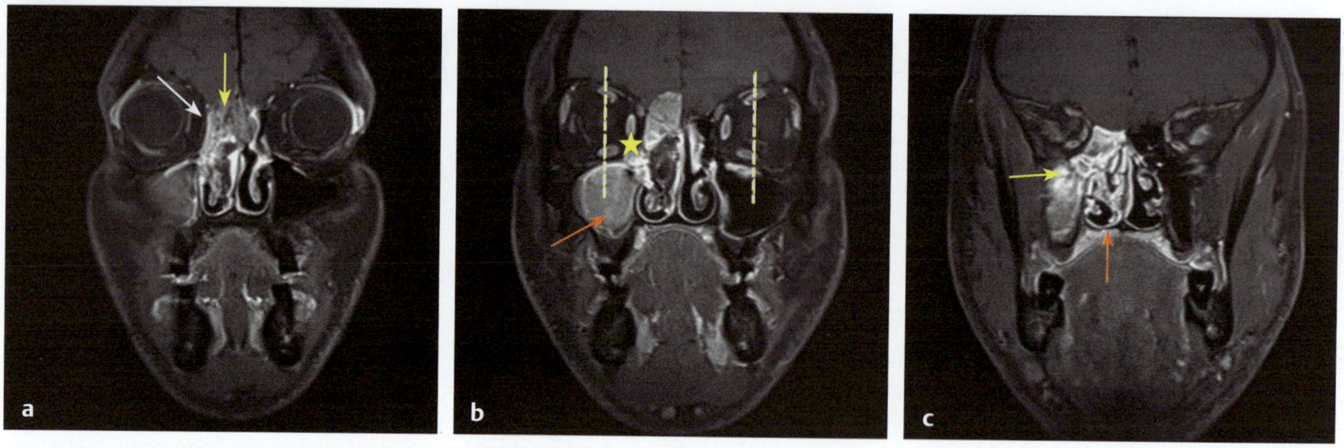

Fig. 14.1 Coronal images. **(a)** *White arrow*, lamina propria intact; *yellow arrow*, erosion of cribriform. **(b)** *Yellow interrupted lines* indicate *midpupillary lines*; *yellow star* indicates intraorbital contents which are uninvolved, *orange arrow* shows the maxillary sinus with inspissated secretions. **(c)** *Yellow arrow* shows the pterygopalatine fossa, and the *orange arrow* shows the intact palate.

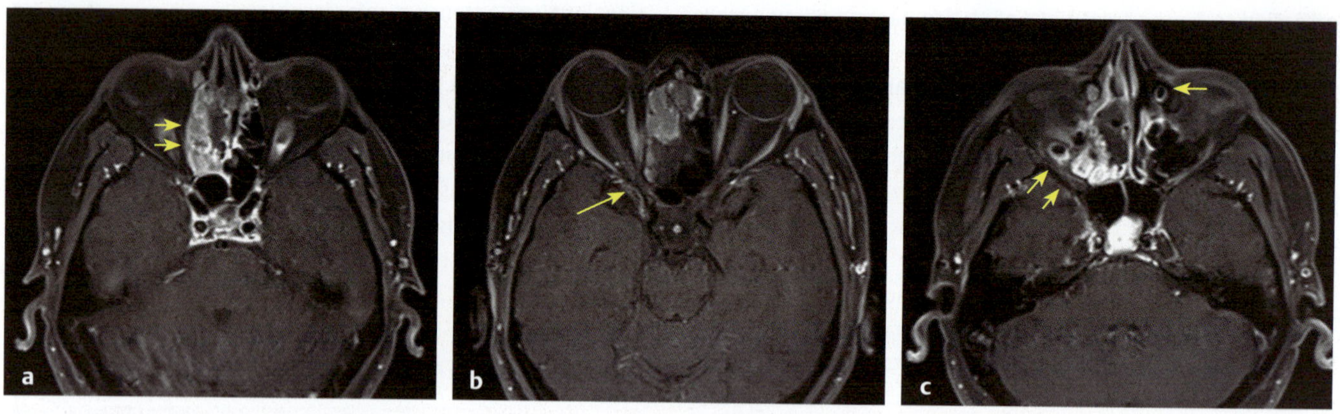

Fig. 14.2 Axial images. **(a)** *Arrows* show the intact lamina papyracea. **(b)** *Arrow* indicates the orbital apex. **(c)** *Single yellow arrow* shows the nasolacrimal duct, while the *two yellow arrows* show the pterygopalatine fossa.

well as involvement of the planum sphenoidale and intracranial spread (**Fig. 14.3**).

Contraindications

The contraindications for a conventional surgical removal of tumors in this region are:

- Bilateral optic nerve involvement.
- Internal carotid artery involvement.
- Extensive dural and brain involvement.
- Extensive dural enhancement.

Steps of Resection

For sinonasal tumors, which have breached the anterior skull base and involved the dura, the endoscopic endonasal trajectory is suitable for access as well as to encompass the tumor with margins. For an oncological clearance, we need to remove the nasal component and the intracranial component with adequate margins.

Central Debulking

The tumor in the nasal cavity usually involves the septum and ethmoids (**Fig. 14.4**). To achieve lateral margins, the lamina papyracea needs to be resected. In tumors breaching the lamina papyracea, the periorbita needs to be resected as the lateral margin. To visualize the lateral margin, central debulking is carried out either with bipolar cautery or using a microdebrider (**Fig. 14.5b**).

Devascularization

The main issue in paranasal sinus tumour surgery is bleeding, which can sometimes be torrential. To reduce the bleeding, the dissection should begin inferiorly along the lateral

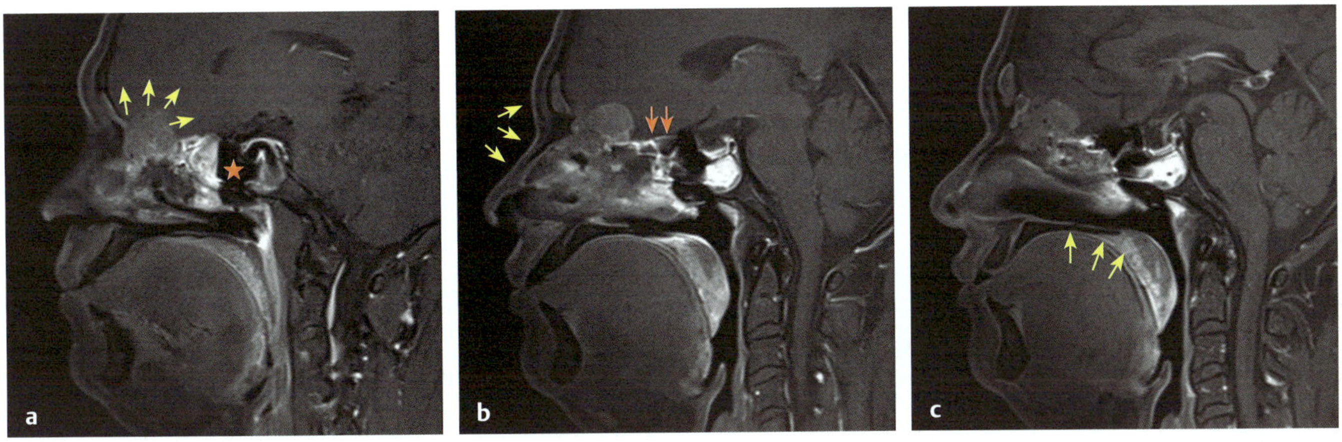

Fig. 14.3 Sagittal images. **(a)** *Yellow arrows* indicate tumor involvement of the brain, and the *orange star* shows the uninvolved sphenoid. **(b)** *Yellow arrows* show the facial skeleton being free, and the *orange arrows* indicate uninvolved planum dura. **(c)** *Yellow arrows* show the intact palate.

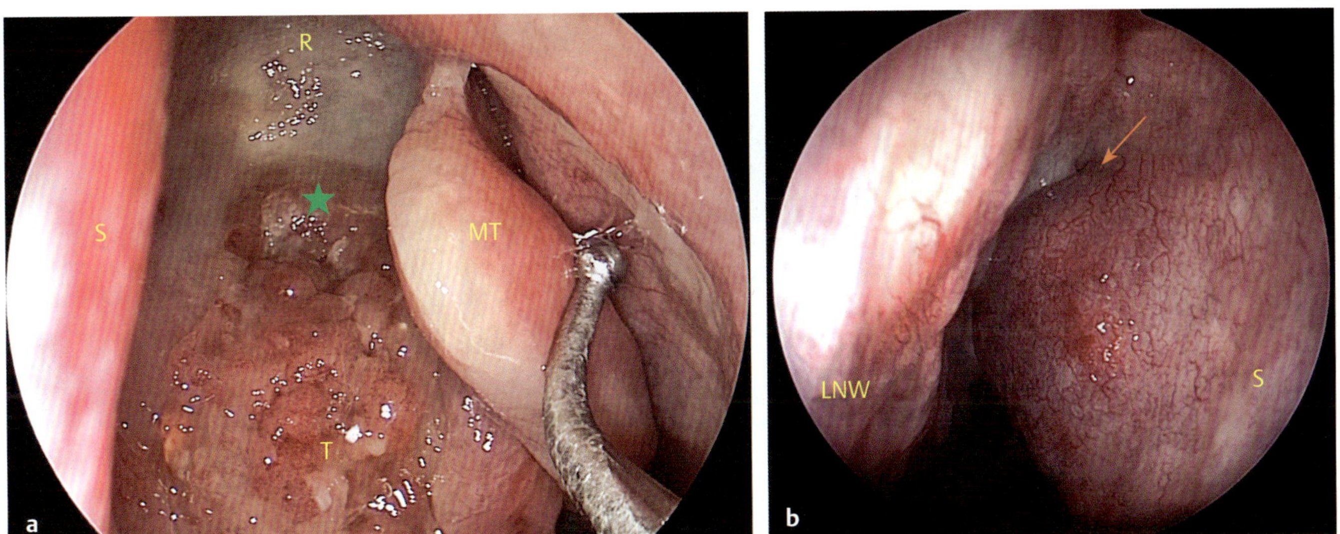

Fig. 14.4 **(a)** Tumor (T) in the left nasal cavity and olfactory groove (*). **(b)** Extension of the tumor through the septum into right olfactory groove (*arrow*).

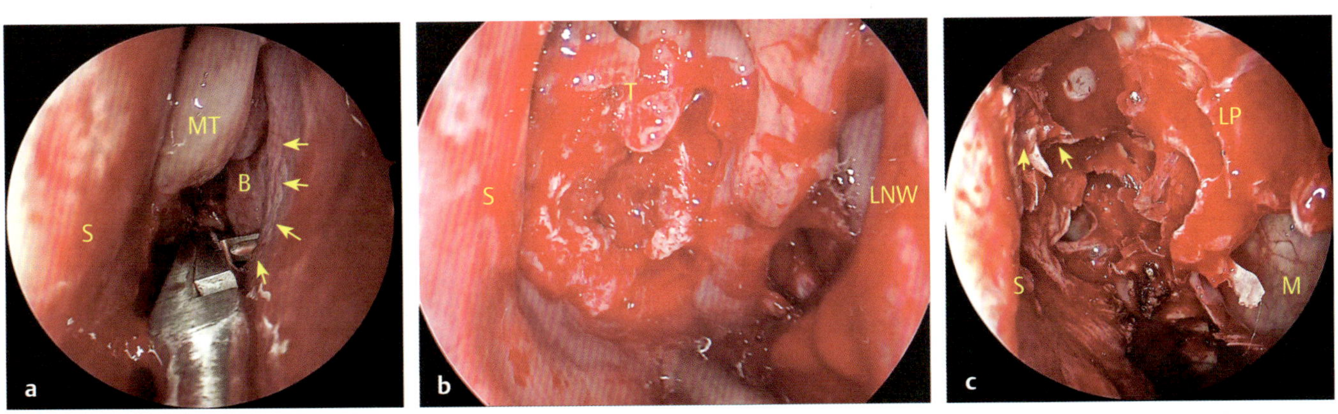

Fig. 14.5 **(a)** Uncinectomy with a back-biting forceps at the junction of horizontal and vertical limb of uncinate process (*yellow arrows*) in left nasal cavity. **(b)** Debulking of the tumor mass (T) in left nasal cavity. **(c)** Ethmoidectomy on left nasal cavity after removal of middle turbinate. Yellow arrows show cut attachment of the middle turbinate.

nasal wall and proceed toward the ethmoid crest onto the sphenopalatine fossa. The branches of the sphenopalatine vessels are identified and controlled either with electrocautery or Ligaclips. This is done bilaterally. As the dissection proceeds, the anterior and posterior ethmoidal vessels are identified and cauterized (**Fig. 14.6**).

Ethmoidectomy

The ethmoids are resected bilaterally exposing the skull base from frontonasal recess anteriorly till the sphenoid posteriorly. The maxillary sinus ostia are widened (**Fig. 14.5a, c**).

Septal Resection

The nasal septum is resected from the maxillary crest inferiorly up to the perpendicular plate of the ethmoid superiorly preserving only a small strut anteriorly to prevent saddling. Posteriorly, the vomer is resected and the rostrum is exposed (**Fig. 14.7**).

Rostrum Resection

The anterior wall of the sphenoid is either drilled or osteotomized along the articulation of the rostrum with the vomer. The rostrum is removed and the intersphenoid septa are drilled gently with a diamond burr up to the planum sphenoidale (**Fig. 14.8**).

Draf III (Modified Lothrop Procedure)

The frontal sinuses are exposed and joined in midline exposing the posterior frontal wall adequately. It is vital to achieve a wide opening of the frontonasal recess to facilitate proper resection of the cribriform as well as placement of the fascia lata grafts during reconstruction (**Fig. 14.9**).

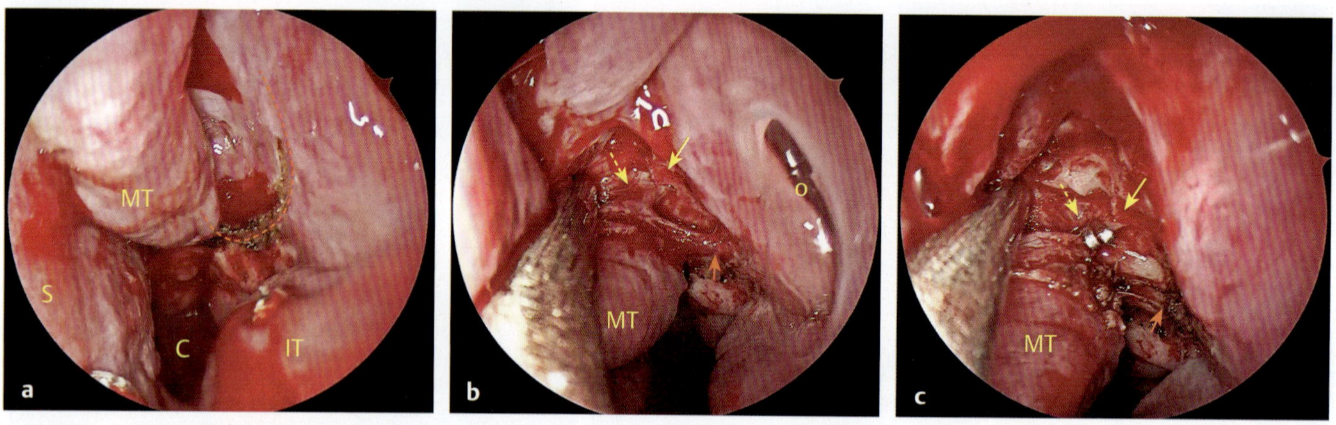

Fig. 14.6 **(a)** For identification of the sphenopalatine artery, a "U" shaped incision (*orange dots*) is made just anterior to posterior end of middle turbinate (MT). **(b)** Exposure of ethmoid crest (*yellow solid arrow*), sphenopalatine artery (*broken yellow arrow*), and branch to middle turbinate (*orange arrow*). **(c)** Sphenopalatine artery is clipped (*broken yellow arrow*). Artery to middle turbinate is cauterized (*orange arrow*).

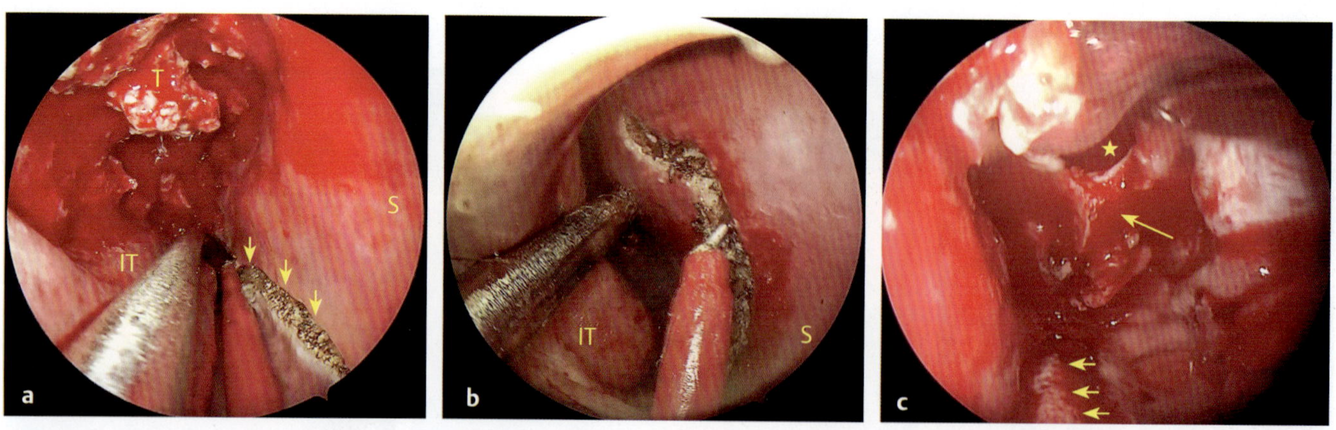

Fig. 14.7 **(a)** Horizontal incision (*arrows*) along the inferior border of septum near the maxillary crest. **(b)** Vertical incision at the anterior end of septum (S) leaving an inverted L-shaped strut of the cartilage about 1 cm wide for stability of the tip of the nose. **(c)** Exposure of keel of vomer and rostrum of sphenoid (*yellow arrow*). Maxillary crest after septectomy (*orange arrows*).

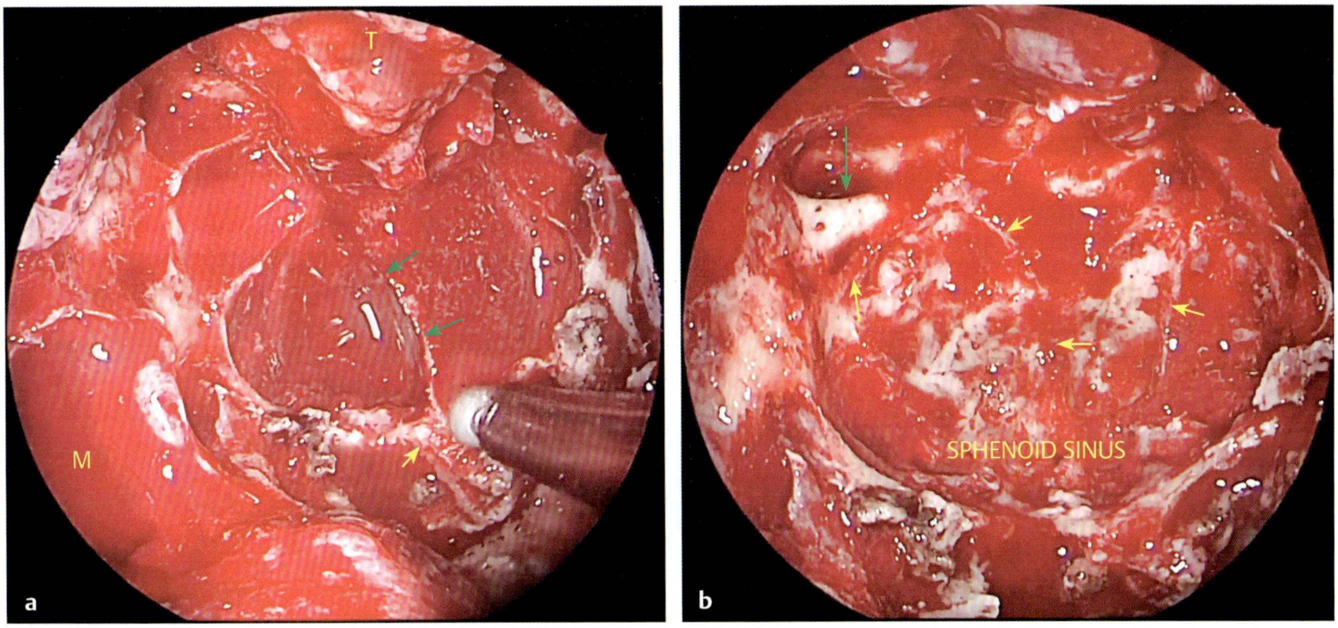

Fig. 14.8 **(a)** Drilling of rostrum (*yellow arrow*) and septae in the sphenoid sinus (*green arrow*). **(b)** View of sphenoid sinus after drilling of rostrum and intrasinus septae (*yellow arrows*). Green arrow represents optic canal.

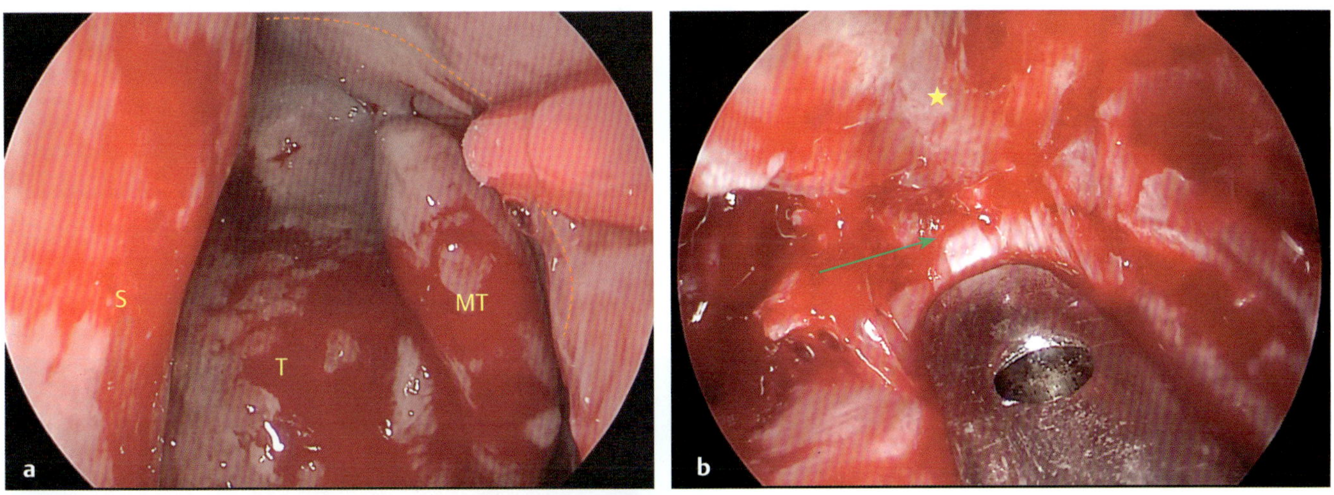

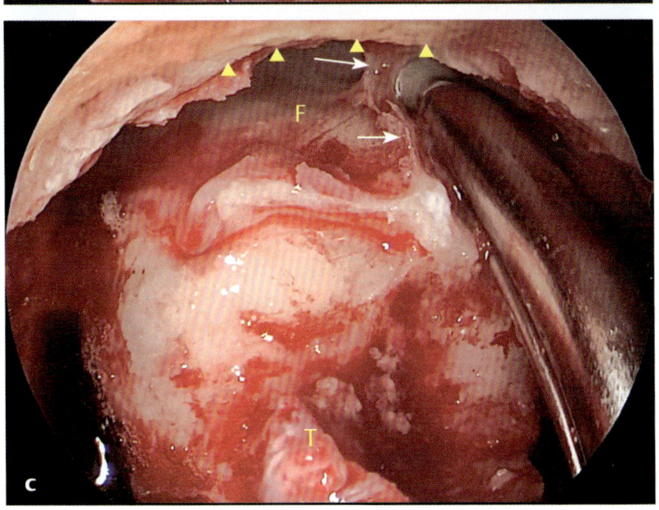

Fig. 14.9 **(a)** Incision on frontonasal mucosa extending to the roof and the septum (*orange dots*). **(b)** Mucosa elevated on nasal roof up to the first olfactory fibrils (*green arrow*). * shows site of frontal sinus for medial approach. **(c)** View of frontal sinus after Draff Type III sinusotomy. Frontal beak (*yellow arrow heads*) and septae (*white arrows*) are drilled out to smoothen the posterior frontal wall.

Devascularization of the Ethmoid Vessels

The lamina papyracea resection is started at its articulation with the orbital process of the palatine bone extending superiorly along its upper margin which articulates with the orbital plate of the frontal bone. This exposes the anterior and posterior ethmoid arteries which are then cauterized as they exit from the orbit (**Fig. 14.10** and **Fig. 14.11**).

Crista Galli

The crista can be kept attached to the cribriform and removed en bloc. However, a better option would be to separate the olfactory filaments and the dura from the cribriform plate and separate the crista galli from the frontal bone before resecting the dura (**Fig. 14.12**).

Cribriform Plate

Once the skull base from frontal bone to sphenoid is exposed and devascularized, the cribriform is drilled with a rough diamond burr exposing the underlying dura. Using small curved elevators, the dura is exposed from the frontal anteriorly to the planum posteriorly (**Figs. 14.13** and **14.14**).

Dural Resection

The dura while intact is elevated from the bone for a distance of 1 cm. This allows the dura to be pliant to form a good seal during reconstruction. Thereafter, using a Cappabianca retractable sharp blade, an incision is made in the dura keeping adequate margins. The cuts are made laterally, and then using fine curved microscissors, the dura is cut anteriorly toward the center. Care should be taken while reflecting the dura to prevent injury to the underlying vessels. Anteriorly, the dura is cauterized before joining the incision in the midline (**Fig. 14.15** and **Fig. 14.16**).

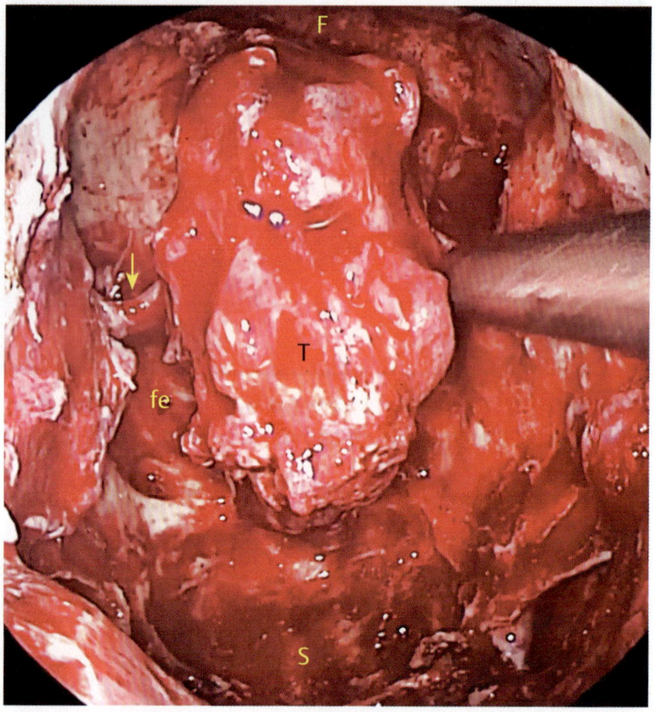

Fig. 14.10 360-degree exposure of the tumor on the cribriform.

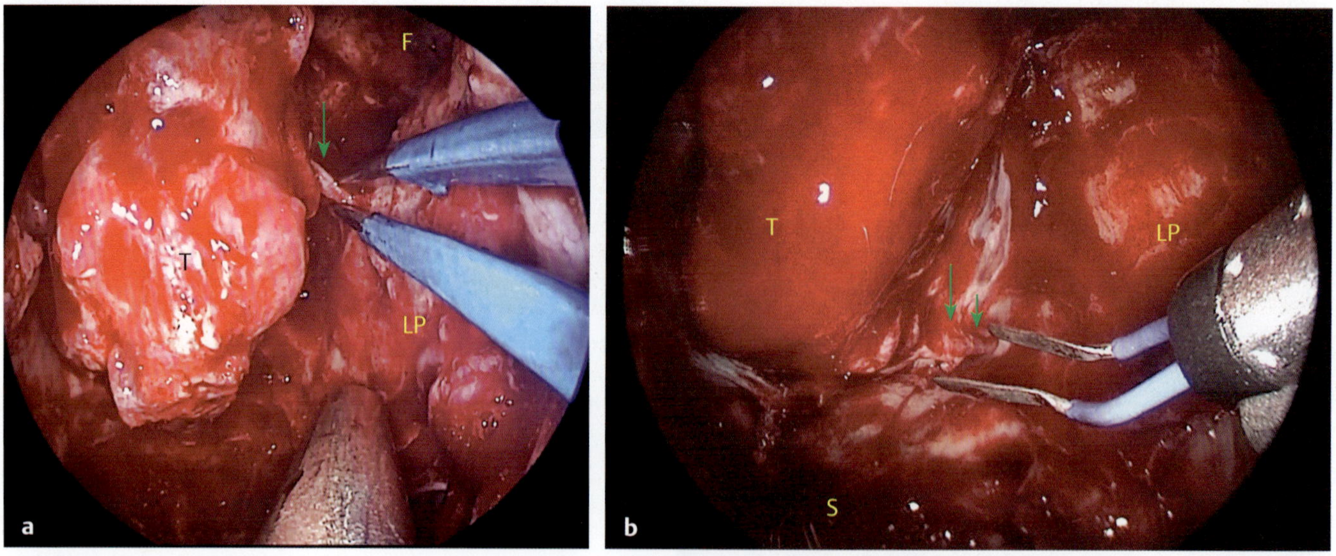

Fig. 14.11 **(a)** Cauterization of left anterior ethmoid artery (*green arrow*). **(b)** Cauterization of left posterior ethmoid artery (*green arrow*).

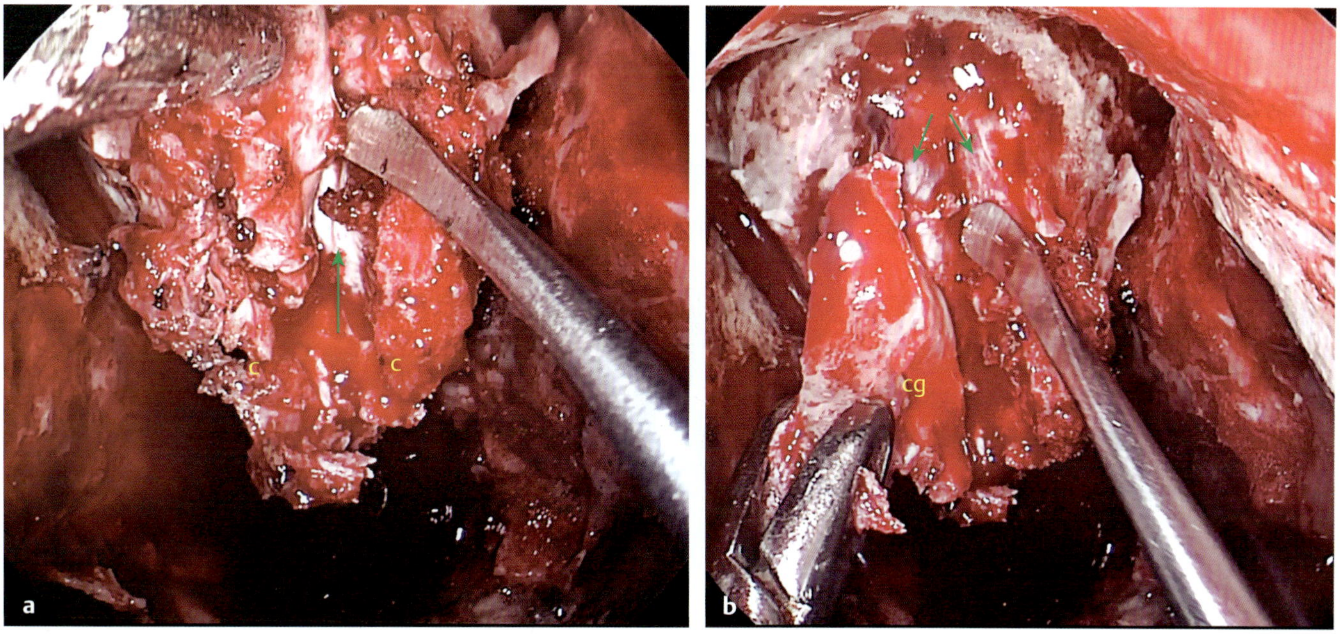

Fig. 14.12 **(a)** Dissection of crista galli (*white arrow*) from the falx (*green arrow*). **(b)** Removal of crista galli (cg). *Green arrows* represent two layers of falx.

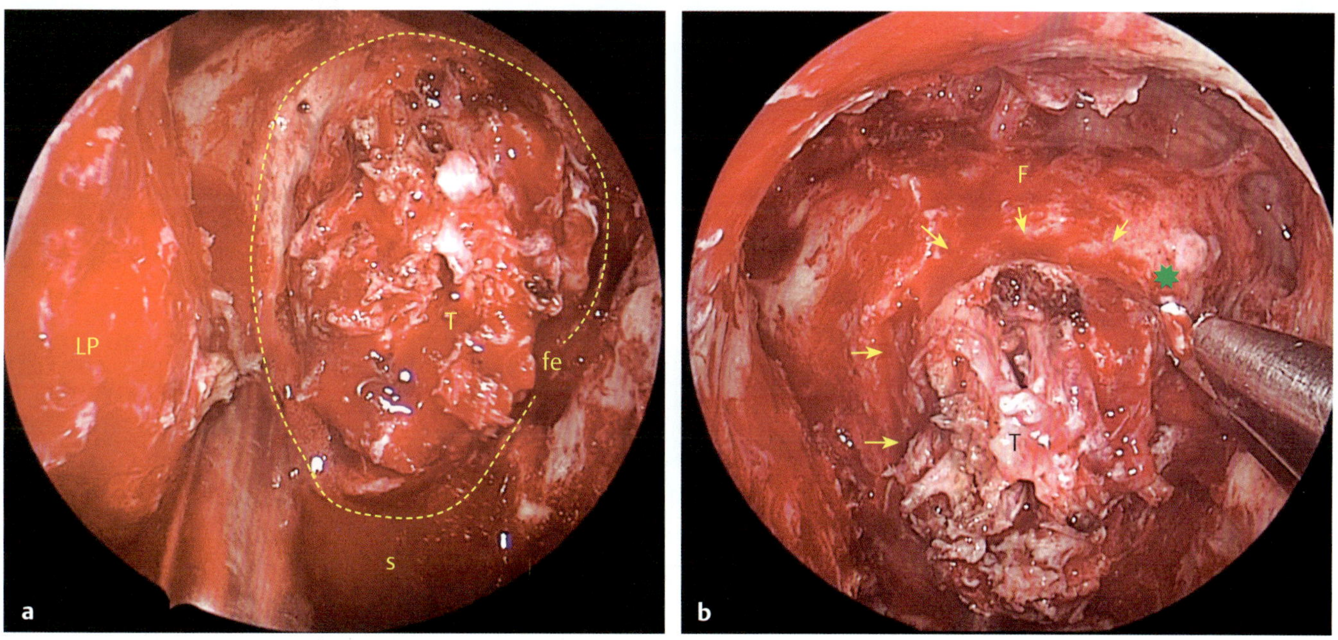

Fig. 14.13 **(a)** Circumferential drilling of the fovea, planum, and posterior frontal wall (*dots*). **(b)** After thinning out the bone (*yellow arrows*), it is punched out (*green star*) with a Kerrison's rongeur to expose the underlying dura.

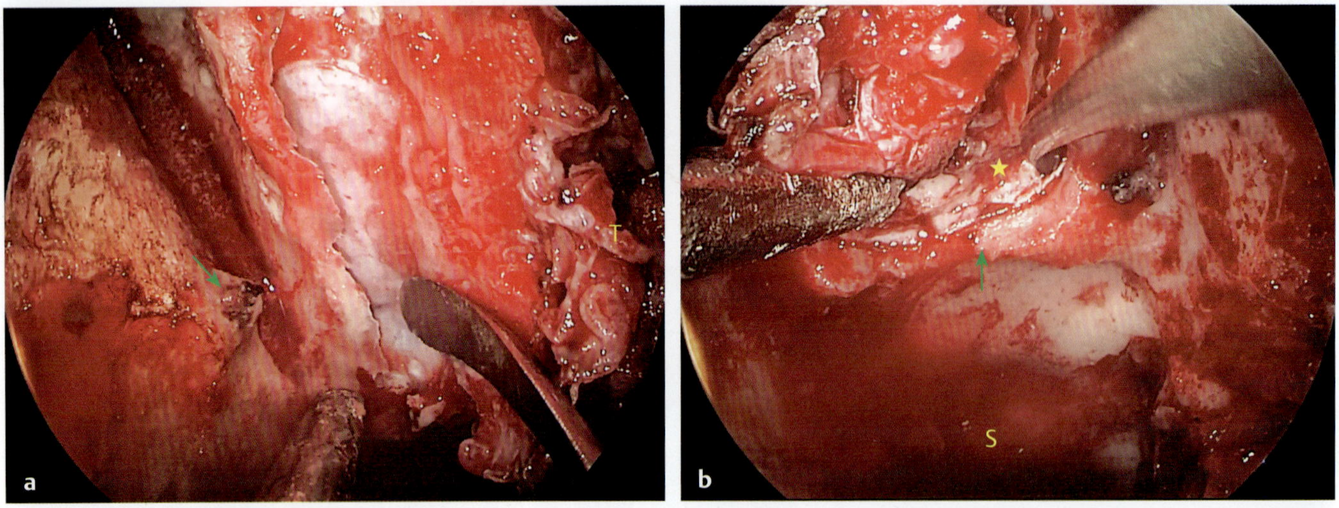

Fig. 14.14 **(a)** Exposed dura is elevated from the bony edges before incision. Green arrow represents cut end of anterior ethmoid artery. **(b)** Dura is elevated posteriorly (*) from the planum sphenoidale (*green arrow*).

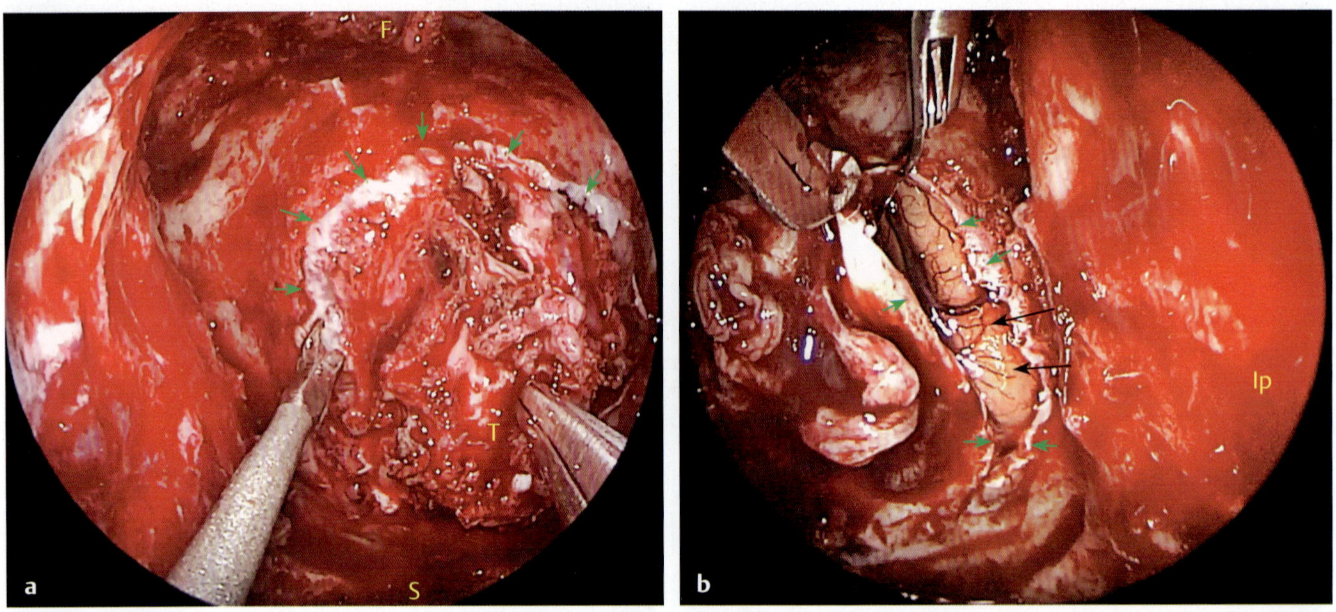

Fig. 14.15 **(a, b)** Incision of the exposed dura (*green arrow heads*). *Black arrows* represent gyrus rectus.

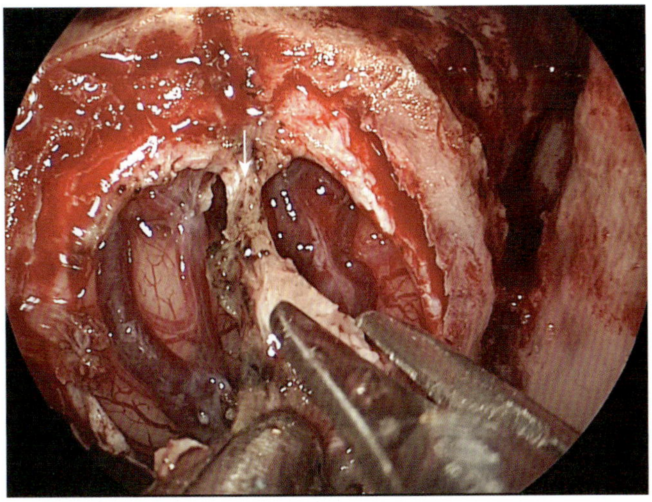

Fig. 14.16 Cutting of falx (*white arrow*) in the midline.

Intradural Dissection

The dura is reflected, and tumor extension into the brain is assessed. The tumor is separated using curved mini bipolar forceps to ensure a bloodless field and avoid contusion of the brain. The falx cerebri is divided in midline, and the two olfactory bulbs are separated. The specimen now hinges on these bulbs and is reflected posteriorly (**Fig. 14.17**).

Olfactory Bulb Division

The olfactory bulbs are cauterized and divided sharply. The posterior dura is then divided under vision, and the specimen is delivered through the nose (**Fig. 14.18**).

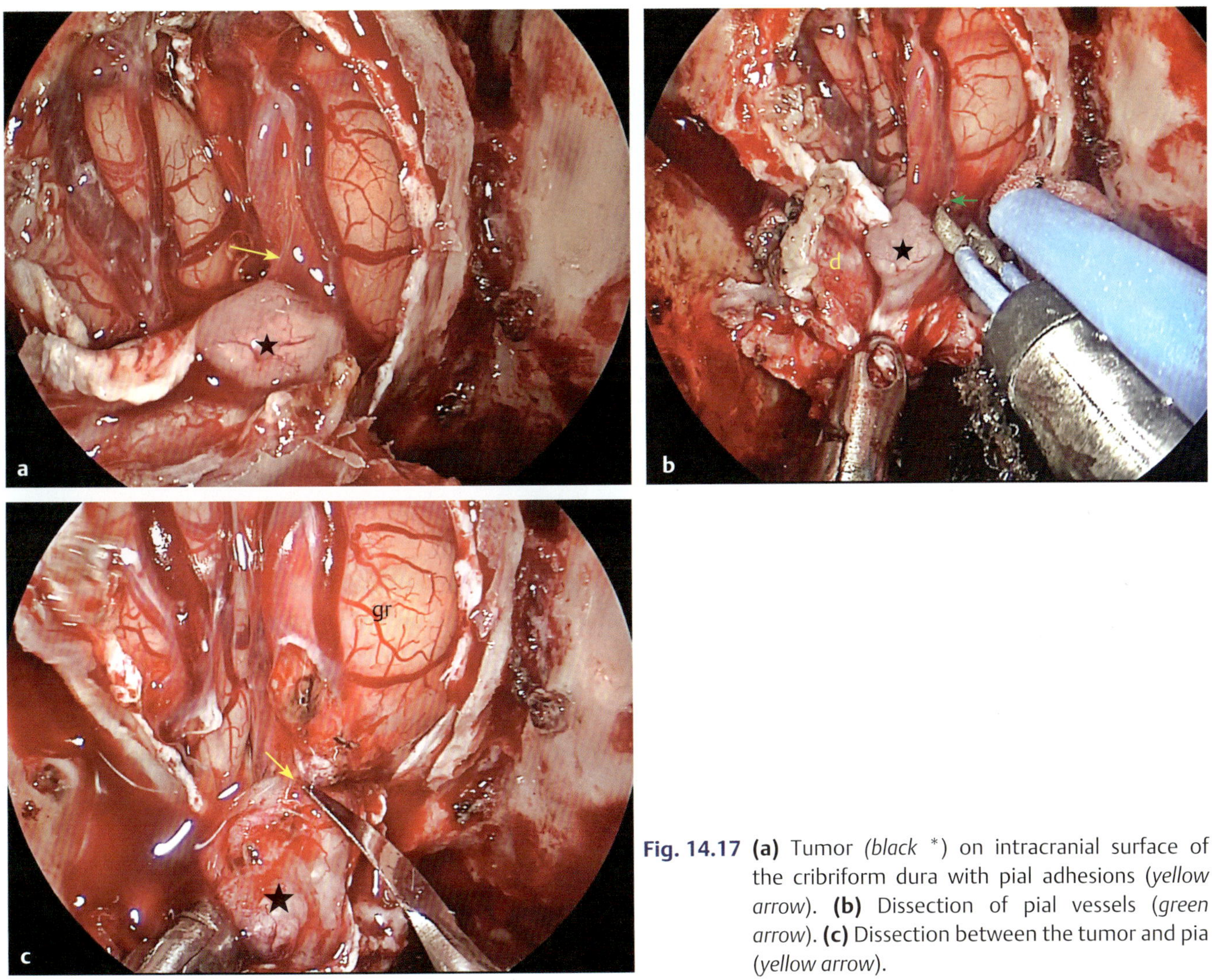

Fig. 14.17 **(a)** Tumor *(black* *) on intracranial surface of the cribriform dura with pial adhesions (*yellow arrow*). **(b)** Dissection of pial vessels (*green arrow*). **(c)** Dissection between the tumor and pia (*yellow arrow*).

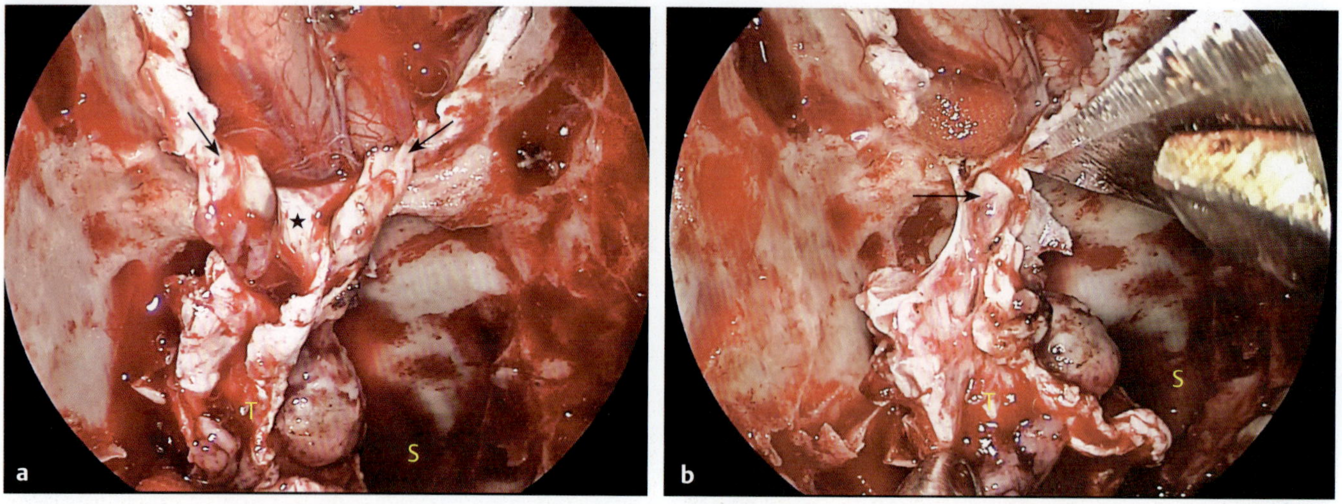

Fig. 14.18 **(a)** Last remaining attachment on the planum (*) with two olfactory bulbs (*black arrows*). **(b)** Cutting planum dura to remove the specimen. Black arrow represents cut olfactory bulb.

Dural Repair

The defect is usually 3 by 3 cm (**Fig. 14.19**). The case selection ensures that a larger defect does not ensue especially toward the planum. In tumors which are lateralized and do not involve the septum, a nasoseptal flap can be used to provide a mucosal cover for the defect. This needs to be planned in advance. The dural defect is covered with either a two- or a three-layer closure (**Fig. 14.20**).

1. *First layer (inlay graft)*: The fascia lata is harvested, and the defect is sized, and appropriate fascia is marked. The fascia lata graft should be at least 1 cm more in both the anteroposterior and the transverse dimensions to accommodate the swelling of the brain which tends to herniate slightly through the defect. Another important issue is the cut made in midline to ensure that the anterior edge of the fascia fits in the two cerebral compartments separated by the falx cerebri. The inner layer adheres with surface tension similar to tympanoplasty (**Fig. 14.21**).
2. *Second layer (overlay graft)*: It is placed over the dura and covering the surrounding bone onto the periorbita on both sides. Care is taken to avoid covering the frontal sinuses (**Fig. 14.22**).

Some groups suggest placing the second layer of fascia as an "interlay" graft between the dural edges and bone followed by fat to smoothen the edges and then a third layer of either fascia lata or Haddad flap.

Final Packing

Surgicel pieces are placed at the edges, and tissue glue is evenly applied all over. After waiting for setting period of the glue, Gelfoam pieces are placed over the assembly. Finally, Merocel pieces are placed strategically to give even pressure and prevent breakdown. The Merocel expands with either antibiotic solution or diluted povidone iodine solution.

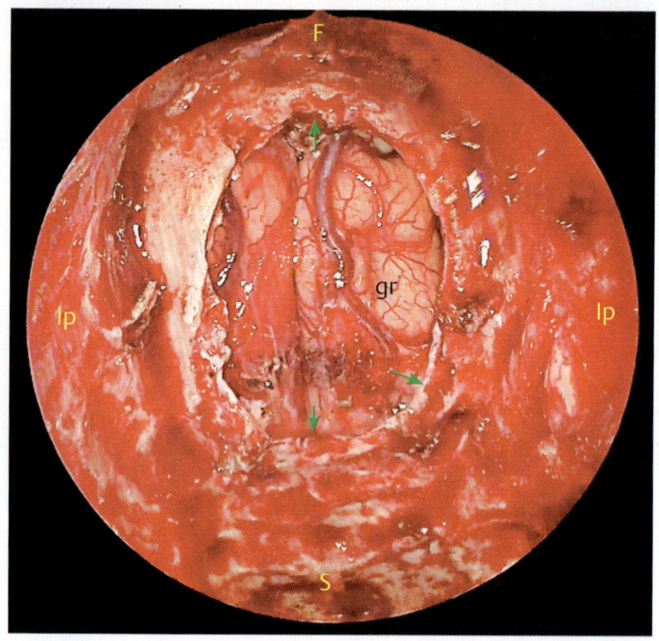

Fig. 14.19 Defect of the dura after the resection. Green arrow heads show dural edges.

Postoperative Care

The patient is given parenteral antibiotics, which cross the blood–brain barrier, head elevation of 15 degrees, complete bed rest, stool softeners, and cough suppressants. These measures prevent sudden rise of intracranial pressure which can potentially destabilize the repair assembly.

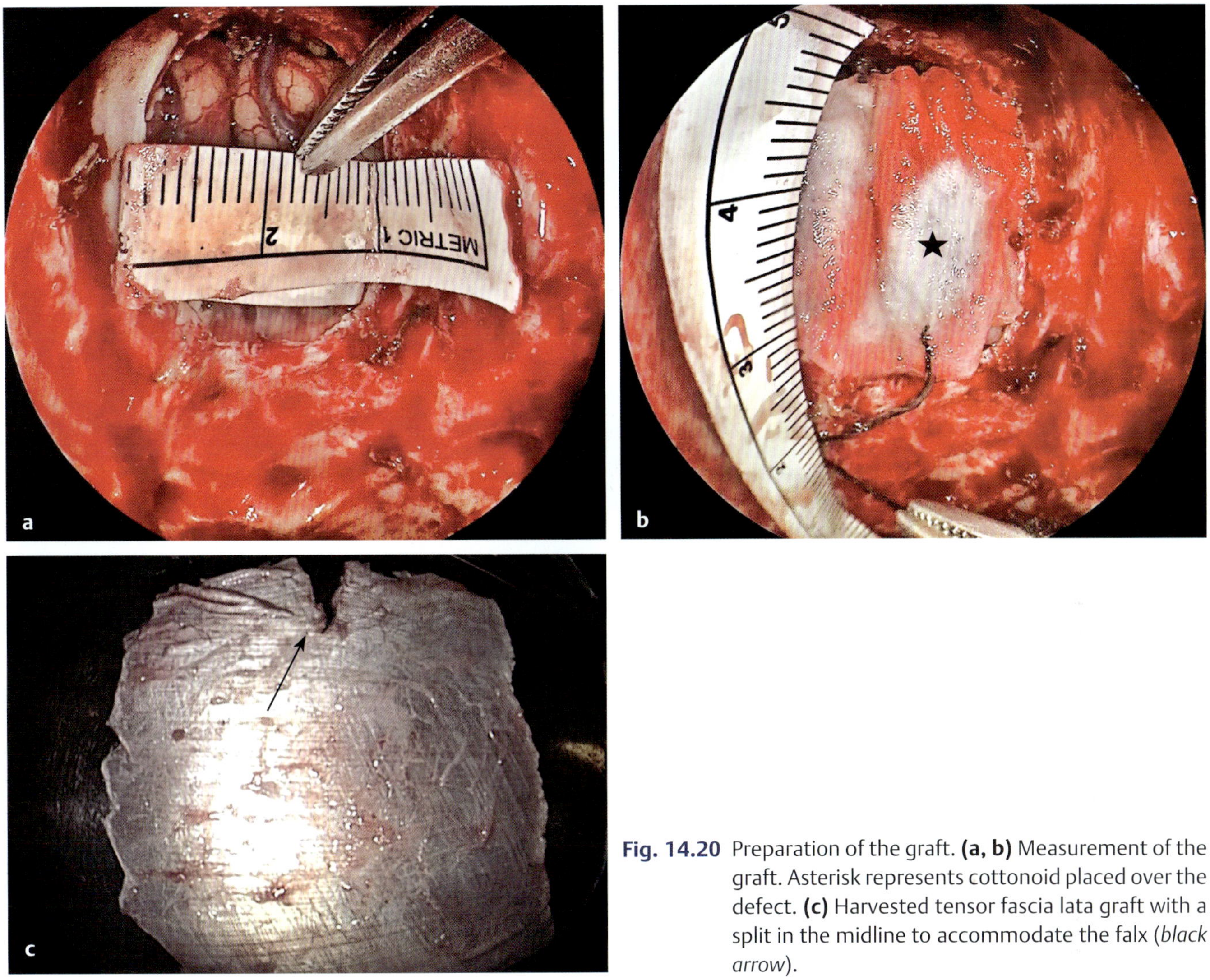

Fig. 14.20 Preparation of the graft. **(a, b)** Measurement of the graft. Asterisk represents cottonoid placed over the defect. **(c)** Harvested tensor fascia lata graft with a split in the midline to accommodate the falx (*black arrow*).

Complications

Cerebrospinal Fluid Leak

It is the most dreaded complication but is extremely rare. Most series report around 5% leak rate. University of Pittsburgh has reduced its complication rate with the use of vascularized flaps both local, such as nasoseptal and lateral nasal flaps, as well as distant, such as pericranial and temporalis fascia flaps.

Meningitis

Meningitis rates are extremely low. In most series it is less than 1%. This should not make us complacent, and all care should be taken to prevent it which otherwise might result in severe morbidity and expense.

Combined Endoscopic and Craniotomy Access (Cranioendoscopic Resection)

Intracranial extension of sinonasal sinuses can be extensive. Tumors with dural involvement, tumors with enhancement laterally beyond the midpupillary line, and tumors reaching the planum sphenoidale are not feasible for endonasal resection and a safe transnasal repair. When there is gross brain involvement not limited to midline, it is not suitable for endonasal resection. In these situations, if the nasal component is amenable for endoscopic resection, then it is addressed transnasally along with a conventional cranial access for the intracranial component.

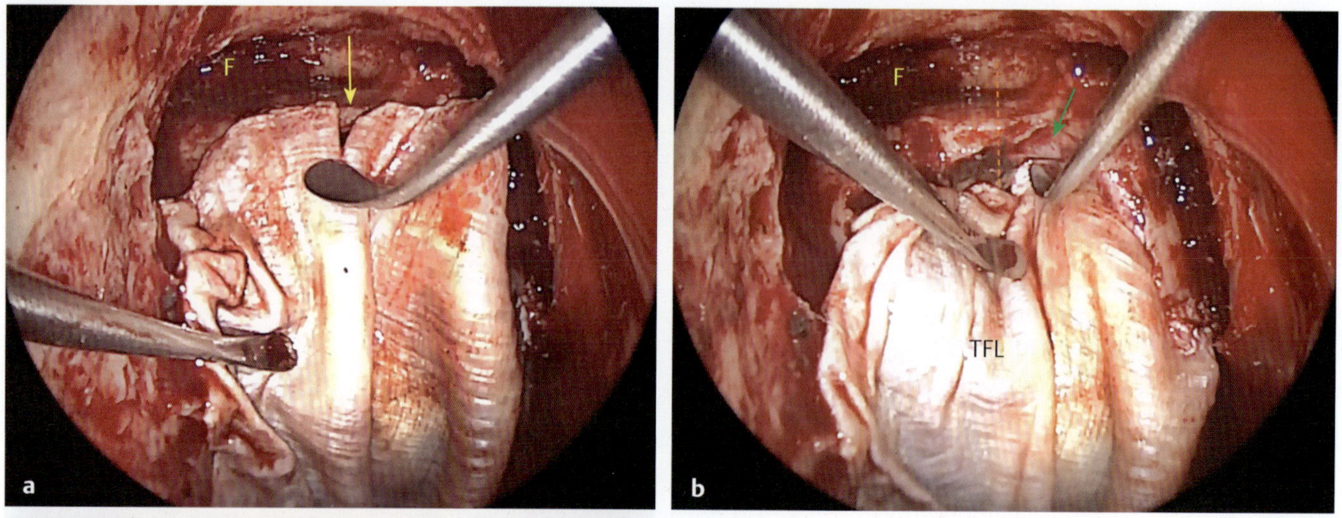

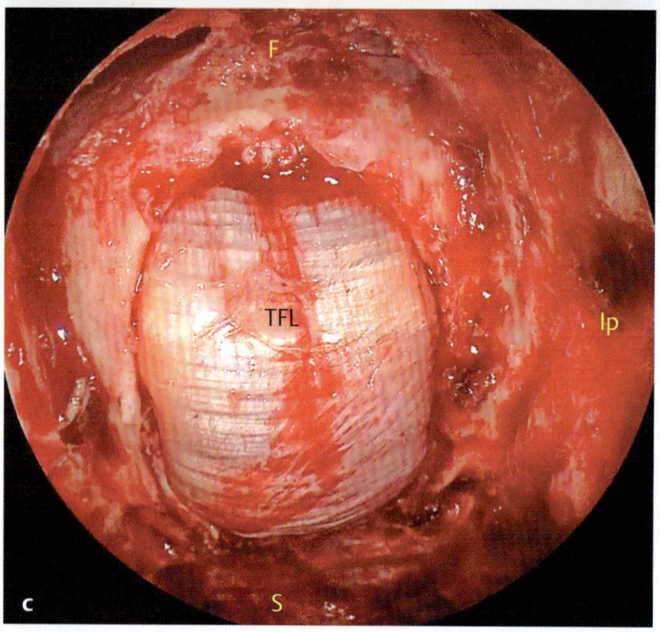

Fig. 14.21 **(a)** Placement of inlay layer. Arrow shows split in the midline. **(b)** Insertion of tensor fascia lata (TFL). Green arrow shows dural edge. **(c)** Inlay after complete insertion of the TFL.

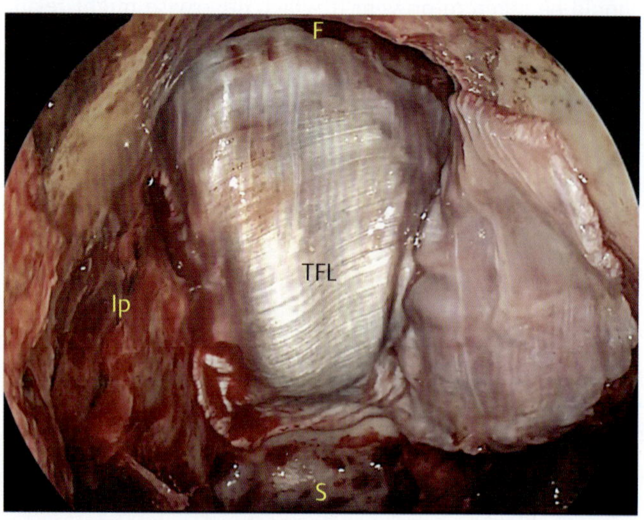

Fig. 14.22 Tensor fascia lata (TFL) placed as overlay layer on the inlay and spread out to cover the left periorbita.

Debate: Endoscopic Surgery versus Conventional Surgery

In our opinion there is no debate about superiority of any single approach. Endoscopic approach is an addition to the existing armamentarium of the surgeon. Depending on the merits of each case the approach should be planned. When contemplating on the approach for resection of a sinonasal/anterior skull base tumor, we need to take into account the training of the surgeon and available resources. A surgeon should be trained in all aspects of conventional skull base surgery before venturing into endoscopic surgery. Endoscopic tumor resection is not an approach for the novice surgeon. The surgeon needs to gain experience in benign endoscopic surgery before venturing to tumor surgery. When dealing with malignant tumors, the first chance is the best chance, and a complete resection regardless of the approach should be achieved. The surgeon needs to be well versed in oncologic management of tumors and more importantly should have the maturity to stop and convert to a conventional approach in adverse situations.

Conclusion

Minimal access surgery for sinonasal and anterior skull base tumors is now an established modality with proven safety. The endonasal access should be used whenever feasible either alone or in combination with external approaches with the sole aim of optimal resection. Before attempting endoscopic endonasal tumor surgery, adequate training with cadaver dissection is essential besides sufficient exposure to routine endoscopic surgical procedures. Malignant tumors are best dealt by a multidisciplinary team with adequate knowledge of tumor biology and experience in conventional surgical techniques.

Suggested Readings

Busquets JM, Hwang PH. Endoscopic resection of sinonasal inverted papilloma: a meta-analysis. Otolaryngol Head Neck Surg 2006;134(3):476–482

Dulguerov P, Allal AS, Calcaterra TC. Esthesioneuroblastoma: a meta-analysis and review. Lancet Oncol 2001;2(11):683–690

Hanna E, DeMonte F, Ibrahim S, Roberts D, Levine N, Kupferman M. Endoscopic resection of sinonasal cancers with and without craniotomy: oncologic results. Arch Otolaryngol Head Neck Surg 2009;135(12):1219–1224

Kassam A, Snyderman CH, Mintz A, Gardner P, Carrau RL. Expanded endonasal approach: the rostrocaudal axis. Part I. Crista galli to the sella turcica. Neurosurg Focus 2005;19(1):E3

Kassam A, Snyderman CH, Mintz A, Gardner P, Carrau RL. Expanded endonasal approach: the rostrocaudal axis. Part II. Posterior clinoids to the foramen magnum. Neurosurg Focus 2005;19(1):E4

Mattavelli D, Schreiber A, Ferrari M, et al. Three-layer reconstruction with iliotibial tract after endoscopic resection of sinonasal tumors. World Neurosurg 2017;101:486–492

Messerklinger W. Technics and possibilities of nasal endoscopy]. HNO 1972;20(5):133–135

Nicolai P, Battaglia P, Bignami M, et al. Endoscopic surgery for malignant tumors of the sinonasal tract and adjacent skull base: a 10-year experience. Am J Rhinol 2008;22(3):308–316

Rosenthal DI, Barker JL Jr, El-Naggar AK, et al. Sinonasal malignancies with neuroendocrine differentiation: patterns of failure according to histologic phenotype. Cancer 2004;101(11):2567–2573

Stamm AC, Draf W, Stamm A. Micro-endoscopic surgery of the paranasal sinuses and the skull base. Berlin: Springer; 2000

Section IV

Clival Region

Chapter 15 Skull Base Chordoma

Saif Al-Zahid, Michel Roethlisberger, Revadi Govindaraju, Yves Brand, Luigi Mariani, Jürgen Hench, Prepageran Narayanan, and Vicknes Waran

Introduction

Chordoma is a rare type of slow-growing, malignant tumor arising from embryonic notochordal tissue within the bone of the axial skeleton. They have a reported incidence of 0.08 per 100,000 and occur evenly in the skull base, spine, and sacrum with a third in each of those sites.[1] Management involves gross total resection (GTR) followed by radiotherapy in the form of fractionated radiotherapy, proton beam therapy, or radiosurgery. Because of the anatomical location, total resection is not always possible with a reported recurrence rate of 31%; thus radiation therapy plays an important role in tumor control.[2]

Chordoma has a poor prognosis in comparison to chondrosarcoma; therefore total tumor resection together with postoperative radiotherapy offers the best chance of cure. An understanding of this challenging area of the posterior to mid skull base anatomy is key for achieving surgical clearance and to minimize morbidity.

Classically, chordomas have been removed through an open craniotomy approach; however, the endonasal endoscopic approach (EEA) is increasingly being utilized.[3] The choice of surgical technique is guided by the extent of lateral tumor involvement, as well as the experience of the surgical team. The focus of this overview lies on the endoscopic management of these lesions.

Anatomical Considerations

The clivus is the commonest site of skull base chordoma and lies within the posterior skull base. An understanding of this anatomical region and its surrounding neurovascular structures is therefore crucial. The clivus forms the anterior part of the occipital bone. It connects to the petrous apex of the temporal bone laterally and to the sphenoid bone anteriorly.

It is useful to anatomically divide the clivus into superior, middle, and inferior divisions when surgically managing tumors in this region (**Fig. 15.1a**)[3]

- *Superior third of the clivus:* The superior clivus is constituted by the sellar floor, dorsum sella, and posterior clinoid. It is laterally associated with the paraclinoid internal carotid artery (ICA) and the third cranial nerve (oculomotor) running within the cavernous sinus.
- *Middle third of the clivus:* The middle clivus starts at the level of the sellar floor to the floor of the sphenoid sinus. Inferolaterally, the lower half of the paraclival carotid lies within the foramen lacerum.[4] Lateral to the paraclival ICA, the cranial nerves IV, V1, V2, and VI traverse the cavernous sinus into their respective foramina, with the latter being at highest risk of injury. The petroclival fissure limits the middle clivus laterally. Above, the Dorello's canal is located containing the abducens nerve entering the cavernous sinus (**Fig. 15.1b**).[5–8] At this midclival level, the vidian canal leads to the lateral aspect of foramen lacerum thus being a useful landmark to find the paraclival ICA in less pneumatized clival bones.[4,9–11] Anterior to the paraclival carotid, Meckel's cave lies laterally and can be exposed to access tumors within this region. Detailed anatomical considerations have been discussed in Chapter 1.
- *Lower third of the clivus:* The inferior clivus is constituted by the basilar part of the occipital bone. This division has a direct relation with the foramen magnum posteriorly. Posterolaterally, it forms the jugular tubercle and corresponding jugular foramen, and anteroinferiorly, the medial condyle of the occipital bone articulates with the C1 condyle. The cranial nerves IX, X, and XI in the jugular foramen and XII in the hypoglossal canal are implicated in lesions of the inferior clivus.[3]

Pathologies and Its Variants

There are various histological entities ranging from low- to high-grade subtypes that pathologists need to be aware of when diagnosing chondroma. Some of those may histologically be mistaken for other pathologies such as chondrosarcoma and chordoid meningioma. Hence, immunohistochemistry and, more robustly, methylome analysis are useful tools when making those distinctions, especially when the biopsy material is of poor quality because of crushing of the specimen. A distinctive immunohistochemical marker is the brachyury protein, which is also expressed in the notochord. Brachyury is not expressed in the histological mimics of chordoma. Chordomas appear macroscopically as grayish-white with areas of central necrosis

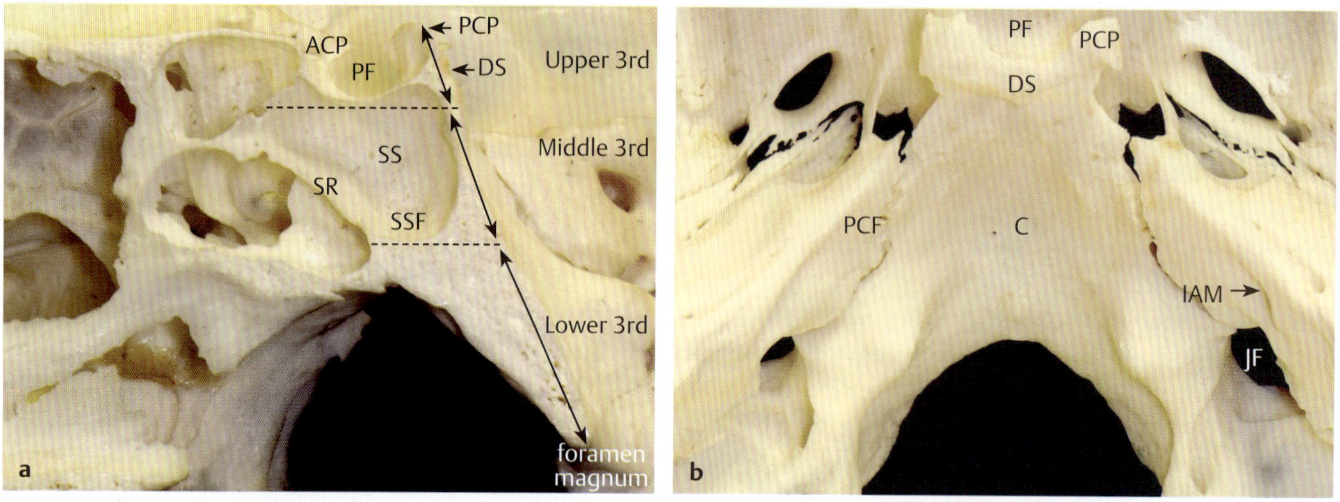

Fig. 15.1 **(a)** Osseous anatomy of the clivus as seen in a sagittal view. The clivus can be arbitrarily divided into a superior third, middle third, and lower third as demonstrated by the transverse *dotted lines* and the *vertical double-ended arrows*. The superior part extends from the posterior clinoid process (PCP) and dorsum sellae (DS) to the level of floor of the sellae. From this junction to the level of the floor is the middle third and from below the sphenoid sinus floor (SSF) to the level of anterior edge of foramen magnum is the lower third. **(b)** In a superior oblique view, the posterolateral relationship of the clivus can be visualized. The inferior petrosal sinus courses through the petroclival fissure (PCF) and forms the lateral boundary. The jugular foramen (JF), hypoglossal canal, and internal acoustic meatus (IAM) are located lateral to the lower third of clivus.

containing mucoid substance and have a pseudocapsule. There are often loose bone fragments because of sequestration. Microscopically, the following pathological entities are recognized:[12]

Conventional Chordoma

The most common type of chordoma consists of chords of tumor cells arranged in lobules within a myxoid matrix and abundant eosinophilic cytoplasm. There are scattered vacuolated cells (physaliphorous cells). According to the literature, approximately 10% of chordoma patients have metastatic disease, while 2 to 8% undergo dedifferentiation or sarcomatous transformation.[12–14]

Chondroid Chordoma

Similar to conventional chordoma, chondroid chordoma consists of chords of tumor cells with the presence of physaliphorous cells, but the matrix resembles that of hyaline cartilage under microscopy. These have a better prognosis than conventional chordoma but can be mistaken for chondrosarcoma because of the similarities in microscopic appearance. Brachyury staining and methylome analysis are distinctive.[15]

Cellular Chordoma

These are also similar to conventional chordoma but lack either a myxoid or chondroid matrix; hence they are more cellular. Thus, they can be mistaken for a carcinoma. Again, brachyury staining and methylome analysis are distinctive. In particular, methylation analysis can readily differentiate a large number of mesenchymal, epithelial, and other neoplasms in a single examination.[15]

Dedifferentiated Chordoma

This rare subtype occurs in less than 4% of chordomas. Microscopically, they appear as tightly packed atypical epithelioid cells lacking physaliphorous architecture. They behave in a highly malignant fashion and have a poor prognosis. Definite distinction from other high-grade soft tissue tumors might only be possible through methylome analysis.

Chordoma should histologically be confirmed by strong nuclear staining for brachyury. Other immunohistochemical markers might be contributive; however, they have been superseded by methylome analysis.[16] At this molecular level, dedifferentiated chordomas are distinct from the remaining histological subtypes and can be distinguished through a public methylation classification platform (www.molecularneuropathology.org). They differ not only by DNA methylation but also in terms of genomic copy number alterations.

Clinical Considerations

The presentation of chordomas relates to the site of clival involvement and its direct relationship to surrounding structures:

- Cavernous sinus involvement implicates cranial nerves IV, V2, V3, and VI.
- Posterosuperior growth exerts pressure onto the intracranial structures and brainstem presenting as headaches.
- Lower clival involvement may affect the cranial nerves IX to XII giving bulbar symptoms thus affecting speech and swallowing. Rarely, far lateral growth into the cerebellopontine angle (CPA) may implicate the cranial nerves VII and VIII.

In a series of 45 skull base chordomas reported by Boari et al., the commonest presenting symptom was diplopia in 27 cases (60%) followed by headache in 13 cases (28.9%).[6] Other presentations included palpebral ptosis in 6 (13.3%); hoarseness/dysphagia with visual loss in 5 (11.1%); and facial numbness/pain because of trigeminal involvement in 4 (8.9%). Less commonly, there was neck pain in 3 (6.7%); nasal obstruction, hearing loss, facial palsy, and tetraparesis in 2 (4.4%); hemiparesis, tongue atrophy, dizziness, dysarthria, and urinary incontinence in 1 (2.2%).[17]

Radiological Features

Chordomas of the skull base are mostly extradural in origin. Similar to other skull base lesions, the main diagnostic radiological tools for chordoma are computed tomography (CT) and magnetic resonance imaging (MRI). Chordoma lesions generally arise from the midline upper clivus. These lesions are differentiated from chondrosarcoma lesions that tend to be more lateral because of their arising from the petroclival junction. Apart from their location, the general radiographic appearances are otherwise very similar. The role of nuclear medicine in the management of chordoma is still being explored and centers on the identification of hypoxic areas to guide radiation therapy.[18]

Computed Tomography

Chordoma on CT appears heterogenous with lytic bone destruction and is generally well circumscribed. The chondroid chordoma can be associated with bony calcification; this makes it difficult to differentiate from chondrosarcoma. Areas of low attenuation are attributable to mucinous content (**Fig. 15.2a, b**).[18]

Magnetic Resonance Imaging

The T1-weighted MRI appearances of chordoma are characteristically a low-to-intermediate signal. Areas of mucous or hemorrhage appear as high intensity (**Fig. 15.2c, d**).[19] On T2-weighted MRI, chordoma is typically of high signal intensity because of fluid content and heterogeneous nature (**Fig. 15.2e, f**). Poorly differentiated chordoma is hypointense on T2-weighted MRI.[18,19] The other important differential is benign notochordal cell tumor that also arises from the axial skeleton. This can be differentiated with contrast, as it does not show postcontrast enhancement compared to chordoma that enhances postcontrast. Additionally, bone destruction is absent.[19]

Surgical Considerations

Surgery is indicated for chordoma as the primary modality of treatment and is generally performed for diagnosis and to reduce the tumor burden prior to adjuvant treatment.[3] Without this, tumors will continue to grow and cause destruction to local and adjacent structures. The main contraindication to surgery is the patient's fitness for general anesthetic. The most important preoperative consideration is the surgical approach, and this should be decided by a skull base multidisciplinary team. Certain tumors may benefit from a combined endoscopic and open technique or a staged procedure to deal with lateral and inferior extension. The EEA to the clivus allows excision of extensive lesions while reducing morbidity, and with similar disease control rates. It is important, however, to consider the limitations of the endoscopic approach given the tumor extent and the skill set of the skull base team.

Preoperative Considerations

Depending on the clinical presentation, parts of the clivus involved (superior third, middle third, lower third), and involvement of anatomical compartments (e.g., cavernous sinus, CP angle, interpeduncular fossa), detailed assessment of neurocranial nerve functions is indicated. This includes neuro-ophthalmological examination and visual acuity, visual field testing and orthoptic measurements, function of the lower cranial nerves (swallowing), and acoustic evoked potentials.

The patient must have a group and save sampling as well as cross-matching of blood in anticipation of heavy bleeding intraoperatively. Fitness for general anesthetic must

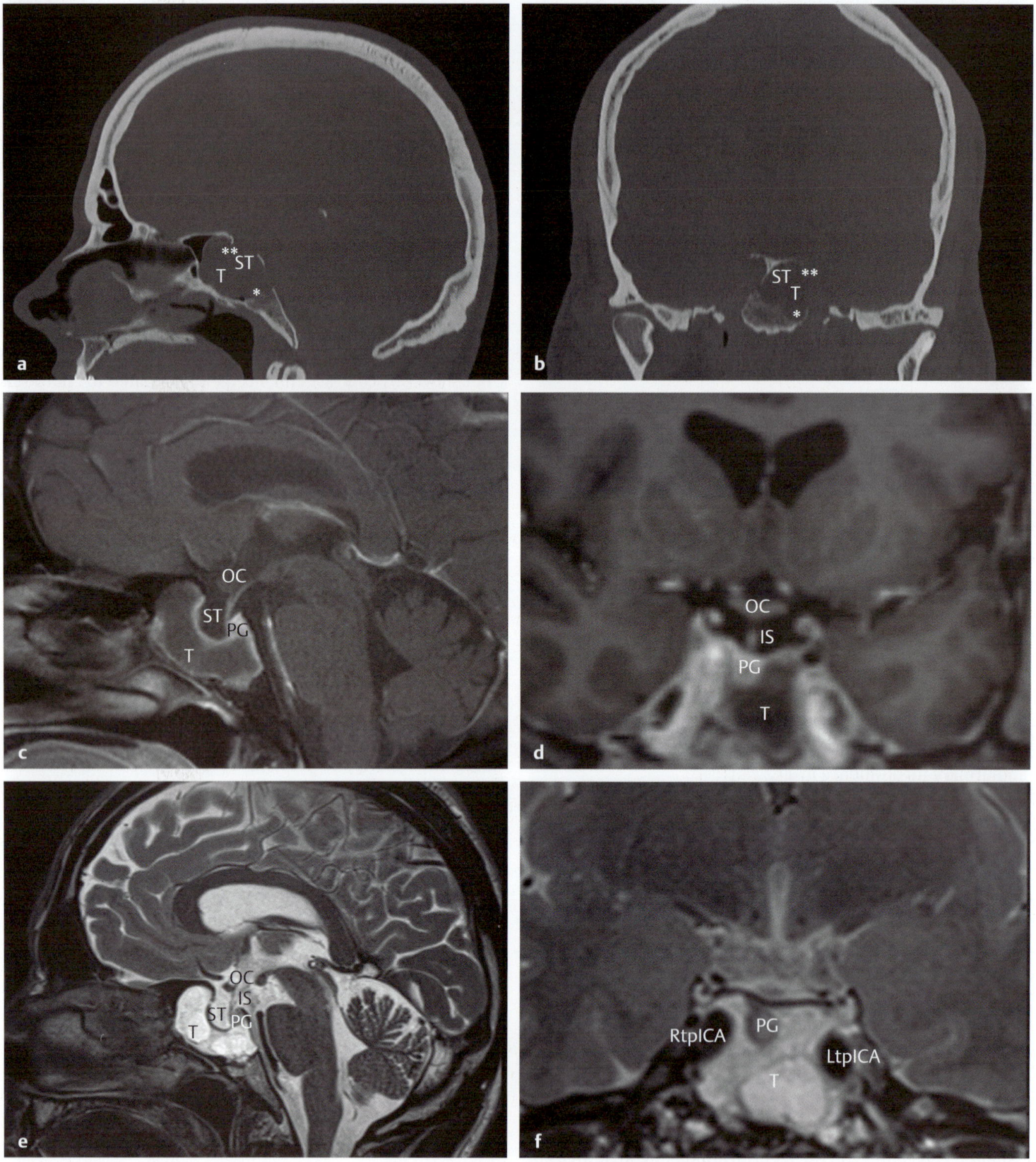

Fig. 15.2 **(a)** Sagittal and **(b)** coronal bone-weighted CT images, demonstrating a midline middle-third clivus chordoma with heterogenous well-circumscribed lytic bone destruction (*). The bone covering (**) the sella turcica (ST) is not visible. **(c)** Sagittal and **(d)** coronal T1-weighted contrast-enhanced MRI images demonstrating the infra-sellar, upper-third clival chordoma with the characteristically low to intermediate signal. **(e)** Sagittal and **(f)** coronal T2-weighted MRI sequences reveal high signal intensity due to fluid content. The sella turcica (ST) appears as "empty sella" with the physiological anterior and posterior pituitary gland (PG) and the infundibular stalk (IS), not affected by the tumorous lesion. The right (RtpICA) and left (LtpICA) paraclival internal carotid are encased by the tumorous lesion (T).

be considered and the patient's medical status be optimized, and postoperative neuro-ICU bed should be booked. Diagnostic information about the lesion can be obtained radiologically with a high degree of accuracy. Histology plays a less important role in the preoperative work-up because of the deep location of the clivus and difficulty in obtaining samples. Thus surgical resection is both diagnostic and curative where possible.

The treatment and management of patients with chordomas of the skull base are interdisciplinary. In larger institutions, the preoperative work-up of these patients involves endocrinologists, ophthalmologists, neurosurgeons, ENT surgeons, and neuroradiologists. Usually, patients are evaluated by multidisciplinary consensus at regularly held tumor boards.

Endocrinological Assessment

Hypothalamic–pituitary hormonal function: Serum prolactin, total or free T4, thyroid-stimulating hormone (TSH), luteinizing hormone (LH), follicle-stimulating hormone (FSH), free testosterone, estrogen and progesterone, morning cortisol 24-hour urinary-free cortisol, and insulin-like growth factor.

Ophthalmological Assessment

Visual acuity and visual field using Goldman's perimetry as well as optometry in cases of double vision.

Neurological Assessment

Focal neurological deficits, cranial nerve deficits, and neuropsychological changes in large lesion with extrasellar extension and relevant brainstem compression.

Rhinological Assessment

Endoscopic examination of the nose to rule out signs of infection, synechiae, or congenital anomalies.

Radiological Investigations

High-resolution (HR) MRI of brain with image-guided surgery (IGS) protocol and HRCT scan for paranasal sinuses, and sphenoid sinus and clival osteolysis involvement are recommended.

Preoperative Radiological Considerations

The surgeon should systematically assess available imaging. This is of special importance when selecting surgical modalities and variations of the available approaches and tailoring the surgical corridor to reach the region of interest:

- *Nasal anatomy:* Signs of upper airway infection, septal deviations, and signs of trauma.
- *Sphenoid anatomy:* Three-dimensional orientation (shelf, divider, wall) and insertion site (cavernous or paraclinoid ICA, opticocarotid recess, or optic nerves) of the sphenoid septations, mucosa, pneumatization pattern (sellar, presellar, or postsellar type), and bone thickness.
- *Clival anatomy:* Clival involvement, extent of erosion and lateral extension, and involvement of the paraclival carotid arteries.
- *Lesion characteristics:* Involvement of the clivus only, extension to the sphenoid cavity, and lateral extension into the orbital apex and orbits. Involvement of the sella turcica, and involvement of the posterior fossa, lower clivus, atlas (C1), odontoid (C1 dens axis) or axis (C2) or lower (C3).
- Neurovascular structures:
    - *Relationship to the cerebral intracranial vessels:* Basilar artery and posterior cerebral artery (PCA), brainstem perforators.
    - *Relationship to the brainstem:* Brainstem compression (medial ventral to posterior), dislocation to one side, compression from lateral.
    - *Relationship to the cranial nerves:* Involvement of cranial nerves (VII–VIII complex, lower cranial nerves, hypoglossal canal).

Recurrent Cases

Chordomas are generally slow-growing lesions. However, their tendency for local invasiveness precipitates a high incidence of local recurrences. If uncontrolled, progressive lesions and recurrent cases potentially result in a high mortality.[20] Observational studies found lower GTR rates for the EEA in previously treated lesions that most likely provide the setting of a recurrent disease when compared to primary chordomas.[20,21]

Selection of the Surgical Approach

Because of the high incidence of local recurrent disease, a GTR should be achieved when resecting chordomas and chondrosarcomas of the skull base.[3,20,21] This goal might be compromised in a significant amount of cases because of local invasiveness and anatomical relationship to critical neurovascular structures. Transcranial (TCA) and transfacial approaches as well as EEAs have been described to treat chordoma and chondrosacroma.[3,20,21] In the past decade, EEA has increasingly being used to treat chordomas of the skull base with promising outcomes.[20,21]

Potential Advantages of the Endonasal Endoscopic Approach

There is a 2B level of evidence favoring the EEA for GTR of chordomas when using a transclival approach.[20,21] Koutourousiou et al. reported 60 patients with 35 (58%) primary and 25 (42%) previously treated chordomas of the skull base. The authors revealed a GTR rate of approximately two-thirds, with a higher rate (83%) in primary and a lower rate (44%) in previously treated patients. They reported a significant impact of the surgeons' learning curve on the surgical outcome in terms of GTR.

- *Approach-related morbidity:* Endonasal endoscopic midline approaches to the clivus result in a midline dissection of the epipharyngeal mucosa and myofascial layer. However, skin incisions, large myocutaneous flaps (e.g., far lateral approach), and highly invasive transfacial approaches can be avoided.

Potential Disadvantages of the Endonasal Endoscopic Approach

The anatomical locations and local invasiveness, potential involvement of critical neurovascular structures, biological behavior, and high recurrence rate are relevant limitations for EEA when treating chordomas.

- *Approach-related morbidity and mortality:* Koutourousiou et al. reported a 20% rate of cerebrospinal fluid (CSF) leakage in their series, with 3.3% eventually resulting in meningitis.[21] In 2 out of 60 patients (3.3%), ICA injuries occurred, of which none resulted in neurological deficits.[21] No operative mortality was reported within this series.[21]
- *Extent of resection:* A tumor volume greater than 20 cm^3, tumor location in the lower clivus with lateral extension, and previously treated disease were found to be relevant limiting factors of GTR in clival chordoma.[21]
- *Neurological morbidity:* Koutourousiou et al found a new-onset cranial nerve deficit rate of 7% and long tract deficits in 2% of chordoma cases treated with EEA.[21]

When to Prefer a Transcranial Approach for Clival Chordoma

The EEA is a competitive alternative to chordomas of the skull base with a good GTR rate and low morbidity and mortality in experienced surgical teams. However, certain features might limit the success for endonasal endoscopic surgery.

- Considerable infratentorial extension (retrosigmoid approach, far lateral approach).
- Significant lateral extension in the lower clivus (far lateral approach).
- Significant extension below the foramen magnum and anterior of C1/C2 (far lateral approach).
- Lateral beyond clinoid portion of the internal carotid (pterional).
- Involvement of the sphenoid wing (pterional).
- Orbital involvement.

Presurgical Phase

Anesthesia, patient positioning, equipment, and ergonomical aspects for the endonasal endoscopic techniques have been described in Chapter 1.

Nasal Phase (Tailored Approach)

Expanded endoscopic endonasal transclival approach: A binostril transclival approach is preferred depending on the extension of the lesion.

1. The floor of the sphenoid sinus is removed as required to improve access for instrumentation (**Fig. 15.3a, b**).
2. The critical landmarks identified include the paraclival ICA bilaterally and the sellar floor. The vidian nerve leads to the lateral surface of the ICA and may assist in identifying the lower limit of the paraclival ICA (**Fig. 15.3a, b**).

Osteodural Exposure (Zonal Dissection)

1. The midclivus bone is drilled, and this approach does cause considerable bleeding from the cancellous bone. This needs to be pre-empted by the anesthetic team (**Fig. 15.3c**).
2. Posteriorly, the dura has two layers, a periosteal and a meningeal layer, with the basilar plexus in between which can also cause significant bleeding (**Fig. 15.3d** and **Fig. 15.4a**).
3. Beneath the periosteal layer, the Dorello's canal and abducens nerve (sixth cranial nerve) can be identified laterally exiting the canal (**Fig. 15.4b**).[5,6,8,24]
4. The lateral limit of the exposure is the paraclival ICA that can be skeletonized and mobilized to improve access laterally.[4]
5. With the dura removed at this level, the neurovascular contents encountered would be the abducens nerve, the basilar artery, the lower pons and far laterally the facial nerve, and the vestibulo-cochlear nerve and the anterior inferior cerebellar artery (**Fig. 15.5**).[7,22,24,25]
6. Superior exposure of the upper third of the clivus requires translocation or transection of the pituitary gland (**Fig. 15.5**).

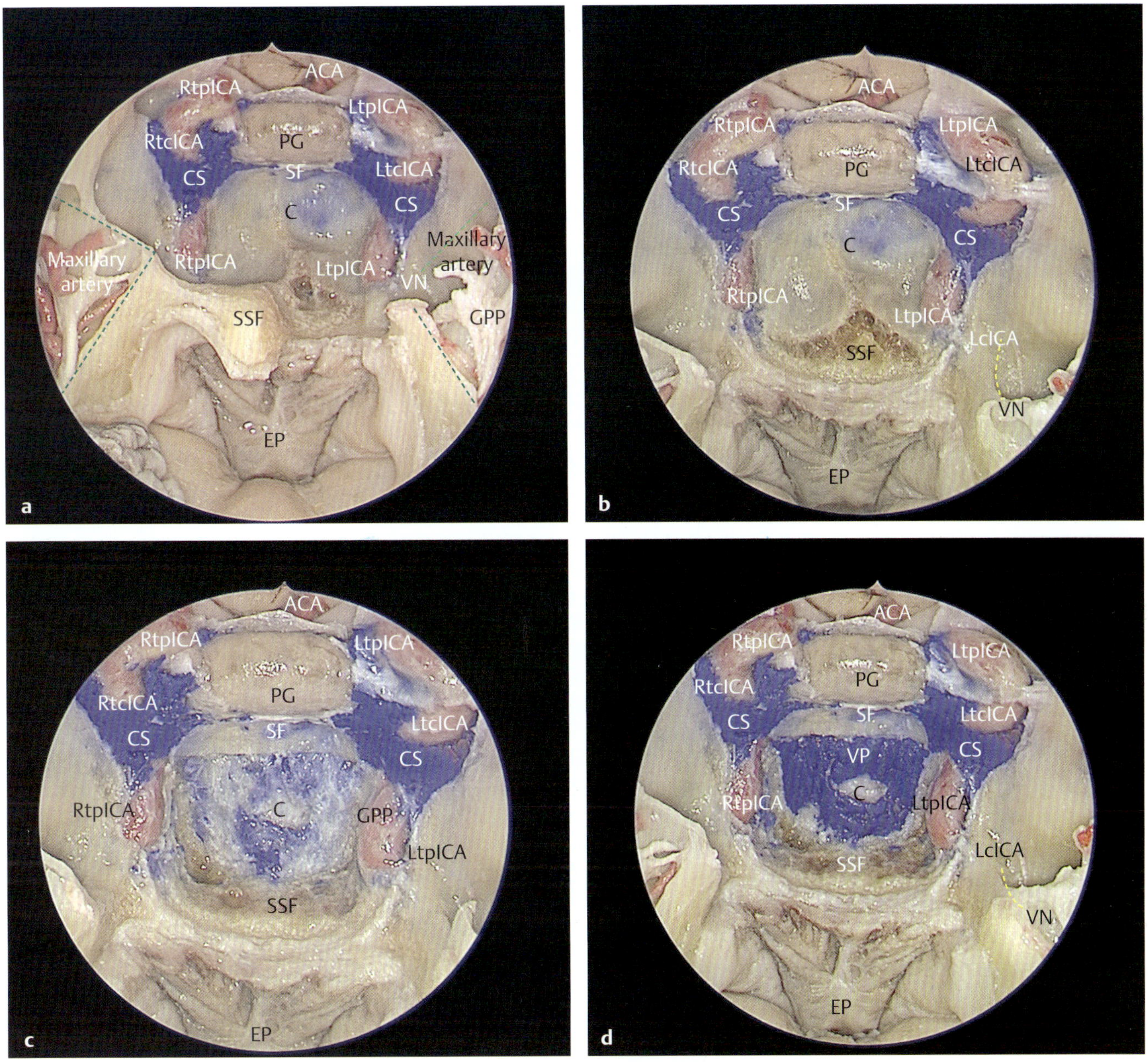

Fig. 15.3 Endonasal endoscopic approach to the midclivus. **(a)** Following posterior septectomy, the sphenoid sinus floor (SSF) is identified and removed. The left side has been drilled, leaving the right aspect intact for the purpose of orientation. The left (LtpICA) and right (RtpICA) paraclival internal carotid artery and the floor of the sella turcica (SF) are identified as they form the superior and lateral limits of the surgical corridor. The pterygopalatine fossa (*green line*), containing the maxillary artery, its branches, and the pterygopalatine ganglion (GPP), has been deliberately exposed to show anatomy of the vidian nerve (VN) as an important landmark for the transition from the lacerum segment of internal carotid artery (LcICA) to the paraclival internal carotid artery (pICA). **(b)** Complete removal of the SSF fully exposes the middle third of the clivus (C). The VN coursing in the vidian canal (*yellow line*) marks the transition from the LcICA to the pICA. **(c)** With the removal of the cancellous bone of the midclivus (C), the periosteal layer of the dura comes into view. **(d)** The basilar venous plexus (VP) of the midclivus (C) is exposed deep to the periosteal layer. The VN coursing in the vidian canal (*yellow line*) marks the transition from the LcICA to the pICA.

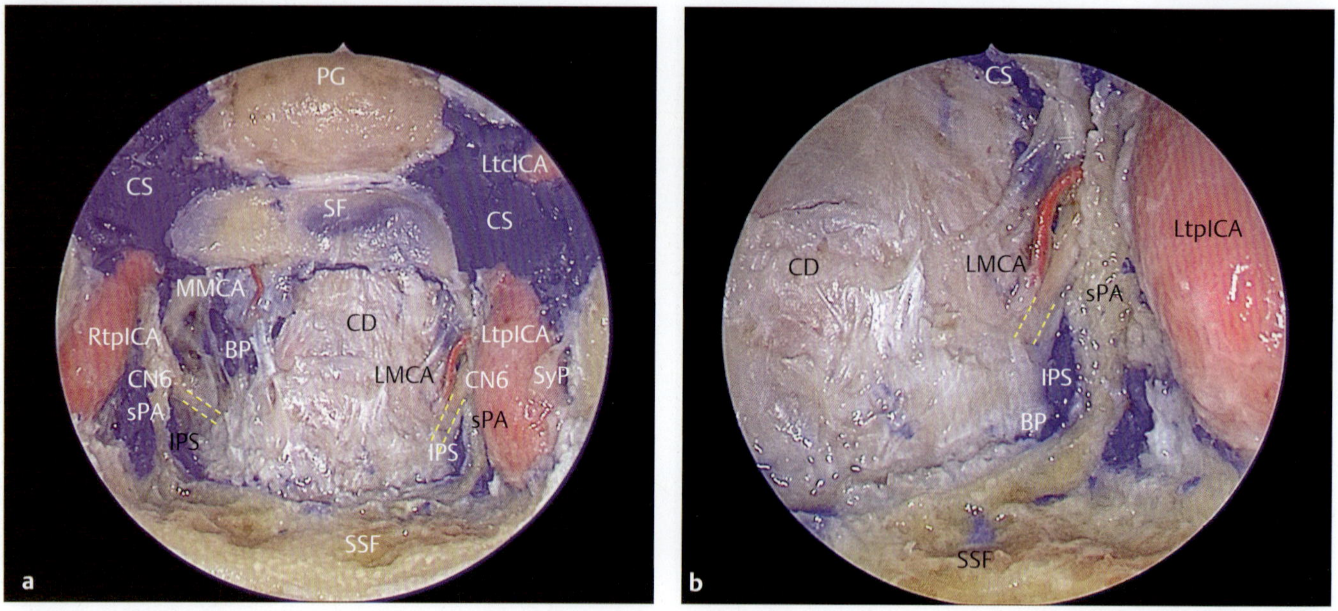

Fig. 15.4 Anatomy of the Dorello's canal and the sixth cranial nerve (abducens nerve). **(a, b)** When removing the venous plexus of the midclivus, the meningeal layer of the dura (CD) is encountered with the exposure of the Dorello's canal (*yellow lines*) and the sixth cranial nerve (abducens nerve) (CN6) as it exits the canal. The Dorello's canal is located medially to the petrous ridge and marks the confluence of the inferior petrosal sinus (IPS), the basilar plexus (BP), and the cavernous sinus (CS).[22] It is formed by the space between the petrous apex, the superolateral portion of the clivus, and superiorly by the petrosphenoidal ligament of Gruber.[5,8] The arterial supply of the Dorello's canal is provided by the meningeal branches of the meningohypophyseal artery, arising from the posterior bend of the cavernous ICA. These meningeal branches can be divided into a medial meningeal clival artery (MMCA) and a lateral meningeal clival artery (LMCA).[5,8] The MMCA generally supplies the dura of the dorsum sellae and the upper clivus. The LMCA supplies the lateral petroclival dura and the dural canal of the CN6.[5,8] The nerve itself receives blood supply from arteries arising in the subarachnoid space penetrating the nerve at its entrance into the dural canal.[6,23] The left (LtpICA) and right (RtpICA) paraclival internal carotid artery, the superior petrous apex (sPA), the basilar plexus (BP), and the inferior petrosal sinus (IPS) form the lateral limitation of the anatomical exposure.

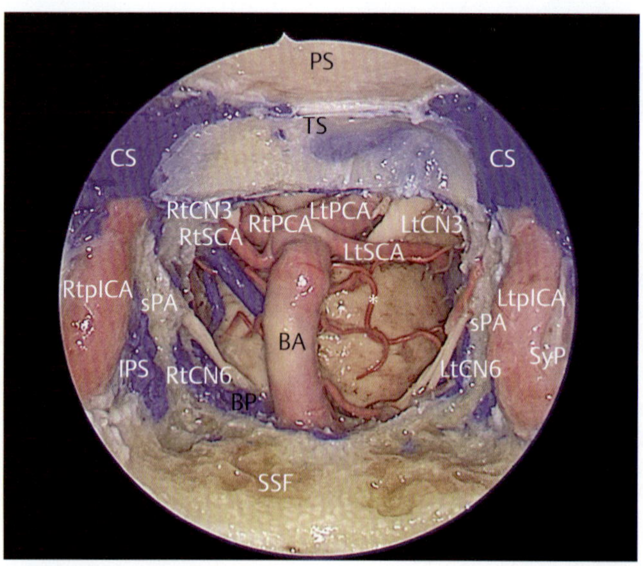

Fig. 15.5 Removal of the dura exposes the left (LtCN6) and right (RtCN6) sixth cranial nerve (abducens nerve), the basilar artery (BA), the basilar bifurcation with the left (LtPCA) and right (RtPCA) posterior cerebral arteries, the left (LtSCA) and right (RtSCA) superior cerebellar arteries with the left (LtCN3) and right (RtCN3) third cranial nerve (oculomotor nerve) exiting the brainstem in between these two vessels. Several perforating arteries to the pons cerebri (*) are visible. The left (LtpICA) and right (RtpICA) paraclival internal carotid artery, the superior petrous apex (sPA), the basilar plexus (BP), and the inferior petrosal sinus (IPS) form the lateral limitation of the anatomical exposure.

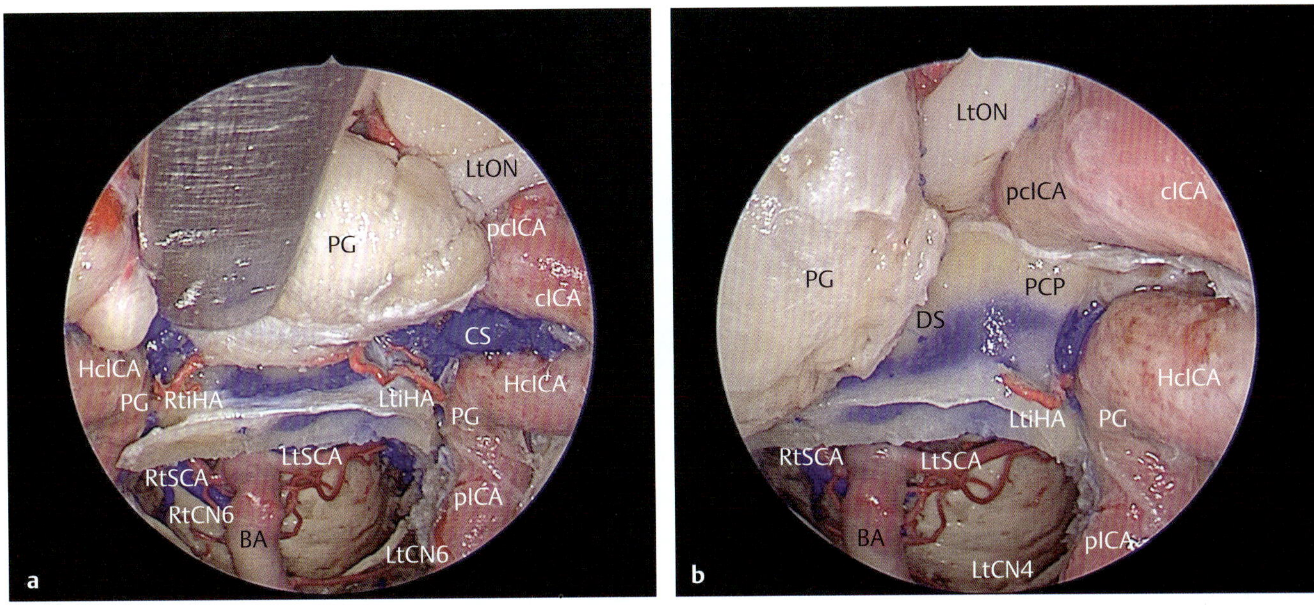

Fig. 15.6 Anatomical relationships of the upper third of the clivus encountered during the pituitary translocation. **(a)** The pituitary gland (PG) is elevated superiorly. The left (LtiHA) and right (RtiHA) inferior hypophyseal artery need to be divided to allow the translocation. **(b)** As the pituitary gland (PG) is retracted medially, the posterior relationship to the dorsum sellae (DS) and posterior clinoid process (PCP) is demonstrated. The PCP is closely related to the paraclinoid ICA (pcICA). Laterally, the DS is adjacent to the cavernous sinus (CS) and the posterior genu (PG) and the horizontal segment (HcICA) of the cavernous internal carotid artery (cICA), which are at risk of injury.

7. Removal of the dorsum sellae and the posterior clinoid process will expose the midbrain, the upper pons, the PCA, the superior cerebellar artery, the oculomotor nerves and the trigeminal nerves laterally (**Fig. 15.6**).
8. The steps in the surgery of the lower clivus are covered in Chapter 18 for craniocervical junction.

Neurosurgical Techniques for Tumor Exposure

- Image-guided surgery (IGS) is crucial to identify the key neurovascular structures, such as the optic nerves and the paraclival carotids, during tumor dissection especially where the bony margins have been eroded.
- These slow-growing tumors tend to erode bone. Following this the tumor might extend to the remaining important neurovascular structures. Thus, bony limitations may be absent.[3]
- Dehiscent or intratumoral vessels (paraclival carotid arteries, basilar arteries) have to be considered.
- Laterally, the sixth cranial nerve (abducens nerve) entering the Dorello's canal causes significant morbidity for this approach.[6,24]

Skull Base Defect Closure

The large dural defects caused by the transclival approach are usually closed using intradural and extradural autologous fat grafts and an artificial dural sealant system. Suture of the myomucosal layer of the epipharynx covering the construct and/or covering by a vascularized nasoseptal or pharyngeal vascularized flaps are recommended.[26–28] Contact to the surrounding bony edges is necessary for an adequate watertight closure and healing of the skull base defect.

Postoperative Care

The nasal packs are usually removed within 24 to 48 hours. They may remain in situ for longer time (72–120 hours) if a CSF leak repair has been performed. The patient is advised to avoid straining (no sneezing, coughing, straining during defecation) if a concomitant intraoperative CSF leak repair was necessary. Endoscopic inspection and toileting are usually performed during the first week after the operation.

Nonsurgical Treatment Modalities

Radiotherapeutic Treatment Options

Because of the anatomical location of the clivus and nearby critical neurovascular structures, achieving complete surgical clearance is difficult, and thus, local recurrence is very common. Radiotherapy therefore plays an important role postoperatively to prolong the disease-free interval when there has been incomplete surgical resection. Conventional two-dimensional external beam radiotherapy techniques cause unacceptably high morbidity from radiation toxicity to the brainstem, spinal cord, optic chiasm, optic nerve, lens, retina, and nearby cranial nerves. Delivery of targeted protons or photons in a three-dimensional pattern designed for the shape of the tumor in the form of intensity-modulated radiation therapy (IMRT), stereotactic radiosurgery (SRS) delivered at one session for smaller tumors, or stereotactic fractionated radiation therapy for larger lesions delivered at multiple sessions, reduces morbidity and increases local control rates.

Despite the importance of radiation therapy, a meta-analysis of 23 studies and 807 patients showed the effect of incomplete surgical resection on outcomes.[29] Patients with incomplete surgical resection were 3.8 times more likely to have recurrence and 5.8 times more likely to die at 5 years compared to the complete resection group. The study found no difference in overall survival between the types of adjuvant radiation therapy (proton beam radiation therapy, carbon ion radiotherapy, stereotactic radiosurgery, and stereotactic fractionated radiation therapy). There was no additional benefit conferred by radiation therapy in overall survival when complete surgical resection has been achieved.

Management of Complications

A neurosurgical high dependency unit is strongly advised postoperatively after complex surgical resections of the skull base. The care received postoperatively will depend on the extent of the surgical resection and managing postoperative complications. As patients can often bleed throughout the procedure, postoperative transfusion may be required, and the patient resuscitated postoperatively. Neurosurgical complications may include CSF leak, meningitis, seizures, and increased intracranial pressure. Antibiotics and lumbar drainage insertion may be required. Lower cranial nerve palsies associated with lesions of the lower clivus can be troublesome and would need care of the upper airway as well as speech and language therapy input. Managing ocular cranial nerve palsies requires ophthalmological input both postoperatively and during future follow-up.

Tips and Pearls

- Chordoma of the clivus can be considered as one of the most challenging areas to treat within the skull base.
- A comprehensive assessment to decide the best surgical approach is paramount.
- A balance between the extent of surgical resection and morbidity from cranial nerve palsies must be sought.
- Complete surgical resection offers the best overall survival and disease-free progression rates.
- Adjuvant radiation therapy plays an important role when surgical resection is incomplete.
- Newer radiation modalities such as proton beam therapy offer reduced toxicity and increased dose delivery to the tumor site.
- Patients should be treated in a tertiary center with ability to manage postoperative general and neurosurgical complications.

Acknowledgments

This chapter was written based on funding from the Martin Allgöwer Foundation, Department of Surgery, University Hospital of Basel (Basel, Switzerland), the Gottfried and Julia Bangerter-Rhyner Foundation (Bern, Switzerland), the Lionel College Travel Fellowship of the Royal College of Surgeons of England (United Kingdom), the Ministry of Health of Malaysia scholarship (Malaysia), and the Adelaide Ear-Nose-Throat Research Institute (Australia). The Department of Neurosurgery of the University Hospital of Basel (Basel, Switzerland) and the Departments of Neurosurgery and Otorhinolaryngology of the University of Malaya (Kuala Lumpur, Malaysia) supported the creation of this chapter.

References

1. McMaster ML, Goldstein AM, Bromley CM, Ishibe N, Parry DM. Chordoma: incidence and survival patterns in the United States, 1973-1995. Cancer Causes Control 2001;12(1): 1–11
2. Fagundes MA, Hug EB, Liebsch NJ, Daly W, Efird J, Munzenrider JE. Radiation therapy for chordomas of the base of skull and cervical spine: patterns of failure and outcome after relapse. Int J Radiat Oncol Biol Phys 1995;33(3):579–584
3. Fernandez-Miranda JC, Gardner PA, Snyderman CH, et al. Clival chordomas: a pathological, surgical, and radiotherapeutic review. Head Neck 2014;36(6):892–906
4. Labib MA, Prevedello DM, Carrau R, et al. A road map to the internal carotid artery in expanded endoscopic endonasal approaches to the ventral cranial base. Neurosurgery 2014;10(Suppl 3):448–471, discussion 471
5. Kshettry VR, Lee JH, Ammirati M. The Dorello canal: historical development, controversies in microsurgical anatomy, and clinical implications. Neurosurg Focus 2013;34(3):E4

6. Ozveren MF, Erol FS, Alkan A, Kocak A, Onal C, Türe U. Microanatomical architecture of Dorello's canal and its clinical implications. Neurosurgery 2007;60(2, Suppl 1): ONS1–ONS7, discussion ONS7–ONS8

7. Reddy RK, Reddy RK, Jyung RW, Eloy JA, Liu JK. Gruber, Gradenigo, Dorello, and Vail: key personalities in the historical evolution and modern-day understanding of Dorello's canal. J Neurosurg 2016;124(1):224–233

8. Umansky F, Elidan J, Valarezo A. Dorello's canal: a micro-anatomical study. J Neurosurg 1991;75(2):294–298

9. Kassam AB, Vescan AD, Carrau RL, et al. Expanded endonasal approach: vidian canal as a landmark to the petrous internal carotid artery. J Neurosurg 2008;108(1):177–183

10. Osawa S, Rhoton AL Jr, Seker A, Shimizu S, Fujii K, Kassam AB. Microsurgical and endoscopic anatomy of the vidian canal. Neurosurgery 2009;64(5, Suppl 2):385–411, discussion 411–412

11. Vescan AD, Snyderman CH, Carrau RL, et al. Vidian canal: analysis and relationship to the internal carotid artery. Laryngoscope 2007;117(8):1338–1342

12. Wasserman JK, Gravel D, Purgina B. Chordoma of the head and neck: a review. Head Neck Pathol 2018;12(2):261–268

13. Hruban RH, Traganos F, Reuter VE, Huvos AG. Chordomas with malignant spindle cell components. A DNA flow cyto-metric and immunohistochemical study with histogenetic implications. Am J Pathol 1990;137(2):435–447

14. Meis JM, Raymond AK, Evans HL, Charles RE, Giraldo AA. "Dedifferentiated" chordoma. A clinicopathologic and immunohistochemical study of three cases. Am J Surg Pathol 1987;11(7):516–525

15. Oakley GJ, Fuhrer K, Seethala RR. Brachyury, SOX-9, and podoplanin, new markers in the skull base chordoma vs chondrosarcoma differential: a tissue microarray-based comparative analysis. Mod Pathol 2008;21(12):1461–1469

16. Capper D, Jones DTW, Sill M, et al. DNA methylation-based classification of central nervous system tumours. Nature 2018;555(7697):469–474

17. Boari N, Gagliardi F, Cavalli A, et al. Skull base chordomas: clinical outcome in a consecutive series of 45 patients with long-term follow-up and evaluation of clinical and biological prognostic factors. J Neurosurg 2016;125(2):450–460

18. Santegoeds RGC, Temel Y, Beckervordersandforth JC, Van Overbeeke JJ, Hoeberigs CM. State-of-the-art imaging in human chordoma of the skull base. Curr Radiol Rep 2018; 6(5):16

19. Meyers SP, Hirsch WL Jr, Curtin HD, Barnes L, Sekhar LN, Sen C. Chordomas of the skull base: MR features. AJNR Am J Neuroradiol 1992;13(6):1627–1636

20. Koutourousiou M, Snyderman CH, Fernandez-Miranda J, Gardner PA. Skull base chordomas. Otolaryngol Clin North Am 2011;44(5):1155–1171

21. Koutourousiou M, Gardner PA, Tormenti MJ, et al. Endoscopic endonasal approach for resection of cranial base chordomas: outcomes and learning curve. Neurosurgery 2012;71(3): 614–624, discussion 624–625

22. Destrieux C, Velut S, Kakou MK, Lefrancq T, Arbeille B, Santini JJ. A new concept in Dorello's canal microanatomy: the petro-clival venous confluence. J Neurosurg 1997;87(1):67–72

23. Ozveren MF, Uchida K, Tekdemir I, et al. Dural and arachnoid membraneous protection of the abducens nerve at the petroclival region. Skull Base 2002;12(4):181–188

24. Barges-Coll J, Fernandez-Miranda JC, Prevedello DM, et al. Avoiding injury to the abducens nerve during expanded endonasal endoscopic surgery: anatomic and clinical case studies. Neurosurgery 2010;67(1):144–154, discussion 154

25. Fernandez-Miranda JC, Zwagerman NT, Abhinav K, et al. Cavernous sinus compartments from the endoscopic endo-nasal approach: anatomical considerations and surgical relevance to adenoma surgery. J Neurosurg 2018;129(2): 430–441

26. Hadad G, Bassagasteguy L, Carrau RL, et al. A novel recon-structive technique after endoscopic expanded endonasal approaches: vascular pedicle nasoseptal flap. Laryngoscope 2006;116(10):1882–1886

27. Kassam AB, Thomas A, Carrau RL, et al. Endoscopic reconstruction of the cranial base using a pedicled nasoseptal flap. Neurosurgery 2008;63(1, Suppl 1):ONS44–ONS52, discussion ONS52–ONS53

28. Moon JH, Kim EH, Kim SH. Various modifications of a vascularized nasoseptal flap for repair of extensive skull base dural defects. J Neurosurg 2019:1–9. doi. https://doi.org/10.3171/2018.10.JNS181556

29. Di Maio S, Temkin N, Ramanathan D, Sekhar LN. Current comprehensive management of cranial base chordomas: 10-year meta-analysis of observational studies. J Neurosurg 2011;115(6):1094–1105

Chapter 16

Transclival Approach to the Skull Base and Posterior Fossa

Rafael Uribe, Vijay K. Anand, and Theodore H. Schwartz

Indications

1. Extradural lesions: chordoma, chondrosarcoma, osteoma/osteosarcoma.[1-7]
2. Intradural lesions: chordoma, meningioma,[8-11] dermoid and epidermoid tumors,[12,13] posterior circulation aneurysms,[14-20] brainstem cavernous malformations,[21-23] and brainstem glioma.[24]

Surgical Steps

1. Patients are placed supine in the operating table with the head fixed using a three-point Mayfield head holder. It is important to reverse the bed so that the base of the operating table does not obstruct the placement of foot pedals or decrease the working space of the surgeon.
2. If the risk for a cerebrospinal fluid (CSF) leak is deemed high, a lumbar drain is inserted prior to the start of the case. Intrathecal fluorescein use is always discussed with patients preoperatively. If there is no contraindication to its use, authors inject it at the time of drain placement. Prior to administration, patients are premedicated with 50 mg of diphenhydramine and 10 mg of dexamethasone. Usually 10 mL of CSF is drawn and then mixed with 0.2 to 0.3 mL of additive-free 10% fluorescein (sodium) solution (10–30 mg dose).
3. Head positioning, like in any other cranial procedure, is paramount to achieve success. Standard transsphenoidal approaches require movement of the head in three axes: extension, lateral rotation, and lateral tilt. Each movement is about 15 degrees with respect to the neutral plane in a way that the patient's chin will point to the foot on the surgeon's side. For transclival approaches, the head is extended slightly more than for a standard transsphenoidal approach to improve visualization of the clivus and to improve instrument maneuverability along the surgical corridor.
4. The video tower and screen are placed at the head of the bed, on the side opposite to the surgeon. The frameless stereotaxic system is placed next to the video tower, at the head of the bed. It is important to make sure that the reference array for the navigation system is placed in such a way that it will not obstruct the surgeon's field. On the side opposite to the surgeon, a support is placed on the bed rail to secure the endoscope holder (**Fig. 16.1**).
5. Neuromonitoring is not generally used for transsphenoidal approaches. However, transclival approaches might require monitoring of cranial nerves depending on the location of the pathology to be treated and its relationship to surrounding structures.
6. Cottonoids soaked in 4 mL of 4% topical cocaine are left inside the nose before the patient is ready to be draped so as to decongest the nasal mucosa.
7. Patients receive a prophylactic dose of antibiotics 1 hour before the start of the case. For extradural cases, cefazolin is sufficient, but for intradural cases, authors prefer vancomycin and a second-generation cephalosporin.
8. After the patient is positioned and the frameless stereotaxic system is registered to a preoperatively acquired magnetic resonance imaging (MRI) and/or computed tomography (CT), the nasal cottonoids are removed, and the patient is prepped and draped in usual sterile fashion. Authors routinely prep the abdomen in case a fat graft needs to be harvested. If the approach involves a very wide bone opening or if there is a high risk for a CSF leak, the leg is prepped in case a fascia lata graft is needed.
9. The nasal mucosa is injected with lidocaine 1% with a 1:100,000 dilution of epinephrine.
10. Under endoscopic visualization using a 0-degree, 18-cm-long, 4-mm-diameter rigid endoscope (Karl Storz), the middle and inferior turbinates are lateralized to identify the sphenoid ostium. Occasionally, a middle or inferior turbinectomy will need to be performed to achieve adequate surgical exposure (**Fig. 16.2**).
11. A vascularized nasoseptal flap is harvested using the standard method described by Hadad[25] and stored in the choanae. In transclival approaches this might obstruct the visual field in which case an antrostomy of the maxillary sinus can be performed and used to store the flap for the duration of the procedure (**Fig. 16.3**).[26]

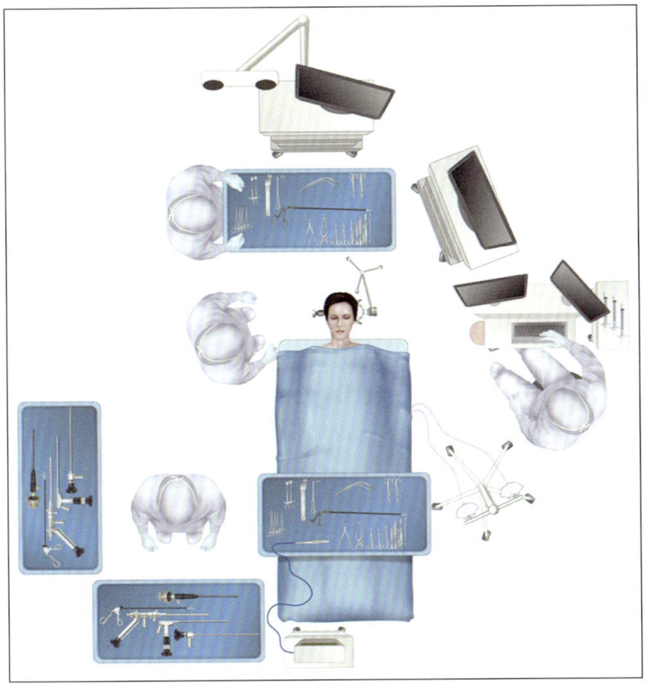

Fig. 16.1 Operating room setup. Notice that the surgeon has an unobstructed view of the screen. The surgical assistant irrigates the endoscope sheath periodically to ensure a clear view throughout the procedure.

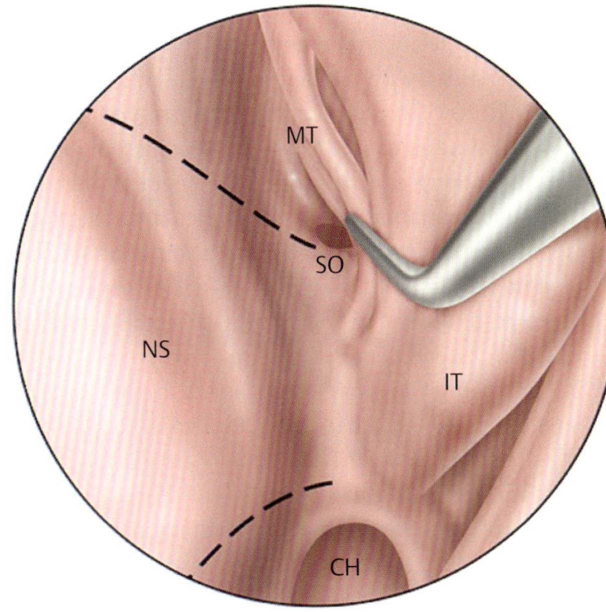

Fig. 16.2 The medial and inferior turbinates are mobilized laterally in order to identify the sphenoid ostium. If necessary, they can be resected partially or totally to improve the surgeon's view. For transclival approaches, it is common to resect the middle turbinate and create a maxillary sinus antrostomy to store the nasoseptal flap during the procedure.

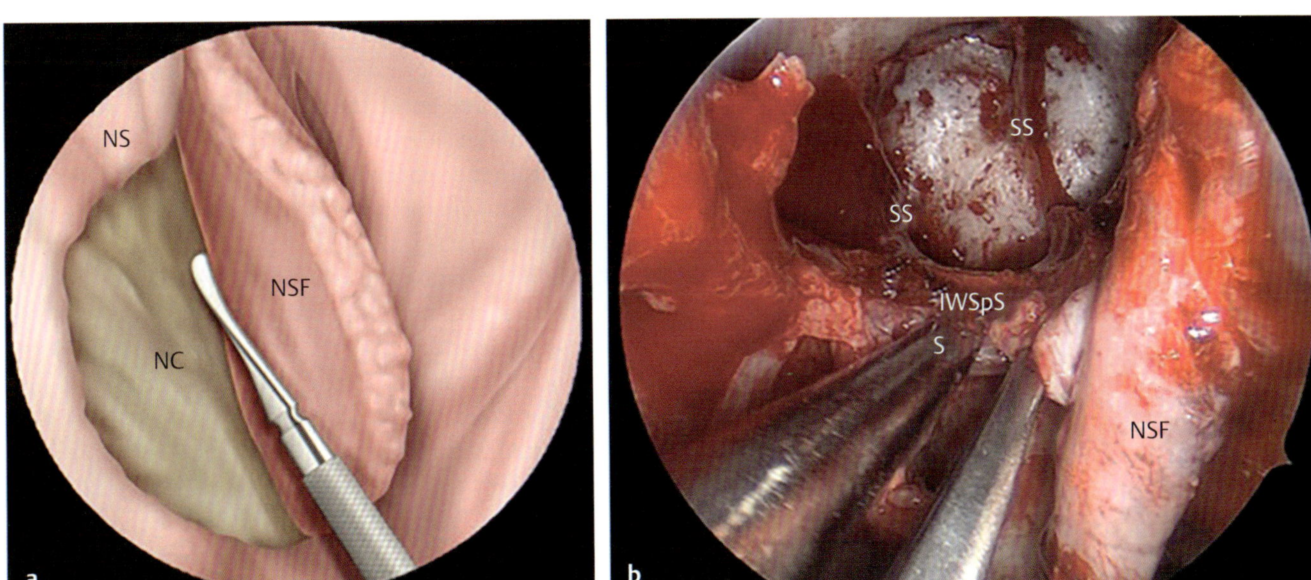

Fig. 16.3 **(a)** A nasoseptal flap is harvested using the standard Hadad technique. The flap is elevated using a periosteal dissector, taking care at all times to preserve the vascular pedicle. **(b)** Intraoperative view demonstrating lateral retraction of the nasoseptal flap while the inferior wall of the sphenoid sinus is removed.

12. A posterior septectomy is performed down to the top of the hard palate. Vomer bone can be harvested at this point to assist with closure; however, authors usually use MEDPOR (Stryker) for a rigid buttress as it can be cut to a desired shape. A wide sphenoidotomy is performed, taking care to protect the septal branches of the sphenopalatine artery that vascularize the nasoseptal flap. This improves visualization of all relevant anatomical landmarks even if the sellar floor does not need to be drilled and aids in nasoseptal flap placement at the end of the procedure.
13. At this point, the scope holder is set in place and the endoscope is switched to a 0-degree, 30-cm-long, 4-mm-diameter rigid endoscope (Karl Storz) with an irrigating sheath. All septations within the sphenoid sinus are smoothed so that the anatomy of the carotid arteries, sella, opticocarotid cisterns, and cavernous sinuses can be clearly visualized (**Fig. 16.4**). The mucosa of the sphenoid sinus is stripped to prevent postoperative formation of a mucocele. Thrombin-soaked Gelfoam (Pfizer) is applied to achieve adequate bone hemostasis.

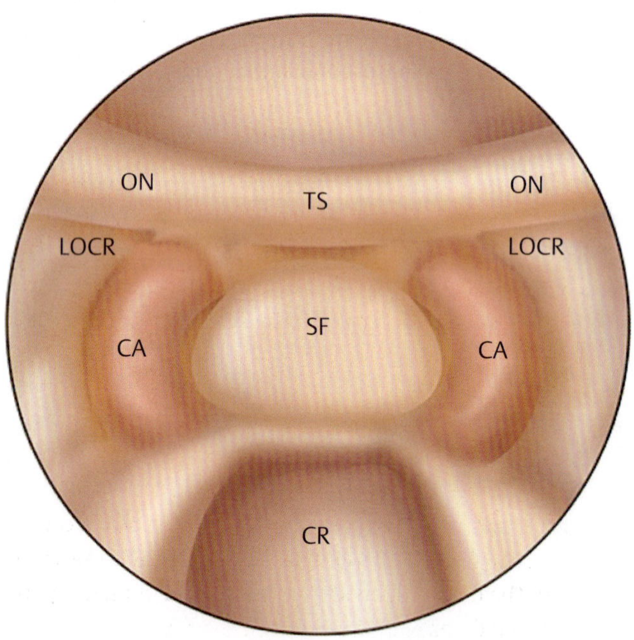

Fig. 16.4 Once the sphenoid sinus is opened widely, inspection of all anatomical structures is performed. It is important to identify the sellar floor, carotid arteries, clival recess, and optic nerves. In transclival approaches, the inferior wall of the sinus must be adequately removed to expose the clivus.

14. Anatomical inspection of all relevant landmarks is performed. Areas of bone dehiscence must be noted and carefully protected to avoid inadvertent injury of relevant structures like the carotid arteries.
15. The posterior skull base and clivus can be anatomically divided into three regions: cranial, middle, and caudal. The cranial part extends from a line that connects the posterior clinoids to the floor of the sella. The middle part extends from the sellar floor to the level of the hypoglossal canals, and the inferior or caudal part extends from the hypoglossal canals to the craniovertebral junction.[26]
16. The amount of bone that needs to be removed depends on the extent of the pathology that is being addressed. Accessing the retrosellar area and removing the posterior clinoids require removal of all the bone over the sella and the medial cavernous sinus. In some circumstances, the pituitary gland can be elevated extradurally to reach the dorsum sella. To remove the clinoid completely, an intradural approach is required with medial mobilization of the gland. This can be done unilaterally or bilaterally.
17. If the lower third of the clivus needs to be accessed, a linear-shaped incision is made in the nasopharyngeal fascia and prevertebral musculature.
18. The amount of bone removal that can be safely performed through a transclival approach is generally limited superiorly by the dorsum sella, inferiorly by the anterior lip of the foramen magnum, and laterally by the internal carotid arteries. The clival bone beneath the sphenoid sinus can be removed inferiorly to the foramen magnum working between the eustachian tubes (**Fig. 16.5**).
19. Neuronavigation and Doppler probes to identify vascular structures are critical for the safety of this approach.
20. Once bone drilling is complete, the dura of the posterior cranial fossa can be opened to address any intradural pathology (**Fig. 16.6** and **Fig. 16.7**). It is important to remember that the basilar plexus lies immediately behind the clivus. Masses in the posterior fossa can compress the plexus; as dissection and resection progress, bleeding can become profuse. This can be controlled using a combination of pressure, hemostatic agents, and bipolar coagulation.

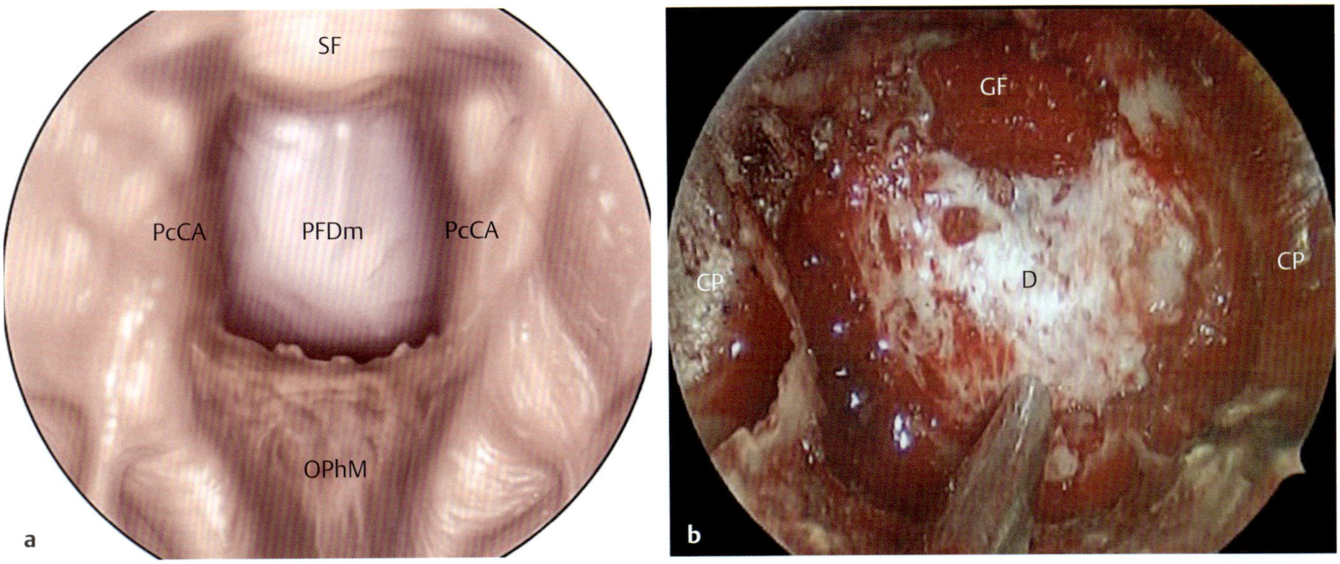

Fig. 16.5 **(a)** After the oropharyngeal mucosa is incised, the clivus is drilled until the posterior fossa dura is exposed. It is important to use neuronavigation and Doppler ultrasound to identify the paraclival carotid arteries at all times. **(b)** Intraoperative view of the posterior fossa dura after the clivus has been drilled. Hemostatic agents (Gelfoam [GF]) are used prior to dural opening.

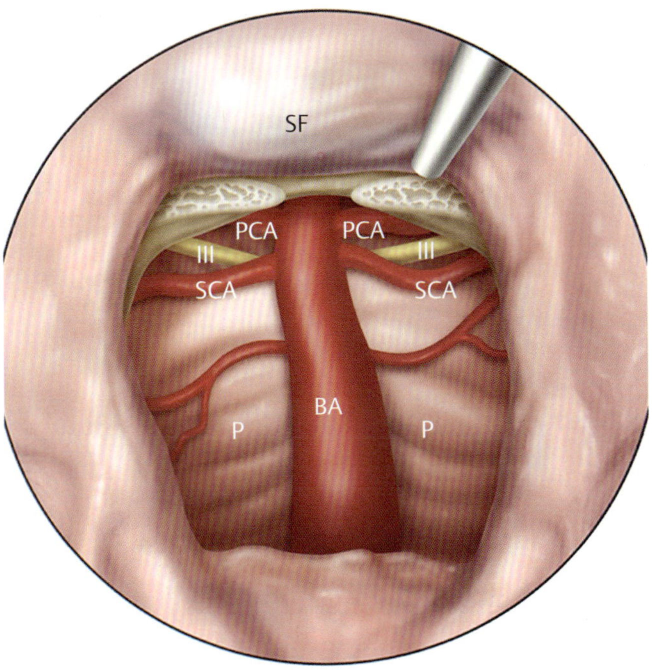

Fig. 16.6 Once the dura mater is open, the contents of the posterior fossa are exposed, including the pons, vertebrobasilar system, and lower cranial nerves. The extent of the exposure is determined by the size and location of the pathology being addressed.

21. On occasion, the carotid arteries have to be skeletonized and mobilized to reach tumor extending posterior to them. The vidian nerve is a useful landmark that can be traced posteriorly to identify the petrous carotid artery.[2,27] Alternatively, the cavernous sinuses can be exposed from the sella working outward, and bone removal can proceed downward on either side to expose the carotid canal.
22. Closure is very straightforward in cases where only bone pathology is addressed. A fat graft can be used in the event of a small dural perforation that occurs with an associated CSF leak. Once adequate hemostasis is achieved, the nasoseptal flap is rotated into place to cover the surgical defect, and a dural sealant is applied.
23. If the dura needs to be opened, authors favor a capital I-shaped incision flapping each leaf of the dura laterally. The dura is opened in a medial-to-lateral direction to avoid damage of the abducens nerve.[2]
24. For cases that require a large dural opening, authors perform a "gasket-seal" closure.[28] A fascia lata graft is harvested, making sure it is larger than the osseous defect. If fascia lata is not available, authors use AlloDerm (Allergan) or bovine pericardium. Once the graft is positioned, a bone graft or a synthetic implant (MEDPOR, Stryker) is used as a buttress which is gently

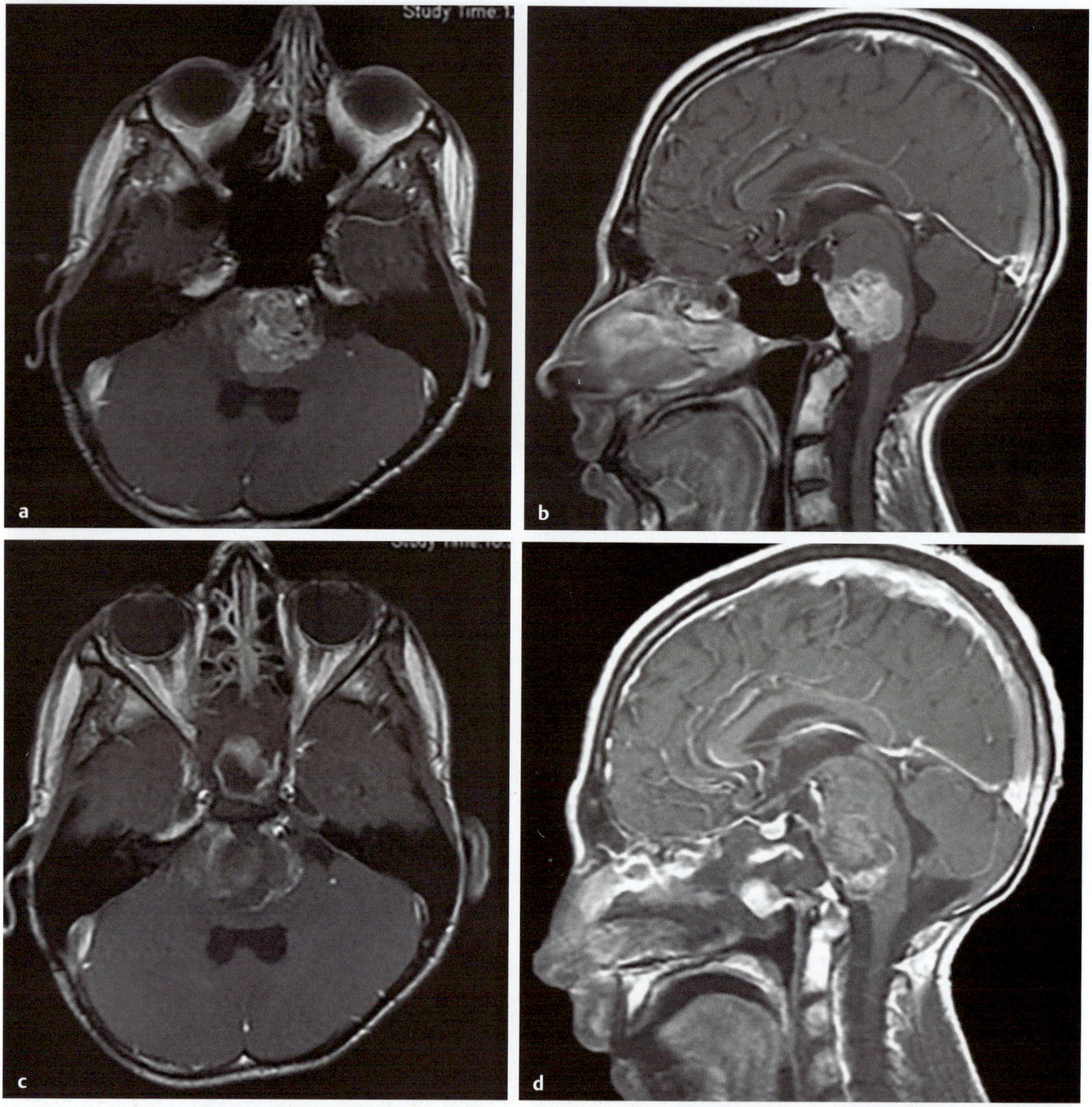

Fig. 16.7 Preoperative **(a)** axial and **(b)** sagittal contrast-enhanced MRI of a pediatric pontine focal glioma addressed through an endoscopic, endonasal, transclival approach. Postoperative **(c)** axial and **(d)** sagittal contrast-enhanced MRI demonstrate near-total tumor resection and adequate skull base reconstruction.

countersunk into the defect (**Fig. 16.8**). This will draw the tissue graft into the defect and create the necessary seal. Hemostasis is obtained, and the rest of closure proceeds as previously described (**Fig. 16.9** and **Fig. 16.10**).

25. Finally, a bioresorbable nasal dressing is placed (NasoPore, Stryker) on each nostril. A moustache dressing can be left in place at the end of the procedure as a wick for any postoperative nasal secretion.

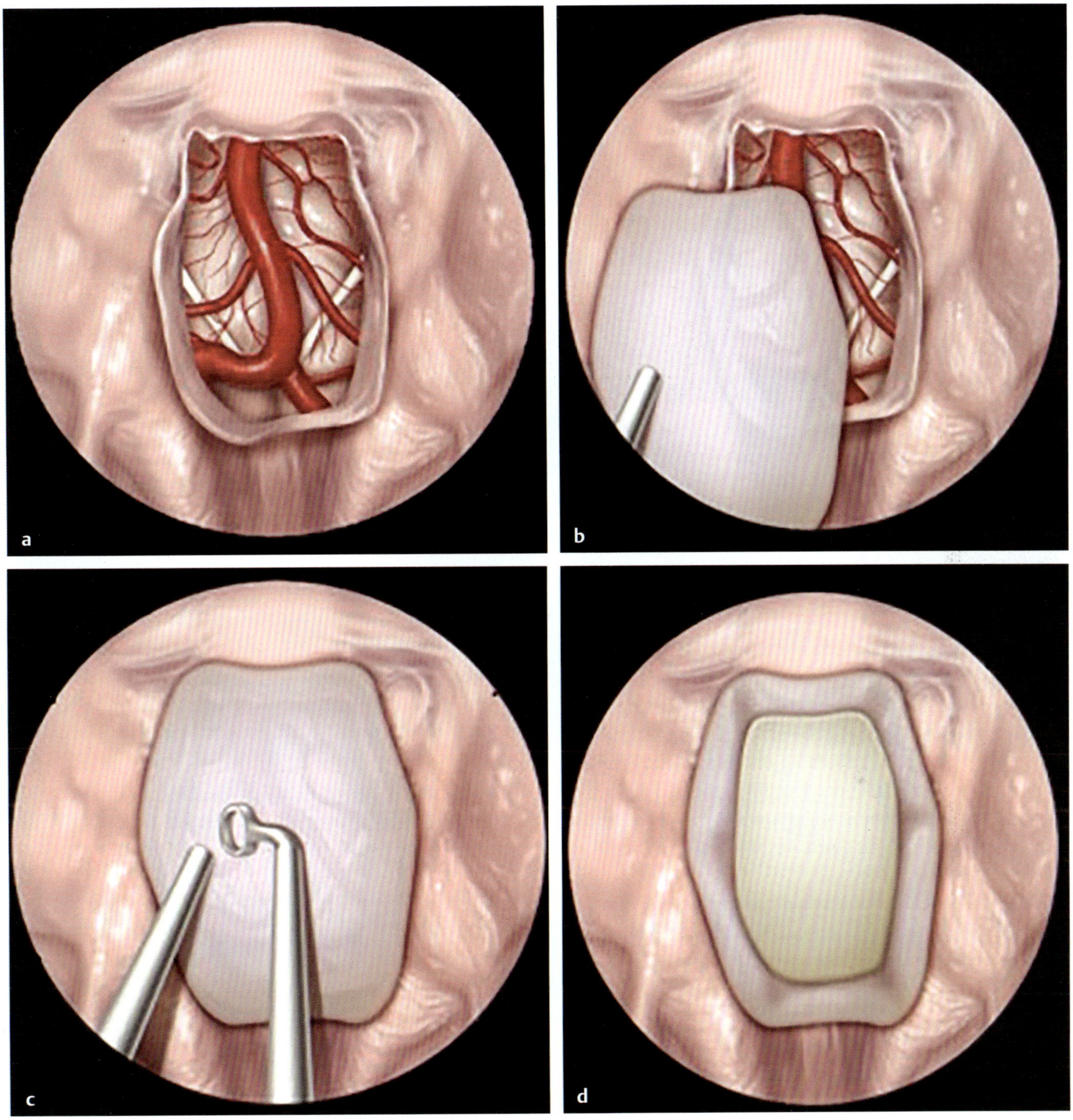

a b c d

Fig. 16.8 For cases with **(a)** intradural involvement, a gasket-seal closure is performed at the end of the case. **(b)** A synthetic dural graft is cut in the shape of the defect. **(c)** Positioned as an inlay, and **(d)** MEDPOR plating is then used to provide a rigid buttress. Once it is determined to be adequately sealed, the nasoseptal flap is positioned in standard fashion and fibrin sealant is sprayed over the graft.

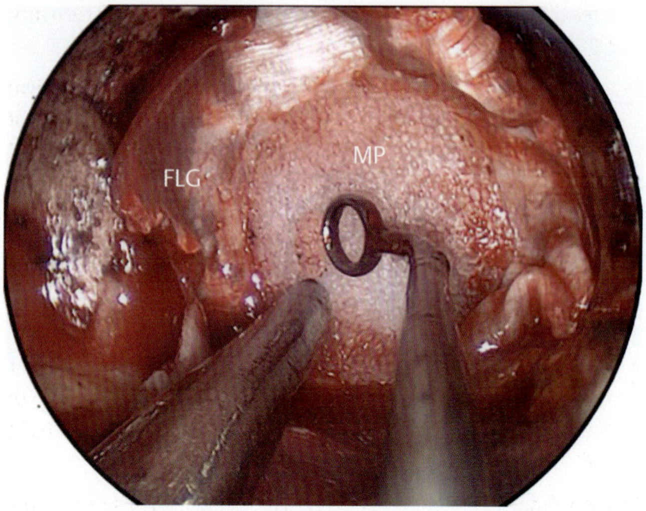

Fig. 16.9 Intraoperative view demonstrating the gasket-seal closure technique. A fascia lata graft was used for this case. MEDPOR plating has been tailored to the defect and is being countersunk against the graft.

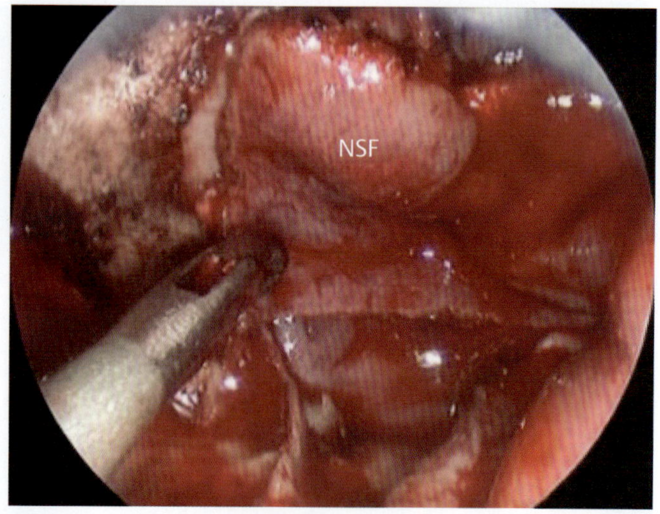

Fig. 16.10 Intraoperative view demonstrating placement of the nasoseptal flap (NSF) over the skull base defect at the end of a transclival approach.

Tips and Pearls

- Mild extension of the head during patient positioning is important to improve the visualization of the clivus.
- A very small intercarotid distance (i.e., "kissing carotids") may preclude the use of the endonasal approach to the skull base depending on the width of the corridor needed to adequately address the pathology.
- A wide bone opening is important to avoid inadvertent injury of intradural structures from a lack of adequate visualization.
- A gasket-seal closure helps reduce the risk of a CSF leak in cases that require a wide dural opening and prevents pontine herniation.[29]

References

1. Fernandez-Miranda JC, Morera VA, Snyderman CH, Gardner P. Endoscopic endonasal transclival approach to the jugular tubercle. Neurosurgery 2012;71:146–158; discussion 158–159
2. Fraser JF, Nyquist GG, Moore N, Anand VK, Schwartz TH. Endoscopic endonasal minimal access approach to the clivus: case series and technical nuances. Neurosurgery 2010;67:ons150-158; discussion ons158
3. Fraser JF, Nyquist GG, Moore N, Anand VK, Schwartz TH. Endoscopic endonasal transclival resection of chordomas: operative technique, clinical outcome, and review of the literature. J Neurosurg 2010;112:1061–1069
4. Holzmann D, Reisch R, Krayenbuhl N, Hug E, Bernays RL. The transnasal transclival approach for clivus chordoma. Minim Invasive Neurosurg 2010;53:211–217
5. Iacoangeli M, Di Rienzo A, di Somma LG, et al. Improving the endoscopic endonasal transclival approach: the importance of a precise layer by layer reconstruction. Br J Neurosurg 2014;28:241–246
6. Shkarubo AN, Koval KV, Dobrovol'skiy GF, et al. [Extended endoscopic endonasal posterior (transclival) approach to tumors of the clival region and ventral posterior cranial fossa. Part 1. Topographic and anatomical features of the clivus and adjacent structures]. Zh Vopr Neirokhir Im N N Burdenko 2017;81:5–16
7. Vellutini Ede A, Balsalobre L, Hermann DR, Stamm AC. The endoscopic endonasal approach for extradural and intradural clivus lesions. World Neurosurg 2014;82: S106–S115
8. Gonzalez-Quarante LH, Ruiz-Juretschke F, Iza-Vallejo B, Scola-Pliego E, Poletti D, Sola Vendrell E. Expanded endoscopic transclival approach for resection of a chordoid meningioma without dural attachment (MWODA) located in the prepontine cistern. World Neurosurg 2016;91:675.e5–675.e10
9. Jean WC, Felbaum DR, Anaizi A, DeKlotz TR. Endoscopic endonasal approach for transclival resection of a petroclival meningioma: a technical note. Cureus 2016; 8:e641
10. Prosser JD, Vender JR, Alleyne CH, Solares CA. Expanded endoscopic endonasal approaches to skull base meningiomas. J Neurol Surg B Skull Base 2012;73:147–156

11. Wang WH, Abhinav K, Wang E, Snyderman C, Gardner PA, Fernandez-Miranda JC. Endoscopic endonasal transclival transcondylar approach for foramen magnum meningiomas: surgical anatomy and technical note. Oper Neurosurg (Hagerstown) 2016;12:153–162

12. Esposito F, Becker DP, Villablanca JP, Kelly DF. Endonasal transsphenoidal transclival removal of prepontine epidermoid tumors: technical note. Neurosurgery 2005; 56:E443; discussion E443

13. Forbes JA, Banu M, Lehner K, et al. Endoscopic endonasal resection of epidermoid cysts involving the ventral cranial base. J Neurosurg 2018;1–10

14. Doan V, Lemos-Rodriguez AM, Sreenath SB, et al. Using the endoscopic endonasal transclival approach to access aneurysms arising from AICA, PICA, and vertebral artery: an anatomical study. J Neurol Surg B Skull Base 2016;77:207–211

15. Drazin D, Zhuang L, Schievink WI, Mamelak AN. Expanded endonasal approach for the clipping of a ruptured basilar aneurysm and feeding artery to a cerebellar arteriovenous malformation. J Clin Neurosci 2012;19:144–148

16. Ensenat J, Alobid I, de Notaris M, et al. Endoscopic endonasal clipping of a ruptured vertebral-posterior inferior cerebellar artery aneurysm: technical case report. Neurosurgery 2011;69:onsE121–E127; discussion onsE127–E128

17. Labib M, Dehdashti AR. Extended endoscopic endonasal transclival clipping of posterior circulation aneurysms—an alternative to the transcranial approach. Acta Neurochir (Wien) 2015;157:2087–2088

18. Lemos-Rodriguez AM, Sreenath S, Unnithan A, et al. A new window for the treatment of posterior cerebral artery, superior cerebellar artery, and basilar apex aneurysm: the expanded endoscopic endonasal approach. J Neurol Surg B Skull Base 2016;77:308–313

19. Sanmillan JL, Lawton MT, Rincon-Torroella J, et al. Assessment of the endoscopic endonasal transclival approach for surgical clipping of anterior pontine anterior-inferior cerebellar artery aneurysms. World Neurosurg 2016;89:368–375

20. Szentirmai O, Hong Y, Mascarenhas L, et al. Endoscopic endonasal clip ligation of cerebral aneurysms: an anatomical feasibility study and future directions. J Neurosurg 2016;124:463–468

21. Linsler S, Oertel J. Endoscopic endonasal transclival resection of a brainstem cavernoma: a detailed account of our technique and comparison with the literature. World Neurosurg 2015;84:2064–2071

22. Nayak NR, Thawani JP, Sanborn MR, Storm PB, Lee JY. Endoscopic approaches to brainstem cavernous malformations: case series and review of the literature. Surg Neurol Int 2015;6:68

23. Sanborn MR, Kramarz MJ, Storm PB, Adappa ND, Palmer JN, Lee JY. Endoscopic, endonasal, transclival resection of a pontine cavernoma: case report. Neurosurgery 2012; 71:198–203

24. Fernandes Cabral DT, Zenonos GA, Nunez M, et al. Endoscopic endonasal transclival approach for resection of a pontine glioma: surgical planning, surgical anatomy, and technique. Oper Neurosurg (Hagerstown) 2018;15: 589–599

25. Hadad G, Roberto R, Demaría JP, et al. The pedicled nasoseptal flap. In: Bernal-Sprekelsen M, Alobid I, Ensenat J, et al, eds. Endoscopic Approaches to the Paranasal Sinuses and Skull Base. Stuttgart, New York, Delhi, Rio: Thieme; 2017:370–377

26. Cavallo LM, Esposito I, Notaris MD, et al. Endoscopic anatomy of the clivus and posterior fossa. In: Stamm AC, ed. Transnasal Endoscopic Skull Base and Brain Surgery. Stuttgart, New York, Delhi, Rio: Thieme; 2011:265–274

27. Kassam AB, Vescan AD, Carrau RL, et al. Expanded endonasal approach: vidian canal as a landmark to the petrous internal carotid artery. J Neurosurg 2008;108: 177–183

28. Leng LZ, Brown S, Anand VK, Schwartz TH. "Gasket-seal" watertight closure in minimal-access endoscopic cranial base surgery. Neurosurgery 2008;62: ONSE342–343; discussion ONSE343

29. Koutourousiou M, Filho FV, Costacou T, et al. Pontine encephalocele and abnormalities of the posterior fossa following transclival endoscopic endonasal surgery. J Neurosurg 2014;121:359–366

Chapter 17 Endoscopic Endonasal Surgeries for Clival Chordomas

Case 17A

Endoscopic Endonasal Excision of a Clival Chordoma

Kong Yew Liew, Michel Roethlisberger, Saif Al-Zahid, Prepageran Narayanan, and Vicknes Waran

History

A 46-year-old female presented with a prolonged history of atypical migraine attacks. A neurocranial magnetic resonance imaging (MRI) was requested to rule out an intracranial pathology. The MRI revealed a heterogeneously enhancing and locally destructive clival mass extending into the sphenoid cavity (**Fig. 17A.1a–d**). A two-surgeon binostril four-handed endoscopic endonasal excision was planned.

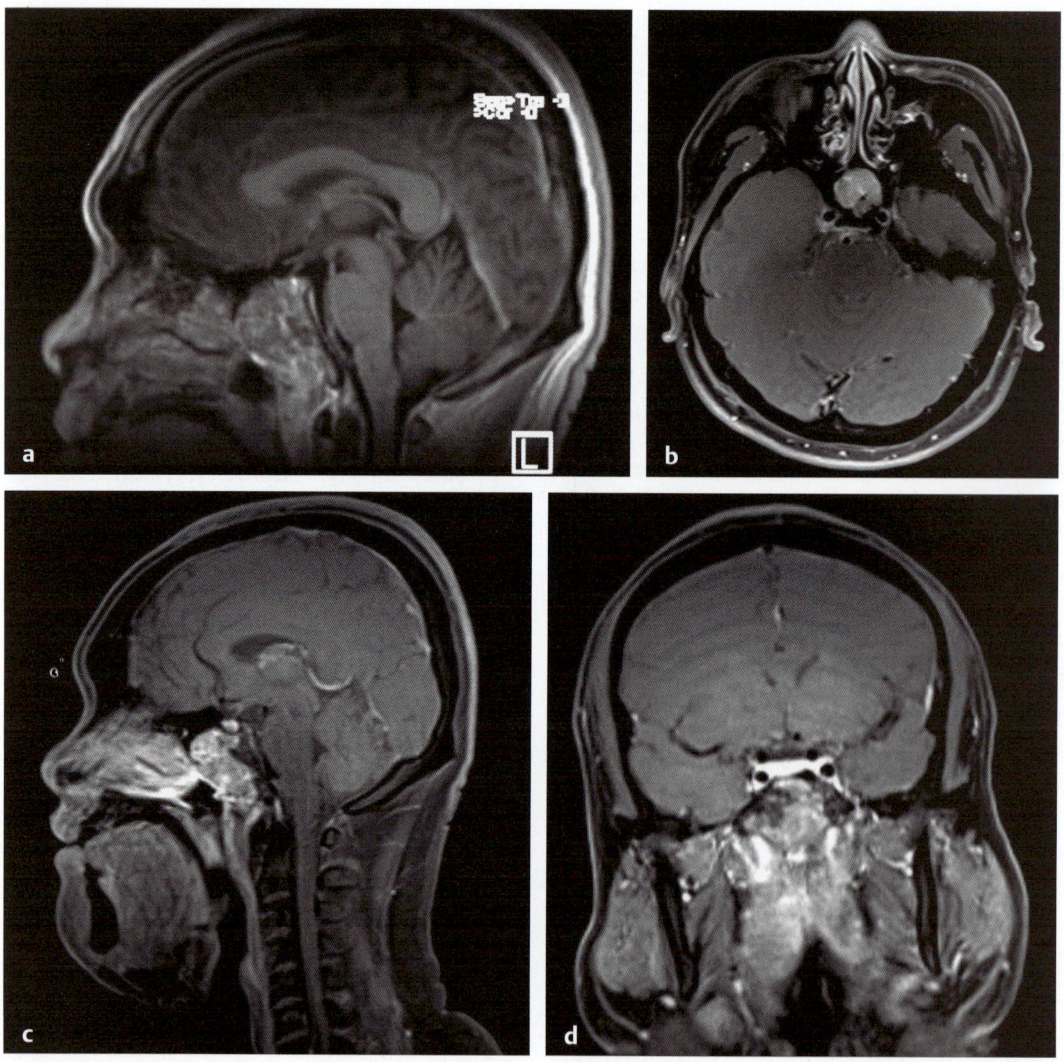

Fig. 17A.1 **(a)** Sagittal, **(b)** axial T1-weighted, **(c)** sagittal, **(d)** coronal T1-weighted contrast enhanced MRI sections revealing a heterogenous mass centered in the upper to midclivus and involving the sphenoid sinus.

Surgical Steps

1. As the tumor involves the upper to midclivus, an endoscopic endonasal binostril approach is used as described in Chapter 1 to expose the sphenoid sinus, utilizing a nasoseptal mucoperichondrial flap on the right and a rescue flap on the left.
2. After removal of the sphenoid rostrum, the remainder of the posterior septum inferiorly is also removed to give full access to the tumor within the sphenoid sinus and nasopharynx (**Fig. 17A.2**).
3. Dissection is started superiorly with an aspirator in a side-to-side fashion, stepwise removing the tumor from its superficial aspects deeper toward the lower clivus, while leaving the sella turcica intact (**Fig. 17A.3** and **Fig. 17A.4**).
4. As the tumor dissection proceeds deeper, a dissector is used to assist with palpation and mobilization of tumor from the unevenly eroded clivus (**Fig. 17A.5**). It is important to be mindful of any focal bony dehiscence that may be present, which should already have been identified on preoperative imaging. Image-guided surgery (IGS) should also be used to reconfirm the depth and direction of dissection and proximity of the paraclival internal carotid arteries.
5. The exposed uneven lower clival bone is then burred to clear any further residual tumor and to resurface the resection margins (**Fig. 17A.6**).

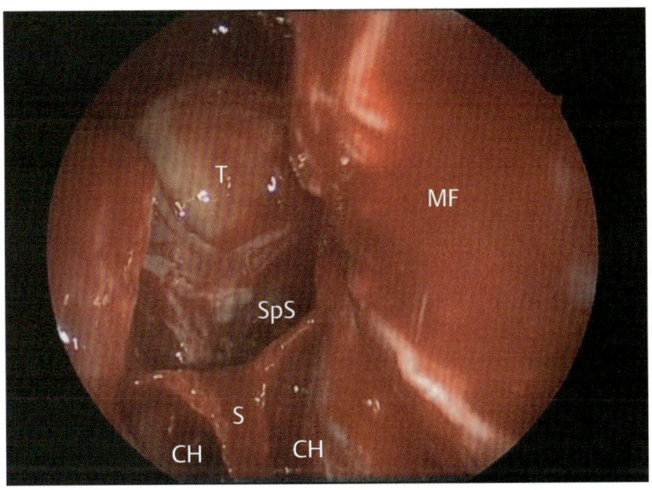

Fig. 17A.2 View after removal of the sphenoid rostrum with tumor (T) visibly occupying the sphenoid sinus (SpS). The remnant posterior septum can be seen (S).

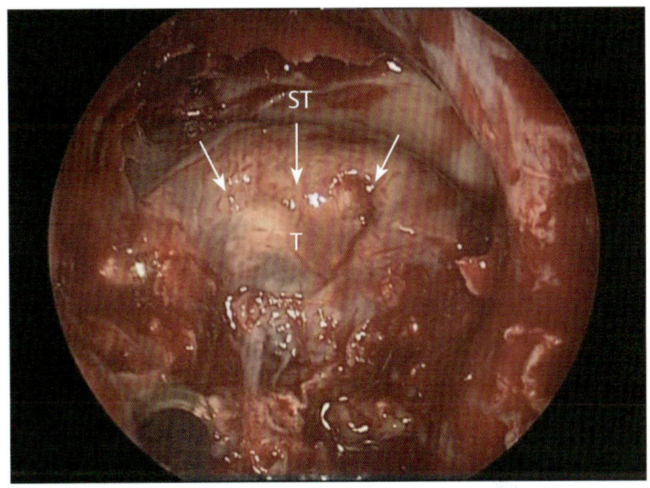

Fig. 17A.3 The fully exposed lesion can be appreciated, originating from the clivus posteriorly and extending anteriorly into the sphenoid sinus and the superior nasopharynx. The white arrows depict the direction of the tumor (T) dissection off the sella turcica (ST).

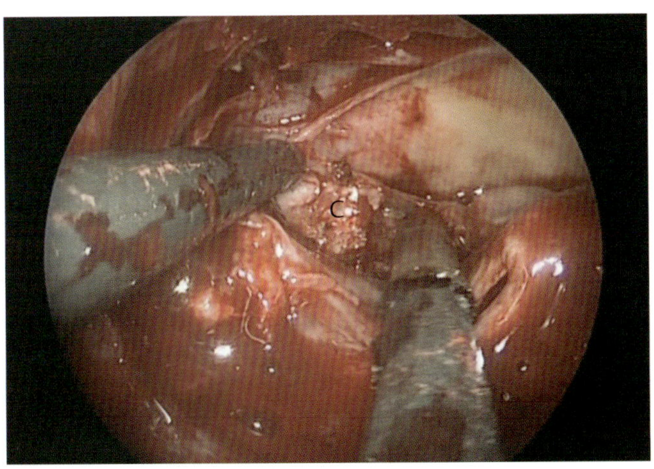

Fig. 17A.4 During the deep central tumor dissection, parts of the clival bone are visualized.

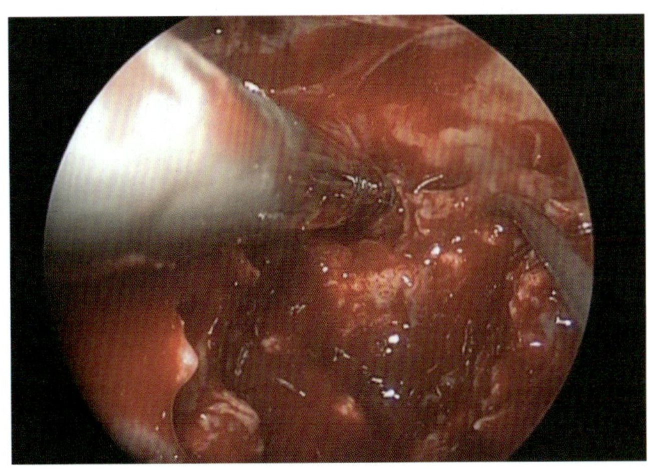

Fig. 17A.5 A dissector is used to palpate and remove tumor off the unevenly eroded surface of the clivus.

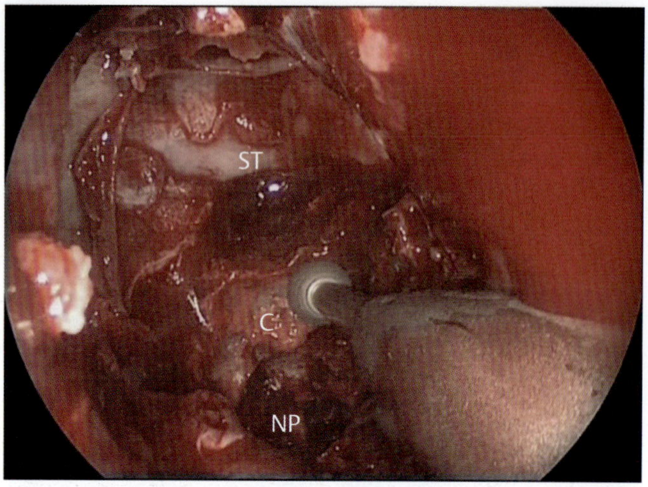

Fig. 17A.6 The exposed bone of the lower clivus (C) is resurfaced using a high-speed drill. The sella turcica (ST) is visible superiorly while the nasopharynx (NP) is seen already opened down to the bone inferiorly.

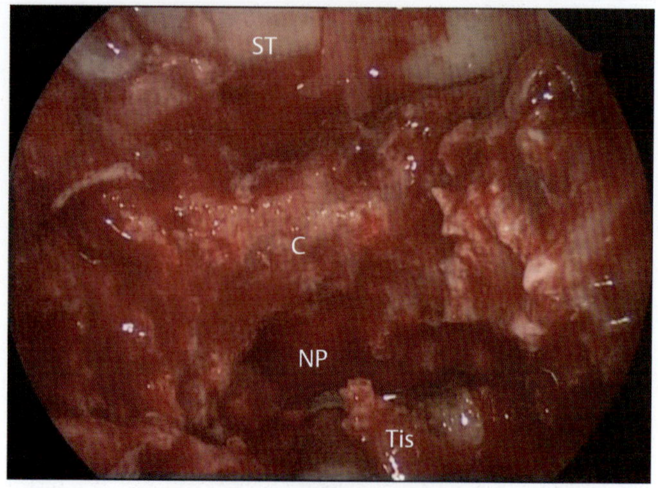

Fig. 17A.7 The completed resection cavity.

6. When there is no breach in the dura or cerebrospinal fluid leak, no skull base defect reconstruction is necessary (**Fig. 17A.7**). The nasopharynx soft tissue is pushed back into place and the exposed bone is covered with absorbable hemostatic sponges and allowed to mucosalize (**Fig. 17A.8**).

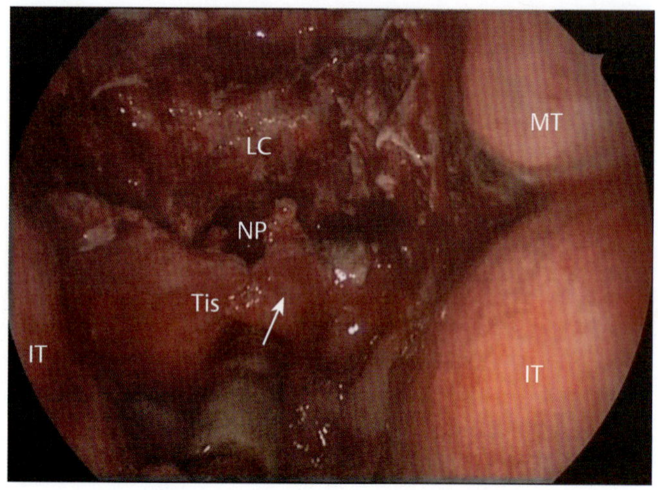

Fig. 17A.8 The soft tissue (Tis) of the nasopharynx (NP) is being pushed back into place (*white arrow*). The inferior turbinates (IT) can be seen on either side.

Case 17B

Endoscopic Endonasal Transclival Approach for the Excision of a Clival Chordoma

Liew Yew Toong, Michel Roethlisberger, Prepageran Narayanan, and Vicknes Waran

History

A 19-year-old man with a 6-month history of unsteady gait and headache presented to the neurosurgical clinic after worsening pain and poor oral intake. A magnetic resonance imaging (MRI) scan revealed a midline-enhancing lesion centered at the clivus region with significant brainstem compression. It measured approximately 6 × 5.5 cm (**Fig. 17B.1** and **Fig. 17B.2**). A binostril endonasal endoscopic excision of the tumor was indicated.

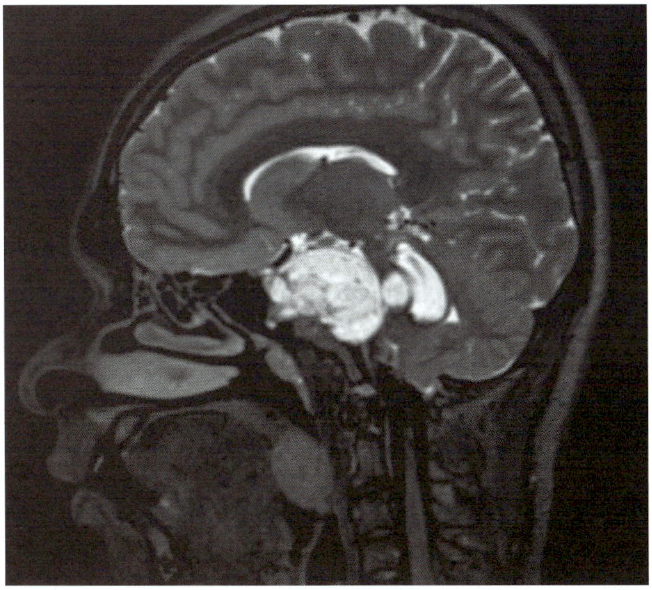

Fig. 17B.1 Sagittal T2-weighted MRI section demonstrating a hyperintense soft erosive clival lesion with relevant brainstem compression.

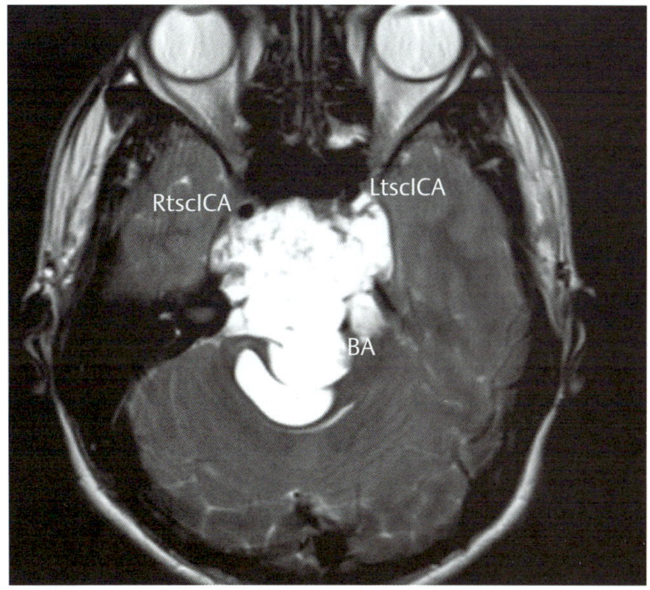

Fig. 17B.2 Axial T2-weighted MRI section demonstrating a hyperintense soft erosive clival lesion with significant brainstem compression.

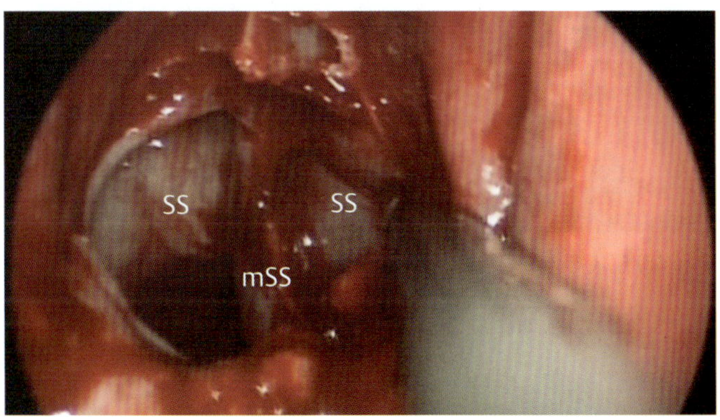

Fig. 17B.3 Endonasal endoscopic view after removal of the sphenoid rostrum bilaterally exposing the sphenoid sinuses (SS).

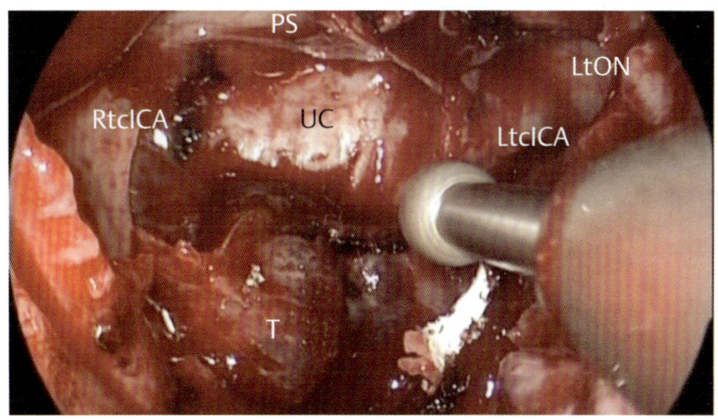

Fig. 17B.4 For a wider access, the sphenoid septations are removed using a high-speed drill.

Surgical Steps

1. A two-surgeon, four-handed binostril endonasal approach is used as described in Chapter 1 to expose the sphenoid sinus (**Fig. 17B.3**), harvesting a right nasoseptal flap for later reconstruction.
2. The anterior wall of the sphenoid sinus is further widened in all directions using a Kerrison punch and a high-speed drill to remove intrasphenoidal septations (**Fig. 17B.4**).
3. The floor of the sphenoid sinus between the midline and the vidian nerves is resected to ensure a wide clival exposure. The inferior extension can be brought down to the second vertebral arch, depending on the exact location of the tumor (**Fig. 17B.5**).
4. The bone of the clivus (**Fig. 17B.6** and **Fig. 17B.7**) is resected using a high-speed drill with wide exposure of the underlying dura.
5. The tumor is removed by sharp and blunt dissection (**Fig. 17B.8**). An ultrasonic surgical aspirator is also used to further remove the tumor mass. Tumor removal is guided with IGS to additionally confirm the location of the paraclival carotid arteries.
6. The tumor is mobilized from the surrounding tissues with a dissector and a suction device taking care not to injure the underlying basilar artery at the posterior limit of the dissection (**Fig. 17B.9**). The underlying dura is exposed (**Fig. 17B.10**).
7. After complete tumor removal, the surgical field is inspected for any bleeding, and hemostasis is

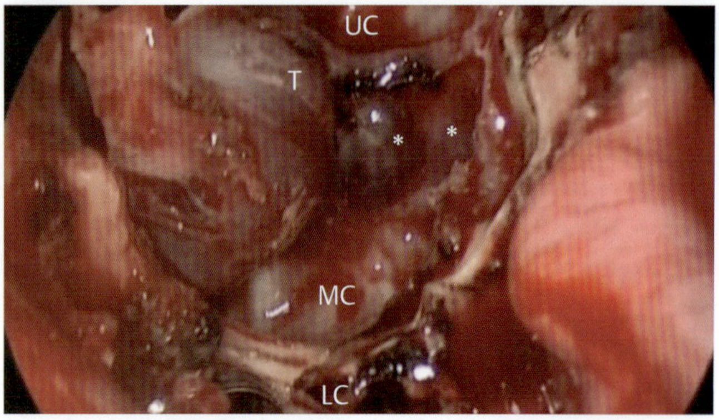

Fig. 17B.5 Endonasal endoscopic view after removal of the anterior sphenoid sinus wall. The encapsulated tumor (T) is evident, partially eroding the clivus (*).

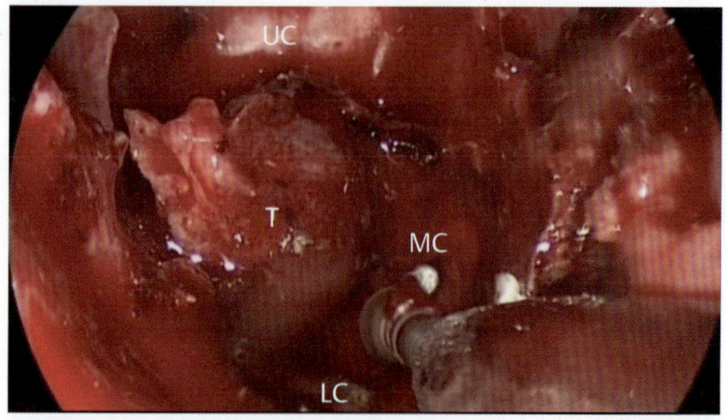

Fig. 17B.6 The clival bone is reduced with a high-speed drill around the cystic tumor compartments (T) for further mobilization and debulking.

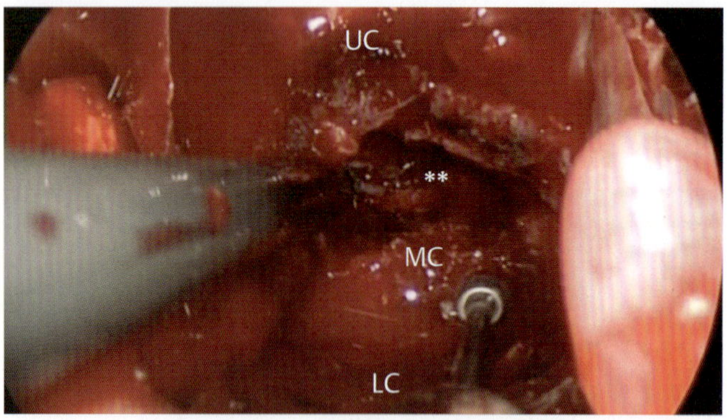

Fig. 17B.7 The floor of the sphenoid sinus is removed from the midline to the vidian nerves bilaterally. A defect (**) remains within the clival bone where the cystic tumor was located.

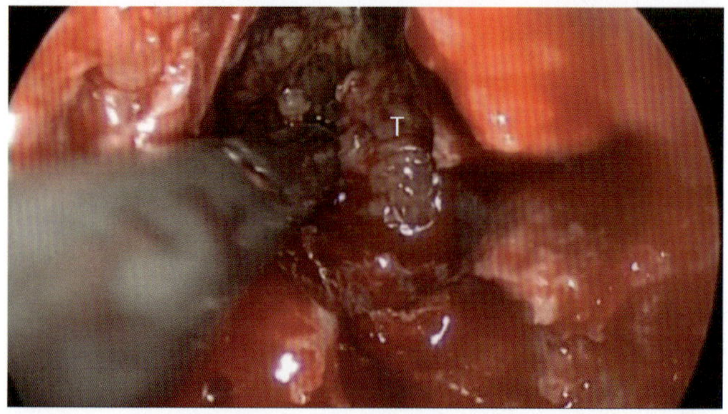

Fig. 17B.8 The tumor (T) is removed using sharp and blunt dissection.

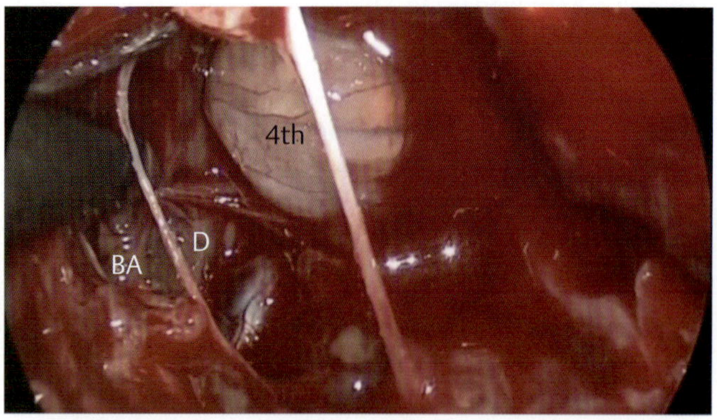

Fig. 17B.9 After removal of the posterior margin of the lesion, the fourth ventricle (4th) and the cerebellum are visible through an intact arachnoid layer. The basilar artery (BA) is located under the suction device.

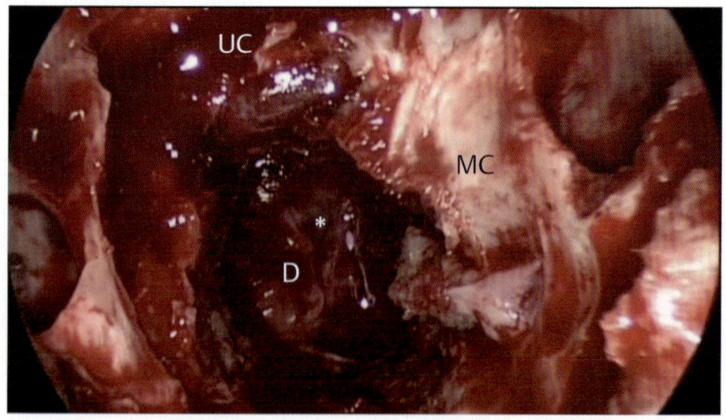

Fig. 17B.10 Endonasal endoscopic view of the final resection cavity with clival dura (D) as the posterior limit of the resection and a dural tear (*) toward the fourth ventricle.

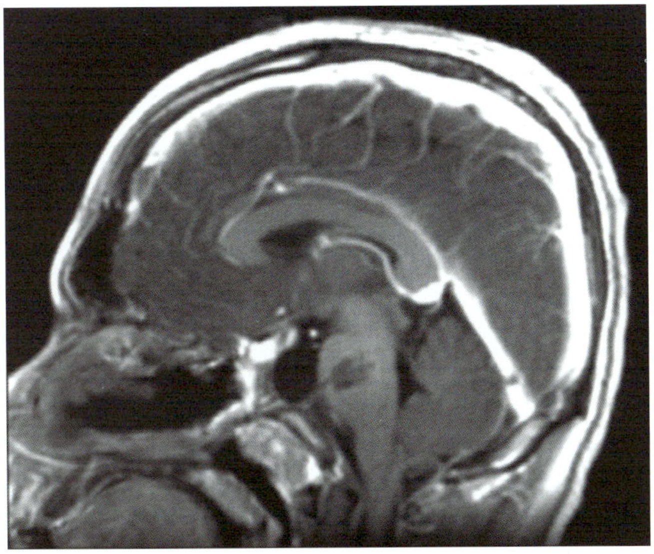

Fig. 17B.11 Intraoperative MRI shows significant reduction of tumor volume.

diligently secured. Intraoperative MRI is performed to assess extent of resection, revealing adequate tumor debulking with sufficient brainstem decompression (**Fig. 17B.11**).

8. After complete removal of the tumor, the defect is reconstructed with an abdominal fat graft. The edges are tucked in to ensure a watertight closure without iatrogenic compression of the underlying vital structures (**Fig. 17B.12**).
9. The multilayer reconstruction is stabilized with vomerine bone harvested during the initial exposure, abdominal fat, Surgicel (Ethicon, USA), and the vascularized Hadad-Bassagasteguy flap. The construct is covered with a synthetic dural sealant or tissue glue (**Fig. 17B.13, Fig. 17B.14,** and **Fig. 17B.15**).
10. The nasal cavity is packed with Nasopore (synthetic biodegradable foam) making sure to provide an adequate airway along the nasal floor.

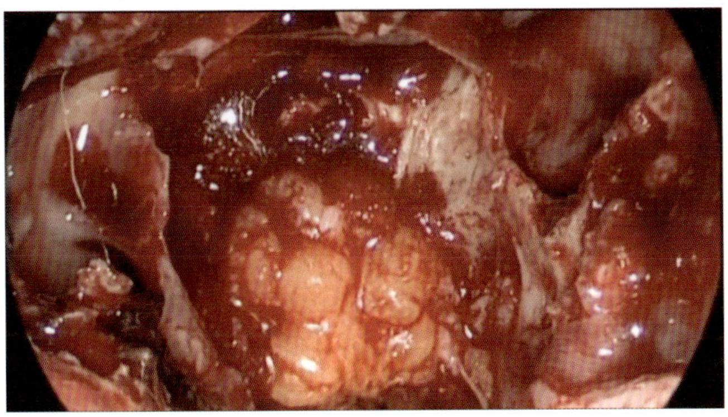

Fig. 17B.12 The dural tear is repaired with an abdominal fat graft.

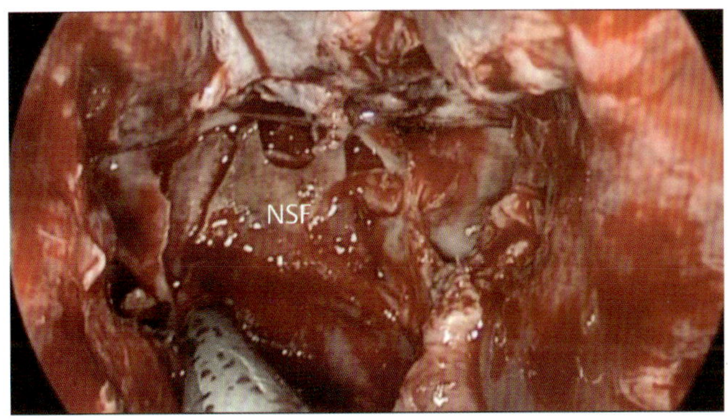

Fig. 17B.13 A nasoseptal flap (NSF) is used to cover the skull base defect.

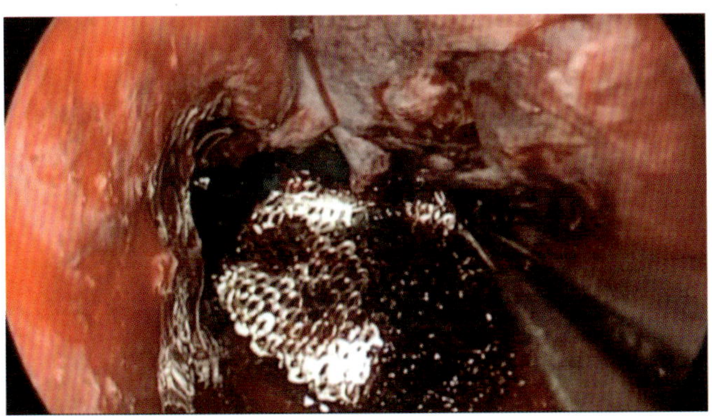

Fig. 17B.14 Multilayer reconstruction: Surgicel (Ethicon, USA) is placed over the dural sealant.

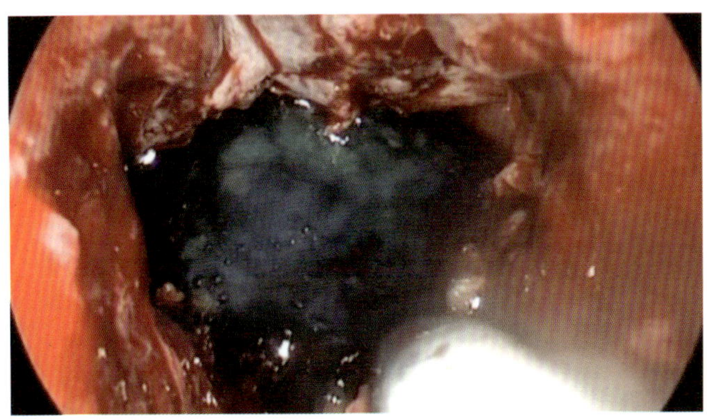

Fig. 17B.15 A further layer of dural sealant has been applied.

Section V

Cranio-cervical Junction

Chapter 18 Pathologies of the Craniocervical Junction

Revadi Govindaraju, Michel Roethlisberger, Prepageran Narayanan, and Vicknes Waran

Introduction

The craniocervical junction (CCJ) is a complex anatomical site with pathologies being peculiar to this region. Hence, its diagnosis and surgery are challenging for a number of reasons. The complexity is given by the anatomical location deep in the center of the base of skull, in close relationship to the brainstem and adjacent critical neurovascular structures. The access is generally limited, and the selection of the appropriate approach is determined by the anatomical extension, variants, potential complications, and biomechanical considerations including joint stability among other factors.

Anatomy

The CCJ is present in the transition zone between the neurocranium and the cervical spine and consists of two important joints: atlantooccipital (OC1) and atlantoaxial joints (C1C2; **Fig. 18.1**).[1] Central to the CCJ are the osteoligamentous structures and the two joints covering the neurovascular structures while allowing specific mobility (cranial flexion, extension, and axial rotation).

Superiorly, the CCJ is bounded by the foramen magnum and lower clivus, and inferiorly, it extends to the level of the axis (C2 vertebra). The petroclival fissure, which extends from the foramen lacerum to the jugular foramen, separates the clivus from the petrous bone laterally. The occipital condyles are located on the anterior half of the foramen magnum and define its lateral border. They articulate with the superior facet of the atlas (C1 vertebra). Lateral to the occipital condyles, the jugular foramina are located (**Fig. 18.1**).[2]

The atlas (C1 vertebra) is devoid of a vertebral body and consists of two lateral masses which are interconnected by a small anterior and a larger posteriorly curved bony arch. The lateral masses have a medial tubercle for the attachment of the transverse ligament. Laterally, the transverse process arises from the lateral mass. The odontoid peg of the axis arises as a perpendicular projection from the body of the axis and articulates with the posterior surface of the anterior arch of the atlas (**Fig. 18.2**). The posterior surface of the odontoid peg also articulates with the cartilaginous facet of the cruciform ligament. Its tip is approximately at the level of the OC1 joint.[2] The apical ligament attaches the peg to the basion and the alar ligaments to the anterolateral part of the foramen magnum or the condyles.[1] The transverse ligament and

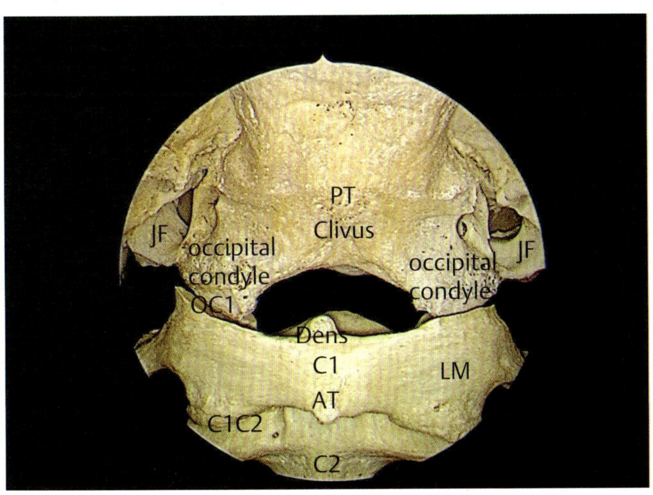

Fig. 18.1 Endoscopic endonasal view of the bony anatomy of the craniocervical junction. The lower third of the clivus, anterior part of the foramen magnum, atlas, and upper part of the axis are seen.

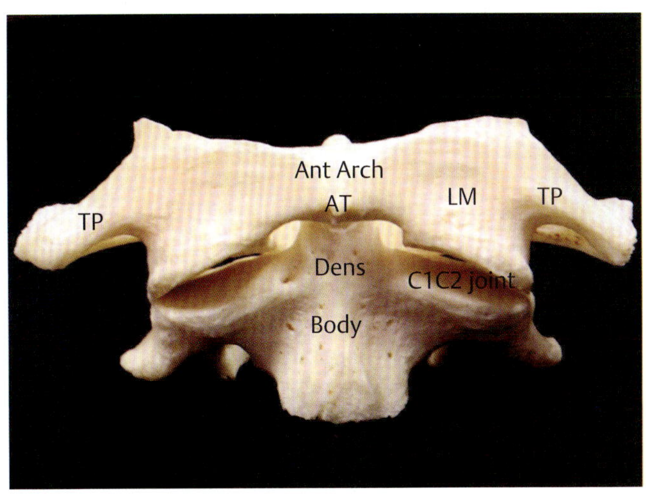

Fig. 18.2 Anterior view of the atlas and axis.

alar ligaments are considered the most important ligaments providing stability to the atlantoaxial joint. The transverse ligament divides the atlas ring into two compartments: the anterior extradural segment containing the osteoligamentous structures and a posterior intradural compartment.[1] Opening the tectorial membrane and dura posterior to the cruciform ligaments at the level of foramen magnum exposes the intradural contents, the cervicomedullary junction defined as the level of exit of the C1 ventral rootlets and the intradural segment of the vertebral arteries (VAs). The exposure of the basilar artery, the proximal segments of the posterior inferior cerebellar artery (PICA), the cranial nerves IX to XII, the olives, and the medullary pyramids is achieved with further removal of the lower clivus (**Fig. 18.3a–l**).[2]

The neck musculature also plays an important role in the anatomy of the CCJ, as it is often mobilized to make way for access. For an endoscopic endonasal approach, the nasopharynx lies anterior to the CCJ. Deep under the mucosa and basiopharyngeal fascia lies the longus capitis muscle with a median raphe in the midline. It attaches to the clivus lateral to the pharyngeal tubercle. The rectus capitis anterior muscle arises behind the longus capitis and inserts near the groove on the anterior surface of the condyles.[3] During a transoral approach, the superior constrictor muscle will be encountered first and deeper to the longus colli and longus capitis muscle (**Fig. 18.3a–l**).

The muscles of the posterior compartment are important for both the lateral and posterior approaches and are more elaborate in their anatomy. They can be divided into a superficial, intermediate, and a deep layer. The superficial layers consist of the sternocleidomastoid and the trapezius muscles. The intermediate layer is formed by the splenius capitis and semispinalis capitis. The muscles in the deeper layer occupy the suboccipital triangle and are formed by the rectus capitis posterior major, superior oblique, and inferior oblique.[2]

The suboccipital triangle is an important landmark for the posterior and lateral approaches and it is crucial to identify the horizontal segment of the VA here. Other important landmarks include the C2 ganglion (related to the C1C2 joint) and rectus capitis lateralis muscle.[2]

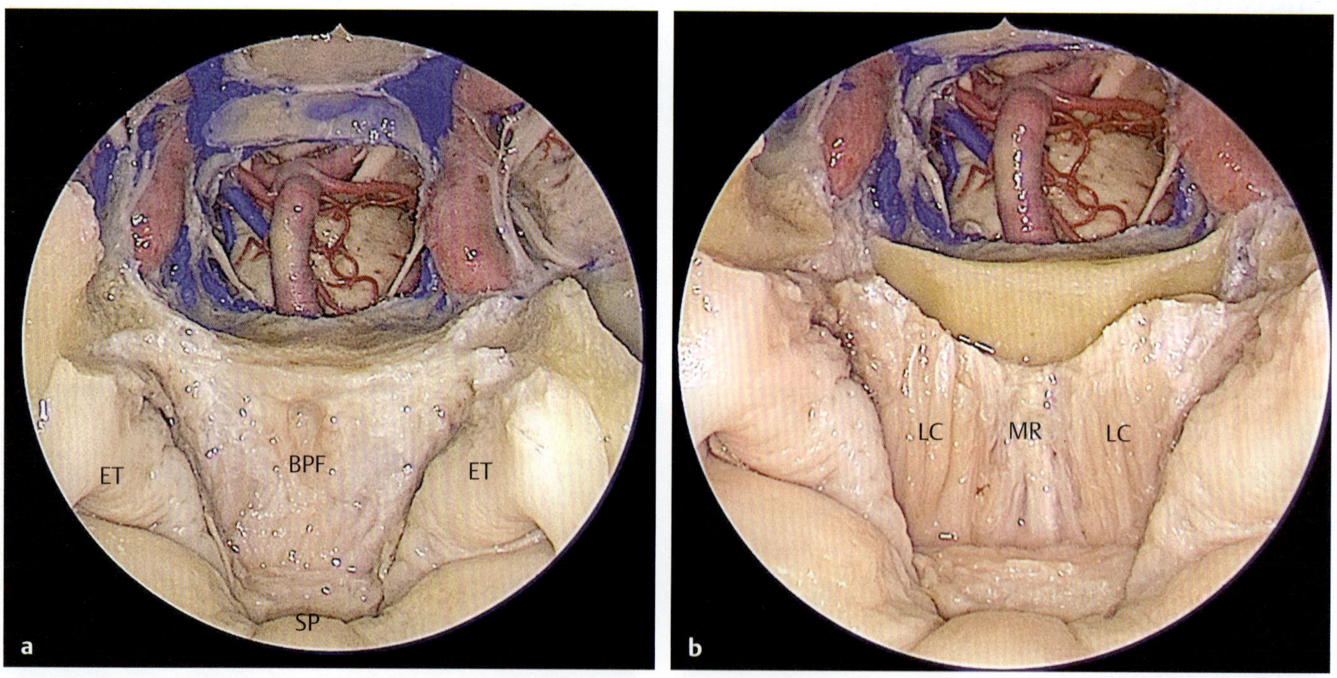

Fig. 18.3 Serial cadaveric dissection images showing the anatomy of the craniocervical junction during the endoscopic endonasal approach. The adjacent neurovascular structures have also been dissected to demonstrate the relationship between related anatomical sites. **(a)** The midclivus has been drilled and the mucosa of the nasopharynx has been removed to expose the basiopharyngeal fascia (BPF). The eustachian tube (ET) opening is seen laterally and the soft palate (SP) inferiorly. **(b)** Deeper to the BPF is the longus colli (LC) muscle on both sides separated by a median raphe (MR) attached to the pharyngeal tubercle.

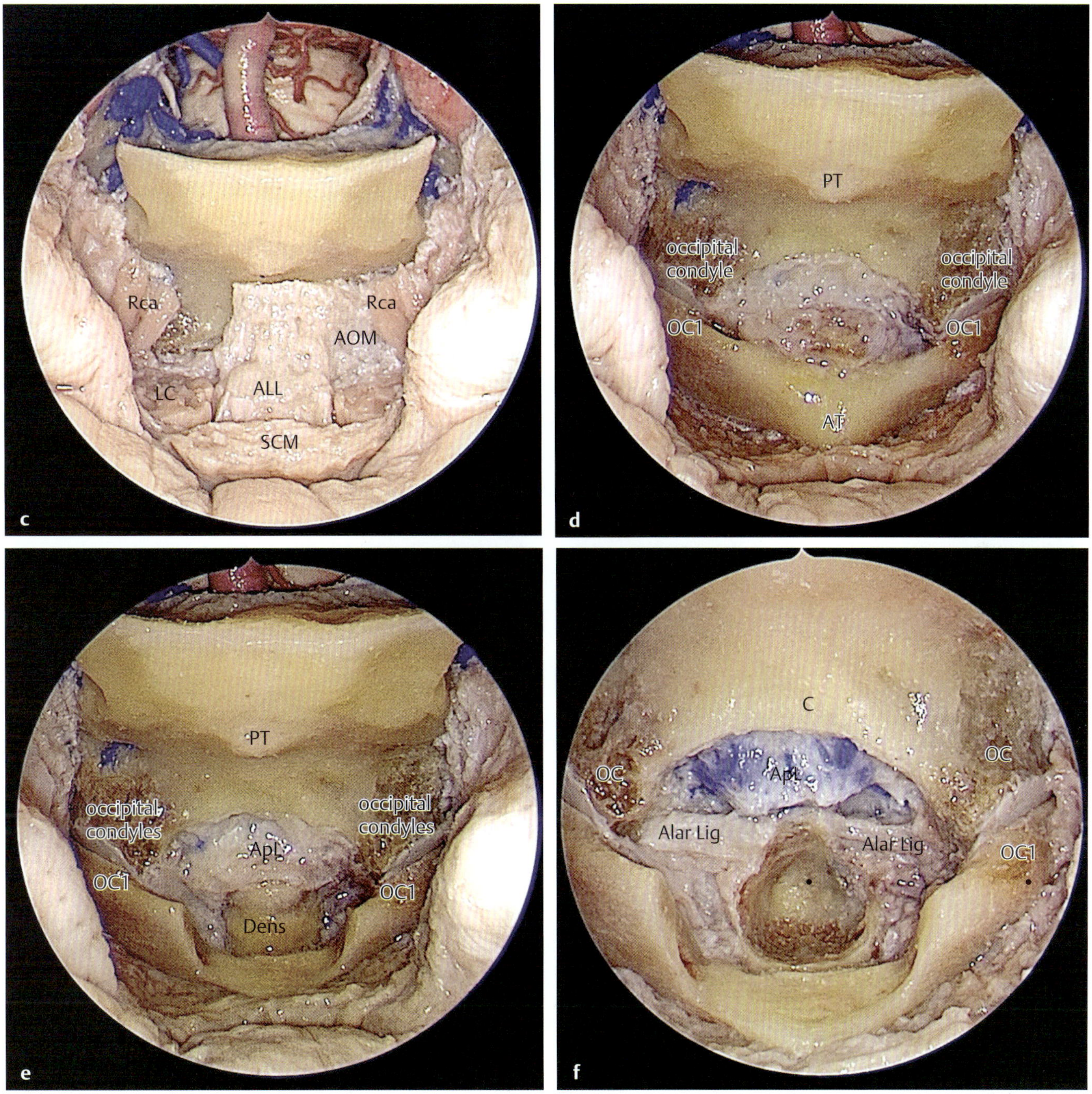

Fig. 18.3 *(Continued)* **(c)** The longus colli (LC) muscle has been resected to expose the rectus capitis anterior (Rca) muscle and the atlanto-occipital membrane (AOM). The anterior longitudinal ligament (ALL) is attached to the anterior tubercle of atlas and is continuous with the median raphe. The upper edge of the superior constrictor (SCM) is visible as the SP has been pushed inferiorly. **(d)** The LC and Rca muscles and the AOM have been removed to expose the lower clivus, occipital condyles and the atlanto-occipital joint (OC1). **(e)** The anterior arch of the atlas has been drilled to expose the dens located on its posterior surface. The apical ligament (ApL) arises from the apex of the dens and is attached to the anterior border of the foramen magnum. **(f)** The dens has been drilled leaving a thin shell of bone. The alar ligaments (Alar Lig.) can be seen arising from the posterolateral part of the dens attaching to the medial side of the condyle. *(Continued)*

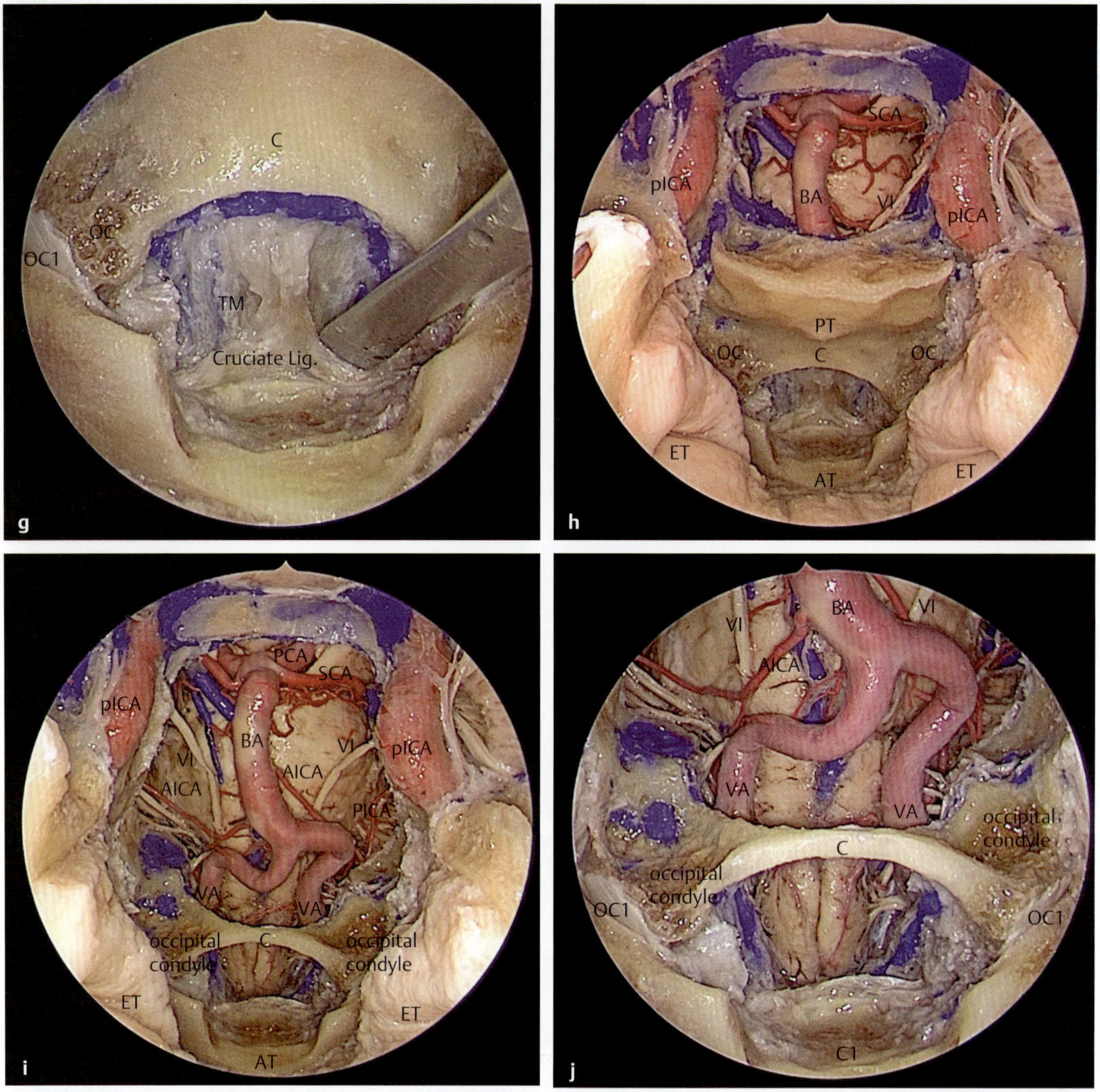

Fig. 18.3 *(Ccontinued)* **(g)** The dens has been completely removed exposing the cruciate ligament (Cruciate Lig.) which has a vertical and transverse component. The transverse ligament arises posterior to the dens and is attached to the medial side of the lateral mass. The tectorial membrane (TM) and dura mater are located posterior to the ligament. The postodontoid region **(h)** after removal of the tectorial membrane/dura **(i)** exposes the neurovascular structures posterior to the lower clivus and below the foramen magnum, structures including the two vertebral arteries (VA), the inferior posterior cerebellar artery (PICA), the basilar artery (BA), the anterior inferior cerebellar artery (AICA) and the sixth cranial nerve (abducens nerve) arising ventrally at the ponto-medullary junction. A bridge of bone which corresponds to the anterior border of the foramen magnum has been left intact. **(j)** Close-up view to show the formation of the basilar artery (BA) by the two vertebral arteries (VA).

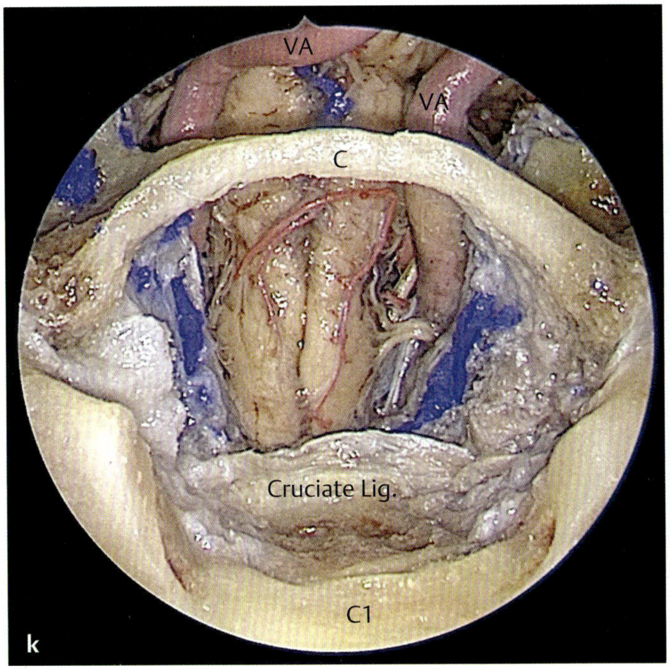

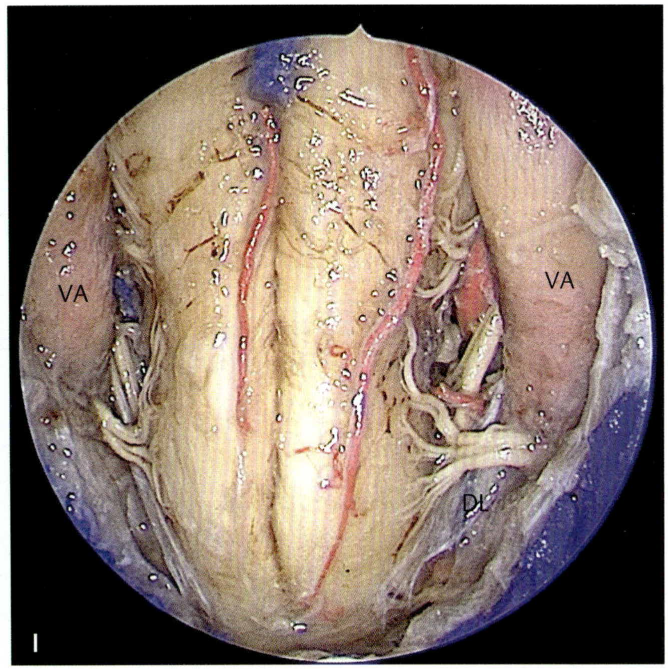

Fig. 18.3 *(Continued)* **(k–l)** Close-up views demonstrating the cervicomedullary junction, the first and second cervical ventral roots, and the dentate ligaments (DL).

Pathologies and Its Variants

A variety of disorders affect the CCJ and include both congenital and acquired lesions. Acquired pathologies involve traumatic, degenerative, infective/inflammatory, metabolic, and neoplastic disorders. A comprehensive list of pathologies with their classifications is available in the literature with some classifications incorporating the biomechanics and the embryology of the CCJ.[4,5] A brief overview of these pathologies are outlined below.

Congenital malformations may affect a specific part of the occipital bone, atlas, axis, or odontoid peg either as a solitary anomaly or involving a few subsites. They further can generally involve the CCJ or appear as anomalies at multiple anatomical sites.

Platybasia is a condition involving flattening of the skull base. It is characterized by an increase in the Welcher basal angle of more than 140 degrees, an asymptomatic condition unless associated with basilar invagination.[5]

Basilar invagination is a common developmental anomaly of the CCJ where the odontoid process prolapses into the foramen magnum.[6] It has been classified into two types: Type A is associated with atlantoaxial instability, characterized by an increase in the atlantodental or clivodental interval. Type B is not associated with atlantoaxial instability.[7] Smith et al. suggested that if this radiological finding is present, an underlying etiology should be sought, where possible.[6] Common CCJ disorders causing basilar invagination include basioccipital hypoplasia, occipital condyle hypoplasia, atlas hypoplasia, incomplete ring of C1 with spreading of the lateral masses, achondroplasia, atlantooccipital assimilation and fused upper vertebrae.[5,6,8] Chiari malformation, syringomyelia, syringobulbia, and hydrocephalus are neurological conditions that may accompany basilar invagination.[8]

Atlas assimilation or occipitocervical fusion may be complete or partial and is associated with Klippel–Feil syndrome if it is accompanied by C2–C3 nonsegmentation.[9] Arch anomalies are rare and most commonly represented by the midline posterior arch rachischisis (posterior arch defect).[5,9]

Axis and odontoid anomalies may be identified as aplasia or hypoplasia of the dens, persistent ossiculum terminale, and os odontoideum. The os odontoideum is an independent osseous structure lying cephalad to the body of C2. Two variations exist, orthotropic and dystrophic; the orthotropic type is located at the anatomical site of dens and moves in unison with C1 and C2. The dystrophic type, on the other hand, is located near the clivus with potential fusion, eventually moving with the clivus.[5,9]

Traumatic injuries of the CCJ have a high mortality rate and are usually associated with high-energy blunt traumas.

Clival fracture may occur as a transverse, longitudinal, or oblique fracture causing cranial nerve VI and VII injuries.[5] Occipital condyle fractures may cause lower cranial nerve deficits. These fractures are classified into three types based on the mechanism and extent of the injury; the disruption or preservation of the alar and tectorial membrane, and the consequent stability of the joint.[5] If accompanied by a ligamentous disruption, the atlas osseous fracture leads to an atlantooccipital or atlantoaxial dislocation. An atlantooccipital dislocation may cause anterior or posterior displacement of the occiput in relation to C1 or a longitudinal distraction of the occiput from C1.[5] Displacement of the lateral mass of C1 over C2 on anteroposterior imaging of more than 7 to 8 mm or an atlantodental space of more than 3 mm is considered pathological.[10] The Jefferson's fracture describes an anterior and a posterior arch fracture with or without disruption of the supporting ligaments.[5] A fracture of the axis may involve the odontoid and cause either an avulsion of the tip, a fracture of the junction of the body and dens, or a fracture of the superior body and superior facet with further subtypes described in association with a ligamental avulsion.[5,10] The Hangman's fracture or traumatic spondylolisthesis of the axis refers to the vertical or oblique fracture through the pars interarticularis of C2 with three subtypes classified based on the displacement of the body and the facet joints.[5,10]

Apart from trauma, a diverse group of acquired diseases may affect craniocervical stability or cause neurovascular compression. A basilar impression is an acquired form of basilar invagination occurring secondary to pathologies causing bone softening diseases such as Paget's disease, osteomalacia, severe osteoporosis, osteogenesis imperfecta, rickets, hyperparathyroidism, renal osteodystrophy, skull base infection, or Hurler's syndrome.[4,8] Another important acquired abnormality at the level of the foramen magnum is a spinal canal and foraminal stenosis caused by underlying disease such as achondroplasia.

Atlantoaxial instability can also result from other acquired diseases such as infection (e.g., Grisel's syndrome, tuberculosis), Down's syndrome, metabolic disorders (e.g., Morquio's syndrome), inflammatory disorders (e.g., rheumatoid arthritis), and neoplasms.[4]

Rheumatoid arthritis is the most common inflammatory disorder of the CCJ causing ligament, bone, and joint destruction. Basilar invagination, atlantoaxial instability, and/or subaxial subluxation have been reported as major manifestations of this disease in the CCJ region. Pannus formation may occur at the superoposterior part of odontoid and worsen brainstem compression. Inflammatory activity in the region of the transverse ligament potentially destroys the joint space and leads to instability.[11]

Neoplasms or tumor-like lesions may also affect the CCJ either from an extradural or an intradural extramedullary origin. Tumors may also be secondary to distant metastasis or extension from a local tumor. Neoplasms of extradural origin include chordoma, benign bony lesions (fibrous dysplasia, osteoid osteoma, and aneurysmal bone cyst; **Fig. 18.4**), and malignant bony tumors (chondrosarcoma, plasmacytoma/multiple myeloma). Those arising from the intradural extramedullary sites are tumors such as meningioma, nerve sheath tumors, arachnoid cyst, and epidermoid cyst.[5]

Chordoma is a low-grade midline tumor believed to arise from remnants of the notochord. However, it has a tendency to be locally aggressive and cause bony destruction with compression of adjacent neurovascular structures. Chondrosarcoma originates from primitive mesenchymal cells in the synchondroses of the base of skull with a predilection for petroclival synchondrosis, and is hence frequently located off midline.[12] Nasopharyngeal carcinoma is a common malignancy in South East Asia and may invade and metastasize to the skull base. In an analysis of 101 patients with invasion (n = 17) and metastasis (n = 84) of the skull base, 42.9% (36/84) had clival invasion and 64.7% (11/17) metastasized to the jugular foramen[13] (**Fig. 18.5**). Meningiomas are believed to be the most commonly observed tumor of foramen magnum arising from the dura mater of the foramen magnum, located anteriorly anywhere from the lower third of the clivus and to the upper edge of the body of C2, laterally from the jugular tubercle and the upper aspect of the C2 lamina, and posteriorly from the anterior edge of the squamous occipital bone and C2 spinous process.[14]

Clinical Features

Pathologies of the CCJ may lead to dysfunction of the brainstem, cerebellum, cervical spinal cord, lower cranial nerves and upper cervical nerves, vasculature, and also the cerebrospinal fluid (CSF) system.[15,16] The mechanism of neurological disturbances is thought to be caused by traction or direct compression of adjacent tissues, blood flow interruption resulting in ischemia or stroke, and disturbances in CSF dynamics leading to hydrocephalus and syrinx formation.[15] The clinical features may have an insidious onset as seen in slow-growing tumors or rapid in cases of trauma. The preexisting condition might manifest itself clinically after a trauma and less frequently as a rapid neurological progression in certain patients.

Pain arising from the suboccipital region with radiation to the vertex has been observed to occur in about 85% of children less than 16 years.[16] Children with congenital

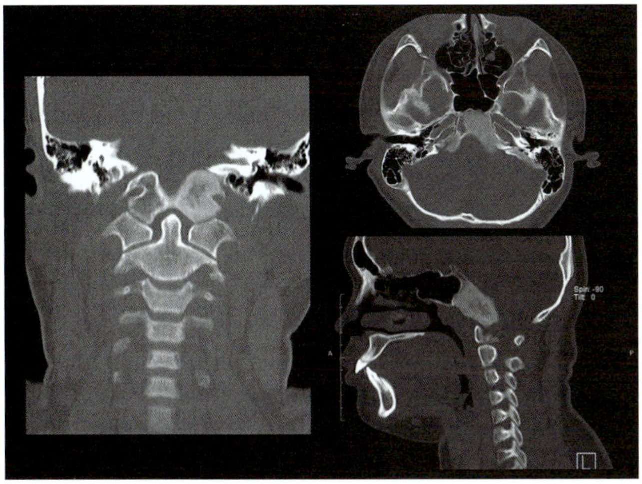

Fig. 18.4 Axial, coronal and sagittal bone-weighted computed tomography images of a 15-year-old child diagnosed with fibrous dysplasia demonstrating an asymmetric hyperdensity of the lower clivus and occipital condyle.

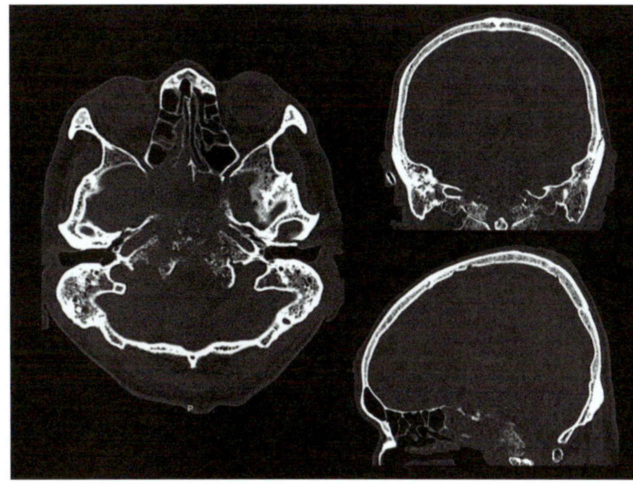

Fig. 18.5 Axial, coronal and sagittal bone-weighted computed tomography images demonstrating an erosion of the lower clivus in a 70-year-old man diagnosed with nasopharyngeal carcinoma who presented with CN VI palsy and right hemiparesis.

CCJ anomalies may as well demonstrate abnormal physical appearances such as a short neck with a low hairline as seen in Klippel–Feil syndrome, dwarfism (achondroplasia), and scoliosis.

Traumatic injury may cause a spectrum of neurological deficits ranging from absent voluntary motor control and slight sensory preservation in the lowest sacral dermatomes to only mild motor and sensory deficits. Bell's cruciate paralysis and acute central cord syndrome are different pathologies described to have disproportionate weakness of the upper extremities.[15]

Neck pain in the C2 dermatome is reported to be the most frequent initial neurological symptom of tumors arising from the CCJ. Other symptoms include weakness and clumsiness of the hands with spasticity in the upper and the lower extremities, myelopathy, dissociated sensory loss, and clockwise progression of neurological symptoms, specifically in paramedian tumors of the foramen magnum and the CCJ. In the presence of syringomyelia, the patient may demonstrate upper extremity muscle atrophy, Charcot's joints, and sensory disturbances.[15]

Brainstem and lower cranial nerve dysfunction usually express symptoms of dysphagia, aspiration pneumonia, and sleep apnea. Vascular symptoms were seen in 20% of children manifesting as altered consciousness, transient loss of visual fields, vertigo, and confusional states, and may be provoked by head movements.[16]

Occlusion of the vertebrobasilar vessels may also lead to consecutive cerebral infarction associated with a myriad of symptoms related to the vessel and the region of blood supply. PICA occlusion results in lateral medullary syndrome (Wallenberg's syndrome) characterized by ipsilateral pain and temperature loss in the face and contralateral loss of pain and temperature in the body. Other features include dizziness, loss of taste, dysphagia, and Horner's syndrome. VA and PICA occlusion may also cause infarction of the inferior cerebellum giving rise to cerebellar symptoms (ataxia, nystagmus, dysarthria, and intention tremor). The medial medullary syndrome may result from an occlusion of the VA or the anterior spinal artery, with symptoms of ipsilateral tongue weakness, contralateral hemiparesis, and dysfunction in vibration and proprioception. Oculomotor symptoms such as internuclear ophthalmoplegia and conjugate gaze palsy may be present in context with an occlusion of the basilar artery along with other signs. Compression of the fourth ventricle and development of hydrocephalus may be accompanied by symptoms such as agitation, nausea, vomiting, and headaches.[16]

Chiari I malformation is characterized by a downward displacement of the cerebellar tonsils through the foramen magnum. A patient may be asymptomatic or present, in adulthood, with occipital or neck pain worsened by straining and the Valsalva maneuvers. Other associated features relate to brainstem, cerebellar, and cervical cord dysfunction. A Chiari II malformation usually presents earlier in infancy. In older children, this malformation is usually associated with myelomeningocele and syringomyelia. The presence of a syrinx may produce scoliosis, hand weakness, wasting of intrinsic hand muscles, dissociated sensory loss, hyperactive reflexes (lower > upper), long-tract symptoms, and cranial nerve palsies.[15,17]

Radiological Features

Computed tomography (CT) and magnetic resonance imaging (MRI) are indispensable to investigate and further characterize pathologies of the CCJ. This includes the extent of involvement of the adjacent bone, soft tissues, neurovascular structures, brain, and paranasal sinus; variations in the skull base anatomy; and resulting complications. Radiological investigations are inevitable for the selection of an appropriate surgical approach.[18]

The normal osseous topographical relationships and anatomical reference lines of the CCJ are presented in **Fig. 18.6** and **Fig. 18.7**. The measurements defining basilar invagination are described in the section "Radiological Considerations." Bony abnormalities such as dislocation, subluxation, and fractures are usually evident on CT scan imaging (**Fig. 18.8**). Lytic lesions, calcifications, and osteosclerotic changes on CT may need further evaluation by dynamic X-rays or other investigations to characterize the disease. MRI sequences are often helpful to identify and differentiate pathologies of the soft tissue. A brief summary of characteristic CT and MRI findings in common lesions of the CCJ is presented in **Table 18.1**.

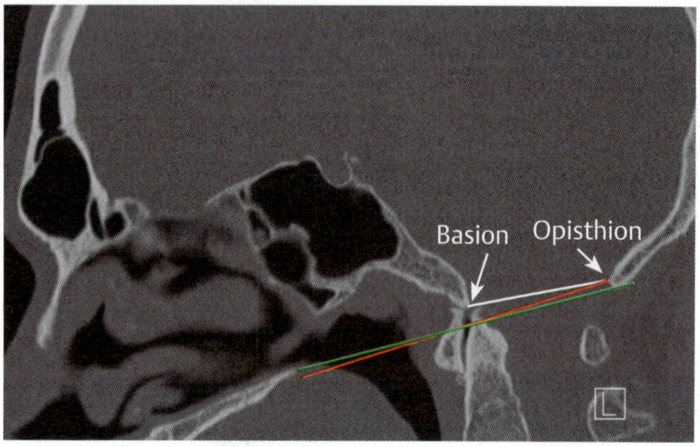

Fig. 18.6 The sagittal view of a CT scan in bony window is used to demonstrate the landmarks necessary to draw the McRae line (*white line*), McGregor line (*green line*), and Chamberlain line (*red line*), which are useful to assess basilar invagination.

Surgical Approaches

The selection of the optimal surgical corridor for the CCJ is of paramount importance. **Table 18.2** summarizes both direct and oblique approaches. The details of endoscopic approach are outlined in the section "Surgical Techniques."

Surgical Procedure—General Considerations

Anesthesia, patient positioning, equipment, and ergonomics are described in general considerations for pituitary adenoma surgery (Chapter 1).

Preoperative Assessment and Evaluation[11,20]

- Assess for vocal cord paresis or palsy and the need for elective tracheostomy.
- Assess potential risk for dysphagia or exacerbation after surgery.
- Neck range of motion should be checked to assess restrictions and instability that may affect surgical positioning.
- Comorbidities in particular patients with rheumatoid arthritis who may have extra-articular disease involving cardiorespiratory system.

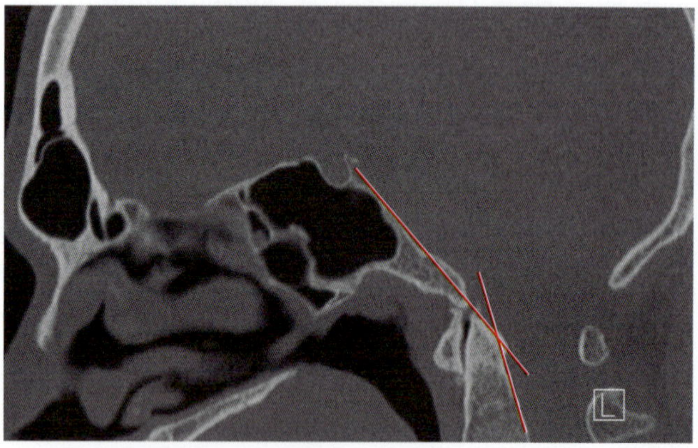

Fig. 18.7 The angle formed by *red lines* in this sagittal view CT scan in bone window represents the cervicomedullary angle.

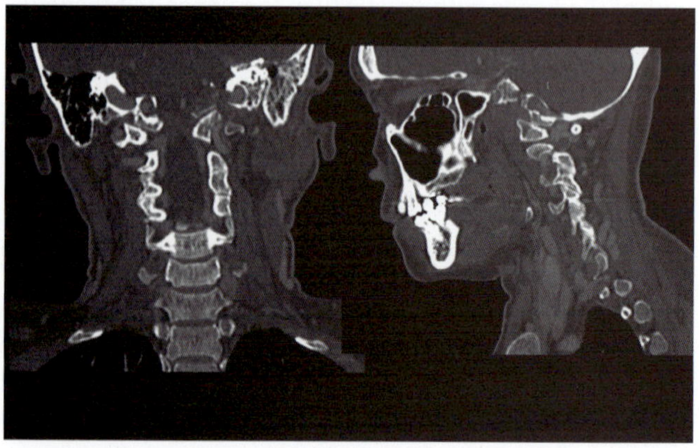

Fig. 18.8 CT imaging showing a subluxed right atlanto-occipital joint in a middle-aged woman treated for skull base osteomyelitis.

Table 18.1 CT and MRI features of common pathologies affecting the CCJ[5,12,18]

CCJ pathology	CT	MRI
Chordoma	Clival midline soft tissue lesion with bone destruction, margin between bone and tumor nonsclerotic and sharp, radiodensities/calcifications are usually present May involve jugular fossa, foramen magnum and cause erosion of C1 and other vertebrae	T1W: hypo/isointense Small hyperintense foci (hemorrhage/mucus) T2W: hyperintense, heterogenous enhancement
Chondrosarcoma	Paramedian lesion, commonly located at the petroclival synchondrosis; bone destruction and stippled calcifications	T1W: low to intermediate signal intensity T2 and FLAIR: hyperintense
Metastasis	Centered within the clivus	T1W, T2W: hypointense
Plasmacytoma/myeloma	Arise from the clivus, cervical vertebrae Show bone invasion without sclerotic borders	T1W: isointense T2W: moderately hyperintense with intense homogenous enhancement
Fibrous dysplasia	Ground glass appearance (56%), homogenously dense (23%), cystic (21%)	T1W, T2W: hypointense Variability exist: T1W: intermediate signal T2W: low to high signal Contrast enhancement may be present
Nasopharyngeal carcinoma	Centered in the nasopharynx, with bony invasion, retropharyngeal adenopathy	T1W, T2W: Intermediate signal intensity with homogenous enhancement
Meningioma	Hyperostosis of bone (90%)	T1W, T2W: iso to hypointensity Uniform intense enhancement with contrast
Rheumatoid arthritis	Erosion of dens with pencil-tip appearance	Erosion of dens, widening of atlantodental space, subluxation, reactive osteophytes
Osteomyelitis	Bony erosion	Ligament destruction leading to instability, phlegmon or abscess formation in the paravertebral and epidural regions

Table 18.2 Surgical approaches to the CCJ

Direct approaches	Oblique approaches
Transnasal anterior approach (endoscopic)	Anterolateral (extreme lateral)
Transoral anterior approach (endoscopic assisted/microscopic)	Posterolateral (far lateral)
Combined transnasal and transoral approach	
Suboccipital midline approach	

Adapted from Visocchi 2019.[19]

Radiological Considerations

- Nasal anatomy: Signs of upper airway infection, septal deviations, signs of trauma.
- Pharyngeal anatomy: Adenoid, congenital anomalies, signs of infection.
- Lesion: Involvement of the lower clivus and foramen magnum (C0), atlas (C1), odontoid (C2 dens axis), or body of the axis (C2).
- Signs of instability (X-ray radiographs, bone CT, MRI):
  - Thickened odontoid capsule (pannus formation).
  - Retroflexed odontoid (loose ligaments).
  - Chiari malformation (downward displacement of the cerebellar tonsils).
  - Cranial settling.
  - Basilar invagination (tip of the odontoid process projects above the foramen magnum):
    - McRae's line (< −19 mm).
    - McGregor's line (> 4.5–6 mm).
    - Chamberlain's line (> 5 mm).
    - Medullocervical angle (< 135°).

- ➢ C1 fractures: Assessed in bone CT (coronal, sagittal) and anterior–posterior radiographs (open mouth):
  - Spread of C1 ring fragments.
  - Spreading or widening of the lateral masses.
  - Asymmetry of the odontoid process from the lateral masses.
- Osteoligamentous structures: Are the anterior longitudinal and the atlanto-occipital ligament distinguishable? Are the tectorial membrane, the apical ligament, and the cruciate ligament distinguishable? Is there evident dural involvement?
- Neurovascular structures: Involvement of the spinal canal through the lesion itself or a dislocated odontoid process. Myelocompression, myeloedema. Involvement of basilar artery and posterior cerebral artery (PCA), brainstem perforators, internal carotid artery (ICA) course in the nasopharynx. Assess with fine-cut CT angiography for bony and vascular imaging; MRI T1, T2 postcontrast for neural and pannus formation.[20]

Surgical Techniques

- Patient positioning: Supine, neutral, or slightly flexed. Caution in patients with neural compression and spinal canal stenosis.
- Endoscopic endonasal: Binostril approach along the nasal floor with posterocaudal resection of the nasal septum.
- Expanded endoscopic endonasal: Trans C1 approach (anterior arch) and resection of ligaments and membranes depending on the pathology and extension.
- Neurosurgical techniques for tumor exposure (**Fig. 18.3 a–l**):
  - ➢ Neuronavigation is crucial to define the superior, lateral, and inferior extensions of the lesion and the odontoid peg.
  - ➢ Step 1: Splitting of the epipharyngeal soft tissue (mucosa and epipharyngeal muscles) with a Y-shaped incision.
  - ➢ Step 2: The inferior end of the clivus (C0) as well as the anterior arch of C1 should be identified. The subperiosteal dissection technique with a monopolar electrocautery should be used to clarify the plane.
  - ➢ Step 3: Removal of the C1 arch with a high-speed diamond drill.
  - ➢ Step 4: Removal of the inferior lip of C0 and identification of the dura mater are mandatory to define a dissection plane.
  - ➢ Step 5: Remove the anterior longitudinal and atlanto-occipital ligament, as well as the tectorial membrane, if necessary, to continue the dissection plane.
  - ➢ Step 6: Define the extension of the odontoid peg (C2) and core using a high-speed diamond drill.
  - ➢ Step 7: Collapse of the remaining shell inward and piecemeal removal of odontoid parts.
  - ➢ Step 8: Follow the plane between the dura mater and the lesion caudally using neuronavigation until the inferior extension of the lesion is reached.

Limitations and Contraindications of the Endoscopic Transnasal Approach[2,20]

- Tortuous or medially displaced pharyngeal ICA if pathology is situated more laterally.
- Inferiorly located pathology below C2.
- Medially or ventrally located critical neurovascular structures.
- Active sinus infection.

When to Prefer a Classical or Alternate Approach[2,3]

- Lesions of the lower clivus to C3 body: **Transoral** may be used but it can be combined with transnasal procedure as a complimentary procedure.
- Pathologies related to dorsal brainstem cerebellum and spinal cord, jugular foramen, foramen magnum, OC1 junction, and C1C2: **Posterior approach**.
- Joint manipulation, fixation, or instrumentation: **Posterior approach**.
- Lateral or lesion behind occipital condyles: **Lateral or posterior approach**.
- Lesions of anterolateral margin of foramen magnum: **Far lateral approach**.

Skull Base Defect Closure

- Hemostasis with Surgicel.
- Suturing of the epipharyngeal muscle and mucosa with single stitches.

Postoperative Care

- Saline nasal spray.
- Oxymetazoline spray for 1 week, if required.
- Nasogastric tube (to be placed only under endoscopic guidance).

- Pneumatic compression stocking.
- If there is a dural breach, avoid positive-pressure mask ventilation, incentive spirometry, drinking straws, nose blowing, sneezing, bending down, and lifting.
- Gentle debridement at 2 and 6 to 8 weeks later.
- Rehabilitation.

Complications[20–22]

- General: Deep vein thrombosis, pneumonia, urinary tract infections.
- Specific: Vascular injury (ICA), transient velopharyngeal insufficiency, CSF leak and meningitis, dysphagia in particular with occipitocervical fixation, epistaxis, infection, osteomyelitis and risk of damage to the lower cranial nerves and brainstem.

Acknowledgments

This chapter was written based on funding from the Martin Allgöwer Foundation, Department of Surgery, University Hospital of Basel (Basel, Switzerland), the Gottfried and Julia Bangerter-Rhyner Foundation (Bern, Switzerland), the Ministry of Health of Malaysia scholarship (Malaysia), and the Adelaide Ear-Nose-Throat Research Institute (Australia). The Department of Neurosurgery of the University Hospital of Basel (Basel, Switzerland) and the Departments of Neurosurgery and Otorhinolaryngology of the University of Malaya (Kuala Lumpur, Malaysia) supported the creation of this chapter.

References

1. Tubbs RS, Hallock JD, Radcliff V, et al. Ligaments of the craniocervical junction. J Neurosurg Spine 2011;14(6):697–709
2. Jhawar SS, Nunez M, Pacca P, Voscoboinik DS, Truong H. Craniovertebral junction 360°: a combined microscopic and endoscopic anatomical study. J Craniovertebr Junction Spine 2016;7(4):204–216
3. Seker A, Inoue K, Osawa S, Akakin A, Kilic T, Rhoton AL Jr. Comparison of endoscopic transnasal and transoral approaches to the craniovertebral junction. World Neurosurg 2010;74(6):583–602
4. Menezes AH. Pathology encountered at the craniocervical junction. Oper Tech Neurosurg. 2005;8:116–124
5. Chen YF, Liu HM. Imaging of craniovertebral junction. Neuroimag-ing Clin N Am 2009;19(3):483–510
6. Smith JS, Shaffrey CI, Abel MF, Menezes AH. Basilar invagination. Neurosurgery 2010;66(3, Suppl):39–47
7. Goel A, Jain S, Shah A. Radiological evaluation of 510 cases of basilar invagination with evidence of atlantoaxial instability (group A basilar invagination). World Neurosurg 2018;110: 533–543
8. Pinter NK, McVige J, Mechtler L. Basilar invagination, basilar impression, and platybasia: clinical and imaging aspects. Curr Pain Headache Rep 2016;20(8):49
9. Sankhe SS, Kumar SK. Neuroimaging in craniovertebral anomalies as seen in the tropics. Neuroimaging Clin N Am 2011; 21(4):879–895, ix
10. Debernardi A, D'Aliberti G, Talamonti G, Villa F, Piparo M, Collice M. The craniovertebral junction area and the role of the ligaments and membranes. Neurosurgery 2015;76(Suppl 1): S22–S32
11. Krauss WE, Bledsoe JM, Clarke MJ, Nottmeier EW, Pichelmann MA. Rheumatoid arthritis of the craniovertebral junction. Neurosurgery 2010;66(3, Suppl):83–95
12. Neelakantan A, Rana AK. Benign and malignant diseases of the clivus. Clin Radiol 2014;69(12):1295–1303
13. Han J, Zhang Q, Kong F, Gao Y. The incidence of invasion and metastasis of nasopharyngeal carcinoma at different anatomic sites in the skull base. Anat Rec (Hoboken) 2012; 295(8):1252–1259
14. Bruneau M, George B. Classification system of foramen magnum meningiomas. J Craniovertebr Junction Spine 2010;1(1):10–17
15. Benglis D, Levi AD. Neurologic findings of craniovertebral junction disease. Neurosurgery 2010;66(3, Suppl):13–21
16. Menezes AH. Craniovertebral junction database analysis: inci-dence, classification, presentation, and treatment algorithms. Childs Nerv Syst 2008;24(10):1101–1108
17. George TM, Higginbotham NH. Defining the signs and symptoms of Chiari malformation type I with and without syringo-myelia. Neurol Res 2011;33(3):240–246
18. Kunimatsu A, Kunimatsu N. Skull base tumors and tumor-like lesions: a pictorial review. Pol J Radiol 2017;82:398–409
19. Visocchi M. Why the craniovertebral junction? Acta Neurochir Suppl (Wien) 2019;125:3–8
20. Gardner PA, Tormenti MJ, Kassam AB, et al. Endoscopic endonasal approach to the odontoid and craniocervical junction. In: Kassam AB, Gardner PA, eds. Endoscopic Approaches to the Skull Base. Prog Neurol Surg Basel, Karger 2012;26:152–167
21. Goldschlager T, Härtl R, Greenfield JP, Anand VK, Schwartz TH. The endoscopic endonasal approach to the odontoid and its impact on early extubation and feeding. J Neurosurg 2015;122(3):511–518
22. Kshettry VR, Thorp BD, Shriver MF, et al. Endoscopic approaches to the craniovertebral junction. Otolaryngol Clin North Am 2016;49(1):213–226

Chapter 19 Endonasal Endoscopic Surgeries of the Craniocervical Junction

Case 19A

Combined Endoscopic Endonasal and Transoral Debridement of Cervical C1–C2 Osteoradionecrosis

Liew Yew Toong, Prepageran Narayanan, and Vicknes Waran

History

A 56-year-old lady presented with chronic oronasal discharge with neck pain occurring during the last 6 months. She was treated for nasopharyngeal carcinoma, NPC T3N0M0 (according to TNM staging 7th edition, American Joint Committee on Cancer, AJCC), 10 years ago, where she received 70 Gy of radiation at the nasopharynx. Endoscopic examination showed exuberant granulation tissues at the nasopharynx and the posterior pharyngeal wall of the oropharynx with exposed bone (**Fig. 19A.1** and **Fig. 19A.2**). Computed tomography revealed an exophytic mass at C1–C2 vertebrae with erosion of the anterior arch of the atlas bone (**Fig. 19A.3** and **Fig. 19A.4**). An endonasal endoscopic debridement of necrotic bone with biopsy under general anesthesia was indicated, followed by craniocervical fusion later on. Histopathological examination revealed granulation without evidence of malignancy.

Surgical Steps

1. The patient is positioned supine under general anesthesia, with indwelling catheter, invasive blood pressure monitoring, intraoperative prophylactic antibiotics, and the head fixed slightly retroflexed within a NORAS frame for intraoperative magnetic resonance imaging (iMRI). Registration for neuronavigation (Brainlab, Munich, Germany) is performed.
2. The nose is prepared with cophenylcaine applied topically with 1-inch ribbon gauzes.
3. A zero-degree rigid endoscope (Karl-Storz, 4 mm) is introduced into the right nasal cavity for a proper examination of the nasopharynx under anesthesia (**Fig. 19A.5**).
4. A posterior septectomy brought up to 2 cm from the choana allows to place the endoscope in the midline for better visualization of the surgical site (**Fig. 19A.6**).

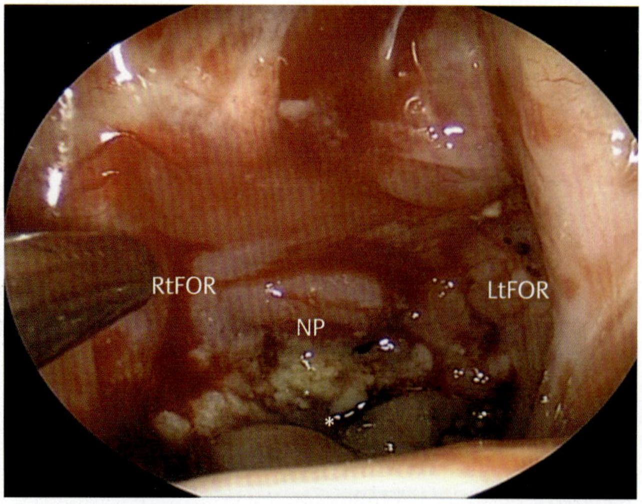

Fig. 19A.1 Endonasal endoscopic visualization of the midline lesion with exposed bone (*).

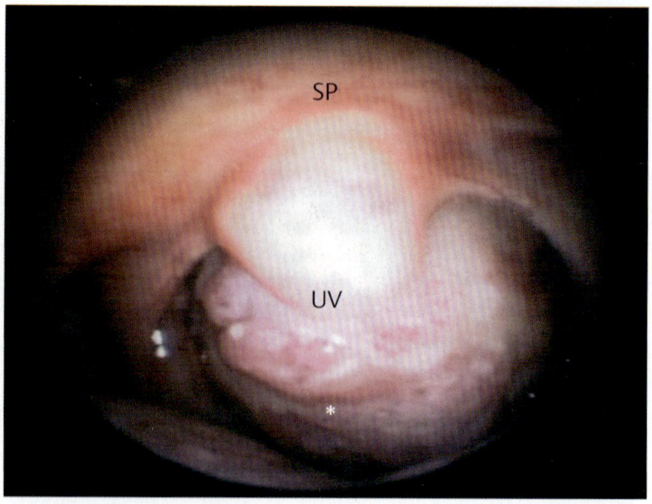

Fig. 19A.2 A protruding mass along the pharyngeal wall next to the oropharynx is visible (*).

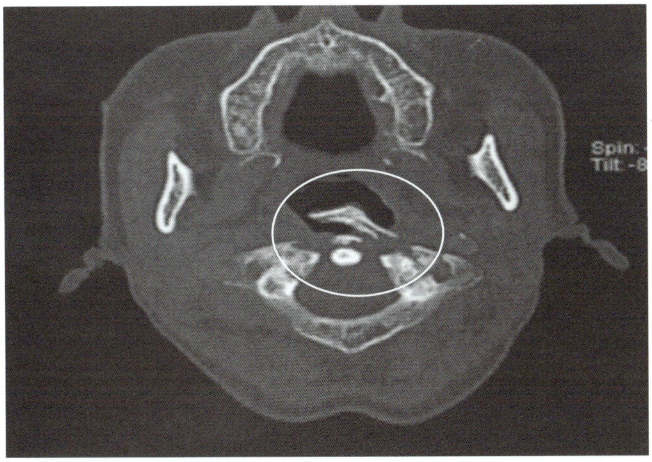

Fig. 19A.3 Axial bone-weighted CT section revealing a dislocated anterior arch of atlas (C1) (*white circle*).

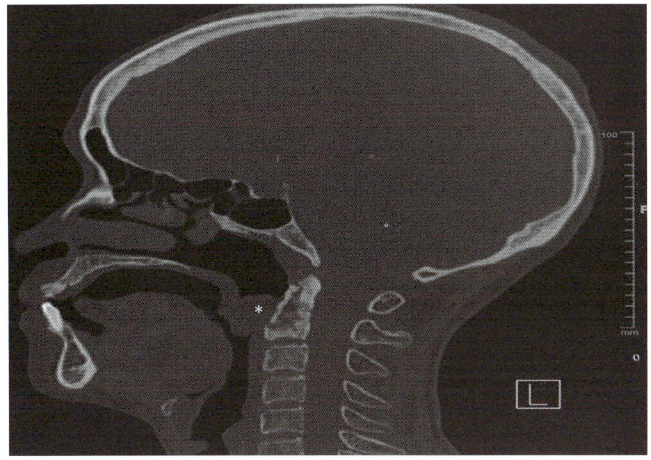

Fig. 19A.4 Sagittal bone-weighted CT section showing a mass anterior to the C1/C2 junction with bony erosion (*).

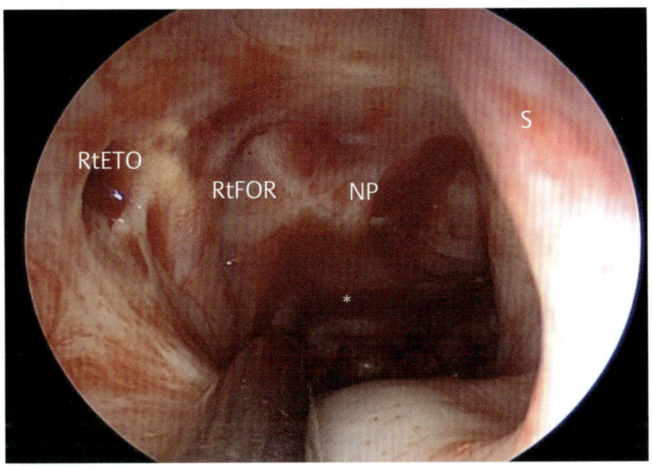

Fig. 19A.5 Endoscopic view of the right nasal cavity and the nasopharynx harboring the midline lesion (*).

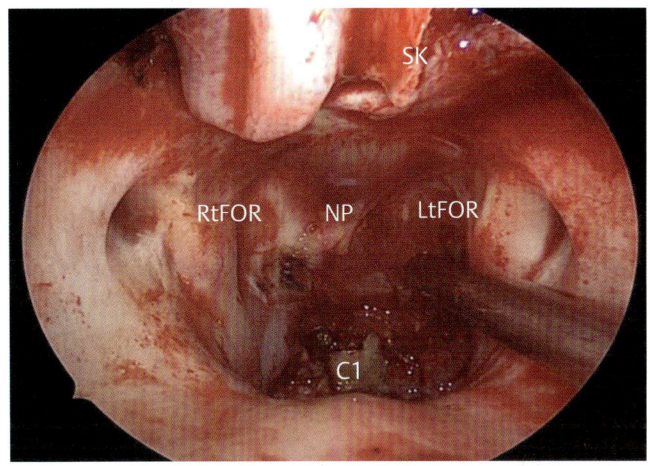

Fig. 19A.6 Following posterior septectomy, a wider exposure allows to visualize the exposed anterior arch of atlas (C1) and facilitates surgical manipulation of the lesion.

5. Mucosa surrounding abnormal granulation is diathermized using a monopolar suction diathermy (**Fig. 19A.7**).
6. The exposed anterior arch of the atlas (C1) and part of the body of axis (C2) are removed with high-speed diamond drill and a Kerrison punch. This is performed up to the point where the odontoid process is visible and fully exposed (**Fig. 19A.8, Fig. 19A.9, Fig. 19A.10**).
7. The mass at the posterior pharyngeal wall of the oropharynx is then removed transorally with a ring curette and monopolar suction diathermy (**Fig. 19A.11**).
8. Flap reconstruction is not used for the defect at the end of the surgery since there is still a thin layer of soft tissue at the base of the defect (**Fig. 19A.12**).
9. The defect healed well without any complications as showed by the endoscope at 6 months, postoperatively (**Fig. 19A.13**).

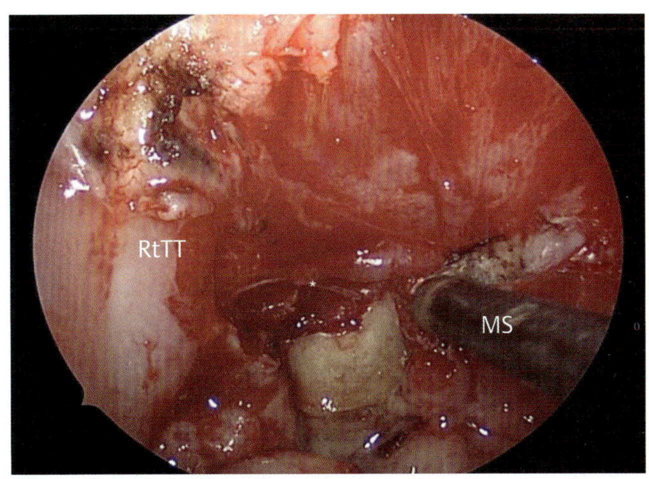

Fig. 19A.7 A monopolar diathermy is used to excise the mass (*).

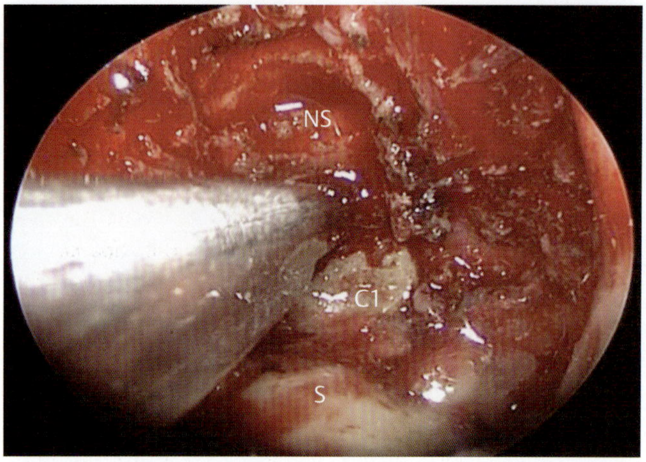

Fig. 19A.8 A Kerrison punch is used to partially remove the anterior arch of atlas (C1).

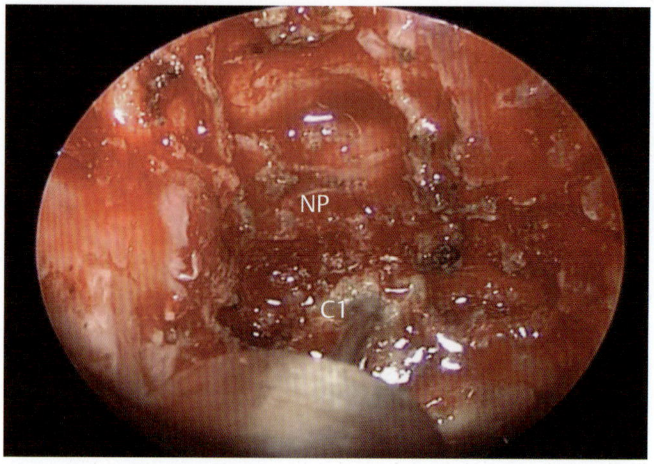

Fig. 19A.9 A high-speed diamond drill is used concurrently with a Kerrison punch to remove the anterior arch of atlas (C1) completely.

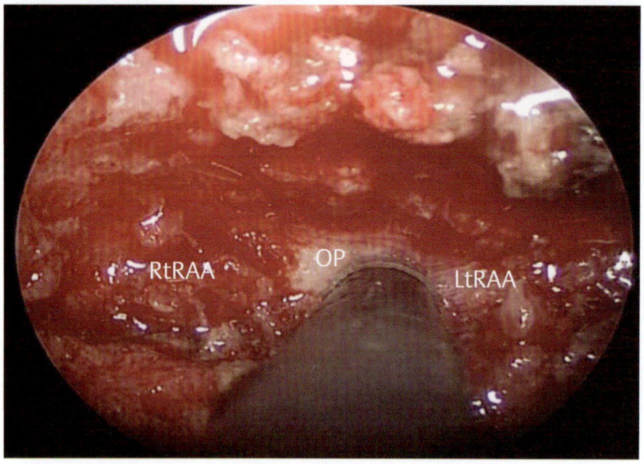

Fig. 19A.10 After removal of the C1 anterior arch of atlas, the odontoid process (OP) is exposed.

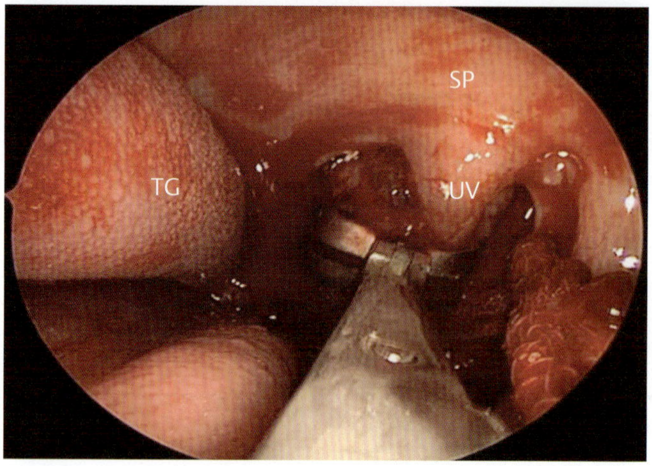

Fig. 19A.11 Removal of the oropharyngeal mass (*) with a ring curette.

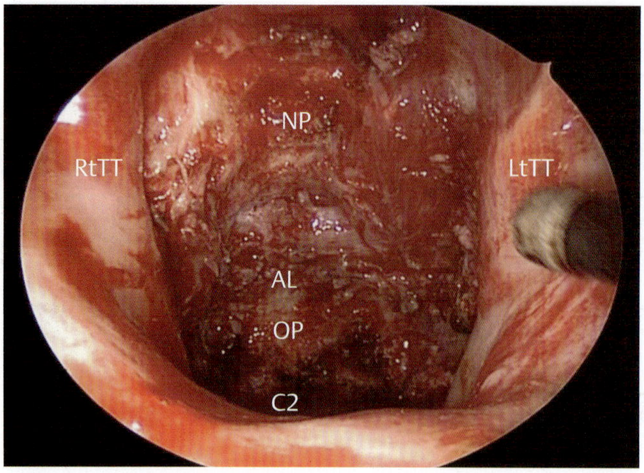

Fig. 19A.12 Final endoscopic view after removal of the necrotic mass.

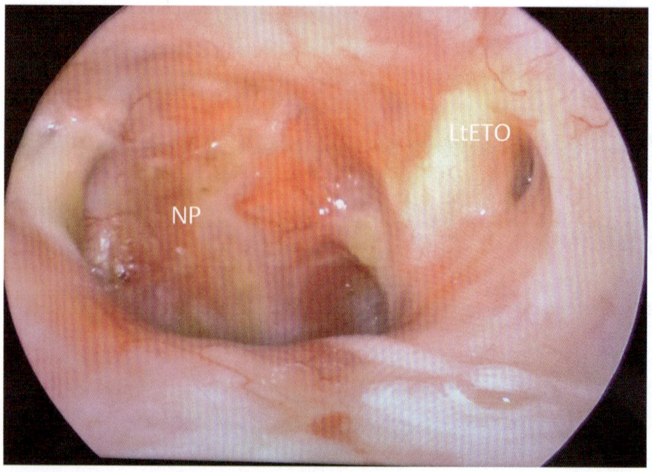

Fig. 19A.13 Well-healed nasopharynx and oropharynx.

Case 19B

Endoscopic Transatlas Decompression of a Basilar Invagination with Syringomyelia

Adzreil Bakri, Michel Roethlisberger, Prepageran Narayanan, Vicknes Waran, and Liew Yew Toong

History

A 13-year-old Chinese boy with a known Chiari malformation Type I treated with posterior fossa decompression presented with upper limb weakness, headache, and limited neck movement for the last 3 months. A computed tomography (CT) scan and magnetic resonance imaging (MRI) revealed a basilar invagination with a prominent odontoid peg narrowing the foramen magnum, medullary compression along with syringomyelia of the cervical spinal cord (**Fig. 19B.1** and **Fig. 19B.2**). A posterior craniocervical spinal fusion and endonasal endoscopic dual nostril approach to the craniocervical junction with resection of the odontoid peg was indicated.

Surgical Steps

1. Local anesthesia is infiltrated into the posterior septum to raise the mucoperichondrium away from the bony septum.
2. The septum is incised with a no. 15 blade and the mucoperichondrial flap is raised up to the choana.
3. Transformation into a vascularized nasoseptal flap is for defect reconstruction is possible at this stage. However, it is not required for this case, and a posterior septectomy is performed. The mucoperichondrial flaps bilaterally and the exposed septum were removed from the level of the sphenoid ostium up to the floor of the nasal cavity allowing a wide exposure of the nasopharynx and the anterior wall of the sphenoid sinus (**Fig. 19B.3**).
4. Meticulous hemostasis is performed with either bipolar cautery or monopolar suction cautery to arrest any bleeding arising from the borders of the septectomy (**Fig. 19B.4**).
5. Once the sphenoid rostrum is fully exposed, the ostia are widened inferomedially using a Kerrison punch in a V shape manner towards the midline (**Fig. 19B.5**).
6. The sphenoid ostia are connected in the midline, and the sphenoid rostrum and the keel is removed (**Fig. 19B.6**).
7. Using a monopolar cautery, the nasopharynx is split in the midline from the basisphenoid superiorly down to the level just above the floor of the nasal cavity inferiorly (**Fig. 19B.7**).
8. The clivus, atlas (C1), and axis (C2) are then exposed via dissection of the anterior atlanto-occipital ligament

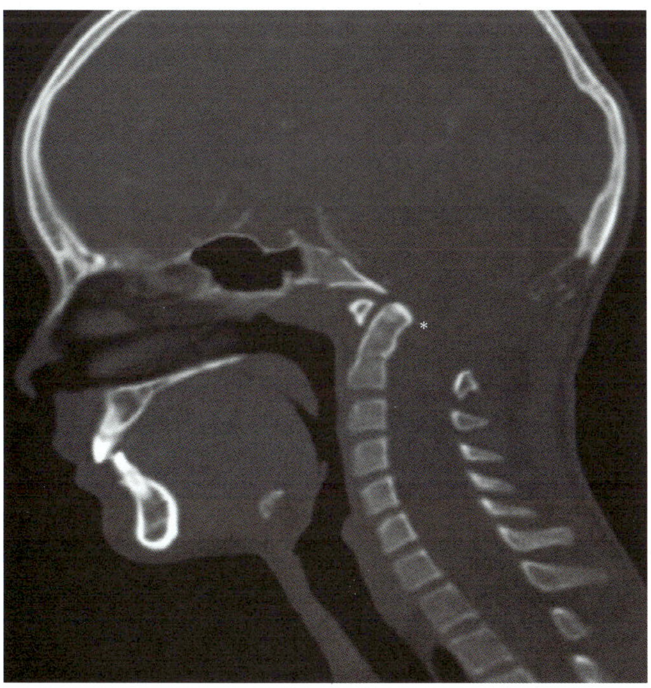

Fig. 19B.1 Sagittal bone-weighted CT section showing a basilar invagination with a prominent odontoid peg (*).

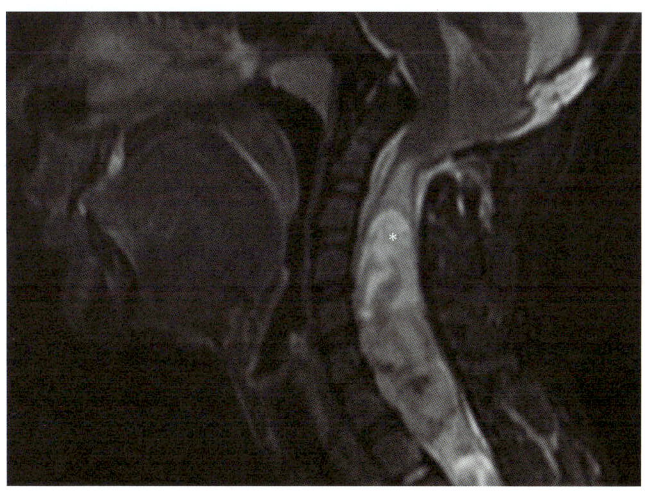

Fig. 19B.2 Sagittal T2-weighted MRI section revealing the odontoid peg causing medullary compression and a cervical syringomyelia (*).

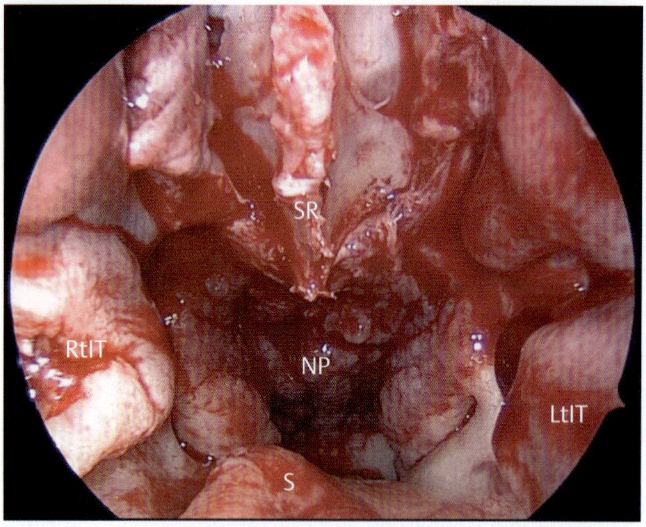

Fig. 19B.3 Endoscopic view of the nasopharynx after posterior septectomy.

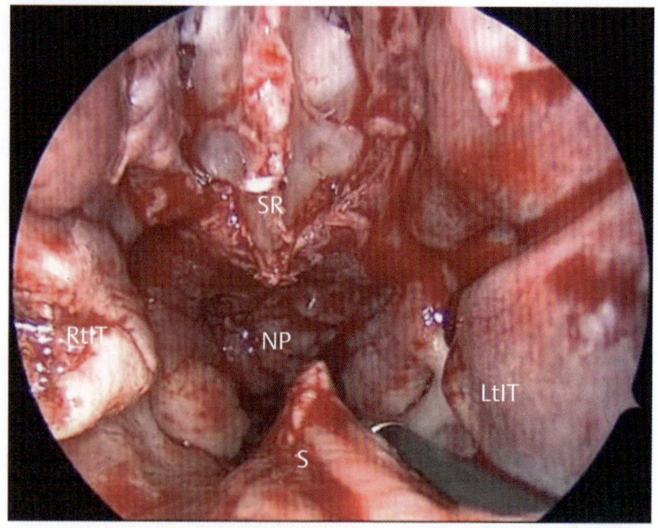

Fig. 19B.4 Meticulous hemostasis along the borders of the posterior septectomy.

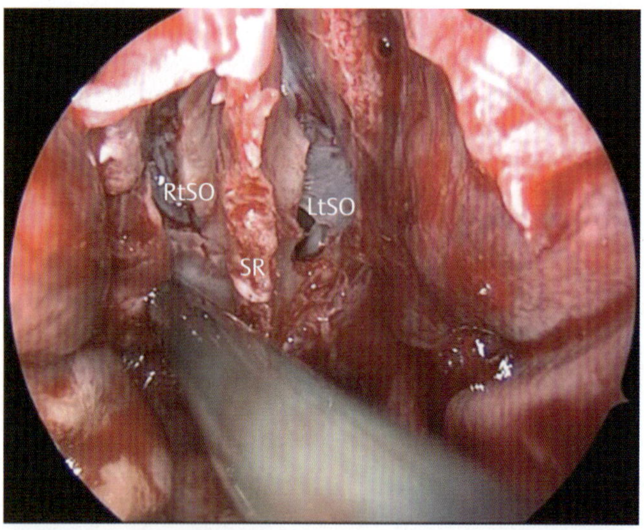

Fig. 19B.5 Widening and connection of the sphenoid ostia in an inferomedial direction.

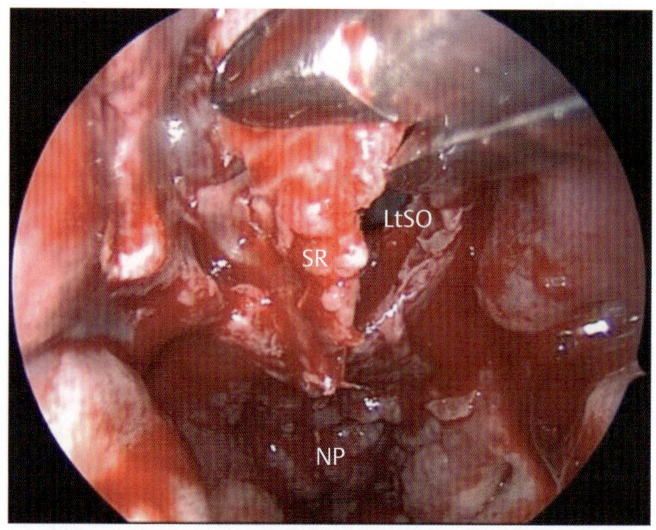

Fig. 19B.6 Removal of the sphenoid rostrum (SR).

and prevertebral fascia off the bone with a monopolar cautery combined with a microdebrider (**Fig. 19B.8** and **Fig. 19B.9**).

9. The anterior arch and tubercle of C1 are fully exposed (**Fig. 19B.10**).
10. To expose the odontoid peg, the tubercle and the anterior arch of C1 are drilled using a diamond high-speed burr (**Fig. 19B.11**).
11. Once the odontoid peg is identified, its anterior cartilaginous surface is fully exposed bilaterally by removing the anterior arch of C1 (**Fig. 19B.12**).
12. The odontoid peg is then drilled and shelled out in an anterior to posterior fashion (**Fig. 19B.13** and **Fig. 19B.14**).
13. The odontoid peg is dissected and freed off its ligamentous attachments laterally and superiorly (**Fig. 19B.15**).
14. Posterior drilling of the peg is stopped once the transverse bands of the cruciform ligaments are identified (**Fig. 19B.16**).
15. The odontoid peg is removed in a piecemeal fashion after it is released and dissected away from its ligamentous attachments.

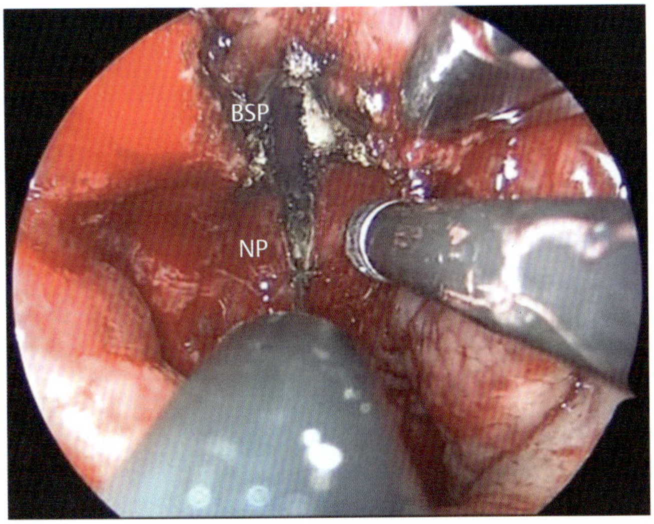

Fig. 19B.7 The nasopharynx is split in the midline from the basisphenoid to the floor of the nasal cavity using monopolar cautery.

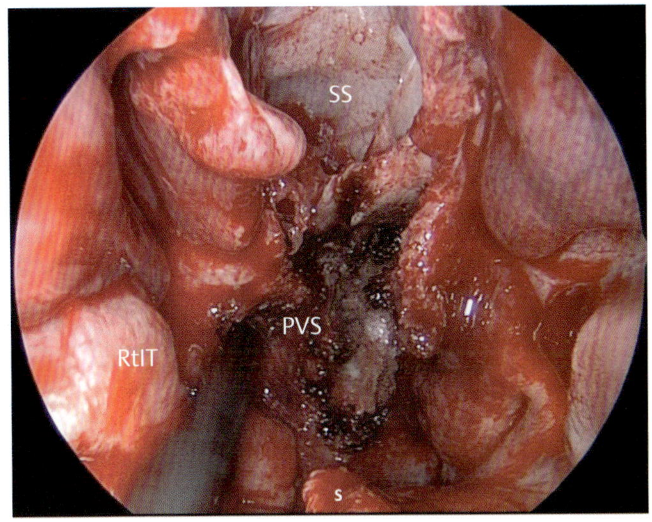

Fig. 19B.8 Dissection of prevertebral soft tissue using monopolar cautery.

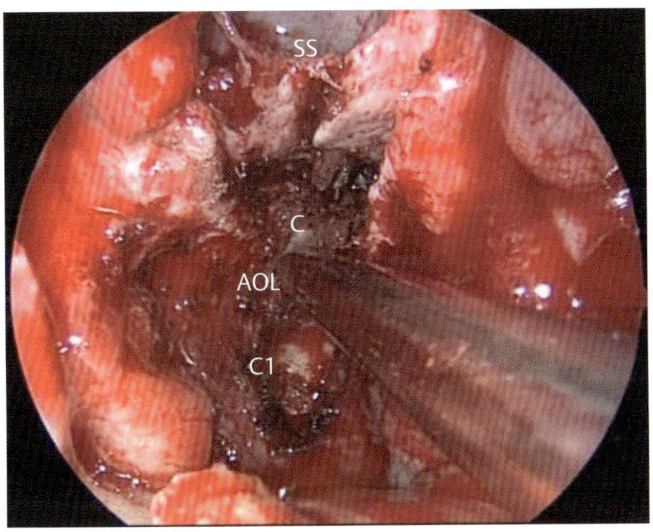

Fig. 19B.9 Dissection of the firm anterior atlanto-occipital ligament (AOL) and anterior longitudinal ligament between the clivus (C) and anterior arch of C1 (C1) using a microdebrider.

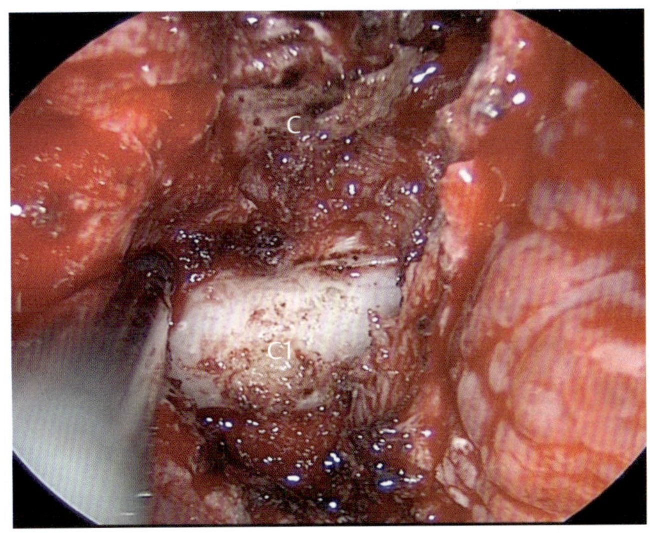

Fig. 19B.10 Exposure of the tubercle and anterior arch of C1 (C1).

16. Complete removal of the odontoid peg is achieved once the transverse bands of the cruciform ligaments are in full view (**Fig. 19B.17**).
17. After careful hemostasis, the edges of the surgical incision are reapproximated and closed with absorbable sutures. No nasal packing is required.
18. A postoperative CT scan reveals sufficient decompression of the craniocervical junction (**Fig. 19B.18** and **Fig. 19B.19**).
19. A nasal endoscopy at 3 months' postoperation revealed a well-healed scar at the surgical site with minimal crusting.

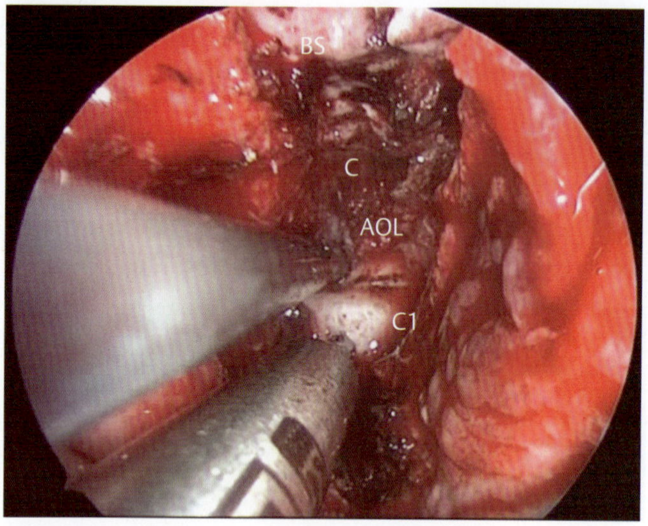

Fig. 19B.11 Drilling over the tubercle and anterior arch of C1 (C1).

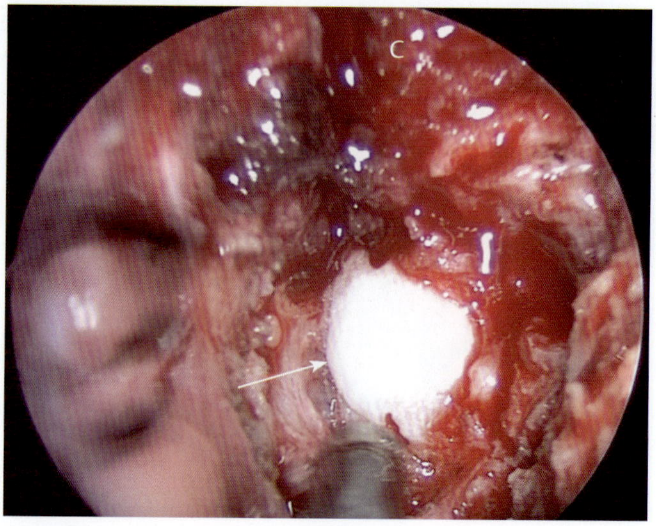

Fig. 19B.12 Exposure of the odontoid peg (*white arrow*).

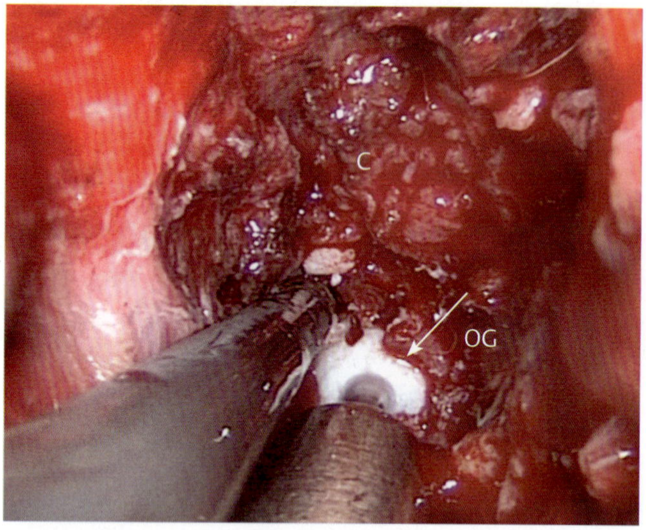

Fig. 19B.13 Drilling (*white arrow*) of the odontoid peg (OG) with a diamond burr.

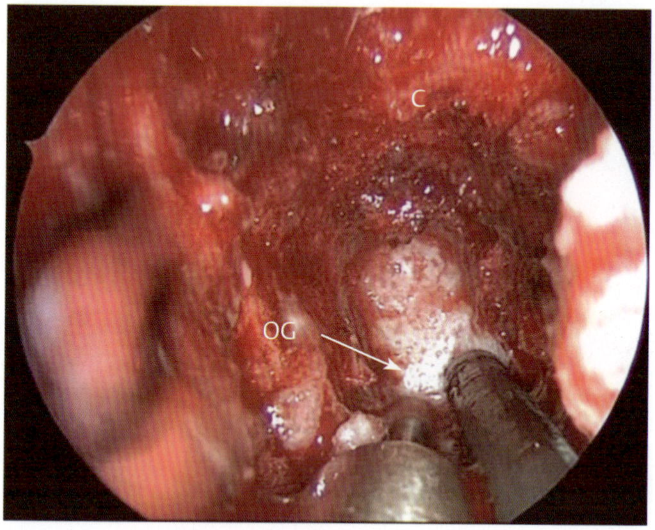

Fig. 19B.14 Drilling (*white arrow*) of the odontoid peg (OG) using the "egg-shell" technique.

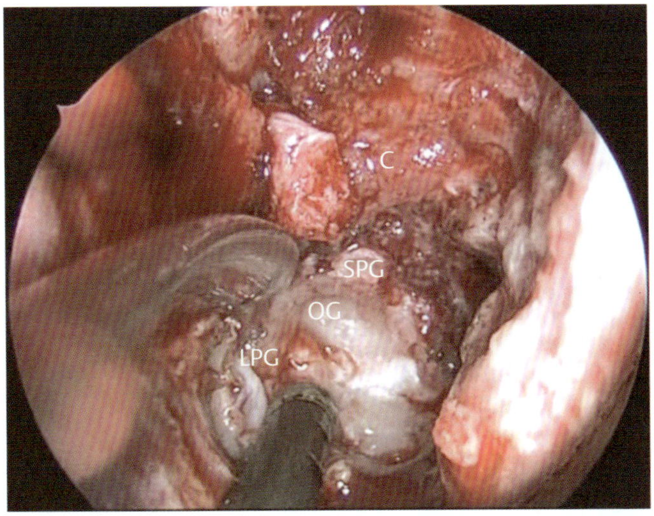

Fig. 19B.15 Dissection of the odontoid peg (OG) from its ligamentous attachments superiorly and laterally.

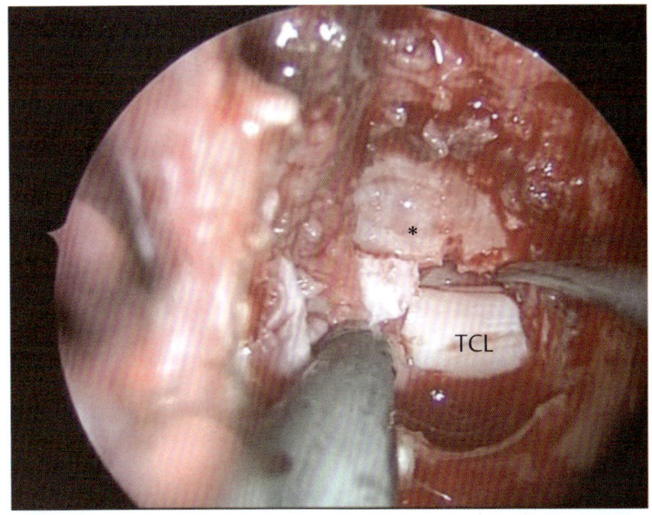

Fig. 19B.16 The posterior limitation of drilling is reached when the transverse band of the cruciform ligament (TCL) is encountered. Shelled-out posterior odontoid peg (*).

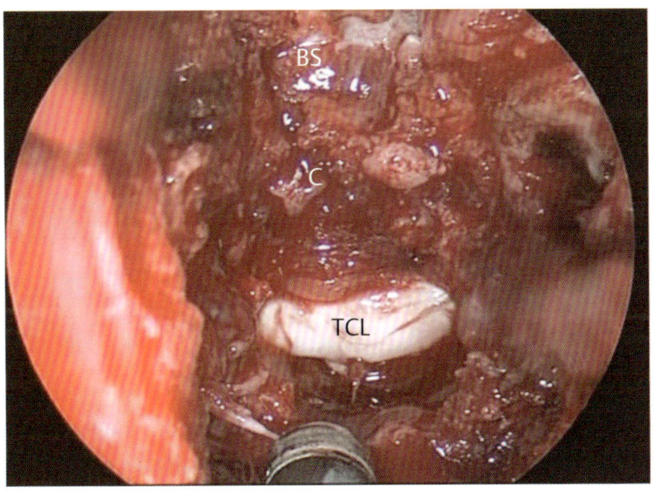

Fig. 19B.17 Complete removal of the odontoid peg is achieved with the transverse band of the cruciform ligament seen in full view.

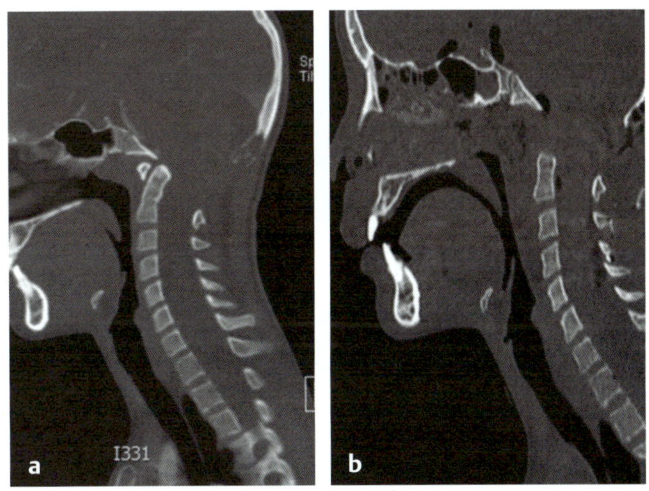

Fig. 19B.18 Preoperative **(a)** and 1-week postoperative **(b)** sagittal bone-weighted CT sections demonstrating sufficient decompression of the craniocervical junction.

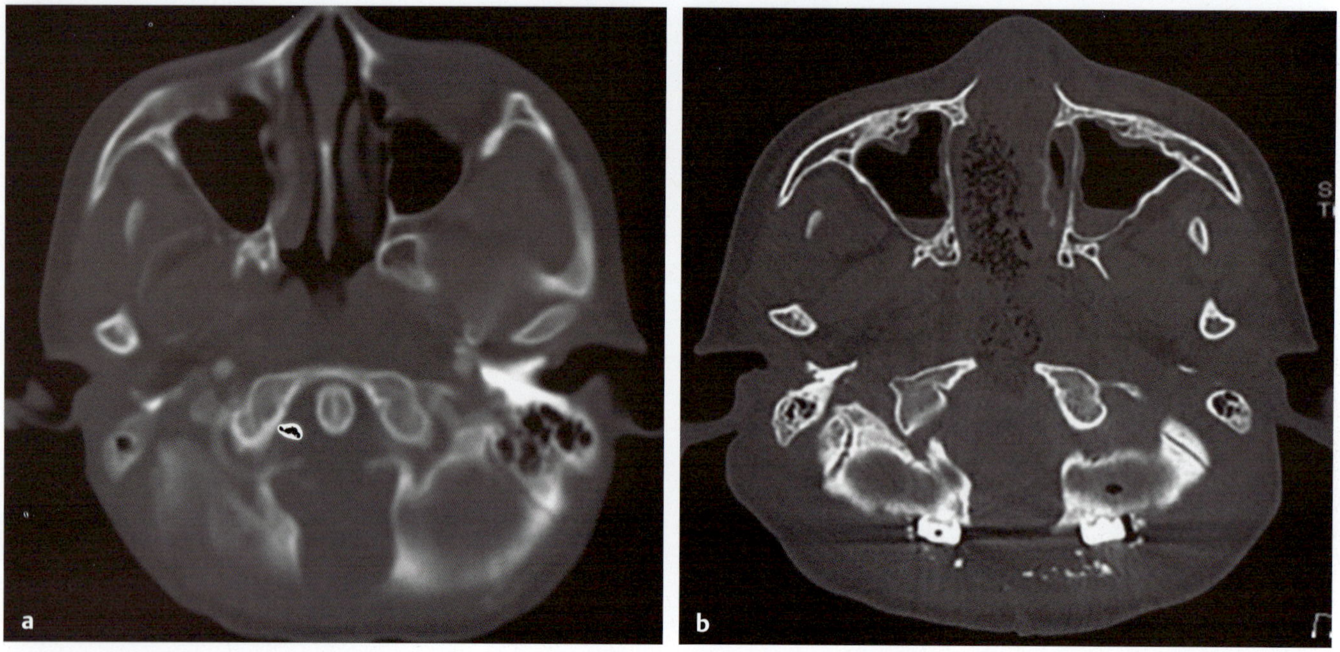

Fig. 19B.19 Preoperative **(a)** and 1-week postoperative **(b)** sagittal bone-weighted CT sections demonstrating sufficient decompression of the cranio-cervical junction and the occipital anchor for the occipito-cervical fusion.

Case 19C

Endoscopic Trans C1/C2 Decompression of Basilar Invagination

Adzreil Bakri, Michel Roethlisberger, Prepageran Narayanan, and Vicknes Waran

History

A 29-year-old lady presented with headache and limited neck movement for the last 6 months. A computed tomography (CT) and magnetic resonance imaging (MRI) revealed a basilar invagination with an atlanto-axial arthrosis and an odontoid peg narrowing the foramen magnum (**Fig. 19C.1, Fig. 19C.2, Fig. 19C.3**). A posterior occipito-cervical fusion and an endonasal endoscopic dual nostril approach to the craniocervical junction to remove the odontoid peg was indicated.

Surgical Steps

1. Local anesthesia is infiltrated into the posterior septum prior to the elevation of the mucoperichondrium away from the bony septum.
2. The septum is incised with a no. 15 blade and the mucoperichondrial flap is raised up to the choana.
3. The plane can be further developed into a nasoseptal flap for skullbase defect reconstruction; however, it was not required for this case and a posterior septectomy was performed. The bilateral mucoperichondrial flaps and the exposed septum were removed from the level of the sphenoid ostium up to the floor of the nasal cavity allowing a wide exposure of the nasopharynx and the anterior wall of the sphenoid sinus.
4. Meticulous hemostasis is performed with either a bipolar cautery or a monopolar suction cautery to arrest any bleeding from the septectomy edges.
5. Once the sphenoid keel is fully exposed, the ostia are interconnected through a wide inferomedial opening toward the midline using a Kerrison punch in a V-shaped manner.
6. After interconnection of the sphenoid ostia, the sphenoid keel is removed.
7. An optional turbinectomy can be performed on either side of the nasal cavity to allow for an adequate surgical access (**Fig. 19C.4**).

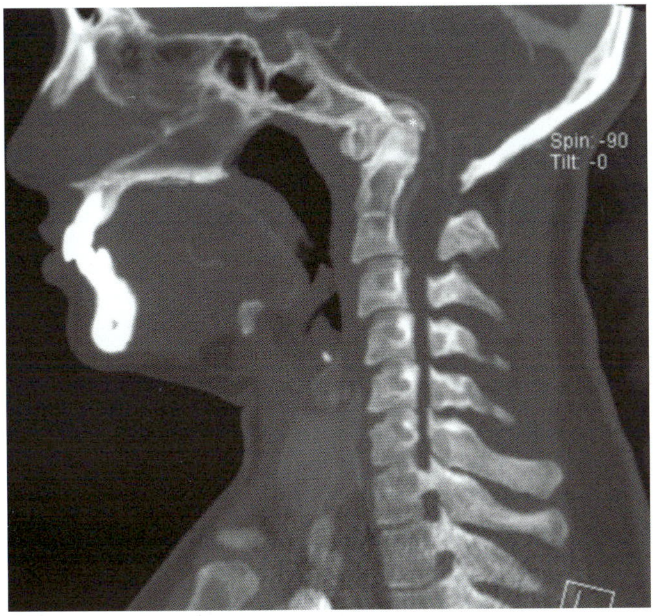

Fig. 19C.1 Sagittal bone-weighted CT scan demonstrating a prominent odontoid peg invaginating into the foramen magnum (*).

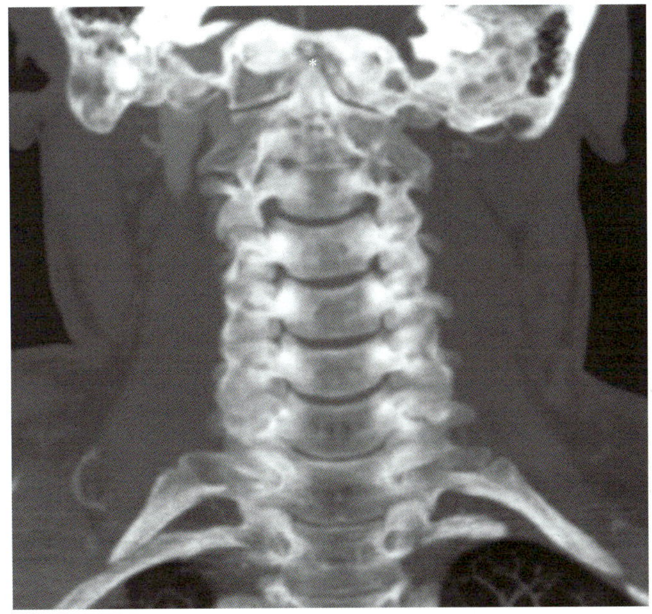

Fig. 19C.2 Coronal bone-weighted CT scan demonstrating degenerative atlanto-dental changes with joint narrowing (*).

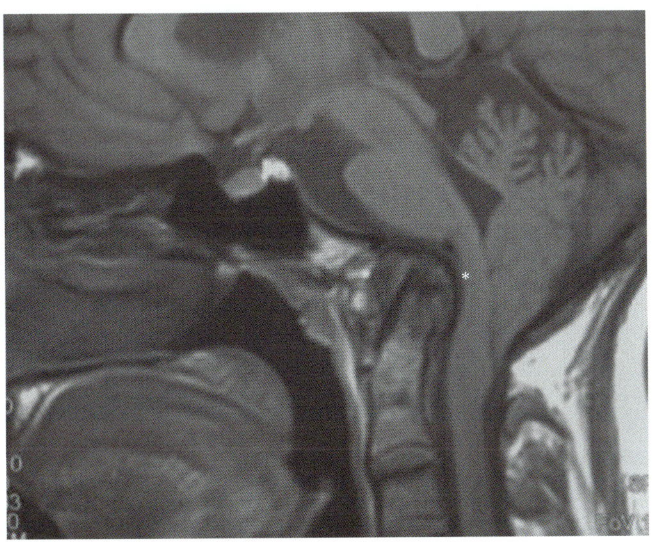

Fig. 19C.3 Sagittal T1-weighted non-contrast enhanced MRI section showing a typical basilar invagination (*).

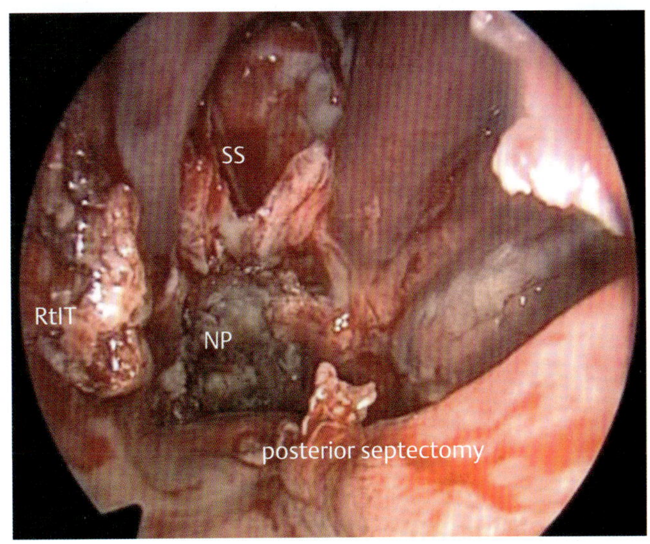

Fig. 19C.4 Endonasal endoscopic view of the nasopharynx (NP) after posterior septectomy, right inferior turbinectomy (RtIT), and removal of the sphenoid rostrum.

8. Using a monopolar cautery, the nasopharynx is split in the midline from the basisphenoid superiorly down to the level just above the floor of the nasal cavity inferiorly.
9. The clivus, atlas (C1), and axis (C2) are then exposed via dissection of the anterior atlanto-occipital ligament and prevertebral fascia off the bone with a monopolar cautery combined with a microdebrider (**Fig. 19C.5**).
10. The anterior arch and tubercle of C1 are fully exposed.
11. Drilling is then commenced with a diamond burr over the tubercle and the anterior arch of C1 to expose the odontoid peg (**Fig. 19C.6**).
12. Once the odontoid peg is identified, its anterior face is fully exposed by further removing the bone of the anterior arch of C1 laterally using image-guided surgery as verification.

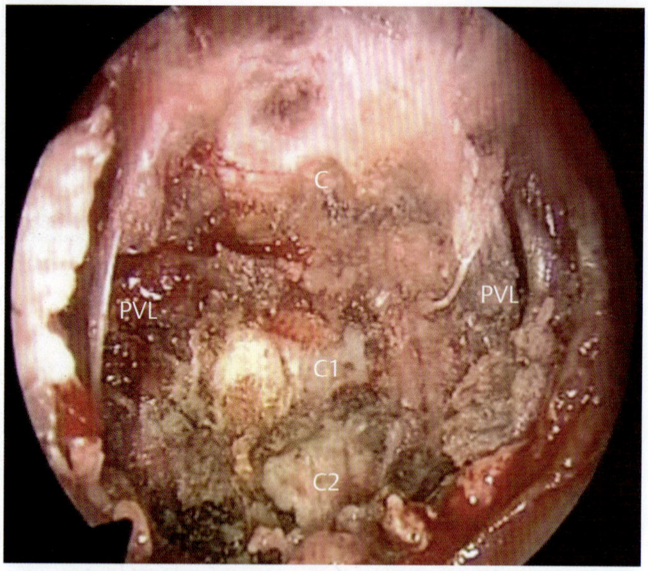

Fig. 19C.5 The dissection of the prevertebral muscles and ligaments (PVL) exposes the lower clivus (C).

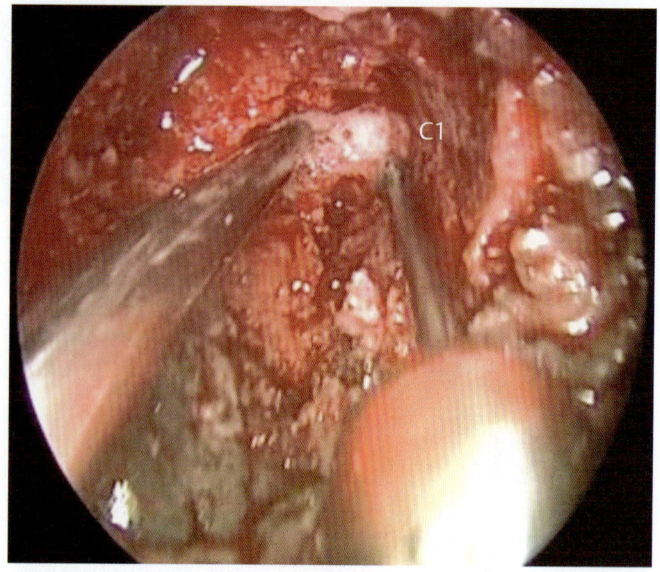

Fig. 19C.6 Drilling of the anterior arch of C1 (C1).

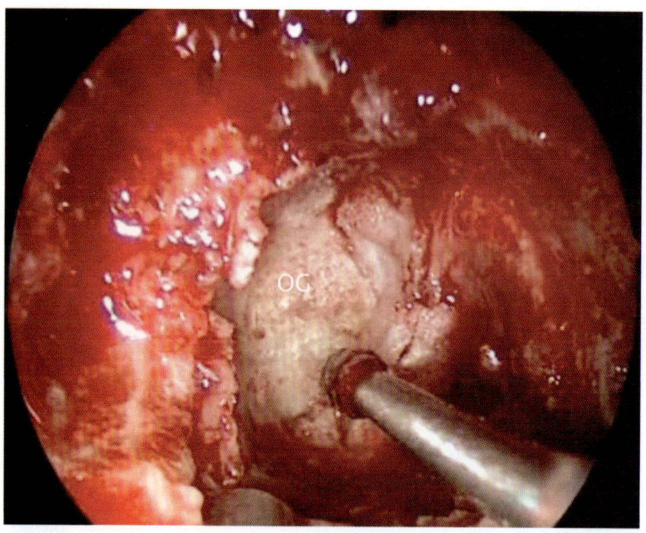

Fig. 19C.7 The odontoid peg (OG) is shelled out using a high-speed diamond burr.

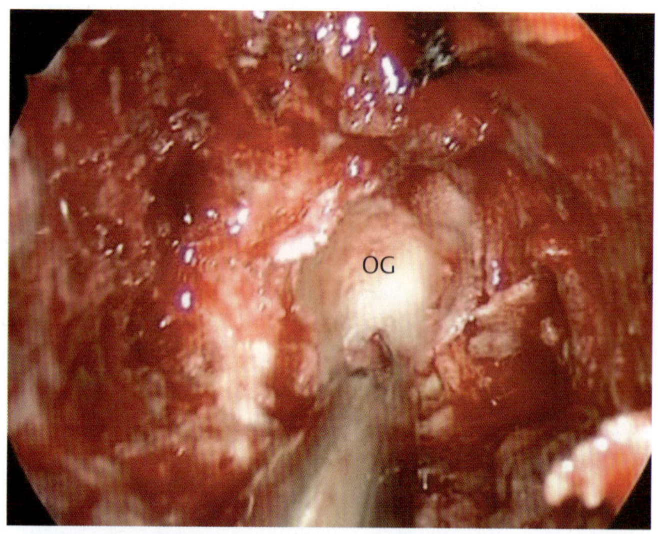

Fig. 19C.8 Removal of the outer shell of the odontoid peg (OG) using a Kerrison punch.

13. The odontoid peg is shelled out using a high-speed drill (egg-shell technique) in an anterior to posterior direction in a wide fashion (**Fig. 19C.7**).
14. The posterior limitation of bone removal are the transverse bands of the cruciform ligaments.
15. The odontoid peg's outer shell is removed in a piecemeal fashion after it is released and dissected away from its ligamentous attachments (**Fig. 19C.8**).
16. Complete removal of the odontoid peg is achieved with small Kerrison punches along a plane between the transverse bands of the cruciform ligaments (**Fig. 19C.9**).
17. After careful hemostasis, the edges of the surgical incision are reapproximated and closed with absorbable sutures. No nasal packing is required.
18. A postoperative CT scan should be performed to demonstrate sufficient bony resection of the invaginated odontoid peg (**Fig. 19C.10** and **Fig. 19C.11**).
19. A nasal endoscopy performed at 3 months' postoperation confirmed a well-healed surgical site (**Fig. 19C.12**).

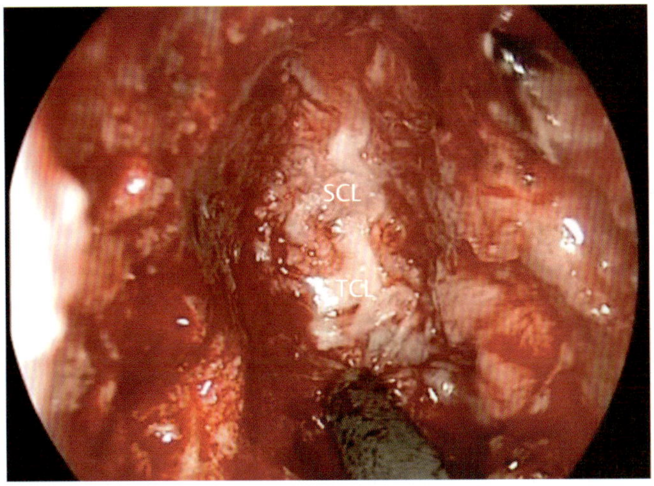

Fig. 19C.9 Endoscopic view after full removal of the odontoid peg. The superior longitudinal band of the cruciform ligament (SCL) and the transverse band of the cruciform ligament (TCL) are identifiable.

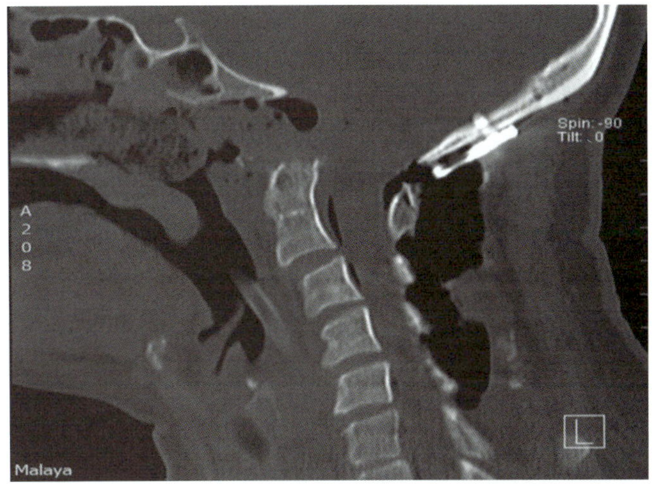

Fig. 19C.10 Sagittal bone-weighted CT section 1 week postoperatively demonstrating sufficient bony removal of the invaginated odontoid peg with postoperative changes.

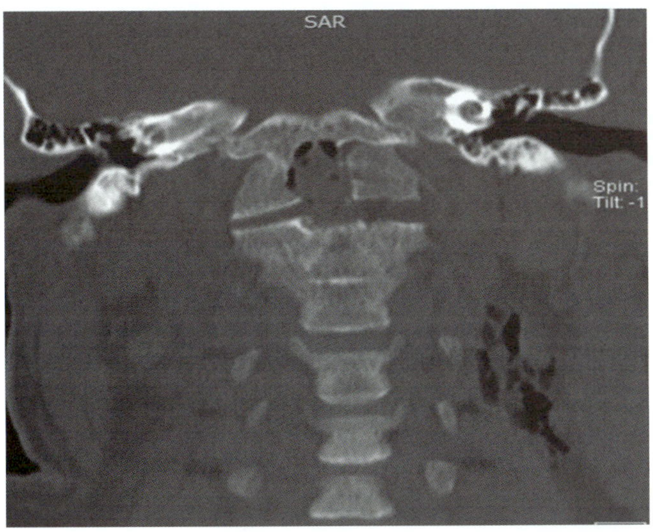

Fig. 19C.11 Coronal bone-weighted CT section 1 week postoperatively demonstrating sufficient bony removal of the invaginated odontoid peg with postoperative changes.

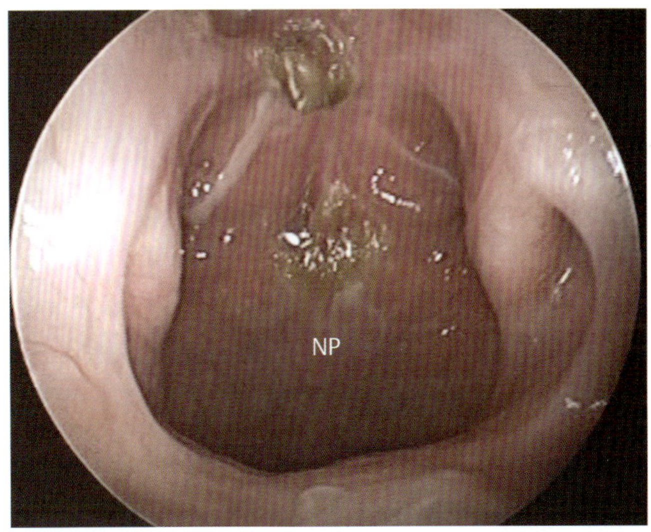

Fig. 19C.12 Endoscopic view of the nasopharynx (NP) 3 months following surgery.

Case 19D

Endoscopic Endonasal Approach for a Foramen Magnum Meningioma

Kong Yew Liew, Michel Roethlisberger, Adzreil Bakri, Prepageran Narayanan, and Vicknes Waran

History

A 65-year-old Chinese female without other underlying medical conditions presented with recurrent headaches, disequilibrium, and progressive lower limb weakness. Neuroimaging revealed an extra-axial enhancing mass at the anterior aspect of the foramen magnum compressing the brainstem and abutting the left vertebral artery (**Fig. 19D.1**).

Surgical Steps

1. Local anesthesia is infiltrated into the posterior septum to raise the mucoperichondrium away from the bony septum (**Fig. 19D.2** and **Fig. 19D.3**).
2. The septum is incised with a no. 15 blade and the mucoperichondrial flap is raised up to the choana.
3. The elevated mucoperichondrial flap can be further developed into a nasoseptal flap if reconstruction

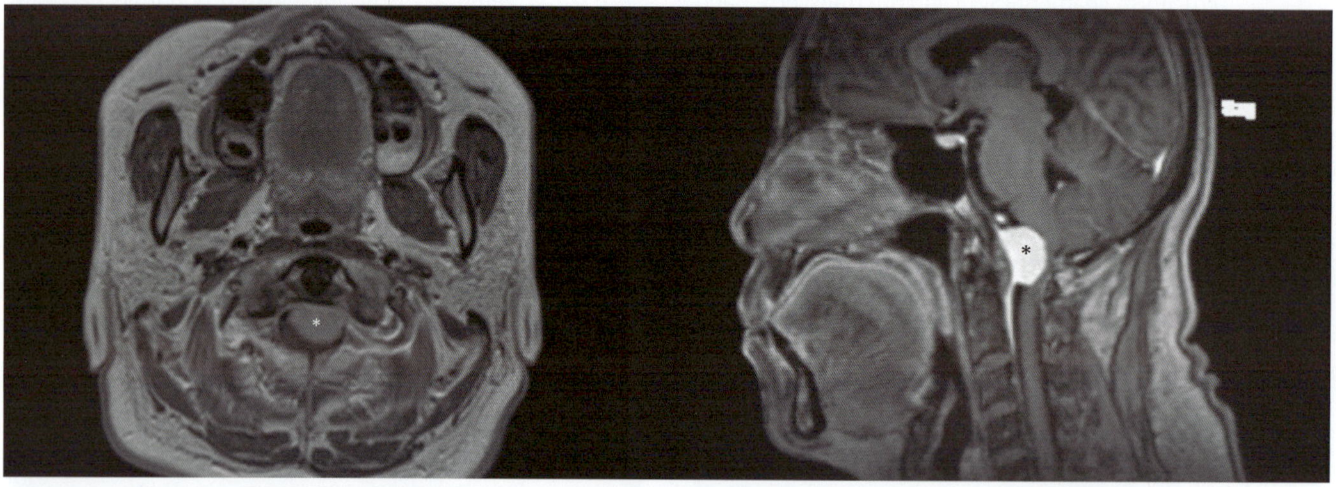

Fig. 19D.1 Axial and sagittal T1-weighted contrast enhanced MRI sections demonstrating an extraaxial enhancing mass (*) at the foramen magnum with significant brainstem compresssion.

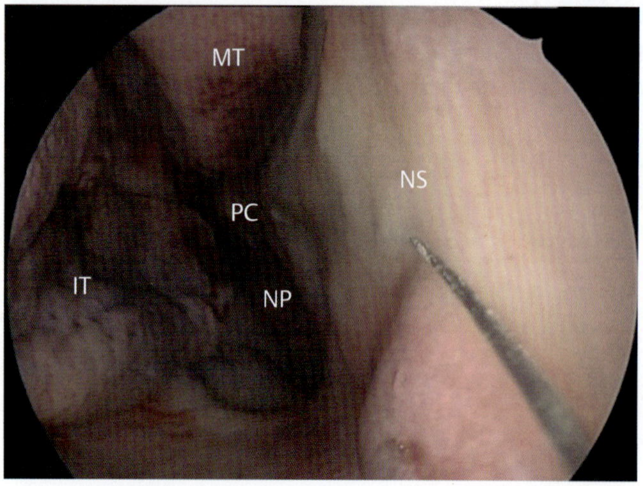

Fig. 19D.2 Administration of local anethesia confirmed by bleaching of the septal mucosa posteriorly up to the superior aspect of the choana.

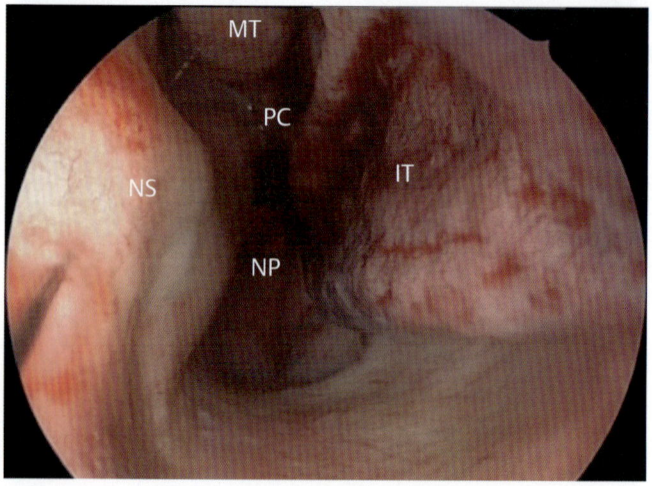

Fig. 19D.3 Administration of local anethesia along the left nasal septum with blanching of the mucosa.

is necessary; however, it was not required for this case and a posterior septectomy was performed. The bilateral mucoperichondrial flaps are stored and the exposed posterior septum removed up to the level of the choanal roof down to the floor of the nasal cavity, thus allowing for a two-handed technique during tumor resection (**Fig. 19D.4 and Fig. 19D.5**).

4. Meticulous hemostasis is performed with either bipolar cautery or monopolar suction cautery to control any bleeding arising from the septectomy borders.
5. A Y-shaped incision along the midline nasopharynx is performed using a monoplar cautery, carrying the incision down along the clivus (**Fig. 19D.6**).
6. The bone of the clivus and the C1-C2 junction are exposed using blunt dissection with a Freer elevator through the soft tissue and prevertebral fascia (**Fig. 19D.7**).
7. The odontoid process is exposed by removing the lower clivus and the C1-C2 junction using a high-speed diamond burr. Care is taken at this step as there may be brisk bleeding from the clival plexus, which can be controlled with cautery. As the bony removal is brought inferiorly, the anterior arch of the atlas will be removed partially or completely for sufficient exposure of the lesion.
8. The odontoid process is shelled out, dissected free, and can be removed with a bone rongeur or a Kerrison punch (**Fig. 19D.8** and **Fig. 19D.9**).
9. Remnant soft tissue and bony ledges are cleared laterally to expand the exposure of the cruciate ligament (**Fig. 19D.10**).
10. The cruciate ligament is incised sharply in the midline (**Fig. 19D.11**).
11. The underlying fibrous tissue is dissected away using a right-angle dissector to prevent inadvertent injury. The incision is carried superiorly and inferiorly to enhance exposure. The cruciate ligament is then dissected away laterally and the dura with the underlying pathology is visualized directly (**Fig. 19D.12**).
12. Tumor resection is carried out using an ultrasonic aspirator, with resection of the central compartments first. This decompresses the lesion and the extracapsular dissection is hence facilitated (**Fig. 19D.13**).
13. After careful circumferential extracapsular arachnoidal dissection the lesion can be removed safely (**Fig. 19D.14, Fig. 19D.15, Fig. 19D.16**).
14. Hemostasis is achieved with neurosurgical patties and the resection cavity is inspected for remnant tumor.
15. The skull base defect is reconstructed with an abdominal fat graft. The edges are tucked intradurally to ensure a watertight seal but not packed tightly to prevent brainstem compression. This is then reinforced with a layer of absorbable hemostat (**Fig. 19D.17**).
16. The borders of the nasopharyngeal incision are reapproximated and closed with absorbable sutures (**Fig. 19D.18**).
17. The construct is further reinforced with a layer of synthetic dural sealant or tissue glue. No nasal packing is required (**Fig. 19D.19**).
18. Postoperatively, an MRI can be used for for further long-term tumor follow-up (**Fig. 19D.20** and **Fig. 19D.21**).

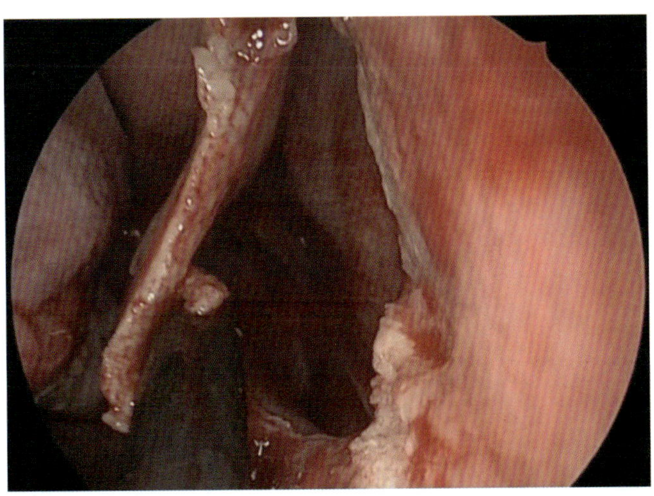

Fig. 19D.4 Right septal mucoperichondrial flap is being elevated from the septum. The choana is visible within under the flap.

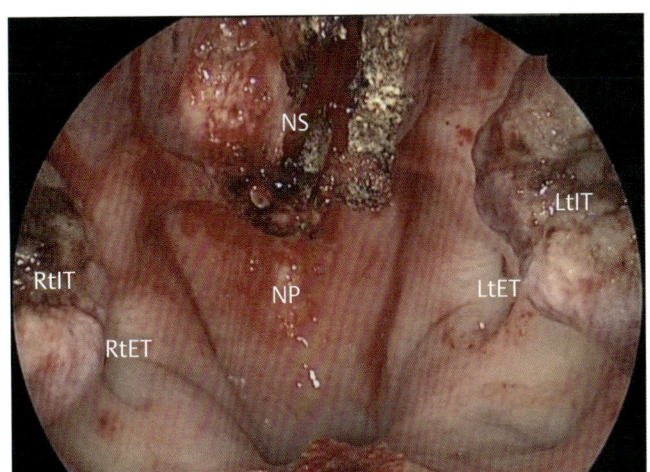

Fig. 19D.5 View of the nasopharynx after posterior septectomy.

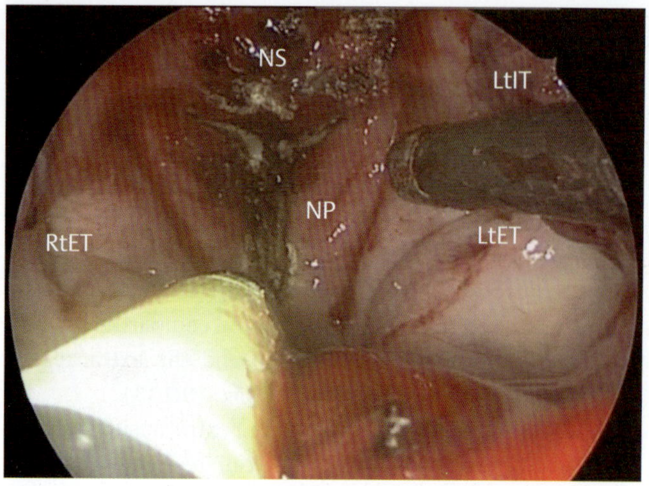

Fig. 19D.6 Y incision on the nasopharynx with monopolar cautery is done to bone.

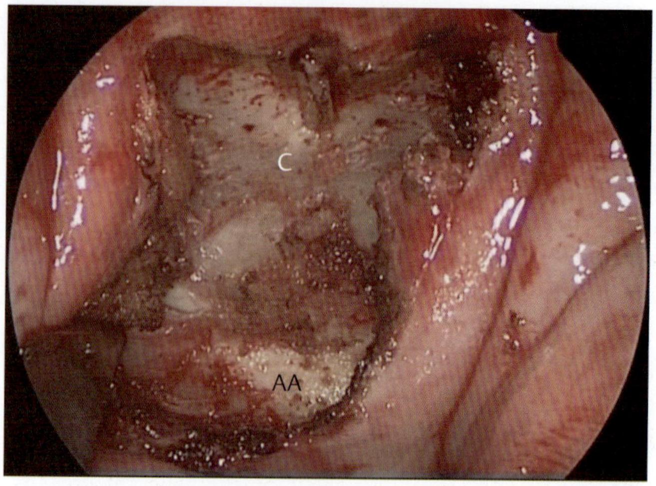

Fig. 19D.7 Exposure of the clivus (CL). The arch of the atlas (AA) is visible inferiorly.

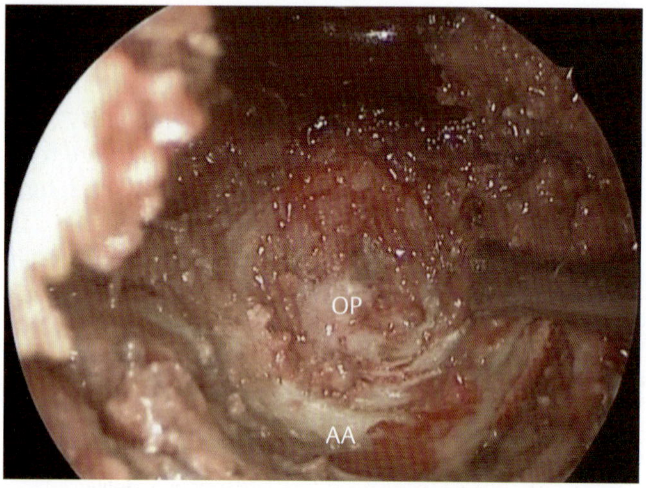

Fig. 19D.8 The odontoid process (OP) and the arch of atlas (AA) are partially drilled.

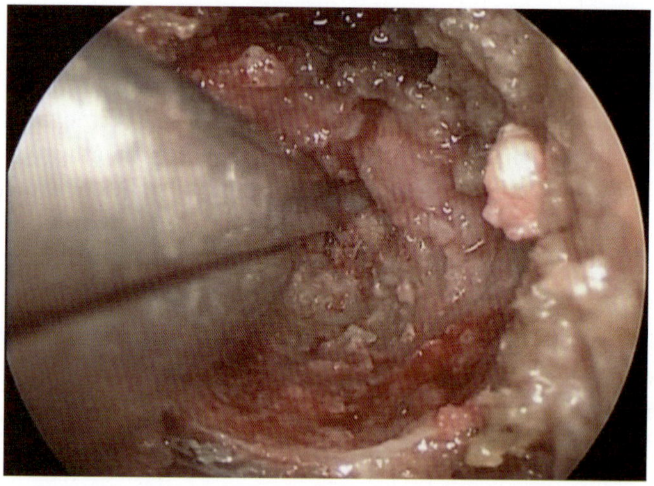

Fig. 19D.9 Odontoid process (OP) is being removed with a Kerrison punch.

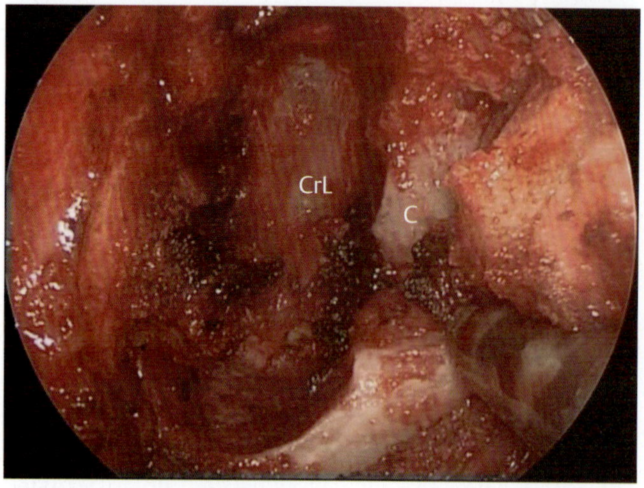

Fig. 19D.10 Complete exposure of the cruciate ligament (CrL).

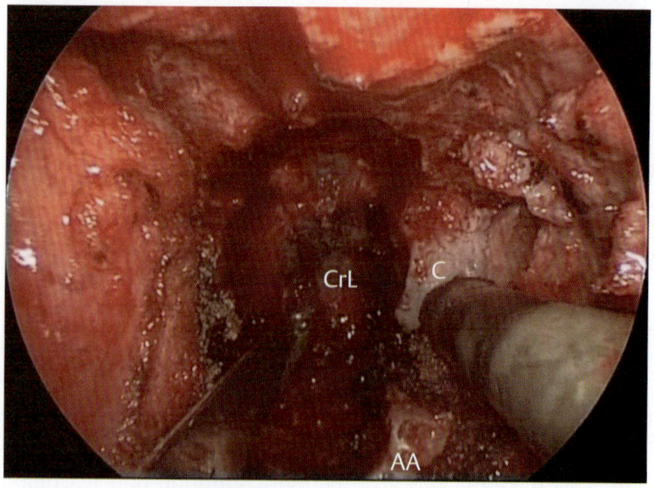

Fig. 19D.11 The incision is done directly on the cruciate ligament (CrL).

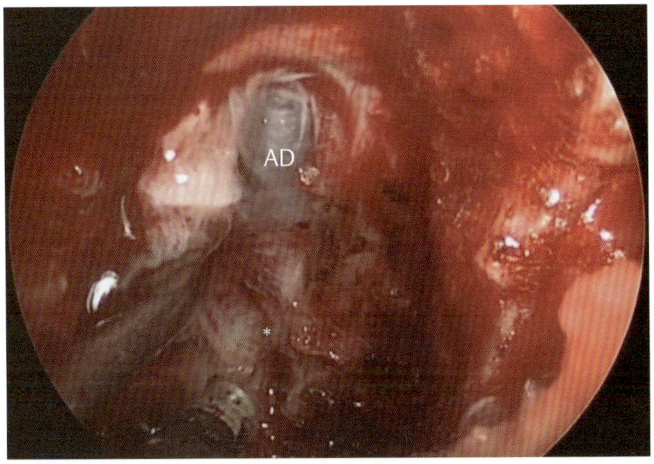

Fig. 19D.12 The superior arachnoidal plane along the arachnoidal dura (AD) and the meningioma (*) are identified.

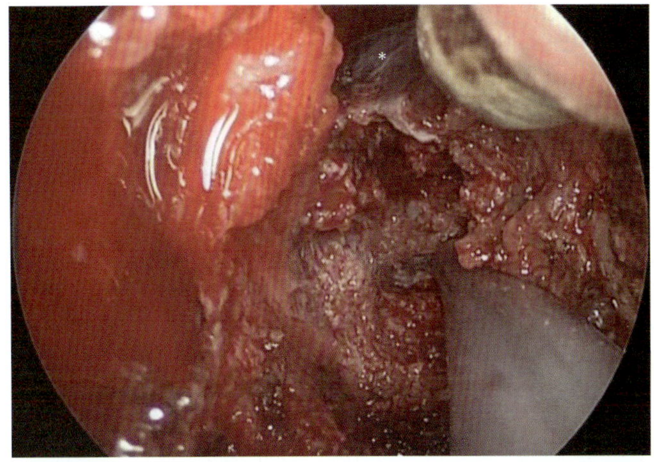

Fig. 19D.13 Central tumor debulking is achieved using an ultrasonic aspirator, facilitating capsular dissection of the lesion (*).

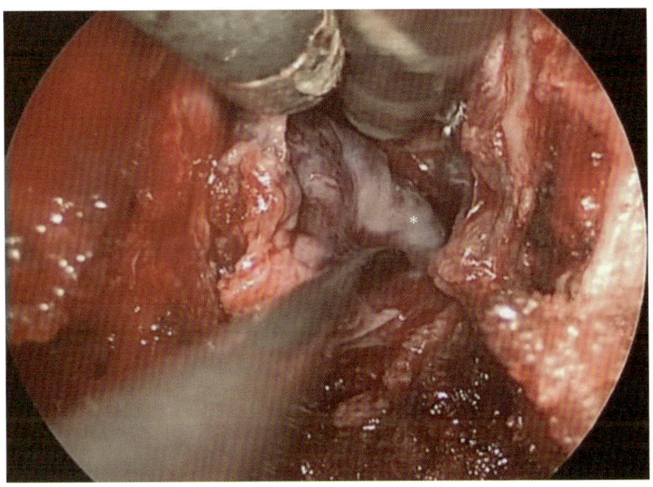

Fig. 19D.14 Extracapsular dissection along the left lateral border (*) of the meningioma by mobilization with a microdissector.

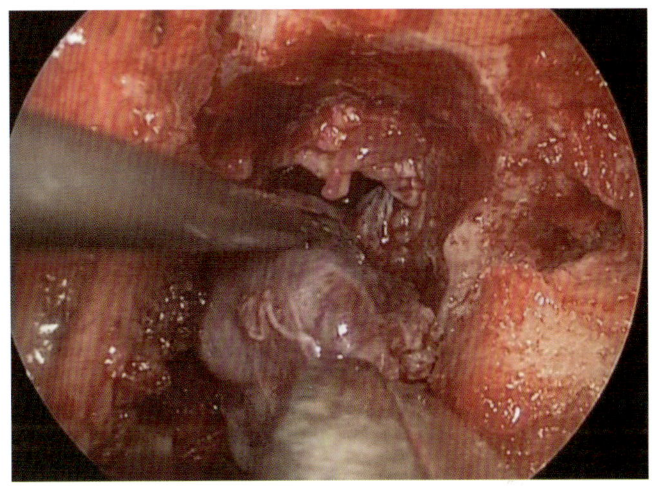

Fig. 19D.15 The superior aspect of the tumor is delivered.

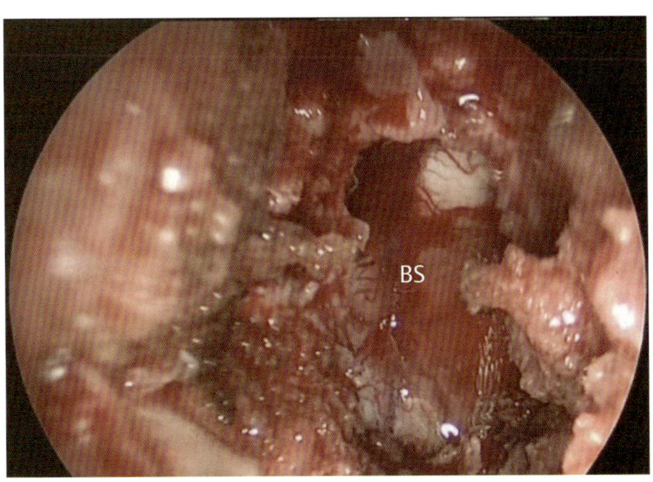

Fig. 19D.16 After complete removal of the tumor, the brainstem (BS) is visible posterior to the resection cavity.

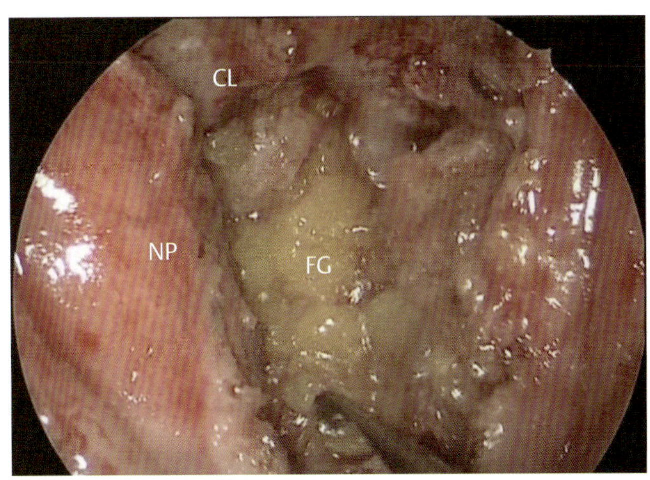

Fig. 19D.17 Skull base defect reconstruction using an abdominal fat graft (FG).

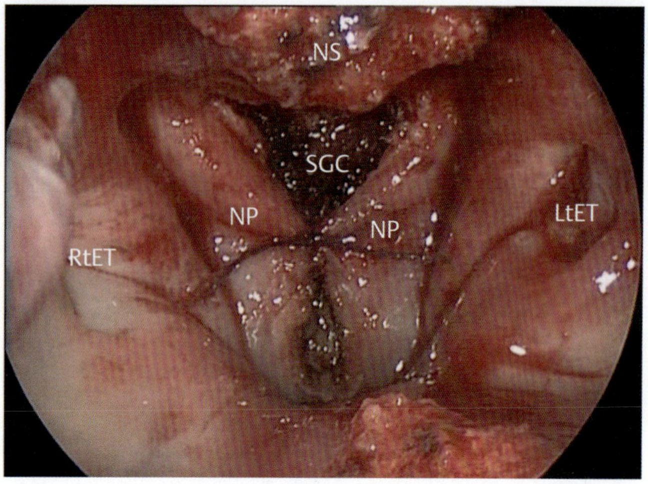

Fig. 19D.18 The medially split nasopharynx is closed with absorbable sutures.

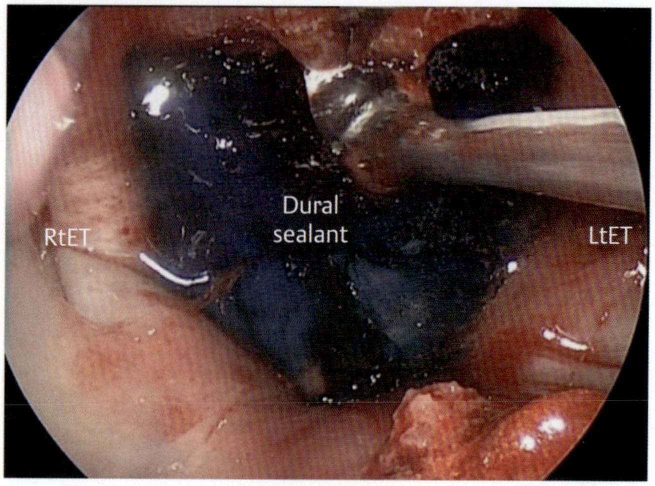

Fig. 19D.19 Superficial application of an artificial dural sealant.

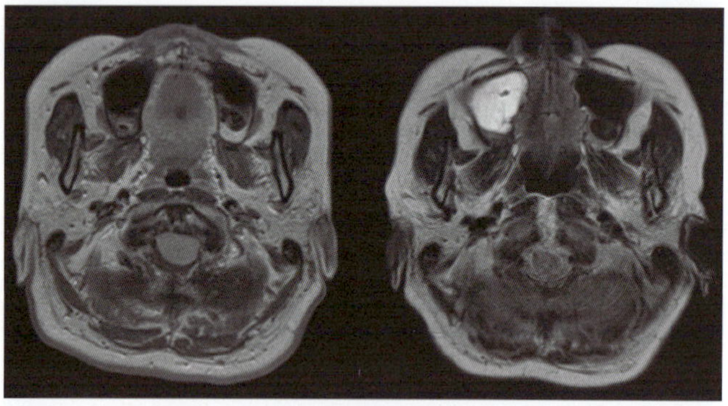

Fig. 19D.20 Axial preoperative (*left*) and 2 months' postoperative (*right*) T1-weighted contrast-enhanced MRI sections demonstrating complete excision of the foramen magnum meningioma with resolution of the brainstem mass effect.

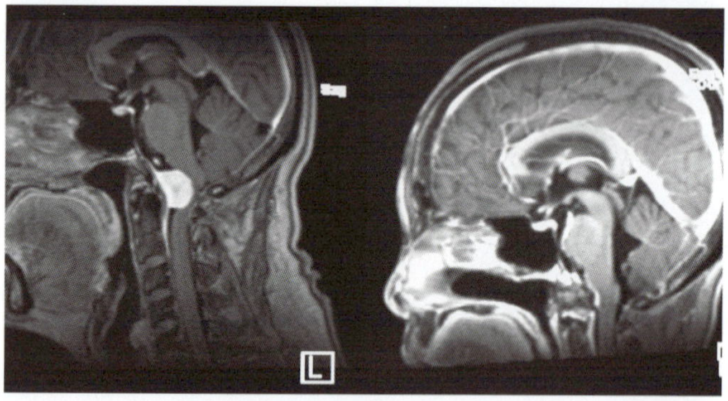

Fig. 19D.21 Sagittal preoperative (*left*) and 2 months' postoperative (*right*) T1-weighted contrast-enhanced MRI sections demonstrating complete excision of the foramen magnum meningioma with resolution of the brainstem mass effect.

Case 19E

Endoscopic Endonasal Approach for a Teratoma of the Craniocervical Junction

Adzreil Bakri, Prepageran Narayanan, and Vicknes Waran

History

A 3-year-old boy presented with sudden weakness of the lower limbs. A magnetic resonance imaging (MRI) revealed a soft tissue tumor arising from the posterior part of the clival bone and compressing on the brainstem just above the foramen magnum (**Fig. 19E.1** and **Fig. 19E.2**). An endoscopic transnasal dual nostril approach to the foramen magnum to remove the tumor was performed.

Surgical Steps

1. The patient is positioned supine with the head slightly extended under general anesthesia.
2. The nose is packed as per standard protocol.
3. Local anesthesia is infiltrated into bilateral inferior turbinates.
4. Bilateral inferior turbinectomy is performed to provide adequate space for access (**Fig. 19E.3**).
5. Local anesthesia is then infiltrated on the nasal septum bilaterally to raise the mucoperichondrium away from the bony septum.
6. At the area opposite the anterior end of the middle turbinate, the septum is then incised with a no. 15 blade and a mucoperichondrial flap is raised until the sphenoid ostia and posterior choana are visible (**Fig. 19E.4**).
7. The nasoseptal flap is then freed with a microscissors superiorly and inferiorly aiming for the sphenoid ostia and posterior choana, respectively (**Fig. 19E.5**).
8. The pedicled flap can then be stored in the nasopharynx until reconstruction is required.
9. The exposed cartilaginous septum is fractured through to the contralateral side and removed piecemeal, all the while freeing it from the overlying contralateral septal mucoperichondrium. This is continued until the sphenoid keel is exposed with the sphenoid ostia visible bilaterally. At this point, a contralateral nasoseptal flap is created in the same manner as described in the previous steps.

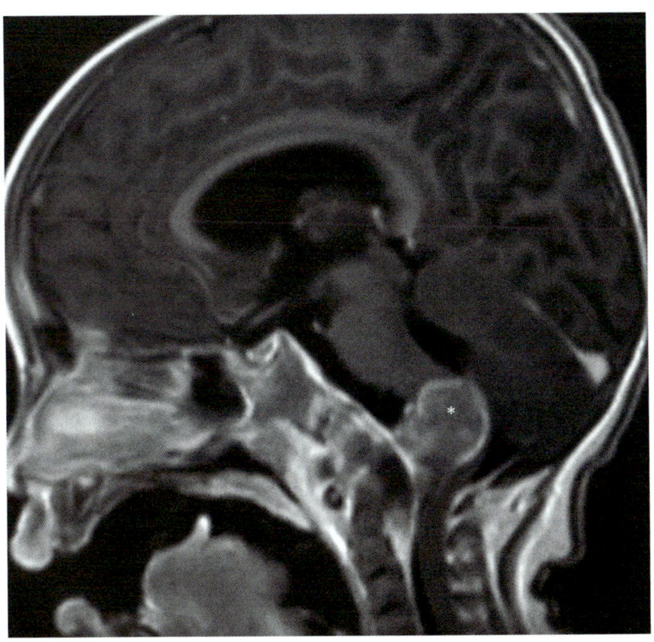

Fig. 19E.1 A sagittal view of the T1-weighted MRI with contrast showing a soft tissue tumor (*) arising from the posterior clival bone compressing on the brainstem and foramen magnum.

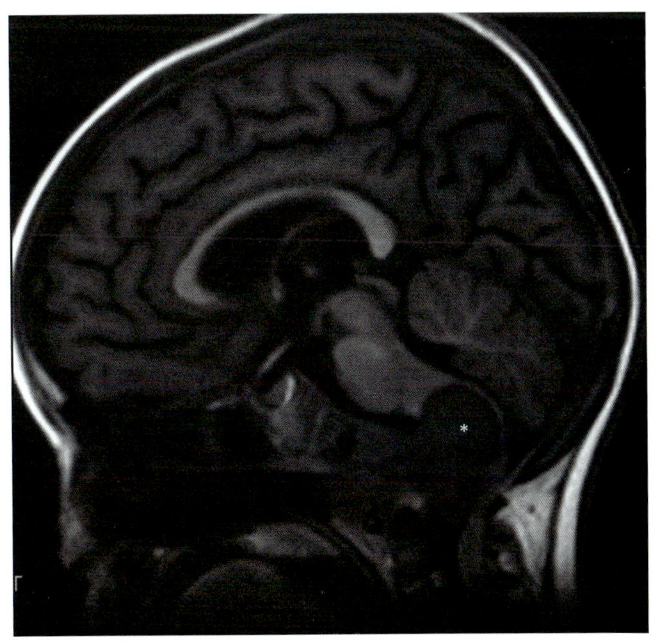

Fig. 19E.2 A sagittal view of the T1-weighted MRI without contrast tumor (*).

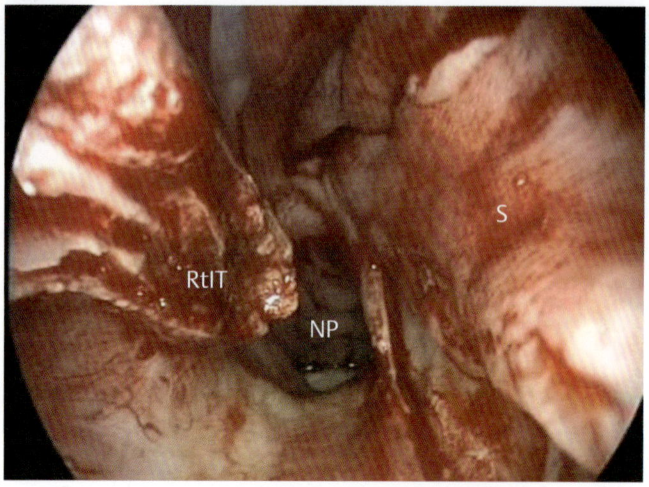

Fig. 19E.3 View of the right nasal cavity after right inferior turbinectomy (RtIT).

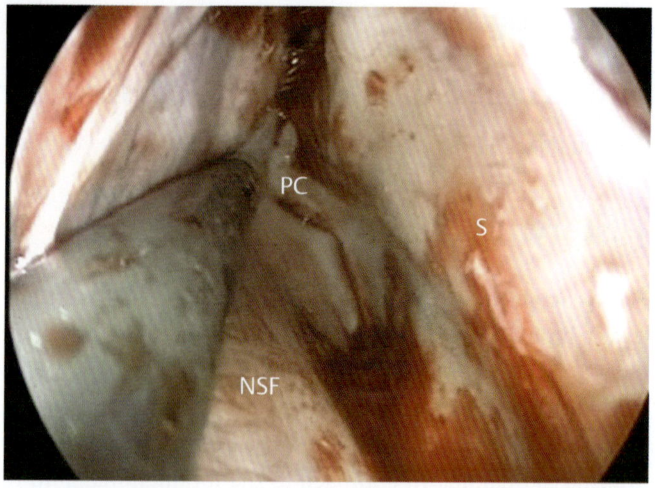

Fig. 19E.4 Raising of the right nasoseptal flap (NSF) with the bony posterior choana (PC) in view.

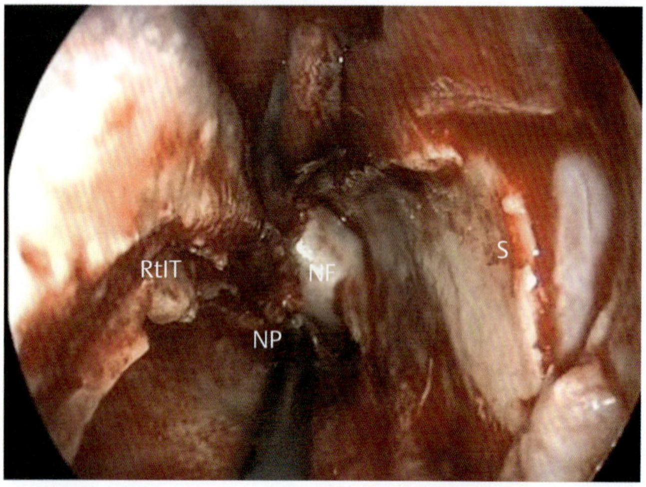

Fig. 19E.5 The right nasoseptal flap (NSF) cut and stored down the nasopharynx (NP) for later use.

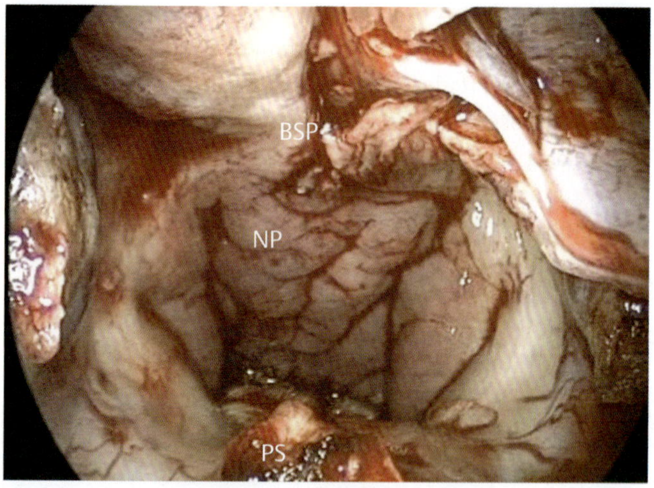

Fig. 19E.6 Full view of the nasopharynx (NP) after preparation of bilateral nasoseptal flaps and posterior septectomy.

10. Remaining bony septum is removed posteriorly, thus completing a posterior septectomy. This provides unobstructed access to the nasopharynx. Meticulous hemostasis is performed with either bipolar cautery or monopolar suction cautery to arrest any bleeding from the septectomy edges (**Fig. 19E.6**).
11. Using a monopolar cautery, the nasopharynx is split in the midline from the basisphenoid superiorly down to the level just above the floor of the nasal cavity inferiorly (**Fig. 19E.7**).
12. The clivus is then exposed via dissection of the anterior atlanto-occipital ligament and prevertebral fascia off the bone with a monopolar cautery combined with a microdebrider.
13. The location of the tumor is confirmed by neuronavigation prior to the commencement of drilling.
14. Drilling is then commenced with a diamond burr over the exposed clival bone (**Fig. 19E.8**).
15. Once the clivus is thinned out and tumor is encountered, the tumor is dissected off gently using a combination of suction and Rhoton or right-angle dissector (**Fig. 19E.9, Fig. 19E.10,** and **Fig. 19E.11**).
16. Once tumor removal is complete, the area is inspected for any residual disease (**Fig. 19E.12** and **Fig. 19E.13**).

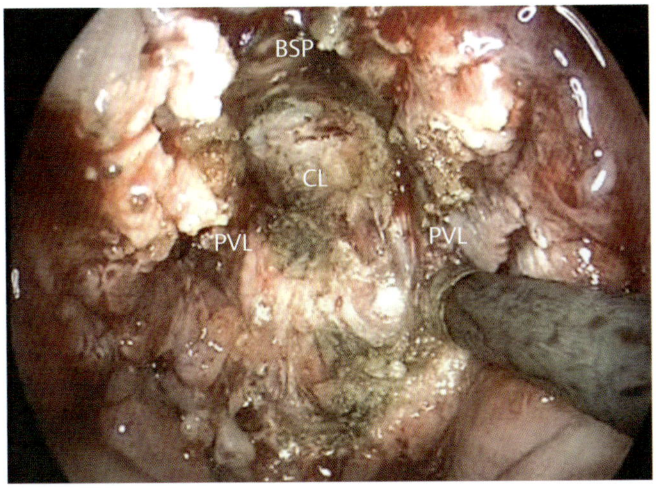

Fig. 19E.7 The nasopharynx is split in the midline from the basisphenoid (BSP) to the level just above the floor of the nasal cavity using monopolar cautery. Prevertebral muscle and ligaments are dissected laterally and deep until the clivus (CL) is encountered.

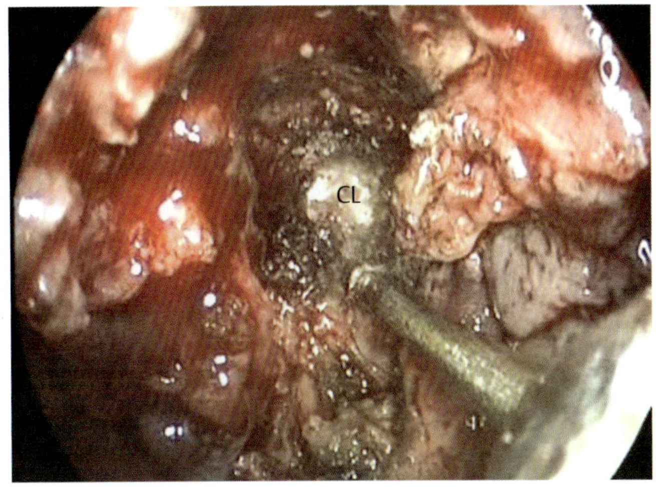

Fig. 19E.8 Drilling of clivus (CL).

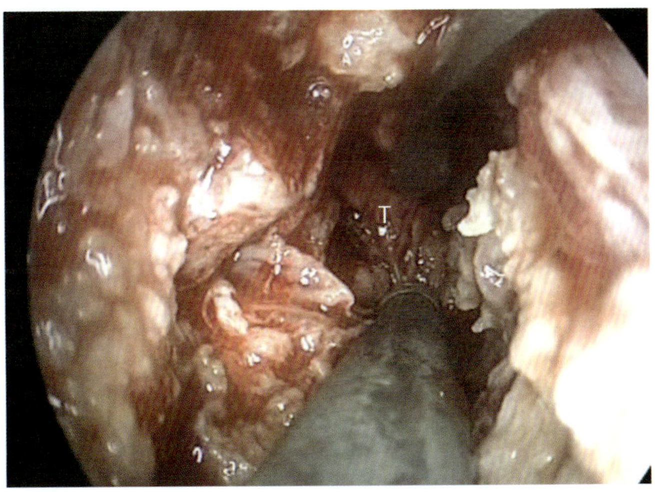

Fig. 19E.9 Tumor (T) encountered and dissected with a suction probe and Rhoton dissector.

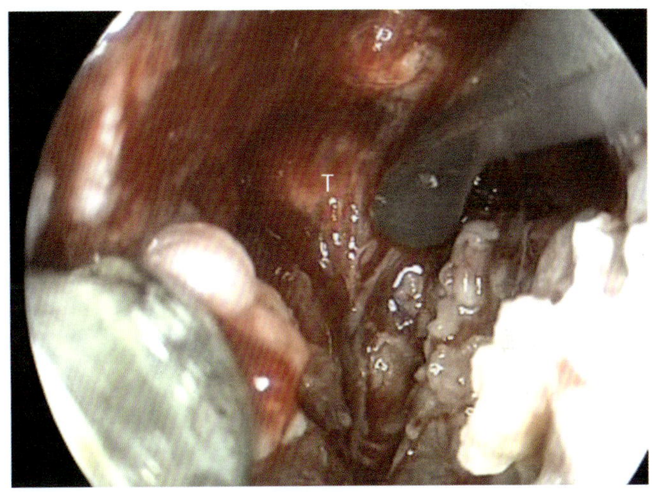

Fig. 19E.10 Tumor (T) dissection with a suction probe and Rhoton dissector.

17. The defect is closed in layers with absorbable gelatin sponges (Gelfoam), fascia lata, oxidized cellulose polymer (Surgicel), and tissue glue (**Fig. 19E.14** and **Fig. 19E.15**).
18. A Valsalva maneuver is performed to assess patency of the first layer of repair.
19. The initial layers of repair are further reinforced with pieces of septal bone and cartilage, fascia lata, bilateral nasoseptal flaps, and tissue glue (**Fig. 19E.16**).
20. The nasal cavity is loosely packed with absorbable foams (Nasopore).

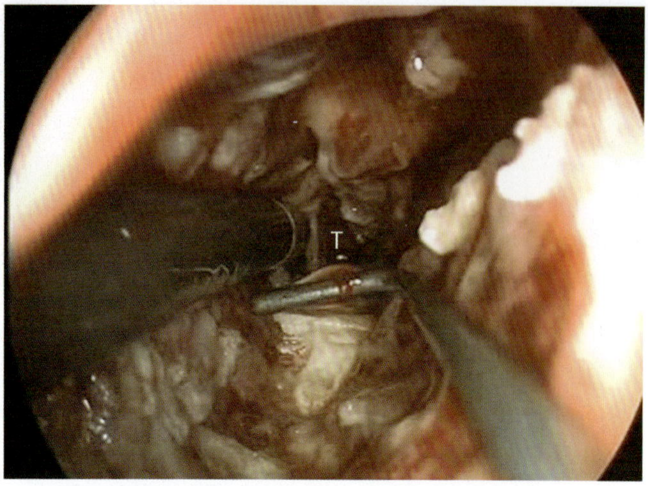

Fig. 19E.11 Tumor dissection with a suction probe and a right-angled dissector.

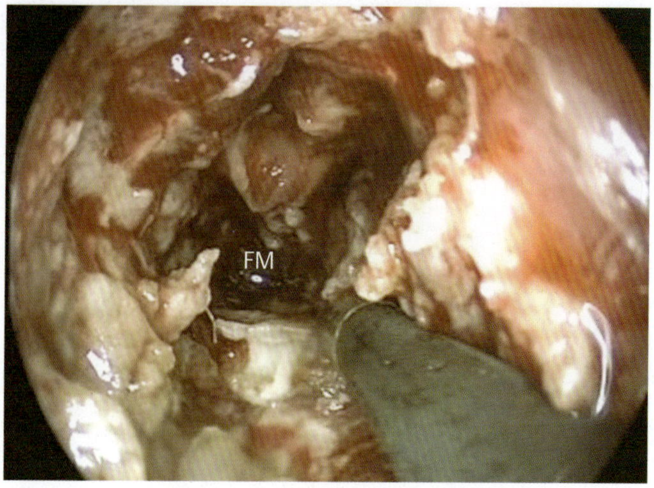

Fig. 19E.12 Final view 1 after tumor removal.

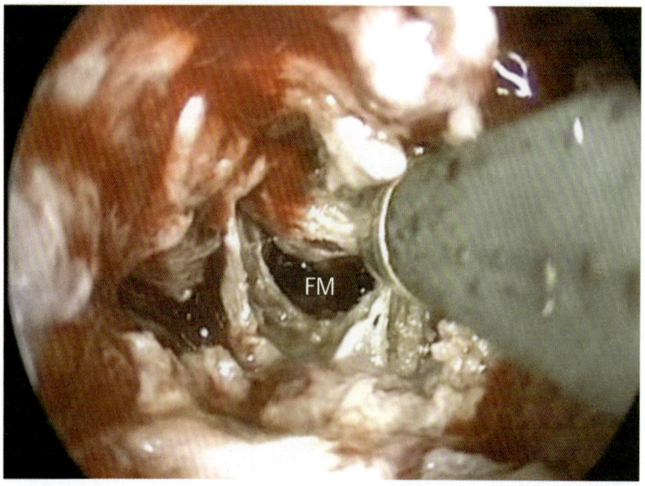

Fig. 19E.13 Final view 2 after tumor removal.

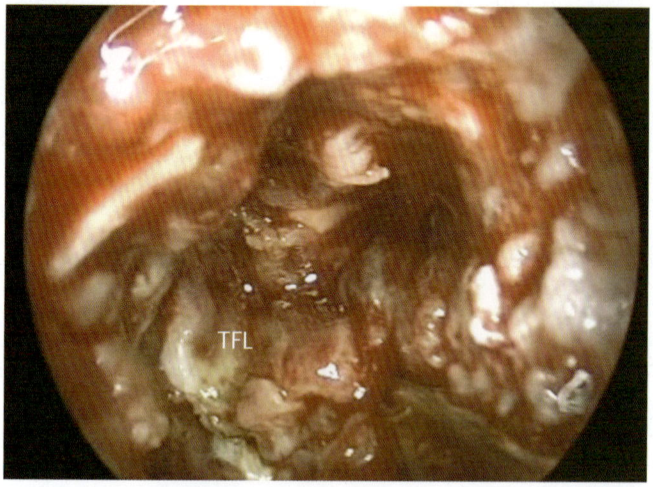

Fig. 19E.14 Tensor fascia lata (TFL) in situ.

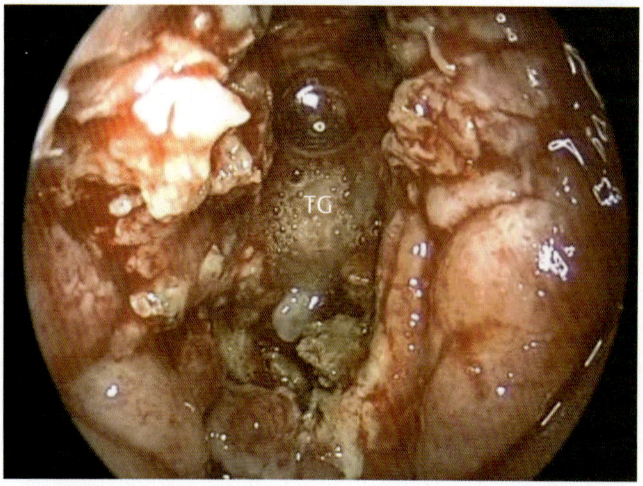

Fig. 19E.15 Application of tissue glue (TG) over the layers of repair.

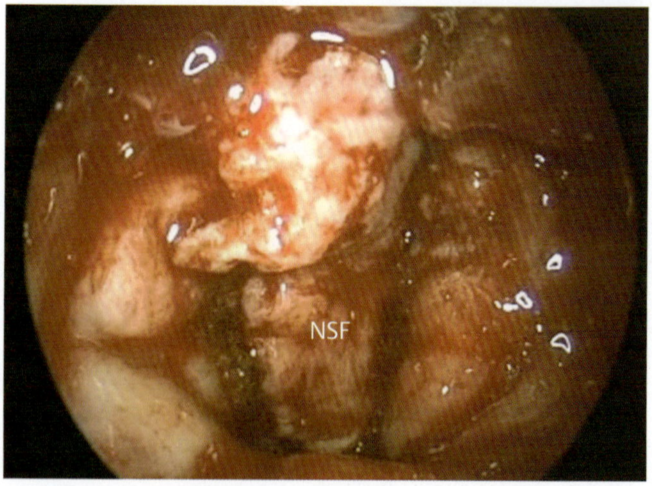

Fig. 19E.16 Bilateral nasoseptal flaps repositioned over defect prior to the application of the second layer of tissue glue.

Section VI

Orbital Region

Chapter 20 Approach to Orbital Lesions: Intraconal and Extraconal

Sarina K. Mueller and Benjamin S. Bleier

Anatomy

Extra- and Intraconal Space

The intraconal space is defined as the conical space within the musculofascial cone formed by the extraocular muscles and their surrounding fascia. The apex of the cone converges posteriorly at the orbital apex in a tendinous ring called the annulus of Zinn. The extraconal space is defined as the intraorbital space outside of the musculofascial cone. The intraconal space contains the ophthalmic artery, cranial nerves (CNs) II, III, VI (e.g., nasociliary nerve), and VI as well as orbital fat. The extraconal space contains lacrimal gland and sac, a portion of the superior ophthalmic vein, the lacrimal and frontal branches of cranial nerve VI as well as fat.

Extraocular Muscles

All extraocular muscles, except the inferior oblique muscle, originate in the orbital apex. The rectus muscles (superior, medial, lateral, and inferior recti) originate in the annulus of Zinn. The superior rectus and levator muscles are innervated by the superior division of CN III (oculomotor nerve). The inferior rectus, medial rectus, and inferior oblique muscles are innervated by the inferior division of CN III. The lateral rectus is innervated by CN VI (abducens nerve). The cranial nerves to the rectus muscles enter the orbit posteriorly through the superior orbital fissure.

Neurovascular Supply

Considerable variability of the neurovascular supply to the medial and inferior rectus muscles is evident in the intraconal space. A mean of 1.5 arterial branches (range 1–4) was identified at a mean of 8.8 mm (range 4–15 mm) from the sphenoid face. The oculomotor nerve inserts at the level of the sphenoid face branching out with a large proximal trunk 5.5 ± 1.1 mm in length and multiple branches extending 13.2 ± 2.7 mm from the sphenoid face. The most anterior neurovascular pedicle extends anteriorly 17 mm (nerve) and 15 mm (artery), respectively.[1] However, these general branching patterns of the inferior division of the oculomotor nerve and inferomedial muscular trunk of the ophthalmic artery enable a conceptualization of the medial intraconal space into three zones. As lesions move from the anterior inferior to posterior superior zones, the complexity of the dissection and risk of neurovascular injury increase. These zones provide a guideline for safe medial rectus muscle (MRM) retraction relative to fixed landmarks of the sphenoid face.[1]

Advantages of Endoscopic Approaches

- Avoidance of scars.
- Improved visualization of certain landmarks.
- Enhanced visualization and illumination of posterior inferomedial orbit.
- Reduced morbidity and avoidance of globe/brain retraction.
- Surgery of concomitant sinonasal pathology or optic nerve decompression.

Indications

- Medial extraconal tumors.
- Inferomedial intraconal tumors.
- Intraconal tumors medial to the optic nerve and inferior to the "plane of resectability."
- Selected inferolateral tumors.

Contraindications

- Lateral extraconal tumors.
- Superolateral intraconal tumors above the "plane of resectability."
- Lateral intraconal tumors.

Key Principles

- Functional sinus surgery.
- Posterior septectomy.
- Orbital decompression.
- Resection of orbital process of palatine bone.
- Medial rectus retraction.
- Blunt dissection of tumor.
- In appropriate cases, preservation of inferomedial bony strut.
- In appropriate cases, reconstruction of medial orbit.

Surgical Approach

Preoperative Preparation

- Computed tomography (CT) scan to verify the bony anatomy of the orbit and surrounding sinonasal structures. Three-dimensional reconstruction is useful to assess the relationship of the lesion to the long axis of the optic nerve.
- Magnetic resonance imaging (MRI) scan, particularly fat-suppression sequences to identify and characterize the intraorbital tumor. Contrast enhancement may facilitate the localization of the ophthalmic artery, which should be avoided during intraconal surgery because of its position adjacent to the optic nerve (**Fig. 20.1a, b**).
- Angiography may be useful when ruling out dolichoectatic ophthalmic artery aneurysms.

Operative Technique

Functional Endoscopic Sinus Surgery

- The first step is a functional endoscopic sinus surgery (FESS) to gain access to the lamina papyracea, the maxillary sinus, and the optic canal. Like in any other sinonasal surgery, decongestion and optimization of hemostasis are important before starting the procedure. We recommend elevation of the head and topicalization using 1:1,000 fluorescein-labeled epinephrine-soaked neuropatties. A local anesthetic may also be injected into the axilla of the middle turbinate to minimize bleeding from the anterior ethmoid arterial region. This part of the surgery may be performed with a 0-degree endoscope. Septoplasty or middle turbinate resection may be performed as needed. Middle turbinate resection should only be performed when necessary, as removal carries the risk of olfactory disruption, frontal sinus obstruction, and postoperative epistaxis. The uncinate process is resected at its insertion on the maxillary line. Unlike in traditional endoscopic sinus surgery, the superior insertion of the uncinate process is left in place. This protects the frontal recess from the secondary obstruction by orbital fat prolapse.

The maxillary sinus should be opened in all cases to prevent the sinus from iatrogenic maxillary obstruction. The ethmoid bulla, basal lamella, and posterior ethmoid cells are removed completely. It is important to extend the dissection to the entire skull base. A wide opening of the sphenoid sinus and a partial resection of the superior turbinate should be performed as a maximal orbital apex decompression is necessary.

Medial Orbital Decompression

The mucosa may be stripped from the lamina papyracea to the lateral skull base to avoid postoperative mucocele formation. The resection of the lamina papyracea may be performed by creating a fracture and then removing the thin bony fragments with a Blakesley forceps or a ball-tipped probe (**Fig. 20.2**). The sphenoid suture line may be identified as the transition of the thinner lamina papyracea to the thicker sphenoid bone. After removal of the lamina papyracea, the periorbital fascial layer can be identified. With a close look, the medial rectus muscle and several venous structures might be identified through the periorbita. These should be spared during the following periorbital incision.

Orbital Process Palatine Bone

The bony limitation to the inferomedial orbital access and inferolateral retraction vector is caused by the orbital process of the palatine bone. This process contributes to the floor of the orbit and is bordered anteriorly by the sphenopalatine

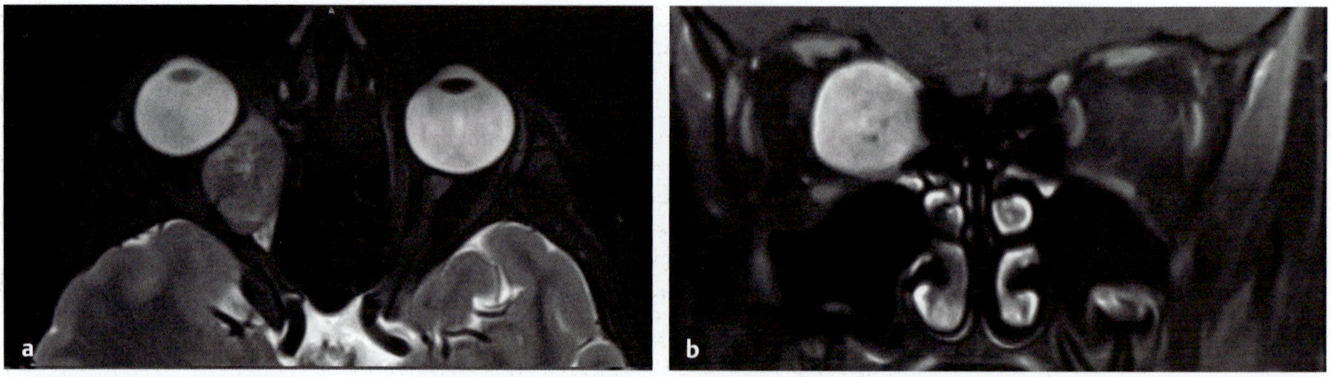

Fig. 20.1 **(a)** Axial and **(b)** coronal preoperative MRI scans of a right intraconal tumor. Histology showing an orbital schwannoma.

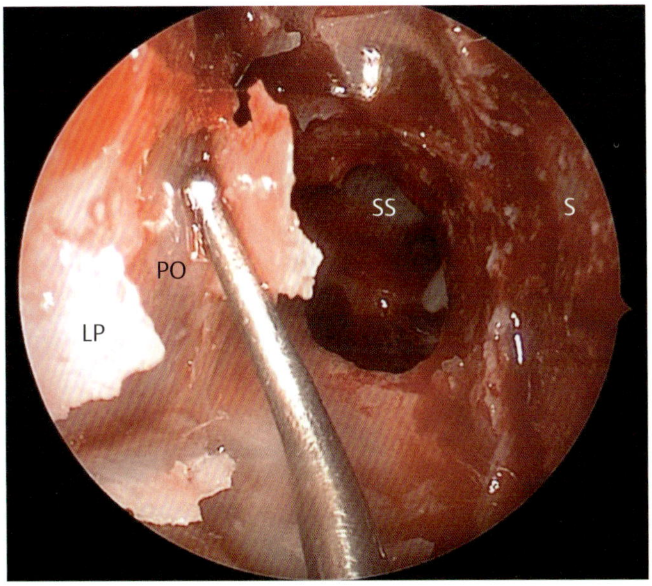

Fig. 20.2 Removal of the right lamina papyracea (LP) using a ball-tipped probe. The periorbita (PO) can be identified beneath.

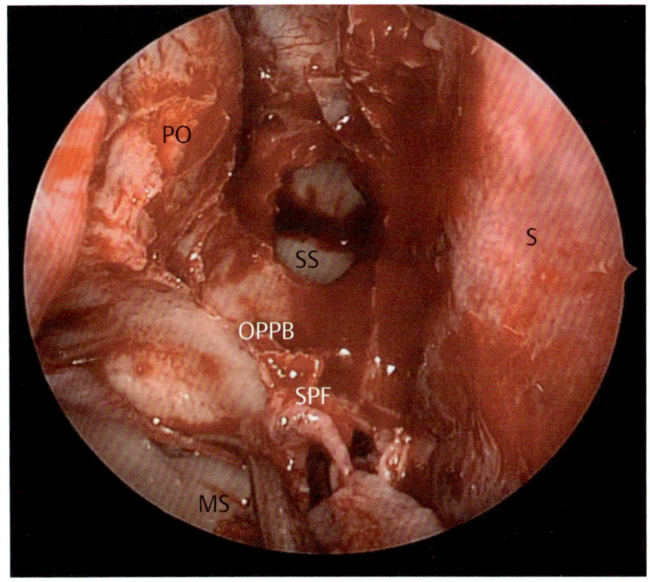

Fig. 20.3 Stripping of the maxillary sinus (MS) mucosa using a ball-tipped probe before resection of the orbital process of the palatine bone (OPPB). The process is located supero-antero-laterally to the sphenopalatine foramen (SPF).

foramen, posterior superiorly by the maxillary wall, and laterally by the infraorbital canal (**Fig. 20.3**). The superior maxillary sinus mucosa may be reflected laterally before bone resection and may be redraped afterward. This procedure facilitates remucosalization, reduces postoperative crusting, and expedites postoperative healing.[2] The thick process may be drilled via a transmaxillary approach with a high-speed drill to thin the bone. Downfracturing of the residual bone in an anterior inferior vector enables resection while avoiding injury to the sphenopalatine neurovascular bundle and infraorbital nerve.[3]

Posterior Septectomy

A posterior septectomy may be performed to allow a four-handed approach with bimanual dissection to the orbit and orbital apex and an improved surgically accessible area (**Fig. 20.4**). The septal mucosa may be bilaterally incised in a vertical fashion approximately 2 cm anterior of the epipharynx. A Cottle elevator may be used to outfracture parts of the vomer and the lamina perpendicularis of the ethmoid bone to create a window of 2 × 2 cm into the bony septum. The superior, inferior, anterior, and posterior bones may be preserved. This transseptal approach is advocated for all intraconal tumors. A conceptual two-dimensional plane may be drawn between the contralateral nare and the long axis of the optic nerve. Tumors that originate medial and/or inferior to this plane are candidates for endoscopic resection regardless of their inferolateral extent.

Medial Rectus Muscle Retraction

The medial rectus muscle represents the doorway to the intraconal space. To provide sufficient access to the intraconal space, several retraction techniques have been described in the literature. These include retraction at the globe insertion point using a vessel loop, static transseptal and retrochoanal retraction using a vessel loop, and dynamic four-handed transseptal retraction using an instrument such as a ball-tipped probe.[4–7] The four-handed transseptal approach with medial rectus muscle retraction with a ball tip probe allows for the greatest intraconal space exposure while ensuring protection of the neuromuscular inputs to the MRM[6] (**Fig. 20.5**). The dissection may be carried out bluntly with a ball probe and a neuropatty. Depending on the location of the tumor, retraction may be carried out inferiorly or superiorly. During resection of the tumor, tonic MRM retraction should be relieved intermittently to prevent neurovascular traction injury and to allow perfusion of the globe and other orbital contents.[7]

Tumor Resection

Resection of the intra- or extraconal tumor may be performed using blunt instruments like the ball probe and

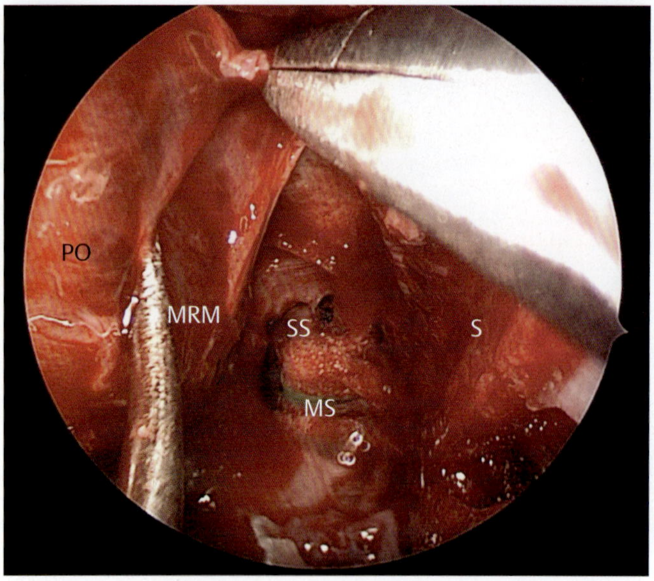

Fig. 20.4 Bimanual dissection of the surgeon in a four-handed approach after creation of a posterior septectomy. Sphenoid sinus (SS) is covered with a neuropatty.

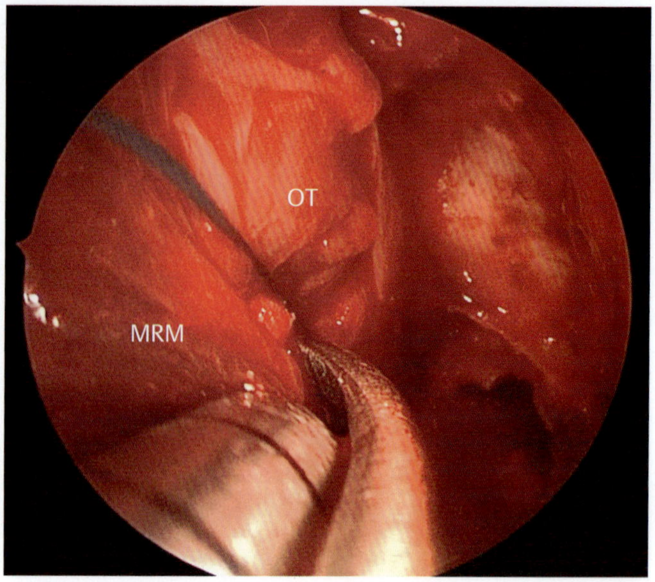

Fig. 20.5 Medial rectus muscle (MRM) retraction using a ball-tipped probe, the suction, and a neuropatty. The MRM is carefully separated from the orbital tumor (OT) assuring to preserve the neurovascular supply to the muscle.

angled Penfield dissector. The capsule of the tumor should be identified and carefully followed. The suction may be used as a second dissecting instrument as are neuropatties (**Fig. 20.6**). A major advantage of this technique may be the simultaneous dissection and improvement of vision because of hemostasis control. The four-handed approach enables bimanual dissection while providing good visualization with the endoscope. Depending on the location of the tumor, 0-degree or angled scopes may be used. An angled scope may be more useful for more anterior and lateral lesions. Cauterization should be avoided to avoid injury to the ophthalmic trunk and/or optic nerve.

Multidisciplinary Team Approach

The multidisciplinary team approach is critical for surgical planning and implementation. Depending on the location of the tumor, a combined resection with ophthalmic, plastic-, or neurosurgeons may be necessary. A multidisciplinary approach may facilitate dissection of tumors that reach too anterior, superior, or lateral for a solely endoscopic approach. The second surgical access vector, for example, through a transcaruncular approach, may also be used to relocate the tumor more medially or posteriorly using a cotton swab to protect the optic nerve with a retractor and to facilitate lateral dissection using blunt instruments (**Fig. 20.7a, b**).

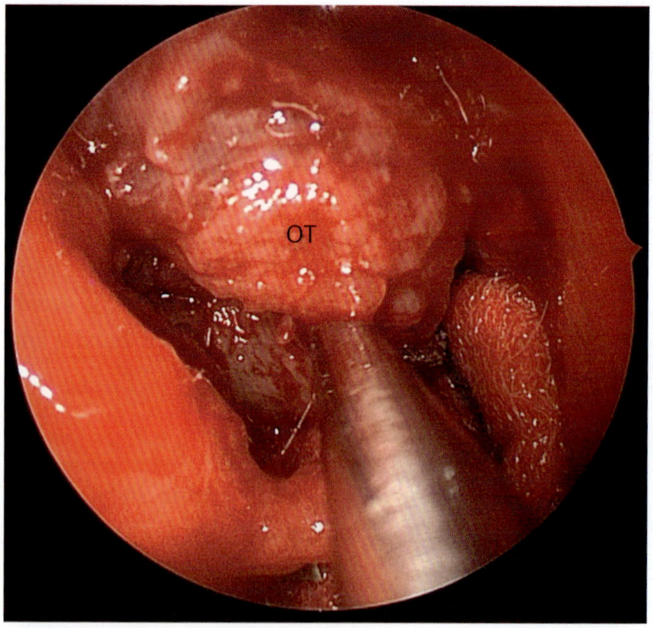

Fig. 20.6 Blunt dissection of the orbital tumor (OT) using an angled Penfield dissector and a neuropatty.

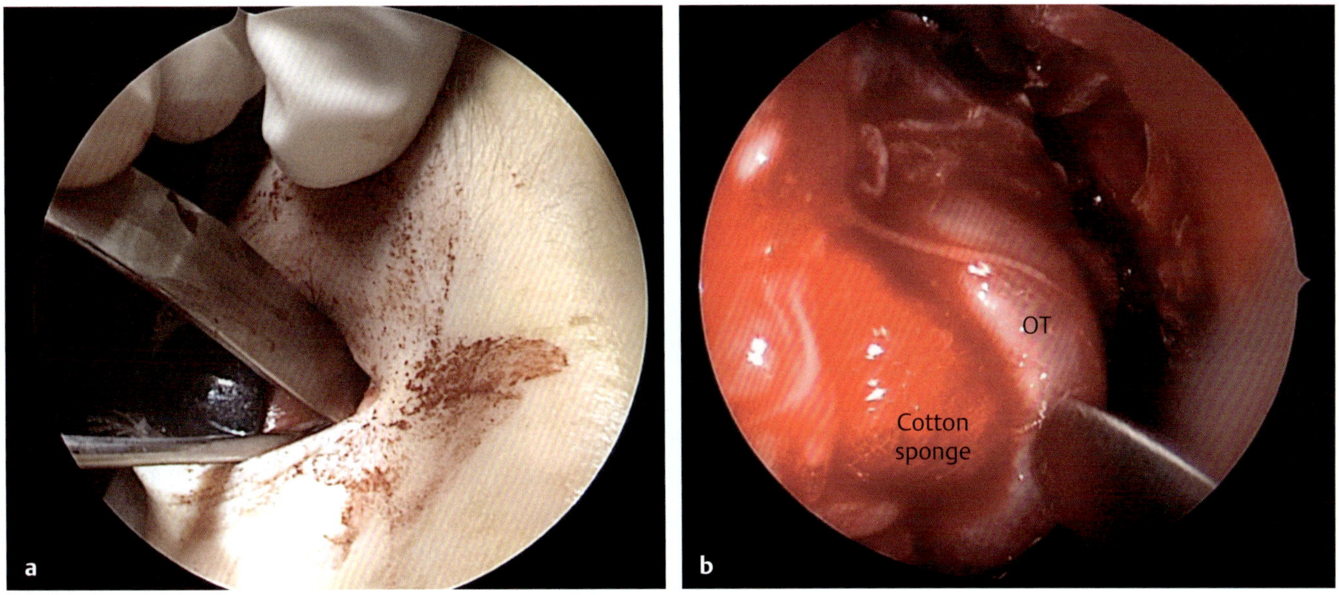

Fig. 20.7 Multidisciplinary, six-handed approach combining a **(a)** transcaruncular approach by the oculoplastic surgeon with **(b)** endoscopic, transnasal approach by the rhinologist. To facilitate endoscopic resection, the orbital tumor (OT) is pushed posteriorly and medially by the oculoplastic surgeon using a cotton sponge.

Medial and Inferior Orbital Reconstruction

Intraconal tumor resection is associated with a higher risk of postoperative diplopia and enophthalmos than extraconal lesions.[8] Therefore, a higher rate of immediate medial and inferior orbital reconstruction is needed. For the majority of extraconal lesions, a formal reconstruction is not required. A nasoseptal flap has been shown to be capable of providing complete coverage of the entire medial and inferior orbit.[9,10] The flap comprises nasal septum mucoperichondrium and mucoperiosteum and is pedicled on the nasoseptal artery, a branch of the posterior septal artery. The flap may be raised using a needle-tipped Bovie and Cottle elevator and may be carried out as far anteriorly as needed[11] (**Fig. 20.8**). This technique has the advantage of providing a “delayed” or soft reconstruction as the flap contracts around the orbitotomy. This provides for immediate blood egress and resolution of edema while avoiding the development of an orbital compartment syndrome, which could occur with immediate rigid reconstruction. However, reconstruction with a half-rigid, self-dissolving material (Gelfilm, Pfizer, 0.075 mm) may be used alternatively.

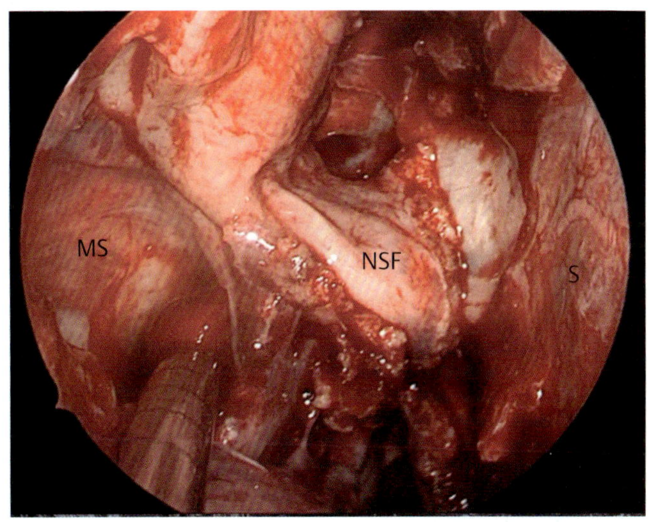

Fig. 20.8 Example of mucosal flap reconstruction using an ipsilateral nasoseptal flap (NSF) to the left orbit following binarial, transseptal resection of an extraconal cavernous hemangioma.

Tips and Pearls

- Early uncontrolled incision of the periorbita should be avoided as herniated orbital fat may obscure visualization of the surgical field.
- Cauterization within the orbit should be avoided to prevent thermal damage to the sensitive orbital structures.
- Packing should be avoided intra- and postoperatively to minimize pressure on the orbit and allow drainage of accumulated blood.
- Patients should avoid nose blowing for 3 weeks.

- Patients should sneeze and cough with an open mouth for 3 weeks to minimize intrasinonasal pressure and reduce the risk of orbital emphysema. Similarly, continuous positive airway pressure (CPAP) should be avoided for 4 weeks.
- The affected eye should never be patched after orbital surgery to not obscure the detection of postoperative vision loss or hemorrhage.

Postoperative Care

- Discharge medications may include an oral antistaphylococcal antibiotic and steroid taper if considered necessary.
- The first postoperative follow-up visit should be scheduled within 1 week after surgery. Nasal saline irrigations may be started after the first follow-up visit independent of medial orbit reconstruction.
- At 1 week, the inferior airway may be carefully debrided to assist with breathing and mucosal healing. Clot adjacent to the orbit or optic nerve should be left in place to be irrigated out by the patient over the subsequent 3 to 4 weeks.
- Patients should have limited activity for 2 weeks and should not resume anticoagulant medications until several days after the surgery.
- A postoperative MRI scan may be performed at 3 months after the surgery to ensure complete resection of the tumor.

Complications

- Similar to complications of routine endoscopic sinus surgery including bleeding, infection (e.g., meningitis), cerebrospinal fluid (CSF) leak, mucocele formation, orbital ecchymosis, hematoma, and epiphora.
- Vision loss to blindness may occur from physical damage of the globe or the optic nerve including direct trauma, thermal/electrical damage from cautery, hemorrhage, or aggressive intraoperative retraction. Intravenous high-dose steroids may be administered in these cases to decrease perineural edema and associated neural injury.
- Diplopia may be caused by direct injury to the muscle belly, damage to the muscular neurovascular inputs, changes of the extraocular muscle vectors, or globe malposition. Strabismus surgery may be considered in stable and nonrecurrent disease 8 to 10 months after the surgery.
- Enophthalmos and hypoglobus may result from extensive orbital decompression and tumor resection. Medial orbital wall reconstruction may minimize enophthalmos in selected cases, especially after intraconal tumor resection.
- Incomplete resection is more likely to be associated with intraconal than extraconal lesions (31.25 vs. 14.29%, respectively).

References

1. Bleier BS, Healy DYJ Jr, Chhabra N, Freitag S. Compartmental endoscopic surgical anatomy of the medial intraconal orbital space. Int Forum Allergy Rhinol 2014;4(7):587–591
2. Palmer N, Chiu A. Atlas of endoscopic sinus and skull base surgery. Philadelphia, PA. Elsevier; 2013;255
3. Mueller S, Freitag S, Bleier B. Morphometric analysis of the orbital process of the palatine bone and its relationship to endoscopic orbital apex surgery. Ophthal Plast Reconstr Surg 2018;34(3):254–257
4. Lenzi R, Bleier BS, Felisati G, Muscatello L. Purely endoscopic trans-nasal management of orbital intraconal cavernous haemangiomas: a systematic review of the literature. Eur Arch Otorhinolaryngol 2016;273(9):2319–2322
5. Yao WC, Bleier BS. Endoscopic management of orbital tumors. Curr Opin Otolaryngol Head Neck Surg 2016;24(1):57–62
6. Lin GC, Freitag SK, Kocharyan A, Yoon MK, Lefebvre DR, Bleier BS. Comparative techniques of medial rectus muscle retraction for endoscopic exposure of the medial intraconal space. Am J Rhinol Allergy 2016;30(3):226–229
7. Shafi F, Zaidi S, Mehta P, Ahluwalia HS, Ahmed SK. Endoscopic medial rectus sling: a window into the intraconal orbital apex. Ophthal Plast Reconstr Surg 2016;32(3):233–236
8. Bleier BS, Castelnuovo P, Battaglia P, et al. Endoscopic endonasal orbital cavernous hemangioma resection: global experience in techniques and outcomes. Int Forum Allergy Rhinol 2016;6(2):156–161
9. Chhabra N, Healy DY, Freitag SK, Bleier BS. The nasoseptal flap for reconstruction of the medial and inferior orbit. Int Forum Allergy Rhinol 2014;4(9):763–766
10. Healy DY Jr, Lee NG, Freitag SK, Bleier BS. Endoscopic bimanual approach to an intraconal cavernous hemangioma of the orbital apex with vascularized flap reconstruction. Ophthal Plast Reconstr Surg 2014;30(4):e104–e106
11. Hadad G, Bassagasteguy L, Carrau RL, et al. A novel reconstructive technique after endoscopic expanded endonasal approaches: vascular pedicle nasoseptal flap. Laryngoscope 2006;116(10):1882–1886

Chapter 21 Endonasal Endoscopic Surgeries of the Orbit

Sien Hui Tan, Adzreil Bakri, and Prepageran Narayanan

Case 21A

Endoscopic Transnasal Approach to a Sharp Intraconal Foreign Body

History

A 42-year-old man presented with an intraconal sharp foreign body in his right eye secondary to an alleged industrial accident. His preoperative vision was light perception in his right eye. A computed tomography scan revealed a right intraconal foreign body (**Fig. 21A.1, Fig. 21A.2, and Fig. 21A.3**). Postoperatively, he showed improvement in vision to finger counting. In this case, it was particularly crucial that the foreign body was successfully removed to prevent the eye from being sacrificed for infection control. This was a challenging procedure because of the deep location of the foreign body within the intraconal space of the eye, its close proximity to the optic nerve, and the sharp nature of the object.

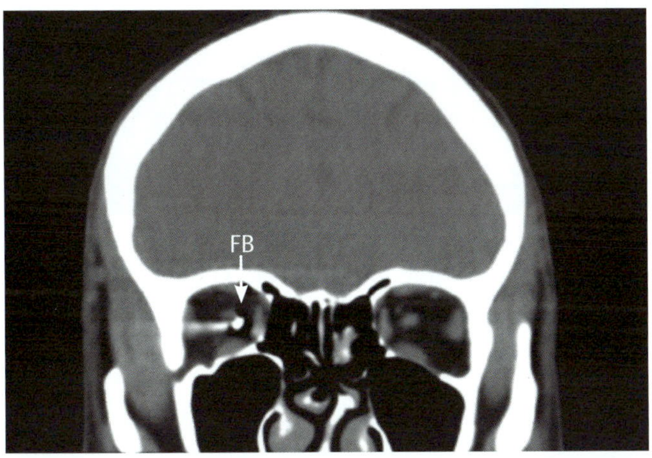

Fig. 21A.1 Coronal CT scan showing a right intraconal foreign body (FB).

Surgical Steps

1. The patient is positioned supine under general anesthesia.
2. The nose is decongested with nasal packing as per the institution's standard methods.
3. The medial rectus muscle is isolated and a traction suture is placed. This is to allow intraoperative identification and elevation to provide adequate intraconal access and exposure (**Fig. 21A.4**).
4. Local anesthesia is infiltrated to the axilla of the middle turbinate.
5. The middle turbinate is gently medialized. An uncinectomy and a wide middle meatal antrostomy are performed.

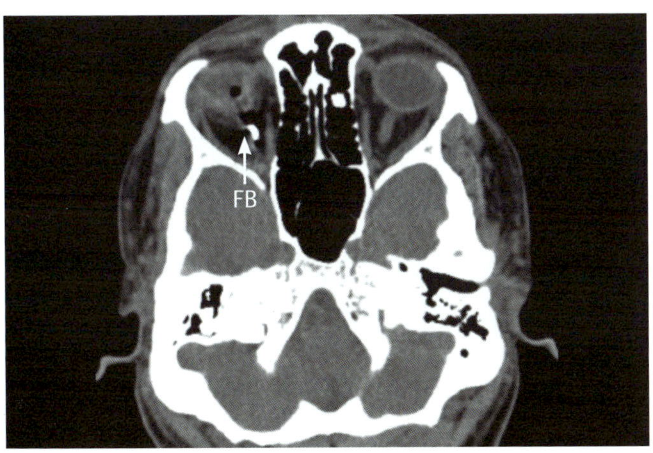

Fig. 21A.2 Axial CT scan showing a right intraconal foreign body (FB) in close proximity to the optic nerve.

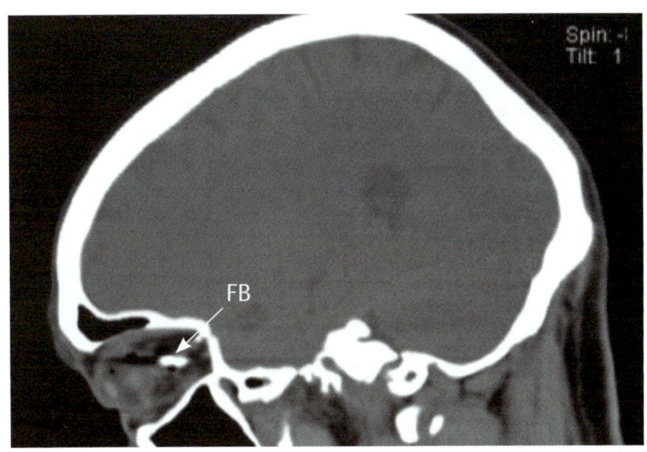

Fig. 21A.3 Sagittal CT scan demonstrating a right intraconal foreign body (FB).

6. Next, both anterior and posterior ethmoidectomy are carried out to expose the medial orbital wall.
7. A sphenoidectomy is performed for visualization of the optic canal and internal carotid artery (**Fig. 21A.5**).
8. The lamina papyracea is removed with a Freer elevator to expose the periorbita. Entry into the lamina papyracea should be below the level of the ethmoid foramina to prevent injury to the ethmoidal arteries. This is to lessen the risk of retrobulbar bleeding and subsequently vision loss.
9. The periorbita and extraconal fat are carefully dissected to expose the medial rectus muscle (**Fig. 21A.6**). The extraconal fat can sometimes be reduced with bipolar cautery to allow easier identification of the medial rectus muscle.
10. The medial rectus muscle is elevated to reach into the intraconal orbital space. Intraconal lesions present a greater challenge, and it is imperative that the dissection is not through the muscle fibers but between the medial and inferior rectus muscles (**Fig. 21A.7**).

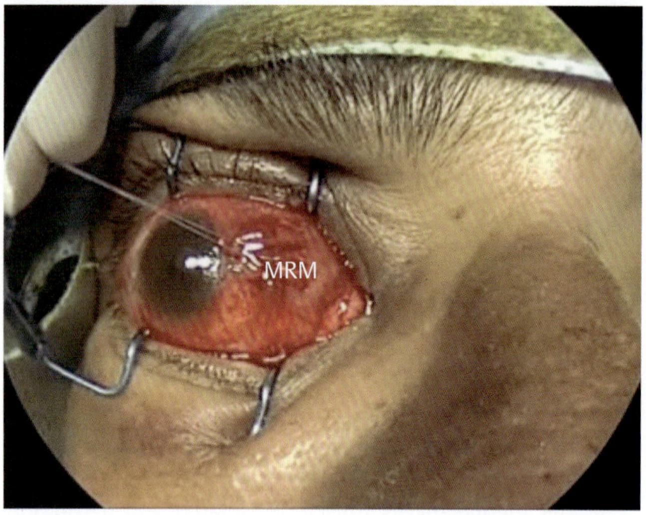

Fig. 21A.4 The medial rectus muscle (MRM) is placed with a suture.

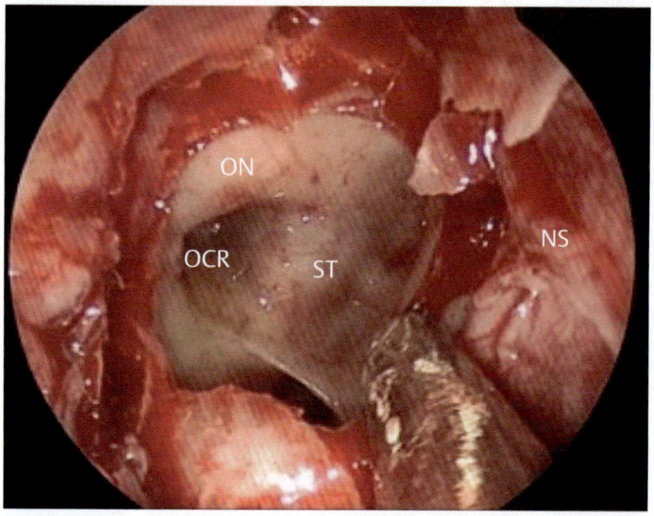

Fig. 21A.5 Endoscopic view of the optic nerve (ON) and opticocarotid recess (OCR) in the right sphenoid sinus.

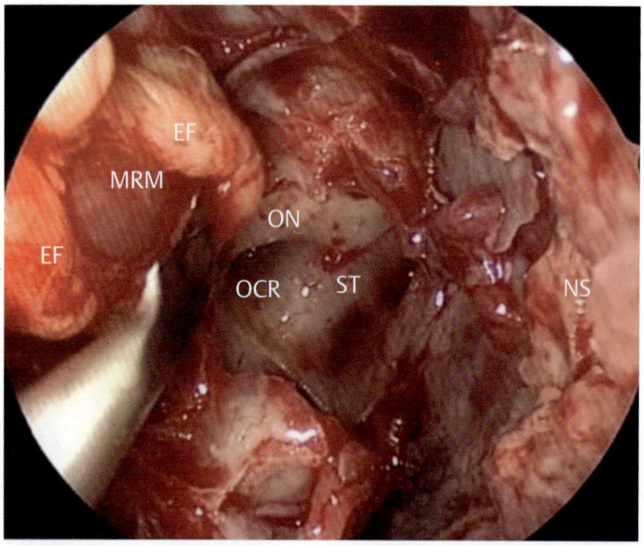

Fig. 21A.6 Endoscopic view of the medial rectus muscle (MRM) after careful dissection of the periorbita and extraconal fat (EF).

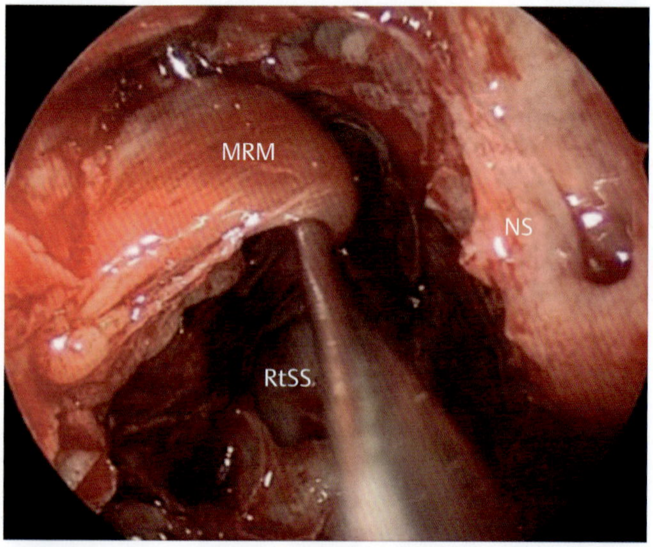

Fig. 21A.7 Elevation of the medial rectus muscle (MRM) to gain intraconal access.

11. The intraconal fat is gently debrided with a microdebrider and meticulously explored. The foreign body was eventually identified near the optic nerve and dissected out with a squint hook (**Fig. 21A.8** and **Fig. 21A.9**).
12. The surgeon should be thorough but prudent in his or her exploration to avoid injury to the optic nerve and the extraocular muscles. The lateral border of the dissection is the optic nerve, and it is crucial to avoid crossing the plane of the optic nerve.
13. Upon successful removal of the foreign body, the intraorbital optic nerve is identified and preserved (**Fig. 21A.10**).
14. A middle turbinate flap is then utilized to cover the orbit area and keep the middle rectus muscle in position (**Fig. 21A.11**).
15. Meticulous hemostasis is secured with adrenaline-soaked gauze, bipolar cauterization, and Surgicel.
16. An X-ray was performed postoperatively to confirm removal of the foreign body (**Fig. 21A.12a, b**).

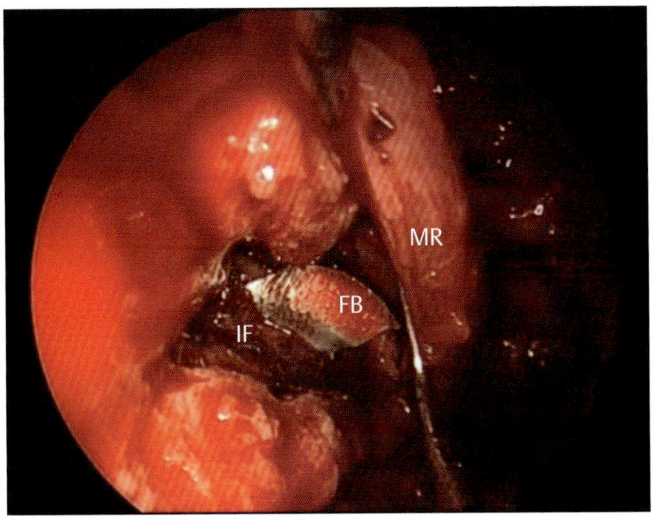

Fig. 21A.8 Foreign body (FB) identified after gentle debridement of the intraconal fat (IF) with a microdebrider and dissected out with a squint hook.

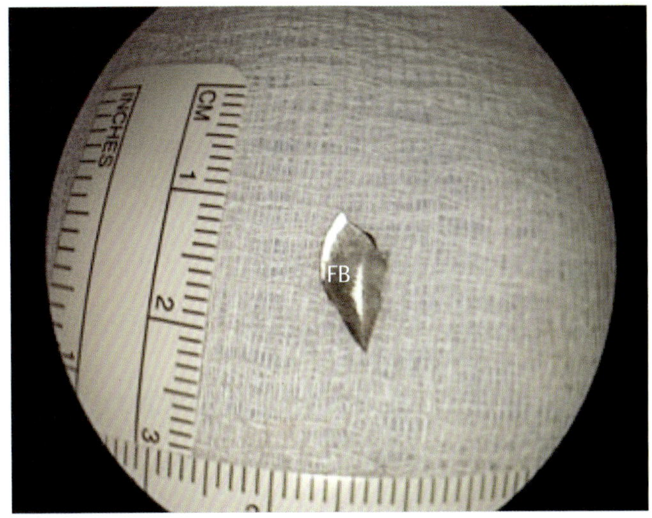

Fig. 21A.9 A sharp foreign body (FB) measuring 1 × 0.5 cm.

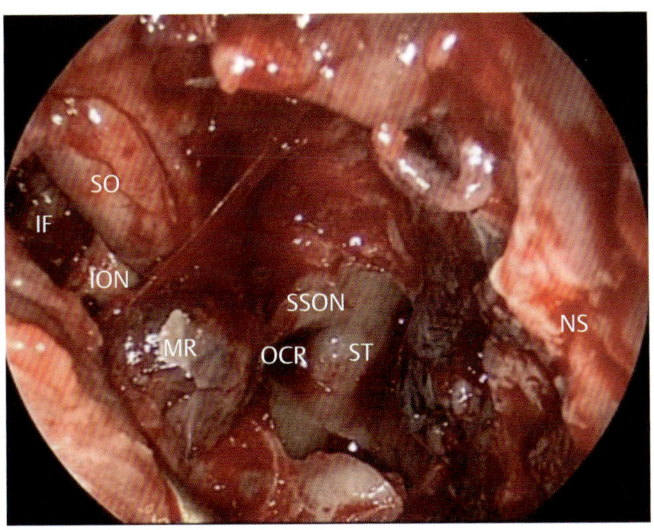

Fig. 21A.10 Postoperative view of the intact intraconal optic nerve (ION).

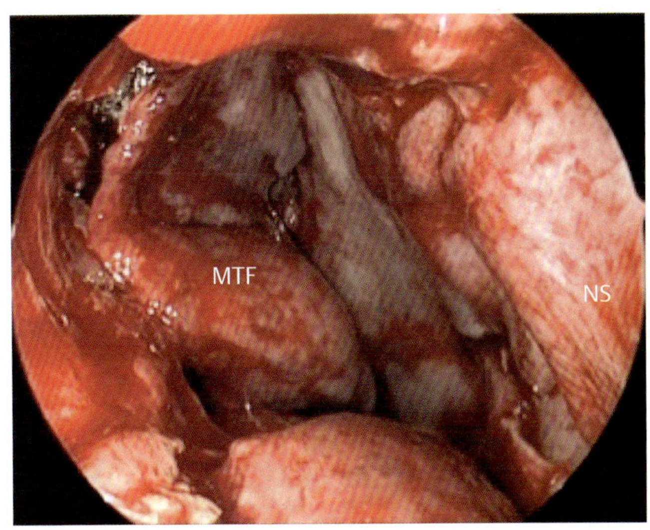

Fig. 21A.11 A middle turbinate flap (MTF) placed over the middle rectus muscle for support.

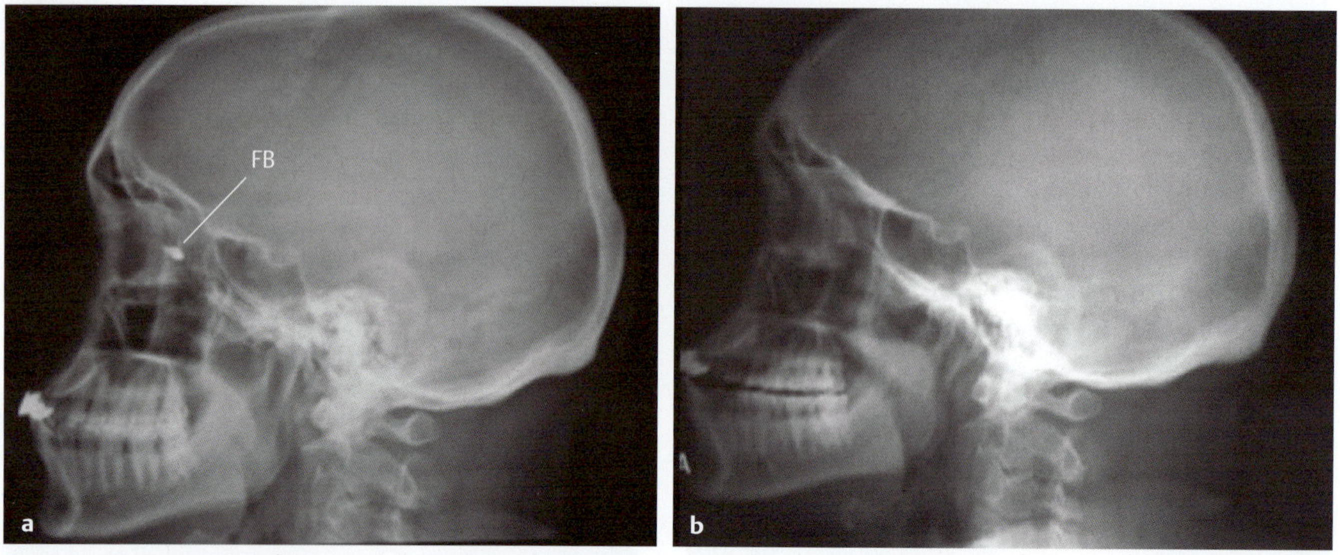

Fig. 21A.12 Comparison between **(a)** preoperative **(b)** and postoperative X-rays showing successful removal of the foreign body (FB).

Case 21B

Endoscopic Transnasal Approach to Superomedial Intraconal Tumors

History

A 9-year-old boy presented with diplopia and reduced eye movements secondary to an intraconal tumor in his right eye. His preoperative vision was 6/12 in his right eye. A magnetic resonance imaging (MRI) scan revealed a right superomedial intraconal tumor (**Fig. 21B.1, Fig. 21B.2, and Fig. 21B.3**). Postoperatively, he showed improvement of vision to 6/6. Intraconal lesions present a greater challenge as they are situated inside the muscle cone. The portal of surgical access depends on the location of the lesion. For superomedially located intraconal lesions, the surgical corridor between the middle rectus muscle and superior oblique muscle is utilized to gain access.

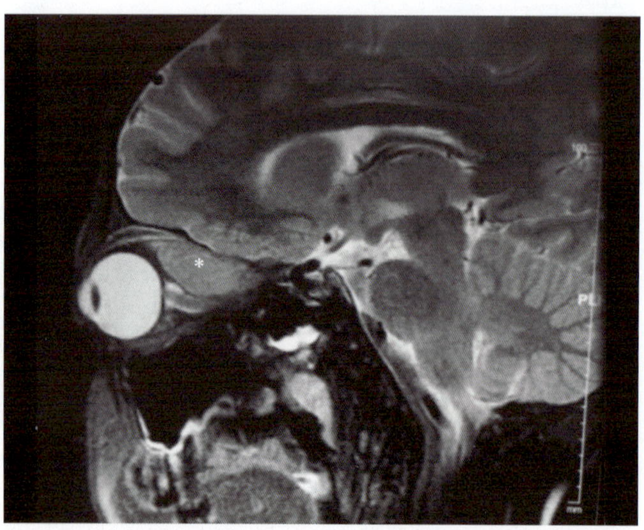

Fig. 21B.1 Sagittal MRI scan showing a right superior intraconal tumor (*).

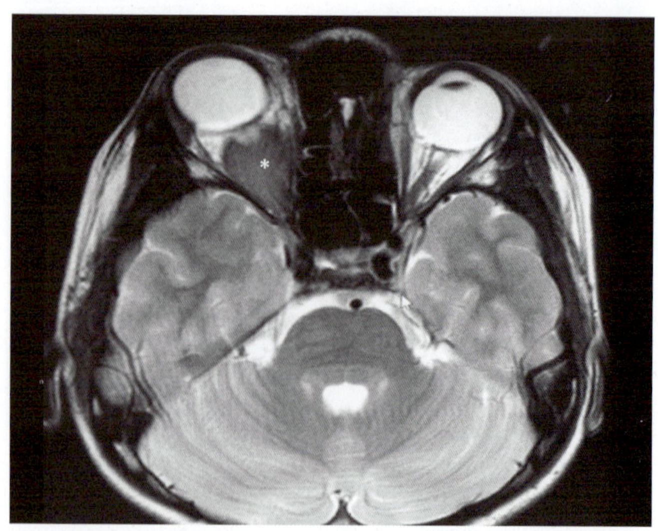

Fig. 21B.2 Axial MRI scan showing a right intraconal lesion (*).

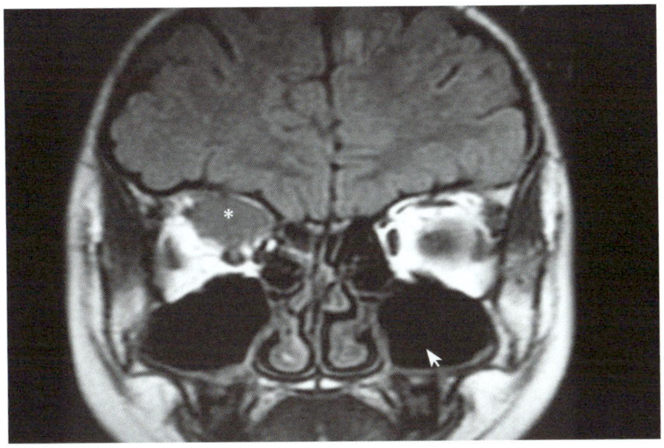

Fig. 21B.3 Coronal MRI scan demonstrating a right superomedial intraconal mass (*).

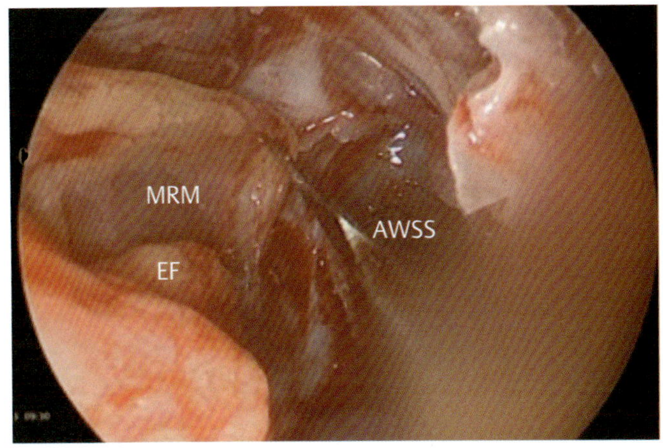

Fig. 21B.4 Endoscopic view of the right medial rectus muscle (MRM) after careful dissection of the periorbita and extraconal fat (EF).

Surgical Steps

1. The patient is positioned supine under general anesthesia.
2. The nose is decongested with nasal packing as per the institution's standard methods.
3. The medial rectus muscle and superior oblique muscle are first isolated. Traction sutures are then placed to aid in intraoperative identification.
4. Local anesthesia is infiltrated to the axilla of the middle turbinate.
5. The middle turbinate is gently medialized. An uncinectomy and a wide middle meatal antrostomy are performed.
6. Next, both anterior and posterior ethmoidectomy are carried out to expose the medial orbital wall.
7. A sphenoidectomy is performed for visualization of the optic canal and internal carotid artery.
8. The lamina papyracea is removed with a Freer elevator to expose the periorbita. Entry into the lamina papyracea should be below the level of the ethmoid foramina to prevent injury to the ethmoidal arteries. This is to lessen the risk of retrobulbar bleeding and subsequently, vision loss.
9. The periorbita and extraconal fat are then carefully dissected with a sickle knife to expose the medial rectus muscle (**Fig. 21B.4**). The extraconal fat can sometimes be reduced with bipolar cautery to allow easier identification of the medial rectus muscle.
10. Intraconal lesions are particularly challenging, and it is imperative that the dissection is not through the muscle fibers. In this case, the medial rectus muscle and superior oblique muscle are separated to access the intraconal space (**Fig. 21B.5**).

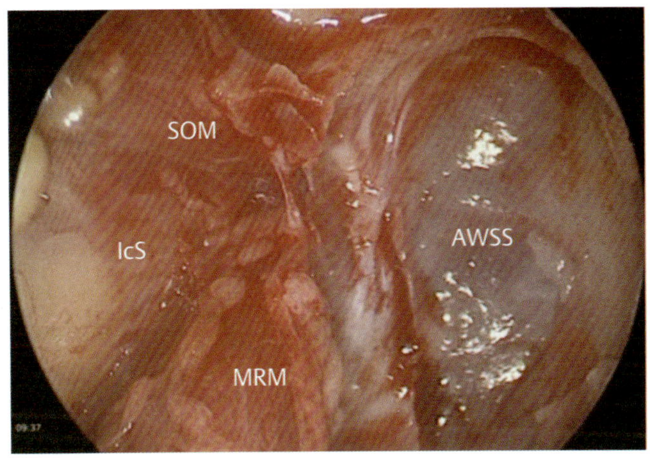

Fig. 21B.5 Separation of the medial rectus muscle (MRM) and superior oblique muscle (SOM) to gain access to the intraconal space (IcS).

11. The intraconal tumor is exposed and a biopsy is performed. Removal of the tumor is then carried out carefully with a Blakesley forceps (**Fig. 21B.6** and **Fig. 21B.7**).
12. The surgeon should be thorough but prudent in his or her exploration to avoid injury to the optic nerve and the extraocular muscles. The lateral border of the tumor dissection is the optic nerve, and it is imperative to avoid crossing the plane of the optic nerve.
13. Upon successful removal of the tumor, the intraorbital optic nerve is identified and preserved (**Fig. 21B.8** and **Fig. 21B.9**).
14. Meticulous hemostasis is secured with adrenaline-soaked gauze, bipolar cauterization, and Surgicel.
15. Packing is generally not advisable because of the potential for causing a rise in the intraocular pressure when there is a large orbital defect.

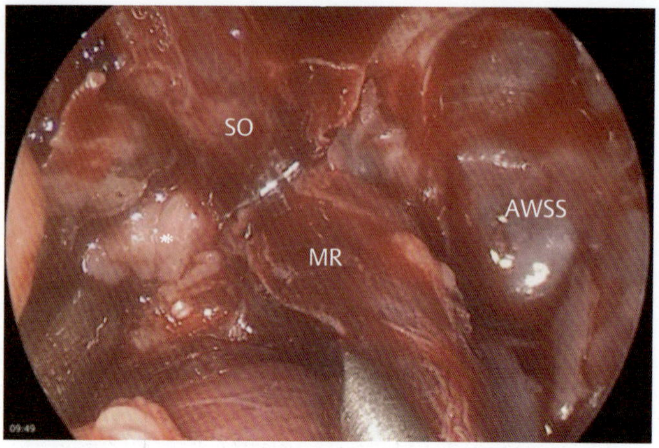

Fig. 21B.6 Tumor (*) exposed in the intraconal space.

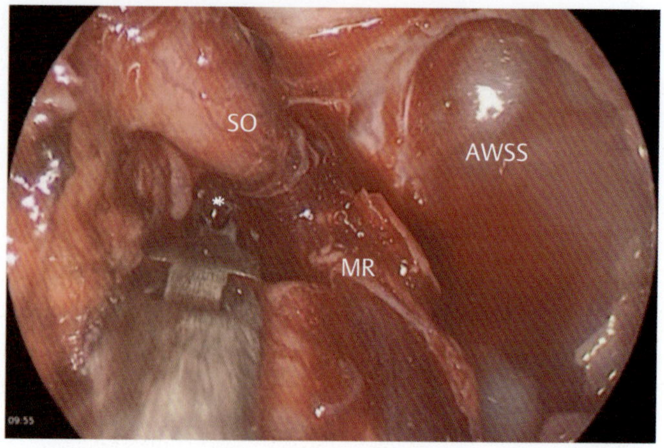

Fig. 21B.7 A Blakesley forceps is used to remove the intraconal tumor (*).

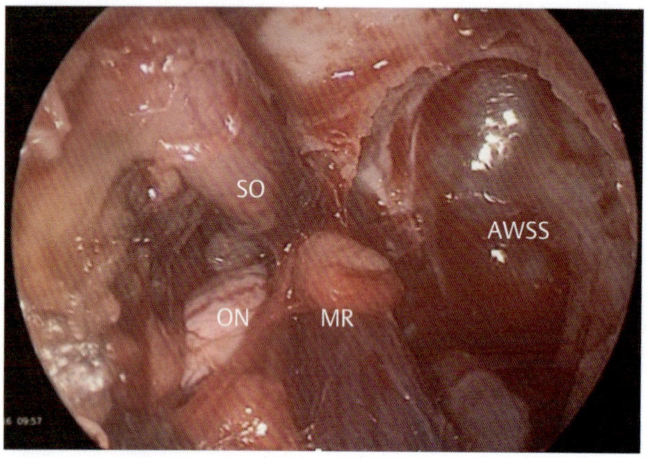

Fig. 21B.8 Endoscopic view of the intraconal optic nerve (ON).

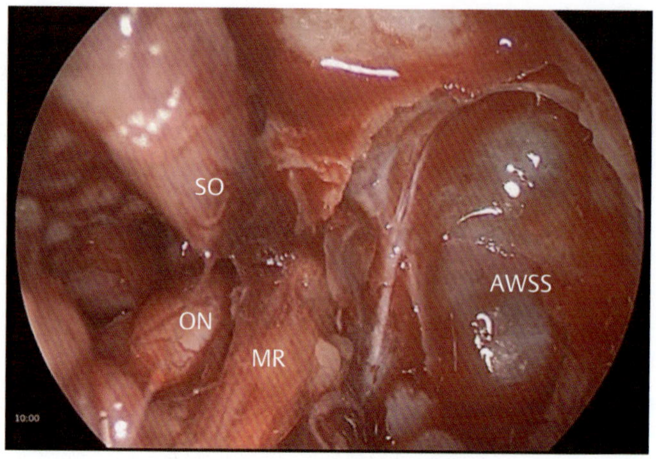

Fig. 21B.9 Postoperative view after complete removal of the tumor.

Case 21C

Endoscopic Transnasal Approach to Inferomedial Intraconal Tumors

History

A 36-year-old man presented with near-total vision loss secondary to an intraconal tumor in his right eye. A computed tomography (CT) scan revealed a right inferomedial intraconal tumor (**Fig. 21C.1, Fig. 21C.2, and Fig. 21C.3**). His preoperative vision was light perception only in his right eye. Postoperatively, he showed improvement of vision. Intraconal lesions render a greater challenge as they are situated inside the muscle cone. The portal of surgical access will depend on where the lesion is located. For inferomedially located intraconal lesions, the surgical corridor between the middle rectus muscle and inferior rectus muscle is utilized to gain access.

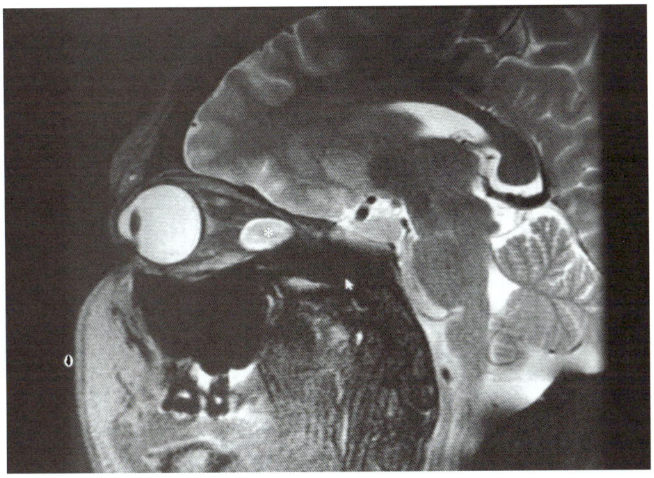

Fig. 21C.1 Sagittal MRI scan showing a right intraconal tumor (*).

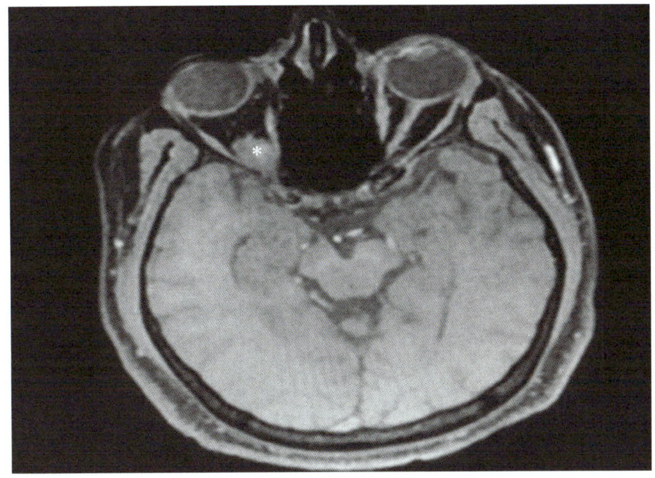

Fig. 21C.2 Axial MRI scan showing a right intraconal lesion (*).

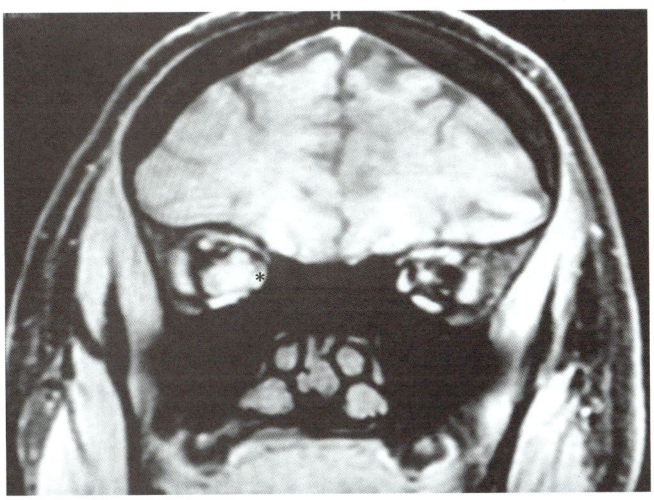

Fig. 21C.3 Coronal MRI scan demonstrating a right inferomedial intraconal mass (*).

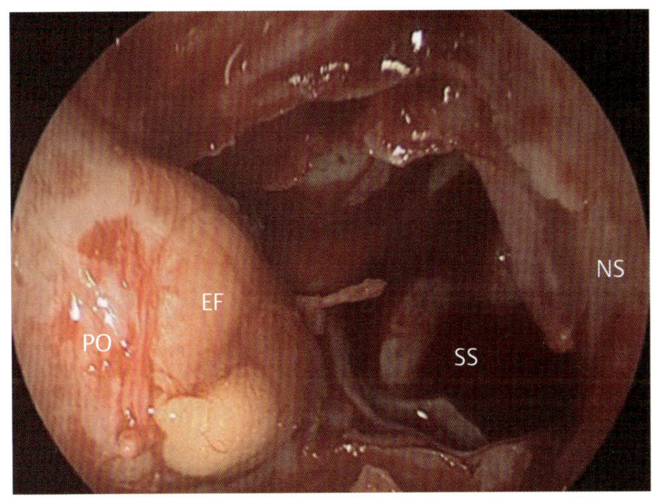

Fig. 21C.4 Endoscopic view of the extraconal fat (EF) after careful dissection of the periorbita (PO).

Surgical Steps

1. The patient is positioned supine under general anesthesia.
2. The nose is decongested with nasal packing as per the institution's standard methods.
3. The medial rectus muscle and inferior rectus muscle are first isolated. Traction sutures are then placed to aid in intraoperative identification.
4. Local anesthesia is infiltrated to the axilla of the middle turbinate.
5. The middle turbinate is gently medialized. An uncinectomy and a wide middle meatal antrostomy are performed.
6. Next, both anterior and posterior ethmoidectomy are carried out to expose the medial orbital wall.
7. A sphenoidectomy is performed for visualization of the optic canal and internal carotid artery.
8. The lamina papyracea is removed with a Freer elevator to expose the periorbita. Entry into the lamina papyracea should be below the level of the ethmoid foramina to prevent injury to the ethmoidal arteries. This is to lessen the risk of retrobulbar bleeding and subsequently, vision loss.
9. The periorbita and extraconal fat are then carefully dissected with a sickle knife to expose the medial rectus muscle (**Fig. 21C.4**).

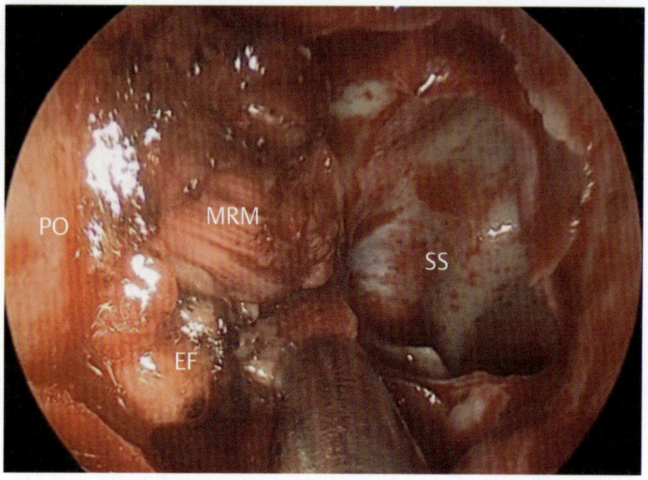

Fig. 21C.5 Endoscopic view of the medial rectus muscle (MRM) after removal of the extraconal fat (EF).

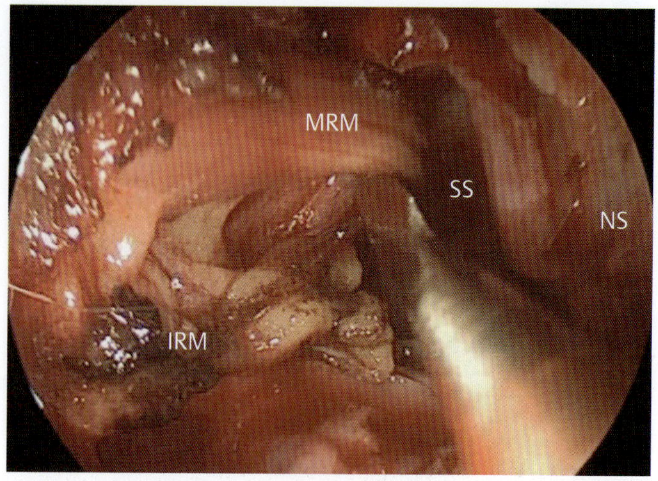

Fig. 21C.6 Separation of the medial rectus muscle (MRM) and inferior rectus muscle (IRM) to gain intraconal access.

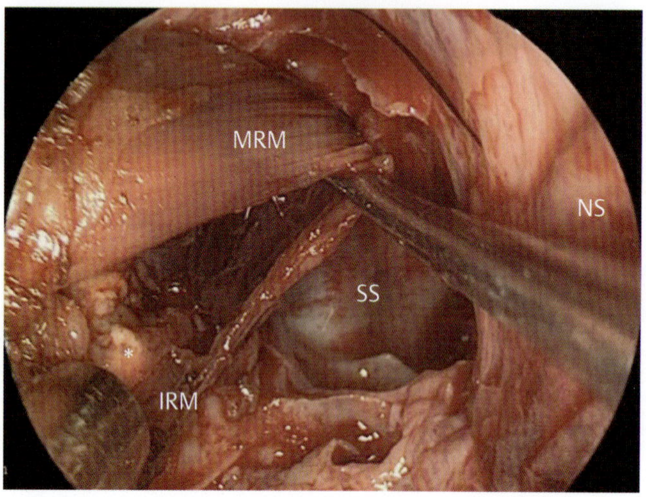

Fig. 21C.7 Tumor (*) is exposed in the intraconal space.

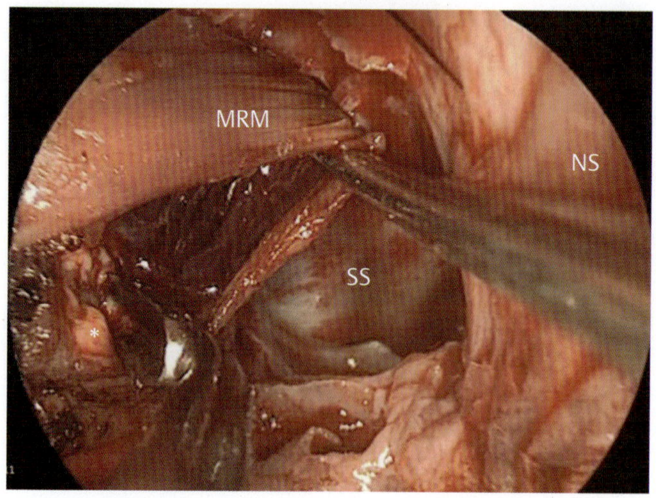

Fig. 21C.8 A curette is used to remove the intraconal tumor (*).

10. The extraconal fat is then gently dissected and the medial rectus muscle comes into view (**Fig. 21C.5**). The extraconal fat can sometimes be reduced with bipolar cautery to allow easier identification of the rectus muscles.
11. Intraconal lesions are particularly challenging, and it is important that the dissection is not through the muscle fibers. In this case, the medial rectus muscle and inferior rectus muscle are separated to access the intraconal space (**Fig. 21C.6**).
12. The intraconal tumor is exposed and a biopsy is performed. The tumor is then removed carefully with a curette (**Fig. 21C.7 and Fig. 21C.8**).
13. The surgeon should be thorough but prudent in his or her exploration to ensure successful removal of the tumor without injury to the optic nerve and the rectus muscles. The lateral border of the tumor dissection is the optic nerve, and it is vital to avoid crossing the plane of the optic nerve.
14. Meticulous hemostasis is secured with adrenaline-soaked gauze, bipolar cauterization, and Surgicel.
15. Packing is typically not advisable because of the potential for causing an increase in the intraocular pressure when there is a large orbital defect.

Case 21D

Endoscopic Transnasal Approach to Extraconal Tumors

History

A patient presented with visual impairment secondary to an extraconal tumor in his right eye. His preoperative vision was 6/36 and color vision was 0/17 in his right eye. A computed tomography scan revealed a right extraconal tumor (**Fig. 21D.1**). Fundoscopic examination of his eye demonstrated disc swelling (**Fig. 21D.2**). Postoperatively, he showed improvement of vision to 6/9 and color vision to 16/17. This approach may be used for all cases of extraconal tumors.

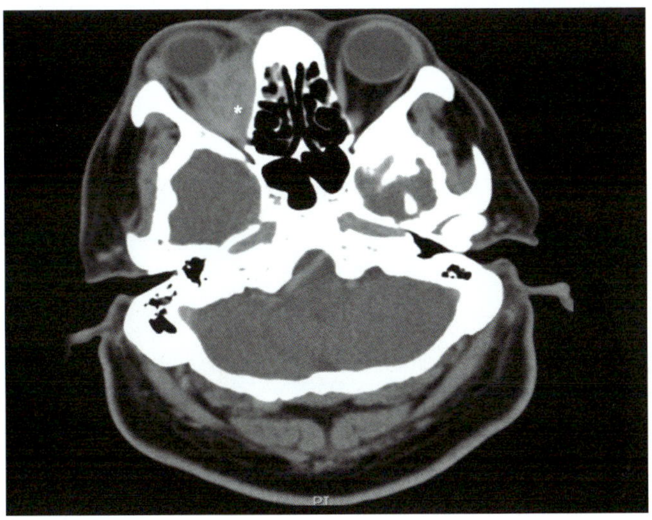

Fig. 21D.1 Axial CT scan showing a right extraconal tumor (*).

Surgical Steps

1. The patient is positioned supine under general anesthesia.
2. The nose is decongested with nasal packing as per the institution's standard methods.
3. Local anesthesia is infiltrated to the axilla of the middle turbinate.
4. The middle turbinate is gently medialized. An uncinectomy and a wide middle meatal antrostomy are performed.
5. Next, both anterior and posterior ethmoidectomy are carried out.
6. A sphenoidectomy is performed for visualization of the optic canal.
7. The lamina papyracea is removed with a Freer elevator to expose the periorbita (**Fig. 21D.3** and **Fig. 21D.4**).
8. The floor of the orbit is then removed cautiously using a curette (**Fig. 21D.5**).
9. The periorbita is incised with a sickle knife to expose the extraconal tumor (**Fig. 21D.6**).

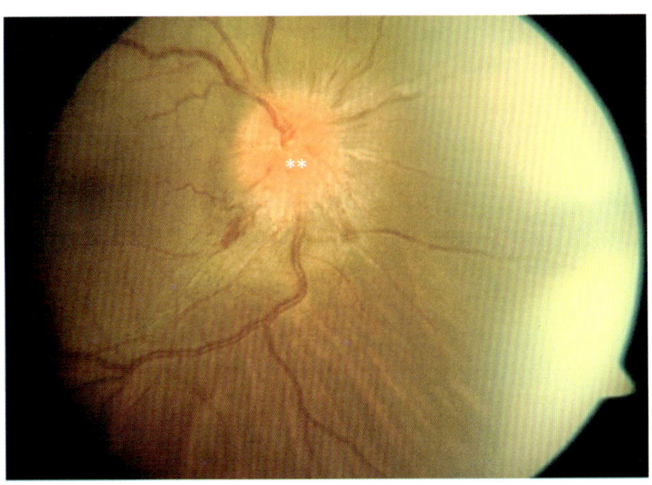

Fig. 21D.2 The fundus of the right eye showing disc swelling (**). There is blurring of the edges of the disc with obscuration of the disc blood vessels and hemorrhage.

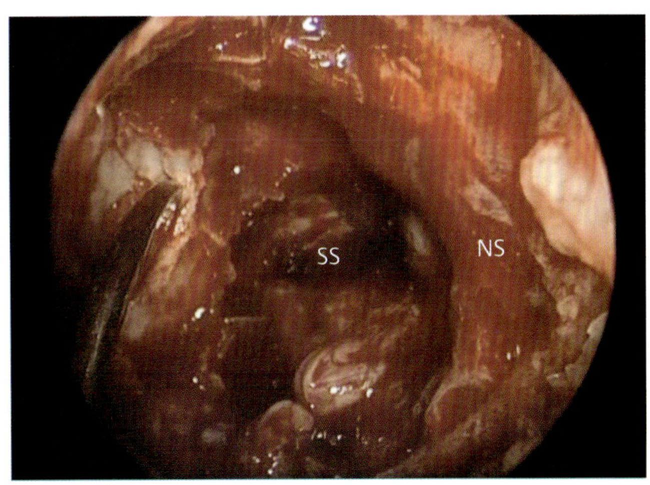

Fig. 21D.3 Removal of lamina papyracea (LP) is carried out with a Freer elevator.

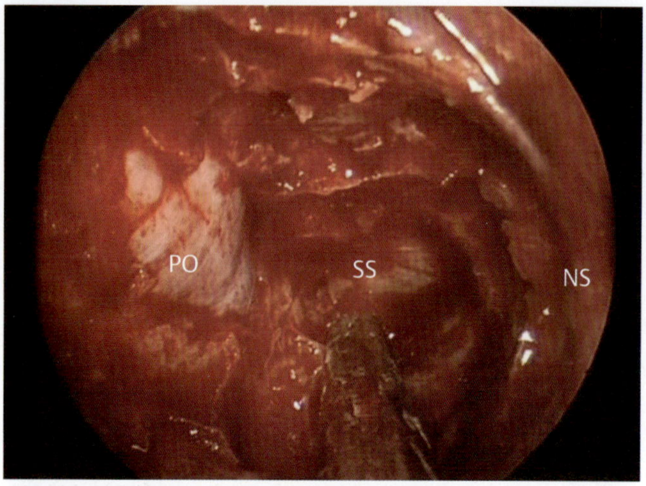

Fig. 21D.4 Exposure of the periorbita (PO) after removal of the lamina papyracea.

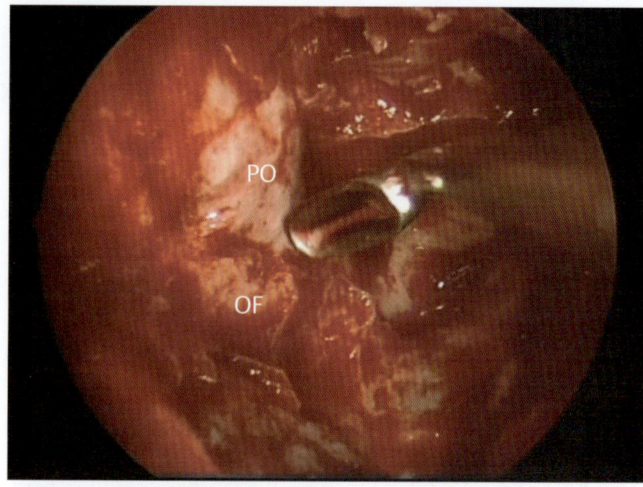

Fig. 21D.5 Removal of the orbital floor (OF) with a curette.

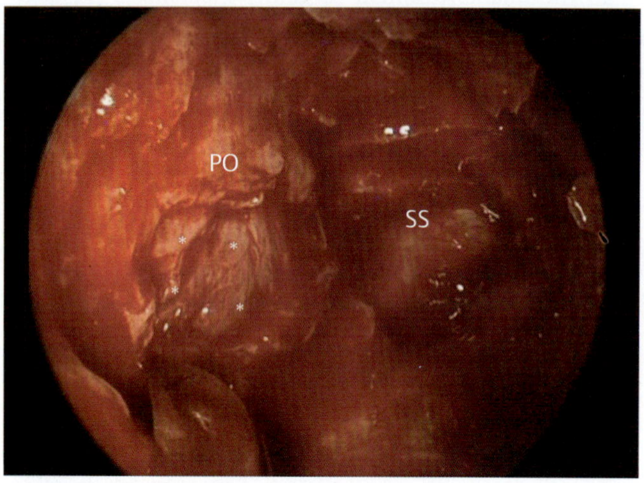

Fig. 21D.6 Extraconal tumor (*) comes into view after opening up the periorbita (PO).

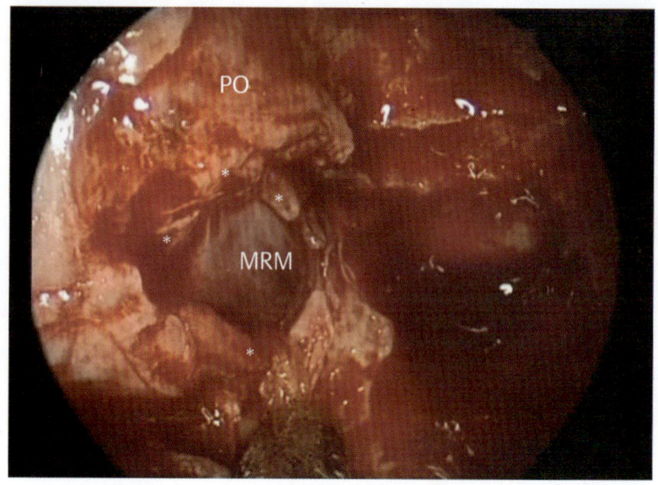

Fig. 21D.7 Endoscopic view of the medial rectus muscle (MRM) after removal of the tumor (*).

10. As the tumor is being removed, the medial rectus muscle becomes visible and becomes the lateral border of dissection (**Fig. 21D.7**).
11. The tumor is then carefully dissected from the orbit with a sickle knife and around the medial rectus muscle with a ball probe (**Fig. 21D.8** and **Fig. 21D.9**).
12. Removal of the final part of the extraconal tumor is performed superomedially with a Blakesley forceps and ball probe (**Fig. 21D.10**).
13. The surgeon should be thorough but prudent in his or her exploration to ensure successful removal of the tumor without injury to the rectus muscles (**Fig. 21D.11**).
14. Meticulous hemostasis is secured with adrenaline-soaked gauze, bipolar cauterization, and Surgicel.

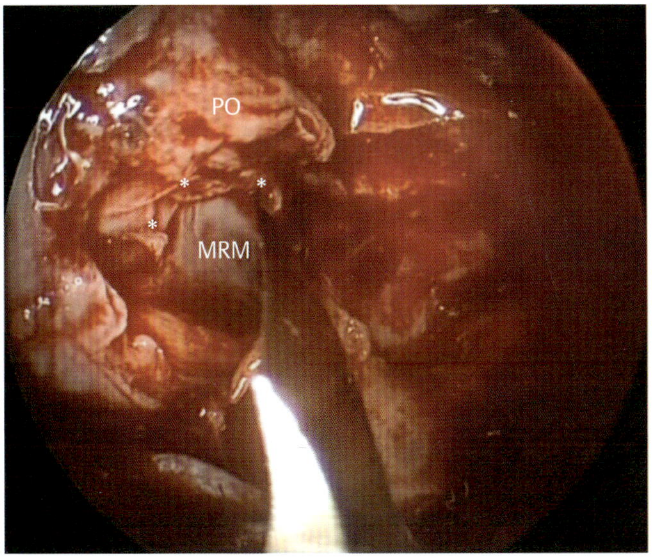

Fig. 21D.8 Tumor (*) dissection from the orbit with a sickle knife.

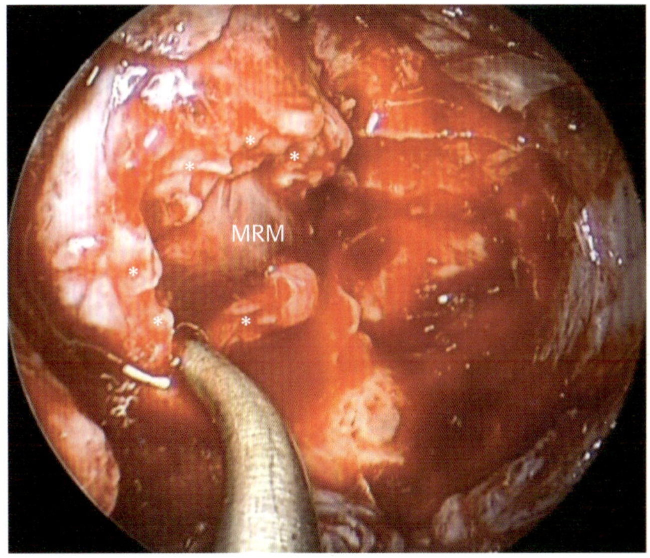

Fig. 21D.9 The extraconal tumor (*) is dissected around the medial rectus muscle (MRM).

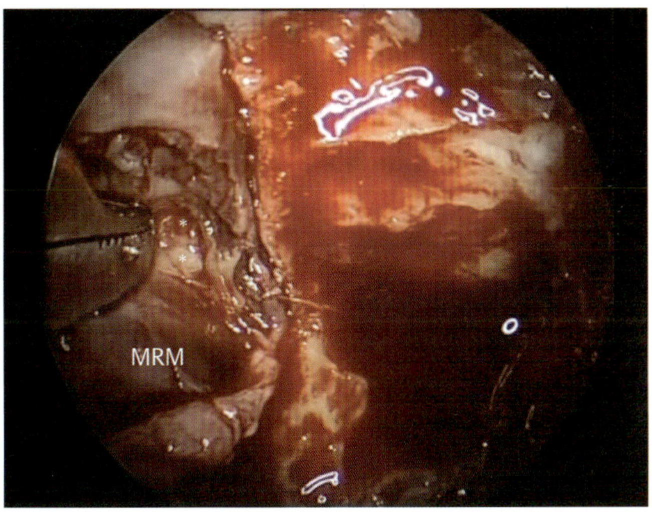

Fig. 21D.10 The extraconal tumor (*) is being removed superomedially with a Blakesley forceps. The medial rectus muscle (MRM) can be seen inferiorly.

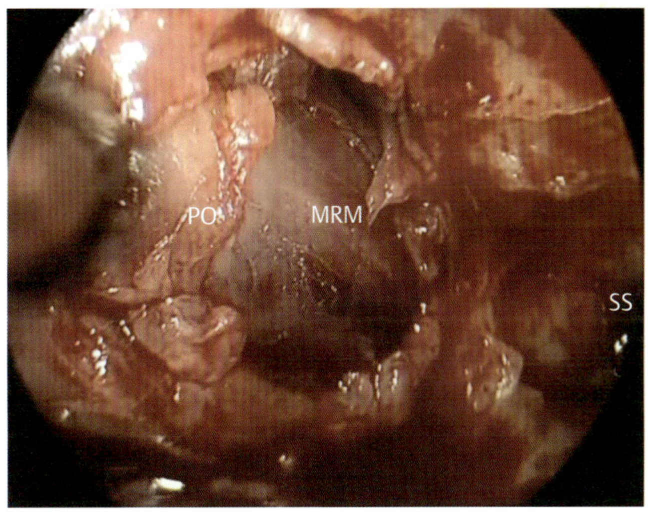

Fig. 21D.11 Postoperative view after complete removal of the tumor. The medial rectus muscle (MRM) is seen.

Section VII

Orbital Apex and Optic Nerve

Chapter 22 Pathologies of the Orbital Apex and Optic Nerve

Revadi Govindaraju, Michel Roethlisberger, and Prepageran Narayanan

Introduction

Pathologies related to the region of the orbital apex can present with a varying combination of signs and symptoms. This is explained by the closely packed bundle of neurovascular structures within a shared bony boundary formed by the paranasal sinuses, the orbit, and the middle cranial fossa. To understand the pathologies and surgical concepts of this region, it is crucial to identify the anatomical landmarks in preoperative radiological imaging and during surgery, many of which have been well defined by cadaveric studies. This overview attempts to present a summary of the available knowledge from literature with regard to the anatomy, pathologies, and options of surgical approaches accompanied by our cadaveric dissection images.

Anatomy

The orbital apex region connects the orbit and the middle cranial fossa via the superior orbital fissure (SOF) and the optic canal (OC). The neurovascular structures passing through this site are bundled together. Anatomical studies have elucidated certain helpful landmarks to reliably identify important neurovascular structures. Particularly relevant for skull base surgeons are recently performed studies identifying such landmarks for endonasal endoscopic surgeries.

The SOF is a space between the lesser wing of the sphenoid (LWS) superiorly and greater wing of sphenoid (GWS) inferiorly. It is typically described as being thin superolaterally and bulbous inferiorly, with the inferior part being directly anterior to the cavernous sinus (**Fig. 22.1a, b**).[1] There are, however, variances concerning the morphological form of the fissure and the arrangement of the neurovascular structures within the orbital apex.[2] Nevertheless, this morphological variability is believed to be less important during endonasal endoscopic surgeries. From an endoscopic point of view, the degree of sphenoid sinus pneumatization is believed to be more important for the ease of access and identification of the relevant landmarks of the skull base.[3] The SOF is divided into either two or three compartments; 1. the superolateral compartment containing the trochlear, frontal, and nasociliary nerves and the superior ophthalmic vein; 2. the inferomedial/medial compartment containing the superior and inferior branches of the oculomotor nerve, the nasociliary nerve, the abducens nerve, and the sensory and sympathetic roots of the ciliary ganglion; 3. the inferior compartment located below the annulus of Zinn containing adipose tissue and the inferior opthalmic vein in certain cases (**Fig. 22.2, Fig. 22.3**). Known anatomical variations include the location of the ophthalmic artery (lateral, superolateral, inferomedial, inferolateral, inferior) and the superior ophthalmic vein (superolateral or lower).[2,4] Studies have

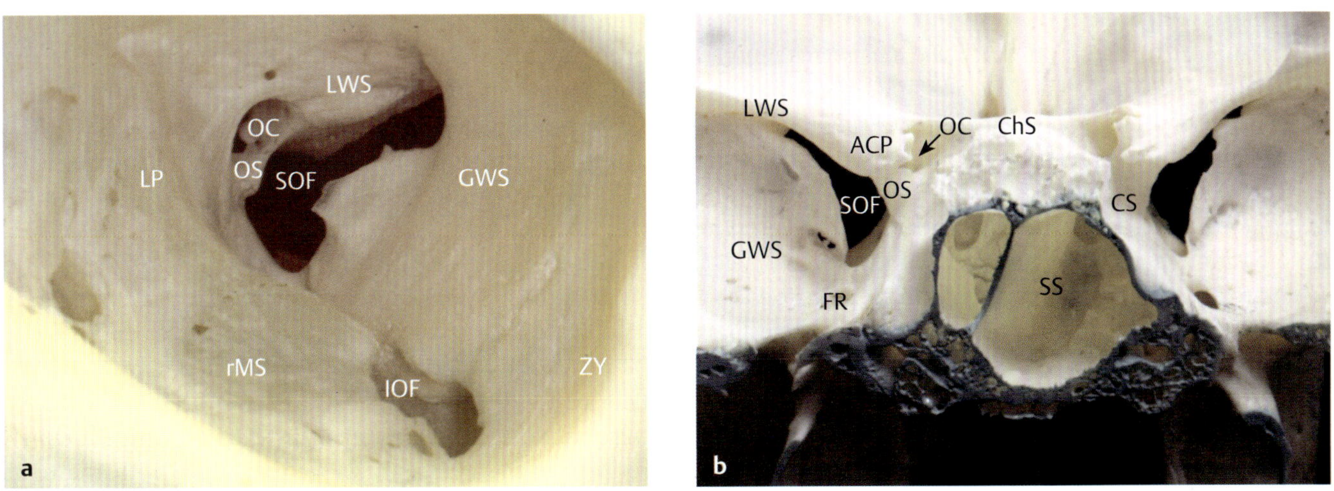

Fig. 22.1 Osseous anatomy of the superior orbital fissure, inferior orbital fissure, and the optic canal. **(a)** Anterior view of the left orbit. **(b)** Posterior view.

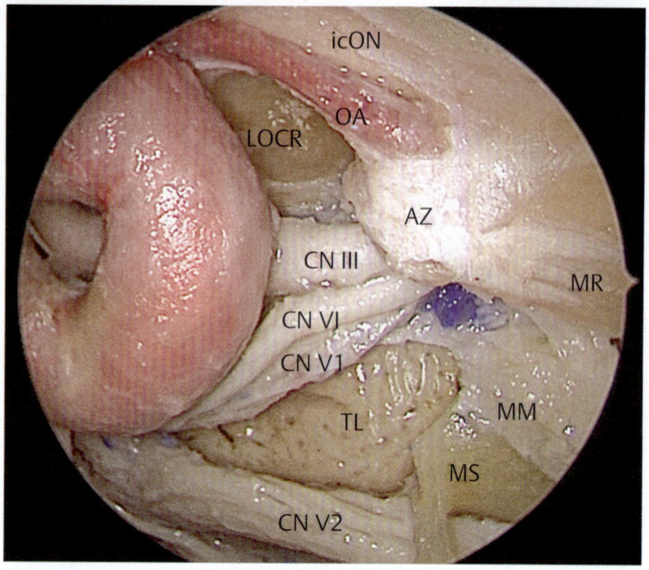

Fig. 22.2 Endonasal endoscopic view of the left orbital apex region and the intracanalicular optic nerve (icON). The bony wall has been removed followed by the orbital fat extending posteriorly, the dura covering the medial cavernous sinus, and the dura covering the maxillary nerve (CN V2) and the temporal lobe (TL). This exposes the medial aspect of the cavernous sinus, the intracavernous ICA, the oculomotor nerve (CN III), the abducens nerve (CN VI), and the ophthalmic branch of the trigeminal nerve (CN V1). The lateral opticocarotid recess (LOCR) corresponds to a pneumatized optic strut. The ophthalmic artery (OA) can be seen coursing inferomedial to the optic nerve in its intracanalicular segment (icON).

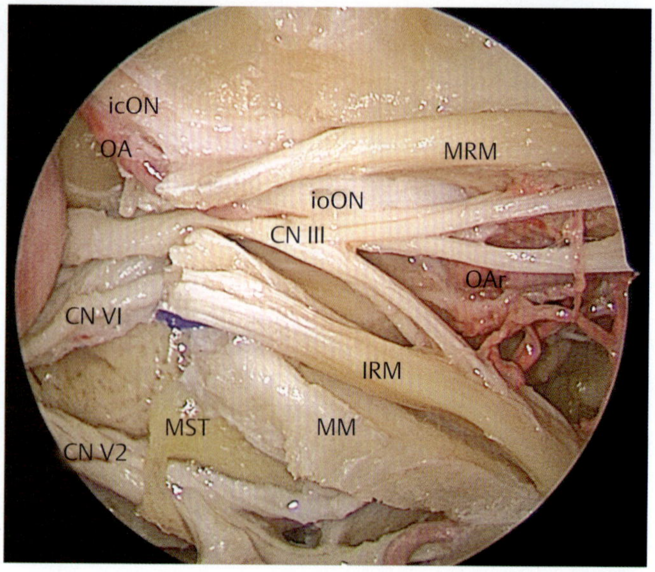

Fig. 22.3 The annulus of Zinn has been divided between the medial rectus muscle (MRM) and inferior rectus muscle (IRM). This exposes the division of the oculomotor nerve into upper and lower division, the intraorbital optic nerve (ioON), and the ophthalmic artery (OA) inferomedially. The Muller's muscle (MM) spans the entire infraorbital fissure (IOF) inferior to the inferior rectus (IRM) and inferior oblique muscle, and passes posteromedially above the maxillary strut (MST), inferior to the annulus of Zinn, to the anterior venous confluence of the cavernous sinus.

also identified a medial orbital or ophthalmic vein located in the extraconal space medial to the annulus of Zinn that drains into the medial cavernous sinus. This vein is easily recognizable during endoscopic endonasal surgery once the periorbita is removed.[3]

The annular tendon from which the four rectus muscles arise is formed by the blend of the periorbita, the optic nerve (ON) sheath, and the dural lining of the SOF and the OC, and is located around the anterior end of the optic foramen and the adjacent SOF. It is attached to the lateral edge of the fissure at the junction of its upper and lower halves.[5] The periorbita forms a continuous layer with the lateral sellar compartment and is in continuation with the fascia covering the infraorbital fissure (IOF) and the pterygopalatine fossa (PPF) anteroinferiorly.[3]

The superior wall of the SOF is located below the LWS, the anterior clinoid process (ACP), and the optic strut (OS). The medial margin is formed by the lateral surface of the OS superiorly and the body of the sphenoid bone inferiorly, with the carotid sulcus just behind it. Inferiorly, it extends to the lower edge of the cavernous sinus and the floor of the middle cranial fossa (**Fig. 22.1b**). The lower part of the SOF merges with the posterior end of IOF.[5] Superiorly, the OS separates the SOF from the OC and inferiorly the maxillary strut forms the boundary between SOF and foramen rotundum (FR; **Fig. 22.1, Fig. 22.4**).[1,3] These are two important bony landmarks when accessing the medial aspect of the SOF during endonasal endoscopic surgery.[3] A pneumatized OS also corresponds to the lateral opticocarotid recess in the sphenoid sinus with the anterior bend of the intracavernous internal carotid artery (ICA) resting posterior to the strut (**Fig. 22.2, 22.4**).[3]

The IOF can be used as a reliable landmark to reach the SOF due to its close topoanatomical relationship. It forms an oblique fissure with an angle of 45 degrees in the sagittal plane and is located between the lateral wall and the floor of the orbit.[1] Three segments have been described for this fissure; 1. the posteromedial segment, where foramen rotundum, the PPF, and SOF communicate with the orbit and the cavernous sinus; 2. the middle segment, which communicates with the infratemporal fossa; 3. the anterolateral segment that communicates with the temporal fossa

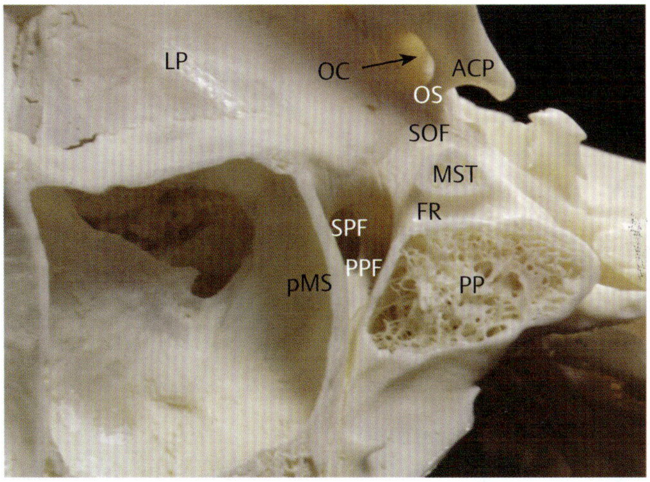

Fig. 22.4 Lateral view of the orbital apex region in a parasagittally transected dry bone specimen at the level of the infraorbital fissure. The view clearly shows the optic strut (OS) forming the boundary between the optic canal (OC) and the superior orbital fissure (SOF). The maxillary strut (MST) separates the SOF from the foramen rotundum (FR).

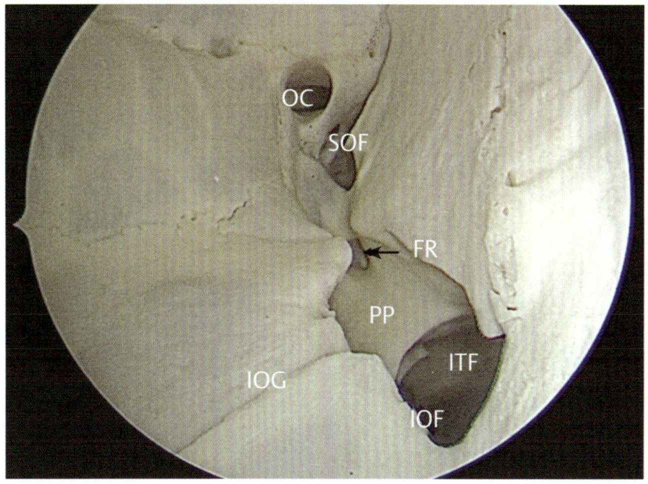

Fig. 22.5 This endoscopic view is deliberately angled inferiorly to show the communication between the superior orbital fissure (SOF), infraorbital fissure (IOF), foramen rotundum (FR), pterygopalatine fossa (PPF), and infratemporal fossa (ITF).

(**Fig. 22.5**).[6] Muller's muscle is a smooth muscle spanning the entire IOF inferior to the inferior rectus and inferior oblique muscle. The muscle passes above the maxillary strut, inferior to the annulus of Zinn to the anterior venous confluence of the cavernous sinus posteromedially (**Fig. 22.3**). The zygomatic nerve is intimately associated with this muscle.[6] Endoscopically, the muscle is identified as another critical surgical landmark to reach the SOF.[3]

Anatomical studies of the ON have identified four different segments along its course: intradural, intracanalicular, intraorbital, and intraocular (**Fig. 22.6**). The intradural course has been further divided into the distal cisternal segment and the proximal preforaminal segment (**Fig. 22.6a–c**).[7] The intracanalicular segment lies within a canal described as an oblique cylinder with an ovoid shape. The lateral opticocarotid recess (LOCR) is a landmark to identify the ON within the sphenoid sinus. It is bounded superiorly by the intracanalicular ON, inferomedially by the paraclinoid ICA, inferolaterally by the SOF, and laterally by the orbital apex.[7] The medial opticocarotid recess (MOCR) is a teardrop-shaped recess corresponding to the junction of the paraclinoid ICA and preforaminal segment of ON. Endonasally, the preforaminal segment thus is estimated to lie between the MOCR and the most medial and posterior parts of LOCR. The intracanalicular segment extends along the length of the LOCR up to its most anterior limitation. Intracranially, the preforaminal segment is located below the falciform ligament attached to the ACP and limbus sphenoidale (**Fig. 22.7**). In their study, Abhinav et al. further recorded that[7] the OA is often located inferomedial or inferior to ON within the OC and in an inferolateral position at the intraorbital opening.[8]

Pathology

Pathologies of the orbital apex region are rare and diverse. Therefore, making a correct diagnosis becomes a challenging process. In the past, the disorders in this region have been classified either as orbital apex syndrome, cavernous sinus syndrome, or SOF syndrome. Recent publications perceive this classification as just anatomical divisions. The actual diseases in these groups seem to share the same etiology, diagnostic evaluation, and management.[9–11]

Disease confined to the orbital apex may present with ophthalmoplegia, proptosis, fixed dilated pupil, ptosis, and hypoesthesia of the forehead, upper eyelid or the cornea, and visual impairment due to ON involvement. The cavernous sinus syndrome additionally presents with paresthesia of the cheek due to the cranial nerve (CN) V2 involvement and possible Horner's syndrome secondary to oculosympathetic paresis. The SOF syndrome on the other hand shares similar characteristics as the orbital apex syndrome, but without ON involvement.[10] These distinct clinical features may be helpful to localize the anatomical region involved. However, there is a remarkable variation concerning the presence and absence of clinical signs and symptoms, especially within the context of disease progression and evolvement.

A myriad of disorders affecting the orbital apex has been described. Most authors agree that besides clinical

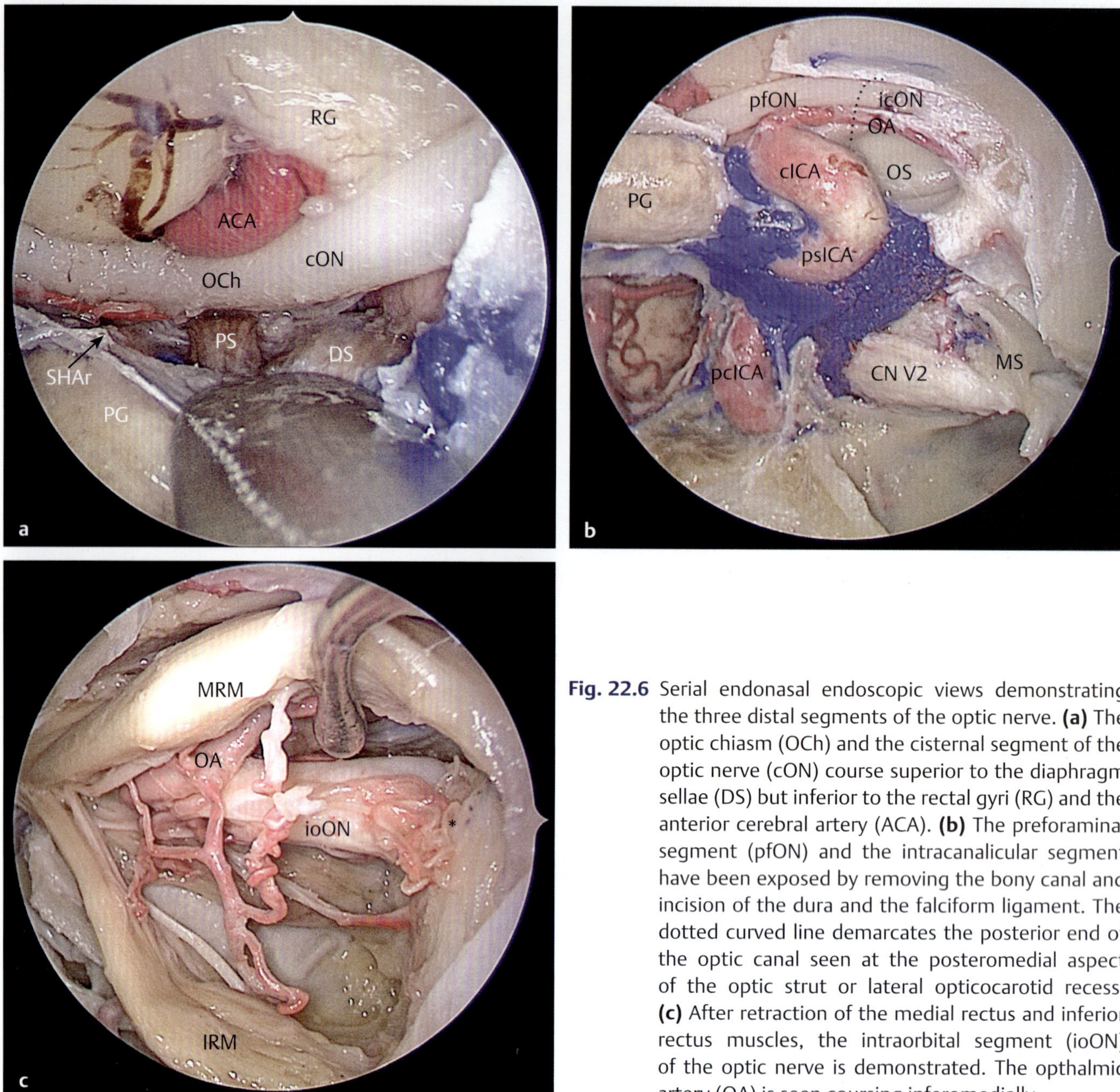

Fig. 22.6 Serial endonasal endoscopic views demonstrating the three distal segments of the optic nerve. **(a)** The optic chiasm (OCh) and the cisternal segment of the optic nerve (cON) course superior to the diaphragm sellae (DS) but inferior to the rectal gyri (RG) and the anterior cerebral artery (ACA). **(b)** The preforaminal segment (pfON) and the intracanalicular segment have been exposed by removing the bony canal and incision of the dura and the falciform ligament. The dotted curved line demarcates the posterior end of the optic canal seen at the posteromedial aspect of the optic strut or lateral opticocarotid recess. **(c)** After retraction of the medial rectus and inferior rectus muscles, the intraorbital segment (ioON) of the optic nerve is demonstrated. The opthalmic artery (OA) is seen coursing inferomedially.

assessment and imaging, a biopsy is required in most cases to properly diagnose conditions that potentially mimic other diseases when inconclusive radiological findings are present. This additionally avoids delay in the management of critical diseases such as malignancies or intracranial infections leading to irreversible loss of function when cranial nerves are involved.[12] Hence, a multidisciplinary evaluation is imperative and involves ophthalmology, neurosurgery, radiology, and otolaryngology specialists.

Neuroimaging is the preferred method of assessment after clinical assessment and evaluation. High-resolution magnetic resonance imaging (MRI) is superior to computed tomography (CT) in delineating the contents and pathology affecting the orbital apex. Yeh and Foroozan et al. recommend neurocranial MRI and orbit sequences with contrast enhancement and fat-suppressed sequences to assess the cavernous sinus and orbital apex, reserving CT scan for patients with contraindications for MRI and the evaluation of orbital and skull base fractures when trauma is present.[11] Additionally, a magnetic resonance angiography (MRA) or CT angiography may be useful if a vascular lesion or injury is suspected. A detailed summary of the MRI, CT, and post-contrast enhancement features specifically for various pathologies has been well outlined by Goyal et al.[9] A report

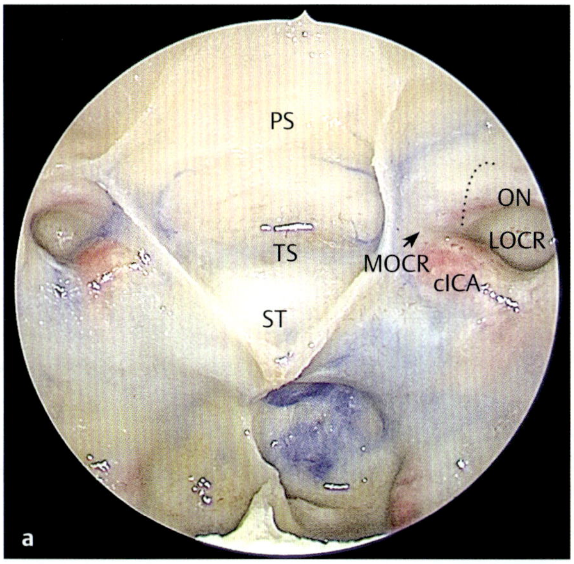

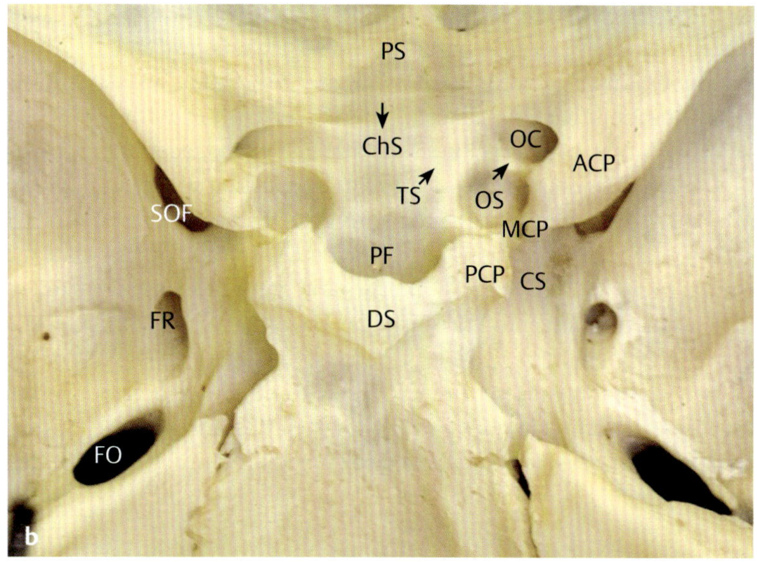

Fig. 22.7 **(a)** Endonasal endoscopic ventral anatomy of the posterior wall of the sphenoid sinus: the dotted curved line represents the posteromedial end of the optic canal. The preforaminal segment is estimated to lie between the medial opticocarotid recess (MOCR) and the most posteromedial part of the lateral opticocarotid recess (LOCR). The intracanalicular segment lies between the posterior part of the LOCR and extends anteriorly. **(b)** Superior oblique intracranial view demonstrating the intracranial location of the optic canal (OC) and its topoanatomical relationship to the adjacent neurovascular structures in a dry bone specimen. The falciform ligament attaches laterally to the anterior clinoid process (ACP) and medially to the limbus sphenoidale.

by Ettl et al. provides detailed images captured from high-resolution MRI sections, and is considered as a landmark study of the normal anatomy of the orbital apex and the cavernous sinus.

Most studies predominantly reported tumors causing an orbital apex or the cavernous sinus syndrome.[11,12,14–18] The incidence of specific histology varied widely between series with a large number of patients. In an analysis of 151 patients with cavernous sinus syndrome, Keane et al. reported nasopharyngeal carcinoma as the most common neoplasm followed by metastases, lymphoma, pituitary adenoma, meningioma, and chordoma.[16] Another series involving 126 patients, however, reported pituitary adenoma and meningioma as the largest tumorous entities.[17] Aryasit et al. reported lymphoma and meningioma as the most frequent neoplasms.[19] Other malignant tumors reported include plasmacytoma, hemangiopericytoma, neuroblastoma, melanoma, sinonasal adenocarcinoma and undifferentiated carcinoma, osteoblastoma, chondrosarcoma, and rhabdomyosarcoma. Local invasion, perineural spread, or distant metastasis from squamous cell carcinoma, renal cell carcinoma, prostate carcinoma, and breast carcinoma have been reported as well.[12,14,15,20,21] Besides meningioma, benign tumors such as histiocytosis, schwannoma of the cavernous sinus or the superior orbital fissure, ossifying fibroma, fibrous dysplasia, neuroma, cavernous hemangioma, and juvenile angiofibroma have to be considered in this region.[12,14,15,17,22–24] In an analysis of 126 patients diagnosed with cavernous sinus syndrome, the absence of pain, V2 involvement, and male sex, appeared to be independently associated with the presence of a tumor.[17]

Vascular disorders including aneurysms and carotid-cavernous fistula were found to be a relevant cause of cavernous sinus syndrome in a series of 80 (n=30, 37.5%) and 126 patients (n=25, 19.8%) patients, respectively.[17,19] Additional specific clinical features including tortuous epibulbar vessels, bruit, pulsatile proptosis, and a history of head trauma might support the diagnosis of a carotid-cavernous sinus fistula. However, in a low-flow fistula, clinical onset is reported to be insidious with milder symptoms.[19]

In a report on SOF syndrome including 130 published cases, an inflammatory etiology made up to 71% of cases presenting with painful ophthalmoplegia.[25] The Tolosa-Hunt syndrome, characterized as painful opthalmoplegia, is an idiopathic inflammatory disease of the cavernous sinus syndrome and a diagnosis of exclusion. It accounts for 8 to 13% of patients in reported case series.[16,17,19] Other inflammatory causes need to be considered during the diagnostic work-up, including sarcoidosis, systemic lupus erythematosus, Churg–Strauss syndrome, Wegener's granulomatosis, giant cell arteritis, orbital inflammatory pseudotumor, and thyroid orbitopathy.[11]

Fungal infections such as aspergillosis or fungal balls, bacterial infections including tuberculosis and that caused by *Staphylococcus aureus*, and viral infections with herpes zoster virus, have been reported to cause orbital apex and cavernous sinus syndrome.[10,12,14,15,17,26,27] The orbital apex syndrome from bacterial sinusitis may occur with or without concurrent orbital cellulitis.[10,26] Pfeiffer et al. recently reported a case of an aggressive bacterial infection without orbital cellulitis, which presented with good vision but consecutive rapid deteriorations to no light perception and other cranial nerve palsies. Surgical intervention and intravenous (IV) antibiotics prevented the further intracranial extension of the infection but the neurologic deficits remained.[26]

Less common causes of the SOF syndrome are trauma, mucocele, and foreign body in the orbit.[11,16] A recent report by Levin et al. revealed a metallic foreign body in the orbital apex following an industrial accident. The visual acuity was preserved in this patient, but the patient suffered from intractable diplopia due to a CN III, IV, VI palsy.[28]

Pathologies of the ON may be divided according to the four previously described segments; the intraocular segment is affected by a myriad of known diseases including papilledema and anterior ischemic neuropathy; the intraorbital segment may be affected by dysthyroid optic neuropathy, optic neuritis, ON sheath meningiomas, and ON gliomas; traumatic optic neuropathy is seen to occur in the intracanalicular part; and lastly, the intracranial part may be affected by ophthalmic artery aneurysm, pituitary tumors, and suprasellar tumors.[29]

Key Principles of Surgery

Orbital Apex

The orbital apex was traditionally approached via external approaches (e.g., transcutaneous, transconjunctival, and transcaruncular). These external approaches provide limited space for instrumentation and cause significant retraction of the orbital contents.[15,24] Transcranial approaches are necessary when pathologies involve the compartments superior and posterior to the ON, and when intracranial involvement is present. In their cadaveric study, Tepedino et al. proposed a division of the orbit into quadrants to determine the choice of access for the differently located pathologies. The supero- and inferomedial aspects are deemed amenable to transnasal surgery, whereas the exposure for the inferolateral part is better achieved with combined transnasal and transmaxillary approaches. However, the superolateral region is not recommended for a transnasal route.[4] Stokken et al. hence suggested the transconjunctival and transcaruncular approaches for this specific location.[15] Nevertheless, there is a report of a rhabdomyosarcoma located at the lateral aspect of the orbital apex in a child that was removed successfully via an endonasal endoscopic transmaxillary, transpterygoid approach; however, the authors cautioned to use this method for small soft tumors only.[21]

The surgical steps for the transcranial and external routes have extensively been described in the literature. This overview aims to focus on the endonasal endoscopic approaches.

The initial steps for the endonasal endoscopic approach of the orbit apex include a complete sphenoethmoidectomy followed by removal of the lamina papyracea, incision of the periorbita, and blunt dissection of the surrounding fat. If the pathology is extraconal, the fat is retracted to expose the lesion; however, if the lesion is intraconal, the fat is removed using a bipolar cautery to expose the medial rectus muscle (MRM), which is then retracted superiorly or inferiorly.

The space between the MRM and the inferior rectus muscle (IRM) at the inferior part of the orbital apex has been recommended as the safest trajectory to the intraconal space.[15] Other principles of safe surgery to reach pathologies of the orbit apex are: 1. entering the orbit below the ethmoidal foramina; 2. avoidance of dissection through the extraocular muscles; 3. avoidance of crossing the ON.

Apart from Muller's muscle, the OS, and the maxillary strut, which have been proposed as landmarks to reach the SOF and OC, further landmarks have recently been described in cadaveric studies. Tepedino et al. found consistent measurements between the ethmoidal crest and the choanal arch to the inferior most point of the OC and SOF, which can be used for the identification of landmarks irrespective of the degree of sphenoid pneumatization.[4] For intraconal dissection of the orbital apex, another cadaveric and radiological study has demonstrated a consistent course of the ON along the superior part of the MRM. Hence, the ON potentially guides the medial dissection with inferior retraction of this muscle.[30]

Several reports have published suggestions and recommendations to improve the technical aspects of the approach and surgery of the orbital apex region: this includes the use of navigation, two-surgeon, four-handed surgery to allow retraction, suctioning, and bimanual dissection, posterior septectomy or modified septoplasty approach, middle turbinectomy, accessory incisions, combined approaches via a transcaruncular route allowing a broader range of maneuvers for the second surgeon, and the use of an endoscope holder.[14,15,20,21]

The main advantages of the endonasal endoscopic approach are an improved cosmetic outcome, less pain, less trauma to orbital structures, the avoidance of morbidities associated with transcranial surgery (cerebral edema, stroke, seizures, cerebrospinal [CSF] leakage), and earlier adjuvant therapies for selected cases.[14,15] Reported disadvantages of the endonasal endoscopic approach to the orbital apex include poor access for more anteriorly located lesions and the need for specialized equipment.[14] Generally, there are few complications associated with this approach, however, reported complications include reduced postoperative visual acuity, worsening diplopia, and CSF leakage and rectal gyrus contusion.[14]

Optic Nerve

The surgical approach to the intraorbital ON is covered in Section IV, Chapter 20. Within this chapter, the endoscopic approach to the intracanalicular and intracranial segment of the ON is described. The endonasal endoscopic approach is suitable for pathologies of the OC medially and inferiorly. The transcranial route allows unroofing of the OC for superior and lateral decompression.[31]

If an endonasal endoscopic route is used, a wide sphenoidotomy is necessary to safely identify critical anatomical landmarks of the base of skull: the lateral and medial opticocarotid recess, the OC, and the paraclival and cavernous ICAs. Drilling of the optic canal is performed using a diamond burr with copious irrigation until an eggshell thin layer of bone is left. The bone can then be removed from distal to proximal using specialized instruments. A circumferential decompression of the optic nerve between 160 and 180 degrees is relatively easy to achieve. However, achieving a 270-degree decompression is deemed to be technically more challenging. If an incision of the optic nerve sheath is required, a superomedial location in relation to the optic nerve is recommended to reduce the risk of arterial injury.[7] A dural incision starting at the sella continuing superiorly across the superior intercavernous sinus, tuberculum sellae, chiasmatic sulcus, and laterally toward the limbus and planum sphenoidale detaches the falciform ligament and allows exposure of the cisternal and preforaminal parts of the ON.[7]

Acknowledged advantages of the endonasal endoscopic approach are less invasiveness while allowing a good exposure of the OC and orbital apex. A safe decompression of the ON is achieved up to approximately 160 to 180 degrees using endonasal endoscopic techniques. If an increased range of decompression up to a total of 360 degrees is necessary, combined transorbital and endoscopic endonasal approaches are necessary, as revealed in cadaveric studies.[32] Other advantages include bilateral early decompression of ON and good access to the preforaminal part of the ON (**Fig. 22.8** and **Fig. 22.9**).[7]

Potential complications of the endonasal endoscopic approach to the intracanalicular and intracranial ON include CSF leakage, injury of the opthalmic artery, and visual impairment.

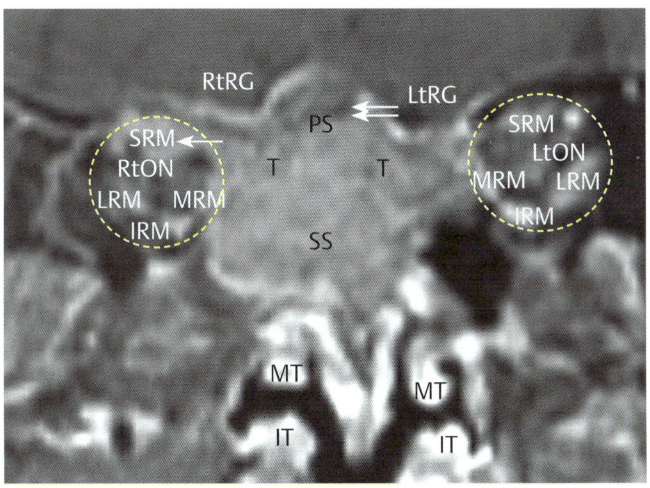

Fig. 22.8 Coronal T1-contrast-enhanced MRI sequence demonstrating a sino-nasal carcinoma (T) of the sphenoid sinus (SS), with invasion (*white arrow*) of the orbit apex (*yellow line*) on the right side, the superior rectus muscle (SRM), the planum sphenoidale (PS), and the anterior cranial fossa dura (*double arrow*). Right (RtGR) and left (LtGR) rectal gyrus, right (RtON) and left (LtON) optic nerve, lateral rectus muscle (LRM), medial rectus muscle (MRM), inferior rectus muscle (IRM), middle turbinate (MT), inferior turbinate (IT).

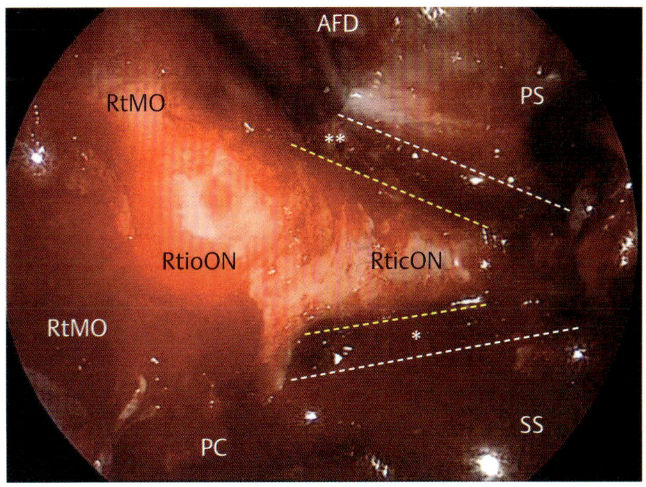

Fig. 22.9 Endonasal endoscopic view after extradural decompression 90 degrees superior (*superior yellow and white line*) and 90 degrees inferior (*inferior yellow and white line*) of the right intra-canalicular optic nerve (RticON) with complete macroscopic removal of a sino-nasal carcinoma of the sphenoid sinus (SS) inferior to the nerve (*) and residual tumor superior to the nerve (**). Anterior cranial fossa dura (AFD), planum sphenoidale (PS), right intraorbital nerve (RtioON), right medial orbit (RtMO), posterior ethmoidal cells (PC).

Acknowledgments

This chapter was written based on funding from the Martin Allgöwer Foundation, Department of Surgery, University Hospital of Basel (Basel, Switzerland), the Gottfried and Julia Bangerter-Rhyner Foundation (Bern, Switzerland), the Ministry of Health of Malaysia scholarship (Malaysia), and the Adelaide Ear-Nose-Throat Research Institute (Australia). The Departments of Neurosurgery of the University Hospital of Basel (Basel, Switzerland) and the Departments of Neurosurgery and Otorhinolaryngology of the University of Malaya (Kuala Lumpur, Malaysia) supported the creation of this chapter.

References

1. Daniels DL, Mark LP, Mafee MF, et al. Osseous anatomy of the orbital apex. AJNR Am J Neuroradiol 1995;16(9):1929–1935
2. Reymond J, Kwiatkowski J, Wysocki J. Clinical anatomy of the superior orbital fissure and the orbital apex. J Craniomaxillofac Surg 2008;36(6):346–353
3. Dallan I, Castelnuovo P, de Notaris M, et al. Endoscopic endonasal anatomy of superior orbital fissure and orbital apex regions: critical considerations for clinical applications. Eur Arch Otorhinolaryngol 2013;270(5):1643–1649
4. Tepedino MS, Pinheiro-Neto CD, Bezerra TF, Gardner PA, Snyderman CH, Voegels RL. Endonasal identification of the orbital apex. Laryngoscope 2016;126(1):33–38
5. Natori Y, Rhoton AL Jr. Microsurgical anatomy of the superior orbital fissure. Neurosurgery 1995;36(4):762–775
6. De Battista JC, Zimmer LA, Theodosopoulos PV, Froelich SC, Keller JT. Anatomy of the inferior orbital fissure: implications for endoscopic cranial base surgery. J Neurol Surg B Skull Base 2012;73(2):132–138
7. Abhinav K, Acosta Y, Wang WH, et al. Endoscopic endonasal approach to the optic canal: anatomic considerations and surgical relevance. Neurosurgery 2015;11(Suppl 3):431–445, discussion 445–446
8. Caporlingua A, Prior A, Cavagnaro MJ, et al. The intracranial and intracanalicular optic nerve as seen through different surgical windows: endoscopic versus transcranial. World Neurosurg 2019;124:522–538
9. Goyal P, Lee S, Gupta N, et al. Orbital apex disorders: imaging findings and management. Neuroradiol J 2018;31(2):104–125
10. Warburton RE, Brookes CC, Golden BA, Turvey TA. Orbital apex disorders: a case series. Int J Oral Maxillofac Surg 2016; 45(4):497–506
11. Yeh S, Foroozan R. Orbital apex syndrome. Curr Opin Ophthalmol 2004;15(6):490–498
12. Unadkat SN, Rennie CE, Grant WE. Endoscopic transnasal image-guided approach to diagnosis in orbital apex and optic canal lesions. J Laryngol Otol 2019;133(6):501–507
13. Ettl A, Zwrtek K, Daxer A, Salomonowitz E. Anatomy of the orbital apex and cavernous sinus on high-resolution magnetic resonance images. Surv Ophthalmol 2000;44(4):303–323
14. Murchison AP, Rosen MR, Evans JJ, Bilyk JR. Endoscopic approach to the orbital apex and periorbital skull base. Laryngoscope 2011;121(3):463–467
15. Stokken J, Gumber D, Antisdel J, Sindwani R. Endoscopic surgery of the orbital apex: outcomes and emerging techniques. Laryngoscope 2016;126(1):20–24
16. Keane JR. Cavernous sinus syndrome. Analysis of 151 cases. Arch Neurol 1996;53(10):967–971
17. Fernández S, Godino O, Martínez-Yélamos S, et al. Cavernous sinus syndrome: a series of 126 patients. Medicine (Baltimore) 2007;86(5):278–281
18. Bhatkar S, Goyal MK, Takkar A, et al. Cavernous sinus syndrome: a prospective study of 73 cases at a tertiary care centre in Northern India. Clin Neurol Neurosurg 2017; 155:63–69
19. Aryasit O, Preechawai P, Aui-Aree N. Clinical presentation, aetiology and prognosis of orbital apex syndrome. Orbit 2013;32(2):91–94
20. Healy DY Jr, Lee NG, Freitag SK, Bleier BS. Endoscopic bimanual approach to an intraconal cavernous hemangioma of the orbital apex with vascularized flap reconstruction. Ophthal Plast Reconstr Surg 2014;30(4):e104–e106
21. Dziedzic TA, Anand VK, Schwartz TH. Endoscopic endonasal approach to the lateral orbital apex: case report. J Neurosurg Pediatr 2015;16(3):305–308
22. Yoshimura K, Kubo S, Yoneda H, Hasegawa H, Tominaga S, Yoshimine T. Removal of a cavernous hemangioma in the orbital apex via the endoscopic transnasal approach: a case report. Minim Invasive Neurosurg 2010;53(2):77–79
23. Sia DI, Chan WO, Wormald PJ, Davis G, Selva D. Decompression of benign orbital apex lesion via medial endoscopic approach. Orbit 2012;31(5):344–346
24. Ruiz D, Rebeiz EE. Endoscopic approach for excision of venous malformation of the orbital apex. J Craniofac Surg 2018; 29(3):733–734
25. Lenzi GL, Fieschi C. Superior orbital fissure syndrome. Review of 130 cases. Eur Neurol 1977;16(1-6):23–30
26. Pfeiffer ML, Merritt HA, Bailey LA, Richani K, Phillips ME. Orbital apex syndrome from bacterial sinusitis without orbital cellulitis. Am J Ophthalmol Case Rep 2018;10:84–86
27. Lim JJ, Ong YM, Wan Zalina MZ, Choo MM. Herpes zoster ophthalmicus with orbital apex syndrome-difference in outcomes and literature review. Ocul Immunol Inflamm 2018;26(2):187–193

28. Levin B, Goh ES, Ng YH, Sethi DS. Endoscopic removal of a foreign body in the orbital apex abutting the optic nerve. Singapore Med J 2019;60(5):265–266

29. Selhorst JB, Chen Y. The optic nerve. Semin Neurol 2009; 29(1):29–35

30. Petrov D, Craig J, Thawani J, et al. Relationship of the optic nerve to the medial rectus muscle during endonasal dissection of the medial intraconal orbital apex. Oper Neurosurg (Hagerstown) 2017;13(1):131–137

31. Güler TM, Yılmazlar S, Özgün G. Anatomical aspects of optic nerve decompression in transcranial and transsphenoidal approach. J Craniomaxillofac Surg 2019;47(4):561–569

32. Oh HJ, Yeo DG, Hwang SC. Surgical treatment for traumatic optic neuropathy. Korean J Neurotrauma 2018;14(2):55–60

Chapter 23 Endonasal Endoscopic Surgeries of the Orbit Apex and Optic Nerve

Case 23A

Endoscopic Endonasal Excision of a Left Orbital Apex Tumor with Extension to the Cavernous Sinus

Adzreil Bakri, Michel Roethlisberger, Prepageran Narayanan, and Vicknes Waran

History

A 57-year-old female presented with a history of pleomorphic adenocarcinoma of the left lacrimal gland, which was excised 2 years ago. Margins of the excised tumor were positive and she subsequently underwent and completed 66 Gy of radiotherapy. Consecutively, the patient presented with blurring of vision for the past few months and new onset blindness of the left eye. A magnetic resonance imaging (MRI) scan showed an ill-defined enhancing lesion at the left orbital apex with extension to the cavernous sinus and lateral part of the optic nerve. It measured approximately 2 × 1 cm (**Fig. 23A.1**). A dual nostril endoscopic excision of the lesion was indicated.

Surgical Steps

1. The patient is placed under general anesthesia in supine position and the head slightly extended fixed within a NORAS frame for intraoperative MRI (iMRI). Registration for image-guided surgery (Brainlab, Munich, Germany) is performed.
2. The nose is decongested with nasal packing as per the institutions' standard methods.
3. Local anesthesia is infiltrated into both sides of the septum to raise the septal mucoperichondrium (**Fig. 23A.2**).
4. After bipolar diathermy, the septum is incised with a no. 15 blade at the area opposite to the anterior part of the middle turbinate on one side, and the mucoperichondrial flap is raised up to the choana (**Fig. 23A.3** and **Fig. 23A.4**).
5. A nasoseptal flap is developed by incising the superior part of the mucoperichondrial flap with microscissors directed toward the sphenoid ostia. About 1 cm of septal mucosa superior to the flap is preserved to maintain the olfactory function.
6. Inferiorly, the nasoseptal flap is freed by cutting it parallel just above the nasal floor posteriorly toward the choana. The flap is then dissected over the choana and stored in the nasopharynx for later use.
7. A second nasoseptal flap or rescue flap is developed on the contralateral side of the septum and stored in the nasopharynx.

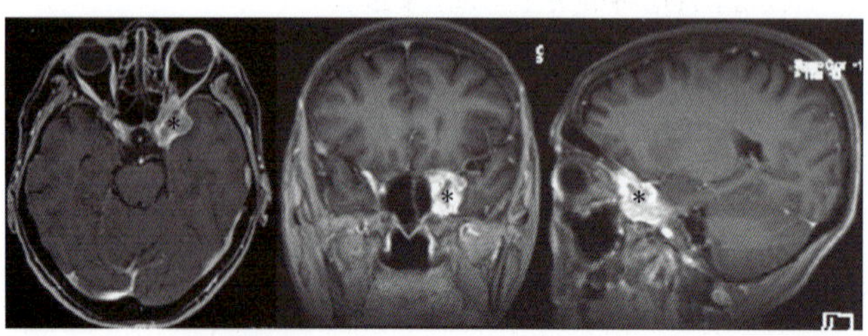

Fig. 23A.1 Preoperative axial, coronal and sagittal T1 contrast-enhanced MRI sections. The tumor (*) is seen at the orbital apex with extensions to the cavernous sinus, optic nerve, and infratemporal fossa.

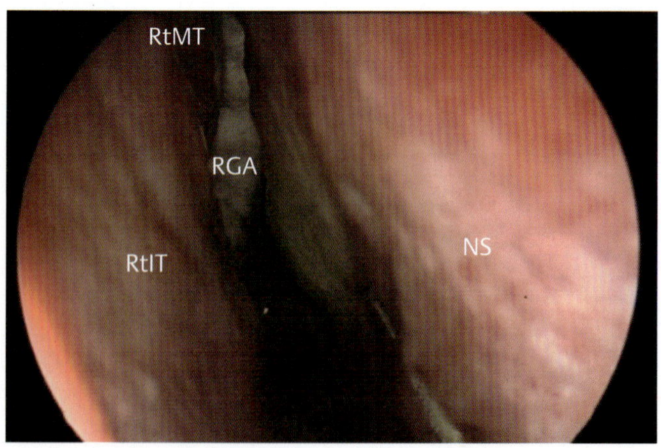

Fig. 23A.2 Local anesthesia infiltration into the nasal septum of the right nasal cavity. A ribbon gauze soaked in adrenaline (1 mg diluted in 10 mL saline) (RGA) is packed between the right middle turbinate (RtMT) and the nasal septum (NS).

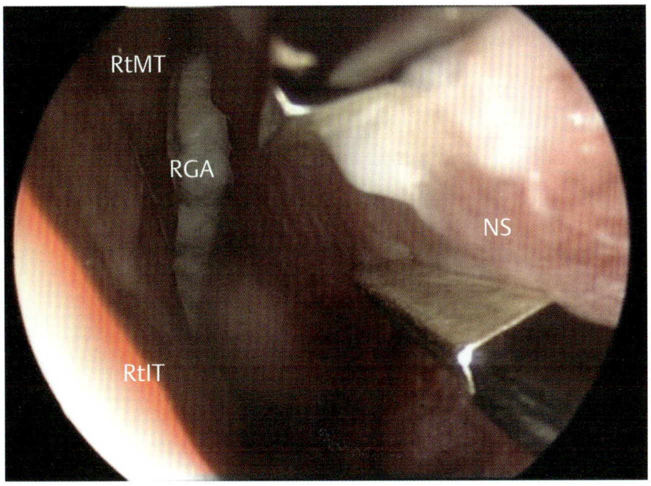

Fig. 23A.3 Bipolar diathermy prior to incision on the nasal septum (NS) of the right nasal cavity opposite to the anterior part of the right middle turbinate (RtMT).

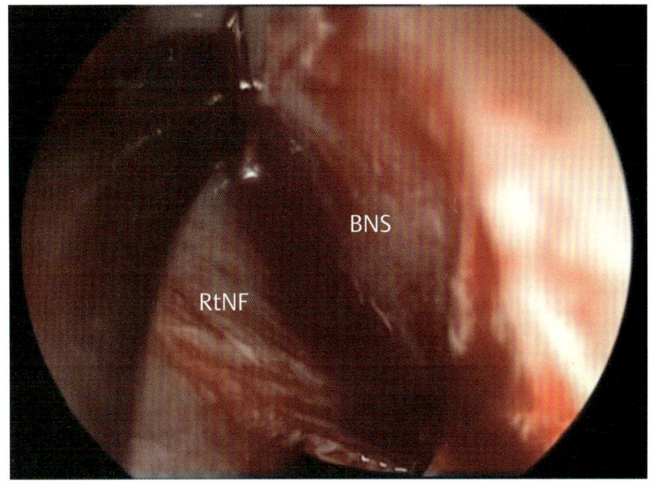

Fig. 23A.4 Raising of bilateral nasoseptal flaps.

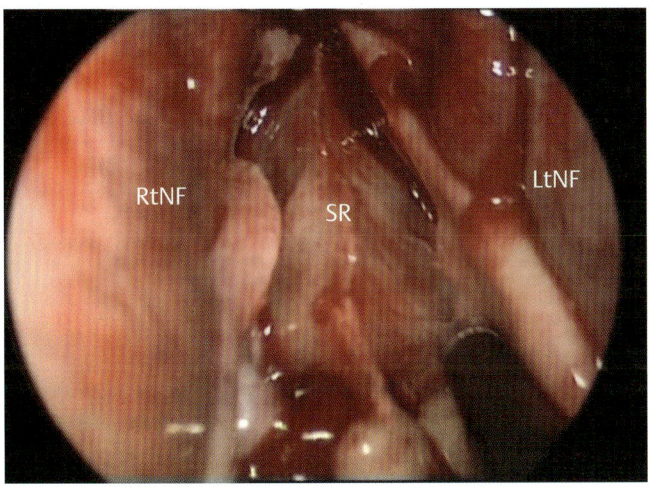

Fig. 23A.5 Exposure of the sphenoid rostrum (SR) after creation of bilateral nasoseptal flaps.

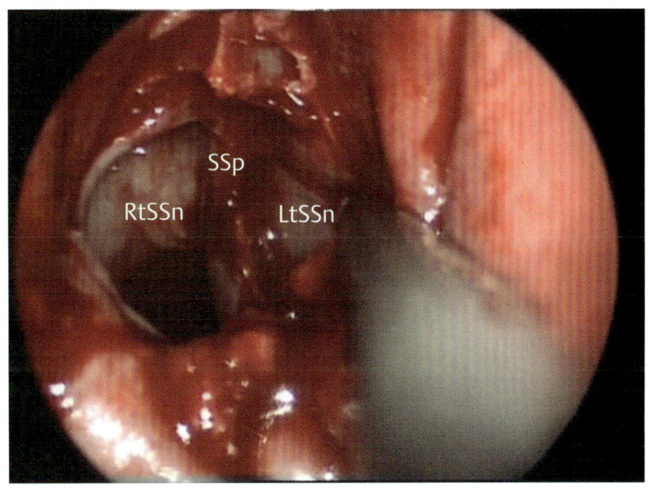

Fig. 23A.6 Removal of the sphenoid rostrum and bilateral exposure of the sphenoid sinuses.

8. Both cartilaginous and bony parts of the septum are removed completely to expose bilateral sphenoid ostia and the sphenoid rostrum (**Fig. 23A.5**).
9. The sphenoid ostia are identified bilaterally and widened inferomedially in a V shape with a Kerrison punch, and once bony removal is sufficient, the sphenoid keel is removed with a pituitary rongeur forceps.
10. After removal of the sphenoid rostrum, any residual mucosa or bony septation is removed to make the bilateral sphenoid sinus a single common cavity (**Fig. 23A.6**).
11. After the creation of bilateral nasoseptal flaps, removal of the nasal septum, sphenoid rostrum, and exposure of the sphenoid sinus, a full-house endoscopic sinus surgery of the left nasal cavity is performed. This includes an uncinectomy, middle meatal antrostomy, anterior and posterior ethmoidectomy, and exposure of the orbit and optic nerve creating a wide surgical view (**Fig. 23A.7** and **Fig. 23A.8**).
12. A left middle turbinate flap is also performed by cutting the first part of the middle turbinate up to its horizontal segment and the flap is pushed down out of the surgical field for later use (**Fig. 23A.9, Fig. 23A.10,** and **Fig. 23A.11**).
13. After a wide surgical exposure, the tumor is peeled off the medial part of the optic nerve and anterior to the cavernous sinus with suction and blunt elevator (**Fig. 23A.12** and **Fig. 23A.13**).
14. Dissection is consistently checked and confirmed with neuronavigation.

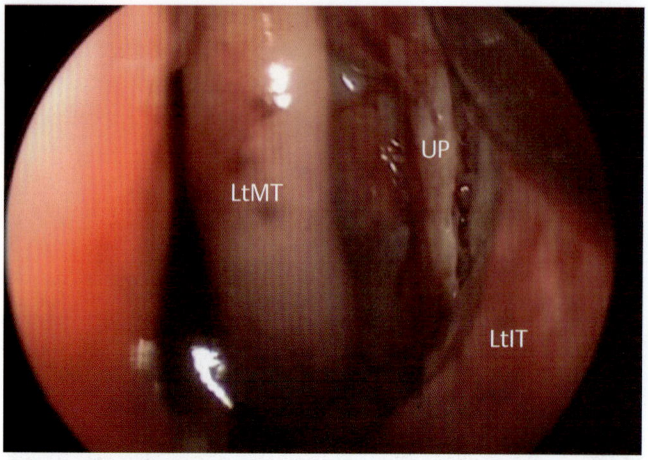

Fig. 23A.7 A full-house endoscopic sinus surgery on the left nasal cavity is performed starting with an uncinectomy.

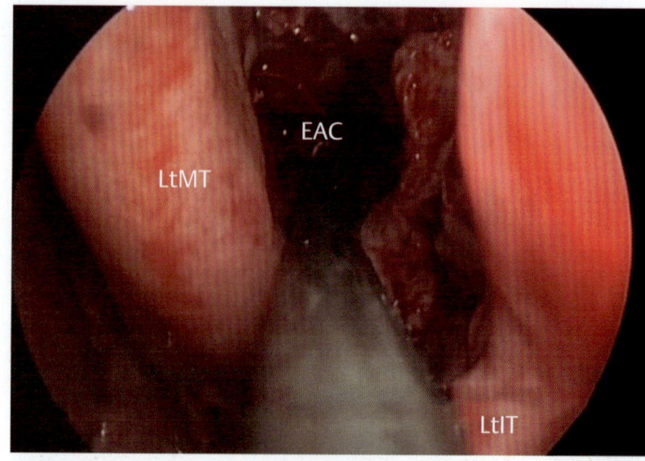

Fig. 23A.8 Anterior and posterior ethmoidectomy are performed.

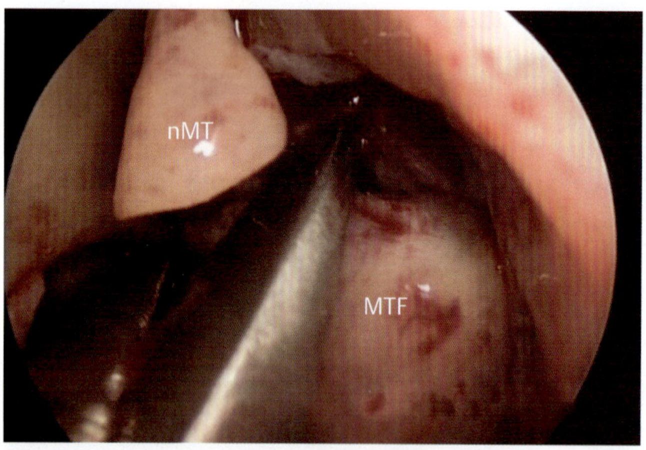

Fig. 23A.9 Creation of a middle turbinate flap (MTF).

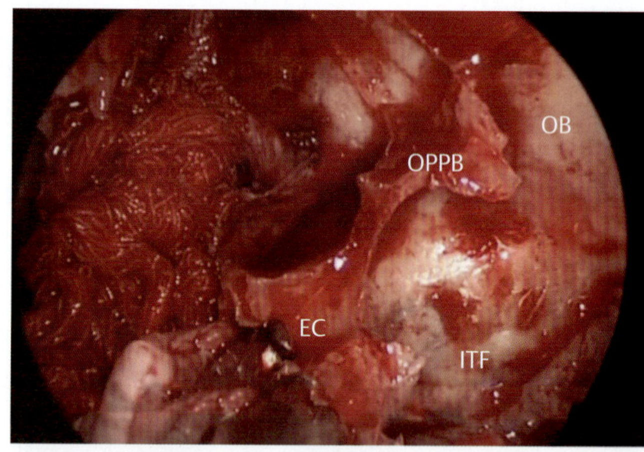

Fig. 23A.10 Removal of the ethmoidal crest (EC) and orbital process of the palatine bone (OPPB) improves the access to the orbital apex and the infratemporal fossa (ITF).

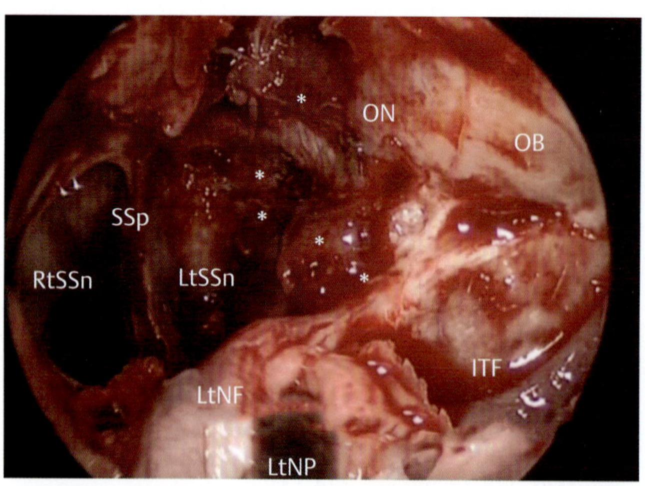

Fig. 23A.11 Creation of a wide surgical view with exposure of the tumor (*), orbit (OB), optic nerve (ON), and infratemporal fossa (ITF).

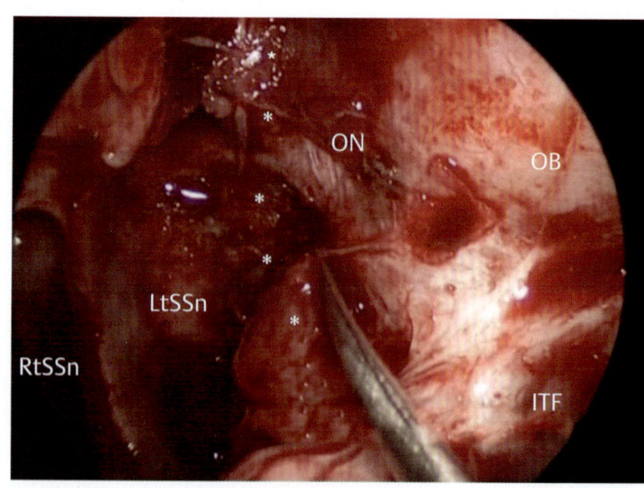

Fig. 23A.12 Dissection of tumor (*) over medial part of the left orbital apex.

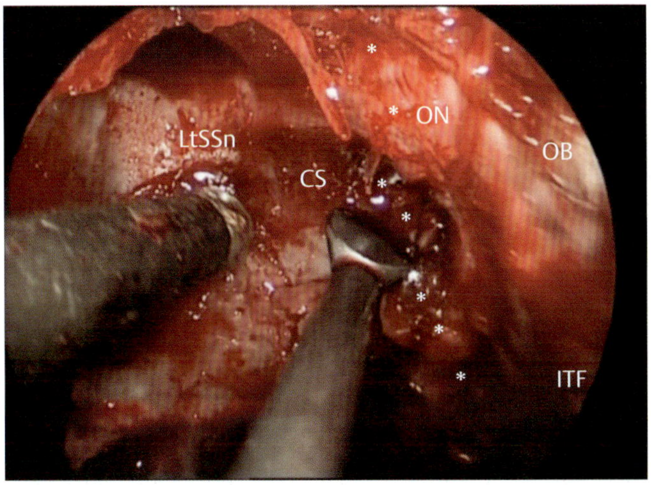

Fig. 23A.13 Mircosurgical tumor (*) dissection from the anterior wall of the left cavernous sinus (CS).

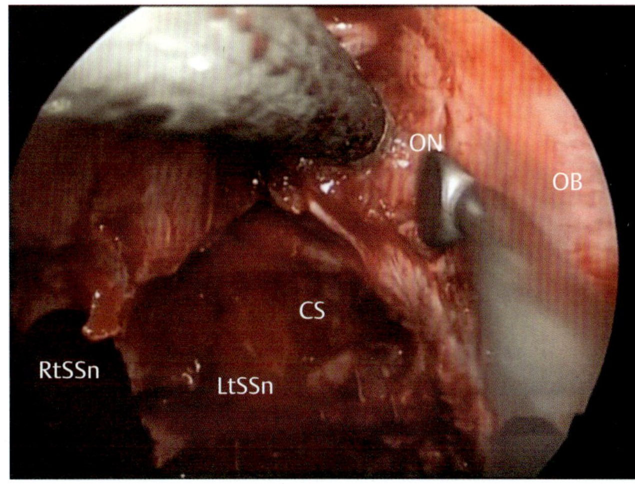

Fig. 23A.14 Dissection of the superior and lateral parts of the tumor (*) in relation to the optic nerve (ON).

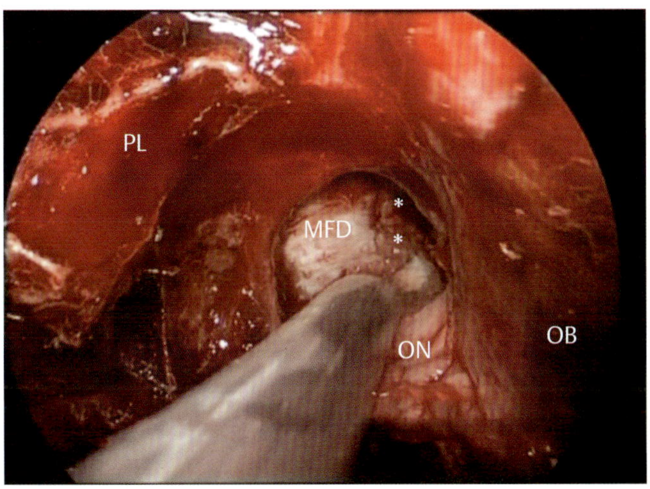

Fig. 23A.15 An ultrasonic surgical aspirator is used to remove loose tumor parts (*) dissected away from the underlying middle fossa dura (MFD).

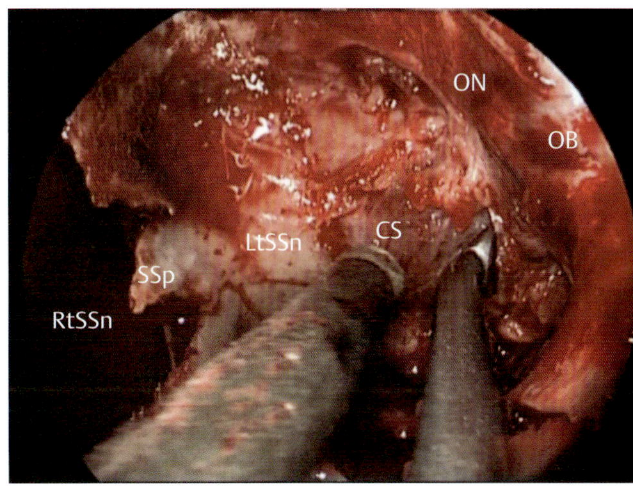

Fig. 23A.16 Dissection of the tumor (*) away from the lateral part of the cavernous sinus (CS).

15. The superior and lateral part of the tumor in relation to the optic nerve is peeled off the underlying dura and loose parts are dissected away with an ultrasonic surgical aspirator (**Fig. 23A.14** and **Fig. 23A.15**).
16. Dissection is now focused on the lateral aspect of the cavernous sinus, again with a combination of blunt dissection and ultrasonic surgical aspirator. The maxillary nerve is exposed in this dissection (**Fig. 23A.16** and **Fig. 23A.17**).
17. After complete tumor removal, the surgical field is inspected for any bleeding, and hemostasis is diligently secured (**Fig. 23A.18**).
18. The surgical field is washed copiously with saline and the defect is closed with layers of Surgicel (oxidized cellulose polymer, Ethicon) and Gelfoam (absorbable gelatin sponge, Pfizer) and covered with the nasoseptal flaps and middle turbinate flap (**Fig. 23A.19**).
19. The nasal cavity is then packed with Nasopore (synthetic biodegradable foam, Stryker, USA) making sure to provide an adequate airway along the nasal floor.

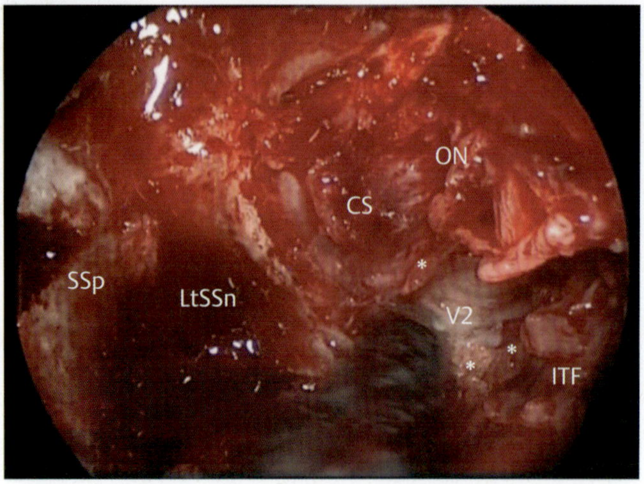

Fig. 23A.17 Exposure of left maxillary nerve (V2) at the tip of the suction device. The tumor (*) is visible on either side.

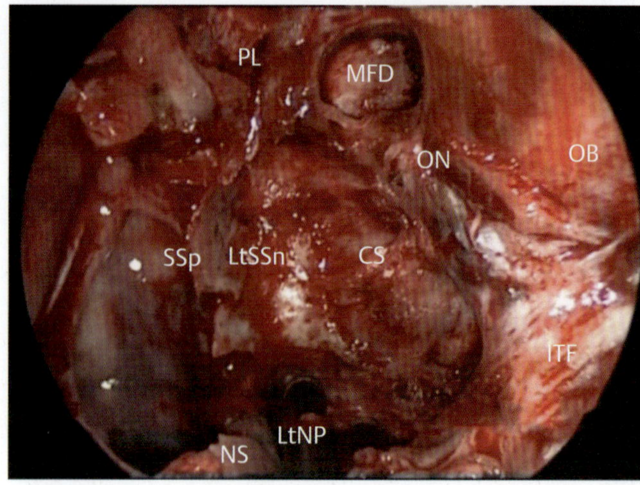

Fig. 23A.18 Final surgical field after tumor removal.

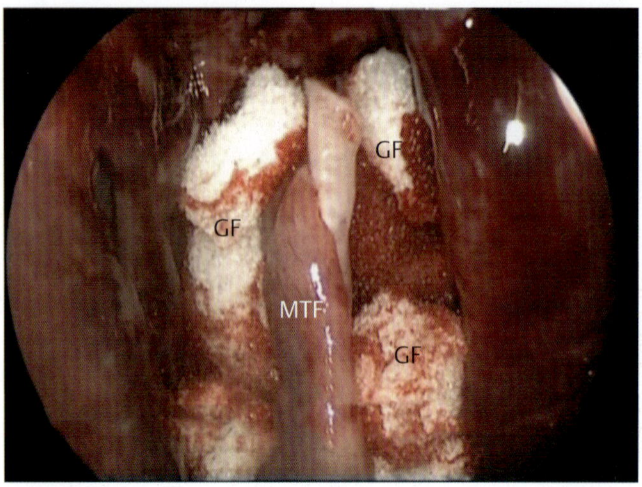

Fig. 23A.19 Placement of Surgicel, Gelfoam (GF), and naso-septal and middle turbinate flaps (MTF) onto the surgical site.

Case 23B

Endoscopic Transnasal Optic Nerve Decompression in a 4-Year-Old Child

Sien Hui Tan, Adzreil Bakri, and Prepageran Narayanan

History

A 4-year-old boy had an alleged fall at home. The patient presented with right near-complete ptosis, hand motion vision in his right eye, and positive relative afferent pupillary defect. His extraocular movement showed restrictions on upward gaze and abduction. A computed tomography (CT) scan revealed right optic nerve compression and pneumo-orbita (**Fig. 23B.1** and **Fig. 23B.2**). This is a particularly challenging case because the sphenoid sinus is not yet pneumatized (**Fig. 23B.3**). Postoperatively, he showed improvement in vision to 6/45 and right partial ptosis. This approach may be used for all cases requiring optic nerve decompression.

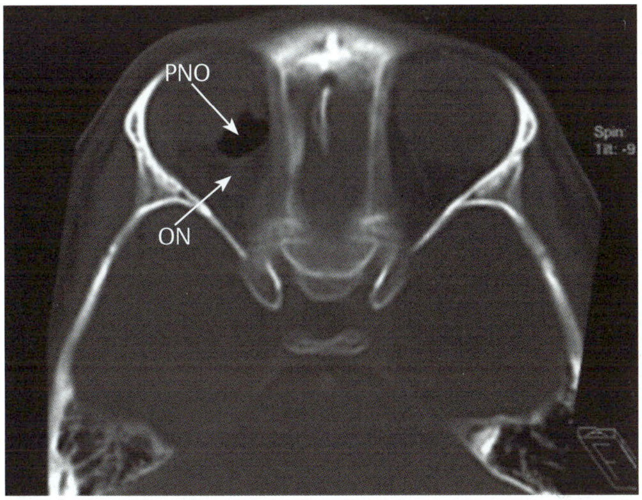

Fig. 23B.1 Preoperative axial CT scan showing right optic nerve (ON) involvement with right pneumo-orbita (PNO).

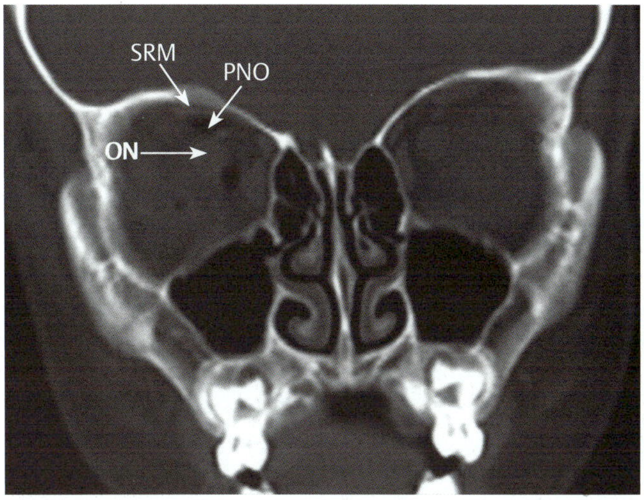

Fig. 23B.2 Preoperative coronal CT scan demonstrating right optic nerve (ON) and superior rectus muscle (SRM) involvement with right pneumo-orbita (PNO).

Surgical Steps

1. The patient is positioned supine under general anesthesia.
2. The nose is decongested with nasal packing as per the institution's standard methods.
3. Local anesthesia is infiltrated to the axilla of the middle turbinate.
4. The middle turbinate is first gently medialized. An uncinectomy and a wide middle meatal antrostomy are performed.
5. Next, both anterior and posterior ethmoidectomy are carried out to expose the medial orbital wall.
6. A sphenoidectomy is usually performed for visualization of the optic canal and internal carotid artery. This case is especially challenging, as the sphenoid sinus is not yet pneumatized at 4 years of age. The surgeon must take extra precautions because of the increased risk of optic nerve damage.
7. The lamina papyracea comes into view and is removed with a Freer elevator to expose the periorbita (**Fig. 23B.4** and **Fig. 23B.5**). Entry into the lamina papyracea should be below the level of the ethmoid foramina to prevent injury to the ethmoidal arteries. This is to lessen the risk of retrobulbar bleeding and, subsequently, vision loss. Care must also be taken to avoid injuring the periorbita and the underlying extraocular muscles.
8. After removal of the posterior lamina papyracea, the periorbita is followed posteriorly to where they converge at the orbital apex.

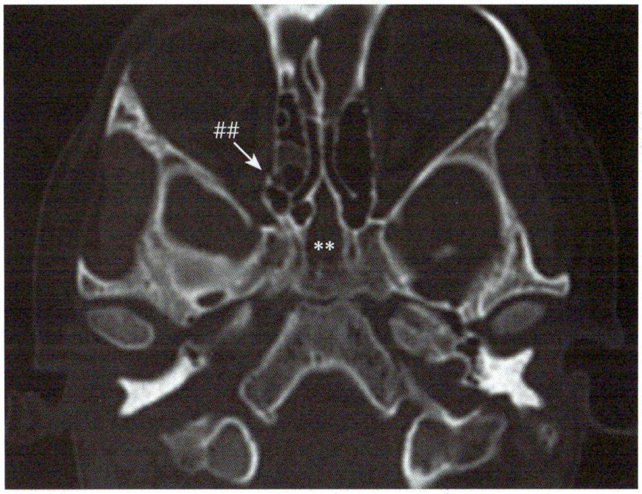

Fig. 23B.3 Preoperative axial CT scan showing right optic nerve compression with fracture at posterior part of lamina papyracea (##) and nonpneumatized sphenoid sinuses (**).

9. The annulus of Zinn is exposed after complete resection of the lamina papyracea. The optic canal is identified in the sphenoid sinus, and part of the overlying bone is removed with a Freer elevator to expose the optic nerve sheath (**Fig. 23B.6**).
10. The optic nerve sheath is incised along the optic nerve and through the annulus of Zinn (**Fig. 23B.7** and **Fig. 23B.8**). It is important to avoid the inferomedial quadrant as the ophthalmic artery is located there.
11. Meticulous hemostasis is secured with adrenaline-soaked gauze, bipolar cauterization, and Gelfoam (Pfizer).

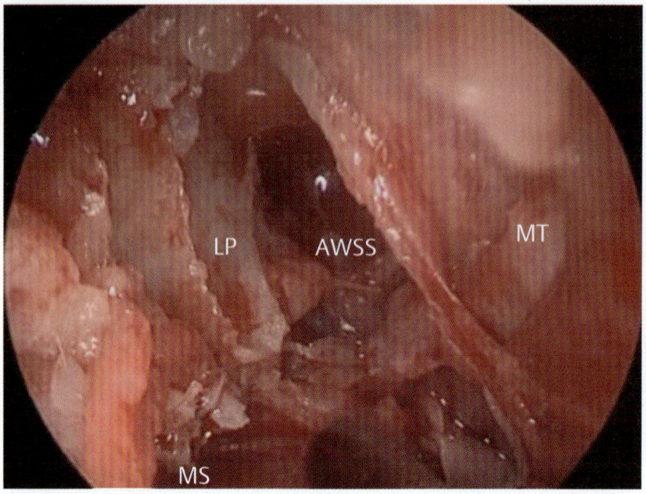

Fig. 23B.4 The lamina papyracea (LP) is exposed after complete ethmoidectomy.

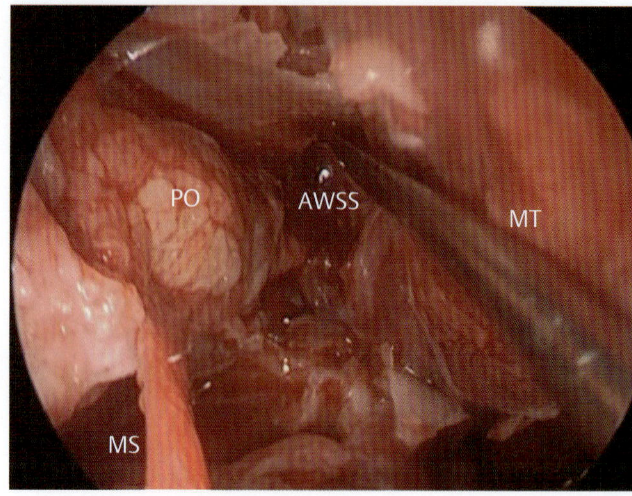

Fig. 23B.5 The lamina papyracea is removed with a Freer elevator and Blakesley forceps to expose the periorbita (PO).

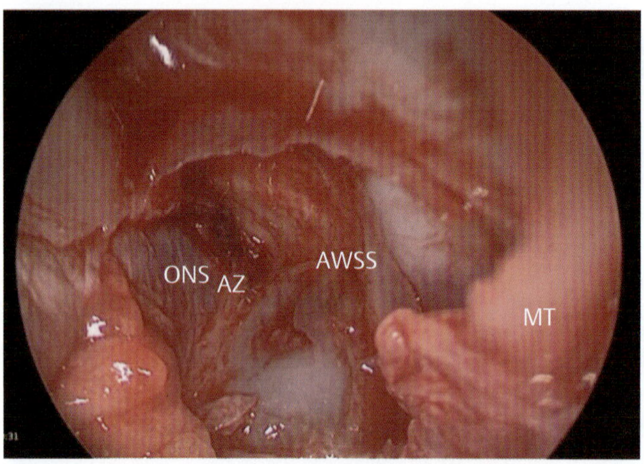

Fig. 23B.6 The Annulus of Zinn (AZ) and the optic nerve sheath (ONS) are exposed after complete removal of the lamina papyracea and part of the overlying bone of the optic canal.

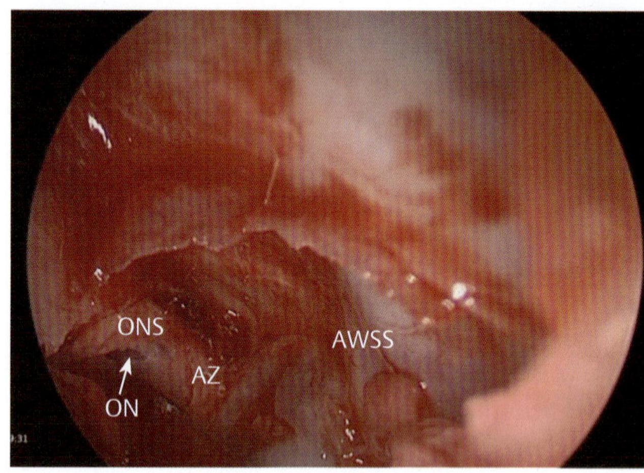

Fig. 23B.7 An incision is made on the optic nerve sheath (ONS) at the superomedial quadrant along the optic nerve (ON) and through the annulus of Zinn (AZ).

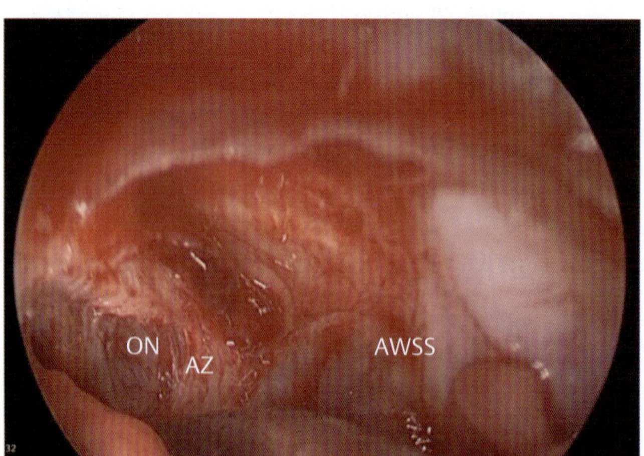

Fig. 23B.8 The exposed optic nerve (ON) after incision of the optic nerve sheath.

Case 23C

Endoscopic Endonasal Excision of Recurrent Optic Nerve Glioma

Kong Yew Liew, Saif Al-Zahid, Michel Roethlisberger, Prepageran Narayanan, and Vicknes Waran

History

A 22-year-old female patient presented with increasing headaches and inability to concentrate in class. She had a history of an optic nerve glioma that underwent previous transcranial excisions and a permanent cerebrospinal fluid (CSF) diversion because of chronic hydrocephalus. The patient had documented blindness. Clinical examination revealed lower limb weakness. A magnetic resonance imaging (MRI) revealed a mixed solid and cystic mass occupying the sellar and suprasellar compartment measuring approximately 4.5 × 4 × 3 cm with significant brainstem and optic chiasm compression (**Fig. 23C.1a–d**).

Surgical Steps

1. A binostril four-handed technique is utilized to give wide access to the planum, tuberculum, sella, and clivus as described in Chapter 1, with harvesting of a left-sided nasoseptal flap for reconstruction of the subsequent defect (**Fig. 23C.2**).
2. Drilling is commenced over the sella with a diamond burr to thin the bone (**Fig. 23C.3**). Care should be taken to remain in the midline to avoid accidental injury in the carotid siphons or cavernous sinuses bilaterally. Positioning should be confirmed with image-guided surgery (IGS) at regular intervals. The anterior intercavernous sinus may also be encountered as the drilling proceeds deeper. Any remnant ledges should also be smoothened to allow easier removal in a later stage.
3. When the bone is sufficiently thinned out, it can be flaked off to reveal the underlying dura. The surrounding dura is then dissected free from the bone with a right-angle dissector (**Fig. 23C.4**).
4. A Kerrison punch can then be insinuated between the bone and the dura to remove the bone (**Fig. 23C.5**). Access to the dura can be widened carefully, making sure to free the underlying dura prior to bone removal. Dural exposure should be extended laterally until the blue color of the cavernous sinus is visible, and superiorly and inferiorly as much as required for removal of the lesion, confirmed by IGS (**Fig. 23C.6**).
5. A cruciate incision is made (**Fig. 23C.7**). The dura is first incised horizontally. Any underlying tissue is dissected away from the dura with a right-angle dissector. A horizontal incision is made to complete the cruciate incision.
6. The anterior intercavernous sinus may be encountered at the inferior limb of the incision and should be controlled with bipolar cautery prior to the incision.
7. Excision is commenced with debulking of the central component of the lesion with an ultrasonic aspirator (**Fig. 23C.8**). Removal of the central component allows the edges of the lesion to collapse inward (**Fig. 23C.9**), aiding the surgeon to visualize and dissect free the margins of the tumor before removal.
8. As debulking proceeds posteriorly, the inferior edge of the lesion is brought into view and delivered into the central dissection zone with a combination of blunt dissection and aspiration (**Fig. 23C.10**).
9. Care is taken as debulking of the inferior component proceeds posteriorly because of the basilar artery and its branches (**Fig. 23C.11**), injury of which can lead to catastrophic consequences.
10. Removal of the cystic component within the central zone of dissection reveals the third ventricle that had been splayed open by the tumor (**Fig. 23C.12**). Further dissection of the thin tumor capsule off the third ventricle wall reveals the foramina of Monro and right mammillary body (**Fig. 23C.13**).
11. The branches of the basilar artery divide the resection cavity into a superior component where the third ventricle is the posterior-most limit (**Fig. 23C.14**) and an inferior component where the midbrain is seen (**Fig. 23C.15**).
12. The resection cavity is then inspected for remnant tumor. Positioning is confirmed on IGS.
13. Meticulous hemostasis is achieved with cottonoids and absorbable hemostats.
14. Completeness of resection is assessed on intraoperative MRI.
15. The defect is then reconstructed with abdominal fat as a first layer (**Fig. 23C.16**). The fat is tucked under the bone edges to ensure a watertight seal but not packed tightly enough to cause compression.

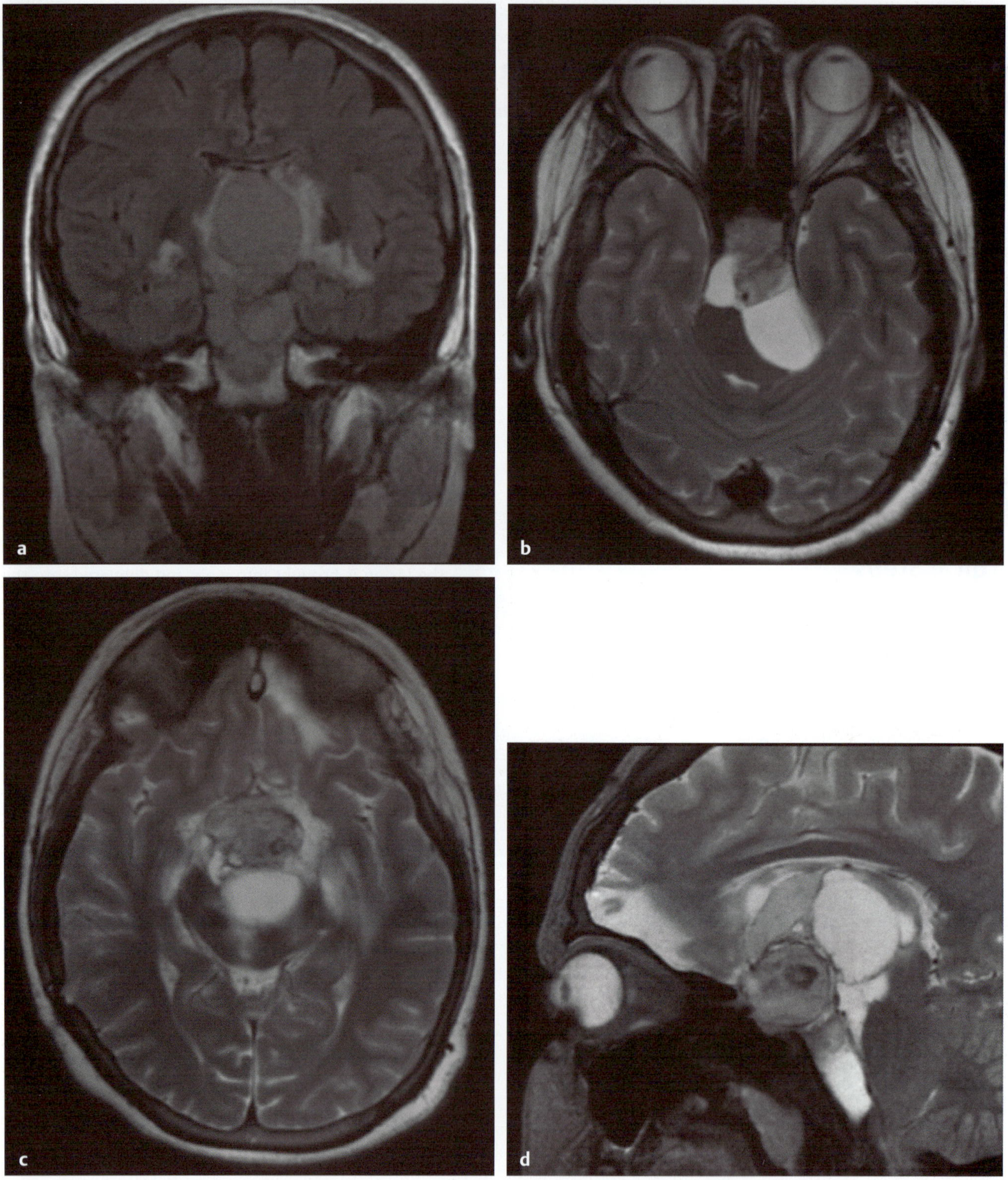

Fig. 23C.1 **(a)** T1-weighted coronal MRI section revealing an iso- to hyperintense mass compressing the lateral ventricles. **(b)** T2-weighted axial MRI section demonstrating extensive brainstem shift to the right side due to a compressive mass lesion. **(c)** T2-weighted axial MRI section revealing splaying of the midbrain by mass effect. **(d)** Parasagittal T2-weighted section revealing the solid component of the tumor mainly occupying the sellar/suprasellar compartment.

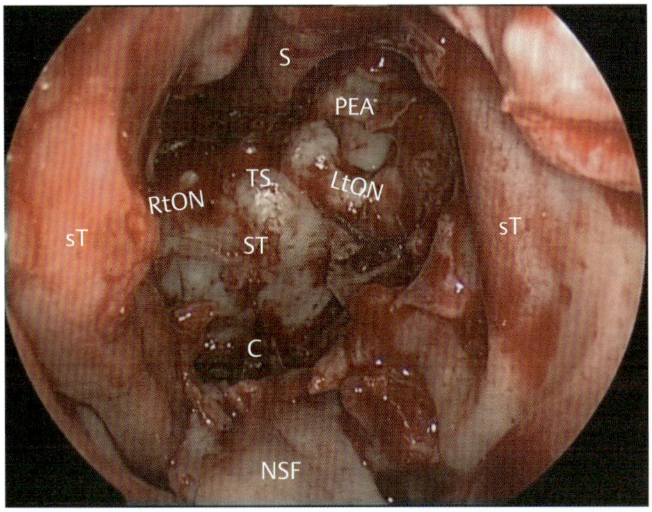

Fig. 23C.2 Endonasal endoscopic view after removal of sphenoidal mucosa and septations. The superior turbinates (sT) can be seen bilaterally, with the nasoseptal flap (NSF) pedicle seen inferiorly and the remnant nasal septum (S) superiorly. Note the hyperpneumatization of the sphenoid sinus allowing direct identification of the left posterior ethmoid artery (PEA).

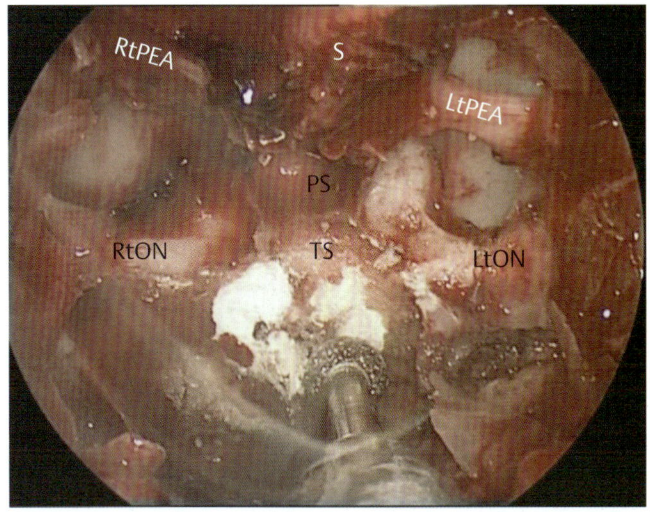

Fig. 23C.3 Commencement of drilling over the sella and tuberculum sellae (TS). The bone is thinned centrally and expanded outward. Hyperpenumatization of the sphenoid sinus allows appreciation of the right (RtsPEA) and left posterior ethmoid arteries (LtPEA).

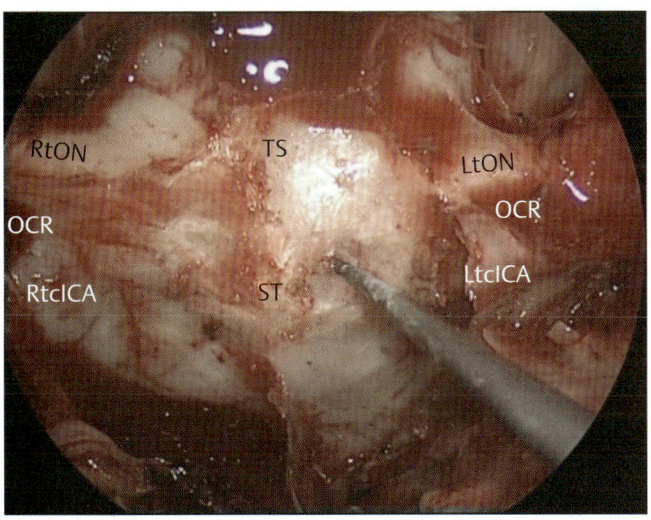

Fig. 23C.4 A right-angle dissector sweeping the underlying dura away from the bone. Note that the bone is thin enough to see through as the dura is dissected away.

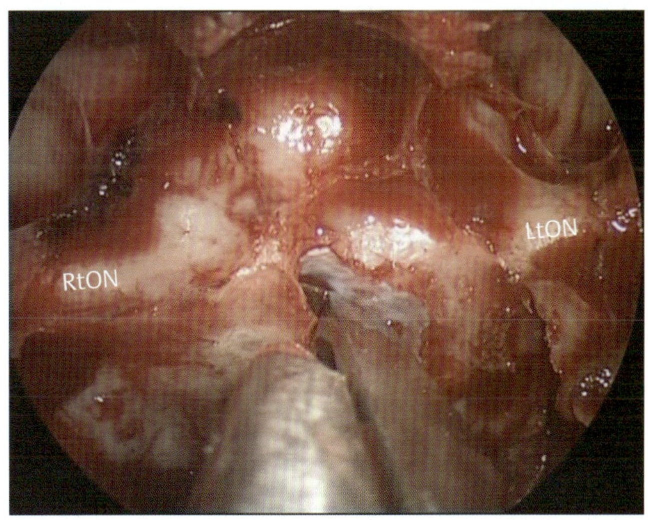

Fig. 23C.5 A Kerrison punch engaged to remove the bone overlying the sella. Dura is visible beneath it.

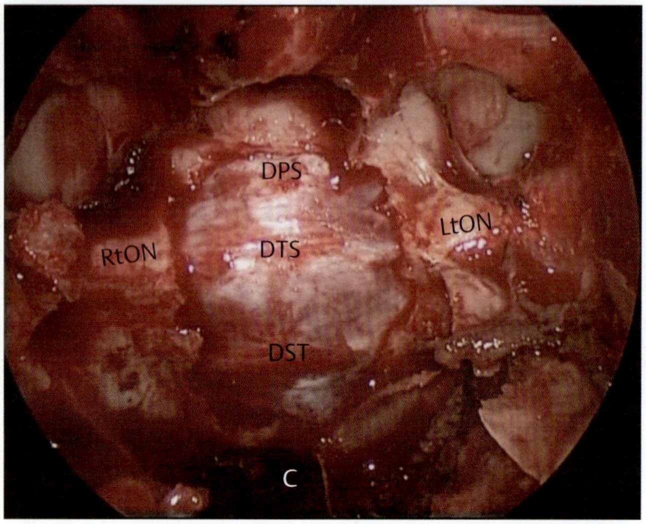

Fig. 23C.6 Final bony exposure before opening of the dura. In this case, the bone overlying the clival recess (C) (inferiorly at the location of the aspirator) did not have to be removed. Dura of planum sphenoidale (DPS), tuberculum sellae (DTS), and sella turcica (DST) exposed.

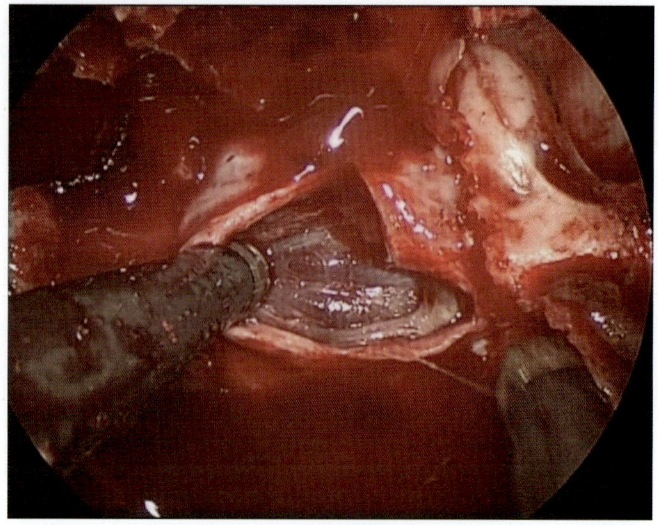

Fig. 23C.7 Completed cruciate incision with the lesion visible beneath. A biopsy can be taken at this stage prior to the commencement of formal excision.

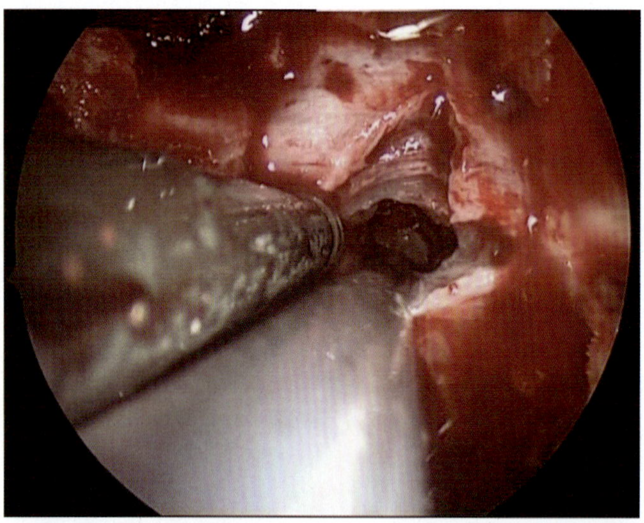

Fig. 23C.8 Commencement of debulking of the lesion with an ultrasonic aspirator.

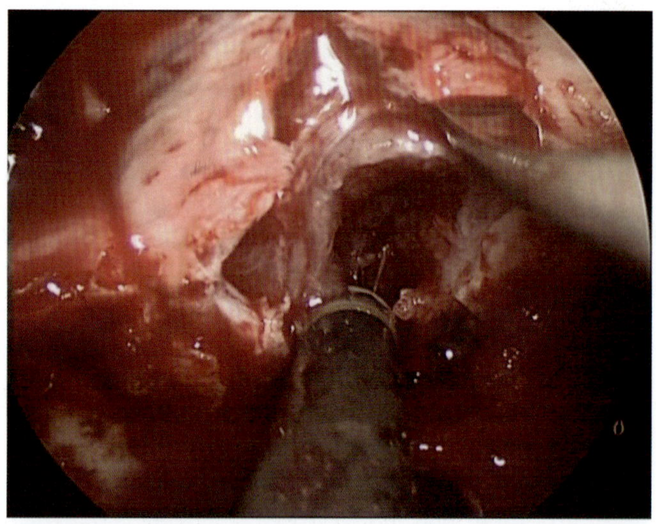

Fig. 23C.9 The visible edges of the lesion coming into view as they collapse into the central dissection zone after debulking of the central component.

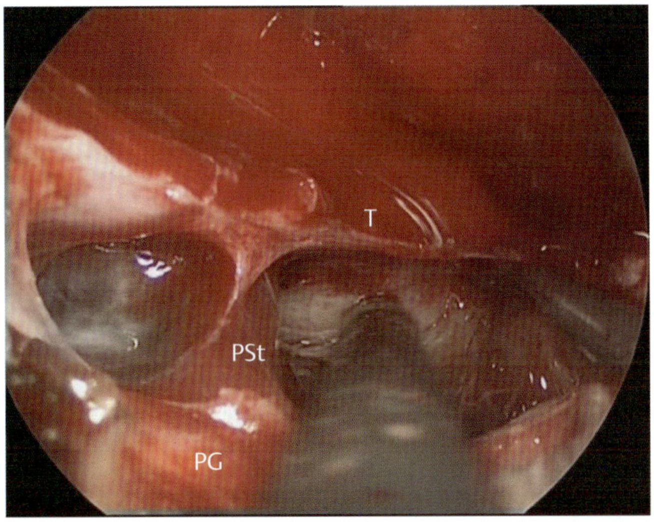

Fig. 23C.10 The inferior edge of the lesion (T) is being pulled upward with a dissector and freed using an aspirator (center). The pituitary stalk (PSt) is now visible.

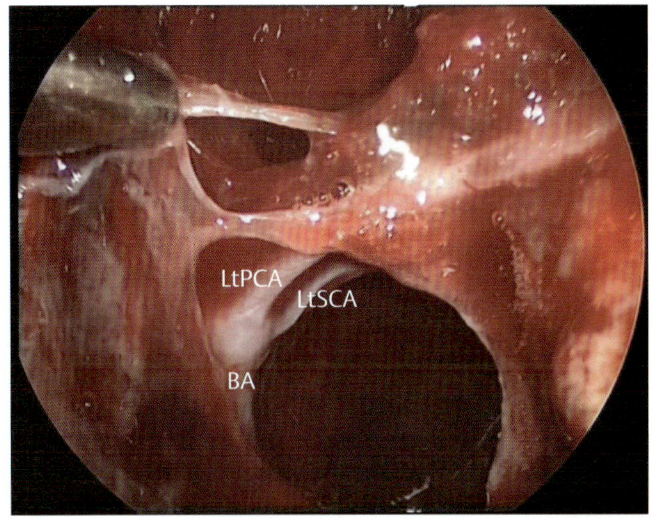

Fig. 23C.11 The left posterior cerebral artery (LtPCA) and left superior cerebellar artery (LtSCA) are seen coming from the basilar artery (BA). The central resection zone is seen superiorly.

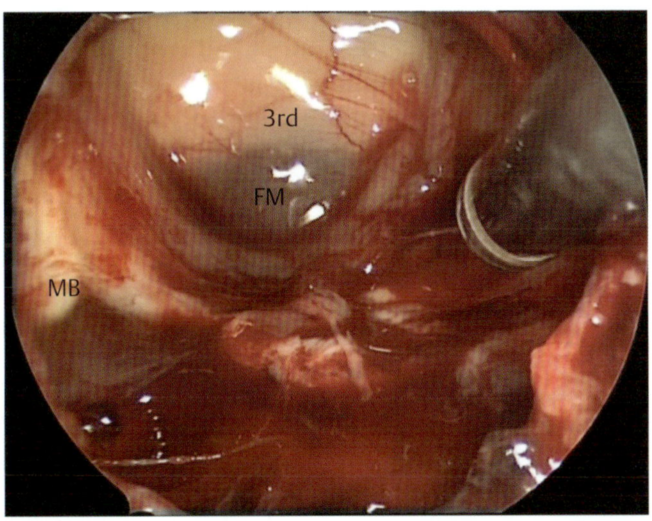

Fig. 23C.12 Endoscopic endonasal view after removal of the posterior cystic component. The third ventricle (3rd) is splayed open revealing the right mammillary body (MB) and tumor capsule still covering the foramina of Monro (FM).

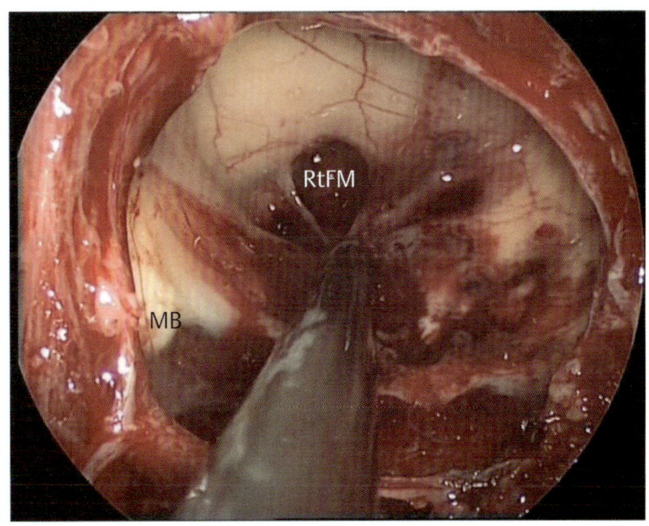

Fig. 23C.13 The right foramen of Monro (RtFM) is seen after removal of the tumor capsule posteriorly.

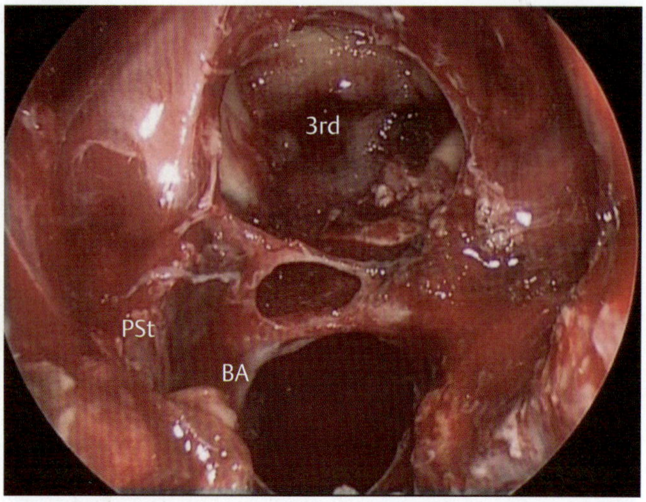

Fig. 23C.14 Final view of the resection cavity. The third ventricle (3rd) is visible superiorly, separated from the inferior cavity by the branches of the basilar artery. The pituitary stalk (PSt) is seen adjacent to the basilar artery (BA).

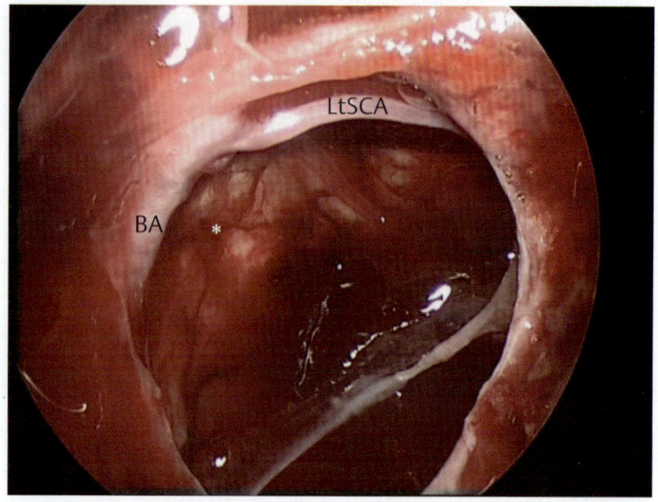

Fig. 23C.15 View of the midbrain (*) deep within the posterior limit of the inferior resection cavity.

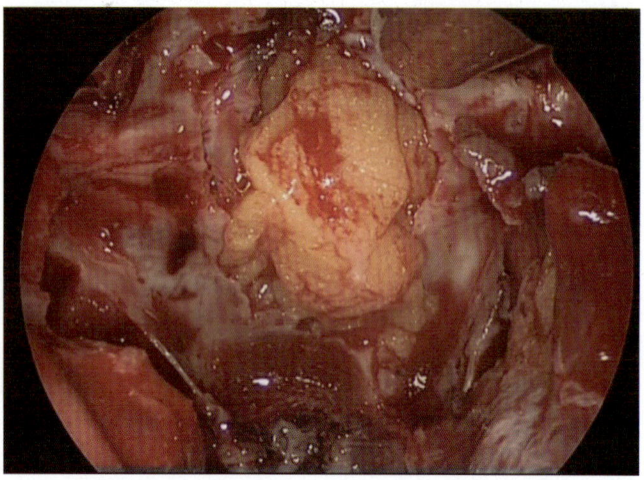

Fig. 23C.16 The first layer of the skull base defect reconstruction consisting of an intradurally plugged abdominal fat graft.

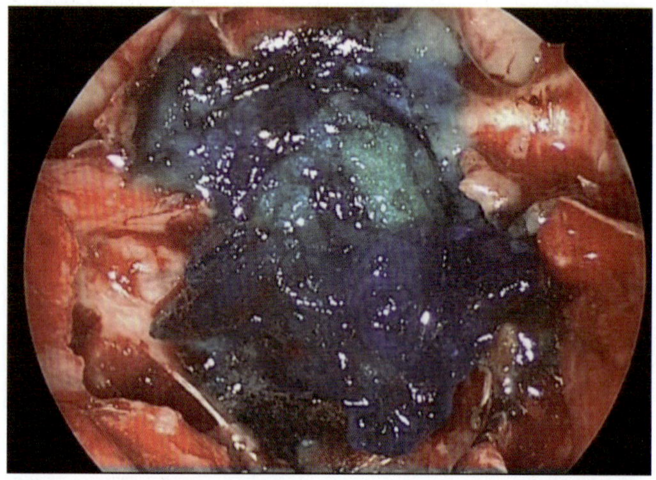

Fig. 23C.17 Fat graft covered with a synthetic dural sealant.

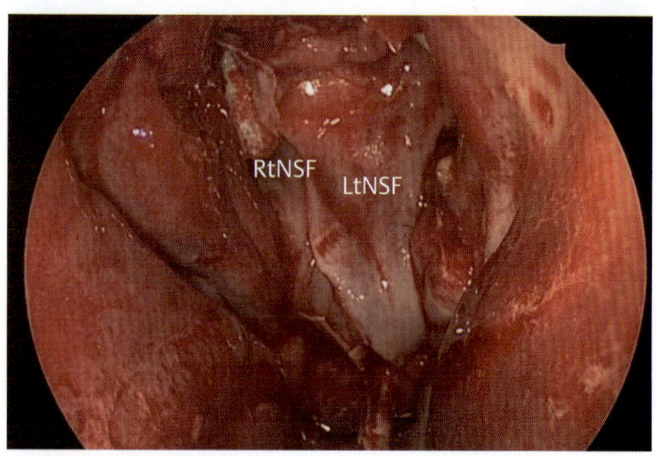

Fig. 23C.18 Bilateral nasoseptal flaps (NSF) reinforcing the defect.

16. This is then covered with synthetic dural sealant or tissue glue (**Fig. 23C.17**).
17. The nasoseptal flap is then rotated in place to reinforce the repair. The construct is stabilized with absorbable sponges and packing (**Fig. 23C.18**).
18. A MRI scan is performed postoperatively to confirm the extent of resection and brainstem decompression. (**Fig. 23C.19**).

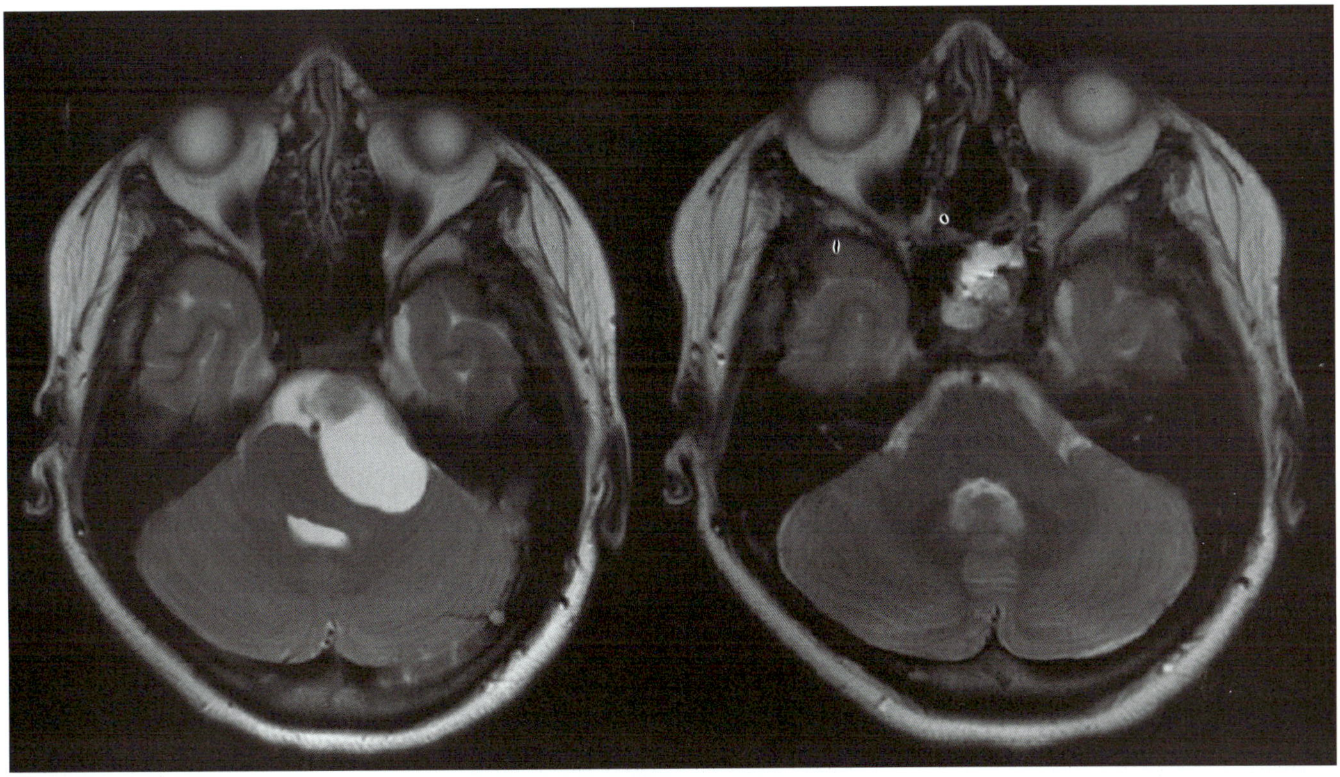

Fig. 23C.19 Comparison between the preoperative axial MRI (*left*) and the postoperative axial MRI (*right*) showing resolution of the brainstem compression.

Section VIII

Infratemporal Fossa and Parapharyngeal Space

Chapter 24 Endoscopic Transpterygoid Approaches to the Coronal Plane

Kyle VanKoevering, Nyall London, Daniel M. Prevedello, and Ricardo L. Carrau

Introduction

Expanded endonasal approaches have radically changed the surgical treatment paradigms for lesions across the ventral skull base. The use of high-definition nasal endoscopy with a two-surgeon, four-handed technique has allowed for minimally invasive, low morbidity approaches. Deep knowledge of the complex anatomy is critical to understand the indications, technical nuances, and limits of these endonasal approaches. Dividing the various approaches and access techniques into anatomical corridors is a key tenant in planning a surgical technique. The sagittal plane corridors include approaches to the "median" skull base from the frontal sinus outflow tracts, back along the cribriform plate and fovea ethmoidalis, planum sphenoidale, sella and pituitary gland, and down the clivus to the craniocervical junction. Conversely, the coronal plane corridors include approaches to the "paramedian" ventral skull base, including the orbit and orbital roof, lateral recess of the sphenoid sinus, infratemporal and pterygopalatine fossae, middle cranial fossa and Meckel's cave, and petrous apex.[1]

Paramedian approaches (apart from the orbit) utilize the pterygoid process as a key anatomical landmark and as a gateway for the corridor. As the pterygoid process is typically transgressed to access the coronal plane anatomy, it is thus termed the "transpterygoid approach."

Pertinent Anatomy

The maxillary sinus serves as the access to the pterygopalatine fossa and pterygoid process. Just behind the posterior maxillary wall sits the pterygopalatine fossa and its soft tissue contents: the pterygopalatine ganglion, V2, and the distal internal maxillary artery; the removal of the lateral wall provides access to the masticator space, including the internal maxillary artery, buccal fat pad, V3, and pterygoid musculature.

Just posterior to the pterygopalatine fossa sits the pterygoid process, descending from the basisphenoid at the junction of the body and greater wing of the sphenoid bone. It comprises a medial and a lateral plate that project inferiorly and posteriorly, joined by a common wall anteriorly. Two foramina and their canals, namely vidian and rotundum, mark the anterior aspect of the pterygoid process and provide anatomical reference to structures in the infratemporal and middle cranial fossa, as well as the nasopharynx.

The vidian nerve is a combined sympathetic/parasympathetic nerve that travels in the vidian or pterygoid canal, along the floor of the sphenoid at the junction of the medial pterygoid plate, and then enters the pterygopalatine ganglion. When following this canal posteriorly, the anterior genu of the internal carotid artery (ICA) can be reliably identified just superior to foramen lacerum. Laterally, the foramen rotundum and its corresponding maxillary nerve run along the lateral wall of the sphenoid sinus, traversing the inferomedial aspect of the middle cranial fossa before emptying into the pterygopalatine fossa. Between the pterygoid plates one can identify the tensor veli palatini muscle. The mandibular nerve exits the foramen ovale just posterolateral to the lateral pterygoid plate, and serves as a good landmark for the distal pharyngeal ICA.[2] Understanding these key anatomical structures is critical to planning and safely performing transpterygoid approaches to the paramedian skull base.

Preoperative Considerations

Patients with lesions located laterally (i.e., in the coronal plane) present with a wide variety of problems, ranging from cerebrospinal fluid (CSF) leaks in the lateral recess of the sphenoid to cranial neuropathies in the maxillary nerve or hypoglossal nerve for malignant processes. Whatever the initial presenting symptoms are, a comprehensive clinical evaluation is critical. In-office nasal endoscopy can provide a potential view of the lesion, as well as demonstrating the nasal anatomy that may be at play (including septal deviations, tumor vascularity, etc.). A detailed neurologic examination should include all cranial nerves and functional testing of the eye. Depending on the degree of orbital involvement, a formal ophthalmologic evaluation may be valuable. Optimization of the patient's comorbidities is ideal if time permits. A biopsy of the lesion allows for histopathologic diagnosis and greatly aids in treatment planning.

Coupled with the histologic diagnosis, cross-sectional imaging with both computed tomography (CT) and contrasted magnetic resonance imaging (MRI) is critical to evaluate the tumor extent and the bony and soft tissue anatomy, respectively. A complete evaluation of the carotid artery's course should be performed with imaging studies, and a CT angiography may be utilized if the anatomy is not well delineated with the MRI. A detailed study of both imaging modalities is complementary. Evidence of bony erosion and relative locations of various skull base foramina can be appreciated on a high-resolution CT, along with the course of the carotid artery. Conversely, the MRI helps delineate the extent of the tumor, soft tissue invasion, intracranial extension, brain or orbital invasion, and perineural spread, and helps distinguish inspissated mucous or inflamed sinuses from the primary lesion.

Compiling the histology, imaging, and clinical data, the surgeon can begin to plan the approach. Lesions located lateral to the vidian nerve are likely to require some component of a transpterygoid approach for comprehensive exposure. Frequently, these tumors will require multidisciplinary care including otolaryngologists, neurosurgeons, ophthalmologists, radiation oncologists, and medical oncologists among others. A dedicated tumor board is an invaluable resource in developing a comprehensive treatment algorithm. Under the direction of the tumor board, the goals of surgical treatment can be discussed. The tumor may only be amenable to subtotal or gross total resection if an extensive perineural spread is noted, or if the carotid is encased. Adjuvant treatment is frequently required for both benign and especially malignant pathologies.

Contraindications

Similar to other skull base procedures, significant cardiopulmonary morbidity must be considered before offering a transpterygoid procedure. During these cases, significant intraoperative bleeding from the tumor bed or internal maxillary artery can result in hemodynamic instability. In spite of being "minimally invasive," this procedure is still analogous to traditional craniofacial approaches to the paramedian skull base. Encasement or invasion of the ICA is not an absolute contraindication for surgery. However, the risk of debulking this tumor is high. If an "oncologic" resection is required, preoperative coil embolization or even bypass may be required. It should be noted that for head and neck malignancies encasement of the carotid artery is generally regarded as an "unresectable" tumor. Even if the tumor is resected after embolization, the prognosis remains grim.

Tumors extending posterior to the carotid artery cannot be safely accessed via this route. Lastly, active sinonasal infection is a relative contraindication to intradural procedures, given a risk of seeding intracranial infection.

Surgical Techniques

To better understand, plan, and communicate transpterygoid techniques, the approaches can be classified into five stages depending on the extent of exposure required.[3] This classification is based on the depth of exposure and the trajectory superior or inferior to the horizontal plane of the vidian nerve:

Type A—Partial removal of the medial and/or lateral pterygoid plates, such as that required to tunnel a temporoparietal fascia flap through the pterygomaxillary fissure.[4]

Type B—Removal of the anteromedial aspect of the base of the pterygoid process, indicated for lesions in the lateral recess of the sphenoid sinus above the level of the vidian canal. This is an extradural approach such as that used for a lateral recess encephalocele or CSF leak.

Type C—Dissection of the vidian canal removing the base of the pterygoid plates to reach the petrous apex (infra- or retropetrous), Meckel's cave, or cavernous sinus. This is indicated for intradural approaches to the middle fossa, and the vidian helps define the anterior genu of the petrous carotid to facilitate safe dissection.

Type D—Provides access to the infratemporal fossa and requires a variable removal of the plates. The infratemporal fossa is lateral to the pterygoid plates and extended endoscopic lateral exposure can often be facilitated by a sublabial (Caldwell-Luc) maxillectomy, Denker's maxillectomy, or transseptal approach.

Type E—Removal of the medial pterygoid plate or even the entire pterygoid process and medial third of the eustachian tube to expose the lateral nasopharynx (fossa of Rosenmüller) or the lateral aspect of the craniocervical junction. This would be indicated for an endoscopic nasopharyngectomy.

Preoperative Setup

After a thorough preoperative workup is complete, a safe and successful transpterygoid approach requires a significant preprocedural setup. Stereotactic navigation is an extremely valuable tool for safely navigating this complex surgical corridor. Unless a limited transpterygoid approach is planned (Type A or B), most patients are secured in a Mayfield head holder with pins. The high-resolution preoperative CT (or CT angiogram) is then registered to the patient's anatomy. This can be fused with the MRI to demonstrate the vasculature, bony anatomy, and soft tissue planes.

In addition to stereotactic navigation, neuromonitoring is a critical adjunct to monitor for cranial nerve or intracranial complications. Given the proximity of the ICA, virtually all patients should be monitored with somatosensory-evoked potentials, along with pertinent cranial nerve electromyography including III, IV, V3, VI, and XII. This would require the patient not to be paralyzed during the case, further supporting the necessity of the Mayfield pins. Preoperative broad-spectrum antibiotics are utilized, and anticoagulation is generally avoided if there is any potential for intradural extension or a vascular lesion is anticipated (such as a juvenile nasopharyngeal angiofibroma).

In addition to preparing the nasal cavity with topical decongestant (oxymetazoline 0.05% or epinephrine 1:10,000 topical pledgets), many cases will require a fat graft to assist with the reconstruction, and the abdomen should be prepped accordingly. Lastly, given the inherent danger in dissecting the petrous ICA, consideration for prepping the thigh for rapid access to a muscle patch (or tensor fascia lata) should be given.

Preparing the Nasal Corridor

The endoscopic approach is initiated with a 0-degree nasal endoscope. The inferior turbinates are out fractured, and the middle turbinate on the ipsilateral side is typically resected to facilitate wide access. Next, an endoscopic uncinectomy is performed. It is imperative to take the uncinate flush to the lateral nasal wall to maximize lateral exposure. With the middle meatus exposed, a complete anterior and posterior ethmoidectomy is done to facilitate wide exposure of the nasal cavity. This can be performed with a combination of cutting instruments such as the Kerrison rongeur or the Blakesley rongeur, as well as a powered microdebrider. The anterior ethmoidectomy should be completed up to the frontal outflow to avoid frontal synechia and delayed obstruction. The posterior ethmoidectomy is taken to the level of the skull base and the orbit is cleared of septations for maximal exposure. Next, the superior turbinate can be partially resected to expose the natural ostium of the sphenoid sinus, and a wide sphenoidotomy is performed.

With the nasal cavity opened, attention is now focused on the lateral (coronal) exposure. Having completed an uncinectomy, the natural ostium of the ipsilateral maxillary sinus is identified and then generously widened posteriorly.

Reconstructive Preparation

Before proceeding with a transpterygoid approach, the surgeon must prepare and plan a reconstructive algorithm. As previously discussed, a fat graft may be required and should be planned in advance. Additionally, a pedicled buccal fat flap can also be used as the infratemporal fossa is exposed and the buccal fat is mobilized from the buccal space. Furthermore, anticipating exposure of the ICA and possible CSF leak, a robust nasoseptal flap to resurface the skull base is advised. Given the anatomical disruption of the transpterygoid approach, an ipsilateral nasoseptal flap is generally not possible as the vascular supply is disrupted when the sphenopalatine vessels are transected to mobilize the pterygopalatine fossa.

Thus, a contralateral nasoseptal flap is generally preferred and is elevated in a standard fashion, pedicled on the posterior septal artery, and is gently placed into the nasopharynx or sphenoid cavity.[5] Depending on the planned approach, the contralateral sphenoid sinus should also be opened and a posterior septectomy be performed to create a common sphenoid cavity and to maximize the visualization of both internal carotid arteries and optic nerves. At this point, the posterior bony and cartilaginous septum are removed. It is imperative to preserve the anterior septal strut back to the attachment on the premaxilla, to prevent saddle deformity. Lastly, the ipsilateral septal mucosa can then be incised superiorly, inferiorly, and posteriorly to perform a reverse septal flap, covering the denuded remnant anterior septum.[6] This allows wide binarial access and a transseptal angle to the transpterygoid corridor.

Preparing the Maxillary Corridor

With the nasal cavity widely exposed and the reconstruction preserved, the maxillary sinus now serves as the window to the pterygopalatine fossa and pterygoid process. For approaches above the vidian (Types A, B, and C), a simple nasoantral window is required. The maxillary antrostomy is widened from the nasolacrimal duct anteriorly to the posterior maxillary wall posteriorly, and from the orbit superiorly to the inferior turbinate inferiorly. This can be performed with a cutting Blakesley, Kerrison, or microdebrider.

However, for a more inferior trajectory (Types D and E), the entire height of the antrum and posterior maxillary wall must be accessed. This requires an endoscopic medial maxillectomy. To perform this, the posterior two-thirds of the inferior turbinate must be resected. The examination of the middle meatus should help one identify the valve of Hasner, the opening of the nasolacrimal duct. This should, if possible, be preserved to prevent epiphora. With the posterior turbinate resected, the medial maxillary wall is then fractured and removed from the valve of Hasner anteriorly back to the posterior wall. A drill can be used to take this resection down to the floor of the nose inferiorly for a wide medial maxillectomy window. With most transpterygoid approaches, this technique and a transseptal window from the prior septectomy allow adequate lateral exposure. However, if the lateral aspects of the infratemporal fossa are to be accessed, a Denker maxillectomy (removal of the pyriform aperture and remaining medial maxilla, transection of the nasolacrimal duct) or sublabial (Caldwell-Luc) maxillectomy may be required to provide the necessary lateral exposure (working around the pyriform aperture and nasolacrimal duct both sublabially and endonasally).

Exposing the Pterygopalatine Fossa

The key to accessing the pterygopalatine fossa is the sphenopalatine foramen. This is the natural corridor from the pterygopalatine fossa into the nasal cavity, carrying the sphenopalatine artery. The artery can be identified with a submucosal dissection just posterior to the posterior wall of the maxillary sinus and the crista ethmoidalis (**Fig. 24.1a**). Once identified, the artery (or arteries) should be cauterized or clipped to maintain hemostasis. Using a 1-mm Kerrison rongeur, the footplate is then placed into the foramen and used to open the posterior wall of the maxillary sinus (**Fig. 24.1b**). As the posterior wall of the maxillary sinus is opened, the pterygopalatine fossa is exposed, ideally maintaining the periosteum around the contents to prevent fat herniation. Following this subperiosteal plane, the posterior wall is resected with the Kerrison and angled instruments to the full exposure of the maxillary sinus. Laterally, the posterior wall should be resected to reach the level of the inferior orbital fissure, where the infraorbital nerve should be identified exiting the pterygopalatine fossa. Notably, for inferior exposures (Types D and E), the inferomedial portion of the posterior wall, where the greater palatine canal and its contents (descending palatine artery, greater and lesser palatine nerves), is found at the junction of the palatine bone and posterior maxilla. Preservation of this neurovascular bundle should be attempted unless transection is required for exposure or tumor extirpation (**Fig. 24.1c, d**).

At this point, removal of the orbital process and perpendicular plate of the palatine bone allows full access to the anterior and medial aspects of the pterygopalatine fossa. Next, the sphenoid process of the palatine bone is also removed heading posteromedially to expose the palatovaginal canal, which is found at the junction of the sphenoid and palatine bones. The palatovaginal artery (i.e., pharyngeal artery) is cauterized and divided and with this maneuver, the pterygopalatine fossa can be mobilized laterally. As the fossa is lateralized, the vidian nerve and canal are then at the trifurcation of the medial pterygoid plate with the lateral wall and floor of the sphenoid sinus.

The Transpterygoid Access

Further dissection is now directed by the anatomical requirements of the tumor. For a simple Type A approach, the periosteum of the pterygopalatine fossa and infratemporal fossa can be incised to allow a tunnel to be created for the passage of a temporoparietal fascia flap. For a Type B approach, the remaining components of the lateral recess of the sphenoid sinus can generally be accessed with this approach. However, depending on the pneumatization pattern, the vidian nerve may need to be sacrificed to allow more complete lateralization of the pterygopalatine fossa and full exposure of the lateral recess in the pterygoid base. With this approach, the foramen rotundum and the maxillary nerve can be visualized in the lateral wall of the sphenoid as it enters the pterygopalatine fossa after the sacrifice of the vidian nerve.

For access to the middle fossa, Meckel's cave, and the petrous apex, either transection or mobilization of the vidian artery and nerve is required. The vidian artery is then followed posteriorly, drilling the inferior portion of the vidian canal, until the anterior genu of the petrous ICA can be identified (**Fig. 24.1e**). A Doppler probe can help confirm the anatomical location along with navigation. The carotid artery is then exposed, as needed, with a high-speed diamond drill.[7] With the internal carotid artery defined, lateralization of the pterygopalatine fossa allows the identification of foramen rotundum and the maxillary artery (after transecting or mobilizing the vidian nerve). This maneuver exposes the base of the pterygoid process. Using foramen rotundum and the vidian canal, the pterygoid base between these canals can be carefully drilled to define the petrous apex and carefully expose the petrous ICA. Similarly, the foramen rotundum can be carefully drilled including the lateral wall of the sphenoid sinus to access the medial portion of the middle fossa, and the maxillary nerve can be followed posteriorly over the anterior genu of the carotid artery and into Meckel's cave.[8]

For a Type D approach, after transecting the vidian nerve, the internal maxillary artery should be controlled as it enters the pterygopalatine fossa. The maxillary nerve is then identified as the exiting foramen rotundum and is isolated and mobilized from the pterygopalatine fossa by dividing the contributions to the pterygopalatine ganglion. Preserving the maxillary nerve, the rest of the pterygopalatine fossa can now be aggressively mobilized laterally and inferiorly, exposing the entire pterygoid process. The anterior face of the pterygoid process is then removed with a high-speed drill, exposing the tensor veli palatini between the pterygoid plates. Depending on the exposure needed to the infratemporal fossa, the medial and lateral plates can be drilled and removed. It is best to detach the pterygoid muscles from the lateral plate in a subperiosteal plane before fully drilling the plates to minimize bleeding. As the lateral plate is followed posteriorly, the mandibular nerve (V3) can be identified exiting the foramen ovale, and the pharyngeal segment of the ICA is usually identified just posterior to this landmark (**Fig. 24.2a–c**). This allows access to the lateral and posterior

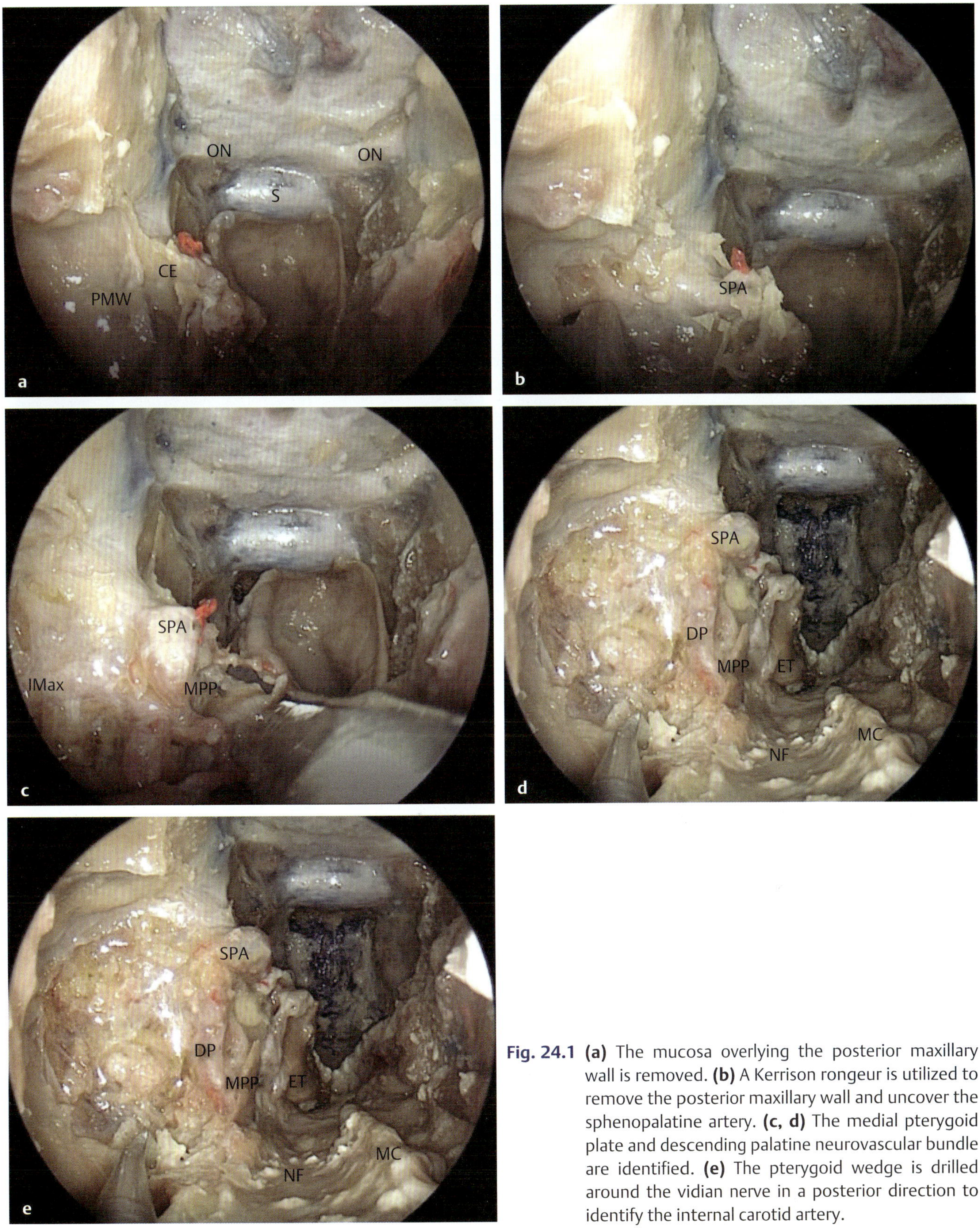

Fig. 24.1 **(a)** The mucosa overlying the posterior maxillary wall is removed. **(b)** A Kerrison rongeur is utilized to remove the posterior maxillary wall and uncover the sphenopalatine artery. **(c, d)** The medial pterygoid plate and descending palatine neurovascular bundle are identified. **(e)** The pterygoid wedge is drilled around the vidian nerve in a posterior direction to identify the internal carotid artery.

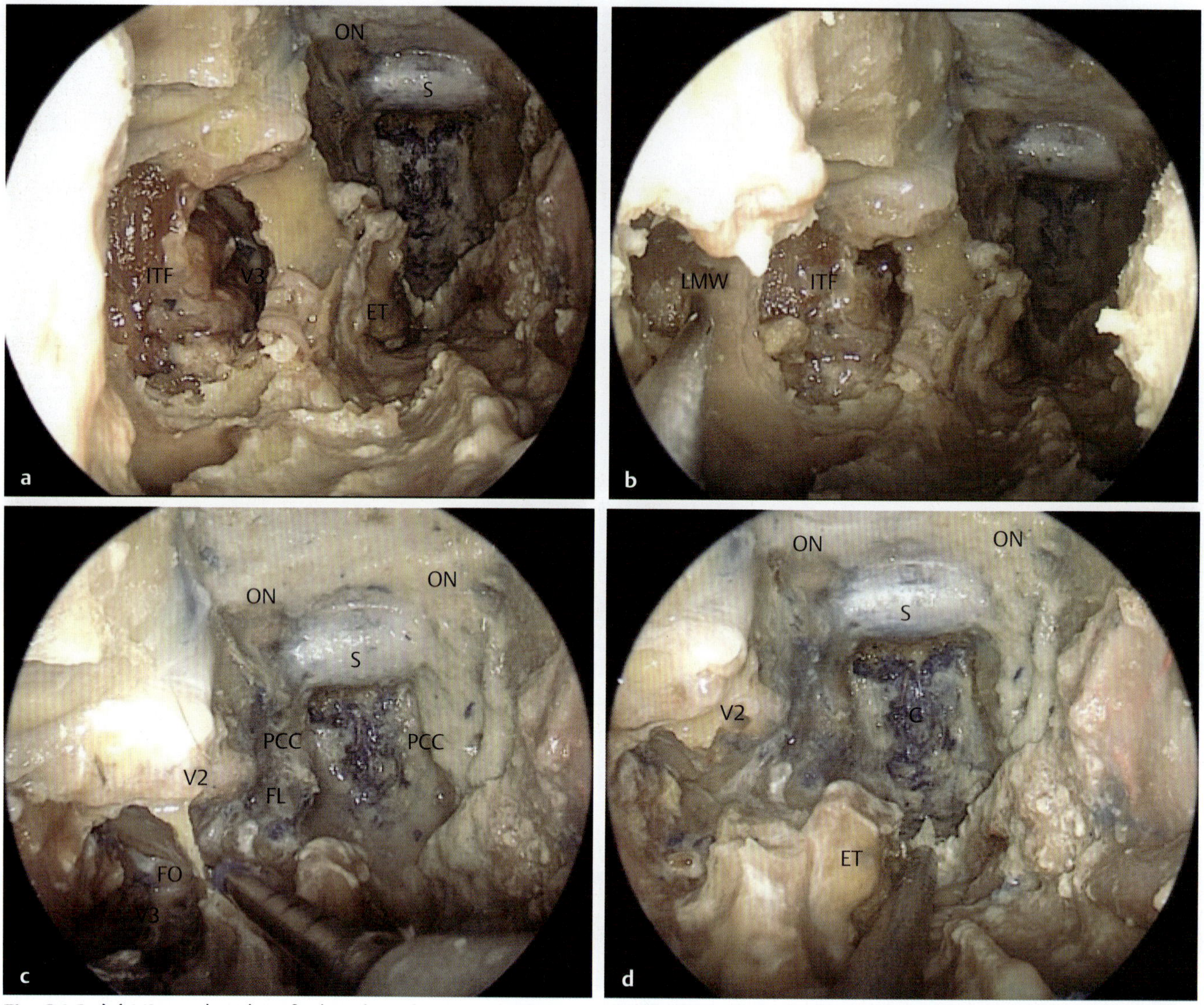

Fig. 24.2 **(a)** V3 can be identified in the infratemporal fossa lateral to the lateral pterygoid plate. **(b)** A Denker maxillectomy can increase the ability to reach the lateral maxillary wall and infratemporal fossa. **(c)** After tracing the vidian nerve, the foramen lacerum can be identified. Inferolateral dissection can uncover the foramen ovale and V3. **(d)** Complete resection of the pterygoid wedge allows the identification of key anatomical structures and resection of the cartilaginous eustachian tube.

compartments of the infratemporal fossa, but extreme caution must be utilized when mobilizing the maxillary artery and working around the carotid artery to avoid uncontrollable bleeding.

A Type E approach requires the same exposure and involves the removal of the entire pterygoid base. The medial plate is then followed back to the eustachian tube (**Fig. 24.2d** and **Fig. 24.3a, b**). The medial one-third of the eustachian tube is cartilaginous and can be gently mobilized and then transected to allow mobilization of the nasopharynx. Following the eustachian tube into the levator palatini muscle, the surgeon must work slowly to identify the carotid artery using the above mentioned landmarks, navigation, and the Doppler probe. The levator muscle can be transected allowing access into the parapharyngeal space and mobilization of the entire fossa of Rosenmüller, facilitating a nasopharyngectomy (**Fig. 24.3c**). Notably, in addition to this exposure, the completion of a nasopharyngectomy requires the mobilization of the nasopharyngeal soft tissues from the cartilaginous plug in foramen lacerum, a meticulous process given the location of the carotid artery and the abundance of fascial attachments (**Fig. 24.4**).[9]

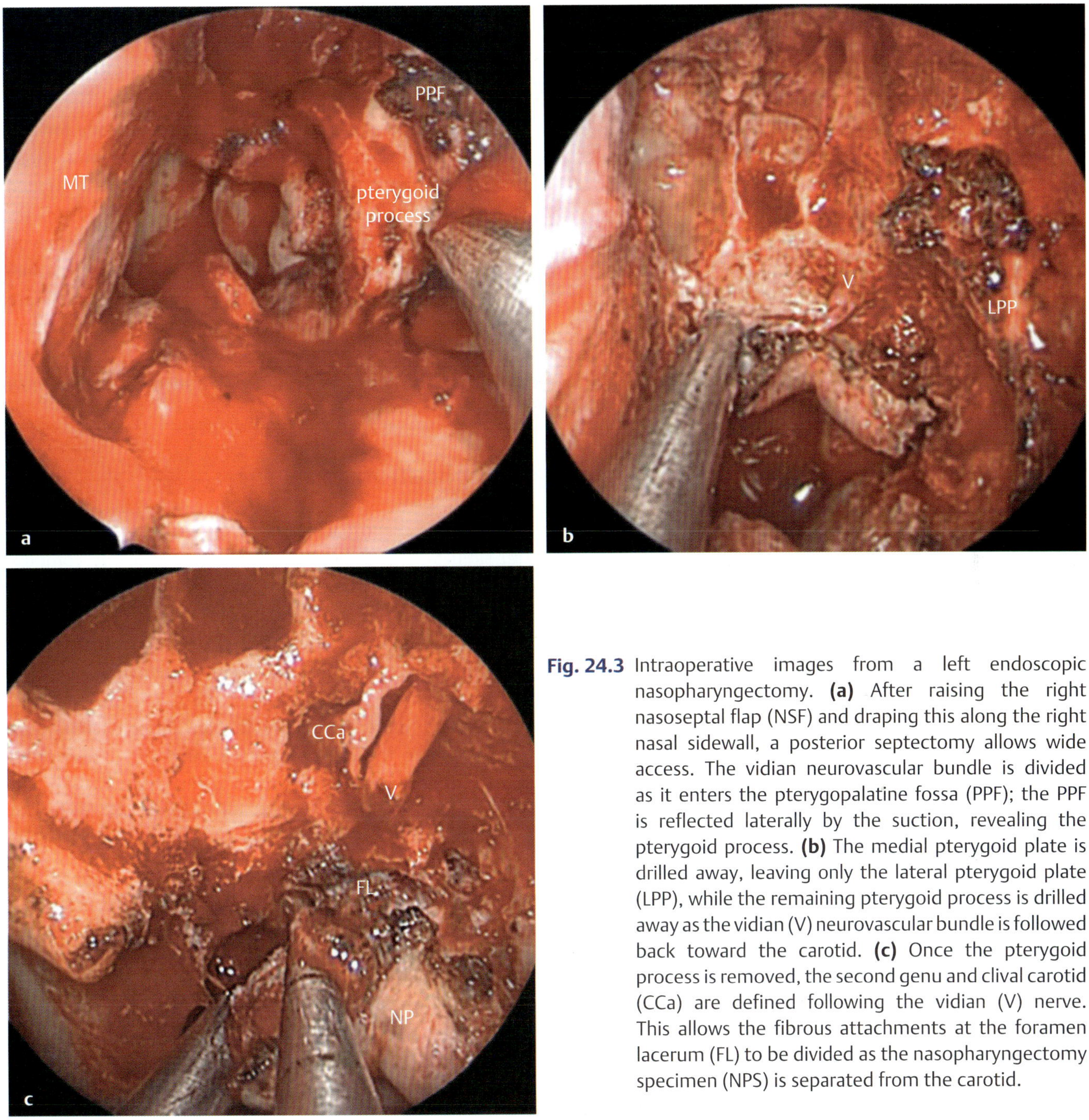

Fig. 24.3 Intraoperative images from a left endoscopic nasopharyngectomy. **(a)** After raising the right nasoseptal flap (NSF) and draping this along the right nasal sidewall, a posterior septectomy allows wide access. The vidian neurovascular bundle is divided as it enters the pterygopalatine fossa (PPF); the PPF is reflected laterally by the suction, revealing the pterygoid process. **(b)** The medial pterygoid plate is drilled away, leaving only the lateral pterygoid plate (LPP), while the remaining pterygoid process is drilled away as the vidian (V) neurovascular bundle is followed back toward the carotid. **(c)** Once the pterygoid process is removed, the second genu and clival carotid (CCa) are defined following the vidian (V) nerve. This allows the fibrous attachments at the foramen lacerum (FL) to be divided as the nasopharyngectomy specimen (NPS) is separated from the carotid.

Reconstruction

After the transpterygoid approach is completed, the lesion of interest is addressed with standard microsurgical tenants and a two-surgeon, four-handed approach. After tumor resection, definitive reconstruction is imperative to cover the exposed ICA and reconstruct any potential CSF leak. A free fat graft, typically harvested from the abdomen, can serve to fill the clival recess or ablate a cavity from extensive drilling. Dural defects can be repaired with a multilayered approach, including a fat graft, tensor fascia lata or synthetic collagen matrix inlay, and nasoseptal flap onlay reconstruction. The contralateral-based nasoseptal flap should also drape across any exposed aspects of the ICA. Notably, the previously resected middle turbinate can be used as a free mucosal graft donor. Lastly, the buccal fat pad can be mobilized from the infratemporal fossa to assist with the reconstruction. After opening the periosteum of the infratemporal fossa, buccal fat

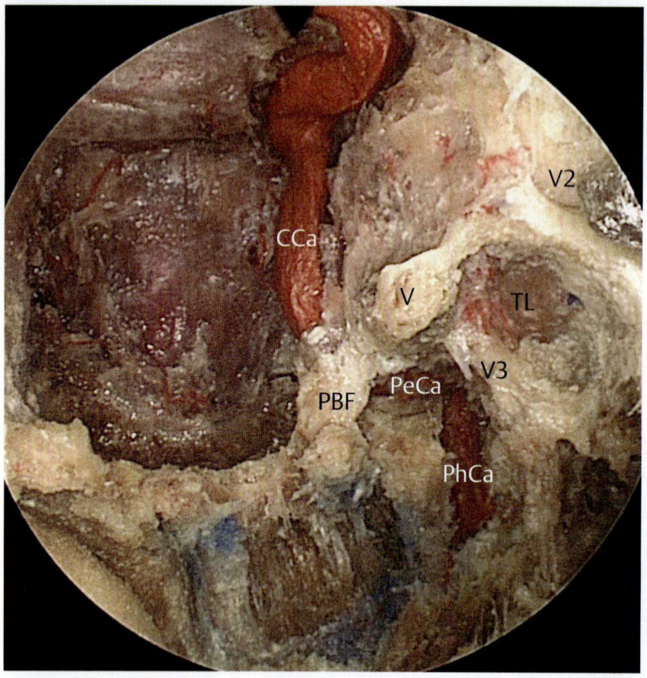

Fig. 24.4 Cadaveric depiction of the key coronal plane anatomy. The entire pterygoid process has been drilled away, and the entire carotid anatomy has been dissected to delineate the anatomy. The pharyngobasilar fascia (PBF) traverses from the nasopharyngeal soft tissues up toward the vidian (V) neurovascular bundle, crossing the second genu of the carotid artery. The pharyngeal (PhCa), petrous (PeCa), and clival (CCa) segments of the carotid artery are visualized. The maxillary nerve (V2) can be seen exiting foramen rotundum adjacent to the dissecting instrument, and having drilled away the lateral pterygoid plate, the mandibular nerve (V3) can be seen leaving the foramen ovale. Drilling between V2 and V3, one finds the dura of the temporal lobe (TL).

starts herniating into the maxillary window. Using a gentle dissection technique to mobilize the buccal fat, its vascular supply can be preserved; thus, yielding a 3- to a 4-cm long pedicled flap that can be mobilized to close the defect.

Postoperative Care

After the completion of the case, the patient is usually taken to the neurosurgical intensive care unit for close neuromonitoring. Routinely, a postoperative CT scan is performed to evaluate the extent of pneumocephalus and confirm the absence of intracranial complications. The patient should be monitored for CSF leak and challenged appropriately. Depending on the extent of surgery, most patients progress within 2 to 4 days for their discharge from the hospital, but this is highly contingent on the patient's comorbidities. The diet and activity levels are slowly advanced to match the patient's clinical progress until the patient is ready for discharge. The patient is usually maintained on intravenous broad-spectrum antibiotics postoperatively and transitioned to oral antibiotics as the diet is advanced. If the postoperative course is uncomplicated, the nasal packing is removed and the nose is debrided approximately 1 week after surgery, often on an outpatient basis. Serial debridements are performed every 2 to 3 weeks depending on the progress of the nasal healing, until well mucosalized. Nasal saline irrigations are instituted after the initial debridement to maximize nasal hygiene.

Complications

Transpterygoid approaches to the coronal plane of the ventral skull base require detailed knowledge of the complex anatomy and necessitate a meticulous dissection across high-risk territories of the skull base. Even in the most experienced hands, complications can occur. Sinonasal synechiae and sinusitis are common postoperative sequelae. Epiphora resulting from accidental injury of the nasolacrimal duct is encountered more frequently in conventional sinus surgery. Injury to the pterygopalatine ganglion, or disruption of the vidian nerve, will result in reduced lacrimation and the inability to generate emotional tears in the ipsilateral eye. Mobilization or injury to the descending palatine nerve can cause numbness in the palate, which is often readily adjusted by the patient. Injury to the proximal maxillary nerve can result in ipsilateral cheek and maxillary numbness, including the dentition. Injury to V3 similarly can result in lower facial numbness, including the ipsilateral mandible, as well as difficulties with mastication and wasting of the ipsilateral masticatory musculature. Postoperative hemorrhage can occur from a poorly controlled internal maxillary artery or the pterygoid plexus and can result in significant bleeding. Postoperative CSF leak is a possible complication if the dissection is extended intradurally. Many patients with postoperative leaks will require surgical reexploration versus diversion with a lumbar drain and conservative management. Orbital injury or VI nerve palsy may cause diplopia or even vision loss. Intracranial injury or hemorrhage is a rare but potentially serious complication. Injury to the ICA intraoperatively can result in catastrophic hemorrhage or ischemic stroke and can be fatal if not managed quickly. A crushed muscle patch can be secured to assist with hemostasis, and the patient should undergo angiography for potential stenting or sacrifice.

Conclusions

The endoscopic transpterygoid approach provides extended access to the paramedian ventral skull base in the coronal plane. It is a complex anatomical region that requires detailed knowledge of the boundaries and techniques. The pterygopalatine fossa and pterygoid process serve as the gateway to accessing lesions from Meckel's cave and the lateral recess of the sphenoid to the petrous apex and middle fossa, infratemporal fossa, and parapharyngeal space lateral to the nasopharynx. Using the described classification system, preoperative planning, and a two-surgeon approach, this corridor can be safely navigated to access a wide variety of skull base lesions.

Suggested Readings

Al-Sheibani S, Zanation AM, Carrau RL, et al. Endoscopic endonasal transpterygoid nasopharyngectomy. Laryngoscope 2011;121(10):2081–2089

Caicedo-Granados E, Carrau R, Snyderman CH, et al. Reverse rotation flap for reconstruction of donor site after vascular pedicled nasoseptal flap in skull base surgery. Laryngoscope 2010;120(8):1550–1552

Fortes FS, Carrau RL, Snyderman CH, et al. Transpterygoid transposition of a temporoparietal fascia flap: a new method for skull base reconstruction after endoscopic expanded endonasal approaches. Laryngoscope 2007; 117(6):970–976

Fortes FS, Sennes LU, Carrau RL, et al. Endoscopic anatomy of the pterygopalatine fossa and the transpterygoid approach: development of a surgical instruction model. Laryngoscope 2008;118(1):44–49

Hadad G, Bassagasteguy L, Carrau RL, et al. A novel reconstructive technique after endoscopic expanded endonasal approaches: vascular pedicle nasoseptal flap. Laryngoscope 2006;116(10): 1882–1886

Hardesty DA, Montaser AS, Carrau RL, Prevedello DM. Limits of endoscopic endonasal transpterygoid approach to cavernous sinus and Meckel's cave. J Neurosurg Sci 2018;62(3):332–338

Kasemsiri P, Solares CA, Carrau RL, et al. Endoscopic endonasal transpterygoid approaches: anatomical landmarks for planning the surgical corridor. Laryngoscope 2013;123(4): 811–815

Kassam AB, Vescan AD, Carrau RL, et al. Expanded endonasal approach: vidian canal as a landmark to the petrous internal carotid artery. J Neurosurg 2008;108(1):177–183

Snyderman CH, Pant H, Carrau RL, Prevedello D, Gardner P, Kassam AB. What are the limits of endoscopic sinus surgery?: the expanded endonasal approach to the skull base. Keio J Med 2009;58(3):152–160

Chapter 25 Endonasal Endoscopic Surgeries of Lesions Occupying the Infratemporal Fossa and the Parapharyngeal Space

Case 25A

Endoscopic Transoral Approach to Parapharyngeal Tumors

Sien Hui Tan, Adzreil Bakri, and Prepageran Narayanan

History

A 70-year-old man presented with progressive dysphagia for 2 years. Flexible nasoendoscopy examination revealed a submucosal mass arising from the lateral wall of the oropharynx on the right side displacing the soft palate and right anterior tonsillar pillar anteromedially. The mass extended superiorly from the nasopharynx to the level of the epiglottis. Cranial nerves IX, X, XI, XII were intact. A computed tomography (CT) scan revealed a right parapharyngeal tumor (**Fig. 25A.1, Fig. 25A.2, Fig. 25A.3**). The histopathological diagnosis was reported as a schwannoma. This approach may be used for cases of parapharyngeal tumors.

Surgical Steps

1. The patient is positioned supine with the neck extended.
2. Tracheostomy under local anesthesia is performed electively prior to the procedure for airway protection.
3. A Boyle–Davis gag is placed in the patient's oral cavity to allow adequate visualization of the surgical field (**Fig. 25A.4**).
4. A transoral endoscopic surgery is performed using a rigid-rod endoscope 4 mm in diameter with a lens angle of 0 degree. The endoscope provides wide-angled, closed-up views and excellent visualization through a narrow surgical corridor.
5. Under endoscopic magnification, a vertical incision is made on the posterolateral wall of the oropharynx where the mass is most prominent with a bipolar diathermy (**Fig. 25A.5**).
6. A tonsillar retractor is used to provide better exposure, and a careful dissection of the pharyngeal constrictor muscles is performed until the tumor is visible (**Fig. 25A.6**).

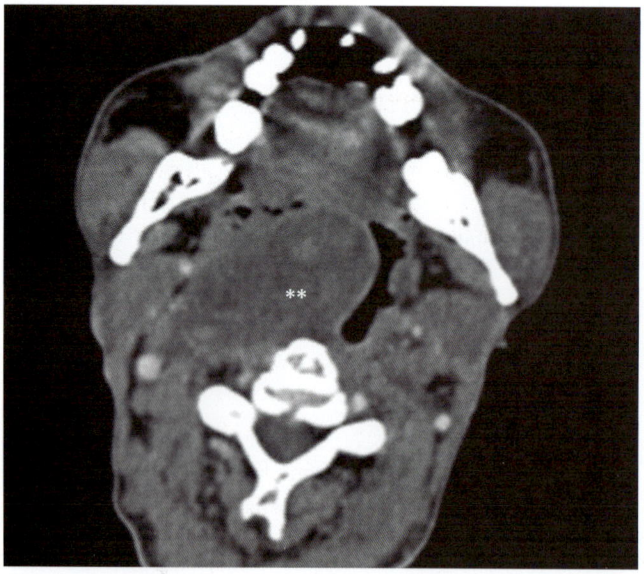

Fig. 25A.1 Axial CT scan showing a right parapharyngeal tumor (**).

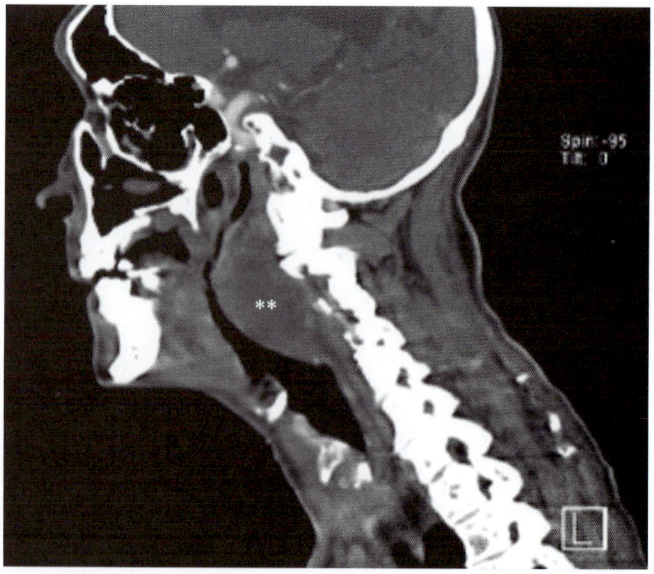

Fig. 25A.2 Sagittal CT scan showing a right parapharyngeal tumor (**) extending to the level of epiglottis.

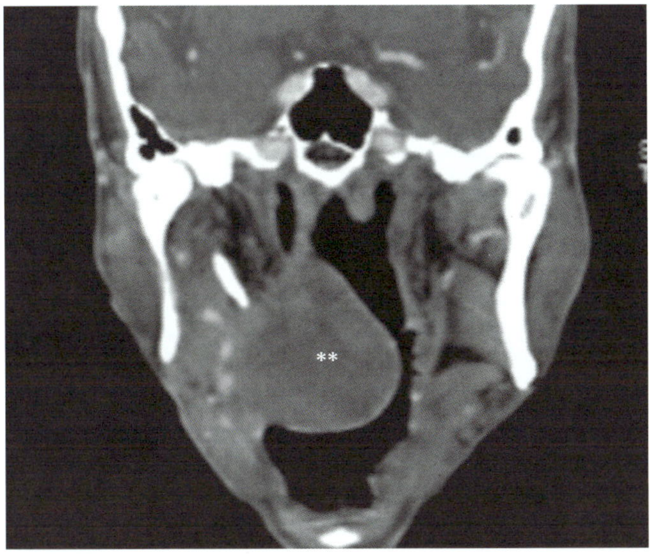

Fig. 25A.3 Coronal CT scan demonstrating a right parapharyngeal tumor (**).

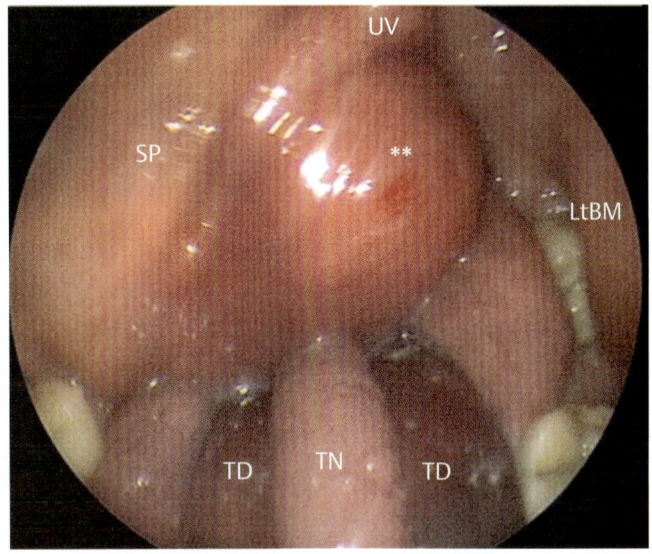

Fig. 25A.4 Endoscopic transoral view of the submucosal mass (**) arising from the lateral wall of the oropharynx on the right side.

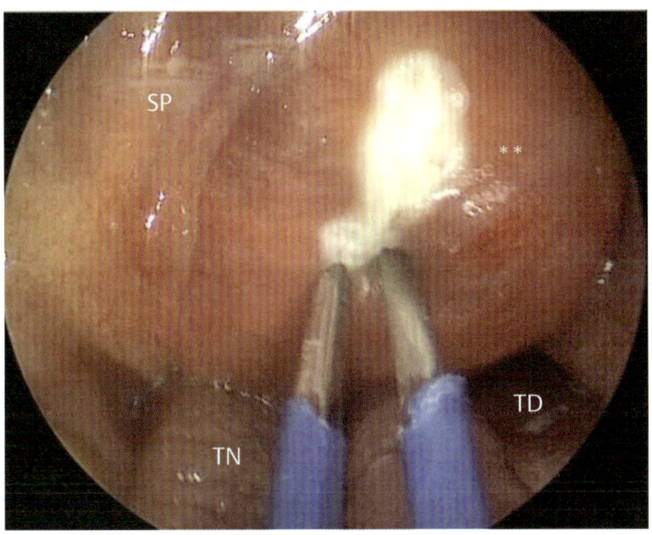

Fig. 25A.5 Intraoperative endoscopic view. A vertical incision is made on the mass (**) at the posterolateral wall of the oropharynx with bipolar diathermy.

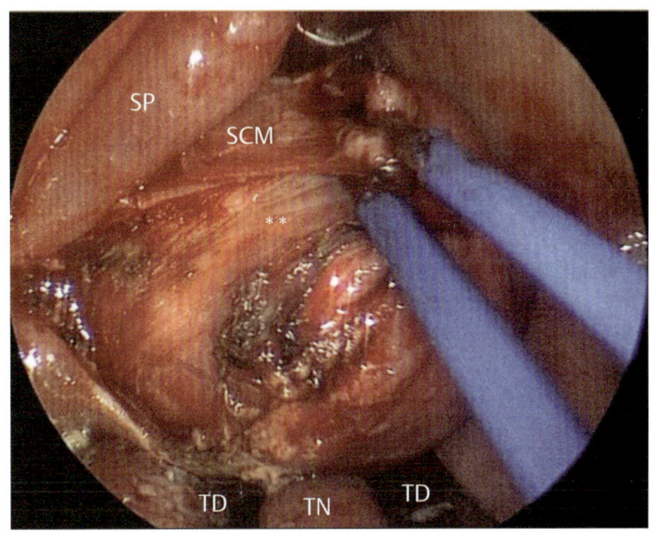

Fig. 25A.6 Intraoperative endoscopic view. Dissection is carried through the superior constrictor muscles (SCM) to reach the tumor (**) in the parapharyngeal space.

7. Blunt finger dissection is carried out cautiously to free the tumor, which is then delivered and removed transorally (**Fig. 25A.7, Fig. 25A.8, Fig. 25A.9**).
8. Meticulous hemostasis is secured with bipolar cauterization and Surgicel.
9. The transoral incision is closed in layers with absorbable sutures Vicryl 3–0 (**Fig. 25A.10**).
10. The tumor specimen is sent for histopathological examination (**Fig. 25A.11**).
11. Postoperatively, the patient is decannulated prior to discharge from the hospital.

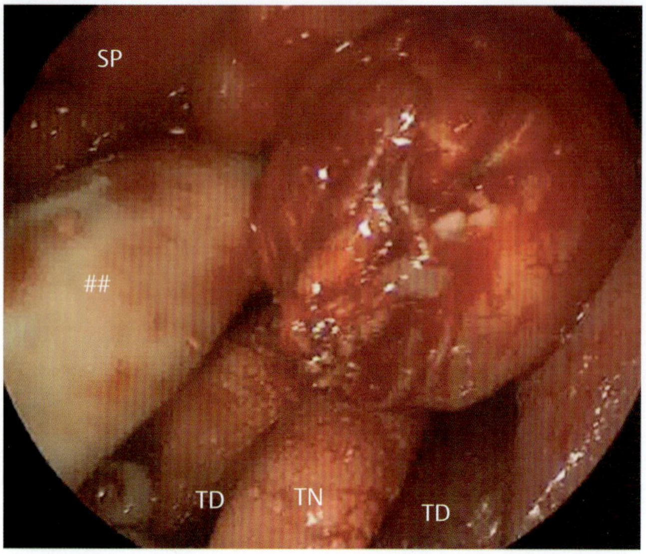

Fig. 25A.7 Intraoperative endoscopic view. The tumor (**) is dissected out via the blunt finger (##) dissection.

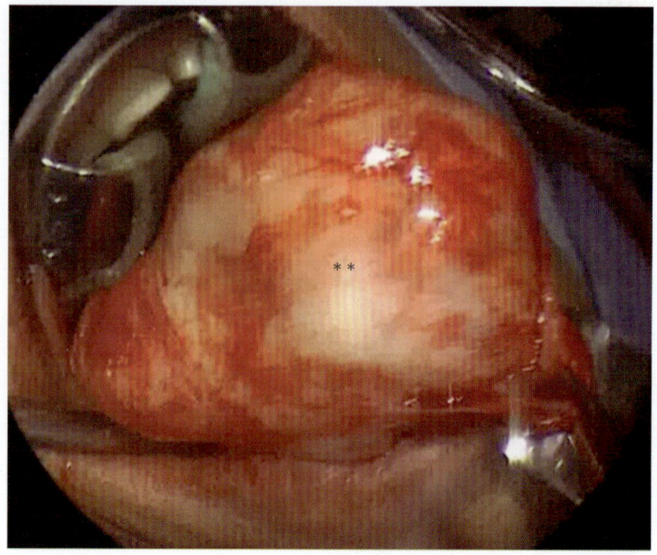

Fig. 25A.8 The whole tumor (**) is delivered en bloc transorally.

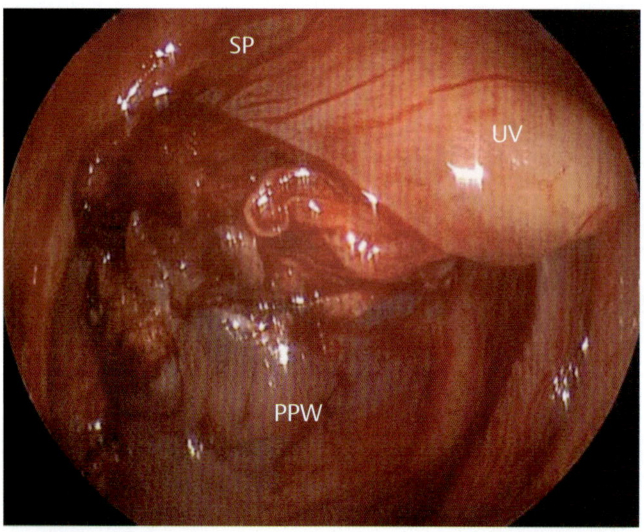

Fig. 25A.9 Postoperative view after complete removal of the tumor.

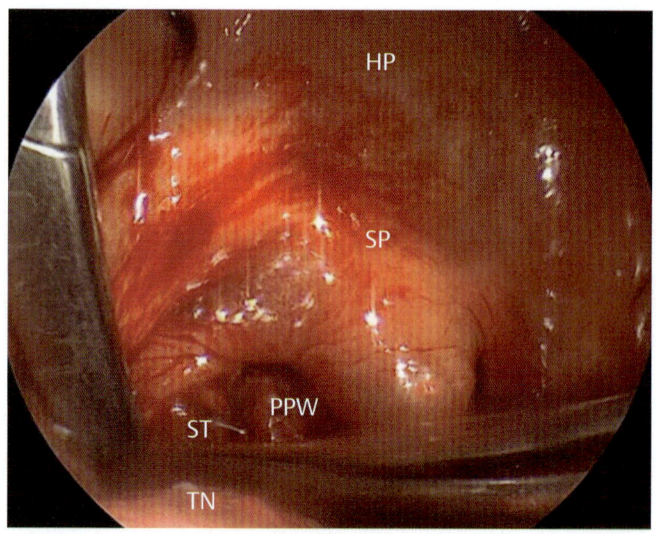

Fig. 25A.10 The incision is closed in a layered fashion with 3–0 absorbable sutures (ST).

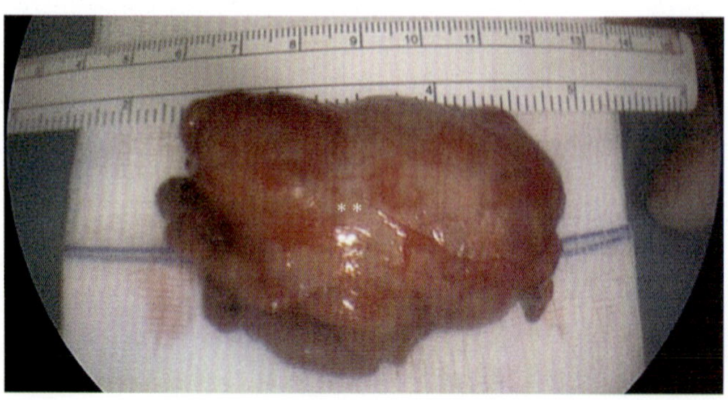

Fig. 25A.11 Tumor specimen (**). Histopathological examination confirmed a schwannoma.

Case 25B

Recurrent Trigeminal Schwannoma—Transcervical Approach for Excision of Complex Giant Tumor and Endoscopic-Assisted Excision of the Intracranial Component

Asiya Kamber Zaidi, Jeyanthi Kulasegarah, Vicknes Waran, and Prepageran Narayanan

History

A 20-year-old female was referred for evaluation of left-sided painless swelling over the parotid region, which recurred after two previous excisions at a different institution. She also reported vague left-sided facial pain with mild hyperesthesia along the distribution of mandibular branch of the trigeminal nerve (CNV3).

Clinical evaluation revealed a well-circumscribed mass involving the left parotid region. The overlying skin was normal with no discoloration. On palpation, the mass was firm and nonfluctuant with no thrill. Intraorally, on the left, there was medialization of the soft palate and lateral pharyngeal wall.

Magnetic resonance imaging (MRI) revealed a large well-defined, encapsulated, and multilobulated mass involving the left parapharyngeal space with its epicenter in the left masticator space. The mass was heterogeneously hyperintense on T2-weighted sequence with multiple cystic degenerative areas within it (**Fig. 25B.1**). The postcontrast study revealed heterogeneous peripheral enhancement with central nonenhancing necrotic areas.

On the coronal MRI sequence, superiorly, the mass extends into the middle cranial fossa via the foramen ovale along CNV3. Widening of the foramen ovale is seen with indentation of the inferior aspect of the temporal lobe. Superomedially, the mass closely abuts the lateral wall of the cavernous sinus, while inferomedially, there is obliteration of the left parapharyngeal space causing medialization of the lateral pharyngeal wall. Laterally, the mass extends into the parotid space compressing the parotid gland (**Fig. 25B.2**).

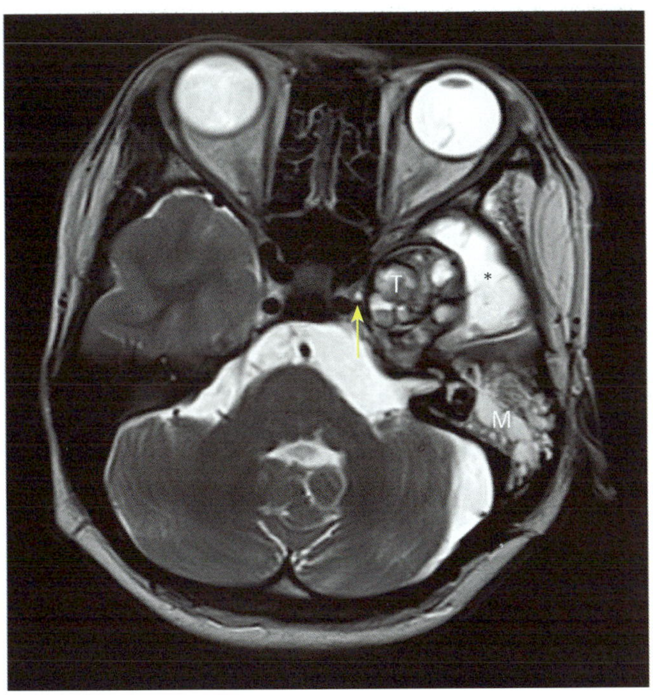

Fig. 25B.1 MRI T2-weighted axial image showing tumor (T) with necrotic areas within, abutting the left cavernous sinus (*solid yellow arrow*) and the lateral orbital wall. Cystic changes are evident in the middle cranial fossa (*black* *). Fluid is seen in the mastoid (M) air cells.

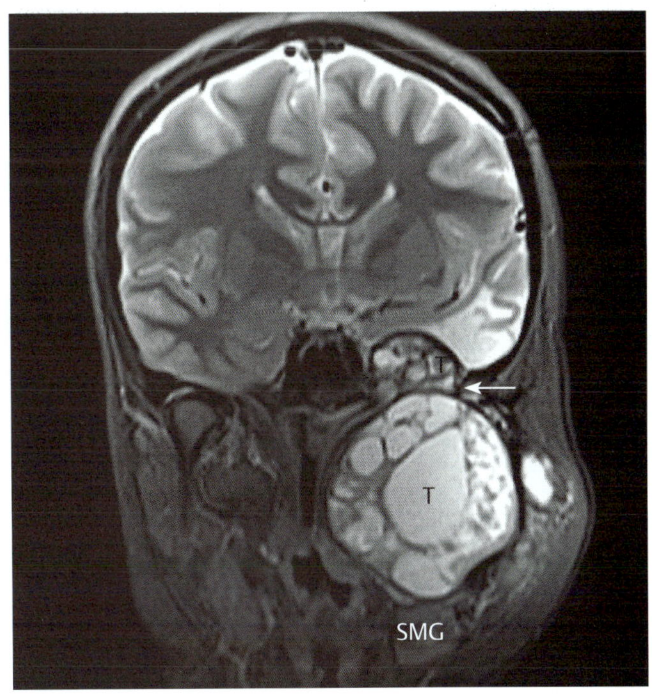

Fig. 25B.2 MRI T2-weighted coronal image showing the tumor (T) with its intracranial component in the middle cranial fossa widening the foramen ovale (*white arrow*) and the extracranial component in the left parapharyngeal space, displacing the pharyngeal mucosa medially and the submandibular gland (SMG) inferiorly.

On the axial MRI sequence, further inferiorly, there is bowing of the posterior wall of the left maxillary sinus (**Fig. 25B.3a**) and alveolar aspect of the maxilla (**Fig. 25B.3b**); however, there is no erosion of the wall. Posteriorly, there is obliteration of the carotid artery and the internal jugular vein (**Fig. 25B.3a, b**). A diagnosis of cystic schwannoma arising from CNV3 was made radiologically. The patient underwent a combined approach for excision of the tumor.

Surgical Steps

1. General anesthesia is induced, and oral intubation is done. Muscle relaxant is avoided as eliciting movement on mechanical or electrical stimulation assists in locating and preserving the cranial nerves (marginal mandibular nerve, hypoglossal nerve, and spinal accessory nerve) during dissection.
2. The patient is placed in a supine position with the neck extended and rotated away from the surgeon, toward the contralateral side. The head is fixed within a NORAS frame for intraoperative MRI (iMRI). Registration for neuronavigation (Brainlab, Munich, Germany) is performed.
3. The site is marked for a modified Blair incision with the transcervical extension (**Fig. 25B.4**). The mastoid tip is also marked for orientation during the surgery (**Fig. 25B.4**).
4. Surgical site is prepped and draped.
5. Local anesthesia 1% lignocaine with 1:1000,000 parts adrenaline is used.
6. Incision is made through the skin, subcutaneous tissue, and platysma. Subplatysmal flaps are elevated and secured with 2-0 silk stitch. The sternocleidomastoid muscle is delineated and retracted posteriorly. Parotid tissue, masseter muscle along with the soft tissue, was retracted superiorly. A well-defined, firm, encapsulated, and smooth pale yellow mass is visualized (**Fig. 25B.5**).
7. The tumor is addressed in two stages in sequence:
   - Stage 1 en bloc resection of the parapharyngeal component of the tumor via the modified Blair incision with a transcervical incision (as described above).
   - Stage 2 direct endoscopic excision of the intracranial component of the tumor through the same incision.

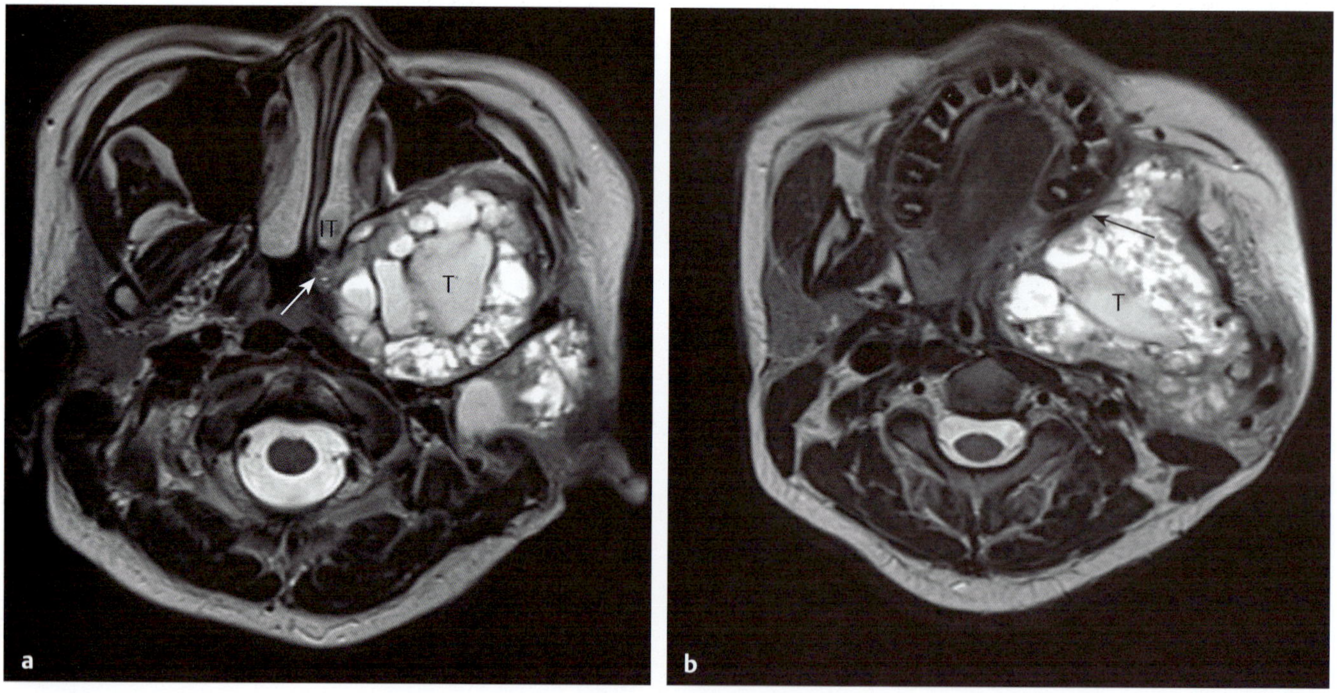

Fig. 25B.3 **(a)** MRI T2-weighted axial image showing tumor (T) pushing forward the posterior wall of the maxillary sinus. The tumor is also abutting the posterior aspect of the inferior turbinate (IT) and obliterating the fossa of Rosenmuller and the eustachian tube (*solid white arrow*). Posteriorly, there is obliteration of the carotid artery and the internal jugular vein. **(b)** MRI T2-weighted axial image showing the tumor (T) displacing the alveolar aspect of maxilla medially (*solid black arrow*).

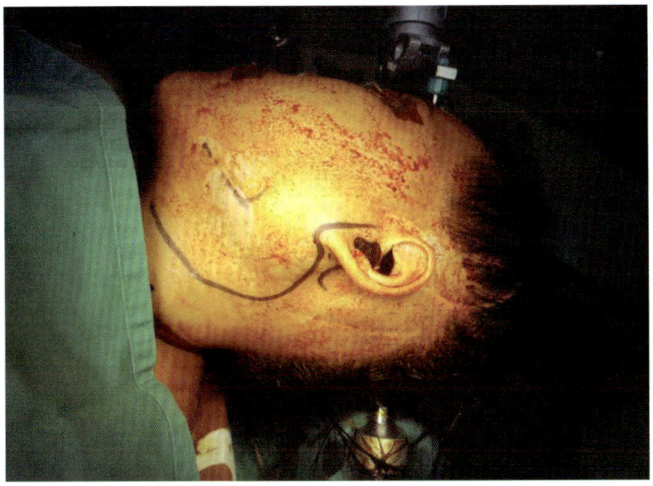

Fig. 25B.4 The patient is positioned, pinned, and prepared for surgery. Marking for a modified Blair incision with transcervical extension is done. The mastoid tip and mandible edge are also marked for intraoperative surgical orientation.

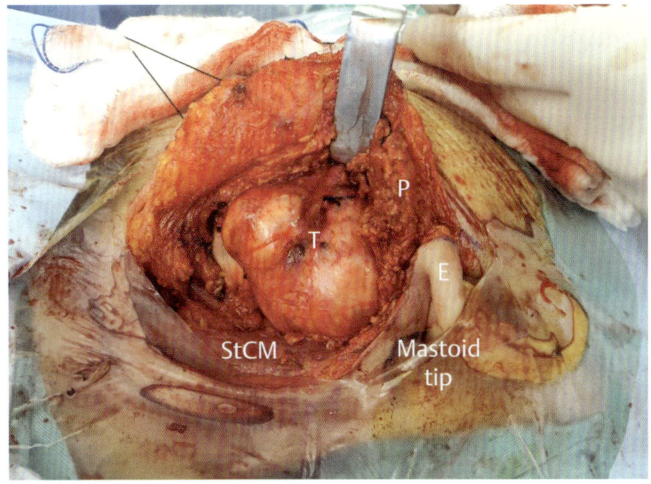

Fig. 25B.5 Subplatysma flap is secured with 2–0 silk stitch and the following are identified: tumor (T), sternocleidomastoid muscle (StCM), parotid tissue (P), and ear lobule (E).

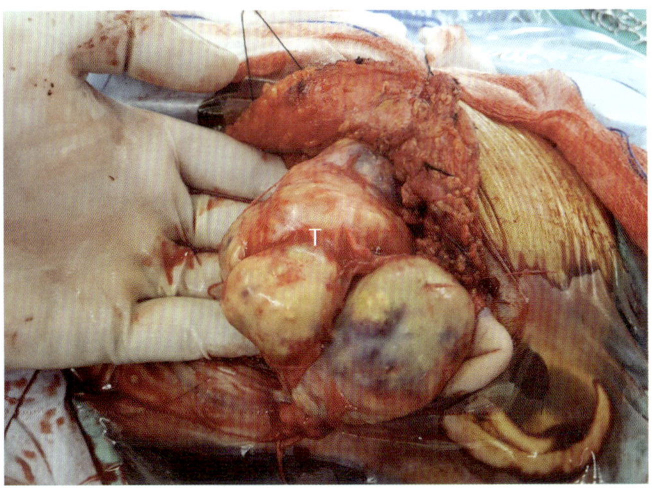

Fig. 25B.6 The tumor (T) is dissected out from the surrounding soft tissue structures with blunt finger dissection.

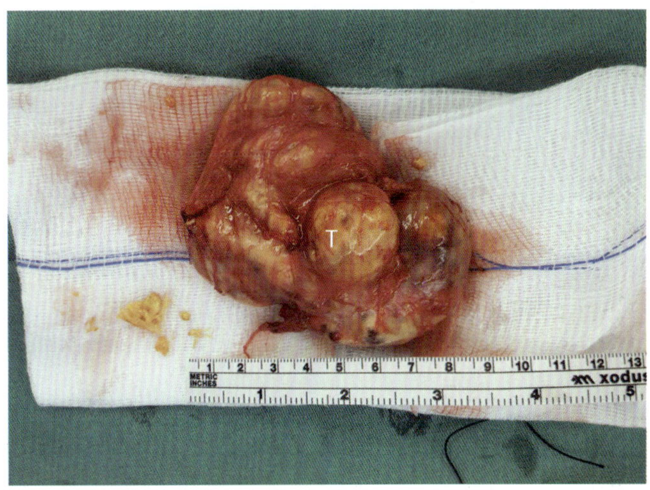

Fig. 25B.7 The excised specimen shows a well-encapsulated, lobulated, firm yellowish tumor (T).

8. Stage 1
   a. Extracapsular dissection (ECD) is done using the finger dissection technique to detach the tumor from the surrounding structures (**Fig. 25B.6**).
   b. The posterior belly of digastric muscle, the styloglossus muscle, and the stylomandibular ligament can be resected or cranially retracted for wider exposure.
   c. The resected specimen was sent for histopathological examination (**Fig. 25B.7**).
9. Stage 2
   a. A zero-degree, 4-mm rigid Hopkins rod endoscope attached to a high-definition camera is held by the assistant surgeon to visualize the intracranial component of the tumor abutting the left cavernous sinus (**Fig. 25B.8**).
   b. The tumor is delineated medially (**Fig. 25B.9**) and laterally (**Fig. 25B.10**) following the excision of the majority of the intracranial component (**Fig. 25B.11**).

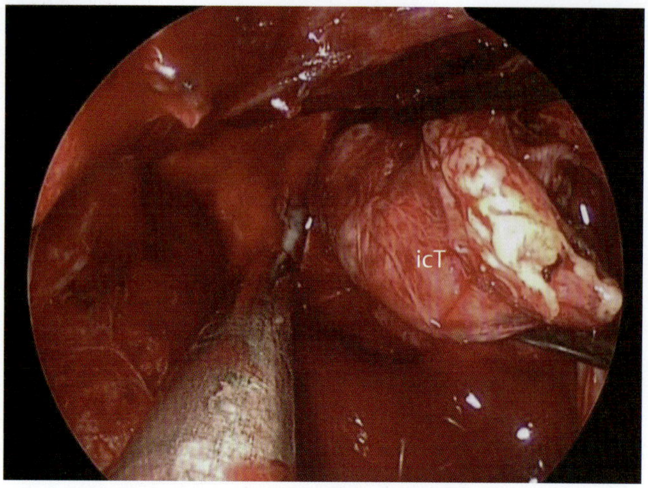

Fig. 25B.8 Endoscopic picture of the intracranial component of the tumor (icT).

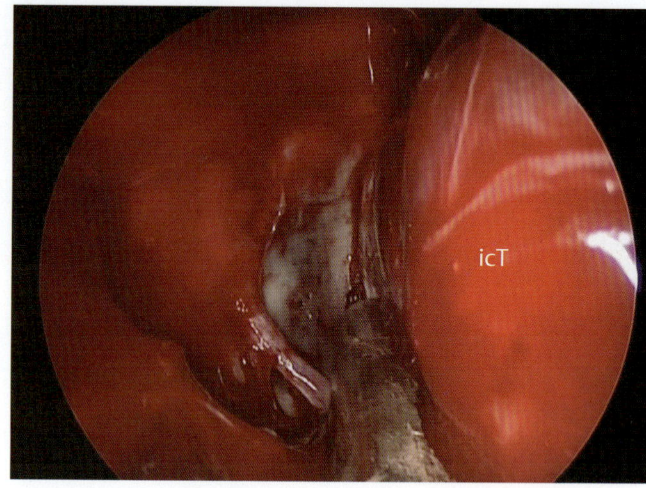

Fig. 25B.9 Endoscopic picture of the tumor (icT) delineation medially.

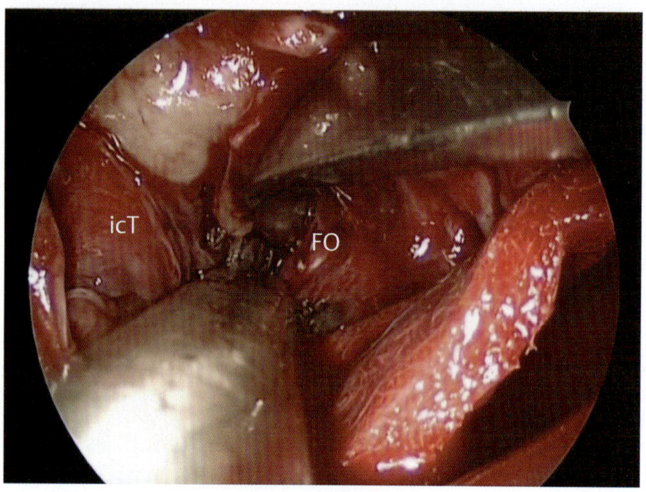

Fig. 25B.10 Endoscopic picture of the tumor (icT) delineation laterally and exposure of the foramen ovale (FO).

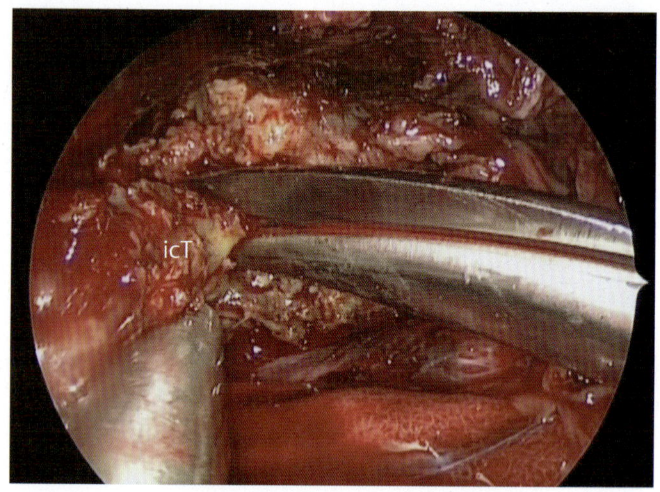

Fig. 25B.11 Intracranial component of the tumor (icT) is debulked.

c. Debulking of the tumor remnant over the dura is done using an ultrasonic aspirator (**Fig. 25B.12**), and the capsule of the tumor is separated from the overlying dura (**Fig. 25B.13**).

10. After the extirpation of the tumor, endoscope-aided inspection of the surgical bed along the entire anatomical corridor created through the transcervical incision confirmed the completeness of the resection (**Fig. 25B.14a, b**).
11. Suction drain is placed.
12. The divided and retracted muscles were reapproximated and the wound is closed in layers.
13. Postoperative computed tomography (CT) scan demonstrated complete excision of the tumor (**Fig. 25B.15a, b**).

No postoperative complication was noted. Histopathological examination showed features consistent with schwannoma.

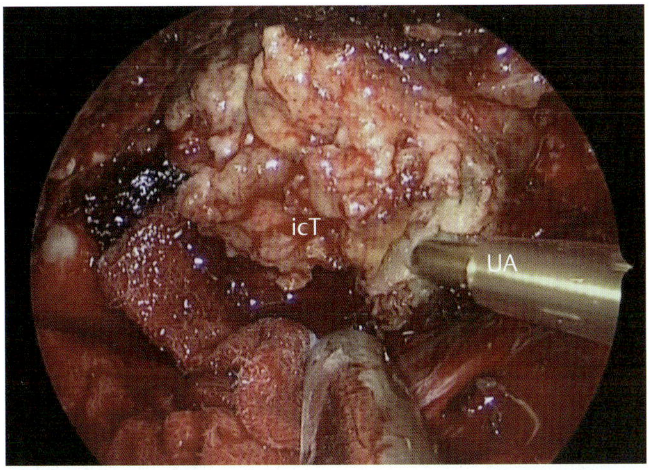

Fig. 25B.12 Further debulking of the tumor (icT) remnant is done on the dura (D) using ultrasonic aspirator (UA) and suction (S) intermittently.

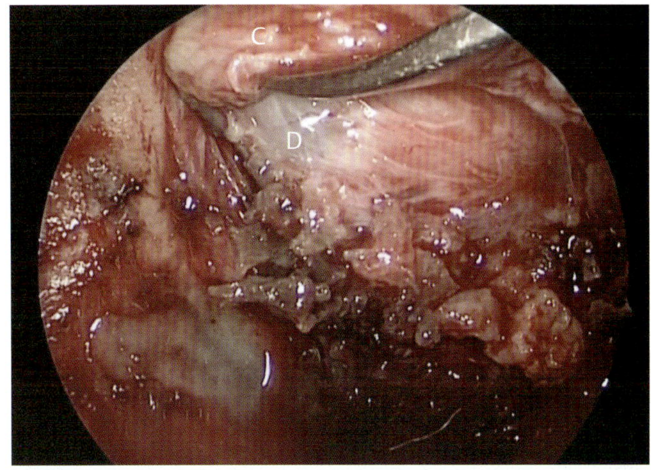

Fig. 25B.13 The capsule (C) of the tumor is separated from the overlying dura (D) of the temporal lobe.

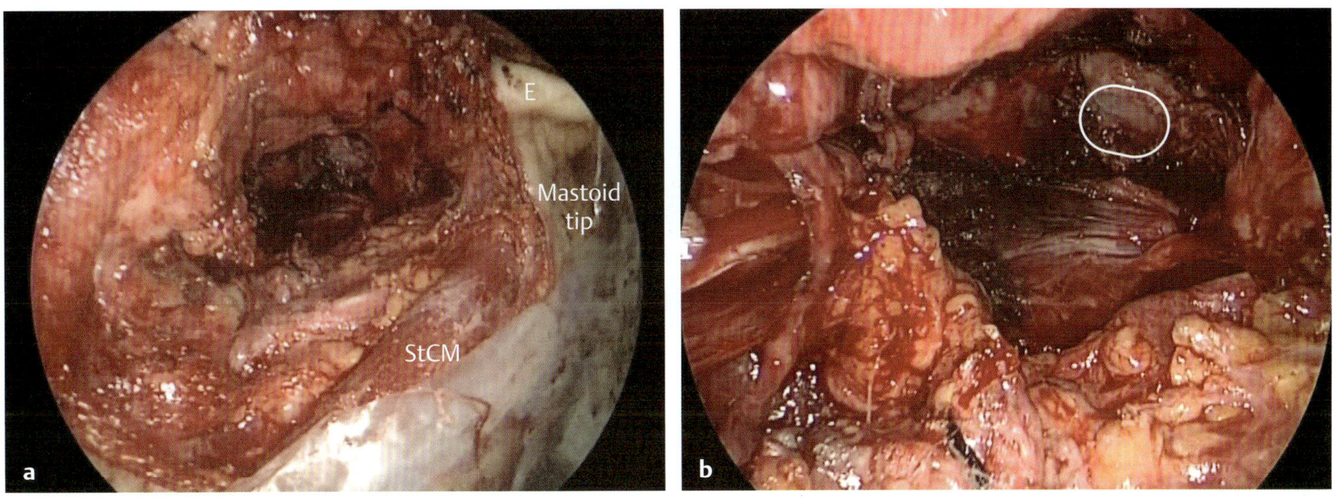

Fig. 25B.14 **(a)** Inspection of the surgical bed along the entire anatomical corridor created through the transcervical incision confirmed the completeness of the resection of sternocleidomastoid muscle (StCM), mastoid tip, and ear lobule (E). **(b)** A zoomed view showing widened foramen ovale (*white oval*).

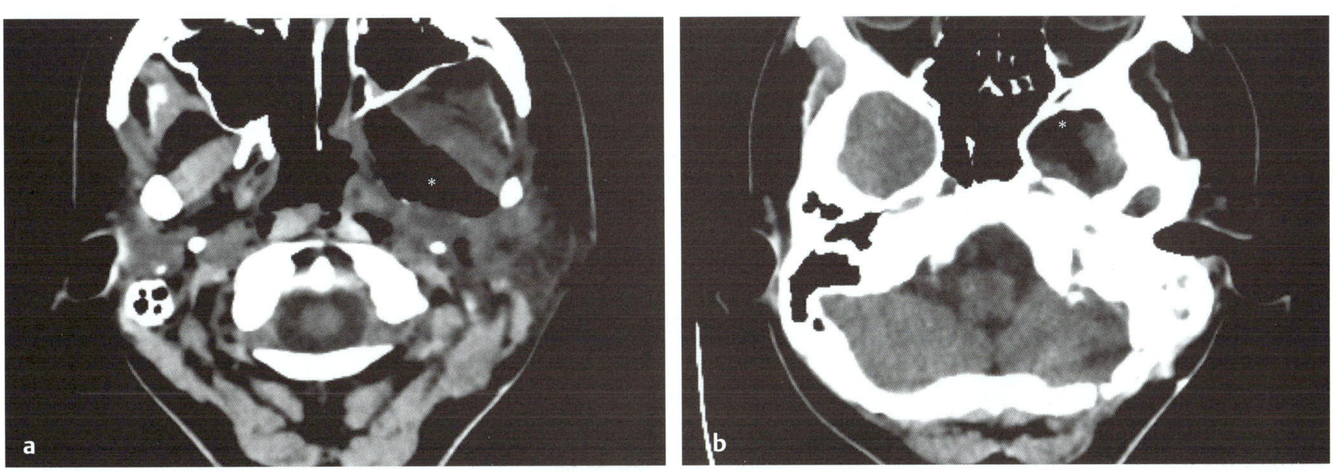

Fig. 25B.15 **(a)** Postoperative CT scan axial image demonstrating complete resection of the tumor in the parapharyngeal space (*). **(b)** Postoperative CT scan axial image demonstrating complete resection of the tumor in the middle cranial fossa (*).

Case 25C

Endoscopic Transoral Approach to Parapharyngeal Neurofibroma

Sien Hui Tan, Adzreil Bakri, and Prepageran Narayanan

History

A 28-year-old patient presented with progressive dysphagia for 2 years. Flexible nasoendoscopy examination revealed a submucosal mass arising from the lateral wall of the oropharynx on the left side displacing the soft palate and left anterior tonsillar pillar anteromedially. The mass extended superiorly from the nasopharynx to the level of the supraglottis. A magnetic resonance imaging (MRI) scan revealed a left parapharyngeal tumor (**Fig. 25C.1, Fig. 25C.2, Fig. 25C.3**). The histopathological diagnosis was reported as a neurofibroma. This approach may be used for cases of large parapharyngeal tumors.

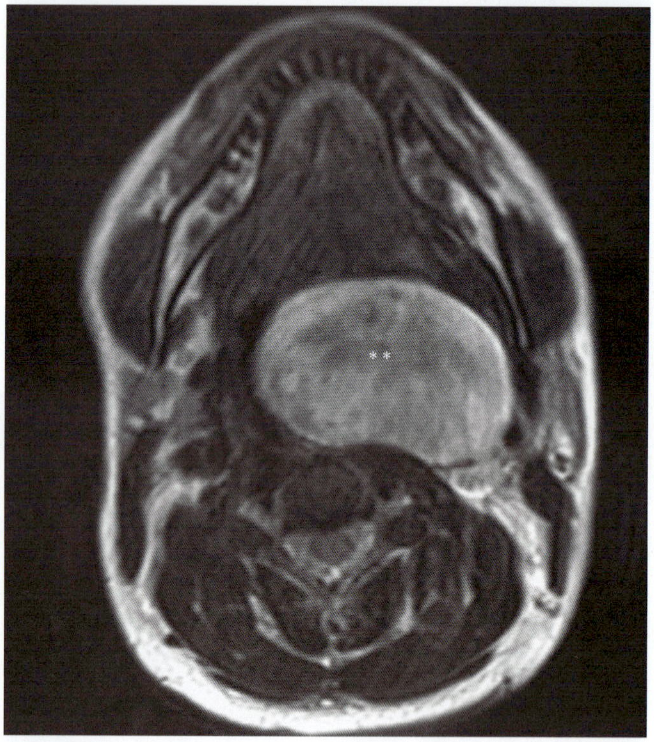

Fig. 25C.1 Axial MRI scan showing a left parapharyngeal tumor (**).

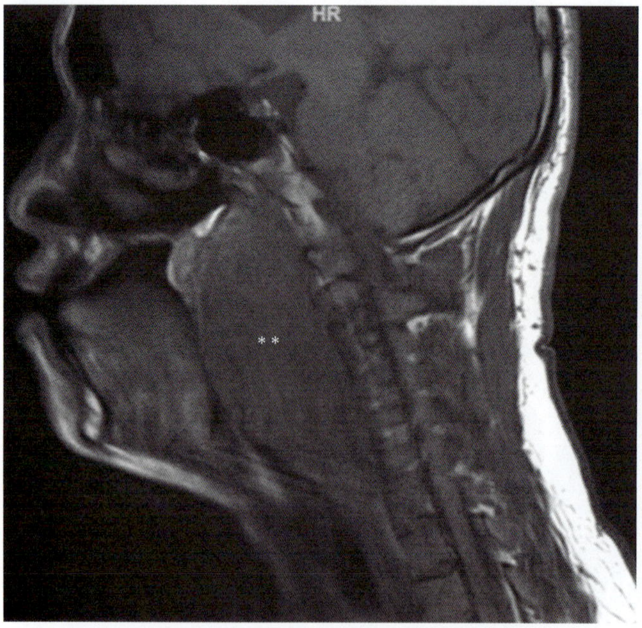

Fig. 25C.2 Sagittal MRI scan showing a left parapharyngeal tumor (**) extending to the level of supraglottis.

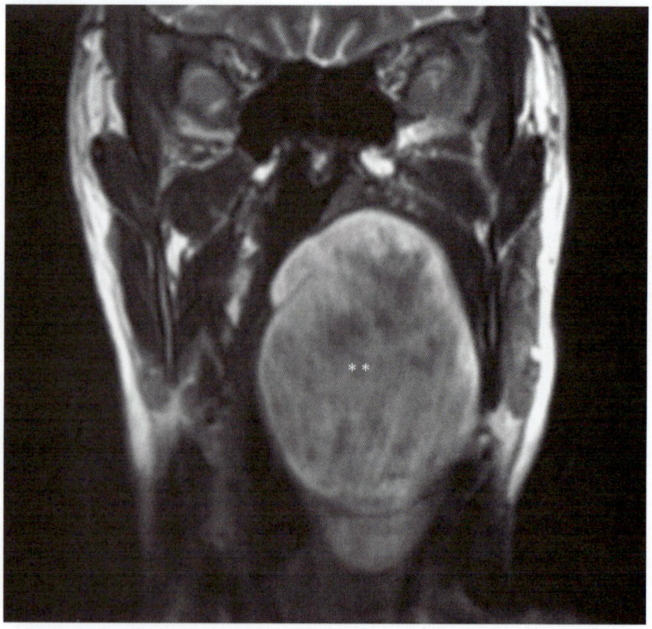

Fig. 25C.3 Coronal MRI scan demonstrating a left parapharyngeal tumor (**).

Surgical Steps

1. The patient is positioned supine with his neck extended.
2. Tracheostomy under local anesthesia is performed electively prior to the procedure for airway protection.
3. Good exposure of the oropharynx is achieved with a Boyle–Davis mouth gag and a stitch is placed in the uvula for upward retraction (**Fig. 25C.4**).
4. A transoral endoscopic surgery is performed using a rigid-rod endoscope 4 mm in diameter with a lens angle of 0 degree. The endoscope provides wide-angled, closed-up views and excellent visualization through a narrow surgical corridor.
5. Under endoscopic magnification, a vertical incision is made on the posterior wall of the oropharynx where the mass is most prominent (**Fig. 25C.5**).
6. Careful dissection of the pharyngeal constrictor muscles is performed with monopolar diathermy until the tumor is visible (**Fig. 25C.6**).
7. A dissector is used to bluntly release the mass from the surrounding loose connective tissue (**Fig. 25C.7**).

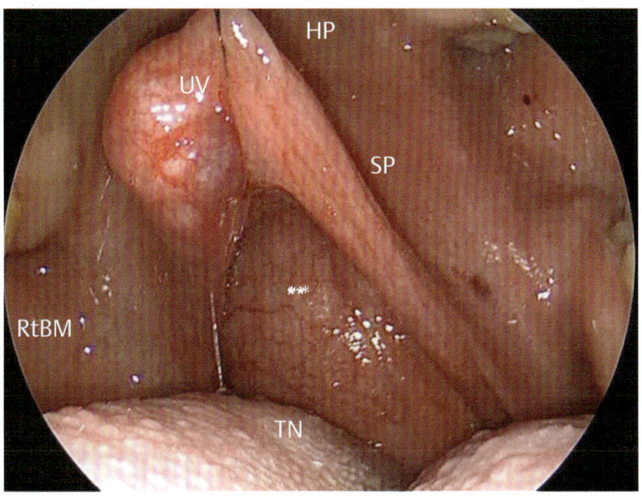

Fig. 25C.4 Upward retraction of the uvula (UV) allows adequate exposure of the submucosal mass (**) arising from the lateral wall of the oropharynx on the left side.

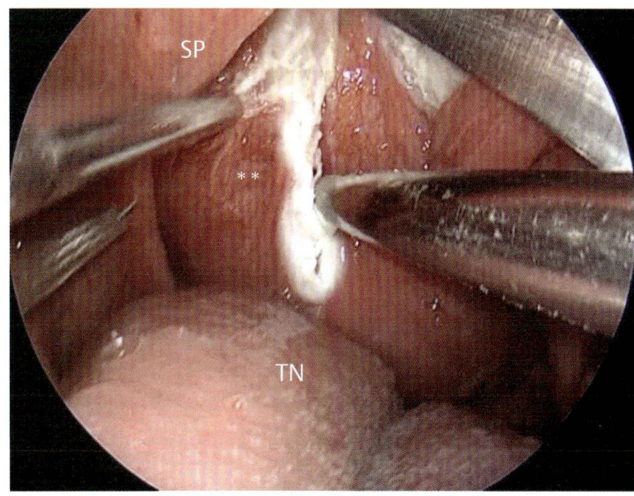

Fig. 25C.5 Intraoperative endoscopic view. A vertical incision is made on the posterior wall of the oropharynx.

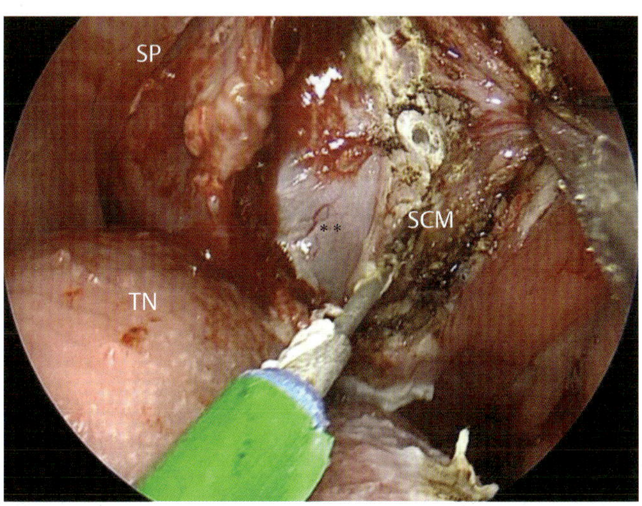

Fig. 25C.6 Intraoperative endoscopic view. Dissection is carried through the superior constrictor muscles (SCM) to reach the tumor (**) in the left parapharyngeal space.

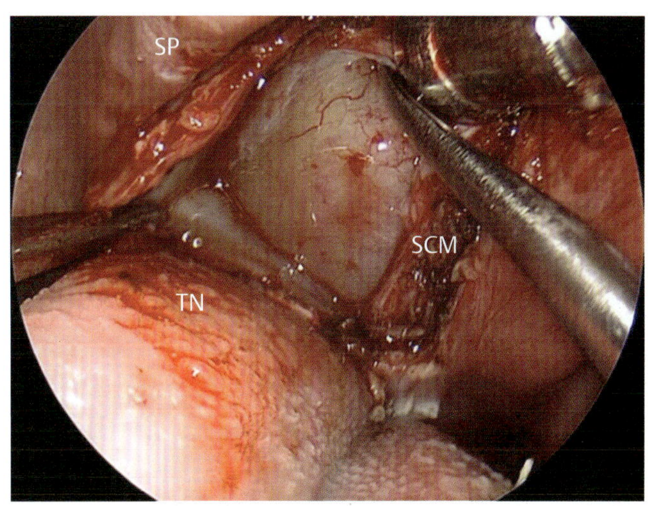

Fig. 25C.7 Intraoperative endoscopic view. Blunt dissection of the tumor (**).

8. Because of the large size of the tumor, an incision is made over the soft palate lateral to the uvula to allow sufficient space for removal of the tumor (**Fig. 25C.8**).
9. Blunt dissection is carried out cautiously to free the tumor, which is then delivered and removed transorally (**Fig. 25C.9**).
10. Meticulous hemostasis is secured with bipolar cauterization and Surgicel.
11. Both oropharyngeal and soft palate incisions are closed in layers with Vicryl suture 3–0. The suture placed on the uvula for retraction is removed (**Fig. 25C.10**).
12. The tumor specimen is sent for histopathological examination (**Fig. 25C.11**).
13. Postoperatively, the patient is decannulated prior to discharge from hospital.

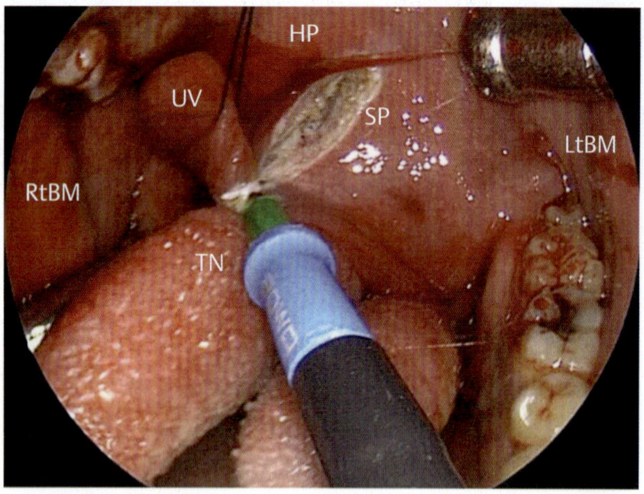

Fig. 25C.8 Intraoperative endoscopic view. An incision is made over the soft palate (SP) with a monopolar cautery.

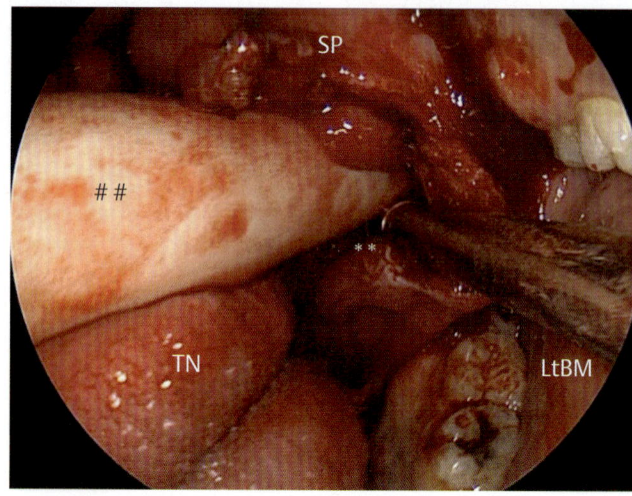

Fig. 25C.9 Intraoperative endoscopic view. The tumor (**) is dissected out via blunt finger (##) dissection.

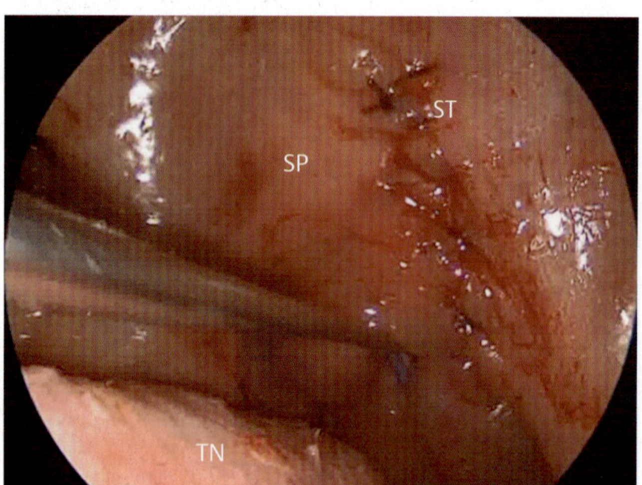

Fig. 25C.10 The soft palate (SP) incision is closed in a layered fashion with 3–0 absorbable sutures (ST).

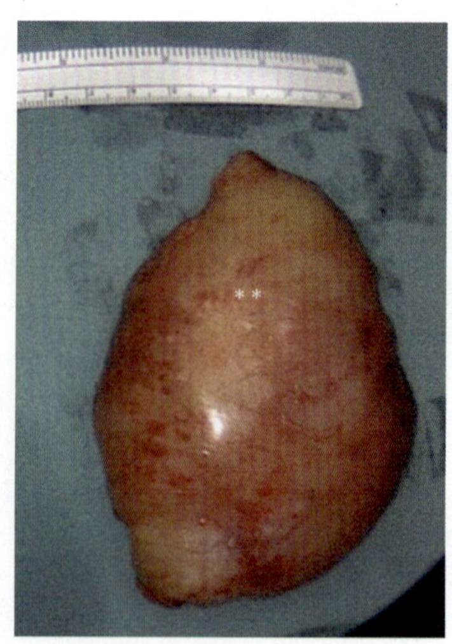

Fig. 25C.11 Tumor specimen (**). Histopathological examination confirmed a neurofibroma.

Case 25D

Endoscopic Transoral Approach to Parapharyngeal Pleomorphic Adenoma

Sien Hui Tan, Adzreil Bakri, and Prepageran Narayanan

History

A 74-year-old patient presented with progressive dysphagia for 6 years. Flexible nasoendoscopy examination revealed a left peritonsillar fullness pushing the uvula to the opposite side. A computed tomography (CT) scan revealed a left parapharyngeal tumor (**Fig. 25D.1, Fig. 25D.2, Fig. 25D.3**). The histopathological diagnosis was reported as a pleomorphic adenoma. This approach may be used for cases of parapharyngeal tumors.

Surgical Steps

1. The patient is positioned supine with the neck extended.
2. Tracheostomy under local anesthesia is performed electively prior to the procedure for airway protection.
3. Good exposure of the oropharynx is achieved with a Boyle–Davis mouth gag (**Fig. 25D.4**).

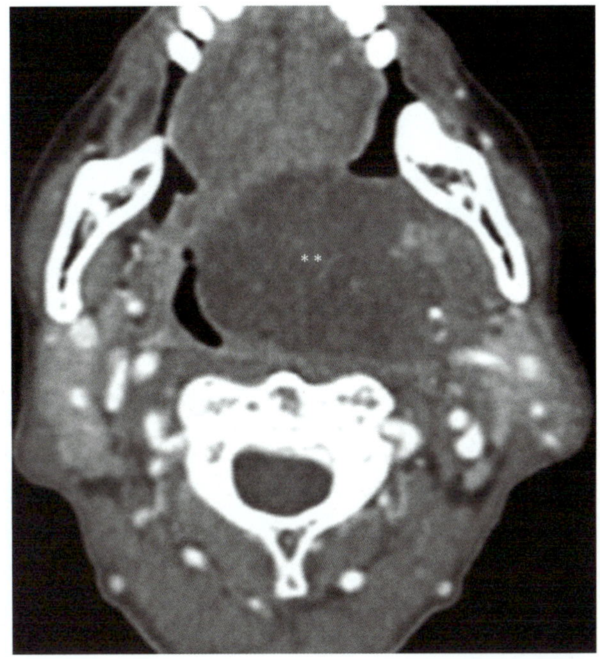

Fig. 25D.1 Axial CT scan showing a left parapharyngeal tumor (**).

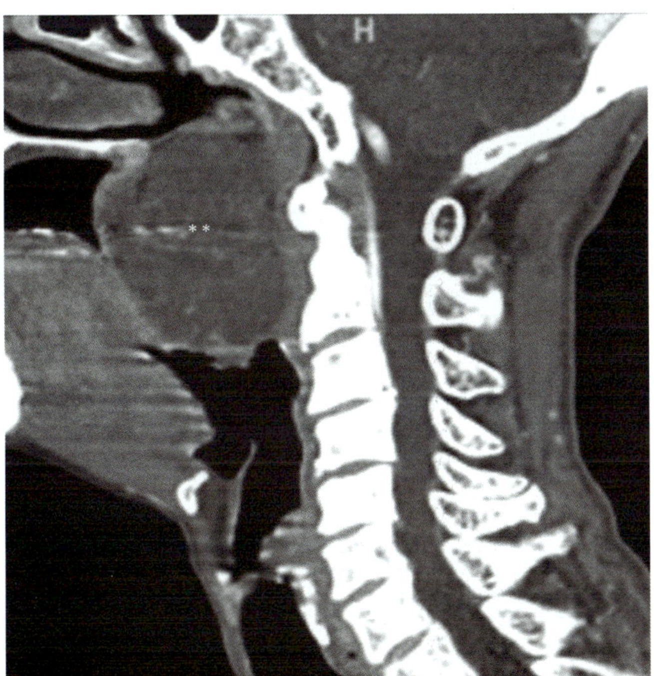

Fig. 25D.2 Sagittal CT scan showing a left parapharyngeal tumor (**).

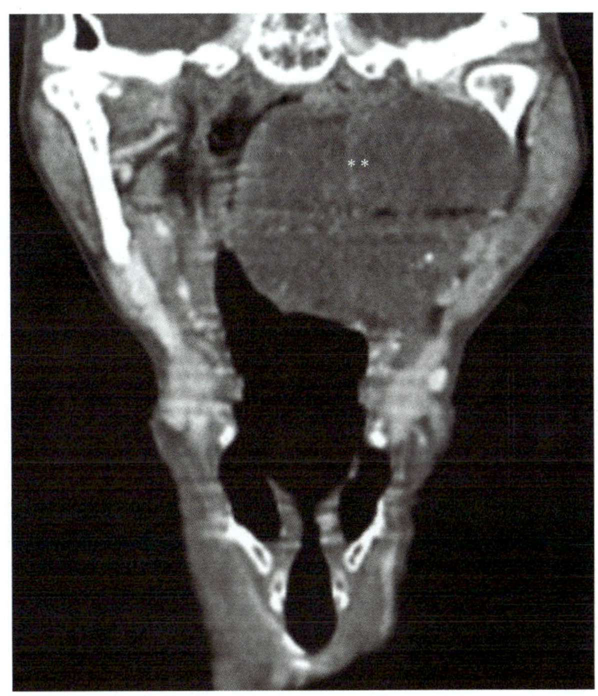

Fig. 25D.3 Coronal CT scan demonstrating a left parapharyngeal tumor (**).

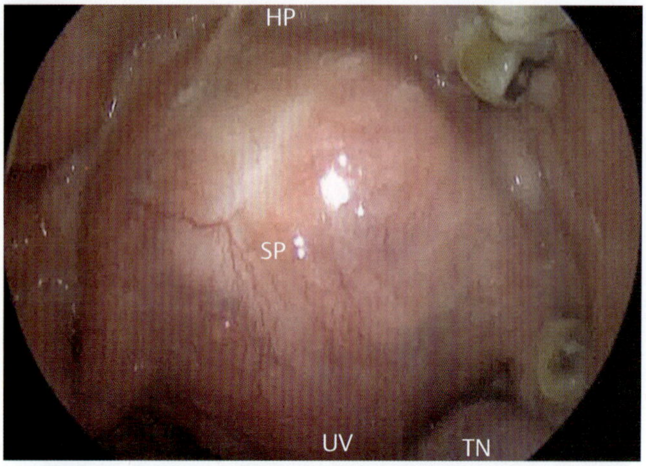

Fig. 25D.4 Exposure of the soft palate (SP) fullness caused by the left parapharyngeal mass.

4. A transoral endoscopic surgery is performed using a rigid-rod endoscope 4 mm in diameter with lens angle of 0 degree. The endoscope provides wide-angled, closed-up views and excellent visualization through a narrow surgical corridor.
5. Under endoscopic magnification, local anesthetic infiltration is done and a transverse incision is made on the soft palate where the mass is most prominent (**Fig. 25D.5** and **Fig. 25D.6**).
6. Careful dissection of the palatoglossus and pharyngeal constrictor muscles is performed with monopolar diathermy until the tumor is visible (**Fig. 25D.7**).
7. Blunt dissection is carried out cautiously to free the tumor, which is then delivered and removed transorally (**Fig. 25D.8, Fig. 25D.9, Fig. 25D.10**).

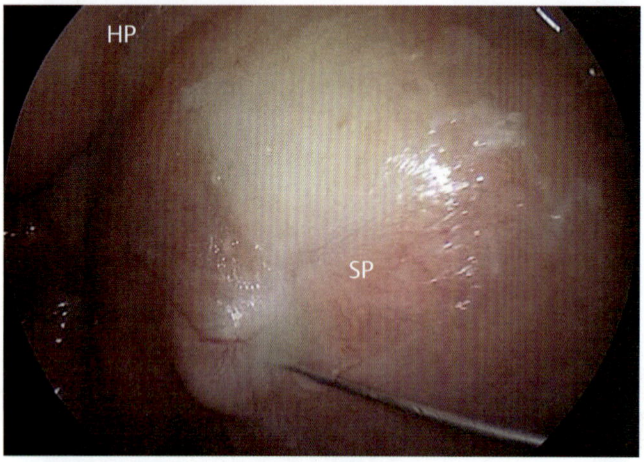

Fig. 25D.5 Intraoperative endoscopic view. Local anesthetic infiltration is carried out on the soft palate (SP).

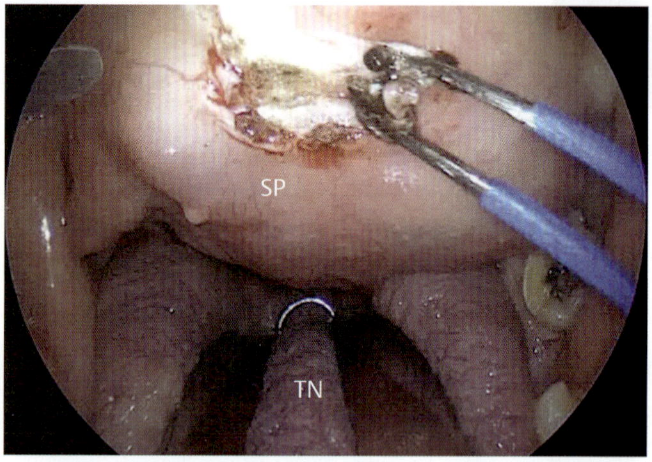

Fig. 25D.6 Intraoperative endoscopic view. A horizontal incision is made on the soft palate (SP).

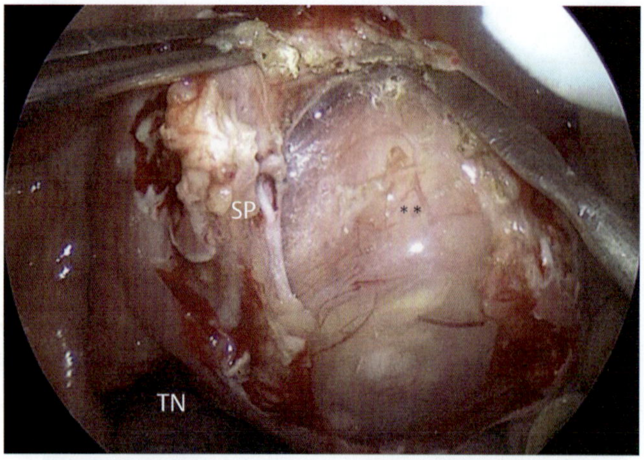

Fig. 25D.7 Intraoperative endoscopic view. Dissection is carried through the deep to soft palate (SP) to reach the tumor (**).

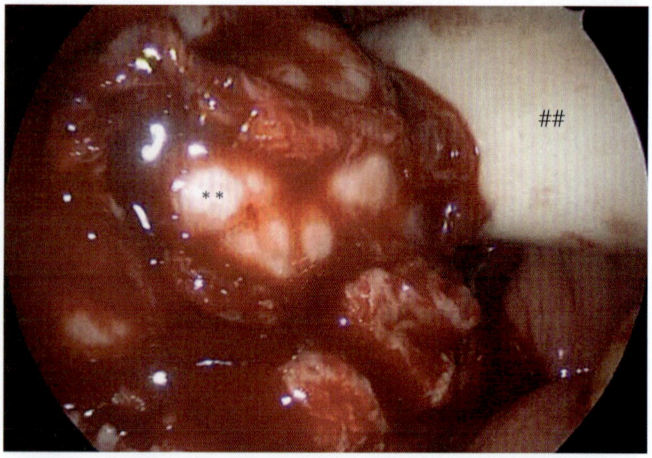

Fig. 25D.8 Intraoperative endoscopic view. The tumor (**) is dissected out via blunt finger dissection (##).

8. Meticulous hemostasis is secured with bipolar cauterization and Surgicel.
9. The soft palate incision is closed in layers with Vicryl suture 3–0 (**Fig. 25D.11**).
10. The tumor specimen is sent for histopathological examination (**Fig. 25D.12**).
11. Postoperatively, the patient is decannulated prior to discharge from the hospital.

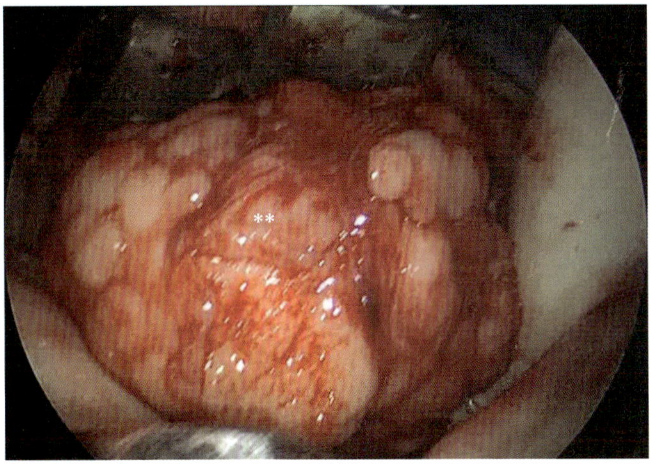

Fig. 25D.9 The tumor (**) is removed transorally.

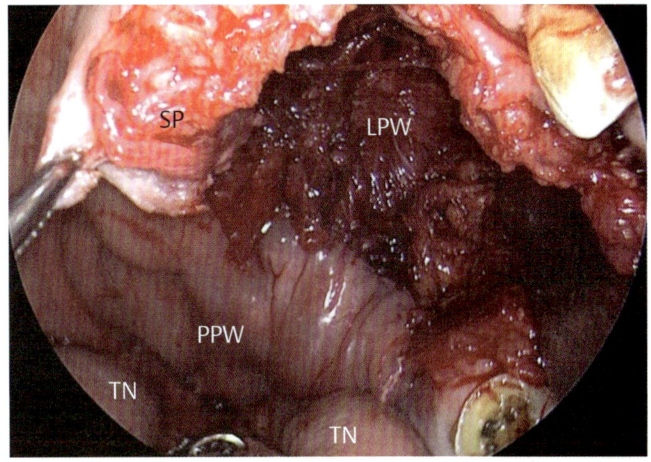

Fig. 25D.10 Postoperative view after complete removal of the tumor.

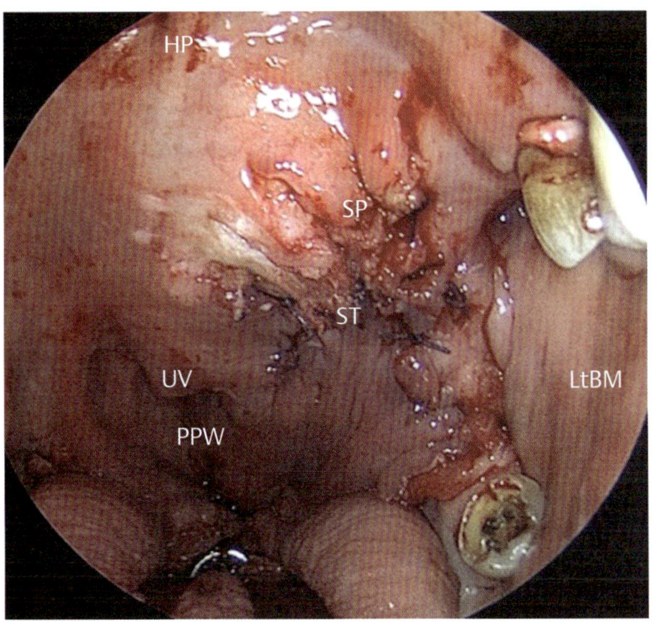

Fig. 25D.11 The soft palate (SP) incision is closed in a layered fashion with 3–0 absorbable sutures (ST).

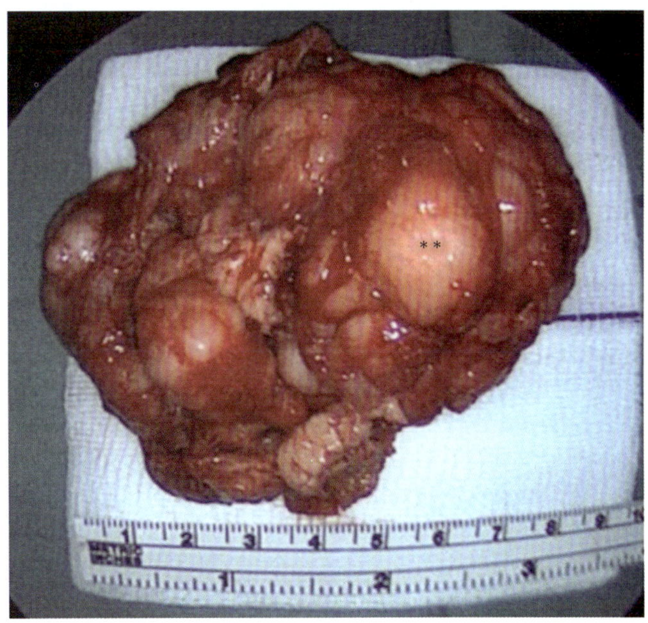

Fig. 25D.12 Tumor specimen (**). Histopathological examination confirmed a pleomorphic adenoma.

Case 25E

Endoscopic Endonasal Transpterygoid Nasopharyngectomy

Ing Ping Tang, Revadi Govindaraju, and Prepageran Narayanan

Introduction

The primary treatment for untreated nasopharyngeal carcinoma (NPC) is radiotherapy for early-stage lesion and concurrent chemoradiation for advanced tumors. The reported incidence of local recurrence is approximately 8 to 58%.[1–3] Local recurrent NPC can be treated with salvage reirradiation or surgery.[4] Ridge et al.[5] recommended that the resection of locally discrete recurrent NPC should be considered unless the patient is not fit for operation. Surgery should be considered for patients presenting with residual or recurrent tumor after radiotherapy or chemoradiotherapy, and for patients with glandular or mesenchymal differentiation tumors, which are poorly responsive to radiotherapy.[6] Furthermore, high-dose reirradiation may result in severe complications like osteoradionecrosis, brain necrosis, radiation-induced myelitis, hypopituitarism, and trismus.[7,8]

Endoscopic endonasal transpterygoid nasopharyngectomy (EETN) has then emerged as a viable treatment option for locally recurrent NPC with minimal invasiveness, avoiding morbidity from external approaches and facial scar. A literature review by Emanuelli et al revealed that endoscopic method attained a higher negative surgical margin of 93.75% than external approach (71.6%).[9]

Patient Selection

Patient selection is perhaps the most important aspect of effectively treating patients with EETN. Generally speaking, patients categorized as rT1, those categorized as rT2 with minimal parapharyngeal extension, and selected patients categorized as rT3 (involvement of the floor of the sphenoid sinus) can be treated with EETN. Exclusion criteria for patients can be based on disease factors and patient factors. Disease factors for exclusion include significant parapharyngeal space extension, internal carotid artery (ICA) involvement, cavernous sinus with involvement of multiple cranial nerves, brain parenchymal involvement, and the presence of distant metastasis. Patient factors include those patients who are medically unfit to tolerate surgery and undergo general anesthesia.

Preoperative Work-Up

The preoperative work-up for patients undergoing EETN includes clinical factors, radiological factors, and pathological factors.

For clinical factors, patients require a thorough medical examination including nasopharyngoscopy to delineate the tumor extension. The patients must also be investigated to determine their fitness and eligibility for general anesthesia. For radiological factors, a radiological examination is essential to ascertain the extent of the primary tumor, assess for regional lymph node involvement, and rule out distant metastatic disease. Investigational techniques include computed tomography, magnetic resonance imaging (MRI), and occasionally, positron emission tomography. For pathological factors, histopathological examination of the suspected local recurrence or residual tumor and confirmation of the type of tumors must be done before any surgical intervention.

Surgical Technique

The surgery is done under general anesthesia with the patient lying in a supine position. The nasal cavities are decongested with Moffett's solution[10] for 30 minutes. The solution contains 1-mL of adrenaline (1:1,000), 2 mL of 10% cocaine, 4 mL of 8.4% sodium bicarbonate, mixed with 13 mL of water for injection. Following general anesthesia, there is often widespread vasodilation, producing hyperemic mucosa. A topical decongestant of Moffett's solution could reduce the nasal blood flow, optimizing the surgical field. Infiltration of both middle turbinates and nasal septum with a solution of lidocaine 1% and epinephrine 1/100,000 enhances hemostasis. Surgery proceeds via a purely endoscopic endonasal approach using 0 and 30 degrees rod lens endoscope. A fundamental premise of the endonasal endoscopic approach is that the two surgeons work concomitantly, using a bimanual, three-/four-handed technique via both nostrils and nasal cavities. This facilitates dynamic visualization as well as bimanual dissection, which is vital for depth perception, traction, and counter traction and for maintenance of a blood-free surgical field.[6]

Nasoseptal Flap

First, the Hadad–Bassagasteguy nasoseptal flap (HBF) should be harvested from the contralateral side of the tumor.[10,11] It is critical to harvest the HBF from the contralateral side because its pedicle and proximal blood supply would be surrendered ipsilateral to the transpterygoid dissection. Later, a Caicedo reverse flap is transposed from the contralateral side to cover the HBF donor defect.[12,13] Clinical harvesting of these septal flaps presumes that the tumor does not involve this area. If the tumor involves the nasal septum, other vascularized flaps can be considered (**Fig. 25E.1, Fig. 25E.2**).

Sinonasal Corridor

Later, the surgery continues with enlarging the natural sinonasal corridor ipsilateral to the lesion by removing the inferior half of the right middle turbinate and completing an uncinectomy, large mid-meatal nasomaxillary window, and anterior and posterior ethmoidectomies. This increases the working space and exposes the entire posterior wall of the antrum. A medial maxillectomy is performed to expose the entire height of the posterior wall of the maxillary sinus and allow an extended dissection of the pterygopalatine fossa. This medial maxillectomy is limited anteriorly by the nasolacrimal duct, which acts as a fulcrum point, preventing free movement of the scope laterally. Endoscopic Denker's approach can be performed to further increase the lateral angle of exposure and optimize instrument maneuverability.[14] Endoscopic Denker's approach is a procedure to remove the piriform aperture, as well as the anterior maxillary wall, until the lateral wall of the antrum is in direct and full view, particularly the entire infratemporal fossa (**Fig. 25E.3**).

Additional lateral control is obtained by bringing the instruments from the contralateral side of the nose through a posterior septectomy. A generous posterior bony septectomy allows a bimanual technique traversing both sides of the nasal cavity. This extensive posterior septectomy allows visualization of the entire posterior wall of the maxillary sinus using a 0-degree endoscope that crosses over the contralateral side of the nose.

Inferior Sphenoidectomy

The anterior face of the sphenoid sinus is often opened early during the approach, enlarging the sphenoid ostium after completing the ethmoidectomies. As the superior part of the sphenoid crest is removed, the floor of sella turcica and intersinus and intrasinus septations, as well as the lateral walls of the sphenoid sinus, come into direct view. The lateral walls of the sphenoid and the medial pterygoid plates (lateral wall of the posterior choana) form a vertical strut that intersects the floor of the sphenoid sinus. After the complete removal of the vomer, the intersinus septum, and the sphenoid sinus floor, sphenoidectomy should extend superiorly to be in

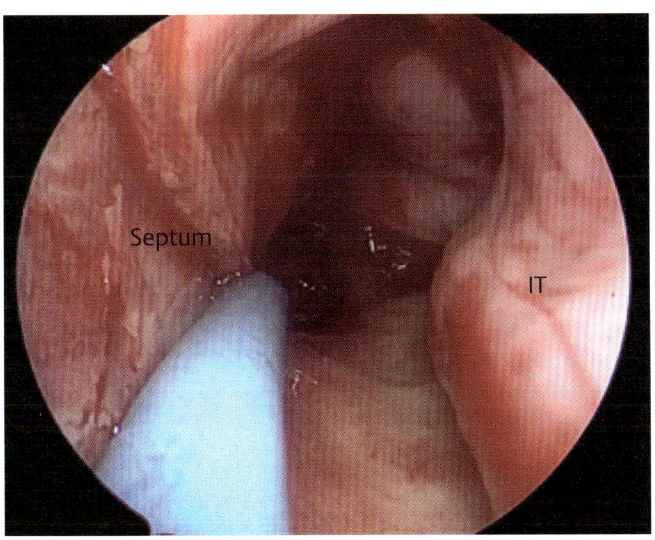

Fig. 25E.1 Creating HB nasoseptal flap.

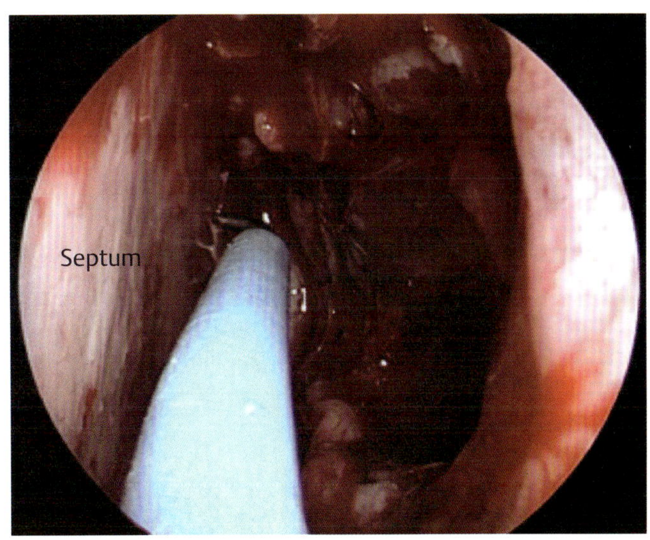

Fig. 25E.2 Creating Caicedo's flap.

plane with the roof of the nose and laterally to be in plane with the laminae papyracea bilaterally.[15] Complete removal of the sphenoid sinus floor is performed until the cavity is flush with the clivus (**Fig. 25E.4**).

Transpterygoid Dissection

Transpterygoid dissection starts with the identification of the vidian nerve proximal to the pterygopalatine ganglion, as it exits from the vidian canal. The vidian nerve can be localized following the palatovaginal canal laterally or by drilling its canal starting at the pterygoid wedge. The vidian nerve, within the pterygoid canal, courses toward the second genu of the ICA between the horizontal and vertical segments. For the most part, the vidian canal remains inferior to the second genu of the ICA; therefore, initial drilling in a 3 to 9 o'clock orientation helps to prevent injury to the ICA. In some cases, the superior aspect of the canal is covered just with a very thin bone or may even be dehiscent, thus exposing the nerve in the floor of the sphenoid sinus.[15]

The maxillary division of the trigeminal nerve passes through the foramen rotundum as it courses from Meckel's cave into the pterygopalatine fossa.[18] The maxillary nerve can also be identified in its canal coursing the lateral wall of the sphenoid sinus. The pharyngeal end of the eustachian tube or torus tubarius is just posterior to the pterygoid process. The removal of the pterygoid process exposes the cartilaginous eustachian tube. The parapharyngeal segment of the ICA is posterior to the eustachian tube in most of the cases.

All these landmarks are crucial to identify during the transpterygoid approach before tumor extirpation (**Fig. 25E.5, Fig. 25E.6**).

Tumor Extirpation

Tumor removal begins by marking out at least 1-cm margin if technically possible around the tumor. The mucosal cuts are made with needle point electrocautery, which helps with hemostasis. The superior and posterior dissection occurs by elevating the mucoperiosteum from the floor of the sphenoid sinus and the clivus posteriorly. The dissection proceeds inferiorly to the level of the soft palate, the prevertebral musculature deep to the pharyngobasilar fascia, and prevertebral fascia are encountered.[16] Both electrocautery and Kerrison's rongeurs can be used and are effective at removing portions of the prevertebral muscle and fascia, as these structures are quite resilient. The muscles are included in the en bloc resection if involved with the malignancy.

Laterally, the medial pterygoid plate and pterygoid process are exposed, above which lies the sinus of Morgagni, through which pass the eustachian tube and tensor veli palatine muscle. These structures can be excised along with the levator palatini muscle to expose the parapharyngeal tissues.[17] The eustachian tube cartilage laterally is identified and included in the specimen. Following complete tumor removal, margin status is confirmed by sending circumferential and deep margins for frozen section analysis (**Fig. 25E.7, Fig. 25E.8**).

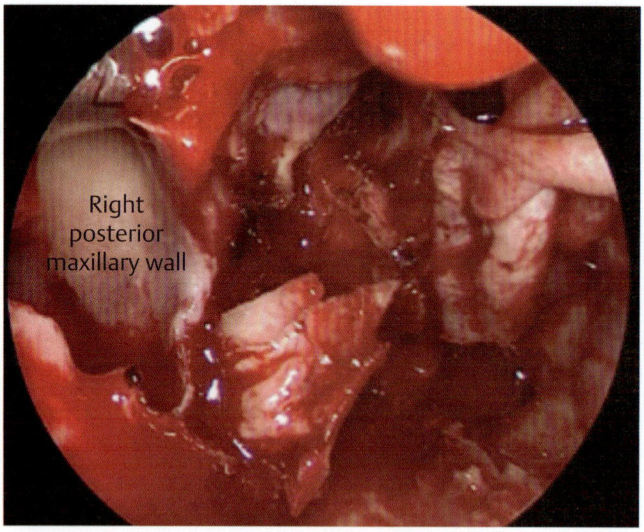

Fig. 25E.3 Right medial maxillectomy performed as part of the transpterygoid approach.

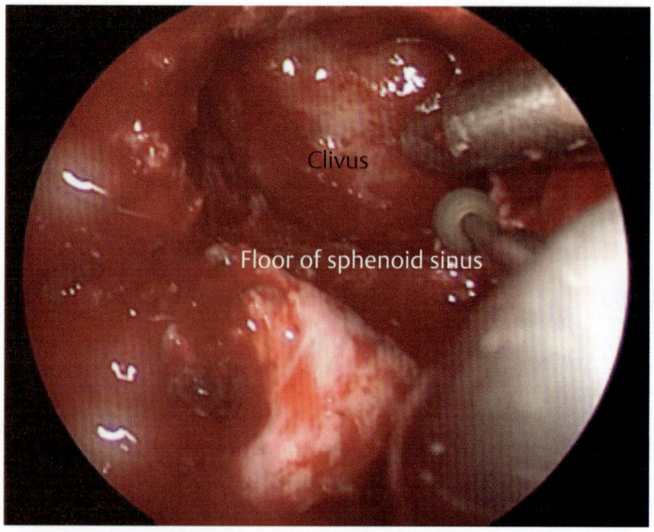

Fig. 25E.4 Drilling of the anterior wall and floor of the sphenoid sinus.

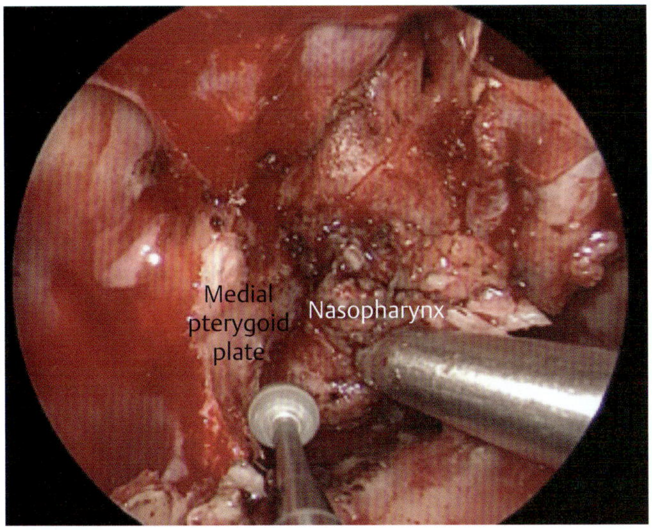

Fig. 25E.5 Drilling of the pterygoid base and the medial pterygoid plate.

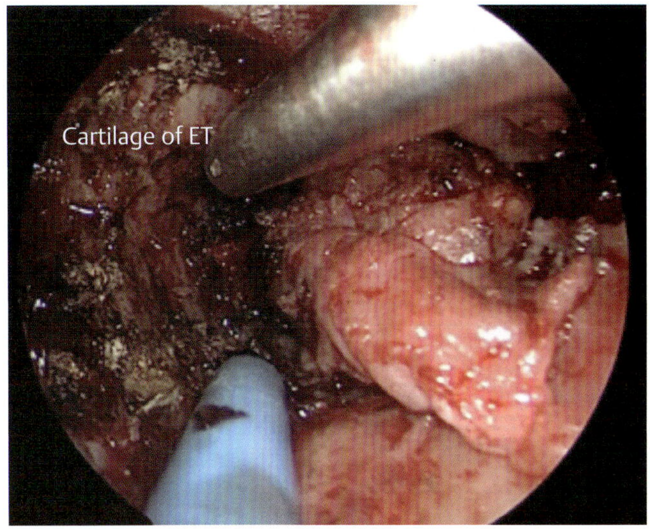

Fig. 25E.6 Resection of cartilage part of the eustachian tube.

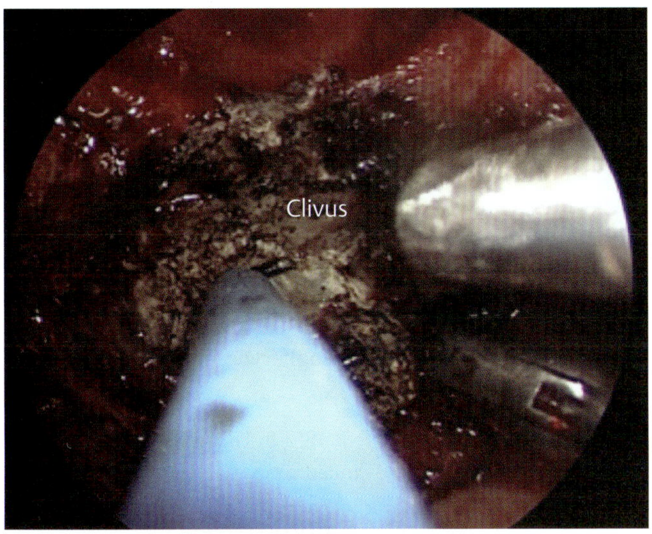

Fig. 25E.7 Resecting posteriorly at prevertebral muscle.

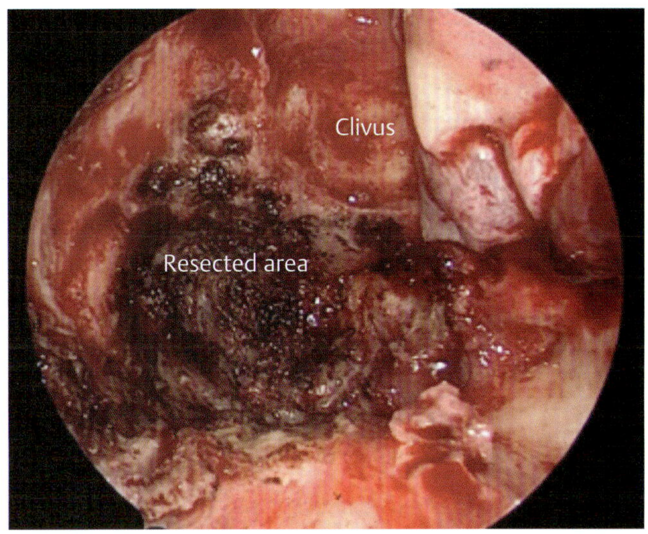

Fig. 25E.8 Final view of resection of right fossa of rosenmuler of nasopharynx.

Nasopharyngeal Reconstruction

Reconstruction with a vascularized pedicle flap at the nasopharyngeal defect facilitates the healing of the defect, resists irradiation, and protects the ICA against exposure and blowout.[6,18] The nasoseptal flap or HBF is rotated into the nasopharyngeal defect. The edges of the flap are allied well to cover the bare area, especially the exposed bony portion at the clivus. Absorbable gelatin sponges are placed on the flap, and a Foley catheter is used to support the nasoseptal flap against the nasopharyngeal defect. In cases where nasoseptal flaps are unavailable, a lateral nasal wall flap can be harvested for reconstruction. Other reconstructive options include healing by secondary intention or using regional flaps such as pedicled temporoparietal fascia flap (**Fig. 25E.9, Fig. 25E.10**).

Following reconstruction, the nasal cavity is thoroughly inspected for hemostasis followed by careful suction of the nasopharyngeal cavity.

Postoperative Care and Complications

The patient is admitted to a standard ward unit and is usually discharged from hospital within 2 to 3 days. After discharge from the ward, the patients are generally seen every 1

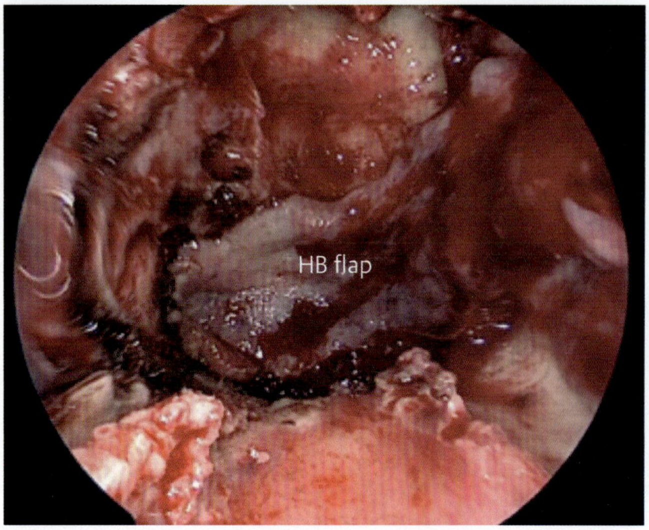

Fig. 25E.9 Placing of HB flap onto the resected area.

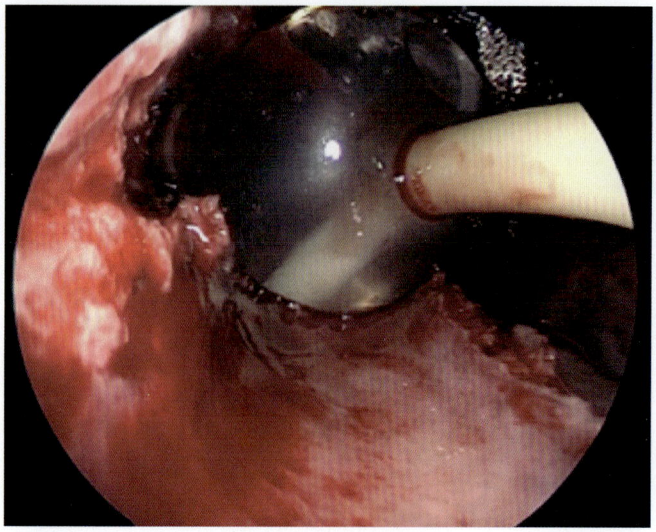

Fig. 25E.10 Catheter tube with a balloon to hold the flap in place.

to 2 weeks to undergo endoscopic examination. During these clinic visits, decrusting is performed, paying careful attention not to disrupt the nasoseptal flap or any other flaps that were laid on. Patients are asked to liberally use sodium bicarbonate mixed with mupirocin nasal rinse every 4 hours. The re-epithelialization process at the operation site can take up to 3 or more months, even with a nasoseptal flap. Postoperative headache is a common complaint following EETN because of the exposed bone. Covering the exposed bone with pedicled nasoseptal flap can reduce this incidence significantly.

Serous otitis media is another common complication encountered in the postoperative period. This can be managed by myringotomy with tympanostomy tube insertion or amplification with hearing aids.[16]

Postoperative epistaxis can occur secondary to bleeders, which are not secured during the surgery, especially when a nasoseptal flap is not used, and secondary to bleeding from the posterior septal artery. Other possible surgical sequelae include xerophthalmia secondary to injury of the vidian nerve, numbness in the V2 distribution, skull base injury including cerebrospinal fluid leak, and injury to the ICA in either its parapharyngeal, petrous, or clival portions.

Conclusion

In conclusion, EETN is a feasible approach for the surgical treatment of selected primary and recurrent nasopharyngeal malignancy tumors. The surgical technique requires a trained and experienced team with specialized equipment. This technique has relatively low morbidity with promising preliminary outcomes and local control of the disease that is comparable to conventional techniques.

References

1. Suárez C, Rodrigo JP, Rinaldo A, Langendijk JA, Shaha AR, Ferlito A. Current treatment options for recurrent nasopharyngeal cancer. Eur Arch Otorhinolaryngol 2010; 267(12):1811–1824
2. Ma J, Mai HQ, Hong MH, et al. Results of a prospective randomized trial comparing neoadjuvant chemotherapy plus radiotherapy with radiotherapy alone in patients with locoregionally advanced nasopharyngeal carcinoma. J Clin Oncol 2001;19(5):1350–1357
3. Lin JC, Liang WM, Jan JS, Jiang RS, Lin AC. Another way to estimate outcome of advanced nasopharyngeal carcinoma—is concurrent chemoradiotherapy adequate? Int J Radiat Oncol Biol Phys 2004;60(1):156–164
4. You R, Zou X, Hua YJ, et al. Salvage endoscopic nasopharyngectomy is superior to intensity-modulated radiation therapy for local recurrence of selected T1-T3 nasopharyngeal carcinoma—a case-matched comparison. Radiother Oncol 2015;115(3):399–406
5. Ridge JA. Squamous cancer of the head and neck: surgical treatment of local and regional recurrence. Semin Oncol 1993;20(5):419–429
6. Al-Sheibani S, Zanation AM, Carrau RL, et al. Endoscopic endonasal transpterygoid nasopharyngectomy. Laryngoscope 2011;121(10):2081–2089
7. To EW, Lai EC, Cheng JH, Pang PC, Williams MD, Teo PM. Nasopharyngectomy for recurrent nasopharyngeal carcinoma: a review of 31 patients and prognostic factors. Laryngoscope 2002;112(10):1877–1882

8. Chang JTC, See LC, Liao CT, et al. Locally recurrent nasopharyngeal carcinoma. Radiother Oncol 2000;54(2): 135–142
9. Emanuelli E, Albu S, Cazzador D, Pedruzzi B, Babighian G, Martini A. Endoscopic surgery for recurrent undifferentiated nasopharyngeal carcinoma. J Craniofac Surg 2014;25(3):1003–1008
10. Al-Sheibani S, Zanation AM, Carrau RL, et al. Endoscopic endonasal transpterygoid nasopharyngectomy. Laryngoscope 2011;121(10):2081–2089
11. Hadad G, Bassagasteguy L, Carrau RL, et al. A novel reconstructive technique after endoscopic expanded endonasal approaches: vascular pedicle nasoseptal flap. Laryngoscope 2006;116(10):1882–1886
12. Prosser JD, Figueroa R, Carrau RI, Ong YK, Solares CA. Quantitative analysis of endoscopic endonasal approaches to the infratemporal fossa. Laryngoscope 2011;121(8): 1601–1605
13. Caicedo-Granados E, Carrau R, Snyderman CH, et al. Reverse rotation flap for reconstruction of donor site after vascular pedicled nasoseptal flap in skull base surgery. Laryngoscope 2010;120(8):1550–1552
14. Benjamin E, Wong DK, Choa D. 'Moffett's' solution: a review of the evidence and scientific basis for the topical preparation of the nose. Clin Otolaryngol Allied Sci 2004;29(6):582–587
15. Hosseini SM, Razfar A, Carrau RL, et al. Endonasal transpterygoid approach to the infratemporal fossa: correlation of endoscopic and multiplanar CT anatomy. Head Neck 2012;34(3):313–320
16. Monteiro E, Witterick I. Endoscopic nasopharyngectomy: patient selection and surgical execution. Oper Tech Otolaryngol Head Neck Surg 2014;25:284–288
17. Kassam AB, Prevedello DM, Carrau RL, et al. The front door to meckel's cave: an anteromedial corridor via expanded endoscopic endonasal approach- technical considerations and clinical series. Neurosurgery 2009;64(3, Suppl):ons71–ons82, discussion ons82–ons83
18. Yip J, Macdonald KI, Lee J, et al. The inferior turbinate flap in skull base reconstruction. J Otolaryngol Head Neck Surg 2013;42:6

Chapter 26

Management of Juvenile Nasopharyngeal Angiofibroma

Renuka Bradoo, Madhu Sudhan V., and Tejal Patel

Introduction

Juvenile nasopharyngeal angiofibroma (JNA) remains an enigmatic and difficult tumor to treat in the nasal cavity and surrounding regions. Although the incidence of this tumor is low (0.05–0.5%) of all the head and neck tumors,[1,2] there are tertiary care centers that have a high-volume load of these cases. Angiofibromas are different from the other nasal tumors because of the following points: (1) They are one of the most vascular tumors of the nasal cavity. (2) They grow through the foramina and fissures without destroying the intervening bone. Hence, they are often called "dumbbell-shaped" tumors. (3) Because of their vascularity, they cannot be removed piecemeal with a microdebriber or cold instruments. Hence, unlike other tumors, the JNA cannot be made to collapse upon itself and later be peeled off gently from the surrounding important neurovascular structures.

Epidemiology

JNA occurs most commonly in the age group of 10 to 18 years with an average age of around 14 years.[3] The youngest case reported in the literature was a newborn infant.[4] The oldest patient to harbor a JNA was a 79-year-old male.[5] Although JNA occurs almost exclusively in males, it can very rarely occur in females as well. The highest incidence of 16% in female patients was reported by Handousa in Egypt.[6] Chromosomal studies should be advised in female patients.

Etiopathogenesis

The first description of JNA probably dates back to the fourth century BC when Hippocrates first observed nasal polyps. It was only in 1847 that Chelius described JNA as "a tumor which commonly occurred in a person about the time of puberty." Friedberg first used the term "angiofibroma" in 1940.[7] The first successful excision of a probable JNA is credited to Liston in 1841 at University College Hospital in London.

In spite of the numerous theories proposed to explain the origin of JNA, the exact histogenesis of the tumor remains debatable. The tumor is most commonly believed to arise at the site where the sphenoidal process of the palatine bone articulates with the base of the sphenoid and the horizontal ala of the vomer.[8] This area forms the superior border of the sphenopalatine foramen (SPF) and lies just above the posterior end of the middle turbinate.

Speculations on the tissue's origin were first made in the 19th century by Nelatori,[9] Verneuil,[10] and Tillaux,[11] who defined angiofibroma as a fibrous neoplasm arising from the periosteum or embryonic fibrocartilage of the skull base. Martin et al[12] and Dane[13] focused on a hormonal imbalance as the cause of these tumors. In 1942, Brunner[14] described endothelium-lined vascular spaces in the fascia basalis and proposed that angiofibromas originated from this tissue. Similarities to nasal erectile tissue were noted by Osborn.[15] Schiff[16] suggested that angiofibroma was ectopic vascular tissue that grew as a result of alterations in pituitary activity. Maurice and Milad[17] interpreted angiofibromas as hamartomas resulting from misplaced genital erectile tissue. In addition to these fibrous or vascular origins, many other hypotheses have been proposed. One such theory proposes that these tumors originate from nonchromaffin paraganglionic cells present at the terminal end of the maxillary artery.[18] Recent studies also suggest that these tumors arise from the vidian canal (pterygoid canal).[19] However, the author has seen cases in which the vidian canal was not involved.

The last decade has seen numerous studies being conducted in an attempt to understand the underlying deranged molecular mechanisms that lead to the formation of this tumor, most commonly in adolescent boys. Immunocytochemical techniques have shown androgen receptors in both vascular and stromal elements of the tumor. In contrast, few progesterone receptors and no estrogen receptors have been found.

The role of factors such as transforming growth factor β1 (TGF-β1) and vascular endothelial growth factor (VEGF) has been studied.[20] Nagai et al. found that TGF-β1 and insulin-like growth factor 2 (IGF-2) show statistically increased expression in these tumors than in controls suggesting that they may be growth regulators of nasopharyngeal angiofibromas. It is thought that the overexpression of IGF-2 might be associated with recurrence and poorer prognosis.[21] Mutations in the adenomatous polyposis coli (APC) gene on chromosome 5q might be involved in the pathogenesis of sporadic juvenile angiofibromas. Platelet-derived growth factor subunit B

(PDGF-B) can contribute, at least in part, to neovascularization and fibrosis.[22]

Recent evidence suggests that angiofibromas are extracolonic manifestations of familial adenomatous polyposis (FAP).[23,24] JNA has been reported to occur more commonly among patients with FAP, suggesting that it is a true neoplasm with alterations of the APC/β-catenin pathway.[25] Schick et al. studied sex chromosome structure in JNA. They found a significant loss of chromosome Y in combination with a gain of chromosome X.[26]

Even as extensive research to discover the etiological factors in this tumor continues, a widely accepted theory of origin is yet to be established.

Pathology

The tumor ranges from a very soft, highly vascular one to a firm, lobulated, nonencapsulated mass (**Fig. 26.1**). The firmness of the tumor depends on the relative proportions of the vascular and fibrous components. It is generally noted that the fibrous component and nodularity increase with the age of the patient.

Microscopically, the tumor is composed of thin-walled vessels of varying caliber interspersed in a mature connective tissue stroma. The vessels typically have a single endothelial cell lining without a muscularis layer (**Fig. 26.2**). This explains the propensity of the tumor to bleed profusely as the vessels do not constrict on being cut. The tumor cells show features of both fibroblasts and smooth muscle cells and are termed as myofibroblasts.

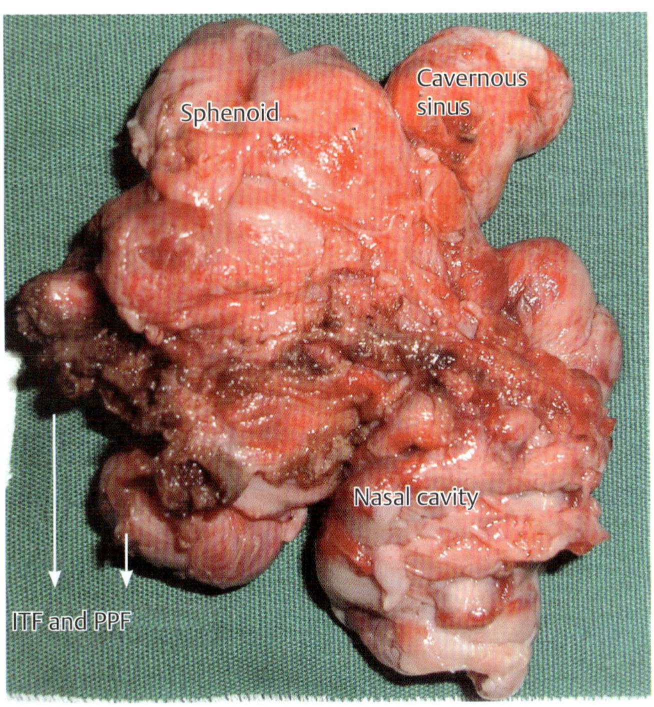

Fig. 26.1 Postoperative tumor specimen showing tumor extensions.

Mode of Spread

The use of high-quality contrast-enhanced computed tomography (CT) scans and nasal endoscopes has led to a greater understanding of the mode of spread of the JNA. There are numerous foramina, fissures, and canals into which the tumor spreads. It takes the path of least resistance and does not destroy the intervening bone. Large tumors are usually multilobulated or dumbbell shaped. The large component of the nasal and nasopharyngeal tumor continues into the other extensions as pseudopodia with an intervening constriction. This constriction corresponds to the foramen or fissure through which the tumor has spread. **Fig. 26.3** shows the different modes of spread. This figure is comprehensive, but every now and then, the authors are surprised to discover yet another new mode of spread.

The tumor originates where the perpendicular plate of the palatine bone articulates with the body of the sphenoid bone to form the SPF. The tumor grows medially into the nasal cavity. It may then grow anteriorly, but more commonly extends posteriorly through the posterior choana into the nasopharynx. If the nasopharyngeal component is very large, it pushes the soft palate downward and can even appear as an oropharyngeal mass behind the soft palate. It can also block the posterior choana of the opposite nasal cavity. Such a large tumor can cause difficulty in breathing and obstructive sleep apnea. The authors have been compelled to do a tracheostomy in a few patients to establish a stable airway prior to the surgery.

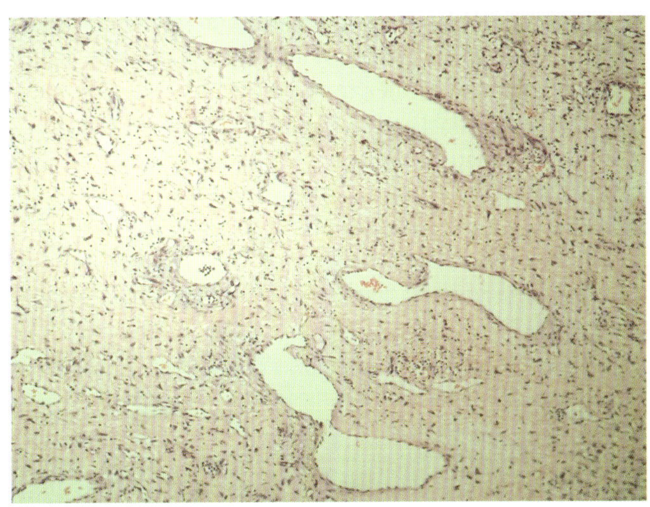

Fig. 26.2 Histological section (H & E, original magnification × 100) showing vascular channels of varying caliber amid dense fibrocollagenous stroma.

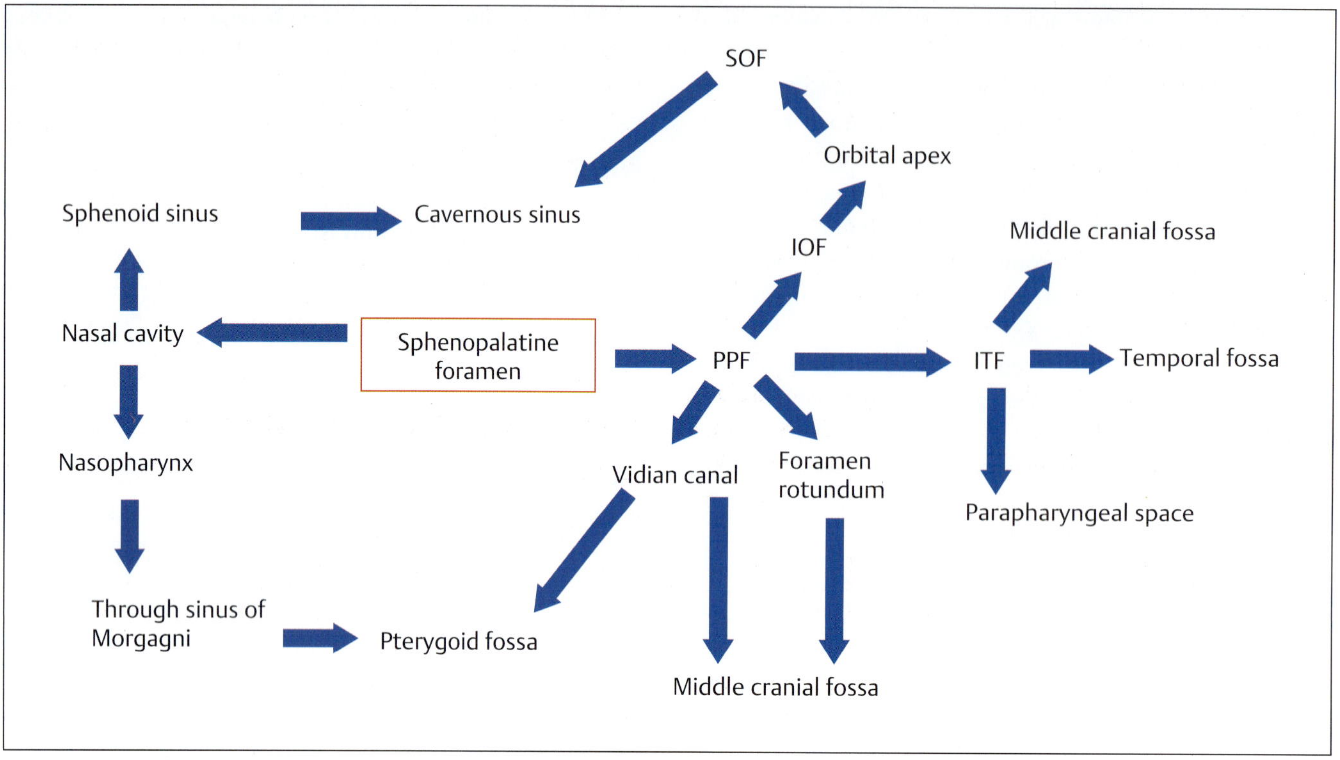

Fig. 26.3 Mode of spread of JNA originating from the sphenopalatine foramen (SPF).

At the level of posterior choana, the tumor may spread superiorly eroding the floor of the sphenoid sinus to lie within it. As it does so, it lifts the mucosa of the sphenoid sinus. Because it lies submucosally, it does not adhere to the roof or lateral wall of the sphenoid sinus.

The lateral spread occurs in two different planes:

1. Anterior to the pterygoid plates. The tumor grows laterally from the SPF anterior to the pterygoid process to lie in the pterygopalatine fossa (PPF). The anterior wall of PPF is formed by the posterolateral wall of the maxilla. The posterior wall is formed by the pterygoid base that has two openings: the vidian canal and the foramen rotundum. The vidian vessels and vidian nerve pass through the vidian canal. The foramen rotundum transmits the maxillary nerve (V2) from the intracranial cavity to the PPF. The maxillary nerve turns laterally in the PPF to continue as the infraorbital nerve. The medial wall of the PPF is formed by the perpendicular plate of the palatine bone and SPF. Laterally, the PPF communicates with the infratemporal fossa (ITF) through the pterygomaxillary fissure. Inferiorly, PPF tapers into a canal transmitting the descending palatine artery. Superiorly, it is continuous with the inferior orbital fissure (IOF). The tumor in PPF spreads into the ITF through the pterygomaxillary fissure. The tumor in ITF can grow to become quite large and multilobulated. It may extend under the zygomatic arch to enter the temporal fossa. It may also grow inferiorly to involve the parapharyngeal space. Rarely, it can grow through the descending palatine canal to appear as a bulge in the hard palate. Anteriorly, it may grow to cause a bulge in the cheek.

The tumor can grow superiorly from the PPF through the IOF to cause proptosis of the eyeball. It can grow posteriorly from the orbit through the superior orbital fissure (SOF) into the cavernous sinus.

The tumor can also spread through the posterior wall of PPF into the vidian canal and foramen rotundum. A noodle-like tumor bit can extend into the palatovaginal canal that lies just medial to the vidian canal.

2. Posterior to the pterygoid plates. The pterygoid fossa is the space behind and between the two pterygoid plates. The nasopharyngeal component of the tumor may grow laterally through the sinus of Morgagni above the superior constrictor muscle and come to lie in the pterygoid fossa. The tumor can also erode the pterygoid base and grow inferiorly into the pterygoid fossa.

The intracranial spread of the tumor mainly occurs through the following routes:

- From the orbit via the SOF.
- By eroding the greater wing of the sphenoid.
- Through the foramen ovale.

- Through the lateral wall of the sphenoid, compressing the medial wall of the cavernous sinus.
- Through the roof of the sphenoid sinus.
- Through the junction of the lateral wall of the sphenoid sinus and greater wing of the sphenoid, at the level of the foramen lacerum.
- Through the vidian canal, up to the paraclival carotid.
- Through the foramen rotundum into the middle cranial fossa.
- Rarely, through the cribriform plate of the ethmoid into the anterior cranial fossa.

Extranasopharyngeal angiofibroma is extremely rare and generally occurs in older patients and females where it tends to be less vascular and aggressive. There have been reports of angiofibromas on the nasal septum, middle turbinate, hard palate, and alveolar ridge.[27–30]

Spontaneous regression of the tumor remains a debatable issue and has been reported in residual tumors.[31,32]

Classification

Although there are numerous classifications described in the literature, the Andrew–Fisch classification,[33] Radkowski (revised sessions) classification,[34] University of Pittsburgh Medical Center (UPMC) classification,[35] and Janakiram classification[36] are particularly useful in planning management and predicting prognosis.

Andrew–Fisch Classification

Stage I—Tumor limited to the nasopharynx and nasal cavity. Bone destruction is negligible or limited to the SPF.

Stage II—Tumor involving the PPF or the maxillary, ethmoid, or sphenoid sinus with bone destruction.

Stage IIIa—Tumor involving the ITF or orbital region without intracranial involvement.

Stage IIIb—Tumor involving the ITF or orbital region with intracranial, extradural (parasellar) involvement.

Stage IVa—Intracranial, intradural tumor without infiltration of the cavernous sinus, pituitary fossa, or optic chiasma.

Stage IVb—Intracranial, intradural tumor with infiltration of the cavernous sinus, pituitary fossa, or optic chiasma.

Radkowski Classification

Stage Ia—Tumor limited to posterior nares and/or nasopharyngeal vault.

Stage Ib—Extension into one or more paranasal sinuses (PNS).

Stage IIa—Minimal lateral extension into the PPF.

Stage IIb—Full occupation of the PPF with or without superior erosion of orbital bones.

Stage IIc—Extension into the ITF or extension posterior to pterygoid plates.

Stage IIIa—Erosion of the base of skull (middle cranial fossa/base of pterygoids).

Stage IIIb—Erosion of the skull base with extensive intracranial extension with or without extension into the cavernous sinus.

University of Pittsburgh Medical Center Staging

Stage I—Nasal cavity, medial PPF.

Stage II—PNS, lateral PPF; no residual vascularity.

Stage III—Skull base erosion, orbit, ITF; no residual vascularity.

Stage IV—Skull base erosion, orbit, ITF; residual vascularity.

Stage V—Intracranial extension, residual vascularity.

M—Medial extension.

L—Lateral extension.

Janakiram Classification

Stage Ia—Pterygoid wedge and/or PNS.

Stage Ib—With extension to the nasopharynx.

Stage IIa—With extension in the nasal cavity and minimal involvement of PPF.

Stage IIb—Involvement of ITF.

Stage IIc—Involvement of ITF with extension to cheek/pterygoid fossa/IOF/laterally along the greater wing of the sphenoid.

Stage IIIa—Involvement of quadrangular space/Meckel's cave.

Stage IIIb—Involvement of cavernous sinus/engulfing carotid artery.

Stage IVa—Prestyloid parapharyngeal tumor extension above the lower border of the mandible.

Stage IVb—Intracranial intradural extension.

Stage V—Massive parapharyngeal, maximal intracranial extensions, and bilateral JNA.

Blood Supply

The major portion of the blood supply to the tumor comes from the ipsilateral maxillary artery. As the tumor grows in size, it derives blood supply from the adjacent structures and blood vessels including the branches of the internal carotid artery (ICA). The other major feeding blood vessels are the contralateral maxillary artery, ascending pharyngeal artery, and the artery of the vidian canal. ICA blood supply is usually seen in the tumors involving the basisphenoid and pterygoid wedges, in tumors with intracranial extension, or in recurrent tumors where the external carotid artery has been ligated during the first surgery.

Clinical Features

The most common presentation of JNA is unilateral nasal obstruction and epistaxis in a young adolescent male. The epistaxis is profuse, recurrent, and usually from a single nostril. A large nasopharyngeal extension causes snoring, mouth breathing, adenoid facies, rhinolalia clausa, and signs of eustachian tube blockage such as ear fullness, autophony, otalgia, and conductive hearing loss. The patient may have complaints of unilateral facial fullness, though headache is not very common. A small tumor extension into the PPF or ITF does not cause any specific symptoms. However, a large mass may present with a bulge in the cheek and proptosis if the orbit is involved (**Fig. 26.4**).

The tumor may have a large extension intracranially, but usually symptoms of a space-occupying lesion, such as headache, projectile vomiting, and blurring of vision, are typically not present. This is probably because of the slow-growing nature of the tumor. The intracranial extension of the tumor is usually an incidental finding on radiological examination. However, cases of meningitis, diabetes insipidus, proptosis, and ptosis have been noted by the authors because of the involvement of meninges, compression of the pituitary gland, involvement of the orbit, and involvement of the cavernous sinus, respectively. Symptoms suggestive of direct optic nerve compression are relatively rare. The authors have noted two such cases, one of them presenting with bilateral blindness.

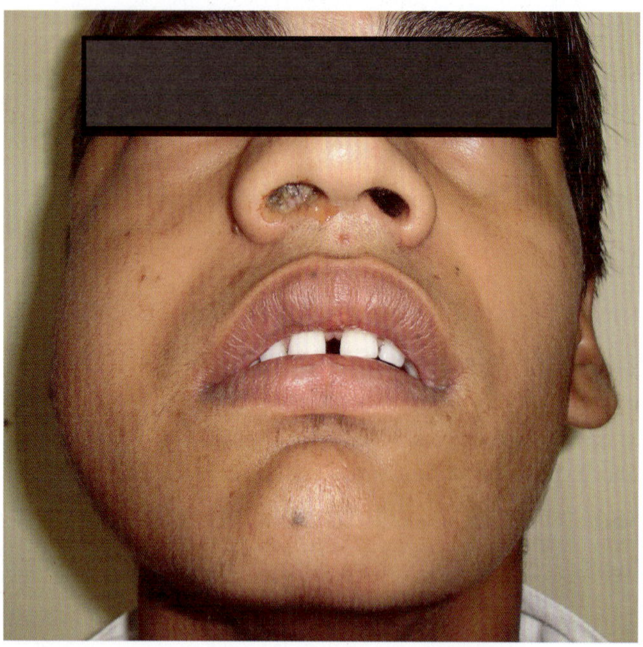

Fig. 26.4 Patient of JNA presenting with a nasal mass and a bulge on the cheek on the right side.

Investigations

A good clinical history and examination can give us a tentative diagnosis, which can be confirmed on nasal endoscopy and radiological evaluation. The gold standard investigation is a CT scan of the PNS with contrast injection. The contrast-enhanced scans show different extensions of the tumor. The bony windows show the bones that have been eroded or remodeled because of the tumor.

A CT scan helps us to identify the mode of spread of the tumor, which is instrumental in planning the surgical steps for excision of the tumor. To map the tumor in its entirety, it is necessary to have all three views: coronal, axial, and sagittal preferably in 1-mm slice thickness (**Fig. 26.5**). Tumors that have an intraorbital or intracranial spread require magnetic resonance imaging (MRI) scan with contrast. This is especially important in case of the encasement of the ICA. A contrast-enhanced CT scan shows the enhancement of both the tumor and the ICA. Therefore, the demarcation of the tumor from the artery is not well seen. A contrast-enhanced MRI shows enhancement of the tumor, while the ICA shows a flow void making the artery black in color. Thus, it is easier to demarcate the artery separately from the enhancing tumor (**Fig. 26.6**). MR angiography may be done to identify branches from the internal carotid system.

The role of X-ray PNS is now redundant. Holman Miller's sign, that is, the anterior bowing of the posterolateral wall of the maxilla, and the Handousa sign, that is, increased maxilla–coronoid distance can be appreciated on the CT scan itself.

A patient who has either partial or complete encasement of the ICA must undergo a balloon occlusion test to ensure that good contralateral blood supply is present via the circle of Willis. Prior knowledge of this is important in case the ICA is damaged during surgery. It is also necessary that the interventional radiology team be informed and kept on standby during the excision of intracranial tumors.

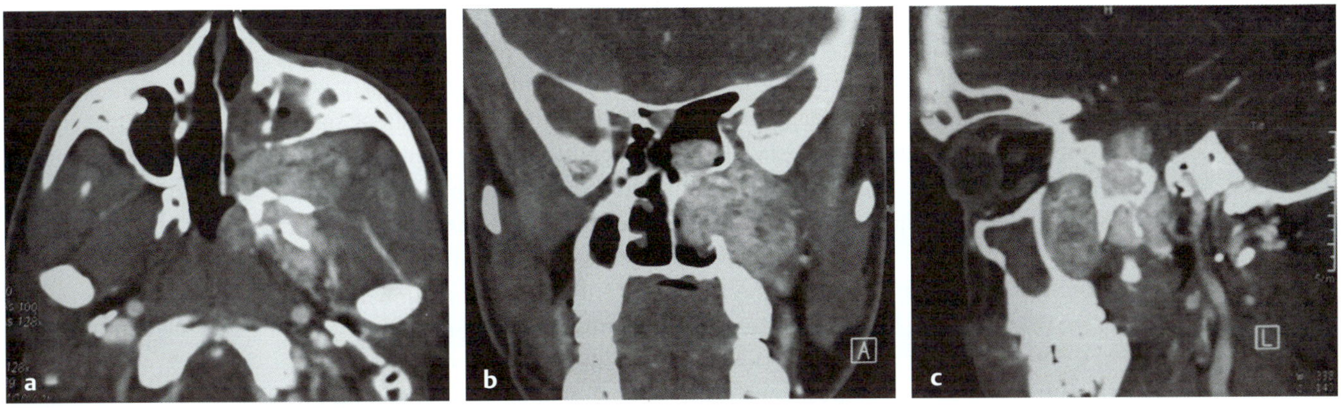

Fig. 26.5 Contrast-enhanced CT scan. **(a)** Axial, **(b)** coronal, and **(c)** sagittal views.

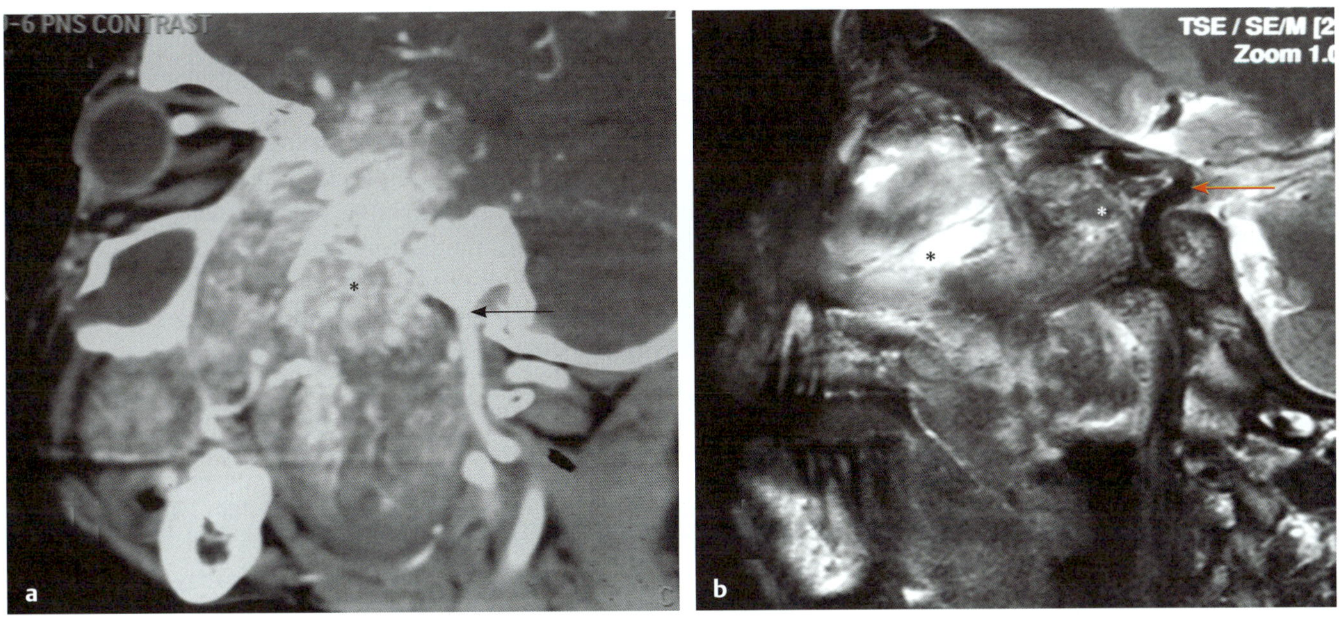

Fig. 26.6 **(a)** Contrast-enhanced CT scan showing the enhancement of both the tumor (*) and ICA (*black arrow*). **(b)** A contrast-enhanced MRI showing the tumor (*) and ICA (*red arrow*).

Because of the risk of hemorrhage, a biopsy is advisable only in those cases where the histopathological diagnosis seems doubtful, for example, in the rare event of a female patient of JNA. The evaluation of the patient is not complete without an otoscopy, tuning fork tests, evaluation of the central nervous system, and an ophthalmological examination. Tuning fork tests may uncover a serous otitis media with conductive hearing loss.

Treatment

Surgical excision remains the mainstay of treatment of JNA. The other treatment modalities include hormonal therapy, radiotherapy using external beam radiation or gamma knife, cryotherapy, electrocoagulation, and coblation.

Surgical Management

The two major approaches to excision of JNA are the open surgical approach and the endoscopic approach. The open surgical approach includes transpalatal, lateral rhinotomy, Weber Ferguson approach, midfacial degloving, maxillary swing, facial translocation, transhyoid and transmandibular approaches.

The basic underlying surgical principles for the removal of this tumor are wide exposure of the tumor, subperiosteal dissection, and en bloc removal wherever possible.

Open Surgical Approach

The description of so many open surgical approaches in literature bears testimony to the fact that no single approach has been found ideal for the management of all stages of the tumor. Weber Fergusson, transpalatal, and the midfacial degloving approaches are three of the most commonly used open approaches.

The Weber Fergusson incision is an extension of the lateral rhinotomy approach. The advantage is that it offers good exposure of the lateral limit of the tumor. Its major disadvantage is a disfiguring facial scar. It also offers only a unilateral approach to the tumor. Anesthesia of the cheek is a frequent occurrence with this approach.

The transpalatal approach[37] offers good exposure of the nasopharynx and the posterior nasal cavity. The advantage of this approach is the absence of an external scar, but there is limited access to the tumor. Large lateral extensions of the tumor are difficult to access. One of the complications of this approach is a palatal perforation.

The midfacial degloving[38,39] approach gives a wide bilateral exposure to the nasal cavity, nasopharynx, and the ITF. This approach is the only open approach that offers wide exposure of the tumor bed without leaving a facial scar. It can occasionally cause vestibular stenosis.

Combined Endoscope-Assisted Open Approach

For those surgeons who have not yet adapted to the endoscopic approach, a combined open and endoscopic approach may be the answer. This involves removing the gross tumor by an open approach and then examining the tumor bed with an endoscope for remnants of the tumor that can then be excised endoscopically.

Endoscopic Approach

Kamel[40] described the first endoscopic excision of JNA in 1996. With advanced imaging studies, safer and selectively targeted embolization, better optics, and increasing surgical experience, endoscopic excision of angiofibromas is now an accepted modality of treatment. Initially, endoscopic attempts were limited to tumors with minimal involvement of ITF. However, a number of tertiary referral centers across the world are now reporting endoscopic excision of much larger tumors and intracranial tumors.

The opinion is divided on whether preoperative embolization is a prerequisite for endoscopic excision of JNA. The authors believe that early in the learning curve of endoscopic excision, preoperative embolization greatly assists the surgeon to achieve complete resection. However, as one's experience grows, it is possible to operate tumors involving the nose, nasopharynx with minimal involvement of ITF without embolization. Large extracranial tumors are better handled if preoperative embolization has been done. A recurrent tumor with primarily ICA supply will not benefit from embolization. The authors usually embolize the tumor 48 hours before the surgery. Highly selective embolization with microcatheters and polyvinyl alcohol particles (150–250 µm) has significantly reduced the possibility of complications following embolization.

Surgical Steps

Refer to **Fig. 26.7** and the following steps for the description of surgical steps:

1. **Decongestion of the nasal cavity.** This is done sequentially with two sets of patties soaked in saline adrenaline. The author uses a solution of 30 mL of saline with 3 ampoules of adrenaline. The first set shrinks the

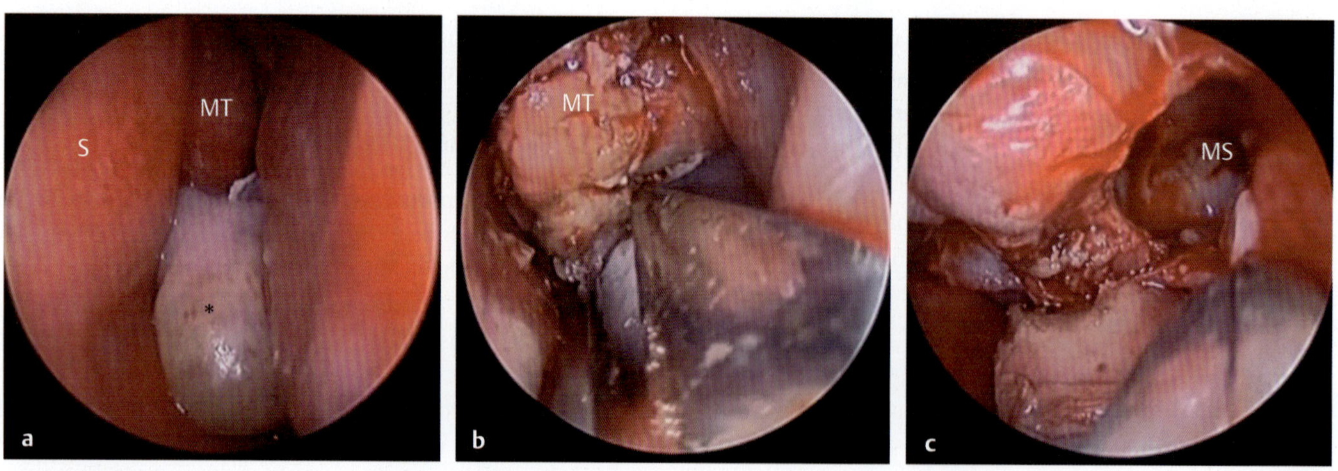

Fig. 26.7 (a) Tumor (*) in the nasal cavity. **(b)** Middle turbinate (MT) is trimmed. **(c)** Maxillary sinus ostium is widened after uncinectomy.

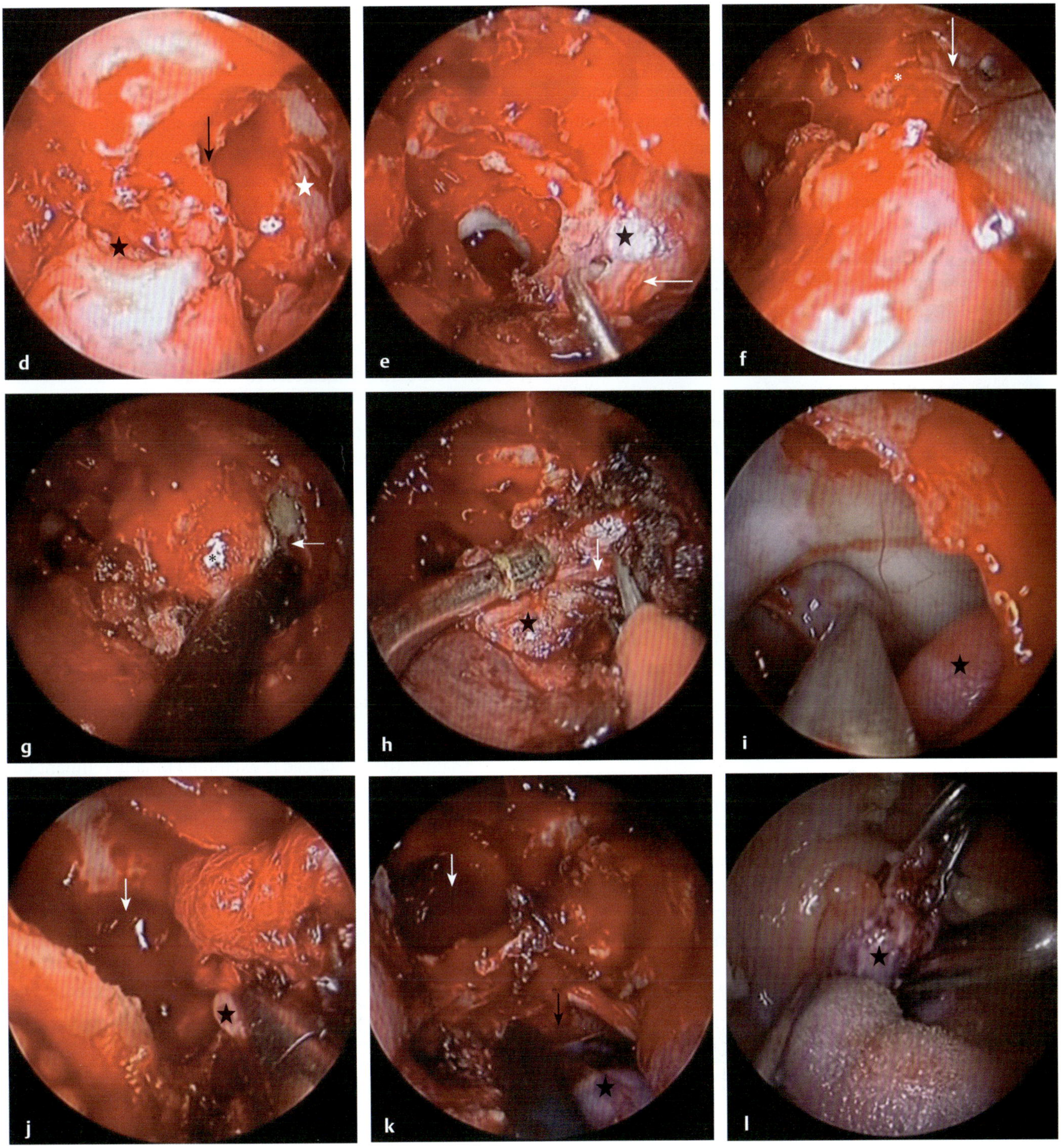

Fig. 26.7 *(Continued)* **(d)** Picture showing nasal part of tumor (*black* *), ITF part (*white* *), and intervening perpendicular plate of palatine bone (*black arrow*). **(e)** The orbital process of the palatine bone (*white arrow*) is removed to release the dumbelling of the tumor (*) at SPF. **(f)** The posterolateral wall (*white arrow*) of the maxillary sinus is removed and bulge of the tumor (*) is seen. **(g)** The periosteum (*white arrow*) just lateral to the lateral extent of the tumor (*) is cauterized and incised. **(h)** The tumor (*) in ITF is dissected and delivered into the nasal cavity, and the ipsilateral maxillary artery (*white arrow*) supplying the tumor is identified and cauterized. **(i)** Tumor (*) seen in the sphenoid sinus that has entered the sinus by eroding its floor. **(j)** The tumor (*) is delivered from the sphenoid sinus (*white arrow*). **(k)** The tumor (*) is delivered from the nasopharynx (*black arrow*); adjacent sphenoid sinus (*white arrow*) is visualized. **(l)** The tumor (*) is delivered through the oral cavity.

mucosa of turbinates and allows better visualization of the tumor. The second set is gently inserted around the tumor to open up spaces around the tumor.

2. **Examination of the tumor.** An attempt is made to visualize the adhesions of the tumor to its surrounding structures. This is done by gently retracting the tumor with a suction elevator, taking care not to traumatize the tumor. The examination is carried out with a zero-degree endoscope, first in the ipsilateral nostril and then the contralateral nostril. The nasopharyngeal portion of the tumor can be studied by inserting a 70-degree endoscope in the oral cavity behind the soft palate and looking upward.
3. **Trimming the middle turbinate.** The tumor almost always adheres to the posterior end of the middle turbinate. This adhesion is cauterized and cut. Cauterization is always done on the normal tissue, 1 to 2 mm away from the tumor. This prevents part of the tumor from being left behind accidentally on one of the normal structures. The middle turbinate is then trimmed to gain better access to the SPF.
4. **Posterior septectomy.** The posterior part of the nasal septum is removed to gain better access to the tumor from both nostrils for the four-handed approach.
5. **Uncinectomy.** The lower half of the vertical part as well as the complete horizontal part of the uncinate process is removed.
6. **Excision of the medial wall of the maxillary sinus.** The entire medial wall is removed superoinferiorly from the orbit up to the attachment of the inferior turbinate and anteroposteriorly from the nasolacrimal duct to where it continues as the posterolateral wall of the maxillary sinus. The orbital process of the palatine bone is removed to expose the sphenopalatine bundle exiting from the PPF into the nasal cavity via the SPF. The vertical part of the palatine bone is also removed to release the dumbelling of the tumor between the nasal cavity and PPF. The author does not trim the inferior turbinate unless absolutely necessary, such as in a large parapharyngeal extension of the tumor. .
7. **Cauterizing the periosteum.** The posterolateral wall of the maxilla is then completely removed. The periosteum covering the tumor in the PPF and ITF is gently cauterized and incised to expose the tumor.
8. **Dissecting the tumor from the ITF and identifying the maxillary artery.** The fat in the ITF is dissected and removed. The lateral extent of the tumor can now be seen. The maxillary artery, which usually enters the ITF from its inferolateral part, can be seen supplying the tumor. The artery is either clipped or cauterized and cut. The extension of the tumor into the ITF is gradually pulled into the nasal cavity. At this stage, the tumor invading the pterygoid base can usually be seen. Gentle and meticulous dissection is carried out to deliver the tumor from within the bone. The vidian artery may bleed at this stage and needs to be cauterized. The infraorbital nerve should be identified and peeled off the tumor.
9. **Removing the sphenoid extension.** The tumor usually erodes the floor of the sphenoid sinus and lies submucosally within the sinus. The bony floor of the sphenoid sinus is removed to release the tumor. It is then gently delivered into the nasal cavity using a Blakesley forceps.
10. **Removing adhesions to the lateral nasal wall.** The tumor has dense adhesions to the lateral nasal wall just above and behind the posterior end of the inferior turbinate extending up to the eustachian tube opening. The eustachian tube itself is never involved.
11. **Dissection of tumor from the nasopharynx.** There are usually dense adhesions at the roof of the posterior choana, the roof of the nasopharynx, and in the fossa of Rosenmuller. These are cauterized and cut.
12. **Delivery of the tumor.** Once the tumor is completely separated from the surrounding adhesions, it is gently pulled out through the oral cavity with all its extensions intact.
13. **Base skull drilling.** After giving washes of warm saline, the tumor bed is examined for any remnant bits of the tumor. The skull base is then drilled to remove any hidden pieces of tumor in the marrow spaces.
14. **Intraorbital and intracranial tumors.** These are removed using the basic principles of tumor excision. The lamina papyracea, the medial wall of the SOF, and the lateral wall of the sphenoid sinus are removed to release dumbelling of the tumor. The tumor is excised gently after the orbital periosteum and the medial wall of the cavernous sinus have been incised.
15. If the tumor has eroded bone to invade intracranially, the bony margins of the eroded bone are drilled to widen the bony defect. Most tumors are extradural in location. The tumor is then gently pulled out. It is dissected off the dura using a two-suction technique. A fascia lata patch is placed over the exposed dura as it is usually thinned out. Intradural spread is rare. In such a case, the surgery is performed along with a neurosurgeon.

Bradoo et al. have devised newer methods of dealing with JNA extending far laterally into the temporal fossa and parapharyngeal space namely "push–pull technique"[41] and "multiport technique."[42]

1. The push–pull technique: This technique is used for endoscopic excision of JNA with infratemporal and parapharyngeal extensions without resorting to open surgery.

An incision approximately 1-inch long is made in the upper gingivobuccal sulcus at the level of the third molar tooth. An assistant introduces the index finger through this incision to "push" the tumor toward the nasal cavity while the operating surgeon applies a simultaneous "pull" on the extension endoscopically (**Fig. 26.8**). This facilitates delivery of the extension into the nose for final removal. The assistant does not dissect with his or her finger as the maxillary artery would be at a risk of being torn. He or she simply stabilizes the tumor so that it does not keep falling back laterally as the primary surgeon works endoscopically through the nostrils to deliver it.

2. The four-port Bradoo technique: This is a new approach by which tumors with very large far lateral extensions can be operated endoscopically without disruption of the anterior facial skeleton.

Steps of Surgery

The structure of the midface is primarily maintained by 3 pillars:

1. The septum (P1)
2. The frontonasal process of the maxilla (P2)
3. The lateral edge of the maxilla (P3) (**Fig. 26.9**)

The frontonasal process protects the nasolacrimal duct.

After decongestion of the nose, the septum is infiltrated with 2 percent xylocaine and adrenaline and a posterior septectomy is performed by removing parts of the vomer and the perpendicular part of the ethmoid bone. Care is taken not to destabilize the quadrangular cartilage. The two nostrils thus become port A and port B. The buccogingival sulcus in the region of the canine fossa is infiltrated with 2% xylocaine adrenaline solution. An incision of approximately 1 inch is made to expose the anterior wall of the maxilla. An antral window is created in the canine fossa by removing enough bone to allow free access for a scope and an instrument, approximately 2 × 2 cm. Care is taken not to damage the frontonasal process of the maxilla or the infraorbital nerve. This becomes port C. A fourth port of access is then created. After infiltrating with 2% xylocaine adrenaline, a second incision of 1 inch is made in the buccogingival sulcus at the level of the last molar. This becomes port D. Thus, the angiofibroma could be accessed anteriorly through any one of these four ports (**Fig. 26.9**).

1. The contralateral nostril after doing a posterior septectomy - port A
2. The ipsilateral nostril - port B.
3. An antral window in the canine fossa - port C.
4. An incision of 1 inch in the buccogingival sulcus adjacent to the last molar. This has been previously described by the author in the push–pull approach - port D.

These ports significantly improve lateral access to the tumor and its feeding vessel—the maxillary artery—without removal of the frontonasal process or the nasolacrimal duct. This is an important advantage of this approach. The scope and various instruments can be passed interchangeably through two or more of these ports, at various stages of the surgery to ensure maximum visualization as well as reach of the instruments by diverse trajectories.

After creating these ports, the nasal portion of the tumor is first excised using ports A and B to create space in the nasal cavity. Port D is used primarily by an assistant surgeon

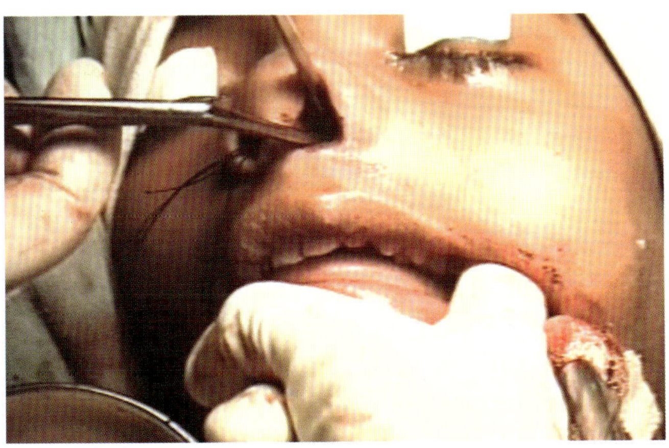

Fig. 26.8 Intraoperative image of the patient showing the push–pull technique.

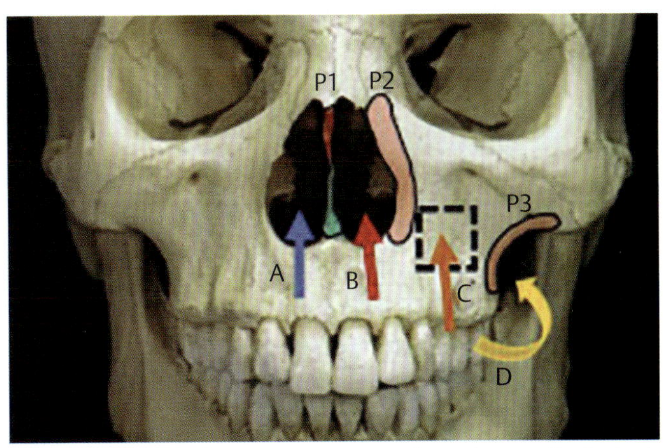

Fig. 26.9 Ports of access. A, contralateral nostril; B, ipsilateral nostril; C, antral window; D, incision in buccogingival sulcus next to last molar; P1, septum; P2, frontonasal process of maxilla; P3, lateral edge of the maxilla.

to insert a finger into the ITF although it could also be used to pass instruments. Dissection in the ITF is similar to the push-pull approach described earlier.

The maxillary artery is ligated. The infraorbital nerve is separated. This is done primarily using ports B and C. Once the tumor is separated from all its adhesions, it is pushed medially into the nasal cavity and delivered out. The access to the intraorbital and the intracranial parts of the tumor thus becomes easier. This technique allows for the maximum access to the angiofibroma while maintaining the anterior facial skeleton, thus ensuring complete removal with minimal morbidity to the patient.

Radiotherapy

Very few centers advocate radiation therapy as the primary modality of treatment today.[43] The authors believe that this is too radical an approach for benign tumors in a young patient, especially where an accepted alternative mode of treatment is available. The long-term complications of radiotherapy may be far worse than the disease itself such as growth retardation, panhypopituitarism, temporal lobe necrosis, cataracts, radiation keratitis, skin, thyroid, nasopharyngeal malignancies, and sarcomatous transformation of the tumor. Radiotherapy acts by arresting the growth of the tumor, and this stabilization takes 2 to 3 years. Although a reduction in the size of the tumor is seen, residual tumor persists. Radiation treatment should therefore be reserved for unresectable residual and recurrent tumors. A dose of 3,600 to 4,000 cGy in 14 to 26 fractions is given over 3 to 6 weeks. Modern techniques such as intensity-modulated radiation therapy should increase the efficacy and safety of this treatment. Targeted radiation with a gamma knife can be given for residual intracranial tumors. Long-term results on this therapy are awaited.

Medical Treatment

There is no consensus on a truly effective medical line of treatment for JNA. Medical treatment is mainly used prior to surgery to reduce the vascularity and the volume of the tumor. The response of the tumor to both androgens and estrogens has been demonstrated. They have also been used as adjunctive therapy in recurrent and inoperable tumors.[44,45] Antiandrogen drugs such as cyproterone acetate and flutamide have been used as they have a dual antiandrogenic effect of target organ inhibition and suppression of plasma testosterone. Hormonal therapy should be restricted only to tumors not resectable by surgery, as the administration of these drugs, particularly during puberty, can significantly interfere with psychophysical development of the patient.

Complications

The tumor itself may be associated with various complications such as severe hemorrhage, facial disfigurement, proptosis, diplopia, intracranial extension, and recurrence. Since the surgery is associated with various complications, excision of JNA should be attempted only by surgeons who have significant experience in endoscopic and open surgery. The surgery can lead to minor complications such as palatal perforation, paresthesia of the face, vestibular stenosis, nasal synechiae, and epiphora. More serious complications include hemorrhage from the tumor itself, the cavernous sinus or rarely the ICA, cranial nerve injuries, and dural tears with cerebrospinal fluid leaks.

Prognosis and Follow-Up

Various factors influence the long-term prognosis of these patients. A primary tumor has a better prognosis than a previously operated one. Recurrence rates of 55% in extensive tumors,[46,47] 25% in moderate size tumors,[48] and 15% in small tumors[49] have been quoted. However, in the authors' experience, the mere size of the tumor is not the only prognostic factor. The regions involved also play a major role in deciding the prognosis. Certain sites such as the foramen lacerum area are more difficult to approach, and there is a greater chance of recurrence if these areas are involved. A large intracranial component would naturally worsen the prognosis. A previous history of early recurrence with rapid regrowth of the tumor suggests an aggressive lesion. Very friable tumors and those with a significant residual postembolization blush are also difficult to manage.

Certain surgical factors also affect prognosis. A relatively bloodless surgery where all the extensions of the tumor have been dissected under direct vision and delivered en bloc has a good prognosis with a low chance of recurrence. Good preoperative planning to decide on a customized treatment plan in every individual case also goes a long way in improving the prognosis.

An immediate postoperative contrast-enhanced CT scan is done in all cases (**Fig. 26.10**). At the end of each surgery, the surgeon makes a note of whether the whole tumor was removed and recurrence is unlikely. In such a case, the patient is included in the low-risk category. These patients are followed up with a contrast-enhanced CT scan and nasal endoscopy once a year for the next 4 years, after which these patients are discharged from care. If the surgeon feels that the residual tumor has accidentally or intentionally been left behind and recurrence is likely, such patients are included in the high-risk category. These patients are followed up every

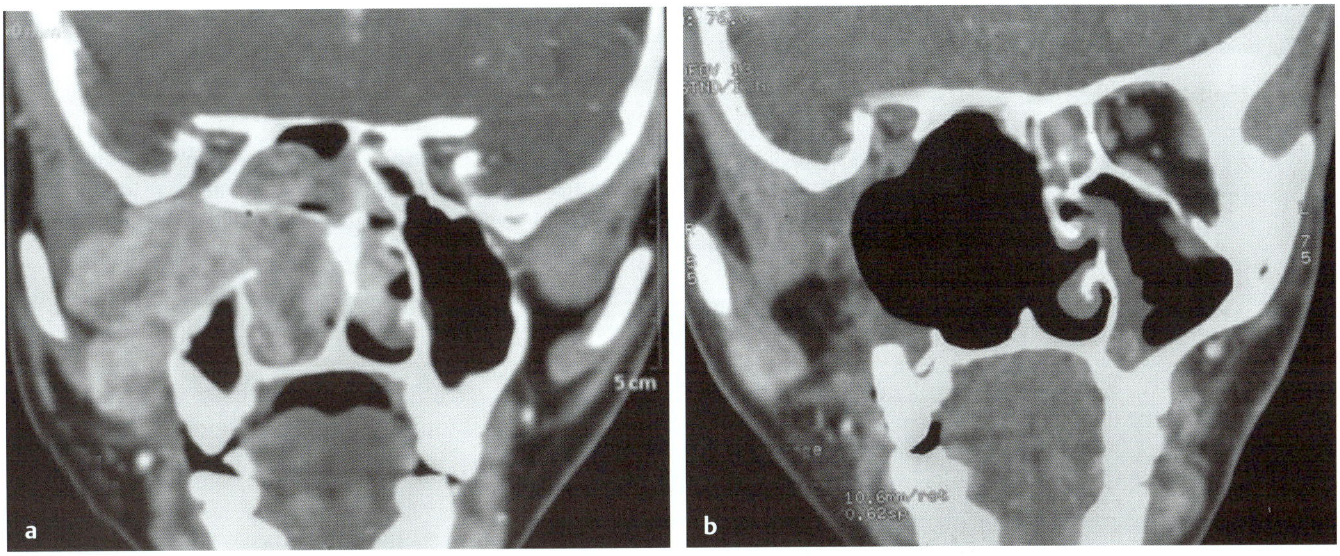

Fig. 26.10 **(a)** Preoperative CT scan of the patient showing tumor with its extensions. **(b)** Postoperative CT scan of the same patient after endoscopic excision showing complete removal of the tumor.

6 months with a contrast-enhanced CT scan and a nasal endoscopy for the next 4 years.

There is increasing evidence that endoscopic/endoscope-assisted open approaches have overcome many of the limitations of conventional approaches. Endoscopy allows meticulous subperiosteal dissection of tumor extensions under direct vision, thus minimizing the possibility of recurrence. Blood loss is minimum, thereby requiring fewer transfusions. Tight nasal packs are not necessary, and hence, postoperative morbidity is significantly decreased. There is no facial disfigurement. It lessens the duration of hospital stay, and endoscopic monitoring on the follow-up of the patients is possible.

In conclusion, endoscopic excision of JNA is a technically challenging surgery which should be undertaken only after the surgeon has had considerable experience in endoscopic surgery.

References

1. Sivanandan R, Fee Jr WE. Benign and malignant tumors of the nasopharynx. In: Cummings CW, Flint PW, Harker LA, et al, eds. Cummings Otolaryngology Head and Neck Surgery. 4th ed. New York, NY: Elsevier, Mosby; 2005:1669–1972
2. Batsakis JG. Tumors of the head and neck: clinical and pathological considerations. 2nd ed. Baltimore, MD: Williams & Wilkins; 1979:296–300
3. Bensch H, Ewing J. Neoplastic disease. 4th ed. Philadelphia, PA: Saunders and Co.; 1941.
4. Chaikovski VK. Angiofibroma of the nose in a 14-day-old infant girl. Zh UshnNos Gorl Bolezn 1967;27(5):103–104
5. Fu YS, Perzin KH. Non-epithelial tumors of the nasal cavity, paranasal sinuses, and nasopharynx: a clinicopathologic study. I. General features and vascular tumors. Cancer 1974;33(5):1275–1288
6. Handousa, Farid H, Elwi AM. Nasopharyngeal fibroma: a clinico-pathological study of seventy cases. J Laryngol Otol 1954;68(10):647–666
7. Friedberg SA. Vascular fibroma of the nasopharynx (nasopharyngeal fibroma). Arch Otolaryngol 1940;31:313–326
8. Neel HB 3rd, Whicker JH, Devine KD, Weiland LH. Juvenile angiofibroma. Review of 120 cases. Am J Surg 1973; 126(4): 547–576
9. Nelatori M. Polypefibreux de la base du crane considerations generals. Gaz Hop 1853;26:22
10. Verneuil V. Seances de la SocieteChirurgie de Paris pendant l'annee. Bull Soc Chir 1861
11. Tillaux P. Traité d'anatomie topographique avec applications à la chirurgie. edition 2. Paris P Asselin 1878:348–349
12. Martin H, Ehrlich HE, Abels JC. Juvenile nasopharyngeal angiofibroma. Ann Surg 1948;127(3):513–536
13. Dane WH. Juvenile nasopharyngeal angiofibroma in state of regression. Ann Otol Rhinol Laryngol 1954;63:997–1014
14. Brunner H. Nasopharyngeal fibroma. Ann Otol Rhinol Laryngol 1942;51:30–65
15. Osborn DA. The so-called juvenile angiofibroma of nasopharynx. Journal of Laryngology and Otology 1959;73: 295–295
16. Schiff M. Juvenile nasopharyngeal angiofibroma. Laryngoscope 1959;908–1016

17. Maurice M, Milad M. Pathogenesis of juvenile nasopharyngeal angiofibroma. Braz J Otorhinolaryngol 1981;95:1121–1126
18. Girgis IH, Fahmy SA. Nasopharyngeal fibroma: its histopathological nature. J Laryngol Otol 1973;87:1107–1123
19. Liu ZF, Wang DH, Sun XC, Wang JJ, Hu L, Li H, Dai P. The site of origin and expansive routes of juvenile nasopharyngeal angiofibroma (JNA). Int J Pediatr Otorhinolaryngol 2011;75: 1088–1092
20. Ferrara N, Houck K, Jakeman L, Leung DW. Molecular and biological properties of the vascular endothelial growth factor family of proteins. Endocr Rev 1992;13(1):18–32
21. Coutinho-Camilfo CM, Brentani MM, Butugan O, et al. Relaxation of imprinting of IGF II gene in juvenile nasopharyngeal angiofibromas. Diagn Mol Pathol 2003;12:57–62
22. Nagai MA, Butugan O, Logullo A, Brentani MM. Expression of growth factors, proto-oncogenes, and p53 in nasopharyngeal angiofibromas. Laryngoscope 1996; 106(2 Pt 1): 190–195
23. Ferouz AS, Mohr RM, Paul P. Juvenile nasopharyngeal angiofibroma and familial adenomatous polyposis: an association? Otolaryngol Head Neck Surg 1995;113: 435–439
24. Giardiello FM, Hamilton SR, Krush AJ, Offerhaus JA, Booker SV, Petersen GM. Nasopharyngeal angiofibroma in patients with familial adenomatous polyposis. Gastroenterology 1993; 105:1550–1552
25. Abraham SC, Montgomery EA, Giardiello FM, Wu TT. Frequent β-catenin mutations in juvenile nasopharyngeal angiofibromas. Am J Pathol 2001;158:1073–1078
26. Schick B, Rippel C, Brunner C, Jung V, Plinkert PK, Urbschat S. Numerical sex chromosome aberrations in juvenile angiofibromas genetic evidence for an androgen-dependent tumor? Oncol Rep 2003;10(5):1251–1255
27. Capodiferro S, Favia G, Lacaita MG, Muzio LL, Maiorano E. Juvenile angiofibroma: report of a case with primary intraoral presentation. Oral Oncol Extra 2005;41:1–6
28. Antoniades K, Antoniades DZ, Antoniades V. Juvenile angiofibroma report of a case with intraoral presentation. Oral Surg Oral Med Oral Pathol Oral Radiol Endod 2002;94(2):228–232
29. Handa KK, Kumar A, Singh MK, Chhabra AH. Extra nasopharyngeal angiofibroma arising from the nasal septum. Int J Pediatr Otorhinolaryngol 2001;58(2):163–166
30. Huang RY, Damrose EJ, Blackwell KE, Cohen AN, Calcaterra TC. Extranasopharyngeal angiofibroma. Int J Pediatr Otorhinolaryngol 2000;56(1):59–64
31. Neel HB, Whicker JH, Devine KD, Weiland JH. Juvenile angiofibroma review of 120 cases. Am J Surg 1973;126:547–558
32. Stansbie JM, Phelps PD. Involution of residual juvenile nasopharyngeal angiofibroma (a case report). J Laryngol Otol 1986;100(5):599–603
33. Andrews JC, Fisch U, Valavanis A, Aeppli U, Makek MS. The surgical management of extensive nasopharyngeal angiofibromas with the infratemporal fossa approach. Laryngoscope 1989;99(4):429–437
34. Radkowski D, McGill T, Healy GB, Ohlms L, Jones DT. Angiofibroma. Changes in staging and treatment. Arch Otolaryngol Head Neck Surg 1996;122(2):122–129
35. Snyderman CH, Pant H, Carrau RL, Gardner PA. New endoscopic staging system for angiofibromas. Arch Otolaryngol Head Neck Surg 2010;136(6):588–594
36. Janakiram TN, Sharma SB, Kasper E, Deshmukh O, Cherian I. Comprehensive preoperative staging system for endoscopic single and multicorridor approaches to juvenile nasal angiofibromas. Surg Neurol Int 2017;8:55
37. Wilson CP. Observations on the surgery of the nasopharynx. Ann Otol Rhinol Laryngol 1957;66(1):5–40
38. Casson PR, Bonanno PC, Converse JM. The midface degloving procedure. Plast Reconstr Surg 1974;53(1):102–103
39. Conley J, Price JC. Sublabial approach to the nasal and nasopharyngeal cavities. Am J Surg 1979;138(4):615–618
40. Kamel RH. Transnasal endoscopic surgery in juvenile nasopharyngeal angiofibroma. J Laryngol Otol 1996;110(10): 962–968
41. Bradoo RA, Joshi AA, Pahtan FA, Kalel KP. The push-pull technique in the management of giant JNAs. Bombay Hosp J 2008; 50(2):220
42. Bradoo R, Joshi A, Shah K, Patel T, Lohiya T. The four-port Bradoo technique: an alternative to the modified endoscopic Denker's approach for giant JNA. Indian J Otolaryngol Head Neck Surg 2017;69(3):277–281
43. Briant TD, Fitzpatrick PJ, Book H. The radiological treatment of juvenile nasopharyngeal angiofibromas. Ann Otol Rhinol Laryngol 1970;79(6):1108–1113
44. Martin H, Ehrlich HE, Abels JC. Juvenile Nasopharyngeal Angiofibroma. Ann Surg 1948 Mar;127(3):513–536
45. Patterson CN. Juvenile nasopharyngeal angiofibroma. Otolaryngol Clin North Am 1973;6(3):839–861
46. Economou TS, Abemayor E, Ward PH. Juvenile nasopharyngeal angiofibroma: an update of the UCLA experience, 1960-1985. Laryngoscope 1988;98(2):170–175
47. McCombe A, Lund VJ, Howard DJ. Recurrence in juvenile angiofibroma. Rhinology 1990;28(2):97–102
48. Roger G, Tran Ba Huy P, Froehlich P, et al. Exclusively endoscopic removal of juvenile nasopharyngeal angiofibroma trends and limits. Arch Otolaryngol Head Neck Surg 2002;128(8): 928–935
49. Scholtz AW, Appenroth E, Kammen-Jolly K, Scholtz LU, Thumfart WF. Juvenile nasopharyngeal angiofibroma management and therapy. Laryngoscope 2001;111(4 Pt 1): 681–687

Section IX

Petrous Region

Chapter 27

Pathologies of the Petrous Apex

Eugene Hung Chih Wong, Revadi Govindaraju, Michel Roethlisberger, and Prepageran Narayanan

Introduction

The diagnosis and management of petrous apex lesions represent a challenging subset of pathologies due to their anatomical location at the medial most aspect of the temporal bone with close proximity to critical local neurovascular structures. Therefore, it is important to strike a balance between the risks and benefits of aggressive management of petrous apex lesions.[3] A good understanding of the natural history of common differential diagnosis located in this anatomical region is essential to establish realistic therapeutic goals.[3]

Anatomy

The lateral skull base comprises the petrous part of the temporal bone and the adjacent bones of the middle and posterior cranial fossa.[4] The apex of this bone forms the anterior foramen lacerum.[4]

The petrous apex forms the medial most part of the temporal bone[2] and is described as a pyramid with an anteromedial apex, bordered anteriorly by the foramen lacerum and posteriorly by the inferior petrosal sinus, and a posterolateral base, formed by the otic capsule[5]; **Fig. 27.1**).

The superior surface of the petrous apex is formed by the floor of the middle fossa, extending from the arcuate eminence to the Meckel's cave.[2] The inferior border is formed by the jugular fossa, vertical petrous carotid canal, and the inferior petrosal sinus.[2]

The posterior surface of the petrous bone extends from the endolymphatic duct operculum to the clivus.[2] The lateral surface of the petrous apex is formed by the otic capsule, the petrous internal carotid artery (peICA), and the semicanal of the tensor tympani muscle.[2]

The superior petrosal sinus defines the border between the middle and posterior fossa surface of the petrous apex, while the internal auditory canal divides the petrous apex into anterior and posterior segments.[2]

The ICA traverses the petrous apex and exits the petrous bone through the anterior foramen lacerum, where it curves superiorly to the cavernous sinus.[4] Lesions in the petrous apex potentially involve the ICA in this anatomical region[4] and affect critical adjacent structures such as the brainstem, temporal lobe, and multiple cranial nerves.[3]

Pathologies and Their Variants

The commonest entity identified on petrous apex imaging is asymmetric pneumatization.[2] The commonest lesion in the petrous apex is the cholesterol granuloma (CG),[1,2] representing up to 40% of all benign lesions within this region[6] with an estimated incidence of 0.6 cases per 1 million population,[7] and being 10 times more common than petrous

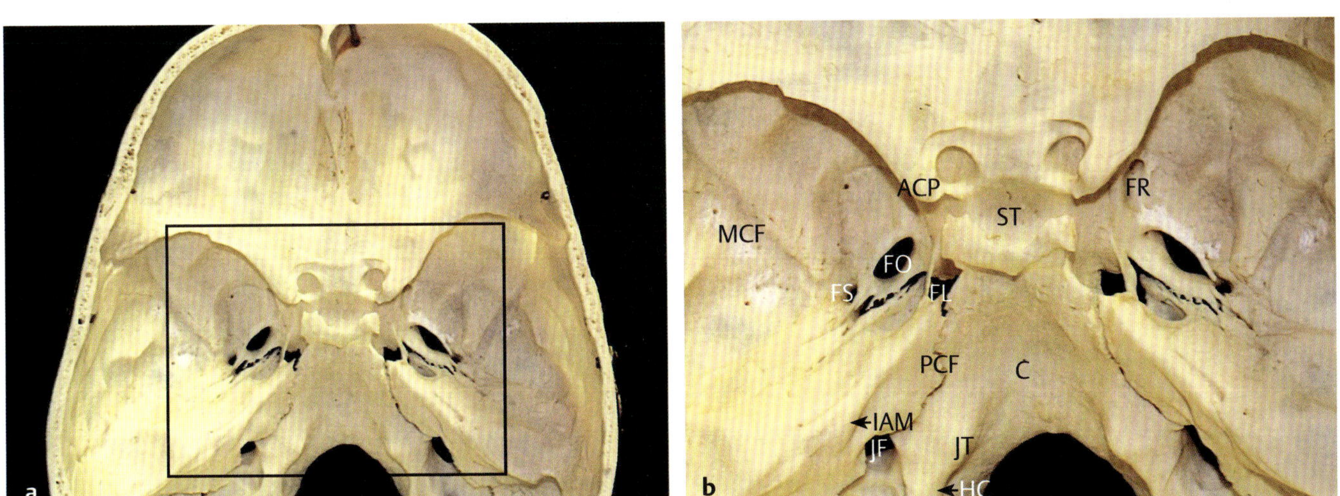

Fig. 27.1 **(a)** Superior view of the skull base of a dry bone specimen and **(b)** an enlarged view of the region of petrous apex and related anatomy.

apex cholesteatomas.[8] Other common pathologies include mucocele, epidermoid or cholesteatoma, and benign or malignant tumors[9] such as meningioma, neuroma, chemodectoma, sarcoma, chordoma, and metastatic lesions.[10]

Petrous apex lesions can also be divided into cystic and solid types. The commonest cystic lesion is CG, followed by cholesteatoma, whereas the commonest solid lesion is chondrosarcoma.[6]

Cholesterol Granuloma of the Petrous Apex

CGs of the petrous apex are expansile cystic lesions containing thick, brown mucoid fluid and cholesterol crystals surrounded by foreign body giant cells, chronic inflammation, and fibrous tissue reaction.[11,12] They are benign, slow-growing[13] lesions that can remain radiographically and clinically stable for an average of 46 months.[3] Two theories for the origin of CG in petrous apex were described. The first theory, the so-called "obstruction-vacuum" theory," postulates that mucosal swelling and gas resorption causes negative pressure and hemorrhage into the temporal bone air cells, resulting in formation of the CG.[14,15] A more recent theory describes over pneumatization of the temporal bone causing coaptation of the marrow and mucosa with a tendency for hemorrhage and clot formation, leading to obstruction of the petrous apex outflow tract.[16] The degradation of hemosiderin and cholesterol leads to an inflammatory granulomatous reaction.[16] Either way, CG contain cholesterol crystals due to anaerobic degradation of blood, which triggers an inflammatory reaction mediated by foreign body giant cells.[17]

Clinical Features

Since lesions in the petrous apex are not accessible to direct clinical detection, a high index of suspicion based on recognition of early signs and symptoms of an expanding tumorous mass is essential.[18]

Petrous apex CG may be asymptomatic when small and are often found incidentally on radiography for unrelated symptoms.[2,9,13] These benign lesions remain stable[3] or present with a varying degree of compressive symptoms depending on the lesion's extent.[19] The commonest presenting features are hearing loss and vestibular symptoms,[4,20,21] followed by tinnitus, headache, facial twitching, facial paresthesia, diplopia, and facial weakness.[2,4,13,20,21]

The majority of these symptoms are directly related to the pressure on one or multiple cranial nerves, including cranial nerves V, VI, VII, or VIII.[2,4] One common clinical feature is pain, paresthesia, or anesthesia mediated by compression or irritation of the ipsilateral mandibular division (V3) of the trigeminal nerve. This phenomenon is observed in about 20% of patients with CG[20] and is most likely caused by a compression of the branch in the foramen ovale,[18] or through irritation of the cisternal segment of the Gasserian ganglion.[20] Patient may also have a rare initial presentation of isolated remitting relapsing sixth nerve palsy with painless unilateral diplopia.[13]

Facial spasm or weakness can be present in up to 20% of patients with petrous apex CG due to an irritation or compression of the facial nerve in the internal auditory canal, cerebellopontine angle, or the fallopian canal.[20] Ear fullness, sensorineural hearing loss, tinnitus, and dizziness can result from compression of the eighth cranial nerve or erosion into the otic capsule due to involvement of the internal auditory canal or the lateral extension of petrous apex CG.[20] However, unilateral hearing loss can also be caused by arterial compression with transient ischemia or mediated by toxins produced by the CG.[22]

Patients may present with severe headache centered around the ipsilateral ear, which usually does not resolve with medication.[18] This may be caused by dural stretching of an expanding tumor in the petrous apex[4,18] or secondary to muscle tension or migraine that is unrelated to the lesion.[2]

Patients can also present with a varying degree of eustachian tube occlusion or compression causing otitis media with effusion and conductive hearing loss.[4,18] Symptoms from direct ICA compression including blurring of vision on head turning and dizziness have also been described.[18] Extensive tumors of the petrous apex can potentially cause multiple cranial nerve palsies when involving the base of skull, in particular, the jugular foramen (cranial nerves IX, X, XI) and hypoglossal foramen (cranial nerve XII)[18] causing dysphagia, hoarseness, and pain or weakness.[2]

The majority of patients experience more than one symptom, with some of them being very nonspecific and nonregular such as ear pressure, facial paralysis, and epileptic attacks.[4] Rapid growth of the lesion leading to carotid artery injury, cyst rupture, and sudden neurological injury is very uncommon.[3]

Radiological Features

Accurate preoperative diagnosis of petrous apex lesions is important to guide the surgeon's decision when selecting the correct approach.[8] Historically, conventional X-rays of the petrous bone and skull base were used showing evidence of osteolytic lesion of the petrous apex. However, the lesions are frequently too small to be detected with this imaging modality.[18]

Petrous apex lesions can be accurately diagnosed using computed tomography (CT) and magnetic resonance imaging (MRI) scans.[6] The accuracy of the diagnosis of primary petrous apex lesions is improved when used in conjunction with each other, e.g. CT with contrast and MRI with or without gadolinium contrast enhancement.[8]

CT scans can provide detailed information on the osseous anatomy of the skull base, which includes the otic capsule, carotid canal, jugular foramen, fallopian canal, semicanal of the tensor tympani muscle, eustachian tube, and other skull base foramina.[2] CT scans also delineate the petrous apex lesions in relation to adjacent structures within the temporal bone and potentially detect intralesional calcifications, which can be useful in narrowing down the differential diagnosis.[2] It is also important to assess the degree of erosion and expansion of the lesion as well as the presence of rim enhancement on CT scan.[23] This information is helpful when deciding on the surgical approach to access lesions of the petrous apex.[2] Furthermore, CT scans can be used to follow up asymptomatic patients and to monitor recurrence or progression in patients that underwent surgical resection of CGs.[2]

CG usually appears nonenhancing, expansile, sharply marginated, and sometimes erosive with consecutive loss of internal bony septations on CT scan.[4,24,25] CG have attenuation values similar to the brain (isodense).[4,10] On the other hand, cholesteatomas have lower attenuation values (isodense with cerebrospinal fluid [CSF] rather than brain).[10] In cases where a CG has eroded into the carotid canal or jugular foramen causing vascular compression, CT angiography or venography may be required to gather more information on the distorted vascular anatomy prior to surgery.[2]

MRI scans can help to significantly narrow the differential diagnosis of petrous apex lesions, obviating the need for tissue biopsies to establish a diagnosis in most cases. MRI is also frequently used to follow-up asymptomatic patients or to monitor disease progression.[2]

Petrous apex CG present themselves as hyperintense in both T1- and T2-weighted MRI imaging whereas most other petrous apex lesions do not follow this pattern.[24] Fragments of bone and solid material within a CG often appear as heterogenous on MRI.[2] MRI is also better in illustrating any extraosseous extension of CG.[2]

The radiological differential diagnosis for CG of the petrous apex includes petrous apex marrow, petrous apex effusion, mucocele, cholesteatoma, arachnoid cyst, cephalocele, and petrous apicitis.[11] **Table 27.1** illustrates the radiological features of various common lesions in the petrous apex region. It is important to note that asymmetric pneumatization and retained secretions can provide a false-positive diagnosis of lesions in the petrous apex.[6]

Table 27.1 Radiological features of different common lesions in the petrous apex[2,3,11]

Diagnosis	CT	MRI (Intensity)			
		T1	T2	FLAIR	DWI
Cholesterol granuloma	• Expansile • Nonenhancing • Erosion (smooth)	High	High	High	Low
Marrow	• Nonexpansile • Nonenhancing	Iso (to fat)	Iso (to fat)	-	Low
Effusion	• Nonexpansile • Nonenhancing • No erosion	Low	High	High	Low
Mucocele	• Expansile • Nonenhancing • Erosion (destruction of septations)	Low to intermediate	High	High	High
Cholesteatoma	• Expansile • Nonenhancing • Bony erosion	Low	High	High	Low
Arachnoid cyst	• Nonenhancing	Low	High	Low	Low
Cephalocele/CSF cyst	• Nonenhancing • Bony erosion (smooth)	Low	High	Low	High
Petrous apicitis	• Enhancing • Bony erosion (irregular)	Low	High	-	-

Abbreviations: cerebrospinal fluid (CSF); computed tomography (CT); diffusion-weighted imaging (DWI); fluid-attenuated inversion recovery (FLAIR).

Note: This list is not exhaustive.

Key Principles of Surgery

Based on the topo-anatomical relationships of the petrous apex, complete removal of lesions in this area is rarely possible.[18] Hence, lesions in this area always represent a challenge for surgeons to navigate around critical structures such as the internal auditory canal, facial nerve, and ICA.[2] One of the advantages of surgical excision is the potential reduction of disease recurrence, however, this is associated with an increased risk of postoperative seizure, intracranial hemorrhage, and CSF leakage.[2] On the other hand, marsupialization does not require craniotomy and can allow decompression of the expanding symptomatic lesion;[2] therefore, surgical exploration usually aims at diagnostic exploration with biopsy and fistulation of the expanding mass.[18]

The petrous apex region can be approached either via a transcranial route such as the middle fossa, transmastoid, infracochlear, infralabyrinthine, translabyrinthine, infratemporal fossa approach, or via endoscopic endonasal techniques.[9,26] The choice of surgical approach needs to be balanced between the ease of access to this complex anatomical area, the surgeon's experience, the need to preserve functions, as well as achieving complete resection of the lesion while minimizing complications.

Transcranial Approaches

Many of the transcranial approaches involve lateral skull base surgery which exposes delicate auditory structures to damage, with hearing loss being one of the common complications.[27]

Middle Fossa Extradural Approach

The petrous apex is approached via the middle cranial fossa.[18] This approach is usually used in patients with good hearing ability,[4] and it allows diagnostic biopsy of solid tissue mass and aspiration of any cystic lesion such as CGs and epidermoid cysts.[18] The labyrinthine function can also be preserved.[18]

CGs can be marsupialized via this approach with drainage catheters inserted from the cyst into the mastoid,[2] although maintenance of a permanent fistulization is often challenging,[18] and resulting in disease progression.[2] An alternative method of drainage by drilling a tract between the petrous apex CG into the anterior epitympanic space above the tensor tympani muscle has also been described.[28]

Hearing Preservation in Transtemporal Approaches

The infra- or subcochlear approach is performed via a postauricular transcanal exposure, where a tympanomeatal flap is elevated, followed by lowering of the medial inferior tympanic bone along with the osseous annulus to the level of the floor of the hypotympanum.[2,29] The key landmarks within the medial wall of the meso- and hypotympanum are the osseous wall of the inferior basal turn of the cochlea the jugular bulb, and the petrous carotid artery.[2]

More medially located CG need extensive drilling, which may be limited by the presence of a large jugular bulb or a posteriorly positioned petrous carotid artery.[2] Occasionally, larger or more laterally based CGs extend to the lateral aspect of the infracochlear tract and can hence be exteriorized readily into the middle ear without extensive bone removal.[2] Therefore, a wide opening of the CG wall is created to reduce postoperative obstruction.[29]

The transcanal endoscopic infracochlear technique provides a minimally invasive approach via the ear canal with a wide superiorly based tympanomeatal flap, where the limits of dissection are the petrous carotid artery, the jugular bulb and inferior cochlear turn.[2] This approach provides a wide-angle view, allowing surgeons to see inside the CG itself to remove any loculations, with reduced intraoperative bleeding and less postoperative pain.[30] However, this technique uses one hand for instrumentation and is associated with loss of depth of the field perception and difficulty in hemostasis control.[30]

The infralabyrinthine approach uses a postauricular transmastoid exposure where a complete mastoidectomy is performed and the posterior semicircular canal, the sigmoid sinus, the jugular bulb and the vertical facial nerve are identified.[2] The CG is then marsupialized with a wide opening within the wall to reduce the risk of tract obstruction.[2]

The subarcuate, sinodural angle and supracochlear approaches are usually reserved for the management of acute petrositis due to their narrow access to the petrous apex,[5] where a postauricular transmastoid exposure is used.[2]

Nonhearing Preservation in Transtemporal Approach

The translabyrinthine approach to the petrous apex involves a wide-field mastoidectomy with the removal of the cochlea and the vestibular labyrinth. This creates a wide bony fistula into the petrous apex via exenteration of bone from the carotid canal anteriorly to the descending facial nerve posteriorly, and from the middle cranial fossa superiorly to the jugular bulb inferiorly.[18] This approach allows for a complete evacuation of the lesion or a diagnostic biopsy of solid tissue.[18] The bony fistula can then be lined with split-thickness skin grafts, followed by 10 to 14 days of packing to hold the skin graft in place.[18]

However, this method causes loss of labyrinthine function[18] and is usually reserved for patients with preoperative absent or severe hearing loss.[4,31] Some authors have reported preservation and even improvement or partial restoration of hearing when a partial labyrinthectomy was performed. The hypothesis behind this phenomenon might be potential reversal of neurovascular compression and elimination of toxins produced by the CG.[22]

This approach usually requires the obliteration of the eustachian tube due to a high frequency of CSF leakage during cochlectomy.[2]

Endonasal Endoscopic Approach

Over the past years, the endonasal endoscopic approach has gained popularity due to improved surgical instrumenation and a broader availability of intraoperative image guidance[1] especially for CG, where a drainage path into the sphenoid sinus can be established.[32]

There are three ways to access the petrous apex endoscopically:

Transsphenoidal Transclival Approach[33]

This approach involves an initial wide bilateral sphenoidectomy, followed by a posterior nasal septectomy using backbiting rongeurs to fully expose the sphenoid rostrum. A wide sphenoidotomy with removal of the rostrum and sphenoid sinus septations is then performed. Important landmarks to be identified are the planum sphenoidale, the sella turcica, the carotid eminences, the optic canal, the medial and the lateral optic-carotid recess, the clival recess, and the paraclival ICAs. The sphenoid floor is then drilled back to the clival recess, followed by a subsequent transclival approach, where the bone between the paraclival ICAs is thinned out to fully expose the clival dura. (**Fig. 27.2a–c**).

Transsphenoidal Transclival Approach with Internal Carotid Artery Lateralization[33]

The second way to access the petrous apex is through an extension of the transclival approach, where the bone covering the paraclival ICA is removed from its medial to its lateral surface to allow the vessel to be gently mobilized laterally. This is followed by removal of the bone posterior to the paraclival ICA to gain access to the petroclival fissure and the most medial aspect of the petrous apex. To maximize the surgical access to the superior petrous apex, the petrous bone between the paraclival ICA and the inferior petrosal sinus is removed as well. During these steps, the sixth cranial nerve (abducent nerve) coursing superiorly along its petrous segment is at risk of injury. (**Fig. 27.2d, e**).

Transpterygoid Infrapetrous or Sublacerum Approach[33]

The initial step of this approach is a maxillary antrostomy followed by removal of the posterior wall of the maxillary sinus to expose the pterygopalatine fossa. Medially, the palatosphenoidal (palatovaginal) artery (a terminal branch

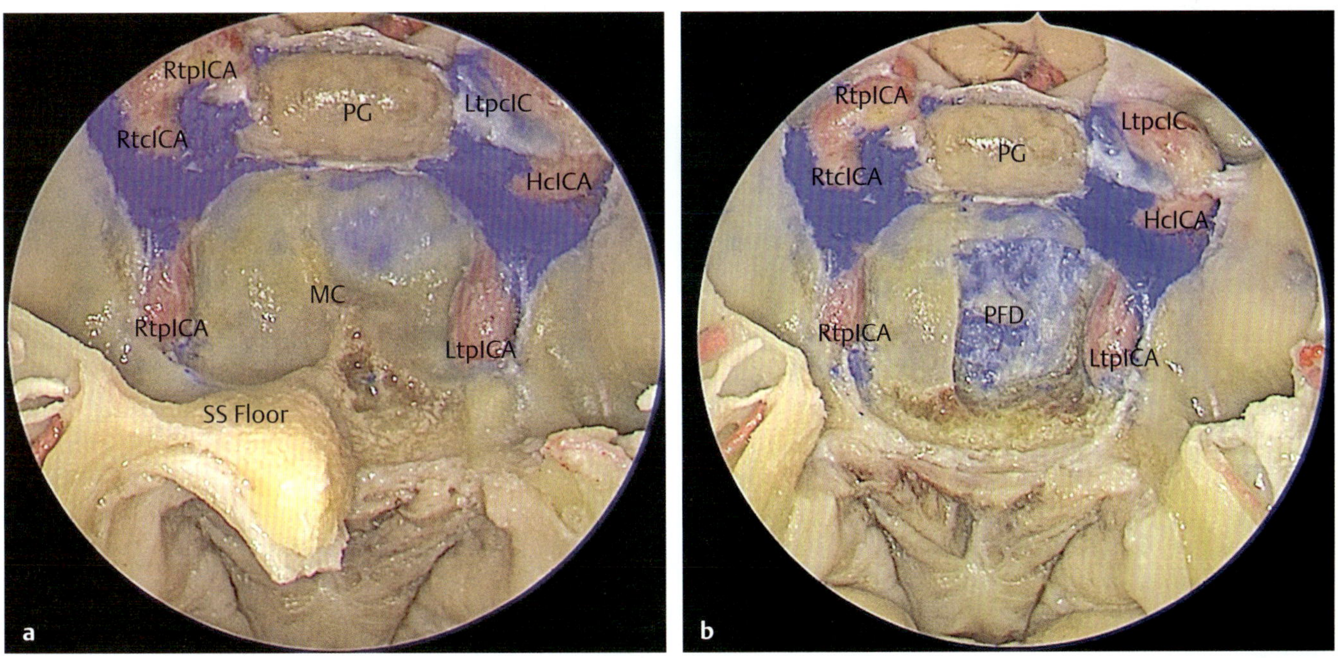

Fig. 27.2 **(a)** Endoscopic endonasal view after a wide sphenoidectomy and removal of the floor of sphenoid sinus on the left side in a cadaveric specimen. The ICA and pituitary gland have been exposed to demonstrate the anatomy. **(b)** Complete removal of the sphenoid sinus floor and midclivus on the left side. *(Continued)*

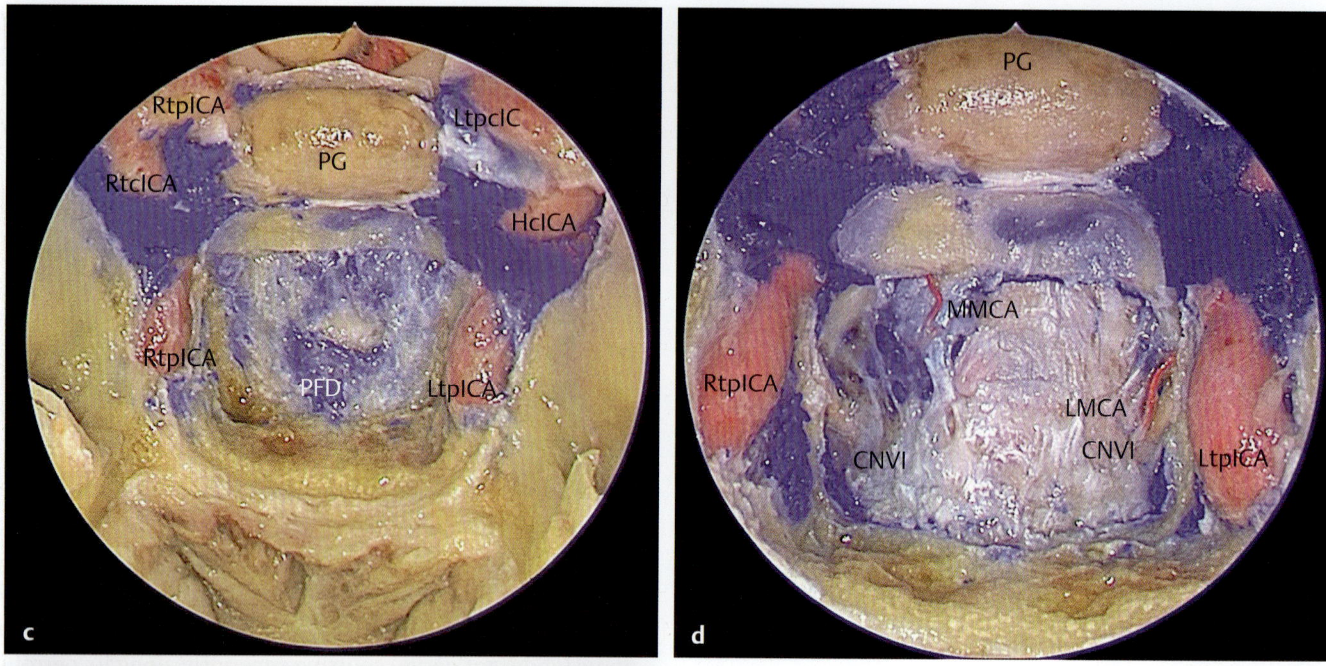

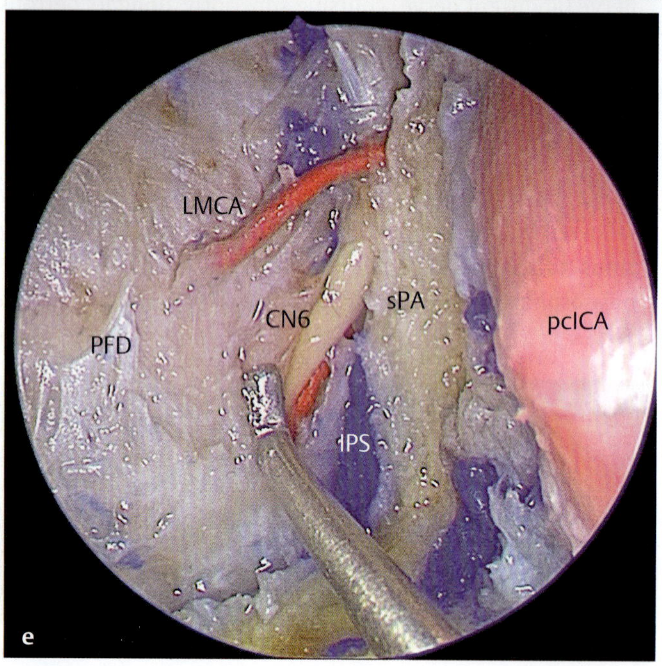

Fig. 27.2 *(Continued)* **(c)** The periosteal layer of the posterior fossa dura (PFD) is exposed after the complete removal of the midclivus bone. **(d)** With the removal of the periosteal layer and the basilar plexus in between, the meningeal layer of the posterior fossa dura is exposed together with the sixth cranial nerve, or abducent nerve (CN6), within the Dorello canal. **(e)** A close-up view of the sixth cranial nerve (CNVI) and the Dorello canal and the superior petrous apex (spA) region. The arterial supply of the Dorello's canal is provided by the meningeal branches of the meningohypophyseal artery, arising from the posterior bend of the cavernous ICA. These meningeal branches can be divided into a medial meningeal clival artery (MMCA) and a lateral meningeal clival artery (LMCA).

of maxillary artery) can be transected with lateral mobilization of the soft tissues in the pterygopalatine fossa to facilitate identification of the vidian nerve.[34] The pterygoid base is then drilled out to reach the foramen lacerum soft tissue and the anterior genu of the ICA eventually.[34] The sublacerum route into the anterior-inferior petrous apex is completed with the transsection of the foramen lacerum soft tissue and drilling of the bone between the horizontal petrous ICA and the eustachian tube (**Fig. 27.3a–e**).

Epidermoid cysts of the petrous apex region can be drained via the ethmoid or the sphenoid sinus[18] due to their close relationship to the posterior wall of the sphenoid sinus.[4] However, since CGs lack an epithelial lining, the aim of surgery is not to remove the entire cyst.[35] It is therefore crucial to drain the lesion and aerate the air cells,[36,37] as well as to maintain a permanent outflow drainage pathway to prevent symptom recurrence.[11] Long-term success of treatment relies on the maintenance of the drainage to prevent the expansion of the cyst, and on a gradual reduction of the cavity size when fibrosis and neoosteogenesis occur.[11] Stent placement after drainage may prolong the drainage patency and reduce the likelihood of symptomatic recurrence.[11]

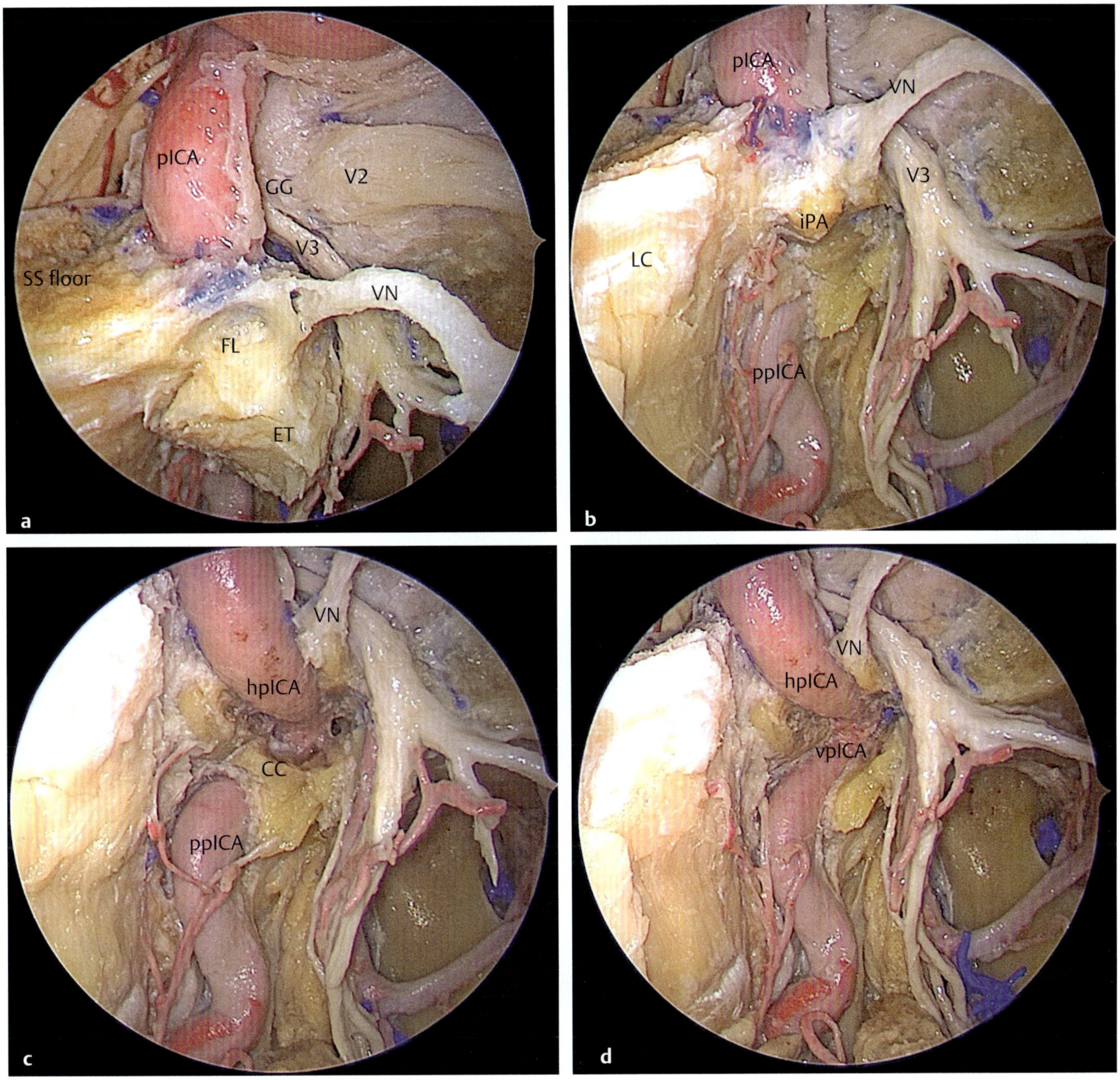

Fig. 27.3 Endonasal endoscopic cadaveric dissection for an inferior petrous approach demonstrating important anatomical landmarks. **(a)** The transpterygoid access has been gained and the eustachian tube has been partially transected. The gasserian ganglion and trigeminal nerve branches are seen lateral to the paraclival ICA. **(b)** The soft tissues of the foramen lacerum have been removed to expose the inferior part of the petrous bone. **(c)** Removal of the inferior petrous bone reveals the horizontal petrous segment of ICA. **(d)** Further removal of carotid canal bone exposes the vertical petrous segment of ICA. *(Continued)*

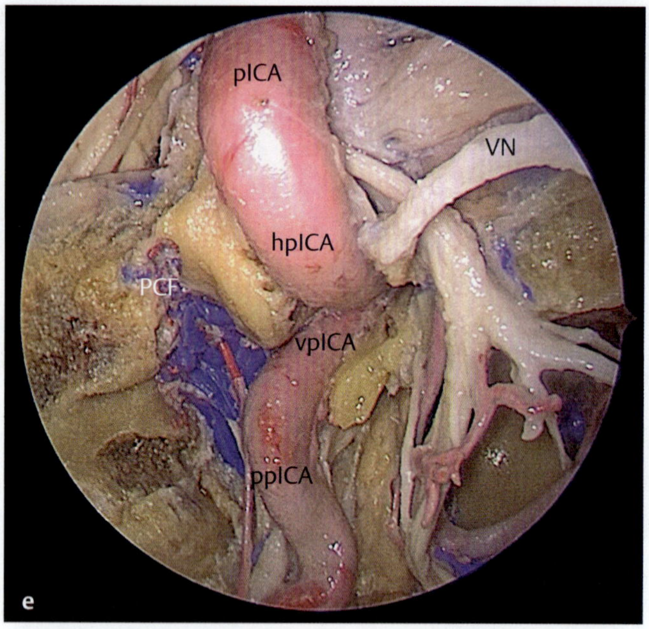

Fig. 27.3 *(Continued)* **(e)** The lower clivus has partially been drilled out to show the petroclival fissure and its relation with the ICA and the petrous apex.

Many advantages of the endonasal endoscopic approach have been mentioned in the literature. The endoscope extends the surgeon's view, allowing for anterior access as far as the sphenoid and an inferior access as far as the atlas. The endoscope also facilitates the identification of neurovascular structures and is allows for a better confirmation of complete resection when placed several millimeters away from the site of resection.[38,39] The superior vision provided by the endoscope further helps to prevent the risk of injury to the vertical segment of the ICA and the facial nerve, with a better functional outcome.[40] Moreover, the endonasal endoscopic approach is less invasive and has the potential to preserve patient's hearing[22] or even totally restore auditory function.[35] Several authors have reported reduced operating time, reduced risk to structural and nerve damage, faster recovery, shorter hospital stay, and better cosmetic outcome using the endonasal endoscopic approach.[17,41,42] They have also reported easier clinical follow-up using a fiberscope, where the cyst can be redrained on-site if necessary.[31]

However, the endonasal endoscopic approach has its limitations in accessing the petrous apex when lesions involve the brainstem and the anterior vertical segment of the ICA, or if a poor sphenoid pneumatization is present.[33] It may also be challenging to maintain a permanent fistula or to evacuate a keratin-filled mass through the nasal cavity, in addition to a higher risk of ascending infections from contaminated areas such as the nasopharynx.[18] Another well-known limitation with the use of endoscope is the provided monocular vision with less information on depth. However, dynamic vision (movement of the endoscope) can provide a more precise depth perception.[40]

In cases of large petrous apex lesions, a combined endoscopic and microscopic approach can be used to compensate the limitations provided by each of both techniques.[40] Complex cases can also be optimized by surgical planning using augmented reality and three-dimensional (3D)-printed anatomical simulation with concurrent navigation, however, further studies are warranted to prove the efficacy on the patient's safety and outcome.[43]

Preoperative Work-up

All patients with complex skull base pathology should have a complete history and physical examination as part of their initial evaluation.[2] It is also essential to have a thorough examination of the cranial nerves, focusing especially on ocular motility, facial sensation, facial function, hearing, and balance.[2]

Otological examination should include otoscopy to look for the middle ear effusion or retrotympanic mass and tuning fork to rule out conductive or sensorineural hearing loss.[2] Pure tone and speech audiometry can help provide objective information on the extent of middle ear and eighth nerve involvement and is important to help in selecting the correct surgical approach for the excision of petrous apex lesions.[2] On the other hand, a head impulse test is useful to assess vestibular deficit involving the lateral semicircular canal.[2]

Postoperative Care

Routine postoperative care such as monitoring of vital signs, wound sites as well as screening for any signs of bleeding and infection should be part of the postoperative care. Clinical examination to look for any cranial nerve dysfunctions including facial nerve and vestibulocochlear nerve should also be carried out postoperatively.

Patients should undergo hearing assessment after surgery to check for resolution or improvement of symptoms and to rule out any worsening of hearing. Postoperative CT and MRI scans can also be performed at 1 year postoperatively if there is no recurrence of symptoms.[4]

Indications and Contraindications

For petrous apex CG, asymptomatic patients are usually managed with observation and serial annual imaging.[2,3,44,45]

Studies have shown an immediate[46] and long-term[20] persistence of symptoms after surgical excision in patients with headaches and dizziness, which were not clearly related to the presence of the cyst. Therefore, these patients should be managed conservatively with close monitoring of symptoms and yearly clinical examinations and serial imaging to demonstrate stable disease.[19,21] MRI is often used in these patients because of better soft tissue resolution and absence of radiation exposure.[2]

Surgical management should be considered in patients with objective symptoms including sensorineural hearing loss attributable to large cysts involving the cochlea and the internal auditory canal[3] or in patients with impending complications including vestibular dysfunction from otic capsule erosion.[2]

Factors that affect the choice of a surgical approach include the topo-anatomical location of the lesion, histopathological examination, inner ear function, cranial nerve status, and the surgeon's experience.[47] Proposed anatomical criteria favoring an endonasal endoscopic approach include pneumatization of the concha,[48] a lateral pneumatization beyond the vidian nerve,[49] and a wide area between the petrous carotid artery and the optic nerve.[50] Pneumatization of the temporal bone plays an important role in determining the surgical approach. A poor pneumatization of the sphenoid sinus will make a transnasal approach more difficult, whereas the need to drill through dense underpneumatized bone makes the lateral approach more challenging.[1]

Complications

Transcranial excision of CG necessitates brain retraction and is therefore associated with encephalomalacia and seizures, as well as an increased risk of intracranial hemorrhage, CSF leakage and therefore longer hospitalization time.[2]

The transtemporal approach has a complication rate of 24.3% (ranged from 0 to 60%) with hearing loss and CSF leakage being the most common complications.[2]

The infra- or subcochlear approach is associated with tympanic membrane perforation during tympanomeatal flap elevation and drilling, CSF leakage when the bone drilling is directed posteriorly toward the posterior fossa dura and cochlear aqueduct, hearing loss and vertigo when the otic capsule or the vein of the cochlear aqueduct are injured, venous bleeding from the jugular bulb, and injury of the internal carotid artery in rare cases.[2] The infralabyrinthine approach is also associated with vertigo and hearing loss if the posterior semicircular canal and the vein of the cochlear aqueduct are injured.[2] Bone drilling angled posteriorly toward the posterior fossa dura can cause CSF leakage.[2] On the other hand, the translabyrinthine and transotic approaches carry a higher risk of facial nerve injury, CSF leakage, vestibular dysfunction, and hearing loss.[2] Severe complications of transtemporal approach are rare but include seizures, meningitis, and injury of the petrous ICA with severe hemorrhage, occlusion and subsequent death.[2]

The endonasal endoscopic approach to the petrous apex has an overall complication rate of 13.3%. This includes restenosis of the drainage pathway, epistaxis, chronic serous otitis media due to injury of the eustachian tube requiring grommet therapy, chronic sphenoid sinusitis, transient sixth nerve palsy causing diplopia, CSF leakage, dry nose, dry eyes from vidian nerve injury, facial anesthesia and in rare cases, ICA and brain inujry.[2,33] However, these risks can be reduced with good surgical anatomy knowledge and the use of image guidance.[51]

Tips and Pearls

- The petrous apex is the medial most part of the temporal bone described as a pyramid with an anteromedial apex and a posterolateral base.
- The most common petrous apex lesion is the CG.
- It is important to understand the natural history of common petrous apex lesions in order to establish a realistic therapeutic goal for patients.
- Petrous apex lesions may be asymptomatic or present with common clinical features including hearing loss, dizziness, tinnitus, headache, facial twitching, diplopia, facial paralysis, and facial weakness.
- Complete history and clinical examination including neurological, hearing, and vestibular examination and investigation are important prior to surgical management.
- CT and MRI imaging can accurately diagnose petrous apex lesions and can be used in following up asymptomatic patients and to monitor disease progression or recurrence in surgically treated patients.
- The choice of surgical approach needs to be balanced between the ease of access to this complex anatomical area, the surgeon's experience, preservation of function, and maximizing the extent of resection while minimizing surgical morbidity.
- Hearing assessment should be performed postoperatively to check for resolution or improvement of symptoms. Serial postoperative CT and MRI imaging is recommended to rule out recurrent disease.

Acknowledgments

This chapter was written based on funding from the Martin Allgöwer Foundation, Department of Surgery, University Hospital of Basel (Basel, Switzerland), the Gottfried and Julia Bangerter-Rhyner Foundation (Bern, Switzerland), the Ministry of Health of Malaysia scholarship (Malaysia), and the Adelaide Ear-Nose-Throat Research Institute (Australia). The Departments of Neurosurgery of the University Hospital of Basel (Basel, Switzerland) and the Departments of Neurosurgery and Otorhinolaryngology of the University of Malaya (Kuala Lumpur, Malaysia) supported the creation of this chapter.

References

1. Malone A, Bruni M, Wong R, Tabor M, Boyev KP. Pneumatization patterns of the petrous apex and lateral sphenoid recess. J Neurol Surg B Skull Base 2017;78(6): 441–446
2. Isaacson B. Cholesterol granuloma and other petrous apex lesions. Otolaryngol Clin North Am 2015;48(2):361–373
3. Sweeney AD, Osetinsky LM, Carlson ML, et al. The natural history and management of petrous apex cholesterol granulomas. Otol Neurotol 2015;36(10):1714–1719
4. Bruchhage KL, Wollenberg B, Leichtle A. Transsphenoidal and infralabyrinthine approach of the petrous apex cholesterol granuloma. Eur Arch Otorhinolaryngol 2017;274(7): 2749–2756
5. Chole RA. Petrous apicitis: surgical anatomy. Ann Otol Rhinol Laryngol 1985;94(3):251–257
6. Muckle RP, De la Cruz A, Lo WM. Petrous apex lesions. Am J Otol 1998;19(2):219–225
7. Lo WW, Solti-Bohman LG, Brackmann DE, Gruskin P. Cholesterol granuloma of the petrous apex: CT diagnosis. Radiology 1984; 153(3):705–711
8. Arriaga MA, Brackmann DE. Differential diagnosis of primary petrous apex lesions. Am J Otol 1991;12(6):470–474
9. Isaacson B, Kutz JW, Roland PS. Lesions of the petrous apex: diag-nosis and management. Otolaryngol Clin North Am 2007; 40(3):479–519, viii
10. Roland PS, Meyerhoff WL, Judge LO, Mickey BE. Asymmetric pne-umatization of the petrous apex. Otolaryngol Head Neck Surg 1990;103(1):80–88
11. Hoa M, House JW, Linthicum FH, Go JL. Petrous apex cholesterol granuloma: pictorial review of radiological considerations in diagnosis and surgical histopathology. J Laryngol Otol 2013;127(4):339–348
12. Mafee MF, Kumar A, Heffner DK. Epidermoid cyst (cholesteatoma) and cholesterol granuloma of the temporal bone and epi-dermoid cysts affecting the brain. Neuroimaging Clin N Am 1994;4(3):561–578
13. Roemer S, Maeder P, Daniel RT, Kawasaki A. Sixth nerve palsy from cholesterol granuloma of the petrous apex. Front Neurol 2017;8:48
14. Ojala L. Pneumatization of the bone and environmental factors; experimental studies on chick humerus. Acta Otolaryngol Suppl 1957;133:3–28
15. Beaumont GD. The effects of exclusion of air from pneumatized bones. J Laryngol Otol 1966;80(3):236–249
16. Jackler RK, Cho M. A new theory to explain the genesis of petrous apex cholesterol granuloma. Otol Neurotol 2003;24(1):96–106, discussion 106
17. Oyama K, Ikezono T, Tahara S, Shindo S, Kitamura T, Teramoto A. Petrous apex cholesterol granuloma treated via the endo-scopic transsphenoidal approach. Acta Neurochir (Wien) 2007;149(3):299–302, discussion 302
18. Gacek RR. Diagnosis and management of primary tumors of the petrous apex. Ann Otol Rhinol Laryngol 1975;84(1 Pt 2, Suppl 18):1–20
19. Mosnier I, Cyna-Gorse F, Grayeli AB, et al. Management of cho-lesterol granulomas of the petrous apex based on clinical and radiologic evaluation. Otol Neurotol 2002;23(4):522–528
20. Brackmann DE, Toh EH. Surgical management of petrous apex cholesterol granulomas. Otol Neurotol 2002;23(4):529–533
21. Sanna M, Dispenza F, Mathur N, De Stefano A, De Donato G. Otoneurological management of petrous apex cholesterol granuloma. Am J Otolaryngol 2009;30(6):407–414
22. Hagr AA. Hearing improvement after partial labyrinthectomy: resection of petrous apex cholesterol granuloma. Sultan Qaboos Univ Med J 2010;10(2):249–254
23. Solodnik P, Som PM, Shugar JM, et al. Intraosseous petrous apex neuroma: CT findings. J Comput Assist Tomogr 1986; 10(6):1027–1029
24. Bockmühl U, Khalil HS, Draf W. Clinicoradiological and surgical considerations in the treatment of cholesterol granuloma of the petrous pyramid. Skull Base 2005;15(4): 263–267, discussion 267–268
25. Jackler RK, Parker DA. Radiographic differential diagnosis of petrous apex lesions. Am J Otol 1992;13(6):561–574
26. Park KC, Wong G, Stephens JC, Saleh HA. Endoscopic trans-sphenoidal drainage of an aggressive petrous apex cholesterol granuloma: unusual complications and lessons learnt. J Laryngol Otol 2013;127(12):1230–1234
27. McLaughlin N, Kelly DF, Prevedello DM, Shahlaie K, Carrau RL, Kassam AB. Endoscopic endonasal management of recur-rent petrous apex cholesterol granuloma. Skull Base Rep 2011;1(1):27–32

28. Kamiguchi H, Kawase T, Toya S, Inoue Y. Cholesterol granuloma of the petrous apex: establishment of a drainage route into the superior tympanic cavity—technical note. Neurol Med Chir (Tokyo) 1996;36(9):662–665

29. Ghorayeb BY, Jahrsdoerfer RA. Subcochlear approach for cholesterol granulomas of the inferior petrous apex. Otolaryngol Head Neck Surg 1990;103(1):60–65

30. Presutti L, Nogueira JF, Alicandri-Ciufelli M, Marchioni D. Beyond the middle ear: endoscopic surgical anatomy and approaches to inner ear and lateral skull base. Otolaryngol Clin North Am 2013;46(2):189–200

31. Samadian M, Akbari Dilmaghani N, Ahmady Roozbahany N, Farzin N, Bahadoram M. Endoscopic transnasal approach for cholesterol granuloma of the petrous apex. Case Rep Neurol Med 2015;2015:481231

32. Kassam AB, Gardner P, Snyderman C, Mintz A, Carrau R. Expanded endonasal approach: fully endoscopic, completely transnasal approach to the middle third of the clivus, petrous bone, middle cranial fossa, and infratemporal fossa. Neurosurg Focus 2005;19(1):E6

33. Scopel TF, Fernandez-Miranda JC, Pinheiro-Neto CD, et al. Petrous apex cholesterol granulomas: endonasal versus infracochlear approach. Laryngoscope 2012;122(4): 751–761

34. Prevedello DM, Pinheiro-Neto CD, Fernandez-Miranda JC, et al. Vidian nerve transposition for endoscopic endonasal middle fossa approaches. Neurosurgery 2010;67(2, Suppl Operative):478–484

35. Radonjic A, Moldovan ID, Kilty SJ, Schramm DR, Alkherayf F. Complete recovery of sensorineural hearing loss following endoscopic transsphenoidal surgery for a petrous apex cholesterol granuloma: case report. Am J Case Rep 2019; 20:335–339

36. Paluzzi A, Gardner P, Fernandez-Miranda JC, et al. Endoscopic endonasal approach to cholesterol granulomas of the petrous apex: a series of 17 patients: clinical article. J Neurosurg 2012;116(4):792–798

37. Prabhu K, Kurien M, Chacko AG. Endoscopic transsphenoidal approach to petrous apex cholesterol granulomas. Br J Neurosurg 2010;24(6):688–691

38. Iannella G, Savastano E, Pasquariello B, Re M, Magliulo G. Giant petrous bone cholesteatoma: combined microscopic surgery and an adjuvant endoscopic approach. J Neurol Surg Rep 2016;77(1):e46–e49

39. Cazzador D, Favaretto N, Zanoletti E, Martini A. Combined surgical approach to giant cholesteatoma: a case report and literature review. Ann Otol Rhinol Laryngol 2016;125(8):687–693

40. Patron V, Humbert M, Micault E, Emery E, Hitier M. How to perform microscopic/endoscopic resection of large petrous apex lesions. Eur Ann Otorhinolaryngol Head Neck Dis 2018; 135(6):443–447

41. Korbmacher D, Lehmann M, Gehl HB, Ebmeyer J, Sudhoff H. Petrous apex cholesterol granuloma involving the sphenoid sinus. Ear Nose Throat J 2011;90(11):E23–E25

42. Georgalas C, Kania R, Guichard JP, Sauvaget E, Tran Ba Huy P, Herman P. Endoscopic transsphenoidal surgery for cholesterol granulomas involving the petrous apex. Clin Otolaryngol 2008;33(1):38–42

43. Barber SR, Wong K, Kanumuri V, et al. Augmented reality, surgical navigation, and 3d printing for transcanal endoscopic appro-ach to the petrous apex. OTO Open 2018; 2(4):X18804492

44. Thorne MC, Gebarski SS, Telian SA. Rapid expansion in a previously indolent cholesterol cyst: a need for lifelong follow-up. Otol Neurotol 2006;27(1):124–126

45. Lorenz KJ, Hamer G, Sator W, Maier H. [Cholesterol granuloma of the petrous apex—etiology, diagnosis and therapy]. Laryngorhinootologie 1996;75(12):775–782

46. Castillo MP, Samy RN, Isaacson B, Roland PS. Petrous apex cholesterol granuloma aeration: does it matter? Otolaryngol Head Neck Surg 2008;138(4):518–522

47. Meneses MS, Moreira AL, Bordignon KC, Pedrozo AA, Ramina R, Nikoski JG. Surgical approaches to the petrous apex: distances and relations with cranial morphology. Skull Base 2004;14(1):9–19, discussion 19–20

48. Hamid O, El Fiky L, Hassan O, Kotb A, El Fiky S. Anatomic variations of the sphenoid sinus and their impact on transsphenoid pituitary surgery. Skull Base 2008;18(1):9–15

49. Iseli TA, Yahng J, Leung R, Briggs RJ, King JA, Phal PM. Anatomic comparison of nasal versus lateral surgical access to the petrous apex. Clin Anat 2013;26(6):682–687

50. Wang J, Bidari S, Inoue K, Yang H, Rhoton A Jr. Extensions of the sphenoid sinus: a new classification. Neurosurgery 2010; 66(4):797–816

51. Zanation AM, Snyderman CH, Carrau RL, Gardner PA, Prevedello DM, Kassam AB. Endoscopic endonasal surgery for petrous apex lesions. Laryngoscope 2009;119(1):19–25

Chapter 28 Endonasal Endoscopic Surgeries for Petrous Apex Lesions

Case 28A

Endoscopic Transsphenoidal Excision of a Large Petrous Apex Cholesteatoma

Jeyanthi Kulasegarah, Vicknes Waran, and Prepageran Narayanan

History

A 48-year-old woman presented with double vision in the right eye, imbalance, right-sided hearing loss, and headache. On examination, the right eye had lateral rectus palsy, and audiogram confirmed a right profound sensorineural hearing loss. MRI (**Fig. 28A.1a–c**) revealed a large right petrous apex cholesteatoma enveloping and displacing the petrous internal carotid artery (ICA) anteriorly, and the lesion extending intracranially involving the temporal lobe with the displacement of the midbrain and compression of the lateral ventricle and the third ventricle. Conventionally, these lesions are removed using a transtemporal approach with significant comorbidity. However, more recently, using a multidisciplinary approach with a neurosurgeon and improved endoscopic techniques, it was possible to excise this endoscopically.

Surgical Steps

1. The patient is placed under general anesthesia in a supine position and the head is fixed slightly retroflexed within a NORAS frame for intraoperative magnetic resonance imaging (iMRI). Registration for neuronavigation (Brainlab, Munich, Germany) is performed.
2. The nose is decongested with nasal packing as per the institution's standard methods.
3. A posterior septectomy and a wide sphenoidotomy are performed (**Fig. 28A.2**).
4. The cholesteatoma sac is visible at the midclival region, which is continuous with the component lateral to the paraclival ICA (**Fig. 28A.3**). Neuronavigation is used to confirm the displaced ICA.

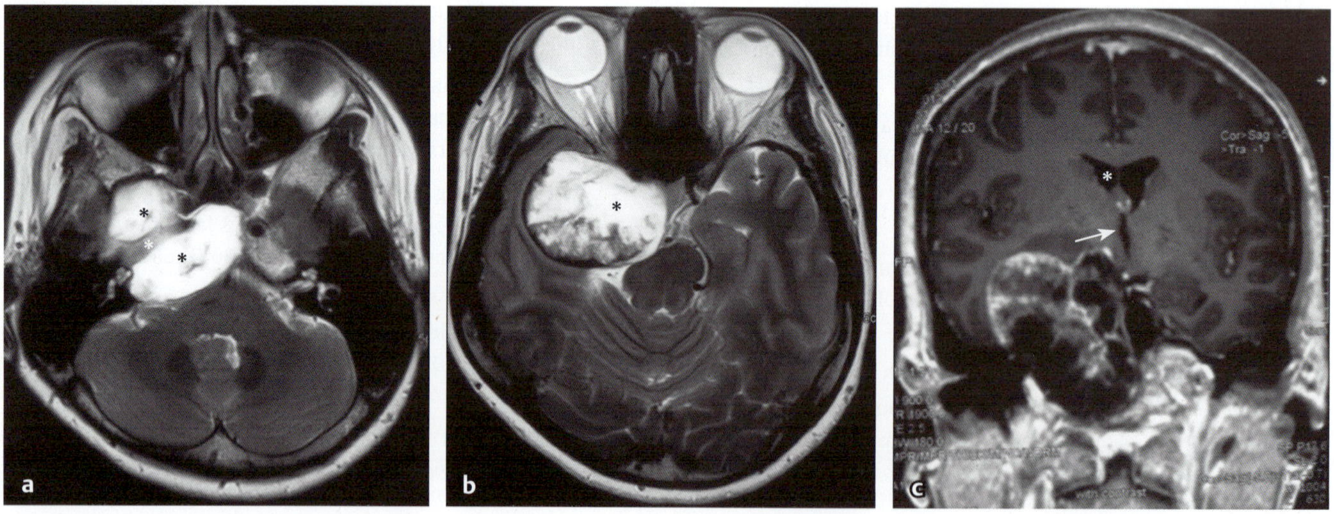

Fig. 28A.1 **(a)** Axial cut of a T2-weighted MRI sequence showing a large petrous apex cholesteatoma (*black* *) enveloping and displacing the petrous internal carotid artery (*white* *) anteriorly. **(b)** The lesion (*black* *) extends intracranially involving the temporal lobe with displacement of the midbrain. **(c)** Coronal cut of a T1-weighted with gadolinium MRI sequence showing the lesion causing compression of the lateral ventricle (*white* *) and third ventricle (*white arrow*).

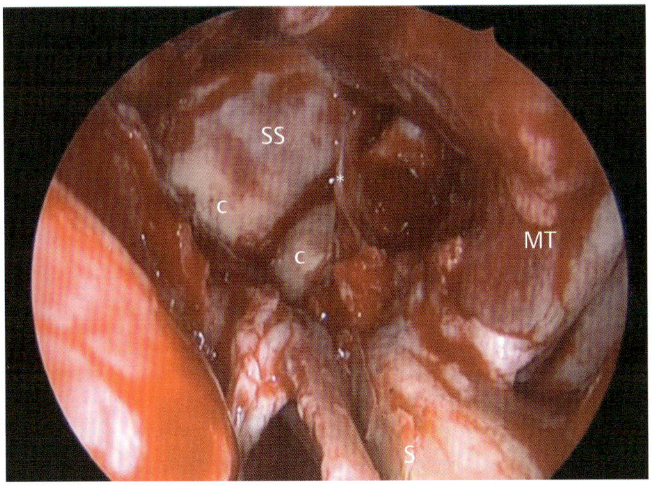

Fig. 28A.2 A posterior septectomy and a wide sphenoidotomy revealing the cholesteatoma sac (c), sphenoid sinus (SS), septum (S), middle turbinate (MT), and intersphenoid septum (*white* *).

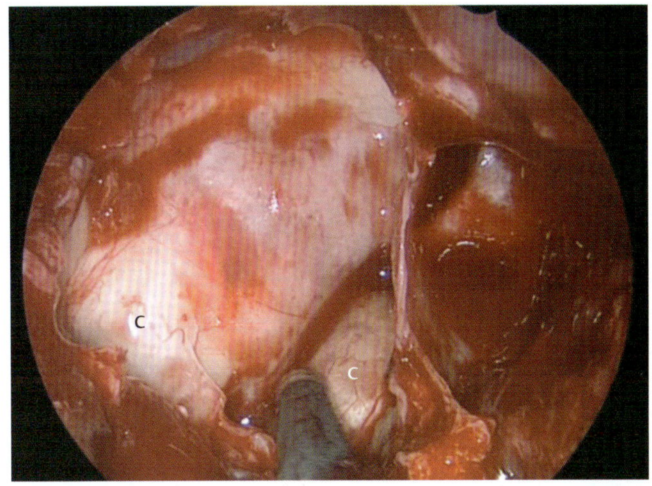

Fig. 28A.3 The cholesteatoma sac is visible at the midclival region (c in *white*), which is continuous with the component lateral to the paraclival internal carotid artery (c in *black*).

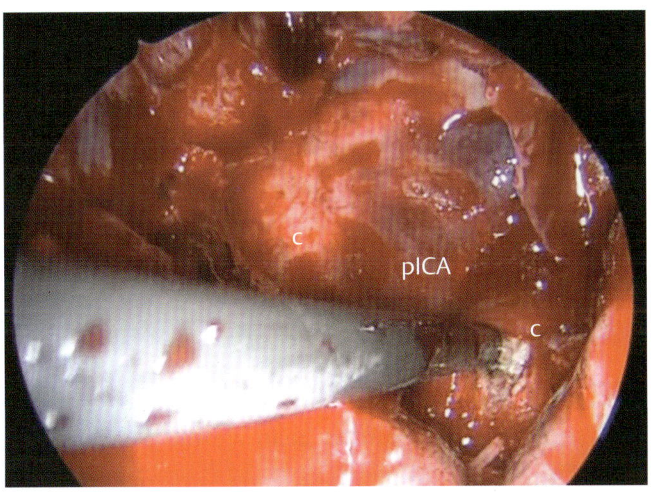

Fig. 28A.4 The cholesteatoma sac (c) medial to the paraclival internal carotid artery (pICA) is opened.

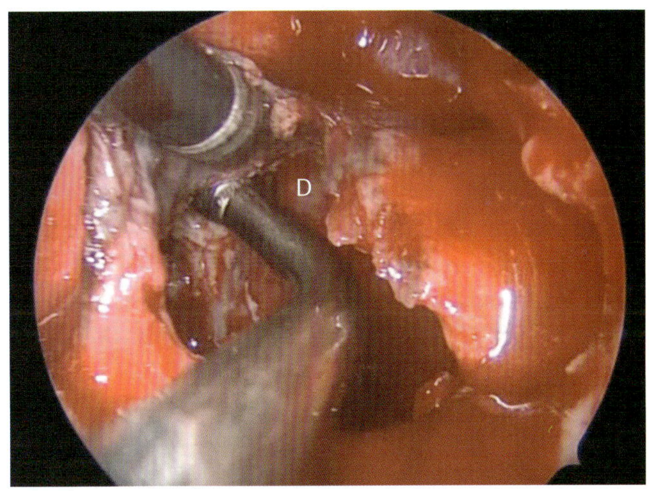

Fig. 28A.5 Using an angled suction, the more lateral component of the matrix is removed and the dura of the temporal lobe (D) is decompressed.

5. The sac at the midclivus is opened with a sickle knife, and the matrix of the cholesteatoma is suctioned (**Fig. 28A.4**).
6. Using an angled suction, the more lateral component of the matrix is removed and the dura of the temporal lobe is decompressed (**Fig. 28A.5**).
7. At the end of cholesteatoma removal, the following structures were identified: right petrous apex, right dura of the right temporal lobe, petrous and paraclival parts of the right ICA, and midclivus (**Fig. 28A.6**).

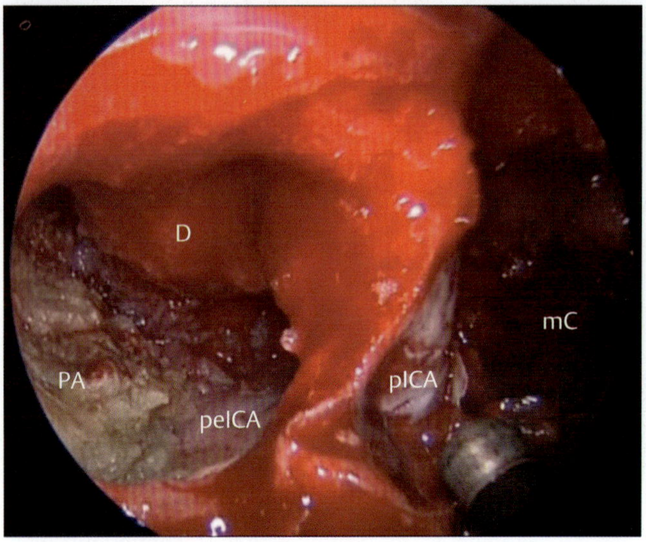

Fig. 28A.6 The following structures were identified at the end: right petrous apex (PA), right dura of the right temporal lobe (D), petrous internal carotid artery (peICA) and paraclival parts of the right internal carotid artery (pICA), and midclivus (mC).

Case 28B

Endoscopic Transsphenoidal Excision of a Left Petrous Apex Cholesterol Granuloma

Jeyanthi Kulasegarah, Michel Roethlisberger, Vicknes Waran, and Prepageran Narayanan

History

A 33-year-old man presented with sudden onset of double vision. He denied any hearing or balance problems, and there were no other associated otological symptoms. On physical examination, a left-sided cranial nerve VI (CN VI) palsy was identified. Other cranial nerves and ENT examinations were normal. Pure tone audiometry showed normal hearing bilaterally. Magnetic resonance imaging (MRI; T2-weighted sequences) revealed a hyperintense lesion involving the left petrous apex (**Fig. 28B.1**). T1-weight sequence with gadolinium showed enhancement of the lesion in the left petrous apex (**Fig. 28B.2**). MRI findings were consistent with a cholesterol granuloma (CG). The patient underwent endoscopic transsphenoidal excision of the lesion. Three months post-surgery, there was complete resolution of the CN VI palsy.

Surgical Steps

1. The patient is placed under general anesthesia in a supine position and the head is fixed slightly retroflexed with NORAS frame for intraoperative MRI (iMRI). Registration for neuronavigation (Brainlab, Munich, Germany) is performed.
2. The nose is decongested with nasal packing as per the institutions' standard methods.
3. A posterior septectomy and a wide sphenoidotomy are performed (**Fig. 28B.3**).
4. The lesion is visible in the midclival region, medial to the paraclival internal carotid artery (ICA; **Fig. 28B.4**). Image-guided surgery (IGS) is used to confirm the paraclival ICA.
5. An angled probe is used to delineate the lesion (**Fig. 28B.5**) and also to delineate the paraclival ICA (**Fig. 28B.6**).
6. A Kerrison punch is used to remove the bone over the paraclival ICA to expose the artery (**Fig. 28B.7**).
7. Following that, the Kerrison punch is used to remove the bone medial to the lesion over the pons (**Fig. 28B.8**).
8. The lesion is decompressed using suction (**Fig. 28B.9**).
9. The capsule of the cyst is seen adherent to the paraclival ICA and midclival dura (**Fig. 28B.10**).
10. A curette is used to remove the capsule that is adherent to the midclival dura and the paraclival ICA (**Fig. 28B.11**).
11. Hyaline crystals are visible within the cavity (**Fig. 28B.12**).
12. The cavity is irrigated with 0.9% normal saline using a suction catheter (**Fig. 28B.13**).
13. In the end, the left petrous apex (**Fig. 28B.14**) and the skull base are inspected (**Fig. 28B.15**).

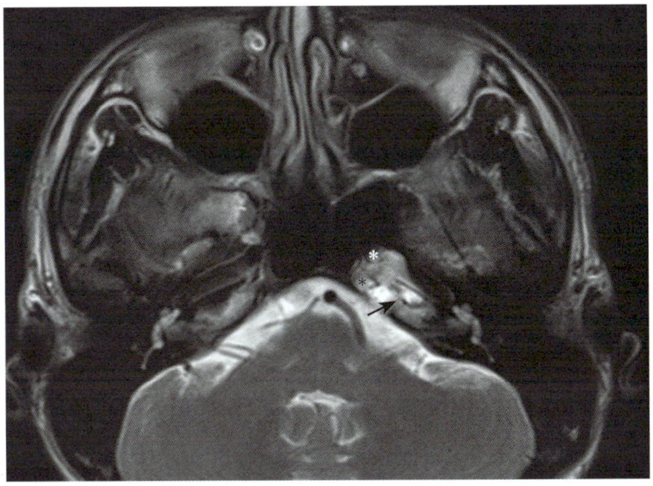

Fig. 28B.1 Axial T2-weighted MRI section demonstrating a hyperintense lesion in the left paraclival region (*black* *) enveloping the paraclival internal carotid artery (*white* *) anteriorly and extending into the left petrous apex (*black arrow*).

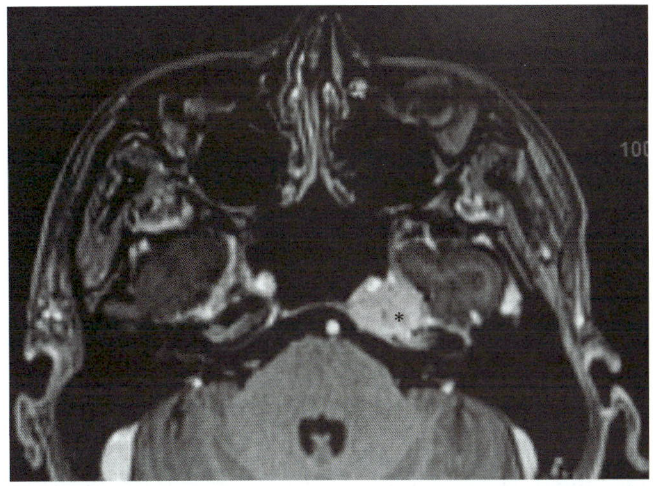

Fig. 28B.2 Axial T1-weighted gadolinium enhanced MRI section demonstrating enhancement of the lesion in the left petrous apex (*black* *).

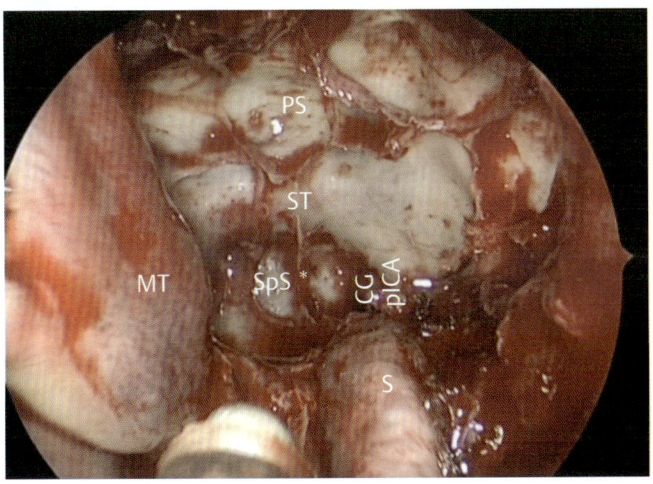

Fig. 28B.3 A posterior septectomy and a wide sphenoidotomy expose the sella turcica (ST), cholesterol granuloma (CG), sphenoid sinus (SpS), septum (S), middle turbinate (MT), inter-sphenoid septum (*white* *), planum sphenoidale (PS), and paraclival ICA (pICA).

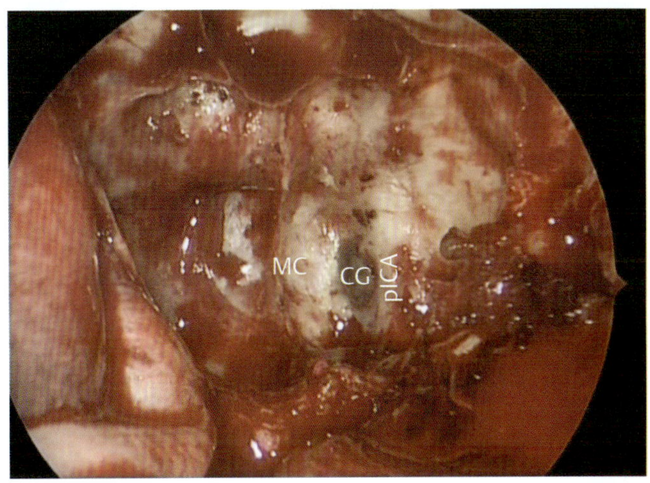

Fig. 28B.4 A closer endoscopic picture of the cholesterol granuloma (CG) at the midclival (MC) region adjacent to the paraclival internal carotid artery (pICA).

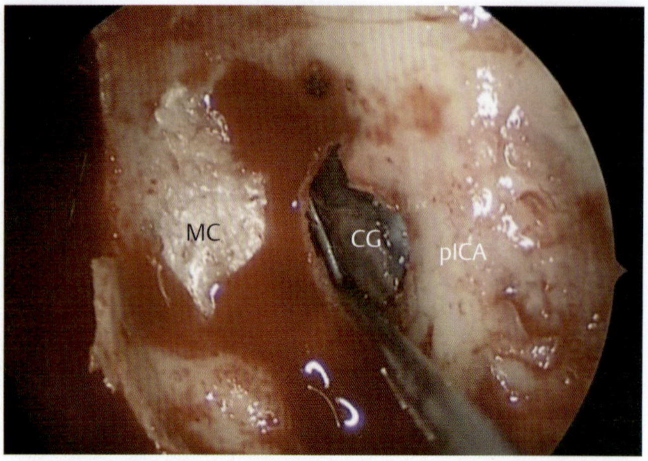

Fig. 28B.5 An angled probe is used to delineate the cholesterol granuloma (CG) at the midclival (MC) region adjacent to the paraclival internal carotid artery (pICA).

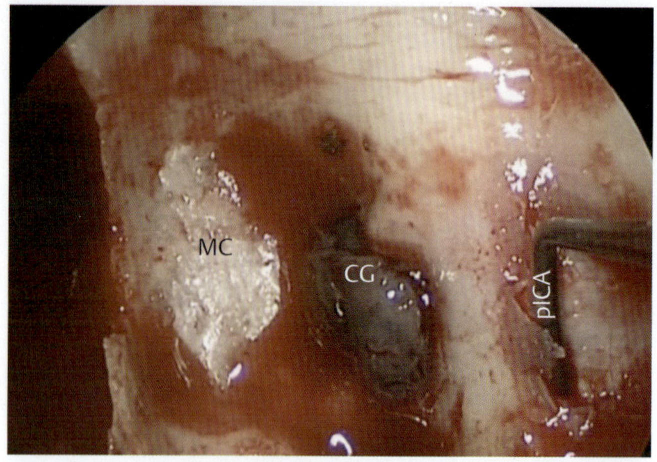

Fig. 28B.6 An angled probe is used to delineate the paraclival ICA (pICA) laterally to the cholesterol granuloma (CG) at the midclival (MC) region.

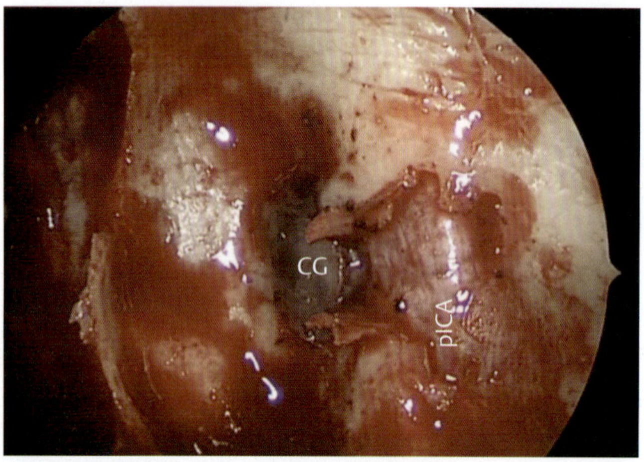

Fig. 28B.7 The bone is removed using a Kerrison punch to expose paraclival ICA (pICA) adjacent to the cholesterol granuloma (CG).

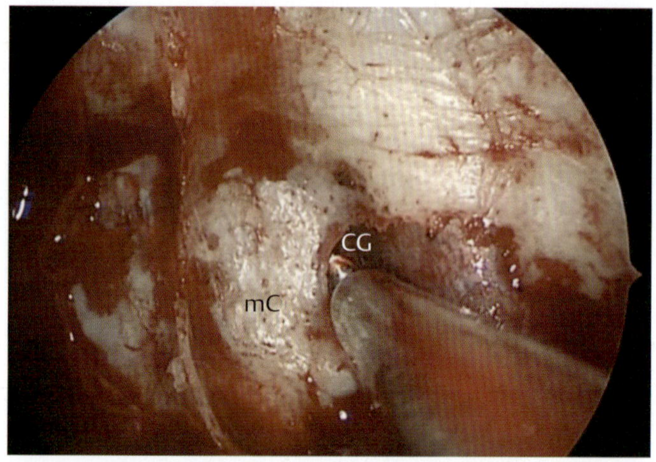

Fig. 28B.8 A Kerrison punch is used to remove the bone medial to the lesion (CG) at the midclivus (mC).

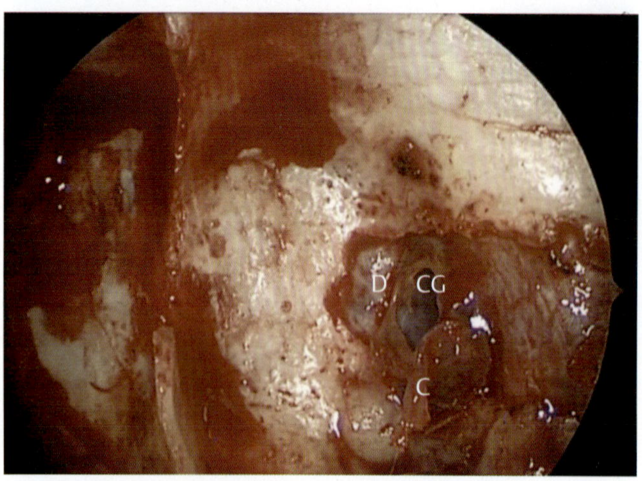

Fig. 28B.9 The capsule (C) is marsupialized lateral to the midclival dura (D) and the cholesterol granuloma (CG) decompressed.

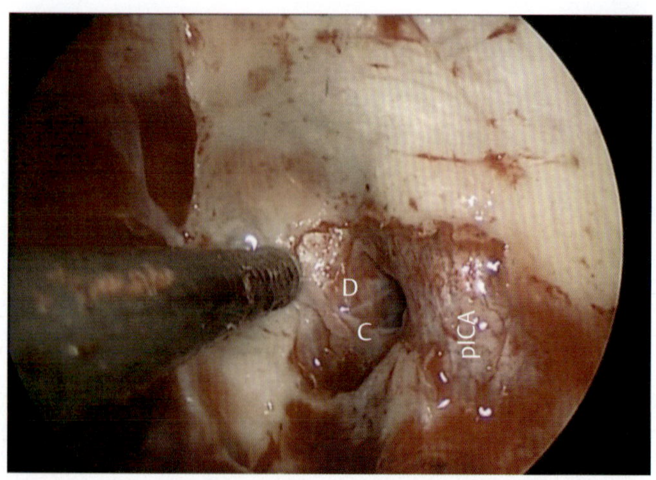

Fig. 28B.10 The capsule (C) is adherent to the paraclival ICA (pICA) and the midclival dura (D).

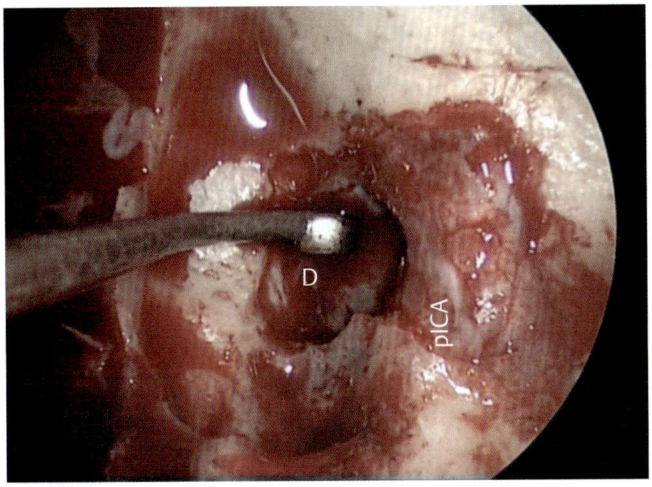

Fig. 28B.11 The adherent capsule is removed with a curette between the dura (D) and paraclival ICA (pICA).

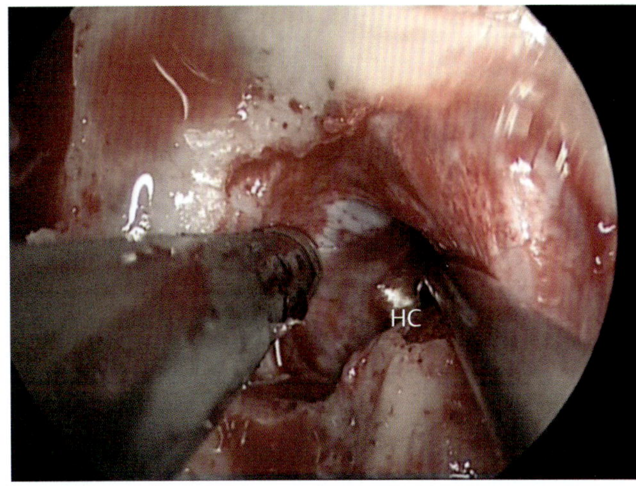

Fig. 28B.12 Hyaline crystals (HC) are detected within the cavity of the lesion.

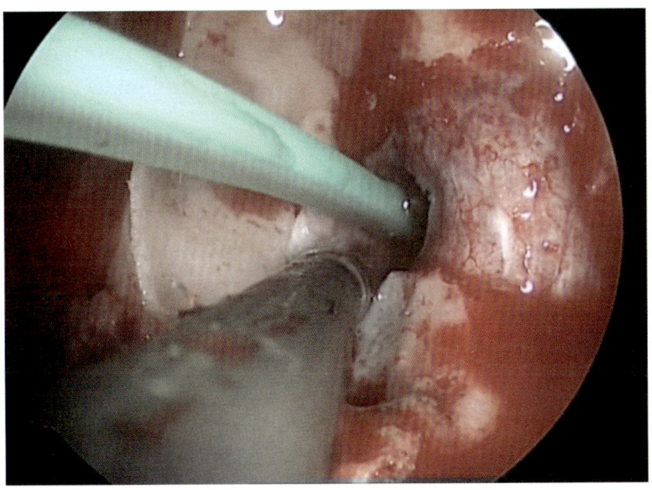

Fig. 28B.13 A suction catheter is used to irrigate the cavity with 0.9% normal saline.

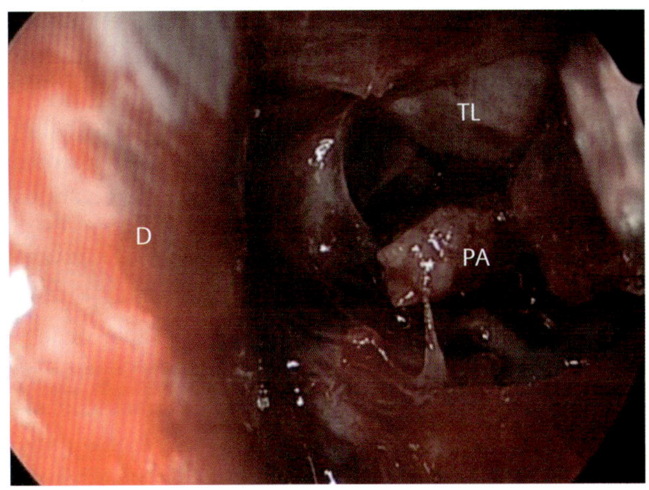

Fig. 28B.14 Final view of the left petrous apex (PA) demonstrating the exposed midclival dura (D) and the temporal lobe (TL).

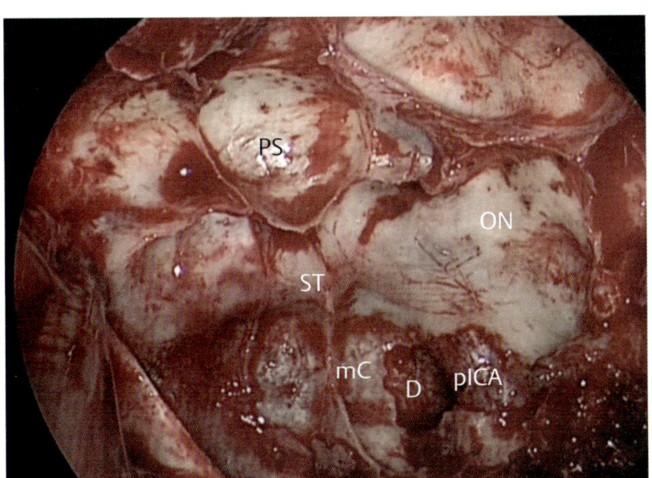

Fig. 28B.15 Final view of the skull base: midclivus (mC), sella turcica (ST), planum sphenoidale (PS), midclival dura (D), paraclival ICA (pICA), optic nerve (ON).

Chapter 29 Endoscopic Petroclival Approach

Jun Muto, John Clemente de Leon, and Yuichi Hirose

Introduction

The petroclival area is an intricate zone of the central skull base formed by the apex of the petrous temporal bone, the posteroinferior surface of the sphenoid, and the clival process of the occipital bone. This area is surrounded by many critical vascular, cranial nerve, and brainstem structures, thus increasing the complexity of procedures that address any lesions that arise in the area.

The horizontal line of the petrous internal carotid artery (peICA) segment, the paraclival ICA segment, and the abducens nerves are the main landmarks used for planning the approach to the petroclival region.[1] Craniotomy techniques for accessing the petrous apex and petroclival area have been described and include anterior petrosectomy, posterior transpetrosal, retrosigmoid, and presigmoid retrolabyrinthine approaches. Recent advancements in endoscopic procedures have allowed neurosurgeons to treat various regional lesions, including deep-seated intradural or extradural cysts or tumors. Endoscopic endonasal approaches (EEAs) have been proposed, such as the medial transsphenoidal, transpterygoid infrapetrous, and transclival approaches.

EEAs to lesions of the petrous apex include the transpterygoid infrapetrous approach and the medial transsphenoidal approach. The former can be performed with or without vidian nerve transposition, while the latter can be achieved with a partial clivectomy, with or without ICA lateralization. Selecting the safest surgical approach depends on the position of the lesion relative to the ICA, degree of tumor extension, and pathology. EEAs are ideal for lesions that abut the lateral recesses of the sphenoid sinus. Their advantages over the transcranial approaches include a shorter operative time, avoidance of craniotomy, easier follow-up in the clinic, and faster recovery. This chapter provides stepwise descriptions of both surgical approaches.

Surgical Anatomy

The petroclival fissure is present at the junction between the petrous apex (PA) and the petrous process of the sphenoid. This fissure lies directly behind the paraclival segment of the ICA, which is the portion of ICA from the upper border of the foramen lacerum to the posterior bend. At the top of the fissure lies the abducens nerve, where it turns from a vertical direction at the interdural segment to a more horizontal direction at the cavernous segment. As the fissure runs downward, it turns more laterally and heads toward the jugular foramen.

Surgical Techniques

The PA is located in the petrous temporal bone, an angular bone located at the confluence of the greater wing of the sphenoid and basilar portion of the occipital bones (**Fig. 29.1a–c**). Several methods for accessing the PA region have been proposed, including the anterior transpetrosal,[1,2] transsphenoidal, and translabyrinthine (in the case of hearing loss) approaches.[3] The description of the techniques begins at the point of completion of total ethmoidectomies and wide sphenoidotomies.

Medial Transsphenoidal Approach

If the PA lesion is small and expands into the sphenoid sinus, a medial transsphenoidal approach can be performed. This approach is defined within the boundary of the paraclival ICA anteriorly, lacerum ICA inferiorly, and the abducens nerve superiorly, as depicted in **Fig. 29.2a**. After ethmoidectomies and wide sphenoidotomies (**Fig. 29.2a**), the floor of the sphenoid sinus is drilled posteriorly with a 3-mm coarse diamond burr until it is flush with the clivus, and a partial clivectomy is performed. Once the medial aspect of the paraclival ICA and the lesion are opened, thin, small pieces of bone are removed with a 1- or 2-mm Kerrison rongeur to avoid injuring the dura mater. In cystic lesions such as cholesterol granulomas, authors advocate drainage of the cystic component into the sphenoid sinus and nasopharynx via a silicone stent (**Fig. 29.2b**) and marsupialization for 3 to 6 months.

When the lesions are located posterior to the ICA or are hard to access because of poor pneumatization, a medial transsphenoidal approach with ICA lateralization is required. A transpterygoid approach is used to identify the vidian nerve and artery, and to follow these structures to the anterior genu of the ICA. The posterior nasal and sphenopalatine arteries are dissected and transected, and the pterygopalatine ganglion is exposed. The soft tissues are dissected laterally until the vidian artery and nerve can be visualized coming from the vidian canal (**Fig. 29.2c**), which can be identified as a petrosal part of ICA. The region medial and

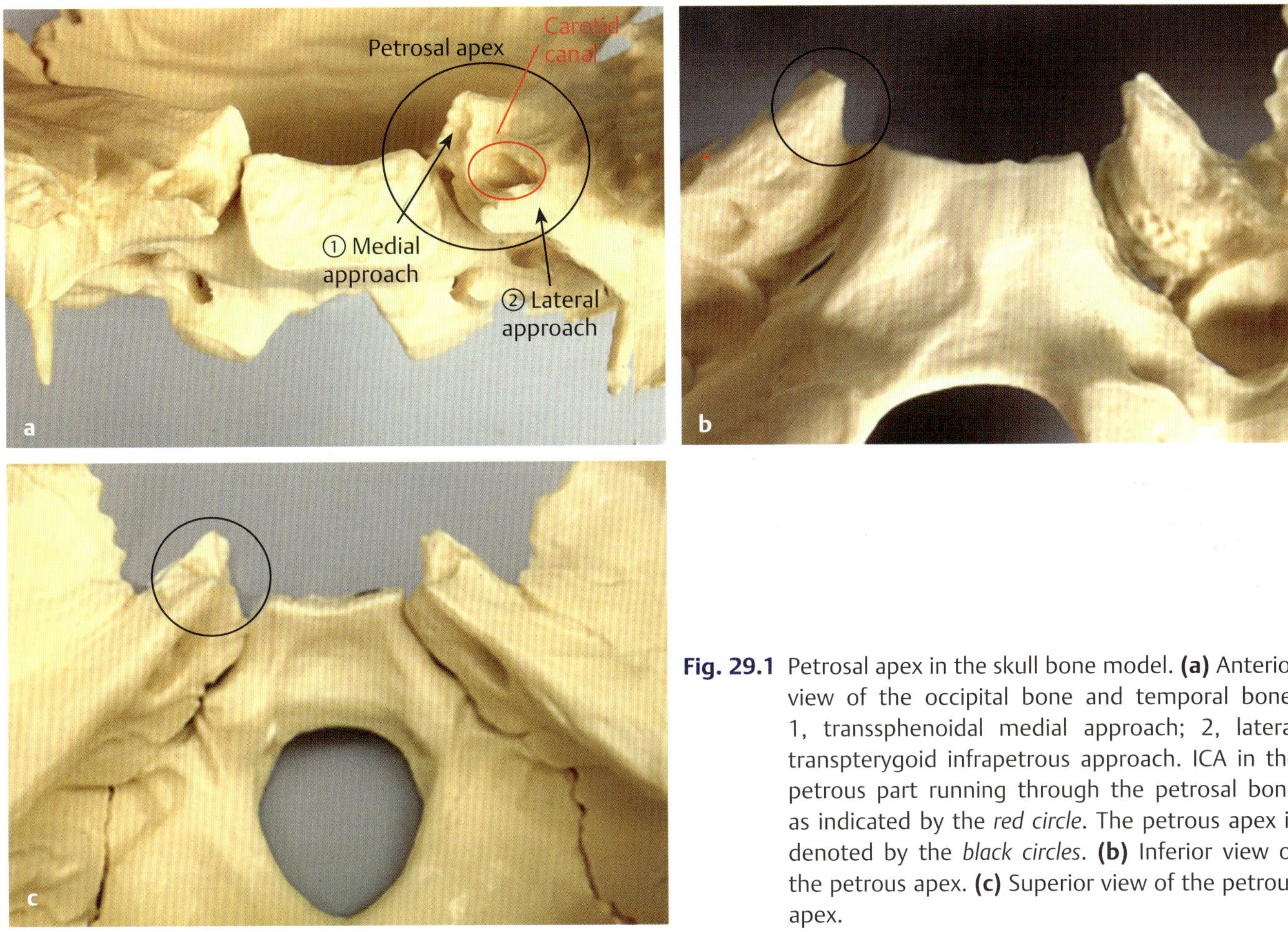

Fig. 29.1 Petrosal apex in the skull bone model. **(a)** Anterior view of the occipital bone and temporal bone. 1, transsphenoidal medial approach; 2, lateral transpterygoid infrapetrous approach. ICA in the petrous part running through the petrosal bone as indicated by the *red circle*. The petrous apex is denoted by the *black circles*. **(b)** Inferior view of the petrous apex. **(c)** Superior view of the petrous apex.

inferior to the vidian canal is skeletonized with a high-speed drill from anterior to posterior to reach the cartilage of the foramen lacerum (**Fig. 29.2d**). This landmark is crucial for avoiding damage to the ICA. The bone over the carotid artery is thinned with the drill and carefully removed with a combination of drilling and elevation with the Kerrison rongeurs to expose the periosteum that surrounds the vertical and horizontal segments of the ICA (**Fig. 29.2e**). The dura of clivus and the entire medial part of the paraclival ICA are exposed to provide adequate space to access the lesion (**Fig. 29.2f**). This allows the lateralization of the paraclival ICA by several millimeters, thus allowing more lateral access to the lesion.

Transpterygoid Infrapetrous Approach

The transpterygoid infrapetrous approach is defined by the lacerum foramen synchondrosis anteriorly, and jugular foramen inferiorly, internal acoustic canal posteriorly, and petrous ICA superolaterally. After performing wide bilateral sphenoidectomies (**Fig. 29.3a**), it is possible to visualize the natural ostium of the maxillary sinus, and the wide antrostomy can help visualize the posterior wall of the maxillary sinus. This posterior wall is removed to expose the contents of the pterygopalatine fossa. The sphenopalatine artery can be followed into the pterygopalatine fossa and ligated. The pharyngobasilar fascia is dissected from the roof of the choana and the pterygoid bone is exposed (**Fig. 29.3b**). The soft tissues of the pterygopalatine fossa are dissected inferiorly and laterally until the vidian canal and foramen rotundum are identified. Drilling around these structures is performed from anterior to posterior, effectively removing the base of the pterygoid process (**Fig. 29.3c**). Initially, the floor of the sphenoid sinus is drilled flush with the clivus. The vidian canal is skeletonized to drill the base of pterygoids and the superior aspect of medial and lateral pterygoid plates from medial to lateral and from inferior to superior. Thus, the vidian nerve is followed posteriorly until the cartilage that shields the anterior face of the foramen lacerum and the anterior genu of the ICA in its transition from the petrous to the paraclival segments are reached (**Fig. 29.3d**). Drilling the lower part of the vidian canal to reach the ICA is safer because the vidian nerve marks the lower limit of the petrosal ICA. After drilling the pterygoid process, the medial part of the foramen ovale and the proximal segment of the

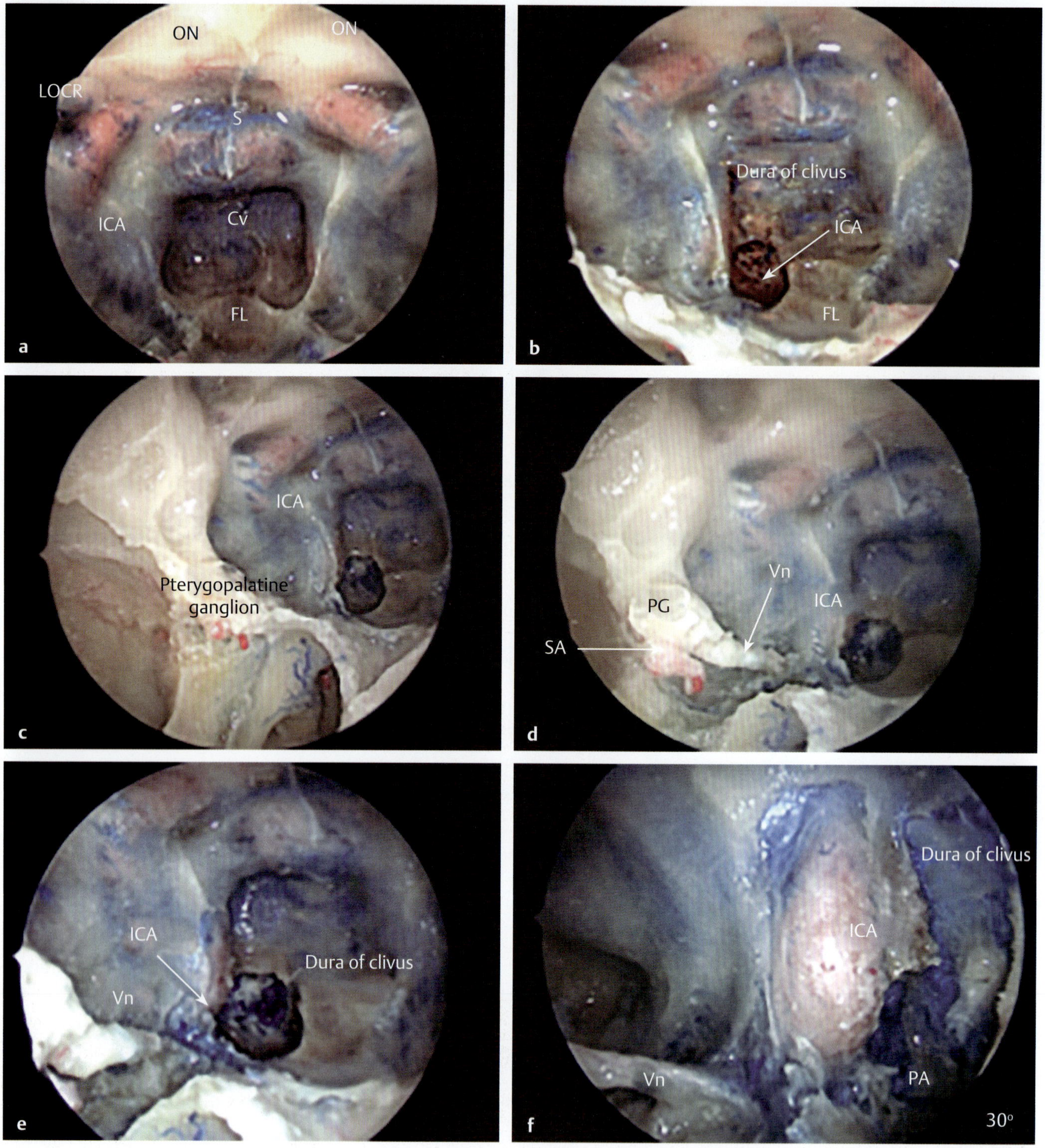

Fig. 29.2 Stepwise transsphenoidal approach to the petrous apex using EEA. **(a)** Wide sphenoidotomy and ethmoidectomy with a posterior septectomy. **(b)** Direct access to the medial part of the lesions in cases of a small tumor. **(c)** In a larger lesion, the overlaying mucosa is stripped to expose the vidian nerve and subsequently identify the pterygopalatine ganglion. **(d)** The pterygoid bone is partially drilled. The vidian nerve is transected to identify the anterior genu of the ICA. **(e)** Exposure of the clivus dura and the entire paraclival ICA. **(f)** Close-up view of the petrosal apex and paraclival ICA (30-degree angled scope).

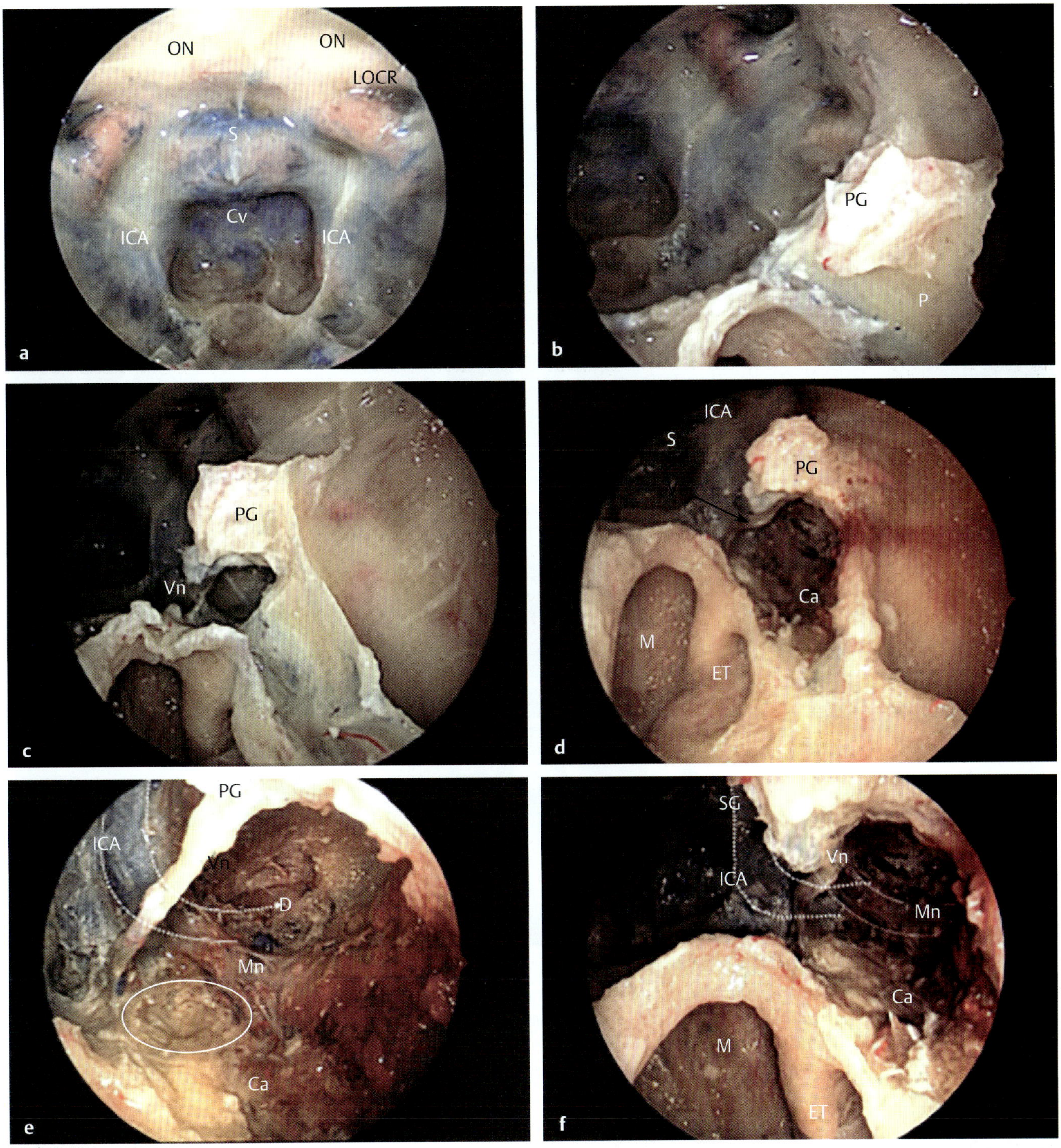

Fig. 29.3 Stepwise lateral transpterygoid infrapetrous approach to the petrous apex using EEA. **(a)** Wide sphenoidectomy is done similarly as in the transsphenoidal medial approach. **(b)** The pterygoid bone is exposed and the pterygopalatine ganglion is identified. **(c)** Following the pterygopalatine ganglion posteriorly, the vidian nerve is identified emerging from the vidian canal. Initially, the inferior and medial halves of the vidian canal are drilled and the vidian nerve is skeletonized. **(d)** Skeletonization of the vidian nerve up to the cartilage of the foramen lacerum. The vidian nerve is followed posteriorly up to the cartilage. **(e)** The white circle is the trajectory of the transpterygoid infrapetrous approach. The *white dotted line* shows the paraclival and petrous ICA. Infrapetrous access to the petrous apex. **(f)** General view of the access by transpterygoid infrapetrous approach. The *white dotted line* shows the paraclival and petrous ICA. The white line shows the mandibular nerve. Whenever possible, authors preserved the vidian nerve as shown here (30-degree angled scope).

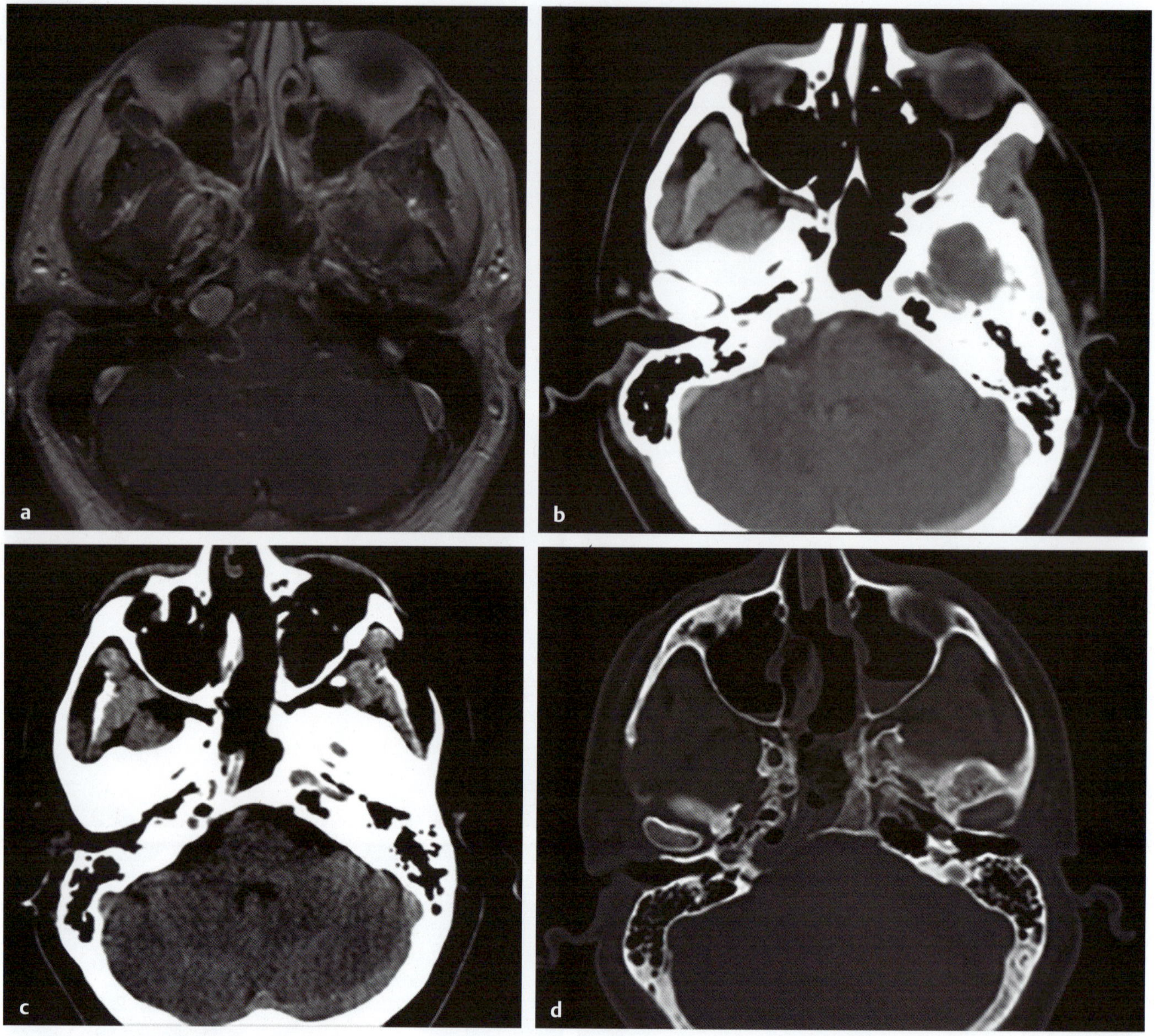

Fig. 29.4 Cholesterol granuloma at the petrous apex. **(a)** Axial contrast-enhanced magnetic resonance imaging showing the cholesterol granuloma at the petrous apex. The tumor enhanced homogenously. **(b)** CT scan showing the erosion of the bone at the right petrosal apex. **(c, d)** Postoperative axial CT scans showing the tube inserted from the tumor cavity draining into the sphenoid sinus.

mandibular nerve anterior to the petrosal part of the ICA are exposed (**Fig. 29.3e, f**). The inferior surface of the petrosal apex can be reached in the petrous ICA, eustachian tube, and the mandibular nerve. The tumors located in the PA are epidural that can compress the surrounding neurovascular structures, especially the ICA and mandibular nerve. As previously mentioned, in cases of cholesterol granuloma, a silicone stent is inserted into the cavity to allow drainage of the cyst fluid.

Case Example

A 42-year-old woman initially presented to her primary care physician with symptoms including dizziness, headache, and right facial numbness. A contrast magnetic resonance imaging (MRI) of the brain revealed a lesion inferomedial to the right internal auditory canal. The lesion was hyperintense on both T1 and T2 images, suggesting a benign cholesterol granuloma (**Fig. 29.4**). Drainage and marsupialization of the lesion were achieved via EEA as described in this chapter. She tolerated the procedure well and postoperative imaging showed a stable lesion.

References

1. Kawase T, Shiobara R, Toya S. Anterior transpetrosal-transtentorial approach for sphenopetroclival meningiomas: surgical method and results in 10 patients. Neurosurgery 1991;28(6):869–875, discussion 875–876
2. Muto J, Kawase T, Yoshida K. Meckel's cave tumors: relation to the meninges and minimally invasive approaches for surgery: anatomic and clinical studies. Neurosurgery 2010; 67(3 Suppl Operative):ons291–298; discussion ons298–299
3. Samii M, Tatagiba M, Carvalho GA. Retrosigmoid intradural suprameatal approach to Meckel's cave and the middle fossa: surgical technique and outcome. J Neurosurg 2000; 92(2):235–241

Section X

Meckel's Cave

Chapter 30 Meckel's Cave Lesions

A.B. Zulkiflee, Michel Roethlisberger, and Prepageran Narayanan

Introduction

The trigeminal nerve is the fifth cranial nerve (V) that provides somatosensory fibers to the three main regions of the face: forehead and periocular region (ophthalmic nerve or V1), cheek and maxillary region (maxillary nerve or V2), and jaw (mandibular nerve or V3). However, V3 also provides somatomotoric fibers eventually innervating eight skeletal muscles, including the four muscles of mastication: the masseter, the temporal, the medial, and the lateral pterygoids. The other four muscles are the tensor veli palatini, the mylohyoid, the anterior belly of the digastric, and the tensor tympani.

The nerve trifurcates via three openings: the superior orbital fissure (V1), the foramen rotundum (V2), and the foramen ovale (V3). The Gasserian or semilunar ganglion, also named Gasser's ganglion, consists of the pseudounipolar ganglia cells of the sensory radix. The ganglion is located within a dural cavity called trigeminal or Meckel's cave. The nerve fibers continue distally via the trigeminal porus.

Anatomy

The Meckel's cave is located at the posterolateral aspect of the cavernous sinus laterally to the sphenoid bone. Medially, it is bounded by the paraclinoid internal carotid artery in the posterior portion of the cavernous sinus. Inferiorly, it is bounded by the motor root of the trigeminal nerve and the petrous apex of the petrous temporal bone with the internal carotid artery traversing the carotid canal.

The cave is formed by the endosteal and meningeal layers of dura mater that are part of an evagination of the cerebellar tentorium near the apex of the petrous part of the temporal bone. It is bounded by four structures:

- Superolateral: cerebellar tentorium
- Superomedial: the lateral wall of the cavernous sinus
- Medial: clivus
- Inferolateral: posterior petrous face.\

The subarachnoid space continues along the posterior aspect of Meckel's cave, representing a continuation of the cerebral basal cisterns.[1]

Pathologies and Its Variants

Pathologies of Meckel's cave are generally divided into:

- **Intrinsic:** Originating within Meckel's cave with an outward expansion:
  - Trigeminal schwannoma
  - Meningioma
  - Rarely, lymphoma or vascular tumors
- **Extrinsic:** Originating outside Meckel's cave and invading the cavity:
  - Bony metastasis
  - Chordoma
  - Chondrosarcoma

Clinical Features

The main clinical presentation of Meckel's cave pathologies is maxillary numbness or trigeminal neuralgia (TN). Some patients may complain of hemifacial pain, frontal and mandibular numbness, or reduced sensation. The classical TN presents with an intense, short and sharp pain usually triggered by minimal stimulation in ≥ 1 branches. An atypical TN, however, presents with a dull constant pain intermittently accompanied by sharp paroxysmal painful episodes. The majority of TN cases have no structural etiology (idiopathic TN). An etiology is found in up to 15% of cases with a correlating structural imaging finding (symptomatic TN).

Extensive Meckel's cave lesion may present with meningeal pain and other focal neurological deficits.

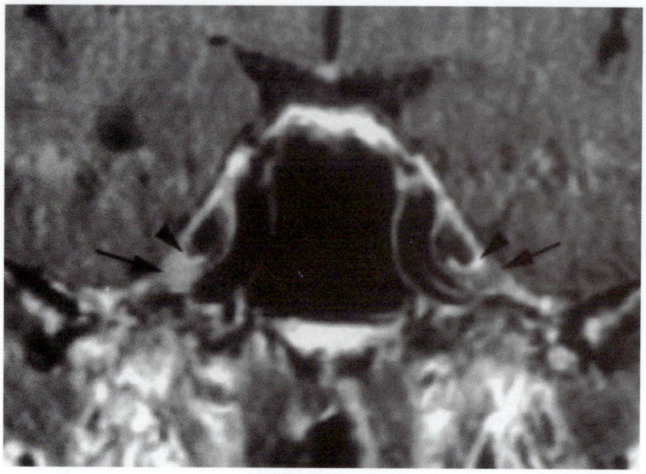

Fig. 30.1 A coronal gadolinium-enhanced T1-MRI section illustrating a slightly less enhancing right trigeminal ganglion (right arrow) as compared to the perineural venous plexus (right arrowhead). This appearance is thought to be caused by an obscuration of the ganglion by an unusually extensive perineural venous plexus. On the contralateral side, the typical appearance of the trigeminal ganglion (left arrow) and the adjacent venous plexus (left arrowhead) is delineated.

Radiological Features

A gadolinium-enhanced magnetic resonance imaging (MRI) is the mainstay radiological modality to assess the nerve and lesions involving Meckel's cave.[3]

In gadolinium-enhanced T1-weighted MRI sections, the trigeminal ganglion usually enhances together with the perineural venous plexus, thus not allowing to identify these structures separately (**Fig. 30.1**).

References

1. Burr HS, Robinson GB. An anatomical study of the gasserian ganglion with particular reference to the nature and extend of Meckel's Cave (MC). Anat Rec 1925;29:269–282
2. Sundararajan S, Loevner LA, Mohan S. Mandibular myalgia and miniscule Meckel's caves ORL J Otorhinolaryngol Relat Spec 2018;80(2):103–107
3. Williams LS, Schmalfuss IM, Sistrom CL, et al. MR imaging of the trigeminal ganglion, nerve, and the perineural vascular plexus: normal appearance and variants with correlation to cadaver specimens. AJNR Am J Neuroradiol 2003;24(7):1317–1323

Chapter 31 Endonasal Endoscopic Surgeries at Meckel's Cave

Revadi Govindaraju, Michel Roethlisberger, A.B. Zulkiflee, Prepageran Narayanan, and Vicknes Waran

Case 31A

Endoscopic Transnasal Biopsy of Meckel's Cave Tumor

History

A 60-year-old man presented to the outpatient clinic complaining of pain in the left cheek and an inability to whistle and to chew for the past 3 months. He had no other comorbidities. On examination, he had a reduced sensation over the left forehead, cheek, and chin (V1, V2, and V3). His facial muscular movements were normal. Other cranial nerves and general neurologic examinations revealed no significant findings.

Magnetic resonance imaging (MRI) demonstrated an ill-defined lesion with heterogenous contrast enhancement at the left Meckel's cave extending into the infratemporal fossa (**Fig. 31A.1 a–e**). Hence, an endonasal endoscopic transpterygoidal biopsy was performed.

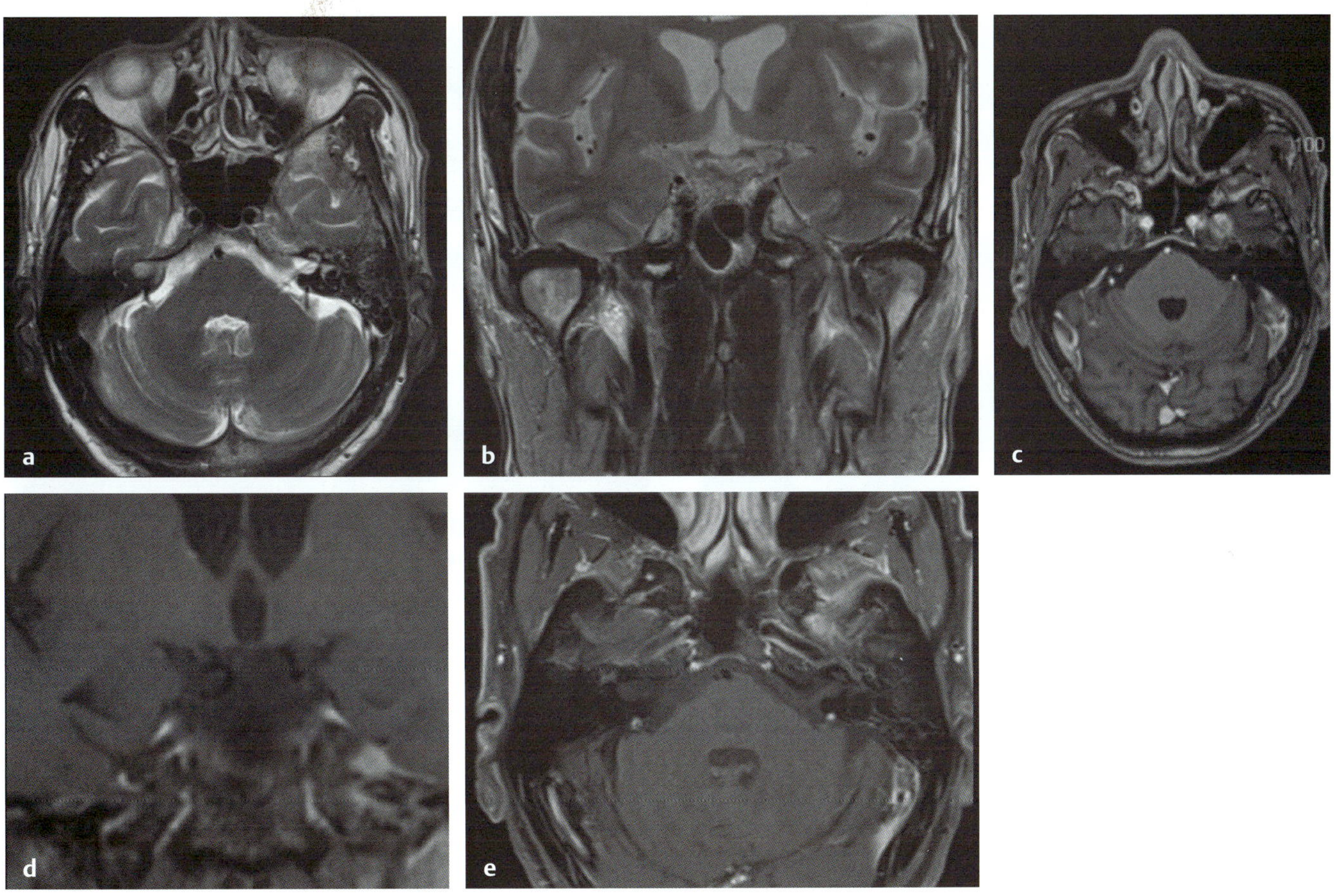

Fig. 31A.1 **(a, b)** Axial and coronal T2-weighted MRI sections demonstrating an ill-defined isointense mass located within the left Meckel's cave. **(c)** Axial T1-weighted contrast-enhanced fat-supressed MRI section demonstrating enhancement of the mass and extension into the infratemporal fossa. **(d, e)** Coronal and axial T1-weighted fat-supressed sequences revealing a contrast-enhancing lesion at Meckel's cave with extension into the infratemporal fossa.

Surgical Steps

1. The patient is placed under general anesthesia in the supine position and the head is fixed slightly retroflexed within a NORAS frame for intraoperative MRI. Registration for image-guided surgery (IGS) is performed.
2. The nose is decongested with adrenaline 1:1,000 units soaked in cotton pledgets and mucosal infiltration is done with local anesthetics and adrenaline 1:1,000 units.
3. A left middle meatal antrostomy, a complete ethmoidectomy, and a middle turbinectomy are performed.
4. Local anesthesia is also infiltrated into the septum to raise the mucoperichondrial/mucoperiosteal flaps bilaterally, and the posterior aspect of the cartilaginous and bony septum is removed.
5. The pedicled nasoseptal flaps are raised and are stored in the nasopharynx.
6. Once the sphenoid keel is fully exposed, the ostia are widened inferomedially using Kerrison's punch in a V shape toward the midline, and the anterior wall of the left sphenoid sinus is widened laterally.
7. The septal window and wide sphenoidotomy allow for a four-handed technique as well as good access and view to the lateral aspect of the sphenoid sinus (**Fig. 31A.2**).
8. The sphenoid cavity is demucosalized, and the crucial neurovascular landmarks of the bony skull base are identified.
9. The most anterior and lateral extensions of the lesion are identified using intraoperative image-guided surgery (IGS).
10. Drilling of the bone overlying the anterior part of the trigeminal ganglion and lateral aspect of the paraclival internal carotid artery is done using a high-speed diamond burr (**Fig. 31A.3**).
11. Once the bone has been sufficiently thinned, a right-angle dissector can be insinuated between the bone and the dura, and the bone is flaked off.

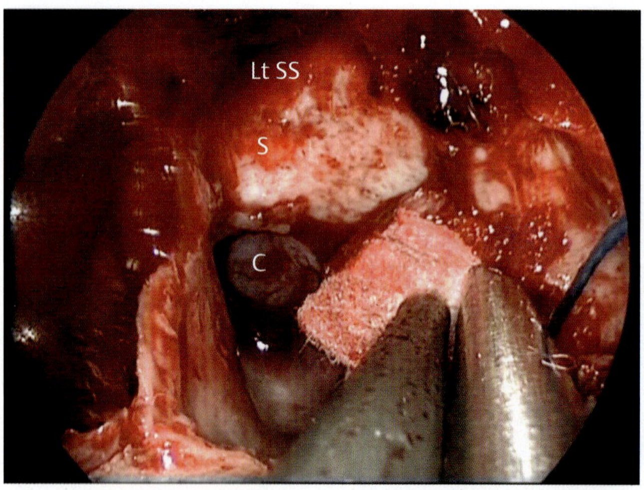

Fig. 31A.2 Endonasal endoscopic view and instrumentation of the site of pathology made possible by the septal window and the four-handed technique.

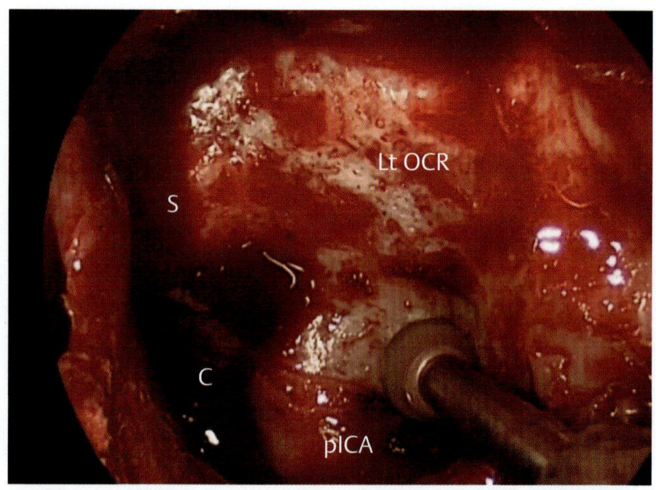

Fig. 31A.3 Drilling is performed on the lateral aspect of the paraclival internal carotid artery (pICA) using a high-speed diamond burr to access the trigeminal ganglion.

12. After an adequate amount of bone is removed with drilling (**Fig. 31A.4**), the bony exposure is completed with Kerrison's punch (**Fig. 31A.5**). This should allow the identification of important landmarks such as the maxillary nerve, the dura overlying Meckel's cave, and the lateral aspect of the paraclival internal carotid artery (**Fig. 31A.6**).
13. The incision of the dura covering Meckel's cave is performed with a microknife. (**Fig. 31A.7**).

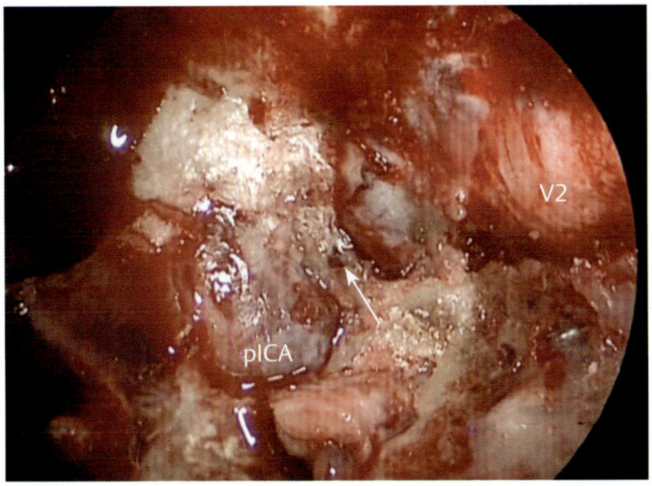

Fig. 31A.4 The dura covering the maxillary nerve and the anteroinferior part of the paraclival internal carotid artery (pICA) is exposed after drilling, leaving the bone of the lingual recess (*white arrow*) in between Meckel's cave and the pICA.

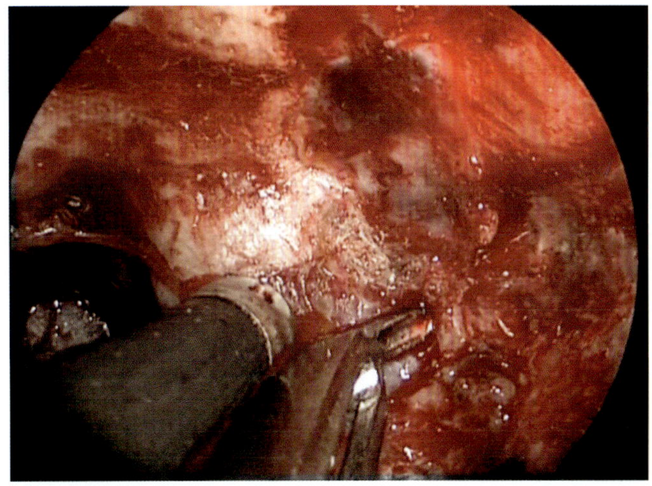

Fig. 31A.5A Kerrison's punch is used to completely remove the bone overlying the Meckel's cave.

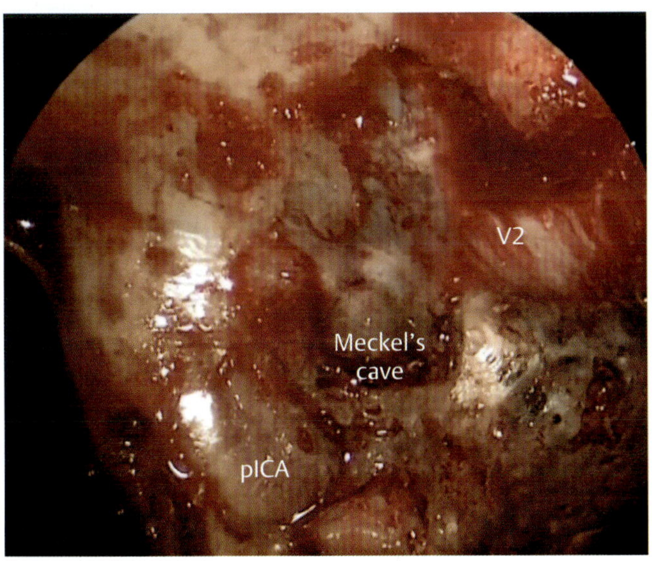

Fig. 31A.6 The dura covering the Meckel's cave is exposed, and the maxillary nerve is seen coursing anteriorly.

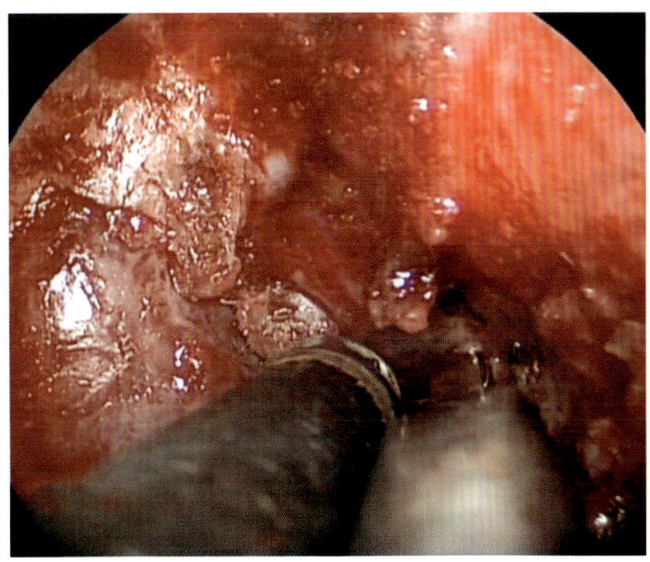

Fig. 31A.7 The incision of the dura covering the Meckel's cave.

14. Bleeding occurring from the inferior part of the cavernous sinus is controlled with hemostats such as Floseal and Surgicel (**Fig. 31A.8**).
15. The trigeminal ganglion (TGG) is then skeletonized and retracted using a right-angled probe (**Fig. 31A.9**).
16. The tumor lateral to the TG is carefully biopsied using a microcurette (**Fig. 31A.10**).
17. The defect is then covered with the nasoseptal flap raised earlier (**Fig. 31A.11**).

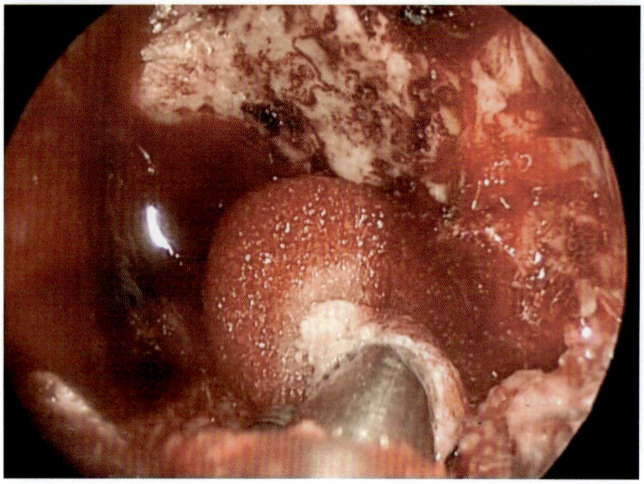

Fig. 31A.8 Floseal is delivered using the Taming sari device to control bleeding from the inferior cavernous sinus.

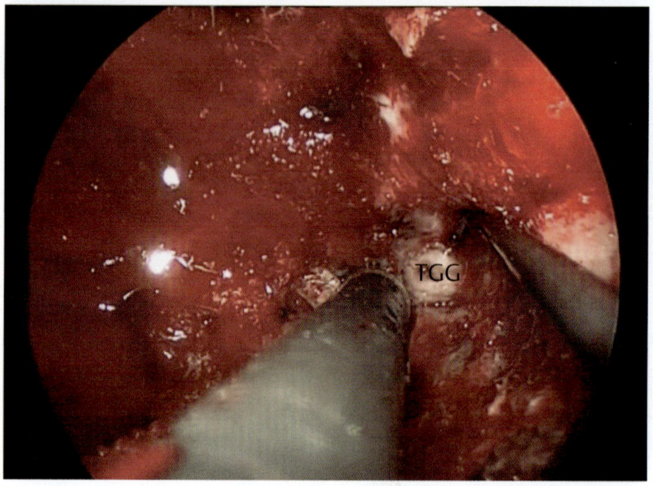

Fig. 31A.9 The trigeminal ganglion (TGG) is well skeletonized and retracted medially with an angled probe.

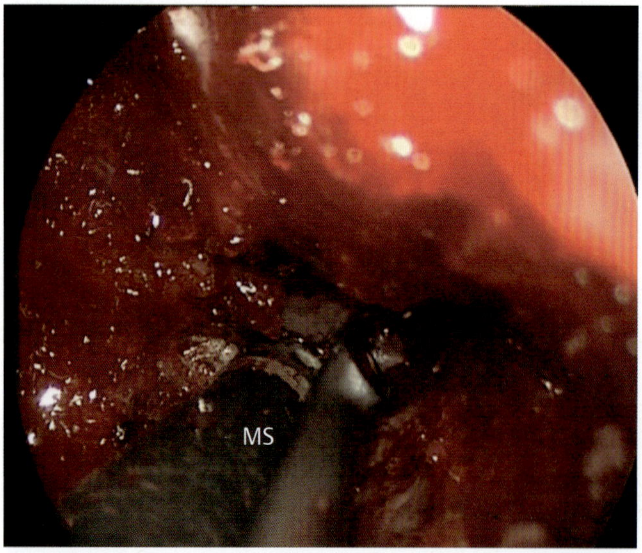

Fig. 31A.10 The tumor is biopsied using a small curette.

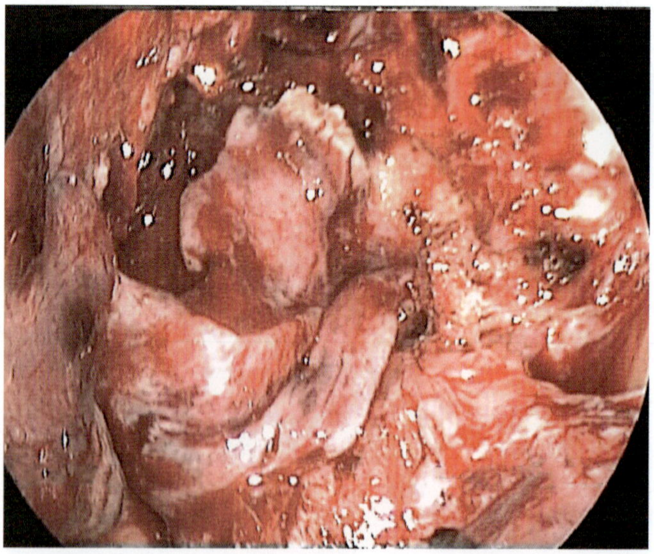

Fig. 31A.11 The nasoseptal flap is used to reconstruct the skull base defect.

Case 31B

Endoscopic Transnasal Excision of a Giant Ancient Meckel's Cave Trigeminal Schwannoma

History

A 35-year-old man presented to the ENT outpatient clinic with a 9-month history of right-sided facial numbness. He had no other complaints or comorbidities. On examination, there was reduced sensation over the right forehead, cheek and chin (V1, V2, and V3). Other cranial nerves and general neurologic examinations revealed no significant findings. Endoscopic examination of the right nasal cavity revealed a mass in the middle meatus (**Fig. 31B.1**).

Magnetic resonance imaging (MRI) was performed and revealed a huge mass occupying the maxillary sinus, pterygoid and infratemporal fossa, and the region of Meckel's cave (**Figs. 31B.2 and 31B.3**). An endonasal endoscopic excision of the tumorous mass via a transpterygoid approach was recommended. Histopathological examination revealed giant ancient trigeminal schwannoma.

Surgical Steps

1. The patient is placed under general anesthesia in the supine position, and the head is fixed slightly retroflexed within a NORAS frame for intraoperative MRI and registration performed for neuronavigation.
2. The nose is decongested with adrenaline 1:1,000 units soaked in cotton pledgets, and mucosal infiltration of the lateral nasal wall and the septum are done with local anesthetics and adrenaline 1:1,000 units.
3. A septal window is created for the purpose of utilizing the two-surgeon three-handed technique, which allows the assistant to perform retraction and suctioning (**Fig. 31B.4**).
4. A medial maxillectomy and a middle turbinectomy are performed for the maximum exposure of the tumor and to allow adequate surgical access (**Fig. 31B.4**).

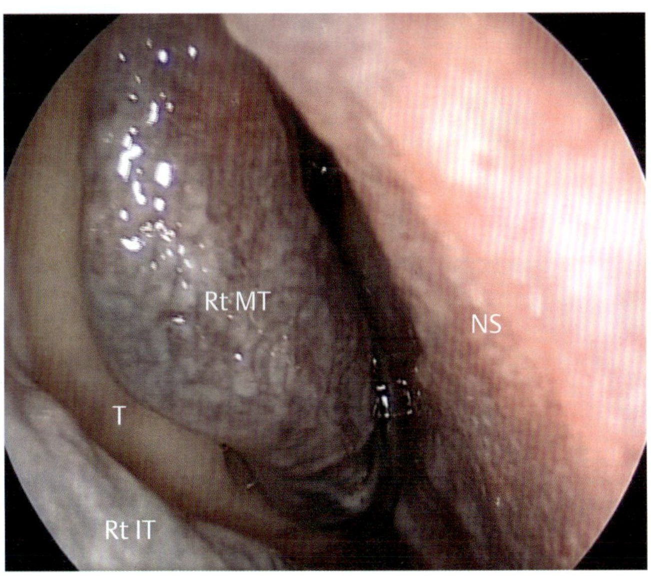

Fig. 31B.1 Endoscopic endonasal view of the right nasal cavity revealing the tumor (T) in the middle meatus.

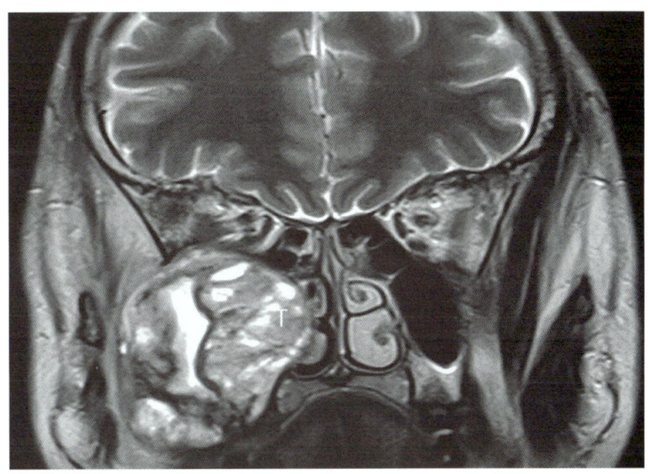

Fig. 31B.2 Coronal T2-weighted MRI section demonstrating a heterogenous lobulated mass occupying the maxillary sinus, extending into the infratemporal fossa laterally, bulging into the nasal cavity medially, and abutting the orbit superiorly.

5. The soft core of the tumor is first removed, allowing the capsule to collapse and to help delineate the deeper extent of the tumor (**Fig. 31B.5**).
6. Once the tumor is removed from the infratemporal fossa and the Meckel's cave region, the remaining capsule attached to the lateral wall of the maxillary sinus is removed (**Fig. 31B.6**).
7. With the complete removal of the tumor, the cavity created by expansion of the tumor comes into view. The pterygoid base, pterygoid plates, and petrous apex have been eroded by the tumor, leaving the infratemporal fossa exposed (**Fig. 31B.7**). The paraclival and petrous segments of the internal carotid artery, the dura covering the cavernous sinus, and Meckel's cave are identified consecutively (**Fig. 31B.8**).

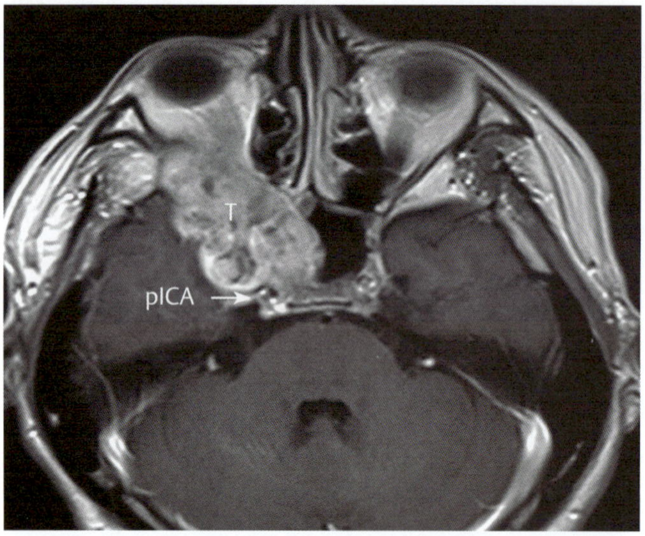

Fig. 31B.3 Axial T1-weighted contrast-enhanced MRI section demonstrating the superior extent of the tumor into the middle cranial fossa and its posterior relationship with the paraclival internal carotid artery.

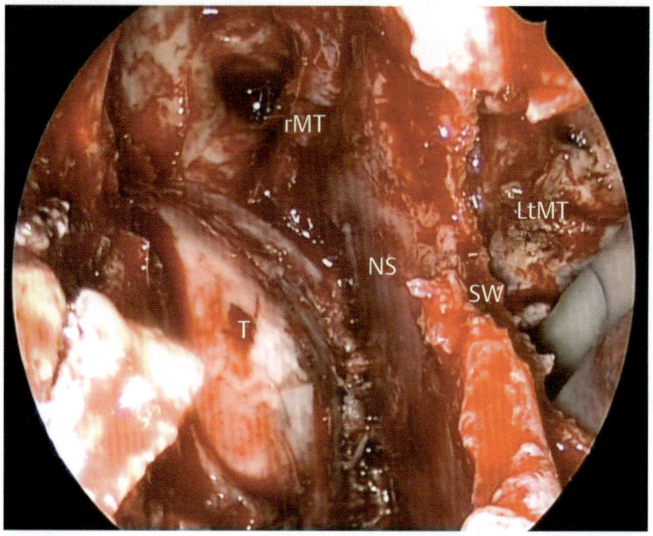

Fig. 31B.4 Endonasal endoscopic view of the tumor in the maxillary antrum after medial maxillectomy. The septal window and stump of the middle turbinate are also seen.

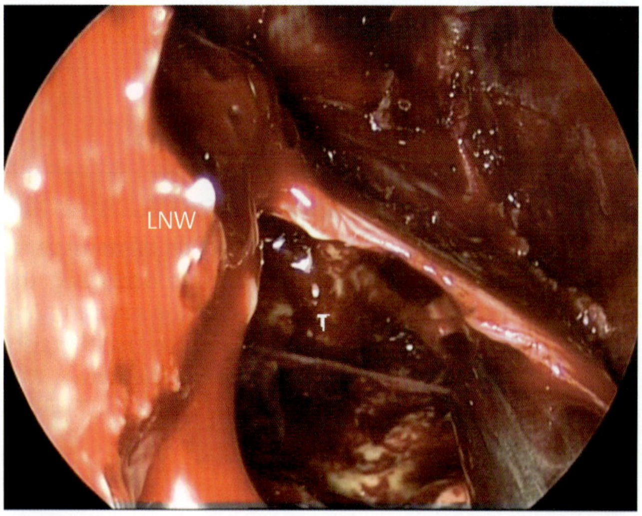

Fig. 31B.5 The core of the tumor that is soft is removed with a suction device.

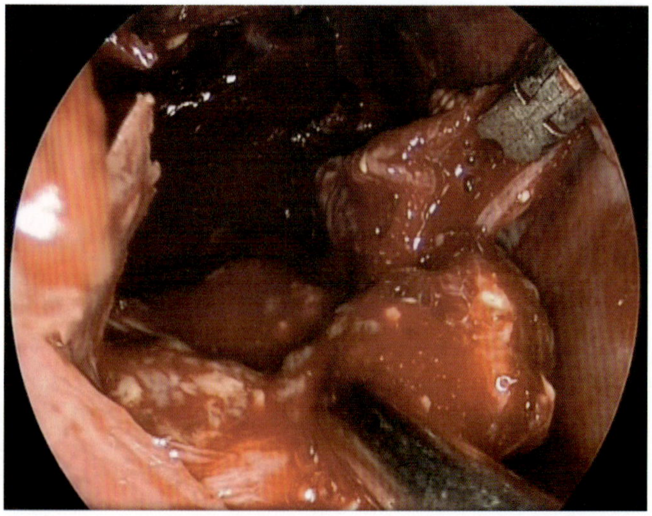

Fig. 31B.6 The capsule and the remaining tumor attachment to the lateral wall of the maxillary sinus are removed.

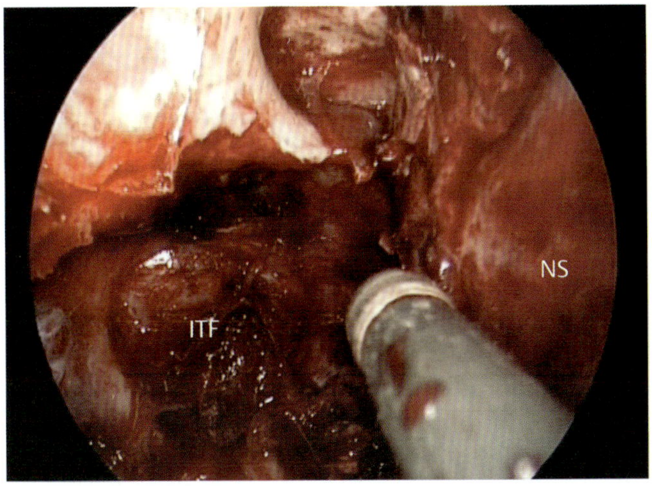

Fig. 31B.7 Final view after tumor excision reveals the exposed infratemporal fossa (ITF) cavity.

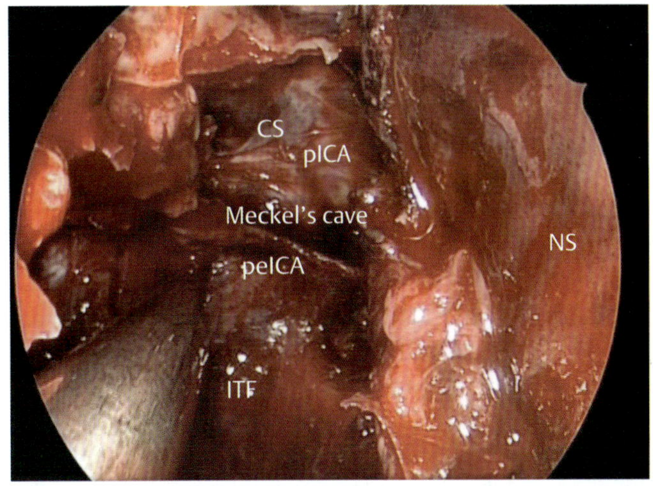

Fig. 31B.8 A close-up view reveals the dura covering the cavernous sinus, Meckel's cave, and paraclival (pICA) and petrous (peICA) segments of the internal carotid artery, exposed by the posterosuperior extension of the tumor.

Chapter 32 Trigeminal Schwannomas

Alexandre B. Todeschini, Bradley A. Otto, Ricardo L. Carrau, and Daniel M. Prevedello

Introduction

The first reported case of a trigeminal schwannoma was by Dixon in 1846.[1,2] They are seldom reported, being rare tumors of the cranial base. The first case series would only be reported in 1952 by Cuneo and Rand.[3] Initial reviews and case series, such as the study by Schisano and Olivecrona, reported a very high 1-year mortality rate (41%).[4] They are histologically benign tumors and can arise from any point of the trigeminal nerve, from the root near the brainstem to the distal extracranial branches.[5–7] It is the second most common intracranial schwannoma (after vestibular lesions), representing 0.5 to 1.5% of all intracranial lesions and 0.8 to 8% of all intracranial schwannomas. There is a slight female predominance, with a peak incidence between the third and fifth decades.[1,2,5–7]

Clinical Presentation

The natural history of these tumors is not well known, with variable presentations, depending on tumor location.[8] Oftentimes, it is an incidental finding in an imaging examination for unrelated issues. Small and asymptomatic lesions may be treated conservatively, with serial imaging.[7,8] There is not a specific interval recommended between examinations. In the authors' institution, they repeat the imaging examination within 3 months after diagnosis to ensure that the lesion is not growing rapidly, which would suggest the need for surgical management. The second imaging follow-up should be at 9 months after diagnosis and then yearly. If, at any time, the patient presents with symptoms, an earlier imaging study should be done.

As mentioned before, the clinical presentation depends on the location of the tumor, with no specific clinical findings associated with this type of lesion.[1,5,6] As expected, the most common symptom referred by patients is trigeminal nerve dysfunction (hypoesthesia, motor deficit, or facial pain), which may involve one or more trigeminal branches, present in 70 to 95% of cases.[1,2,5,6] It has been suggested that complete anesthesia in all three division is an indicator of invasion of the trigeminal ganglion. Headaches (different from facial pain) are identified in 28% of patients.[1] Diplopia is present in 10 to 52% of cases, being higher in dumbbell-shaped lesions. The main nerve related to extrinsic eye movement affected is the sixth cranial nerve, followed by the fourth and the third cranial nerves, respectively.[1,2,5,6] Other symptoms that may be present are vertigo and hearing loss, facial palsy, and ataxia.[1,2,7] It is uncommon, but large tumors can also lead to dysfunction of lower cranial nerves.[1,5]

Imaging Studies

Trigeminal schwannomas tend to appear as isodense or hypodense to brain parenchyma on computed tomography (CT), with avid enhancement after contrast administration. On magnetic resonance imaging (MRI) they are iso- to hypointense lesions on T1-weighted images and hyperintense on T2-weighted images, with significant enhancement after gadolinium injection. Cystic and necrotic changes are present in up to 54% of tumors.[1] A high-quality, high-powered field (3T) MRI complemented with computed tomography angiography (CTA) offers excellent information on type of tumor, relationship to neighboring neural and vascular structures, and bone changes (e.g., enlargement of the superior orbital fissure [SOF], foramen *rotundum*, foramen *ovale*, and erosion of the middle fossa and petrous apex).[8,9] The position of the internal carotid artery (ICA) in relation to the tumor is a key factor on the approach selection.[10–12] The use of modern MRI acquisition sequences (fast imaging employing steady-state acquisition [FIESTA] diffusion tension imaging [DTI]) also offers a reliable method of identifying the position of nerves surrounding the tumor.[13–14] The pre- and postoperative images illustrating the case examples at the end better demonstrate these characteristics.

Classifications

These tumors can be intradural, interdural, or extradural, possibly involving multiple anatomical compartments: posterior fossa, middle fossa, Meckel's cave, extending along the ophthalmic division of the trigeminal nerve (V1; into the orbit), maxillary division of the trigeminal nerve (V2; into the pterygopalatine fossa [PPF]), or mandibular division of the trigeminal nerve (V3; into the infratemporal fossa).[10] Different classifications for trigeminal schwannomas have been created to describe the affected compartments, according to imaging studies.

The earliest classification by Jefferson in 1953[15] divided tumors in three types: type A (of the gasserian ganglion in the middle fossa), type B (of the root of the nerve in the posterior fossa), and type C (dumbbell shaped in the posterior and middle fossae). Day and Fukushima[16] added the type D (of the peripheral branches in the extracranial space). A more recent classification by Yoshida and Kawase[17] divides the tumors in type P (posterior fossa tumors in the subdural space), type M (middle fossa tumors in the interdural space), type E (extracranial tumors in the epidural space), type E1 (tumor in the orbit), type E2 (tumor in the pterygopalatine and infratemporal fossae), type MP (dumbbell-shaped tumor in the middle and posterior fossae), type ME (dumbbell-shaped tumor in the middle fossa and extracranial space), and type MPE (tumor involving the posterior fossa, middle fossa, and extracranial space).[8,18] **Table 32.1** summarizes and relates the different classifications mentioned.

Surgical Anatomy

Careful preoperative imaging of these lesions enables the treatment team to have a clear understanding of the anatomy surrounding the tumor to plan the best approach to these complex, multicompartmental lesions.[7–9] The trigeminal nerve is formed by axons originating from four nuclei: the mesencephalic nucleus (in the mesencephalon and upper pons; pressure and proprioception); the principal sensory nucleus (in the upper pons; tactile and pressure sense); the spinal trigeminal nucleus (in the midpons extending caudally into the upper cervical medulla; pain, temperature, and tactile sensation); and the motor nucleus (in the tegmentum of the pons).[18]

At the cisternal segment (**Fig. 32.1**), the trigeminal root emerges from the lateral surface of the midpons extending anteriorly in the prepontine cistern, along the medial aspect of the petrous apex. It is formed by a large sensory root and a smaller motor root, which lies on the anterosuperomedial side of the sensory root. The nerve passes through the *porus trigeminus*, located at the trigeminal depression of the petrous apex, formed by the posterior petroclinoid ligament and the base of the posterior clinoid process (**Fig. 32.2**).

Through the *porus trigeminus*, it reaches Meckel's cave in the middle fossa (**Fig. 32.3**). Meckel's cave is a space between the meningeal and periosteal layers of dura mater, from the posterior fossa into the posteromedial portion of the middle fossa. These two layers of dura mater form the basis of the peeling of the middle fossa for surgical approaches, which the authors will discuss momentarily. From Meckel's

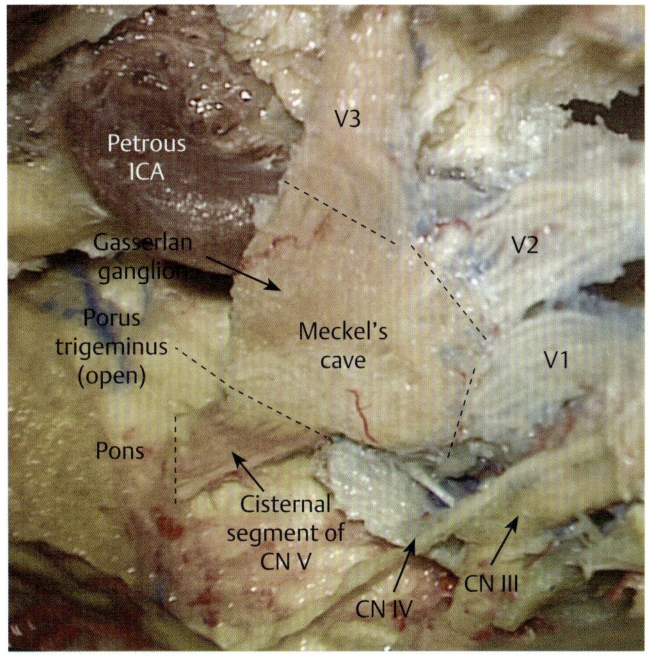

Fig. 32.1 Cadaveric specimen dissection showing the trigeminal ganglion in Meckel's cave, the cisternal segment of the trigeminal nerve emerging from the pons, and the three divisions: ophthalmic (V1), maxillary (V2), and mandibular (V3). The petrous bone was drilled to expose the posterior fossa and the petrous internal carotid artery (peICA).

Table 32.1 Different classifications described for trigeminal schwannomas

Yoshida and Kawase	Description	Jefferson/Day and Fukushima
P	Posterior fossa tumor in the subdural space	B
M	Middle fossa tumor in the interdural space	A
E	Extracranial tumor in the epidural space	D
E1	Tumor invading the orbit	
E2	Tumor in the pterygopalatine and infratemporal fossae	
MP	Dumbbell-shaped tumor in the middle and posterior fossae	C
ME	Dumbbell-shaped tumor in the middle fossa and extracranial space	
MPE	Tumor involving the posterior fossa, middle fossa, and extracranial space	

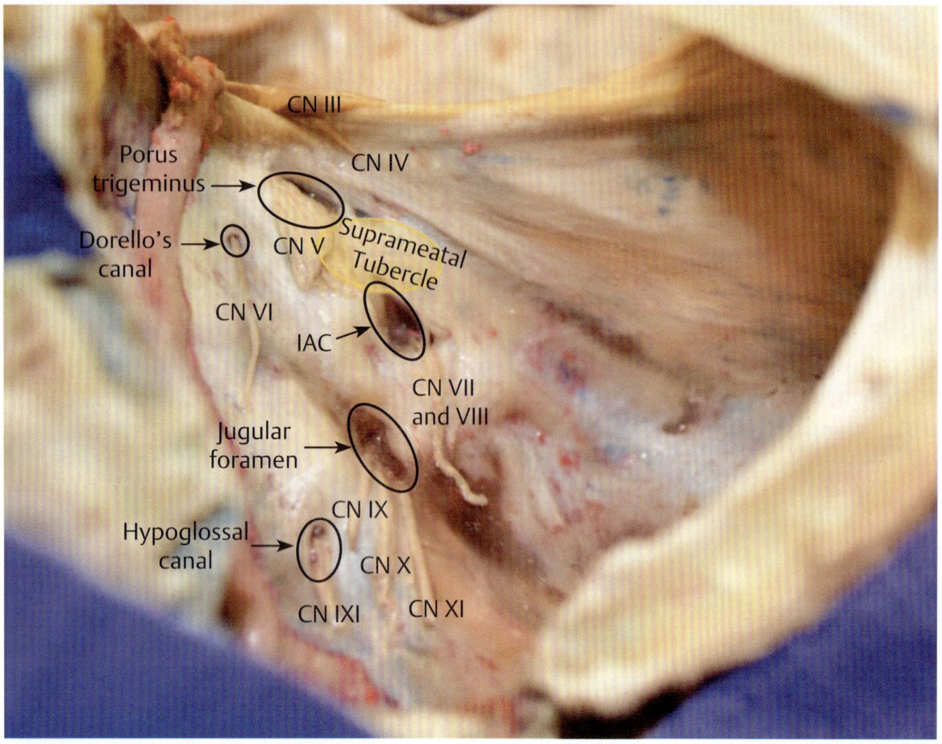

Fig. 32.2 Cadaveric specimen with the cerebellum removed and only the cranial nerves preserved to show their respective foramens.

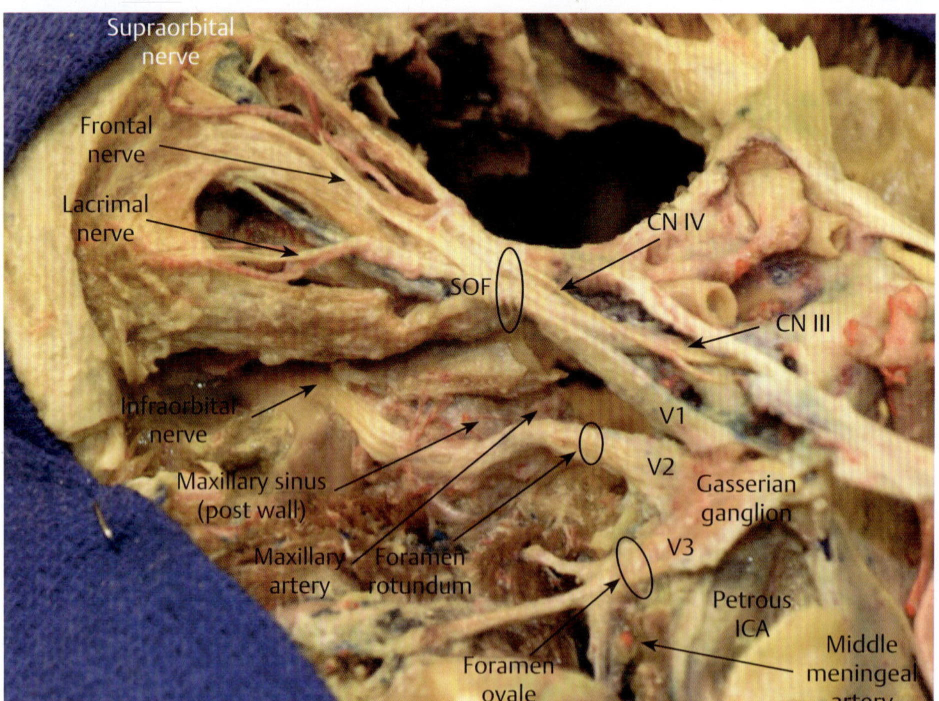

Fig. 32.3 Cadaveric specimen extensive dissection of the cranial base, showing the peripheral anatomy of the trigeminal divisions into the orbit (V1), the pterygopalatine fossa (V2), and the infratemporal fossa (V3) from a lateral view.

cave, the three main divisions of the trigeminal nerve emerge anteriorly.

The ophthalmic division (V1) courses upward and travels anteriorly in the lower portion of the lateral wall of the cavernous sinus to reach the SOF, after which it branches into the lacrimal, nasociliary, and frontal nerves (**Fig. 32.3**).

The maxillary division (V2) emerges anteriorly as the intermediate division of the three. It travels beneath the dura of the middle fossa below the junction of the lateral and medial walls of the cavernous sinus to foramen *rotundum* to enter the PPF. The PPF is embedded in fat, with the pterygopalatine ganglion and its branches and the maxillary artery and its branches. When approaching this area, it is important to remember that the neural structures lie posterior to the vascular (maxillary artery and branches). From the PPF, it enters the infraorbital canal and becomes the infraorbital nerve, running below the floor of the orbit on the roof of the maxillary sinus until it emerges on the face through the infraorbital foramen (**Fig. 32.3** and **Fig. 32.4**). Along its course, it gives of the zygomatic nerve, posterior superior alveolar nerves, the palatine nerves, the nasopalatine nerve, the pharyngeal nerve, the middle and anterior superior alveolar nerves, and the inferior palpebral and the superior labial branches.

The mandibular division (V3) is the largest and most caudal of the three. It emerges from Meckel's cave in an anteroinferior direction passing through foramen *ovale* into the infratemporal fossa (**Fig. 32.3**). The motor fibers travel in the small motor root, passing under the trigeminal ganglion (or semilunar ganglion), to join the sensory fibers after crossing foramen *ovale*. In the infratemporal fossa, V3 passes between the *tensor veli palatini* (medial) and the medial pterygoid (lateral) muscles. It gives a meningeal branch (sensory), which passes through the foramen spinosum with the middle meningeal artery to innervate the middle fossa dura, and a medial pterygoid (motor), *tensor veli palatini* (motor), and *tensor timpani* (motor) nerves. Then, it divides into anterior (smaller) and posterior (larger) divisions. From the anterior division of V3 emerges the buccal (sensory), masseteric (motor), deep temporal (motor), and lateral pterygoid (motor) nerves; from the posterior division emerges the auriculotemporal (sensory), inferior alveolar (sensory and motor to the mylohyoid muscle and the anterior belly of the digastric muscle), and lingual (sensory) nerves.

Surgical Approaches

With a clear understanding of the anatomy of the trigeminal nerve and careful analysis of the imaging examinations, the best surgical approach can be planned. While early surgical series reported very high mortality (41%),[4] more recent series report a low morbidity/mortality associated with surgery and complementary treatments. This change is largely attributed to the advances in neuroimaging, electrophysiological monitoring, microsurgical techniques, and newer skull base approaches.[2,5,6,10,19]

When planning surgery, different surgical corridors may be used to reach the tumor and Meckel's cave: the posterior corridor through a retrosigmoid craniotomy; the lateral corridor through a temporal craniotomy; the anterolateral corridor through orbitozygomatic (O-Zy) or transorbital approach; and the anteromedial corridor through an endoscopic endonasal approach (EEA; **Fig. 32.5**). These approaches and their limitations and indications are discussed in detail.

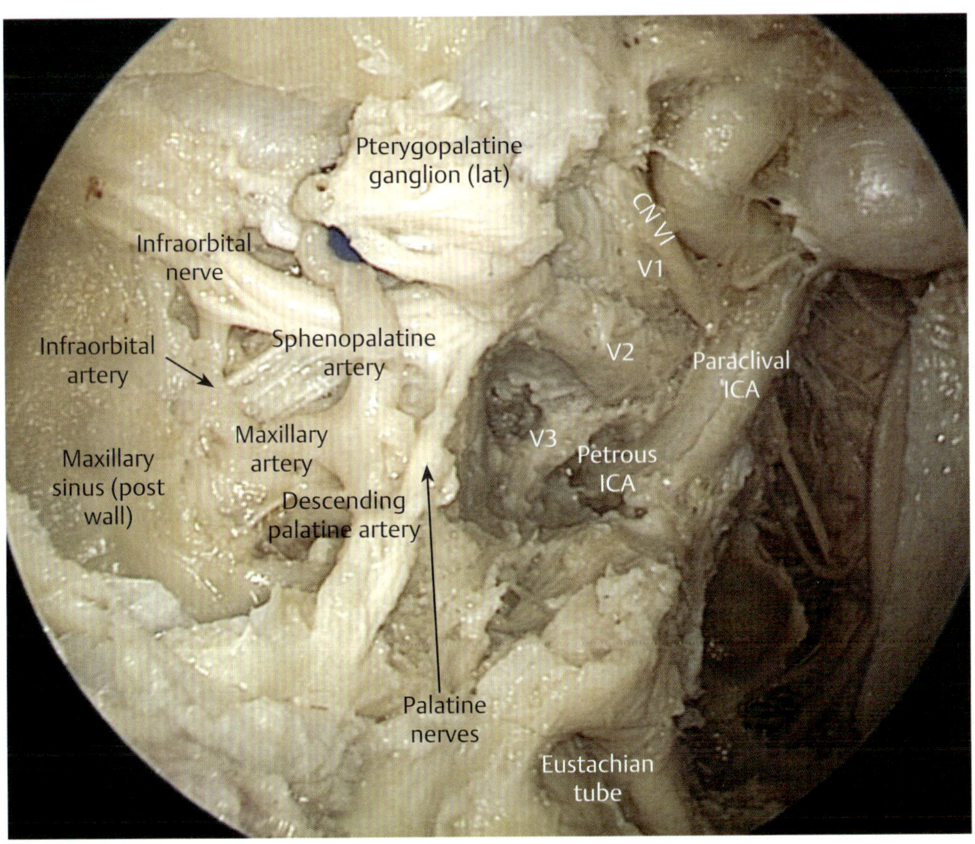

Fig. 32.4 Cadaveric specimen endonasal endoscopic dissection after a transpterygoid approach to show the anatomical structures involved. ICA, internal carotid artery.

Posterior Corridor

This corridor is optimal for "B" tumors[15,16] or "P" tumors.[17] Some of the "MP" lesions[17] may be reached through this corridor by drilling the suprameatal tubercle.[20] The retrosigmoid approach is recommended for lesions that are mainly located in the posterior fossa. This approach offers direct access to the posterior fossa and to the entire lateral aspect of the brainstem and cerebellum, from the tentorium to the foramen magnum and the cranial nerves III through XI.[21–24]

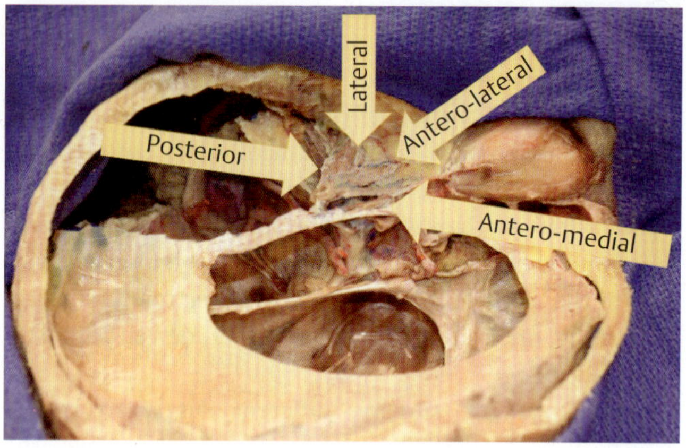

Fig. 32.5 Cadaveric specimen (encephalon removed) illustrating the different corridor to reach Meckel's cave.

The patient can be positioned supine with a shoulder bump and the head rotated to the contralateral side, or lateral, in the park bench position, when the neck does not allow rotation of the head, or in the sitting position. The sitting position offers a clearer surgical field with blood and cerebrospinal fluid (CSF) draining easily; however, it is associated with a higher incidence of air embolism (symptomatic or not).[25]

The head is supported and fixed by a three-pin fixation head holder. The authors do not routinely use a lumbar drain. The incision is placed 2 fingerbreadths behind the pinna (**Fig. 32.6a**). During this phase, image guidance helps place the incision as close as possible to the junction of the sigmoid and transverse sinuses. Careful planning of the incision helps prevent injury to the sinuses. The transverse sinus is located beneath the imaginary line between the external occipital protuberance and the origin of the zygomatic arch. The sigmoid sinus is identified by drawing a line 2 fingerbreadths

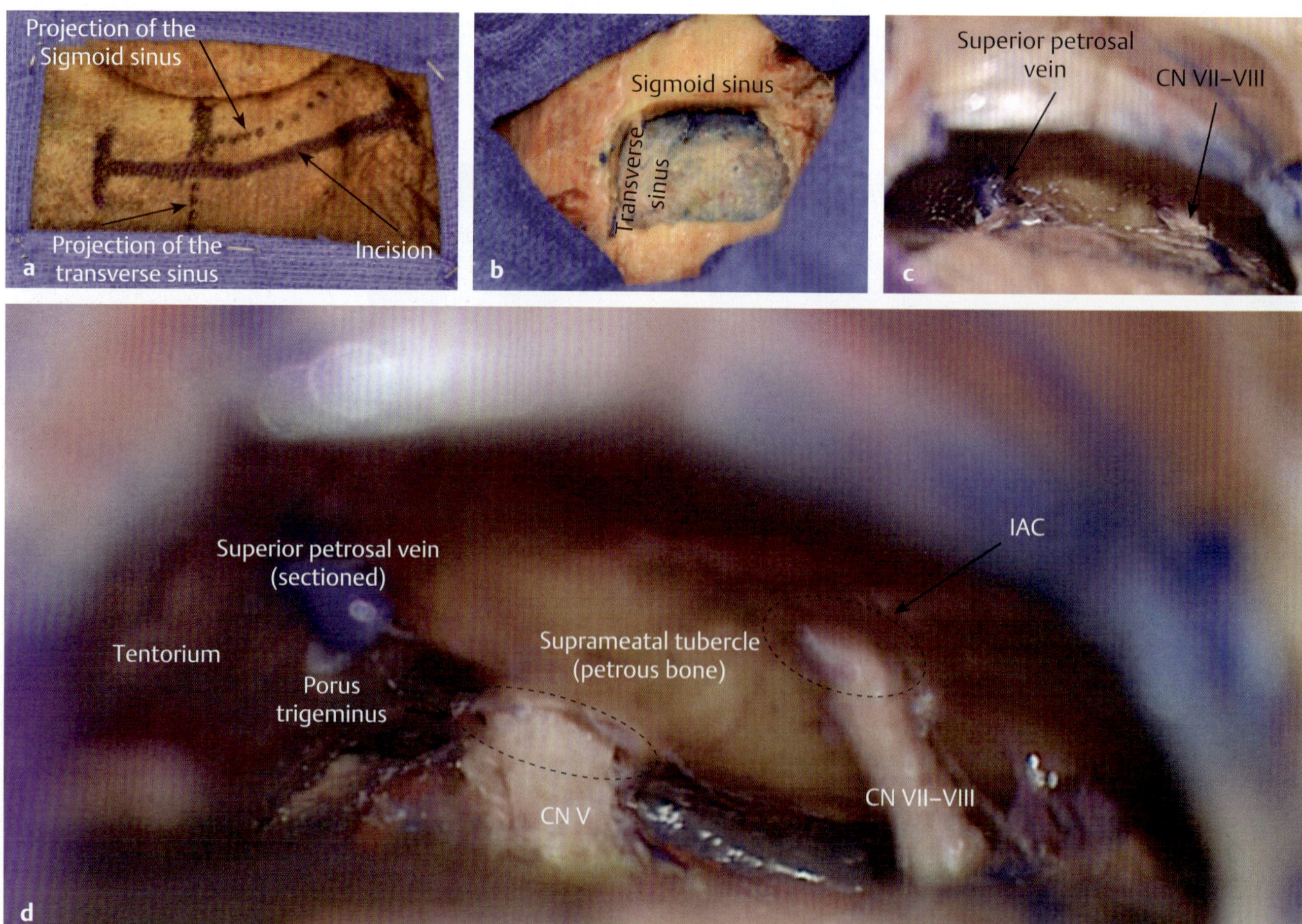

Fig. 32.6 (a–d) A retrosigmoid approach performed in a cadaveric specimen.

behind the ear aimed toward the mastoid tip.[22,23] After incision and elevation of the muscles, the asterion (junction of the lambdoid, parietomastoid, and occipitomastoid sutures) is used as a reference point to where the transverse and sigmoid sinus meet, and the sigmoid sinus is usually under the projection of an imaginary line from the parietomastoid suture to the mastoid tip.[22,23]

The craniotomy should expose the edge of both sinuses in the anterior and superior border (**Fig. 32.6b**). Mastoid air cells opened during the craniotomy should be carefully waxed. The dura is opened in a semicircular fashion with the base facing the sigmoid sinus.[21] Early after dural opening, the authors gently retract the inferior part of the cerebellum and open the cisterna magna to drain CSF, which relaxes the cerebellum making retractors seldom necessary to expose the lateral surface of the posterior fossa and identify the cranial nerves (**Fig. 32.6c, d**). The cerebellar surface is covered and protected.

Tumor exclusively in the posterior fossa can be resected without extending the approach using careful microsurgical dissection, in the lateromedial direction. If access to Meckel's cave and the middle fossa is also required, a *retrosigmoid intradural suprameatal approach (RISA)* (**Fig. 32.7**) can be done.[20] Once the tumor in the cerebellopontine angle (CPA) has been resected or debulked, the cranial nerves VII and VIII as well as the internal auditory canal (IAC; **Fig. 32.7a**) can be identified. The dura above the IAC is incised and elevated, exposing the suprameatal tubercle of the petrous bone (**Fig. 32.7b**), forming the superior lip of the porus, which can be drilled toward the middle fossa (**Fig. 32.7c**), dorsolateral to the trigeminal nerve and *porus trigeminus*. Meckel's cave can then be reached and the tumor followed into the middle fossa to expose the lateral margin of the trigeminal nerve in Meckel's cave and to complete resection (**Fig. 32.7d**). This drilling is a complex maneuver and should be performed by surgeons experienced in drilling the petrous bone. Anatomy laboratory practice is always recommended.[19,20]

When tumor removal is no longer possible using the microscope, an endoscope can be used to increase the extent of resection or even to complete it. The endoscope is inserted parallel to the posterior petrous ridge above the IAC, directed to Meckel's cave and the already enlarged *porus trigeminus*.[19] The endoscope can be used handheld by the surgeon or using a pneumatic arm to keep it steady. Different angled endoscopes can be used to carefully inspect Meckel's cave and to complete removal. The authors recommend that the endoscope be introduced into the surgical field not using its own image as guidance but looking through the microscope to avoid contact and damage to any delicate structures in the posterior fossa. Once the target is reached, the endoscope's image is used to complete the resection. Removing the endoscope from the surgical field should be equally careful to

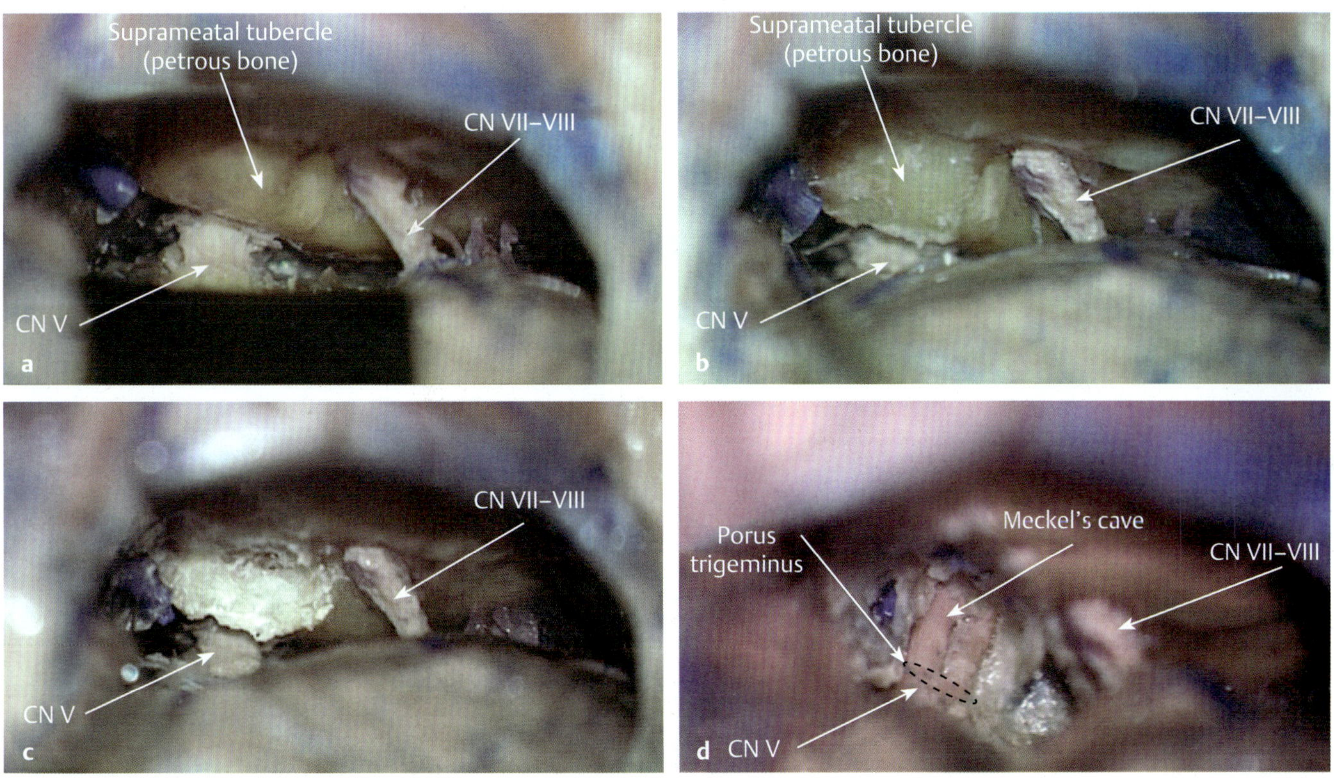

Fig. 32.7 (a–d) After the standard retrosigmoid approach, the suprameatal tubercle was drilled to gain access to Meckel's cave and even the middle fossa.

avoid damage to the peripheral limits of the narrow endoscopic corridor.[26] After tumor resection, reconstruction is performed in a standard fashion.

Lateral Corridor

The lateral corridor to Meckel's cave is done through a *middle fossa approach*, in a subtemporal extradural fashion (**Fig. 32.8**). Tumors ideally suited for this approach are the A type[15,16] or M type.[17] Extending the approach by drilling the petrous bone and the floor of the middle fossa may also allow the resection of lesion types MP, ME, and MPE,[17] but the middle fossa component is best to be approached through the lateral corridor.

A straight temporal incision usually allows sufficient exposure for the approach, but a curved frontotemporal incision behind the hair line can also be used. The craniotomy is usually 5 × 5 cm centered on the posterior origin of the zygomatic arch (**Fig. 32.8a**). According to the size of the lesion, a larger or more anterior craniotomy may occasionally be necessary. The inferior margin should be at the level of the floor of the middle fossa. Since this is an extradural approach, no cisterns can be tapped to remove CSF and reduce the retraction to the temporal lobe. A lumbar drain to remove 30 to 40 mL of CSF can reduce the traction and pressure applied to the temporal lobe and should be considered in a case-by-case basis. The dura is elevated of the floor of the middle fossa to expose its landmarks (**Fig. 32.8b**). The first landmark is the foramen *spinosum*, from which the middle meningeal artery emerges. After dissecting the artery, coagulating, and sectioning it, elevation of the dura can proceed to identify foramen *rotundum* with V2 entering it and foramen *ovale* with V3 entering it. Posterior to foramen *ovale* the lesser (lateral) and greater (medial) superficial petrosal nerves (GSPN) are identified. Carefully, using a sharp blade, the outer layer of the dura can be incised from the lateral side of foramen *rotundum* to foramen *ovale*, which allows the outer layer to be peeled, preserving the medial structures and separating the two layers of dura from posterior to anterior. During this stage, traction on the GSPN should be avoided, as it can lead to traction injury to the facial nerve. The authors recommend always striving to preserve GSPN to avoid postoperative dry eye and its ensuing complications; however, to preserve the facial nerve, GSPN can be sacrificed early in the peeling to avoid any traction to the geniculate ganglion. At this point, the resection of M-type tumors[17] from the middle fossa and cavernous sinus is possible, without entering the CSF space (**Fig. 32.8b**).[2,18,27–29]

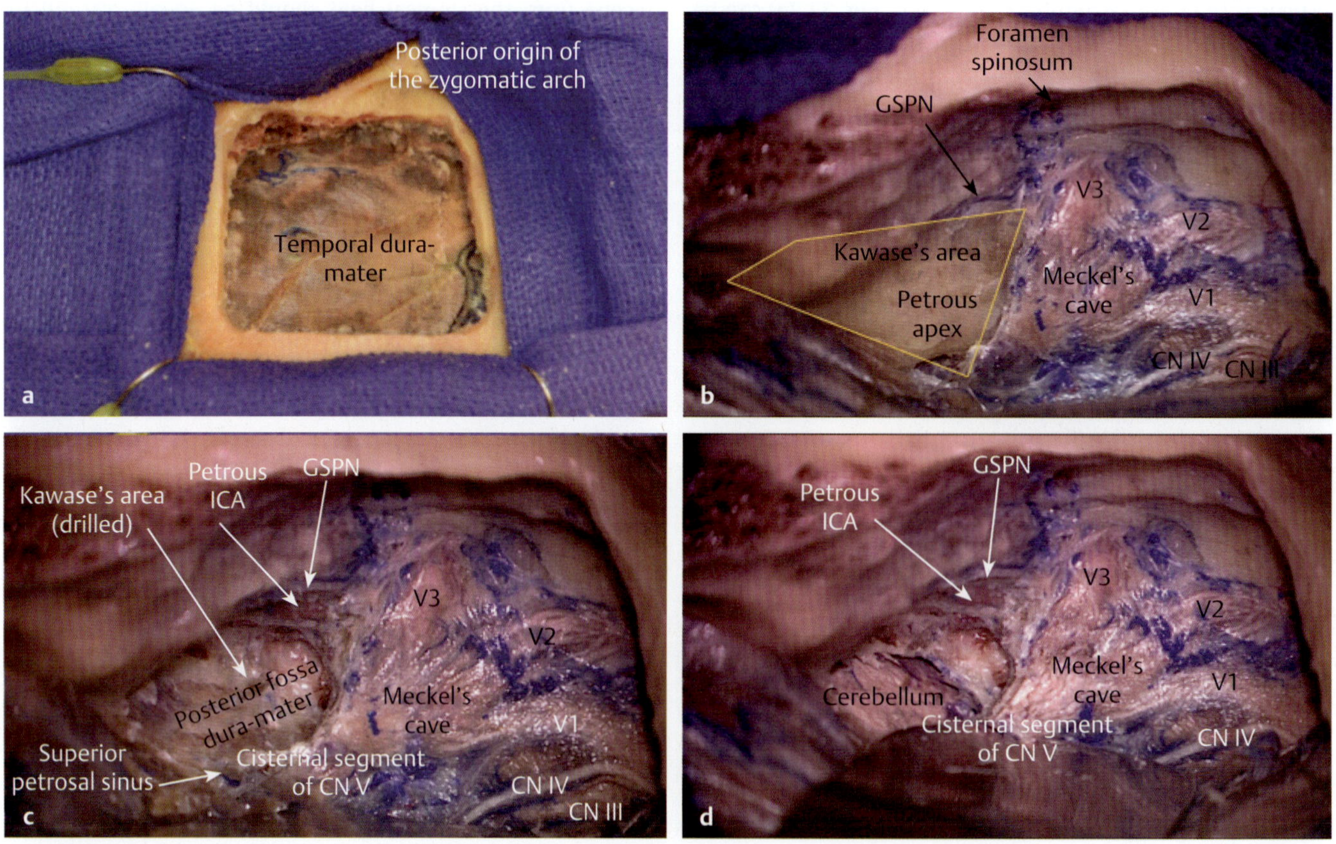

Fig. 32.8 (a–d) A middle fossa approach and peeling of the middle fossa done in a cadaveric specimen. Kawase's area was also drilled to expose the posterior fossa.

Larger tumors, extending into the posterior fossa (e.g., MP-type tumors[17]) can be reached through the middle fossa, using the *Shiobara–Kawase approach* (anterior petrosectomy).[30] Once the floor of the middle fossa is exposed, its landmarks and the important anatomical structures they delineate should be clearly identified. Anteriorly, Glasscock's triangle, underneath which the petrous ICA passes, is formed by the GSPN medially, V3 (foramen *ovale*) at the base, and laterally a line between foramen spinosum and the facial hiatus. Posteriorly, Kawase's triangle is limited by the arcuate eminence (an elevation on the floor of the middle fossa created by the superior semicircular canal); GSPN, laterally; and the petrous ridge medially. The IAC is located in the posterior part of Kawase's triangle, under the meatal plane, usually described as located in a 60-degree angle with the arcuate eminence or by bisecting the angle between GSPN and the arcuate eminence.[2,28,31]

Drilling these areas is a time-consuming process and requires high surgical skills with the drill, but once it is done, it offers a corridor into the posterior fossa to remove tumor extending to the CPA and the lateral and ventral areas of the brainstem (**Fig. 32.8c, d**).[18] When tumor resection using the microscope cannot be safely done anymore for lack of visualization, the endoscope can be brought into the surgical field to complete or maximize resection, using the same technique described for vestibular schwannomas.[27]

Tumor types ME and some select MPE,[17] extending into the infratemporal fossa, may also be removed through the middle fossa approach by drilling and removing the floor of the middle fossa until the margin of the tumor can be identified. Removal of the zygomatic arch may be required for this extended approach. For tumors with larger components in the extracranial space, other approaches may be better suited for it.[18]

Anterolateral Corridor

This corridor can be used to resect tumor types M, MP, ME, and MPE[17]; however, the reach into the posterior fossa is limited. It can be done through an anterior petrosectomy as described above, but to perform this drilling from this angle is challenging. When the posterior fossa component is small, it can be done, but if large, it is safer to combine this approach with a posterior corridor as detailed above. The same can be said about large extracranial components. Oftentimes, staging the approach through different corridors is safer for the patient, maximizes resection, and decreases morbidity, as it is true with other lesions involving multiple compartments.[9,29,32–34]

The objective of this corridor for these tumors is to reach the anterolateral portion of Meckel's cave and the trigeminal nerve. This can be achieved through different craniotomies, with more or less exposure and surgical trauma, according to the size of the tumor and the requirements of each case. Smaller lesions may even be treated using minimally invasive approaches through the orbit, with or without the assistance of the endoscope, or even a purely endoscopic approach. The efficacy and benefit of a purely endoscopic approach are not yet well established, but cadaveric studies are promising, including an ongoing cadaveric study at the authors' institution in the Anatomical Laboratory for Visuospatial Innovations in Otolaryngology and Neurosurgery (ALT-VISION).[35–38]

Access to the parasellar area, cavernous sinus, Meckel's cave, and the posterior fossa through a *lateral orbital approach* is achieved by drilling the lateral and superior walls of the orbit to create a route to these areas of the skull base (**Fig. 32.9** and **Fig. 32.10**).[38]

This approach is done through a transeyelid incision (**Fig. 32.9a**), which follows its curvature and is placed in the superior eyelid crease. The incision runs from the midpupillary line to approximately 1 cm beyond the lateral orbital ridge along the superior border of the zygomatic arch. Care must be taken to avoid perforating the orbital septum, which separates the skin and *orbicularis oculi* muscle from the postseptal orbit. A plane is developed between the *orbicularis oculi* muscle and the septum, toward the superior orbital rim, where it starts. Once exposed, the periosteum is divided sharply from the supraorbital notch to the zygomaticotemporal foramen and elevated from the orbit in a subperiosteal fashion. Avoiding injury to the periorbit is crucial to protect the eye and reduce complications. The temporalis muscle fascia is cut along the orbital rim, allowing the anterior part of the muscle to be elevated to expose the lateral wall of the orbit, the sphenoid wing, and *pterion*. To prevent injury to the *frontalis* branch of the facial nerve, neither the incision nor the dissection should extend more than 1.5 cm beyond the lateral orbital ridge (**Fig. 32.9b**). The lateral orbitotomy is then done using a combination of high-speed drill and reciprocating saw from the frontozygomatic suture to the zygomatic angle and, posteriorly, to the inferior orbital fissure (IOF; **Fig. 32.9c**). More recently, authors have been using ultrasonic bone scalpel to perform the lateral orbitotomy. At this point, the sphenoid ridge on the lateral surface can be used as a guide to bone drilling, to expose the frontal dura, temporal dura, and the orbit. The IOF is the caudal limit of the drilling and the pterion is the posterior limit. The dura is elevated up to the SOF, exposing the frontotemporal dural fold, which can be sectioned and the two layers of dura (periosteal dura and dura propria) can be separated, performing a peeling of the middle fossa to expose the cavernous sinus and Meckel's cave (**Fig. 32.10**).

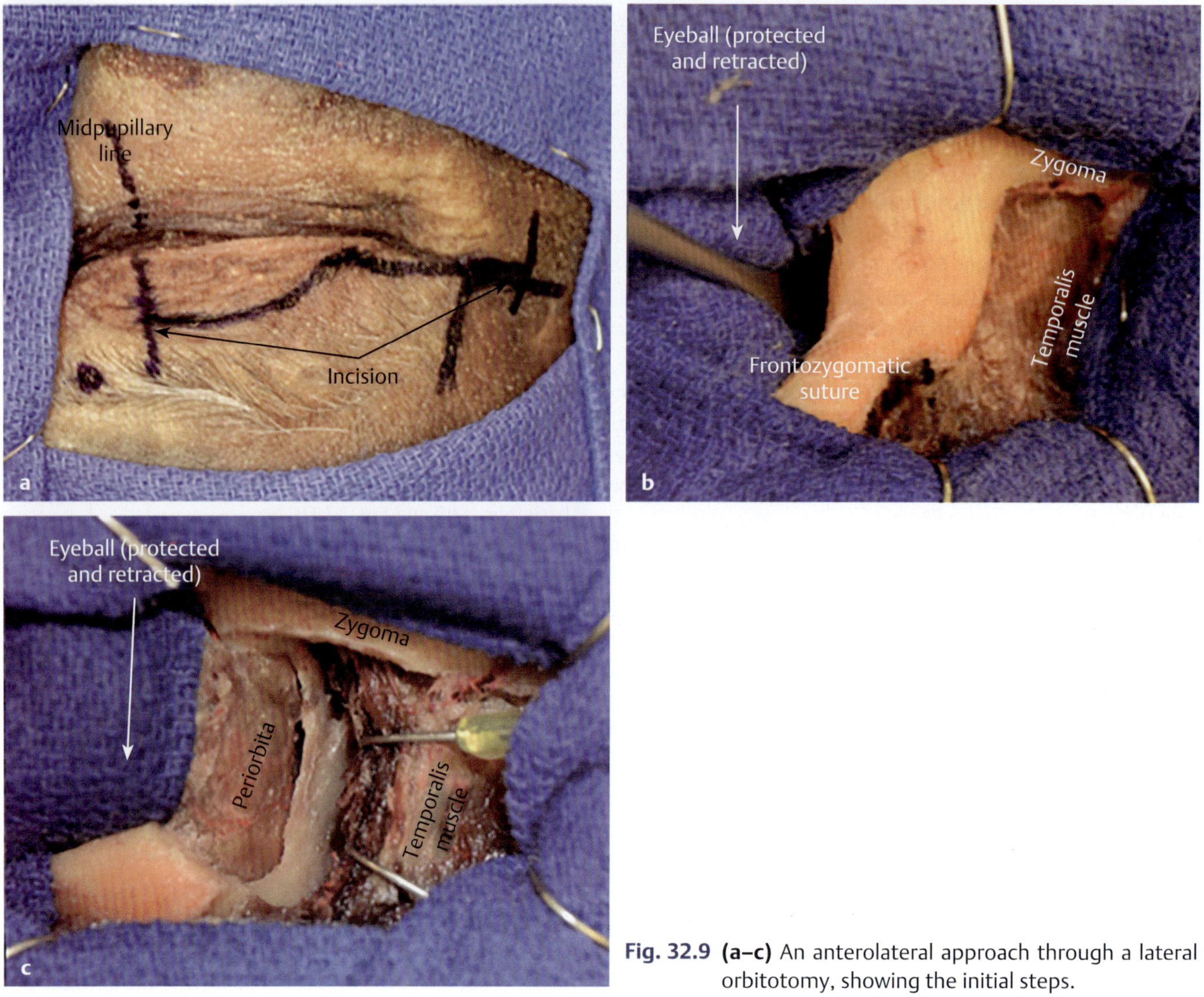

Fig. 32.9 (a–c) An anterolateral approach through a lateral orbitotomy, showing the initial steps.

This minimally invasive technique allows resection of lesions with minimal disruption of normal tissue or brain retraction; however, it is ill suited for large lesions, when a wider corridor is needed. In such cases, a frontotemporal craniotomy is recommended, usually extended with orbital rim, zygomatic arch, or orbital-zygomatic osteotomies. The authors will describe the steps to an *orbital-zygomatic approach* (**Fig. 32.11** and **Fig. 32.12**) as it is the wider approach, but it should be noted that this approach can be modulated and smaller approaches can be used in select cases to minimize normal tissue disruption.[23,34,39,40]

The O-Zy starts with a frontotemporal (hemicoronal), curved incision behind the hairline, or, for maximal exposure, a bicoronal incision may be used. The skin flap is elevated subperiosteally past the orbital rim. Lateral to the supraorbital notch, the periorbita is gently released from the orbital rim and extended down to the zygoma, fully exposing the zygomatic arch. Care must be taken to avoid injury to the frontal branch of the facial nerve by utilizing an interfascial dissection plane (**Fig. 32.11a**). Authors recommend the two-piece craniotomy, beginning with a frontotemporal craniotomy. Once a complete exposure is achieved (**Fig. 32.11b**), three burr holes are created at the keyhole (junction of the frontal, temporal, and sphenoid bones), at the junction of the superior temporal line and coronal suture, and at the level of the floor of the middle fossa. A wide craniotomy (first piece) exposes the frontal and temporal lobes, protected by the dura mater (**Fig. 32.11c**), which is elevated from the orbital roof from anterolateral to posterior. Next, protecting the temporal lobe, the sphenoid wing and ridge are drilled exposing the lateral orbit, the SOF, and anterior clinoid process. Next, an orbitozygomatic osteotomy is performed to remove the orbital rim, body of the zygoma, and zygomatic arch en bloc (second piece). The first cut is through the orbital rim and

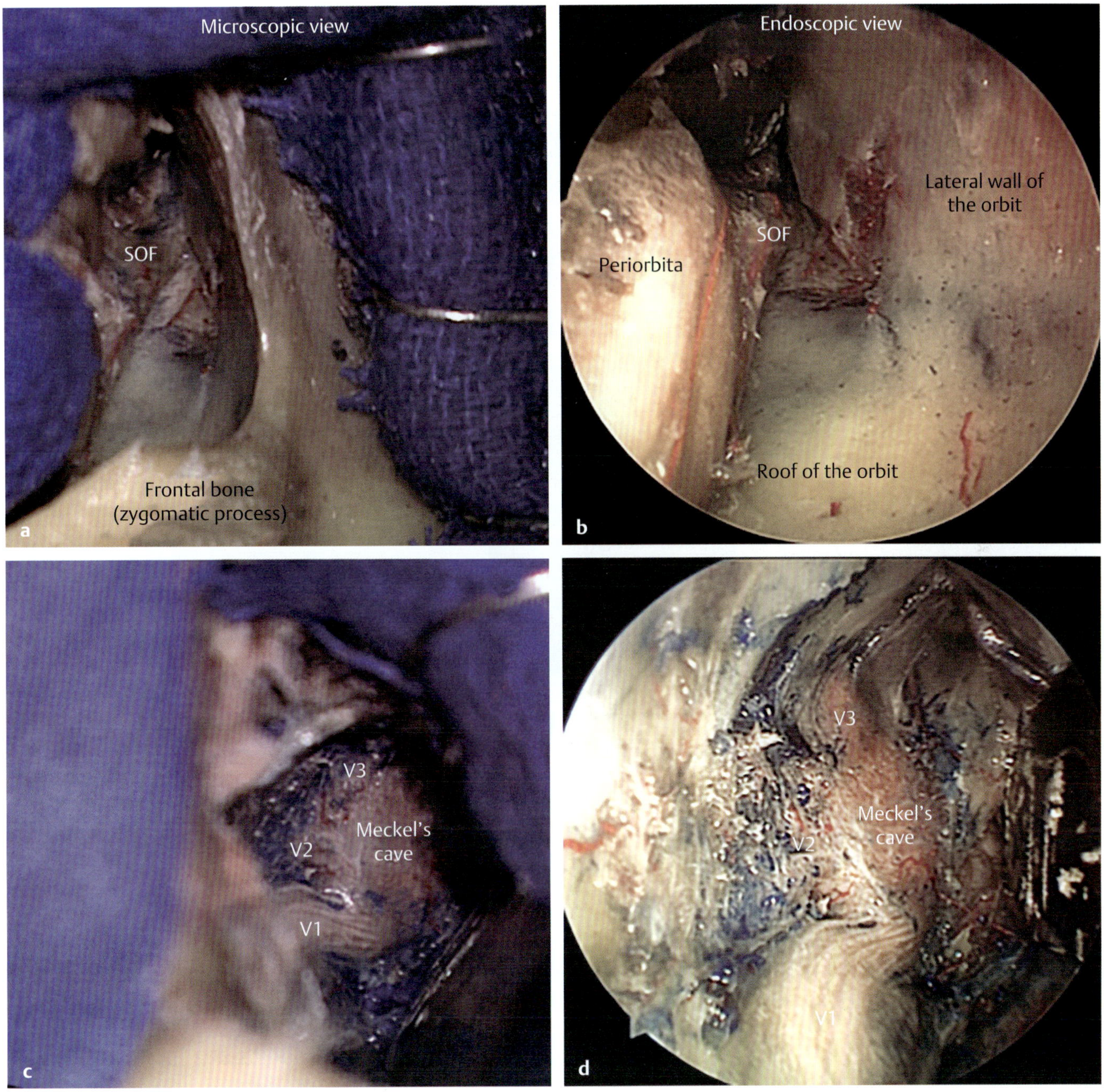

Fig. 32.10 Once the initial steps of the lateral orbitotomy, including the removal of the orbital rim, the lateral wall of the orbit and the greater sphenoid wing are drilled to reach Meckel's cave. Compare the visualization that the microscope affords us **(a, c)** with the endoscopic view **(b, d)**.

roof, lateral to the supraorbital notch extending posteriorly toward the SOF. The second cut is through the lateral wall of the orbit toward the IOF, which cannot be directly seen but can be identified using a small dissector (**Fig. 32.11d**). The third osteotomy extends from the IOF, through the anterior aspect of the zygomatic bone, and ends above the zygomaticofacial foramen. The final osteotomy releases the posterior edge of the zygomatic process from the temporal bone (**Fig. 32.11e**).[23,34,39–41]

With this exposure (**Fig. 32.12a**), the dura can be peeled from the floor to the middle fossa, exposing the cavernous sinus, Meckel's cave and all the landmarks mentioned in the lateral and anterolateral corridor, offering an excellent view and reach to remove the tumor (**Fig. 32.12b, c**). Even tumors in the extracranial space can be reached through this approach as it exposes the foramen ovale and the infratemporal fossa. The orbit is already exposed, requiring only the opening of the periorbita to remove the tumor from it.

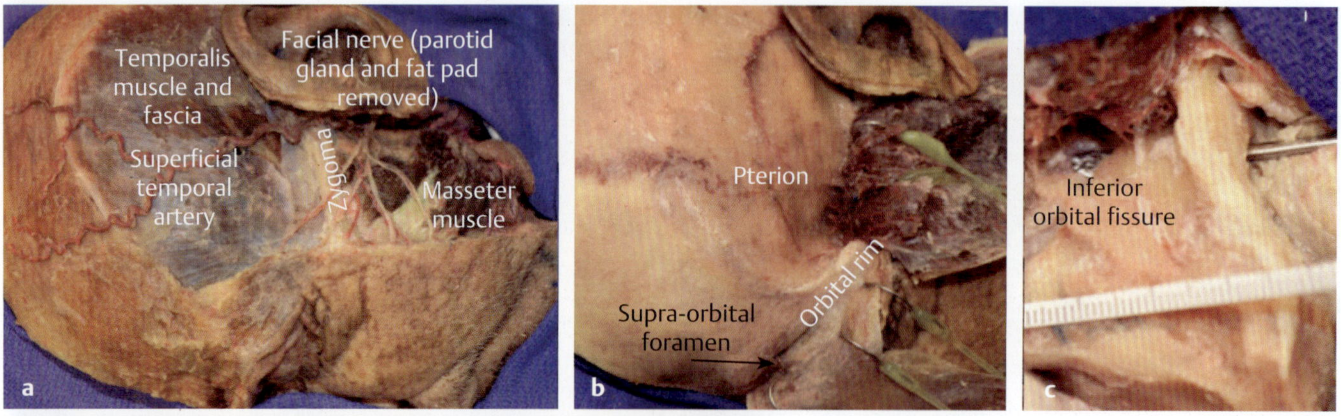

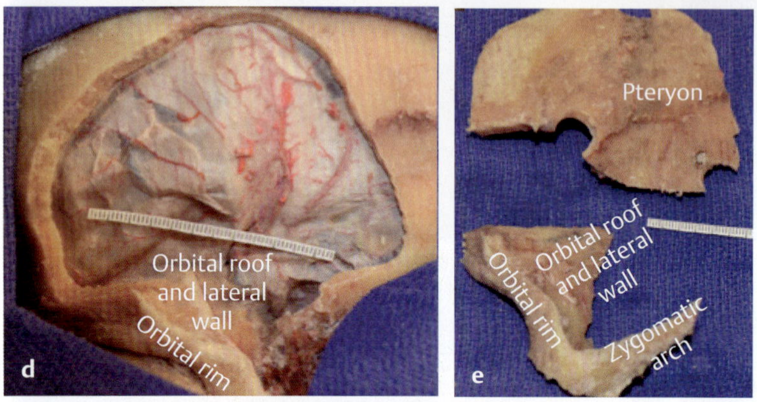

Fig. 32.11 An orbitozygomatic approach in a cadaveric specimen. **(a)** An interfacial dissection was done and the branches of the orbital nerves were isolated and the fat pad was removed to show the position of the frontalis branch to the zygomatic arch. To completely expose the facial nerve the parotid gland was also removed. **(b–e)** Steps in a two-piece orbitozygomatic approach.

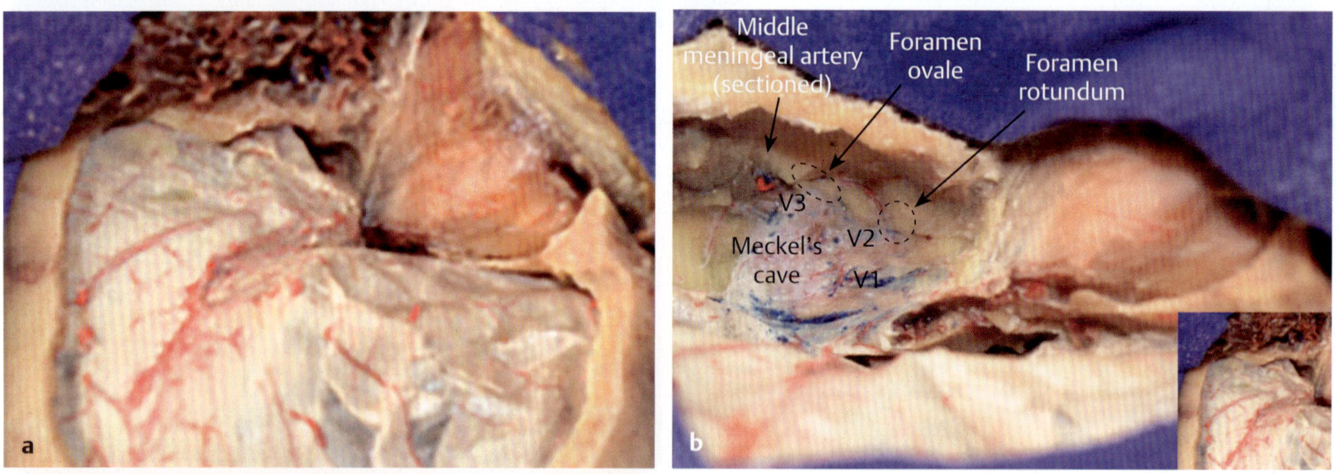

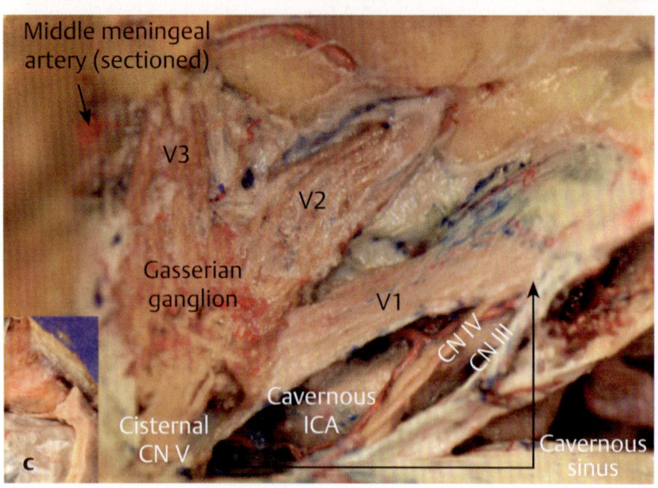

Fig. 32.12 (a–c) After the orbitozygomatic approach is done, excellent access to the middle and anterior fossa, cavernous sinus, Meckel's cave, and orbit is obtained.

The PPF, infratemporal fossa, and sinonasal space can be reached by drilling the anteromedial triangle (between V1 and V2), the anterolateral triangle (between V2 and V3), and the floor of the middle fossa.

When the extracranial component cannot be removed by expanding one of the previous approaches, nor by an EEA, it may be necessary to use a direct approach to the infratemporal fossa. The *preauricular (subtemporal) infratemporal fossa approach* can be added to either the anterior or lateral surgical corridors, by adding a preauricular extension to the incision. Type E tumors[17] can be resected using only this approach. Adding this approach can put the facial nerve at risk as it emerges from the stylomastoid foramen.[42–44] This lateral approach to the infratemporal fossa, for trigeminal schwannomas, can frequently be replaced by an EEA, which can explore the infratemporal fossa more safely and with less morbidity by an anteromedial corridor.

Anteromedial Corridor

The sinonasal or antero-medial corridor was not a viable choice for the resection of trigeminal schwannomas and other lesions on the coronal plane until the introduction of the endoscope. The limited lateral vision and reach of this approach with the microscope did not allow its use. When the endoscope was introduced to the transsphenoidal technique, it had a better lateral view and reach, allowing the development of the transpterygoid approach to the coronal plane.[11,45–47] Bolger and Osenbach were the first to describe a clinical application of the lateral reach of the endoscope by treating a CSF leak into the lateral sphenoid recess using a purely endoscopic technique.[48] The EEA (**Fig. 32.13** and **Fig. 32.14**) can be used to resect tumor types M, ME, MP, MPE, E1, and E2.[17] Tumors that grow and project into the sphenoid sinus are particularly well suited for this approach. When analyzing preoperative images, the main concern for this approach should be the position of the ICA. When the tumor lies posterior to the ICA, "protected" by it, the risk of a carotid injury may be too great, and a middle fossa approach is likely a safer choice. However, if the tumor lies anterior to the ICA, even if not protruding into the sphenoid, the EEA is a good choice for resection.

We will review the main aspects of the EEA related to trigeminal schwannomas, which may include an approach to the orbit and a transpterygoid approach.[11,45–47,49–54]

The nasal cavity is prepared with cottonoids soaked in a vasoconstricting agent (oxymetazoline) to decrease bleeding. The ipsilateral middle turbinate is usually removed followed by a wide sphenoethmoidectomy to expose the skull base and lamina papyracea. The lamina papyracea is normally thin and can be removed using a periosteal elevator, without disrupting the periorbita. If not, drilling should

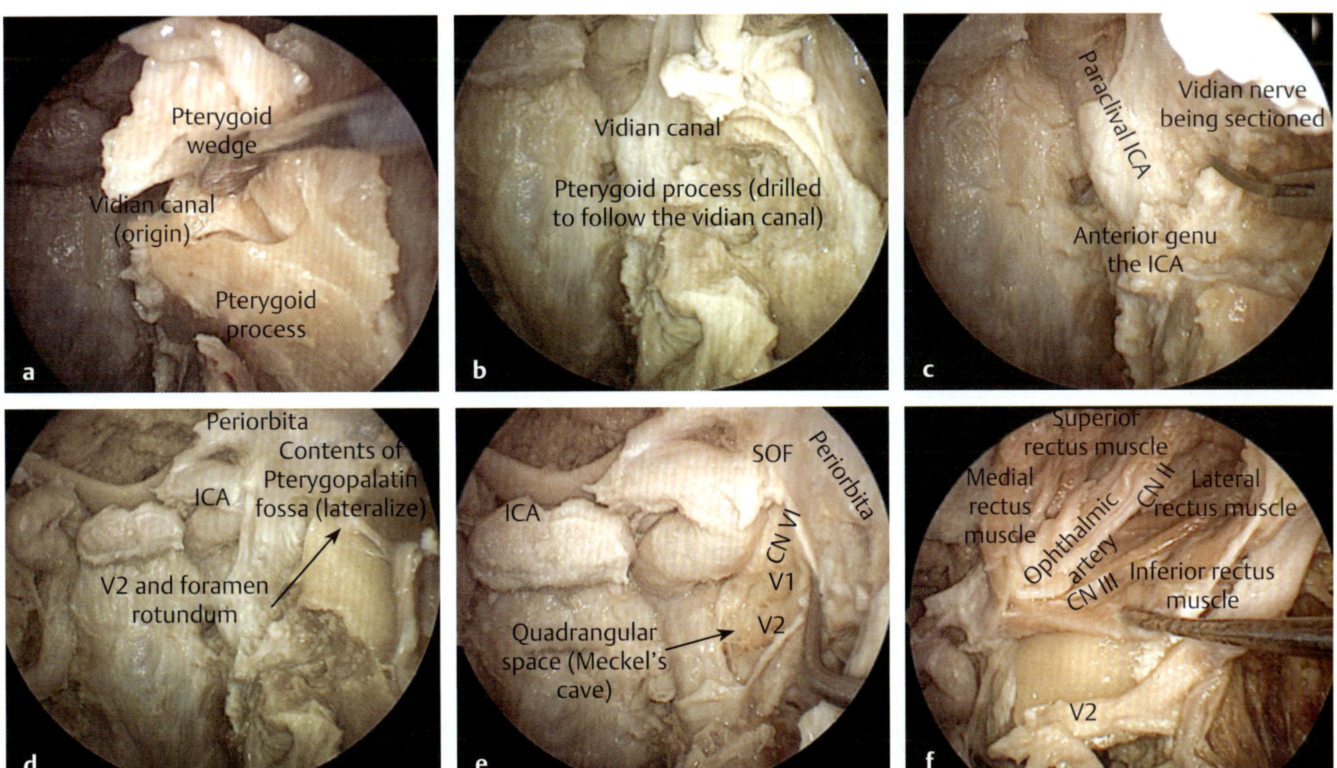

Fig. 32.13 (a–f) Stepwise endoscopic endonasal transpterygoid approach and to the orbit—part 1.

be used to thin the lamina to eggshell thickness, allowing it to be removed. If needed, an endoscopic dacryocystorhinostomy can be performed to maximize this exposure.[51] It allows access from the lacrimal sac to the orbital apex and SOF, when the tumor follows V1 path. A sickle or 90-degree knife can be used to open the periorbita, with care to avoid the medial rectus muscle which lies 1 to 2 mm deep to the periorbita. Extraconal lesions require minimal dissection. Intraconal lesions demand careful dissection between the medial rectus muscle and the inferior or superior rectus muscle (**Fig. 32.13f**).[55] Once the lesion is identified, it must be delicately dissected from the orbital contents, avoiding excessive traction which may injure the fragile nerves, vessels, and muscles in the orbit. Once resection is completed, reconstruction is usually not needed as the mucosa typically recovers well, and no opening into the CSF space has been done.[53] The authors recommend that this approach be used only for lesions medial or inferior to the optic nerve. If the tumor has extended beyond the optic nerve, a combined strategy would be safer to decrease morbidity to the optic nerve.

When the tumor is located exclusively in the orbit, the aforementioned exposure will suffice. However, as most lesions also have a cavernous, Meckel's cave, pterygopalatine fossa, or infratemporal fossa component, a transpterygoid approach is required.

The exposure for a transpterygoid approach to Meckel's cave begins by preparing the nasal cavity and the reconstruction. The right middle turbinate is resected and the left is lateralized. Authors recommend elevating a pedicled nasoseptal flap for reconstruction at the end of the case. This must be elevated from the contralateral side of the approach to make sure the arterial pedicle will be preserved.[46,56] A posterior nasal septectomy, wide bilateral sphenoidotomies, posterior and anterior ethmoidectomies, and a maxillary antrostomy are completed. The sphenopalatine foramen and the sphenopalatine and posterior nasal arteries are identified. The arteries are isolated and coagulated. The posterior wall of the maxillary sinus is removed exposing the contents of the PPF, which are lateralized preserving the periosteum intact. To allow the lateralization of the PPF, the palatovaginal vessels and nerves are transected. At this point, the vidian canal can be identified originating at the PPF (**Fig. 32.13a**), usually at the insertion of the middle pterygoid plate on the pterygoid process of the sphenoid bone. The basopharyngeal fascia is elevated from the undersurface of the sphenoid floor to allow drilling of the floor down to the level of the clival recess (**Fig. 32.13b**). Knowing the position of the petrous ICA is crucial for a safe surgery, and it can be identified following the vidian canal; drilling along the inferior and medial margin is done to identify the lacerum segment of the ICA, which lies along the superior margin of the vidian canal (**Fig. 32.13c**).[1–12,45–47]

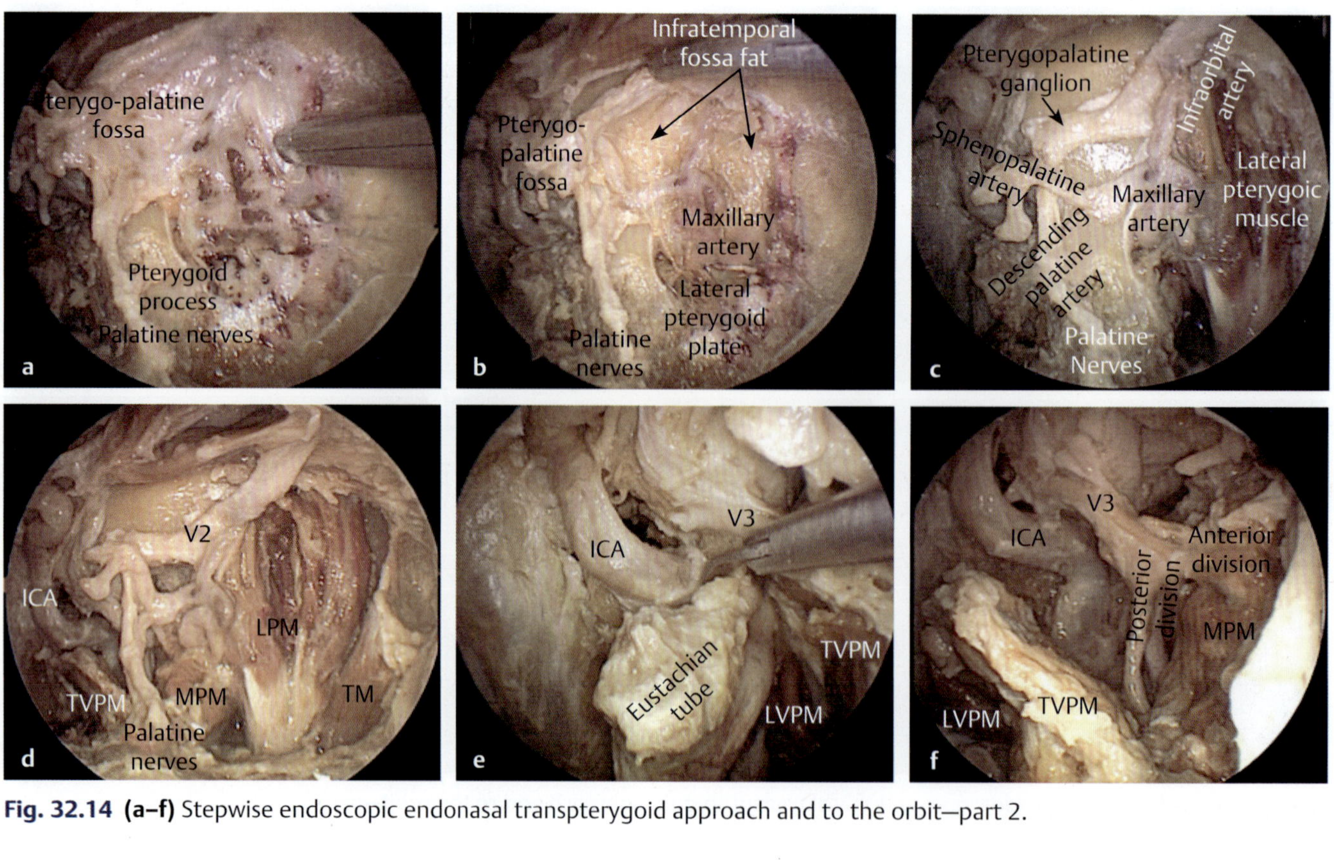

Fig. 32.14 (a–f) Stepwise endoscopic endonasal transpterygoid approach and to the orbit—part 2.

Once the anterior genu of the ICA is identified, the bone overlaying the horizontal segment can be drilled to eggshell thinness and removed with exquisite care to avoid injuring the carotid. If needed, the maxillary antrostomy can be further widened to identify V2 in the posterior and superior wall of the maxillary sinus and can be followed posteriorly to foramen rotundum (**Fig. 32.13d**). The bone between V2 and the vidian canal, all the way posteriorly to foramen rotundum and down to the horizontal segment of the ICA should be removed to expose the quadrangular space, the front door to Meckel's cave (**Fig. 32.13e**). The quadrangular space is limited by the paraclival ICA medially, the horizontal segment of the petrous ICA inferiorly, the dura mater of the middle fossa and V2 laterally, and the abducens nerve superiorly. The angle of the ICA varies between individuals; therefore this space may be wider or narrower.[10,12,57]

At this point, tumors in Meckel's cave can be resected, in a posterior and lateral trajectory, below the abducens nerve (upper limit of the quadrangular space). The remaining cranial nerves in the cavernous sinus are cranial to the cranial nerve VI, therefore using it as the upper limit of the approach ensures the preservation of all nerves, which should be monitored throughout the surgery (cranial nerves III, IV, VI, and motor V3).

When access to the infratemporal fossa is necessary, further exposure is required. If the tumor is readily identifiable in the maxillary sinus from the infratemporal fossa, resection can be done through the corridor created by the tumor. When this is not the case, the medial pterygoid plate and the posterior wall of the maxillary sinus have not been removed, they should be drilled (**Fig. 32.14a**) to expose the convoluted terminal branches of the maxillary artery so they can be isolated and ligated (**Fig. 32.14b, c**). At this point, the lateral pterygoid plate should be identified (**Fig. 32.14c**) and drilled flush with the middle cranial fossa and foramen *ovale* (**Fig. 32.14d**) to expose V3 and the muscles in the infratemporal fossa (**Fig. 32.14e, f**), which can be dissected and the tumor was removed with minimal disruption to normal tissues when compared to the preauricular approach.

Multimodal Management

Choosing the ideal treatment for a trigeminal schwannoma is not always simple, particularly when considering that added to the different surgical corridors, these tumors may also be observed with serial imaging or treated with radiation. The treatment of these usually benign lesions can have a devastating impact on the quality of life because of their proximity to neural and vascular structures. Tumors should be discussed and followed by a multidisciplinary team involving neurosurgery, head-and-neck surgery, otolaryngology, radiology, and radiation oncology. The ideal management will vary according to each tumor, patient, and local resources.[7,8,18,32]

As mentioned above, The authors believe small, asymptomatic, incidentally discovered lesions with a typical MRI and CT appearance can be followed clinically with serial imaging. A short interval (3 months) between the diagnosis and first follow-up should be used to ensure this is not a fast-growing lesion, which would raise concern for other diagnoses. If atypical characteristics are observed, unusual growth or symptomatic progression, a histopathological diagnosis should be pursued. A tissue sample should be obtained through a percutaneous biopsy of Meckel's cave or a microscopic or endoscopic approach particularly for patients with other comorbidities (i.e., elderly people).[7]

The different approaches described above may be used. The most direct approach to the lesion, avoiding crossing the planes of nerves, should be used. When involving a single compartment (M, P, or E type lesions[17]), the decision is usually simpler. However, when multiple compartments are involved (MP, ME, and MPE type lesions[17]), the decision becomes more challenging. It may require combined approaches through more than one corridor, at the same moment or as multiple, staged procedures.

Furthermore, the use of stereotactic radiosurgery (SRS) has been a useful complementary tool in the treatment of schwannomas. In selected cases, a subtotal resection to preserve neurological function should be done and then complemented with SRS, which offers high tumor control with a low rate of radiation-associated complications, particularly for moderate volume lesions.[7,8] In a 4 to 8 years follow-up, control rate was between 79 and 93%, with few adverse effects from radiation which were mainly related to the trigeminal nerve (facial pain or hypoesthesia).[8,58,59]

Illustrative Cases

Case 1: Posterior Corridor (RISA)

A 43-year-old female presented to our clinic with progressive headaches for the past 3 months. MRI revealed a large, heterogeneous lesion centered on Meckel's cave, with a large component in the posterior fossa (**Fig. 32.15a**). The size of the posterior fossa component made a middle fossa approach less favorable. A retrosigmoid approach would successfully remove the posterior fossa lesion; however, the portion in the middle fossa and Meckel's cave would not be accessible. Therefore, the authors decided to do a retrosigmoid craniotomy, expanded by the drilling of the suprameatal tubercle (RISA) as described previously. When presented with this option, the patient agreed to proceed with surgery. Through a standard retrosigmoid approach, the authors identified the

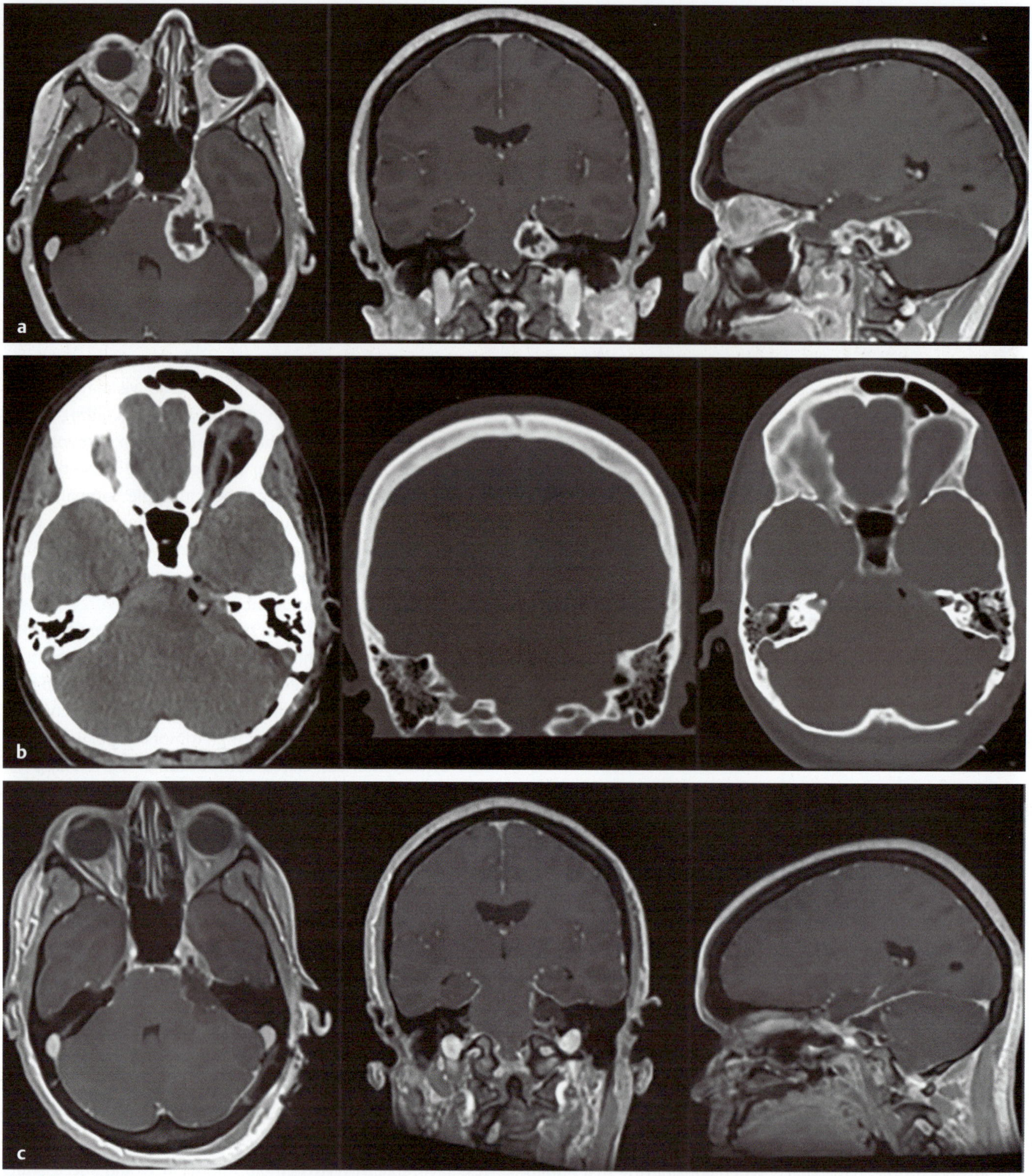

Fig. 32.15 Illustrative case 1. **(a)** Preoperative T1, gadolinium-enhanced MRI in the axial, coronal, and sagittal planes. **(b)** Postoperative CT in axial brain window (notice air is present in Meckel's cave, confirming that it was accessed), bone window in the coronal and axial planes. **(c)** Postoperative T1, gadolinium-enhanced MRI in the axial, coronal, and sagittal planes.

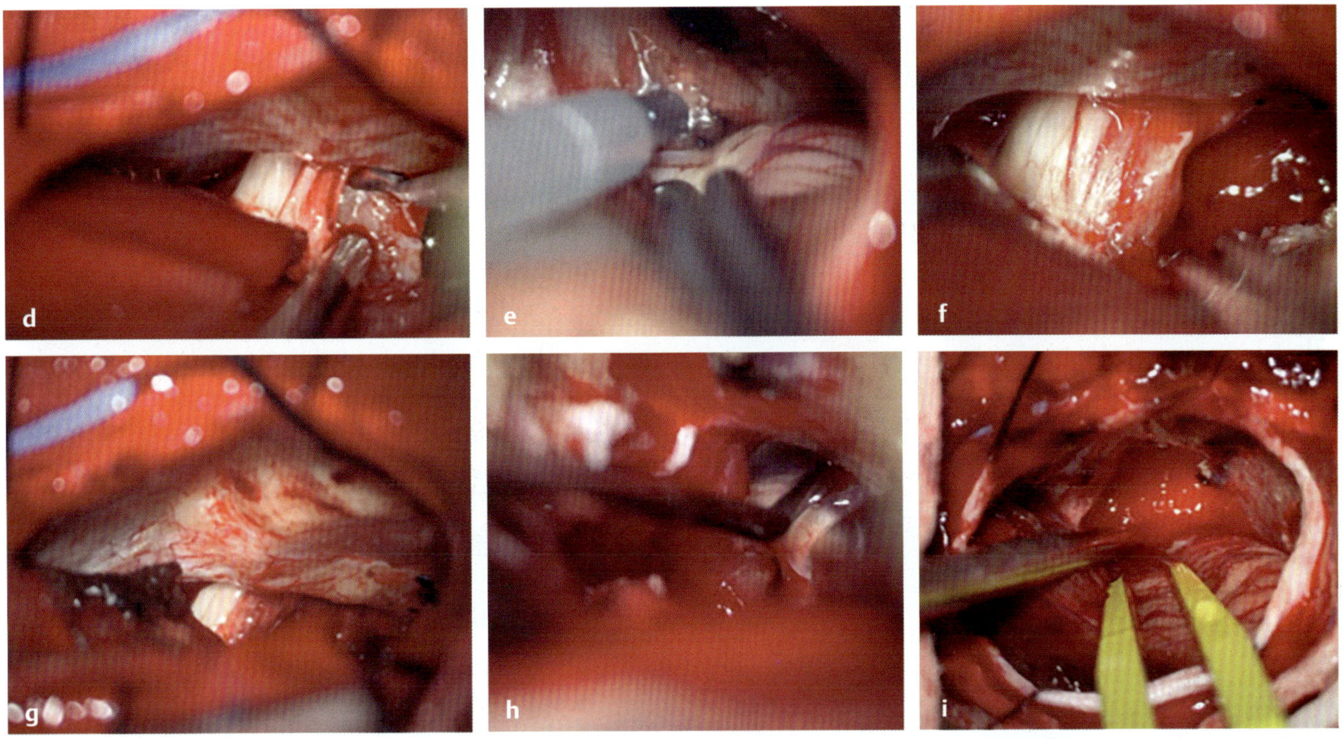

Fig. 32.15 *(Continued)* **(d–i)** Intraoperative images showing the cisternal segment of the trigeminal nerve and the tumor being debulked with the ultrasonic aspirator until further tumor resection is blocked by the suprameatal tubercle, which is then drilled to allow a complete resection.

cranial nerves V, VII, and VIII and the posterior fossa lesion, and a debulking of the lesion using ultrasonic aspirator was done (**Fig. 32.15d–f**). No further tumor could be removed because of the suprameatal tubercle obstructing the corridor (**Fig. 32.15g**). After drilling the tubercle, the authors were able to remove the tumor from Meckel's cave and complete resection (**Fig. 32.15h, i**). The patient postoperative course was uneventful and she was discharged on postoperative day 3 with no new neurological deficits. Postoperative CT suggests a complete removal of the tumor and shows the drilling of the petrous bone through the posterior fossa (**Fig. 32.15b**). MRI confirmed a complete resection (**Fig. 32.15c**). At 1-year follow-up, the patient's recovery has been very satisfactory, with no recurrences or complications and no further treatments.

Case 2: Middle Fossa Approach

A 57-year-old female presented to our clinic with progressive facial pain affecting mainly V2's territory. MRI imaging showed a lesion centered on Meckel's cave with avid enhancement after gadolinium administration and a small component in the posterior fossa (**Fig. 32.16a**). Careful analysis of the images showed that the lesion was posterior to the ICA. This position relative to the ICA made an approach through the anteromedial corridor (EEA) ill suited, requiring extensive manipulation of the ICA and with an increased risk of injury. Therefore, the authors opted for a middle fossa, subtemporal extradural approach. The small component in the posterior fossa was removed by drilling Kawase's triangle, which allowed a complete resection. Postoperative MRI confirmed a gross total resection (**Fig. 32.16b**). The patient had an uneventful postoperative course and was discharged on postoperative day 5 with hypoesthesia on V2 and V3 territories. At 6 months' follow-up, sensation returned to normal. At last follow-up, 3 years after surgery, no recurrences or complications have been observed and no further treatments were needed.

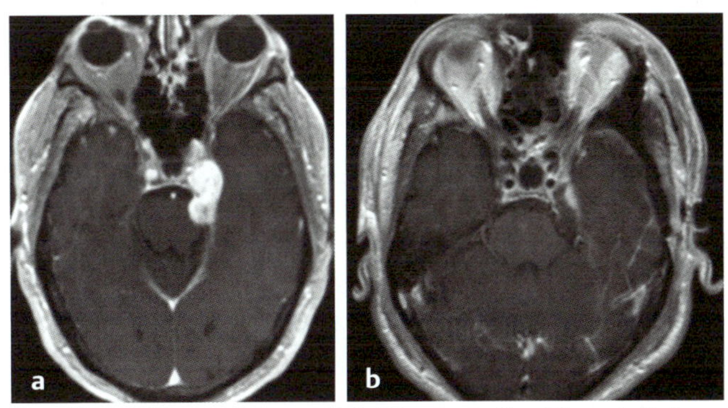

Fig. 32.16 Illustrative case 2. **(a)** Preoperative T1, gadolinium-enhanced MRI in the axial plane. **(b)** Postoperative T1, gadolinium-enhanced MRI in the axial plane.

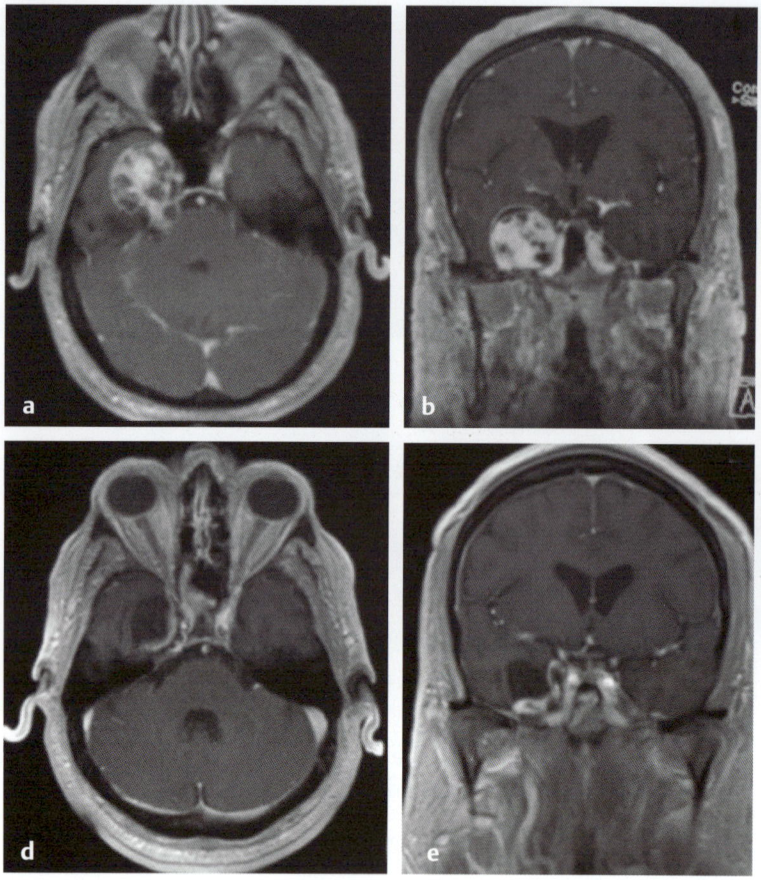

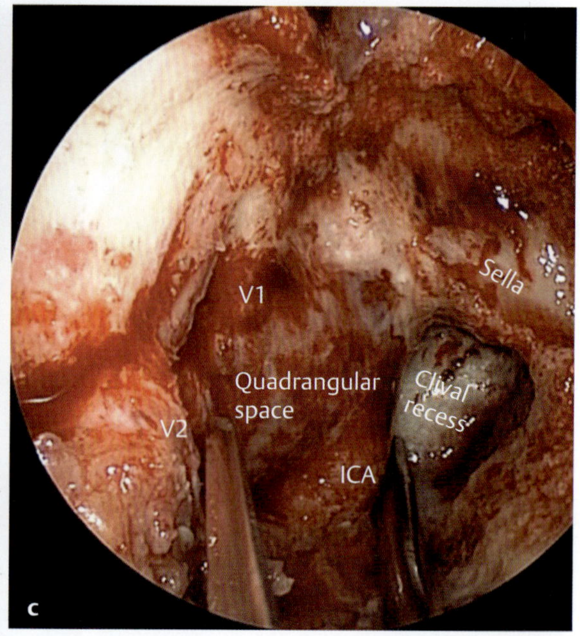

Fig. 32.17 Illustrative case 3. **(a, b)** Preoperative T1, gadolinium-enhanced MRI in the axial and coronal planes. **(c)** Intraoperative endoscopic endonasal approach. **(d, e)** Postoperative T1, gadolinium-enhanced MRI in the axial and coronal planes.

Case 3: Anteromedial Corridor (EEA)

A 59-year-old patient presented to our clinic with facial numbness for 3 weeks. MRI revealed a large heterogeneous, contrast-enhancing lesion centered on Meckel's cave (**Fig. 32.17a, b**). The ICA was displaced posteriorly and the anteromedial triangle of the middle fossa was enlarged. Despite the large size, these made the anteromedial corridor (EEA) an ideal approach, avoiding the risk to the ICA and without requiring brain retraction, as it would have been needed for a complete resection through a middle fossa approach. Intraoperatively, using the vidian canal as a guide, the authors located the ICA, V2, and V1 (**Fig. 32.17c**). After using neurostimulation to make sure no motor fibers were damaged, the dura was opened, and Meckel's cave was accessed through the "front door," the quadrangular space. Following the tumor posteriorly the authors removed the entire lesion in Meckel's cave and the small component protruding into the posterior fossa. Postoperative MRI confirmed a complete resection. The patient was discharged with unchanged facial hypoesthesia, which progressively improved and, after 4 months, it was back to normal. In 3.5 years of follow-up, no complications or recurrences have been observed.

Conclusion

Trigeminal schwannomas are complex lesions for which gross total resection is still the ideal treatment. However, the main goal of treatment nowadays should be the patient's quality of life, preserving and recovering neurological function. A subtotal resection to preserve the patient neurologically intact is often preferred over a complete resection and a permanent sequela. Small remnants can be safely treated using radiation therapy.

The combination of microscopic approaches, endoscopic approaches, or microscopic approaches assisted by endoscopic visualization can improve the extent of resection and outcomes, particularly when using combined surgical corridors. Therefore, these patients should be treated in a specialized Skull Base Center by a team well versed in multiple surgical approaches adopting a tailored treatment strategy to each patient.

References

1. Ocak PE, Ocak U, Dinc C, Baskaya MK. Trigeminal schwannomas: part I—anatomy, clinical presentation, and radiology. Contemp Neurosurg 2018;40(1):1–6

2. Al-Mefty O, Ayoubi S, Gaber E. Trigeminal schwannomas: removal of dumbbell-shaped tumors through the expanded Meckel cave and outcomes of cranial nerve function. J Neurosurg 2002;96(3):453–463
3. Cuneo HM, Rand CW. Tumors of the gasserian ganglion; tumor of the left gasserian ganglion associated with enlargement of the mandibular nerve; a review of the literature and case report. J Neurosurg 1952;9(5):423–431
4. Schisano G, Olivecrona H. Neurinomas of the gasserian ganglion and trigeminal root. J Neurosurg 1960;17(2): 306–322
5. Samii M, Migliori MM, Tatagiba M, Babu R. Surgical treatment of trigeminal schwannomas. J Neurosurg 1995;82(5): 711–718
6. McCormick PC, Bello JA, Post KD. Trigeminal schwannoma. Surgical series of 14 cases with review of the literature. J Neurosurg. 1988;69(6):850–860
7. Makarenko S, Ye V, Akagami R. Natural history, multimodal management, and quality of life outcomes of trigeminal schwannomas. J Neurol Surg B Skull Base 2018;79(6): 586–592
8. Niranjan A, Barnett S, Anand V, Agazzi S. Multimodality management of trigeminal schwannomas. J Neurol Surg B Skull Base 2016;77(4):371–378
9. Todeschini AB, Otto BA, Carrau RL, Prevedello DM. Endoscopic endonasal approaches for the management of skull base meningiomas: selection criteria and clinical outcomes. J Neurosurg Sci 2018;62(6):617–626
10. Raza SM, Amine MA, Anand V, Schwartz TH. Endoscopic endonasal resection of trigeminal schwannomas. Neurosurg Clin N Am 2015;26(3):473–479
11. Prevedello DM, Pinheiro-Neto CD, Fernandez-Miranda JC, et al. Vidian nerve transposition for endoscopic endonasal middle fossa approaches. Neurosurgery 2010;67(2, Suppl Operative):478–484
12. Kassam AB, Prevedello DM, Carrau RL, et al. The front door to Meckel's cave: an anteromedial corridor via expanded endoscopic endonasal approach- technical considerations and clinical series. Neurosurgery 2009;64(3 Suppl):ons71–82; discussion 82–83
13. Mikami T, Minamida Y, Yamaki T, Koyanagi I, Nonaka T, Houkin K. Cranial nerve assessment in posterior fossa tumors with fast imaging employing steady-state acquisition (FIESTA). Neurosurg Rev 2005;28(4):261–266
14. Hodaie M, Quan J, Chen DQ. In vivo visualization of cranial nerve pathways in humans using diffusion-based tractography. Neurosurgery 2010;66(4):788–795; discussion 795–796
15. Jefferson G. The trigeminal neurinomas with some remarks on malignant invasion of the gasserian ganglion. Clin Neurosurg. 1953;1:11–54
16. Day JD, Fukushima T. The surgical management of trigeminal neuromas. Neurosurgery 1998;42(2):233–240; discussion 240–241
17. Yoshida K, Kawase T. Trigeminal neurinomas extending into multiple fossae: surgical methods and review of the literature. J Neurosurg 1999;91(2):202–211
18. Ocak PE, Ocak U, Dinc C, Baskaya MK. Trigeminal schwannomas: part II—classification, pathology, and treatment. Contemp Neurosurg 2018;40(2):1–7
19. Samii M, Alimohamadi M, Gerganov V. Endoscope-assisted retrosigmoid intradural suprameatal approach for surgical treatment of trigeminal schwannomas. Neurosurgery 2014;(10, Suppl 4):565–575; discussion 575
20. Samii M, Tatagiba M, Carvalho GA. Retrosigmoid intradural suprameatal approach to Meckel's cave and the middle fossa: surgical technique and outcome. J Neurosurg. 2000;92(2): 235–241
21. Rhoton AL Jr. The cerebellopontine angle and posterior fossa cranial nerves by the retrosigmoid approach. Neurosurgery 2000;47(3 Suppl):S93–S129
22. Reis CV, Arantes AA, Nicolato A, Gusmão S. Delimitação dos acessos cranianos. Arq Bras Neurocir 2012;31(3):135–145
23. Gusmao S, Silveira RL, Arantes A. [Landmarks to the cranial approaches]. Arq Neuropsiquiatr 2003;61(2A):305–308
24. Ebner FH, Dimostheni A, Tatagiba MS, Roser F. Step-by-step education of the retrosigmoid approach leads to low approach-related morbidity through young residents. Acta Neurochir (Wien) 2010;152(6):985–988; discussion 988
25. Feigl GC, Decker K, Wurms M, et al. Neurosurgical procedures in the semisitting position: evaluation of the risk of paradoxical venous air embolism in patients with a patent foramen ovale. World Neurosurg 2014;81(1):159–164
26. Kurucz P, Baksa G, Patonay L, Thaher F, Buchfelder M, Ganslandt O. Endoscopic approach-routes in the posterior fossa cisterns through the retrosigmoid keyhole craniotomy: an anatomical study. Neurosurg Rev 2017;40(3):427–448
27. Montaser AS, Prevedello DM, Otto BA, Carrau RL. Endoscopic endonasal multimodular approach for resection of concomitant trigeminal schwannoma and pituitary adenoma: a single corridor for different pathologies. J Neurol Surg B Skull Base 2018;79(S 01):S1–S18862
28. Glasscock ME 3rd. Middle fossa approach to the temporal bone. An otologic frontier. Arch Otolaryngol 1969;90(1): 15–27
29. Mohyeldin A, Prevedello DM, Jamshidi AO, Ditzel Filho LF, Carrau RL. Nuances in the treatment of malignant tumors of the clival and petroclival region. Int Arch Otorhinolaryngol 2014;18(Suppl 2):S157–S72
30. Kawase T, Shiobara R, Toya S. Middle fossa transpetrosal-transtentorial approaches for petroclival meningiomas. Selective pyramid resection and radicality. Acta Neurochir (Wien) 1994;129(3-4):113–120

31. Miller CG, van Loveren HR, Keller JT, Pensak M, el-Kalliny M, Tew JM Jr. Transpetrosal approach: surgical anatomy and technique. Neurosurgery 1993;33(3):461–469; discussion 469
32. Montaser AS, Todeschini AB, Harris MS, Adunka OF, Prevedello DM. The role of endoscopy in resection of intracanalicular vestibular schwannoma via middle fossa approach: technical nuances. World Neurosurg 2018;120: 395–399
33. Beer-Furlan A, Vellutini EA, Balsalobre L, Stamm AC. Endoscopic endonasal approach for posterior fossa tumors. In: Couldwell WT, ed. Skull Base Surgery of the Posterior Fossa; Springer; 2018:75–86
34. Sindou M, Emery E, Acevedo G, Ben-David U. Respective indications for orbital rim, zygomatic arch and orbito-zygomatic osteotomies in the surgical approach to central skull base lesions. Critical, retrospective review in 146 cases. Acta Neurochirurgica 2001;143(10):967–975
35. Abdel Aziz KM, Bhatia S, Tantawy MH, et al. Minimally invasive transpalpebral “eyelid” approach to the anterior cranial base. Neurosurgery 2011;69(2 Suppl Operative):ons195–206; discussion 206–207
36. Balakrishnan K, Moe KS. Applications and outcomes of orbital and transorbital endoscopic surgery. Otolaryngol Head Neck Surg 2011;144(5):815–820
37. Locatelli D, Pozzi F, Turri-Zanoni M, et al. Transorbital endoscopic approaches to the skull base: current concepts and future perspectives. J Neurosurg Sci 2016;60(4):514–525
38. Laleva L, Spiriev T, Dallan I, et al. Pure endoscopic lateral orbitotomy approach to the cavernous sinus, posterior, and infratemporal fossae: anatomic study. J Neurol Surg B Skull Base; 2019;80(3):295–305
39. Hakuba A, Liu S, Nishimura S. The orbitozygomatic infratemporal approach: a new surgical technique. Surg Neurol 1986;26(3):271–276
40. Inoue T, Rhoton AL Jr, Theele D, Barry ME. Surgical approaches to the cavernous sinus: a microsurgical study. Neurosurgery 1990;26(6):903–932
41. van Furth WR, Agur AM, Woolridge N, Cusimano MD. The orbitozygomatic approach. Neurosurgery 2006;58(1 Suppl): ONS103–107; discussion ONS103–107
42. Sekhar LN, Janecka IP, Jones NF. Subtemporal-infratemporal and basal subfrontal approach to extensive cranial base tumours. Acta Neurochir (Wien) 1988;92(1-4):83–92
43. Mansour OI, Carrau RL, Snyderman CH, Kassam AB. Preauricular infratemporal fossa surgical approach: modifications of the technique and surgical indications. Skull Base 2004;14(3):143–151; discussion 151
44. Isolan GR, Rowe R, Al-Mefty O. Microanatomy and surgical approaches to the infratemporal fossa: an anaglyphic three-dimensional stereoscopic printing study. Skull Base 2007; 17(5):285–302
45. Kassam AB, Gardner P, Snyderman C, Mintz A, Carrau R. Expanded endonasal approach: fully endoscopic, completely transnasal approach to the middle third of the clivus, petrous bone, middle cranial fossa, and infratemporal fossa. Neurosurg Focus 2005;19(1):E6
46. Kasemsiri P, Solares CA, Carrau RL, et al. Endoscopic endonasal transpterygoid approaches: anatomical landmarks for planning the surgical corridor. Laryngoscope 2013; 123(4):811–815
47. Cavallo LM, Messina A, Gardner P, et al. Extended endoscopic endonasal approach to the pterygopalatine fossa: anatomical study and clinical considerations. Neurosurg Focus 2005;19(1):E5
48. Bolger WE, Osenbach R. Endoscopic transpterygoid approach to the lateral sphenoid recess. Ear Nose Throat J 1999;78(1): 36–46
49. Kennedy DW, Goodstein ML, Miller NR, Zinreich SJ. Endoscopic transnasal orbital decompression. Arch Otolaryngol Head Neck Surg 1990;116(3):275–282
50. Metson R,Dallow RL, Shore JW. Endoscopic orbital decompression. Laryngoscope 1994;104(8 Pt 1):950–957
51. Sprekelsen MB, Barberan MT. Endoscopic dacryocystorhinostomy: surgical technique and results. Laryngoscope 1996; 106(2 Pt 1):187–189
52. Metson R, Pletcher SD. Endoscopic orbital and optic nerve decompression. Otolaryngol Clin North Am 2006;39(3): 551–561, ix
53. Healy DY Jr, Lee NG, Freitag SK, Bleier BS. Endoscopic bimanual approach to an intraconal cavernous hemangioma of the orbital apex with vascularized flap reconstruction. Ophthalmic Plast Reconstr Surg 2014;30(4):e104–e106
54. Pai SB, Nagarjun MN. A neurosurgical perspective to approaches to the orbit: a cadaveric study. Neurol India 2017;65(5):1094–1101
55. Bleier BS, Healy DY Jr, Chhabra N, Freitag S. Compartmental endoscopic surgical anatomy of the medial intraconal orbital space. Int Forum Allergy Rhinol 2014;4(7):587–591
56. Bossi Todeschini A, Montaser AS, Hardesty DA, Carrau RL, Prevedello DM The limits of the endoscopic endonasal transclival approach for posterior fossa tumors. J Neurosurg Sci 2018; 62(3):322–331
57. Dolci RLL, Ditzel Filho LFS, Goulart CR, et al. Anatomical nuances of the internal carotid artery in relation to the quadrangular space. J Neurosurg 2018;128(1):174–181
58. Ryu J, Lee SH, Choi SK, Lim YJ. Gamma knife radiosurgery for trigeminal schwannoma: a 20-year experience with long-term treatment outcome. J Neurooncol 2018;140(1):89–97
59. Snyder MH, Shepard MJ, Chen CJ, Sheehan JP. Stereotactic radiosurgery for trigeminal schwannomas: a 28-year single-center experience and review of the literature. World Neurosurg 2018;119:e874–e881

Section XI

Cerebrospinal Fluid Rhinorrhea

Chapter 33 Endoscopic Management of Cerebrospinal Fluid Rhinorrhea

Milind Kirtane, Kashmira Chavan, and Achala Kamath

Introduction

Cerebrospinal fluid (CSF) rhinorrhea is the leakage of CSF through a communication of the subarachnoid space with the sinonasal cavity following a defect in the skull base.

With advancements in technology and endoscopic surgical techniques over the last three decades, a large number of cases of CSF rhinorrhea can now be managed via the transnasal endoscopic approach. This chapter deals with the management of such anterior skull base defects.

Physiology of Cerebrospinal Fluid Production

The rate of CSF production is 0.35 to 0.37 mL/min (20 mL/h or 350–500 mL/d), with the total CSF volume in a normal adult ranging between 90 and 150 mL.

CSF produced by the choroid plexus in ventricles (50–80%), the ependymal surface layer (~ 30%), and by capillary ultrafiltration (~ 20%), flows from the lateral ventricles to the third ventricle via the foramen of Monro. It further flows into the fourth ventricle through the aqueduct of Sylvius, and out into the subarachnoid space via the foramina of Magendie and Luschka. CSF resorption takes place at the arachnoid villi and granulations projecting into the dural sinuses. Higher hydrostatic pressure facilitates unidirectional CSF flow into the dural sinuses. Backflow into the subarachnoid space is prevented by the arachnoid villi, which acts like a valve. The process of CSF production and absorption is shown in **Flowchart 33.1**.

CSF turnover occurs about three to five times a day because of continuous production and absorption. Normal CSF pressure in the supine position is 5 to 15 cm H_2O. Neurologic symptoms may be seen when the pressure exceeds 15 to 20 cm H_2O.[1]

Classification of Cerebrospinal Fluid Leaks

The classification of CSF leaks can be based on etiology, anatomic site, or underlying intracranial pressure.

Etiology

Congenital

- Congenital skull base defects with CSF leak.
- Associated with congenital meningocele or meningoencephalocele.
- Congenital hydrocephalus.

Acquired

- Traumatic: Most common reported cause of CSF leak (70–80%).[2–4]
  - ➢ Iatrogenic trauma.
    - Intranasal surgery (e.g., intranasal ethmoidectomy).
    - Endoscopic sinus surgery.
    - Skull base surgery (transnasal endoscopic approach, craniotomy).
  - ➢ Accidental trauma.
    - Head injuries (open/closed).
    - Posttraumatic hydrocephalus.
- Inflammatory:
  - ➢ Sinonasal polyps.
  - ➢ Invasive fungal sinusitis.
  - ➢ Mucoceles.
  - ➢ Osteomyelitis.
- Neoplastic:
  - ➢ Neoplasms involving the skull base.
  - ➢ Sinonasal malignancy.

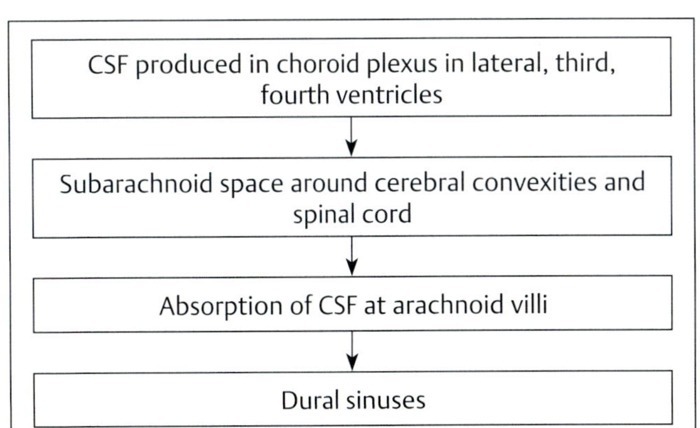

Flowchart 33.1 The process of CSF production and absorption.

    - Nasopharyngeal carcinoma.
    - Intracranial tumors.
- Miscellaneous:
    - Hydrocephalus.
- Spontaneous: CSF leaks occurring in the absence of any distinct etiological factor. Ommaya et al[5] have categorized spontaneous CSF leaks as "nontraumatic CSF leaks" as they were of the opinion that there are no CSF leaks that are truly "spontaneous" in nature. These were further classified into high-pressure and normal-pressure CSF leaks. We are of the opinion that "spontaneous" leaks may actually occur secondary to some old, forgotten injury resulting in a skull base defect. These defects may be potential sites for active CSF leaks in later life because of predisposing factors like osteoporosis or raised intracranial pressure.

In our series of 373 cases of endoscopic CSF rhinorrhea repairs performed in 26 years, 204 (54.69%) cases were spontaneous in origin, 168 (45.04%) cases were secondary to trauma (accidental = 37%, iatrogenic = 8.04%), and one (0.27%) was a congenital defect with an encephalocele (unpublished data).

Sites of Cerebrospinal Fluid Rhinorrhea

The cribriform plate has been reported to be the commonest site of defect in CSF rhinorrhea, followed by the roof of the ethmoid, sphenoid sinus, and the frontal sinus.[2,6,7] In our series (unpublished data), the cribriform plate was the commonest site of defect (76.58%), followed by the sphenoid sinus (16.52%), roof of ethmoid (6%), and the frontal recess and frontal sinus (0.9%).

Frontal sinus CSF leaks operated by an external approach are not included in this series.

Clinical Features

Table 33.1 lists the presenting symptoms and signs of CSF rhinorrhea.

Preoperative Assessment

Nasal Endoscopy

Performed on an outpatient basis after adequate decongestion may reveal the skull base defect or an associated pseudomeningocele or meningoencephalocele.

Biochemical Tests

These are performed to confirm the presence of CSF in nasal secretions.

- Beta-2 transferrin test: Testing for the presence of beta-2 transferrin in nasal fluid is a highly sensitive and specific method to identify CSF.[10] False-negative results may be seen in the presence of high mucus

Table 33.1 Presenting features of CSF rhinorrhea

- Active leakage of clear watery fluid from the nose:
    - Usually unilateral, intermittent, aggravated on bending forward or straining
    - "Teapot sign:" CSF may collect within the sphenoid sinus and drip through the nose when the patient bends forward, seen in sphenoid sinus leaks
    - "Reservoir sign:" Presence of intermittent rhinorrhea as CSF accumulates in the paranasal sinuses and drains externally with changes in head position
    - "Halo sign:" Ring of clear fluid surrounding a central blood stain may be elicited when CSF leaking from the nose mixed with blood is absorbed on a filter paper
- A past history of CSF leak/trauma
- Meningitis—One or more episodes
- Deafness, secondary to meningitis
- Headache
- Persistent "cold"
- Mass in the nose
- Pneumocephalus[8] may occur following a large skull base defect because of transmission of pressure on coughing, sneezing, etc.
- Associated symptoms:
    - Headache and visual disturbances suggesting raised intracranial pressure
    - Pressure-type headaches, pulsatile tinnitus, and balance abnormalities may be seen in "spontaneous" CSF leaks[1,9]

content in the secretions, while false-positive results may be obtained in patients with chronic alcohol abuse, chronic hepatic disorders, certain rare glycoprotein metabolism disorders, rectal carcinomas, or with certain genetic variants of transferrin.[11,12]

- Beta-trace protein: Beta-trace test has a specificity of nearly 100% and a sensitivity of 91.17%.[13]

Radiological Investigations

Precise identification of the size and location of the skull base defect is the first step toward its successful management. Radiological investigations help in localizing the defect, as well as identifying the presence of associated pseudomeningocele, meningoencephalocele, tumors, or any other associated pathology.

- High-resolution computed tomography (HRCT): A high-resolution CT scan may often be sufficient to identify the site of CSF leak.[14] Additional investigations may, however, be required in the presence of skull base defects without an obvious leak (e.g., previous surgical defects). HRCT may also be unable to differentiate between mucosal thickening and a meningocele, or retained secretions and CSF accumulated in a sinus.[7,15] Presence of an empty sella on magnetic resonance imaging (MRI) may be a CSF-filled herniating dura compressing the pituitary gland.[4] In such situations, MRI may be required.
- MRI and magnetic resonance cisternography (MR cisternography): MR cisternography utilizes the inherent bright signal of CSF on T2-weighted images to identify CSF leaks, avoiding radiation exposure. MRI and MR cisternography can help differentiate between inflammatory tissue and meningoencephalocele.[7] However, bony details that are required during surgery cannot be visualized on MRI.
- CT cisternography: CT cisternography with the injection of an intrathecal dye can be used in cases of doubt, when the site of CSF leak is not accurately identifiable. Cotton pledgets can be placed in the nasal cavity in cases of inactive leaks, when the leakage of dye through the defect may not be visualized.[7,15,16] These cotton pledgets are scanned later. If traces of the dye are found on the pledgets, it confirms a leak, even though the site of leak is not identifiable. CT cisternography is relatively contraindicated in the presence of raised intracranial hypertension or active meningitis. It is an invasive procedure and can lead to postprocedure headache or infections.
- Radionuclide cisternogram: During radionuclide cisternography, intranasal pledgets are placed, followed by intrathecal injection of Technetium-99. This modality can be useful in cases of low-volume or intermittent leaks, as the imaging can be completed hours to days after injection of the agent depending on the half-life of the agent used. It is, however, an invasive procedure with a high false-positive rate, variable sensitivity, less spatial resolution, and localizing ability, and is less specific in delineating fine anatomical details as compared to CT cisternography.[17,18]
- Intrathecal fluorescein: Intrathecally injected fluorescein can help diagnose a CSF leak preoperatively, or accurately localize a skull base defect, when injected intraoperatively. A lumbar puncture is performed to inject 0.1 mL of 5% fluorescein diluted in 10 mL of the patient's CSF. Leakage of the green–yellow fluid during endoscopic sinus surgery helps identify the site of CSF leak. Detection can be improved by using a blue light filter. Seizures, dizziness, nausea, vomiting may occur following intrathecal fluorescein. These, however, appear to be dose dependent and are transient at lower concentrations.[19]

Conservative Management

Traumatic CSF leaks often heal with conservative measures over a course of 7 to 10 days. Conservative management of CSF leaks include the following:

- Bed rest with head elevation.
- Avoidance of straining, for example, nose blowing, sneezing, coughing, constipation.
- Diuretics and stool softeners.[6]
- Prophylactic antibiotics: The use of prophylactic antibiotics in the management of CSF leaks is controversial as some authors are of the view that it may lead to an increased risk of developing antibiotic resistance.[1,19]
- Lumbar drain: May be indicated in high-pressure leaks.[20]

Surgical Management

Indications for Surgery

- Failure of conservative management.
- CSF leaks developing days or weeks after trauma.
- Very large postsurgical defects.
- High-pressure leaks which do not heal even on normalizing the intracranial pressure.
- Persistent pneumocephalus despite cessation of leak.

Spontaneous CSF leaks are unlikely to heal, and hence merit surgical repair.

Endoscopic Repair of Cerebrospinal Fluid Rhinorrhea

Endoscopic repair of CSF rhinorrhea, rather than transcranial approach, is now the preferred method, because of comparable success rates and lower morbidity. A careful reading of CT/MRI scans to define the site and size of the skull base defect and preoperatively planning the approach to the defect site is necessary before embarking on the procedure.

Types of Reconstruction

The choice of reconstruction technique for skull base defects should be individualized depending on the etiology, location and size of the bony defect, and underlying intracranial pressure.[21,22] They can be repaired using the underlay technique, overlay technique, or a combination of both (**Fig. 33.1**).

Underlay Technique

Graft is placed between the dura and bone after elevating the dura from the margins of the skull base defect.

Overlay Technique

Graft material is placed over the skull base bone. An overlay graft may be sufficient in cases of small defects (< 5 mm).

Combined Underlay–Overlay Technique

Moderate-sized (5–10 mm) defects and larger defects (>10 mm) would usually require a combined underlay (graft placed between bony defect and dura) and overlay technique of graft placement.[23] A multilayered combined underlay and overlay reconstruction using soft tissue may suffice for moderate-sized defects (≥4 mm) with normal intracranial pressure. However, for large defects, a rigid underlay graft (cartilage or bone) with an overlay soft tissue graft may be required.[1]

The graft size should be slightly larger than the size of the defect[23] with the placement being such that there is no tenting or stretching.[24] Fibrin glue, a combination of fibrinogen, thrombin, and calcium cofactor, is commonly used to ensure that the graft is held in place and to provide an additional barrier to CSF leakage during wound healing. Oxidized cellulose and gelatin sponge may be used to provide additional support. Nasal packs are used to provide temporary support.[4]

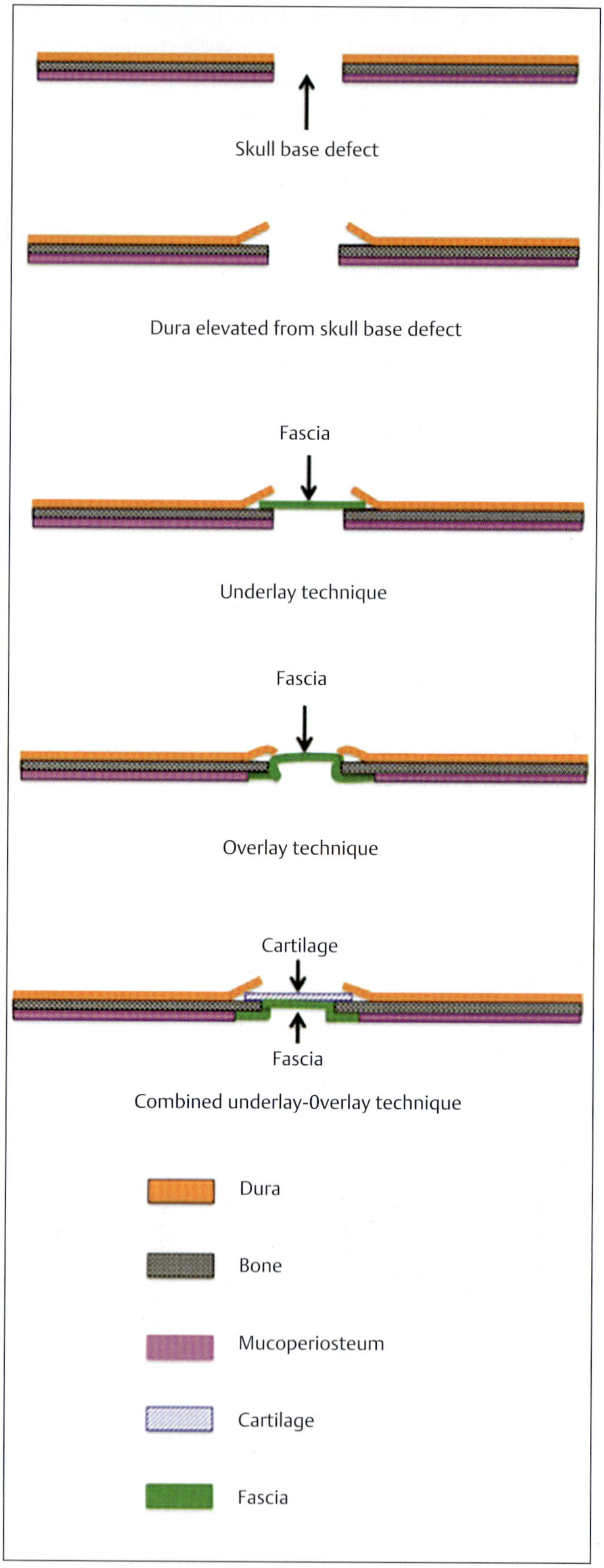

Fig. 33.1 Diagrammatic representation of techniques for repair of skull base defects.

Graft Material

A variety of graft materials have been used for skull base reconstruction.[25–36]

- Local flaps:
  - Middle turbinate osteomucoperiosteal flap.[25]

- Septal mucoperichondrial flap.[26]
- Hadad–Bassagasteguy flap: Neurovascular pedicled flap of the nasal septal mucoperiosteum and mucoperichondrium based on the nasoseptal artery (branch of the posterior septal artery).[27]

- Free grafts from local nasal sites: For example, septal mucoperiosteum, turbinate mucosa, or septal cartilage,
- Free grafts from distant areas: For example, conchal cartilage, temporalis fascia, fascia lata, rectus sheath, abdominal or thigh fat, muscle, radial free forearm flaps,[28] calvarial bone.[29]
- Dermal allograft,[30] lyophilized cadaver dura,[4] bovine pericardium.[4]
- Exogenous materials: For example, hydroxyapatite cement,[31] Vicryl mesh.[32]

Free grafts adhere to bone by 1 week.[33] Integration of vascularized fibrous tissue into free fascial grafts occurs by 2 to 3 weeks, even in the absence of an overlying vascularized flap.[34] About 92 to 96% of skull base defect repairs have been reported to be successful, irrespective of the graft materials used.[10,24,35,36]

Endoscopic repair of anterior skull base defects is carried out under general anesthesia with the patient in supine position. Strict asepsis is followed when preparing and draping the area around the nose and the graft site (thigh or abdomen). Adequate nasal decongestion is performed using saline–adrenaline-soaked pledgets.

Repair of Cribriform Plate Defects

The attachment of the middle turbinate separates the cribriform plate into medial and lateral lamella. Thus, the middle turbinate acts as a useful landmark when approaching medial and lateral lamella defects.

Endoscopic Repair of Medial Lamella Defects

Approach to the Medial Lamella

The middle turbinate is gently lateralized, and the area medial to the middle turbinate adequately decongested with adrenaline-soaked pledgets to approach the medial lamella.

Repair of Medial Lamella Defects

The defect in the medial lamella is identified (**Fig. 33.2**). A pseudomeningocele, prolapsing through the defect, is cauterized with a bipolar cautery (**Fig. 33.3** and **Fig. 33.4**). The mucosa over the bone is abraded to create a raw area (**Fig. 33.5**), and to stimulate osteoneogenesis.[6] A sliver of fat (harvested from the thigh or abdomen) is then placed over the defect (**Fig. 33.6**). This may be further covered with fascia (from thigh or abdomen; **Fig. 33.7**) and oxidized cellulose. However, in our experience, for medial lamellar defects (82 cases), using fat alone has also shown good results with no recurrence of the leak (unpublished data). The fat, fascia, and

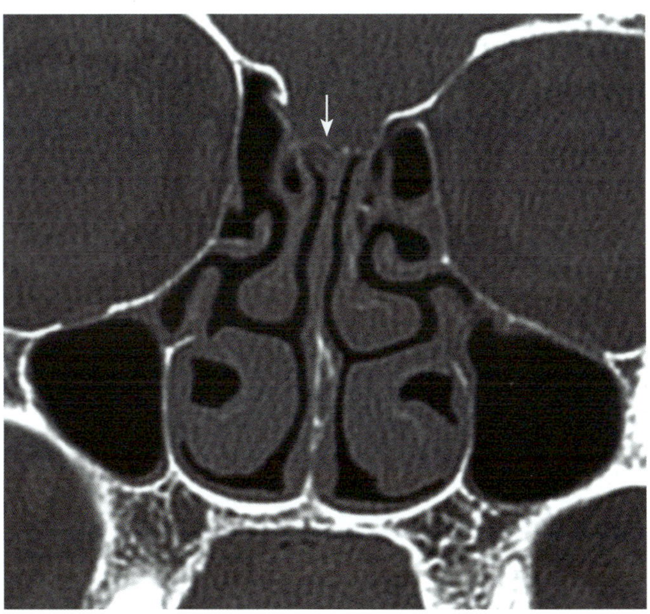

Fig. 33.2 CT scan paranasal sinus (PNS) showing a defect in the right medial lamella and a small pseudomeningocele (*white arrow*).

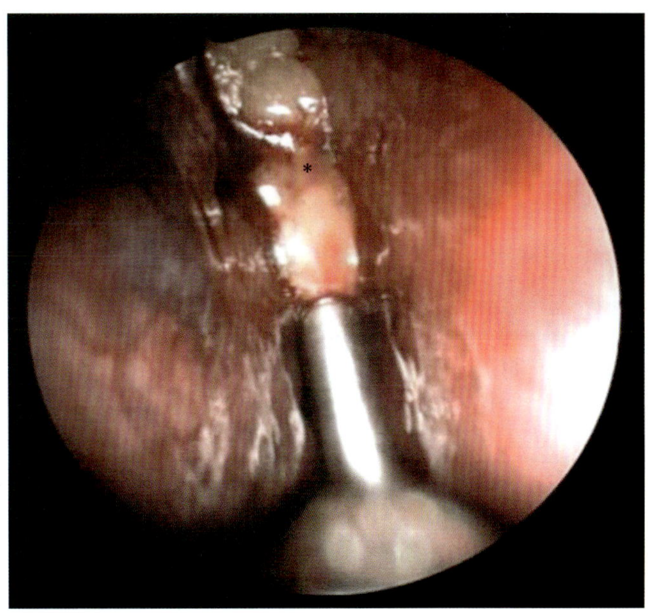

Fig. 33.3 Endoscopic view of pseudomeningocele in the right medial lamella (*).

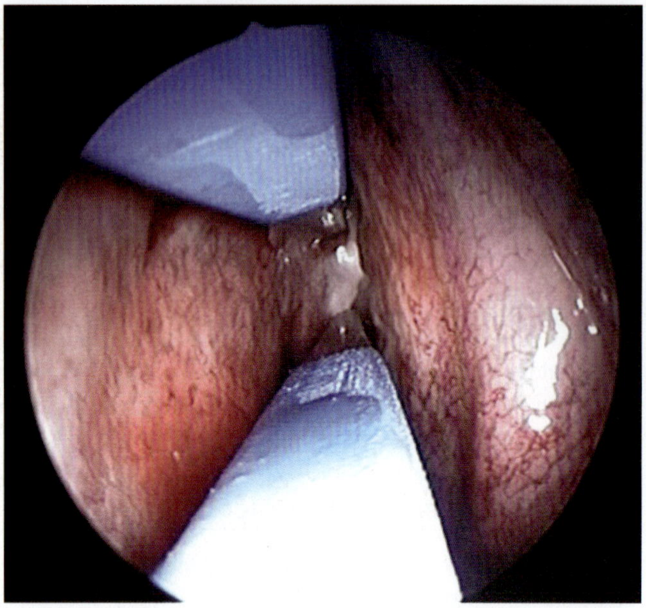

Fig. 33.4 Cauterization of pseudomeningocele with bipolar cautery.

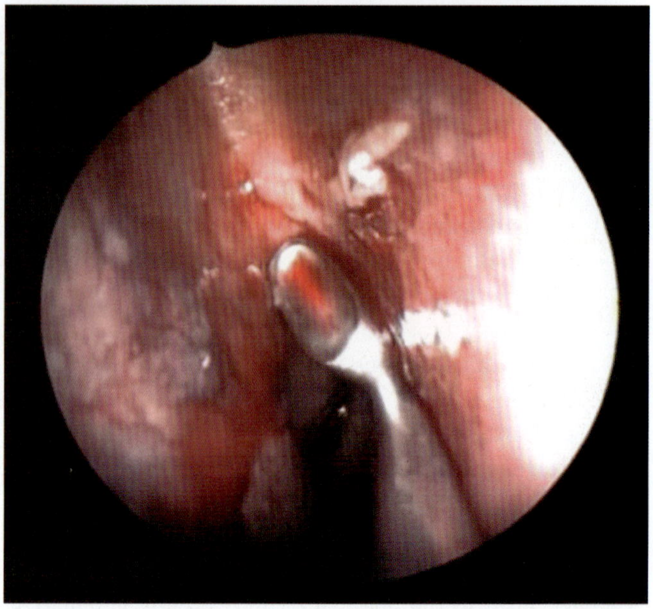

Fig. 33.5 Raw area created around the defect.

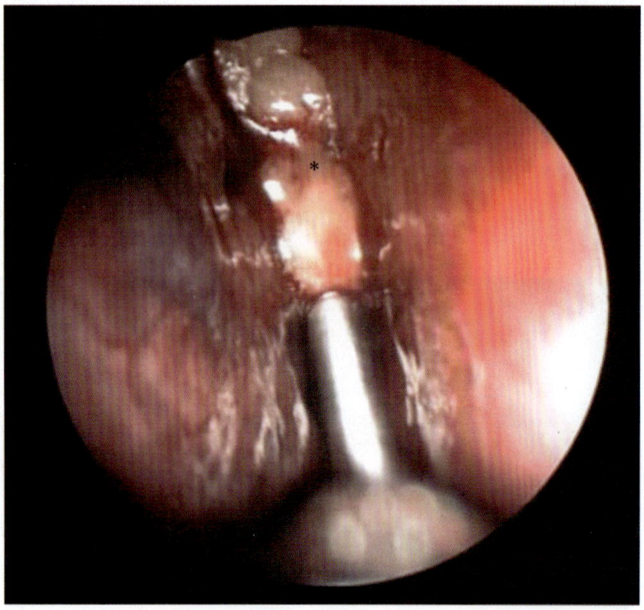

Fig. 33.6 Fat (*black* *) harvested from the thigh being positioned at the defect site.

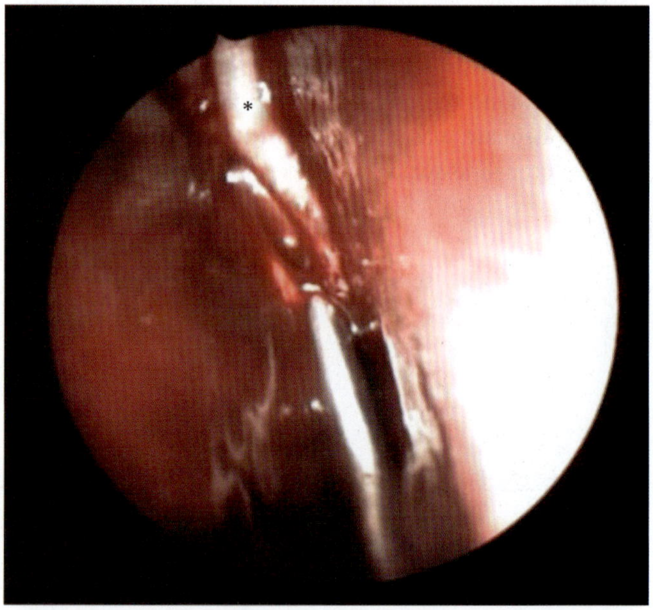

Fig. 33.7 Fat covered with a piece of fascia lata (*black* *) and covered with a layer of fibrin glue.

oxidized cellulose are further covered by a layer of fibrin glue, followed by reinforcement with absorbable gelatin sponge (**Fig. 33.7** and **Fig. 33.8**). The nasal cavity is then packed with nonabsorbable sponge to hold the repair in place (**Fig. 33.9**). The defect is thus sealed with the formation of a thick layer of fibrosis postoperatively (**Fig. 33.10**).

Endoscopic Repair of Lateral Lamella Defects

Approach to the Lateral Lamella

The lateral lamella (**Fig. 33.11**) can be approached by passing the endoscope lateral to the middle turbinate. An ethmoidectomy is usually required to access the defect site.

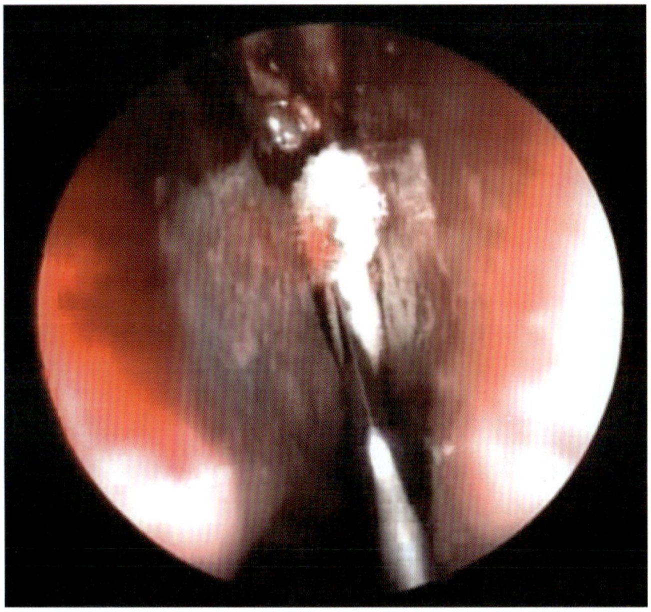

Fig. 33.8 Absorbable gelatin sponge placed over the layer of fibrin glue.

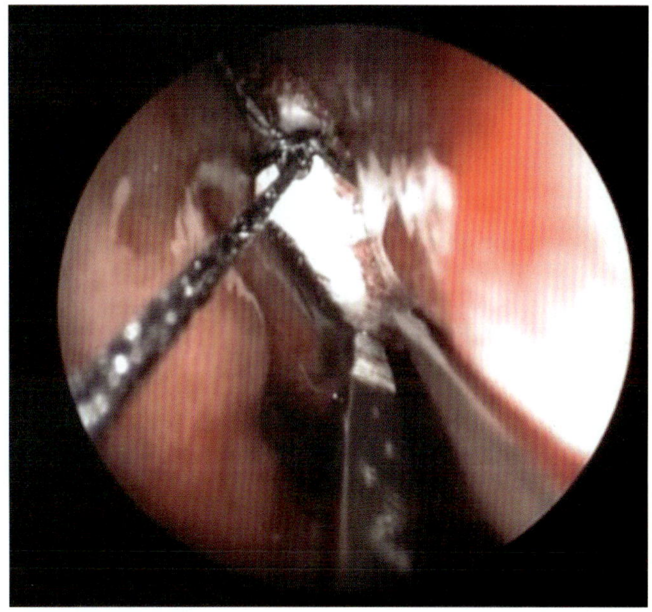

Fig. 33.9 Nasal packing with nonabsorbable sponge.

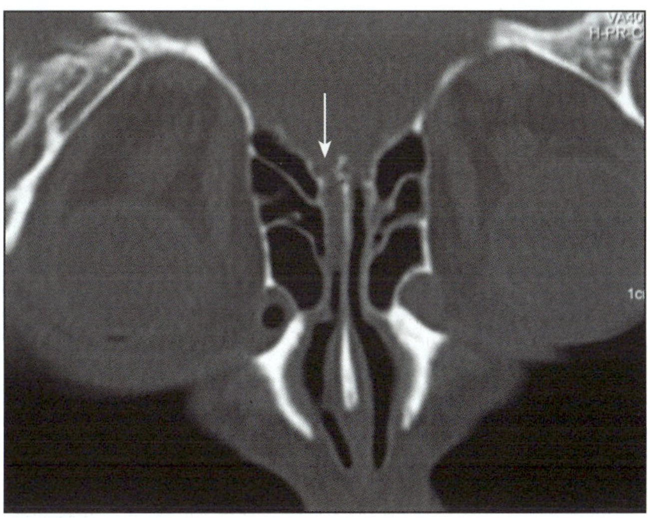

Fig. 33.10 Postoperative CT scan demonstrating the sealed medial lamella defect and a thick layer of fibrosis (*white arrow*).

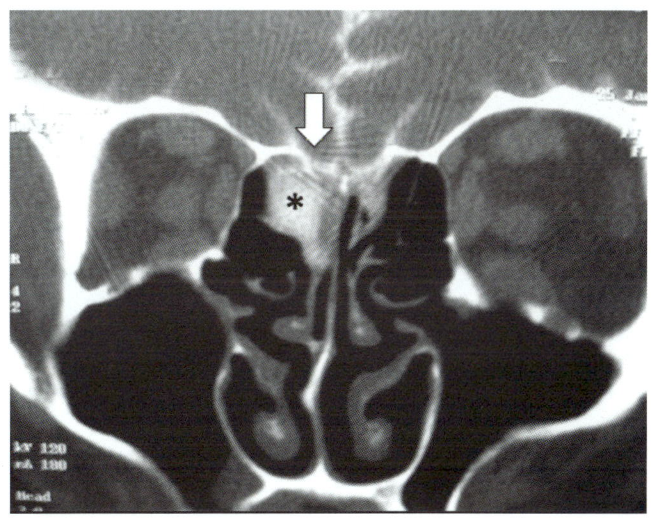

Fig. 33.11 CT cisternogram demonstrating a right lateral lamella defect (*white arrow*) with a pseudomeningocele (*).

Repair of Lateral Lamella Defects

Once the defect is identified (**Fig. 33.12**), the pseudomeningocele or the meningoencephalocele prolapsing through the defect is cauterized with a bipolar cautery and trimmed if needed (**Fig. 33.13**). Once the defect is well-delineated and its size determined (**Fig. 33.14**), it can be sealed with the "bath plug technique" (**Fig. 33.15, Fig. 33.16, Fig. 33.17, Fig. 33.18, Fig. 33.19,** and **Fig. 33.20**). A fat plug larger than the defect is harvested from the abdomen, thigh, or ear lobule. A 3–0 absorbable suture is passed along the length of the fat plug and knotted at one end of the plug. The fat plug is then introduced through the skull base defect and gently pushed through the defect using a blunt instrument. Once the fat plug is completely introduced into the defect, a gentle pull is applied on the absorbable suture so that the fat plug is hitched at the defect to provide a snug fit. A piece of fascia slightly larger in size than the size of the defect is slid along the absorbable suture to cover the fat plug and defect completely. Fibrin glue is used to reinforce the reconstruction,

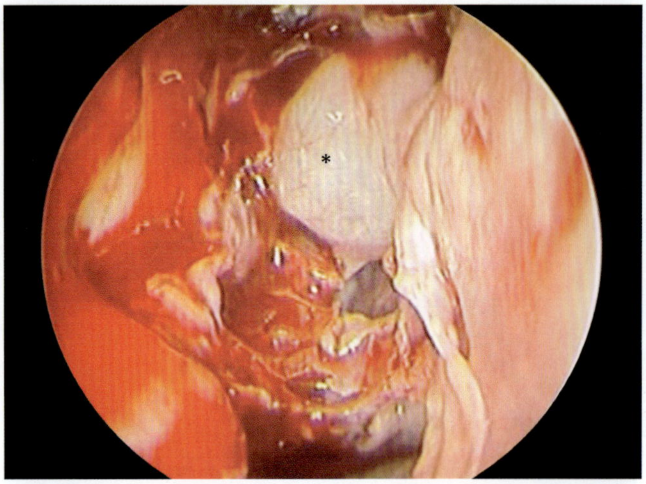

Fig. 33.12 Endoscopic view after dissection showing the pseudomeningocele (*).

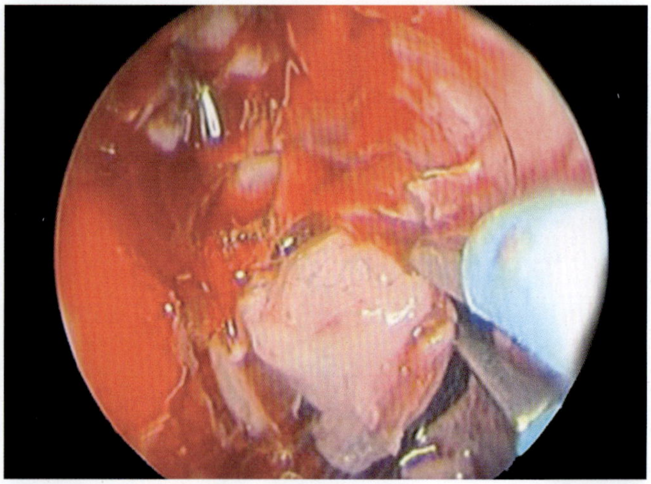

Fig. 33.13 Cauterization of the pseudomeningocele with bipolar cautery.

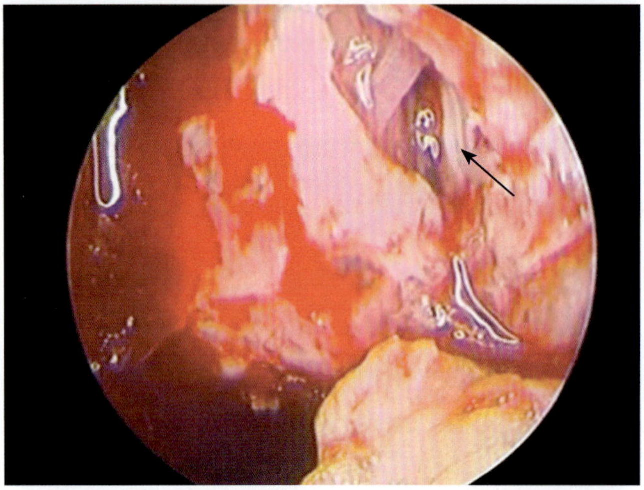

Fig. 33.14 Delineation of the lateral lamella defect with visualization of CSF leaking through the defect (*black arrow*).

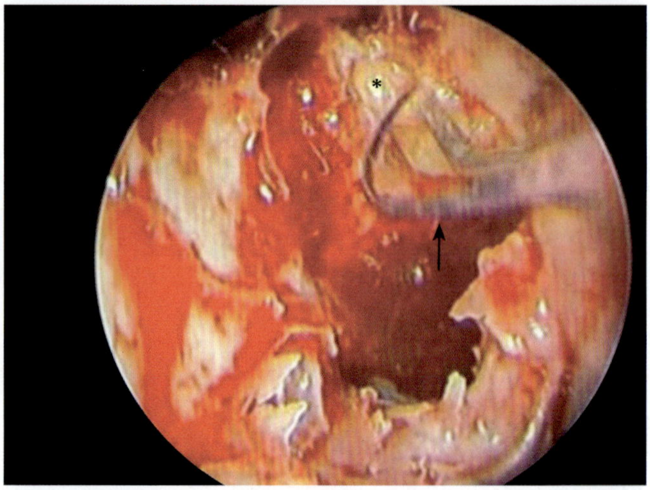

Fig. 33.15 Defect packed using a snug fitting fat plug (bath plug technique)—*black* *. Note the polyglactin thread with which the fat plug is tied (*black arrow*).

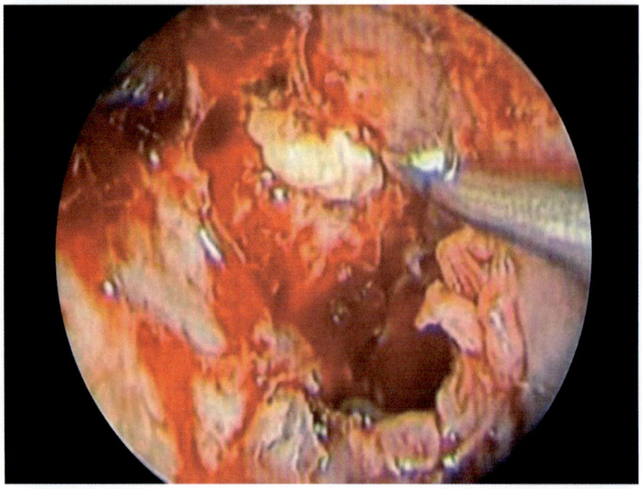

Fig. 33.16 Creation of raw area around the defect.

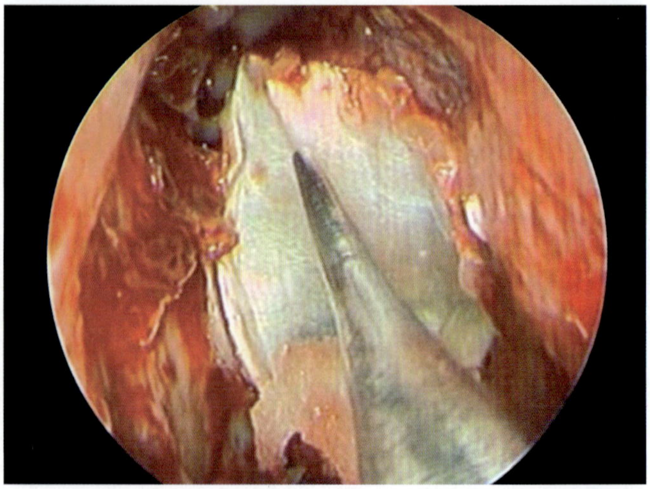

Fig. 33.17 A piece of fascia lata threaded over the polyglactin suture, held in place by the fibrin glue.

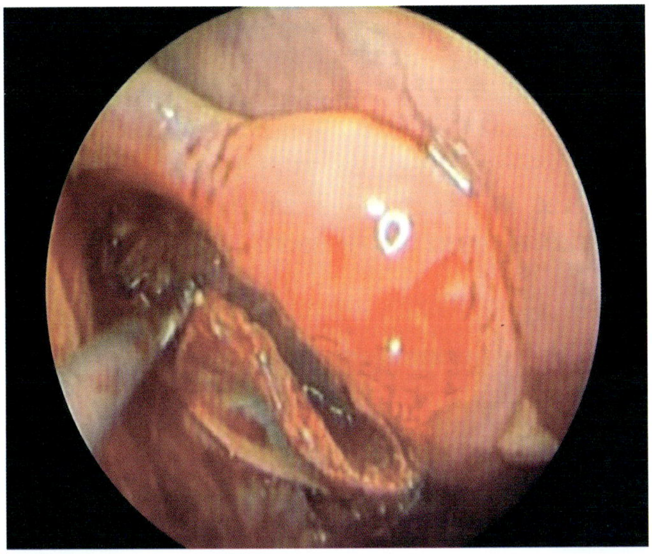

Fig. 33.18 Application of fibrin glue between the fascia and fat.

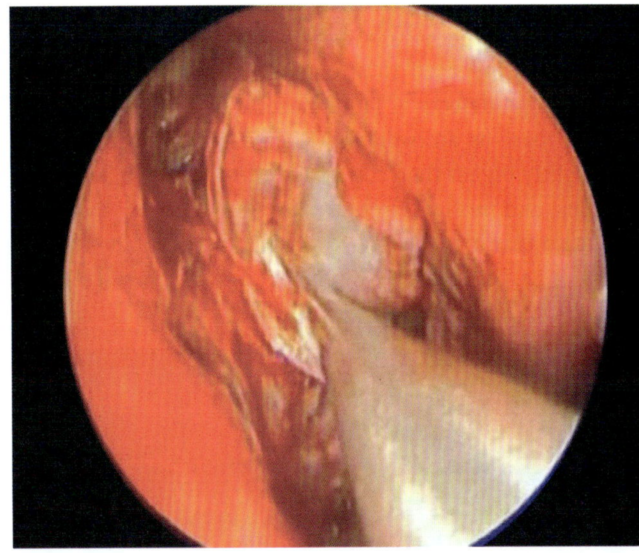

Fig. 33.19 Reposition of the fascia lata.

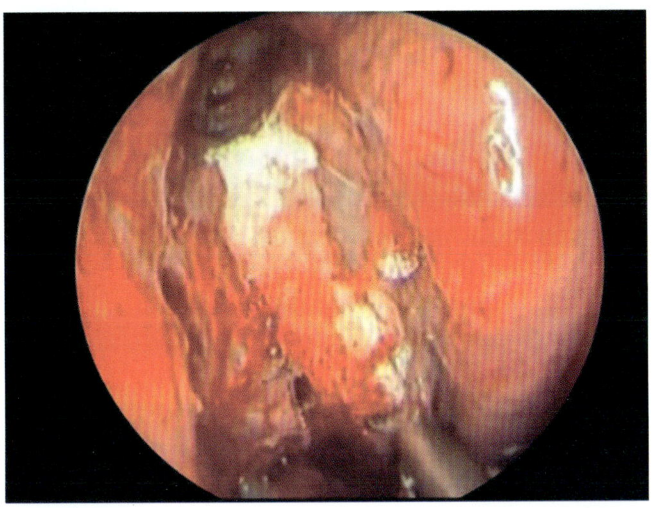

Fig. 33.20 Pieces of absorbable gelatin sponge placed over the fascia for reinforcement.

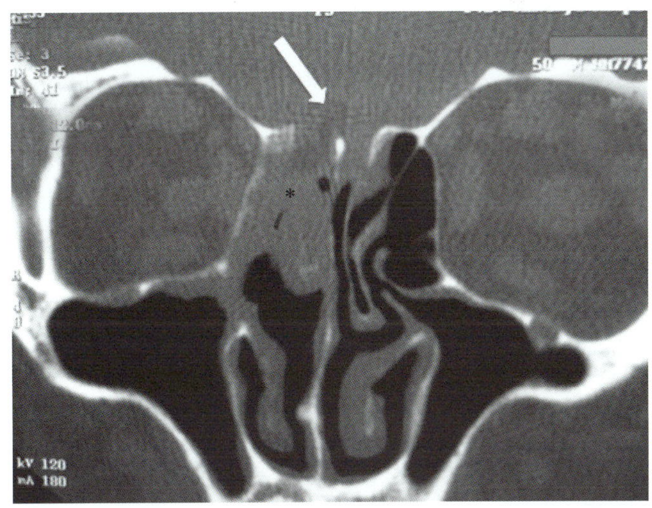

Fig. 33.21 Postoperative CT scan image (3 months postoperative) demonstrating the repair (*). Note the hypodense shadow because of the fat plug used to seal the defect (*white arrow*).

and the absorbable suture is cut. Gelatin sponge is then placed over the fascia for support. **Fig. 33.21** shows a postoperative CT scan image of a lateral lamella defect repaired via the "bath plug technique."

Endoscopic Repair of Roof of Ethmoid Defects—Sandwich Technique

Approach to the Roof of Ethmoids

The roof of ethmoids is approached by passing the endoscope lateral to the middle turbinate. An ethmoidectomy is required to visualize the defect, with occasional trimming of the middle turbinate to improve access.

Repair of Defect in the Roof of Ethmoids

After delineation of the defect, a pseudomeningocele prolapsing through the defect is cauterized with a bipolar cautery and excised. If the sac is not cauterized, intracranial hemorrhage may occur during attempts to reduce or excise the sac. In case of very large defects, the encephalocele may be reduced by gently pushing it intracranially instead of excising it.

Sandwich Technique

Cartilage can be used to strengthen the reconstruction in cases of large defects. A large piece of fascia is placed over the skull base as an overlay. A premeasured piece of cartilage slightly bigger than the size of the defect is placed over the fascia and pushed through the defect, carrying the fascia with it, so that a collar of fascia remains externally, lying in contact with the bone. A second piece of fascia is then placed over the cartilage as an overlay graft. A layer of fibrin glue is used to reinforce the adherence of the fascia to the cartilage and skull base. This is further covered with a gelatin sponge.[37] See **Fig. 33.22, Fig. 33.23, Fig. 33.24, Fig. 33.25, Fig. 33.26, Fig. 33.27, Fig. 33.28, Fig. 33.29, Fig. 33.30, Fig. 33.31, Fig. 33.32,** and **Fig. 33.33.**

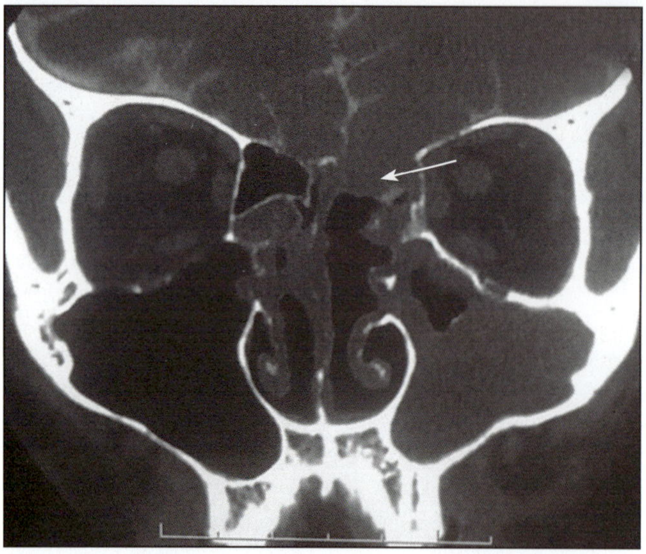

Fig. 33.22 CT PNS showing a large defect in the roof of the ethmoids with an encephalocele prolapsing through the defect (*white arrow*).

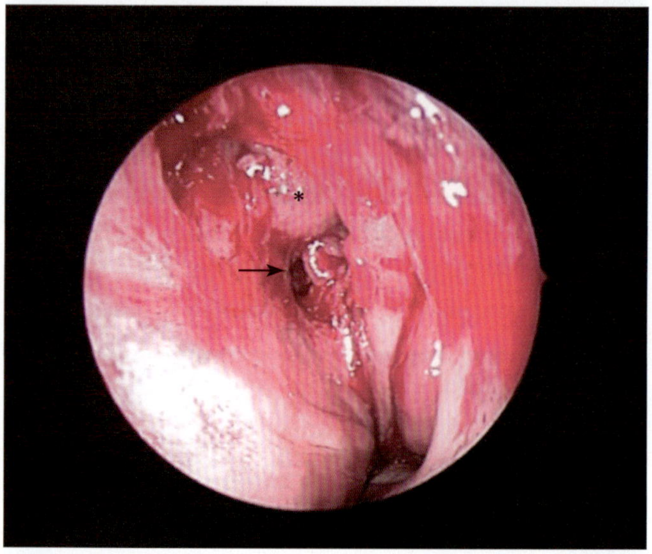

Fig. 33.23 Endoscopic view of the defect showing the encephalocele (*) prolapsing through the defect in the roof of ethmoids (*black arrow*).

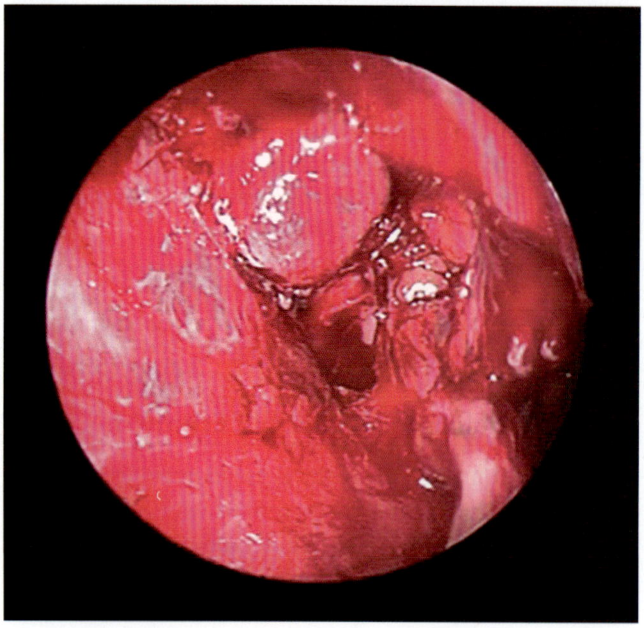

Fig. 33.24 Delineation of the defect and creation of a raw area around the defect.

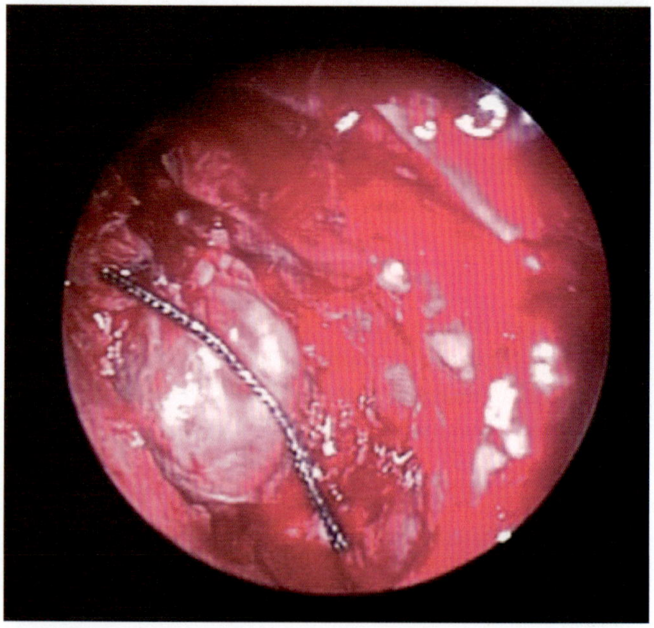

Fig. 33.25 Estimation of the approximate size of the defect using a piece of suture material.

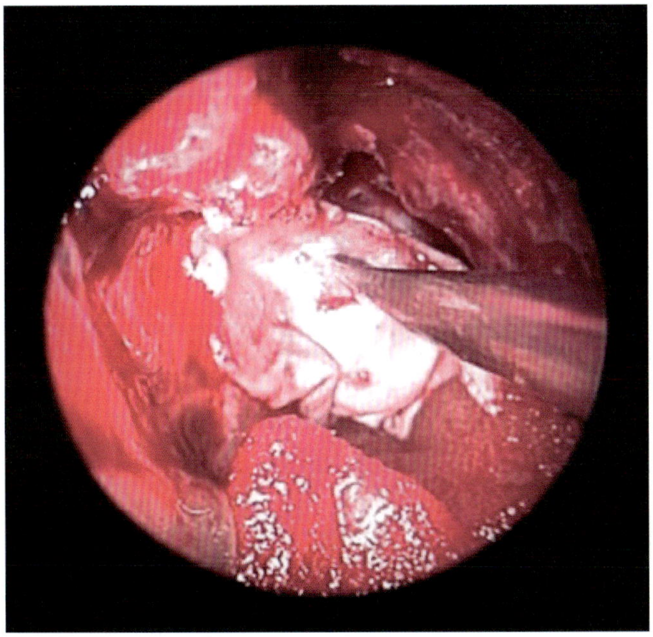

Fig. 33.26 Piece of fascia lata graft placed over the encephalocele.

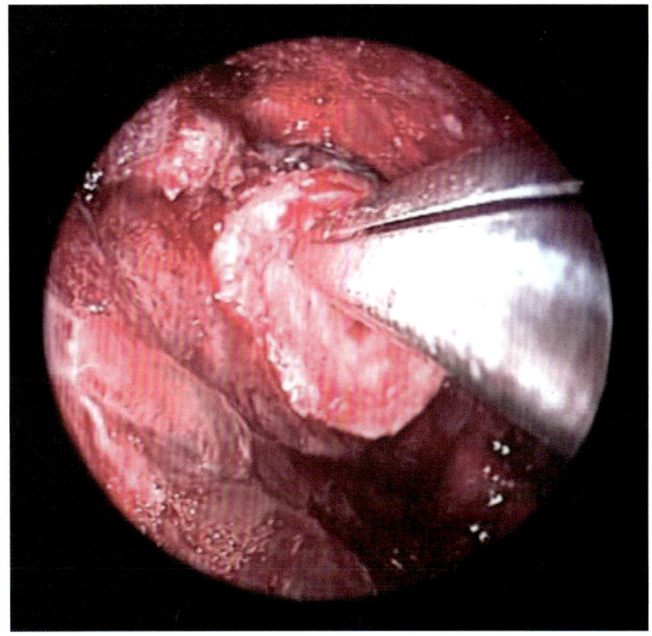

Fig. 33.27 A piece of septal cartilage (slightly larger in dimensions than the size of the defect) placed over the piece of fascia and manipulated so that the encephalocele and the fascia covering it are pushed in through the defect.

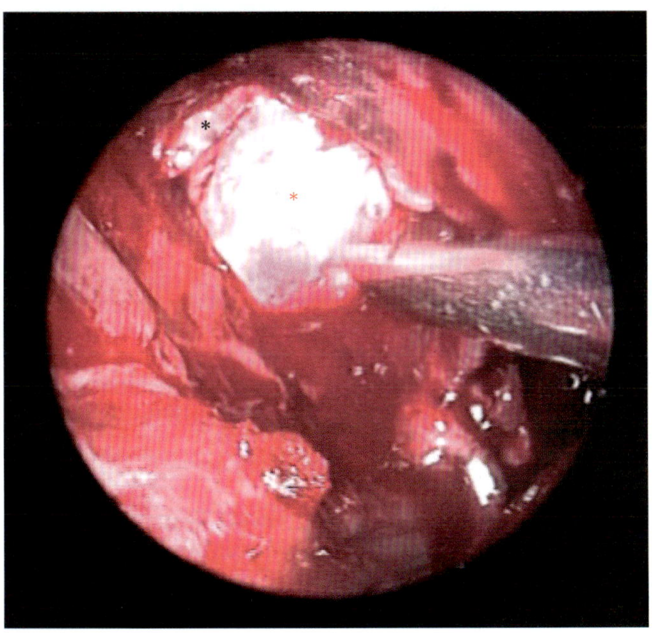

Fig. 33.28 The cartilage (*red* *) is further pushed in gently through the defect so that both the fascia (*black* *) and the cartilage piece are placed in an underlay fashion.

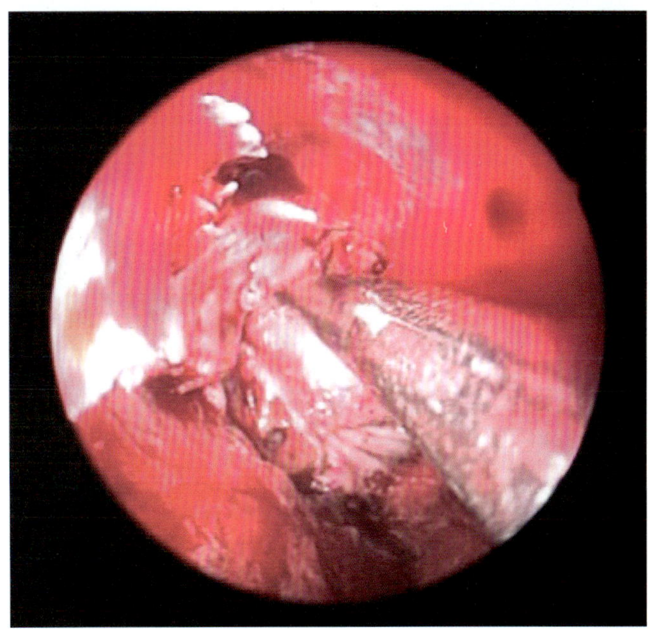

Fig. 33.29 A second piece of fascia is placed over the cartilage piece as an overlay graft.

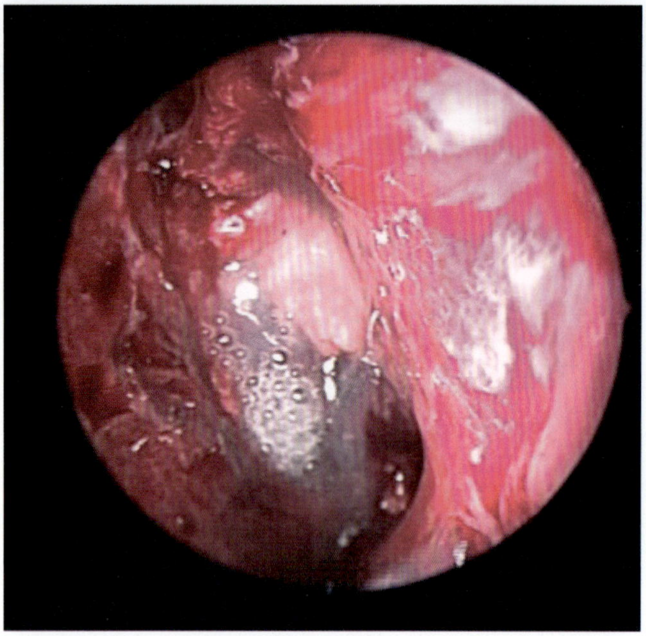

Fig. 33.30 Tissue glue applied over the second layer of fascia.

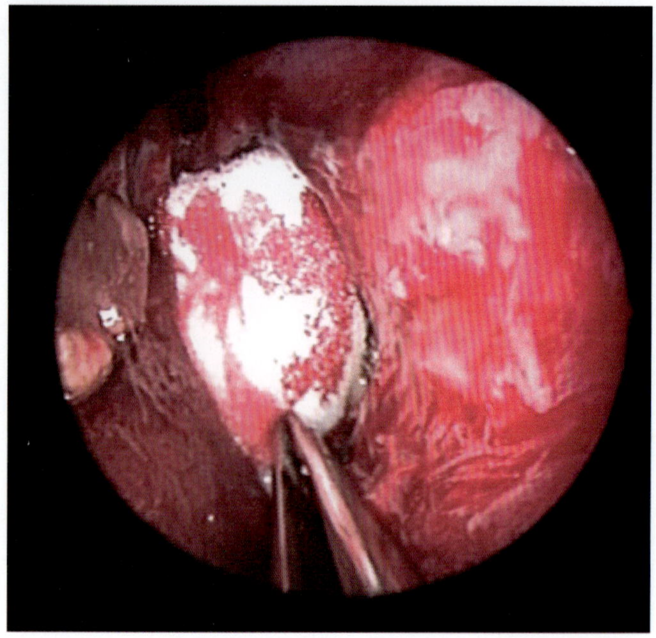

Fig. 33.31 Absorbable gelatin sponge placed over the repair for reinforcement.

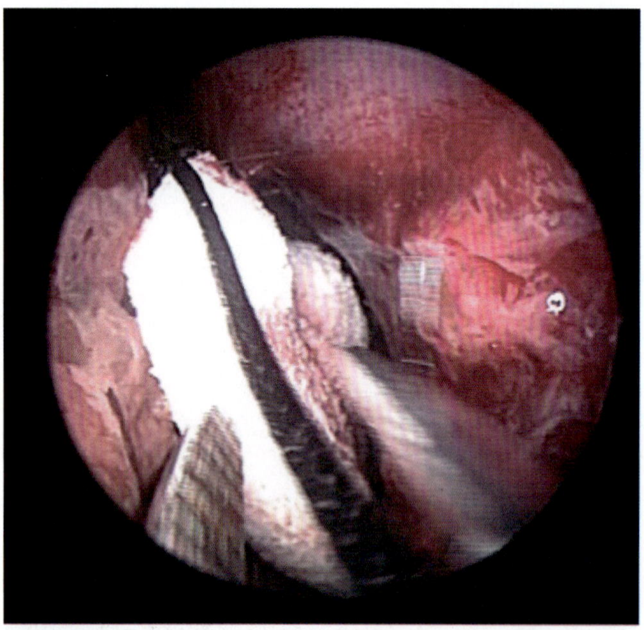

Fig. 33.32 Nasal packing with nonabsorbable sponge.

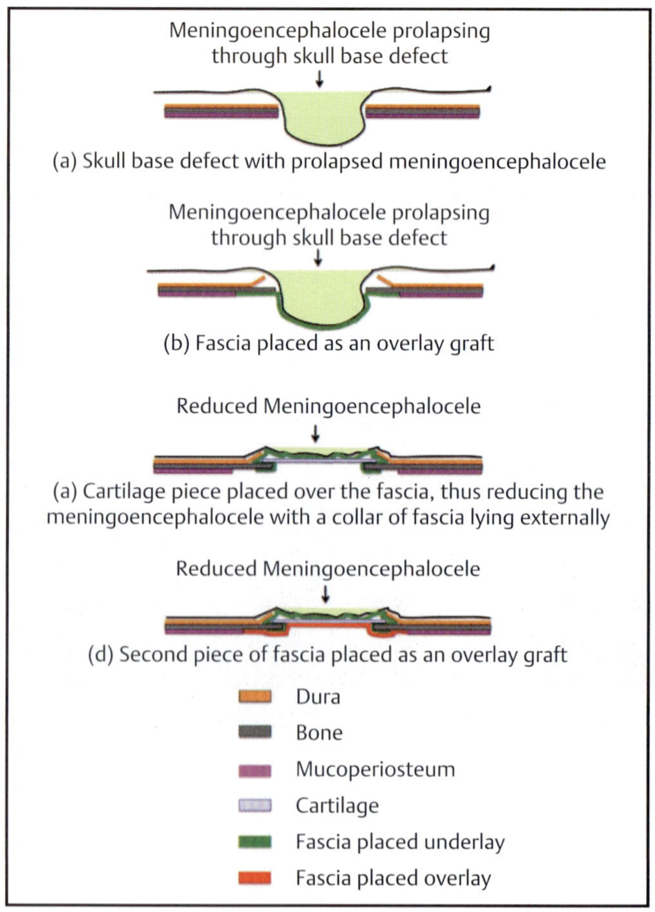

Fig. 33.33 Diagrammatic representation of fascia-cartilage-fascia (sandwich) technique for repair of skull base defects.

Endoscopic Repair of Sphenoid Sinus Defects

Approach to the Sphenoid Sinus Ostium

Transethmoidal approach: A complete anterior and posterior ethmoidectomy is performed, followed by identification of the sphenoid sinus ostium.[38]

Parasagittal approach: The sphenoid ostium is identified medial to the superior turbinate.

Approaching the Pterygoid Recess of the Sphenoid

Defects in the pterygoid recess of the sphenoid sinus can be repaired by various approaches.

The pterygoid recess can be reached by widening the sphenoid ostium laterally.[38] After identifying the sphenoid ostium, a wide exposure is obtained by removing the anterior wall of the sphenoid sinus to visualize the roof and lateral wall of the sphenoid sinus. Widening is continued laterally until the lateral end of the pterygoid recess is reached, and the defect is clearly visualized and identified in all its margins.[38]

An endoscopic transpterygoid approach[39] has also been used. This approach involves performing a posterior ethmoidectomy, followed by identification and widening of the sphenoid sinus ostium. The maxillary ostium is widened and the posterior wall of the maxillary sinus is removed to provide access to the pterygopalatine fossa and to expose the anterior pterygoid aspect of the sphenoid. The anterior aspect of the pterygoid portion of the sphenoid is drilled to enter the lateral sphenoid recess.

Trimming of the posterior end of the middle turbinate may be performed.

Endoscopic Repair of Sphenoid Sinus Defects

The defect in the sphenoid sinus is clearly visualized and identified in all its margins. An encephalocele, if present, is ablated with a bipolar cautery. The mucosa surrounding the defect is removed. It is plugged with a fat plug. The "bath plug" technique can be used for this. The fat is further covered with fascia, fibrin glue, and absorbable gelatin sponge. See **Fig. 33.34, Fig. 33.35, Fig. 33.36, Fig. 33.37, Fig. 33.38, Fig. 33.39, Fig. 33.40, Fig. 33.41, Fig. 33.42, Fig. 33.43,** and **Fig. 33.44**.

In cases where there are multiple potential sites of leaks because of dehiscence in sphenoid sinus walls, the entire sinus mucosa is denuded, and the sinus is packed with fat. This is then supported with a septal mucosal flap such as the Hadad–Bassagasteguy flap[27] based on the sphenopalatine artery.

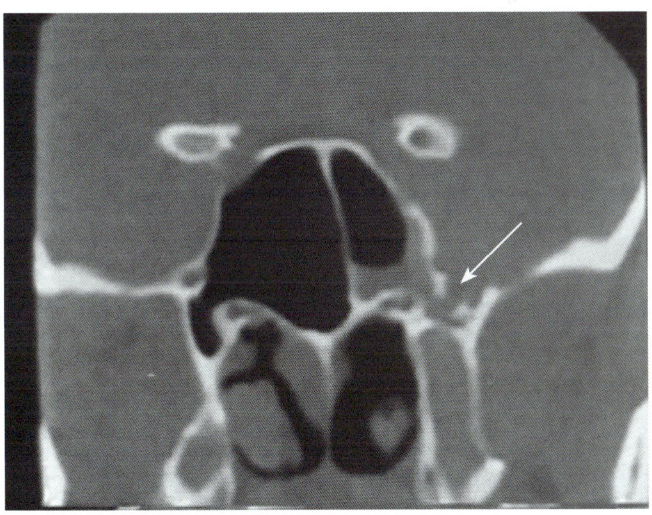

Fig. 33.34 CT scan showing a defect in the pterygoid recess of the left sphenoid sinus (*white arrow*).

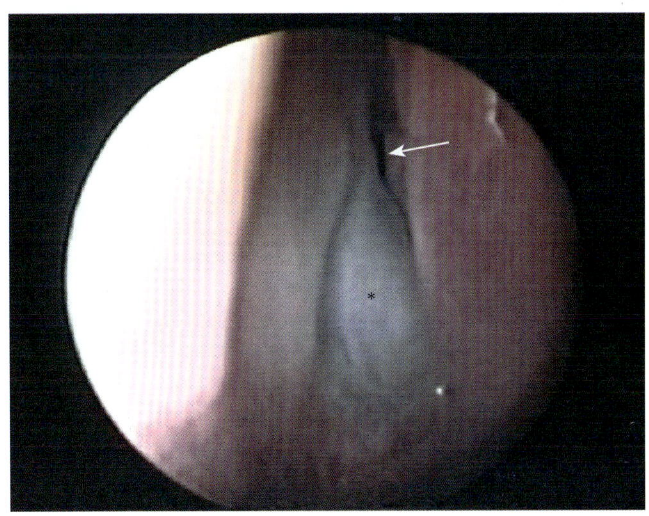

Fig. 33.35 Endoscopic view showing the left sphenoid ostium (*white arrow*) with a meningocele (*).

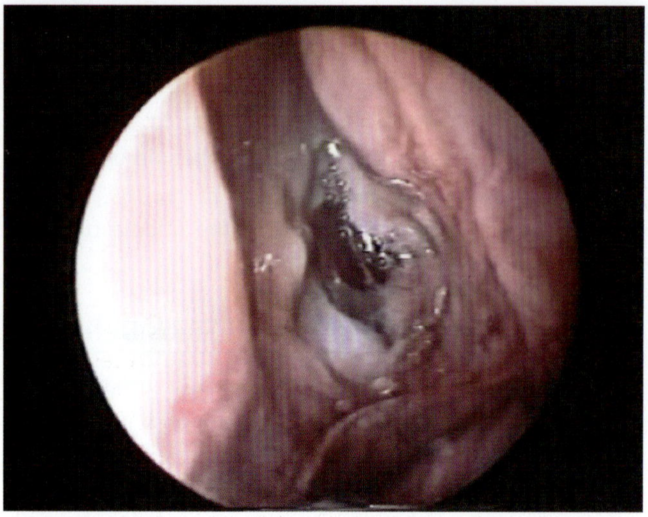

Fig. 33.36 CSF leaking out through the sphenoid ostium.

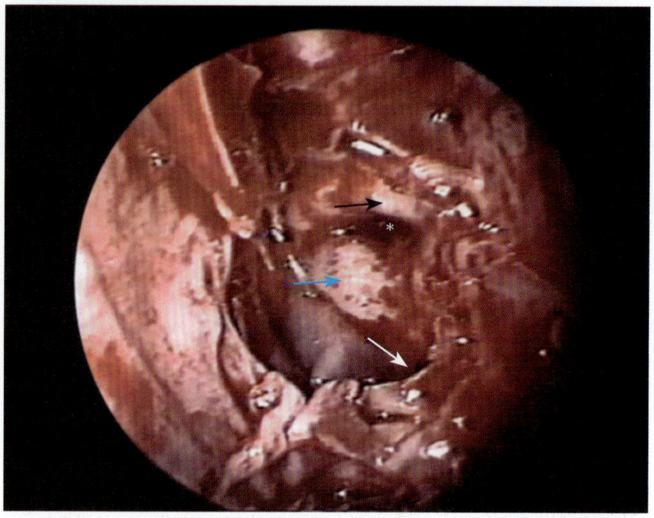

Fig. 33.37 The sphenoid sinus following the widening of the sphenoid ostium (*white arrow*) showing the optic nerve (*black arrows*) and the internal carotid artery (*blue arrow*). The carotico-optico recess is seen between the two (*). The white arrow points toward the pterygoid recess.

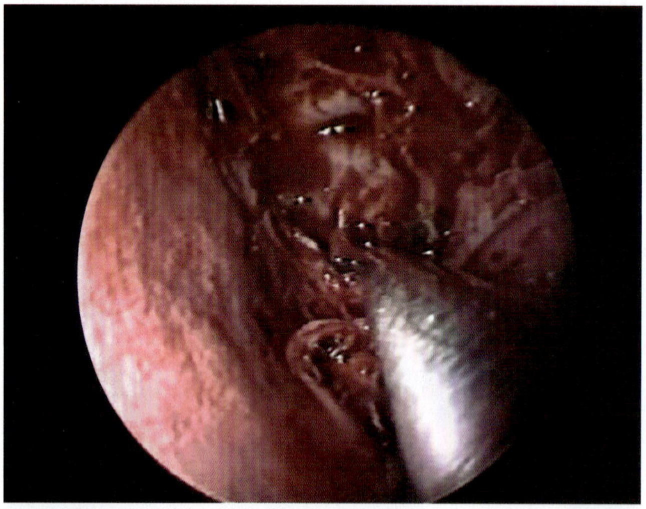

Fig. 33.38 Widening of the sphenoid ostium with a bone punch.

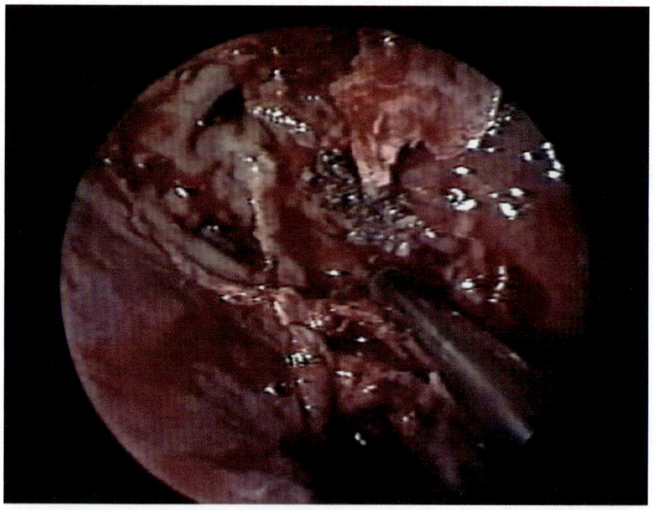

Fig. 33.39 Drilling of the lateral wall of the sphenoid to expose the pterygoid recess.

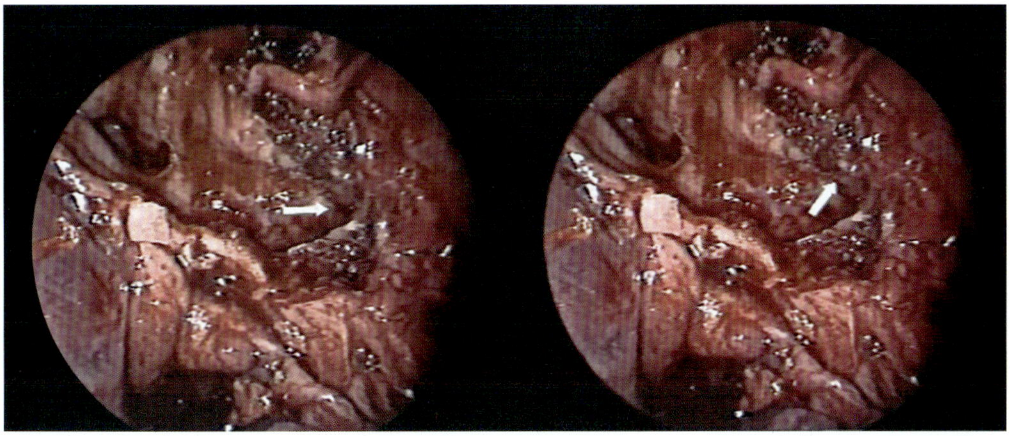

Fig. 33.40 Defect in the lateral recess of the sphenoid (*white arrow*).

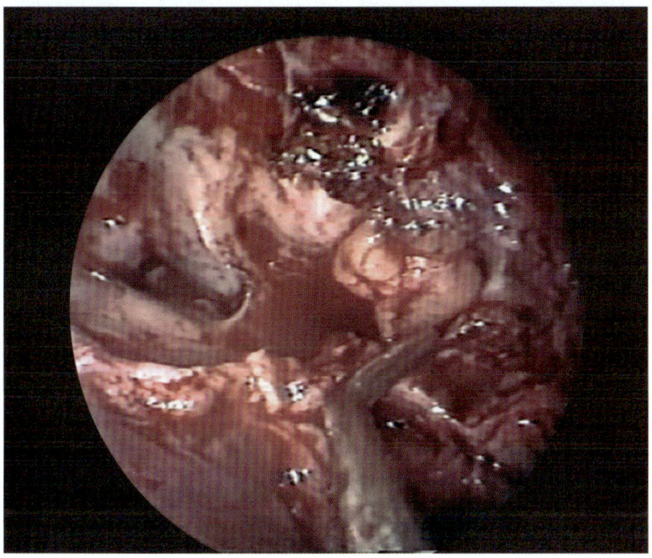

Fig. 33.41 Defect in the pterygoid recess being plugged with fat.

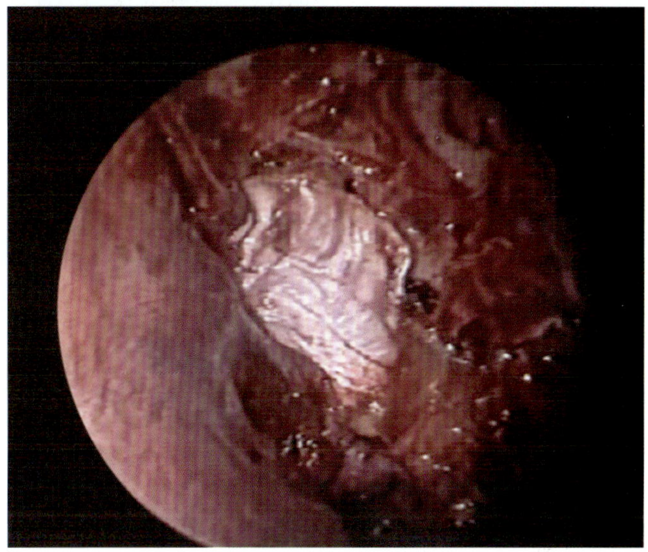

Fig. 33.42 A piece of fascia lata used to cover the layer of fat.

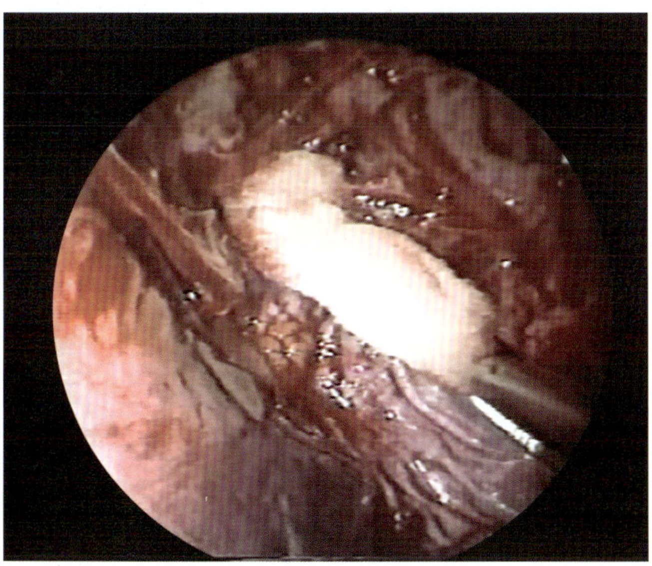

Fig. 33.43 Absorbable gelatin sponge placed over the fascia.

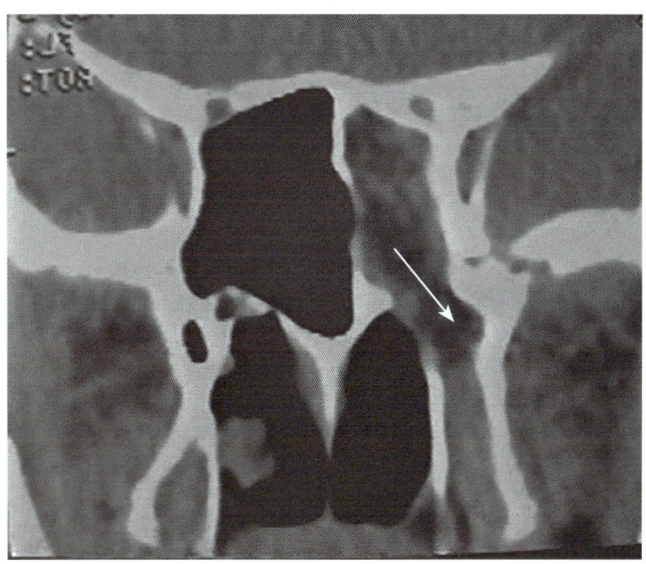

Fig. 33.44 Postoperative CT scan. The hypodense area (*white arrow*) represents the fat used to seal the defect.

Endoscopic Repair of Frontal Recess Defects

The repair of defects in the roof of the frontal sinus requires an external approach. However, frontal recess and accessible frontal sinus defects can be repaired via the transnasal endoscopic approach. **Fig. 33.45, Fig. 33.46, Fig. 33.47,** and **Fig. 33.48** demonstrate endoscopic repair of a frontal recess defect sealed with fat and fascia. Care should be taken to keep the frontal sinus outflow tract patent while performing this procedure.

Endoscopic Repair of Cerebrospinal Leaks from the Clivus

CFS leaks through the clivus are usually posttraumatic or occur secondary to lesions such as chordomas.[40] The clivus is an uncommon site for a primary spontaneous CSF leak.[40] CSF leaks from the clivus can be repaired via an endoscopic transsphenoidal approach.[40] See **Fig. 33.49, Fig. 33.50, Fig. 33.51, Fig. 33.52, Fig. 33.53, Fig. 33.54, Fig. 33.55, Fig. 33.56,** and **Fig. 33.57**.

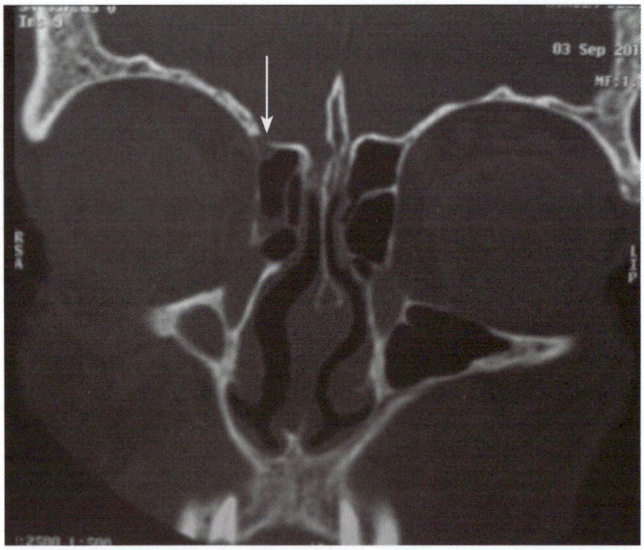

Fig. 33.45 CT scan demonstrating a right frontal recess defect (*white arrow*).

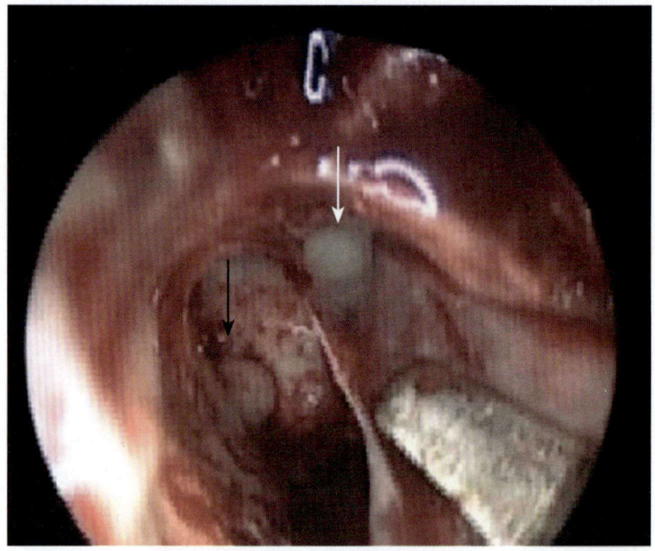

Fig. 33.46 Endoscopic view of the frontal recess defect (*black arrow*). The *white arrow* points toward the frontal ostium.

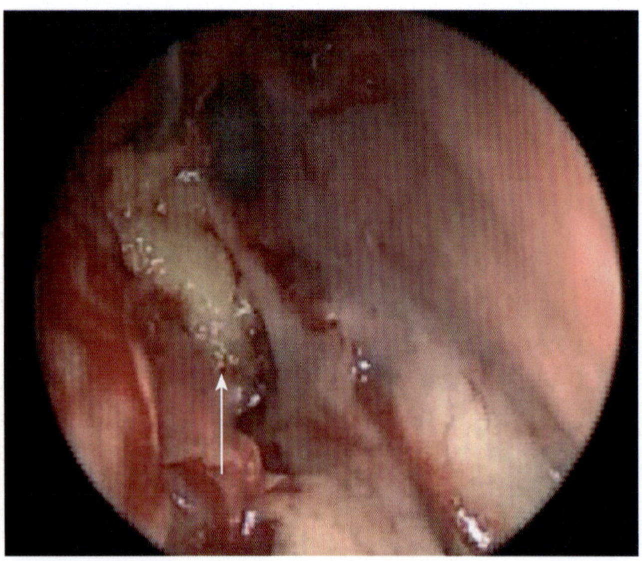

Fig. 33.47 Defect sealed with fat (*white arrow*).

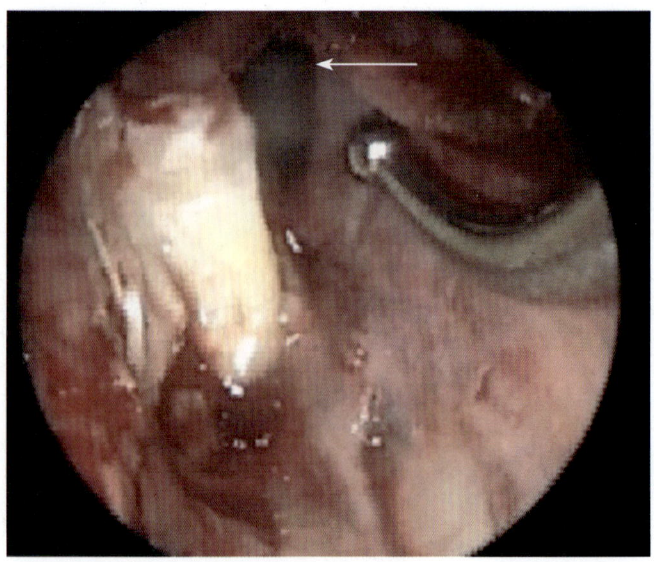

Fig. 33.48 A layer of fascia held over the fat with fibrin glue. Note the patent frontal ostium (*white arrow*).

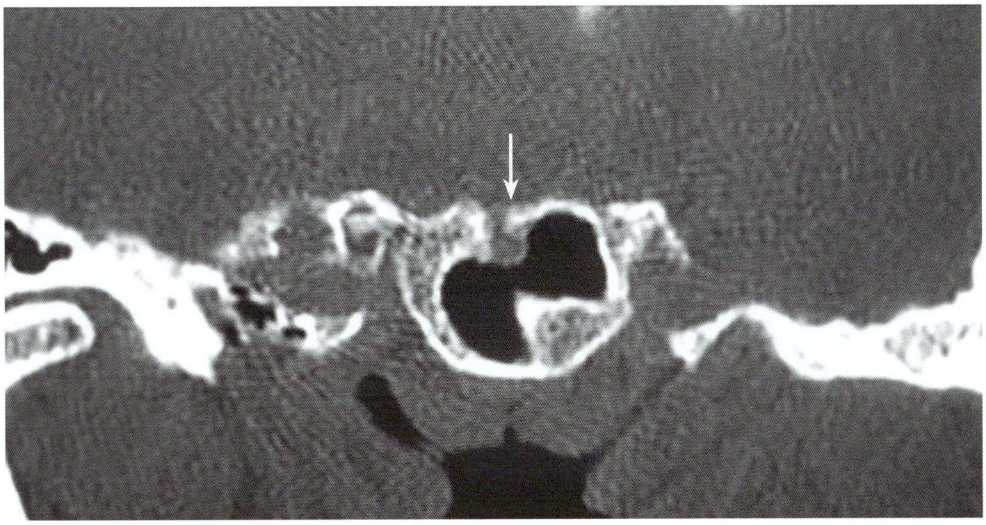

Fig. 33.49 CT scan showing a defect in the clivus with a protruding meningocele (*white arrow*).

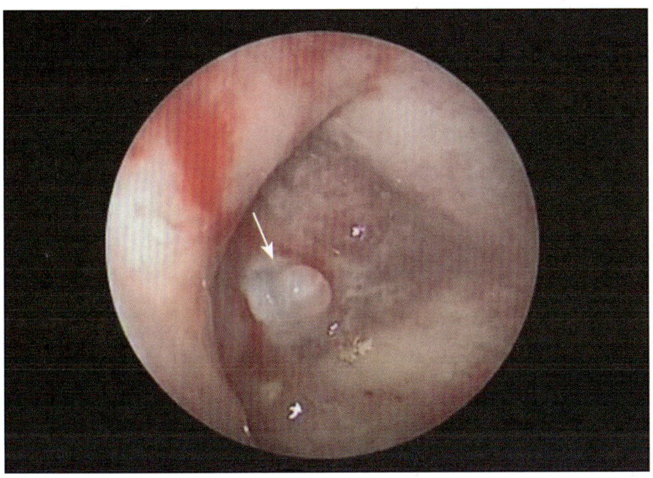

Fig. 33.50 Endoscopic view of the sphenoid sinus with visualization of the protruding meningocele through the clival defect (*white arrow*).

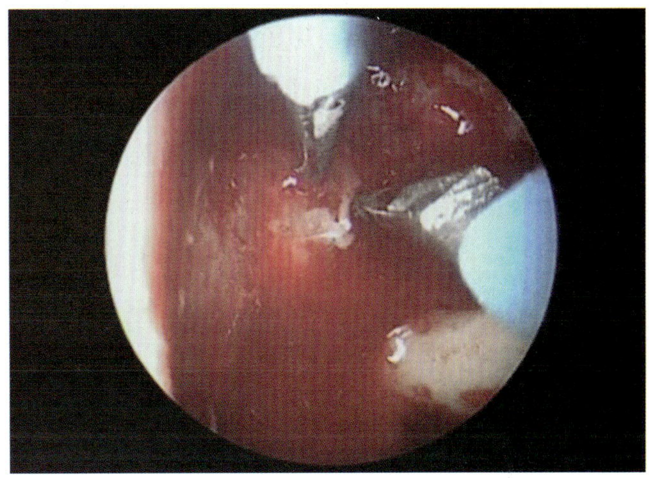

Fig. 33.51 Cauterization of the base of the meningocele with bipolar cautery.

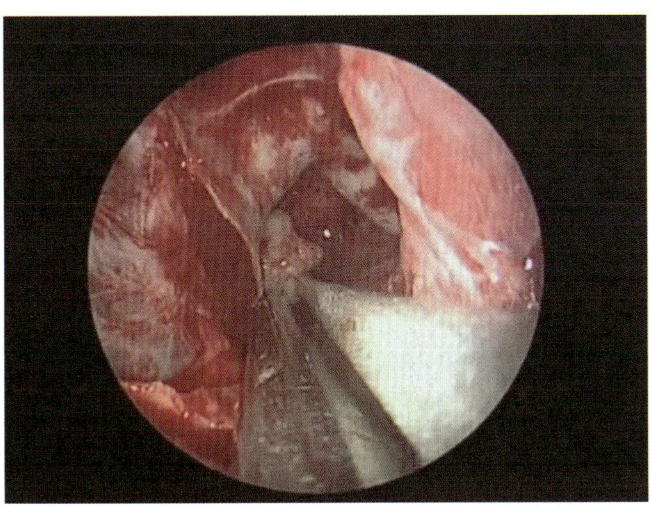

Fig. 33.52 Defect plugged with fat.

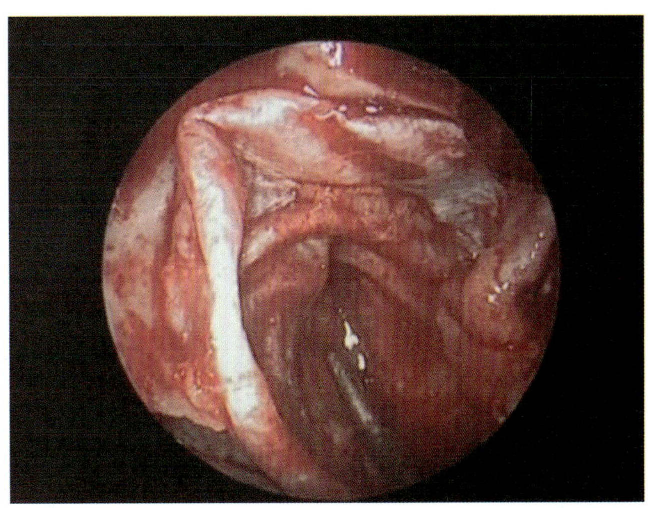

Fig. 33.53 Fascia lata placed over the fat.

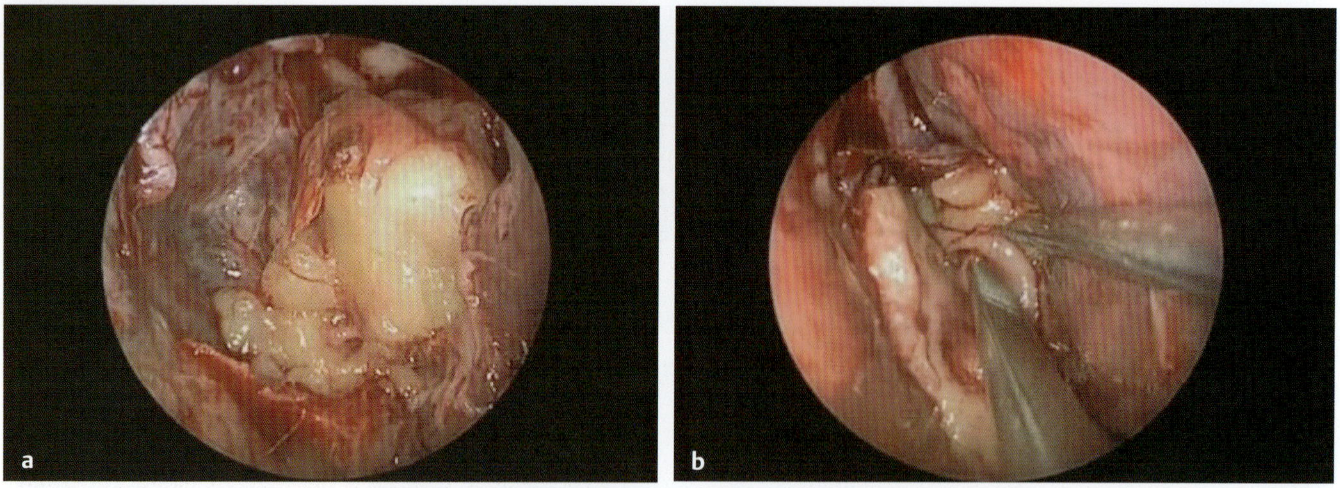

Fig. 33.54 **(a)** Sphenoid sinus packed with fat. **(b)** Sphenoid ostium covered with a nasoseptal flap.

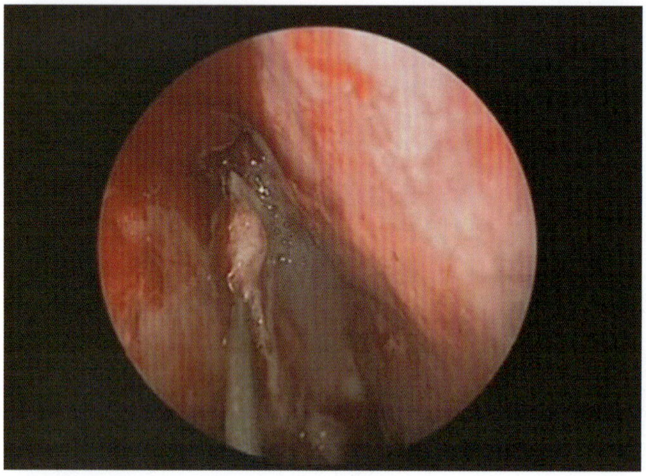

Fig. 33.55 A layer of fibrin glue applied.

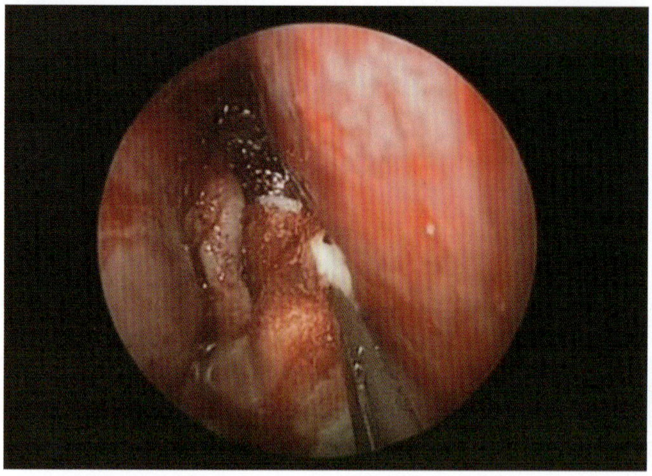

Fig. 33.56 Reinforcement of the repair with oxidized cellulose and absorbable gelatin sponge.

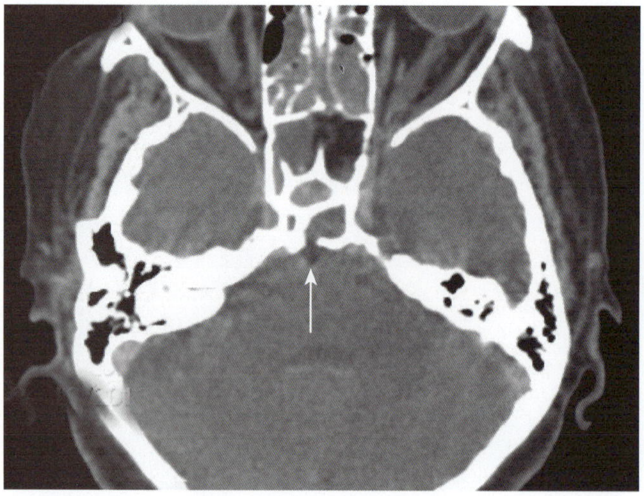

Fig. 33.57 Postoperative CT scan. *Arrow* shows the hypodense shadow created by the fat seal.

Approach to the Clivus

The sphenoid sinus ostium is identified and widened. The clivus is visualized and the defect identified. Any pseudomeningocele protruding through the defect is cauterized, the defect defined, and a raw area created around the defect by denuding the mucosa. The defect can then be plugged using fat in a "bath plug" fashion, covered with a piece of fascia and held in place with fibrin glue. The sphenoid sinus can be completely packed with fat after denuding the mucosa, and covered with a septal flap. This is further reinforced with fibrin glue, oxidized cellulose, and absorbable gelatin sponge.

Postoperative Care

- Complete bed rest with head elevation for a period of 5 days.
- Nonabsorbable nasal packs usually removed on the fifth postoperative day.
- Nose blowing, any strenuous activity, lifting of heavy weights, and bending down should be avoided for about 6 weeks. Constipation, if any, should be treated.
- Antibiotic prophylaxis: May be given in the perioperative period and continued postoperatively till the nasal packs are removed.[6]
- Diuretics: For example, acetazolamide to decrease CSF pressure, especially in cases of raised intracranial pressures and spontaneous CSF leaks. Electrolyte monitoring and potassium supplementation are required with acetazolamide administration.
- Lumbar drain: Some authors recommend routine use of a lumbar drain,[41] while others recommend a lumbar drain only in the presence of raised intracranial pressure or hydrocephalus.[42–45]
- Follow-up CT scan: It is done 3 months postoperatively to look for sinus outflow tract obstruction.

Postoperative Complications

Endoscopic CSF leak repair is associated with a low rate of complications.[41,43] Complications[43] in the postoperative period include the following:

- Meningitis.
- Brain abscess.
- Subdural hematoma.
- Olfactory disorders.
- Headache.
- Failure of previously done CSF repair.

Limitations of Endoscopic Techniques

- Defects located in the roof of the frontal sinus may require an osteoplastic flap with or without obliteration of the frontal sinus.
- Multiple/bilateral/comminuted or large posttraumatic, or very large defects.
- Coexistent tumors with intracranial extension, which cannot be resected endoscopically.

Failure of Endoscopic Repair

Factors that may contribute to the potential failure of endoscopic repair of skull base defects include the following:[30,41,46,47–49,50]

- Unsuccessful localization of the defect.
- Failure to identify coexisting defects.
- Insufficient graft size.
- Graft displacement.
- Inadequate approximation of the graft to the skull base defect.
- Patient noncompliance with postoperative instructions.
- Poor wound healing because of coexisting comorbid conditions.
- Elevated body mass index.
- Prior radiation therapy.
- Infection.
- Very large skull base defects.

Endoscopic repair of CSF rhinorrhea has been reported to be successful in 75.9 to 97% cases at the first attempt, with the success rates increasing to 100% after a second attempt.[36,44,45,47–49,51]

Factors which contribute to a successful endoscopic repair of skull base defects include a proper understanding of the etiology and mechanism of a CSF leak, accurate localization of the defect site, and following the appropriate surgical technique. With better techniques and knowhow, lesser morbidity, and a shorter postoperative recovery period, endoscopic repair is now a preferred surgical approach for most cases of CSF rhinorrhea.

References

1. Schlosser RJ, Bolger WE. Endoscopic management of cerebrospinal fluid rhinorrhea. Otolaryngol Clin North Am 2006;39(3):523–538, ix
2. Lindstrom DR, Toohill RJ, Loehrl TA, Smith TL. Management of cerebrospinal fluid rhinorrhea: the Medical College of Wisconsin experience. Laryngoscope 2004;114(6):969–974
3. Lee TJ, Huang CC, Chuang CC, Huang SF. Transnasal endoscopic repair of cerebrospinal fluid rhinorrhea and skull base defect: ten-year experience. Laryngoscope 2004;114(8):1475–1481
4. Kerr JT, Chu FW, Bayles SW. Cerebrospinal fluid rhinorrhea: diagnosis and management. Otolaryngol Clin North Am 2005; 38(4):597–611

5. Ommaya AK, Di Chiro G, Baldwin M, Pennybacker JB. Non-traumatic cerebrospinal fluid rhinorrhoea. J Neurol Neurosurg Psychiatry 1968;31(3):214–225
6. Lanza DC, O'Brien DA, Kennedy DW. Endoscopic repair of cerebrospinal fluid fistulae and encephaloceles. Laryngoscope 1996;106(9 Pt 1):1119–1125
7. Shetty PG, Shroff MM, Sahani DV, Kirtane MV. Evaluation of high-resolution CT and MR cisternography in the diagnosis of cerebrospinal fluid fistula. AJNR Am J Neuroradiol 1998; 19(4):633–639
8. Wise SK, Harvey RJ, Patel SJ, Frankel BM, Schlosser RJ. Endoscopic repair of skull base defects presenting with pneumocephalus. J Otolaryngol Head Neck Surg 2009;38(4):509–516
9. Rudnick E, Sismanis A. Pulsatile tinnitus and spontaneous cerebrospinal fluid rhinorrhea: indicators of benign intracranial hypertension syndrome. Otol Neurotol 2005; 26(2):166–168
10. PapadeaC,SchlosserRJ.Sensitivedetectionofbeta-2transferrin in cerebrospinal fluid leakage using an automated immunofixation electrophoresis method. Clin Chem 2004;51(2): 464–470
11. Sloman AJ, Kelly RH. Transferrin allelic variants may cause false positives in the detection of cerebrospinal fluid fistulae. Clin Chem 1993;39(7):1444–1445
12. Stibler H. Carbohydrate-deficient transferrin in serum: a new marker of potentially harmful alcohol consumption reviewed. Clin Chem 1991;37(12):2029–2037
13. Bachmann G, Nekic M, Michel O. Clinical experience with beta-trace protein as a marker for cerebrospinal fluid. Ann Otol Rhinol Laryngol 2000;109(12 Pt 1):1099–1102
14. Lloyd MNH, Kimber PM, Burrows EH. Post-traumatic cerebrospinal fluid rhinorrhoea: modern high-definition computed tomography is all that is required for the effective demonstration of the site of leakage. Clin Radiol 1994; 49(2):100–103
15. Shetty PG, Shroff MM, Fatterpekar GM, Sahani DV, Kirtane MV. A retrospective analysis of spontaneous sphenoid sinus fistula: MR and CT findings. AJNR Am J Neuroradiol 2000; 21(2):337–342
16. Chow JM, Goodman D, Mafee MF. Evaluation of CSF rhinorrhea by computerized tomography with metrizamide. Otolaryngol Head Neck Surg 1989;100(2):99–105
17. Stone JA, Castillo M, Neelon B, Mukherji SK. Evaluation of CSF leaks: high-resolution CT compared with contrast-enhanced CT and radionuclide cisternography. AJNR Am J Neuroradiol 1999;20(4):706–712
18. Flynn BM, Butler SP, Quinn RJ, McLaughlin AF, Bautovich GJ, Morris JG. Radionuclide cisternography in the diagnosis and management of cerebrospinal fluid leaks: the test of choice. Med J Aust 1987;146(2):82–84
19. Keerl R, Weber RK, Draf W, Wienke A, Schaefer SD. Use of sodium fluorescein solution for detection of cerebrospinal fluid fistulas: an analysis of 420 administrations and reported complications in Europe and the United States. Laryngoscope 2004;114(2):266–272
20. Stankiewicz JA. Cerebrospinal fluid fistula and endoscopic sinus surgery. Laryngoscope 1991;101(3):250–256
21. Cooper PR. Skull fracture and traumatic cerebro-spinal fluid fistulas in head injury. In: Cooper PR, ed. Head Injury. Baltimore, MD: Williams and Wilkins; 1982
22. Schlosser RJ, Bolger WE. Nasal cerebrospinal fluid leaks: critical review and surgical considerations. Laryngoscope 2004; 114(2):255–265
23. El-Banhawy OA, Halaka AN, Altuwaijri MA, Ayad H, El-Sharnoby MM. Long-term outcome of endonasal endoscopic skull base reconstruction with nasal turbinate graft. Skull Base 2008; 18(5):297–308
24. Mattox DE, Kennedy DW. Endoscopic management of cerebrospinal fluid leaks and cephaloceles. Laryngoscope 1990; 100(8):857–862
25. Yessenow RS, McCabe BF. The osteo-mucoperiosteal flap in repair of cerebrospinal fluid rhinorrhea: a 20-year experience. Otolaryngol Head Neck Surg 1989;101(5):555–558
26. Weisman RA. Septal chondromucosal flap with preservation of septal integrity. Laryngoscope 1989;99(3):267–271
27. Hadad G, Bassagasteguy L, Carrau RL, et al. A novel reconstructive technique after endoscopic expanded endonasal approaches: vascular pedicle nasoseptal flap. Laryngoscope 2006;116(10): 1882–1886
28. Weber SM, Kim J, Delashaw JB, Wax MK. Radial forearm free tissue transfer in the management of persistent cerebrospinal fluid leaks. Laryngoscope 2005;115(6):968–972
29. Bolger WE, McLaughlin K. Cranial bone grafts in cerebrospinal fluid leak and encephalocele repair: a preliminary report. Am J Rhinol 2003;17(3):153–158
30. Lorenz RR, Dean RL, Hurley DB, Chuang J, Citardi MJ. Endoscopic reconstruction of anterior and middle cranial fossa defects using acellular dermal allograft. Laryngoscope 2003;113(3): 496–501
31. Stankiewicz JA, Vaidy AM, Chow JM, Petruzzelli G. Complications of hydroxyapatite use for transnasal closure of cerebrospinal fluid leaks. Am J Rhinol 2002;16(6): 337–341

32. Verheggen R, Schulte-Baumann WJ, Hahm G, et al. A new tech-nique of dural closure—experience with a vicryl mesh. Acta Neurochir (Wien) 1997;139(11):1074–1079
33. Tachibana E, Saito K, Fukuta K, Yoshida J. Evaluation of the healing process after dural reconstruction achieved using a free fascial graft. J Neurosurg 2002;96(2):280–286
34. Fliss DM, Gil Z, Spektor S, et al. Skull base reconstruction after anterior subcranial tumor resection. Neurosurg Focus 2002; 12(5):e10
35. Lund VJ. Endoscopic management of cerebrospinal fluid leaks. Am J Rhinol 2002;16(1):17–23
36. Castelnuovo PG, Delú G, Locatelli D, et al. Endonasal endoscopic duraplasty: our experience. Skull Base 2006;16(1):19–24
37. Kirtane MV, Chavan KP, Satwalekar DR. Endonasal endoscopic repair of cerebrospinal fluid rhinorrhea with meningo-encephalocele: the three-layered 'sandwich' technique. Ann J Otolaryngol Head Neck Surg 2014;22:1–3
38. Kirtane MV, Lall A, Chavan K, Satwalekar D. Endoscopic repair of lateral sphenoid recess cerebrospinal fluid leaks. Indian J Otolaryngol Head Neck Surg 2012;64(2):188–192
39. Bolger WE, Osenbach R. Endoscopic transpterygoid approach to the lateral sphenoid recess. Ear Nose Throat J 1999;78: 36–46
40. Kirtane MV, Chavan KP, Satwalekar DR. Primary spontaneous transclival cerebrospinal fluid leak. Pakistan J Otolarygol Head Neck Surg 2014;30(2):61–63
41. Senior BA, Jafri K, Benninger M. Safety and efficacy of endoscopic repair of CSF leaks and encephaloceles: a survey of the members of the American Rhinologic Society. Am J Rhinol 2001;15(1):21–25
42. Dodson EE, Gross CW, Swerdloff JL, Gustafson LM. Transnasal endoscopic repair of cerebrospinal fluid rhinorrhea and skull base defects: a review of twenty-nine cases. Otolaryngol Head Neck Surg 1994;111(5):600–605
43. Hegazy HM, Carrau RL, Snyderman CH, Kassam A, Zweig J. Transnasal endoscopic repair of cerebrospinal fluid rhinorrhea: a meta-analysis. Laryngoscope 2000;110(7):1166–1172
44. Komisar A, Weitz S, Ruben RJ. Cerebrospinal fluid dynamics and rhinorrhea: the role of shunting in repair. Otolaryngol Head Neck Surg 1983;91(4):399–403
45. Casiano RR, Jassir D. Endoscopic cerebrospinal fluid rhinorrhea repair: is a lumbar drain necessary? Otolaryngol Head Neck Surg 1999;121(6):745–750
46. Marshall AH, Jones NS, Robertson IJ. CSF rhinorrhoea: the place of endoscopic sinus surgery. Br J Neurosurg 2001;15(1):8–12
47. Schick B, Ibing R, Brors D, Draf W. Long-term study of endonasal duraplasty and review of the literature. Ann Otol Rhinol Laryngol 2001;110(2):142–147
48. Wise SK, Harvey RJ, Neal JG, Patel SJ, Frankel BM, Schlosser RJ. Factors contributing to failure in endoscopic skull base defect repair. Am J Rhinol Allergy 2009;23(2):185–191
49. Castillo L, Jaklis A, Paquis P, Haddad A, Santini J. Nasal endoscopic repair of cerebrospinal fluid rhinorrhea. Rhinology 1999; 37(1):33–36
50. Cassano M, Felippu A. Endoscopic treatment of cerebrospinal fluid leaks with the use of lower turbinate grafts: a retrospective review of 125 cases. Rhinology 2009;47(4):362–368
51. Kirtane MV, Gautham K, Upadhyaya SR. Endoscopic CSF rhinor-rhea closure: our experience in 267 cases. Otolaryngol Head Neck Surg 2005;132(2):208–212

Chapter 34 Endonasal Endoscopic Surgeries for Cerebrospinal Fluid Leakage

Case 34A

Endonasal Endoscopic Repair of Spontaneous Cerebrospinal Fluid Leak in the Left Cribriform Plate

Michel Roethlisberger, Wong HT, and Prepageran Narayanan

History

A 41-year-old female person with a high body mass index (BMI) score presented with spontaneous left-sided cerebrospinal fluid (CSF) rhinorrhea. With the suspicion of a spontaneous CSF leak, a computed tomography (CT) scan detected a left-sided skull base defect, suggestive of an encephalocele (**Fig. 34A.1** and **Fig. 34A.2**). An **endoscopic endonasal repair** with an abdominal fat graft was recommended.

Surgical Steps

1. The patient is positioned supine with the head slightly extended under general anesthesia.
2. The nose is packed as per standard protocol.
3. Endoscopic examination of the nose showed the translucent mass at the left middle turbinate (**Fig. 34A.3**).
4. The anterior part of the middle turbinate is transected, and the middle turbinate is preserved for vascularized mucosal flap harvesting. After transection of the middle turbinate, the encephalocele is exposed (**Fig. 34A.4**).
5. The encephalocele is reduced using bipolar cauterization (**Fig. 34A.5**).
6. After reduction of the encephalocele by cauterization the skull base defect can be identified (**Fig. 34A.6**).
7. Surgicel is used for hemostasis and hold the reduced encephalocele in place (**Fig. 34A.7** and **34A.8**).

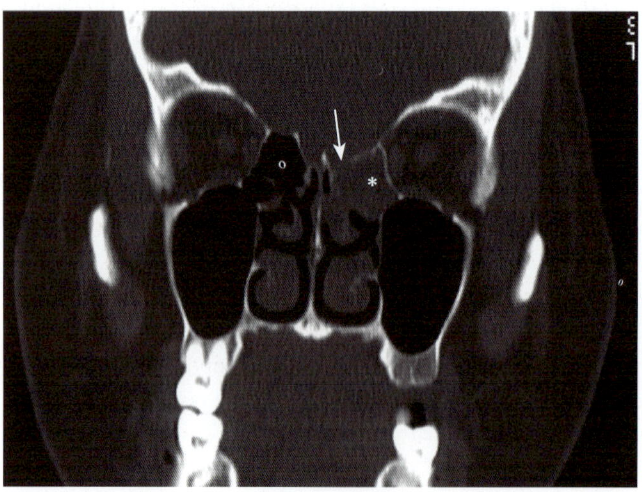

Fig. 34A.1 Coronal bone-weighted CT scan demonstrating a defect (*white arrow*) at the lateral lamella of the left cribriform region with opacity (*) in the sinus directly inferior to the defect, highly suggestive of an encephalocele.

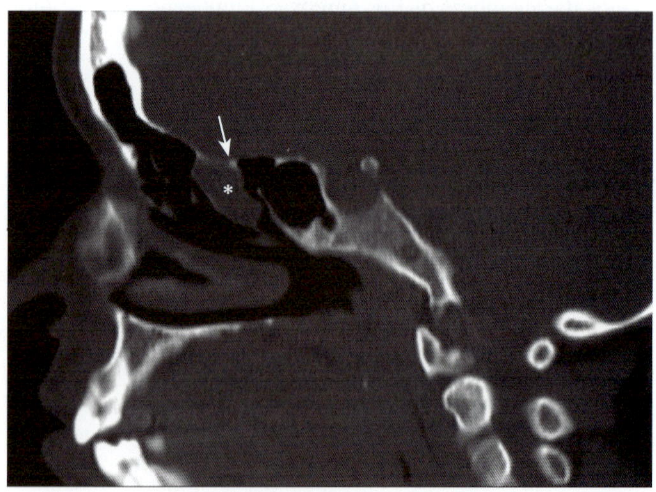

Fig. 34A.2 Sagittal bone-weighted CT scan demonstrating the skull base defect (white arrow). All the sinuses are clear except the region directly inferior to the skull base defect (*).

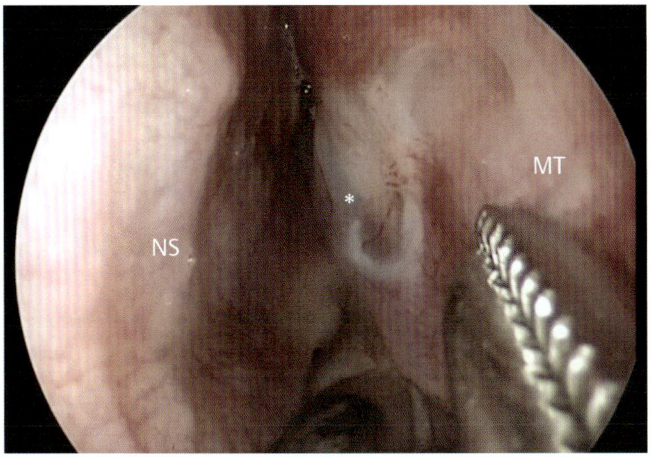

Fig. 34A.3 Endonasal endoscopic view of a translucent mass (*) is suggestive of an encephalocele located medially to left middle turbinate (MT).

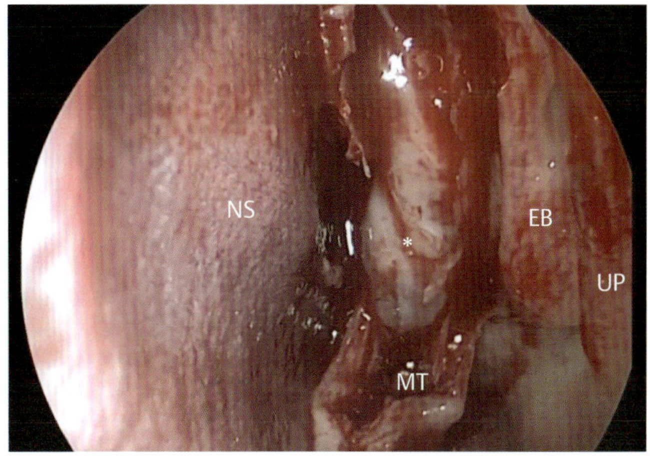

Fig. 34A.4 The anterior part of the middle turbinate (MT) is transected and the encephalocele (*) is exposed.

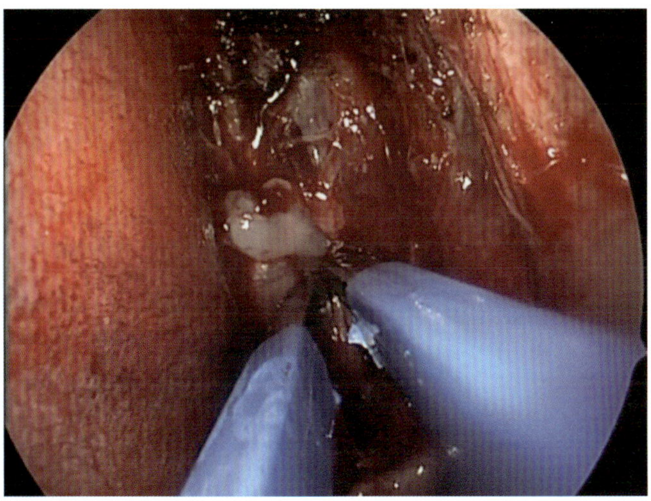

Fig. 34A.5 Bipolar cauterization of the encephalocele.

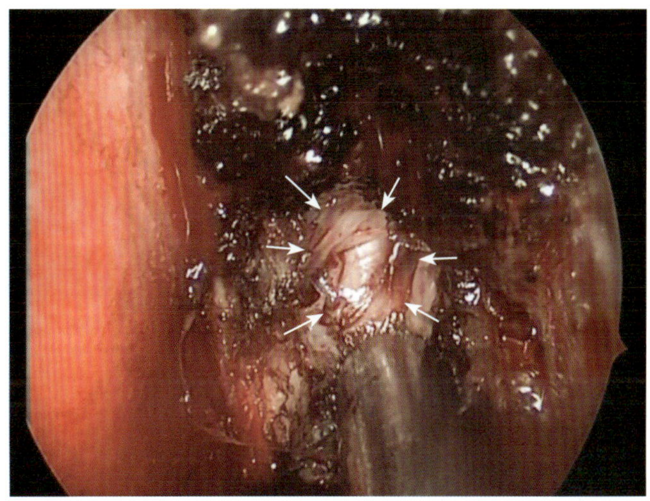

Fig. 34A.6 The bony skull base defect can be clearly visualized (*white arrows*) at the upper part of the encephalocele.

8. An abdominal fat graft is used to repair the skull base defect using the "bath-plug" technique technique (**Fig. 34A.9**).
9. Dural sealant is applied over the first layer of fat (**Fig. 34A.10**).
10. A multilayer of fat and dural sealant are then used to strengthen the reconstruction.
11. The middle turbinate is repositioned back and used as a flap to support the reconstruction (**Fig. 34A.11**).
12. Dural sealant then applied over the middle turbinate flap (**Fig. 34A.12**).

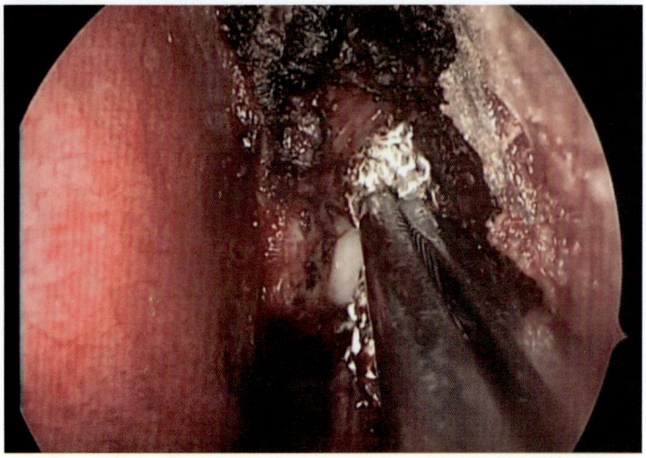

Fig. 34A.7 Surgicel is used to help reduce the encephalocele.

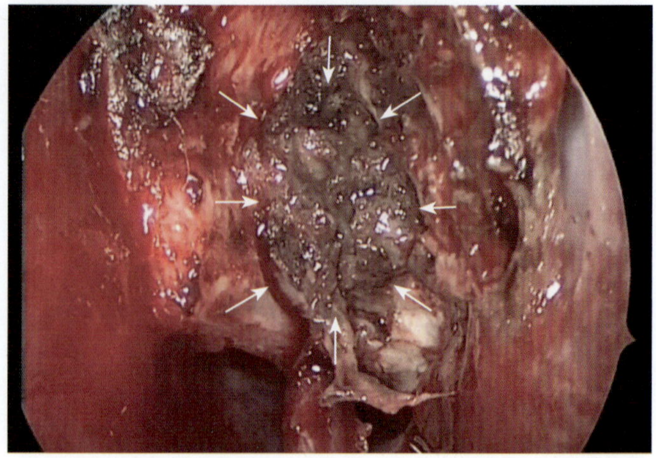

Fig. 34A.8 The skull base defect can be clearly visualized (*white arrows*) after the encephalocele has been reduced.

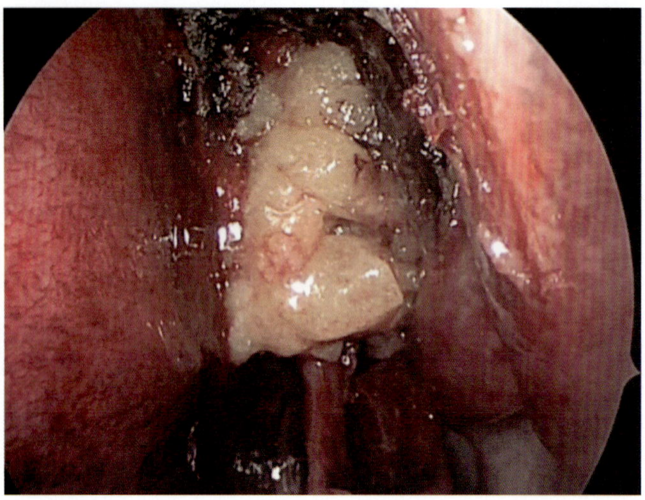

Fig. 34A.9 Abdominal fat is used to repair the skull base defect.

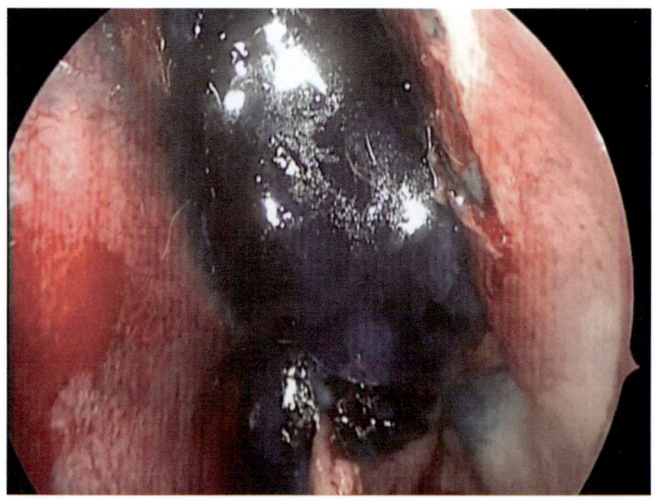

Fig. 34A.10 Dural sealant is applied over the first layer of fat.

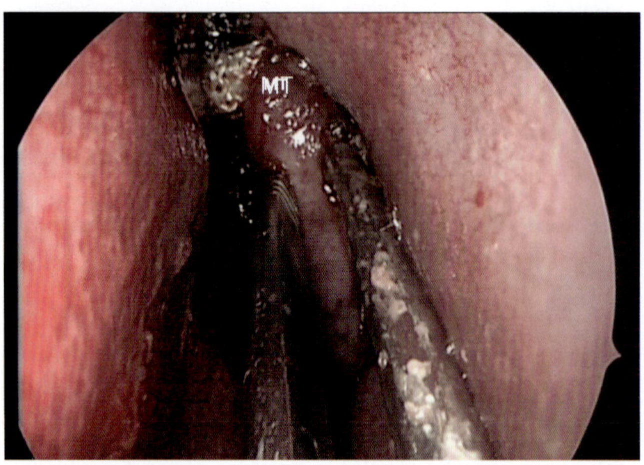

Fig. 34A.11 Middle turbinate (MT) is now repositioned back and used as a flap to strengthen the reconstruction.

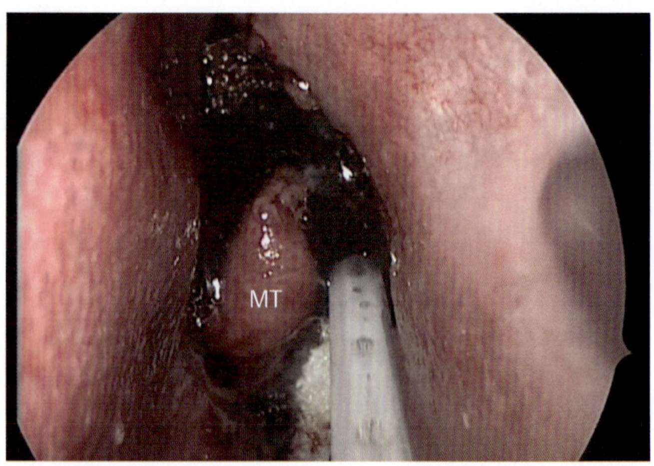

Fig. 34A.12 Dural sealant is applied over the middle turbinate (MT) flap.

Case 34B

Endonasal Endoscopic Repair of a Traumatic Cerebrospinal Fluid Leak

Adzreil Bakri, Michel Roethlisberger, and Prepageran Narayanan

History

A 65-year-old Indian lady presented with a 5-year history of intermittent clear watery discharge from the left nostril which started after she was hit with force by a blunt object at her left forehead. Clinically, there was clear watery rhinorrhea demonstrable when the head is bent forward. A high-resolution computed tomography (HRCT) scan of the paranasal sinuses revealed a bony defect at the left lateral lamella of the ethmoid bone with soft tissue density in the left ethmoid sinuses (**Fig. 34B.1**). A repair of the defect was planned via endoscopic endonasal approach.

Surgical Steps

1. The patient is positioned supine under general anesthesia with the head slightly extended.
2. The nose is decongested with nasal packing as per the institution's usual methods.
3. The nasal cavity is inspected for the potential leakage site.
4. In this case, a smooth pulsatile whitish mass is seen lateral to the left middle turbinate posterior to the uncinate process and occupying the ethmoid air cells in the middle meatus (**Fig. 34B.2**).
5. A middle turbinate flap is produced by cutting the axilla of the middle turbinate and pushing it posteriorly and inferiorly to be stored and used later for reconstruction (**Fig. 34B.3**). This also improves exposure to the leak site.
6. An uncinectomy is also performed to improve exposure to the skull base defect (**Fig. 34B.4**).
7. Adequate exposure to fully visualize the leak site and the edges of the skull base defect and encephalocele is performed by removing the surrounding ethmoid sinuses (**Fig. 34B.5**).
8. The encephalocele is reduced and excised using bipolar diathermy (**Fig. 34B.6**).
9. Once the encephalocele is excised, the defect is repaired with an abdominal fat graft using the "bath-plug" technique. This is further reinforced with a few layers of Surgicel (oxidized cellulose polymer) (**Fig. 34B.7**).
10. A Valsalva maneuver is performed to assess the patency of the repair. If there is no sign of cerebrospinal fluid (CSF) leakage through the repair, the middle turbinate flap is positioned so that it covers the whole skull base defect reconstruction (**Fig. 34B.8**).
11. A dural sealant or tissue glue is then applied over the repaired area (**Fig. 34B.9**).
12. The left nasal cavity is packed loosely with gelatin sponges and synthetic biodegradable foam.

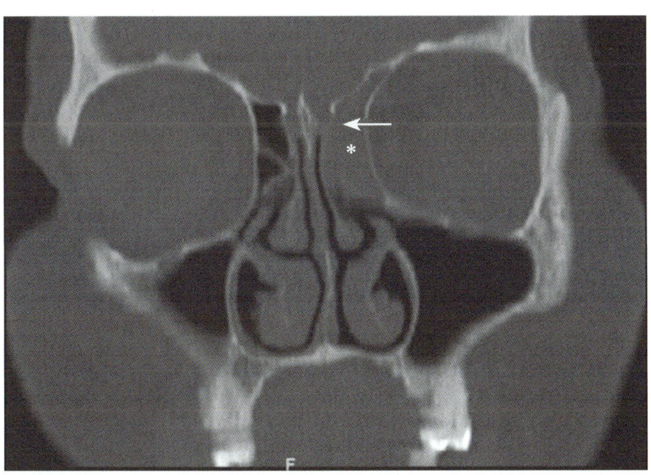

Fig. 34B.1 Coronal high-resolution CT scan of the paranasal sinuses demonstrating a bony defect at the lateral lamella (*white arrow*) and a soft tissue density occupying the left ethmoid sinuses (*).

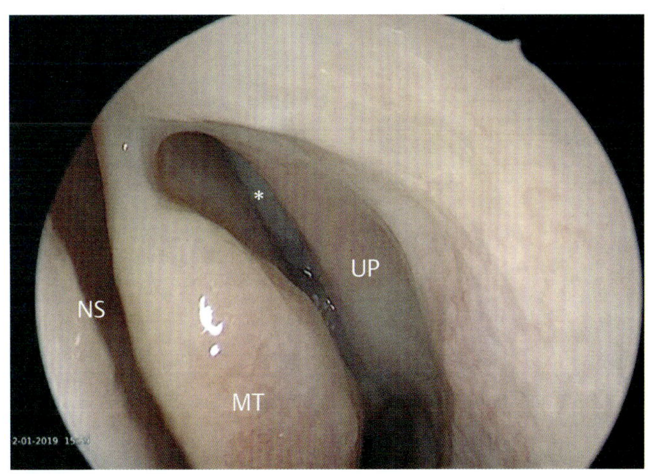

Fig. 34B.2 Endonasal endoscopic appearance of the left nasal cavity. Note a whitish mass (*) located between the middle turbinate (MT) and posterior to uncinate process (UP).

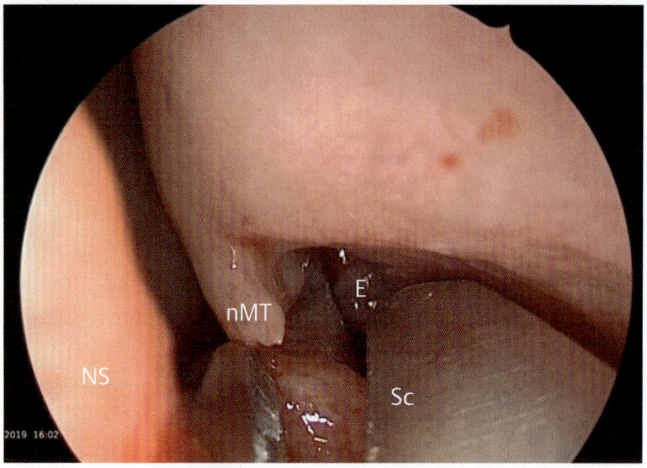

Fig. 34B.3 The middle turbinate is cut at its neck (nMT) with a turbinectomy scissors (Sc) and pushed posteriorly and inferiorly.

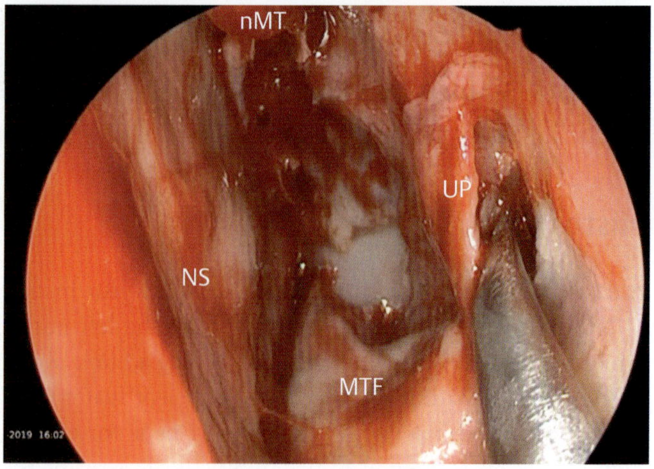

Fig. 34B.4 The uncinate process (UP) is removed to improve exposure to the skull base defect and leak site.

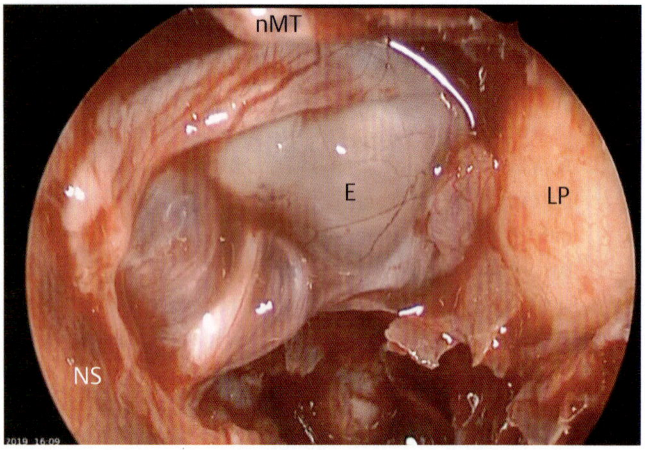

Fig. 34B.5 The skull base defect and an encephalocele (E) are fully exposed and visualized.

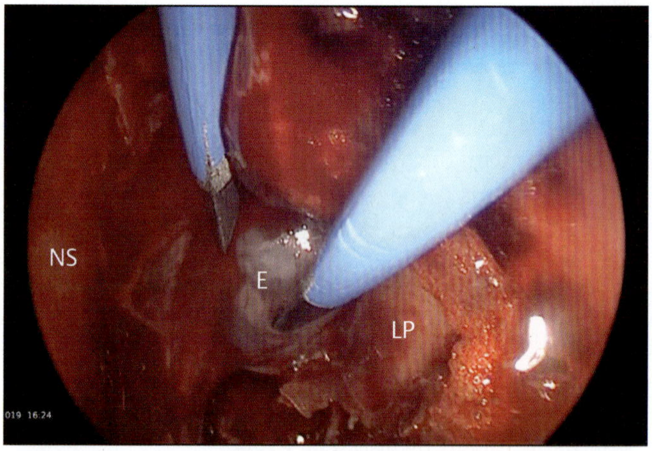

Fig. 34B.6 The encephalocele (E) is reduced and excised using bipolar diathermy.

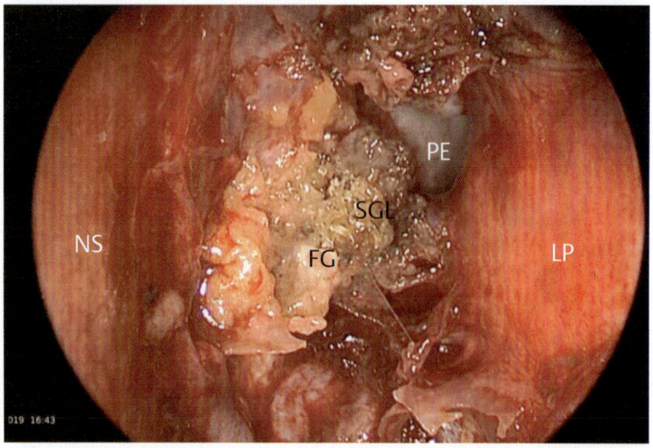

Fig. 34B.7 An abdominal fat graft (FG) is tucked around the edges of the skull base defect and reinforced with Surgicel (SGL).

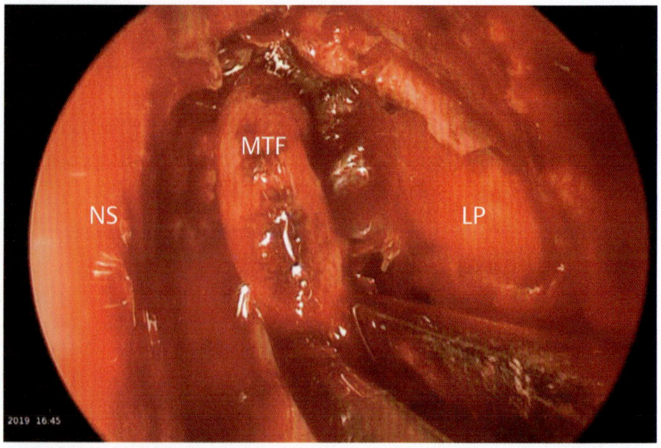

Fig. 34B.8 The middle turbinate flap (MTF) is repositioned over the skull base repair construct.

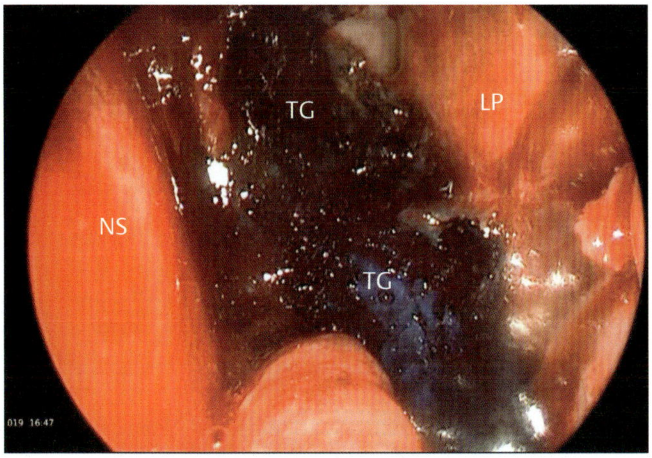

Fig. 34B.9 A dural sealant or tissue glue (TG) is applied over the layers of repair.

Case 34C

Iatrogenic Cerebrospinal Fluid Leak of the Cribriform Plate

Warren O. Bennett, Revadi Govindaraju, Michel Roethlisberger, Prepageran Narayanan, and Vicknes Waran

History

This is the case of a 55-year-old man who was suffering from left-sided cerebrospinal fluid (CSF) rhinorrhea. He has a history of previous endoscopic sinus surgery. Endoscopic examination of the nasal cavity showed evidence of previous surgery with absence of the middle turbinate and a pulsating meningocele from the left olfactory cleft region. The computed tomography (CT) scan imaging confirmed the defect in the skull base at the lateral lamella of the cribriform plate.

Surgical Steps

1. The imaging, MRI and CT, must be carefully reviewed prior to the surgery to inspect the extent of the defect, and also its relations to important surrounding structures.
2. The patient is placed under general anesthesia in supine position.
3. The nose is decongested with adrenaline 1:1,000 units on ribbon gauze.
4. The abdomen is prepared with iodine solution for harvesting of the abdominal fat graft.
5. The nasal cavity is fully examined with the rigid endoscope, and the skull base defect identified (**Fig. 34C.1**).
6. Bipolar diathermy is used to reduce the meningocele (**Fig. 34C.2**). It makes identifying the edges of the defect in the skull base easier and reduces the risk of bleeding into the intracranial cavity.
7. The meningocele is reduced to the level of the defect (**Fig. 34C.3**), and the coagulum is carefully removed with a spatula dissector (**Fig. 34C.4**).
8. The dural and bony edges are identified (**Fig. 34C.5**). A blunt-ended 90-degree hook is used to free the edges from the arachnoid (**Fig. 34C.6**). The defect must be measured with a curette or similar instrument to estimate the size of fat graft required.
9. A piece of oxidized regenerated cellulose such as Surgicel is placed into the defect (**Fig. 34C.7**). We believe this promotes fibrosis, strengthening the repair, and also controls any unwanted bleeding.
10. A piece of abdominal fat is harvested with a small C-shaped incision below the umbilicus. It is important to make sure that enough graft is taken, and it can always be reduced if too large. The abdominal wound is closed with absorbable sutures.
11. The fat graft is placed into the defect slowly and carefully to prevent intracranial injury. The graft must overlap the bony edge intracranially to create a tight seal. There should be no CSF leak at this stage (**Fig. 34C.8**).

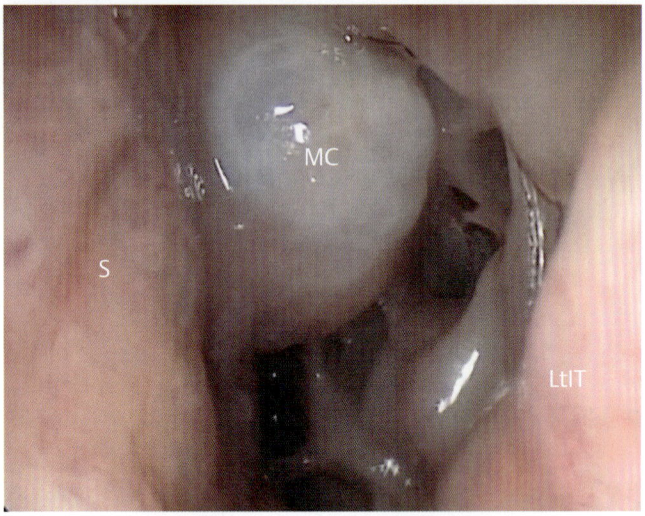

Fig. 34C.1 Endoscopic view of the left nasal cavity shows evidence of previous sinus surgery and a middle turbinate transection. The meningocele is seen protruding from the region of the cribriform plate.

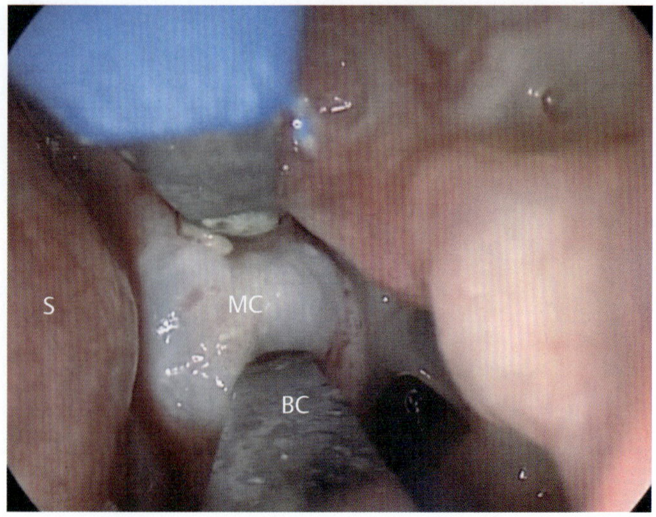

Fig. 34C.2 Bipolar cautery is used to reduce the meningocele.

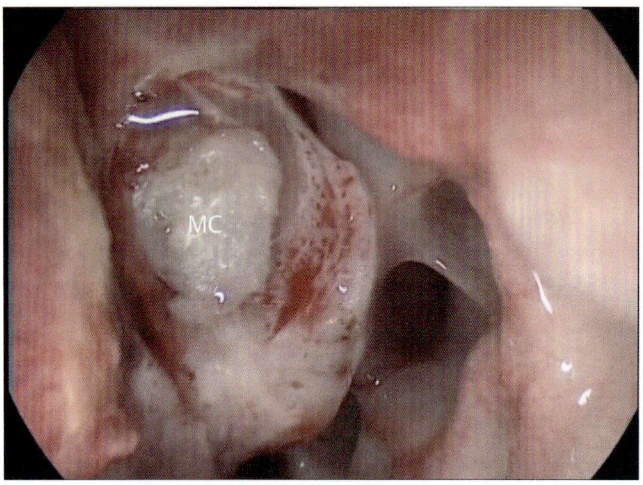

Fig. 34C.3 The meningocele is reduced to the level of the defect, and the coagulum can be seen in the center of the defect.

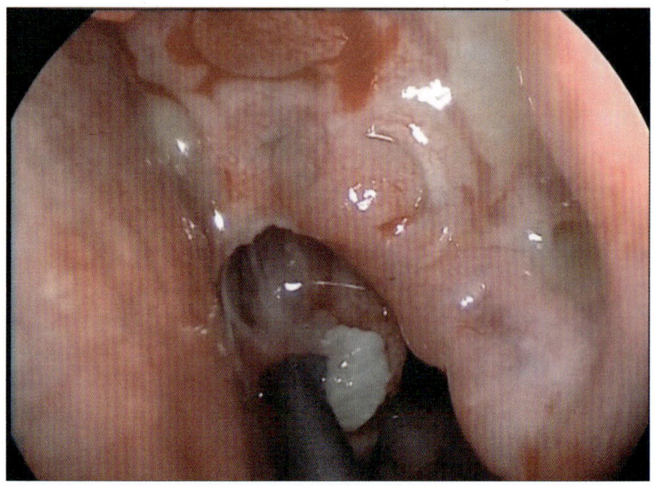

Fig. 34C.4 The coagulated meningocele is carefully removed from the edges of the defect with a spatula dissector.

A Valsalva maneuver can be performed at this point to check the seal.

12. We place oxidized regenerated cellulose in and around the graft to help manipulate the fat and to create further fibrosis (**Fig. 34C.9**).
13. A synthetic dural sealant is placed over the fat and then supported with an absorbable dressing or hemostat (**Fig. 34C.10** and **Fig. 34C.11**).
14. Postoperatively, the patient must be nursed at 45 degrees and have strict bed rest for 48 hours to increase the likelihood of a successful repair.

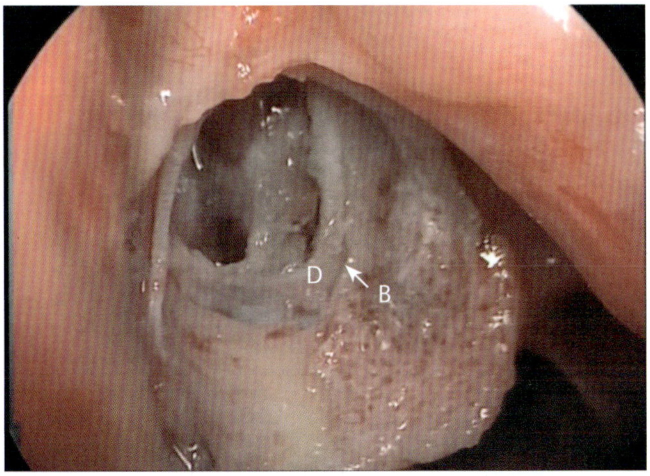

Fig. 34C.5 The dural and The dural (D) and bony (B) edges of the skull base defect (arrow) are identified. of the defect are identified.

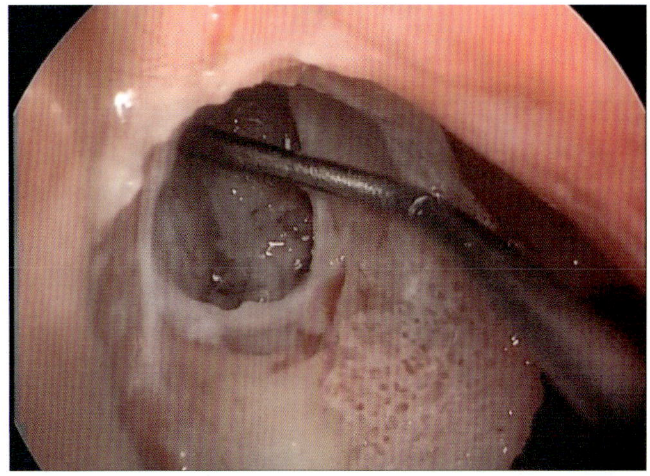

Fig. 34C.6 A blunt-ended 90-degree hook is used to free the edges of defect from the arachnoid.

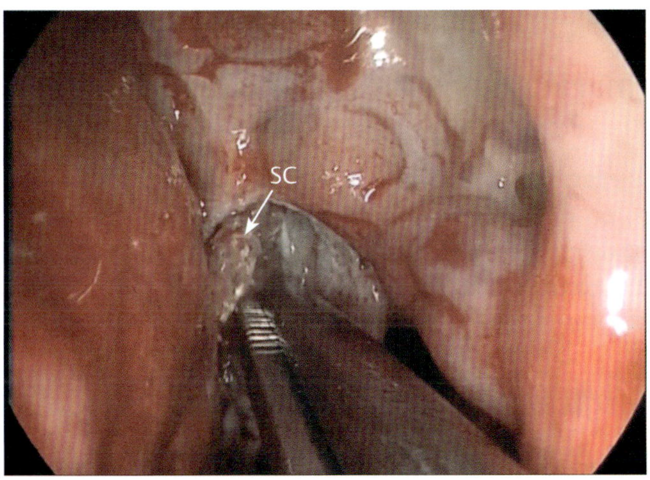

Fig. 34C.7 A piece of oxidized regenerated cellulose such as Surgicel is placed into the defect.

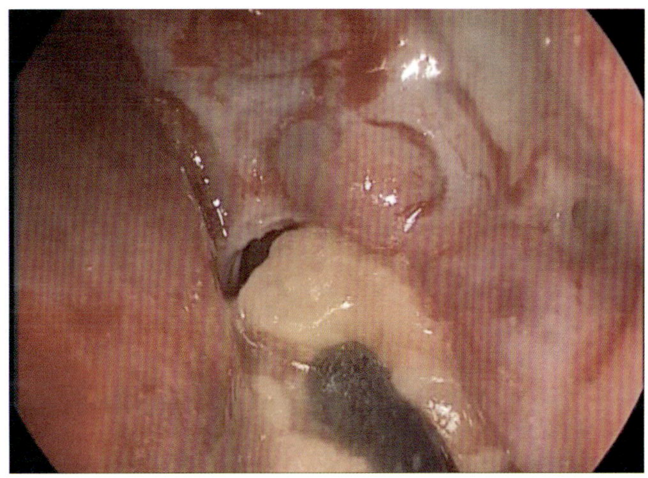

Fig. 34C.8 Abdominal fat is placed into the defect.

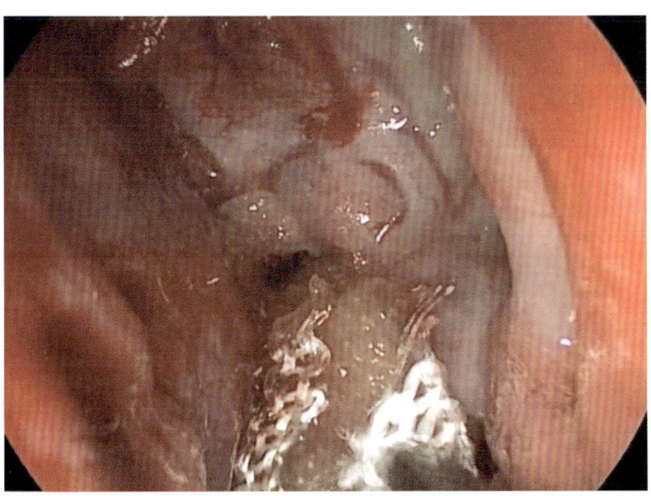

Fig. 34C.9 Further oxidized regenerated cellulose is placed around and inside the fat graft.

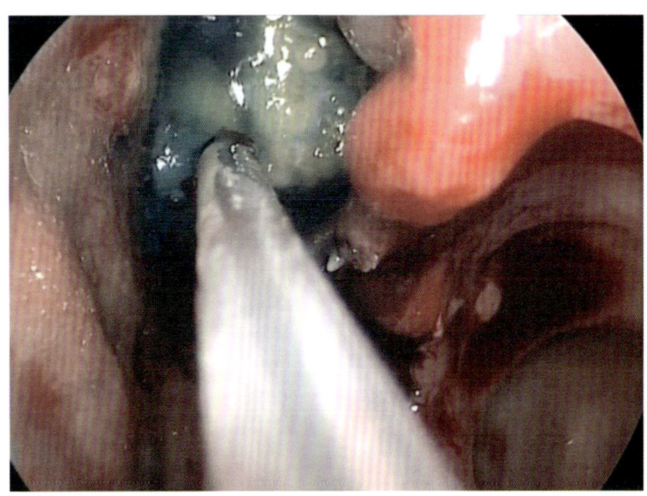

Fig. 34C.10 Synthetic dural sealant is placed over the fat graft.

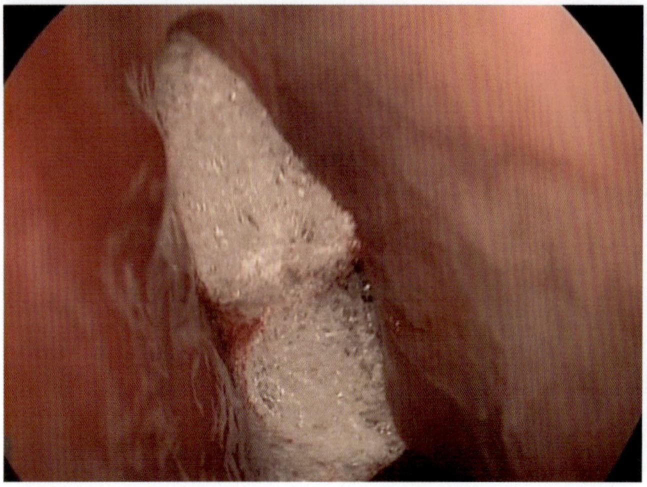

Fig. 34C.11 Absorbable hemostat is placed to support the repair.

Case 34D

Endoscopic Repair of an Iatrogenic Cerebrospinal Fluid Leak after Functional Endoscopic Sinus Surgery

Wong HT, Michel Roethlisberger, Adzreil Bakri, Sien Hui Tan, and Prepageran Narayanan

History

This case describes the endonasal endoscopic repair of an iatrogenic cerebrospinal fluid (CSF) leak postfunctional endoscopic sinus surgery in a 48-year-old lady. The patient experienced an iatrogenic injury to the skull base at the left sphenoid sinus adjacent to the optic nerve. The patient also suffered from left upper quadrantanopia. Hence, the patient was referred into authors' reference center for the repair of the defect. delete these words Coronal and sagittal sections of the computed tomography (CT) scan were used to identify the exact location of the defect (**Fig. 34D.1** and **34D.2**).

Surgical Steps

1. The patient is positioned supine with the head slightly extended under general anesthesia.
2. The nose is packed as per standard protocol.

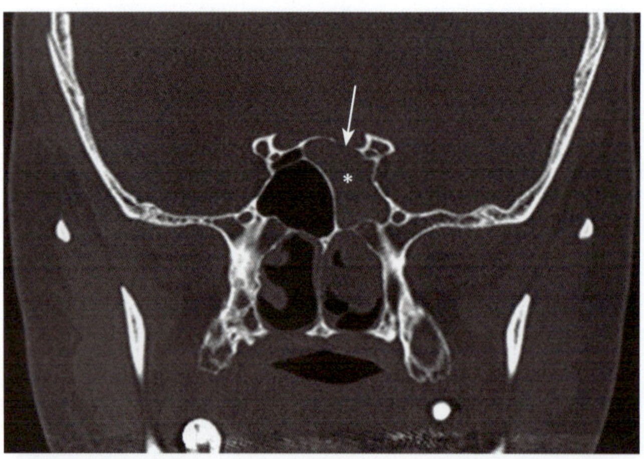

Fig. 34D.1 Coronal bone-weighted CT section demonstrating a bony defect (*white arrow*) at the superior lateral wall of the left sphenoid sinus (*).

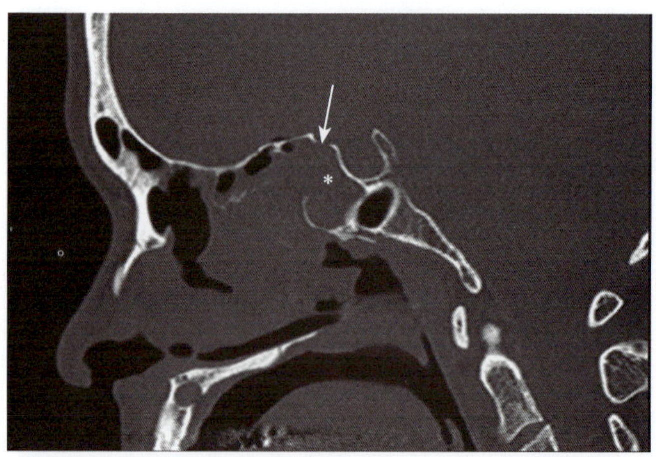

Fig. 34D.2 Sagittal bone-weighted CT section demonstrating the skull base defect (*white arrow*). The asterisk (*) marks the left sphenoid sinus.

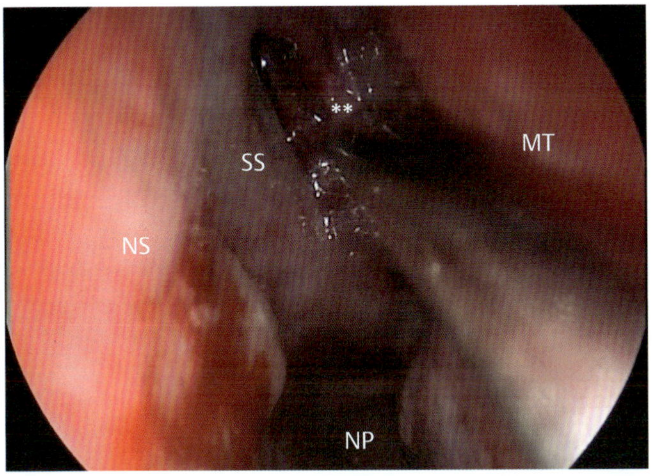

Fig. 34D.3 Endoscopic view of the left nasal cavity showing the packing material (**) from previous surgery being suctioned out.

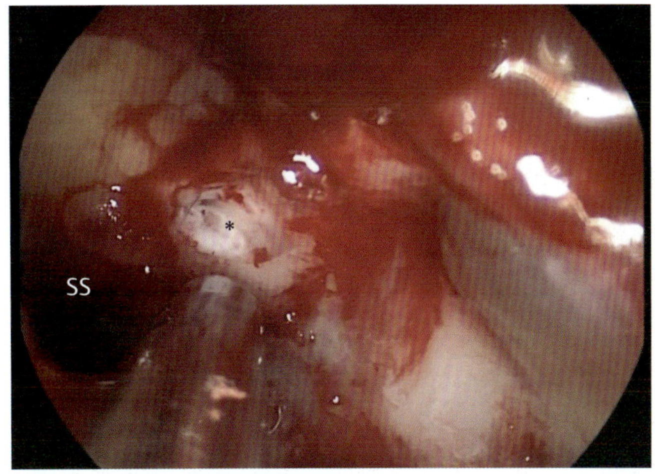

Fig. 34D.4 The skull base defect (*) is seen superior to the suction probe in the figure.

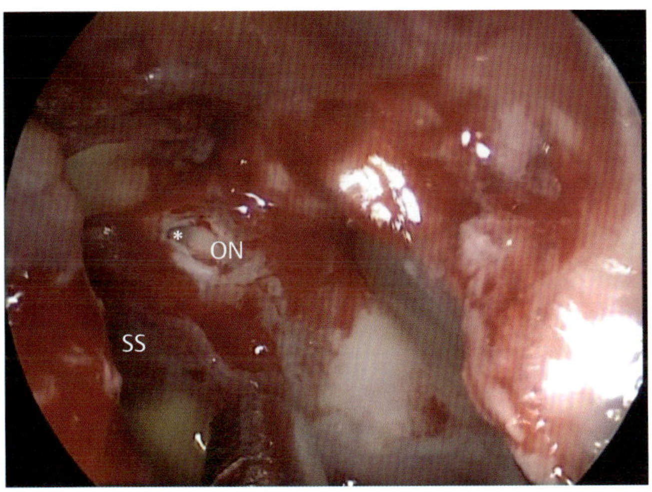

Fig. 34D.5 The optic nerve (ON) is identifiable near the area of the iatrogenic skull base defect (*).

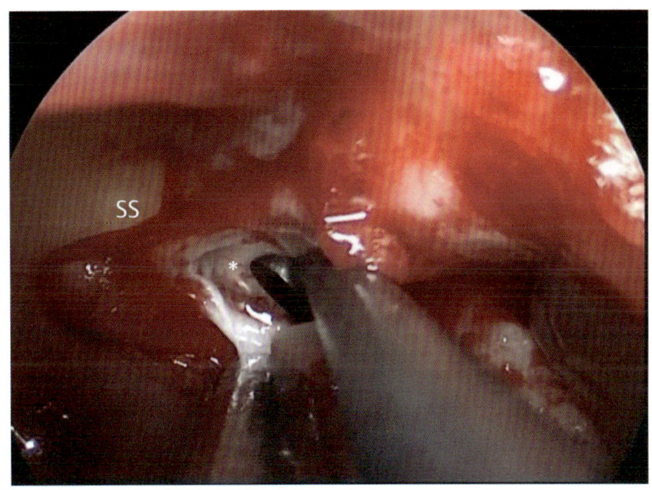

Fig. 34D.6 Refreshening of the edges of the skull base defect (*).

3. Endoscopic examination of the nose showed packing material lateral to the middle turbinate from the previous surgery (**Fig. 34D.3**).
4. After endoscopic removal of the packing material, the bony skull base defect in the superolateral wall of the sphenoid sinus can be clearly visualized. There is evident CSF leakage through the bony defect (**Fig. 34D.4**).
5. On closer examination, the optic nerve can be visualized through the area of the iatrogenic skull base defect (**Fig. 34D.5**).
6. The edges of the defect are refreshened gently and with care as the optic nerve is just nearby (**Fig. 34D.6**).
7. The skull base defect is repaired with an abominal fat graft. The size of the graft is important in this case as an oversized graft might compress on the optic nerve (**Fig. 34D.7a, b**).
8. A dural sealant is applied over the first layer of repair (**Fig. 34D.8**).
9. A second layer of fat is then applied (**Fig. 34D.9**).
10. Absorbable gelatin sponges (Gelfoam) are placed over the repaired site for additional support (**Fig. 34D.10**).

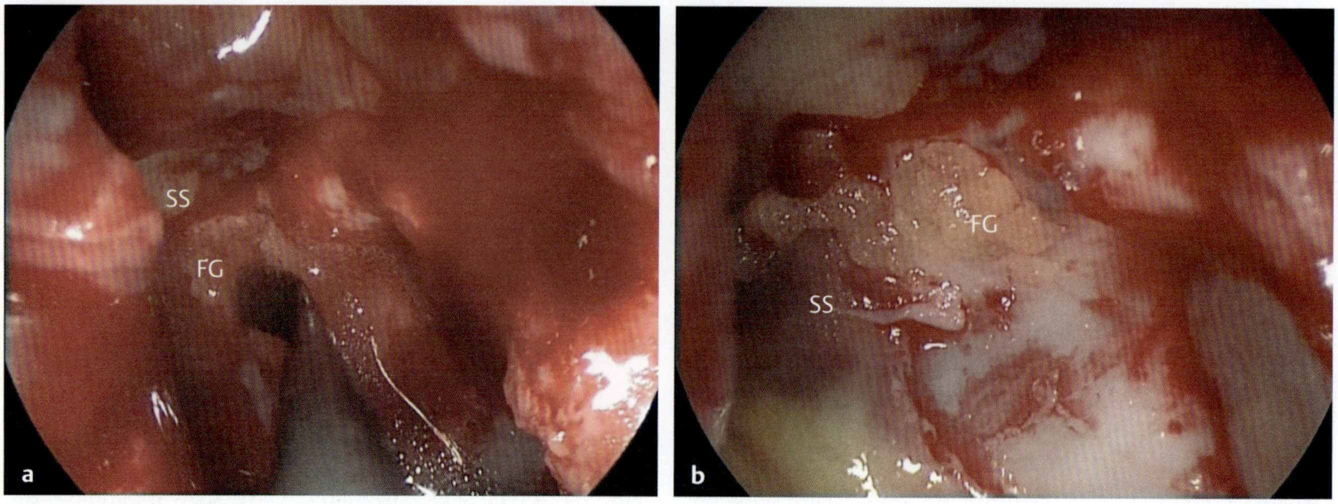

Fig. 34D.7 **(a)** The defect is repaired with abdominal fat graft (FG). The graft is tucked into the defect to create a watertight closure. **(b)** View of the first layer of repair.

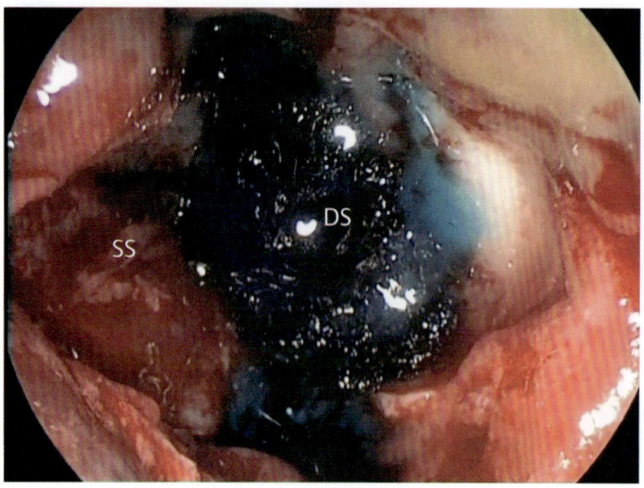

Fig. 34D.8 Dural sealant (DS) is applied over the first layer of repair.

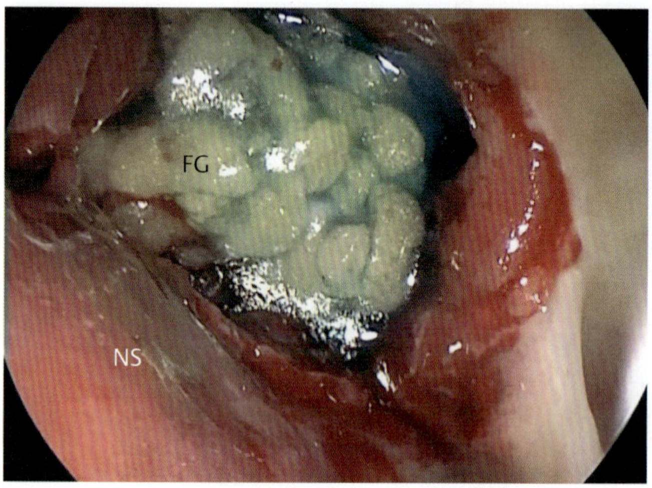

Fig. 34D.9 Second layer of fat graft (FG) is applied over the repaired site.

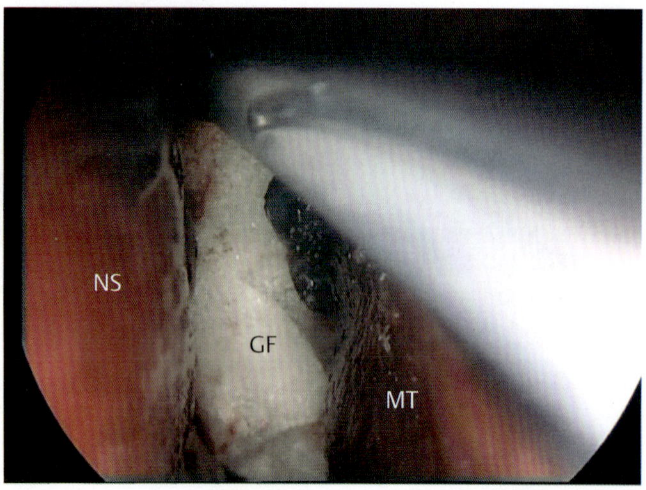

Fig. 34D.10 Gelfoam (GF) is placed over the layers of repair as additional support.

Case 34E

Endoscopic Repair of an Encephalocele in the Cribriform Plate

Michel Roethlisberger, Wong HT, Adzreil Bakri, Vicknes Waran, and Prepageran Narayanan

History

This case describes the surgical steps for an endonasal endoscopic repair of an encephalocele in a 41-year-old lady. She presented with features of meningitis and later was diagnosed to have an encephalocele with cerebrospinal fluid (CSF) leakage. High-resolution computed tomography (CT) and a magnetic resonance imaging (MRI) revealed a defect in the right cribriform plate (**Fig. 34E.1** and **Fig. 34E.2**).

Surgical Steps

1. The patient is positioned supine with the head slightly extended under general anesthesia.
2. The nose is packed as per standard protocol. The packing is done between the septum and the middle turbinate.
3. Endoscopic examination of the nose does not reveal the encephalocele immediately. The anterior part of middle turbinate is transected, and the middle turbinate is preserved for the purpose of a vascularized flap. The encephalocele is exposed after the transection of middle turbinate (**Fig. 34E.3a, b**).
4. The surrounding area is exposed to allow visualization of the whole encephalocele. As this case was done via a single nostril technique and the patient had a deviated nasal septum, a septoplasty was performed to allow adequate surgical access (**Fig. 34E.4a, b**).
5. The encephalocele is then reduced with bipolar cauterization. A part of the encephalocele is truncated and sent for histopathological examination (**Fig. 34E.5**).
6. The edges of the bony skull base defect become more clearly visible as the bipolar cauterization reduces the size of the encephalocele (**Fig. 34E.6a, b**).
7. Eventually, the edges of the bony defect can be clearly visualized after the encephalocele has been cauterized and removed (**Fig. 34E.7**).
8. The size of the skull base defect is then measured and estimated with the aid of a measuring tape or a standard square neuro patty.
9. The defect is then repaired with an abdominal fat graft. The graft is plugged into the defect to create a watertight seal. A Valsalva maneuver is then performed to elicit any CSF leakage (**Fig. 34E.8**).
10. A dural sealant is then applied over the fat (**Fig. 34E.9**).
11. The repair is reinforced with multiple layers of fat and application of dural sealant.
12. The vascularized middle turbinate flap is used to strengthen and support the reconstruction (**Fig. 34E.10**).

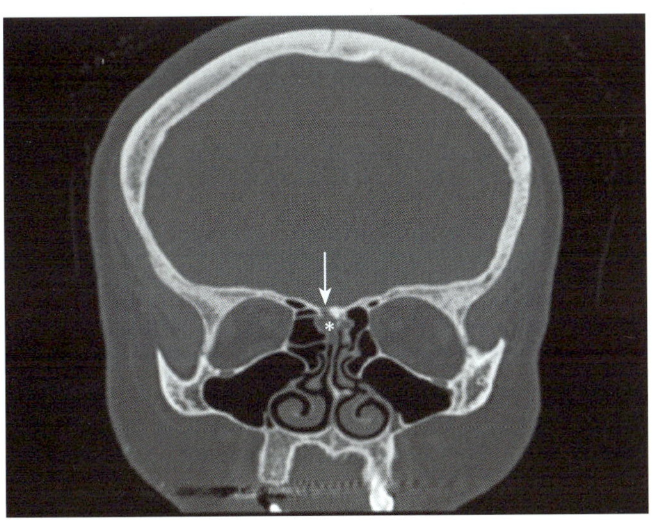

Fig. 34E.1 Coronal bone-weighted CT section demonstrating the skull base defect (*arrow*) at the right cribriform plate. An opacity (*) is seen directly below the defect.

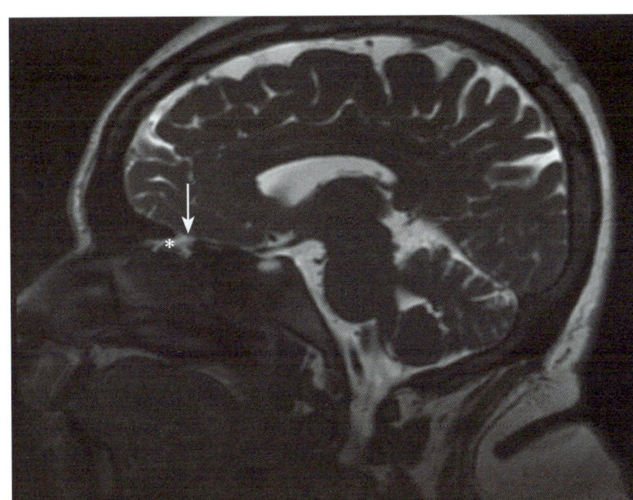

Fig. 34E.2 Sagittal T2-weighted MRI section demonstrating an encephalocele (*) of the cribriform plate. A hyperintense signal of CSF within the ethmoidal mucosa is visible (*arrow*).

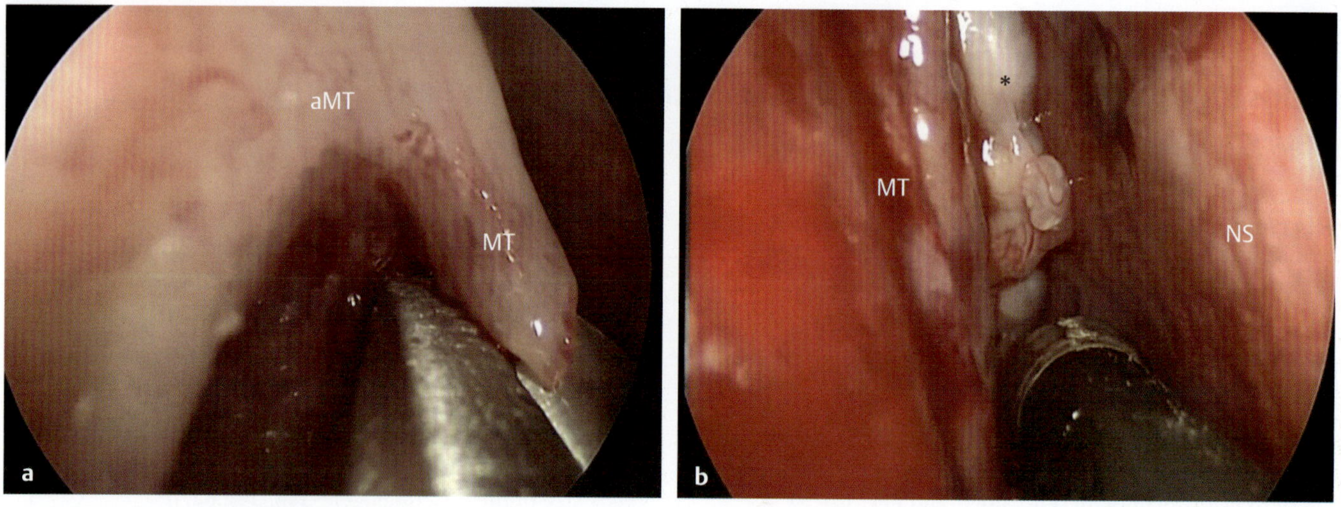

Fig. 34E.3 **(a)** Endonasal endoscopic view of the right nasal cavity. The anterior part the middle turbinate (MT) is transected. **(b)** The encephalocele (*), which is located medially to the right middle turbinate, is clearly visible after transection of the anterior part of the middle turbinate (MT).

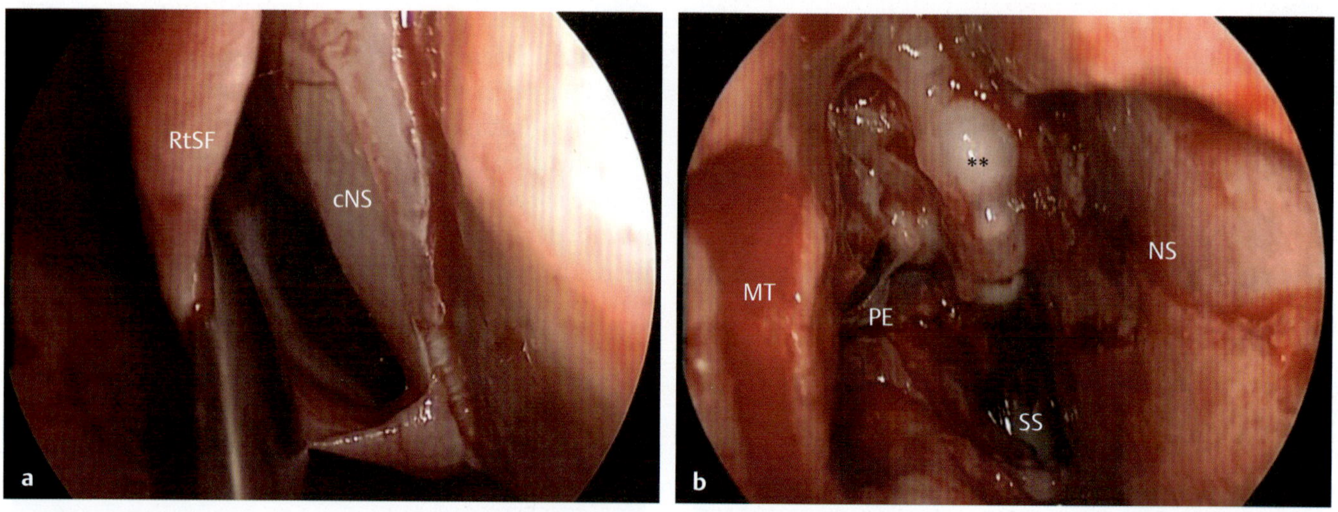

Fig. 34E.4 **(a)** A septoplasty is done to provide adequate surgical access. **(b)** The encephalocele (**) is fully exposed.

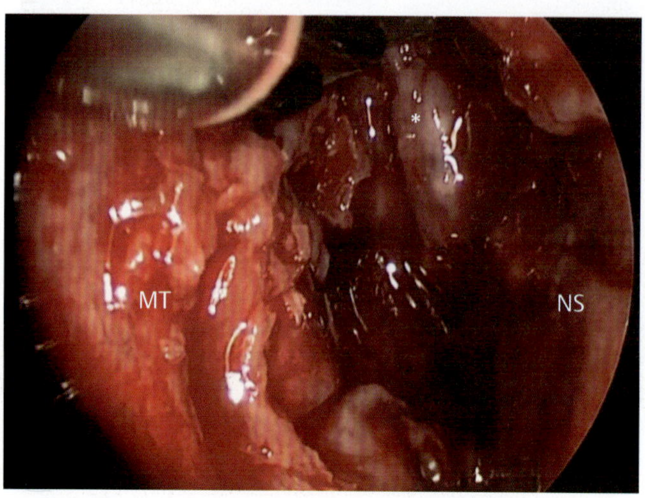

Fig. 34E.5 The encephalocele (*) is reduced with bipolar cautery.

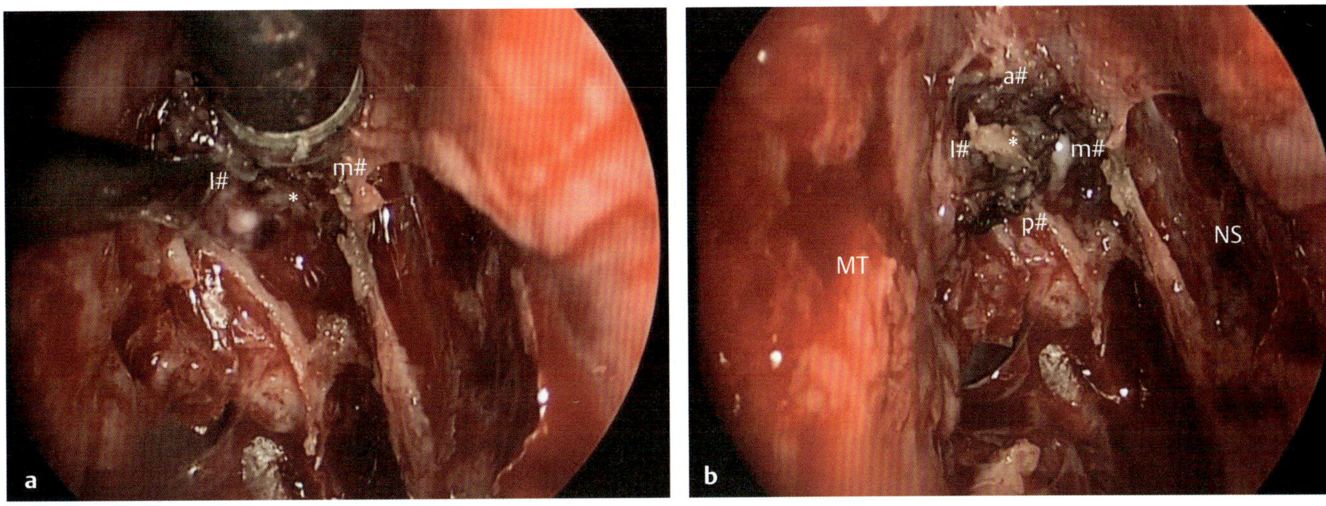

Fig. 34E.6 **(a)** The medial (m#) and lateral (l#) edges of the defect have become clearly visible as cauterization reduces the size of the encephalocele (*). **(b)** As the size of encephalocele (*) reduces, the anterior (a#) and posterior (p#) edges of the skull base defect are clearly visualized.

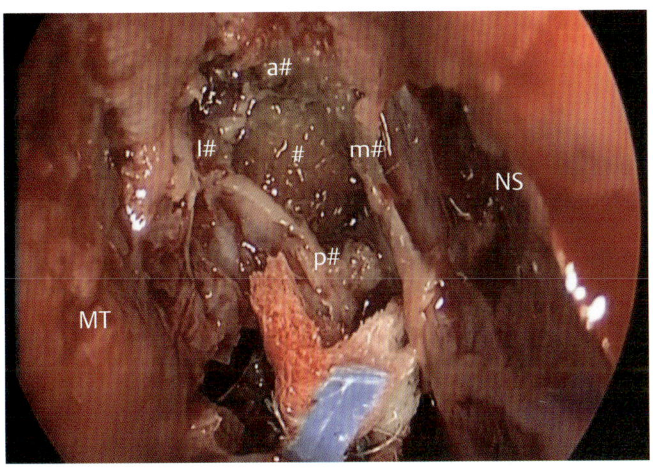

Fig. 34E.7 The bony defect (#) of skull base after cauterization and removal of the encephalocele.

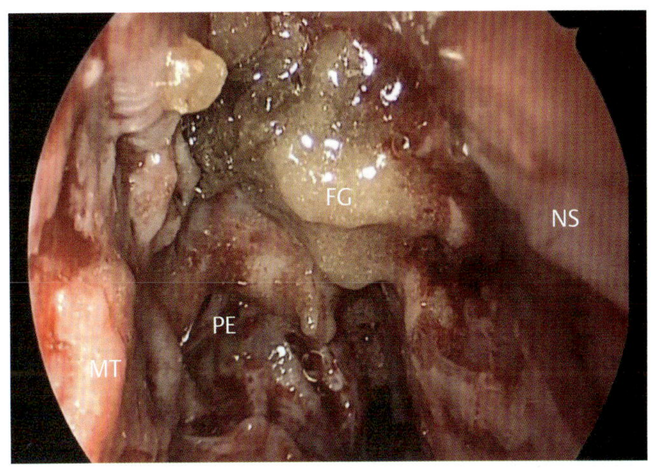

Fig. 34E.8 The skull base defect is plugged with an abdominal fat graft (FG).

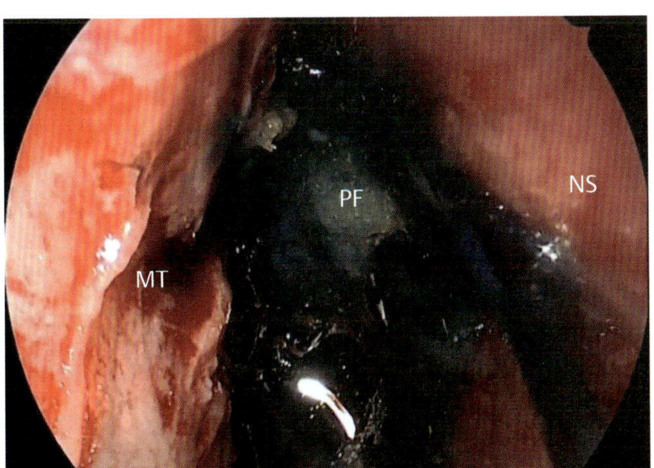

Fig. 34E.9 Application of dural sealant over the fat graft (FG).

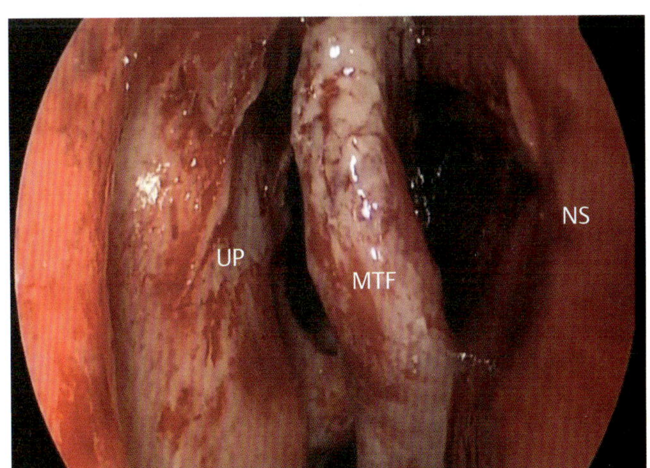

Fig. 34E.10 The middle turbinate is used as a vascularized flap (MTF) for the final reconstruction layer.

Case 34F

Endoscopic Repair of Cerebrospinal Fluid Leaks in the Lateral Sphenoid Sinus Recess

Nishit J. Shah and Viraj J. Kaluskar

Introduction

Cerebrospinal fluid (CSF) fistula from the middle cranial fossa into the sphenoid sinus is a rare condition. Pathology within a lateral recess of a widely pneumatized sphenoid sinus is difficult to access with the use of traditional open surgical approaches. Blind endoscopic packing of the sphenoid sinus without seeing the site of defect cannot be successful. Hence, we recommend the endoscopic transpterygoid approach which can directly access this region.

We present a case of a 38-year-old man who presented with a nontraumatic spontaneous CSF leak from the lateral aspect of the left sphenoid sinus and was successfully treated using an endoscopic transpterygoid approach.

Computed tomography (CT) cisternography showed a CSF fistula 9 mm in superolateral wall of left sphenoid sinus (**Fig. 34F.1**). Magnetic resonance imaging (MRI) suggested soft tissue in sphenoid sinus through defect with medial pulling of left temporal horn (**Fig. 34F.2**).

Surgical Steps

1. Inspection of the nasal cavity with a 0-degree endoscope is done to get familiar with the anatomy of the patient (**Fig. 34F.3**).
2. A unilateral inferior turbinectomy may be done depending on site of the lesion. If the defect is very low, then it is easier to do the inferior turbinectomy. This can be best assessed on the axial scans (**Fig. 34F.4**).
3. This is followed by wide maxillary antrostomy and a medial maxillectomy. We like to save the head of inferior turbinate and start the bone removal just posterior to the pyriform aperture to avoid postoperative alar retraction (**Fig. 34F.5**).
4. Complete ethmoidectomy and wide sphenoidotomy are done to have a view of posterior skull base (**Fig. 34F.6**).
5. Sphenopalatine artery (SPA) is identified and cauterized (**Fig. 34F.7** and **Fig. 34F.8**).

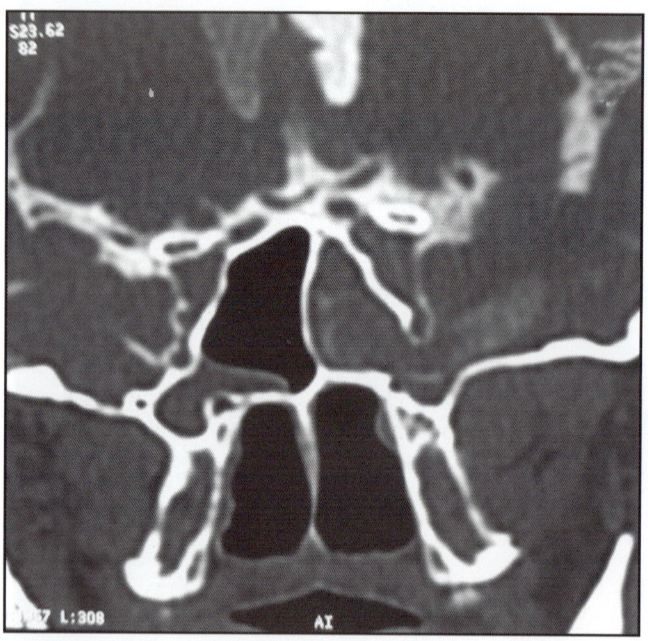

Fig. 34F.1 CT cisternography.

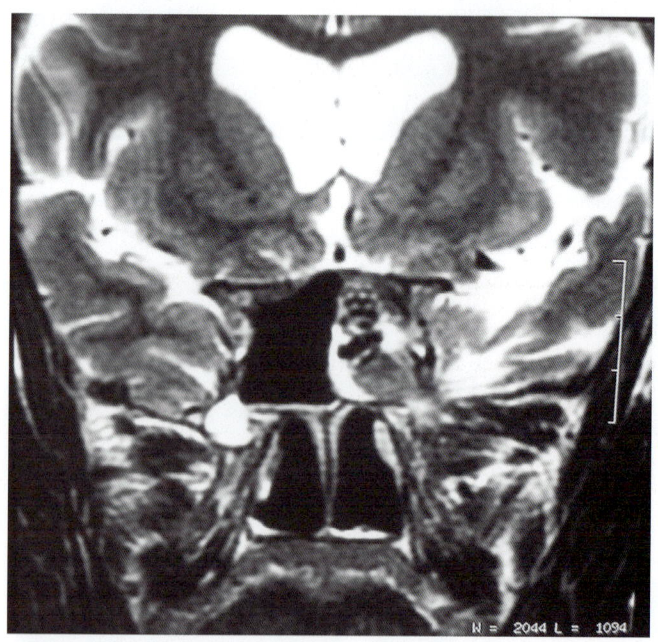

Fig. 34F.2 T2-weighted MRI image.

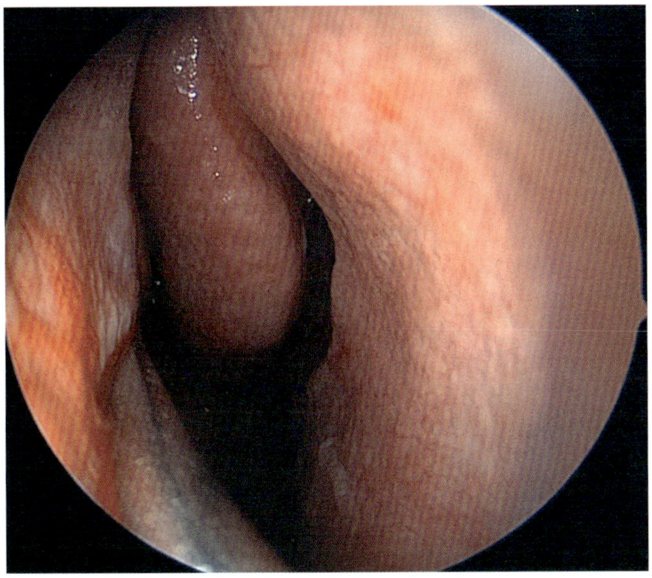

Fig. 34F.3 Left nasal cavity showing middle turbinate and middle meatus.

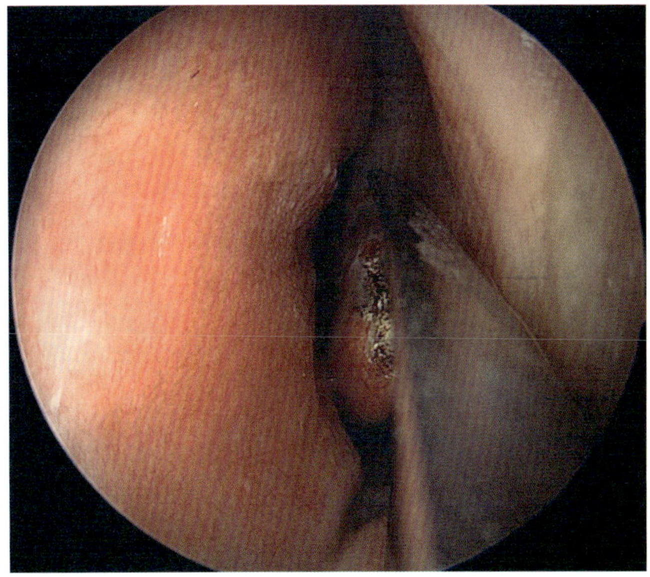

Fig. 34F.4 Cauterized incision on left inferior turbinate for inferior turbinectomy.

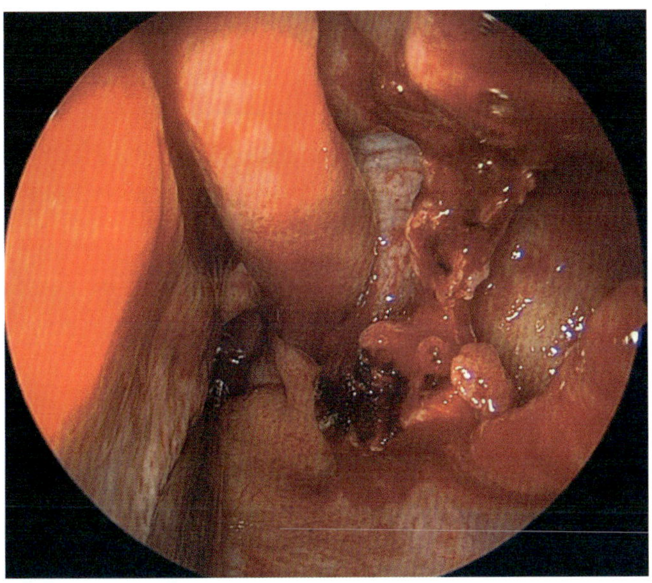

Fig. 34F.5 Complete inferior turbinectomy with widening of medial maxillary wall to expose maxillary sinus.

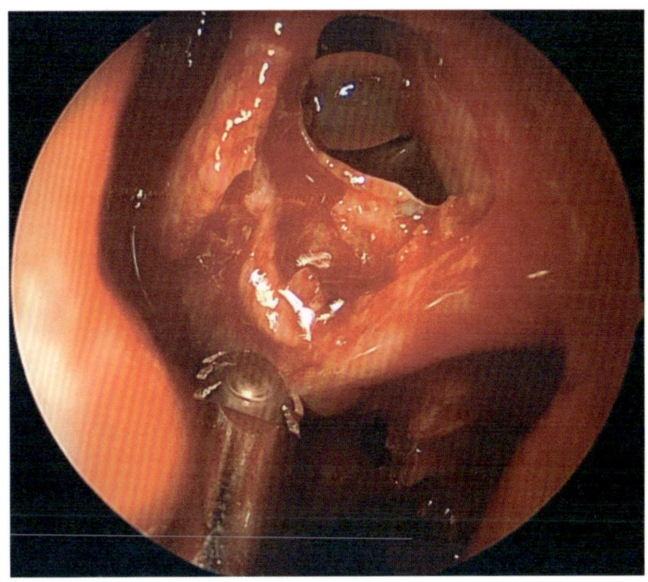

Fig. 34F.6 Clearing ethmoid bulla and opening ground lamella to expose posterior ethmoid cells and posterior skull base.

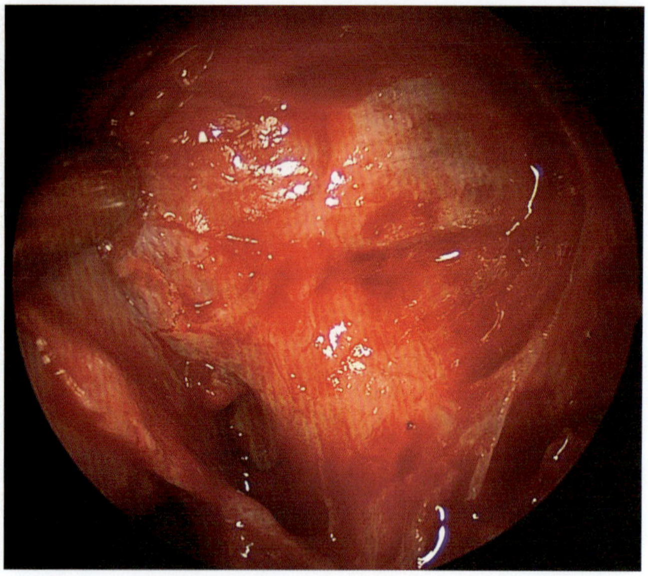

Fig. 34F.7 Exposing sphenopalatine artery and subsequent cauterization.

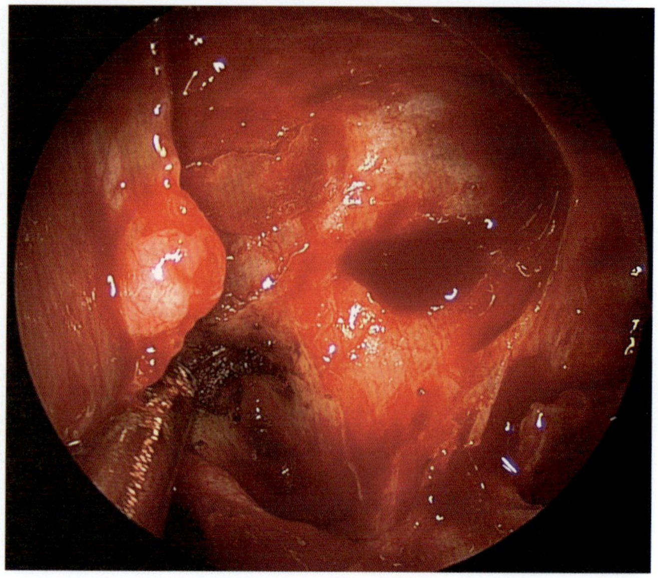

Fig. 34F.8 Cauterization of sphenopalatine artery.

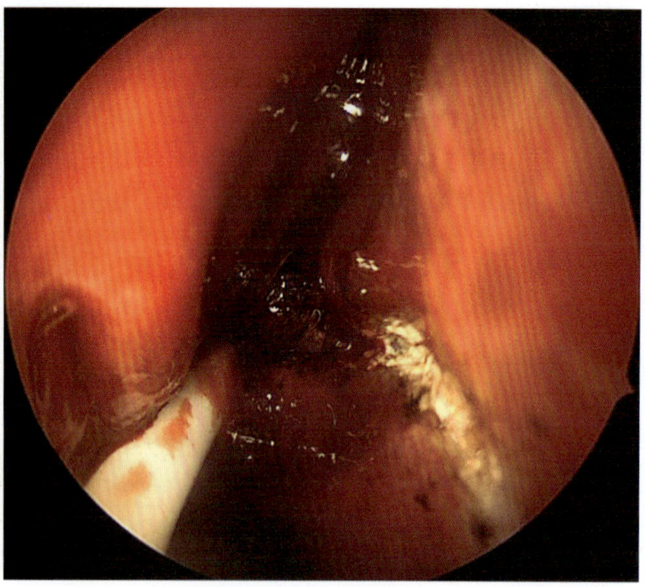

Fig. 34F.9 Harvesting Hadad–Bassagasteguy flap (HBF) of opposite side. It is a vascular pedicled mucosal flap of the nasal septum mucoperichondrium and mucoperiosteum based on the nasoseptal artery.

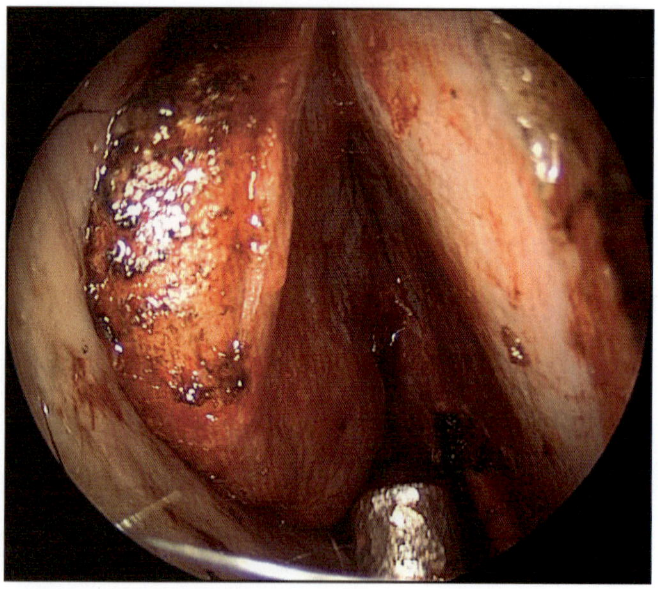

Fig. 34F.10 Elevation of HBF.

6. A contralateral *Hadad–Bassagasteguy* (HB) *flap* is raised. A HB flap is a vascular pedicled mucosal *flap* of the nasal septum mucoperichondrium and mucoperiosteum based on the nasoseptal artery, a branch of posterior septal artery which in turn is a branch of SPA. As authors are going to cauterize the SPA and internal maxillary artery (IMA), the vascular pedicle is compromised, so one cannot take HB flap from the same side. So, a crossover HB flap is used. A free mucoperiosteal flap can also be used for the repair of defect, especially if the defect lies very lateral and one is unsure if the length of the flap would be adequate (**Fig. 34F.9** and **Fig. 34F.10**).

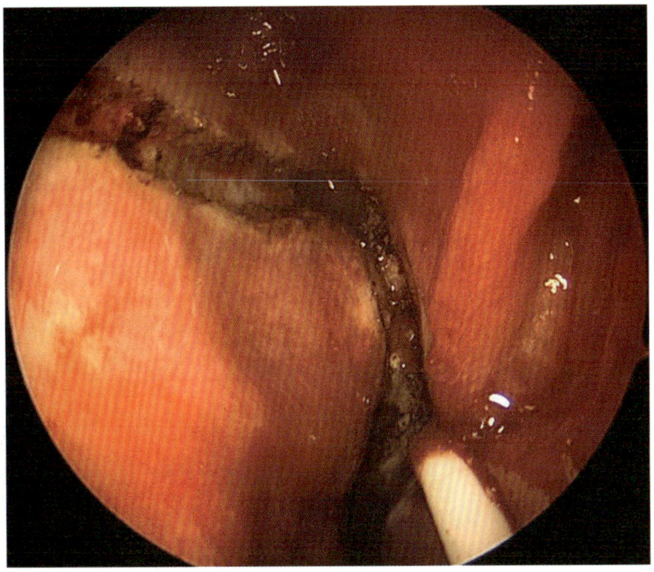

Fig. 34F.11 Elevating left side reverse flap.

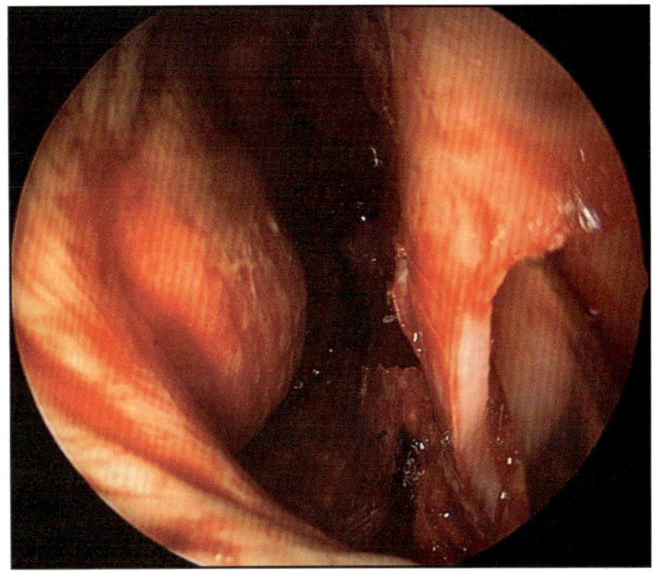

Fig. 34F.12 Harvesting cartilage for subsequent repair of bony deficiency of lateral sphenoid wall along with a posterior septectomy.

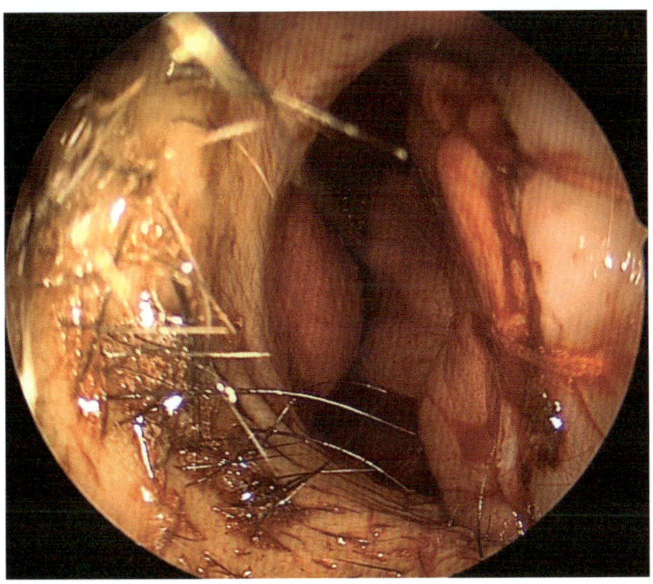

Fig. 34F.13 Suturing of reverse flap on right side.

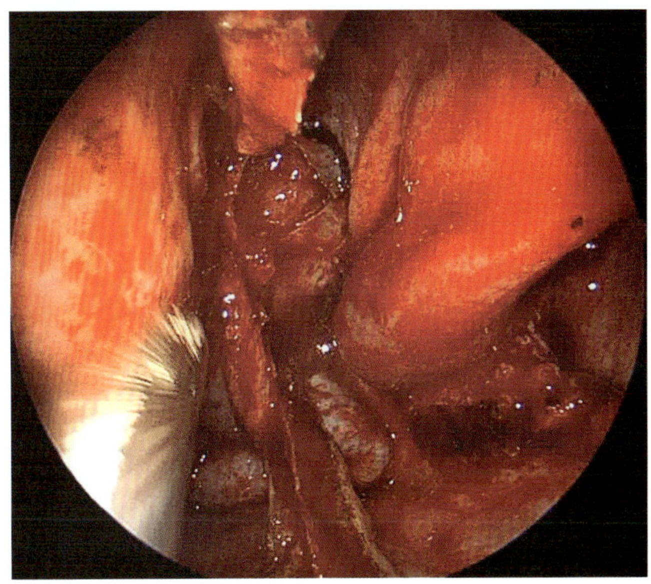

Fig. 34F.14 Post posterior septectomy view from right side. Note the HB flap in nasopharynx, inferolaterally exposed maxillary sinus showing posterior wall of maxilla and superolaterally middle turbinate. Suction is on right inferior turbinate.

7. A unilateral reverse flap is raised so as to cover the exposed septal cartilage of contralateral surface (**Fig. 34F.11**).
8. A posterior septectomy is always done to have a binasal approach. This allows a four-hand approach for drilling of posterior wall of maxilla and subsequent IMA clipping (**Fig. 34F.12**).
9. The reverse flap is sutured so as to cover the exposed cartilage (**Fig. 34F.13**).
10. Adequate posterior septectomy allows visualization of posterior wall of maxillary sinus from opposite nostril (**Fig. 34F.14**).
11. A middle turbinectomy is mandatory to allow access to lateral recess of sphenoid by communicating posterior

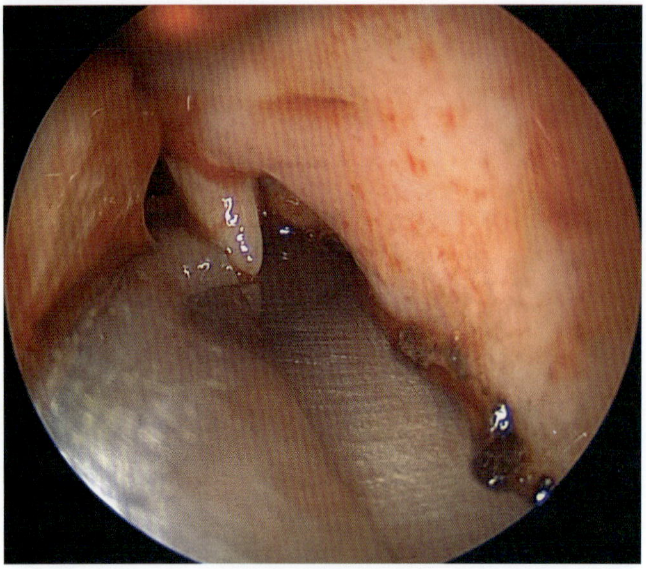

Fig. 34F.15 Left middle turbinectomy and subsequent cauterization of bleeding points.

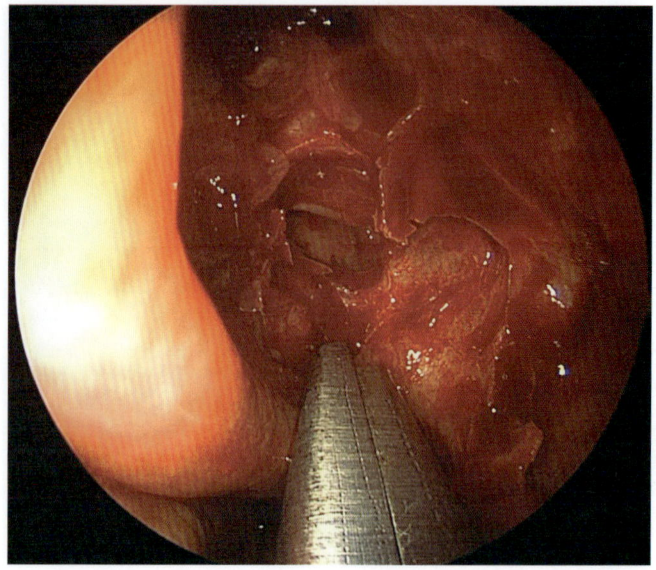

Fig. 34F.16 Punching out posterior wall of maxilla to expose pterygopalatine fossa and infratemporal fossa.

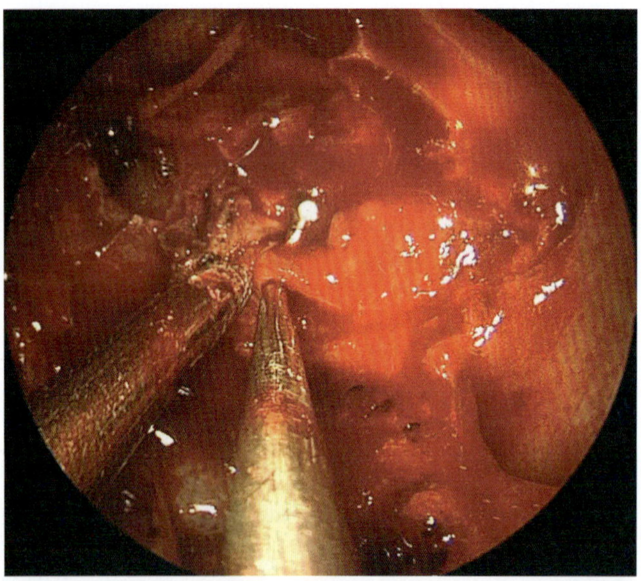

Fig. 34F.17 Exposing IMA and subsequent cauterization and division of artery. Similarly, branches of IMA are separated, cauterized, and divided to allow lateral retraction and exposure.

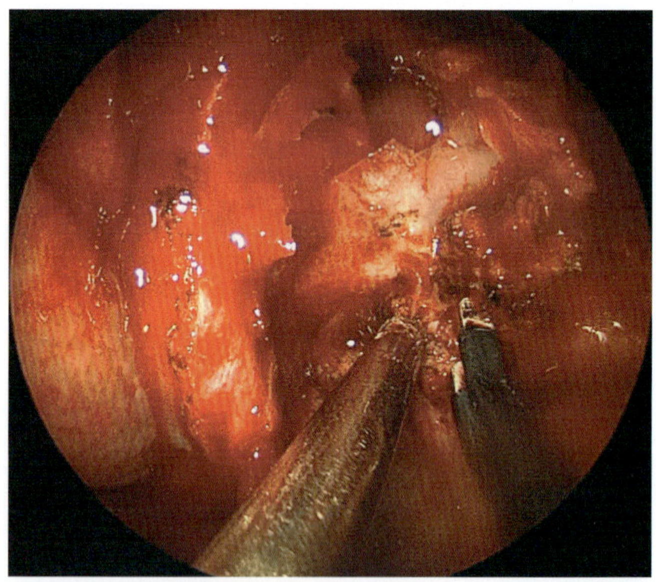

Fig. 34F.18 Exposing vidian nerve and subsequent cauterization. This allows the inferolateral exposure of medial pterygoid.

wall of maxilla with the sphenoid via the transpterygoid approach (**Fig. 34F.15**).

12. The pterygopalatine fossa is exposed either by punching out or by drilling the posterior wall of maxilla. The extent of removal of posterolateral wall of maxilla depends on the lateral extent of the defect (**Fig. 34F.16**).
13. The IMA and its branches are identified and cauterized or Ligaclips are applied. This is optional and can be avoided if extent of lateral exposure to expose the defect is less (**Fig. 34F.17**).
14. The vidian canal is identified and nerve and artery are cauterized and cut as they usually lie in the field of vision. This also allows an increase of lateral exposure. It is always advisable to work with a 0-degree endoscope as instrumentation and repair become easier. This may necessitate a little extra bone removal but is certainly worth it (**Fig. 34F.18** and **Fig. 34F.19**).

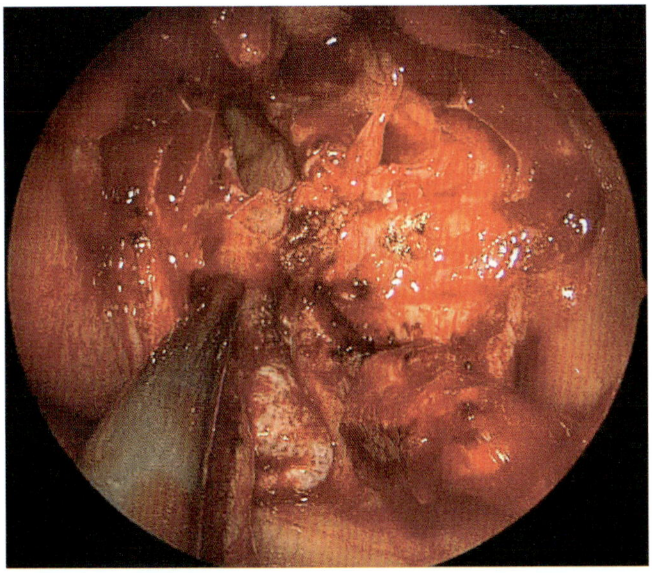

Fig. 34F.19 Removing anterior wall of sphenoid sinus. Note the visualization of meningoencephalocele in sphenoid sinus and exposure of floor of sphenoid sinus and medial pterygoid plate.

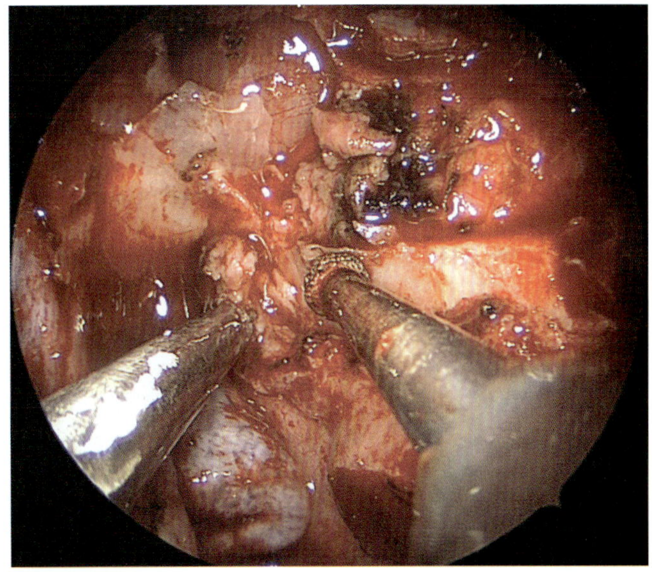

Fig. 34F.20 Drilling of medial pterygoid. This allows attainment of inferolateral limit of defect.

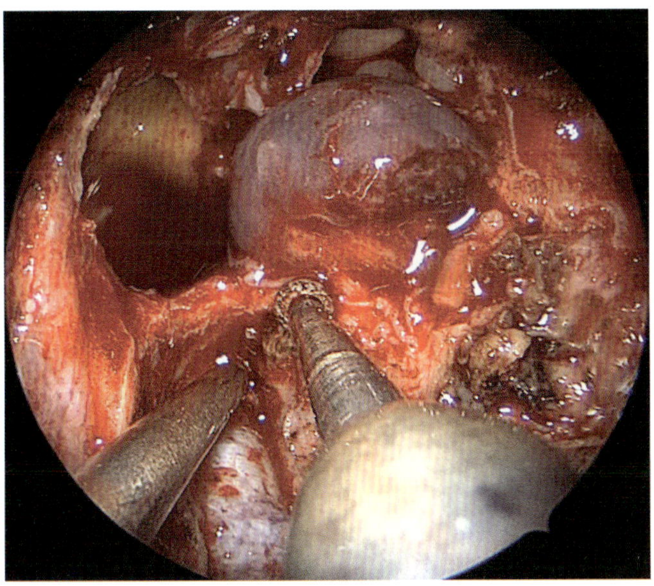

Fig. 34F.21 Drilling of floor of sphenoid.

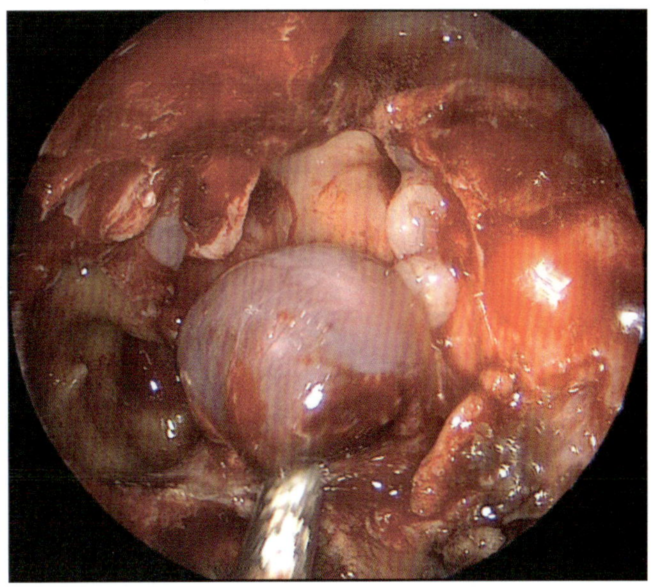

Fig. 34F.22 Exposure of meningoencephalocele arising from lateral recess of sphenoid sinus. Note the widely communicated right sphenoid sinus.

15. The well-exposed medial pterygoid bone is now drilled, so also the floor of sphenoid is lowered. This gradually exposes the lateral recess of sphenoid bone visualized from 0-degree endoscopic view (**Fig. 34F.20** and **Fig. 34F.21**).
16. The pterygoid wedge is drilled until lateral end of defect is seen. Once the exposure is complete, the meningoencephalocele is now reduced by cauterization so that there is no bleeding (**Fig. 34F.22**, **Fig. 34F.23**, and **Fig. 34F.24**).
17. The superolateral limit of drilling is up to identification of foramen rotundum. It is vital to preserve V2 as it has sensory supply to lower eyelid and cheek, the nares and upper lip, the upper teeth and gums, the nasal

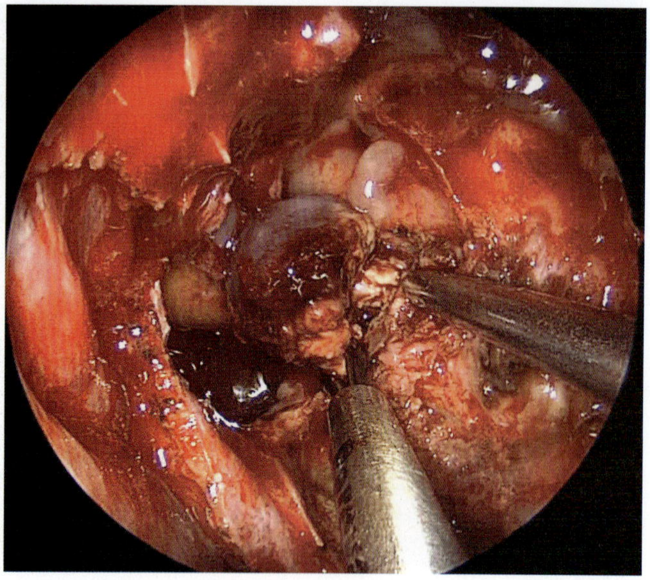

Fig. 34F.23 Cauterization of meningoencephalocele.

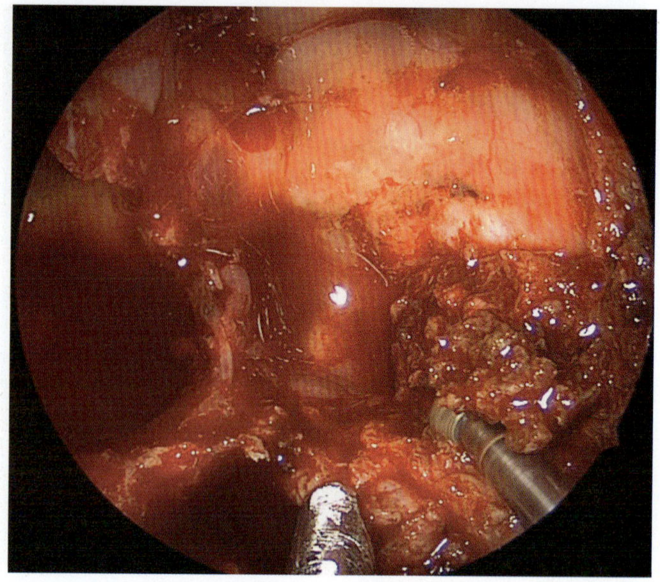

Fig. 34F.24 Further drilling of pterygoid wedge for complete lateral exposure of the defect.

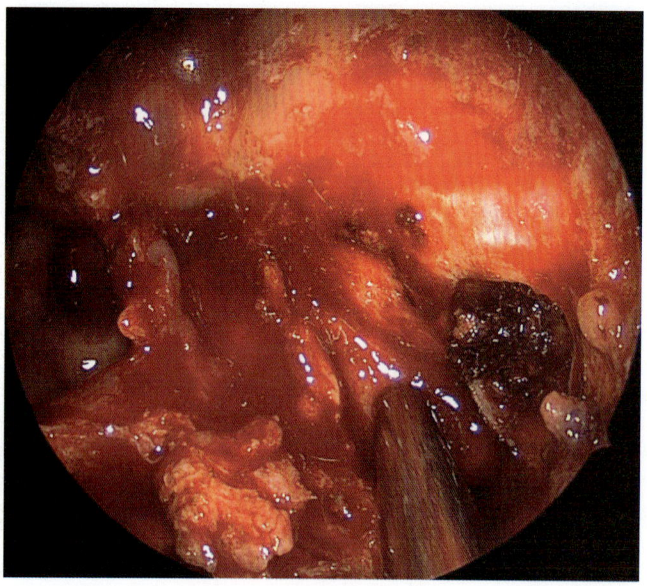

Fig. 34F.25 Complete exposure of defect in lateral recess of left sphenoid. Note the impression of V2 above the defect.

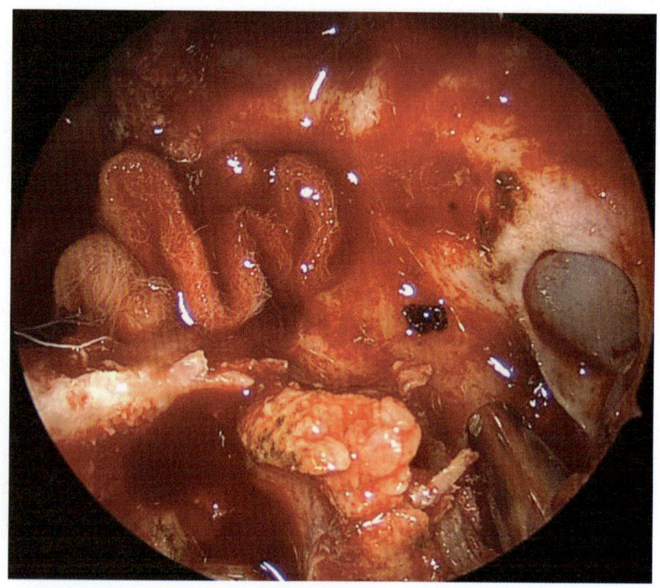

Fig. 34F.26 Cartilage of apt size snuggly fitting in bony defect. Also, note the denuding of surrounding mucosa as a step for preparation of repositioning of crossover HB flap.

mucosa, the palate and roof of the pharynx, the maxillary, ethmoid, and sphenoid sinuses (**Fig. 34F.25**).

18. The mucosa of sphenoid sinus and lateral recess surrounding the defect is completely denuded. It is important to denude the bone completely before laying HB flap as a layer of mucosa between flap and bone can cause failure of uptake of flap. This principle is similar even in case of free flap repair (**Fig. 34F.26**).
19. Prior to putting an overlay graft/HB flap, it is our practice to plug the defect with either cartilage or fat (**Fig. 34F.26**).

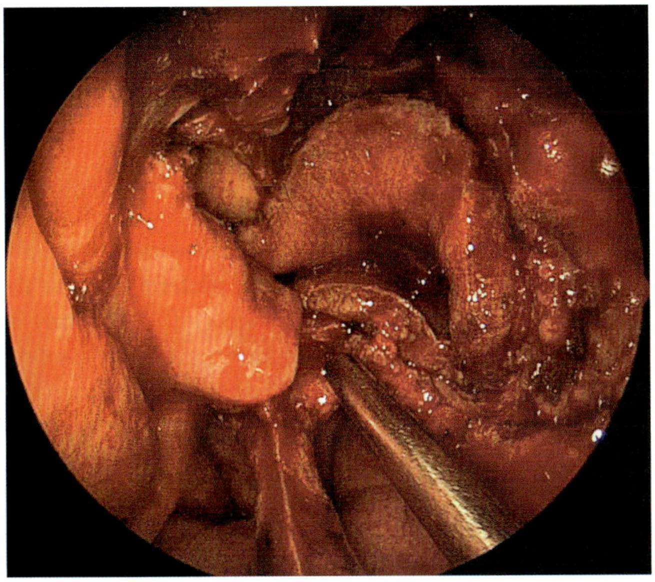

Fig. 34F.27 Repositioning of HB flap to completely cover the defect. The rest of the sphenoid sinuses remains open.

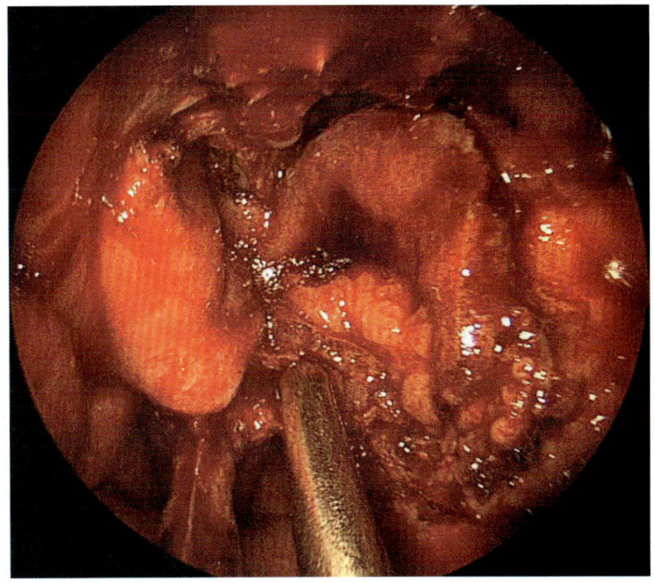

Fig. 34F.28 Layer of fat as a buffer over the HB flap.

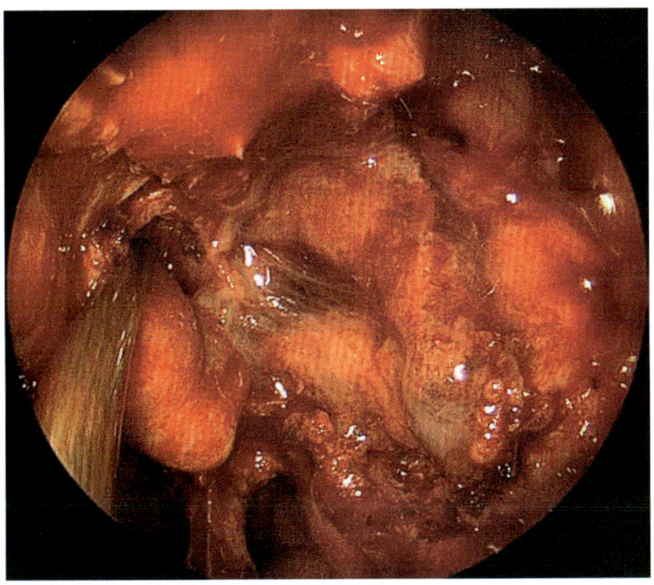

Fig. 34F.29 Layer of tissue glue over the repair. Caution to be taken not to let the glue leak under the HB flap.

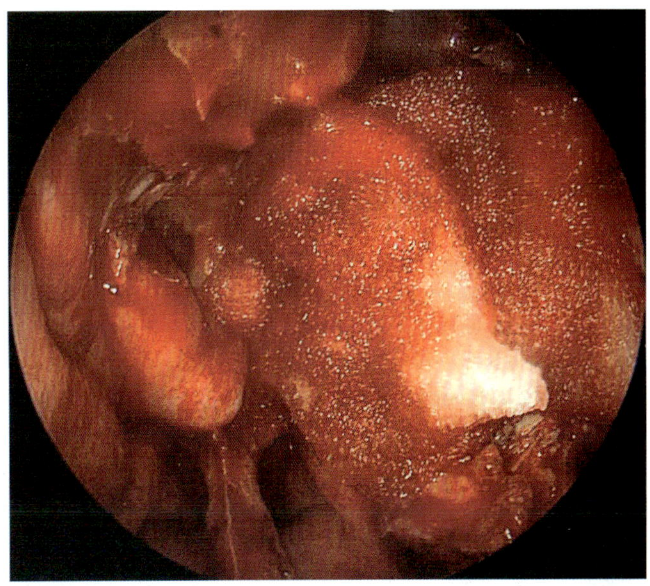

Fig. 34F.30 Final buffer layer of Gelfoam over the repair. A nasal pack is kept over for support for 5 days.

20. The HB flap is repositioned to completely cover the defect keeping rest of the sphenoid sinus open (**Fig. 34F.27**).
21. A layer of fat as a buffer over HB flap is kept (**Fig. 34F.28**).
22. This is followed by application of tissue glue. Authors then put Gelfoam as a buffer to avoid an inadvertent pull on the repair material during pack removal (**Fig. 34F.29** and **Fig. 34F.30**).
23. Merocel pack is kept for 5 days.

Case 34G

Endoscopic Transpterygoid Approach to Repair Sphenoid Sinus Lateral Recess Meningoencephalocele

Revadi Govindaraju, Michel Roethlisberger, and Prepageran Narayanan

History

A 49-year-old lady presented with the occurrence of frequent headaches requiring regular medication intake. Initially treated for migraine, she was later investigated for an intracranial space-occupying lesion. Computed tomography (CT) of the neurocranium revealed an opacity of the right sphenoid sinus. A subsequent high-resolution CT of the paranasal sinuses confirmed a bony defect in the right sphenoid sinus lateral recess. Further history revealed no other complaints of visual, nasal, or otological symptoms; neuro-ophthalmological examination and nasal endoscopy were also normal. She underwent an endoscopic transpterygoid exploration with excision of a meningoencephalocele (ME) and repair of the skull base defect.

Surgical Steps

1. The patient is placed under general anesthesia in supine position and the head in a slightly hyperextended position.
2. The nose is decongested with ribbon gauze soaked in adrenaline 1:1,000 units, and mucosal infiltration is done with lignocaine hydrochloride anhydrous 2% with adrenaline 1:100,000.
3. An endoscopic medial maxillectomy is performed in a standard way. First, an inferior turbinectomy is performed, followed by a middle meatal antrostomy, enlarged to the floor inferiorly, posteriorly up to the posterior wall of the maxillary sinus, anteriorly to the anteromedial wall, and superiorly up to the floor of the orbit. This is done along with the transection of the nasolacrimal duct. The extent of removal of the anterior wall is dictated by the amount of exposure required to allow for a sufficient instrumentation (**Fig. 34G.1**).
4. After the antrostomy, a complete ethmoidectomy and sphenoidotomy follow. (**Fig. 34G.2, Fig. 34G.3,** and **Fig. 34G.4**). The sphenoid opening is enlarged in a medial to lateral direction (**Fig. 34G.5**) until the ME is identified (**Fig. 34G.6**).
5. To gain further access to the sphenoid sinus lateral recess (SSLR), the superior part of the pterygoid process needs to be removed. The sphenopalatine artery is first identified, cauterized, and divided (**Fig. 34G.7** and **Fig. 34G.8**). This allows the rest of the contents of the pterygopalatine fossa to be reflected inferiorly and the superior part of the pterygoid process to be removed until complete exposure of the ME is obtained (**Fig. 34G.9**).
6. Special microdissectors and probes are used to delineate the bony defect (**Fig. 34G.10**) followed by cauterization of the ME with a bipolar diathermy (**Fig. 34G.11**).

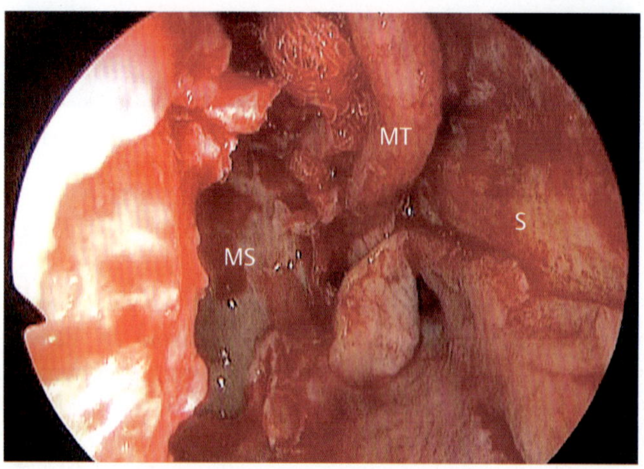

Fig. 34G.1 Endoscopic view of the medial maxillectomy allowing to access the sphenoid sinus lateral recess via a transpterygoid approach.

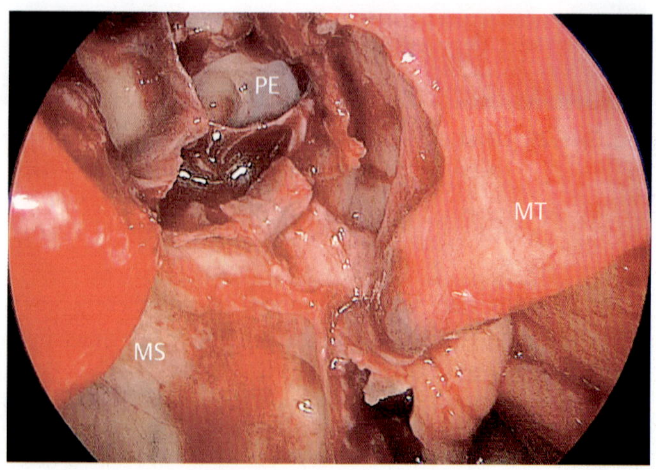

Fig. 34G.2 Anterior and posterior ethmoid cells have been removed to reach the sphenoid sinus.

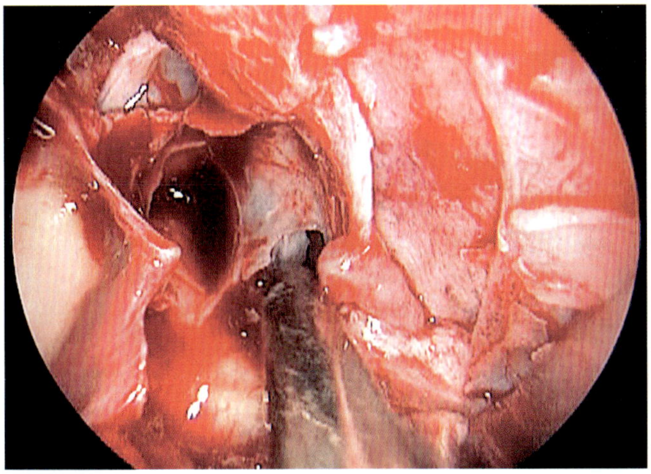

Fig. 34G.3 The thin-walled anterior face of the sphenoid sinus is punctured with a suction device.

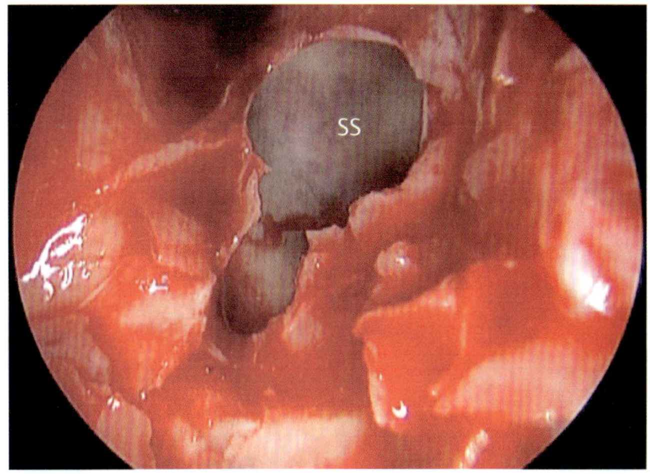

Fig. 34G.4 Endoscopic view of the initial sphenoidotomy.

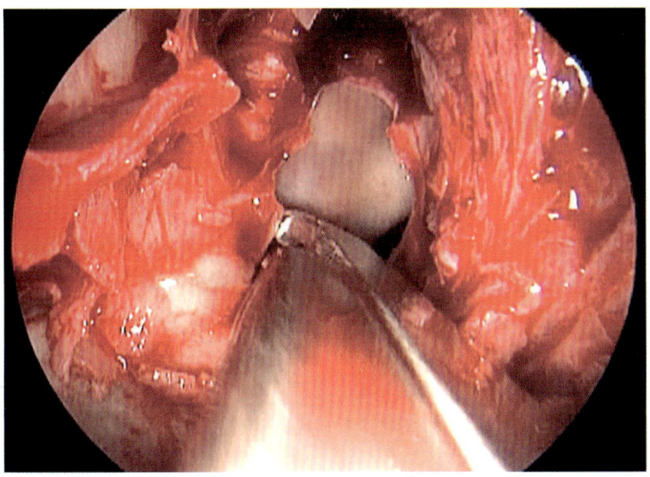

Fig. 34G.5 The sphenoidotomy is enlarged in a medial to lateral direction using a Kerrison's punch.

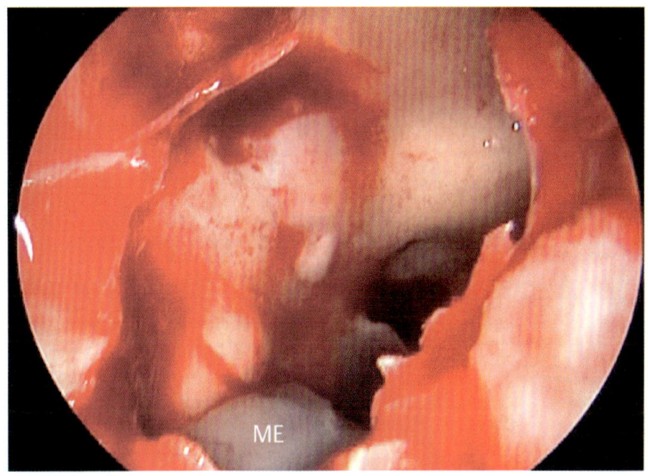

Fig. 34G.6 The superior part of the meningoencephalocele can be visualized through a standard sphenoidotomy.

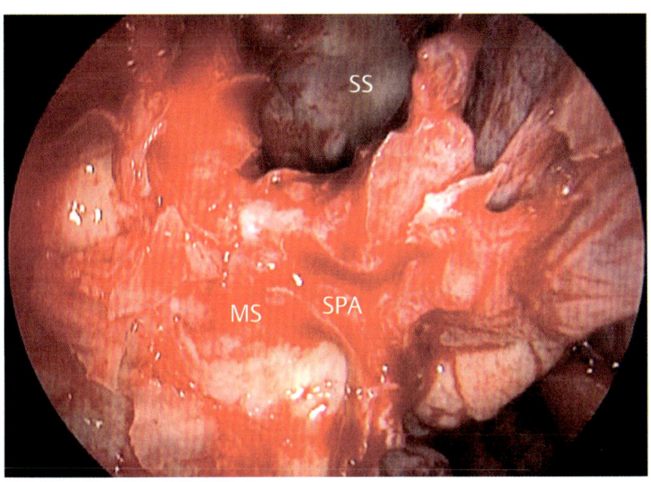

Fig. 34G.7 The sphenopalatine artey (SPA) and its branches are identified as they exit the sphenopalatine foramen.

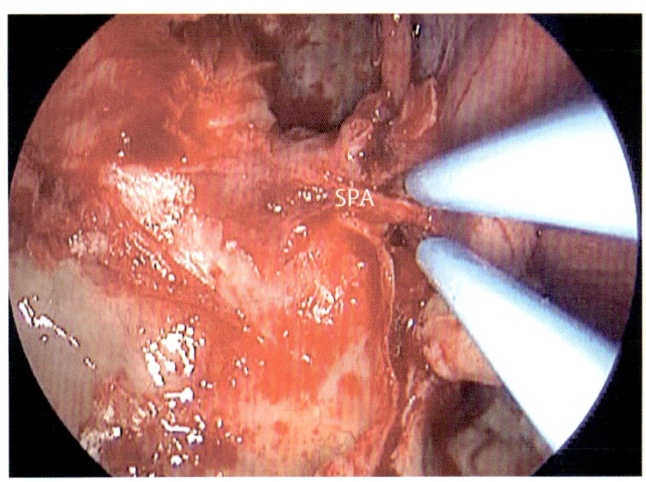

Fig. 34G.8 The sphenopalatine artery (SPA) is cauterized prior to sharp division.

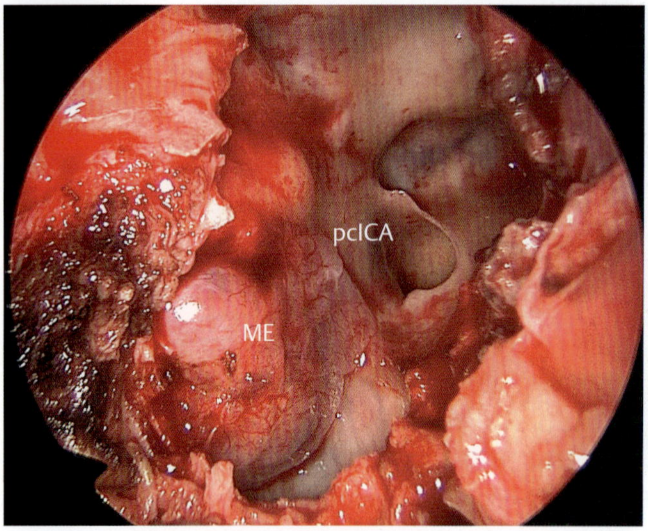

Fig. 34G.9 After removal of the superior part of the pterygoid process, the meningoencephalocele (ME) is completely exposed.

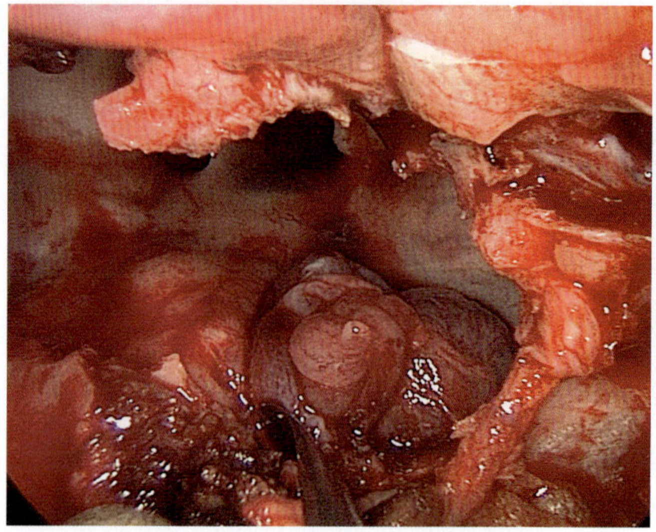

Fig. 34G.10 The bony defect of the meningoencephalocele is delineated using a special microdissector.

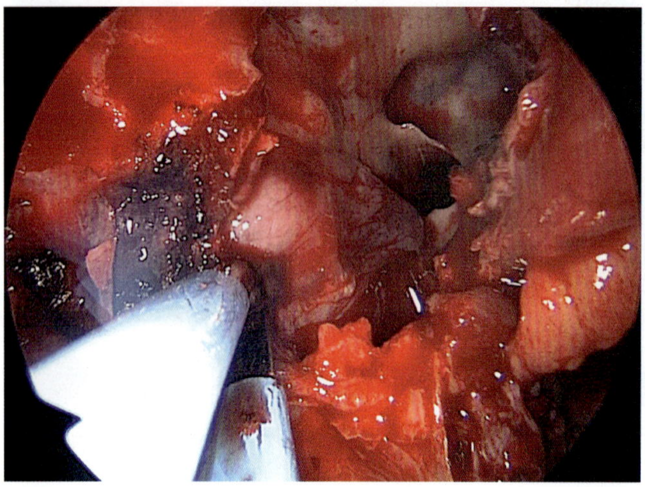

Fig. 34G.11 The meningoencephalocele is reduced using bipolar cauterization.

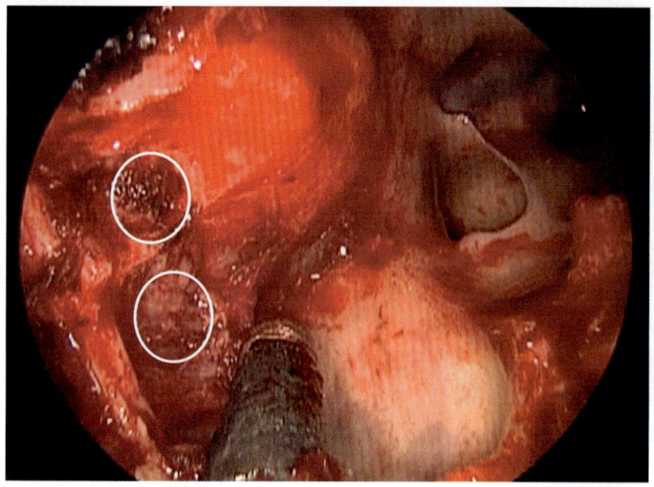

Fig. 34G.12 After reduction of the meningoencephalocele, the bony edges of the defect are visible *(white circles)*.

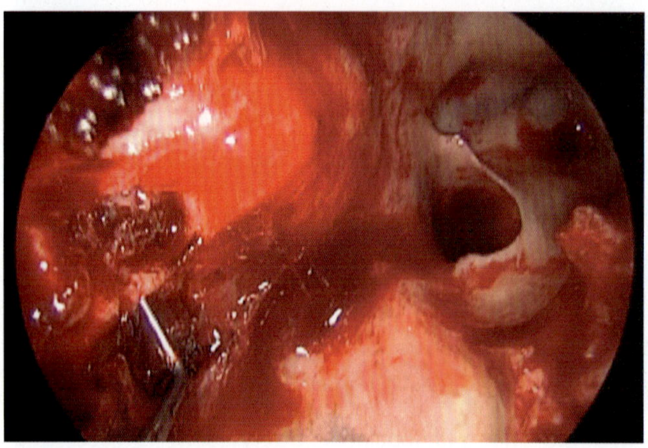

Fig. 34G.13 A probe is placed underneath the ridge of bone separating the two defects.

7. The bony defect is identified and surrounding mucosa is removed (**Fig. 34G.12**). In this case two adjacent defects are separated by a small ridge of bone (**Fig. 34G.13**), hence, the creation of one large single defect is necessary (**Fig. 34G.14**).
8. Bleeding mucosal edges and vessels are meticulously cauterized to secure hemostasis and prevent intracranial hemorrhage (**Fig. 34G.15**).
9. The defect is plugged with an abdominal fat graft followed by a fibrin dural sealant. A multilayer repair follows with a free mucosal graft, more fibrin sealant, absorbable hemostat, finally supported by multiple gelatine foams (**Fig. 34G.16a–d**).

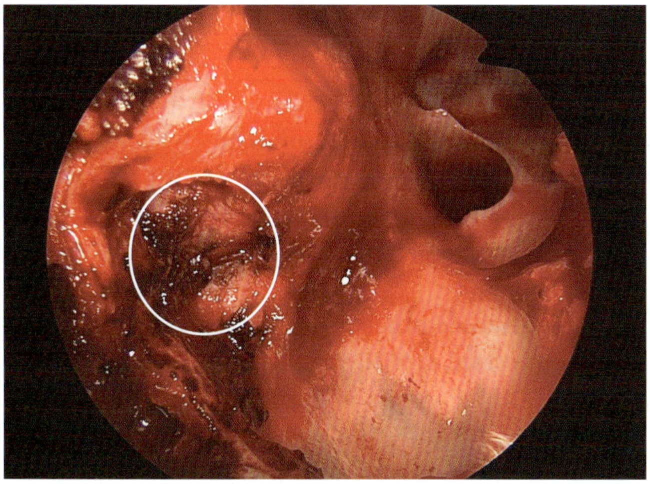

Fig. 34G.14 A single defect (*white circles*) in the sphenoid sinus lateral recess inferior and lateral to the course of the maxillary nerve is created.

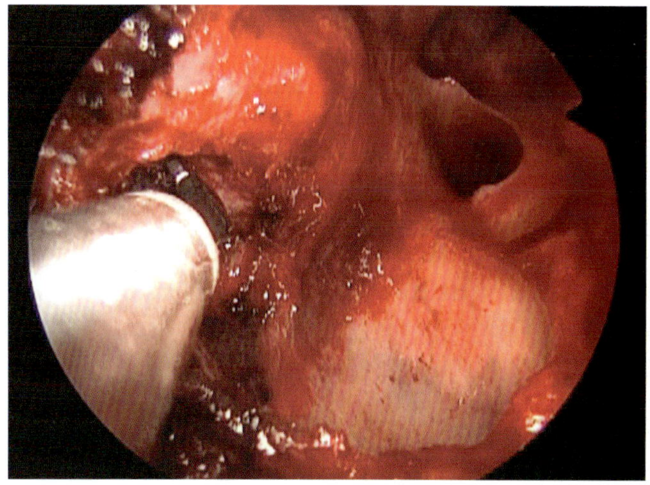

Fig. 34G.15 An angled biploar cautery is used to achieve hemostasis around the skull base defect.

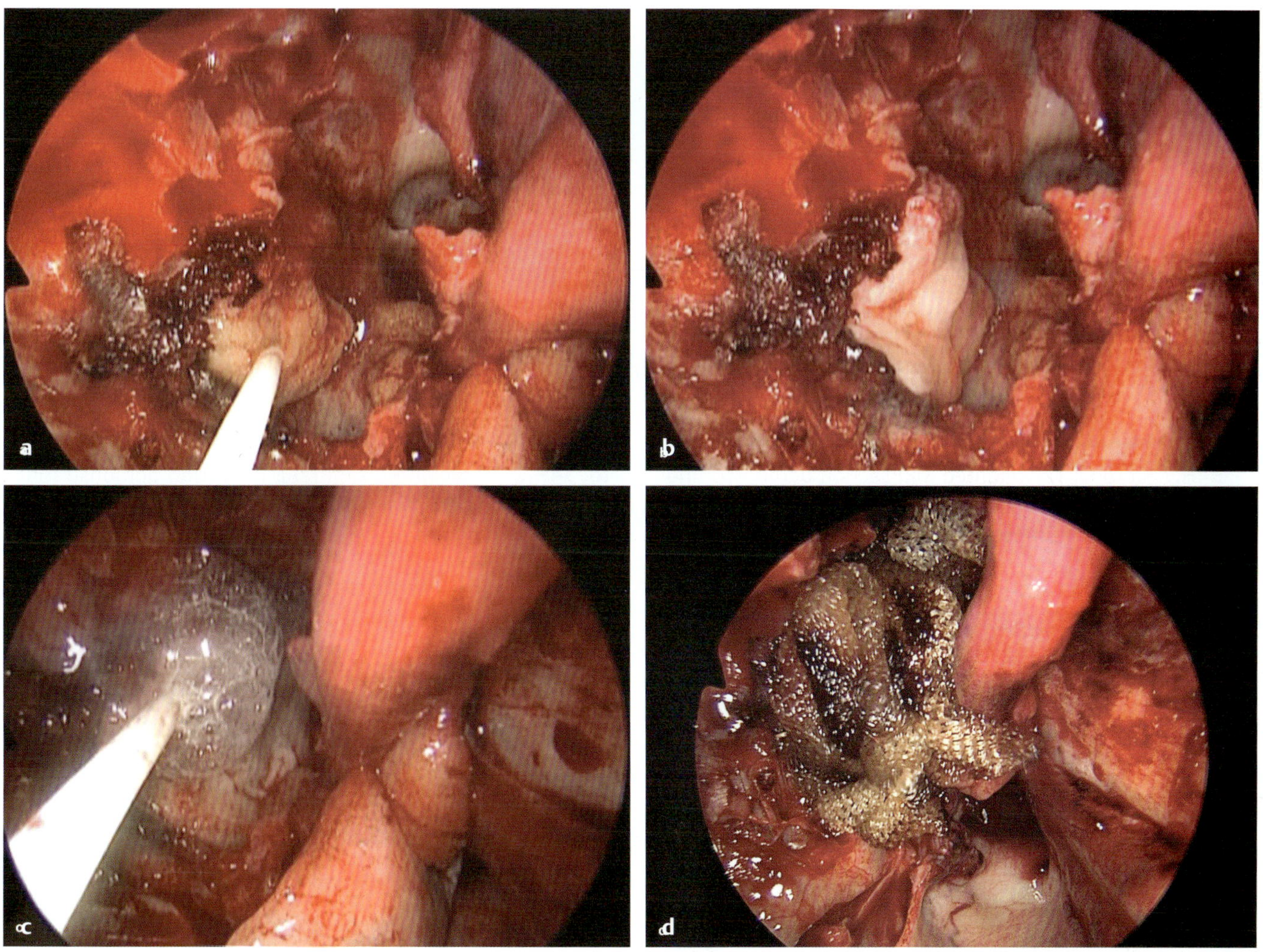

Fig. 34G.16 The multilayer repair is performed using **(a)** an abdominal fat graft, **(b)** a free mucosal graft, **(c)** dural fibrin sealant, and **(d)** absorbable hemostat.

Case 34H

Endonasal Endoscopic Repair of a Pediatric Encephalocele

Wong HT, Michel Roethlisberger, Sien Hui Tan, Saif Al-Zahid, Vicknes Waran, and Prepageran Narayanan

History

The present case describes an endonasal endoscopic repair of an encephalocele in a 9-year-old girl following a one year history of a head trauma. The skull base defect was detected on both coronal and sagittal T2-weighted magnetic resonance imaging (MRI) sections (**Fig. 34H.1** and **Fig. 34H.2**).

Surgical Steps

1. The patient is positioned supine with head slightly extended under general anesthesia.
2. The nose is packed as per standard protocol. The packing is placed between the septum and the middle turbinate.
3. Endonasal endoscopic examination reveals a pulsating mass located medially to the right middle turbinate (**Fig. 34H.3**).
4. The area is exposed to allow visualization of the whole encephalocele. Any bony fragments are removed. In case a wider exposure is needed, the septum is removed partially to allow the endoscopic placement via the contralateral nostril. The lesion is now accessable using a four-hand technique (**Fig. 34H.4a, b**).

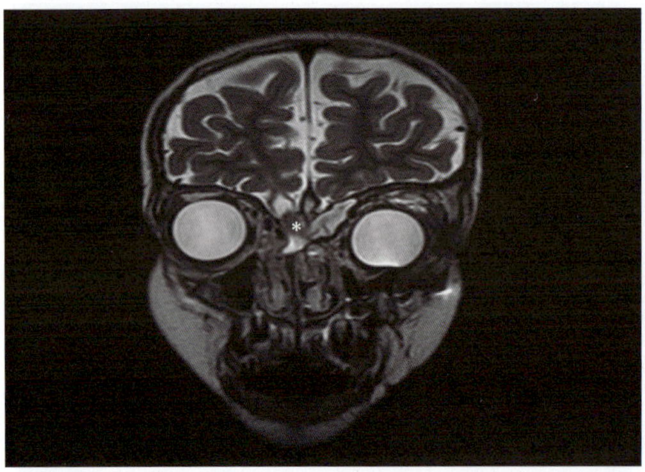

Fig. 34H.1 Coronal T2-weighted MRI section demonstrating an encephalocele (*) located medially to the middle turbinate prolapsing into the right nasal cavity.

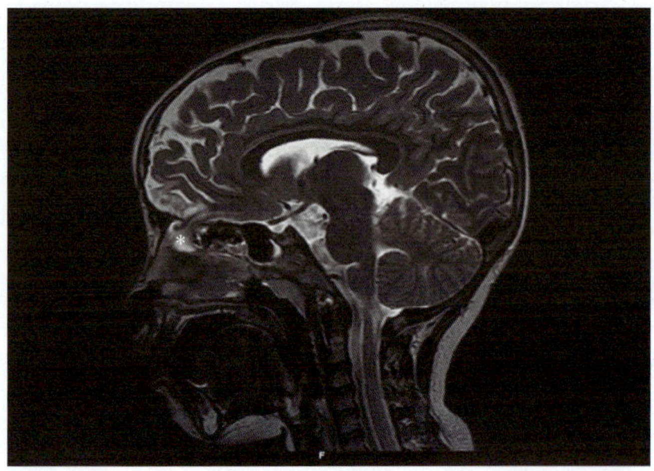

Fig. 34H.2 T2-weighted sagittal MRI section demonstrating an encephalocele (*) within the cribriform region.

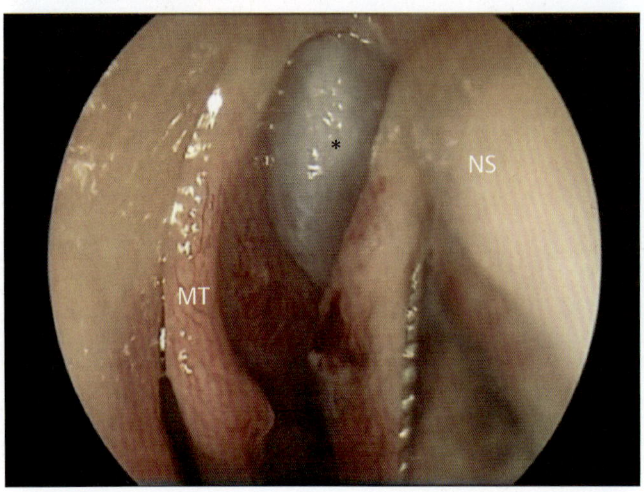

Fig. 34H.3 Endoscopic view of the encephalocele (*) medial to the right middle turbinate (MT).

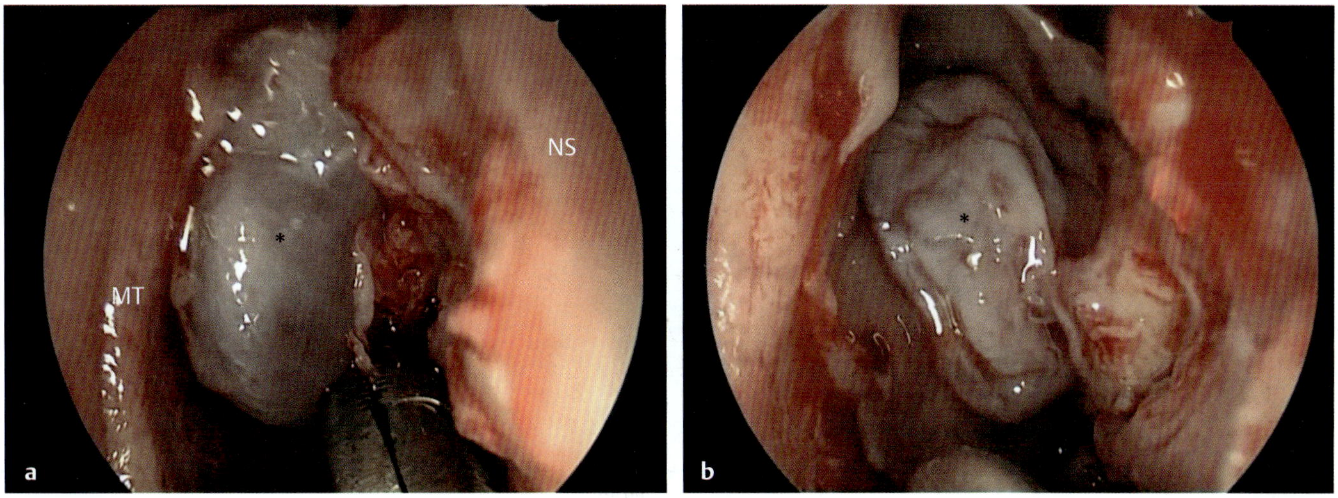

Fig. 34H.4 **(a)** The nasal septum (NS) is removed to allow for a wider exposure and a four-handed technique approach. **(b)** Complete exposure of the encephalocele (*).

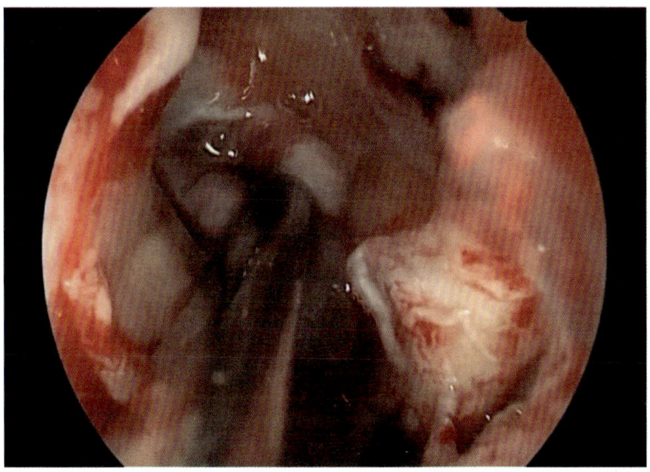

Fig. 34H.5 The encephalocele is compressed and reduced to delineate the skull base defect.

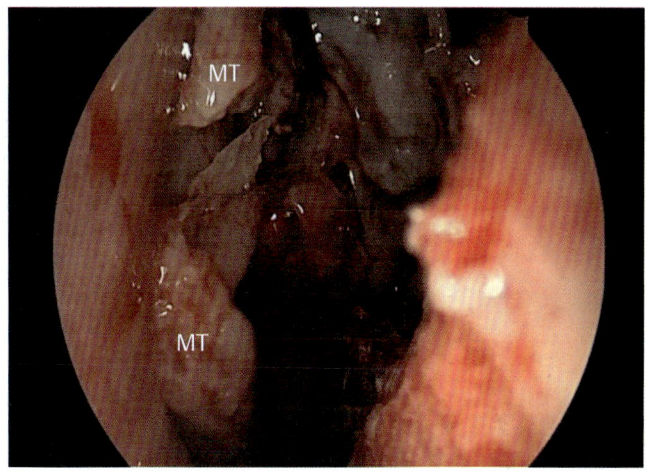

Fig. 34H.6 Parts of the right middle turbinate (MT) are divided anteriorly keeping the posterior attachment intact for blood supply. This allows to use the middle turbinate flap as a vascularized support of the reconstruction.

5. The encephalocele is compressible and can be reduced back to the intracranium to delineate the skull base defect (**Fig. 34H.5**).
6. Part of the middle turbinate is divided anteriorly and reserved for middle turbinate flap reconstruction (**Fig. 34H.6**).
7. The encephalocele is then reduced using bipolar cauterization. Some parts of the encephalocele are truncated (**Fig. 34H.7**).
8. After significant reduction of the encephalocele, the edges of the bony skull base defect are clearly visualized. Bipolar diathermy is used for hemostatis where evident bleeding occurs. In addition, evident CSF leakage will occur after reduction of the encephalocele (**Fig. 34H.8**).
9. The skull base defect can then be measured using a measurement tape, or the size can be estimated with a standard square neuropatty (1 × 1 cm) (**Fig. 34H.9**).
10. The skull base defect is then repaired with an abominal fat graft. in this case. Depending on the size of the defect, additional bone or cartilage can be used for the repair (**Fig. 34H.10**).
11. An artificial dural sealant is then applied over the skull base repair construct (**Fig. 34H.11**).
12. The construct is reinforced using multiple layers of abdominal fat followed by artificial dural sealant.
13. The middle turbinate is used as vascularized flap to support the reconstruction. Additional artificial dural sealant is applied over the middle turbinate flap (**Fig. 34H.12**).

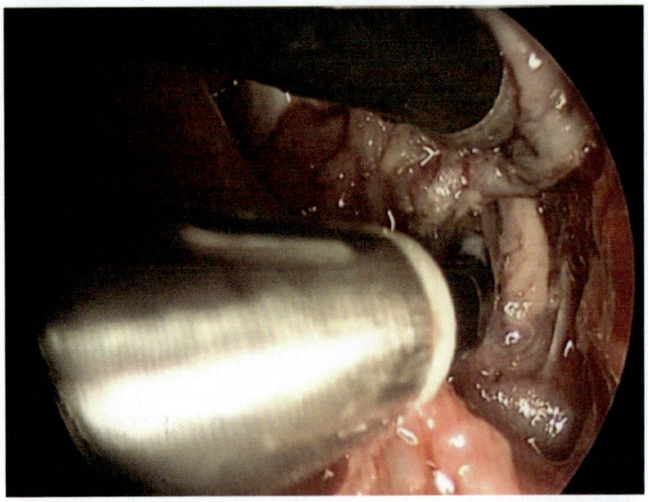

Fig. 34H.7 The encephalocele is reduced using bipolar diathermy.

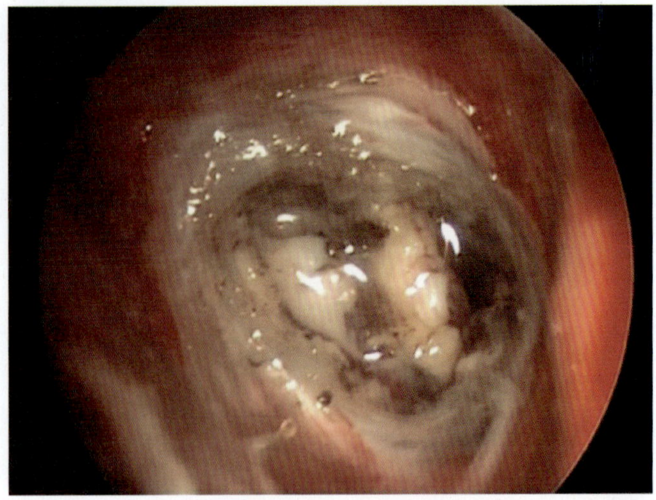

Fig. 34H.8 The edges of the skull base defect are evident after reduction of the encephalocele.

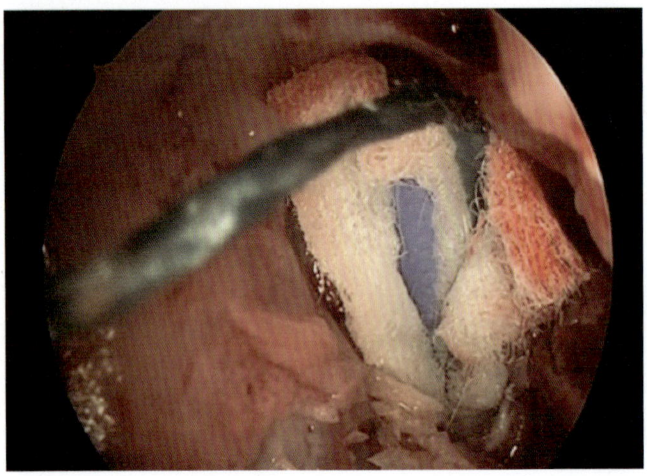

Fig. 34H.9 tight spacing using a standard square 1 × 1 cm neuropatty. In this case, the defect is less than 1 cm.

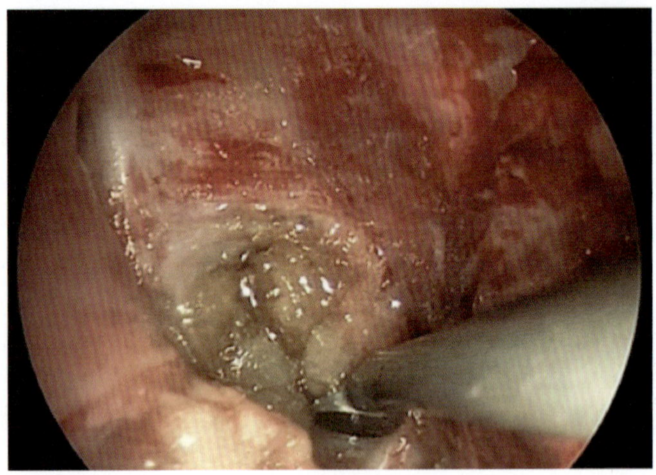

Fig. 34H.10 The skull base defect is repaired with fat.

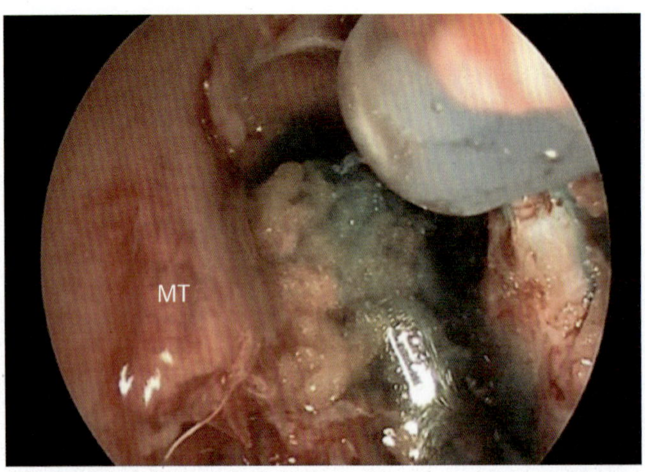

Fig. 34H.11 Applications of the dural sealant over the repaired site.

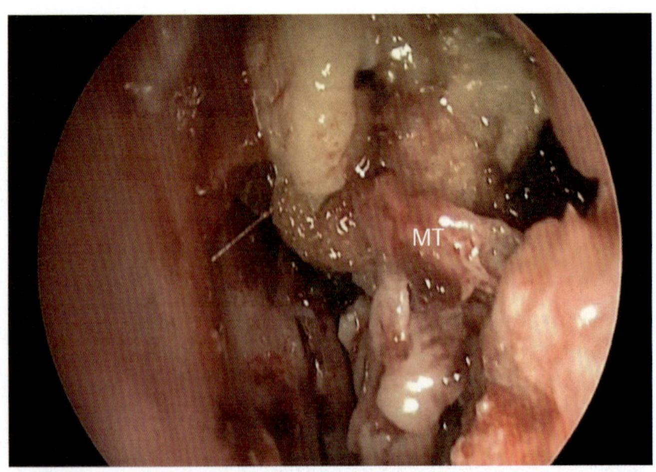

Fig. 34H.12 The lower cut end of the middle turbinate (MT) that is still attached posteriorly is used as a flap for final reconstruction.

Chapter 35 Open Surgical Management of Encephaloceles

Liew Yew Toong, Saif Al-Zahid, Michel Roethlisberger, and Prepageran Narayanan

Case 35

Transmastoid Extradural Approach for a Temporal Lobe Meningoencephalocele

History

A 24-year-old woman presented with 6 months of progressive right ear fullness and intermittent clear otorrhea. She had previously undergone a canal wall down mastoidectomy for cholesteatoma in the same ear in a different institute 3 years prior to presentation and had hearing loss as a result. She had no vertigo or purulent ear discharge. Endoscopic ear examination showed a pulsatile lobulated mass occupying the whole external ear canal. On gentle probing, the mass appeared to be originating from deep within the ear canal (**Fig. 35.1**). High-resolution computed tomography (HRCT) of the temporal bone revealed soft tissue opacity occupying the whole of the right middle ear cleft with an obvious tegmen defect measuring 1.5 cm and a mastoid cavity from previous cholesteatoma surgery (**Fig. 35.2** and **Fig. 35.3**). Magnetic resonance imaging (MRI) of the brain revealed soft tissue in the middle ear cleft in continuity with the right temporal lobe, consistent with a meningoencephalocele (**Fig. 35.4**).

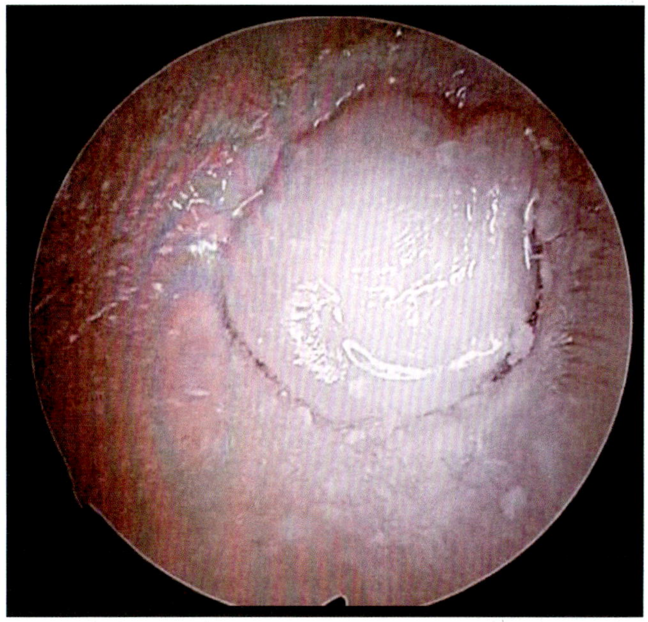

Fig. 35.1 Endoscopic ear examination showing a pulsatile lobulated mass occupying the whole external ear canal.

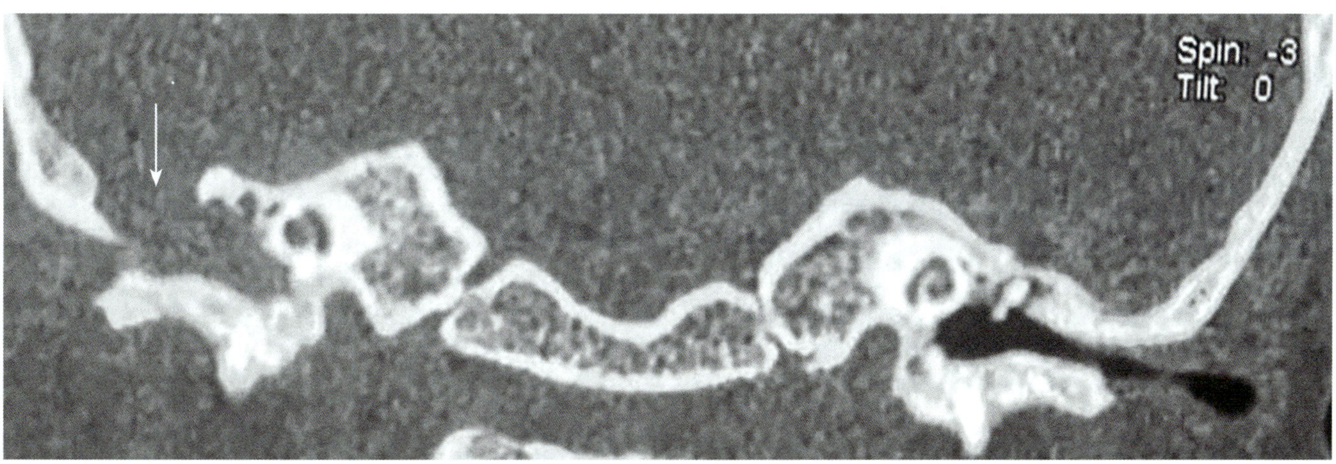

Fig. 35.2 High-resolution computed tomography (HRCT) of the temporal bone (coronal view) demonstrating a soft tissue opacity occupying the whole of the right middle ear cleft with an obvious tegmen defect measuring 1.5 cm (*white arrow*).

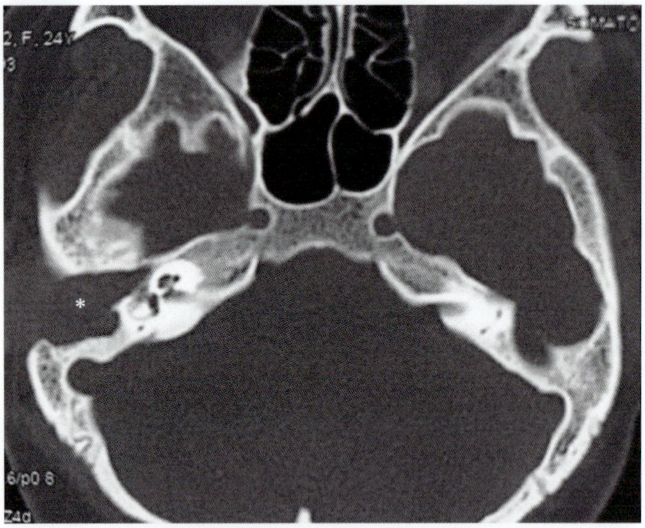

Fig. 35.3 HRCT temporal (axial) showed evidence of a previous mastoidectomy with opacity involving the whole of the mastoid cavity and middle ear cleft (*).

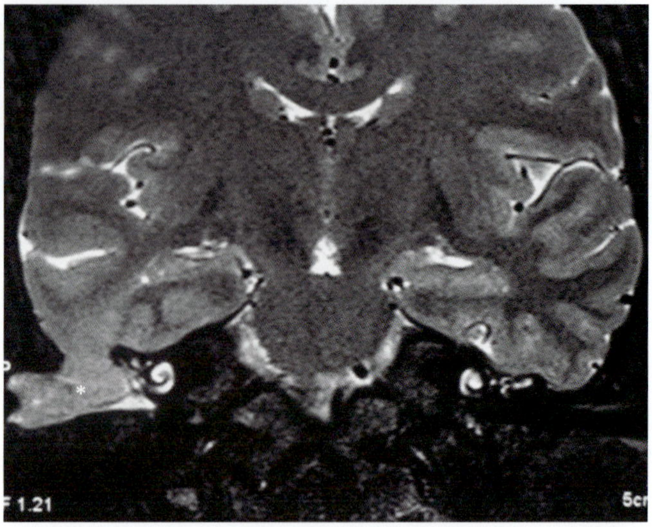

Fig. 35.4 MRI of the brain revealed soft tissue in the middle ear cleft in continuity with the right temporal lobe, findings consistent with meningoencephalocele (*).

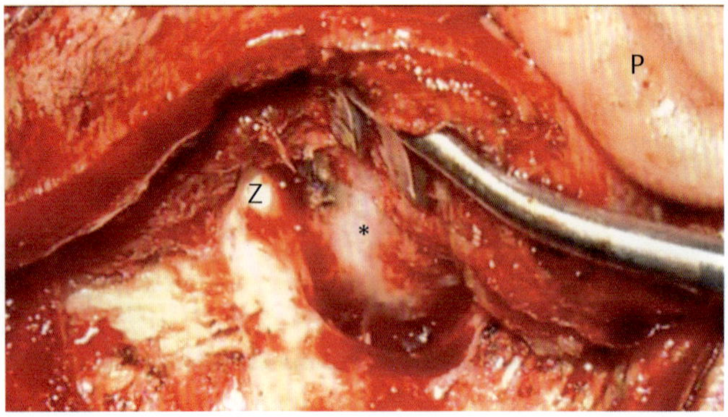

Fig. 35.5 Postauricular approach with the meatal skin retracted anteriorly to provide a wide access to the encephalocele (*).

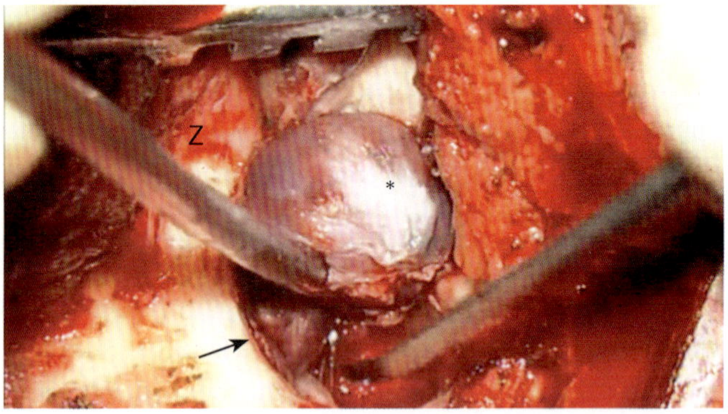

Fig. 35.6 The exposed encephalocele (*) is dissected free from surrounding adhesions with a Rosen knife and suction. The encephalocele, emerging from a defect located within the tegmen, is identified (*black arrow*).

Surgical Steps

1. The procedure is performed under general anesthesia with facial nerve monitoring. The patient is positioned supine with the head slightly extended and turned to the contralateral side.
2. The previous postauricular incision (Wilde's) is reopened and the meatal skin is retracted anteriorly to provide wide access to the encephalocele (**Fig. 35.5**).
3. Granulation tissue and adhesions are dissected off the encephalocele using a Rosen knife and suction to identify its origin from the tegmen defect (**Fig. 35.6**).
4. The tegmen mastoideum is skeletonized and the surrounding bone removed with a diamond burr to expose the base of the stalk (**Fig. 35.7**).
5. The stalk is cauterized and sectioned at its base to amputate the encephalocele. The resected base is further cauterized, allowing it to shrink toward the intracranial compartment. The herniated tissue is usually nonfunctional, and devitalized (**Fig. 35.8**).
6. A Rosen knife is used to refashion the surrounding edges and to create an epidural space for the graft to be laid for repair (**Fig. 35.9**).
7. Two layers of Surgicel followed by a 2-cm piece of temporalis fascia are inserted as an underlay, extradural technique (**Fig. 35.10** and **Fig. 35.11**).
8. Finally, the whole mastoid cavity is filled up and obliterated with soft tissue taken from the postauricular flap.

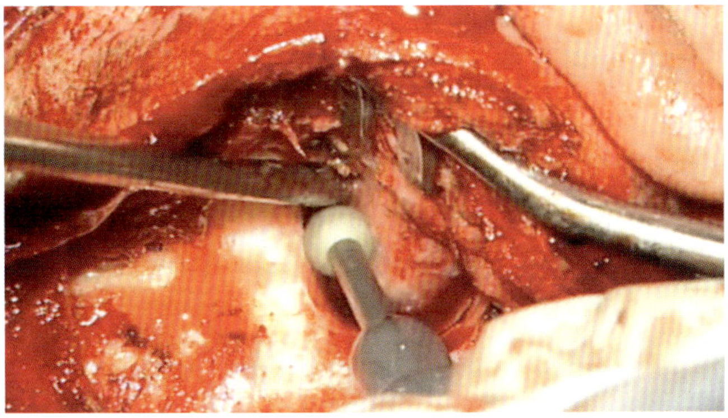

Fig. 35.7 The tegmen mastoideum is skeletonized and the base of the encephalocele is fully exposed by removing the lateral bony edges with a diamond drill.

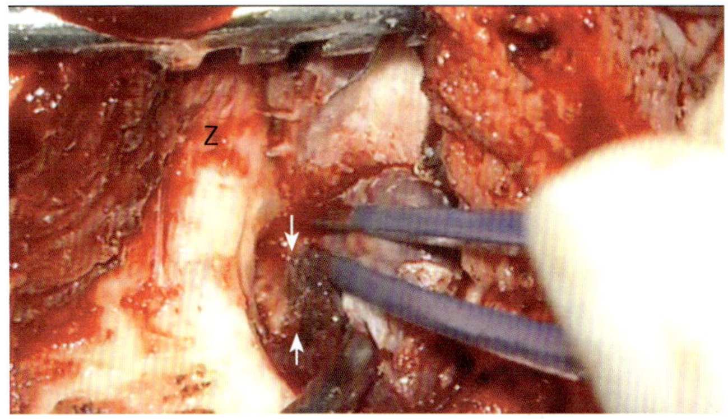

Fig. 35.8 The stalk (*white arrows*) is cauterized and amputated with bipolar diathermy.

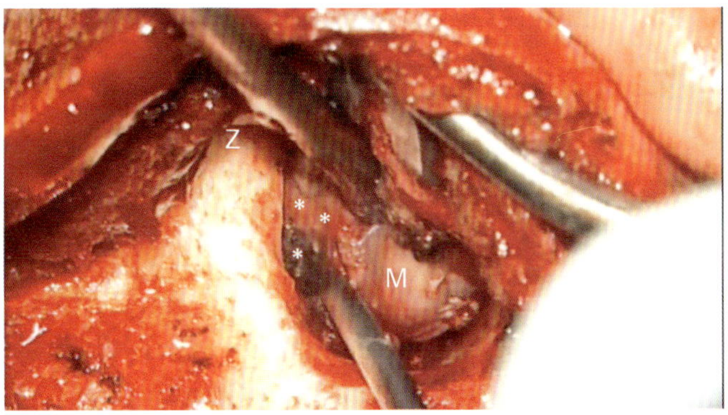

Fig. 35.9 The edges are refashioned with a Rosen knife to create an epidural space for the graft to be laid. The tegmen defect can now be clearly appreciated (*).

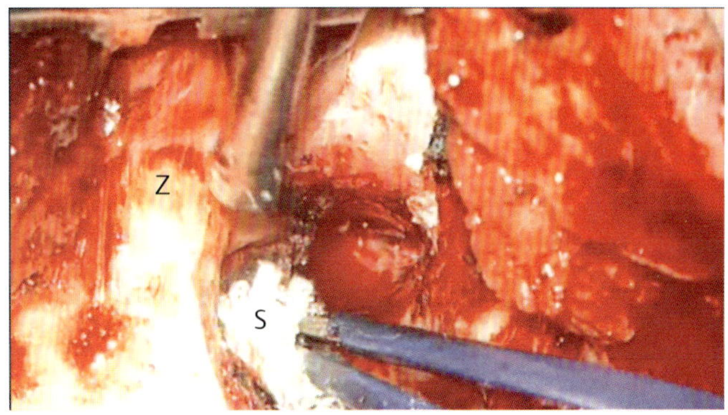

Fig. 35.10 First layers of Surgicel (S) are being laid into the created extradural space.

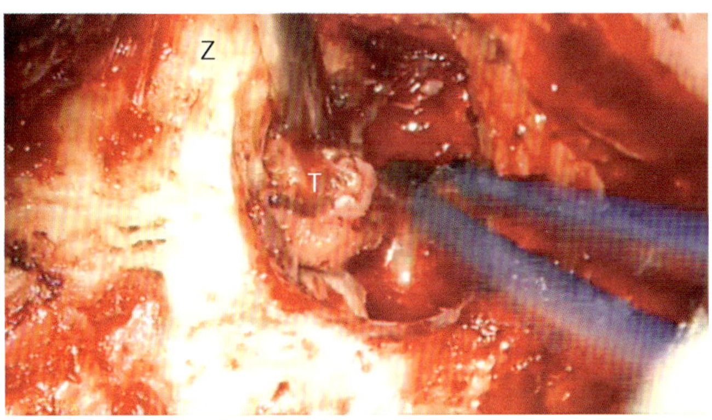

Fig. 35.11 Harvested temporalis fascia (T) is placed into the space following the surgical reduction.

Section XII

Reconstruction in Endoscopic Skull Base

Chapter 36 Principles and Techniques of Reconstruction in Skull Base Defects

Swati Kodur Patil and Narayan Jayashankar

Introduction

Over the past couple of decades, the frontier of endoscopic endonasal sinus surgery has seen great advances. The challenge posing a successful extirpation of the tumor pathology is to reconstruct the open barrier between the cranial cavity and the sinonasal tract. The process of reconstruction of the ventral skull base defects commenced with the use of a number of free tissue nonvascularized grafts which included autologous fascia, allogenic collagen grafts, fat grafts, and free mucosal grafts being used to plug the leak. This led to a high postoperative incidence of cerebrospinal fluid (CSF) leaks of around 58%[1] as reported in the literature for endonasal endoscopic craniopharyngioma surgery, most often leak being due to graft migration and CSF fistula formation in the most dependent areas. The saga of reconstruction using a vascular graft began with Oscar Hirsch,[2] in 1952, describing a septal flap for CSF leaks, which has seen a number of variations and upgradations over the years. Hadad–Bassagasteguy nasoseptal pedicle flap (HBNPF) was first described in 1999 and was initially used to close iatrogenic skull base defects. However, the HBNPF was widely used for large skull base defects after 2005.[3–5] This dramatically decreased the incidence of postoperative CSF leak in endonasal endoscopic craniopharyngioma surgery to 5.56%[6] and was similarly described by others. This was probably one of the most significant contributions to the further expansion of endoscopic endonasal skull base surgery since the ensuing skull base defects could be managed effectively using vascularized pedicle flaps. A number of vascularized pedicle intranasal grafts were then described by various authors which include posterior pedicled inferior turbinate flap, anterior or posterior pedicled lateral nasal flap, and middle turbinate flap.[7] Regional vascularized flaps developed include pericranial flap and temporoparietal fascia flaps.

Principles of Reconstruction

- Choice of reconstructive technique is planned prior to surgery depending on the biology of the lesion, site of the lesion, and the size of the anticipated defect.
- A single large vascularized flap can be used to cover one module or two adjacent modules. For example, transsellar and transplanar, transsellar and transclival, and so on.
- For large defects involving multiple modules a second pedicled flap may be needed.
- It is critical that the dimensions of vascularized pedicle flaps must be at least one and half times the size of the defect so that the flap can be comfortably placed over the bare bone surrounding the defect.
- Care should be taken to avoid having intervening mucosa, nonvascularized tissue, or fibrin glue between the flap and the bare bone surrounding the defect.
- Skull base reconstruction is generally done in a multilayered fashion with vascularized pedicle graft as the final layer covering the defect.
- Always have an alternative reconstruction option in case the first option fails.

Intranasal Vascularized Pedicle Flaps

Hadad–Bassagasteguy Nasoseptal Pedicle Flap

HBNPF is the workhorse of skull base reconstruction in most instances.[3–5]

Vascular Anatomy

It is a vascular pedicled composite flap including the septal mucosa along with its underlying perichondrial and periosteal layers that is based on the posterior nasoseptal branch of the sphenopalatine artery, which is a branch of the internal maxillary artery. This branch of the sphenopalatine artery arises just inferior to the posterior end of middle turbinate, traverses the sphenoethmoidal recess dividing into multiple branches and supplies the nasal septum from posterior to the anterior direction in the submucosal plane, superficial to the septal periosteum and perichondrium (**Fig. 36.1**).

Indications

- Sellar and suprasellar defects.
- Clival defects.
- Lateral sinus CSF leaks.
- Craniocervical junction defects.
- Defects following approaches to the cavernous sinuses/Meckel's cave.

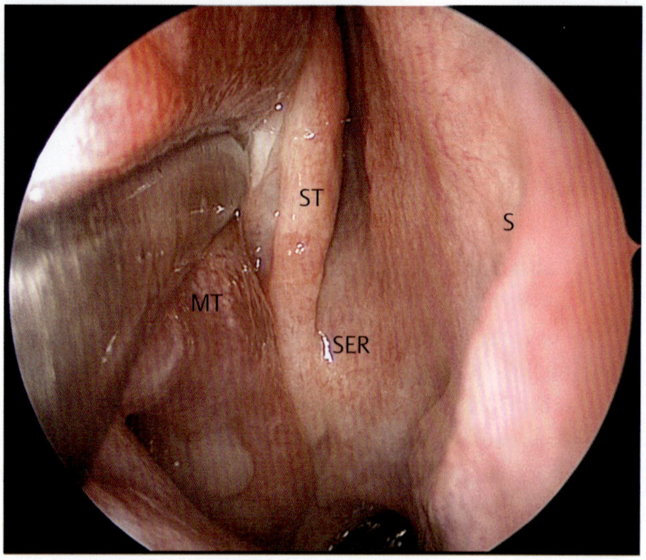

Fig. 36.1 Anatomy of the posterior end of the nasal cavity with pedicle of HB flap.

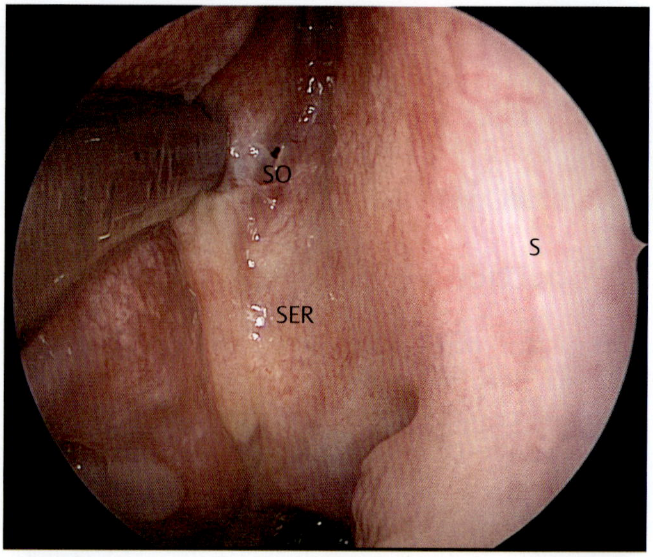

Fig. 36.2 Displacing the superior turbinate laterally exposes the sphenoid ostium and the sphenoethmoidal recess for incisions of the HBNPF.

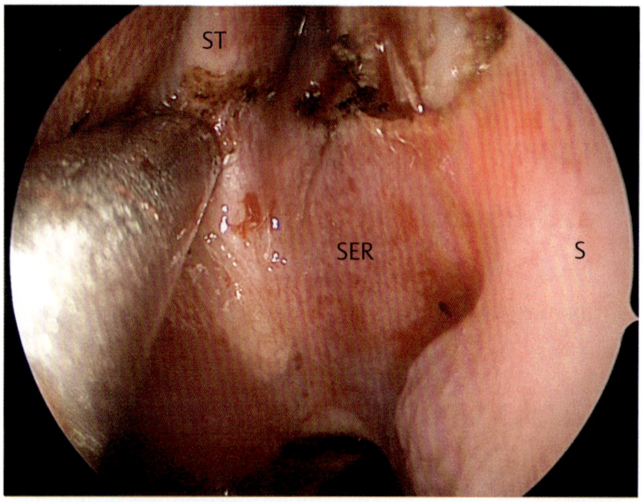

Fig. 36.3 Superior and inferior horizontal incisions to preserve pedicle of HBNPF.

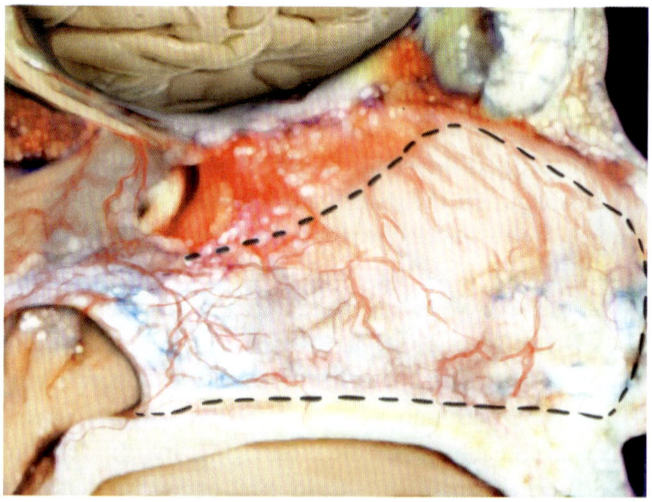

Fig. 36.4 *Dashed line* indicates the incisions taken on the nasal septum. Note preservation of the olfactory area.

Surgical Technique

Two horizontal parallel incisions are taken over the anterior face of the sphenoid bone that constitutes the region of the sphenoethmoidal recess (**Fig. 36.2** and **Fig. 36.3**). The superior horizontal incision is taken at the superior end of sphenoethmoidal recess just inferior to the sphenoid ostia, extending from the posterior end of the middle turbinate to the posterior end of the nasal septum. It is extended horizontally onto the nasal septum at a level corresponding to the lower level of the horizontal limb of the middle turbinate, thereby preventing injury to the vertical olfactory fibers from the cribriform plate and preserving olfaction. After crossing the junction between the horizontal and vertical portion of anterior end of the middle turbinate, it swings upward to reach the superior border of the nasal septum. From here the incision traverses parallel to the superior border of the septum from posterior to anterior direction up to the mucocutaneous junction (**Fig. 36.4**).

The inferior incision starts from the lateral end of the roof of the posterior choana, arches over the roof of the choana toward the floor of the nasal septum (this corresponds to the inferior edge of the sphenoethmoid recess). The incision then traverses anteriorly along the floor of the nasal septum till the mucocutaneous junction (**Fig. 36.4**). A vertical incision at the mucocutaneous junction joins the superior and inferior incisions taken on the septum. Flap elevation starts from this anterior edge and proceeds posteriorly (**Fig. 36.5** and **Fig. 36.6**). The mucoperichondrial and mucoperiosteal flaps are raised as a single composite layer with the pedicle of the flap based on the lateral end of sphenoethmoid recess. If the requirement arises for a broader flap, the inferior incision can be extended to include the mucoperiosteum of the nasal floor. This flap is raised as a composite unit comprising nasal septal mucosa, perichondrium, and periosteum of the nasal septum. The pedicle is raised up to the lateral end of the sphenoethmoidal recess (**Fig. 36.7**). Once the flap is raised, it is carefully preserved in the nasopharynx till required. In approaches inferior to clivus, the flap is preserved in the ipsilateral maxillary sinus.

After removal of the pituitary tumor, if there is no breach of the diaphragm, the sellar cavity is left open (**Fig. 36.8**). However, if there does occur a breach in the diaphragm with resultant CSF leak, we pack the sellar cavity gently with fat harvested from the thigh or abdomen (**Fig. 36.9**). Care is

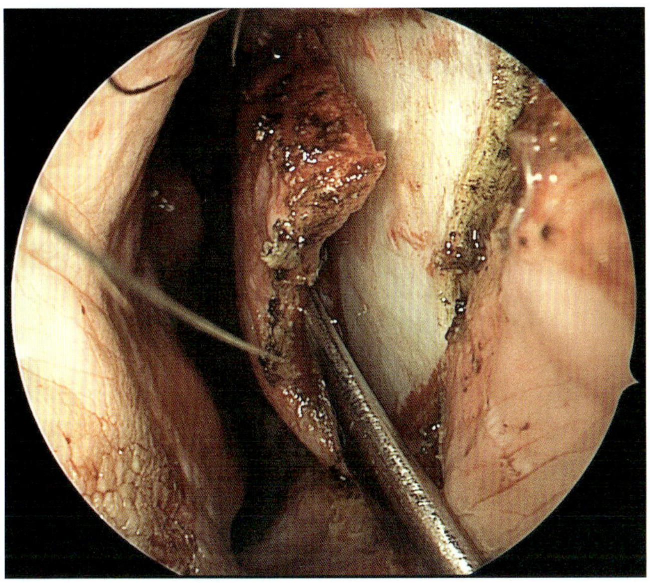

Fig. 36.5 Elevation of the flap commences at the anterior end (mucocutaneous junction of the septum).

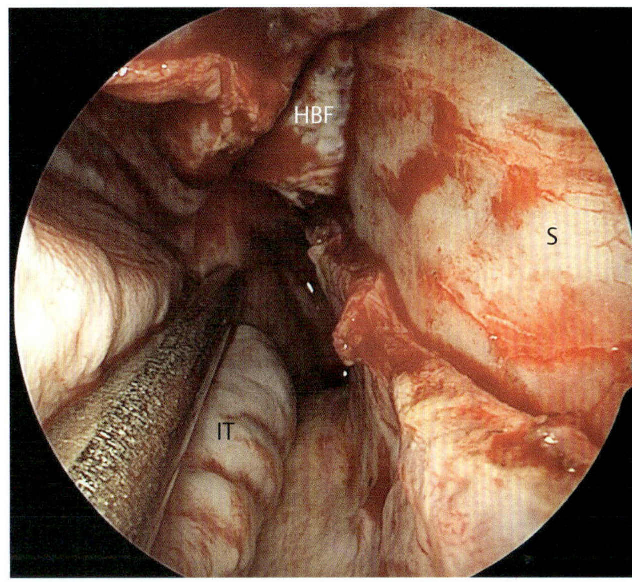

Fig. 36.6 Inferior incision at the floor of the septum, over the maxillary crest.

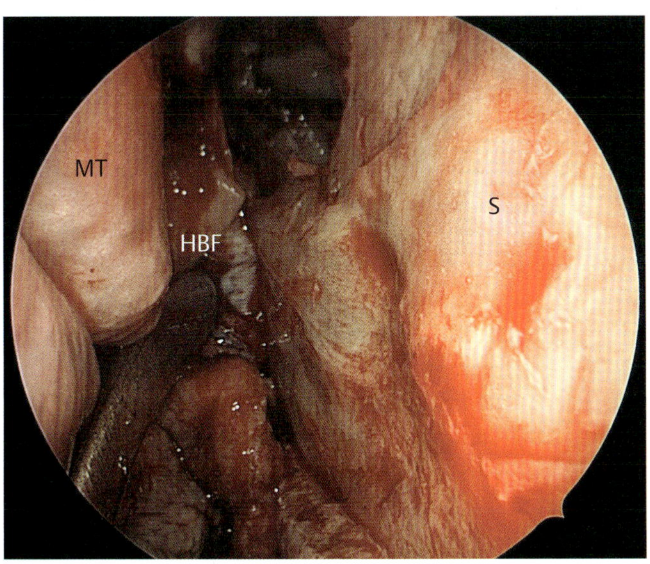

Fig. 36.7 The pedicle of the flap dissected off the rostrum of the sphenoid up to its lateral limit.

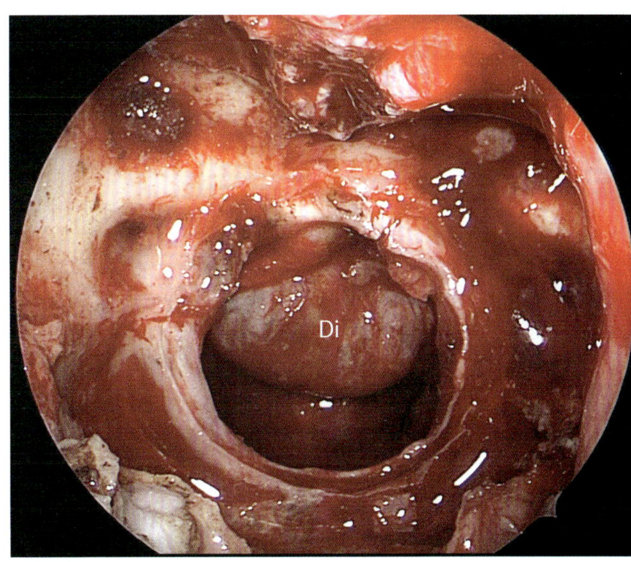

Fig. 36.8 If there is no CSF leak, the sellar cavity is left open.

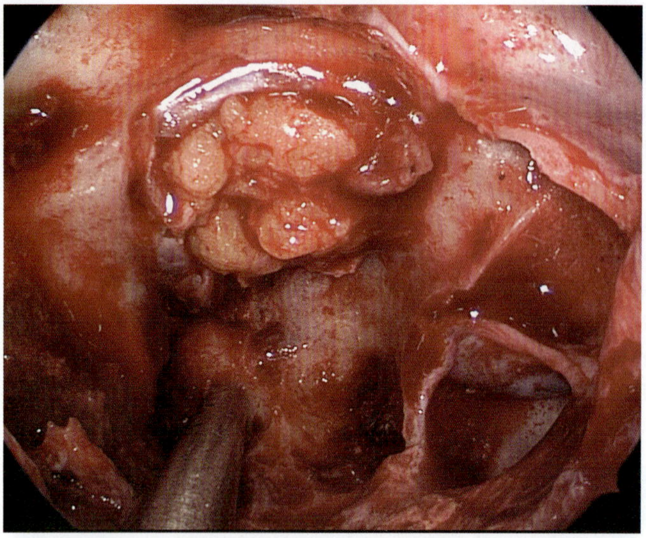

Fig. 36.9 In case of CSF leak, fat is plugged in the sellar cavity to seal the defect in the diaphragm.

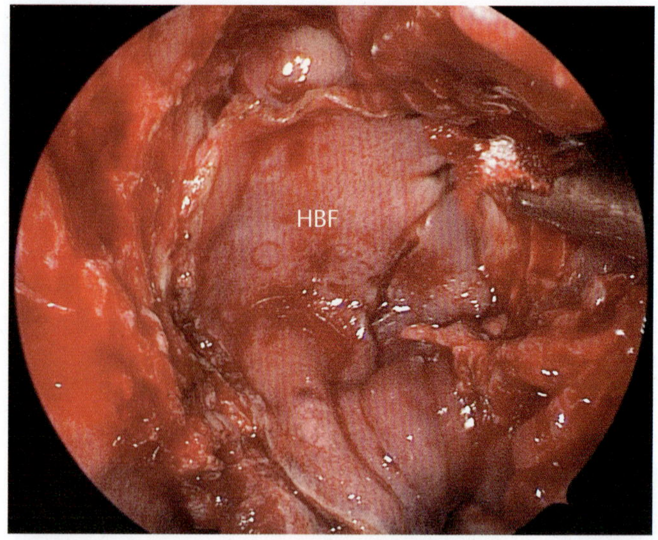

Fig. 36.10 A Hadad–Bassagasteguy flap (HBF) is then placed over the operated area.

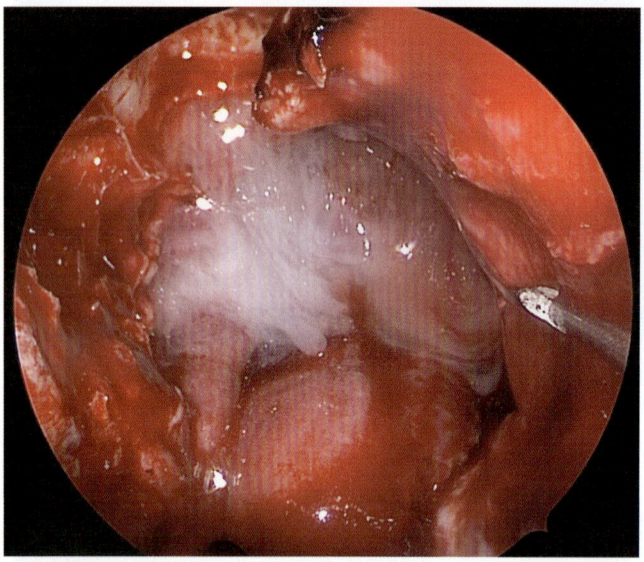

Fig. 36.11 Tissue glue is used over the edges of the flap (never between the flap and bone).

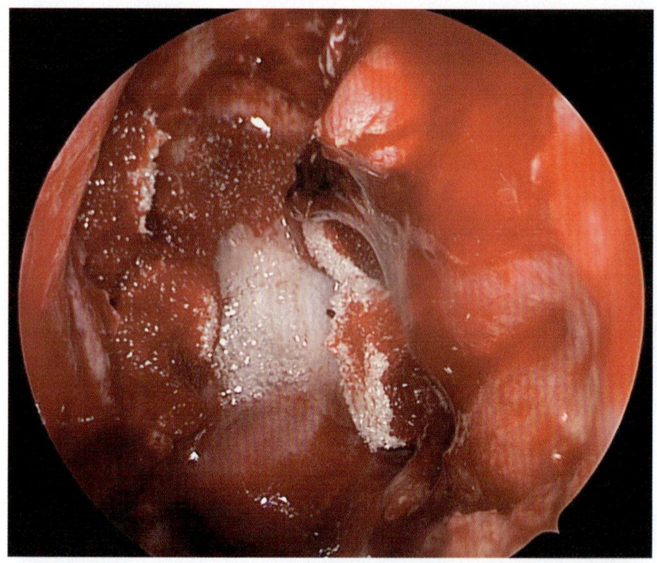

Fig. 36.12 A few layers of Gelfoam is placed over the flap.

taken not to pack the sellar cavity too tightly. An HBNPF is then placed over the defect. The pedicle of the HBNPF lies along the smooth floor of the sphenoid. The flap covers the sellar defect and is placed over the raw bone of the sphenoid sinus surrounding the defect (**Fig. 36.10**). There should not be any intervening material between the flap and bare bone. Tissue glue is sprayed on the edges of the flap (**Fig. 36.11**). A few layers of Gelfoam are placed over the reconstruction (**Fig. 36.12**). Netcell nasal packs are placed in both nasal cavities abutting the Gelfoam thereby giving a gentle support to the reconstruction. The Gelfoam layers also protect against flap displacement when the Netcell nasal packs are removed.

Following transplanar transtubercular surgery, as for example following craniopharyngioma surgery (**Fig. 36.13**), the closure is performed in multilayer fashion as described below. The defect is plugged with a fat plug taking care to see that the fat does not prolapse into the intracranial space (**Fig. 36.14**). A piece of fascia lata is placed over this fat plug (**Fig. 36.15**). The fascia edges should cover the edges of the defect (fascia should be slightly larger than the defect). A piece of bone, harvested earlier from the septum or vomer, is used over the fascia to snugly fit into the edges of the defect similar to a gasket seal technique (**Fig. 36.16**). The HBNPF is then placed over this reconstructed area making sure that the edges of the HBNPF are placed over the raw bone of the

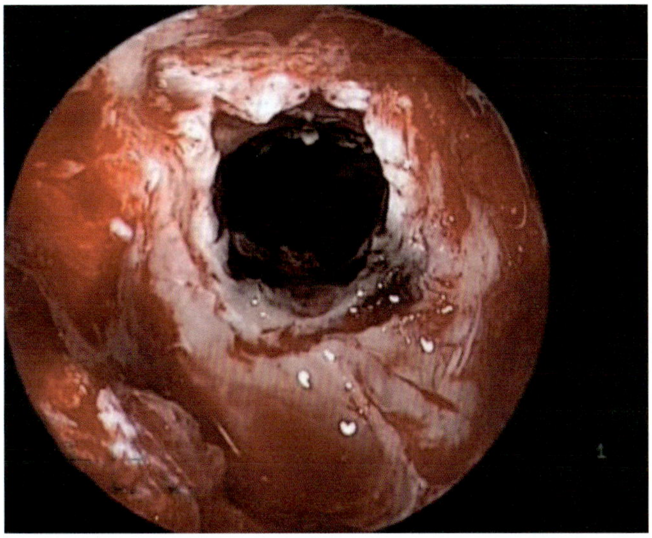

Fig. 36.13 Defect after craniopharyngioma excision.

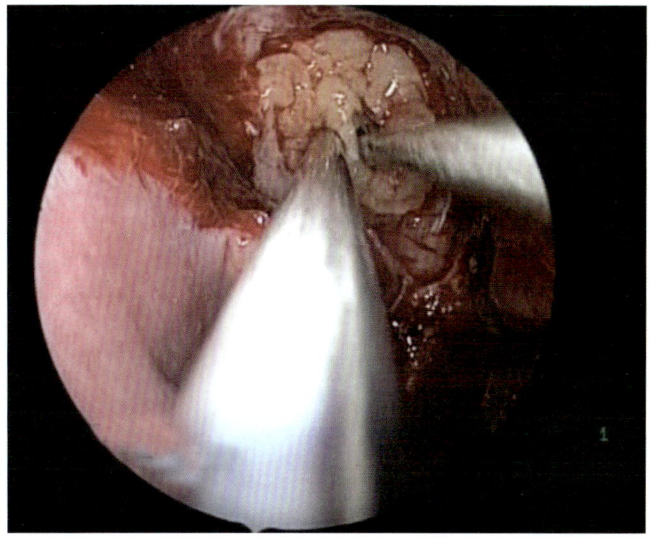

Fig. 36.14 Fat used to plug the defect.

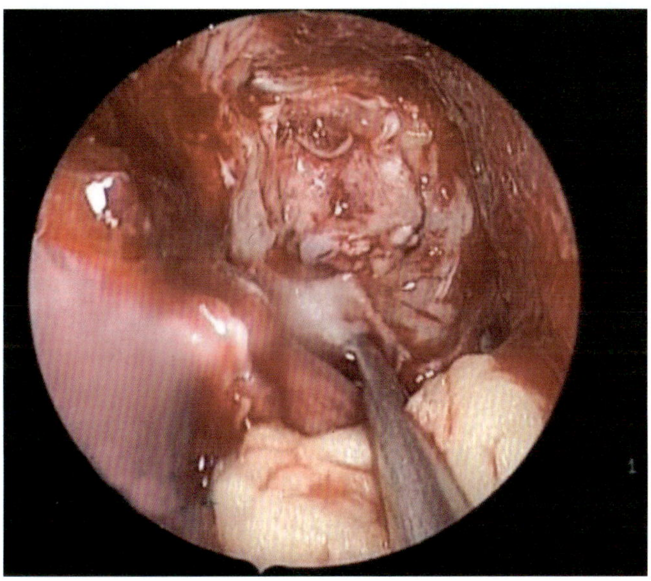

Fig. 36.15 A piece of fascia is placed over the defect overlapping its edges.

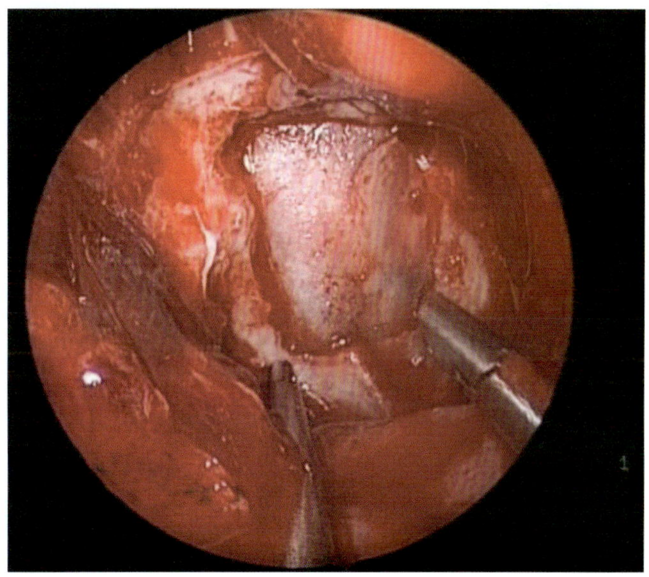

Fig. 36.16 A bone chip is placed snugly fitting the defect edges.

periphery (**Fig. 36.17**). Tissue glue is used over the edges of the flap and reinforced with Gelfoam as described above. A similar technique is used for transclival defects.

Tips and Pearls

- In the presence of a spur, the flap is raised on the opposite site.
- In transpterygoid or infratemporal fossa approaches, ipsilateral sphenopalatine or internal maxillary artery is generally transected and thus the flap needs to be planned on the opposite side.
- In revision cases, the flap can be recycled or reused.

Rescue Flap

It is most logical to briefly describe a rescue flap[8-11] after a detailed description of a HBNPF. A rescue flap is a HBNPF where the pedicle of the flap is preserved for harvesting the flap in the eventuality of a CSF leak. This is done prior to inferior widening of the sphenoid ostia, wherein the possibility of damaging the vascular pedicle exists. The superior incision follows on the same lines as that of the HBNPF, starting from the lateral end of sphenoethmoidal recess extending up to the bony cartilaginous junction of the septum. The inferior incision arches at the superior edge of the posterior choanae (inferior edge of the sphenoethmoidal recess) from lateral

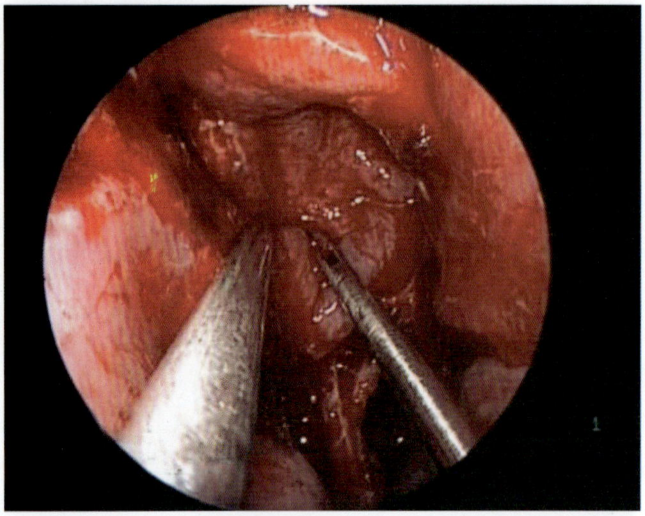

Fig. 36.17 A HBNPF is placed to cover the area.

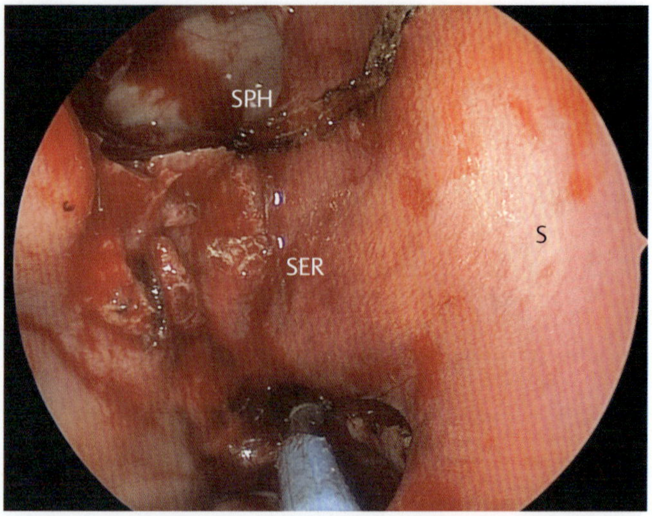

Fig. 36.18 Incisions for the rescue flap.

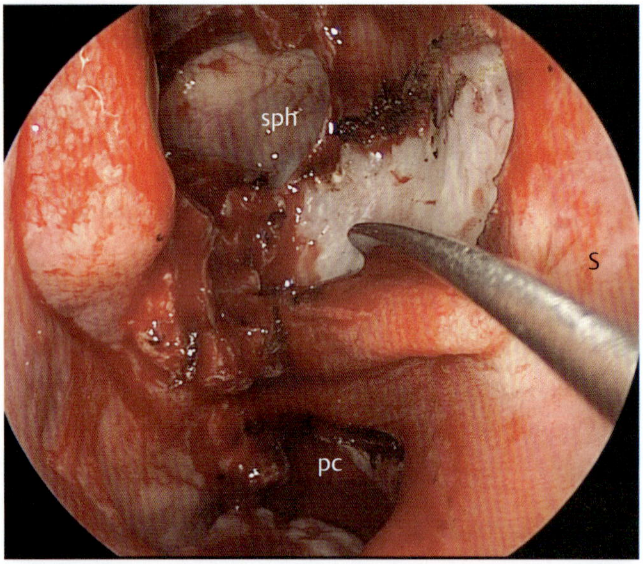

Fig. 36.19 Pedicle dissected off the rostrum of sphenoid and preserved.

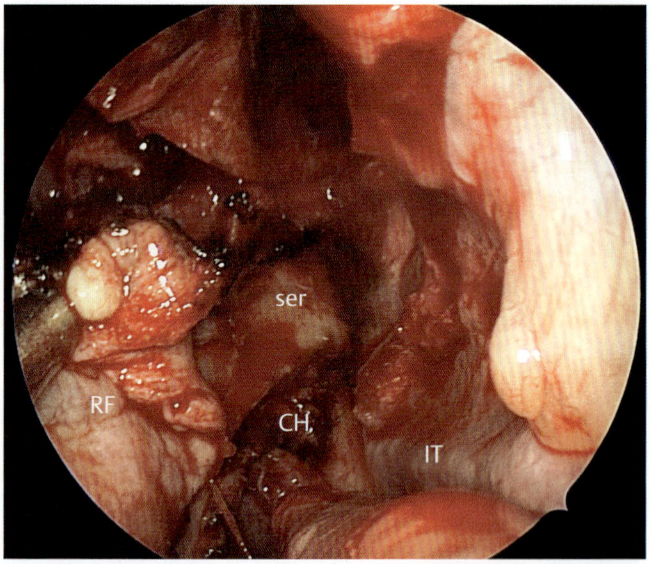

Fig. 36.20 Pedicle transected on left side and flap raised toward the posterior end of the septum.

to medial and then traverses along the floor of the septum posteriorly for a centimeter or so (**Fig. 36.18**). The pedicle of the flap is dissected off the front face of the sphenoethmoidal recess without harvesting the entire flap (**Fig. 36.19**). In case of an inadvertent CSF leak, an HBNPF is raised completely as per the required measurement to close the barrier between the subarachnoid space and the nasal cavity.

The Caicedo Reverse Rotation Flap

The Caicedo reverse rotation flap[12,13] primarily serves the purpose of reconstruction of the donor site of the septum from where the HBNPF has been harvested. This is aimed at remucosalization of the denuded septum and therefore is raised on the other side of the HBNPF (**Fig. 36.20**). Superior and inferior incisions are similar to an HBNPF but extend to the edge of the posterior septectomy (do not extend to the mucocutaneous junction). A vertical incision is taken on the front face of the sphenoid rostrum to divide the pedicle of the flap. Once the flap is elevated anteriorly, it is rotated to the opposite side of the septum and fixed in place with sutures (**Fig. 36.21** and **Fig. 36.22**).

Posterior Pedicled Inferior Turbinate Flap

Described in 2007, the posterior pedicled inferior turbinate flap[14,15] acts as an additional option in managing small defects following endonasal endoscopic posterior fossa surgery in

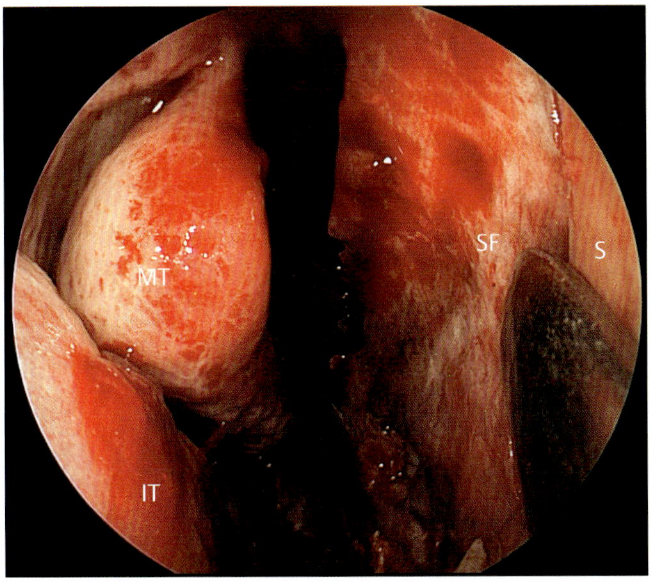

Fig. 36.21 View from the right nasal cavity. Preserved flap of the opposite side (left) that was raised as seen in the step above and is used to cover the donor area of the septum from where HB flap is harvested. Note that posterior septectomy has been performed and cartilage is seen in the anterior half of the septum.

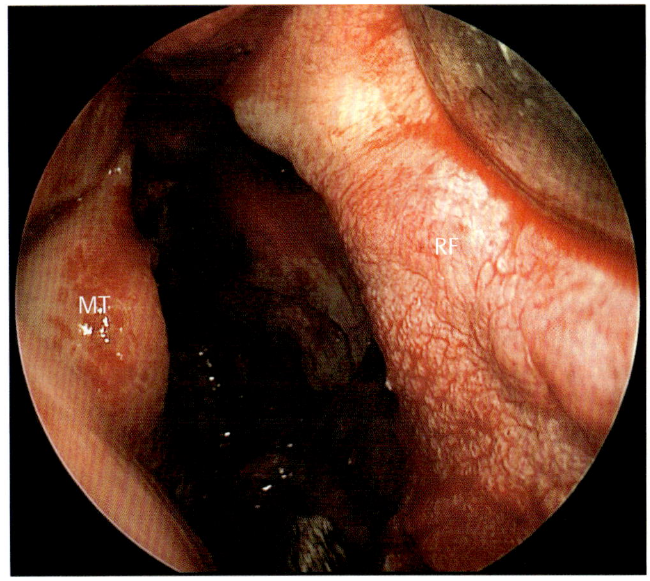

Fig. 36.22 Reverse flap covering the donor area of HBNPF on septum.

situations wherein a classical HBNPF is not feasible or has been accidentally injured during surgery.

Vascular Anatomy

The flap is based on the inferior turbinate artery, a terminal branch of the posterior lateral nasal artery (PLNA), which arises from the sphenopalatine artery. This artery courses anteroinferiorly from the sphenopalatine artery along the perpendicular plate of the ascending process of palatine bone and enters the inferior turbinate at its attachment to the lateral nasal wall posteriorly, around 1 cm approximately from its posterior end.

Indications

- Small defects of the sella.
- Small defects of posterior fossa and clivus.

Surgical Technique

Harvesting the inferior turbinate pedicle flap should ideally start with identification of the sphenopalatine artery exiting the sphenopalatine foramen. This donor pedicle can be identified by two methods. A flap can be raised along the palatine bone under the posterior end of the middle turbinate just posterior to the membranous posterior fontanelle or a wide middle meatal antrostomy is performed with widening of the same posteriorly till the palatine bone is encountered. Delicate dissection submucosally leads to the ethmoidal crest, posterior to which the sphenopalatine artery enters the lateral nasal wall. This artery is then followed distally to identify the PLNA on which the flap will be based. Two parallel incisions are taken. The superior incision starts at the sphenopalatine foramen traverses horizontally along the superior aspect of the inferior turbinate up to its anterior end. The inferior incision follows the inferior margin of the turbinate. A vertical incision, placed over the anterior end of the inferior turbinate, connects the two previous incisions (**Fig. 36.23**). Then, the mucoperiosteum is elevated starting at the anterior aspect of the inferior turbinate, extending posteriorly as per the surgeon's discretion.

Anterior Pedicled Lateral Nasal Wall Flap

A validated, recent technique (2011) presents as an alternative to HBNPF named as Hadad–Bassagasteguy 2 (HB2) flap.[16,17]

Vascular Anatomy

This flap is based on branches of the facial and anterior ethmoidal arteries.

Indications

- Transfrontal defects.
- Transfoveal defects.

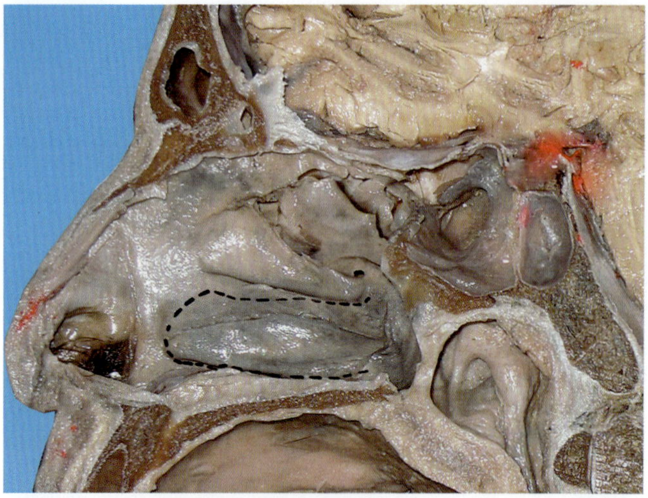

Fig. 36.23 Markings for the posterior pedicled inferior turbinate flap.

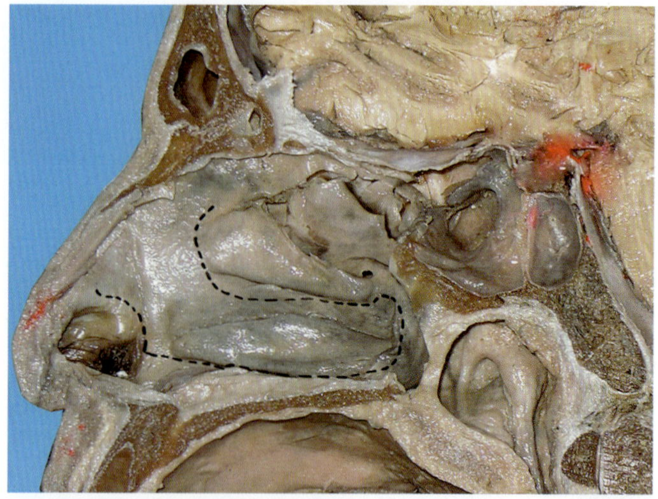

Fig. 36.24 Markings for the anterior pedicled lateral nasal wall flap.

Surgical Technique

An incision starts from the lateral nasal wall just anterior to the axilla of the middle turbinate, traverses down vertically up to the posterior bend of the middle turbinate and runs along the middle meatus. The incision continues horizontally just inferior to the maxillary ostium but can also be arched around it superiorly to incorporate the mucosa of the posterior fontanelle. The incision then traverses posteriorly to the posterior end of the middle turbinate. This incision is then carried on vertically downward toward the nasal floor or the nasal septum. At this juncture, bleeding from anterior branches of the sphenopalatine artery needs to be controlled using bipolar forceps. A second incision starts at the caudal end of the nasal bone, follows the bony edge of the piriform aperture to the head of the inferior turbinate (**Fig. 36.24**). This incision is extended vertically and inferiorly toward the floor of the nose and can be extended further to the nasal septum in case a wider flap is needed. The two vertical incisions are joined by another incision that follows the maxillary crest. In case a wider flap is required, the horizontal incision is taken at the junction of the floor of the nose and nasal septum, connecting the two extended vertical incisions described above.

Posterior Pedicled Lateral Nasal Flap

Described in 2016, the posterior pedicled lateral nasal flap, also called the Carrau–Haddad flap,[18] can be used in large skull base defects wherein the HBNPF is unavailable.

Vascular Anatomy

This flap is based on the posterior branches of sphenopalatine artery.

Surgical Technique

The first incision is taken starting just anterior and superior to the attachment of the middle turbinate to the skull base. The incision is extended vertically going down to a point just anteroinferior to the lower end of uncinate bone. The incision then curves posteriorly and runs along the superior surface of the inferior turbinate, on the lateral nasal wall, till the region of the sphenopalatine foramen.

A second incision is taken, anterior to the first incision described above, starting at the most caudal tip of nasal bone, runs along the bony rim of the piriform aperture toward the head of the inferior turbinate. This incision then runs vertically anterior to the head of the inferior turbinate toward inferiormost level of the lateral nasal wall. In case a wider flap is desired, the incision is extended on to the nasal floor.

A third incision connects the superiormost ends of the first and second incisions, parallel to the nasal vault (**Fig. 36.25**).

A sagittally oriented incision is taken on the nasal floor from the inferiormost point of the anterior incision (second incision) toward the posterior choana.

The mucoperiosteum is then elevated from anterior to posterior. The mucoperiosteum is dissected off the anterior head of the inferior turbinate bone and thereafter the area of the inferior meatus. The bone of the inferior turbinate is resected piecemeal after separating the overlying mucoperiosteum. At a point in the elevation, there will be a tethering of the flap where the nasolacrimal duct opens in the inferior meatus. The mucoperiosteum is carefully trimmed around the opening of the nasolacrimal duct and elevation then proceeds posteriorly. The elevation of the lateral nasal wall flap stops as authors approach the region of the sphenopalatine foramen from where the posterolateral nasal artery supplying the flap can be appreciated.

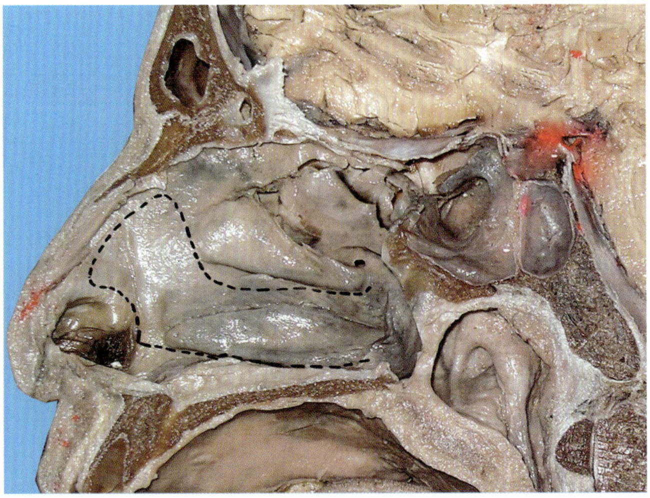

Fig. 36.25 Markings for the posterior pedicled lateral nasal wall flap.

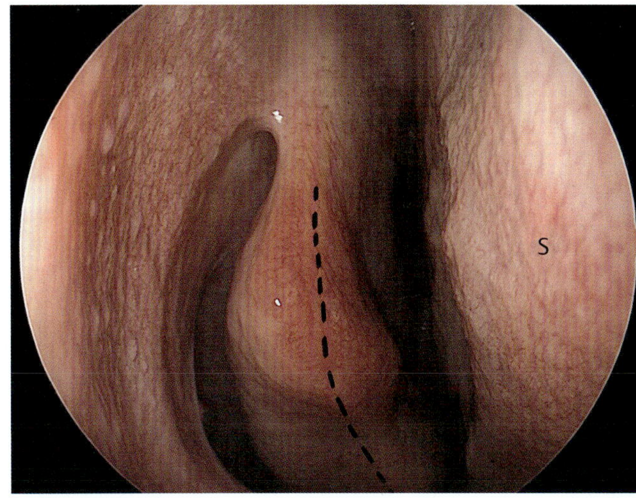

Fig. 36.26 Incision along the length of the middle turbinate.

This flap can then be rotated on its posterior pedicled vascular supply to cover the skull base defect.

Middle Turbinate Flap

The middle turbinate flap[19–21] should be considered as an alternative for the reconstruction of small defects of the fovea ethmoidalis, planum, and sella, particularly for patients for whom a reconstruction with vascularized tissue is desirable but the nasoseptal flap is not available.

Vascular Anatomy

This flap is based on the sphenopalatine artery branch to middle turbinate.

Indications

Small- to medium-sized planar or fovea ethmoidalis defects.

Surgical Technique

First incision in made vertically over the head of the middle turbinate **(Fig. 36.26)**. A horizontal incision is made at the medial aspect of the turbinate mucosa respecting the attachment to the cribriform plate. The mucoperiosteal flaps are raised on both sides of the bone of the middle turbinate (**Fig. 36.27**) which is subsequently excised piecemeal. A horizontal incision is next taken at the axilla of the middle turbinate parallel to the cribriform plate leaving a small tail of attachment of the middle turbinate to the vertical lamella of the cribriform plate (**Fig. 36.28**). The mucoperiosteal flap is opened like a book to create a middle turbinate flap based on sphenopalatine artery.

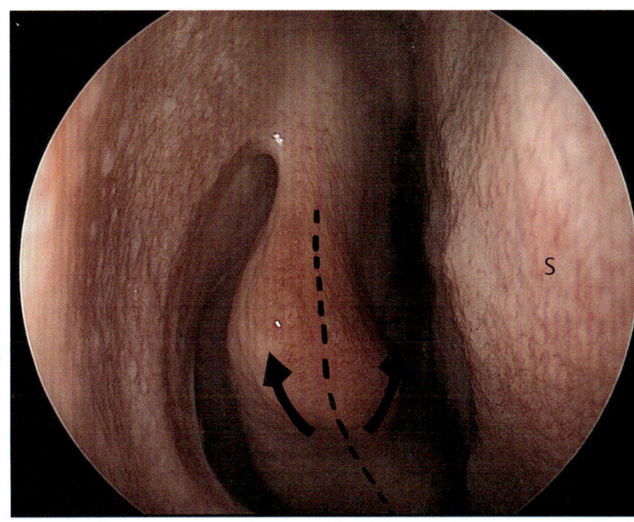

Fig. 36.27 Mucoperiosteum dissected off the middle turbinate bone which is then excised.

Regional Vascularized Flaps

Pericranial Flap

At times, the septal mucosal flap may be unavailable for reconstruction either because of prior surgical resection or involvement of the nasal septum by sinonasal cancer. Endonasal skull base surgery in such cases warrants the use of extranasal regional flaps which are transported into the nasal cavity with a rich vascular pedicle supporting it. These flaps have a superior survival rate than nonvascularized fascial grafts. Pericranial flap[22–24] was first described in 2011 and proves to be an effective addition to the armamentarium of the reconstruction techniques.

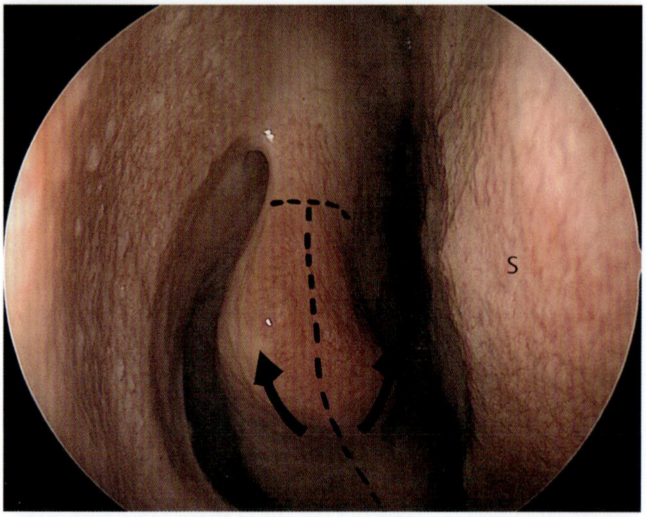

Fig. 36.28 Horizontal incision made at axilla of middle turbinate.

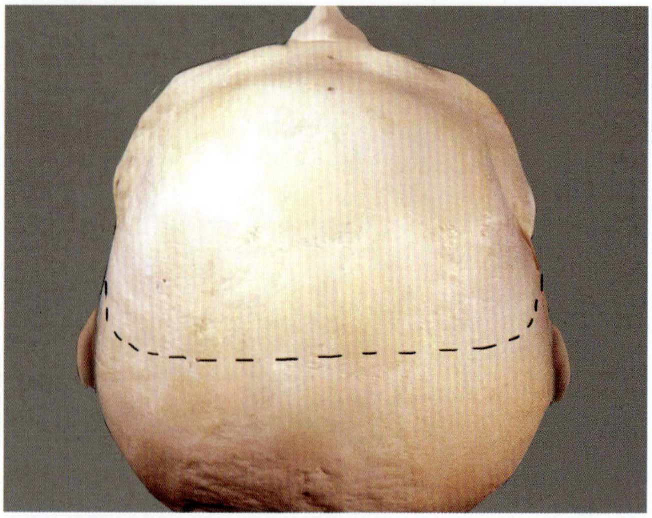

Fig. 36.29 Bicoronal skin incision.

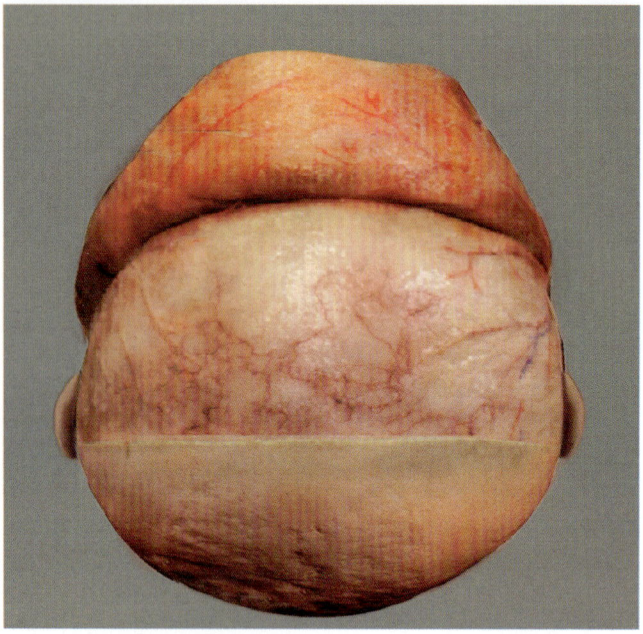

Fig. 36.30 Skin flap elevated.

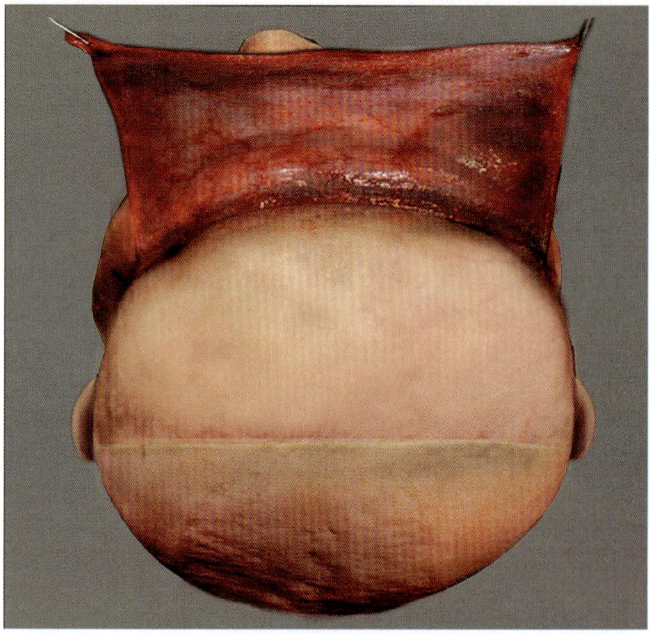

Fig. 36.31 Pericranial flap elevated.

Vascular Anatomy

The flap is based on supraorbital and supratrochlear vessels.

Indications

- Large anterior skull base defects.
- Fovea ethmoidalis defects.

Surgical Technique

The technique basically involves two components. During the first intranasal component, the anterior cranial base is prepared for the grafting. This includes bilateral anterior and posterior ethmoidectomies and bilateral frontal sinusotomy (DRAF 3). The extent of exposure on the anterior skull base could be from the crista galli to the planum of the sphenoid bone. An entry site is drilled at the nasion for the graft delivery into the nasal cavity. The second extranasal component of the technique involves harvesting of the pericranial flap off the frontal bone. The supraorbital and supratrochlear arteries are localized by Doppler ultrasound and marked. A bicoronal incision is taken within the hairline (**Fig. 36.29** and **Fig. 36.30**), raising a pericranial flap after dissection in the subgaleal plane (**Fig. 36.31**). Flap is then introduced into the nasal cavity through the aperture created at the nasion.

The flap is then placed over the cranial base under endoscopic guidance. While covering the cranial base, care should be taken to place the superficial surface of the graft toward the cranial cavity avoiding any torsion at the pedicle.

Temporoparietal Fascia Flap

The temporoparietal fascia flap[25] was described in 2007 for situation prompting a search for an extranasal flap like in patients who have undergone previous sphenoidotomies, posterior septectomies, and postradiation to the area of nasal cavity, those requiring postoperative radiation. This flap has the advantage of having rich and a predictable vascularity.

With an additional leverage of having a long pedicle, an excellent arc of rotation can be achieved. This technique involves transpositioning of the temporoparietal fascia flap into the nasal cavity through a temporal–infratemporal soft tissue tunnel and a transpterygoid window.

Vascular Anatomy

This is a pedicle flap based on the anterior branch of superficial temporal artery, a terminal branch of the external carotid artery (**Fig. 36.32**).

Indications

- Large defects of the posterior cranial fossa.
- Large defects of the middle cranial fossa.
- Other indications include intraoral defects, nasocutaneous fistulas, and oronasal defects.

Surgical Technique

Anterior and posterior ethmoidectomy are performed on both sides. A wide maxillary antrostomy is performed (on the same side as the temporoparietal fascia flap harvest) extending up to the posterior wall of the maxillary sinus. Sphenopalatine artery and posterior nasal artery are identified and clipped. The posterior wall of the maxillary sinus is resected. A part of the lateral wall of the maxillary sinus is also excised to create some space for the transposition of the flap. The internal maxillary artery is preserved. Contents of the pterygopalatine fossa are displaced inferiorly and laterally after dividing the descending palatine artery from the internal maxillary artery and the vidian nerve from the pterygopalatine ganglion, thus exposing the pterygoid plates which are drilled to facilitate the formation of a soft tissue tunnel for the graft transposition.

Temporoparietal fascia flap is then harvested using a hemicoronal incision. The skin and subcutaneous tissue are dissected off to expose the temporoparietal fascia. The superficial part of the temporal fascia is dissected of the underlying temporal muscle, and the extent of the required graft is cut (**Fig. 36.33**).

A wide lateral canthotomy then follows to separate the temporalis muscle from the lateral orbital wall and the pterygomaxillary fissure thus ultimately creating a soft tissue tunnel between the temporal fossa and the infratemporal fossa through a transpterygoid approach.

A guidewire is passed externally through the temporal fossa and visualized endoscopically inside the nasal cavity.

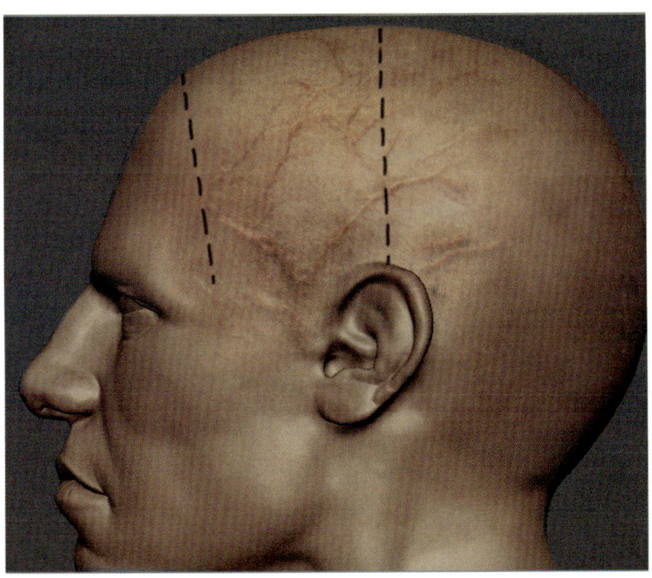

Fig. 36.32 The vascular pedicle of superficial temporal artery with its anterior frontal branch and posterior parietal branch is seen. The *dashed lines* indicate the area from which the temporoparietal fascia can be harvested.

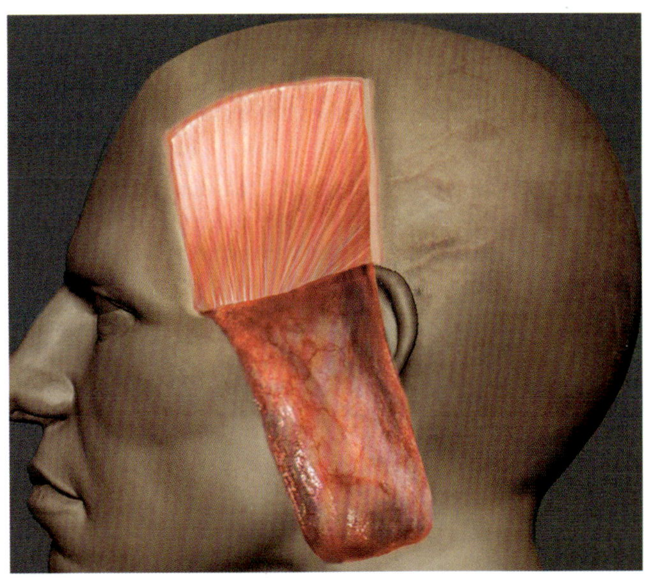

Fig. 36.33 Temporoparietal fascia flap reflected.

This final tunnel is then dilated using dilators till an adequate noncollapsible tunnel is formed. The flap is then tied to the guidewire and delivered intranasally. It is then spread over the previously prepared bed over the skull base defect.

References

1. Gardner PA, Kassam AB, Snyderman CH, et al. Outcomes following endoscopic, expanded endonasal resection of suprasellar craniopharyngiomas: a case series. J Neurosurg 2008;109(1):6–16
2. Hirsch O. Successful closure of cere brospinal fluid rhinorrhea by endonasal surgery. AMA Arch Otolaryngol 1952; 56(1): 1–12
3. Hadad G, Bassagasteguy L, Carrau RL, et al. A novel reconstructive technique after endoscopic expanded endonasal approaches: vascular pedicle nasoseptal flap. Laryngoscope 2006;116(10):1882–1886
4. Kassam AB, Thomas A, Carrau RL, et al. Endoscopic reconstruction of the cranial base using a pedicled nasoseptal flap. Neurosurgery 2008;63(1, Suppl 1):ONS44–ONS52, discussion ONS52–ONS53
5. Zanation AM, Carrau RL, Snyderman CH, et al. Nasoseptal flap reconstruction of high flow intraoperative cerebral spinal fluid leaks during endoscopic skull base surgery. Am J Rhinol Allergy 2009;23(5):518–521
6. Rutka JT. Endonasal resection of craniopharyngiomas. J Neurosurg 2008;109(1):1, reply 3–5
7. Patel MR, Stadler ME, Snyderman CH, et al. How to choose? Endoscopic skull base reconstructive options and limitations. Skull Base 2010;20(6):397–404
8. Rivera-Serrano CM, Snyderman CH, Gardner P, et al. Nasoseptal "rescue" flap: a novel modification of the nasoseptal flap technique for pituitary surgery. Laryngoscope 2011;121(5): 990–993
9. Rawal RB, Kimple AJ, Dugar DR, Zanation AM. Minimizing morbidity in endoscopic pituitary surgery: outcomes of the novel nasoseptal rescue flap technique. Otolaryngol Head Neck Surg 2012;147(3):434–437
10. Otto BA, Bowe SN, Carrau RL, Prevedello DM, Ditzel Filho LF, de Lara D. Transsphenoidal approach with nasoseptal flap pedicle transposition: modified rescue flap technique. Laryngoscope 2013;123(12):2976–2979
11. Kim BY, Shin JH, Kang SG, et al. Bilateral modified nasoseptal "rescue" flaps in the endoscopic endonasal transsphenoidal approach. Laryngoscope 2013;123(11):2605–2609
12. Caicedo-Granados E, Carrau R, Snyderman CH, et al. Reverse rotation flap for reconstruction of donor site after vascular pedicled nasoseptal flap in skull base surgery. Laryngoscope 2010;120(8):1550–1552
13. Kasemsiri P, Carrau RL, Otto BA, et al. Reconstruction of the pedicled nasoseptal flap donor site with a contralateral reverse rotation flap: technical modifications and outcomes. Laryngoscope 2013;123(11):2601–2604
14. Fortes FS, Carrau RL, Snyderman CH, et al. The posterior pedicle inferior turbinate flap: a new vascularized flap for skull base reconstruction. Laryngoscope 2007;117(8):1329–1332
15. Harvey RJ, Sheahan PO, Schlosser RJ. Inferior turbinate pedicle flap for endoscopic skull base defect repair. Am J Rhinol Allergy 2009;23(5):522–526
16. Hadad G, Rivera-Serrano CM, Bassagaisteguy LH, et al. Anterior pedicle lateral nasal wall flap: a novel technique for the reconstruction of anterior skull base defects. Laryngoscope 2011;121(8):1606–1610
17. Lee HY, Kim HU, Kim SS, et al. Surgical anatomy of the sphenopalatine artery in lateral nasal wall. Laryngoscope 2002;112(10):1813–1818
18. Rivera-Serrano CM, Bassagaisteguy LH, Hadad G, et al. Posterior pedicle lateral nasal wall flap: new reconstructive technique for large defects of the skull base. Am J Rhinol Allergy 2011;25(6):e212–e216
19. Prevedello DM, Barges-Coll J, Fernandez-Miranda JC, et al. Middle turbinate flap for skull base reconstruction: cadaveric feasibility study. Laryngoscope 2009;119(11):2094–2098
20. Marks SC. Middle turbinate graft for repair of cerebral spinal fluid leaks. Am J Rhinol 1998;12(6):417–419
21. Simal Julián JA, Miranda Lloret P, Cárdenas Ruiz-Valdepeñas E, Barges Coll J, Beltrán Giner A, Botella Asunción C. Middle turbinate vascularized flap for skull base reconstruction after an expanded endonasal approach. Acta Neurochir (Wien) 2011;153(9):1827–1832
22. Snyderman CH, Janecka IP, Sekhar LN, Sen CN, Eibling DE. Anterior cranial base reconstruction: role of galeal and pericranial flaps. Laryngoscope 1990;100(6):607–614
23. Johns ME, Winn HR, McLean WC, Cantrell RW. Pericranial flap for the closure of defects of craniofacial resection. Laryngoscope 1981;91(6):952–959
24. Zanation AM, Snyderman CH, Carrau RL, Kassam AB, Gardner PA, Prevedello DM. Minimally invasive endoscopic pericranial flap: a new method for endonasal skull base reconstruction. Laryngoscope 2009;119(1):13–18
25. Fortes FS, Carrau RL, Snyderman CH, et al. Transpterygoid transposition of a temporoparietal fascia flap: a new method for skull base reconstruction after endoscopic expanded endonasal approaches. Laryngoscope 2007;117(6):970–976

Section XIII

Cavernous Sinus

Chapter 37 Transcavernous and Anterior Transpetrous Approaches

Ankit S. Shah, Amol Raheja, and Ashish Suri

Introduction

- The transcavernous approach, created by Dolenc et al in 1987, was devised as a means of enlarging the area of exposure around the interpeduncular and prepontine cisterns obtained by the pterional approach. Anterior transpetrosal approach involves expanded bony resection at the petrous apex to expose the upper petroclival region and ventrolateral brainstem. A major portion of these approaches involves extradural dissection and bony work.
- Frontotemporal craniotomy with orbitozygomatic (FTOZ) osteotomy is an adjunct to pterional craniotomy that allows access to the anterior and middle skull base along with a greater rostral trajectory to the midline structures. By removing the superior and lateral bony orbit, one gains a more anterior and inferior starting point for the approach than would be possible with a conventional pterional craniotomy.
- For FTOZ craniotomy, the patient is placed supine on the operating table with head rotation to contralateral side and ipsilateral shoulder elevated (**Fig. 37.1**). After pinning, the head is usually positioned such that the malar eminence is the highest point on the patient's head. This is usually achieved by 15 to 30 degrees contralateral head rotation and a slight neck extension and head elevation. Type of lesion often determines the degrees of head rotation.
- For a temporal craniotomy and its variants, the patient is positioned supine with head angled 90 degrees from the vertical plane and a shoulder roll under the ipsilateral shoulder (**Fig. 37.2**). The head is then tilted approximately 20 degrees toward the floor such that the zygoma is the highest point in the field which allows the temporal lobe to fall with gravity and providing a direct line of view to the tentorium.
- The skin incisions for frontotemporal (**Fig. 37.3**) and temporal (**Fig. 37.4**) craniotomy along with its variants have been graphically depicted.
- Here, we have performed a right-sided two-piece FTOZ craniotomy with the demonstration of transcavernous and anterior transpetrous approaches along with intradural exposure of anterior and middle fossa contents in a formalin-fixed dye-injected cadaver head.

Surgical Steps

1. After positioning, the skin incision is marked (**Fig. 37.5**). The incision begins at the level of the zygoma 1 cm anterior to tragus, curving behind along the upper border of pinna till the posterior border of the pinna to the superior temporal line. From here the incision is curved anteriorly and toward the midline till the widow's peak. It can vary depending on the need of a particular case. Care should be taken to preserve the main trunk of the superficial temporal artery.

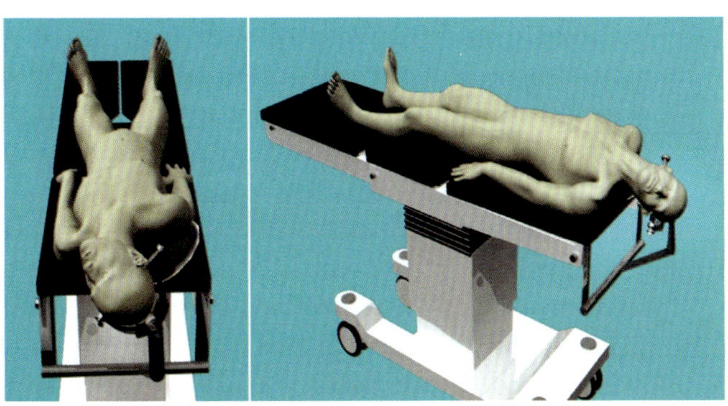

Fig. 37.1 Positioning for frontotemporal orbitozygomatic (FTOZ) craniotomy.

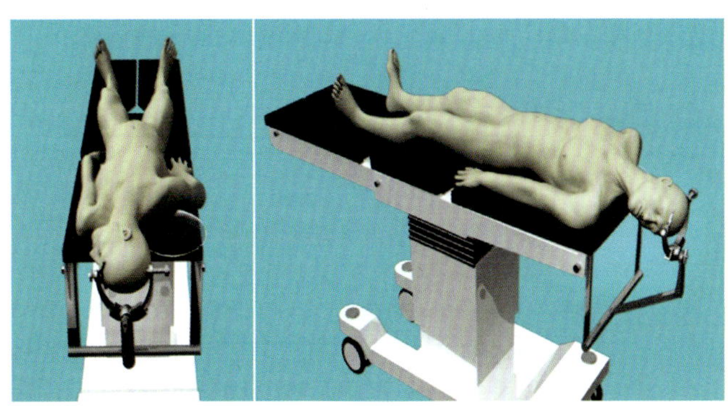

Fig. 37.2 Positioning for extended temporal craniotomy.

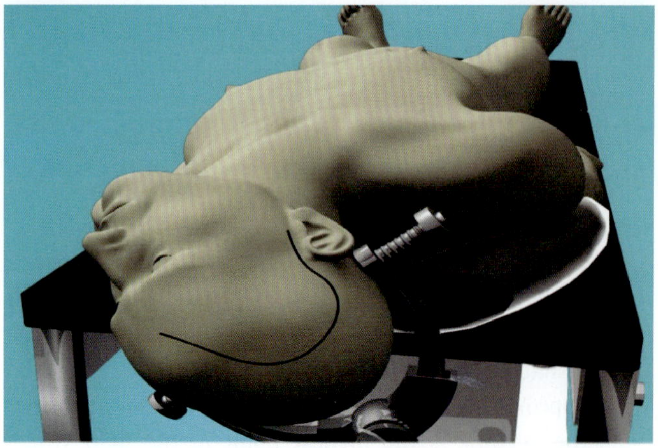

Fig. 37.3 Incision for frontotemporal orbitozygomatic craniotomy.

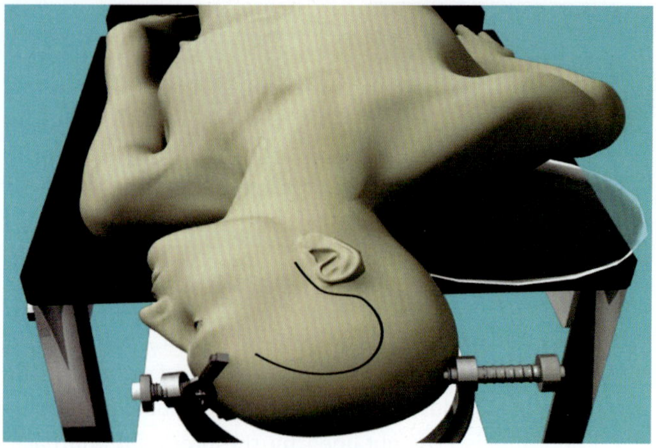

Fig. 37.4 Incision for extended temporal craniotomy.

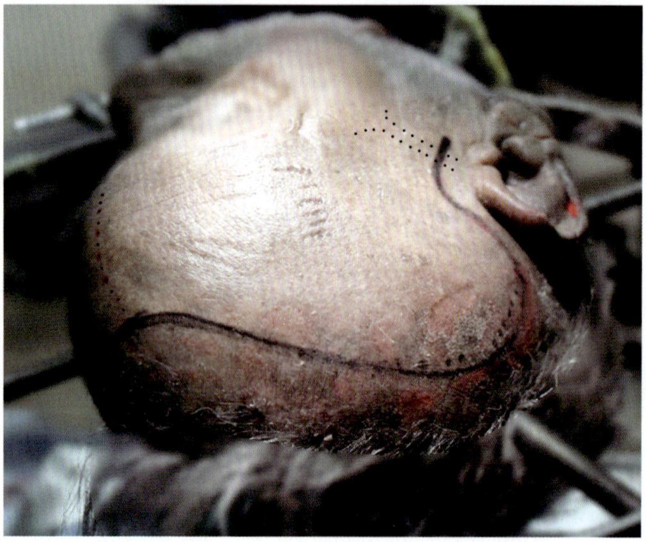

Fig. 37.5 Incision for middle skull base exposure.

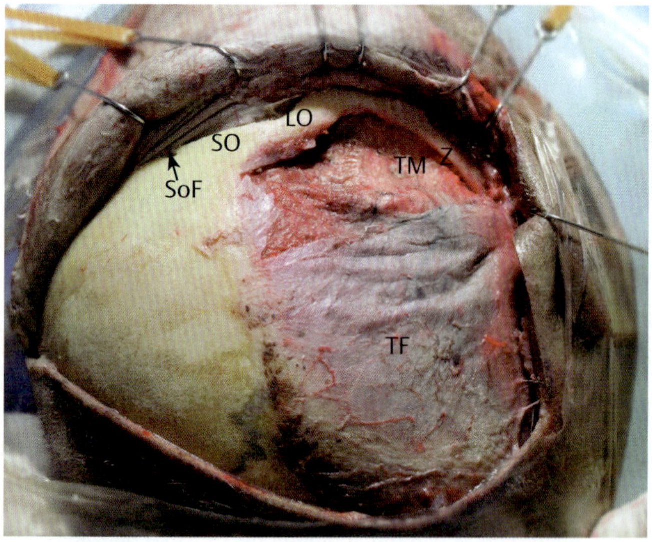

Fig. 37.6 Soft tissue elevation and exposure of bone.

2. The skin flap is elevated along with the temporalis fascia. The frontalis branch of the frontal nerve runs in the subcutaneous fat pad outside the temporalis fascia. Hence, the scalp and fat pad must be reflected anteriorly over the bone either by interfascial or subfascial approach. The superficial layer is elevated leaving behind the deep fascia in **interfascial exposure**. Deep fascia is elevated along with the skin flap for **subfascial exposure**. The frontalis branch of the facial nerve is thus protected. The skin flap is elevated to expose the supraorbital bar, lateral orbit, maxillary buttress, and the contiguous zygomatic arch (**Fig. 37.6**). The muscle and fascia are elevated as a second layer. This procedure is indicated for an extended orbitozygomatic craniotomy.
3. For an orbitozygomatic extension of the craniotomy, periorbita is separated from the inner bony surface of orbit using the rounded edge of periosteum elevator or curved sharp dissector. The separation begins medial to the supraorbital nerve and continues laterally and inferiorly till the inferior orbital fissure (**Fig. 37.7**).
4. The supraorbital nerve and vessels can be encountered at the medial margin of orbitotomy which can be preserved by dilating the supraorbital foramen (**Fig. 37.8**) and elevating nerve with the skin flap.
5. Transcavernous approaches are usually undertaken with pterional or FTOZ craniotomy while anterior transpetrous approaches are usually performed by a temporal or extended temporal craniotomy with removal of the zygomatic arch. Graphical depictions of

craniotomies with removed bone flap are depicted in **Fig. 37.9** and **Fig. 37.10**.

6. A single-piece or two-piece FTOZ osteotomy can be done. A two-piece FTOZ has been done here. For a single-piece FTOZ craniotomy, the first burr hole is placed at the MacCarty keyhole. It is located over the frontosphenoidal suture 1 cm behind the frontozygomatic junction. The upper half of the burr hole should expose the dura mater and its lower half the periorbita, with the bony roof of the orbit separating the two halves. For a two-piece FTOZ craniotomy, the burr hole can even be placed over the pterional keyhole burr described by Dandy. The rest of the burr holes are then placed just above the root of the zygoma and one along the superior temporal line along the route of proposed craniotomy. Dura may be stuck to the undersurface of bone in elderly in which case an extra burr hole might be required for better separation of dura avoiding any dural tears. The size of the craniotomy is varied according to the pathology. Craniotomy is done by connecting the burr holes using a craniotome (**Fig. 37.11**). The free bone flap is carefully separated from the underlying dura and removed. The second piece of orbitozygomatic osteotomy is done by making six cuts with a cutting drill or an osteotome (**Fig. 37.12**). The supraorbital bar, frontal process of zygomatic bone, and zygomatic arch are removed as a single piece (**Fig. 37.13**).
7. The dura is dissected off the sphenoid wing using a Penfield dissector. The sphenoid wing is drilled gradually toward the superior orbital fissure retracting the dura using a brain spatula or suction cannula. The meningo-orbital band (**Fig. 37.14**) is encountered on the lateral most aspect of superior orbital fissure and is devoid of any neural structures. It is coagulated and divided. Its division paves a way to bloodless transcavernous dissection and anterior clinoidectomy.

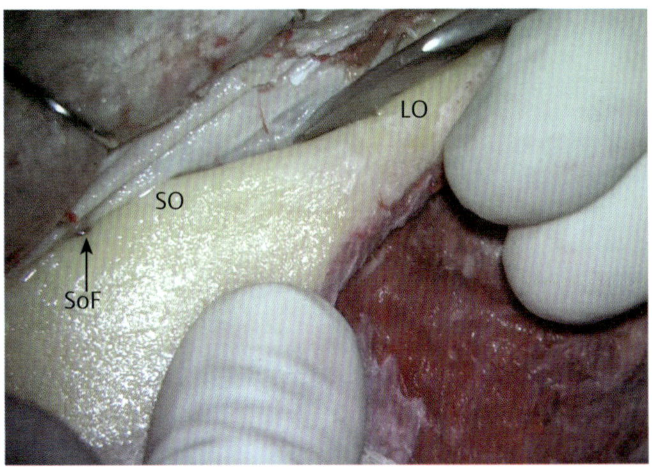

Fig. 37.7 Separation of periorbita.

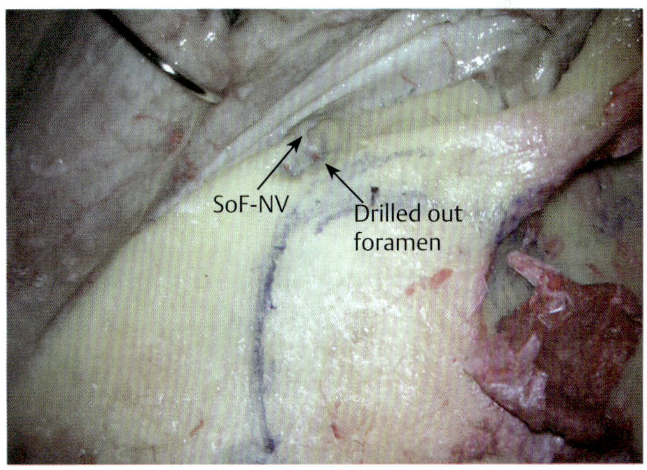

Fig. 37.8 Release of supraorbital nerve.

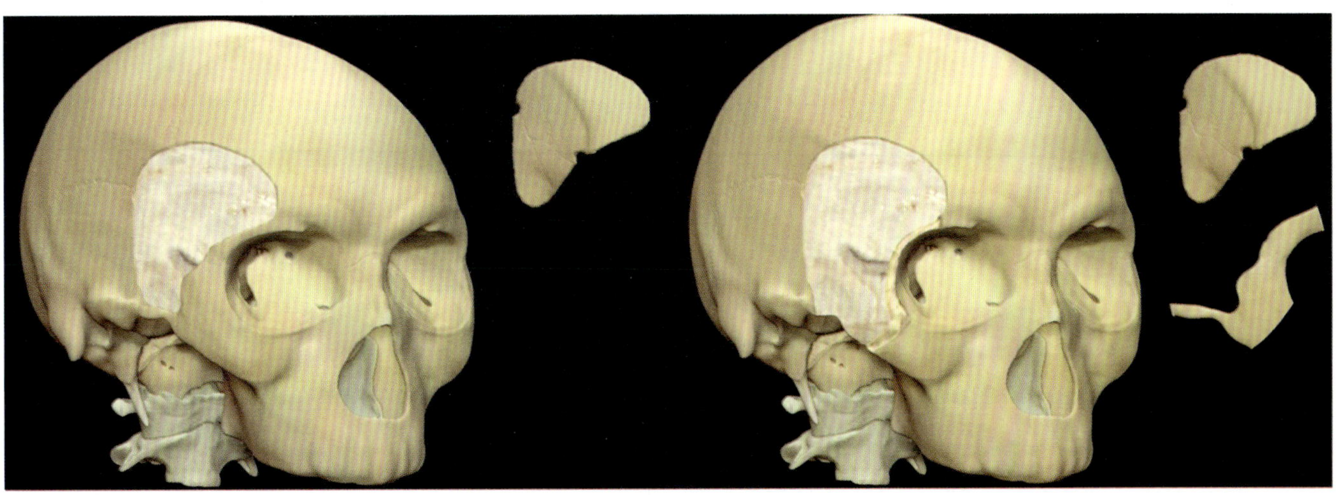

Fig. 37.9 Graphic depiction of pterional and frontotemporal orbitozygomatic craniotomy.

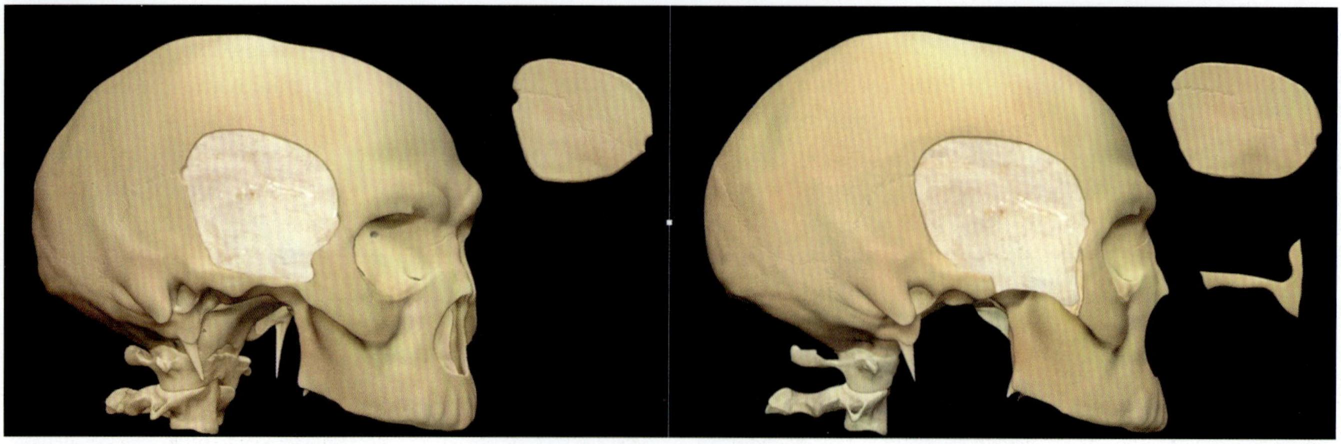

Fig. 37.10 Graphic depiction of temporal and extended temporal craniotomy.

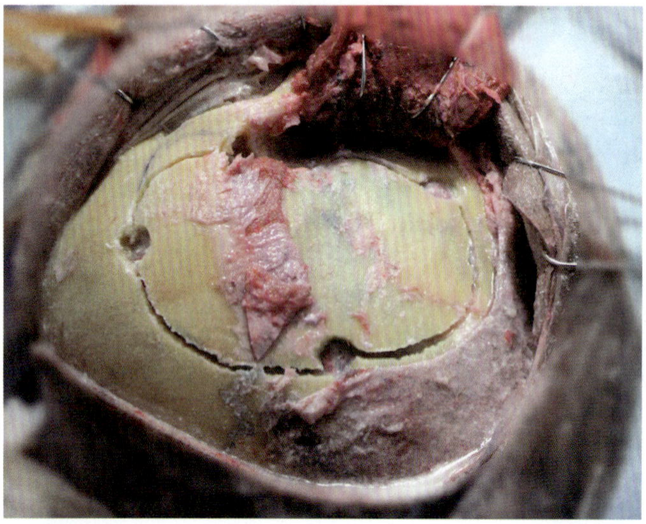

Fig. 37.11 Frontotemporal craniotomy.

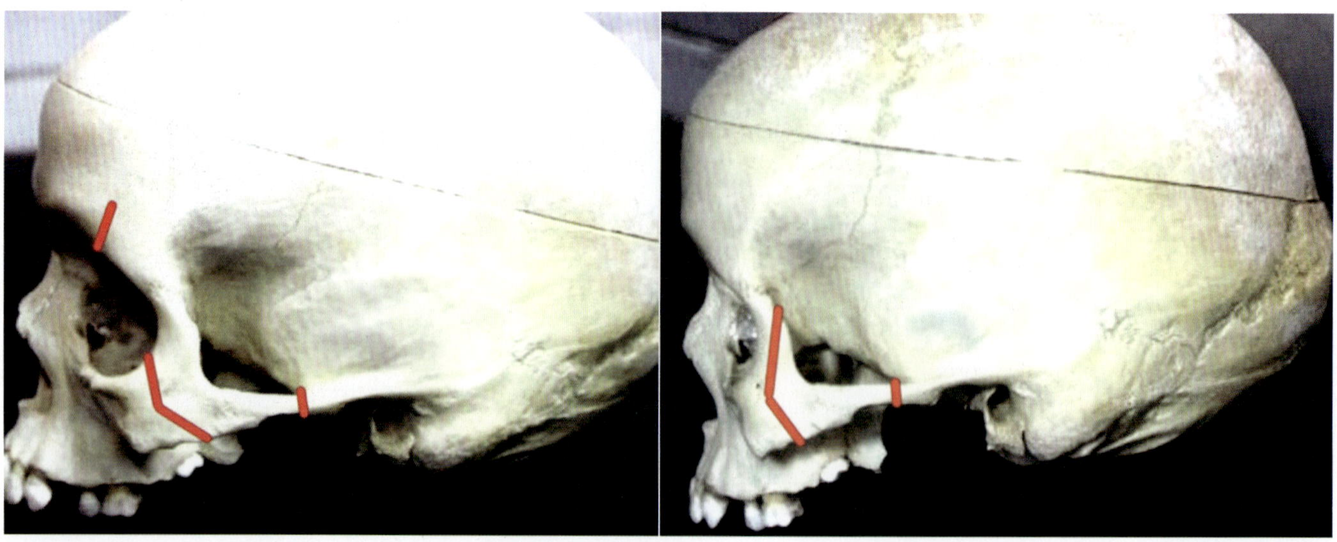

Fig. 37.12 Cuts for orbitozygomatic and zygomatic osteotomy.

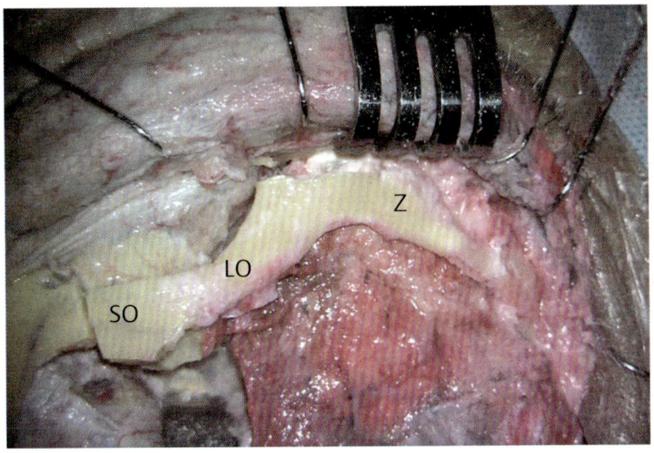

Fig. 37.13 Orbitozygomatic osteotomy.

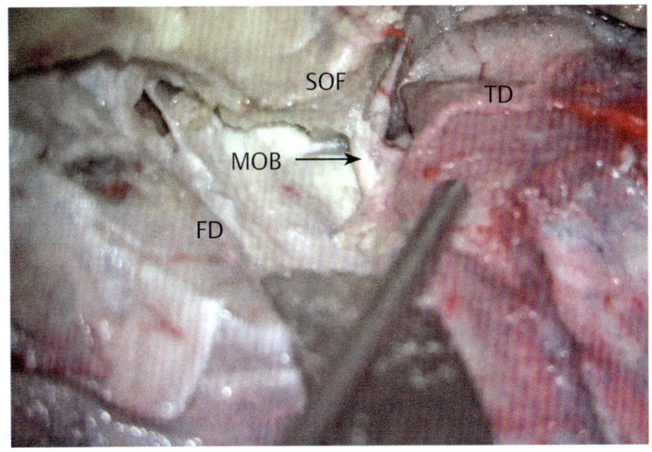

Fig. 37.14 Identification and division of meningo-orbital band.

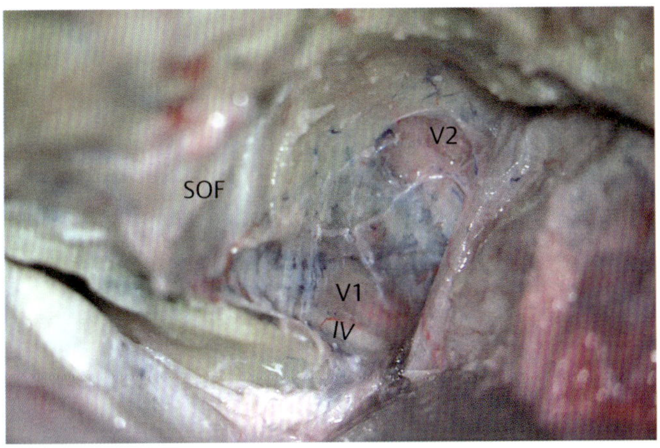

Fig. 37.15 Interdural dissection and exposure of anterior cavernous sinus.

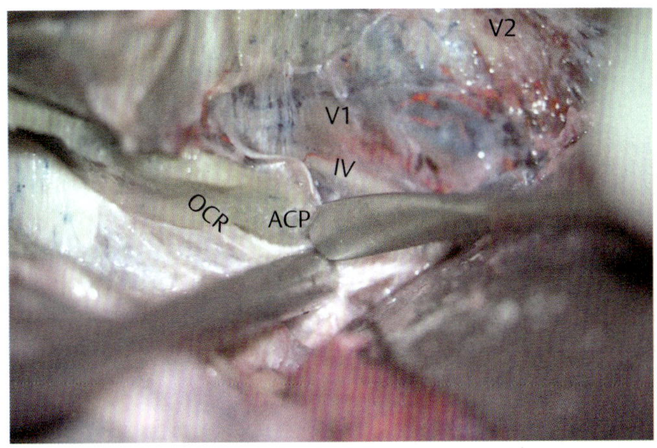

Fig. 37.16 Exposure of the base of the anterior clinoid process.

8. After the meningo-orbital band is cut, the temporal dura is dissected from the outer layer of the cavernous sinus thus commencing the transcavernous approach. Elevation of dura propria reveals the anterior part of cavernous sinus along with cranial nerves III, IV, V1, and V2 (**Fig. 37.15**). The dura medial to the superior orbital fissure is often thin, but with a sharp dissector, it can usually be elevated from the lesser wing of the sphenoid gently exposing the anterior clinoid process (ACP) (**Fig. 37.16**).
9. Clinoidectomy begins by coring out the ACP with a cutting and diamond burr making it hollow and empty followed by the detachment of ACP from the lesser wing of sphenoid, optic canal roof, and optic strut sequentially (**Fig. 37.17**).

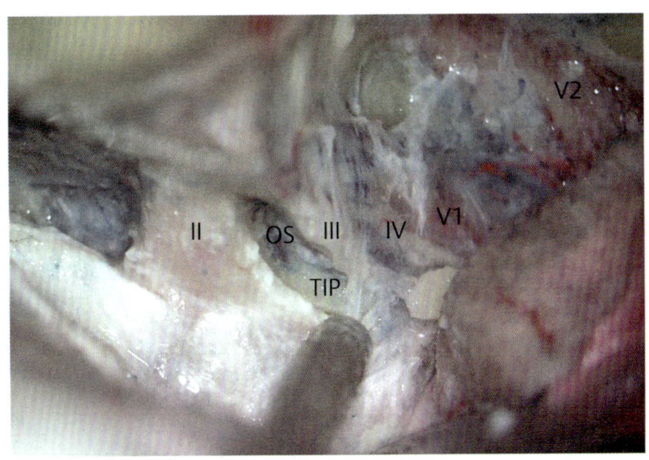

Fig. 37.17 Drilling of anterior clinoid process and optic canal deroofing.

10. Deroofing of the optic canal is done to expose and decompress the optic nerve and for intracranial mobilization (**Fig. 37.17**). Deroofing is started from the orbital side to the falciform ligament.
11. After the ACP is cored out, the tip of ACP is detached with a dissector and removed with the help of forceps or a flat dissector (**Fig. 37.18**). The optic strut (**Fig. 37.19**) is partially drilled for better visualization of the underlying internal carotid artery (ICA) and gives way for increased mobilization of the optic nerve. The drilling of the ACP and the optic canal should be performed very gently with cooling irrigation. **Fig. 37.20** depicts the exposure after completion of anterior clinoidectomy.
12. For transsylvian approaches, the dura is opened in a curvilinear fashion extending over the Sylvian fissure from frontal base to temporal base. For skull base and pretemporal approaches, the "C-shaped" curvilinear incision is converted to a "T-shaped" incision with the vertical limb along the Sylvian fissure extending till falciform ligament (**Fig. 37.21**).

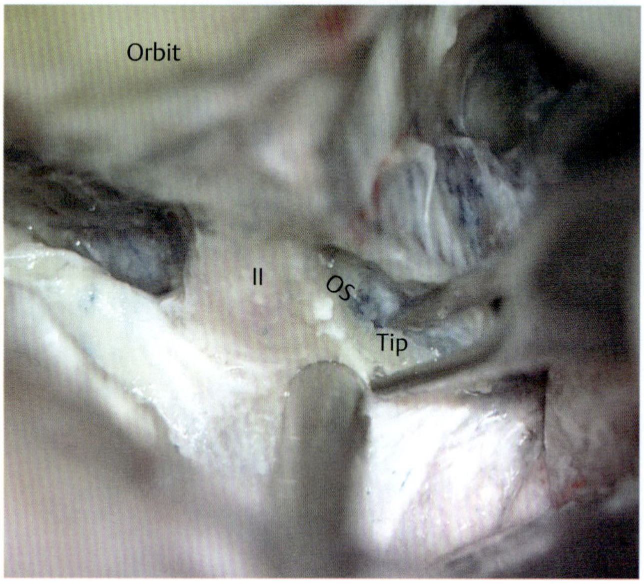

Fig. 37.18 Removal of anterior clinoid process.

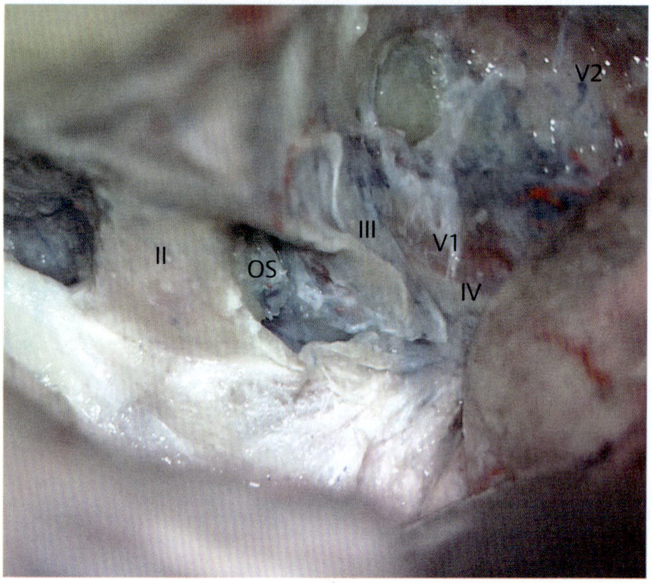

Fig. 37.19 Removal of optic strut.

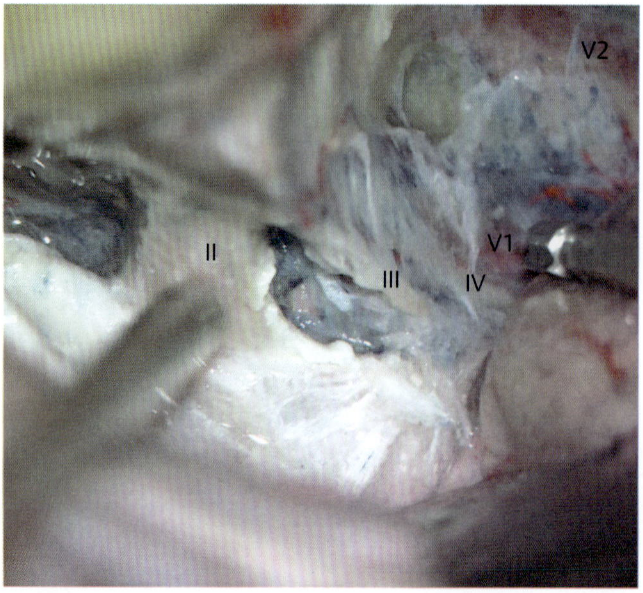

Fig. 37.20 Completion of anterior clinoidectomy.

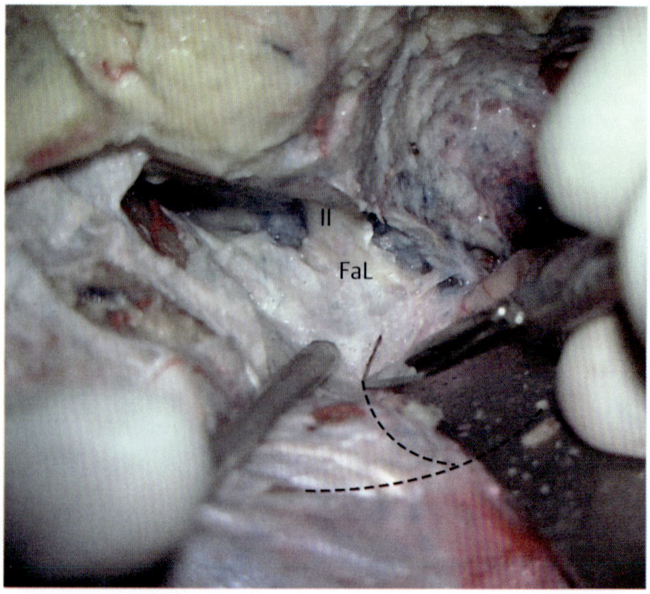

Fig. 37.21 Dural incision.

13. After dural opening, the arachnoid bridging from frontal to temporal lobe over the anterior Sylvian fissure should be meticulously divided using microscissors, dissector, or bipolar cautery, as necessary (**Fig. 37.22**). Arachnoid dissection continues until the frontal and temporal lobes are separated roughly back to the limen insulae. Brain retractors are placed on the frontal and temporal lobes to permit visualization of the basal cisterns.
14. As the Sylvian fissure is opened, the ICA is identified with its bifurcation into the middle cerebral and anterior cerebral arteries. The optic nerve can be seen medial to the ICA (**Fig. 37.23**). The right optic nerve and carotid artery are seen. The carotid cisterns are opened to drain cerebrospinal fluid (CSF), and the A1 anterior cerebral artery is followed to chiasma.
15. After dissecting the ipsilateral optic nerve, the dissection proceeds medially toward the contralateral basal surface. The frontal lobes are elevated and dissected over the optic chiasma exposing the anterior circulation complex and contralateral optic nerve. Ipsilateral hypoplastic A1 and contralateral dominant A1 are seen along with B/L optic nerves (**Fig. 37.24**).
16. Lamina terminalis is a thin sheet of gray mater and pia mater that attaches to the upper surface of the chiasma and stretches upward to fill the interval between the optic chiasma and rostrum of the corpus callosum. Lamina terminalis is opened to relieve CSF from the third ventricle (**Fig. 37.25**).
17. The pituitary stalk is exposed at the undersurface of the optic chiasma attaching superoposteriorly to the hypothalamus and going inferiorly to the pituitary gland (**Fig. 37.26**).

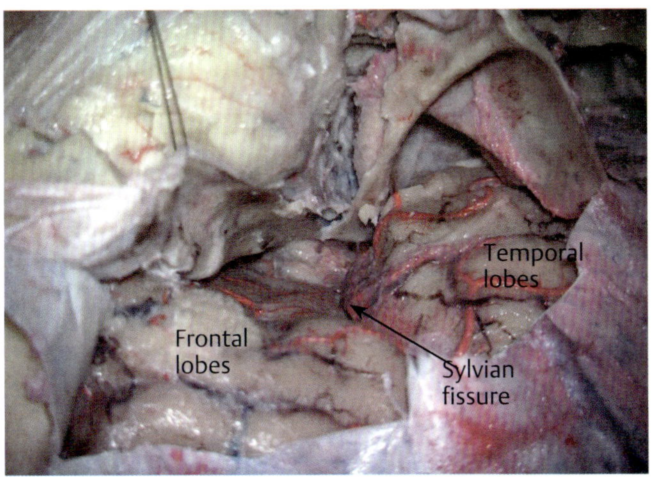

Fig. 37.22 Final exposure after opening the dura. The dissection is begun by opening the Sylvian fissure.

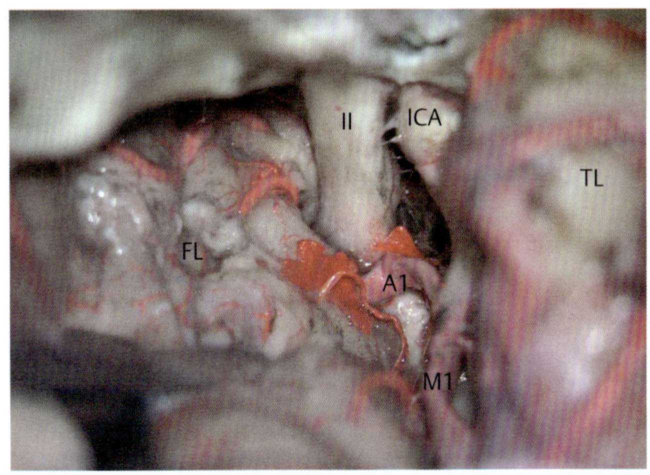

Fig. 37.23 Ipsilateral ICA bifurcation.

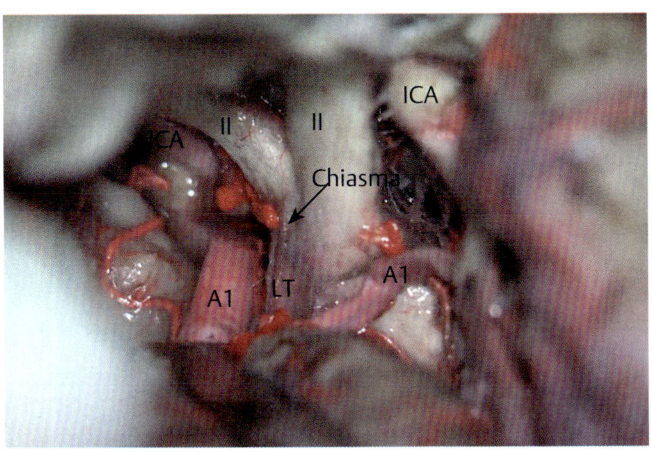

Fig. 37.24 Exposing optic chiasma.

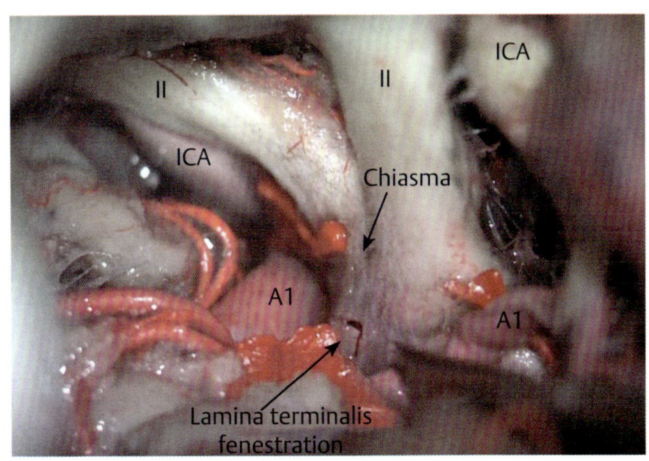

Fig. 37.25 Opening of lamina terminalis.

18. The ICA is carefully followed and dissected to visualize the posterior communicating artery (PCom).
19. The posteromedial structures to the temporal lobe can be visualized by the pretemporal or temporopolar approach. Gentle posterior and lateral retraction of the temporal lobe along with dural reflection exposes the distal ICA and posterior circulation. The PCom and anterior choroidal artery are identified (**Fig. 37.27**). The anterior choroidal artery leads to the choroidal fissure, and careful dissection of this artery separates the deep adhesions between frontal and temporal lobes to maximize temporal lobe mobilization. The PCom emerges from the posteromedial surface of the ICA as the carotid bends upward and laterally toward its bifurcation. The PCom leads to the membrane of Liliequist, which is carefully opened to enter the posterior fossa. PCom can be seen anastomosing to the posterior cerebral artery (PCA) (**Fig. 37.27**).
20. The undersurface of the P1 PCA is followed medially to its intersection with the basilar artery (BA), where the superior cerebral artery (SCA) is also identified. Dissection of the arachnoid around the BA also brings the contralateral P1 and SCA into view. Difficulty in differentiating contralateral PCA and SCA can be determined with certainty by establishing the relationship of the two arteries and oculomotor nerve (CN III) that runs between them (**Fig. 37.28**). The oculomotor nerve can be visualized running between PCA superiorly and SCA inferiorly (**Fig. 37.28** and **Fig. 37.29**).
21. The falciform ligament extends medially from the ACP across the optic nerve to the posterior border of the jugum sphenoidale (**Fig. 37.30**). Length of optic nerve under falciform ligament measures approximately 2.7 cm. The falciform ligament is carefully incised (**Fig. 37.31**) to facilitate mobilization of the optic nerve. Sectioning of the falciform ligament usually

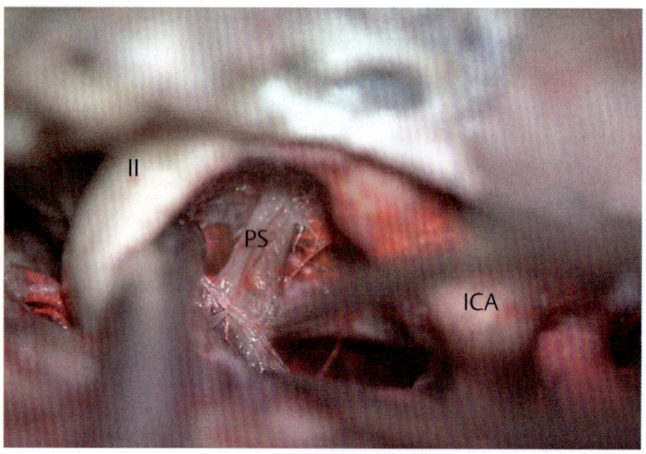

Fig. 37.26 Exposure of pituitary stalk.

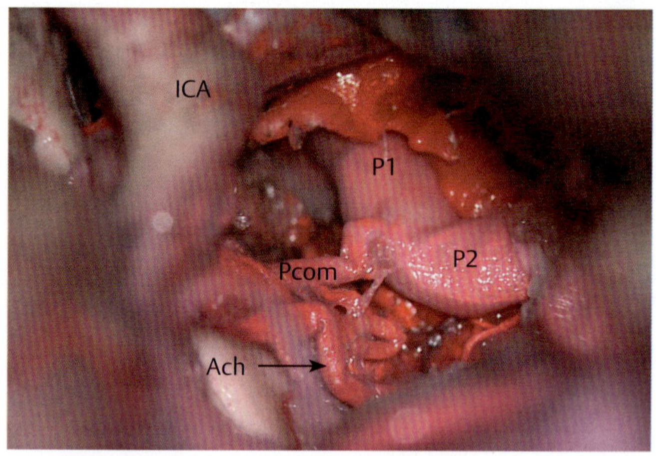

Fig. 37.27 Ipsilateral distal ICA and branches.

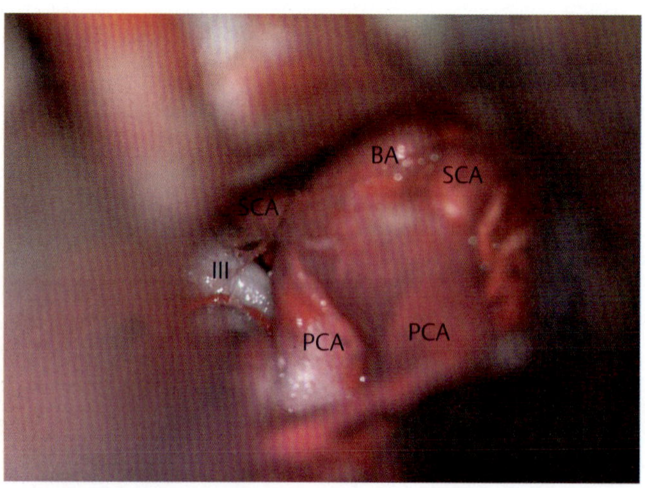

Fig. 37.28 Exposure of upper posterior circulation.

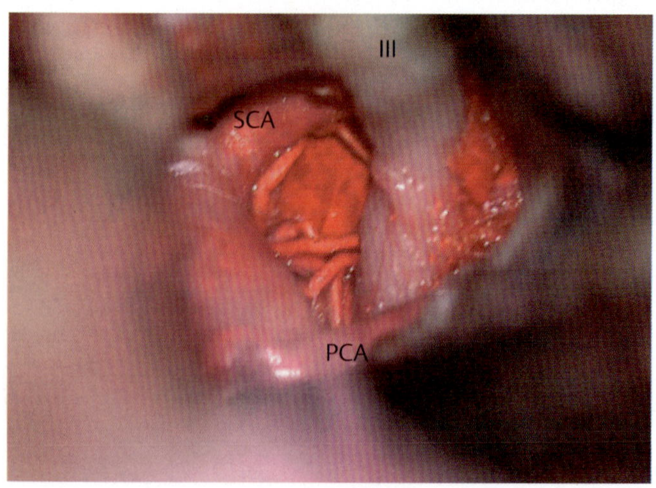

Fig. 37.29 Exposure of ipsilateral upper posterior circulation.

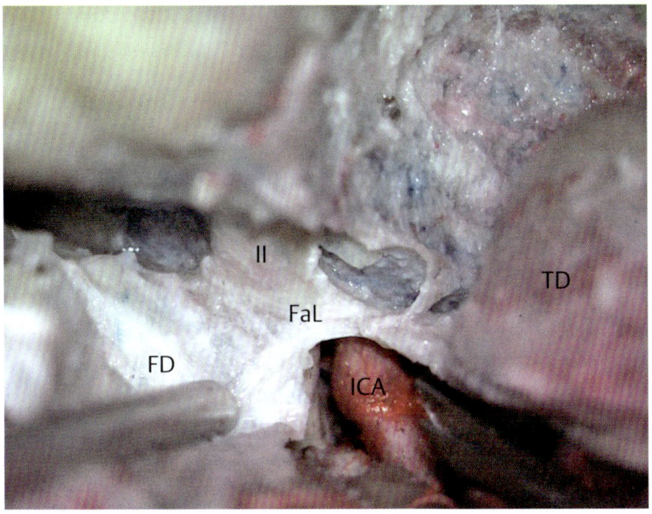

Fig. 37.30 Exposure of falciform ligament.

yields exposure of the origin of the ophthalmic artery (**Fig. 37.32**) and proximal ICA. Extreme care needs to be taken to protect the pial vasculature of the optic nerve.

22. The upper or distal dural ring is part of the dural fold extending from the outer layer of the lateral wall of cavernous sinus to the superior aspect of ACP and ICA (**Fig. 37.33**). It divides ICA into extradural and intradural segments. The layer of dura that lines the lower margin of the ACP and extends medially forms the lower or proximal dural ring and is referred to as the carotico-oculomotor membrane.
23. The segment of the ICA located between the upper and lower dural rings, which is exposed by removing the ACP, is referred to as the clinoidal segment. It may be necessary to divide the dural rings (**Fig. 37.33** and **Fig. 37.34**) to mobilize the carotid artery for dealing

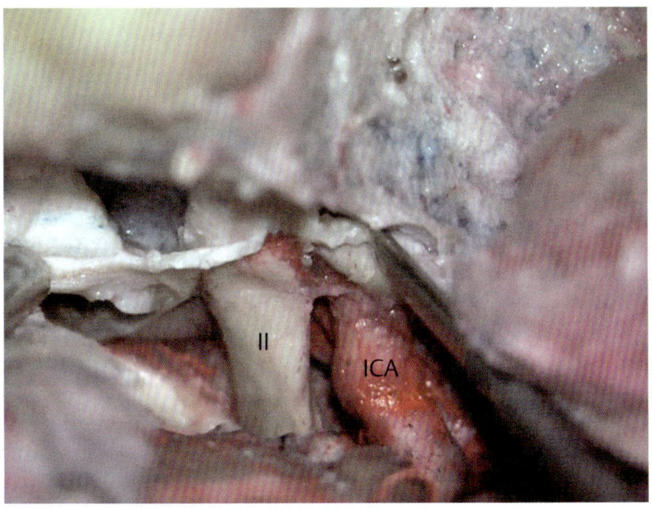

Fig. 37.31 Division of falciform ligament.

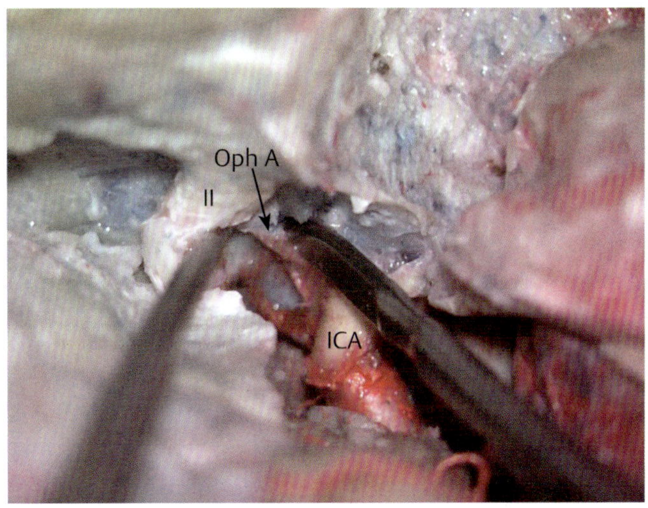

Fig. 37.32 Exposure of ophthalmic artery.

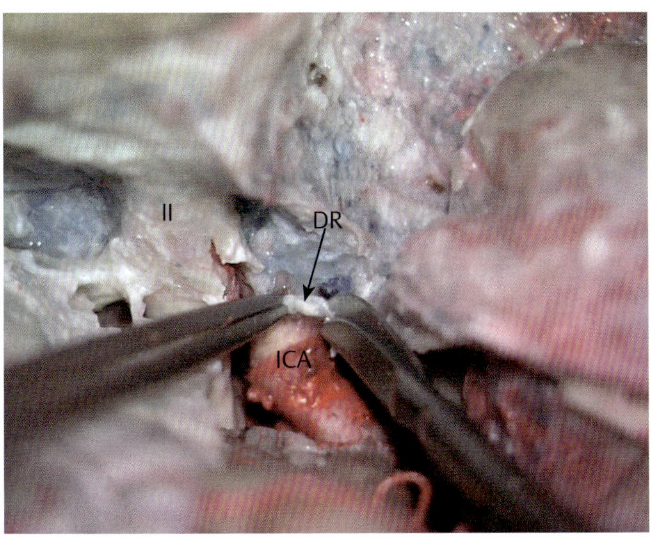

Fig. 37.33 Division of distal dural ring (DR).

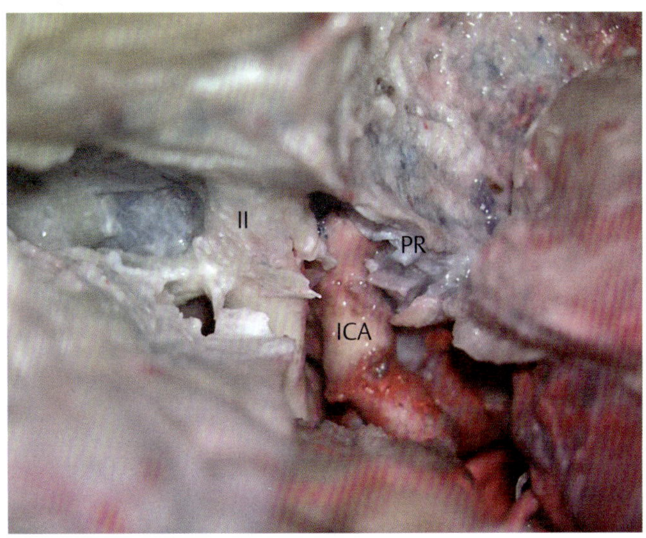

Fig. 37.34 Exposure of clinoidal ICA segment.

with aneurysms arising at the level of the roof of the cavernous sinus from the ICA at the origin of the ophthalmic artery.

24. For an anterior transpetrous approach, either a FTOZ craniotomy or an extended temporal craniotomy is done. After craniotomy, the temporal dura is elevated gently from the temporal base. As the dura is being elevated, the ridges present over the base of the temporal bone are flattened so as not to obstruct the surgeon's view.
25. As we elevate the temporal dura, the middle meningeal artery (MMA) over the dura can be followed to its emergence from the foramen spinosum. The foramen spinosum is usually located at the level of the root of the zygoma (**Fig. 37.35**).
26. The foramen spinosum needs to be drilled and enlarged so as to prevent retraction of the stump of MMA after being cut and avoid any inadvertent bleeding. Hence, as the foramen spinosum is identified, it is drilled (**Fig. 37.36**), and adequate space is made to coagulate the artery and cut it (**Fig. 37.37**). The division of MMA paves way for extradural retraction from the temporal base.
27. Initial separation of the dura propria from the dural covering of cavernous sinus is done with a sharp knife, which is later continued with a blunt flat dissector. The dissection continues to expose the foramen ovale and the mandibular division of the trigeminal nerve (**Fig. 37.38**). At this stage, the greater superficial petrosal nerve (GSPN) is identified at the posterior margin of the mandibular nerve. Its identification is necessary prior to dissection because of the risk of injury from either traction along the dura or thermal injury because of bipolar coagulation of neighboring structures. Interdural dissection continues until the whole gasserian ganglion with its branches exposed.
28. The gasserian ganglion (**Fig. 37.39**) lies at the petrous apex and is contained in a pocket of dura filled with CSF commonly called Meckel's cave.
29. The temporal basal bone is drilled to expose the internal maxillary artery (IMA) in the infratemporal fossa between the maxillary and mandibular divisions of the trigeminal nerve (**Fig. 37.40**). IMA is often used for high-flow bypass surgeries.
30. Middle fossa cavernous sinus triangles can be identified after the completion of interdural dissection and exposure of cavernous sinus in its entirety (**Fig. 37.41**).
31. Kawase's rhomboid (**Fig. 37.42**) is delineated and is bounded anteriorly by the posterior border of the mandibular nerve, posteriorly by arcuate eminence, medially by petrous ridge and superior petrosal sinus, and laterally by the GSPN.
32. Kawase's rhomboid is drilled (**Fig. 37.43**) so as to gain access to the posterior fossa dura.
33. Temporal dura is incised parallel to superior petrosal sinus, and the temporal lobe along with the dura is gently retracted to expose the tentorium (**Fig. 37.44**). Great care is taken to preserve the vein of Labbe, which is accomplished by sharp arachnoidal dissection and avoiding overretraction. Retractors are gradually placed deeper to retract posterior temporal lobe until medial tentorial edge is visualized.

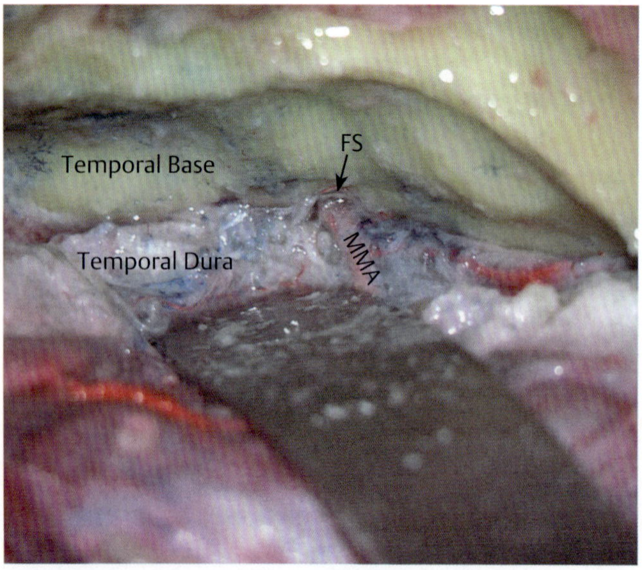

Fig. 37.35 Elevation of temporal dura.

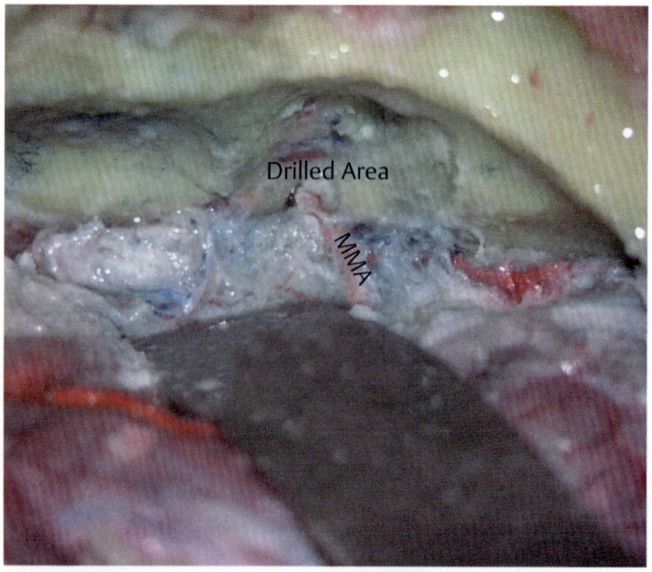

Fig. 37.36 Dilation of foramen spinosum.

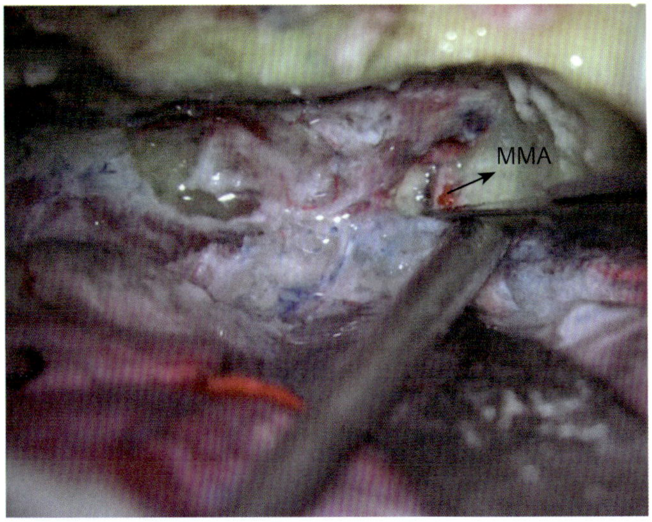

Fig. 37.37 Division of middle meningeal artery (MMA).

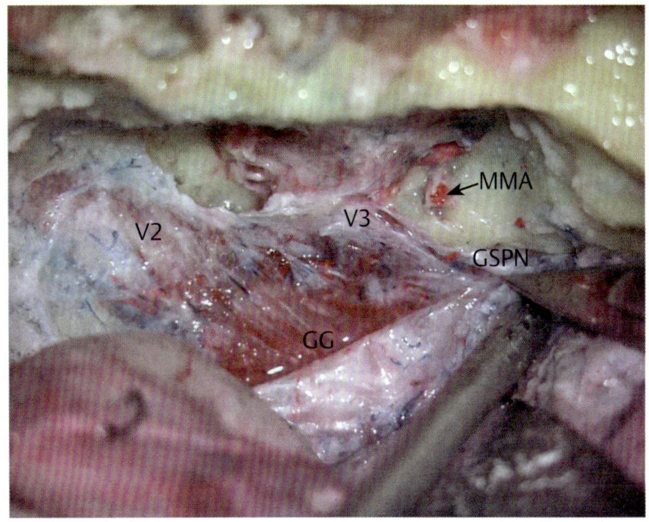

Fig. 37.38 Separation of dura propria from trigeminal branches.

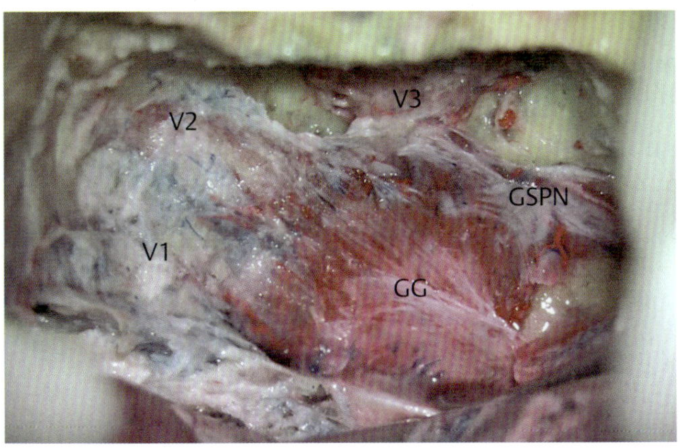

Fig. 37.39 Exposure of the gasserian ganglion.

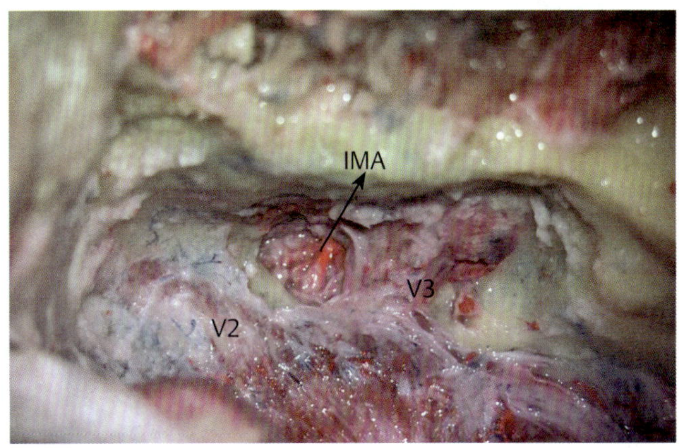

Fig. 37.40 Dissection of internal maxillary artery (IMA).

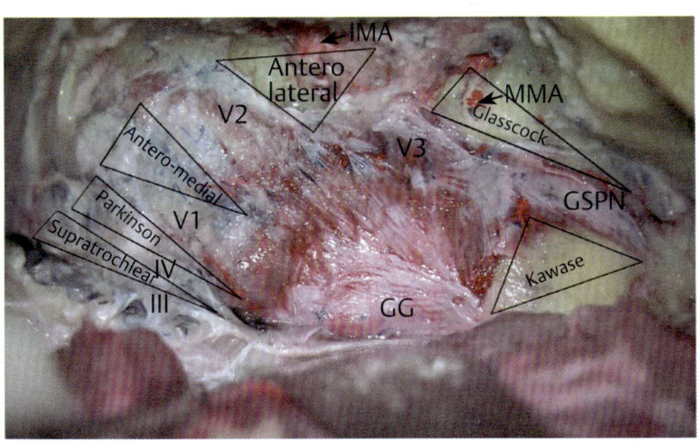

Fig. 37.41 Middle fossa triangles.

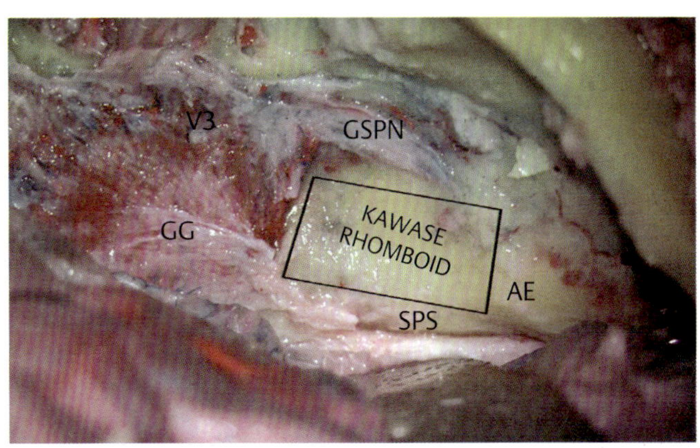

Fig. 37.42 Exposure of Kawase's rhomboid.

34. For gaining access to the pathologies in areas near and around the clivus involving both middle and posterior fossae, both fossae need to be connected. The tentorium is incised in a lateral to medial direction (**Fig. 37.45**). The proposed line of incision is initially cauterized followed by incision with a no. 11 knife. It is usually incised 1 cm behind the trochlear nerve, which runs in the free edge of the tentorial hiatus. Tentorial edges are coagulated so as to control bleeding from the venous sinuses. Similarly, posterior fossa dura is incised anterior to the sigmoid sinus and both middle and posterior fossae are connected by ligation and division of superior petrosal sinus **(Fig. 37.46)**.
35. On retracting the cut tentorial leaf anteriorly, the trigeminal nerve can be seen coursing anteriorly from the brainstem and entering the Meckel cave to form gasserian ganglion (**Fig. 37.47**).
36. The internal auditory canal (IAC) can be identified by imagining a plane that bisects the angle between the arcuate eminence and the GSPN. The plane of the IAC meets the plane of the GSPN or the superior canal at 60 degrees posteriorly. IAC can be drilled to expose the seventh–eighth nerve complex (**Fig. 37.48**).
37. The abducens nerve can be seen after elevating the trigeminal nerve in normal individuals (**Fig. 37.49**). A part of clivus might need to be drilled to see the abducens nerve as it passes through Dorello's canal located at the upper edge of the petroclival fissure.
38. As we move slightly anteriorly along the tentorium, contents of the ambient cistern can be exposed. The oculomotor nerve can be seen traversing anteriorly toward the oculomotor trigone, while SCA can be seen traversing laterally to the brainstem below the oculomotor nerve (**Fig. 37.50**).
39. The contents of the cavernous sinus are being exposed by opening the dura over the anteromedial triangle between V1 and V2 segments of the trigeminal nerve (**Fig. 37.51**). It can also be accomplished by opening infratrochlear or Parkinson's triangle.
40. The nerves in the lateral aspect of the cavernous sinus are being exposed. The course of abducens nerve exiting from the Dorello's canal can be seen. The abducens nerve passes under the petrosphenoidal ligament and courses lateral to the ICA (**Fig. 37.52**) in the cavernous sinus.
41. Complete course of ICA after opening the cavernous sinus can be visualized and is shown in **Fig. 37.53**.
42. Microphotographs of surgical steps of transcavernous and anterior transpetrous approaches are shown in **Fig. 37.54**, **Fig. 37.55**, **Fig. 37.56**, **Fig. 37.57**, **Fig. 37.58**, and **Fig. 37.59**.

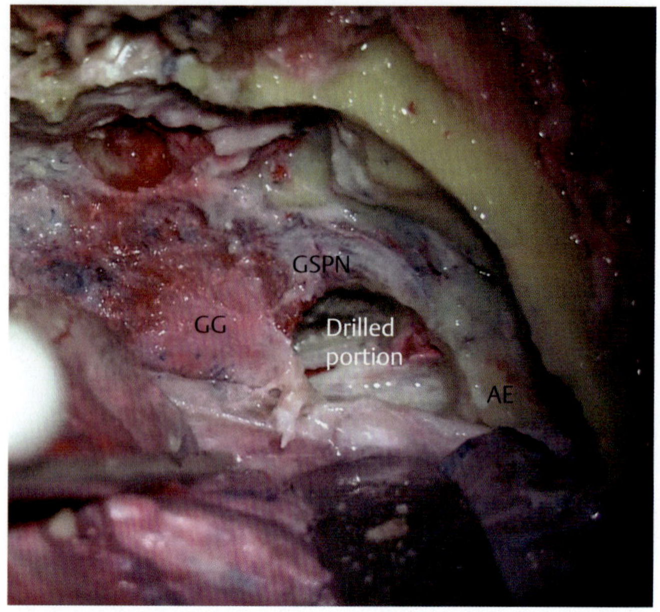

Fig. 37.43 Drilling of Kawase's rhomboid.

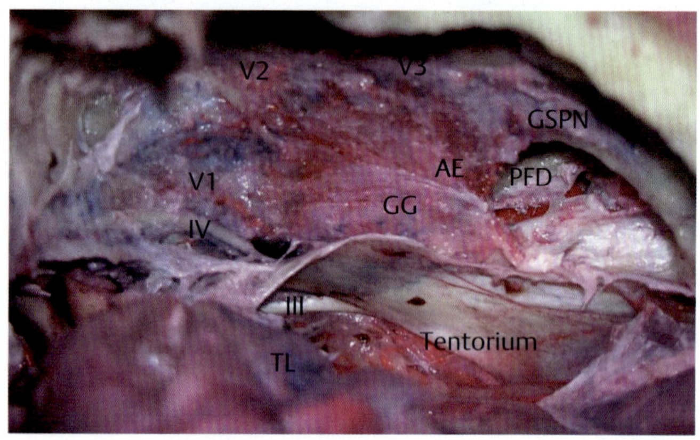

Fig. 37.44 Exposure of tentorium.

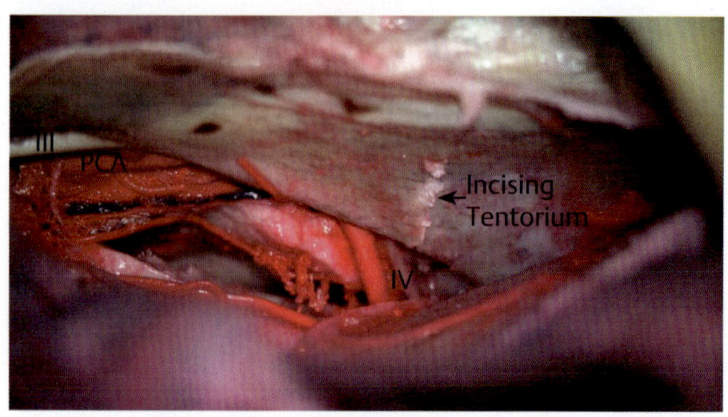

Fig. 37.45 Incision over tentorium.

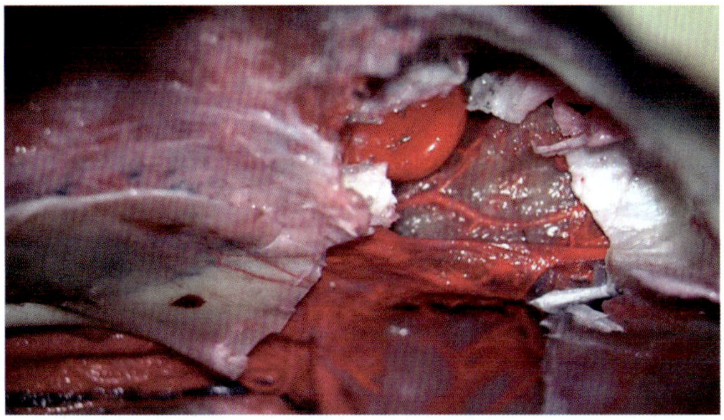

Fig. 37.46 Division of tentorium and superior petrosal sinus.

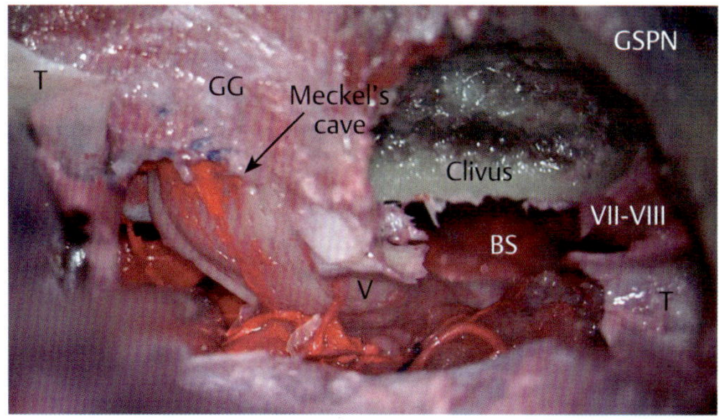

Fig. 37.47 Opening Meckel's cave and trigeminal nerve exposure.

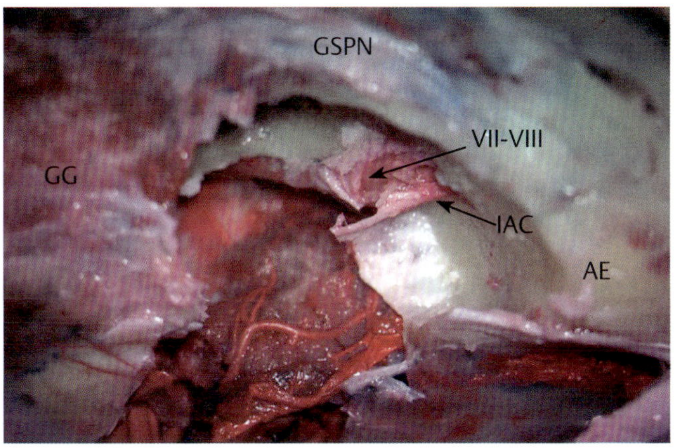

Fig. 37.48 Exposure of seventh and eighth nerves.

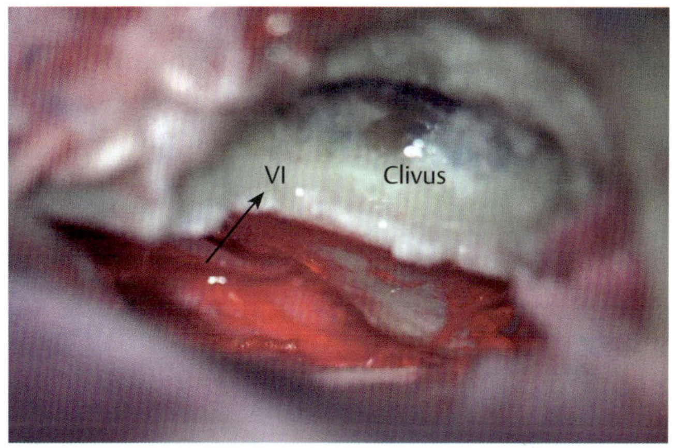

Fig. 37.49 Exposing abducens nerve.

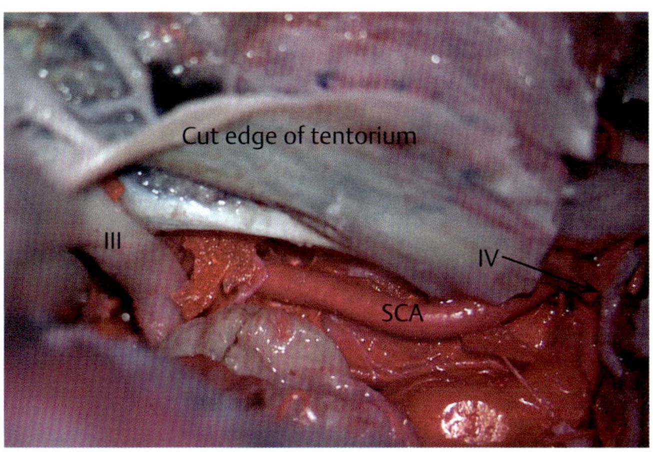

Fig. 37.50 Exposing ambient cistern and its contents.

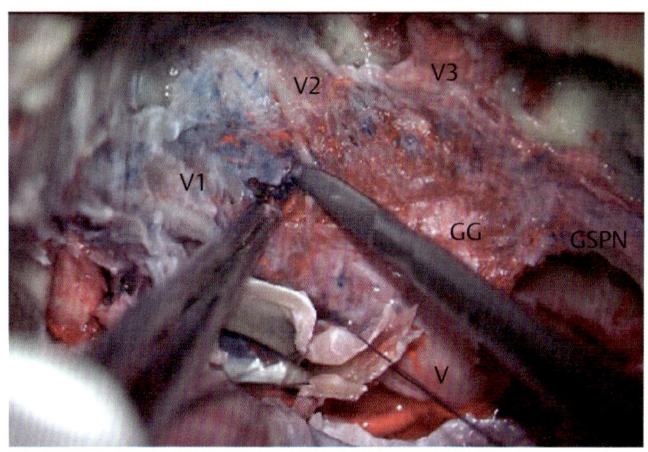

Fig. 37.51 Opening of cavernous sinus.

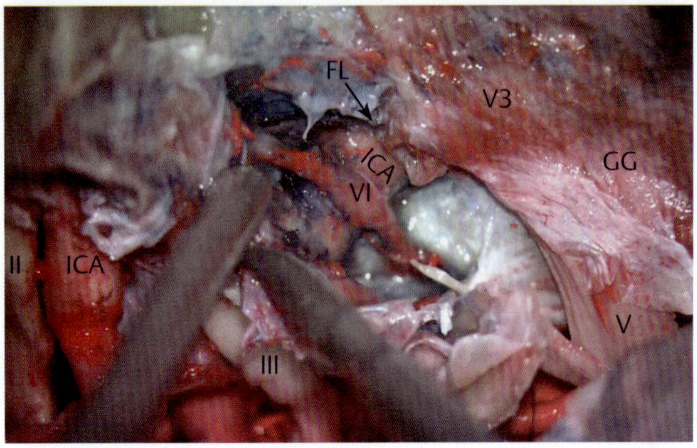

Fig. 37.52 Exposure of abducens nerve.

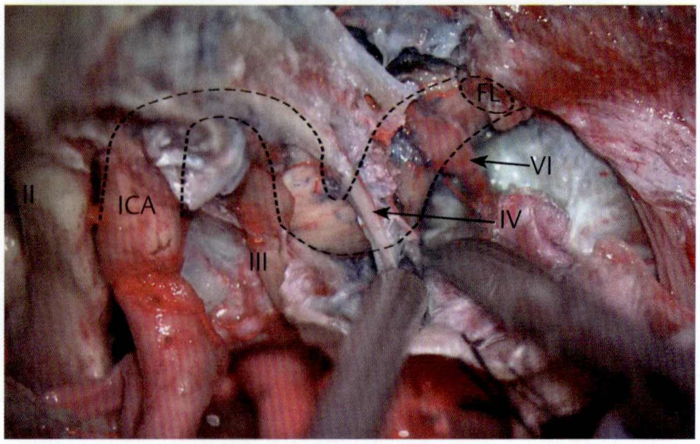

Fig. 37.53 Intracavernous course of ICA.

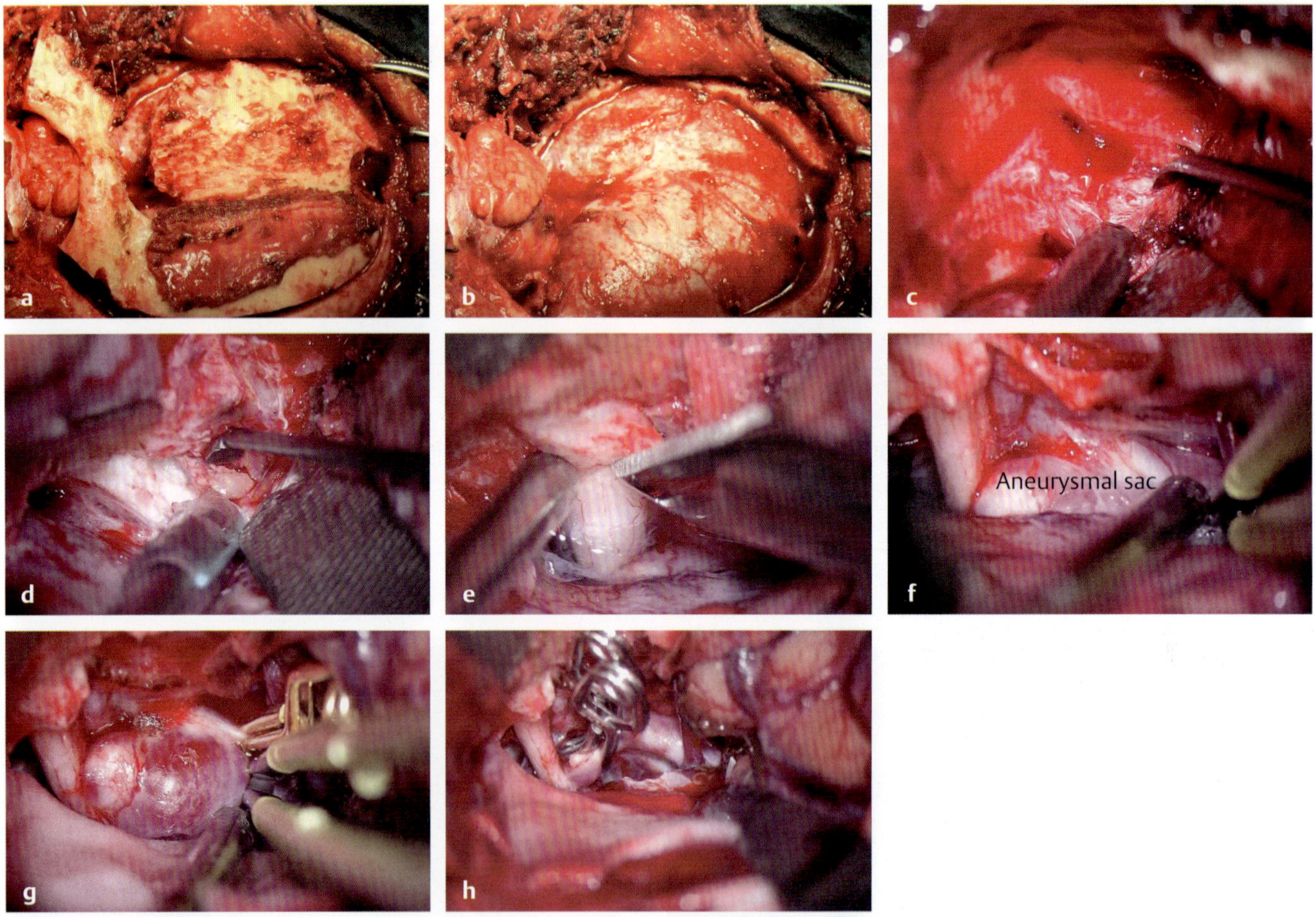

Fig. 37.54 Steps during surgery of paraclinoidal ophthalmic aneurysm. **(a)** Frontotemporal orbitozygomatic (FTOZ) craniotomy. **(b)** Exposure after FTOZ craniotomy. **(c)** Dissection of the anterior cavernous sinus. **(d)** Anterior clinoidectomy. **(e)** Division of the falciform ligament. **(f)** Exposure of aneurysmal sac. **(g)** Defining dome of aneurysm. **(h)** Clipping of aneurysm.

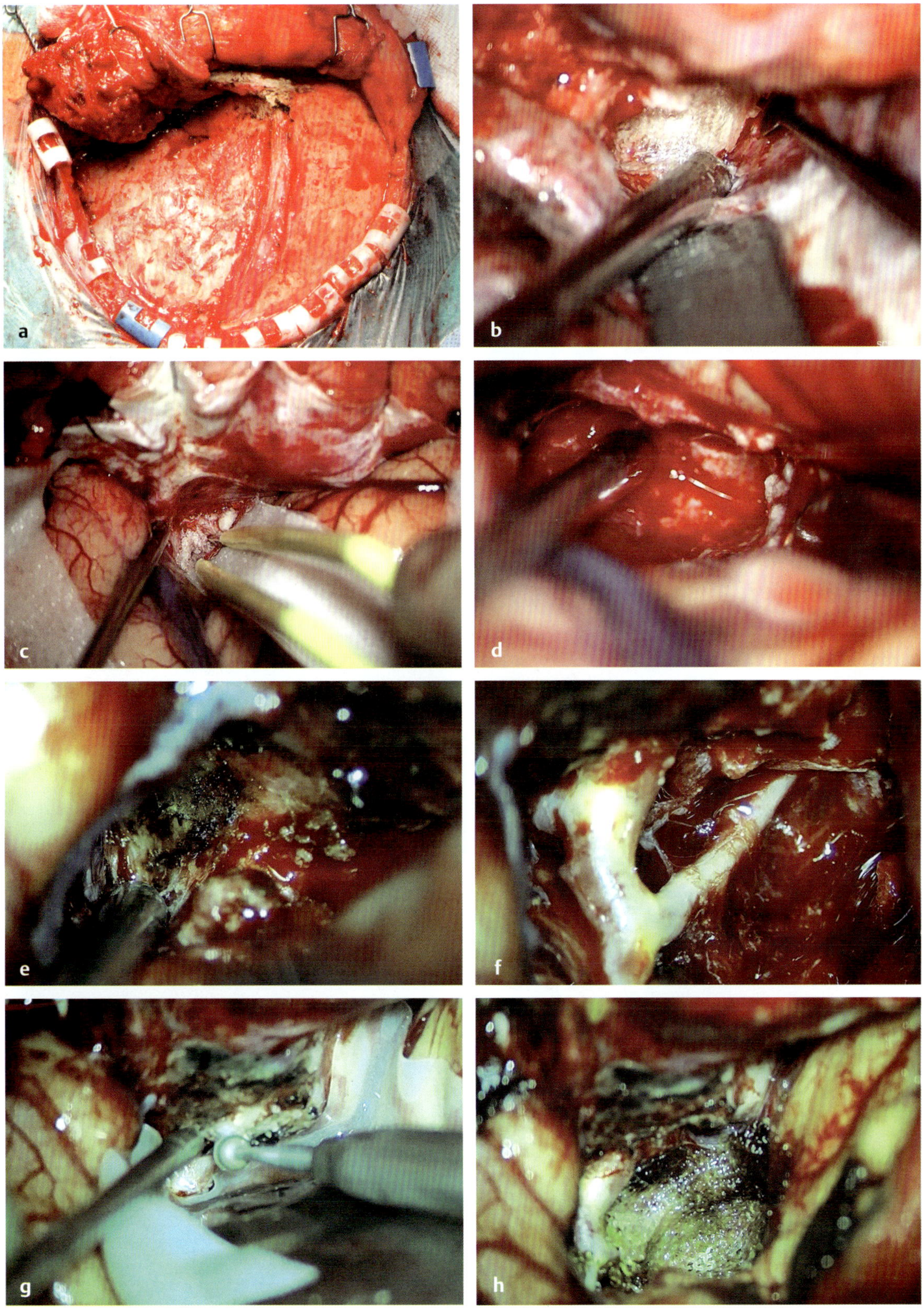

Fig. 37.55 Steps during surgery of medial clinoidal meningioma. **(a)** Exposure for FTOZ craniotomy. **(b)** Extradural anterior clinoidectomy is being done. **(c)** Exposure of tumor after opening Sylvian fissure. **(d)** Tumor debulking. **(e)** Coagulation of basal dura. **(f)** Tumor decompression around ICA. **(g)** Intradural drilling of hypertrophied bone. **(h)** Tumor cavity after gross total excision.

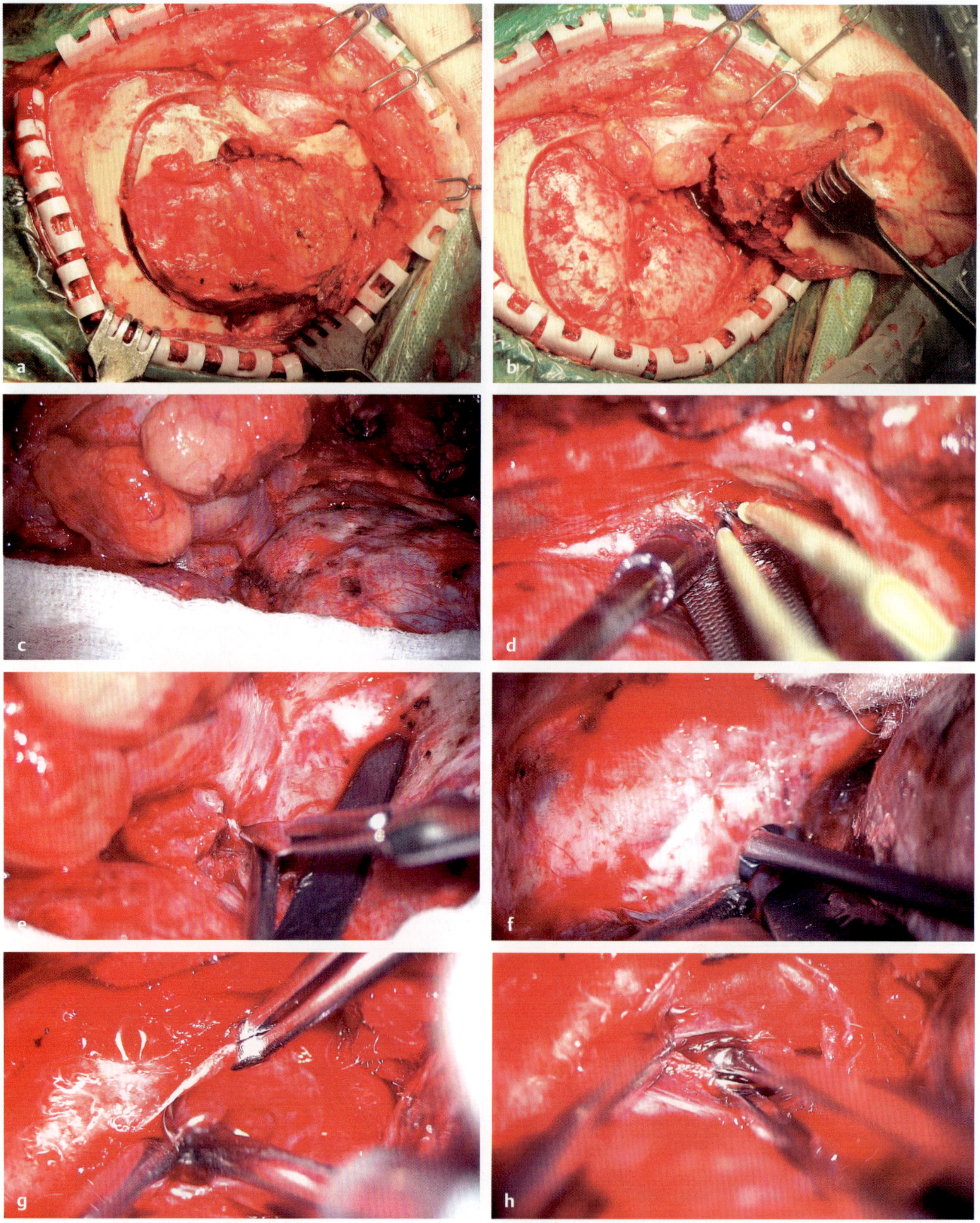

Fig. 37.56 Steps during surgery of cavernous hemangioma. **(a)** Extended temporal craniotomy with the removal of the zygoma. **(b)** Exposure after craniotomy. **(c)** Exposure of superior orbital fissure. **(d)** Coagulation of middle meningeal artery. **(e)** Division of meningo-orbital band. **(f)** Dissecting membranous layer to expose hemangioma in the cavernous sinus. **(g)** Tumor debulking by ultrasonic aspirator. **(h)** Removal of anteromedial part of the tumor.

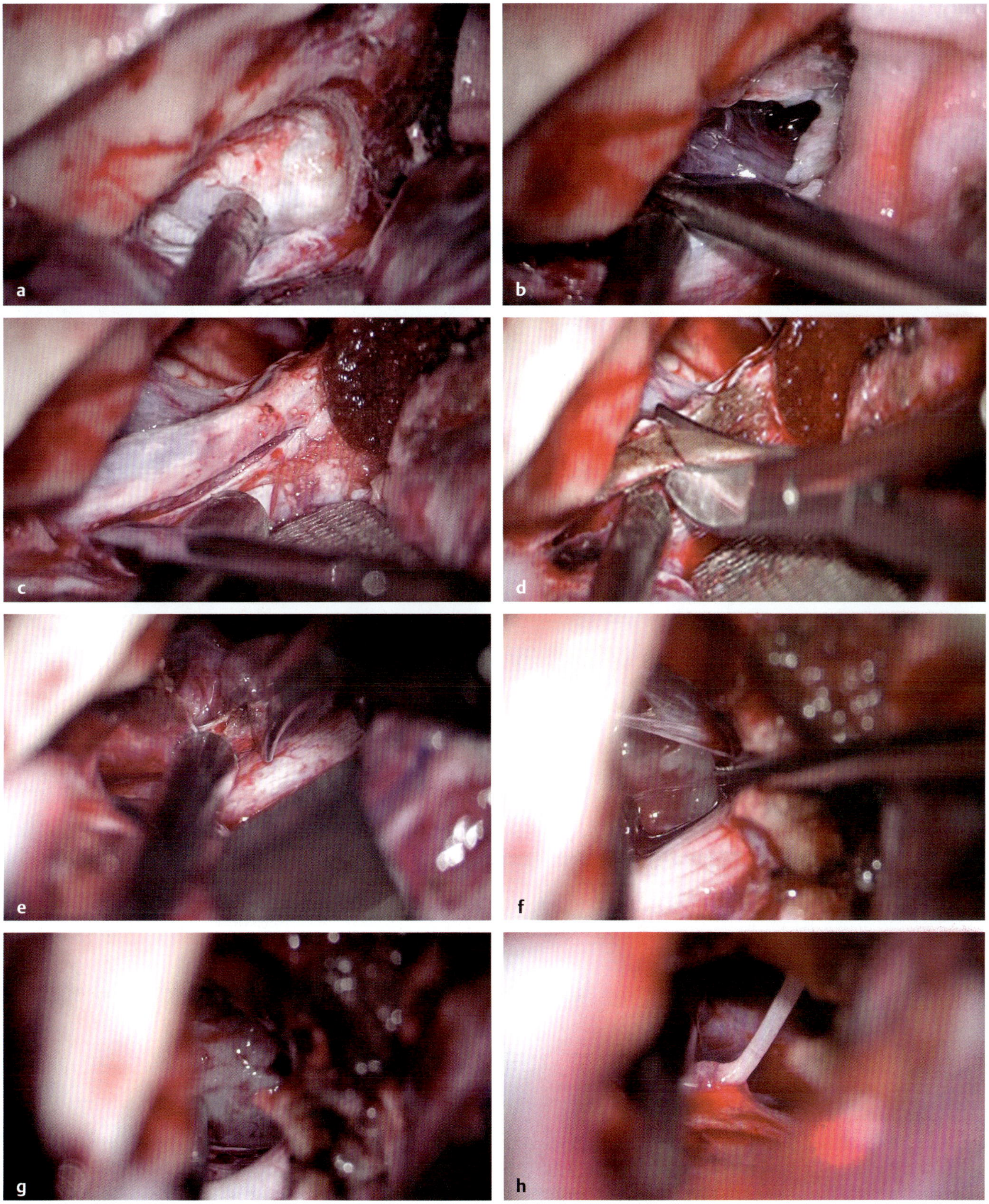

Fig. 37.57 Steps during surgery of clival chordosarcoma. **(a)** Exposure and drilling of Kawase's rhomboid. **(b)** Dural opening over posterior fossa. **(c)** Dural incision over basal temporal dura. **(d)** Coagulation and division of superior petrosal sinus. **(e)** Division of tentorium. **(f)** Tumor decompression is being done. **(g)** Tumor decompression is being done. **(h)** Abducens nerve identified after tumor removal.

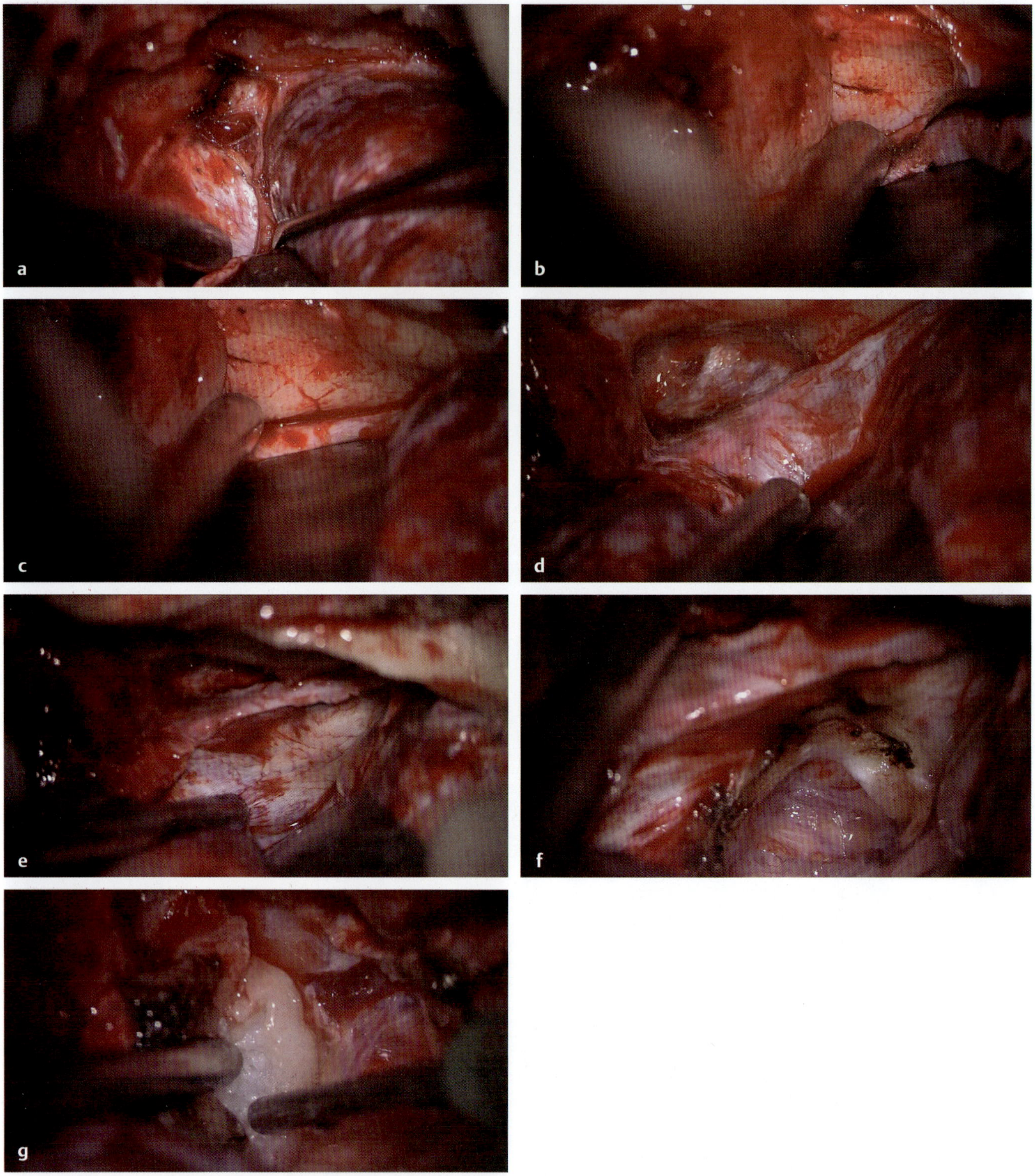

Fig. 37.58 Steps during surgery of trigeminal schwannoma. **(a)** Interdural dissection and transcavernous exposure. **(b)** Interdural dissection for Kawase's rhomboid exposure. **(c)** Exposure of Kawase's rhomboid for transpetrous approach. **(d)** Dural exposure over posterior fossa after drilling Kawase's rhomboid. **(e)** Exposure of tentorium after incising basal temporal dura. **(f)** Division of tentorium. **(g)** Posterior fossa tumor debulking by ultrasonic aspirator.

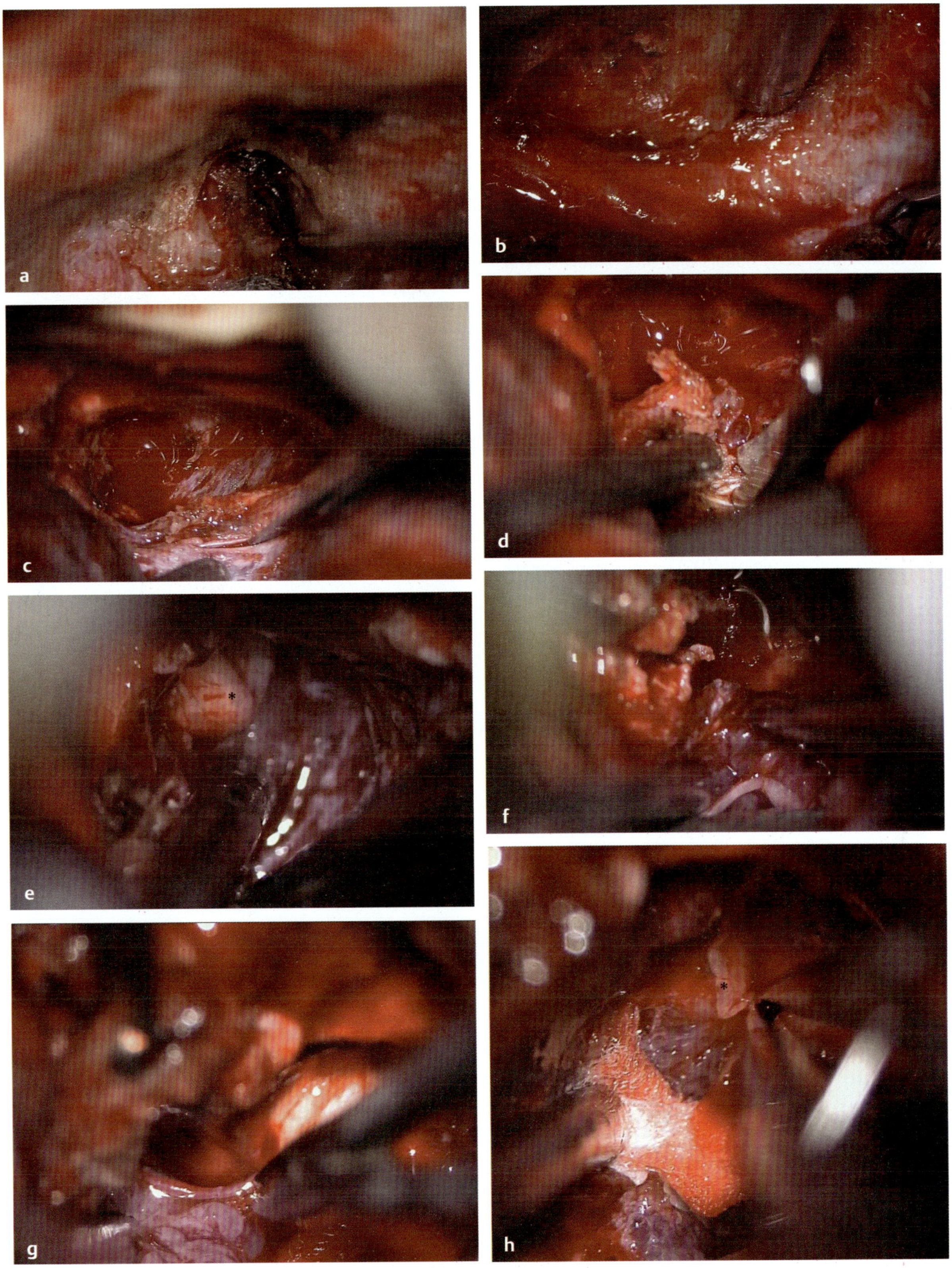

Fig. 37.59 Steps during surgery of petroclival meningioma. **(a)** Drilled out foramen spinosum with division of MMA. **(b)** Interdural dissection for exposure of Kawase's rhomboid. **(c)** Basal temporal dural opening after drilling Kawase's rhomboid. **(d)** Division of tentorium and superior petrosal sinus. **(e)** Visualization and dissection of the trigeminal nerve (*) away from tumor. **(f)** Dissection of the trochlear nerve from the tumor. **(g)** Dissection of the tumor from perforators. **(h)** Dissection of the abducens nerve (*) from the tumor.

Acknowledgments

We would like to express our special gratitude to Mr Shashi Shekhar and Mr Trivendra Yadav from Neurosurgery Education and Training Skills (NETS) Laboratory, AIIMS for the formatting and editing of this manuscript. This manuscript would not have been completed without their hard work and dedication. I am grateful to NETS Lab for providing the adequate facilities needed for completion of this cadaveric dissection. A sincere thanks to Department of Anatomy, body donors and their families, who, through their altruism, contributed to this manuscript.

Financial Disclosures

This manuscript is the result of research projects funded by extramural grants from:

1. Department of Health Research (DHR), Ministry of Health and Family Welfare, Govt. of India. Project Number: V.25011/260-HRD/2016-HR DHR/HRD/Support to Institute/Type-VIII
2. Dept. of Science and Technology (DST), Ministry of Science and Technology, Govt. of India. Project Number: SR/FST/LSII-029/2012
3. Department of Biotechnology (DBT), Ministry of Science and Technology, Govt. of India. Project Number: BT/PR13455/CoE/34/24/2015

Suggested Readings

Dolenc VV, Skrap M, Sustersic J, Škrbec M, Morina A. A transcavernous-transsellar approach to the basilar tip aneurysms. Br J Neurosurg 1987;1(2):251–259

Rhoton AL Jr. The supratentorial cranial space: microsurgical anatomy and surgical approaches. Neurosurgery 2002; 21(suppl 1):375–410

Suri A, Ahmad FU, Mahapatra AK. Extradural transcavernous approach to cavernous sinus hemangiomas. Neurosurgery 2007;60(3):483–488, discussion 488–489

Suri A, Tripathi M, Deo RC. Anterolateral transcavernous extradural petrosectomy approach: 3-dimensional operative video demonstration in cadavers. Neurosurgery 2014;10(Suppl 4): 656, discussion 656

Tripathi M, Deo RC, Damodaran N, et al. Quantitative analysis of variable extent of anterior clinoidectomy with intradural and extradural approaches: 3-dimensional analysis and cadaver dissection. Neurosurgery 2015;11(Suppl 2):147–160, discussion 160–161

Tripathi M, Deo RC, Suri A, et al. Quantitative analysis of the Kawase versus the modified Dolenc-Kawase approach for middle cranial fossa lesions with variable anteroposterior extension. J Neurosurg 2015;123(1):14–22

Wanibuchi M, Friedman A, Fukushima T. Photo Atlas of Skull Base Dissection. New York, NY: Thieme; 2008

Chapter 38

Cavernous Sinus Surgery

Robert Iorga, Amr Mohamed, Fintan Sheerin, Jash Patel, Samuel Mackeith, and Sanjeeva Jeyaretna

Case 38

Interdural Approach to Resect Cavernous Sinus Chondrosarcoma

History

A 65-year-old lady was presented with a right sixth nerve palsy. Her magnetic resonance (MR) scans demonstrated an avidly enhancing lesion occupying the entirety of the right cavernous sinus with compression toward the right optic nerve. A subtemporal interdural approach was employed to access the cavernous sinus with the aim of complete resection. Preoperative magnetic resonance imaging (MRI) is shown in **Fig. 38.1**.

Surgical Steps

1. The patient was positioned in the supine position with a sandbag under the ipsilateral shoulder. The head was fixed in a Mayfield three-pin fixation system. The head was raised above the level of the heart to improve venous drainage, turned 45 degrees to the contralateral side with lateral extension (**Fig. 38.2**).
2. A curvilinear skin incision was performed beginning anterior to the tragus (< 1 cm to avoid injury to the temporal branch of the facial nerve) just above the upper border of the zygomatic arch, extending superiorly toward the superior temporal line, then turning anterior to cross the midline, and ending just on the contralateral side of the midline (**Fig. 38.3**).
The temporalis fascia is kept intact, but the periosteum is included in the incision. Next, the authors performed a subperiosteal dissection of the skin flap anteriorly, followed by a subfascial dissection of the temporalis fascia.
3. The superficial temporal fascia, fat pad, and deep temporal fascia are dissected off the temporalis muscle and reflected anteriorly with the skin flap. This will expose the buccal fat deep to the deep layer of the temporalis fascia. The dissection should continue anteriorly exposing the zygomatic process of the frontal bone (**Fig. 38.4**).
4. The temporalis muscle is detached from the superior temporal line with monopolar cautery and then subperiosteally elevated from the squamous part of the temporal bone using a sharp periosteal elevator. The muscle is reflected inferiorly while the skin flap is reflected anteriorly using fish hook retractors and sharp clips (**Fig. 38.5**).
5. The first burr hole is at the keyhole, just posterior to the zygomatic process of the frontal bone and inferior to the superior temporal line. Authors drill across the

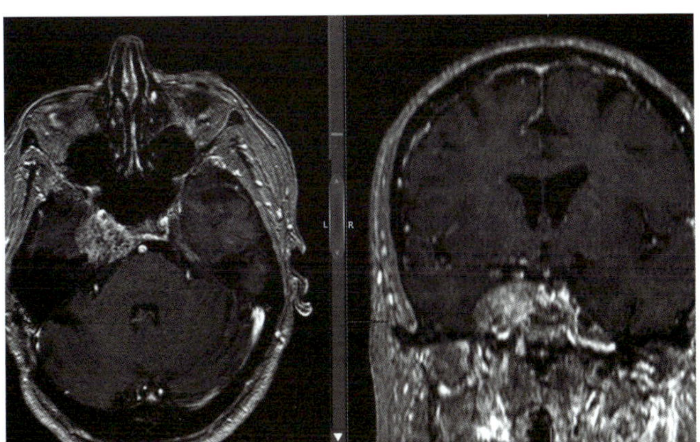

Fig. 38.1 Preoperative MRI with contrast demonstrating the cavernous sinus chondrosarcoma.

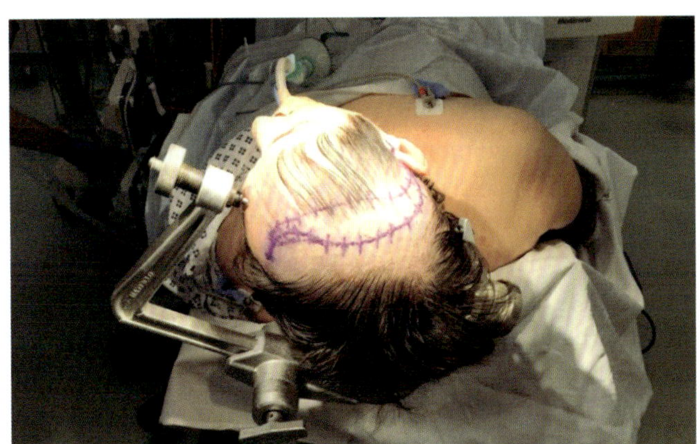

Fig. 38.2 Patient positioning and skin incision. These are two possible incisions (authors favor the posterior incision).

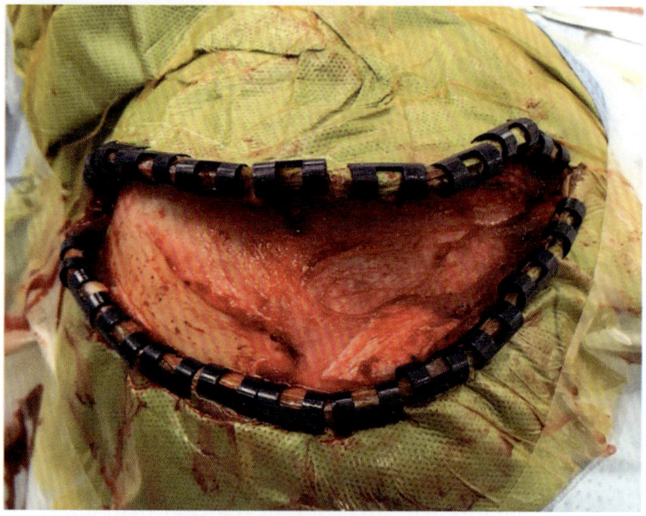

Fig. 38.3 Skin incision: Authors use plastic skin clips on the skin edges for hemostasis.

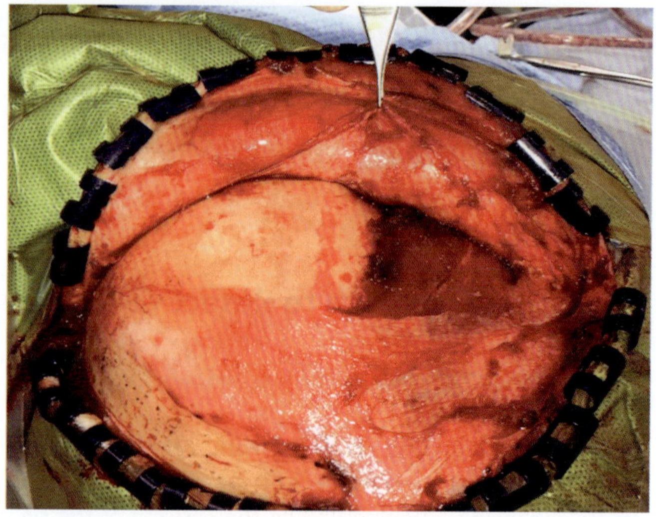

Fig. 38.4 Subfascial dissection of the temporalis fascia.

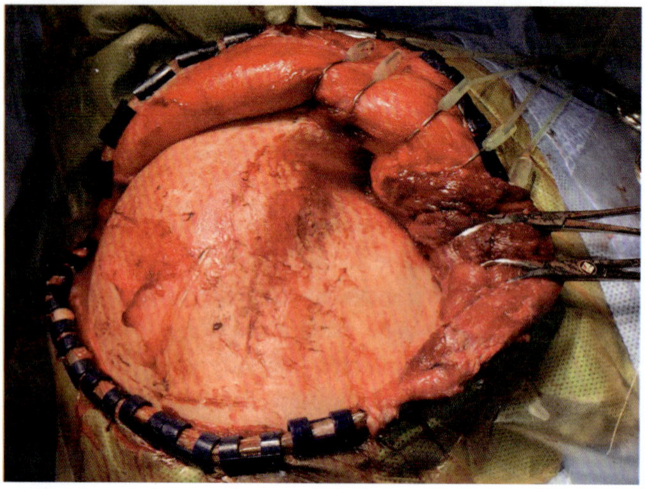

Fig. 38.5 Temporalis muscle dissection.

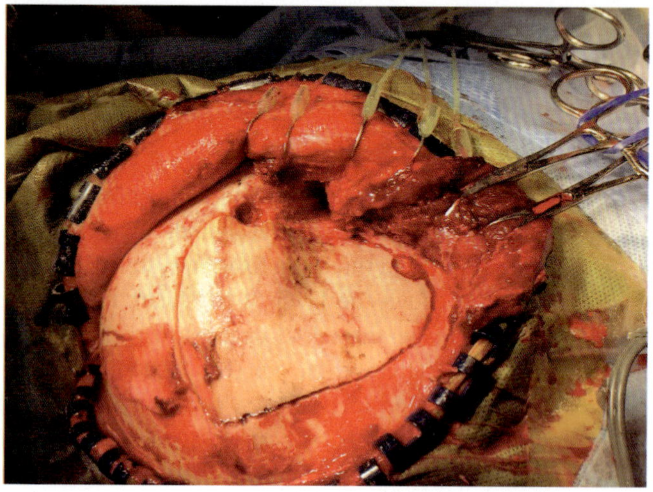

Fig. 38.6 Pterional craniotomy showing the location of the burr holes.

sphenoid ridge using a 4-mm burr or a match head burr to create a trench. The second burr hole is over the temporal lobe. Authors complete the craniotomy by using a craniotome connecting the end of the trench to the keyhole then proceeding posteriorly till the edge of the wound and turn inferiorly to the middle fossa floor then anteriorly to the inferior end of the trench (**Fig. 38.6**).

When lifting the bone flap, authors carefully fracture through the remaining bony attachment at the sphenoid ridge. This is followed by drilling the greater wing of the sphenoid until the lateral edge of the superior orbital fissure is reached. The match head burr is used to flatten the superior surface of the orbital roof, and the authors used a combination of rongeurs and burrs to remove the squamous temporal bone down toward the middle fossa floor.

6. Tumor resection was mainly through an extradural approach. Once the dura is exposed, authors coagulate the meningo-orbital artery (**Fig. 38.7**). An extradural clinoidectomy was not required in this case.
7. After partial transection of the meningo-orbital dural band at the lateral edge of the superior orbital fissure, the dura propria of the temporal lobe is separated from the cavernous sinus dura (**Fig. 38.8**). This exposes the nerves invested in the inner layer as the lateral wall is peeled away.
8. Authors dissected the lateral wall of the cavernous sinus with a Penfield dissector, starting in the area of the sphenoparietal sinus and proceeding

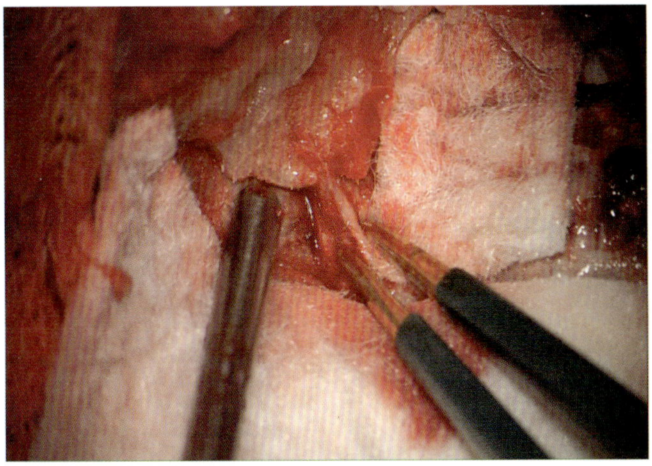

Fig. 38.7 Meningo-orbital artery is shown between the tips of the bipolar.

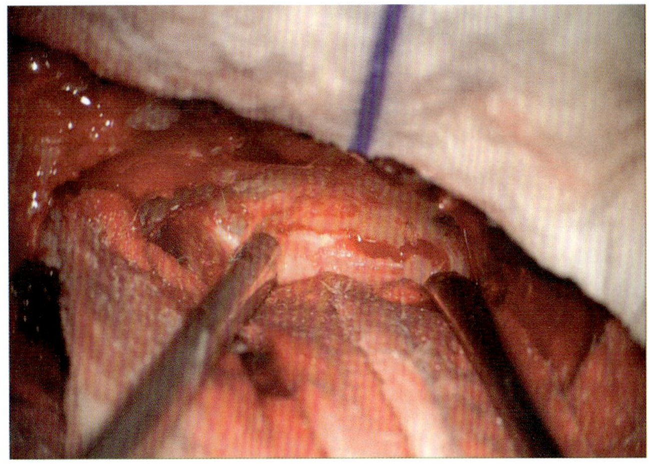

Fig. 38.8 Interdural dissection.

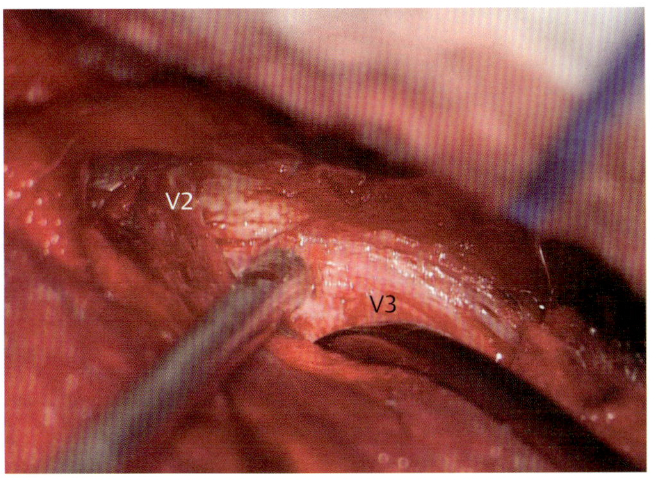

Fig. 38.9 V3 exiting through foramen ovale and V2 exiting through foramen rotundum.

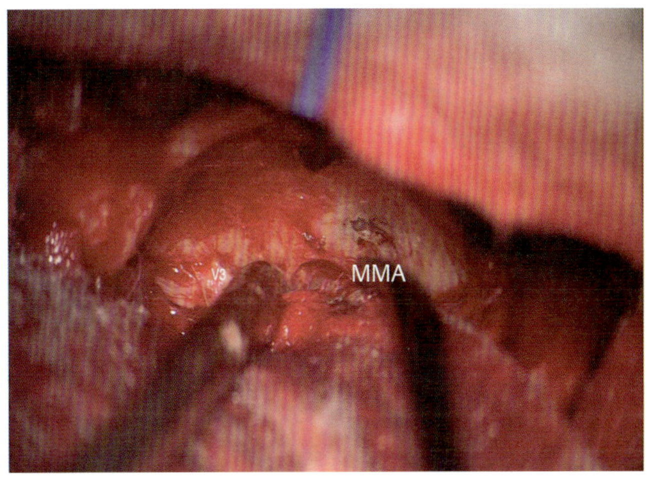

Fig. 38.10 Dissector showing the location of the middle meningeal artery (MMA).

inferolaterally to the regions of V2 and V3 (**Fig. 38.9**) and from anterior to posterior, toward the tentorial edge and Meckel's cave. Foramen rotundum and ovale are identified (**Fig. 38.9**).

9. The middle meningeal artery (MMA) is sacrificed lateral to the posterior edge of V3 (**Fig. 38.10**).
10. The elevation of the middle fossa dura continues posteriorly. Authors identified the cavernous sinus triangles and nerves, such as cranial nerves (CNs) IV and V1 (denoting Parkinson's triangle), the anteromedial triangle (between V1 and V2); the anterolateral triangle (between V2 and V3); the posterolateral triangle, also called Glasscock's triangle (between V3 and the greater petrosal nerve); and the posteromedial triangle, also called Kawase's triangle (lateral to the trigeminal nerve and posterior to the greater petrosal nerve).
11. The petrous carotid is normally exposed under the greater petrosal nerve. In this case, the carotid was pushed inferiorly and anteriorly. A linear incision made in the dura of the cavernous sinus, between and parallel to V1 and V2, unveils the tumor (**Fig. 38.11**).
12. The tumor was soft and grayish-white typical of a chondrosarcoma. The tumor had eroded through the petrous apex creating a corridor to the posterior fossa. The tumor was resected from the cerebellopontine angle and the middle fossa using blunt dissection techniques and suction (**Fig. 38.12**).
13. The authors preserved the adjacent nerves and internally debulked the tumor. Once the bulk was diminished, the authors dissected the tumor capsule from the surrounding cavernous sinus nerves. The bleeding from the cavernous sinus was controlled with Floseal.

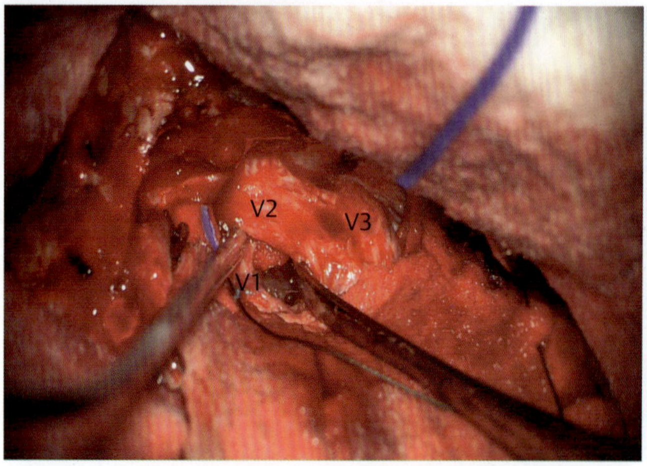

Fig. 38.11 Ophthalmic (V1), maxillary (V2), and mandibular (V3) divisions of the trigeminal nerve.

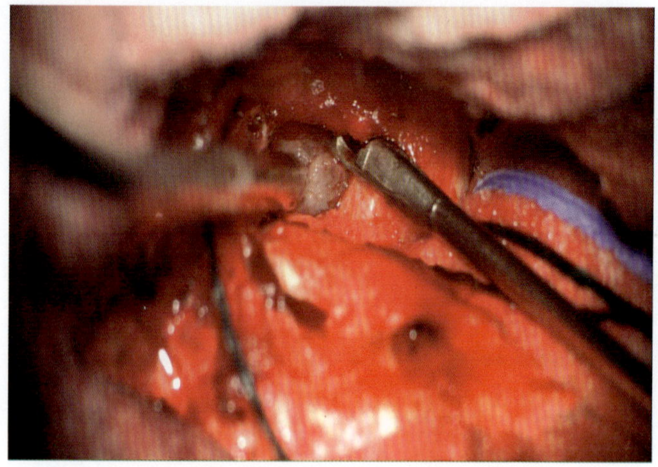

Fig. 38.12 Tumor resection.

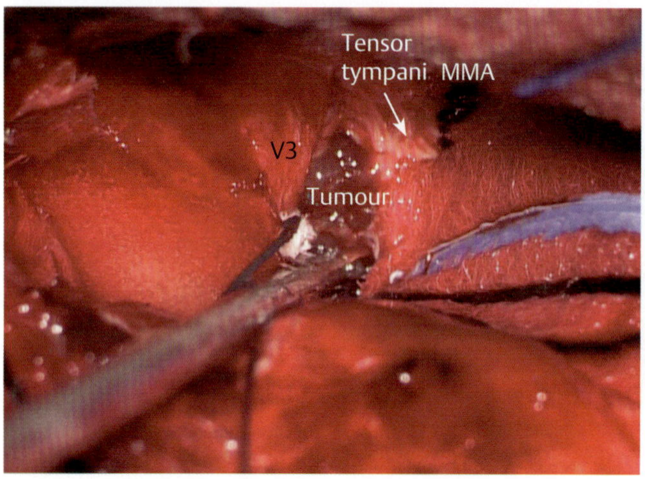

Fig. 38.13 Tumor delivered from Glassock's triangle.

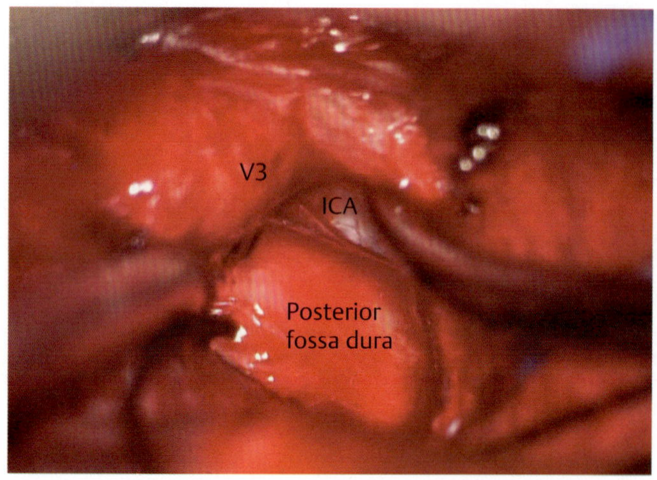

Fig. 38.14 Internal carotid artery (ICA), mandibular branch of trigeminal nerve (V3), posterior fossa dura.

The authors avoided packing the sinus too densely to protect the cranial nerves.

14. The authors identified Glasscock's triangle, which overlies the carotid artery (**Fig. 38.13**).
15. The petrous apex was eroded by the tumor and following tumor removal, the petrous ICA was exposed. The tensor tympani muscle is the posterior limit of the exposure (**Fig. 38.14**).
16. The extent of resection is confirmed using the Stealth navigation (**Fig. 38.15**).
17. After the extradural resection, the authors confirmed that the right optic nerve was decompressed by entering intradurally and splitting the proximal Sylvian fissure (**Fig. 38.16**).
18. The dura is closed in the standard fashion with interrupted sutures. The bone flap is replaced and secured using miniplates (**Fig. 38.17**). The temporalis muscle and its fascial layers are sutured from the superior border of the muscle and affixed at multiple points including to the miniplates.
19. The scalp flap is closed via galea stitches, and the skin is closed using staples (**Fig. 38.18**).
20. Postoperative MRI scan shows gross total resection of the tumor and the patient has made an excellent recovery with the improvement of the sixth nerve palsy and no new neurological deficits (**Fig. 38.19**).

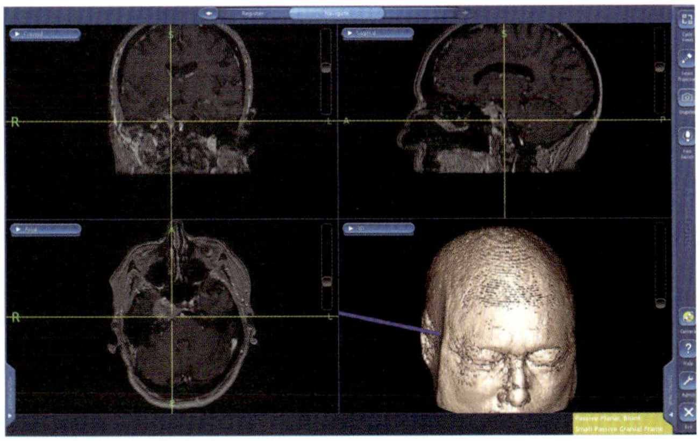

Fig. 38.15 Stealth: Coronal, sagittal, and axial views demonstrating the posterior extent of resection onto the posterior fossa dura.

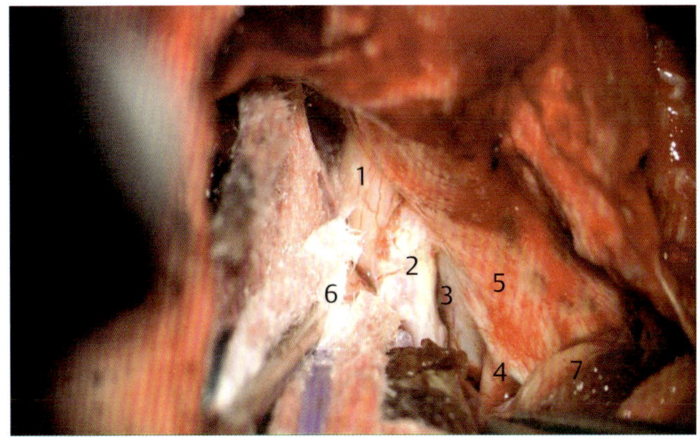

Fig. 38.16 Panoramic view of the intradural cranial nerves and dissected cavernous sinus. 1, optic nerve; 2, internal carotid artery; 3, posterior communicating artery; 4, oculomotor nerve; 5, roof of the cavernous sinus; 6, frontal lobe; 7, temporal lobe.

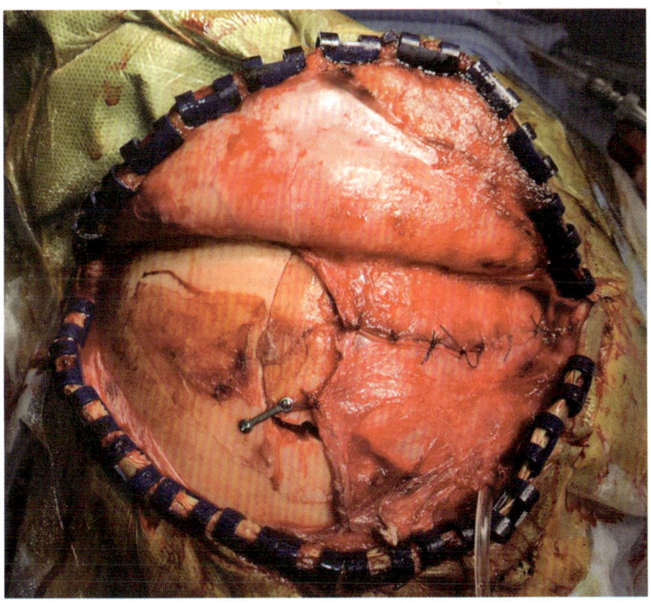

Fig. 38.17 Bone and temporalis fascia closure.

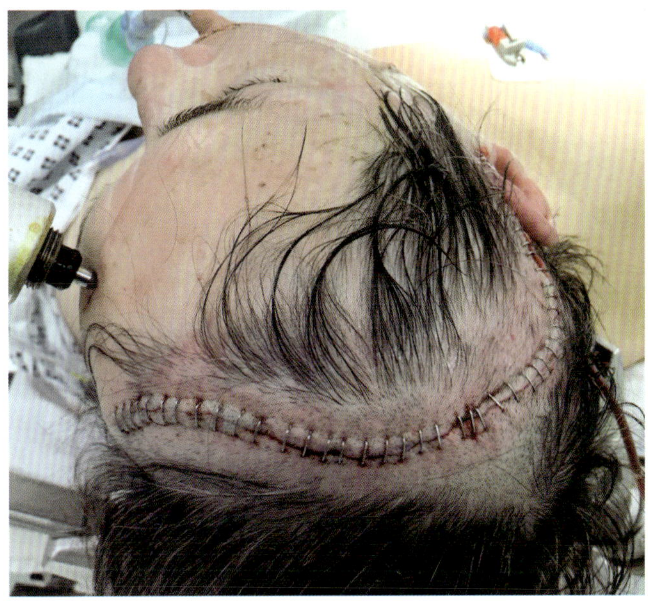

Fig. 38.18 Skin closure.

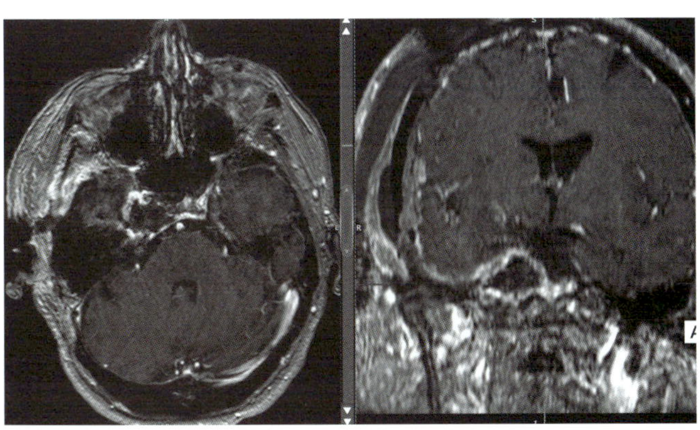

Fig. 38.19 T1 with contrast MRI demonstrating a macroscopic excision of the tumor.

Section XIV

Sinonasal Tumors

Chapter 39 Sinonasal Tumors

Eugene Hung Chih Wong, Revadi Govindaraju, and Prepageran Narayanan

Introduction

Sinonasal mass is a common disease seen by ENT surgeons, which can be either benign or malignant. Malignant sinonasal tumors are rare and account for about 3% of head and neck malignancies.[1] Majority of patients with sinonasal cancer are found to be non-Hispanic white males,[2,3] where most patients present with high T classification without lymph node involvement.[4] This chapter aims to provide some insight into a few of the newer sinonasal tumor entities, focusing more on the malignant types.

Pathologies and Its Variants

There has been a complete overhaul in the fourth edition of the World Health Organization classification of specific tumors related to the nasal cavity, paranasal sinuses, and skull base.[5] Brief descriptions of the major groups of tumors are described below.

Squamous Cell Carcinoma: Keratinizing and Nonkeratinizing

The commonest sinonasal malignancy is squamous cell carcinoma[5] with common variants such as keratinizing (KSCC), nonkeratinizing (NKSCC), spindle cell (sarcomatoid), and lymphoepithelial carcinoma.[6,7] KSCC accounts for 15 to 25% of sinonasal SCC and consists of nests and cords of tumor cells with variable degrees of keratinization and invaginating interconnecting ribbons of squamous epithelium and sharply demarcated epithelial-stromal interface.[5] Necrotic areas and high mitotic activities are also commonly seen in KSCC.[8] Active high-risk human papillomavirus (HPV) is more frequently detected in NKSCC (35–50%) compared to KSCC (0–15%).[5]

NUT Carcinoma

These are high-grade poorly differentiated carcinomas with "round blue cell" morphology and may have foci of mature keratinized squamous cells, brisk mitotic activity, apoptotic bodies, and necrotic areas.[5] Diagnosis usually requires identification of *NUTM1* gene rearrangement (via reverse transcription polymerase chain reaction [RT-PCR] or fluorescence in situ hybridization [FISH])[5] although immunohistochemical nuclear staining for NUT is considered sensitive and specific enough to support this diagnosis as well.[9]

Sinonasal Undifferentiated Carcinoma

These are undifferentiated carcinomas without glandular or squamous features, which are not otherwise classifiable,[8] and are still a diagnosis of exclusion.[5] These tumors are highly aggressive, consist of infiltrating nests of relatively uniform basaloid cells and complete loss of SMARCB1 expression on immunohistochemistry.[5] IDH2 mutations at *R172* were recently identified in 55% of sinonasal undifferentiated carcinomas (SNUCs), suggesting the existence of other genomically defined subsets of SNUCs.[10]

Neuroendocrine Carcinoma: Small Cell and Large Cell Types

Sinonasal neuroendocrine carcinomas (SNECs) are rare (3% of sinonasal tumors) and usually affect middle- to older-aged men.[11–14] They were previously referred to as neuroendocrine tumors using terms such as typical carcinoid, atypical carcinoid, and small cell carcinoma.[5] These are high-grade malignant epithelial neoplasm with morphological and immunohistochemical features of neuroendocrine differentiation.[5] It is important to differentiate SNEC from other sinonasal malignancies with neuroendocrine features such as olfactory neuroblastoma, NUT carcinoma, and SNUC.[5] There is usually a lack of neurofibrillary stroma with no glandular or squamous differentiation, and minimal or absence of lymphoid infiltrate in SNECs.[15,16] Patient tends to present at an advanced stage with local and distant metastases,[14,17] and SNECs generally require multimodality treatment.[11,17,18]

Adenocarcinoma: Intestinal and Nonintestinal Type

Intestinal-type adenocarcinoma (ITAC) is morphologically and immunophenotypically similar to primary adenocarcinomas of the intestines, where the neoplastic cells are positive for markers such as cytokeratin 2–, CDX2, MUC2, and villin.[5] They have a papillary, tubular, solid, or mixed growth pattern, where a minority of cases also showed abundant mucous production.[5] Survival rate of patients with ITAC is variable, depending on the histological grading.[5]

Low-grade nonintestinal-type adenocarcinoma (non-ITAC) have tubular-glandular or papillary architecture, composed of cuboidal to columnar cells with only focal mild atypia, with a histological resemblance to metastatic renal carcinoma and strong positive reaction to CK7 and CAIX.[5] These tumors typically have an excellent prognosis, with rare local recurrence.[5] On the other hand, high-grade non-ITAC is histologically very heterogeneous (both cytologically and architecturally) and commonly shows cellular pleomorphism, brisk mitotic activity, necrosis, and infiltrative growth.[19]

Sinonasal Papilloma: Inverted, Oncocytic, and Exophytic Types

Sinonasal papillomas are benign tumors with three major subtypes: inverted, oncocytic, and exophytic types.[5] Recent updates include its etiological relation to HPV serovars (low and high risk), association with activation of mutation in the *EGFR* gene, unique histological appearance of oncocytic type, and its synchronous malignant associations.[5] Key histological features of sinonasal papillomas are the presence of multilayered epithelium, usually with ciliated columnar epithelial surface layer showing well-developed transepithelial migration of neutrophils and development of microabscesses with mucinous debris.[20–22]

Respiratory Epithelial Lesions

Two rare benign acquired lesions of the sinonasal tracts include the respiratory epithelial adenomatoid hamartoma (REAH) and seromucinous hamartoma (SH).[5] REAH is composed of gland-like structures, arising in continuity with surface epithelium, lined by multilayered ciliated respiratory epithelium, often with admixed mucous-producing cells.[5] Squamous metaplasia, osseous or cartilaginous metaplasia, and inflammatory background can also be present.[5] REAHs have been described in isolation as well as in the setting of concomitant sinonasal disease (from inflammatory polyps to malignancy), which suggests a potential reactive etiology of these lesions.[23]

On the other hand, SH consists of a proliferation of small glands and tubules lined by a single layer of cuboidal cells, organized in clusters and lobules, intermixed with preexisting seromucinous glands of the nasal mucosa.[5] The myoepithelial cells around the proliferating glands are usually not recognized.[5]

Chondromesenchymal Hamartoma

These are benign sinonasal tumors consisting of variably sized nodules of hyaline cartilage within a stromal component of spindle cells[5] where bony trabeculae surrounding the cartilage nodules and epithelial may also be present.[24]

Malignant Soft Tissue Tumors

Biphenotypic Sinonasal Sarcoma

This was formerly known as low-grade sinonasal sarcoma with neural and myogenic features.[5] The distinctive histological features include a bland, spindle cell proliferation arranged in fascicles below an intact, proliferative surface epithelium with elongated and slender nuclei and inconspicuous mitoses.[5] The neoplastic cells also show focal and variable immunoreactivity to S100 protein, smooth muscle actin (SMA), and muscle-specific actin (MSA).[5] It is common to have tumor infiltration into adjacent tissues including bone[25–27] and recurrence is common (50%), although there have not been any reported distant metastases and death from biphenotypic sinonasal sarcoma (BSNS).[25]

Borderline Soft Tissue Tumors

Desmoid-Type Fibromatosis

These are locally infiltrative, nonmetastasizing cytologically bland (myo) fibroblastic neoplasms, associated with *CTNNB1* (β-catenin encoding gene) mutations (for sporadic cases) and *APC* gene mutations (in Gardner's type familial adenomatous polyposis [FAP] syndrome–associated tumors).[5] There is strong immunoreactivity to nuclear β-catenin.[5]

Sinonasal Glomangiopericytoma

These tumors are highly vascularized and unencapsulated with submucosal patternless proliferations and characteristic prominent, thick, acellular peritheliomatous hyalinization.[5] It is also associated with somatic, single nucleotide mutations in the *CTNNB1* gene[28,29] and shows a strong reaction with actins, nuclear β-catenin, and cyclin-D1.[28,30]

Hematolymphoid Tumors

Overall, lymphomas are the third commonest malignancy in the sinonasal tract.[31,32] Hematolymphoid neoplasm with specific predilection for sinonasal tract are referred to as the extranodal natural killer (NK)/T-cell lymphoma nasal type (ENKTLNT).[5,33–36] These tumors have a strong predilection in Latin Americans and East Asians[33,34] and are associated with Epstein–Barr virus (EBV).[5,33–36] There is usually significant geographic necrosis and the neoplastic cells showing irregular contours, fold, and grooves with increased mitoses.[5] The cells are often immunoreactive to CD3 and other cytotoxic markers such as TIA-1, granzyme B, and perforin.[5]

Neuroectodermal/Melanocytic Tumors

Ewing's Sarcoma/Primitive Neuroectodermal Tumors

Ewing's sarcomas are classically defined by the presence of a translocation between *EWSR1* gene on chromosome 22 and the *FLI1* gene on chromosome 11.[37,38] These tumors usually show strong immunoreactivity to CD99.[5]

Olfactory Neuroblastoma

This is a malignant neuroectodermal neoplasm with neuroblastic differentiation, most commonly located at the superior nasal cavity.[5] These tumors usually arise from the cribriform plate of the ethmoid sinus, part of the superior turbinate, or the superior half of the nasal septum.[5] Low-grade tumors usually show the characteristic submucosal, sharply demarcated lobular architecture of small cells with round to oval nuclei and delicate salt and pepper chromatin.[5] On the other hand, high-grade tumors show nuclear pleomorphism, nucleoli, tumor necrosis, increased mitoses, and decreased to absent neuropil.[5] The olfactory neuroblastoma (ONB) cells usually show strong and diffuse immunoreactivity to synaptophysin, chromogranin A, CD56, neurofibrillary protein, and calretinin[39] and the sustentacular cells at the periphery of the cell nests are highlighted by both S100 protein and glial filament acidic protein (GFAP).[5] Hyams' grading system is used to provide prognostic values based on tumor architecture, pleomorphism, neural matrix, mitotic activity, necrosis, and gland/rosette presence.[40,41]

Metastatic Sinonasal Carcinoma

Sinonasal metastases from distant extranasal sites are very rare and about 50% are from renal cell carcinoma.[42] Other common sites of origin are lungs, breasts, colon, prostate, urogenital ridge, gastrointestinal tract, thyroid, and pancreas.[42] The commonest sinonasal site for metastases is the maxillary sinus, followed by sphenoid, ethmoid, frontal sinuses, and nasal cavity.[42] However, different incidences of common primaries in different populations will have different biological behavior for distant metastatic spread.[42] The time from treatment to the development of metastases depends on the presence of metastasis at the initial stage during diagnosis.[42] Diagnosis usually requires a combination of clinical, radiological, and histopathological (specific biomarkers for primary cancers such as carcinoembryonic antigen [CEA] and prostate-specific antigen [PSA]) investigations.[42]

Clinical Features

Sinonasal cancers are usually diagnosed at an advanced stage because patients remain asymptomatic until the tumor has grown large enough to cause symptoms[43] and also because of the fact that early symptoms resemble common sinusitis or rhinitis.[44] For example, SCC frequently presents as unilateral nasal mass, which during the early stages of the disease can appear like benign nasal polyps.[45]

The specific clinical features of some of the newer sinonasal tumor entities have been described in the literature. NUT carcinoma affects patients of all ages with a predilection for young female adults.[5,46,47] These tumors tend to have rapid growth and infiltration with orbital and cranial involvement.[23] Patients usually present with nasal obstruction, epistaxis, and orbital pain.[46,47] Almost 50% of patients have regional or distant metastases at presentation.[46,48] This highly aggressive tumor has a median survival of less than 1 year.[5]

On the other hand, respiratory epithelial lesions (REAH and SH) arise predominantly from the posterior nasal septum and mainly affect adult patients[5] with a male predilection.[23] Patients usually present with nasal congestion, anosmia, and rhinorrhea.[49,50]

Chondromesenchymal hamartoma affects mainly male children with documented local invasiveness involving intracranial extension via the cribriform plate[5] where patients can present with nasal congestion, facial and tooth pain.[45]

Patients with BSNS usually present in the sixth decade with female predilection (2:1)[25–27] and mainly affects the superior nasal cavity and ethmoid sinus.[5] Patients with BSNS present with facial pressure and nasal obstruction.[23]

ENKTLNT commonly present with nonspecific symptoms initially, simulating chronic rhinosinusitis but will eventually progress to perforation, ulceration, and even extension into the soft tissues and facial skin.[5]

In olfactory neuroblastoma, even though there is marked destruction of the olfactory apparatus, only less than 5% of patients reported having anosmia.[5] It usually affects those in the fifth and sixth decades[51–53] with slight male preponderance (1.2:1).[5]

Sinonasal metastatic malignancies usually present with nonspecific symptoms,[54] related to the characteristics of the primary tumor and metastatic sites.[55] For example, RCC is usually highly vascular and patients usually present with epistaxis.[56] Patients with metastases to the nasal cavity may present with epistaxis, increased nasal secretion, and nasal obstruction, whereas maxillary sinus metastases usually present with facial swelling, facial numbness, or eye symptoms.[42] On the other hand, tumors affecting the ethmoid and sphenoid sinus may cause headache, proptosis, diplopia, and vision changes.[42]

In general, there is a relatively low incidence of regional node metastases in sinonasal malignancies during initial diagnosis (ranging from 8.3 to 21.9%),[1,57,58] which could be secondary to the relatively sparse lymphatic drainage in the maxillary sinus, which consists of most of the sinonasal malignancies.[44] The incidence of nodal metastases during follow-up was found to be 13%.[3]

Radiological Features

The fourth edition of the World Health Organization Classification of Head and Neck Tumors described several new and emerging sinonasal tumor entities. Some have a more distinct radiological appearance while others have no pathognomonic findings on imaging alone. Some of the rare emerging entities also lack sufficient published data to draw any conclusion on their radiological features. The imaging review of some of the major new and emerging sinonasal tumors was described in recent literature.

NUT carcinoma can appear as near muscle density on computed tomography (CT) scan with possible bony hyperostosis[23,59] and internal mineralizations.[23] The tumors are hypointense on T1 and heterogenous on T2 magnetic resonance imaging (MRI) scans relative to the cortex, enhancing[60] and are FDG-avid.[25] Positron emission tomography (PET)/CT may play an important role in staging because of the tendency for distant metastases at presentation.[60]

On the other hand, SMARCB1-deficient sinonasal carcinomas (a subtype of SNUC) were reported to be highly aggressive and infiltrative with local skull or brain invasion.[61] On CT scans, these lesions are isodense to muscle, commonly with calcifications and have expansile and erosive patterns involving the skull base.[61] These tumors are isointense on T1 and variable on T2 MRI imaging relative to the cortex, showing FDG avidity in all cases.[61]

REAHs usually appear as well-defined, near muscle density, homogenous mass on CT scan and are isointense on T1 and heterogeneous on T2 with uniform enhancement on MRI scans.[23,62] It is usually not possible to differentiate REAH from SH on imaging alone.[23] Both lesions often give a characteristic half-moon appearance when situated in the olfactory cleft, described as a "crescent sign," on sagittal images without any erosive changes.[23]

Chondromesenchymal hamartomas are often smoothly marginated and expansile with cystic components and calcifications on CT scans.[23] Skull base erosion is often demonstrated on the scans as well.[23] MRI imaging shows solid components that strongly enhance.[63,64]

BSNS usually appears as well-marginated but locally aggressive lesions that can erode through the skull base or into the orbit and may have associated hyperostotic bone formation on CT scans.[23,65] These lesions also avidly enhance and are isointense to hypointense to the cortex on T2 MRI scans.[23]

Olfactory neuroblastomas usually show the classic dumbbell-shaped mass extending across the cribriform plate on imaging.[5]

Key Principles of Surgery

The general treatment strategy is focused on achieving adequate local control while preserving nearby critical structures.[44] Maximal safe surgical resection was found to give the best overall survival in locally advanced sinonasal malignancies.[66]

However, many studies have shown that multimodality approach provides improved treatment survival outcomes,[4,67–69] for example, surgery followed by radiotherapy was shown to be superior to radiotherapy alone.[70,71] Other studies have also demonstrated improved survival in patients receiving preoperative radiotherapy,[70] induction chemotherapy, and adjuvant and neoadjuvant chemoradiotherapy.[4,69] However, the optimum combination and sequencing of radiotherapy and chemotherapy remains controversial,[72] where neither sequences appear to be superior over the other.[4] Neoadjuvant radiotherapy may be preferred in cases where conversion of unresectable disease into resectable disease is required, whereas adjuvant therapy is generally more preferred because of the complexity of operating in a preradiated field.[4] However, there are currently insufficient data to support these hypotheses.

Patients with clinically positive nodes should receive surgery and/or radiotherapy.[1] However, the treatment of patients with N0 neck remains unclear, where some authors stressed the importance of prophylactic neck treatment[73–75] while others concluded that prophylactic irradiation of N0 neck is not indicated because cervical recurrences alone are rare and can be salvaged by neck dissection.[3,76] For carcinoma in the nasal cavity and ethmoid sinus, there is a consensus that prophylactic neck irradiation is not indicated (unless poorly differentiated tumors and tumors involving areas rich in capillary lymphatics) because nodal metastases are very rare and most subsequent neck metastases appeared together with recurrence of the primary tumor.[1] Similarly, for maxillary sinus non-SCC tumor, the rate of lymph node metastases is quite low.[1] On the other hand, a prophylactic neck treatment may be considered in patients with T2 maxillary sinus SCC but not indicated in patients with T3 and T4N0 SCCs.[1] This is because for maxillary sinus SCCs, T2 tumors were found to have a much higher percentage of cervical metastases than T3 and T4 tumor because of their involvement of the floor of maxillary sinus and inferior nasal cavity, which are rich with lymphatic network.[1]

Sinonasal metastatic carcinomas are advanced diseases associated with poor prognosis, therefore usually not treated with curative intent.[42] Surgical resection for palliation may be the only goal for patients with multiple metastatic lesion with close proximity to vital structures.[55] Surgeries are usually performed endoscopically and patients may benefit from preoperative embolization of feeding vessels to reduce intraoperative bleeding.[77] For inoperable tumors, patients can be offered other multimodality treatments such as radiotherapy, chemotherapy, hormone therapy (for urogenital cancer), or iodine ablation therapy (for thyroid cancer) depending on the characteristics of the primary tumor.[42]

Patients with nasal cavity tumors were found to have better OS compared to tumors of other sites of the sinonasal tract.[4] Histology wise, patients with esthesioneuroblastoma were found to have the best OS whereas patients with mucosal melanoma had the poorest OS.[4,78] Negative surgical margin has been shown to be very important in patient survival.[3,4] The initial presence or later development of neck metastases is considered to be an unfavorable prognostic factor.[1,3,73]

Preoperative Work-up

- All patients should have a complete history and thorough ENT examination including any potential complications from tumor extensions to the brain, eye, or oral cavity.
- CT or MRI scans are also crucial before surgical interventions to look for specific features of the tumor as well as its extension.

Postoperative Care

- Routine postoperative care should be carried out especially looking for any signs of bleeding, eye and brain injuries.
- ENT clinic follow-up and postoperative imaging are carried out to ensure no recurrences are necessary.

Indications and Contraindications

Factors to be considered before surgical intervention include disease staging, the extent of the tumor, surgeons' expertise, as well as patients' preference. Contraindications to surgical resection of primary tumor include large intracranial extension with the involvement of the brain, bilateral cavernous sinus, and bilateral optic nerve or chiasma.[1]

Complications

Complications of operation depend on the staging of the tumor and its extension to nearby critical structures. Common complications include epistaxis, injury to orbit and brain, as well as postoperative synechiae and crusting.

Tips and Pearls

- The fourth edition of the World Health Organization Classification of Head and Neck Tumors described several new and emerging sinonasal tumor entities.
- The commonest sinonasal malignancy is SCC. Other pathologies include NUT carcinoma, SNUC, neuroendocrine carcinoma, adenocarcinoma, sinonasal papilloma, respiratory epithelial lesions, chondromesenchymal hamartoma, and BSNS.
- Patients with sinonasal malignancies tend to present late because they either remain asymptomatic or present with nonspecific nasal symptoms initially.
- Some tumors have a distinct radiological appearance while others have no pathognomonic findings on imaging alone.
- The key surgical principle for the management of sinonasal malignancies is maximal safe surgical resection while preserving nearby critical structures. A multimodality approach is found to improve patient survival.
- ENT clinic follow-up and postoperative imaging are carried out to ensure no recurrences are necessary.

References

1. Cantù G, Bimbi G, Miceli R, et al. Lymph node metastases in malignant tumors of the paranasal sinuses: prognostic value and treatment. Arch Otolaryngol Head Neck Surg 2008; 134(2):170–177
2. Danesh-Sani SA, Sarafraz A, Chamani M, Derakhshandeh H. Paranasal sinuses malignancies: a 12-year review of clinical characteristics. Med Oral Patol Oral Cir Bucal 2016;21(5): e626–e630
3. Dulguerov P, Jacobsen MS, Allal AS, Lehmann W, Calcaterra T. Nasal and paranasal sinus carcinoma: are we making progress? A series of 220 patients and a systematic review. Cancer 2001;92(12):3012–3029

4. Robin TP, Jones BL, Gordon OM, et al. A comprehensive comparative analysis of treatment modalities for sinonasal malignancies. Cancer 2017;123(16):3040–3049

5. Thompson LDR, Franchi A. New tumor entities in the 4th edition of the World Health Organization classification of head and neck tumors: nasal cavity, paranasal sinuses and skull base. Virchows Arch 2018;472(3):315–330

6. Kees UR, Mulcahy MT, Willoughby ML. Intrathoracic carcinoma in an 11-year-old girl showing a translocation t(15;19). Am J Pediatr Hematol Oncol 1991;13(4):459–464

7. Kubonishi I, Takehara N, Iwata J, et al. Novel t(15;19)(q15;p13) chromosome abnormality in a thymic carcinoma. Cancer Res 1991;51(12):3327–3328

8. Stelow EB, Bishop JA. Update from the 4th edition of the world health organization classification of head and neck tumours: Tumors of the nasal cavity, paranasal sinuses and skull base. Head Neck Pathol 2017;11(1):3–15

9. Haack H, Johnson LA, Fry CJ, et al. Diagnosis of NUT midline carcinoma using a NUT-specific monoclonal antibody. Am J Surg Pathol 2009;33(7):984–991

10. Jo VY, Chau NG, Hornick JL, Krane JF, Sholl LM. Recurrent IDH2 R172X mutations in sinonasal undifferentiated carcinoma. Mod Pathol 2017;30(5):650–659

11. Patel TD, Vazquez A, Dubal PM, Baredes S, Liu JK, Eloy JA. Sinonasal neuroendocrine carcinoma: a population-based analysis of incidence and survival. Int Forum Allergy Rhinol 2015;5(5):448–453

12. Chai L, Ying HF, Wu TT, et al. Clinical features and hypoxic marker expression of primary sinonasal and laryngeal small-cell neuroendocrine carcinoma: a small case series. World J Surg Oncol 2014;12:199

13. Huang S, Zhao Y, He L, Dan LV, Yang F. [Clinical analysis and review of 8 cases with sinonasal neuroendocrine carcinoma]. Lin Chung Er Bi Yan Hou Tou Jing Wai Ke Za Zhi 2013;27(14): 751–753

14. Qian GH, Shang JB, Wang KJ, Tan Z. [Diagnosis and treatment of 11 cases with sinonasal neuroendocrine carcinoma]. Zhonghua Er Bi Yan Hou Tou Jing Wai Ke Za Zhi 2011;46(12): 1033–1035

15. Weinreb I, Perez-Ordoñez B. Non-small cell neuroendocrine carcinoma of the sinonasal tract and nasopharynx. Report of 2 cases and review of the literature. Head Neck Pathol 2007;1(1):21–26

16. Sugita Y, Kusano K, Tokunaga O, et al. Olfactory neuroepithelioma: an immunohistochemical and ultrastructural study. Neuropathology 2006;26(5):400–408

17. Mitchell EH, Diaz A, Yilmaz T, et al. Multimodality treatment for sinonasal neuroendocrine carcinoma. Head Neck 2012;34(10):1372–1376

18. van der Laan TP, Bij HP, van Hemel BM, et al. The importance of multimodality therapy in the treatment of sinonasal neuroendocrine carcinoma. Eur Arch Otorhinolaryngol 2013;270(9):2565–2568

19. Stelow EB, Jo VY, Mills SE, Carlson DL. A histologic and immunohistochemical study describing the diversity of tumors classified as sinonasal high-grade nonintestinal adenocarcinomas. Am J Surg Pathol 2011;35(7):971–980

20. Barnes L. Schneiderian papillomas and nonsalivary glandular neoplasms of the head and neck. Mod Pathol 2002;15(3): 279–297

21. Rodic N, Maleki Z. Cytomorphologic findings of Schneiderian papilloma: a case report. Diagn Cytopathol 2012;40(12): 1100–1103

22. Sarioglu S. Update on inverted epithelial lesions of the sinonasal and nasopharyngeal regions. Head Neck Pathol 2007;1(1):44–49

23. Dean KE, Shatzkes D, Phillips CD. Imaging review of new and emerging sinonasal tumors and tumor-like entities from the fourth edition of the world health organization classification of head and neck tumors. AJNR Am J Neuroradiol 2019;40(4): 584–590

24. Ozolek JA, Carrau R, Barnes EL, Hunt JL. Nasal chondromesenchymal hamartoma in older children and adults: series and immunohistochemical analysis. Arch Pathol Lab Med 2005;129(11):1444–1450

25. Lewis JT, Oliveira AM, Nascimento AG, et al. Low-grade sinonasal sarcoma with neural and myogenic features: a clinicopathologic analysis of 28 cases. Am J Surg Pathol 2012;36(4):517–525

26. Powers KA, Han LM, Chiu AG, Aly FZ. Low-grade sinonasal sarcoma with neural and myogenic features—diagnostic challenge and pathogenic insight. Oral Surg Oral Med Oral Pathol Oral Radiol 2015;119(5):e265–e269

27. Huang SC, Ghossein RA, Bishop JA, et al. Novel pax3-ncoa1 fusions in biphenotypic sinonasal sarcoma with focal rhabdomyoblastic differentiation. Am J Surg Pathol 2016; 40(1):51–59

28. Lasota J, Felisiak-Golabek A, Aly FZ, Wang ZF, Thompson LD, Miettinen M. Nuclear expression and gain-of-function β-catenin mutation in glomangiopericytoma (sinonasal-type hemangiopericytoma): insight into pathogenesis and a diagnostic marker. Mod Pathol 2015;28(5):715–720

29. Haller F, Bieg M, Moskalev EA, et al. Recurrent mutations within the amino-terminal region of β-catenin are probable key molecular driver events in sinonasal hemangiopericytoma. Am J Pathol 2015;185(2):563–571

30. Thompson LD, Miettinen M, Wenig BM. Sinonasal-type hemangiopericytoma: a clinicopathologic and immunophenotypic analysis of 104 cases showing perivascular myoid differentiation. Am J Surg Pathol 2003;27(6):737–749

31. Hoffman HT, Karnell LH, Funk GF, Robinson RA, Menck HR. The National Cancer Data Base report on cancer of the head

and neck. Arch Otolaryngol Head Neck Surg 1998;124(9): 951–962

32. Cooper JS, Porter K, Mallin K, et al. National Cancer Database report on cancer of the head and neck: 10-year update. Head Neck 2009;31(6):748–758
33. Dubal PM, Dutta R, Vazquez A, Patel TD, Baredes S, Eloy JA. A comparative population-based analysis of sinonasal diffuse large B-cell and extranodal NK/T-cell lymphomas. Laryngoscope 2015;125(5):1077–1083
34. Aoki R, Karube K, Sugita Y, et al. Distribution of malignant lymphoma in Japan: analysis of 2260 cases, 2001-2006. Pathol Int 2008;58(3):174–182
35. Kreisel FH. Hematolymphoid lesions of the sinonasal tract. Head Neck Pathol 2016;10(1):109–117
36. Crane GM, Duffield AS. Hematolymphoid lesions of the sinonasal tract. Semin Diagn Pathol 2016;33(2):71–80
37. Folpe AL, Goldblum JR, Rubin BP, et al. Morphologic and immunophenotypic diversity in Ewing family tumors: a study of 66 genetically confirmed cases. Am J Surg Pathol 2005;29(8):1025–1033
38. Bishop JA, Alaggio R, Zhang L, Seethala RR, Antonescu CR. Adamantinoma-like Ewing family tumors of the head and neck: a pitfall in the differential diagnosis of basaloid and myoepithelial carcinomas. Am J Surg Pathol 2015;39(9): 1267–1274
39. Wooff JC, Weinreb I, Perez-Ordonez B, Magee JF, Bullock MJ. Calretinin staining facilitates differentiation of olfactory neuroblastoma from other small round blue cell tumors in the sinonasal tract. Am J Surg Pathol 2011;35(12):1786–1793
40. Saade RE, Hanna EY, Bell D. Prognosis and biology in esthesioneuroblastoma: the emerging role of Hyams grading system. Curr Oncol Rep 2015;17(1):423
41. Tajudeen BA, Arshi A, Suh JD, St John M, Wang MB. Importance of tumor grade in esthesioneuroblastoma survival: a population-based analysis. JAMA Otolaryngol Head Neck Surg 2014;140(12):1124–1129
42. Chang MH, Kuo YJ, Ho CY, Kuan EC, Lan MY. Metastatic tumors of the sinonasal cavity: a 15-year review of 17 cases. J Clin Med 2019;8(4):8
43. Turner JH, Reh DD. Incidence and survival in patients with sinonasal cancer: a historical analysis of population-based data. Head Neck 2012;34(6):877–885
44. Lee WH, Choi SH, Kim SH, Choi EC, Lee CG, Keum KC. Elective neck treatment in clinically node-negative paranasal sinus carcinomas: impact on treatment outcome. Radiat Oncol J 2018;36(4):304–316
45. Belli S, Yildirim M, Eroglu S, Emre FK. Single-sided sinonasal mass: a retrospective study. North Clin Istanb 2018;5(2): 139–143
46. Bauer DE, Mitchell CM, Strait KM, et al. Clinicopathologic features and long-term outcomes of NUT midline carcinoma. Clin Cancer Res 2012;18(20):5773–5779
47. Kakkar A, Antony VM, Irugu DVK, Adhikari N, Jain D. Nut midline carcinoma: A series of five cases, including one with unusual clinical course. Head Neck Pathol 2018;12(2): 230–236
48. Edgar M, Caruso AM, Kim E, Foss RD. Nut midline carcinoma of the nasal cavity. Head Neck Pathol 2017;11(3):389–392
49. Huang YW, Kuo YJ, Ho CY, Lan MY. Sinonasal seromucinous hamartoma. Eur Arch Otorhinolaryngol 2018;275(3): 743–749
50. Tatekawa H, Shimono T, Ohsawa M, Doishita S, Sakamoto S, Miki Y. Imaging features of benign mass lesions in the nasal cavity and paranasal sinuses according to the 2017 WHO classification. Jpn J Radiol 2018;36(6):361–381
51. Jethanamest D, Morris LG, Sikora AG, Kutler DI. Esthesioneuroblastoma: a population-based analysis of survival and prognostic factors. Arch Otolaryngol Head Neck Surg 2007;133(3):276–280
52. Platek ME, Merzianu M, Mashtare TL, et al. Improved survival following surgery and radiation therapy for olfactory neuroblastoma: analysis of the SEER database. Radiat Oncol 2011;6:41
53. Broich G, Pagliari A, Ottaviani F. Esthesioneuroblastoma: a general review of the cases published since the discovery of the tumour in 1924. Anticancer Res 1997;17(4A):2683–2706
54. Weber AL, Stanton AC. Malignant tumors of the paranasal sinuses: radiologic, clinical, and histopathologic evaluation of 200 cases. Head Neck Surg 1984;6(3):761–776
55. Gottlieb MD, Roland JT Jr. Paradoxical spread of renal cell carcinoma to the head and neck. Laryngoscope 1998;108(9): 1301–1305
56. Aziz SA, Sznol J, Adeniran A, Colberg JW, Camp RL, Kluger HM. Vascularity of primary and metastatic renal cell carcinoma specimens. J Transl Med 2013;11:15
57. Katz TS, Mendenhall WM, Morris CG, Amdur RJ, Hinerman RW, Villaret DB. Malignant tumors of the nasal cavity and paranasal sinuses. Head Neck 2002;24(9):821–829
58. Homma A, Hayashi R, Matsuura K, et al. Lymph node metastasis in t4 maxillary sinus squamous cell carcinoma: incidence and treatment outcome. Ann Surg Oncol 2014; 21(5):1706–1710
59. Bair RJ, Chick JF, Chauhan NR, French C, Madan R. Demystifying NUT midline carcinoma: radiologic and pathologic correlations of an aggressive malignancy. AJR Am J Roentgenol 2014;203(4):W391-9
60. Shaikh F, Pagedar N, Awan O, McNeely P. Sinonasal nut-midline carcinoma—a multimodality approach to diagnosis, staging and post-surgical restaging. Cureus 2015;7(7):e288

61. Shatzkes DR, Ginsberg LE, Wong M, et al. Imaging appearance of smarcb1 (ini1)-deficient sinonasal carcinoma: a newly described sinonasal malignancy. AJNR Am J Neuroradiol 2016;37(10):1925–1929

62. Seol JG, Livolsi VA, O'Malley BW Jr, Chen JY, Loevner LA. Respiratory epithelial adenomatoid hamartoma of the bilateral olfactory recesses: a neoplastic mimic? AJNR Am J Neuroradiol 2010;31(2):277–279

63. Wang T, Li W, Wu X, et al. Nasal chondromesenchymal hamartoma in young children: CT and MRI findings and review of the literature. World J Surg Oncol 2014;12:257

64. Yao-Lee A, Ryan M, Rajaram V. Nasal chondromesenchymal hamartoma: correlation of typical MR, CT and pathological findings. Pediatr Radiol 2011;41(5):675–677

65. Hellquist HB, Lundgren J. Neurogenic sarcoma of the sinonasal tract. J Laryngol Otol 1991;105(3):186–190

66. Resto VA, Chan AW, Deschler DG, Lin DT. Extent of surgery in the management of locally advanced sinonasal malignancies. Head Neck 2008;30(2):222–229

67. Chen NX, Chen L, Wang JL, et al. A clinical study of multimodal treatment for orbital organ preservation in locally advanced squamous cell carcinoma of the nasal cavity and paranasal sinus. Jpn J Clin Oncol 2016;46(8):727–734

68. Corvò R. Evidence-based radiation oncology in head and neck squamous cell carcinoma. Radiother Oncol 2007;85(1): 156–170

69. Lee MM, Vokes EE, Rosen A, Witt ME, Weichselbaum RR, Haraf DJ. Multimodality therapy in advanced paranasal sinus carcinoma: superior long-term results. Cancer J Sci Am 1999;5(4):219–223

70. Guntinas-Lichius O, Kreppel MP, Stuetzer H, Semrau R, Eckel HE, Mueller RP. Single modality and multimodality treatment of nasal and paranasal sinuses cancer: a single institution experience of 229 patients. Eur J Surg Oncol 2007;33(2):222–228

71. Mendenhall WM, Amdur RJ, Morris CG, et al. Carcinoma of the nasal cavity and paranasal sinuses. Laryngoscope 2009;119(5):899–906

72. Khademi B, Moradi A, Hoseini S, Mohammadianpanah M. Malignant neoplasms of the sinonasal tract: report of 71 patients and literature review and analysis. Oral Maxillofac Surg 2009;13(4):191–199

73. Le QT, Fu KK, Kaplan MJ, Terris DJ, Fee WE, Goffinet DR. Lymph node metastasis in maxillary sinus carcinoma. Int J Radiat Oncol Biol Phys 2000;46(3):541–549

74. Jeremic B, Shibamoto Y, Milicic B, et al. Elective ipsilateral neck irradiation of patients with locally advanced maxillary sinus carcinoma. Cancer 2000;88(10):2246–2251

75. Paulino AC, Fisher SG, Marks JE. Is prophylactic neck irradiation indicated in patients with squamous cell carcinoma of the maxillary sinus? Int J Radiat Oncol Biol Phys 1997;39(2):283–289

76. Kim GE, Chung EJ, Lim JJ, et al. Clinical significance of neck node metastasis in squamous cell carcinoma of the maxillary antrum. Am J Otolaryngol 1999;20(6):383–390

77. López F, Devaney KO, Hanna EY, Rinaldo A, Ferlito A. Metastases to nasal cavity and paranasal sinuses. Head Neck 2016;38(12):1847–1854

78. Manolidis S, Donald PJ. Malignant mucosal melanoma of the head and neck: review of the literature and report of 14 patients. Cancer 1997;80(8):1373–1386

Chapter 40 Endonasal Endoscopic Management of Sinonasal Tumors

Case 40A

Endoscopic Excision of an Inverted Papilloma with Extension to the Orbit, Infratemporal Fossa, and the Base of Skull

Adzreil Bakri, Michel Roethlisberger, and Prepageran Narayanan

History

A 71-year-old Indonesian man with a history of inverted papilloma of the left nasal cavity, which was operated on 5 years ago, presented with progressive left nose block for the past 1 year. There were no other complaints. His vision was normal. Endoscopic examination revealed a pinkish fleshy mass occupying the whole left nasal cavity. Biopsies taken in the outpatient clinic reported an inverted papilloma. A computed tomography (CT) scan and magnetic resonance imaging (MRI) revealed a large tumor in the left nasal cavity with extensions to the skull base, the orbit, and the infratemporal fossa (**Fig. 40A.1** and **Fig. 40A.2**).

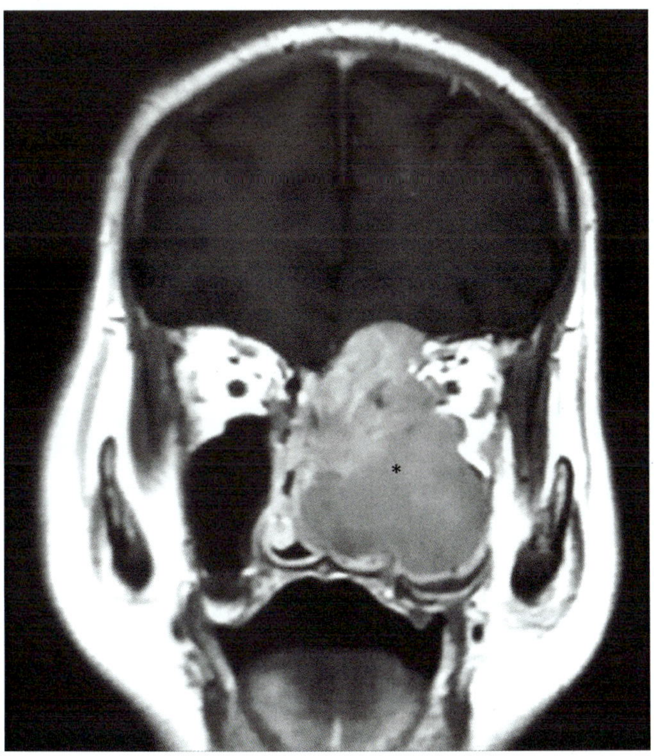

Fig. 40A.1 A coronal view of the T1-weighted MRI section demonstrating a tumorous mass (*) in the left nasal cavity extending intracranially (extradural) and into the left orbit.

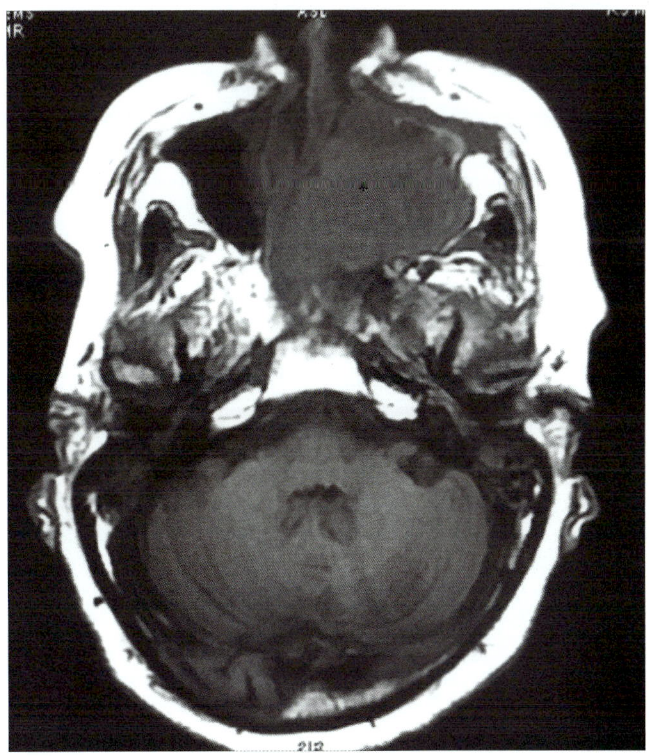

Fig. 40A.2 An axial T1-weighted MRI section demonstrates the gross tumor (*) extension posteriorly to the nasopharynx and laterally to the infratemporal fossa.

Surgical Steps

1. The patient is positioned supine and reverse Trendelenburg (30 degrees) with the neck slightly extended under general anesthesia.
2. The nose is decongested with nasal packing as per the institution's usual method.
3. The nasal packs are removed and the nasal cavity is inspected endoscopically.
4. Tumor extension is assessed endoscopically. In this case, the tumor fully occupies the nasal cavity with extensions superiorly to the skull base, posteriorly to the nasopharynx, and attachments to the lateral wall of the nose (**Fig. 40A.3**).
5. A biopsy is taken from the tumor (**Fig. 40A.4**).
6. The free sides of the tumor are packed with adrenaline-soaked ribbon gauze to reduce the incidence of bleeding.
7. The anterior and inferior bulk of the tumor is removed using a combination of a powered microdebrider and Luc's forceps. This dissection is made to clear the floor of the nasal cavity down to the nasopharynx so that anatomical relations could be established. Excessive bleeding from the tumor during dissection can be reduced and cleared with the help of an assistant holding a suction tube (**Fig. 40A.5** and **Fig. 40A.6**).

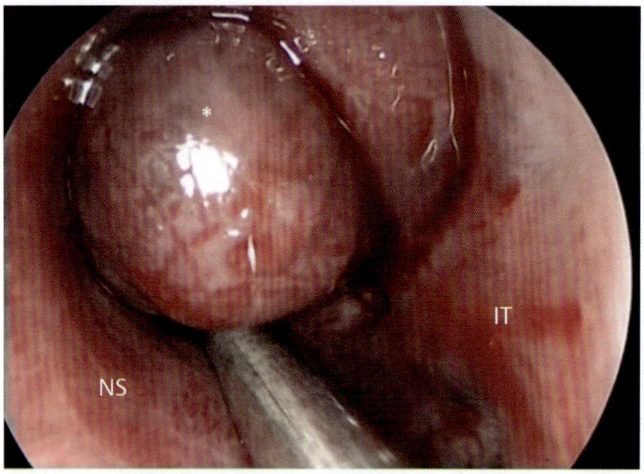

Fig. 40A.3 Main bulk of the tumor (*) occupying the left nasal cavity.

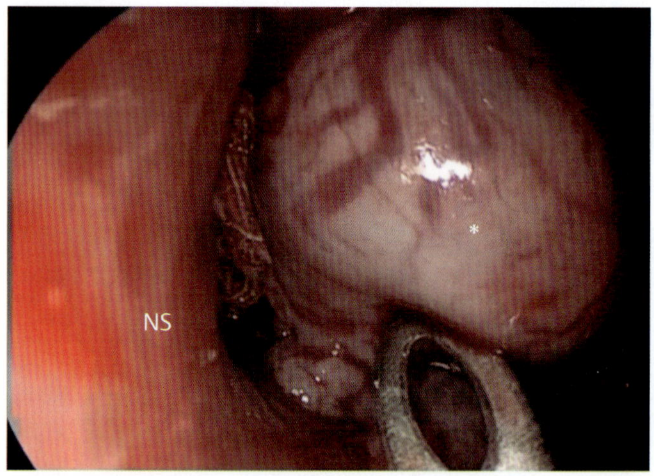

Fig. 40A.4 A biopsy is taken from the tumor (*).

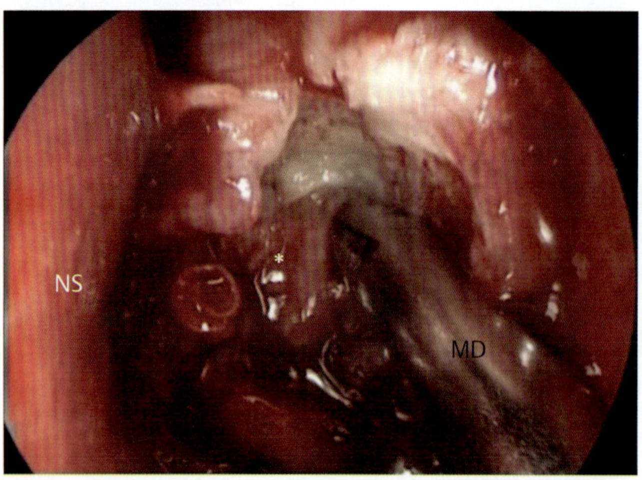

Fig. 40A.5 The tumor (*) is removed with a microdebrider (MD), clearing the floor of the nasal cavity until the nasopharynx.

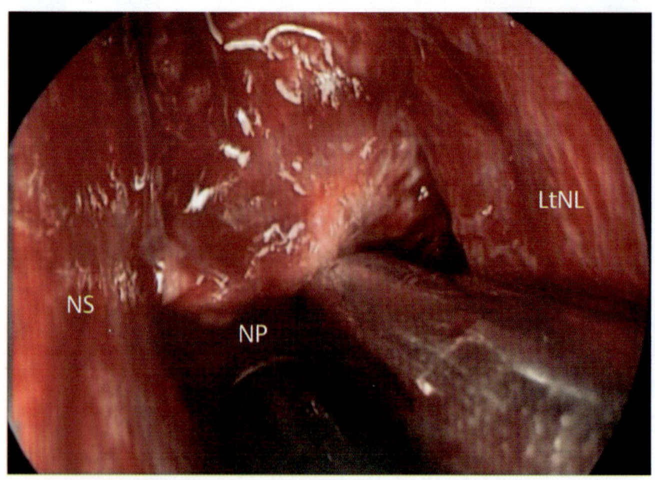

Fig. 40A.6 The left nasopharynx (NP) is visualized at the end of the suction probe.

8. Once the floor of the left nasal cavity and nasopharynx are cleared, attention is given superomedially to where the tumor is loosely attached to the septum and skull base. The tumor is dissected away from these structures gently using a blunt suction tube or a Freer elevator. Tumor which is free or not attached is carefully removed using the microdebrider or forceps (**Fig. 40A.7, Fig. 40A.8, Fig. 40A.9**).

9. The same technique of blunt dissection and suction is used for the tumor parts attaching to the medial orbit, infratemporal fossa, and maxilla. After creating a plane with blunt dissection between these structures, the tumor is debrided away. The use of angled endoscopes (30- or 70 degrees) is necessary to inspect tumor attachments to the lateral or anterior walls of the maxilla (**Fig. 40A.10, Fig. 40A.11, Fig. 40A.12**).

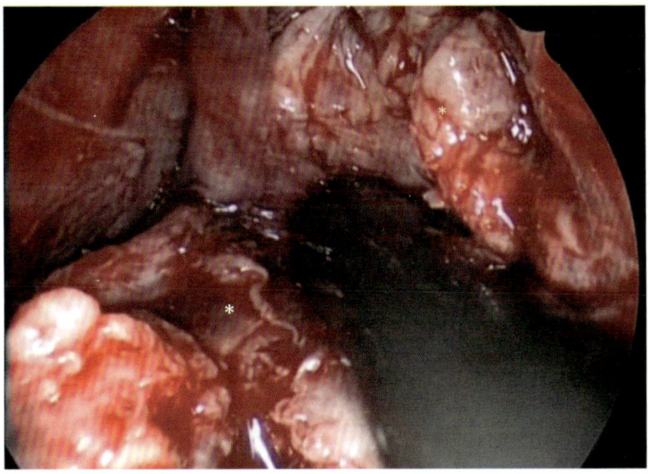

Fig. 40A.7 Blunt dissection creating a plane between the tumor (*) and the skull base.

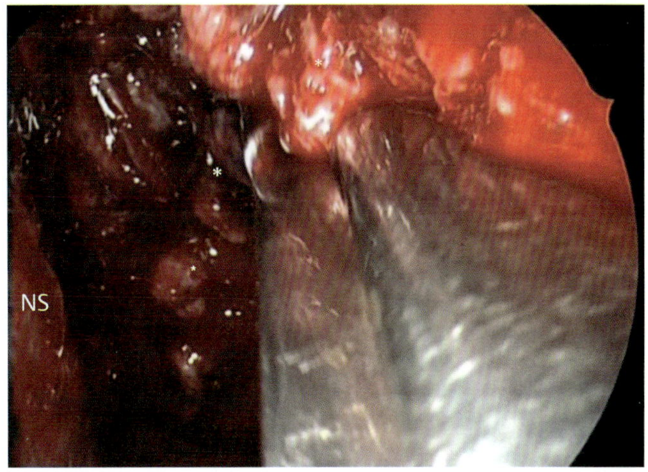

Fig. 40A.8 Loose tumor (*) is removed by a microdebrider or forceps.

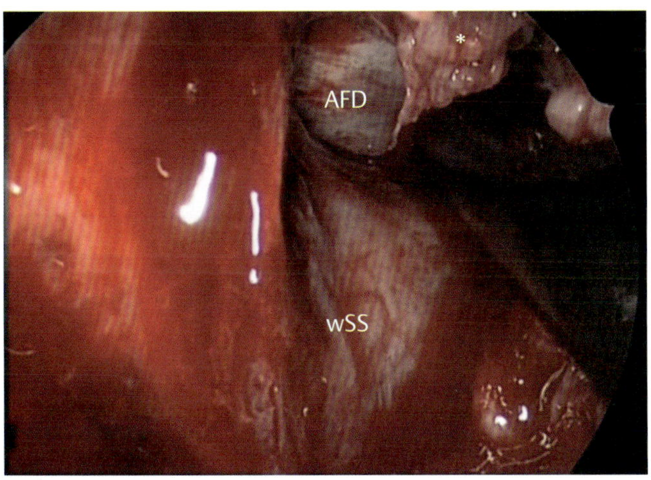

Fig. 40A.9 Peeling of the tumor (*) from anterior fossa dura (AFD).

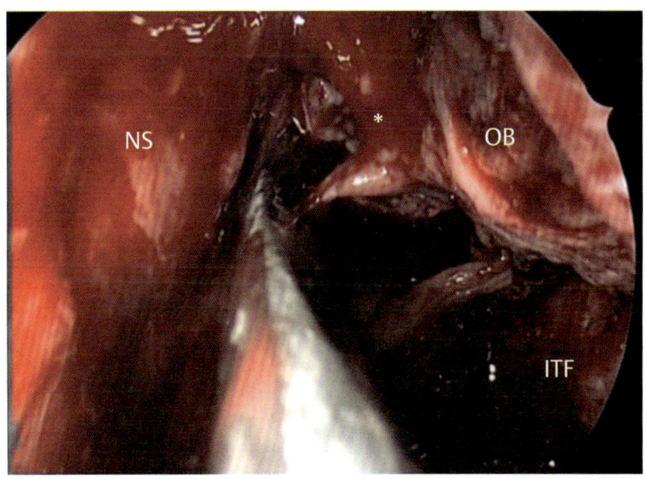

Fig. 40A.10 Blunt dissection creating a plane between the tumor (*) and the left orbit (OB).

10. Once complete tumor clearance has been achieved (**Fig. 40A.13**), the nasal cavity is flushed with normal saline and remaining bleeding points are secured diligently. The raw areas of the nasal cavity are laid with oxidized cellulose polymers (Surgicel® Original Absorbable Hemostat; Ethicon, Johnson&Johnson, USA) and absorbable gelatin sponges (Surgifoam® Absorbable Gelatin Sponge; Ethicon, Johnson&Johnson, USA) and packed with synthetic biodegradable foams (Nasopore®; Stryker, Germany).

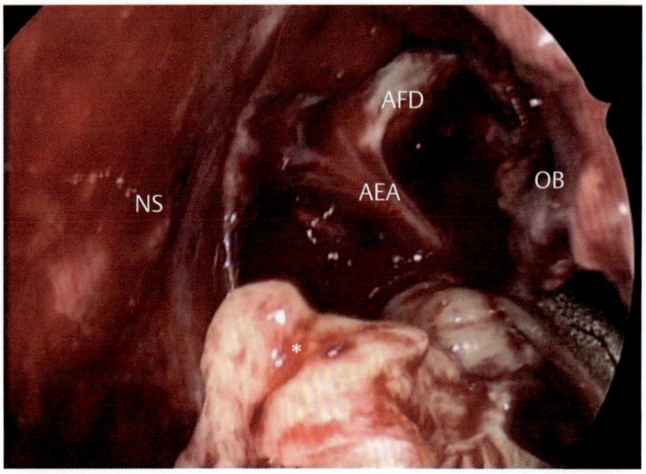

Fig. 40A.11 The tumor (*) is removed from the left orbit (OB) and skull base revealing the anterior ethmoidal artery (AEA) in the background.

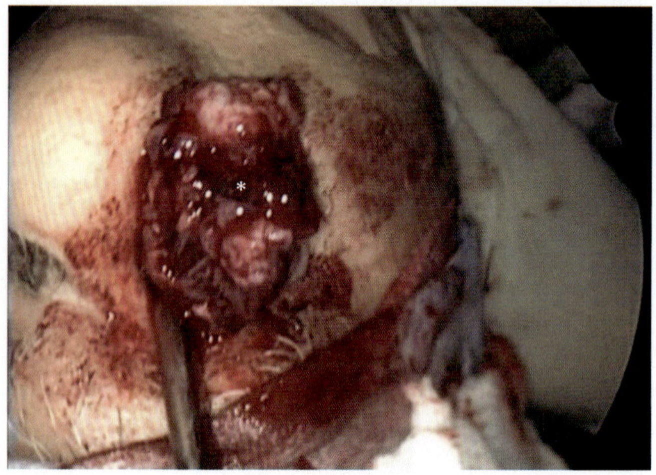

Fig. 40A.12 Loose tumor (*) is removed piecemeal using a combination of microdebrider and Blakesley's or Luc's forceps.

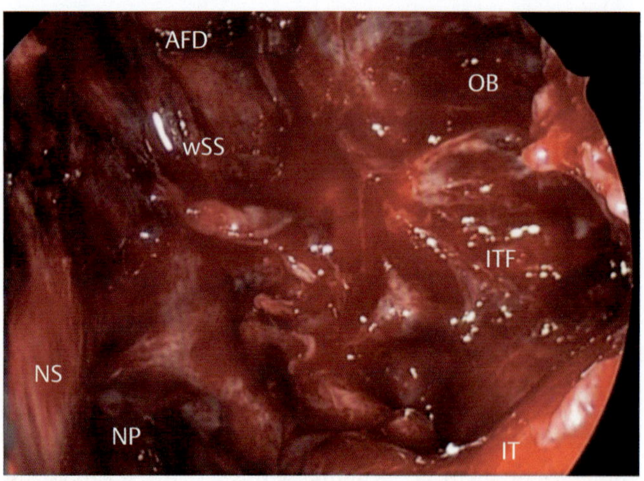

Fig. 40A.13 Final view of the left nasal cavity showing complete tumor removal.

Case 40B

Endoscopic Excision of a Sinonasal Adenoid Cystic Carcinoma

Eugene Hung Chih Wong, Revadi Govindaraju, and Prepageran Narayanan

History

A 47-year-old man presented with nasal block for 3 months associated with recurrent episodes of epistaxis. Nasal endoscopy revealed a tumor in the left nose and posterior part of the right nose. Imaging revealed opacity in all sinuses on the left side and mass in the nasopharynx. Biopsy revealed adenoid cystic carcinoma. He underwent endoscopic excision of the tumor, which was noted to involve the left maxillary sinus, ethmoids, sphenoid sinus, posterior septum, and nasopharyngeal mucosa on the left side.

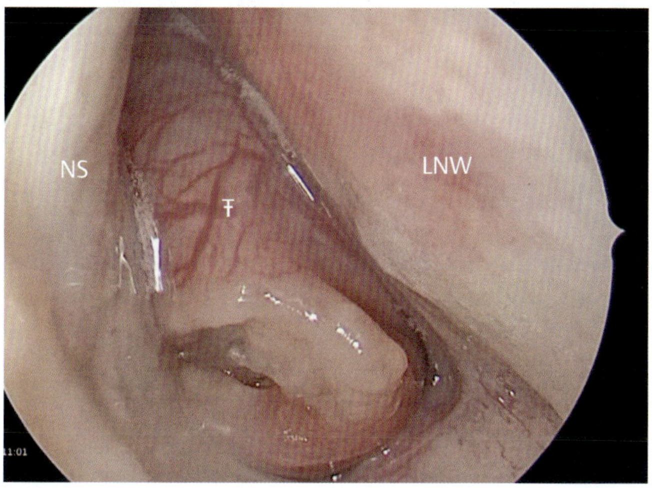

Fig. 40B.1 Preoperative view of the tumor occupying the left nasal cavity.

Surgical Steps

1. The patient is placed under general anesthesia in the supine position with the head in neutral position, in reverse Trendelenburg 30 degrees up.
2. The nasal cavities are packed with a ribbon gauze soaked in co-phenylephrine prior to the surgery to reduce bleeding and to decongest the nose.
3. A microdebrider is used to debulk and remove the tumor occupying the left nasal cavity first (**Fig. 40B.1** and **Fig. 40B.2**).
4. A posterior septectomy is performed to remove the tumor attached to the posterior septum (**Fig. 40B.3**).
5. The lateral nasal wall is cleared off the tumor, with an uncinectomy, a medial maxillary antrostomy, and a turbinectomy (middle and inferior).

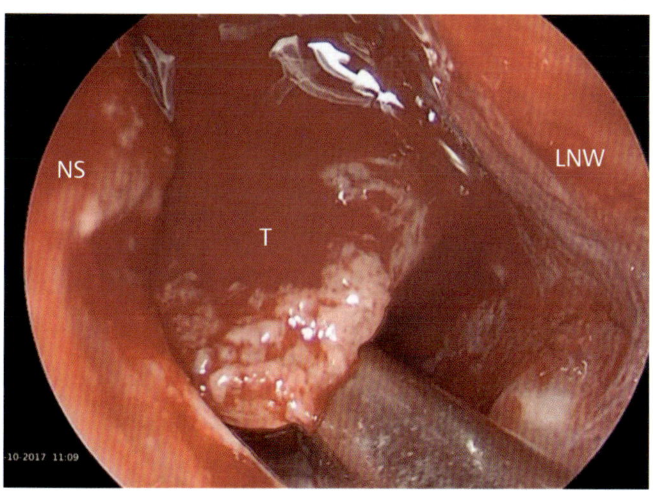

Fig. 40B.2 Debulking of the tumor from the nasal cavity with a microdebrider.

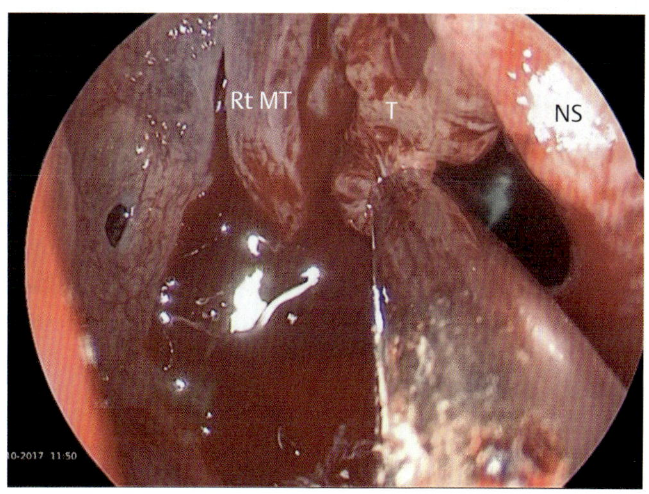

Fig. 40B.3 Removal of tumor attached to the nasal septum.

6. An ethmoidectomy (anterior and posterior) as well as a sphenoidectomy (**Fig. 40B.4**) is performed to remove the remaining of the tumor that extends posteriorly.
7. The tumor in the pterygopalatine fossa is removed and the internal maxillary artery is clipped in this area to minimize bleeding complications (**Fig. 40B.5**).
8. The posterior attachment of the tumor to the nasopharynx is removed, where a monopolar diathermy is used to outline the resection margin and the tumor is dissected off the nasopharyngeal wall starting from a superior to an inferior direction (**Fig. 40B.6** and **Fig. 40B.7**).

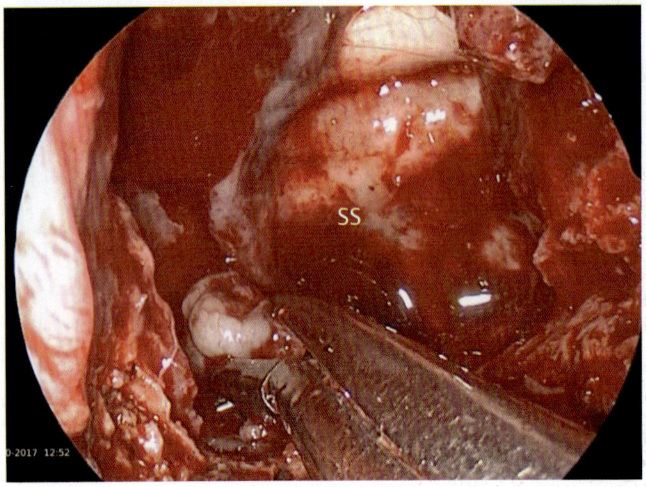

Fig. 40B.4 Dissection of tumor from sphenoid sinus. SS, sphenoid sinus.

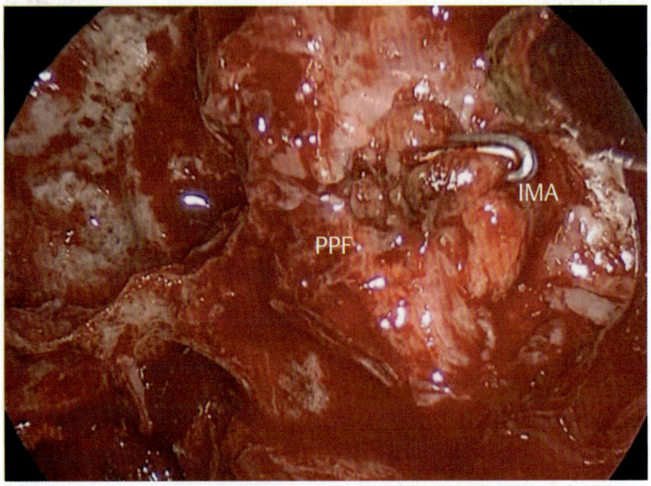

Fig. 40B.5 The internal maxillary artery (IMA) is ligated and divided during dissection of the pterygopalatine fossa (PPF).

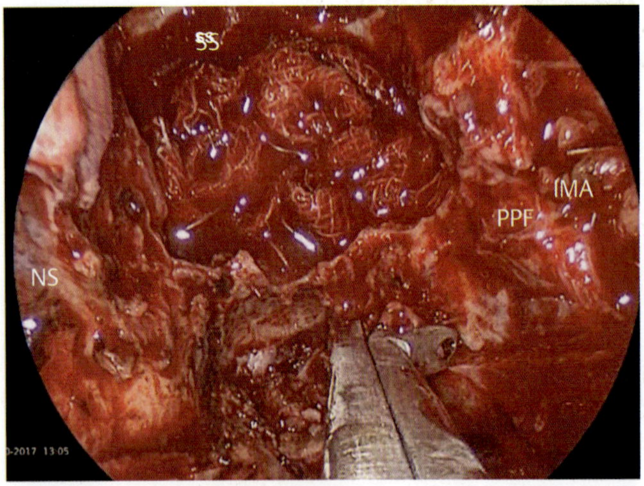

Fig. 40B.6 A left nasopharyngectomy is performed. A ribbon gauze is seen within the sphenoid cavity.

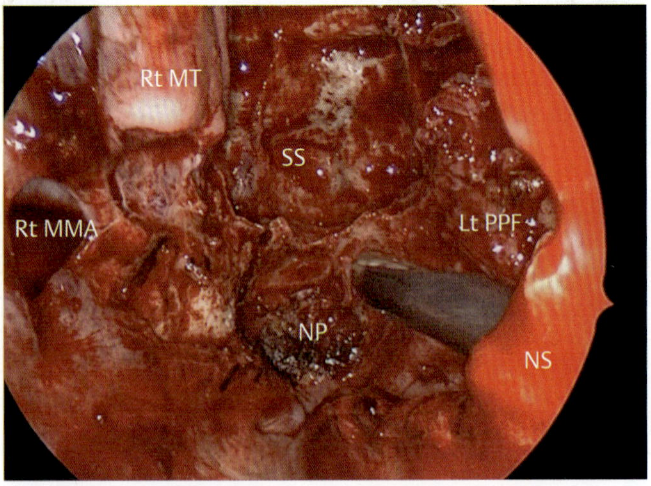

Fig. 40B.7 Final view after removal of the entire tumor.

Case 40C

Endoscopic Excision of Recurrent Olfactory Neuroblastoma with Extension to the Orbit, Infratemporal Fossa, and Cavernous Sinus

Adzreil Bakri, Prepageran Narayanan, and Vicknes Waran

History

A 63-year-old man with an underlying history of recurrent olfactory neuroblastoma of the nasal cavity presented with a history of loss of vision of the left eye associated with paresthesia of the left side of the face. He was operated on 9 years and 6 years ago for an olfactory neuroblastoma and also completed a course of chemotherapy and radiotherapy 6 years ago prior to this presentation. Clinically, there was evidence of previous nasal surgery with the posterior nasal septum being absent and the medial wall of the left maxilla exposed. The tumor was occupying the left nasal cavity at the level just above the inferior turbinate extending superiorly until the skull base, medially until the right nasal cavity, and laterally until the orbit, maxilla, and infratemporal fossa. A magnetic resonance imaging (MRI) revealed the tumor extending deeper posteriorly to the left cavernous sinus and temporal lobe dura with large areas of new bone formation (**Fig. 40C.1**). An endoscopic excision of the tumor was performed.

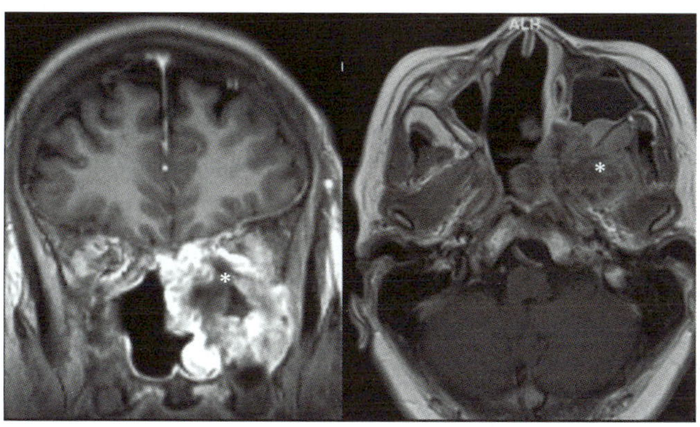

Fig. 40C.1 MRI showing a heterogeneously enhancing lobulated mass (*) eroding the skull base at the clivus, cribriform plate, and ethmoid and sphenoid sinuses. It is extending laterally and posteriorly to the infratemporal fossa and posteriorly and superiorly to the orbital apex, temporal lobe, and cavernous sinus.

Surgical Steps

1. The patient is placed under general anesthesia in supine position and the head slightly extended fixed within a NORAS frame for intraoperative MRI (iMRI). Registration for neuronavigation (Brainlab, Munich, Germany) is performed.
2. The nose is decongested with nasal packing as per the institution's usual method.
3. The nasal packs are removed and the nasal cavity inspected with an endoscope.
4. Tumor extension is assessed endoscopically. In this case, the tumor fully occupies the nasal cavity with extensions superiorly and posteriorly to the skull base, medially to the right nasal cavity, and laterally to the left orbit, maxilla, and infratemporal fossa (**Fig. 40C.2**).
5. An incision is made at the left anterolateral site of the tumor on the lateral nasal wall while dissecting and pushing the tumor medially and opening the space lateral to the tumor and exposing the infratemporal fossa (**Fig. 40C.3** and **Fig. 40C.4**).

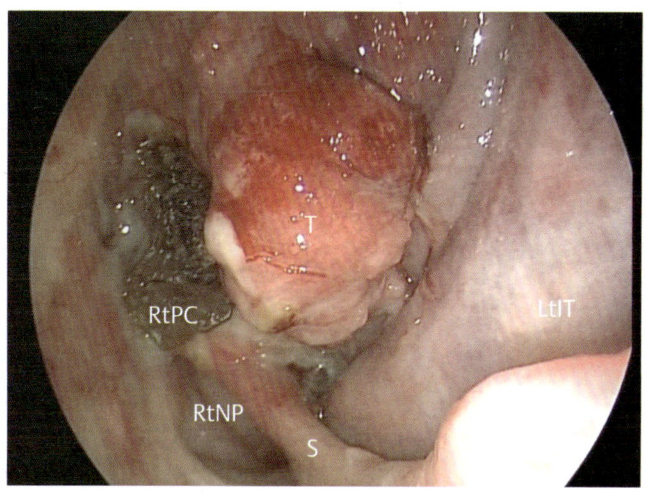

Fig. 40C.2 Endoscopic view of the tumor (T).

6. The anterosuperior site of the tumor is carefully dissected away from the skull base and cut with scissors (**Fig. 40C.5**).
7. The anterior bulk of the tumor is removed and sent for biopsy (**Fig. 40C.6**).
8. The deeper base of the tumor is assessed. Loose and soft parts of the tumor are removed using a microdebrider with care to identify and preserve the underlying normal structures such as the orbit, dura, and cavernous sinus (**Fig. 40C.7**).

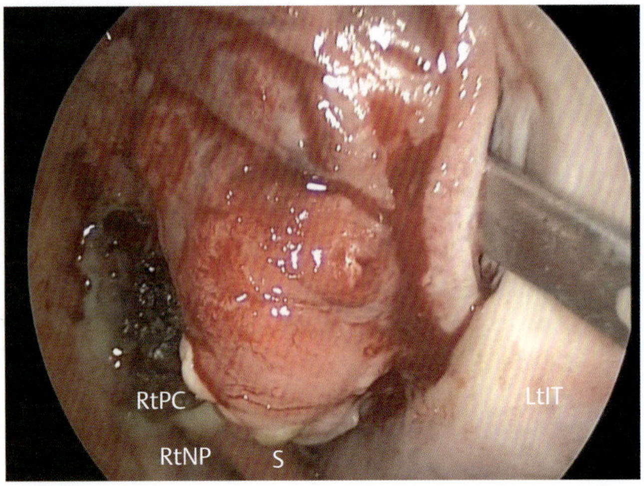

Fig. 40C.3 An incision is made at the lateral nasal wall, slightly anterior and lateral to the tumor (T).

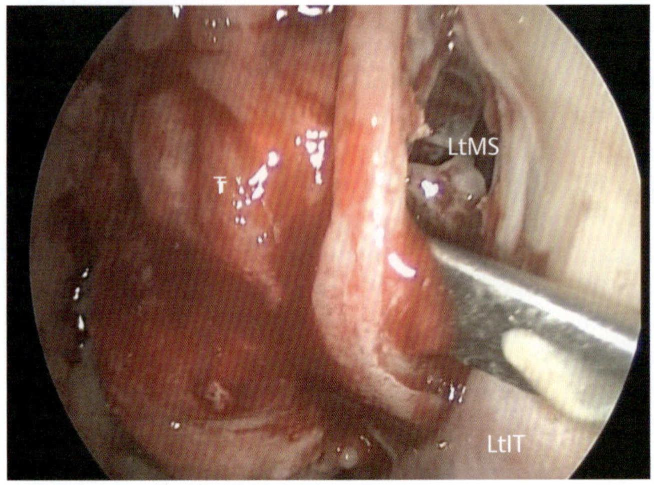

Fig. 40C.4 The tumor (T) is pushed medially after the incision exposing the left maxillary sinus (LtMS), a space that was created from previous surgeries.

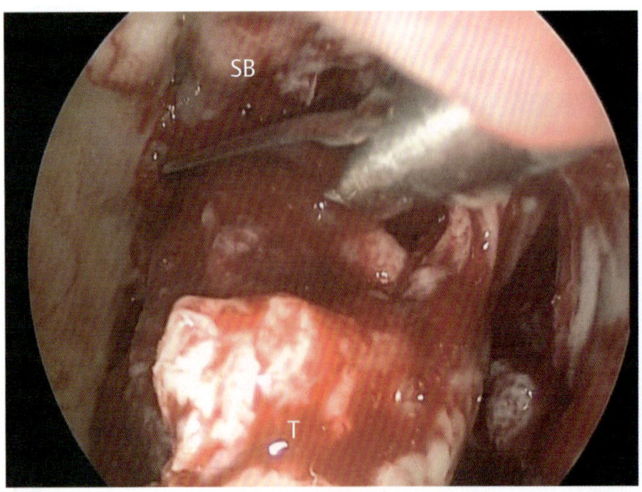

Fig. 40C.5 The anterior bulk of the tumor (T) is dissected away and the superior part is cut with endoscopic nasal scissors.

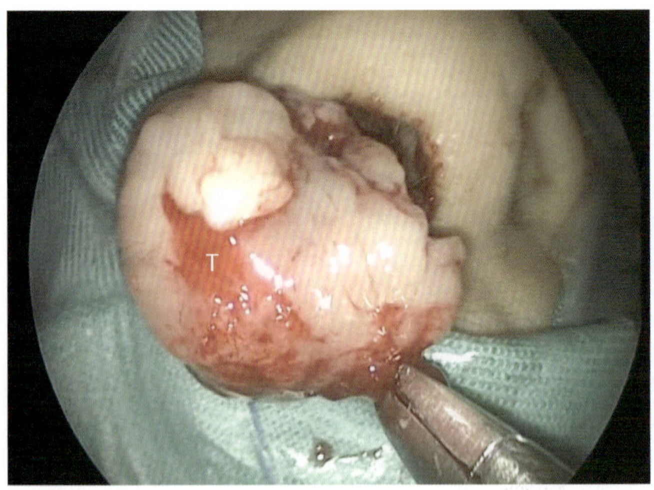

Fig. 40C.6 The anterior bulk of the tumor (T) is delivered.

9. The tumor in the infratemporal fossa is gently peeled off using a dissector and suction probe (**Fig. 40C.8**). It is important to identify and preserve normal-looking structures that are not infiltrated by the tumor.
10. Abnormal bony formation at the body of the sphenoid bone and the pterygoid base is drilled and smoothened down (**Fig. 40C.9**). The drilling is continued posteriorly following the tumor until the cavernous sinus and temporal lobe dura are exposed (**Fig. 40C.10**).
11. The tumor is gently removed from the anterior wall of the cavernous sinus and the temporal lobe dura with a blunt dissector and suction probe (**Fig. 40C.11**). Any loose tumor is carefully removed using a microdebrider or forceps.

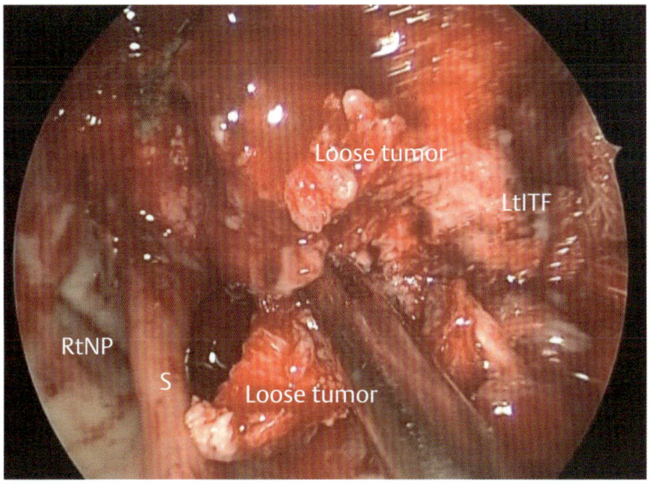

Fig. 40C.7 Loose tumor is removed with a microdebrider.

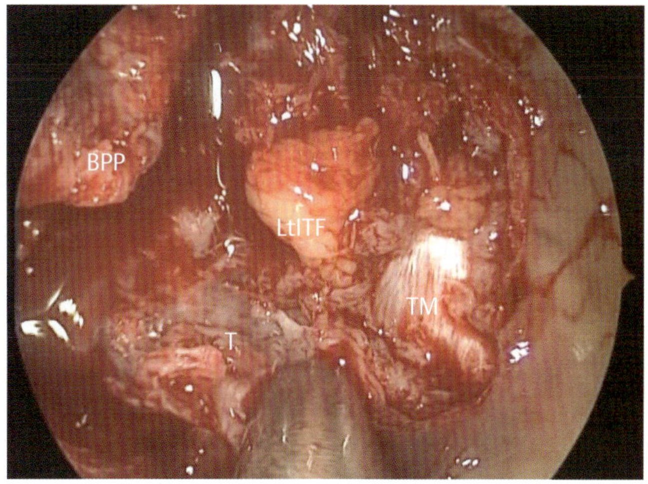

Fig. 40C.8 Blunt dissection of the tumor (T) in the left infratemporal fossa (LtITF).

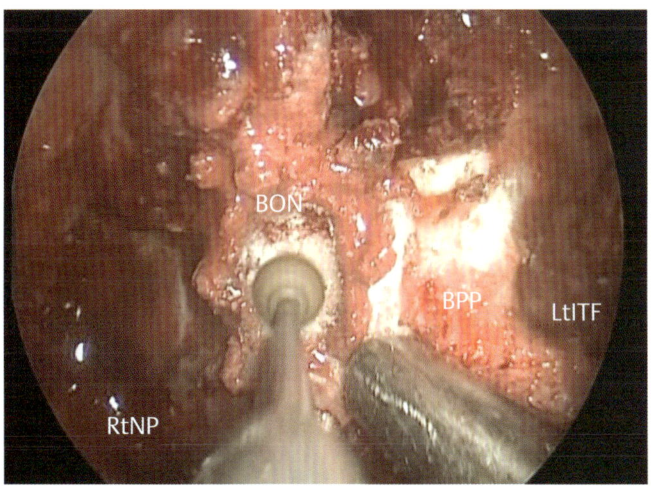

Fig. 40C.9 Drilling of abnormal bone (BON) over the body of sphenoid.

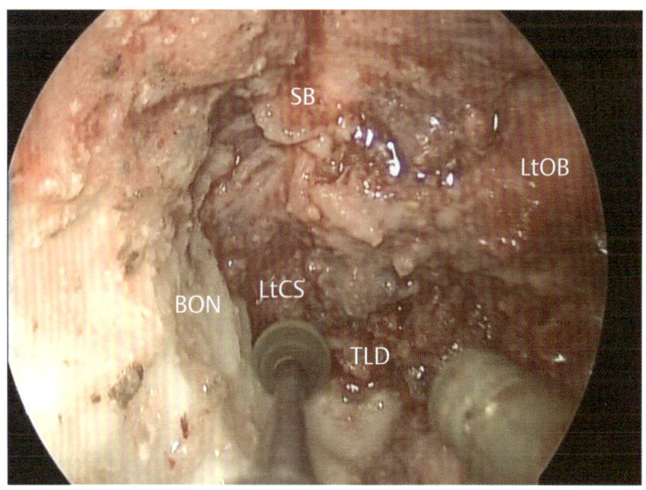

Fig. 40C.10 Drilling and smoothening down of abnormal bone (BON) until the cavernous sinus and temporal lobe dura (TLD) are encountered.

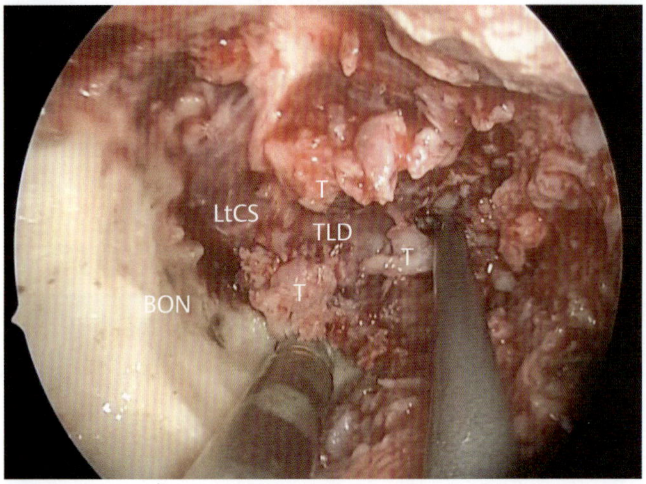

Fig. 40C.11 Blunt dissection of the tumor (T) from the left cavernous sinus (LtCS) and temporal lobe dura (TLD).

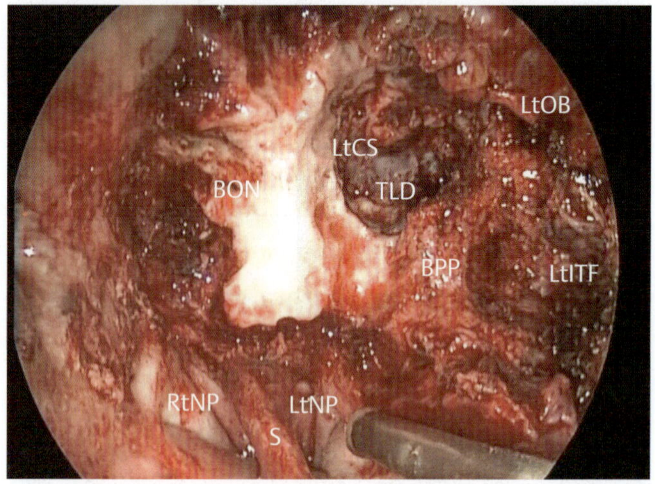

Fig. 40C.12 Final view after the tumor excision.

12. This same technique of blunt dissection and removal of tumor once it is detached is carefully applied throughout the surgery especially when the tumor parts are attached to vital structures such as the orbit, dura, and cavernous sinus (**Fig. 40C.12**).
13. Once complete tumor clearance has been achieved, the nasal cavity is flushed with normal saline and the remaining bleeding points are secured diligently. The raw areas of the nasal cavity are laid with oxidized cellulose polymers (Surgicel® Original Absorbable Hemostat; Ethicon, Johnson&Johnson, USA) and absorbable gelatin sponges (Surgifoam® Absorbable Gelatin Sponge; Ethicon, Johnson&Johnson, USA) and packed with synthetic biodegradable foams (Nasopore®; Stryker, Germany).

Case 40D

Endoscopic Transpterygoid Infrapetrous Approach to Petrous Apex in Recurrent Nasopharyngeal Carcinoma

Liew Yew Toong, Prepageran Narayanan, and Vicknes Waran

History

A 69-year-old gentleman presented with foul-smelling and blood stained discharge for 6 months. He was treated for nasopharyngeal carcinoma 2 years ago with concurrent chemoradiation for a total of 70 Gy at his nasopharynx. His magnetic resonance imaging (MRI) showed an obvious enhancing nasopharyngeal mass (**Fig. 40D.1**), which extended to the right petrous apex. Biopsy of the right fossa of Rosenmuller showed a positive recurrence of the nasopharyngeal carcinoma.

Surgical Steps

1. The patient is positioned supine under general anesthesia, with an indwelling catheter, invasive blood pressure monitoring, intraoperative prophylactic antibiotics, and the head fixed slightly retroflexed within a NORAS frame for intraoperative MRI (iMRI). Registration for neuronavigation (Brainlab, Munich, Germany) is performed.
2. The nose is prepared with co-phenylcaine applied topically with 1-inch ribbon gauzes.

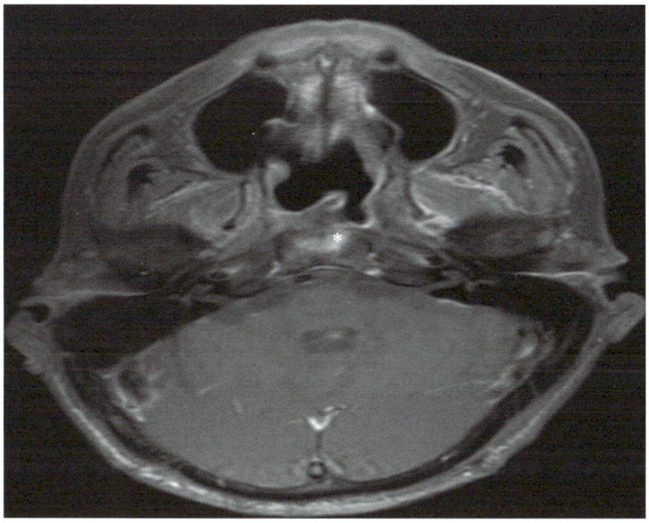

Fig. 40D.1 Contrasted T1-weighted MRI showing an enhancing mass (*) that extends into the right petrous apex.

3. A posterior septectomy is performed up to 2 cm from the posterior choana in order to place the endoscope in the midline, for better exposure and to allow instruments to be inserted by the assistant (**Fig. 40D.2, Fig. 40D.3**).
4. A nasopharyngectomy is performed by excising the right eustachian tube together with the tumor at the fossa of Rosenmuller until the medial pterygoid plate is exposed (**Fig. 40D.4**).
5. Under neuronavigation, the right pterygoid bone is removed with a coarse 3-mm diamond drill to reach the right carotid artery at its second genu (**Fig. 40D.5**).
6. Once the vertical segment of the carotid artery is identified, the artery is lateralized with a rigid suction probe (**Fig. 40D.6**).
7. Further drilling of bone is performed inferomedially down to the junction between the horizontal and the vertical segment of the petrous carotid artery to reach the petrous apex in order to clear any residual tumor (**Fig. 40D.7**).
8. The area of resection is left exposed without flap coverage at the end of the surgery and complete epithelization occurred at 3 months postoperatively.

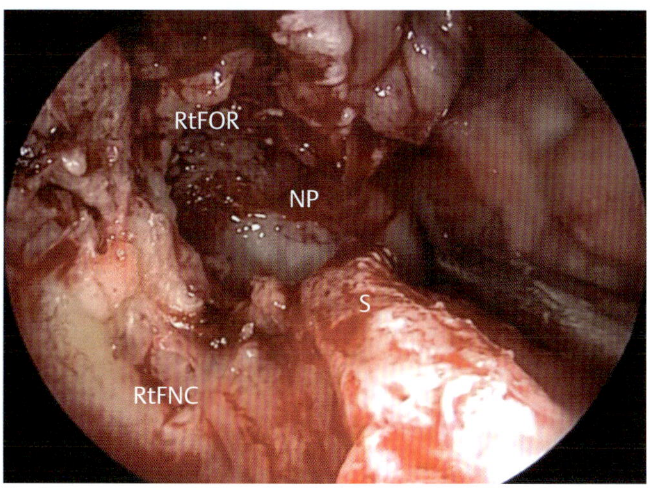

Fig. 40D.2 Endoscopic view after the performed posterior septectomy revealing recurrent tumor at the right fossa of Rosenmuller.

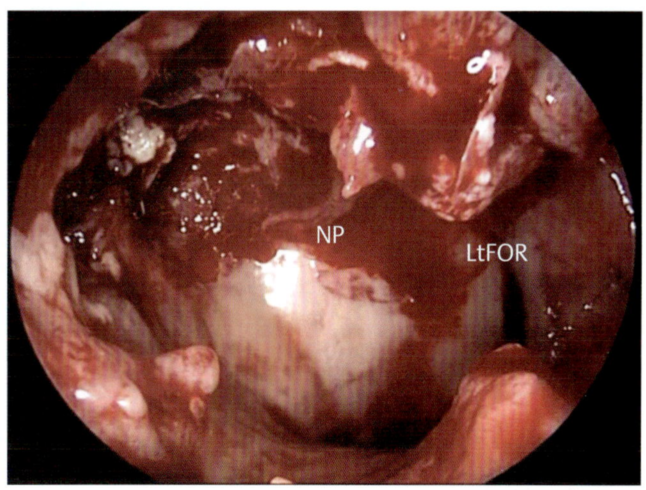

Fig. 40D.3 Closer endoscopic view demonstrating tumor (*) extending into the right petrous apex.

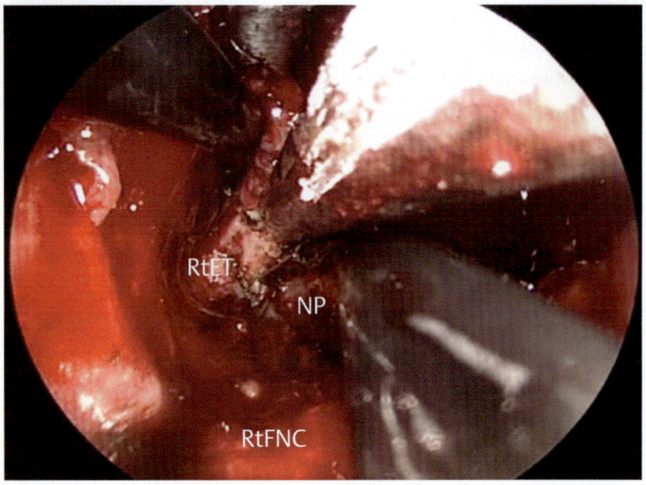

Fig. 40D.4 The right eustachian tube is excised.

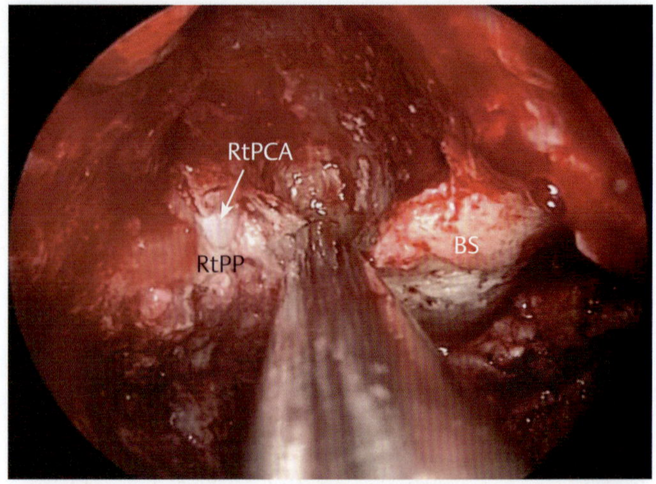

Fig. 40D.5 The right vertical part of the carotid artery is identified using neuronavigation and used as a landmark for the identification of the petrous apex.

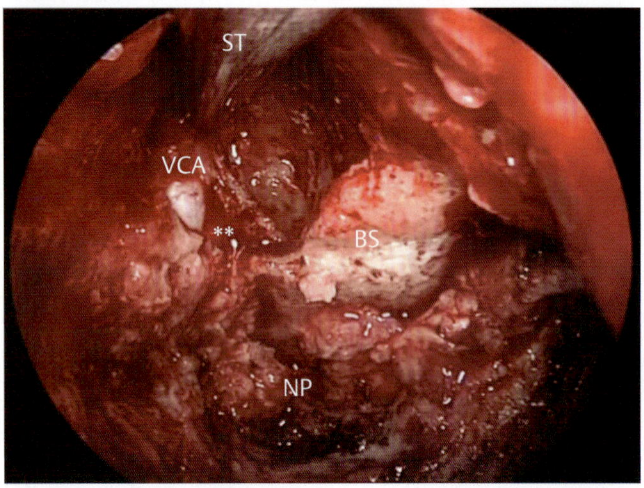

Fig. 40D.6 The carotid artery is lateralized with a rigid suction tube to improve the exposure to the petrous apex, which is located inferiomedially (**) to the vertical segment of the right carotid artery.

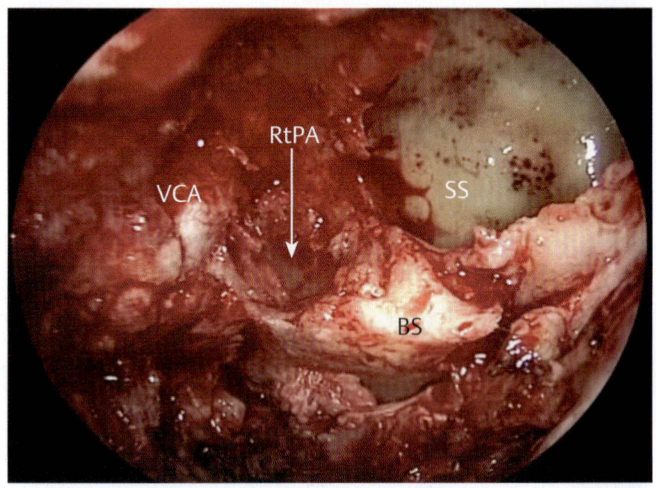

Fig. 40D.7 Drilling of bone is performed in an inferomedial direction to the vertical segment of the carotid artery to expose the petrous apex.

Case 40E

Endoscopic Excision of a Sinonasal Osteosarcoma with Orbital Decompression

Saif Al-Zahid, Revadi Govindaraju, Michel Roethlisberger, and Prepageran Narayanan

History

A 14-year-old female presented with a 1-month history of left-sided nose bleeds and left eye protrusion followed by 1 week of reduced vision in the left eye and double vision. On examination, the patient had proptosis of the left eye and diplopia (**Fig. 40E.1a–c** and **Fig. 40E.2a, b**). Her visual acuity on presentation in the left eye was poor at 6/24. Nasal examination revealed a mass filling the left nasal cavity and septal deviation to the right.

Computed tomography (CT) and magnetic resonance imaging (MRI) revealed an extensive left sinonasal tumor with orbital involvement causing proptosis and mass effect to the left optic nerve (**Fig. 40E.3, Fig. 40E.4a–c, Fig. 40E.5**).

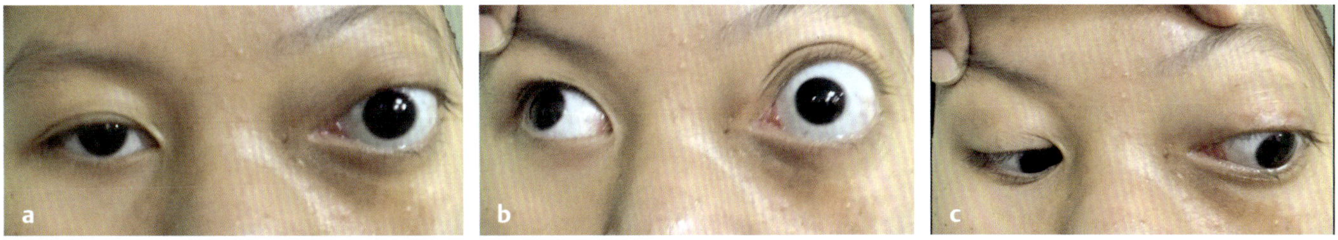

Fig. 40E.1 (a–c) Preoperative eye movements with restricted left eye mobility.

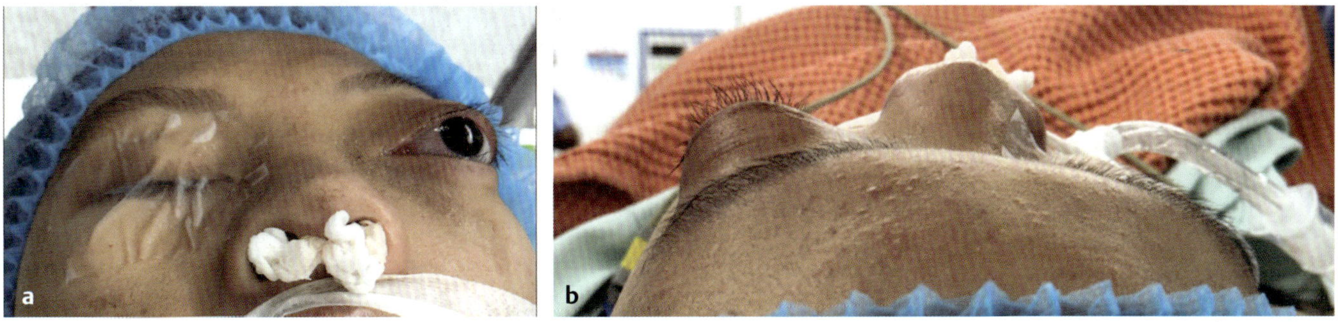

Fig. 40E.2 (a,b) Proptosis is seen intraoperatively prior to tumor excision.

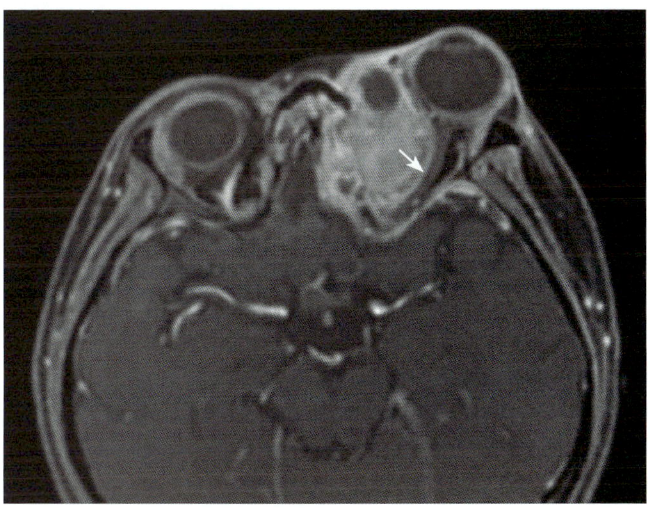

Fig. 40E.3 Three-dimensional fast spoiled gradient echo (3D FSPGR) MRI axial section showing orbital involvement and optic nerve compression by the tumor (*white arrow*).

There was an extension to the dura of the anterior cranial fossa and infratemporal fossa. Initial biopsy revealed fibrous dysplasia with differential of osteoblastoma. The patient underwent an urgent endoscopic excision and decompression of the left orbit. Following excision, the formal histology revealed an osteosarcoma. Her visual acuity returned to normal 48 hours after surgery to 6/6, and proptosis improved significantly. Her eye movements improved apart from some mild restriction to the upper lateral left gaze (**Fig. 40E.6a–d**). The patient was referred to a multidisciplinary team (MDT) for further management. The steps of the surgery are outlined below.

Surgical Steps

1. The patient is placed under general anesthesia in supine position.
2. The nose is decongested with light nasal packing anterior to the tumor as per the institutions' standard methods.
3. The left eye is kept open and protected with chloramphenicol ointment to facilitate balloting of the eye during surgery.
4. After removal of the initial packing, new ribbon gauze soaked with adrenaline is placed superiorly, inferiorly, medial, and lateral to the tumor and pushed with a sucker to dissect the tumor from surroundings and ascertain tumor attachments and its free edges (**Fig. 40E.7**).
5. Following debulking, the tumor was found to be attached to anterior skull base superiorly and orbit laterally.
6. The tumor is peeled off the periorbita using a sharpened sucker (**Fig. 40E.8**). This is facilitated by balloting

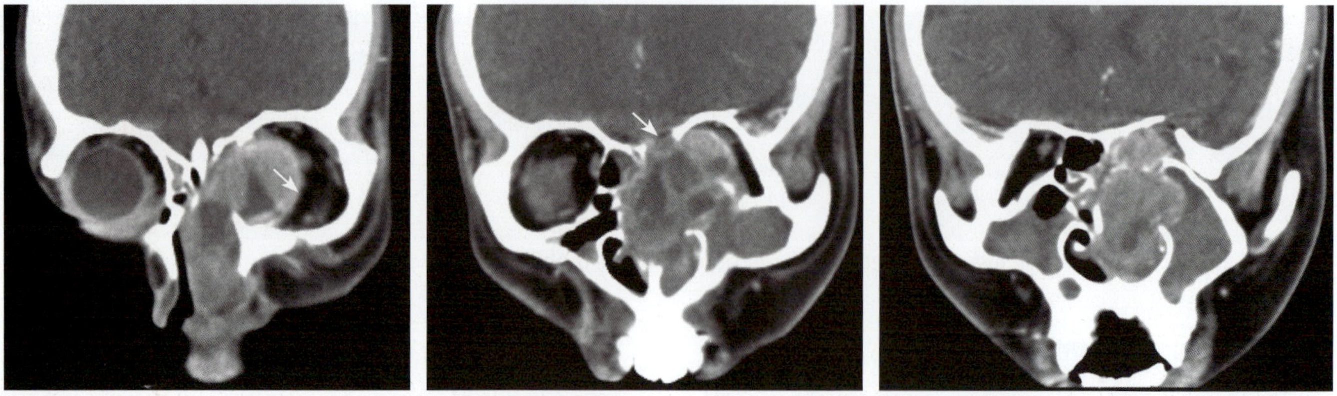

Figs. 40E.4 **(a–c)** Sagittal CT scans showing aneurysmal bone cyst formation into the orbit (*white arrow*) and a skull base defect (*arrow*).

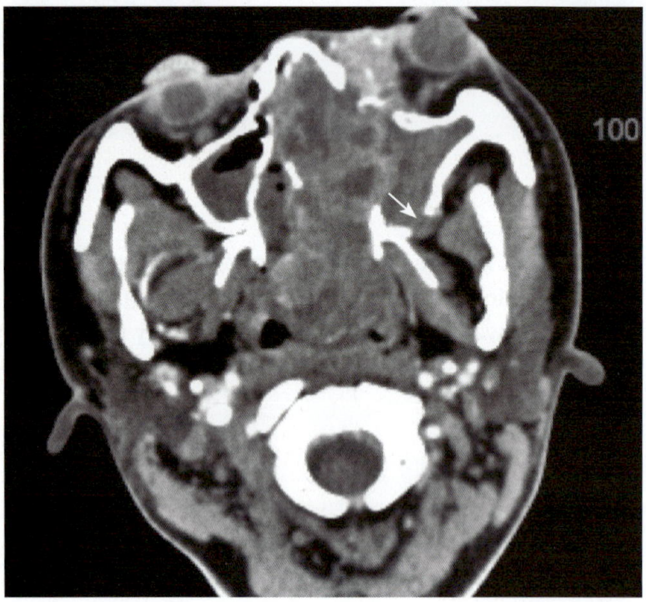

Fig. 40E.5 Axial CT showing extensive tumor with bony erosion and extension into the left infratemporal fossa (*arrow*).

the eyeball during the dissection to evert tumor out of the orbit and into the nasal cavity.

7. In a similar fashion, this dissection is taken more posteriorly to decompress the optic nerve (**Fig. 40E.9**).
8. In this case, the orbital sheath is left intact as the compression was external to the orbital contents.
9. The tumor is then peeled off the skull base where the anterior ethmoidal artery can be seen running lateral to medial at an angle (**Fig. 40E.10**).
10. The tumor is removed further posteriorly from the skull base where a bone defect can be seen with intact dura between the anterior and posterior ethmoidal artery (**Fig. 40E.11**).
11. The nasal cavity is washed and inspected, prior to application of Gelfoam dressings.

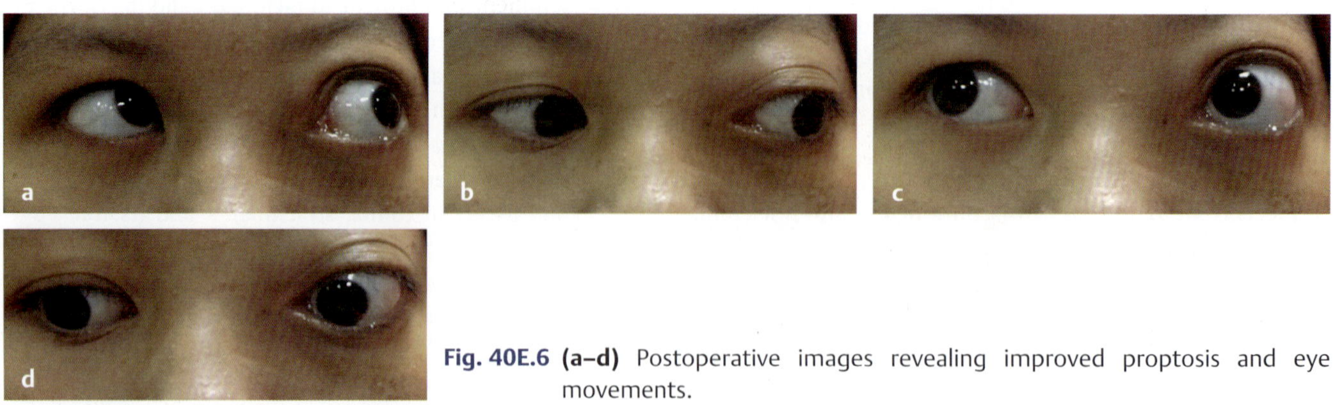

Fig. 40E.6 **(a–d)** Postoperative images revealing improved proptosis and eye movements.

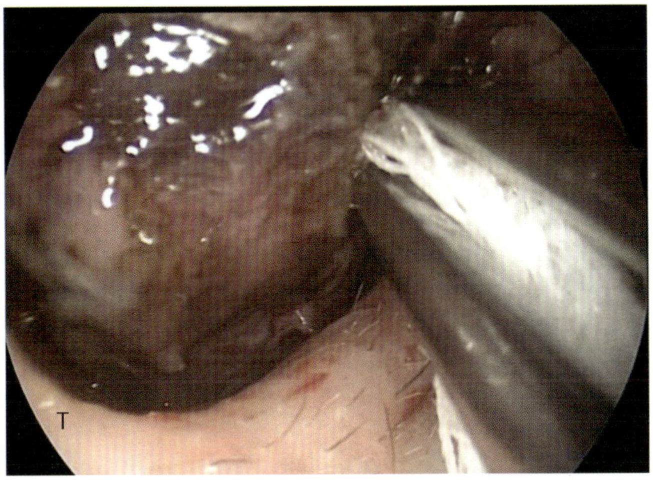

Fig. 40E.7 Packing around the tumor (T) to establish the plane and ascertain attachment to surrounding tissues.

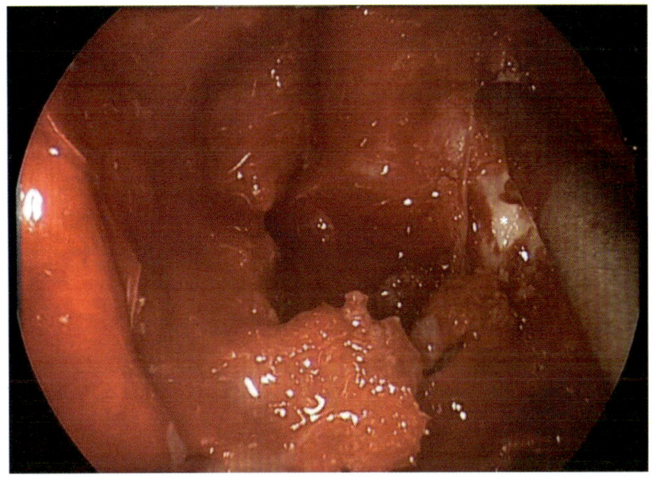

Fig. 40E.8 Endoscopic view of the tumor being peeled off the periorbita using a sharp-ended sucker.

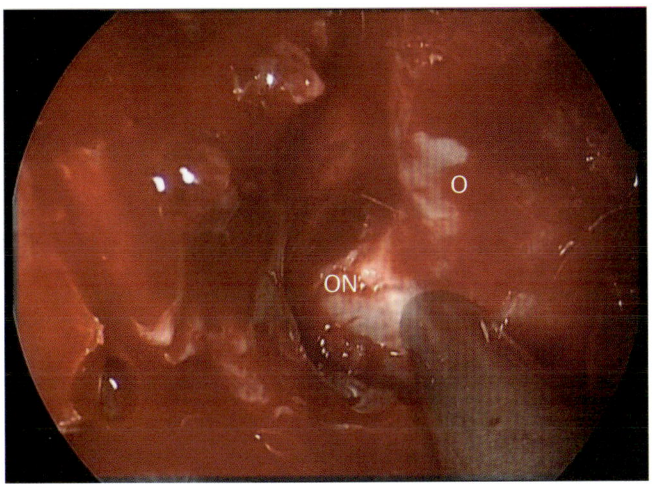

Fig. 40E.9 Endoscopic view of the right optic nerve (ON) and orbit (O) after decompression.

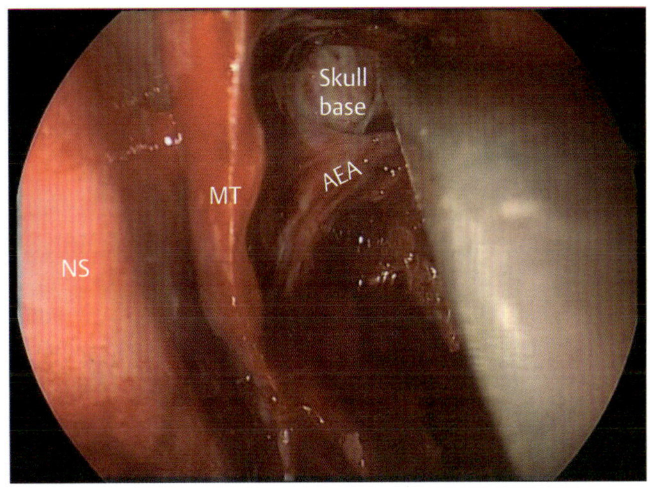

Fig. 40E.10 Endoscopic view of the tumor dissection off skull base, and anterior ethmoid artery (AEA). Remnant of the middle turbinate (MT) can be seen.

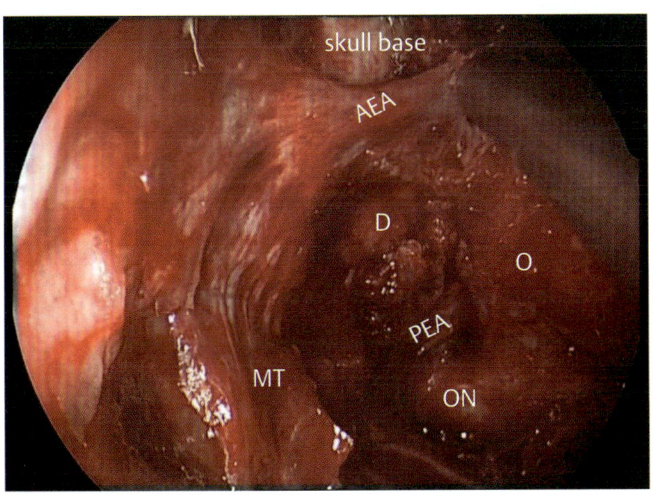

Fig. 40E.11 More posteriorly, a skull base defect can be seen with intact dura (D) where the tumor has eroded bone. The posterior ethmoid artery (PEA) is also identified.

Case 40F

Endoscopic Modified Denker's Approach for Excision of Sinonasal Verrucous Carcinoma

Revadi Govindaraju, Michel Roethlisberger, and Prepageran Narayanan

History

A 53-year-old man presented with a 2-month history of left-sided nasal block associated with intermittent epistaxis. No smell disturbances, facial pain, headache, facial numbness, epiphora, or visual disturbances were noted. Clinical findings were notable for a fleshy mass in the left nasal cavity (**Fig. 40F.1**). Other examinations were normal. A high-resolution paranasal sinus computed tomography (CT) scan revealed an opacity in the left nasal cavity, anterior ethmoids, frontal recess, and maxillary sinus with bony erosion of the medial wall of the maxillary sinus extending to the pyriform aperture. Histopathological examination (HPE) of the biopsy taken revealed a verrucous carcinoma. This patient underwent an endoscopic modified Denker's procedure to address the pyriform aperture involvement.

Surgical Steps

1. The patient is positioned supine in a 20- to 30-degree reverse Trendelenburg's position with slight hyperextension of the head.
2. The nose is decongested with a ribbon gauze soaked in adrenaline 1:1,000 units and mucosal infiltration is performed with lignocaine hydrochloride anhydrous 2% with adrenaline 1:100,000.
3. Initial steps involve tumor debulking with a microdebrider to allow identification of anatomical landmarks prior to further tumor excision (**Fig. 40F.2**).
4. Tumor excision is often interrupted with profuse bleeding from the partially excised tumor. This may require temporary packing with the assistant performing continuous suctioning. Bipolar cautery is used to stop the bleeding from cut surfaces of the tumor (**Fig. 40F.3**). Blood loss will become less the sooner the tumor bulk is reduced, and this can be rapidly performed if the stalk/base/proximal part is identified and the large distal portions are removed with Blakesley's forceps or equivalent instrument (**Fig. 40F.4** and **Fig. 40F.5**). The removed tissue also serves as a specimen for HPE. However, there is a need to exercise caution when the tumorous mass is adjacent to critical structures, for example, the orbit, large blood vessels, the optic nerve, or the skull base. Note that with most tumor debulked, the bleeding has reduced in **Fig. 40F.6** as compared to **Fig. 40F.3**.
5. Prior to the inferior turbinectomy, the mucosa anterior to the head of the inferior turbinate is cauterized (**Fig. 40F.7**).
6. The inferior turbinate is then outfractured, cauterized, and transected (**Fig. 40F.8a–c**). The posterior stump of the inferior turbinate is cauterized and anatomical landmarks are identified (**Fig. 40F.9**).

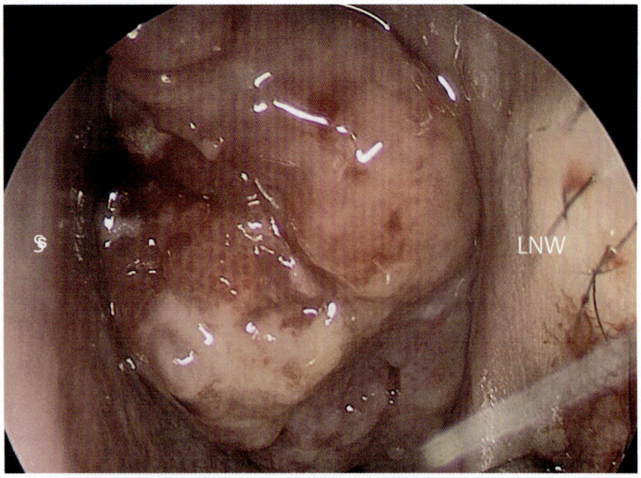

Fig. 40F.1 The large and fleshy tumorous mass is seen occupying the left nasal cavity.

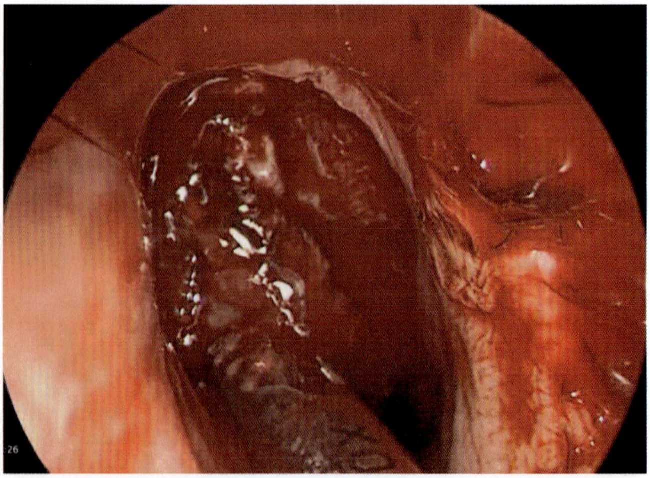

Fig. 40F.2 The tumor is debulked with a microdebrider.

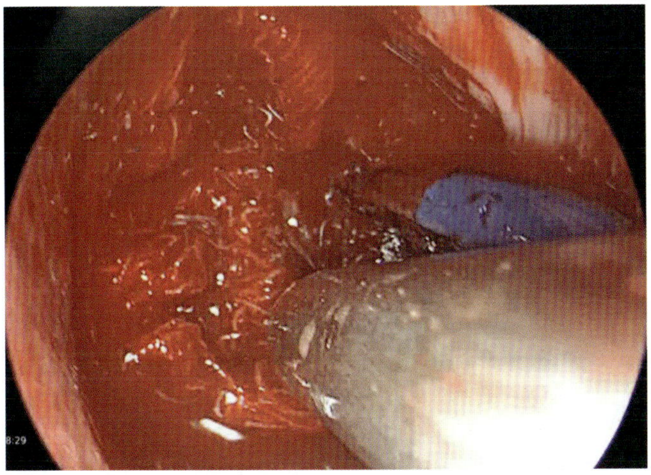

Fig. 40F.3 As the tumor is excised, profuse bleeding is controlled with nasal packing using ribbon gauze continuous suction applied by the assistant, and bipolar cautery of bleeding surfaces.

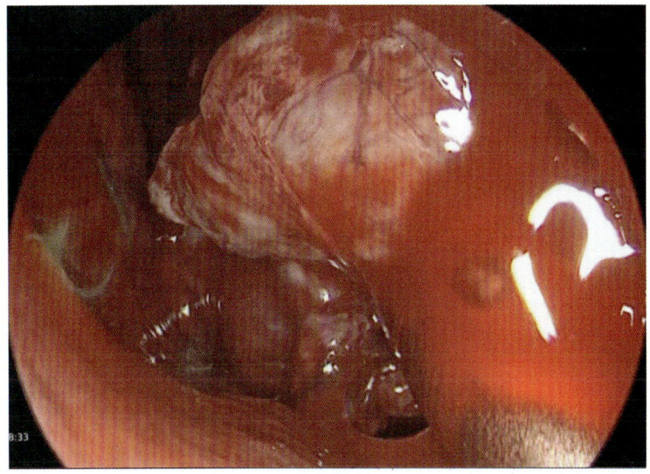

Fig. 40F.4 As the tumorous mass is debulked, attempts are made to identify the tumor base or origin.

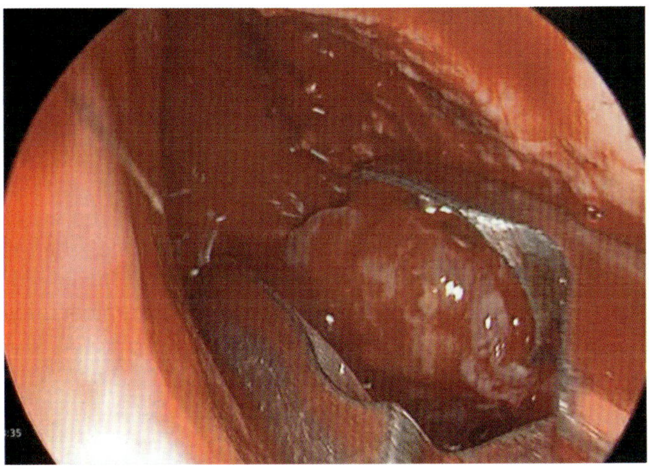

Fig. 40F.5 The proximal tumor portion is removed with Blakesley's forceps.

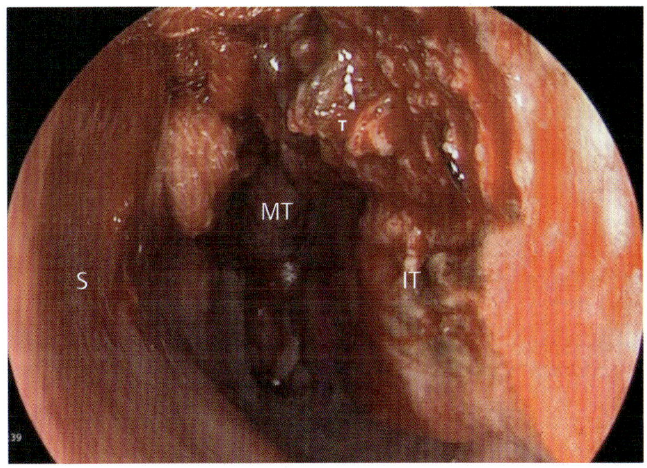

Fig. 40F.6 Tumor remnants are seen on the lateral nasal wall above the inferior turbinate.

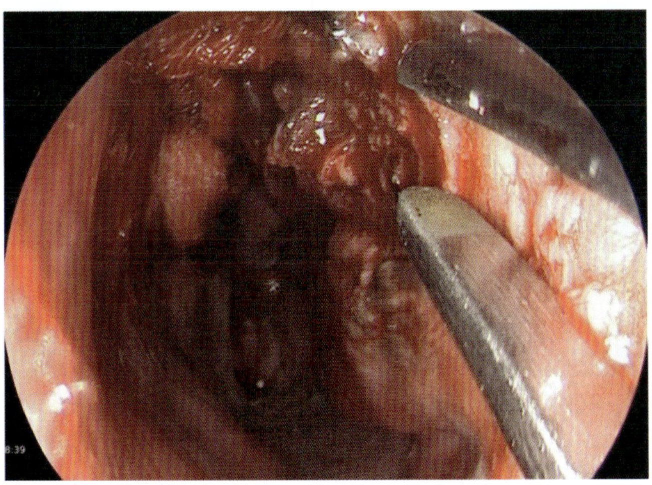

Fig. 40F.7 The mucosa anterior to the head of the inferior turbinate is cauterized.

7. The tumor overlying the pyriform aperture is removed and the pyriform aperture edges are identified (**Fig. 40F.10**).
8. Sharp subperiosteal dissection is performed with an elevator or suction elevator on the anteromedial wall of the maxilla and the infraorbital foramen and its neurovascular structures are identified exiting the foramen (**Fig. 40F.11**).
9. An osteotomy is performed to the inferomedial aspect of the involved pyriform aperture with a 4-mm chisel (**Fig. 40F.12a–c**). This can alternatively be performed with a burr/drill.
10. The step described above (anterior maxillotomy) allows for an excellent view into the maxillary sinus for its anteromedial wall and inspection of the extent of tumor involvement (**Fig. 40F.13**).

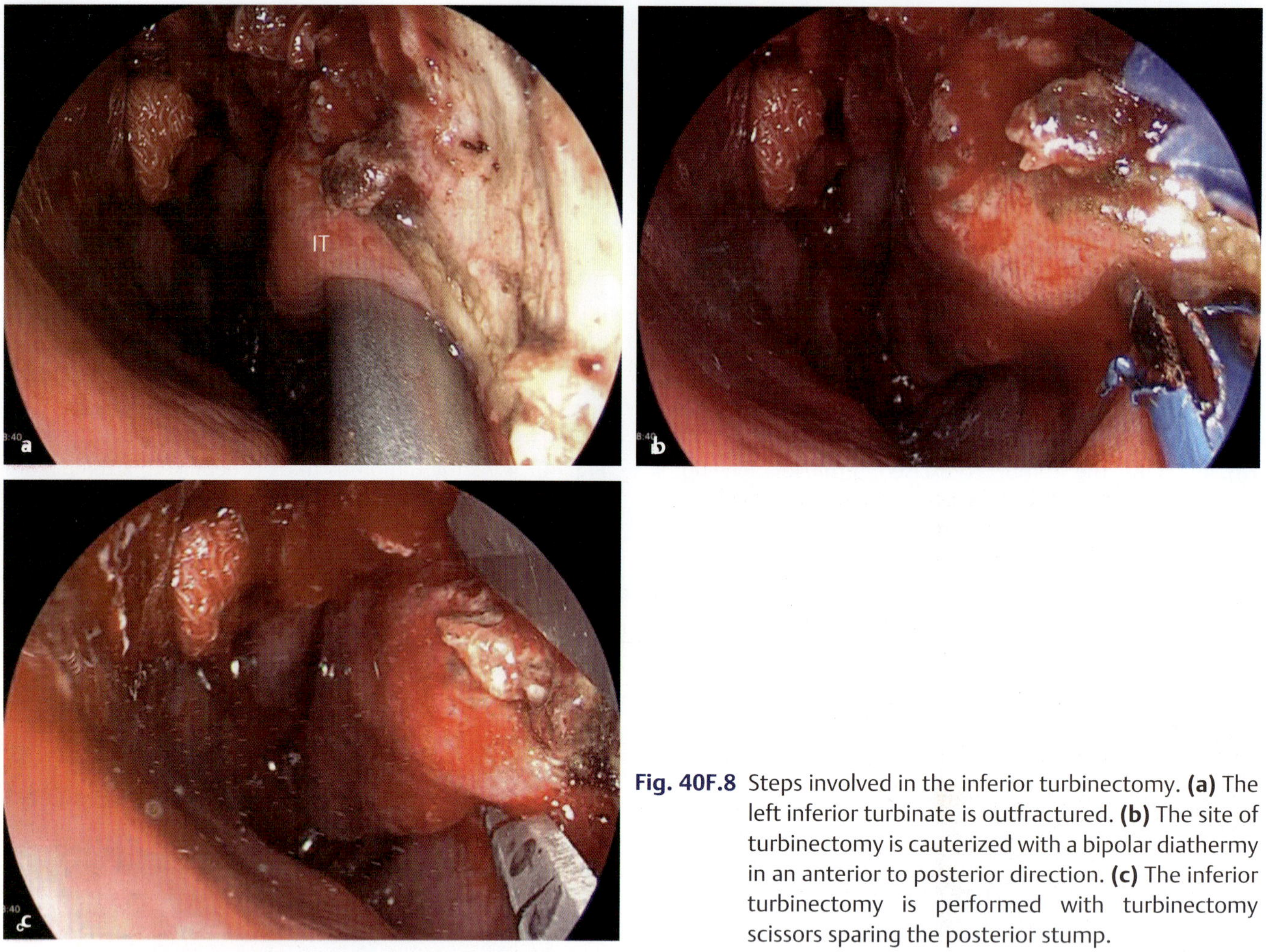

Fig. 40F.8 Steps involved in the inferior turbinectomy. **(a)** The left inferior turbinate is outfractured. **(b)** The site of turbinectomy is cauterized with a bipolar diathermy in an anterior to posterior direction. **(c)** The inferior turbinectomy is performed with turbinectomy scissors sparing the posterior stump.

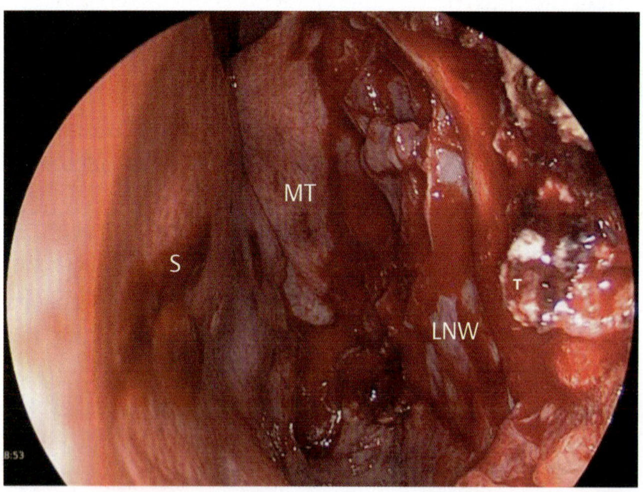

Fig. 40F.9 A view of the lateral nasal wall after inferior turbinectomy; the posterior stump of the inferior turbinate has been cauterized, the middle tubrinate is identified, and the tumor remnant is visible anteriorly.

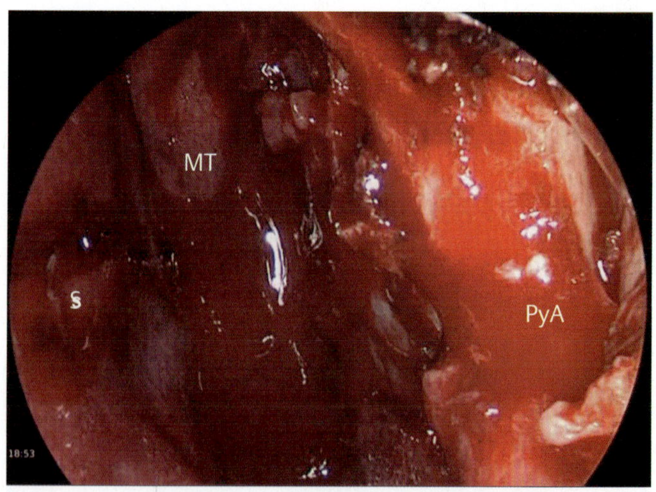

Fig. 40F.10 Dissection has been performed towards the apical end of the inferior turbinate to identify the edges of the pyriform aperture.

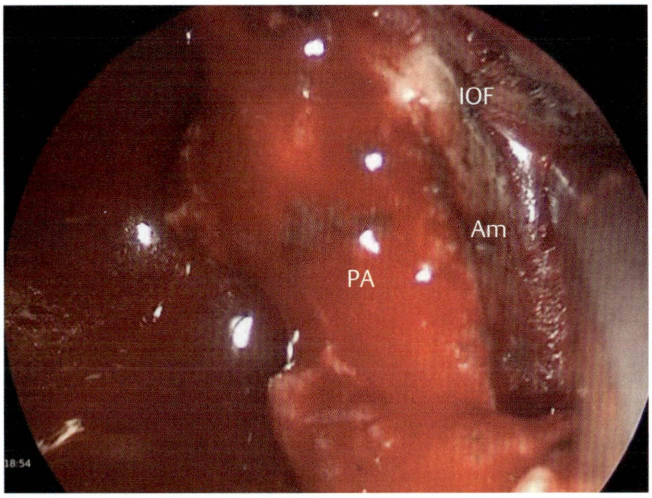

Fig. 40F.11 Subperiosteal dissection of the anteromedial wall of maxilla reveals the IOF and its neurovascular contents exiting the foramen.

11. The remaining medial wall of the maxillary sinus is removed with a microdebrider (**Fig. 40F.14**) followed by the transsection of the nasolacrimal duct. Excision is performed with the orbital floor identified superiorly and greater palatine canal posteroinferiorly on the medial wall. The final view of the endoscopic modified Denker's procedure is shown in **Fig. 40F.15**.

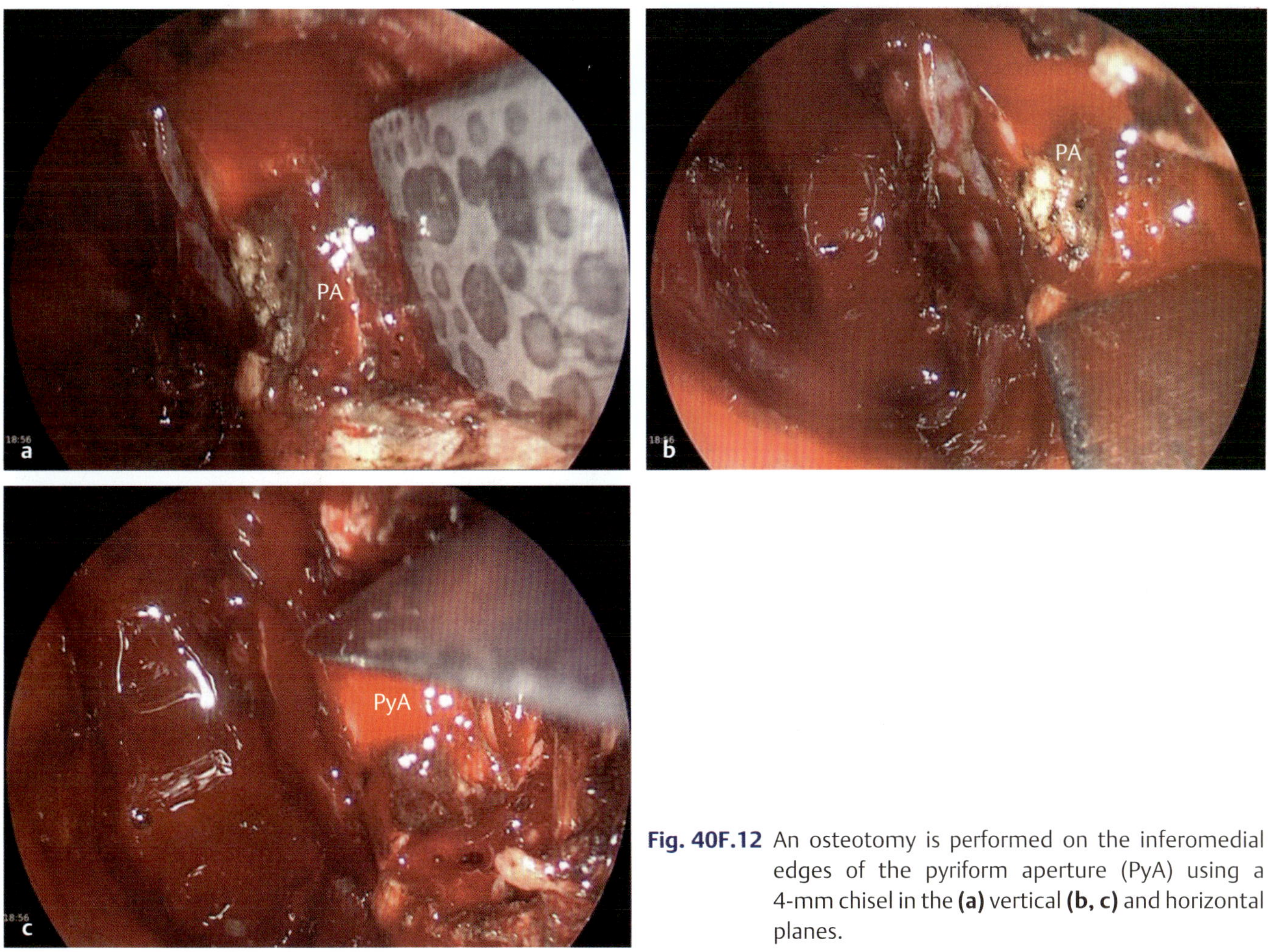

Fig. 40F.12 An osteotomy is performed on the inferomedial edges of the pyriform aperture (PyA) using a 4-mm chisel in the **(a)** vertical **(b, c)** and horizontal planes.

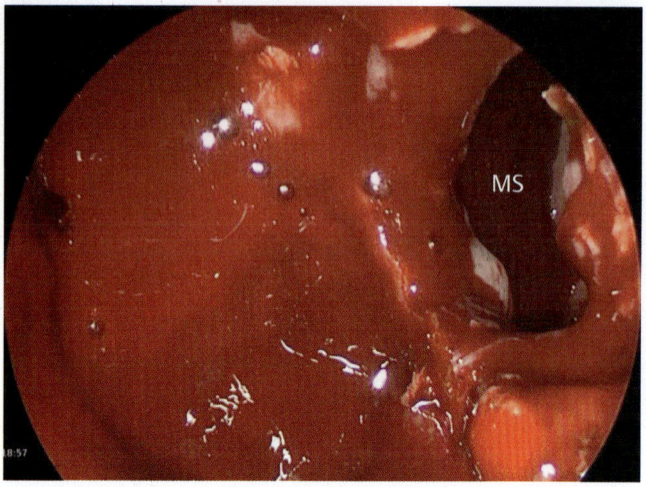

Fig. 40F.13 The osteotomy of the inferior part of anteromedial wall of the maxilla allows for an excellent view into the maxillary sinus.

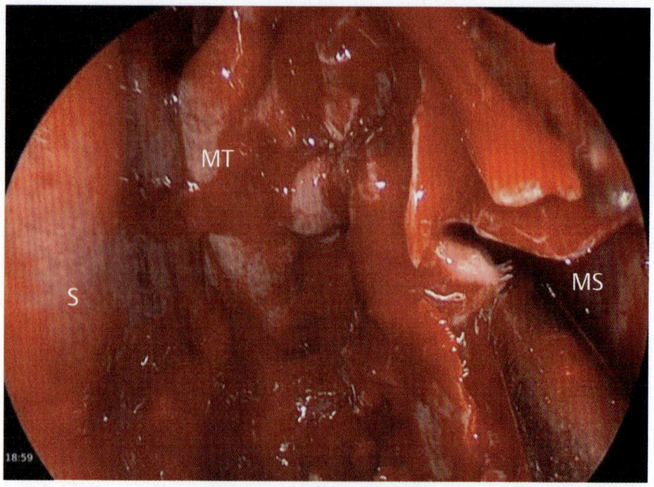

Fig. 40F.14 The remaining medial wall of the maxillary sinus is carefully removed with a microdebrider identifying the orbital floor superiorly and the greater palatine canal posteromedially.

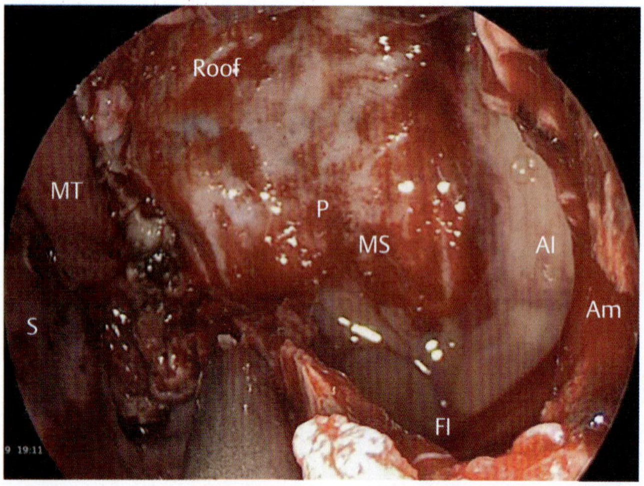

Fig. 40F.15 Final view of the endoscopic modified Denker's procedure.

Suggested Reading

Lee JT, Suh JD, Carrau RL, Chu MW, Chiu AG. Endoscopic Denker's approach for resection of lesions involving the anteroinferior maxillary sinus and infratemporal fossa. Laryngoscope 2017;127(3):556–560

Section XV

Skullbase Fibro-osseous Pathologies

Chapter 41 Skull Base Fibro-osseous Pathologies

Jeyanthi Kulasegarah, Vicknes Waran, and Prepageran Narayanan

Introduction

Skull base fibro-osseous lesions (FOL) are characterized by the replacement of normal bone with variable amounts of connective tissue matrix and this matrix displays varying amounts of focal mineralization.[1] The definitive diagnosis of FOL relies not only on histopathological features of incisional or excisional biopsy material but also on clinical and radiological correlation.[2]

In this chapter, FOL will be reviewed with an emphasis on appropriate diagnosis and management and also highlighting unique aspects of each lesion including histological and radiological features.

Anatomy

Anatomy of the skull base will be covered in depth in Chapter 1. The three main regions of the skull base are the anterior, middle, and posterior cranial fossa.

Anterior cranial fossa boundaries are as follows:

- Anteriorly: Posterior wall of the frontal sinus.
- Posteriorly: Anterior clinoid processes (attachment of tentorium cerebelli), planum sphenoidale (roof of the sphenoid sinus).
- Laterally: Frontal bone.
- Floor: Anterior to posterior:
  - ➢ Foramen cecum.
  - ➢ Crista galli (provides attachment of falx cerebri).
  - ➢ Slit and groove for nasociliary nerve.
  - ➢ Cribriform plate [olfactory nerve fibers' cranial nerve (CN) I passes through and supports olfactory bulb] lateral to the crista galli.
  - ➢ Anterior ethmoid foramen (anterior ethmoidal artery, vein, and nerve).
  - ➢ Posterior ethmoid foramen (posterior ethmoidal artery, vein, and nerve).

The middle cranial fossa is subdivided into a central and two lateral components by the petro-occipital fissure. The boundaries of the middle cranial fossa are as follows:

- Anteriorly: Posterior margins of the lesser wings of the sphenoid bone, anterior clinoid processes, anterior margin of chiasmatic groove.
- Posteriorly: Anterior surface of the petrous temporal bone, dorsum sellae.
- Laterally: Greater wing of the sphenoid; it extends laterally and upward from the sphenoid body to meet the squamous portion of the temporal bone and the anteroinferior portion of the parietal bone.

The central part of the middle cranial fossa is formed by the body of the sphenoid bone and contains the following anteriorly to posteriorly:

- Chiasmatic groove.
- Anterior clinoid processes.
- Tuberculum sellae (anterior wall of sella turcica).
- Hypophyseal fossa (houses the pituitary gland).
- Dorsum sellae (posterior wall of sella turcica).
- Carotid grooves (on either side of sella turcica).
- Posterior clinoid processes.

The lateral part of the middle cranial fossa contains the following anterior to posterior:

- Superior orbital fissure (oculomotor nerve CN III, trochlear nerve CN IV, abducens nerve CN VI, and ophtalmic branch of trigeminal nerve CN V1, inferior ophthalmic veins).
- Foramen rotundum (maxillary branch of trigeminal nerve CN V2, artery of foramen rotundum, emissary veins).
- Foramen ovale (mandibular branch of trigeminal nerve CN V3, accessory meningeal artery, emissary veins, otic ganglion, lesser petrosal nerve).
- Foramen spinosum (middle meningeal artery, middle meningeal vein, nervus spinosus).
- Foramen lacerum (meningeal branch of the ascending pharyngeal artery, emissary veins).
- Carotid canal (internal carotid artery, deep petrosal nerve).
- Pterygoid canal (vidian artery, vidian nerve).

The posterior cranial fossa is bounded anteriorly by the posterior surface of petrous temporal bone, posteriorly by the occipital bone, and laterally by the squamous and mastoid parts of the temporal bone. The following structures are present from anterior to posterior:

- Internal acoustic meatus (facial nerve CN VII, vestibulocochlear nerve CN VIII, vestibular ganglion, labyrinthine artery).

- Foramen magnum (medulla oblongata, meninges, spinal root of accessory nerve CN XI, vertebral arteries, anterior and posterior spinal arteries, tectorial membrane, alar ligaments).
- Groove for superior petrosal sinus.
- Jugular foramen (inferior petrosal sinus, glossopharyngeal nerve CN IX, jugular bulb, vagus nerve CN X, spinal accessory CN XI).
- Hypoglossal canal (hypoglossal nerve CN XII).
- Vestibular aqueduct.
- Condylar foramen (emissary veins, meningeal branch of the occipital artery).

Pathologies and Its Variants

The classification of FOL subtypes has represented a challenge for decades. Various classification systems have been proposed for this diverse group of FOL, most of these aim at distinguishing these lesions into three main groups according to their developmental, reactive, or neoplastic origins.[2] The various classifications of FOL proposed by different authors are listed below:

- Charles Waldron's classification 1985.[3]
- Working classification of FOL 1987.[4]
- Peiter J. Slootweg and Hellmuth Müller classification 1990.[5]
- World Health Organization (WHO) classification 2005.[6]
- Waldron's modified classification 1993.[7]
- Brannon and Fowler classification 2001.[8]
- WHO classification of FOL 2005.[6]
- Paul M. Speight and Roman Carlos classification 2006.[9]
- Eversole et al's classification 2008.[2]

In 2008, Eversole et al[2] gave a comprehensive classification and emphasized that the definitive diagnosis of FOL can rarely be confirmed on histopathology features alone but can be attained by correlation of microscopic, clinical, and imaging features together.

Classification of FOL[2]

- Bone dysplasia:
  - ➢ Fibrous dysplasia (FD):
    - Monostotic.
    - Polyostotic.
    - Polyostotic with endocrinopathy (McCune–Albright).
    - Osteofibrous dysplasia.
  - ➢ Osteitis deformans.
  - ➢ Pagetoid heritable bone dysplasias of childhood.
  - ➢ Segmental odontomaxillary dysplasia.
- Cemento-osseous dysplasia (COD):
  - ➢ Focal cemento-osseous dysplasia.
  - ➢ Florid cemento-osseous dysplasia.
- Inflammatory/reactive processes:
  - ➢ Focal sclerosing osteomyelitis.
  - ➢ Diffuse sclerosing osteomyelitis.
  - ➢ Proliferative periostitis.
- Metabolic disease: Hyperparathyroidism.
- Neoplastic lesions (ossifying fibromas):
  - ➢ Ossifying fibroma not otherwise specified (NOS).
  - ➢ Hyperparathyroidism-jaw lesion syndrome.
  - ➢ Juvenile ossifying fibroma:
    - Trabecular type.
    - Psammomatoid type.
  - ➢ Gigantiform cementoma.

Detailed description of the following FOL.

Fibrous Dysplasia

FD is a benign developmental dysplastic disease that may occur within a single bone (monostotic), multiple bones (polyostotic), or associated with McCune–Albright syndrome. The most common form is the monostotic subtype (70% of cases), occurring typically between ages 20 and 30 years and the lesion usually involves the craniofacial bones. The polyostotic subtype (30% of cases), on the other hand, typically occurs in childhood and tends to cause more severe skeletal and craniofacial involvement.[10] McCune–Albright syndrome (3% of cases) is the most severe subtype and is associated with short stature, endocrine abnormalities, and pigmented cutaneous lesions.[11]

The pathogenesis of FD is not fully understood, but one proposed cause is the disease is mediated by the upregulation of the guanine nucleotide-binding protein alpha-stimulating activity polypeptide 1 (*GNAS1*) gene which results in increased G-protein activity and interference in normal osteoblast maturation.[12,13] The timing of the mutation either during fetal or postnatal life determines the clinical severity of the disease. Mutation of the *GNAS1* gene at early embryonic life results in McCune–Albright syndrome. While the mutation that occurs at later stages of embryonic life results in polyostotic FD. Monostotic FD is a result of mutation occurring during postnatal life.[14]

The craniofacial bones are typically involved in approximately 10% of patients with monostotic form and in 50% of patients with the polyostotic form. Clinically, patients can present with vague symptoms such as headaches and sinonasal symptoms such as nasal obstruction and recurrent sinusitis as FD typically involves the sinuses. Some patients can develop visual changes, such as proptosis and diplopia, because of the preponderance of ethmoid, sphenoid, and frontal bone involvement by FD. Painless swelling is another common presenting symptom, or patients may be completely asymptomatic and the lesion was identified incidentally on imaging for another indication.[10]

Histopathological analysis of FD is characterized by replacement and expansion of medullary and cortical bone with sheets of fibro-osseous tissues with intermixed trabecular bone. The trabecular bone takes on abnormal shapes like "Chinese character" appearance because of osteoclastic activity within the lesion.[2]

Computed tomography (CT) is the study of choice for diagnosis and follow-up because of its superior bony detail, and the extent of the lesion can be assessed more accurately. Distinguishing features of FD include "ground glass" appearance, mixed sclerotic and lytic, sinus involvement, and aneurysmal bone cyst formation, and there is often no clear margin between affected and unaffected bone.[15,16] Magnetic resonance imaging (MRI) is a useful modality to define the extent of soft tissue involvement and the impingement of central nervous system structures. Typically, the lesions are low intensity on T2- and low to moderate intensity on T1-weighted MRI sequence and also shows moderate to marked enhancement with gadolinium.[10]

Surgery remains the mainstay of treatment for FD. However, incidental and asymptomatic lesions can be monitored with serial CT or MRI and serial ophthalmology examination if involving the orbit and the optic canal. If the diagnosis cannot be confirmed by radiological studies, then an open biopsy is warranted.[10] Once the diagnosis is confirmed, if the lesion involves vital structures (cranial nerves, carotid artery), subtotal resection with close follow-up is often adequate to control clinical symptoms. A multidisciplinary approach combining otorhinolaryngology, neurosurgery, ophthalmology, and maxillofacial surgery can help optimize outcomes. Lesions involving sinuses or maxilla can be approached anteriorly either endoscopically[17] or via a more traditional transfacial approach.[18] Radiation therapy is ineffective and contraindicated because of the possibility of malignant transformation.[19] **Table 41.1** highlights the key features of FD.

Osteitis Deformans

Osteitis deformans, also known as Paget's disease, is a benign dysplastic disease characterized by bone remodeling that begins with excessive resorption followed by an increase in bone formation.[2] Three phases have been described: lytic, mixed lytic and blastic, and sclerotic phase. The lytic phase is because of the resorption of normal bone by osteoclasts, followed by the mixed phase characterized by osteoblastic activity causing a rapid increase in abnormal bone formation (woven bone). The ongoing osteoclastic and osteoblastic process leads to a high turnover of bone. The final sclerotic phase is also known as the burned-out phase where bone resorption and formation are minimal.

The exact etiology of Paget's disease is unknown, but genetic and environmental factors have been implicated. Genetic linkage studies have identified several loci associated with Paget's disease. These include the defective function of the osteoprotegerin tumor necrosis factor receptor superfamily member-11A (*TNFRSF11A)* pathway, a molecular regulator of osteoclastogenesis.[20] Secondly, the mutation in *SQSTM1*, the sequestosome gene that encodes a scaffold protein p62 for the nuclear factor kappa-B (NF KappaB) signaling pathway, which is involved in osteoclast differentiation and activation. Thirdly, valosin-containing protein (*VCP*), which is involved in the autophagy process has been linked to Paget's disease.[21–24] Infectious etiology is another leading hypothesis for Paget's disease, and suspected viruses are paramyxoviruses (such as measles), canine distemper viruses, and respiratory syncytial virus.[25,26]

Classical Paget's disease of bone (CPDB) usually is a disease of the elderly causing marked elevation of alkaline phosphatase with a normal calcium and phosphate level.[2] The majority of patients are asymptomatic, however, some present with bone pain, secondary osteoarthritis, bony deformity, or neurological complications. The disease can affect all bones of the skull and facial bones to varying degrees. Bone remodeling can cause narrowing of the neural foramina leading to cranial neuropathies.

Histologically, the bones of the maxillofacial and skull base manifest a ground glass trabecular pattern at early stages of the disease and as the disease progresses, with marked evidence of cell turnover, resting and reversal lines of lamellar compact and trabecular bone are prevalent and haphazardly arranged into a "mosaic" or "jigsaw" pattern.[2] This histological pattern is the hallmark of Paget's disease.

Bisphosphonates (pamidronate, alendronate, risedronate) have been shown to have reversing effects on the osseous lesions in CPDB.[27] It also reduces symptoms and decreases alkaline phosphatase blood levels.

Table 41.1 Key features of fibrous dysplasia[2]

Clinical features	Expansion of bone Unilateral, painless Monostotic, polyostotic, or McCune-Albright syndrome
Histology	"Chinese/Hebrew character" trabecular appearance
Genetic	Upregulation of *GNAS1* gene
Radiology	Diffuse radiolucent or ground glass appearance Blends with unaffected bone
Treatment	Subtotal resection

Among patients with CPDB, two neoplastic processes may occur, namely giant cell tumors and sarcomas; however, the incidence is rare. **Table 41.2** highlights the key features of Paget's disease.

Cemento-osseous Dysplasia

Lesions classified under COD encompass two different subgroups: focal COD and florid COD. Focal COD, also known as periapical COD, is the most common FOL of the jaw. Florid COD is because of an extensive process with multifocal involvement of the jaw.[2] **Table 41.3** highlights the key features of the disease.

Focal COD predominantly occurs in females of Afro-Caribbean origin in fourth or fifth decades of life and the majority of lesions are asymptomatic and nonexpansile.[28] Mandible is the most common site for the lesion. Radiographically, there are three phases: early, intermediate, and late stages. At the early stage, focal COD presents with a well-defined radiolucency of the apices of the mandibular teeth. At the intermediate stage, a mixed radiolucent/opaque pattern with a well-defined radiolucent rim is seen and at the late stage, diffuse radiopacities with ill-defined borders are encountered.[2] The diagnosis of focal COD can be made by clinical and radiographic investigations alone; however, it is important to rule out neoplastic lesion that requires urgent surgical intervention. Histopathology of focal COD exhibits three stages: early, mid, and late stage. The early stage shows multifragmented tissue composed of vascular fibrous stroma with scattered osteoid trabeculae. At mid stage, the lesion consists of progressively more trabeculae with cement-like calcifications. In the late stage, the lesion displays a "ginger-root" pattern of trabeculae with very little fibrotic stroma. The majority of patients with focal COD are treated conservatively with periodic follow-up to ensure no further enlargement or expansion occurs.[29] Complete surgical removal is reserved for cases with a severe facial deformity or symptoms resulting in a reduction in quality of life.

Florid COD is diagnosed when lesions with radiographic and microscopic features similar to focal FOD but involves two or more quadrants of the jaw.[30,31] The majority of cases, the disease affects the mandible bilaterally but may also involve the maxilla. Florid COD mostly affects African females in their mid-forties. Radiographically, the lesions are most commonly found in the mandibular molar or premolar region characterized by multiple nonexpansile radio-opacities, which are confluent and found in all four quadrants of the jaw. Clinically, florid COD causes no symptoms. Occasionally, the lesions can get infected causing pain and swelling. In these patients, radical surgical treatment has a favorable prognosis and allows complete resolution.[32] Histopathology of florid COD shows some mixed stage but mainly late-stage characteristics of focal COD, which is mainly sclerotic.

Table 41.2 Key features of osteitis deformans/Paget's disease[2]

Clinical features	Asymptomatic Expansile lesion Elevated alkaline phosphatase levels Cranial neuropathies Polyostotic
Histology	Trabecular, giant cell lesions, jigsaw or mosaic pattern
Genetic	Adult: *SQSTM1* Childhood: *TNFRSF11A*
Radiology	Ground glass, cotton wool appearance
Treatment	Bisphosphonates

Inflammatory/Reactive Processes

Infections within the craniofacial bones, usually the mandible, are caused by low virulence, pyogenic and anaerobic organisms (*streptococci, Bacteroides, actinomycetes*).[2] These infections can lead to suppurative intraoral lesions, as well as cutaneous sinus tracts. This can lead to destructive osseous lesions because of osteoclastic resorption of bone by infectious organisms and host inflammatory response. On radiographical image, this is seen as "moth-eaten" radiolucencies. **Table 41.4** highlights the key features of inflammatory or reactive processes.

Table 41.3 Features of focal versus florid cemento-osseous dysplasia[2]

	Focal COD	Florid COD
Clinical features	Nonexpansile Painless	Nonexpansile African descent
Histology	Trabecular, cementifying, "ginger root" trabeculae	Trabecular, sclerotic
Radiology	Focal, circumscribed, lucent	Multiquadrant opacities
Treatment	Conservative	Conservative Surgery

Table 41.4 Key features of inflammatory/reactive processes[2]

	Focal sclerosing osteomyelitis	Diffuse sclerosing osteomyelitis
Clinical features	Young adults and children Nonexpansile Painless Carries	Adults Expansile Painful Dental infection
Histology	Trabecular, sclerotic	Trabecular, sclerotic
Radiology	Apical well-demarcated Lucent, target, or opaque	Diffuse ground glass Proliferative periostitis
Treatment	Extraction or endodontic	Medical treatment

Focal sclerosing osteomyelitis, also known as condensing osteitis, is usually a self-limiting disease of the mandible, affecting young adults and children. On radiographical imaging, there is localized but uniform increased radiodensity related to the tooth with widened periodontal ligament space or periapical area. Sometimes an adjacent radiolucent inflammatory lesion may be present. The mainstay of treatment includes the elimination of the source of inflammation by either extraction or endodontic treatment.[2,33,34]

Diffuse sclerosing osteomyelitis is because of chronic intraosseous bacterial infection, which creates a mass of chronic granulation tissue. It arises exclusively in adulthood and primarily occurs in the mandible. Clinically, it can cause severe pain or swelling with cortical osseous expansion. Radiological appearance is characterized by a unilateral diffuse ground glass opacification without define boundaries. Treatment includes antimicrobial therapy, hyperbaric oxygen, steroid or analgesic medication, and surgical debridement.[2,35,36]

Proliferative osteitis, also known as *Garre's osteomyelitis*, is a rare disease characterized by new bone formation with periosteal reaction. It is commonly caused by dental caries, periodontitis, and trauma. This disease entity is managed by eliminating any odontogenic source of infection either by dental extraction or endodontic treatment. Long-term antibiotics have a role to resolve the problem.[2]

Ossifying Fibroma

Ossifying fibroma is a slow-growing, benign FOL, characterized by the substitution of normal bone by fibrous tissues and newly formed calcified products like bone, cementum, or both.[37] Radiologically, the lesion shows bony expansion with well-defined margins.

The subtypes of ossifying fibroma consist of ossifying/cementifying fibroma not otherwise specified, trabecular variant of juvenile ossifying fibroma (TrJOF), psammomatoid variant of juvenile ossifying fibroma (PsJOF), and gigantiform cementoma. This overview will further discuss juvenile ossifying fibroma (JOF).

JOF is a unique entity affecting primarily children and adolescents under the age of 15. Although it is a benign bone tumor, it is locally aggressive with a high tendency for recurrence. The etiology of JOF is unknown, but there is an association of a new tumor suppressor gene, *HPRT2*, that was reported by Pimenta et al.[38] *HPRT2* is a gene that encodes parafibromin protein and mutation of this gene can cause hyperparathyroidism-jaw tumor syndrome leading to OF.

Histologically, JOF is characterized by the presence of a cellular fibrous stroma, garland-like bony strands, and cement particles.[39] Two histopathological variants of JOF are TrJOF and PsJOF.[40] The average age of occurrence of TrJOF is considerably younger than PsJOF with the average being 8 to 12 years as compared to 16 to 33 years age range of PsJOF. With respect to the site, PsJOF occurs mainly in the sinonasal and orbital bones of the skull, whereas TrJOF predominantly affects the jaws with a predilection for the maxilla[41] more so than the mandible.

Clinically, TrJOF can present with a progressive and sometimes rapidly expanding painless lesion involving the jaw. On the other hand, PsJOF can present clinically with nasal symptoms, facial deformity, proptosis, visual complaints including blindness, ptosis, and double vision secondary to orbital extension of the tumor.[42] Radiologically, TrJOF tumor is well circumscribed with cortical thinning and perforation. The lesion can show varying degree of radiolucency depending on the amount of calcified tissue as well as a multilocular honeycomb appearance. Radiographical examination of PsJOF exhibits a well-circumscribed, osteolytic lesion with a cystic appearance. There may be ground glass appearance because of sclerotic changes within the lesion.

Complete excision of JOF is the treatment of choice. Radiotherapy is contraindicated because the tumor is radioresistant. **Table 41.5** highlights the features of JOF.

Table 41.5 Key features of juvenile ossifying fibroma[2]

	Juvenile ossifying fibroma - trabecular variant	Juvenile ossifying fibroma - psammomatoid variant
Clinical features	8–12 years old Expansile Painless Root divergence Aggressive	16–33 years old Expansile Facial bones Aggressive
Histology	Trabecular Giant cell foci Fibroplasia	Psammomatoid
Radiology	Circumscribed/lucent Floccular opacities	Circumscribed Dense floccular opacities
Treatment	Complete surgical resection Infrequent recurrence	Complete surgical resection Higher recurrence rate

References

1. Alawi F. Benign fibro-osseous diseases of the maxillofacial bones. A review and differential diagnosis. Am J Clin Pathol 2002;118(Suppl):S50–S70
2. Eversole R, Su L, ElMofty S. Benign fibro-osseous lesions of the craniofacial complex: a review. Head Neck Pathol 2008;2(3):177–202
3. Waldron CA. Fibro-osseous lesions of the jaws. J Oral Maxillofac Surg 1985;43(4):249–262
4. Makek MS. So called "fibro-osseous lesions" of tumorous origin. Biology confronts terminology. J Craniomaxillofac Surg 1987;15(3):154–167
5. Slootweg PJ, Müller H. Differential diagnosis of fibro-osseous jaw lesions. A histological investigation on 30 cases. J Craniomaxillofac Surg 1990;18(5):210–214
6. Barnes LEJ, Reichart P, Sidransky, D. World Health Organisation classification of tumours: pathology and genetics of head and neck tumours. IARC Press; 2005
7. Waldron CA. Fibro-osseous lesions of the jaws. J Oral Maxillofac Surg 1993;51(8):828–835
8. Cuisia ZE, Brannon RB. Peripheral ossifying fibroma—a clinical evaluation of 134 pediatric cases. Pediatr Dent 2001; 23(3):245–248
9. Speight PM, Carlos R. Maxillofacial fibro-osseous lesions. Curr Diagn Pathol 2006;(12):1–10
10. Lustig LR, Holliday MJ, McCarthy EF, Nager GT. Fibrous dysplasia involving the skull base and temporal bone. Arch Otolaryngol Head Neck Surg 2001;127(10):1239–1247
11. Nager GT, Holliday MJ. Fibrous dysplasia of the temporal bone. Update with case reports. Ann Otol Rhinol Laryngol 1984;93(6 Pt 1):630–633
12. Warner DR, Weinstein LS. A mutation in the heterotrimeric stimulatory guanine nucleotide binding protein alpha-subunit with impaired receptor-mediated activation because of elevated GTPase activity. Proc Natl Acad Sci U S A 1999;96(8):4268–4272
13. Warner DR, Weng G, Yu S, Matalon R, Weinstein LS. A novel mutation in the switch 3 region of Gsalpha in a patient with Albright hereditary osteodystrophy impairs GDP binding and receptor activation. J Biol Chem 1998;273(37):23976–23983
14. Srichinthu KK, Yoithapprabhunath TR, Chitture RT, Yamunadevi A, Potsangbam AD, Singh DN. Fibro-osseous lesions—classifications, pathophysiology and importance of radiology: a short review. Int Biol Biomed J. 2016;2(1): 11–20
15. Unal Erzurumlu Z, Celenk P, Bulut E, Barıs YS. CT imaging of craniofacial fibrous dysplasia. Case Rep Dent 2015;2015: 134123
16. Efune G, Perez CL, Tong L, Rihani J, Batra PS. Paranasal sinus and skull base fibro-osseous lesions: when is biopsy indicated for diagnosis? Int Forum Allergy Rhinol 2012;2(2):160–165
17. Ikeda K, Suzuki H, Oshima T, Shimomura A, Nakabayashi S, Takasaka T. Endonasal endoscopic management in fibrous dysplasia of the paranasal sinuses. Am J Otolaryngol 1997; 18(6):415–418
18. Ferguson BJ. Fibrous dysplasia of the paranasal sinuses. Am J Otolaryngol 1994;15(3):227–230
19. Edgerton MT, Persing JA, Jane JA. The surgical treatment of fibrous dysplasia. With emphasis on recent contributions from cranio-maxillo-facial surgery. Ann Surg 1985;202(4): 459–479
20. Yip KH, Feng H, Pavlos NJ, Zheng MH, Xu J. p62 ubiquitin binding-associated domain mediated the receptor activator

of nuclear factor-kappaB ligand-induced osteoclast formation: a new insight into the pathogenesis of Paget's disease of bone. Am J Pathol 2006;169(2):503–514

21. Candeliere GA, Glorieux FH, Prud'homme J, St-Arnaud R. Increased expression of the c-fos proto-oncogene in bone from patients with fibrous dysplasia. N Engl J Med 1995; 332(23):1546–1551
22. DiCaprio MR, Enneking WF. Fibrous dysplasia. Pathophysiology, evaluation, and treatment. J Bone Joint Surg Am 2005;87(8):1848–1864
23. Marie PJ. Cellular and molecular basis of fibrous dysplasia. Histol Histopathol 2001;16(3):981–988
24. Monfort J, Sala DR, Romero AB, Duró JC, Maymó J, Carbonell J. Epidemiological, clinical, biochemical, and imaging characteristics of monostotic and polyostotic Paget's disease. Bone 1999;24(5, Suppl):13S–14S
25. Mills BG, Singer FR. Nuclear inclusions in Paget's disease of bone. Science 1976;194(4261):201–202
26. Rebel A, Malkani K, Basle M, Bregeon C, Patezour A, Filmon R. Ultrastructural characteristics of osteoclasts in Paget's disease. Rev Rhum Mal Osteoartic 1974;41(12):767–771
27. Hosking D. Pharmacological therapy of Paget's and other metabolic bone diseases. Bone 2006;38(2, Suppl 2):S3–S7
28. Macdonald-Jankowski DS. Focal cemento-osseous dysplasia: a systematic review. Dentomaxillofac Radiol 2008;37(6): 350–360
29. Bhandari R, Sandhu SV, Bansal H, Behl R, Bhullar RK. Focal cemento-osseous dysplasia masquerading as a residual cyst. Contemp Clin Dent 2012;3(Suppl 1):S60–S62
30. Ong ST, Siar CH. Florid cemento-osseous dysplasia in a young Chinese man. Case report. Aust Dent J 1997;42(6):404–408
31. Mangala M, Ramesh DN, Surekha PS, Santosh P. Florid cemento-osseous dysplasia: review and report of two cases. Indian J Dent Res 2006;17(3):131–134
32. Aiuto R, Gucciardino F, Rapetti R, Siervo S, Bianch AE. Management of symptomatic florid cemento-osseous dysplasia: Literature review and a case report. J Clin Exp Dent 2018;10(3):e291–e295
33. Douglass GD, Trowbridge HO. Chronic focal sclerosing osteomyelitis associated with a cracked tooth. Report of a case. Oral Surg Oral Med Oral Pathol 1993;76(3):351–355
34. Ludlow JB, Brooks SL. Idiopathic focal sclerosing osteomyelitis mimicking retained root tip. Oral Surg Oral Med Oral Pathol 1990;70(2):241–242
35. Jacobsson S. Diffuse sclerosing osteomyelitis of the mandible. Int J Oral Surg 1984;13(5):363–385
36. Montonen M, Lindqvist C. Diagnosis and treatment of diffuse sclerosing osteomyelitis of the jaws. Oral Maxillofac Surg Clin North Am 2003;15(1):69–78
37. Khan SA, Sharma NK, Raj V, Sethi T. Ossifying fibroma of maxilla in a male child: report of a case and review of the literature. Natl J Maxillofac Surg 2011;2(1):73–79
38. Pimenta FJ, Gontijo Silveira LF, Tavares GC, et al. HRPT2 gene alterations in ossifying fibroma of the jaws. Oral Oncol 2006;42(7):735–739
39. Keles B, Duran M, Uyar Y, Azimov A, Demirkan A, Esen HH. Juvenile ossifying fibroma of the mandible: a case report. J Oral Maxillofac Res 2010;1(2):e5
40. El-Mofty S. Psammomatoid and trabecular juvenile ossifying fibroma of the craniofacial skeleton: two distinct clinicopathologic entities. Oral Surg Oral Med Oral Pathol Oral Radiol Endod 2002;93(3):296–304
41. Urs AB, Kumar P, Arora S, Augustine J. Clinicopathologic and radiologic correlation of ossifying fibroma and juvenile ossifying fibroma—an institutional study of 22 cases. Ann Diagn Pathol 2013;17(2):198–203
42. Wilson M, Snyderman C. Fibro-osseous lesions of the skull base in the pediatric population. J Neurol Surg B Skull Base 2018;79(1):31–36

Chapter 42

Endoscopic Management of Skull Base Fibro-osseous Pathologies

Saif Al-Zahid, Michel Roethlisberger, Vicknes Waran, and Prepageran Narayanan

Case 42

Endoscopic Excision of a Sinonasal Fibro-osseous Lesion with Intracranial Extension

History

An 8-year-old boy presented with unilateral blurred vision, progressive swelling and epiphora in the right eye. On examination, the right eye had reduced visual acuity to 6/9 and mild proptosis with no diplopia. The nasal examination was normal. A computed tomography (CT) (**Fig. 42.1a-d**) and a consecutive magnetic resonance imaging (MRI) scan (**Fig. 42.2a, b**) revealed an extra-axial fibro-osseous lesion arising from the right ethmoid air cells and extending intracranially. The lesion involved the right supraorbital bone with mass effect onto the right extraconal space. A large proportion of this lesion was considered intracranial and therefore conventionally this would likely have involved a supraorbital

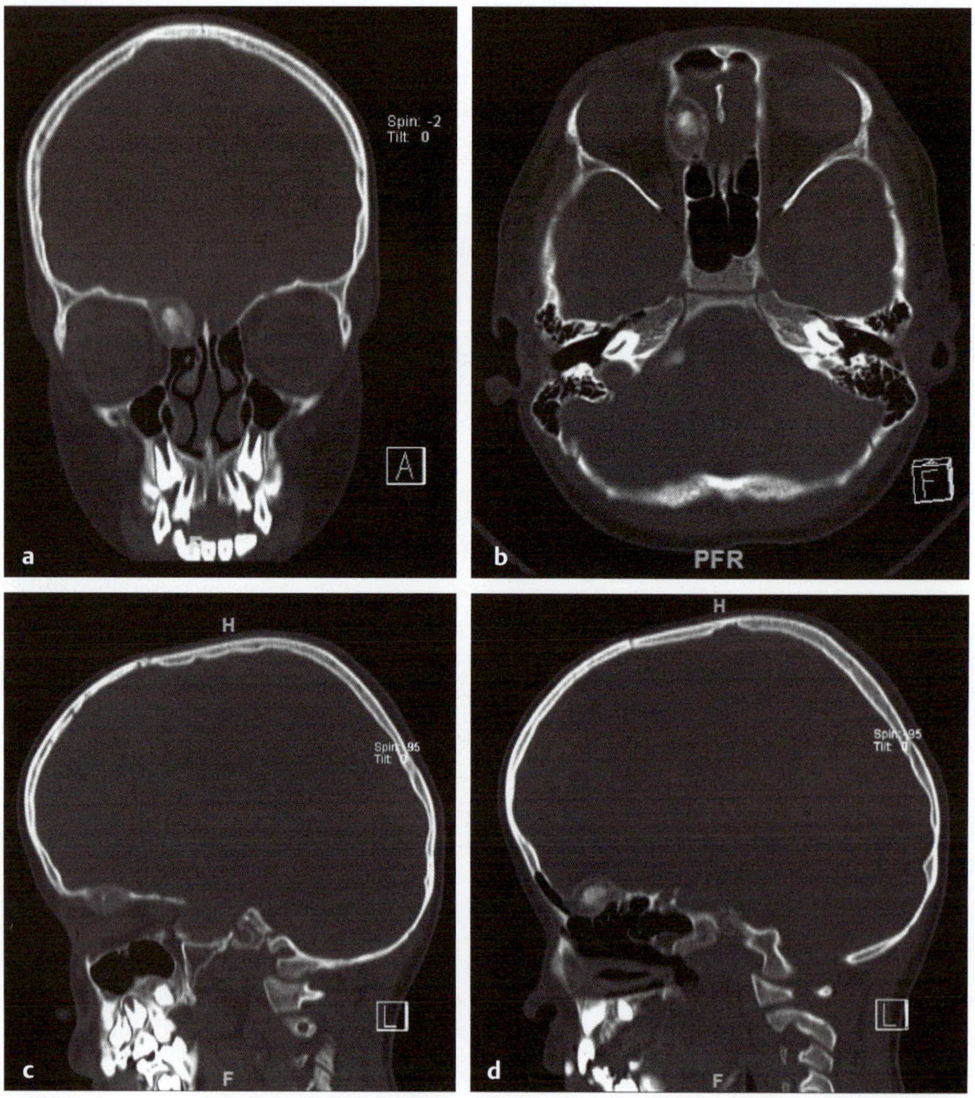

Fig. 42.1 **(a)** Coronal computed tomography (CT) bone-weighted section showing fibro-osseous lesion attached to the right skull base and the right orbital process of the frontal bone. **(b)** Axial bone-weighted CT section showing orbital mass effect. **(c)** Sagittal bone-weighted CT section showing intra-orbital extension. **(d)** Sagittal bone-weighted CT section showing intracranial extension.

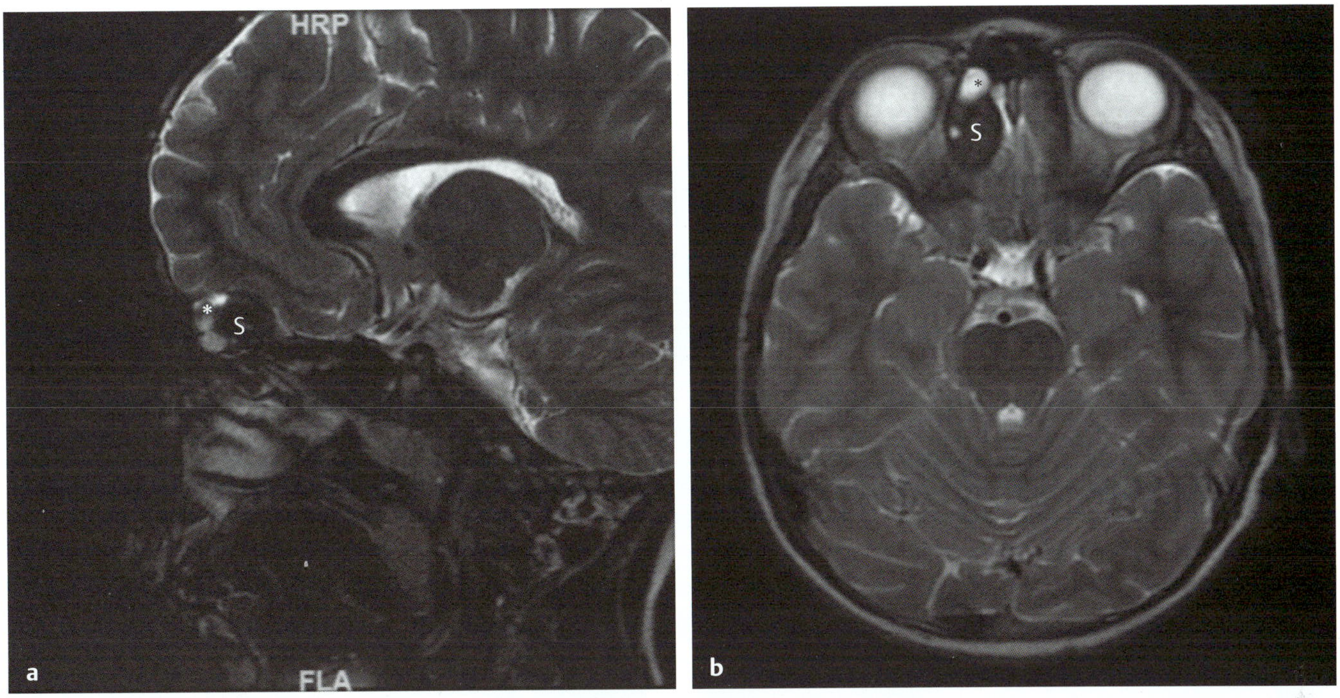

Fig. 42.2 **(a)** Fat-suppressed sagittal T2 MRI showing lesion is centrally solid (S), with cystic surrounding enhancement (*). **(b)** Axial T2 MRI showing solid and cystic elements to the lesion.

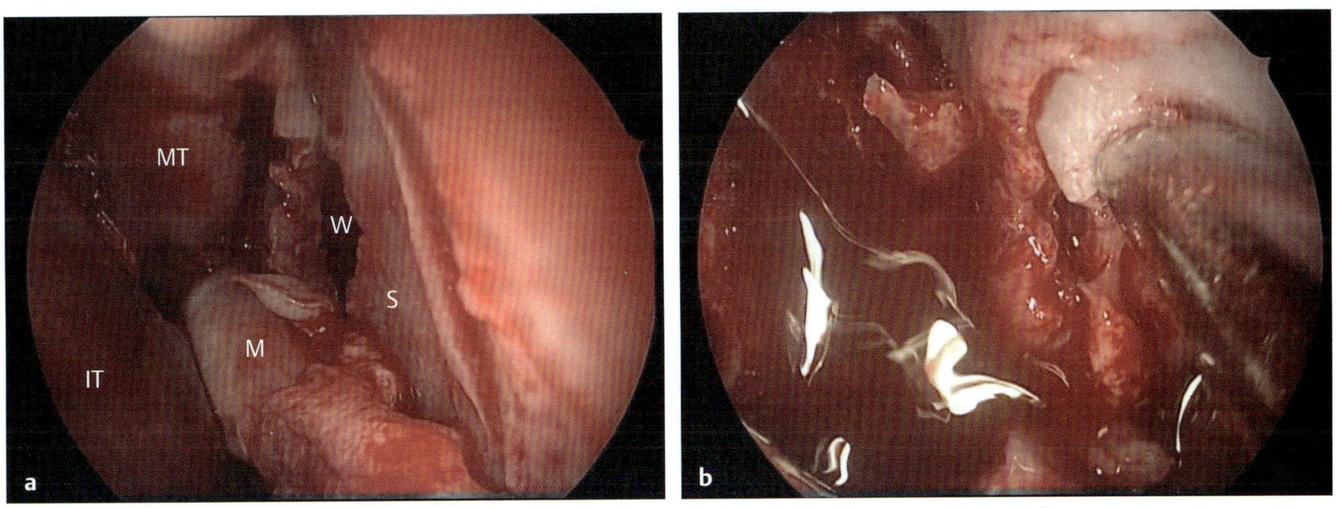

Fig. 42.3 **(a)** Septal window (W) created with an inferiorly based mucosal flap (M). **(b)** The window is widened with a microdebrider.

incision and craniotomy to excise this. With improvement in endoscopic techniques and close cooperation between otolaryngology and neurosurgery, it is possible to excise this endoscopically, thus avoiding morbidity from the former approach.

Surgical Steps

1. The patient is placed under general anesthesia in the supine position and the head is fixed slightly retroflexed within a NORAS frame for intraoperative MRI (iMRI). Registration for image-guided surgery (Brainlab, Munich, Germany) is performed.
2. The nose is decongested with nasal packing as per the institution's usual methods.
3. For improved access, a septal window is performed by raising an inferiorly based mucosal flap and excising a window of cartilage (**Fig. 42.3a**). This can then be widened to improve access with a microdebrider (**Fig. 42.3b**).

4. For adequate exposure, a right-sided uncinectomy, followed by an anterior and posterior ethmoidectomy, is performed.
5. The middle turbinate is divided and pushed inferiorly (**Fig. 42.4**) keeping its posterior attachment intact; this will act as a vascularized pedicled flap later for reconstruction. This exposes the skull base and lamina papyracea where the lesion can be identified in between (**Fig. 42.5**).
6. The mucosa over the lesion is cauterized using monopolar diathermy, and the lesion is uncapped using a Freer elevator and a curette (**Fig. 42.6a, b**).
7. The bone capsule surrounding tumor is identified (**Fig. 42.7**). The anterior ethmoid artery is completely embedded in the tumor and not yet identified.
8. To achieve tumor removal, the abnormal bone attached to lamina papyracea is removed with a cuff of uninvolved lamina papyracea inferior to the tumor to achieve clear margins (**Fig. 42.8**). The AEA is identified after tumor dissection and is later cauterized and divided.
9. Clearance is also obtained medially by removing bone toward the cribriform plate and exposing healthy dura (**Fig. 42.9a**). A plane between bone and dura is dissected with a right-angled dissector, followed by a Kerrison punch to remove bone (**Fig. 42.9b**).
10. Once a cuff of bone has been excised around the mouth of the tumor, access to the tumor bulk becomes much more straightforward (**Fig. 42.10a, b**).
11. Orbital fat protrusion is dealt with by surface bipolar cautery to shrink this and allow further dissection.

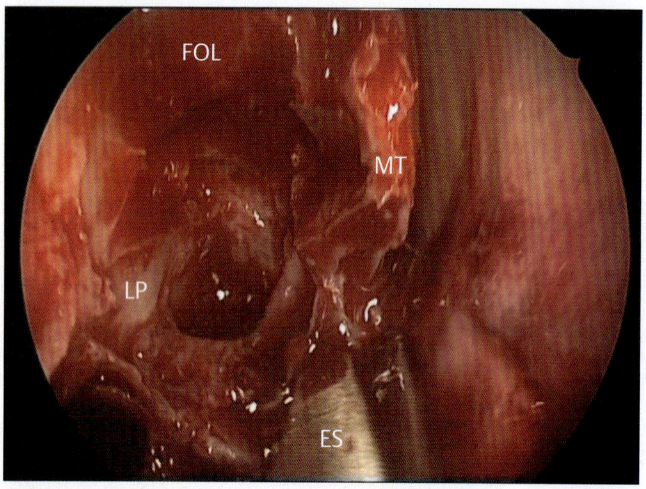

Fig. 42.4 Division of the middle turbinate (MT) to facilitate access to the skull base and the fibro-osseous lesion (FOL).

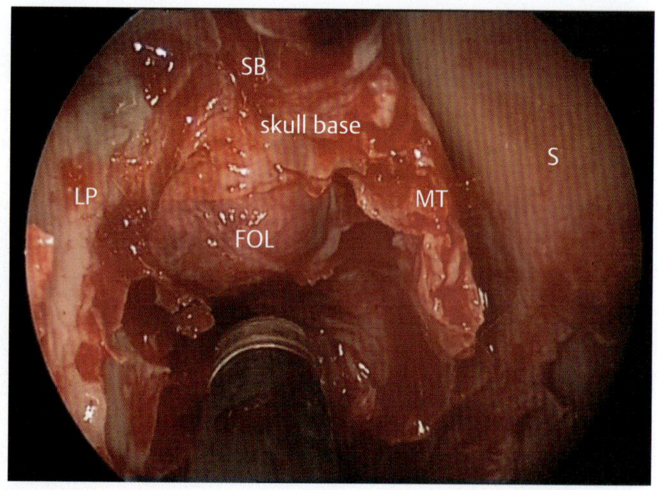

Fig. 42.5 The fibro-osseous lesion (FOL) is seen attached to both the lamina papyracea (LP) and the skull base.

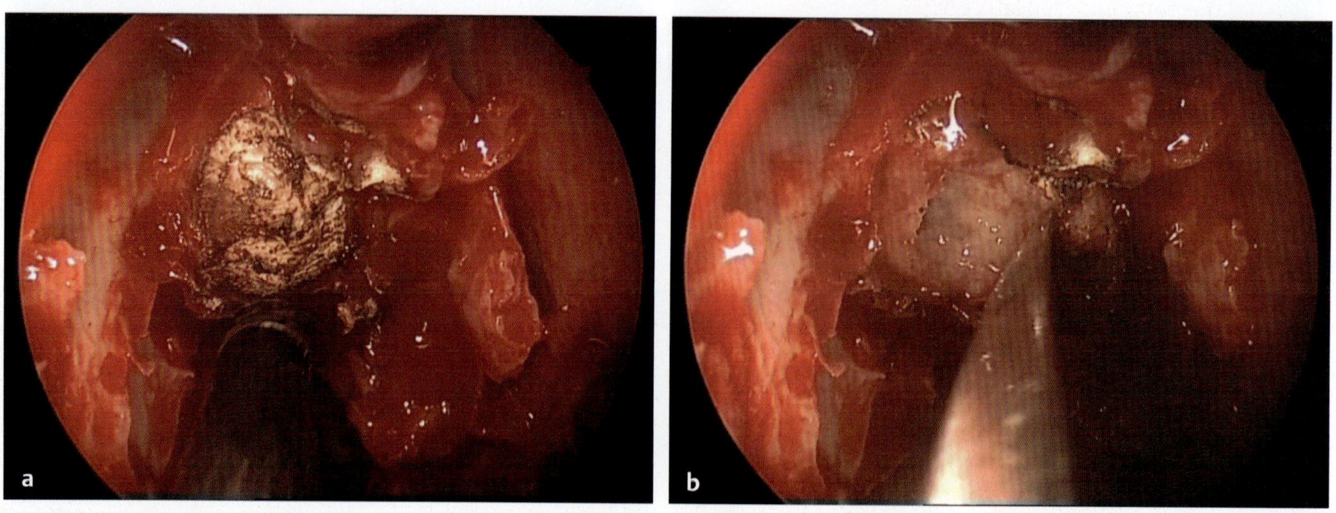

Fig. 42.6 **(a, b)** Monopolar diathermy of the mucosa overlying the fibro-osseous lesion, followed by uncapping with a Freer elevator.

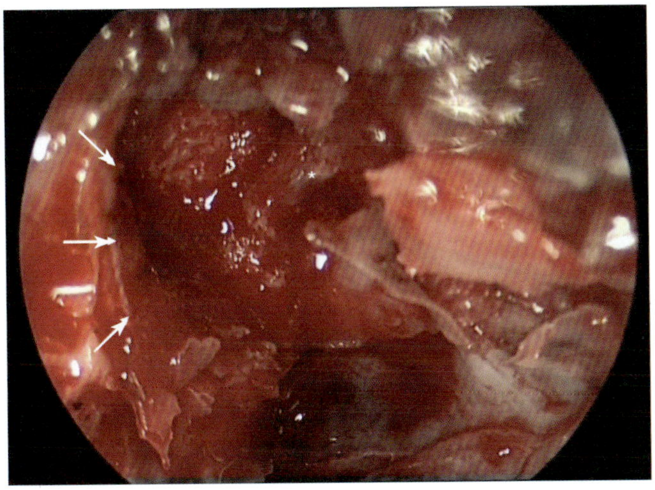

Fig. 42.7 The bone surrounding the tumor capsule is revealed (*white arrows*). The anterior ethmoidal artery is embedded in the tumor and not visible at this stage of dissection.

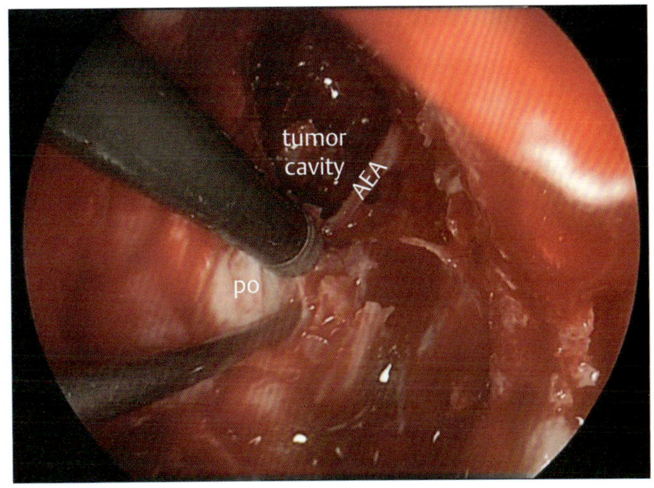

Fig. 42.8 Cuff of healthy lamina papyracea (LP) is removed inferior to the tumor cavity to achieve bony clearance. The anterior ethmoidal artery (AEA) is now visible after dissection of the tumor of the artery.

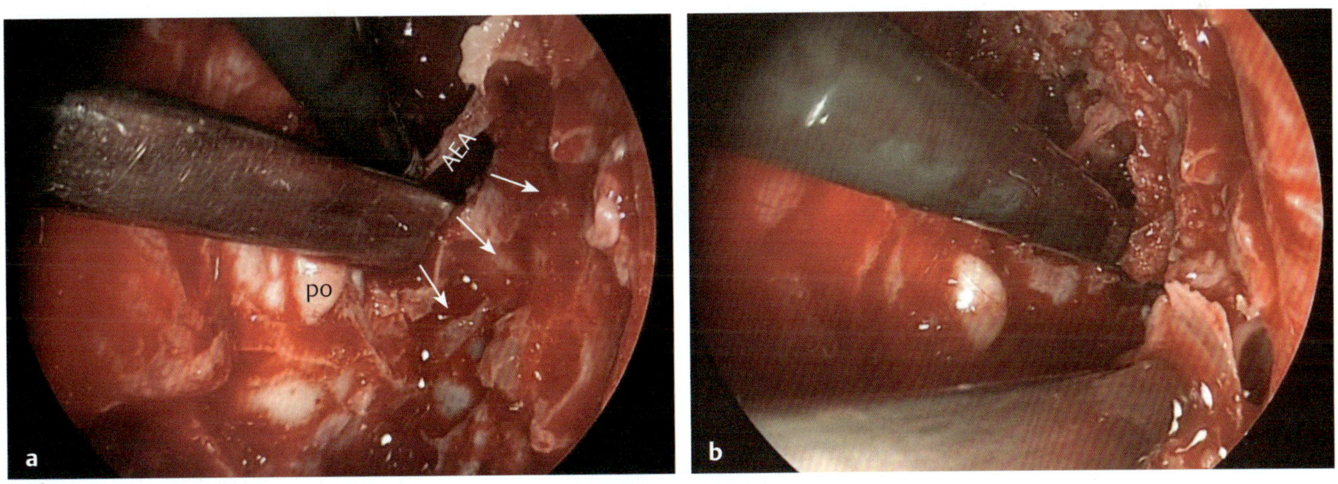

Fig. 42.9 **(a, b)** Dissection around the tumor and removal of bone with healthy resection margins medially (*white arrows*) and the periorbita (po) laterally.

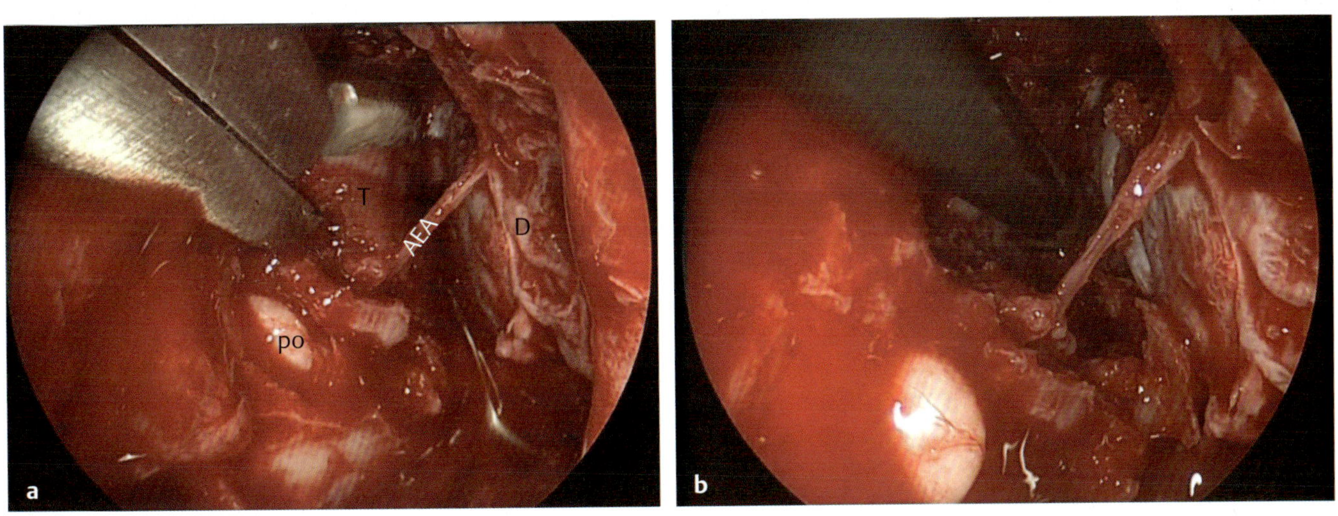

Fig. 42.10 **(a, b)** Medial clearance of the tumor (T) is achieved with dura (D) and periorbita (po) exposed.

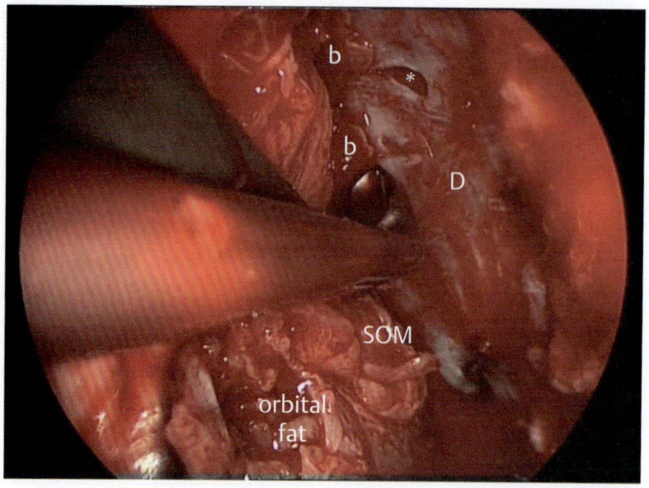

Fig. 42.11 Lateral bone removal along the supraorbital bones (b) with the superior oblique muscles (SOM) visible, along with dura (D) medially, orbital fat laterally, and a dural tear (*) superiorly.

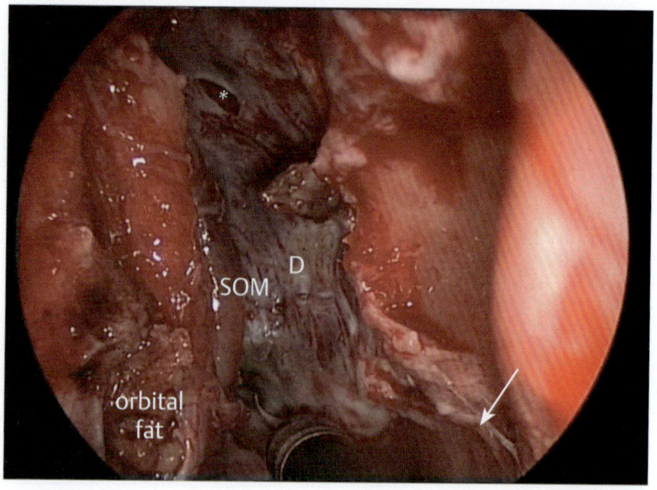

Fig. 42.12 A dural tear is identified (*), medially to the exposed superior oblique muscle (SOM) and the orbital fat. superior oblique muscle is clearly demonstrated. The olfactory fibres (*white arrow*) are visible.

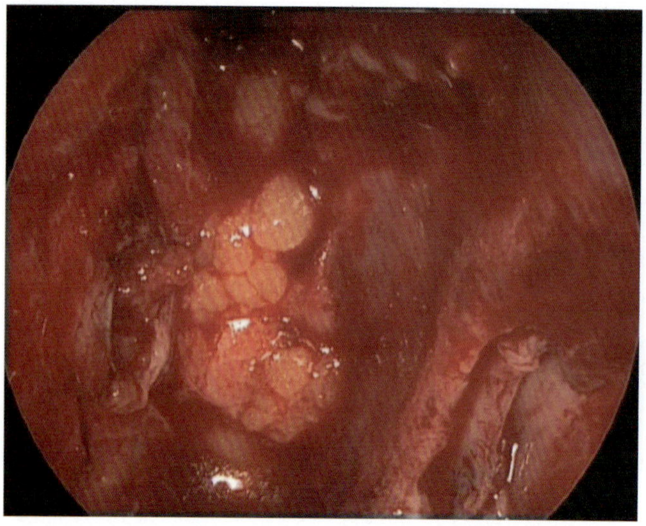

Fig. 42.13 Abdominal fat graft is applied to the defect.

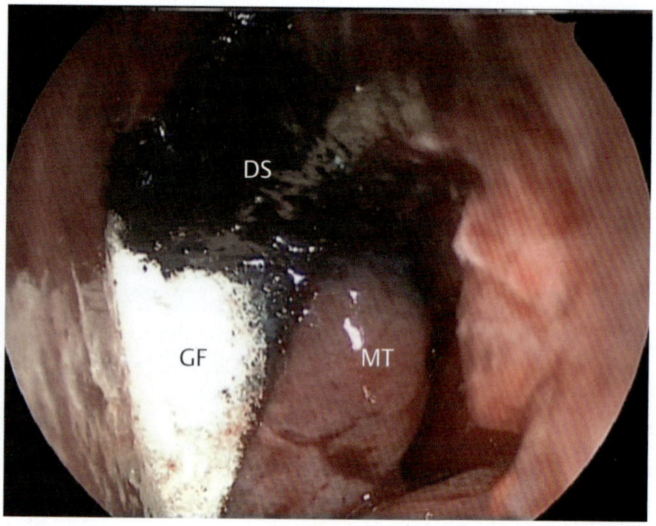

Fig. 42.14 Middle turbinate (MT) is covering reconstruction with DuraSeal (DS).

12. Abnormal bone can now be flicked inward until the healthy bone is reached laterally onto the supraorbital bones. Care has to be taken not to injure the exposed superior oblique muscles (**Fig. 42.11**).
13. Saline wash is performed and bone spicules are removed. Inspection reveals a small dural tear and exposure of olfactory fibers (**Fig. 42.12**).
14. An abdominal autologous fat graft is harvested and used to seal the defect with Dural Sealant System (DuraSeal, Integra Life Sciences) applied on top of this (**Fig. 42.13**).
15. The middle turbinate is placed back on top of the reconstruction to act as a vascularized pedicled flap (**Fig. 42.14**).
16. The nose is packed lightly with Nasopore® (Stryker, Germany).

Chapter 43

Combined Open and Endonasal Endoscopic Management of Skullbase Fibro-osseous Pathologies

Saif Al-Zahid, Malik Ibrahim Malik, Revadi Govindaraju, Michel Roethlisberger, Vicknes Waran, and Prepageran Narayanan

Case 43

Combined Endoscopic and External Excision of an Extensive Ossifying Fibroma

History

A 17-year-old male with biopsy-proven juvenile ossifying fibroma presented with bilateral proptosis, intermittent epistaxis, and bilateral nasal blockage. The patient had three previous endoscopic resections for similar symptoms in the past 4 years. On examination, the patient had severe hypertelorism and remodeling of the facial bones (**Fig. 43.1a, b**). The visual acuity in the right eye was 6/9 and severely reduced in the left eye to 6/60. Both nasal cavities were occupied with the tumor. Magnetic resonance imaging (MRI) scan of the sinuses, orbit, and brain revealed a multiloculated mass occupying the whole of the nasal cavity, with lateral displacement of the orbits and optic nerves (**Fig. 43.2a–c**). The mass extends to the cavernous sinuses, and because of bone resorption there is no discernible sinus anatomy evident on MRI. The tumor exerted a mass effect on both frontal lobes. Surgery is planned as a combined external and endoscopic excision.

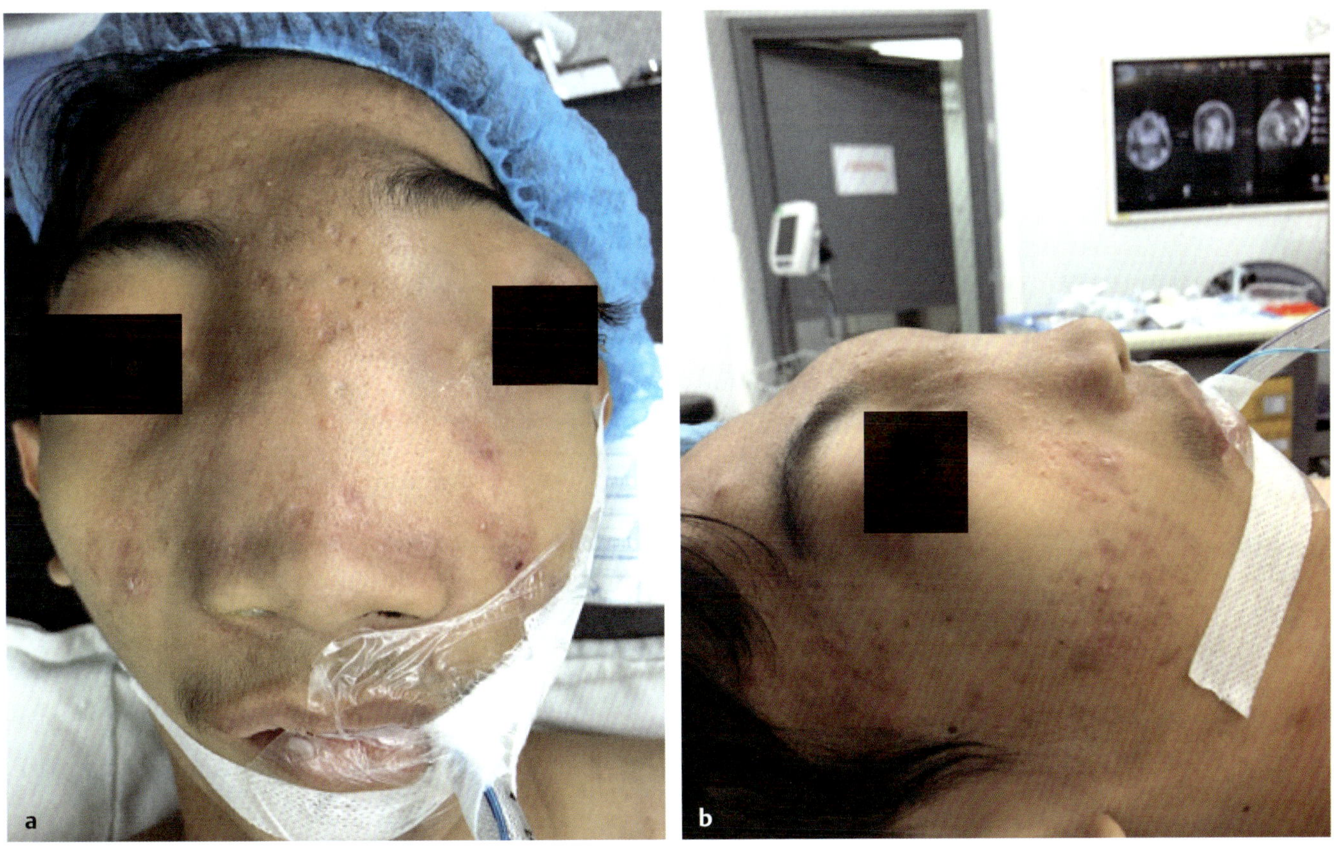

Fig. 43.1 (a, b) Images reveal the degree of hypertelorism and remodeling of facial bones.

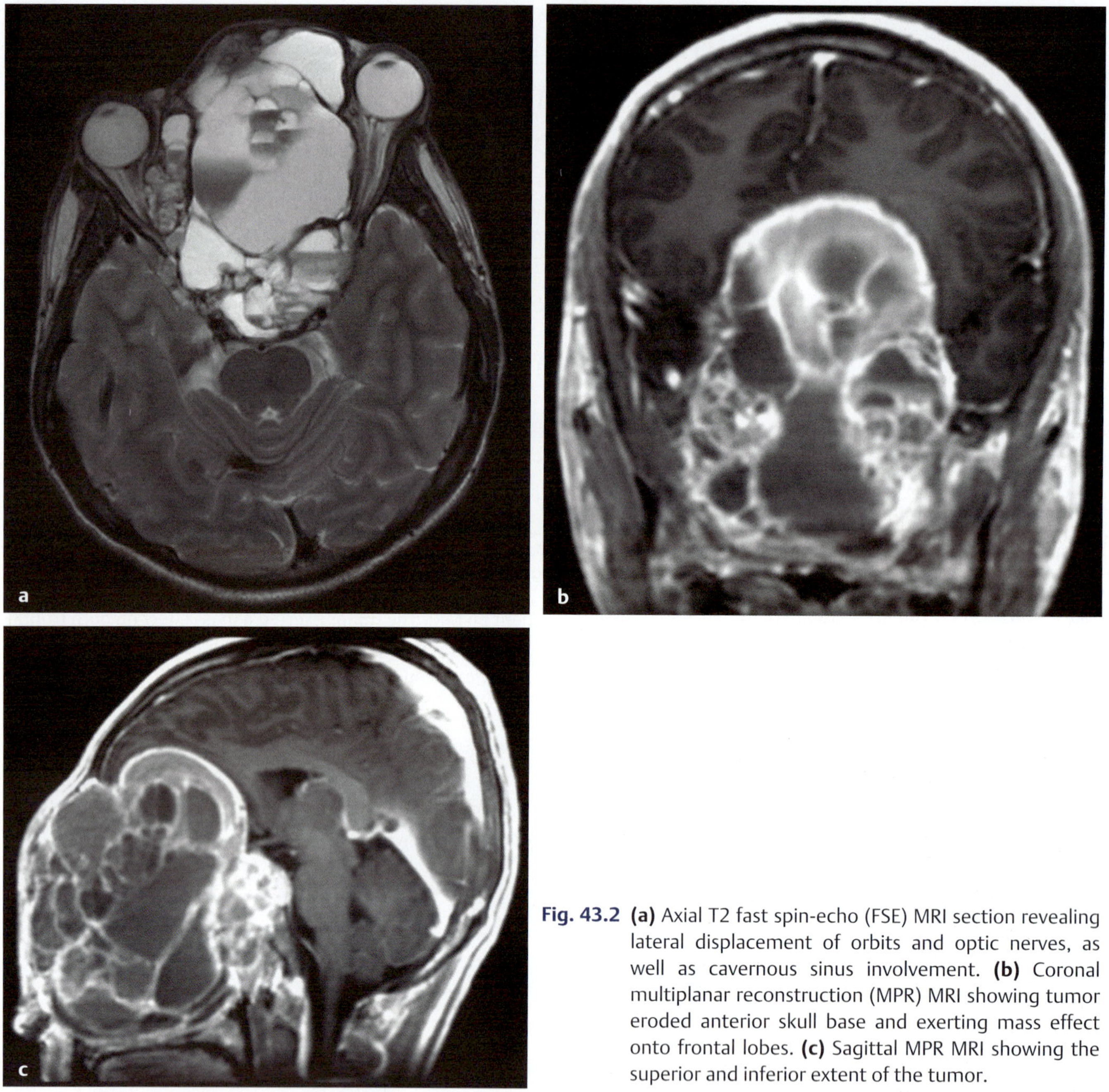

Fig. 43.2 **(a)** Axial T2 fast spin-echo (FSE) MRI section revealing lateral displacement of orbits and optic nerves, as well as cavernous sinus involvement. **(b)** Coronal multiplanar reconstruction (MPR) MRI showing tumor eroded anterior skull base and exerting mass effect onto frontal lobes. **(c)** Sagittal MPR MRI showing the superior and inferior extent of the tumor.

Surgical Steps

1. The patient is placed under general anesthesia in the supine position, and the head is fixed slightly retroflexed within a NORAS frame for intraoperative MRI (iMRI). Registration for neuronavigation (Brainlab, Munich, Germany) is performed (**Fig. 43.3a, b**).
2. Following marking and infiltration, a left lateral rhinotomy incision is performed, and the skin is elevated in a subperiosteal plane with a periosteal elevator. This is complemented with separate incisions of the columella and contralateral alar attachment giving excellent exposure for tumor excision (**Fig. 43.4a–c**).
3. Initially, a plane is established between the tumor and nasal floor with blunt finger dissection. In the same fashion, this dissection is extended laterally and superiorly with the bulk of the tumor delivered out of the nose to facilitate the use of the endoscope for further excision (**Fig. 43.5a, b**).

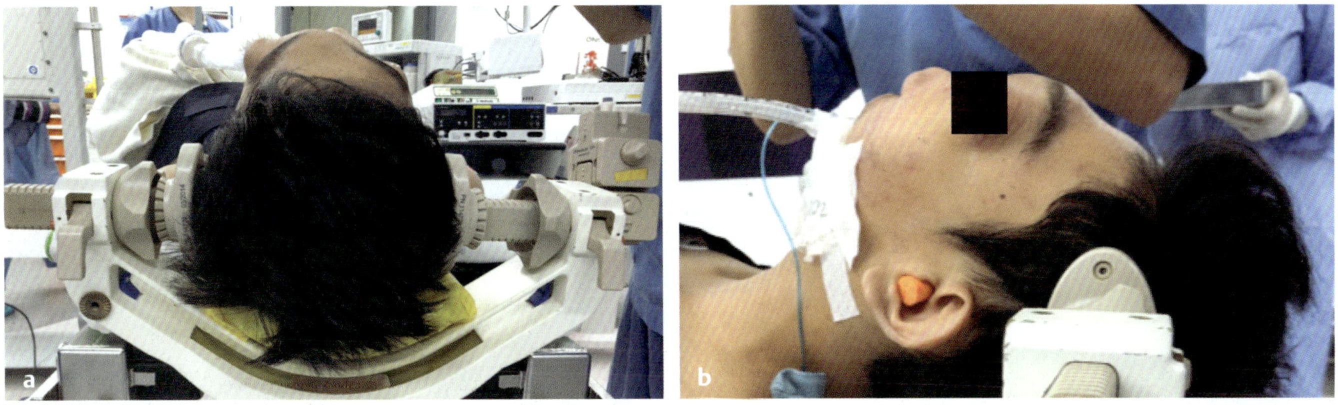

Fig. 43.3 (a, b) Head fixation in a NORAS frame for intraoperative MRI and neuronavigation.

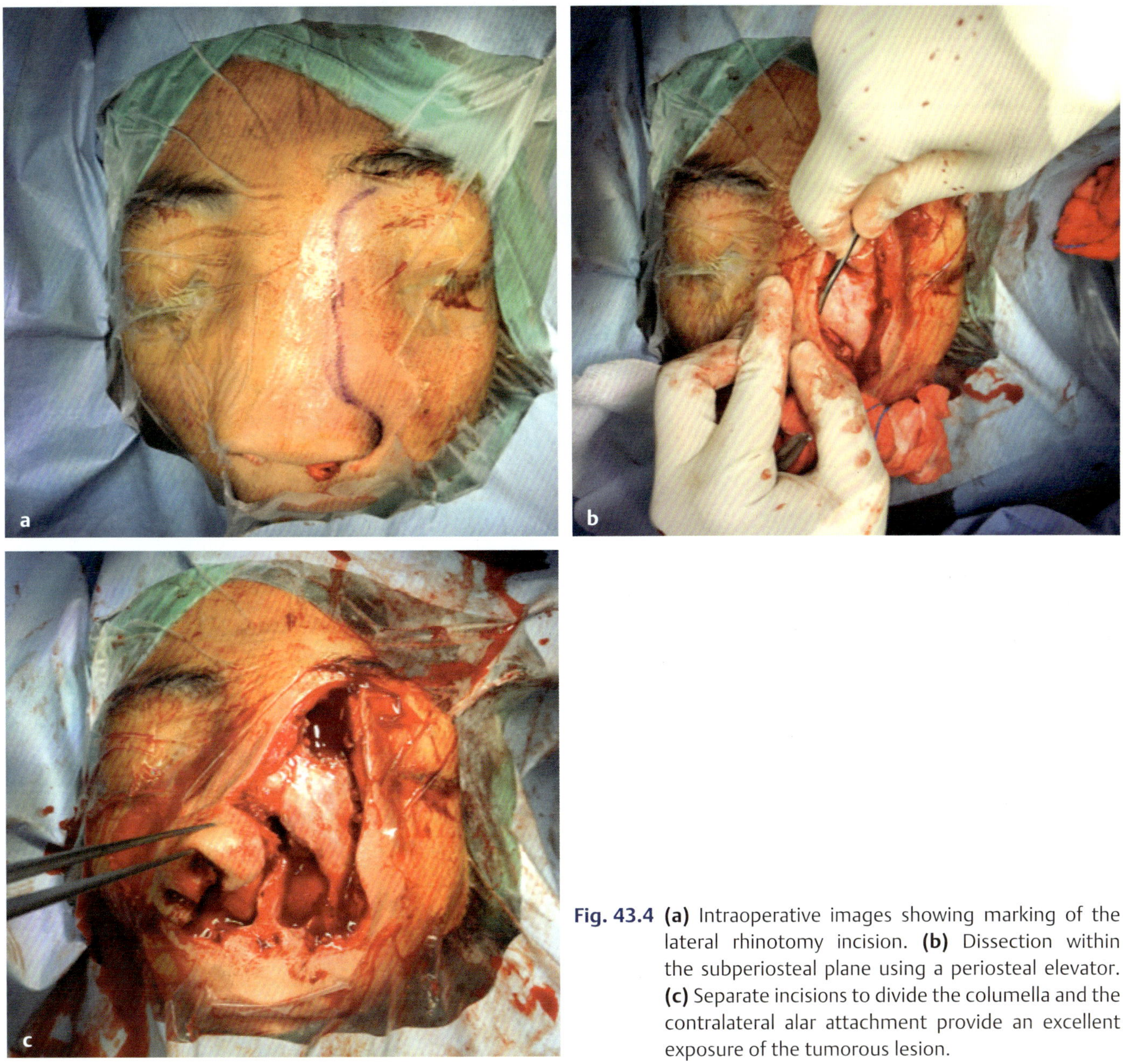

Fig. 43.4 (a) Intraoperative images showing marking of the lateral rhinotomy incision. **(b)** Dissection within the subperiosteal plane using a periosteal elevator. **(c)** Separate incisions to divide the columella and the contralateral alar attachment provide an excellent exposure of the tumorous lesion.

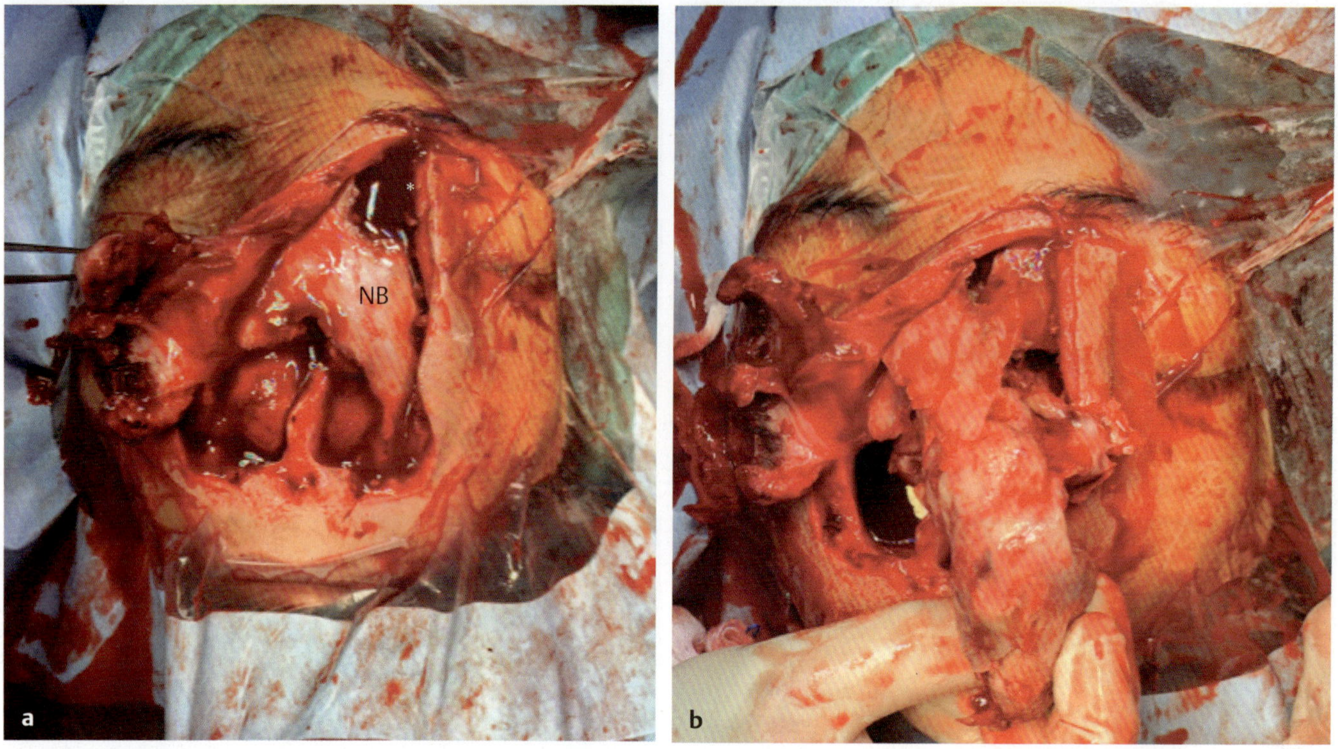

Fig. 43.5 **(a)** Intraoperative views showing areas of thinned-out and mobile nasal bone (NB), as well as deficient bone (*) replaced by tumor capsule. **(b)** Blunt dissection of the bulk of tumor to facilitate endoscopic resection.

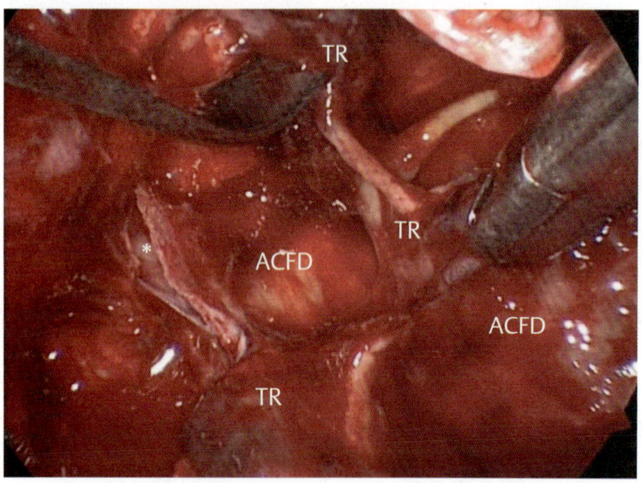

Fig. 43.6 Tumor capsule remnants (TR) adherent to the anterior cranial fossa dura (ACFD) are carefully removed using a Freer and a Debakey forceps. A dural tear is also seen (*).

4. Three-handed endoscopic dissection of tumor remnants from the anterior cranial fossa dura is carefully performed using a Freer and Debakey forceps (**Fig. 43.6**).
5. A dural tear identified is repaired with endoscopic suturing (**Fig. 43.7a–c**). This is covered with autologous abdominal fat followed by DuraSeal Dural Sealant System at the end of the procedure.
6. The tumor capsule is dissected off the left periorbita; this is facilitated by balloting of the eye to identify tissues attached to the orbit (**Fig. 43.8**).
7. The tumor is dissected and removed from the remnant sphenoid sinus, clivus, and petrous apex until the healthy bone is encountered. Knowledge of the important anatomical relationships to vital structures is key for this dissection: orbital apex, left optic nerve, optic chiasm, and the paraclival carotids (**Fig. 43.9a–c**).

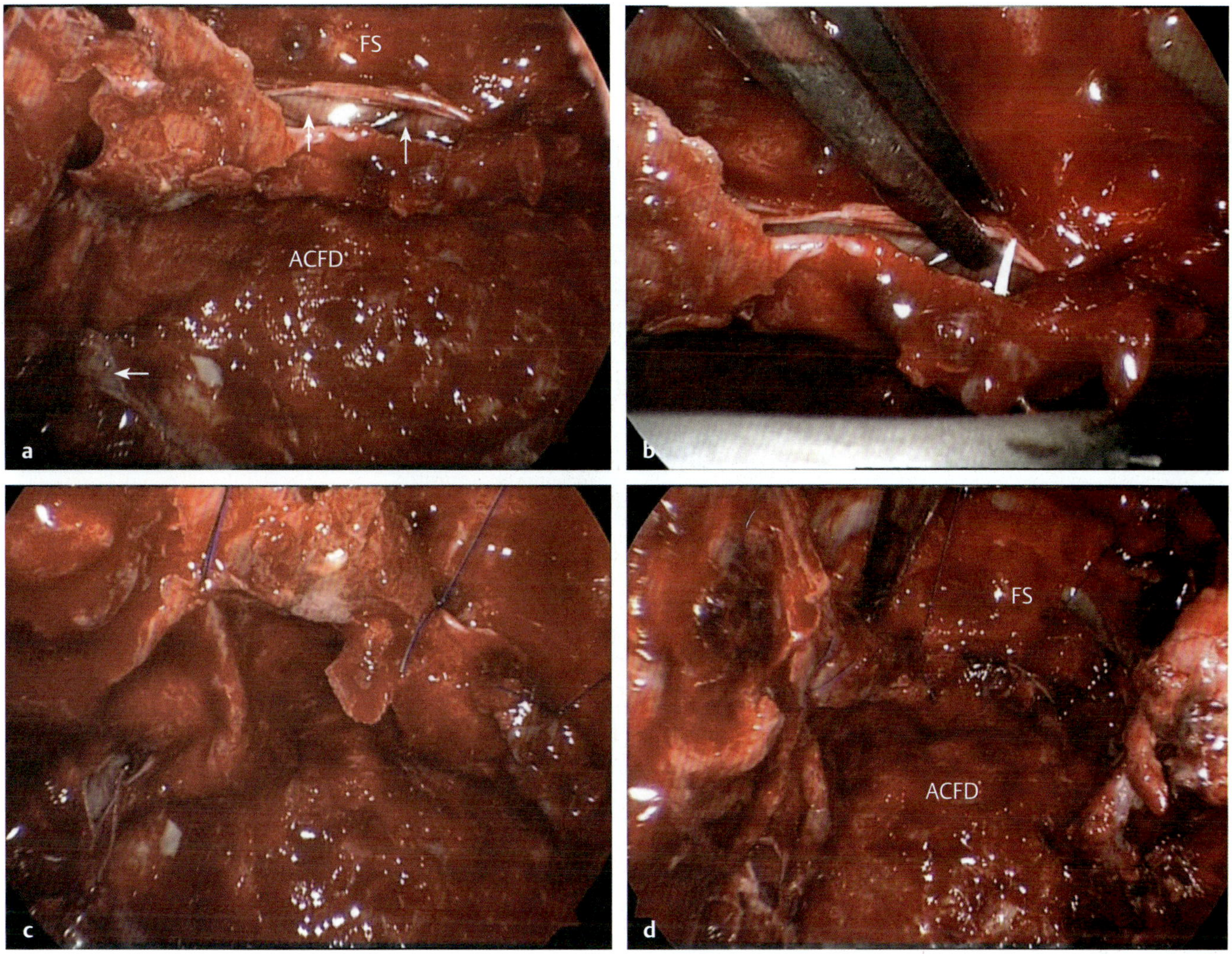

Fig. 43.7 (a) Dural tears (*white arrows*) are seen following tumor dissection from the anterior cranial fossa dura (ACFD). **(b, c)** The tears in the dura are sutured endscopically with nylon. **(d)** The eroded frontal sinus (FS) with a remnant anterior table is intact.

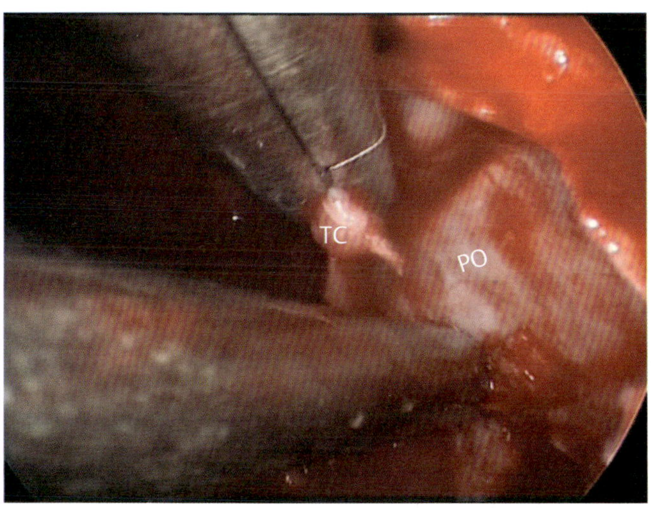

Fig. 43.8 Three-handed endoscopic dissection of the tumor capsule (TC) from the left periorbita (PO).

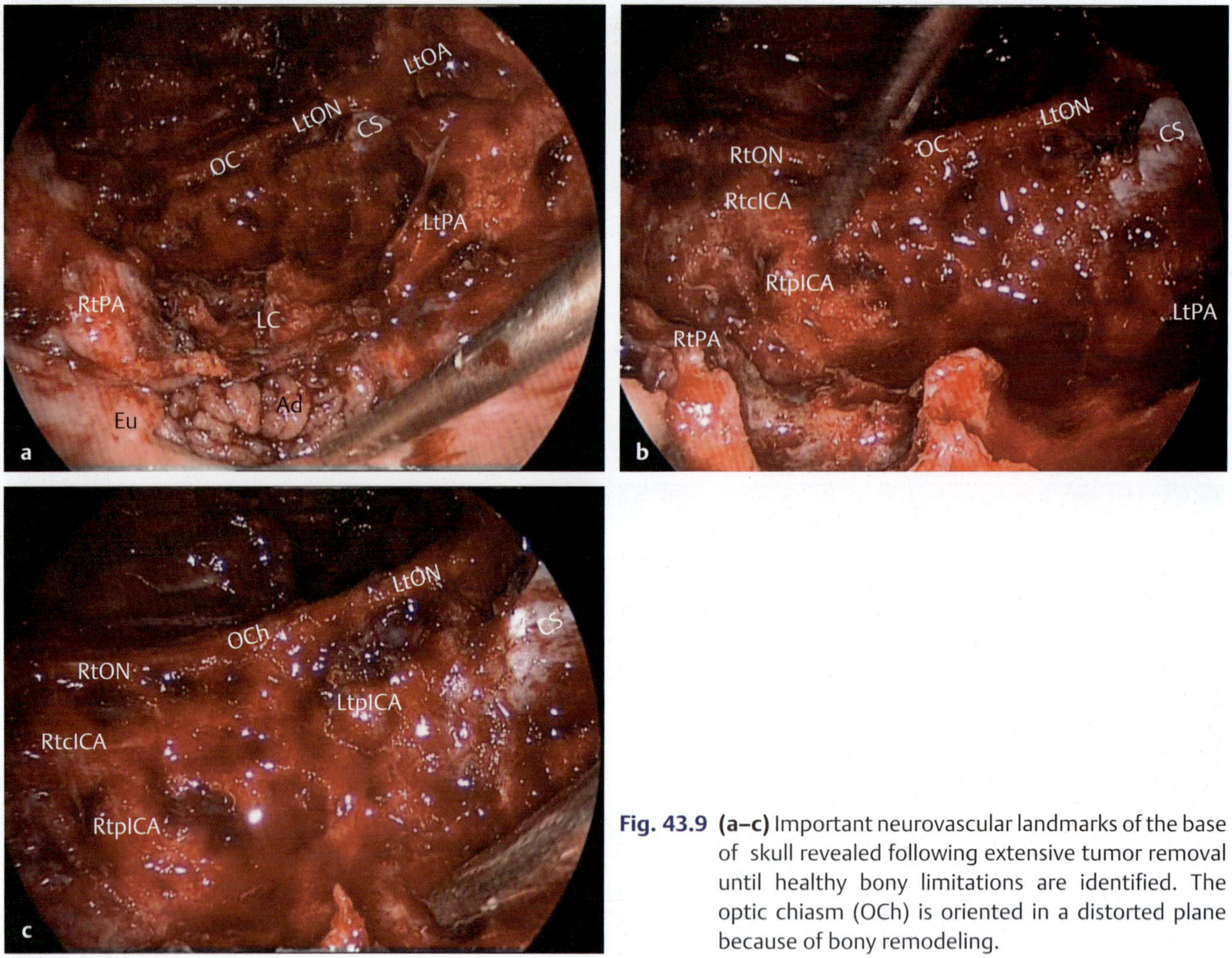

Fig. 43.9 (a–c) Important neurovascular landmarks of the base of skull revealed following extensive tumor removal until healthy bony limitations are identified. The optic chiasm (OCh) is oriented in a distorted plane because of bony remodeling.

Section XVI

Complications

Chapter 44 Complications in Endoscopic Skull Base Surgery

Gaurav Shankar Medikeri and Satish Jain

Introduction

In the ever-evolving field of endoscopic nasal surgery, its use has never been more appreciated than in the management of ventral skull base lesions. Ease of access, reduced morbidity and hospital stay, improved visualization with the advent of angled endoscopes, which help you look around corners, are only some of the numerous advantages of this approach. However, like every other procedure, things could go wrong, and when they do, it could be disastrous. In this chapter, we will be focusing on the prevention and management of the various complications that can occur during or after endoscopic skull base surgery. It is important to remember that a good surgeon not only prevents complications but should be able to manage them when they do occur.

Classification

Complications in endoscopic skull base surgery can be classified in many ways:

- Based on the anatomical structure or system involved
  - ➢ Neurological complications
    - Cerebrospinal fluid (CSF) leak.
    - Cranial nerve injuries.
    - Pneumocephalus.
  - ➢ Infectious complications
    - Meningitis and Encephalitis.
    - Brain abscess.
  - ➢ Endocrine complications
    - Hypopituitarism.
    - Diabetes insipidus (DI).
    - Hyponatremia.
  - ➢ Vascular complications
    - Arterial injuries
      - ○ Internal carotid injury.
      - ○ Circle of Willis injury.
    - Venous injuries
      - ○ Cavernous sinus bleeding.
      - ○ Basilar plexus bleeding.
  - ➢ Orbital complications
    - Intraorbital hemorrhage.
  - ➢ Intranasal complications
    - Synechia formation.
    - Anosmia.
    - Rhinosinusitis.
    - Crusting.
    - Septal perforation.
    - Epistaxis.
    - Flap necrosis.
- Based on the approach
  - ➢ Median sagittal approaches
    - Transcribriform.
    - Transplanum.
    - Transsellar.
    - Transclival.
    - Transodontoid.
  - ➢ Paramedian approaches
    - Pterygopalatine fossa approach.
    - Infratemporal fossa approach.
    - Transorbital approach.
    - Far lateral approach.
- Based on the duration of complication
  - ➢ Temporary complications.
  - ➢ Permanent complications.
- Based on the time of complication
  - ➢ Perioperative (within 1 week).
  - ➢ Early postoperative (1 week–6 months).
  - ➢ Delayed postoperative (after 6 months).

All of the above-mentioned complications can be broadly classified into intraoperative and postoperative complications. Intraoperative complications are those that occur directly as a result of the surgical procedure itself. Postoperative complications are those that occur in the immediate or late postoperative period and usually are a sequela of using the transnasal route—crusting, synechia, sinusitis, epistaxis, hyposmia, etc.

Preoperative Risk Factors in Endoscopic Skull Base Surgery

There are many predictors of complications, both in the intra- and postoperative periods, which can be determined by assessing the risk factors involved.

Patient Factors

- *Age:* There are some studies that indicate that younger age groups (< 65 years) are at a higher risk of complications such as cerebrospinal fluid (CSF) leak, reoperation, and readmission.[1–3] However, it is possible that surgeons tend to be more aggressive with younger patients with regard to surgery, because of a lack of comorbidities and also tend to discharge them earlier from their care, resulting in readmissions. Elderly patients with multiple comorbidities are perhaps offered conservative management rather than surgical options, and hence there might be a bias in terms of complication rates.[1]
- *Race:* Globally, Caucasians were the highest of all ethnicities to have complications followed by African Americans. However, this could be because of a lack of data from other countries. There are very limited data from the Indian population to draw any specific conclusions.
- *Gender:* Some studies show that female patients are at a higher risk of complications.[1,3] Females are also at a higher risk of postoperative hyponatremia after pituitary surgery.[4]
- *Body mass index (BMI):* Overweight (BMI > 25), obese (BMI > 30), and morbidly obese (BMI > 35) patients are at higher risk for CSF leak or reoperation.[1–3,5] According to one study, a 5 kg/m^2 increase in BMI increases the risk of a CSF leak by a factor of 1.61.[3]
- *Comorbidities:* Diabetes mellitus was shown to have higher chances of infection in the postoperative period.[6] In a 6-year retrospective data review by Barber et al consisting of 344 patients, the authors found that patients with preexisting cardiac, renal, or thyroid disorders were more prone to develop postoperative hyponatremia after pituitary surgery.[4]

Tumor-Related Factors

- *Extent of tumor:* Tumors with intraventricular extension have a very high chance of postoperative infection, carotid artery injury, intra- and postoperative CSF leak.[1,2,7] Tumors extending beyond the middle cranial fossa (MCF) into the anterior or posterior cranial fossa had a higher chance of an intracranial bleed and intra- and postoperative CSF leak. Also, extrapituitary tumors predispose to cranial nerve injury.[1]
- *Previous surgery:* According to previous reports, no association was seen between prior surgery being a risk factor for CSF leak.[2,3,8]
- *Previous radiotherapy:* One study found significant increase in the risk of CSF leak with prior radiation therapy, but there were other studies which found no such correlation with previous radiotherapy.[1,2,6] However, prior radiation was a risk factor for carotid bleeds.[1]
- *Tumor size:* According to a study by Cerina et al, when corrected for tumor type, patients with postoperative DI had a mean tumor size of 23 mm when compared to the mean tumor size of 17 mm in those without DI.[8] Hence, larger tumors might be associated with higher chances of complications.
- *Pathology:* Rathke's cleft cyst (RCC) had the highest chance of DI in two studies.[5,9] One study showed a four-time increase in the incidence of DI in RCC cases whereas the other showed a 2.35-time increase in the same.

Neurological Complications

Cerebrospinal Fluid Leak

One of the most common complications and drawbacks of the endoscopic approach to skull base lesions is a CSF leak, which entails CSF leaking through dural and bony skull base defects into the nasal cavity. It is the gateway to some serious complications such as pneumocephalus, meningitis, and intracranial abscess. Risk factors for a CSF leak have already been mentioned before, but most notable are the intraventricular extension of a tumor and a patient with high BMI, both of which increase the risk significantly. Although, in the initial days of endoscopic skull base surgery, the incidence of CSF leak was as high as 40%, this complication has now drastically reduced in the recent past to around 2.3%. CSF leaks are classified into two types based on the volume of leak into high-flow and low-flow leaks.

There are many approaches to improve the success rate of CSF leak repair. These include but are not limited to nursing in head-up position after surgery, lumbar drains, antibiotics, restricted activity, continuous positive airway pressure, nasal packing, etc.[10]

Cranial Nerve Injuries

The risk of cranial nerve injuries in a patient undergoing endonasal endoscopic skull base surgery is on par with that of microscopic surgery.[11] The overall risk of transient (2.5%) and permanent (1.8%) cranial nerve deficit is relatively low when compared to other complications.[12] Preservation of cranial nerves depends on many factors: choosing the right approach, optimal surgical exposure, minimal nerve manipulation, and meticulous dissection to name a few.

In certain approaches, such as the transcribriform approach, the sacrifice of the cranial nerve (olfactory) is inevitable. However, the disease process itself would have already destroyed the nerve in the first place, and hence, it would not matter any further.[12] Optic nerve involvement is quite common in many pathologies such as pituitary lesions extending into the suprasellar cistern and tuberculum sella meningioma. The majority of the tuberculum sella meningiomas involve either one or both optic canals. The opening of the optic canal to remove the intracanalicular portion of the lesion helps improve visual outcomes in these cases.[13] Visual field compromise has been reported in approximately 4% of transsphenoidal surgery cases as per a systematic review and meta-analysis by Muskens et al.[14] Compromise may be either primary, wherein the surgeon causes direct damage to the nerve or to the blood supply of the nerve, or secondary to overenthusiastic packing while sealing a CSF leak or prolapse of the optic nerve or chiasm into an empty sella.[15] Optic nerve involvement must be documented with a swinging flashlight test prior to surgery to document tumor-induced nerve damage (**Fig. 44.1**).

Ocular motility issues occur with pituitary apoplexy with an incidence ranging from 40 to 100%. In the majority of the cases, the third nerve involvement can be explained by the trapping of the third nerve between the tumor and the interclinoid ligament. This is usually seen in larger tumors infiltrating the cavernous sinus. If the tumor extends posteriorly toward the Dorello's canal, sixth nerve palsy can also be found, albeit rare.[16]

A thorough examination of all cranial nerves and documentation prior to surgery is vital to prevent any medicolegal complications and should be standard practice in any endoscopic skull base surgeon's routine evaluation process.

A detailed explanation of every cranial nerve involvement is beyond the scope of this chapter. The cranial nerves at risk during a procedure depend on the type and extent of lesion, approach chosen, and skill of the surgeon. Appropriate consent must be specifically obtained if they are at risk or may need to be sacrificed to obtain complete clearance of the lesion.

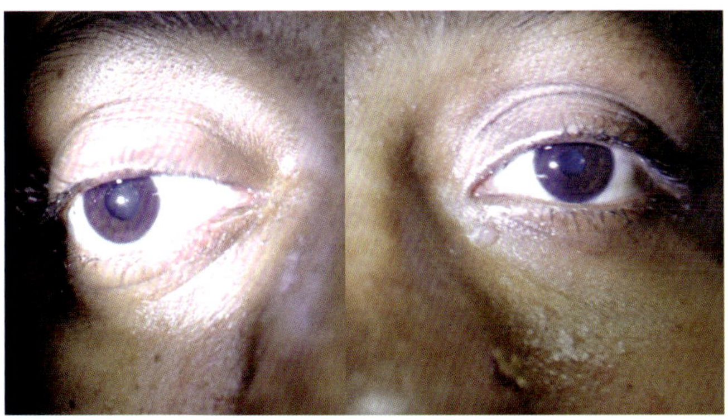

Fig. 44.1 Image showing Marcus Gunn's pupillary defect in a patient with an ossifying fibroma involving the optic nerve on the right side. Note that the pupil is dilated despite the light being shone into the eye whereas the opposite pupil is constricted.

Pneumocephalus

Intracranial collection of air is defined as pneumocephalus. It has been classified as acute (< 72 hours) or delayed (> 72 hours) depending on the time of occurrence after surgery. Some reports have also classified it as early (< 7 days) or late onset (> 7 days) depending on the time of onset.

The mechanism of pneumocephalus has been explained by two hypotheses: (1) the ball valve mechanism of Dandy[17] and (2) the inverted soda can effect by Horowitz.[18] The ball valve mechanism proposes that air gets trapped intracranially because of unidirectional airflow, whereas the soda can theory suggests that negative intracranial pressure secondary to CSF loss because of a CSF fistula sucks air intracranially.

Clinical features include confusion, delirious state, headaches, agitation, seizures, frontal lobe syndrome, and rarely transient hemiplegia. Usually, the air gets trapped in the frontal region or the vertex as it preferentially rises. In some rare instances, if the air is trapped in the posterior cranial fossa, it could result in some disastrous complications such as respiratory or cardiac compromise which could result in death secondary to brainstem dislocation.[19]

The investigation should be based on clinical suspicion in a postoperative case with the above-mentioned features. The gold standard investigation to detect a pneumocephalus is a CT scan, which is highly sensitive as it can pick even 0.55 mL of air in the intracranial space as compared to a radiograph which detects air when more than 2 mL.[20] Air between the two edges of the frontal lobes is the imaging signature of a pneumocephalus and has been described classically as the "Mount Fuji sign."[21] This indicates higher surface tension of air in comparison with CSF between the two frontal lobes. Bilateral compression of the frontal lobes, without separation of the interfrontal space, is called the "peaking sign."[22]

Management options depend on the clinical features, extent and location of the trapped air, and the critical structures at risk of compression. Asymptomatic patients and those with minimal air trapping may be observed clinically for any further deterioration. Any maneuvers which can increase intracranial pressure such as nose blowing or the Valsalva maneuver must be avoided. Conservative management includes the administration of hyperbaric oxygen, which helps not only in symptomatic and radiological improvement but also reduces the duration of hospitalization.[23] Treatment options for symptomatic patients (neurological deterioration, altered consciousness, increasing pressure on serial scans, tension pneumocephalus) include needle aspiration, burr hole evacuation, and/or subdural drain with underwater seal followed by subsequent airtight closure of the skull base and dural defect to prevent further entry of air into the cranium. Patients must be advised not to fly for at least 7 days if they have had a skull base repair as they could have a pneumocephalus because of negative intracranial pressure while flying.[24]

Infectious Complications

Meningitis and Encephalitis

The risk of postoperative meningitis after endonasal skull base surgery ranges from as low as 0.3% to as high as 7%.[25–27] Risk factors include male sex, use of a ventriculoperitoneal shunt intraoperatively, history of the previous craniotomy, or endonasal skull base surgery. The presence of a CSF fistula at the time of surgery increases the risk of meningitis 10.2 times when compared to the absence of the same. The center for disease prevention and control criteria for meningitis include (1) fever (temperature, 38°C), headache, stiff neck, meningeal signs, cranial nerve signs, and/or irritability with no other recognized cause; (2) increased white blood cell count, elevated level of protein and/or decreased level of glucose in the CSF, and/or positive blood cultures.[28] Definitive diagnosis needs the presence of a positive Gram stain or culture. Patients often present with a new-onset or progressive headache, nausea and vomiting, fever, altered mental status, etc.; however, full-blown symptoms of meningitis such as nuchal rigidity and photophobia are less common in this scenario. These symptoms may be masked with postoperative antibiotics, antipyretics, and painkillers which are usually prescribed after surgery.[15,29] The median time of onset of symptoms is around 18 days, and in most cases, symptoms occur after the patient has been discharged from the hospital. Hence, it is very important to warn patients about the clinical features suggestive of meningitis and that they should seek medical help at the earliest possible time, should they have a suspicion.[30]

The most common organisms seen in postsurgical meningitis are *Staphylococcus aureus*, *Streptococcus* sp., *Enterobacteriaceae*, and *Pseudomonas*.[31–33]

Management involves intravenous antibiotics after admission and is usually culture driven. However, empirically, antibiotics must be started as early as possible and different hospitals have different policies regarding the use of empirical antibiotics. The use of prophylactic antibiotics in patients with skull base fractures to avoid meningitis has been studied in the past quite extensively. There is mixed opinion with regard to the routine use of antibiotic prophylaxis. Although there is a potential benefit of reduced infections, there is also the likelihood of antimicrobial resistance, the possibility of adverse reactions to the drug, and the increased cost to deliver the drug intravenously.[10]

At the time of writing this chapter, there is no irrefutable evidence to support the routine prescription of antibiotics in skull base surgery. Of all the meta-analyses on the topic, the majority of them lean toward the notion that there is no benefit to prove that infection risk is reduced with prophylactic antibiotics, whereas only one supports reduced infection.[34–36] High index of suspicion is necessary to identify patients with meningitis.

Brain Abscess

Brain abscess secondary to endoscopic skull base surgery is quite rare. Only 20% of the patients in this group present with the classic triad of headache, fever, and focal neurological deficits as most of their symptoms may be masked by postoperative antibiotics and painkillers. It is also not uncommon to see normal values of C-reactive protein (CRP), erythrocyte sedimentation rate (ESR), and white cell counts in these patients. According to a meta-analysis, about 5% of patients with a brain abscess are initially missed on a computed tomography (CT) scan which can be picked up on magnetic resonance imaging (MRI). In order to differentiate these abscesses from other intracranial pathologies such as tumors or other cystic lesions, diffusion-weighted imaging (DWI) is used. DWI in the case of abscesses shows a hyperintense signal whereas other pathologies seldom do. Imaging also tells us about the extent of the abscess and any sequela such as a midline brain shift caused by the pathology. In the presence of a midline brain shift, a lumbar puncture should not be performed.[37] Depending on the size and location of the abscess, it can either be aspirated or an open drainage may be performed.

Endocrine Complications

Hypopituitarism

Surgical manipulation of the gland or damage to its vasculature during surgery can cause damage to the pituitary gland. This is common in large tumors of the sella with supra- and parasellar extension.[38] Partial dysfunction of the pituitary necessitates supplementation for the deficient hormone depending on which part of the pituitary is affected. In most cases, it is usually a dysfunction of adrenocorticotropic hormone (ACTH) secretion which results in reduced serum cortisol levels. Low levels can lead to dangerously low blood pressures and could result in cerebral hypoperfusion. This needs strict monitoring in patients diagnosed with ACTH deficiency. In extreme cases, if the patients develop panhypopituitarism, they may need lifelong supplementation with hormones and regular monitoring.

Diabetes Insipidus

Fluid and electrolyte imbalances after pituitary surgery are quite common, especially if the neurohypophysis has been manipulated during surgery.[39] In comparison to microscopic pituitary tumor resections, endoscopic resections have a fewer incidence of DI.[40] DI can be classified into two types:

- Transient, which usually presents within 24 to 48 hours postsurgery and resolves by the fourth or fifth day.
- Permanent, wherein the polyuria does not resolve as long as 6 months postsurgery.[41]

DI can present with or without hypocortisolemia and is commonly seen after craniopharyngioma resections. However, they can be present in these patients prior to surgery as well and this must be well documented when a patient is being worked up for surgery.[42–44] Clinically, a diagnosis of postsurgical DI can be made when a patient presents with hypovolemia, polyuria, and polydipsia. A urine output of more than 300 mL for 2 consecutive hours should alert the physician to investigate further. In a patient with DI, the laboratory results would show the following:

- Serum osmolality greater than 300 mOsm/kg.
- Urine osmolality less than 300 mOsm/kg.
- Urine specific gravity less than 1.005.[38]

Permanent DI requires long-term management with desmopressin, a synthetic form of antidiuretic hormone available as a nasal spray or delivered subcutaneously.

Hyponatremia

Postsurgical hyponatremia is diagnosed when the serum sodium drops to less than 120 mmol/L and commonly occurs between 4 and 7 days after surgery. Patients usually present with confusion, seizures, headache, rarely may result in death. There are two mechanisms of hyponatremia:

- *Syndrome of inappropriate antidiuretic hormone secretion (SIADH):* Occurs because of excessive release of antidiuretic hormone from the posterior pituitary, despite hyponatremia. However, the kidneys are still functional in terms of sodium excretion, and hence, the patient is euvolemic as the urine is concentrated.[45]
- *Cerebral salt wasting syndrome:* Occurs because of excess release of natriuretic peptide resulting in urinary loss of sodium as compared to SIADH wherein the hyponatremia is because of free water retention.[46] This leads to hypovolemia as there is increased urine output. It is critical to differentiate between the two conditions as cerebral salt wasting must not be managed with fluid retention.

Strong predictors of postoperative hyponatremia include elderly patients, larger tumor size, ACTH-producing adenomas, Cushing's disease, rate of decline of blood sodium, and female patients. Although the exact mechanism of postoperative hyponatremia has not been clearly understood, it has been hypothesized that it is caused because of excessive release of stored antidiuretic hormone from the posterior pituitary gland during surgical manipulation.[46] A retrospective review of 1,045 patients has shown that tolvaptan is the most efficient method of correction of postsurgical hyponatremia followed by Vaprisol. They state that fluid restriction, hypertonic saline, and sodium supplementation are not as effective.[47] However, the recommendation is to use them in conjunction rather than individually for the best chance of correction.

Vascular Complications

Vascular complications will be discussed under two broad headings: arterial and venous.

Arterial Injuries

Internal Carotid Artery Injury

One of the deadliest complications in endoscopic skull base surgery is a carotid injury, which fortunately is quite low in incidence. A literature search revealed that the incidence is estimated to be between 0.016 and 1% in most high-volume centers.[48] A retrospective review of 2,015 endoscopic skull base cases revealed that the most common pathology involved in carotid injury was chondroid lesions such as chondroma or chondrosarcoma and the most common segment involved was the paraclival segment. Chondroid tumors apparently stand to have a 10 times higher risk for carotid injuries when compared to pituitary tumors.[49] Risk factors which increase the risk of damage to the ICA include the following[50]:

- Tumor invasion into the cavernous sinus.
- Previous trans-sphenoidal surgery.
- Previous radiation therapy.
- Acromegaly.
- Medial displacement of the cavernous carotid artery by tumor/lesion.
- Tumors needing exposure of multiple segments of the ICA.

Tumor invasion into the cavernous sinus and adherence of the tumor to the carotid artery obviously make the surgery more challenging and increase the risk of injury to the carotid artery. In revision surgeries, the neo-osteogenesis alters the shape and pneumatization of the sphenoid sinus and throws the surgeon off track. Previous radiation not only induces radionecrosis to a certain extent but also increases tissue bleeding and makes the bone more fibrotic. The excess bleeding may hamper vision and may cause an unintentional entry into the artery. It also thins out the carotid wall to a certain extent, making it more vulnerable to damage.

The distance of the carotid arteries from the midline is extremely critical during transsphenoidal surgery. A cadaveric microsurgical study by Albert Rhoton Jr revealed that the mean distance between the carotid artery and the pituitary gland is roughly 2.3 mm, but it ranges from abutting onto the pituitary to being as far as 7 mm away from it.[51,52] In patients with acromegaly, this distance is drastically reduced because of bony changes that occur as part of the disease. This further increases the risk of carotid injury in this set of patients.

In most of the papers describing an injury to the carotid artery, the majority of the cases occurred because of the surgeon deviating from the midline. In our opinion, this is an important factor in for the occurrence of a carotid injury. Intraoperative orientation to the midline is of grave significance if a carotid injury is to be avoided. It is prudent to rely on the landmarks which orientate a surgeon and keep him/her in the midline. The following are some of the landmarks which can be used:

- *Nasal septum:* Although the posterior septum is resected in transsphenoidal surgery, traversing along the anterior septum is one of the safest landmarks which helps avoid straying from the midline in most cases.
- *Vidian canal:* Good landmark for the petrous and paraclival carotid segments. Drilling inferomedial to the vidian canal is the safest location to avoid early contact with the petrous carotid segment.[53,54]
- *Eustachian tubes:* Injury to the parapharyngeal carotid is higher once the eustachian tubes are crossed.[44]
- *Rostrum of sphenoid:* If it has not been completely drilled out.
- *Opticocarotid recess:* In most cases, it may be prominent. However, if the clinoid process is not well pneumatized, it may not be prominent and hence is not always a reliable landmark (**Fig. 44.2**).

Landmarks such as sphenoid septa should not be used to identify the midline, as they more often than not deviate from the midline. Another important tool that can be used to trace out the course of the carotid artery intraoperatively is the Doppler. Yamasaki et al have reported the use of a 1-mm microvascular Doppler probe which provides real-time monitoring in a "picture-in-picture" module. This could help in identifying the course of the artery early in the surgery and also provides a constant guide even after major drilling has been done to expose the tumor and bony landmarks are lost. It can also be placed onto the tumor and identify the vessel even if the lesion is encasing it.[55]

Management of a Carotid Injury

The best modality of management of an ICA injury is to avoid one if possible. The ideal profile of the surgeons dealing with cases wherein there is a risk of ICA injury should constitute a rhinologist with good knowledge of the course of the ICA not only in the nose but also with the ability to expose the vessel in the neck–should that is necessary; and a neurosurgeon with extensive exposure in skull base and vascular surgery.

Vascular control of the ICA will be discussed in two components:

- *Proximal control:* Proximal control of the carotid artery is difficult but achievable, more so in the horizontal petrous, paraclival, lacerum, or parapharyngeal segments. This can be achieved by means of a cervical incision on the corresponding side of the tumor and pressure or ligation of the vessel in the neck. This can either be done prophylactically in case of large tumors

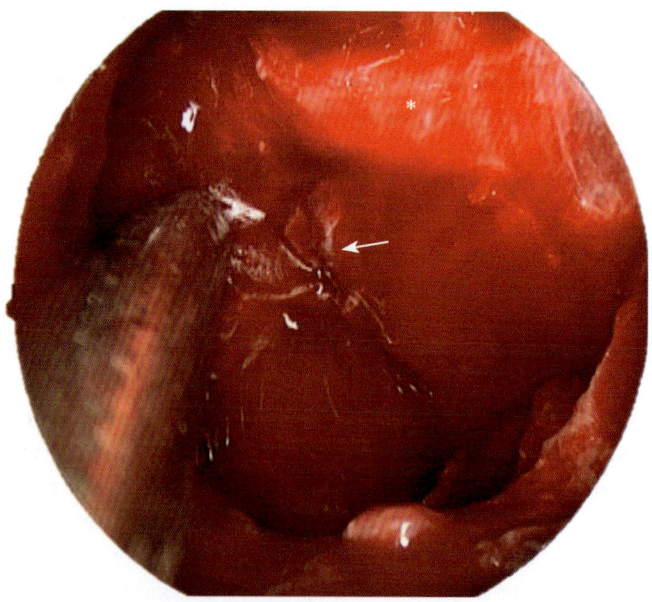

Fig. 44.2 A small stellate-shaped injury to the carotid artery during bone removal in a case of the optic nerve (*) decompression for post-traumatic optic neuropathy. In this case, the ethmoid and sphenoid bones were fractured downward, obliterating the the opticocarotid recess, and hence, the optic nerve was in close proximity to the carotid artery.

involving the carotid or in cases where there is a high risk such as revision surgeries or prior radiation, etc.

- *Distal control:* This is challenging, more so in the paraclival and parasellar regions. Distal control in these regions is more difficult than proximal control given the fact that the vessel is tortuous and there are some critical cranial nerves in the superolateral compartment of the cavernous sinus. Application of an aneurysmal clip, although ideal, is easier said than done in these situations.[44]

Intraoperative Management of Internal Carotid Artery Injury

The first and most important step in the management of an ICA bleed is packing. It is prudent to understand that the surgeon must use the minimal packing necessary to ward off any major bleeding which can ruin the surgical field visibility or even reduce the amount of light transmission through the endoscope. Excessive packing should be avoided as it may lead to compressive neuropathy of the optic or oculomotor nerves (cavernous segment) or compression of the basilar artery (paraclival segment).[56] A wide range of materials have been used in the past for packing, ranging from ribbon gauze to Surgicel. The surgeon must not panic in this given situation, and it would be of great help to use two suctions to manage the extensive amount of blood loss to keep the field as clean as possible. The endoscope must be slightly retracted from the site of bleeding to avoid soiling of the scope as the pressure of the bleeder would be high and the fact that the viewing eye of the scope is at the tip. Wormald and Valentine have recommended the use of the posterior septal edge as a shield to prevent soiling of the endoscope by passing the scope through the nasal cavity contralateral to the injury in the presence of a posterior septotomy.[57] Another good location would be to park the scope near the head of the middle turbinate. A suction caliber of greater than 12 F would be ideal to keep up with the high-volume bleeding that occurs in a closed space (**Fig. 44.3**). It is important to take care not to suck the vessel walls into the suction device as it would only result in an increase in the defect size. One suction could be introduced from the same nostril underneath the endoscope, and a forceps could also be used to apply pressure with hemostatic material.[43] This maneuver necessitates significant dexterity on behalf of the surgeon and simultaneous coordination with the other surgeon in order to provide visualization and access to instruments. A cell saver may also be used to transfuse the blood suctioned from the ICA later on if necessary. Once the rent in the vessel has been identified, again there are many techniques which can be used to manage it as follows:

- *Bipolar forceps:* It can be used if the defect is very small and can be well localized. This technique is not ideal for large defects as it induces clotting and thrombus formation in the lumen of the vessel which could later lead to delayed neurological complications. Although bipolar forceps are easily available in most hospitals, the drawback of this technique is that it does not work well in a wet field and the surgeon may need to attempt many times prior to finding success with this technique, thus wasting valuable time and causing excessive bleeding. The risk of a delayed blow out is also high when thermal energy has been used to create scar tissue to achieve primary hemostasis as the scar tissue is not strong enough to withstand the pressure in the vessel. Bipolar forceps are perhaps not the best tool for a linear trauma to the carotid as per an animal-based study comparing three different techniques of ICA trauma with three different hemostatic techniques.[58]
- *Muscle patching:* It has been reported extensively by many authors with reasonable success in the past.[59,60] A 10 × 10 mm crushed sternomastoid muscle patch when apparently held with a Blakesley forceps over the bleeding site with firm pressure for around 10 minutes, helps reduce bleeding.[51] Advantages of the muscle patch include its easy availability, low chances of rejection as it is autologous, ability to attain initial hemostasis quickly as the patch is large, it does not need precise placement to obtain initial tamponade. However, a muscle patch bears the risk of being blown off (more so with punch injury to the vessel) because of the high pressure within the vessel. This usually happens in the early postoperative period and may necessitate taking the patient back to the theater immediately. It also takes the longest time

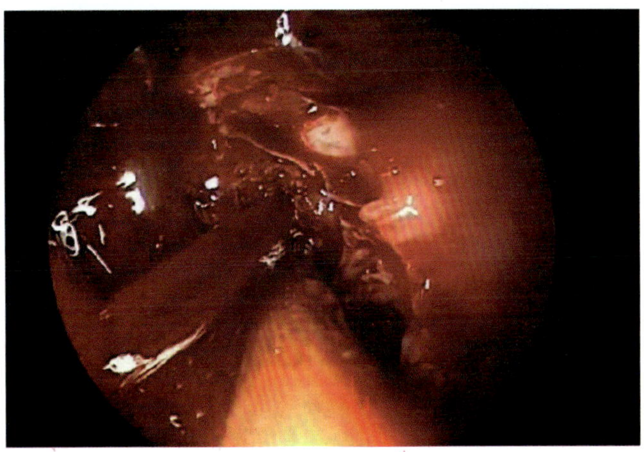

Fig. 44.3 A large rent in the carotid artery showing the force with which the vessel bleeds necessitating the need for the use of a large-bore suction to keep pace with the bleeding vessel to keep the field relatively bloodless.

to attain secondary hemostasis as it has to be held in place for about 10 minutes before all instruments can be removed from the nasal cavity. This is in order to allow the hemostatic factors to work. This technique is also not free of the risk of a pseudoaneurysm as there is no approximation of the tunica intima layer of the vessel.[52] The risk of pseudoaneurysm with this technique has been reported to be between 28 and 60% in the literature.[52,53] It is highly recommended that if a muscle patch is used, then serial angiography should be carried out to monitor the possibility of a pseudoaneurysm formation.[61]

- *Hemostatic clips and sutures:* The Sundt type clip has been described by Laws in one of his cases where it was successfully managed with this hemostatic device. However, further details on the application and parameters to define success had not been discussed.[62] Another device that has been used and reported is called the "U-clip anastomotic device" (Medtronic, Jacksonville, FL). This has been used in the dural reconstruction and coronary artery anastomosis previously and apparently has had success in managing ICA bleeds without sacrificing the vessel. This device is an endoscopic instrument which can be used to suture the vessel without having to tie knots. S20 sutures have been mentioned as the best size for the management of ICA bleeds as they suture only the edges of the ICA wall and do not create significant stenosis of the carotid lumen and neither are they too large to prevent close approximation of the vessel walls.[51]

Neuroradiological Techniques

Occasionally, despite the best efforts of some of the trained surgeons, it may not be possible to stop the hemorrhage primarily or secondarily. In such situations, the patient might have to be shifted to a neuroradiology suite wherein one of the two methods of management will be used.

- *Parent vessel occluding*: This is the more common of the two techniques applied. This is preferred in those patients in whom a balloon occlusion test is negative. A balloon occlusion test involves monitoring clinical neurological parameters and cerebral blood flow. In a patient who is under general anesthesia, clinical monitoring will not be possible and the interventional team may have to rely on the cerebral perfusion alone. The challenge in occluding a high-flow vessel such as the ICA, is the high probability of distal migration of the coil into the ophthalmic artery. One of the ways to combat this would be to apply firm digital pressure onto the cervical segment of the carotid artery to artificially create a low-flow system for a time sufficient enough to place an endovascular coil[63] (**Fig. 44.4**, **Fig. 44.5**).
- *Parent vessel preserving*: This is preferred in those patients who fail to tolerate the 30-minute balloon occlusion test. In such cases, a stent may be used to isolate the pseudoaneurysm from the main parent vessel. The risk of rupturing the pseudoaneurysm is quite high from the compression by the stent graft. The other drawback is that these stents are not always yielding

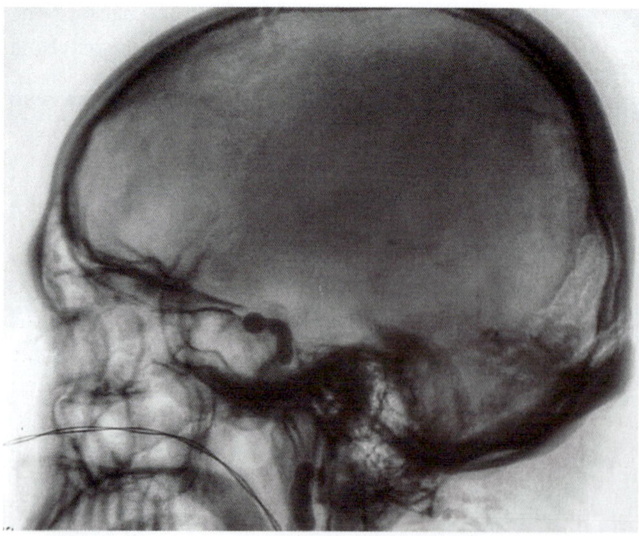

Fig. 44.4 Parent vessel occlusion in a case with cavernous carotid injury with good contralateral blood flow through the circle of Willis. The radiograph shows proximal and distal vessel occlusion with coils.

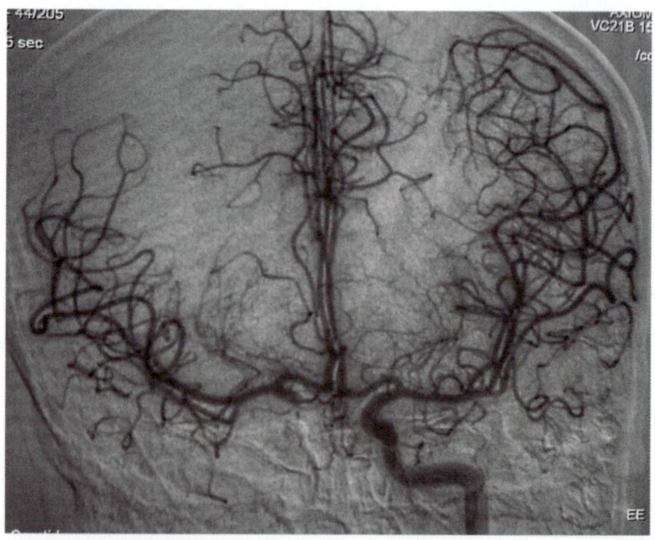

Fig. 44.5 A radiograph showing good collateral blood flow after ipsilateral carotid occlusion. This is one of the safest techniques to prevent a pseudoaneurysm but can only be safely carried out in a patient with good collateral flow.

and hence may be difficult to use in areas like the cavernous carotid. The other option is to use a detachable balloon or coil. This is the lesser preferred of the two methods as most authors believe that a pseudoaneurysm is fragile as there is not a wall, and hence this method of preservation of the vessel patency may lead to a fatal rebleed (**Fig. 44.6**). There is also a significant risk of migration of the coils. The only situation where it might be apt to use a detachable balloon or coil is a cavernous carotid fistula as it is not as urgent as other conditions.[53,64,65]

Circle of Willis Injury

The circle of Willis is named after the English physician Thomas Willis and is constituted by five vessels of the left and right sides (except ACOM which is a single midline vessel):

- Anterior cerebral artery (ACA).
- Anterior communicating artery (ACOM).
- ICA.
- Posterior cerebral artery (PCA).
- Posterior communicating artery (PCOM).

Injury to the vessels constituting the circle of Willis is a possibility in cases involving the parasellar and transplanum/transtuberculum approaches. Injury to any of these vessels is a stressful situation and could result in significant intracranial bleed in the form of a subarachnoid hemorrhage (SAH), intraventricular hemorrhage (IVH), or an intraparenchymal hemorrhage (IPH).

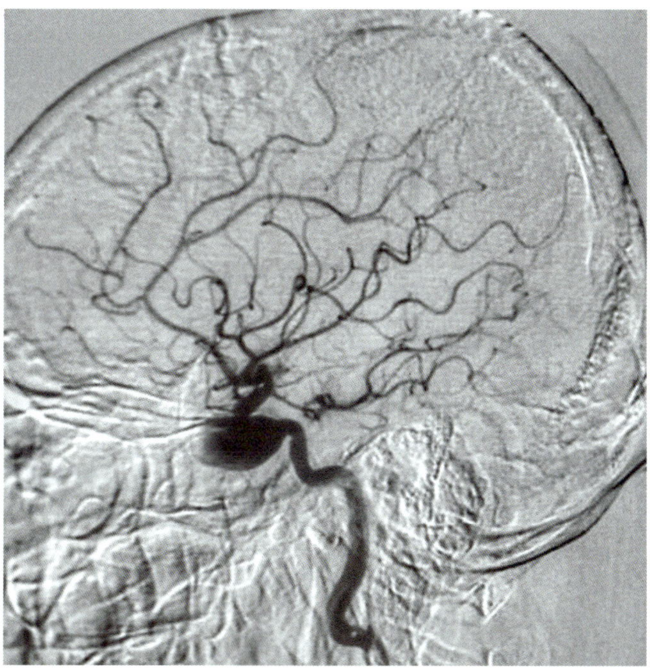

Fig. 44.6 A pseudoaneurysm is seen in a patient with cavernous carotid artery injury. Such a large pseudoaneurysm could lead to a fatal rebleed if not managed with interventional radiological techniques.

Bleeding from these vessels can lead to significant neurological deterioration at a rapid rate and definitely necessitates keeping a close watch on the patient's neurological status. The patient will also need serial angiograms in the postoperative period to rule out the possibility of a pseudoaneurysm or a rebleed from these vessels.

Management is by selective embolization of the pseudoaneurysm, and in case of stenosis of the vessel, a balloon angioplasty may be performed if the vessel is being spared. The most definitive and common method of management is vessel sacrifice as it eliminates the possibility of a pseudoaneurysm, but it is often not feasible as it may leave the patient with significant neurological morbidity. In some cases, a craniotomy may be necessary wherein the bleed is evacuated and a bypass or microanastomosis is performed to restore blood flow to the brain. There are very few reports of such intracranial vessel injury in endoscopic skull base surgery. Most of the patients managed in these reports had poor outcomes; some of them passed away despite best efforts by the team and others had significant neurological morbidity leaving them with a poor quality of life.[38,66–68]

Venous Injuries

Cavernous Sinus Bleeding

The cavernous sinus is a common location for tumor extension and involvement of this site invariably causes significant venous bleeding when the tumor is debulked (**Fig. 44.7**). However, fortunately, the venous ooze from the cavernous sinus can be easily managed with the use of a hemostatic agent like Surgicel (Ethicon, Sommerville, NJ) at the end of neuropatties with firm pressure over the cavernous sinus. Floseal could also be injected into the sinus and the two dural layers of the sinus could be compressed together to reduce bleeding. However, one must not put too much pressure onto the sinus to avoid trauma to the cranial nerves or the carotid artery located within the cavernous sinus. Kim et al have described the use of an angled bipolar instrument to control an intercavernous sinus bleed during transsphenoidal surgery.[69] Gazzeri et al compared the use of flowable gelatin hemostatic with thrombin, without thrombin, and a classic hemostatic agent in 932 intracranial surgeries and found that they had more incidence of thrombus formation in the venous sinuses in the group with flowable gelatin hemostatic matrix without thrombin. They also found that if more than 10 mL of the material was used, the chances of having a thrombus was much higher.[70] Although during a bleed, it is quite tempting to overuse the hemostatic agent,

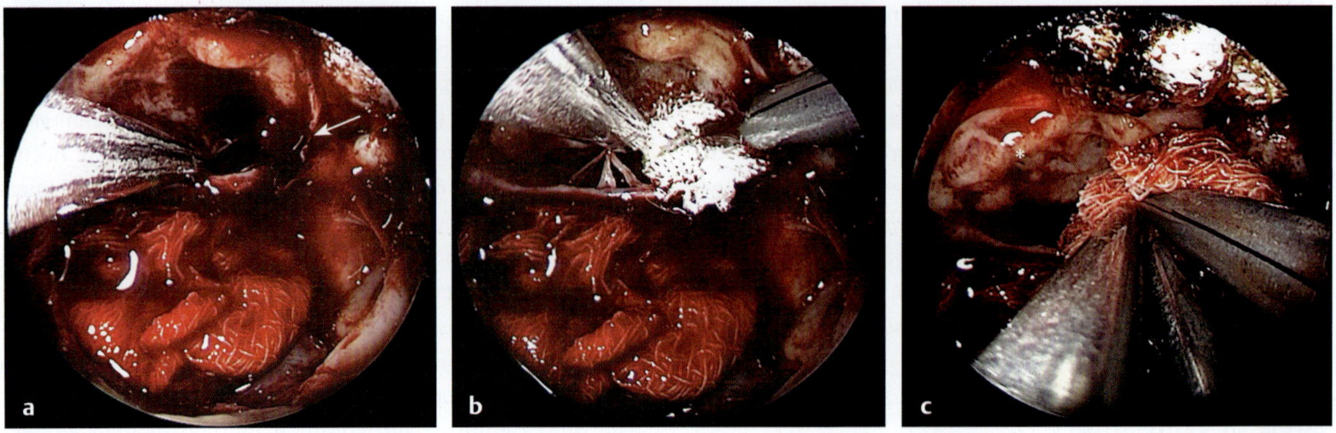

Fig. 44.7 **(a)** Cavernous sinus bleeding (*arrow*) is seen after the intracavernous component of the tumor was debulked; **(b)** this was managed intraoperatively with the use of Surgicel and **(c)** gentle pressure with a piece of gauze. Since it is a venous structure, it gets compressed and bleeding can be managed until the remaining tumor (*) is completely resected.

one must refrain from overenthusiastic use of the same for the fear of thrombus formation.

Basilar Plexus Bleeding

The other situation where one might encounter troublesome venous bleeding is during the management of lesions necessitating the transclival approach. The basilar plexus bleeds voraciously once the dura in this region is opened and takes a while to tame with the help of hemostatic agents. Warm water rinsing in this area also helps reduce bleeding. Occasionally, the team might have to stage the procedure wherein the drilling of the clivus and dural exposure is carried out in the first stage and after a day or two, the dura is opened in the second stage and the bleeding is then managed.[71]

Orbital Complications

Intraorbital Hemorrhage

This complication is usually associated with sinus surgery but may occur in certain situations like optic nerve decompression, orbital decompression, or the transcribriform approach, wherein the anterior or posterior ethmoid vessels are being managed.

Presentation is with orbital proptosis on the table with chemosis of the conjunctiva. In such situations, it is extremely important to involve an oculoplastic surgeon and monitor for pupillary response with a swinging flashlight test and tonometry. If the pressure is significantly high, a lateral canthotomy and cantholysis can be performed. In cases, where this doesn't help, a medial orbital decompression followed by an inferior orbital decompression may be practiced. There is a higher chance that a posterior ethmoid artery bleed into the orbit may go unnoticed. In these cases, the vision is at higher risk because of the conical shape of the orbit and earlier compressive neuropathy of the optic nerve, as space is lesser in the posterior section of the orbit.[72]

Nasal Complications

Synechia Formation

One of the most common complications in endoscopic skull base surgery is the presence of synechia in the postoperative period. This usually happens when two opposing surfaces of the mucosa are damaged leading to adhesions. These adhesions may impact breathing or may create scar bands not allowing surveillance in the postoperative period. They may also prevent sinus outflow tracts from functioning correctly and may thus lead to sinusitis in the long term. Management of these synechiae depends on how they impact postoperative surveillance and breathing. If they do, then they can be cut and a splint be placed between the two edges until the mucosa heals completely. Care must be taken during surgery not to inadvertently damage the mucosa while accessing the skull base lesion.

Anosmia/Hyposmia

Irrespective of the type of endoscopic endonasal skull base surgery, there is apparently a decrease in olfaction postsurgery. A randomized control trial by Tam et al showed that, at the end of 6 months, there is a mean reduction of 20% in the University of Pennsylvania smell identification test (UPSIT) scores when compared to their scores prior to surgery in those patients in whom a nasoseptal flap (NSF) has been raised. In those patients where a NSF has not been raised, there is a drop in the UPSIT scores by a mean of 9%.[73] However, some authors have reported no significant change in olfaction before and after NSF use in endoscopic skull base surgery.[74] The general consensus, however, remains that raising an NSF causes transient hyposmia at the least. Although it may be quite severe in the initial months after surgery, it has been reported to reduce in severity by 9 months postsurgery.[75] The use of monopolar cautery to raise the NSF has been shown to be associated with higher chances of anosmia in the postoperative period.[76] It is now recommended that the NSF should not be raised if a CSF leak is not expected, or a rescue Hadad flap could be raised if necessary. If an NSF must be raised, then ideally a cold steel instrument like a knife would be apt for the superior incisions to reduce chances of hyposmia.[77]

Rhinosinusitis

There is not a lot of evidence to prove that endoscopic skull base surgery causes long-standing rhinosinusitis after surgery. However, there are two authors who conducted a retrospective analysis and assessed quality-of-life (QOL) scores and also assessed CT scans of patients in the postoperative period. One mentions that there is significant mucosal thickening when the middle turbinate is resected and the maxillary antrum is opened up.[78,79] Surgeries carried out with minimal mucosal damage should not result in significant scarring and hence should not cause grave symptoms of sinus disease in these patients.

Crusting

Almeida et al have described in their prospective cohort study that crusting was seen in 98% of patients undergoing skull base surgery and was the most common symptom in their study. They found that there was no difference in crusting whether an NSF was harvested. The mean time to the absence of crusting was around 101 days.[80] Roxbury et al also found in their study that persistent crusting beyond 6 months after surgery was seen in 7.9% of patients undergoing endoscopic skull base surgery, and there was no difference in crusting whether an avascular free graft was used or a vascularized flap was used.[81] The factors which alter the degree of crusting are as follows:

- *Location of tumor*: Anteriorly located tumors are associated with a higher degree of crusting as the resection is in the exposed area of the nose where airflow is higher and results in drying and crusting.[82]
- *Complexity of the lesion*: More complex lesions are associated with a greater degree of crusting since they need a wider exposure and hence more mucosal dissection.[70]
- *Prior radiotherapy*: Patients who have received prior radiotherapy will have greater crusting because of radiation-induced mucosal injury and dryness.[83]

Postoperative debridement and saline rinses can help reduce the amount of dryness and crusting in the follow-up period. The ENT surgeon must be involved in the postoperative care of the patient until the closest point to the physiological normalcy of the nose and paranasal sinuses has been achieved.

Septal Perforation

Posterior septectomy is routinely performed in most skull base surgeries and hence is a natural sequela of endoscopic skull base surgery. However, in certain cases, anterior perforation can also occur because of devascularization of the cartilaginous septum or inadvertent damage to the mucosal lining of the septum on both sides of the cartilage with subsequent necrosis. The incidence of septal perforation in skull base surgery ranges from 0 to 10%.[84–88] It would be prudent for the rhinologist to guide the neurosurgeon with the endoscope all the way to the skull base with the instrument and then change the nasal passage to allow more space for instrumentation. This would minimize unnecessary trauma to the nasal passages, and this reduces the possibility of a perforation anteriorly. In such cases, there might be worsening of QOL scores such as whistling, bleeding, and crusting for a prolonged duration of time. If the symptoms are bothersome, then a second-stage procedure may be performed to fix the septal perforation either surgically or with a septal prosthesis.

Epistaxis

The incidence of epistaxis after endoscopic skull base surgery has been widely reported, and the incidence rates range from 0 to 7% in various studies.[41,89–92] A retrospective review of 5-year data comprising 330 patients showed an epistaxis incidence of 3% in the initial month after endoscopic skull base surgery. Most patients were reported to be male hypertensive patients. Epistaxis was higher in those patients in whom an NSF had been raised during surgery.[93] A small amount of postsurgical bleeding is expected and usually resolves on its own in a few days. Most cases of major epistaxis originate from the nasoseptal branch of the sphenopalatine artery, especially when the flap has been raised. The majority of these cases are managed in the emergency room with nasal packing. In those cases where packing does not resolve the bleeding, a major vessel bleed must be suspected and the patient must be taken to the theater to achieve hemostasis. In the case of torrential bleeding, an intracranial source of bleeding must also be borne in mind.

Flap Necrosis

The vascularized NSF is the workhorse flap for reconstruction of the ventral skull baes in endoscopic skull base surgeries. However, although robust in preventing postoperative CSF leak, it is vulnerable to necrosis as well, albeit rare. Flap necrosis is a very rare complication in endoscopic skull base surgery. In a retrospective data analysis of 1,285 consecutive patients, who underwent endoscopic skull base surgery, Chabot et al documented 8 patients who had developed necrosis of the NSF.[94]

Clinical suspicion of flap necrosis should occur in the presence of symptoms suggestive of meningitis along with the endoscopic picture of a black necrosed flap. The patient may or may not have signs of a CSF leak. The use of a fat graft intraoperatively can significantly increase the risk for the development of flap necrosis. A contrast MRI will reveal a nonenhancing flap on imaging. The presence of all the above-mentioned characteristics in a postsurgical patient entails the need for prompt debridement, and the new skull base defect must be reconstructed either with a free mucosal graft or a vascularized flap. The necrotic tissue must be widely excised prior to application of a new flap lest it may fail too.

References

1. Boling CC, Karnezis TT, Baker AB, et al. Multi-institutional study of risk factors for perioperative morbidity following transnasal endoscopic pituitary adenoma surgery. Int Forum Allergy Rhinol 2016;6(1):101–107
2. Karnezis TT, Baker AB, Soler ZM, et al. Factors impacting cerebrospinal fluid leak rates in endoscopic sellar surgery. Int Forum Allergy Rhinol 2016;6(11):1117–1125
3. Dlouhy BJ, Madhavan K, Clinger JD, et al. Elevated body mass index and risk of postoperative CSF leak following transsphenoidal surgery. J Neurosurg 2012;116(6):1311–1317
4. Barber SM, Liebelt BD, Baskin DS. Incidence, etiology and outcomes of hyponatremia after transsphenoidal surgery: experience with 344 consecutive patients at a single tertiary center. J Clin Med 2014;3(4):1199–1219
5. Senior BA, Ebert CS, Bednarski KK, et al. Minimally invasive pituitary surgery. Laryngoscope 2008;118(10):1842–1855
6. Zhang L, Chen M. Analysis of factors causing intracranial infection after endoscopic resection of pituitary tumors by transnasal-sphenoidal approach. Biomed Res 2014;25(4): 437–440
7. Thawani JP, Ramayya AG, Pisapia JM, Abdullah KG, Lee JY, Grady MS. Operative strategies to minimize complications following resection of pituitary macroadenomas. J Neurol Surg B Skull Base 2017;78(2):184–190
8. Cerina V, Kruljac I, Radosevic JM, et al. Diagnostic accuracy of perioperative measurement of basal anterior pituitary and target gland hormones in predicting adrenal insufficiency after pituitary surgery. Medicine (Baltimore) 2016;95(9):e2898
9. Sigounas DG, Sharpless JL, Cheng DM, Johnson TG, Senior BA, Ewend MG. Predictors and incidence of central diabetes insipidus after endoscopic pituitary surgery. Neurosurgery 2008;62(1):71–78, discussion 78–79
10. Oakley GM, Orlandi RR, Woodworth BA, Batra PS, Alt JA. Management of cerebrospinal fluid rhinorrhea: an evidence-based review with recommendations. Int Forum Allergy Rhinol 2016;6(1):17–24
11. Cappabianca P, Cavallo LM, Solari D, Stagno V, Esposito F, de Angelis M. Endoscopic endonasal surgery for pituitary adenomas. World Neurosurg 2014;82(6, Suppl):S3–S11
12. Kassam AB, Prevedello DM, Carrau RL, et al. Endoscopic endonasal skull base surgery: analysis of complications in the authors' initial 800 patients. J Neurosurg 2011;114(6): 1544–1568
13. Mahmoud M, Nader R, Al-Mefty O. Optic canal involvement in tuberculum sellae meningiomas: influence on approach, recurrence, and visual recovery. Neurosurgery 2010;67(3, Suppl Operative):ons108–ons118, discussion ons118–ons119
14. Muskens IS, Zamanipoor Najafabadi AH, Briceno V, et al. Visual outcomes after endoscopic endonasal pituitary adenoma resection: a systematic review and meta-analysis. Pituitary 2017;20(5):539–552
15. Ciric I, Ragin A, Baumgartner C, Pierce D. Complications of transsphenoidal surgery: results of a national survey, review of the literature, and personal experience. Neurosurgery 1997;40(2):225–236, discussion 236–237
16. Saul RF, Hilliker JK. Third nerve palsy: the presenting sign of a pituitary adenoma in five patients and the only neurological sign in four patients. J Clin Neuroophthalmol 1985;5(3): 185–193
17. Dandy WE. Pneumocephalus (intracranial penumatocele or aerocele). Arch Surg 1926;12:949–982
18. Horowitz M. Intracranial pneumocele. An unusual complication following mastoid surgery. J Laryngol Otol 1964;78:128–134
19. Kuncz A, Roos A, Lujber L, Haas D, Al Refai M. Traumatic prepontine tension pneumocephalus—case report. Ideggyogy Sz 2004;57(9-10):313–315
20. Karavelioglu E, Eser O, Haktanir A. Pneumocephalus and pneumorrhachis after spinal surgery: case report and review of the literature. Neurol Med Chir (Tokyo) 2014;54(5): 405–407

21. Ishiwata Y, Fujitsu K, Sekino T, et al. Subdural tension pneumocephalus following surgery for chronic subdural hematoma. J Neurosurg 1988;68(1):58–61
22. Agrawal A, Singh BR. Mount Fuji sign with concavo-convex appearance of epidural haematoma in a patient with tension pneumocephalus. J Radiol Case Rep 2009;3(1):10–12
23. Dabdoub CB, Salas G, Silveira EdoN, Dabdoub CF. Review of the management of pneumocephalus. Surg Neurol Int 2015;6(1):155
24. Huh J. Barotrauma-induced pneumocephalus experienced by a high risk patient after commercial air travel. J Korean Neurosurg Soc 2013;54(2):142–144
25. Lee TJ, Huang CC, Chuang CC, Huang SF. Transnasal endoscopic repair of cerebrospinal fluid rhinorrhea and skull base defect: ten-year experience. Laryngoscope 2004;114(8):1475–1481
26. van Aken MO, de Marie S, van der Lely AJ, et al. Risk factors for meningitis after transsphenoidal surgery. Clin Infect Dis 1997;25(4):852–856
27. Carrau RL, Snyderman C, Janecka IP, Sekhar L, Sen C, D'Amico F. Antibiotic prophylaxis in cranial base surgery. Head Neck 1991;13(4):311–317
28. Garner JS, Jarvis WR, Emori TG, Horan TC, Hughes JM. CDC definition for nosocomial infections. In: Olmsted RN, ed. APIC Infection Control and Applied Epidemiology: Principles and Practice. 1st ed. St. Louis, MO: Mosby; 1996:A1–A20
29. Kono Y, Prevedello DM, Snyderman CH, et al. One thousand endoscopic skull base surgical procedures demystifying the infection potential: incidence and description of post-operative meningitis and brain abscesses. Infect Control Hosp Epidemiol 2011;32(1):77–83
30. Allen KP, Isaacson B, Kutz JW, Purcell PL, Roland PS. The association of meningitis with postoperative cerebrospinal fluid fistula. J Neurol Surg B Skull Base 2012;73(6):401–404
31. Korinek AM, Baugnon T, Golmard JL, van Effenterre R, Coriat P, Puybasset L. Risk factors for adult nosocomial meningitis after craniotomy: role of antibiotic prophylaxis. Neurosurgery 2006;59:126–133
32. Korinek AM, Golmard JL, Elcheick A, et al. Risk factors for neurosurgical site infections after craniotomy: a critical reappraisal of antibiotic prophylaxis on 4,578 patients. Br J Neurosurg 2005;19(2):155–162
33. Reichert MC, Medeiros EA, Ferraz FA. Hospital-acquired meningitis in patients undergoing craniotomy: incidence, evolution, and risk factors. Am J Infect Control 2002;30(3):158–164
34. Rathore MH. Do prophylactic antibiotics prevent meningitis after basilar skull fracture? Pediatr Infect Dis J 1991;10(2): 87–88
35. Villalobos T, Arango C, Kubilis P, Rathore M. Antibiotic prophylaxis after basilar skull fractures: a meta-analysis. Clin Infect Dis 1998;27(2):364–369
36. Ratilal BO, Costa J, Sampaio C, Pappamikail L. Antibiotic prophylaxis for preventing meningitis in patients with basilar skull fractures. Cochrane Database Syst Rev 2011;(8): CD004884
37. Brouwer MC, Coutinho JM, van de Beek D. Clinical characteristics and outcome of brain abscess: systematic review and meta-analysis. Neurology 2014;82(9):806–813
38. Gardner PA, Kassam AB, Thomas A, et al. Endoscopic endonasal resection of anterior cranial base meningiomas. Neurosurgery 2008;63(1):36–52, discussion 52–54
39. Kristof RA, Rother M, Neuloh G, Klingmüller D. Incidence, clinical manifestations, and course of water and electrolyte metabolism disturbances following transsphenoidal pituitary adenoma surgery: a prospective observational study. J Neurosurg 2009;111(3):555–562
40. Schreckinger M, Walker B, Knepper J, et al. Post-operative diabetes insipidus after endoscopic transsphenoidal surgery. Pituitary 2013;16(4):445–451
41. Berker M, Hazer DB, Yücel T, et al. Complications of endoscopic surgery of the pituitary adenomas: analysis of 570 patients and review of the literature. Pituitary 2012;15(3):288–300
42. Dehdashti AR, Ganna A, Witterick I, Gentili F. Expanded endoscopic endonasal approach for anterior cranial base and suprasellar lesions: indications and limitations. Neurosurgery 2009;64(4):677–687, discussion 687–689
43. Laufer I, Anand VK, Schwartz TH. Endoscopic, endonasal extended transsphenoidal, transplanum transtuberculum approach for resection of suprasellar lesions. J Neurosurg 2007;106(3):400–406
44. Stamm AC, Vellutini E, Harvey RJ, Nogeira JF Jr, Herman DR. Endoscopic transnasal craniotomy and the resection of craniopharyngioma. Laryngoscope 2008;118(7):1142–1148
45. Ransom ER, Chiu AG. Prevention and management of complications in intracranial endoscopic skull base surgery. Otolaryngol Clin North Am 2010;43(4):875–895
46. Cote DJ, Alzarea A, Acosta MA, et al. Predictors and rates of delayed symptomatic hyponatremia after transsphenoidal surgery: a systematic review. [corrected]. World Neurosurg 2016;88:1–6
47. Jahangiri A, Wagner J, Tran MT, et al. Factors predicting postoperative hyponatremia and efficacy of hyponatremia management strategies after more than 1000 pituitary operations. J Neurosurg 2013;119(6):1478–1483
48. Cavallo LM, Briganti F, Cappabianca P, et al. Hemorrhagic vascular complications of endoscopic transsphenoidal surgery. Minim Invasive Neurosurg 2004;47(3):145–150
49. Gardner PA, Tormenti MJ, Pant H, Fernandez-Miranda JC, Snyderman CH, Horowitz MB. Carotid artery injury during endoscopic endonasal skull base surgery: incidence and outcomes. Neurosurgery 2013;73(2, Suppl Operative):ons261–ons269, discussion ons269–ons270

50. Raymond J, Hardy J, Czepko R, Roy D. Arterial injuries in transsphenoidal surgery for pituitary adenoma; the role of angiography and endovascular treatment. AJNR Am J Neuroradiol 1997;18(4):655–665

51. Harris FS, Rhoton AL. Anatomy of the cavernous sinus. A microsurgical study. J Neurosurg 1976;45(2):169–180

52. Rhoton AL Jr. The sellar region. Neurosurgery 2002;51(4, Suppl):S335–S374

53. Vescan AD, Snyderman CH, Carrau RL, et al. Vidian canal: analysis and relationship to the internal carotid artery. Laryngoscope 2007;117(8):1338–1342

54. Kassam AB, Vescan AD, Carrau RL, et al. Expanded endonasal approach: vidian canal as a landmark to the petrous internal carotid artery. J Neurosurg 2008;108(1):177–183

55. Yamasaki T, Moritake K, Nagai H, Kimura Y. Integration of ultrasonography and endoscopy into transsphenoidal surgery with a "picture-in-picture" viewing system—technical note. Neurol Med Chir (Tokyo) 2002;42(6):275–277, discussion 278

56. Kalinin PL, Sharipov OI, Shkarubo AN, et al. [Damage to the cavernous segment of internal carotid artery in transsphenoidal endoscopic removal of pituitary adenomas (report of 4 cases)]. Zh Vopr Neĭrokhir Im N Burdenko 2013;77(6):28–37; discussion 38

57. Valentine R, Wormald PJ. Controlling the surgical field during a large endoscopic vascular injury. Laryngoscope 2011; 121(3):562–566

58. Padhye V, Valentine R, Paramasivan S, et al. Early and late complications of endoscopic hemostatic techniques following different carotid artery injury characteristics. Int Forum Allergy Rhinol 2014;4(8):651–657

59. Gardner PA, Tormenti MJ, Pant H, Fernandez-Miranda JC, Snyderman CH, Horowitz MB. Carotid artery injury during endoscopic endonasal skull base surgery: incidence and outcomes. Neurosurgery 2013;73(2, Suppl Operative):ons261–ons269, discussion ons269–ons270

60. Weidenbecher M, Huk WJ, Iro H. Internal carotid artery injury during functional endoscopic sinus surgery and its management. Eur Arch Otorhinolaryngol 2005;262(8):6 40–645

61. Valentine R, Wormald PJ. Carotid artery injury after endonasal surgery. Otolaryngol Clin North Am 2011;44(5):1059–1079

62. Laws ER Jr. Vascular complications of transsphenoidal surgery. Pituitary 1999;2(2):163–170

63. Park AH, Stankiewicz JA, Chow J, Azar-Kia B. A protocol for management of a catastrophic complication of functional endoscopic sinus surgery: internal carotid artery injury. Am J Rhinol 1998;12(3):153–158

64. Fox AJ, Viñuela F, Pelz DM, et al. Use of detachable balloons for proximal artery occlusion in the treatment of unclippable cerebral aneurysms. J Neurosurg 1987;66(1):40–46

65. Kocer N, Kizilkilic O, Albayram S, Adaletli I, Kantarci F, Islak C. Treatment of iatrogenic internal carotid artery laceration and carotid cavernous fistula with endovascular stent-graft placement. AJNR Am J Neuroradiol 2002;23(3):442–446

66. de Divitiis E, Cavallo LM, Esposito F, Stella L, Messina A. Extended endoscopic transsphenoidal approach for tuberculum sellae meningiomas. Neurosurgery 2007;61(5, Suppl 2):229–237, discussion 237–238

67. Stippler M, Gardner PA, Snyderman CH, Carrau RL, Prevedello DM, Kassam AB. Endoscopic endonasal approach for clival chordomas. Neurosurgery 2009;64(2):268–277, discussion 277–278

68. Zhang Q, Kong F, Yan B, Ni Z, Liu H. Endoscopic endonasal surgery for clival chordoma and chondrosarcoma. ORL J Otorhinolaryngol Relat Spec 2008;70(2):124–129

69. Kim EH, Ahn JY, Chang JH, Kim SH. Management strategies of intercavernous sinus bleeding during transsphenoidal surgery. Acta Neurochir (Wien) 2009;151(7):803–808

70. Gazzeri R, Galarza M, Conti C, De Bonis C. Incidence of thromboembolic events after use of gelatin-thrombin-based hemostatic matrix during intracranial tumor surgery. Neurosurg Rev 2018;41(1):303–310

71. Snyderman CH, Pant H, Gardner PA, Carrau RL, Prevedello DM, Kassam AB. Management of complications of endonasal cranial base surgery. Kassam AB, Gardner PA. Endoscopic Approaches to the Skull Base 2012;26:182–190

72. Borg A, Kirkman MA, Choi D. Endoscopic endonasal anterior skull base surgery: a systematic review of complications during the past 65 years. World Neurosurg 2016;95:383–391

73. Tam S, Duggal N, Rotenberg BW. Olfactory outcomes following endoscopic pituitary surgery with or without septal flap reconstruction: a randomized controlled trial. Int Forum Allergy Rhinol 2013;3(1):62–65

74. Chaaban MR, Chaudhry AL, Riley KO, Woodworth BA. Objective assessment of olfaction after transsphenoidal pituitary surgery. Am J Rhinol Allergy 2015;29(5):365–368

75. Zimmer LA, Shah O, Theodosopoulos PV. Short term quality-of-life changes after endoscopic pituitary surgery rated with SNOT-22. J Neurol Surg B Skull Base 2014;75(4):288–292

76. Greig SR, Cooper TJ, Sommer DD, Nair S, Wright ED. Objective sinonasal functional outcomes in endoscopic anterior skull-base surgery: an evidence-based review with recommendations. Int Forum Allergy Rhinol 2016;6(10):1040–1046

77. Kim SW, Park KB, Khalmuratova R, Lee HK, Jeon SY, Kim DW. Clinical and histologic studies of olfactory outcomes after nasoseptal flap harvesting. Laryngoscope 2013;123(7): 1602–1606

78. Deconde AS, Vira D, Thompson CF, Wang MB, Bergsneider M, Suh JD. Radiologic assessment of the paranasal sinuses after endoscopic skull base surgery. J Neurol Surg B Skull Base 2013;74(6):351–357

79. Langdon C, Enseñat J, Rioja E, et al. Long-term radiological findings after endonasal endoscopic approach to the skull base. Am J Otolaryngol 2016;37(2):103–107

80. de Almeida JR, Snyderman CH, Gardner PA, Carrau RL, Vescan AD. Nasal morbidity following endoscopic skull base surgery: a prospective cohort study. Head Neck 2011;33(4):547–551

81. Roxbury CR, Saavedra T, Ramanathan M Jr, et al. Layered sellar reconstruction with avascular free grafts: acceptable alternative to the nasoseptal flap for repair of low-volume intraoperative cerebrospinal fluid leak. Am J Rhinol Allergy 2016;30(5):367–371

82. de Almeida JR, Witterick IJ, Gullane PJ, et al. Physical morbidity by surgical approach and tumor location in skull base surgery. Head Neck 2013;35(4):493–499

83. Thorp BD, Sreenath SB, Ebert CS, Zanation AM. Endoscopic skull base reconstruction: a review and clinical case series of 152 vascularized flaps used for surgical skull base defects in the setting of intraoperative cerebrospinal fluid leak. Neurosurg Focus 2014;37(4):E4

84. Dolci RLL, Miyake MM, Tateno DA, et al. Postoperative otorhinolaryngologic complications in transnasal endoscopic surgery to access the skull base. Rev Bras Otorrinolaringol (Engl Ed) 2017;83(3):349–355

85. Cheng Y, Xue F, Wang TY, et al. Analyses and treatments of postoperative nasal complications after endonasal transsphenoidal resection of pituitary neoplasms. Medicine (Baltimore) 2017;96(15):e6614

86. Rowan NR, Wang EW, Gardner PA, Fernandez-Miranda JC, Snyderman CH. Nasal deformities following nasoseptal flap reconstruction of skull base defects. J Neurol Surg B Skull Base 2016;77(1):14–18

87. Heo KW, Park SK. Rhinologic outcomes of concurrent operation for pituitary adenoma and chronic rhinosinusitis: an early experience. Am J Rhinol 2008;22(5):533–536

88. Koren I, Hadar T, Rappaport ZH, Yaniv E. Endoscopic transnasal transsphenoidal microsurgery versus the sublabial approach for the treatment of pituitary tumors: endonasal complications. Laryngoscope 1999;109(11):1838–1840

89. Cappabianca P, Cavallo LM, Colao A, de Divitiis E. Surgical complications associated with the endoscopic endonasal transsphenoidal approach for pituitary adenomas. J Neurosurg 2002;97(2):293–298

90. Charalampaki P, Ayyad A, Kockro RA, Perneczky A. Surgical complications after endoscopic transsphenoidal pituitary surgery. J Clin Neurosci 2009;16(6):786–789

91. Dehdashti AR, Ganna A, Karabatsou K, Gentili F. Pure endoscopic endonasal approach for pituitary adenomas: early surgical results in 200 patients and comparison with previous microsurgical series. Neurosurgery 2008;62(5):1006–1015, discussion 1015–1017

92. Harvey RJ, Nogueira JF, Schlosser RJ, Patel SJ, Vellutini E, Stamm AC. Closure of large skull base defects after endoscopic transnasal craniotomy. Clinical article. J Neurosurg 2009; 111(2):371–379

93. Thompson CF, Wang MB, Kim BJ, Bergsneider M, Suh JD. Incidence and management of epistaxis after endoscopic skull base surgery. ORL J Otorhinolaryngol Relat Spec 2012;74(6):315–319

94. Chabot JD, Patel CR, Hughes MA, et al. Nasoseptal flap necrosis: a rare complication of endoscopic endonasal surgery. 2017:1–10

Section XVII

Basics in Otology

Chapter 45 Cortical Mastoidectomy

Narayan Jayashankar

Indications

- It is the first step in various surgeries, for example, endolymphatic sac decompression, cochlear implantation, and the translabyrinthine approach.
- It is performed for single-stage drainage of otogenic brain abscess where the primary etiology is granulation tissue disease in the mastoid cavity.
- Acute coalescent mastoiditis.

Surgical Steps

1. Identify the spine of Henle, Macewen's triangle, and temporal line. The root of the zygoma has two limbs. The inferior limb of the root of the zygoma continues in a posterior direction along the roof of the mastoid and represents the temporal line.
2. Drilling is started along the temporal line from anterior to posterior direction, parallel to the middle fossa plate. Similarly, drilling is performed along the posterior border of the mastoid parallel to the course of the sigmoid sinus till the mastoid tip (**Fig. 45.1** and **Fig. 45.2**). Care is taken to identify the sigmoid sinus, especially when it is forward lying. The position of the sigmoid sinus is identified by the color change as cells are progressively drilled. Anteriorly, drilling is performed from the region of Macewen's triangle to the mastoid tip, parallel to the posterior wall of external auditory canal without damaging it. The cells in between these three borders are cells of the mastoid cortex and can be safely drilled (**Fig. 45.3**). We believe in a wide cortical mastoidectomy which identifies landmarks as drilling proceeds toward the antrum. Drilling in only the Macewen's triangle toward the antrum is to be avoided so as to prevent risk to various surrounding structures like the posterior canal wall and low-lying middle fossa dura as also lateral semicircular canal, second genu of facial nerve, or ossicles.
3. Cells of the mastoid cortex are drilled. The bone is drilled superiorly to identify the tegmen mastoidale. The cells over the sigmoid sinus are exenterated to delineate the sigmoid plate of bone. Similarly, the cells over the posterior canal wall and mastoid tip are exenterated. Antrum is the largest cell and is approximately about 1.25 cm deep to the Macewen's triangle. The lateral semicircular canal will almost immediately come into view as the antrum is opened. The lateral semicircular canal is identified by the color change under the cells (**Fig. 45.4**).
4. The antrum is opened widely to identify the aditus to antrum. The short process of the incus is seen (**Fig. 45.5**). The cells over the lateral, posterior, and

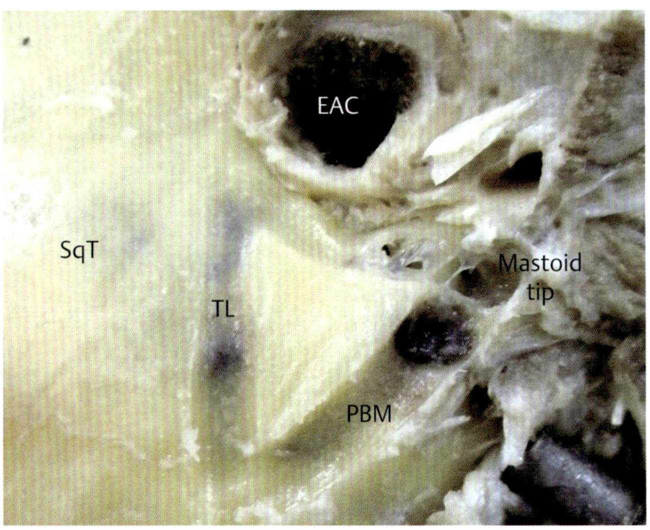

Fig. 45.1 A wide-angle view of the boundaries of the mastoid bone where initial drilling commences.

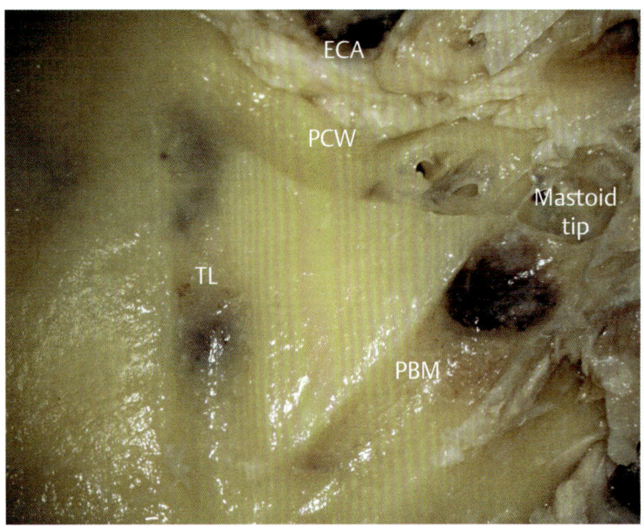

Fig. 45.2 Initial drilling for cortical mastoidectomy.

superior semicircular canal are exenterated. The cells of the sinodural angle are exenterated. Cells in the infralabyrinthine area are also exenterated, the medial limit being the bone covering the jugular bulb. The cells over the mastoid segment of the fallopian canal are also exenterated (**Fig. 45.6**).

5. Although in a cortical mastoidectomy it is not essential to remove all cells and delineate structures as described above, it is good to practice the same in cadaveric dissection and is especially useful in neurotologic procedures.

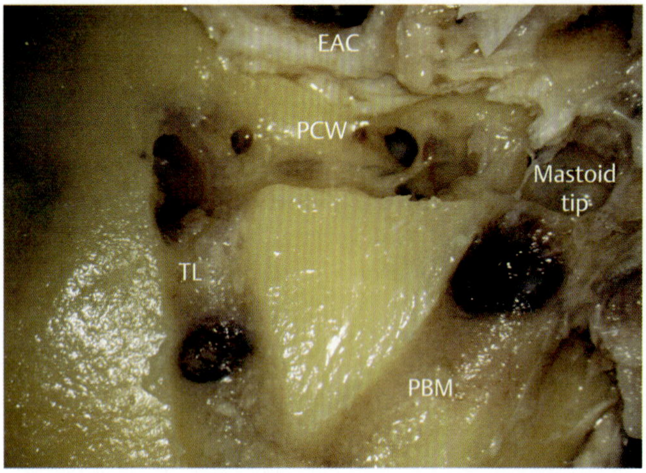

Fig. 45.3 The central triangular bone leads to cells of the mastoid cortex in a pneumatic mastoid. Care is taken to look for a forward-lying sigmoid sinus or low-lying dura.

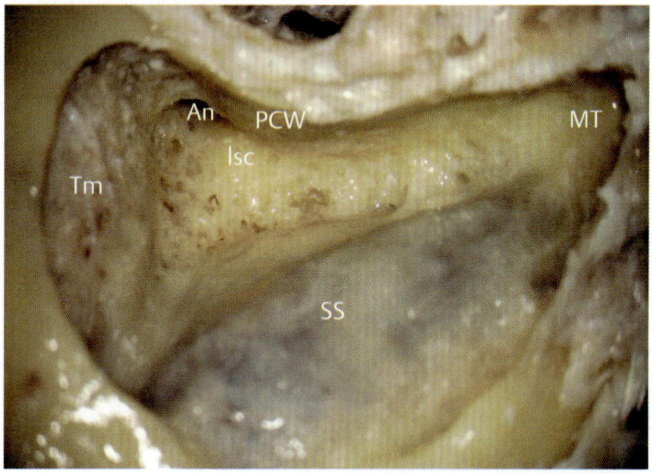

Fig. 45.4 The superior, posterior, and anterior limits are defined and drilling proceeds medially to identify the antrum. Defining the limits helps achieve a wide-based cortical mastoidectomy.

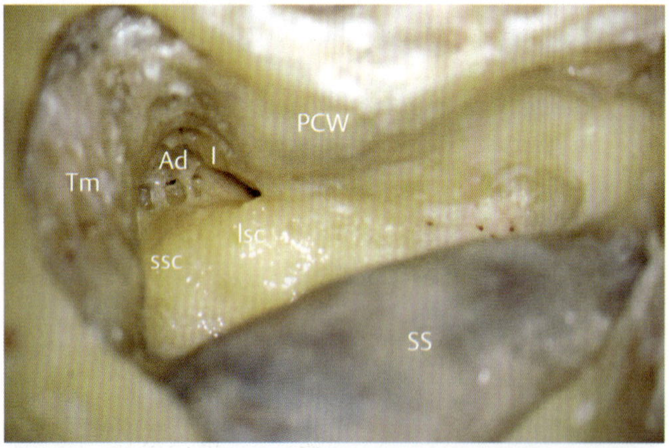

Fig. 45.5 Antrum opened and aditus identified.

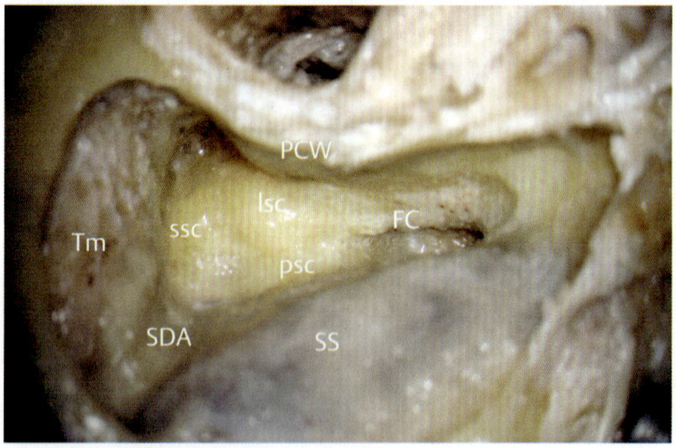

Fig. 45.6 Cortical mastoidectomy.

Chapter 46 Posterior Tympanotomy and Extended Posterior Tympanotomy

Narayan Jayashankar

Posterior Tympanotomy

Indications

- Cochlear implant.
- Facial nerve decompression.

Surgical Steps

1. A good cortical mastoidectomy is performed as described in Chapter 45.
2. The mastoid (vertical) segment of the facial nerve is an important focus in this approach (**Fig. 46.1**). The facial nerve at its second genu runs in a groove on the anterior aspect of the lateral semicircular canal. At the second genu, the facial nerve lies medial (deeper) to the dome of the lateral semicircular canal as also the short process of the incus. It traverses inferiorly toward the stylomastoid foramen where it is perpendicular to the digastric ridge and posterior belly of the digastric muscle. The facial nerve in its mastoid segment courses laterally at a subtle 10- to 15-degree angle from the second genu to the stylomastoid foramen. It should be noted that in posterior tympanotomy, only the mastoid segment needs to be identified and not the second genu of the facial nerve. Drilling begins just inferior to the short process of the incus, parallel to the vertical segment of the facial nerve, using a diamond burr, and is carried inferiorly. The burr diameter is always larger than the diameter of the fallopian canal. Drilling is never perpendicular to the facial nerve. Use good irrigation so that the whitish color change of the facial nerve as we approach the fallopian canal is visible. We should be able to identify the mastoid segment of the facial nerve within a reasonably thin bony covering of fallopian canal, without exposing it.
3. A diamond burr is used again to identify the origin and course of the chorda tympani nerve. The chorda tympani nerve always arises from the inferior half of the mastoid segment of the facial nerve.
4. The cells between the tympanic annulus and the mastoid segment of the facial nerve are exenterated leaving behind a thin bone protecting the short process of incus (fossa incudis).
5. Approach of posterior tympanotomy is triangular shaped. The boundaries are the facial nerve medially, the chorda tympani nerve laterally, and the fossa incudis superiorly (**Fig. 46.2**). We usually find an air cell, even in very sclerotic bones, just lateral to the second genu of the facial nerve. This cell guides us to the middle ear.

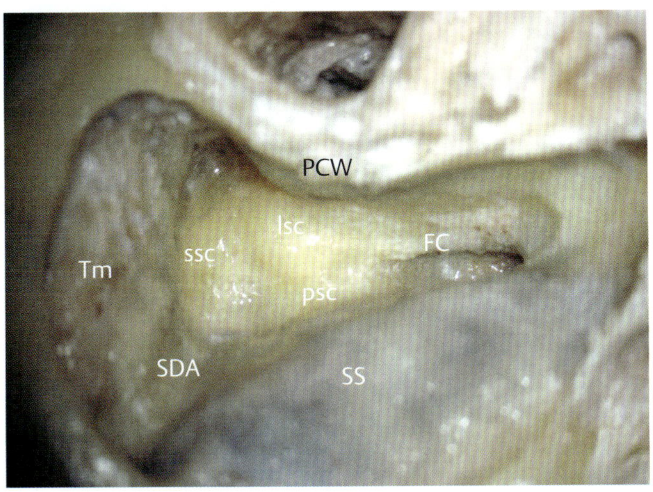

Fig. 46.1 Cortical mastoidectomy and identification of vertical (mastoid) segment of the fallopian canal.

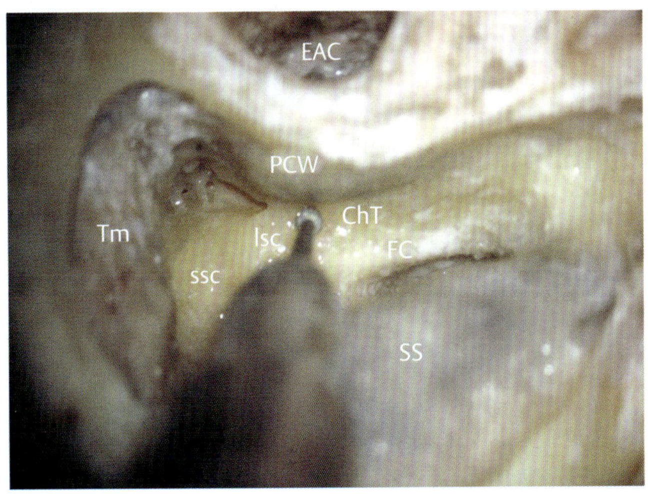

Fig. 46.2 The area where the initial access to the middle ear is obtained during posterior tympanotomy.

6. Once the facial and chorda tympani nerves are identified, smaller burrs can be used to open the facial recess fully. The opening should be started at the superior most part of the triangle—just inferior to the fossa incudis—as that is the widest part of the recess. The direction of the burr should always be toward the incudostapedial joint without touching it inadvertently. The posterior tympanotomy is widened up to the chorda facial angle (**Fig. 46.3**). Bone is also thinned anterior to the mastoid segment of the facial nerve to expose the sinus tympani completely. Care is taken to see that the shaft of the rotating burr does not touch the fallopian canal.
7. At the completion of the facial recess approach we should be able to visualize the pyramidal process, stapedial tendon, stapes superstructure, complete round window, sinus tympani, and promontory (**Fig. 46.4** and **Fig. 46.5**).
8. In cochlear implant surgery, the electrode can be inserted directly through the round window (**Fig. 46.6**) or a separate cochleostomy can be done anteroinferior to the round window. We prefer to use the round window approach. In this approach, the first the anterior and the superior bony overhangs of the round window are drilled to completely expose the intact round window. The round window membrane can then be removed atraumatically with the help of a pick. There is a bony ridge at the posterior inferior margin of the round window. To drill this ridge the burr is used in an inside out fashion so that a minimal amount of bone dust enters the inner ear. The size of the window will depend on the type of implant being used.

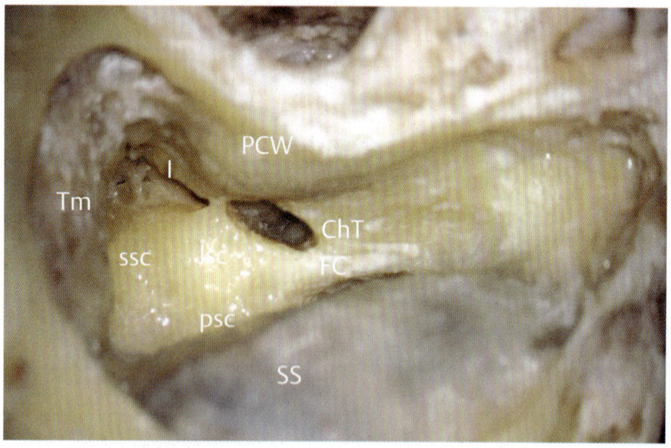

Fig. 46.3 Posterior tympanotomy.

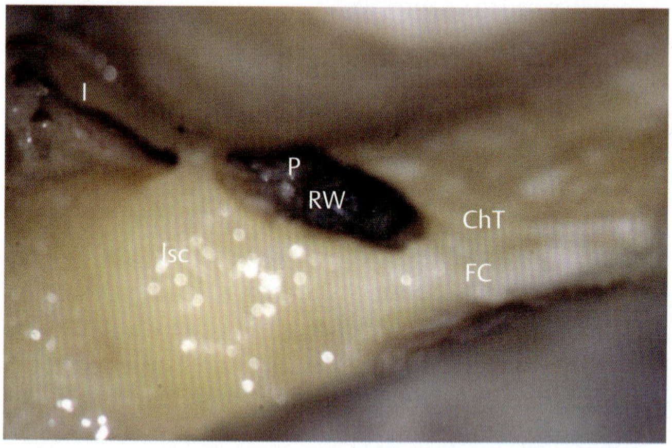

Fig. 46.4 Round window seen through the posterior tympanotomy.

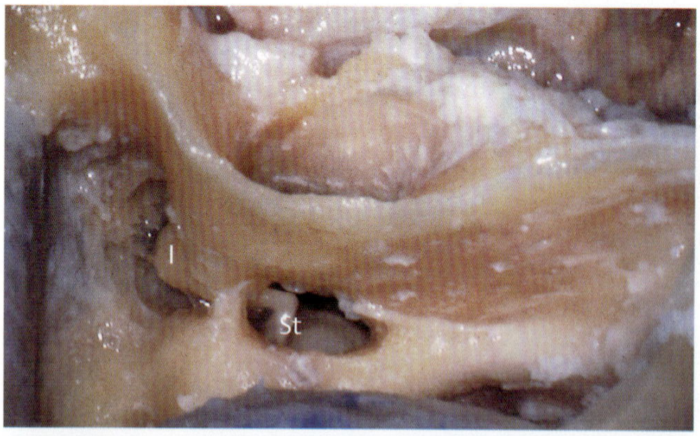

Fig. 46.5 Incudostapedial joint is seen (Courtesy of Dr M. Shaan and Dr S. Bhatia).

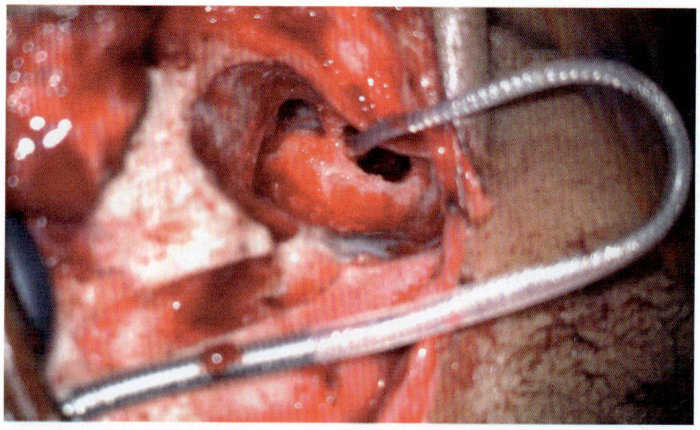

Fig. 46.6 Posterior tympanotomy for cochlear implantation (*right side*).

Extended Posterior Tympanotomy

Indications

Class B glomus tumors.

Surgical Steps

1. A posterior tympanotomy is performed as described above.
2. Thin bone covering the chorda tympani nerve is removed. The chorda tympani nerve is sectioned as far away from its origin as possible with microscissors (**Fig. 46.7**).
3. The sectioned chorda tympani nerve is lifted off from its groove toward its origin (**Fig. 46.8**). The bone between the tympanic annulus and the mastoid segment of the fallopian canal is drilled off to expose the hypotympanum (**Fig. 46.9** and **Fig. 46.10**).

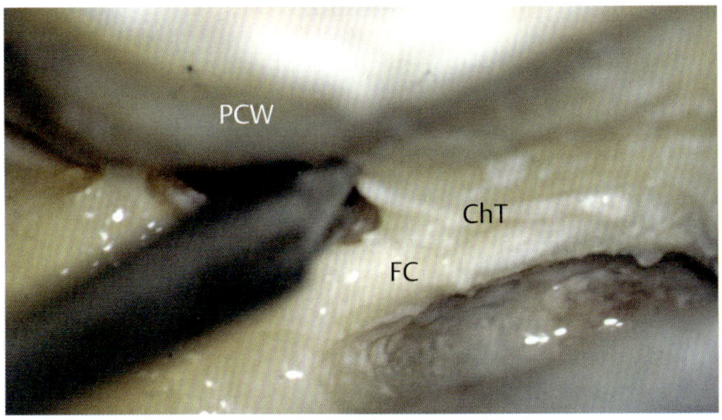

Fig. 46.7 Sectioning of chorda tympani nerve.

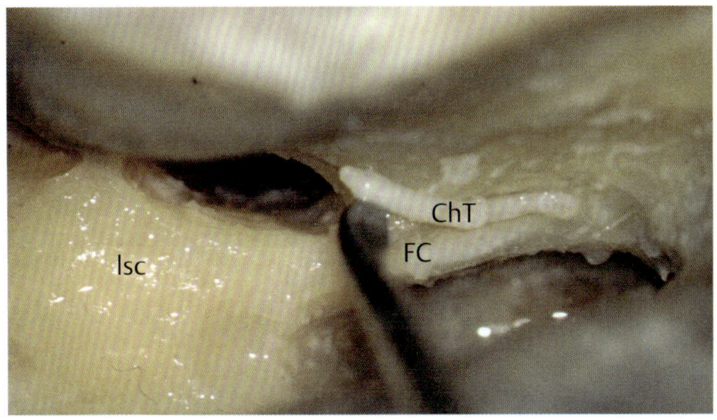

Fig. 46.8 Sectioned chorda tympani nerve is lifted off its groove.

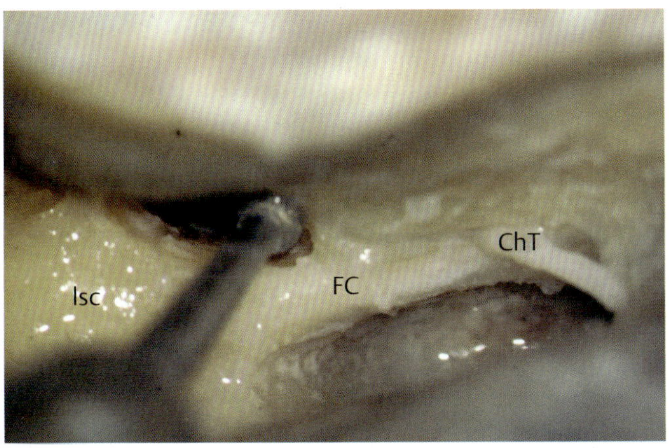

Fig. 46.9 Drilling between the tympanic annulus and the fallopian canal (mastoid segment).

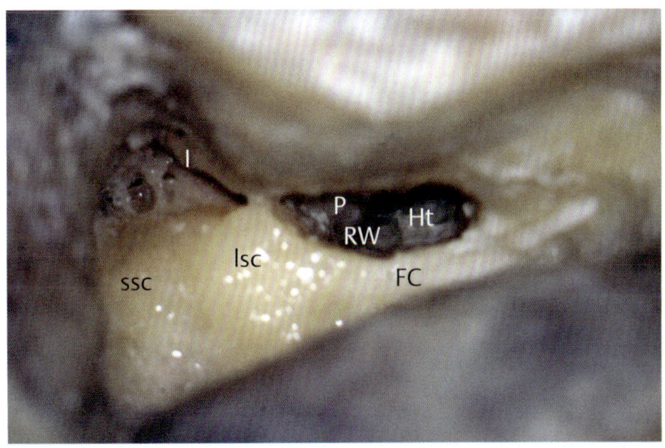

Fig. 46.10 Extended posterior tympanotomy.

Chapter 47

Facial Nerve Anatomy and Relationships

Narayan Jayashankar

The anatomy of the facial nerve is of utmost importance when performing lateral skull base surgery. The anatomy of the facial nerve is described from periphery to origin to orient the reader to the anatomical relationships from surface to depth.

1. The main trunk of the facial nerve at its exit from the stylomastoid foramen is identified (**Fig. 47.1**). A few landmarks have been described to identify the main trunk. The main trunk is located at the perpendicular bisection of a line joining the tragal pointer and the mastoid tip. It lies anteromedial to the posterior belly of the digastric muscle. On palpation with a finger, the stylomastoid foramen area is identified easily between the base of the styloid process and mastoid tip.
2. At the stylomastoid foramen area, the facial nerve is perpendicular to the digastric ridge. As the facial nerve courses in its infralabyrinthine mastoidal (vertical) course, it lies anterior to the ampullary end of the posterior semicircular canal at a variable distance depending on the pneumatization of the mastoid bone. As the facial nerve courses toward the tympanic (horizontal) segment, it takes a bend anteriorly which is called the second genu of the facial nerve. The facial nerve at the second genu runs in a groove on the anteromedial side of the lateral semicircular canal.
3. Drilling is carried out over the area anterior to the ampullary end of the posterior semicircular canal up to the stylomastoid foramen area to identify the fallopian canal in its vertical course (**Fig. 47.2**). Drilling is performed stroke by stroke with a burr whose diameter is larger than the diameter of the fallopian canal. Liberal irrigation is used so that bone dust does not accumulate. As we approach the fallopian canal, we appreciate a color change of the bone to whitish because of the presence of the facial nerve in the fallopian canal.
4. An extended posterior tympanotomy is performed maintaining the chorda intact for demonstration of anatomy (**Fig. 47.3**). The chorda tympani nerve arises from the lower third of the vertical segment of the facial nerve and courses toward the middle ear. Hence, the chorda can also be traced backward to its origin to identify the facial nerve mastoidal (vertical) segment. Also, note that the facial nerve traverses along a line bisecting the jugular bulb that lies deeper to it.
5. The facial recess has been opened up. The bone on the anterior surface of the fallopian canal in its vertical course is thinned out to expose the sinus tympani to understand the surrounding anatomy. The facial nerve in its vertical segment lies posterior and lateral to the round window (**Fig. 47.4**).
6. A canal wall down procedure has been performed. The chorda tympani arises from the mastoidal segment of the facial nerve, runs anteriorly between the incus long process and malleus handle and further anteriorly runs in the petrotympanic fissure (**Fig. 47.5**).
7. At the stylomastoid foramen, the facial nerve is covered over by periosteum (**Fig. 47.6**). The incus and malleus have been removed. At the second genu, the facial nerve is posterior and a little lateral to the base of the pyramidal process (of the stapedial tendon). Also seen

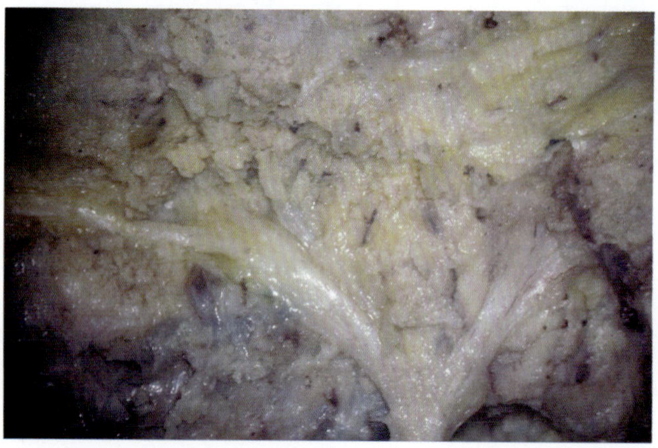

Fig. 47.1 Main trunk of the facial nerve dividing into upper and lower divisions in parotid (*right side*).

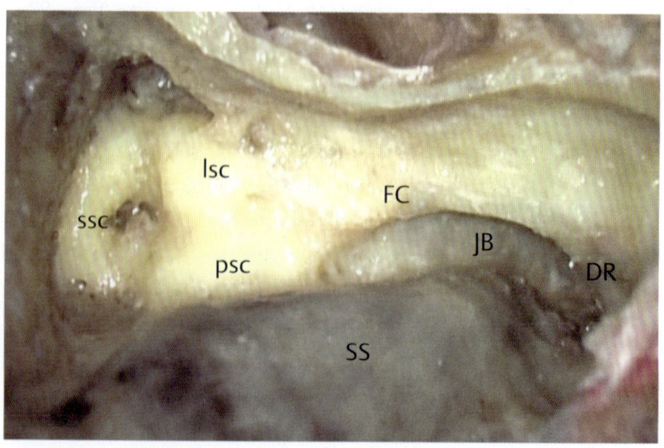

Fig. 47.2 Mastoidal (vertical) segment of the facial nerve.

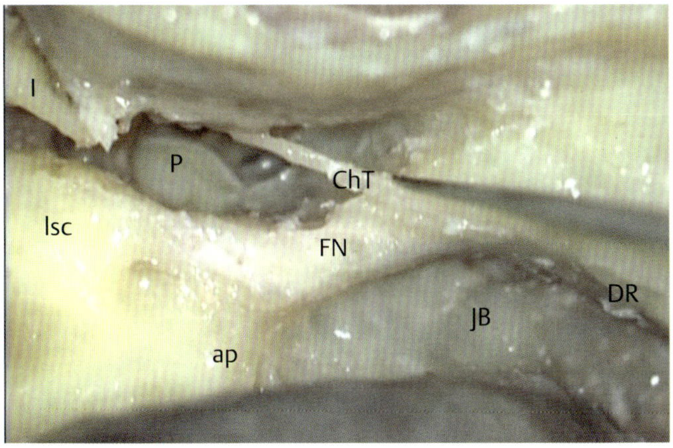

Fig. 47.3 Origin of chorda tympani nerve from the facial nerve.

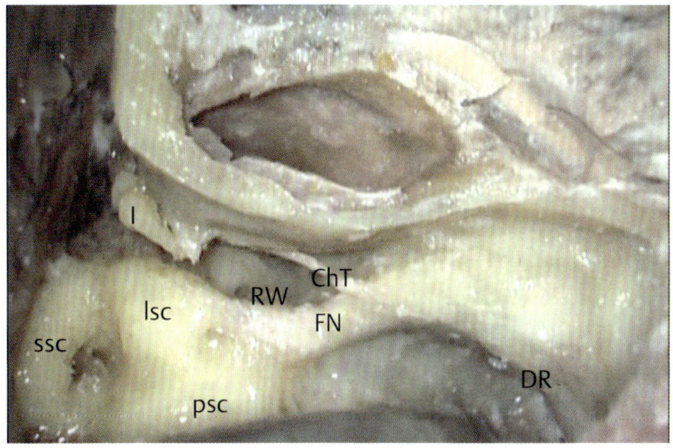

Fig. 47.4 Round window relationship to the facial nerve (mastoidal segment) is seen through an extended posterior tympanotomy keeping the chorda tympani intact for demonstration of anatomy.

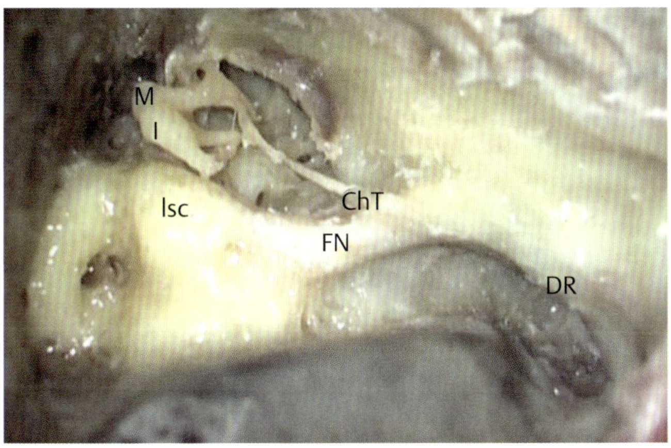

Fig. 47.5 Course of chorda tympani.

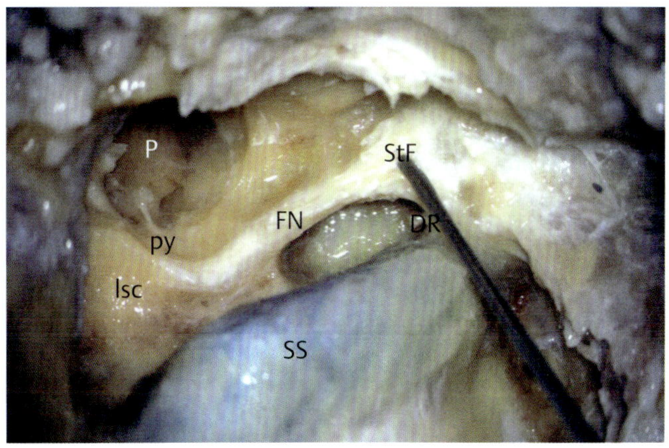

Fig. 47.6 Periosteum at the stylomastoid foramen covering the facial nerve.

is the second genu running in a groove on the anteromedial surface of the lateral semicircular canal. The mastoid tip is excised to demonstrate the continuity of the facial nerve from the mastoidal segment to its extratemporal course in the parotid (**Fig. 47.7**).

8. The tympanic segment of the facial nerve courses medial to the incus and malleus (**Fig. 47.8**). The most anterior lip of the ampullary end of the lateral semicircular canal is adjacent to the tympanic segment of the facial nerve. The tympanic segment of the facial nerve courses superior to the cochleariform process from the second genu to the geniculate ganglion (**Fig. 47.9**).
9. The geniculate ganglion represents the anterior end of the tympanic segment of facial nerve where it takes an acute bend posteriorly and medially as the labyrinthine segment of the facial nerve (**Fig. 47.10**). At the geniculate ganglion, it gives off the greater superficial petrosal nerve.
10. The labyrinthine segment of facial nerve courses toward the ampullary end of the superior semicircular canal. In a fairly pneumatic mastoid, this segment can be traced via a transmastoid route. However, in most cases, the middle fossa approach is ideal to trace this segment of facial nerve.
11. The facial nerve then courses medially in the internal auditory meatus (**Fig. 47.11**). At the lateral end of the internal auditory meatus, it is anterior to the superior vestibular nerve. At the internal auditory meatus, the orientation of the nerves is as follows Facial nerve—anterosuperior, cochlear nerve—anteroinferior, superior vestibular nerve—posterosuperior, and inferior vestibular nerve—posteroinferior. The facial nerve at

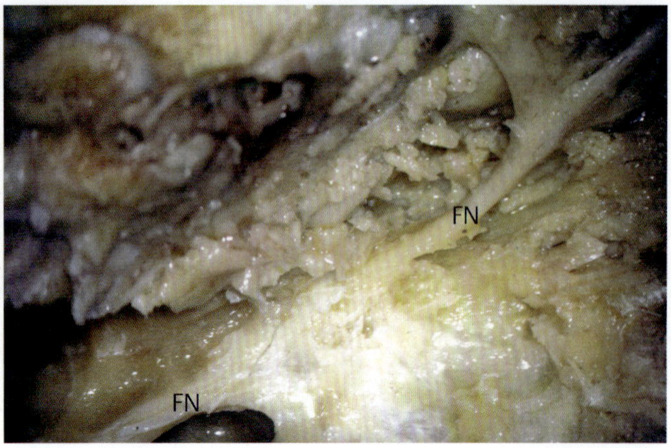

Fig. 47.7 Facial nerve continuity from the mastoidal segment to the main trunk in parotid (mastoid tip excised).

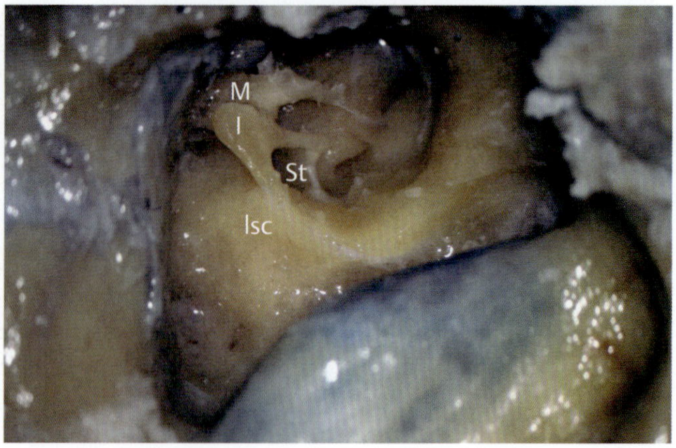

Fig. 47.8 Malleus and incus in position. Tympanic segment lies medial to them.

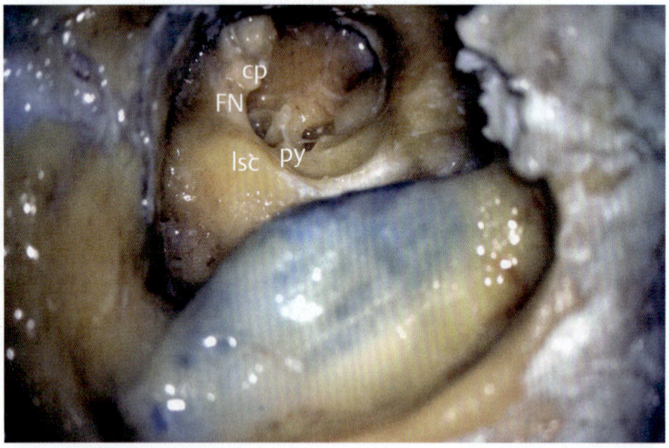

Fig. 47.9 Incus and malleus removed to understand the the course of tympanic segment (horizontal segment) of the facial nerve.

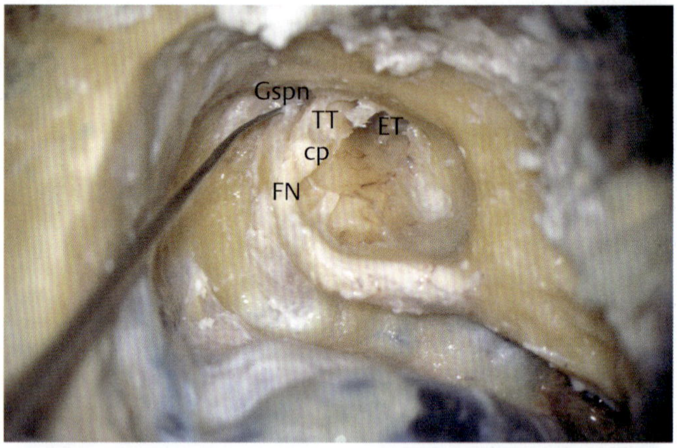

Fig. 47.10 Geniculate ganglion of facial nerve (picture depicts an early stage of the modified transcochlear approach).

the lateral end of the internal auditory meatus is separated from the superior vestibular nerve by the vertical crest, also called Bill's bar. The superior vestibular nerve is separated from the inferior vestibular nerve by the horizontal crest (**Fig. 47.12 and Fig. 47.13).**

12. The facial nerve lies anterior to the vestibulocochlear nerve at the cerebellopontine angle and brainstem areas. The vestibulocochlear nerve needs to be retracted in a translabyrinthine or retrosigmoid approach to identify the facial nerve in the VII–VIII nerve complex (**Fig. 47.14**).
13. The origin of the VII–VIII nerve from the brainstem is seen in **Fig. 47.15**. A loop of the anteroinferior cerebellar artery is located in close proximity to the VII–VIII nerves. The orientation of the lower cranial nerves is also seen in the figures below.
14. The vascular supply to the facial nerve is depicted below (**Fig. 47.16**). The intracranial and internal auditory meatus segments of the facial nerve are supplied by the anterior inferior cerebellar artery (AICA). The AICA arises from the basilar artery, forms a loop over the VII–VIII nerve complex and supplies it. The loop may be in the cerebellopontine angle or may extend toward or partly into the internal auditory meatus. AICA gives out the internal auditory artery. The internal auditory artery gives off fine branches which supply the facial and auditory nerves in the internal auditory meatus. The labyrinthine segment as also the geniculate ganglion are supplied by superficial petrosal branch of the middle meningeal artery (MMA) as also few small twigs directly from the internal carotid artery. The superficial petrosal branch of MMA is given

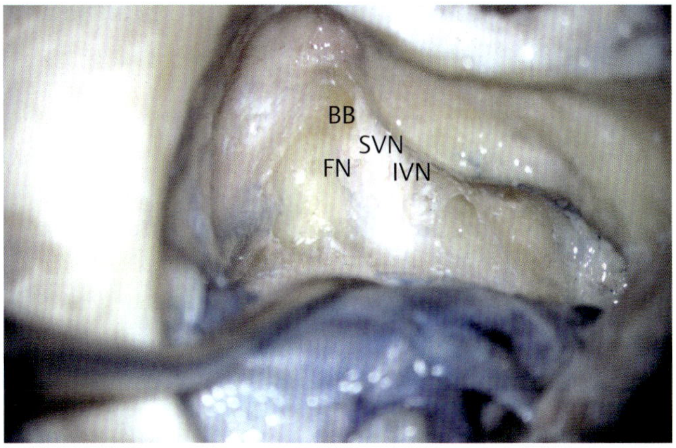

Fig. 41.11 Internal auditory meatus view via a translabyrinthine approach (dura of IAM intact).

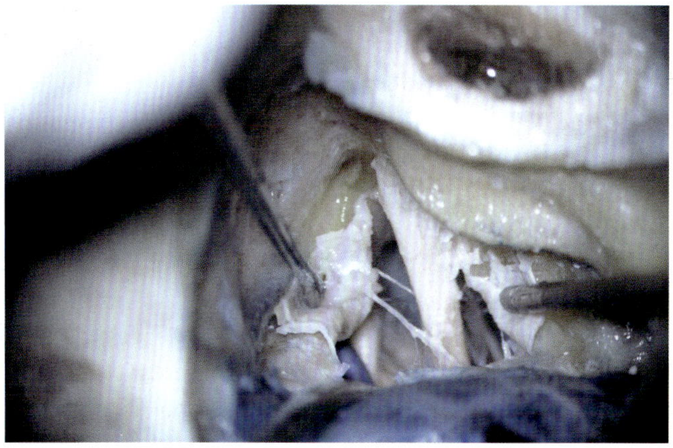

Fig. 47.12 The dura of internal auditory meatus and cerebellopontine angle opened to expose the VII–VIII nerve complex (translabyrinthine approach).

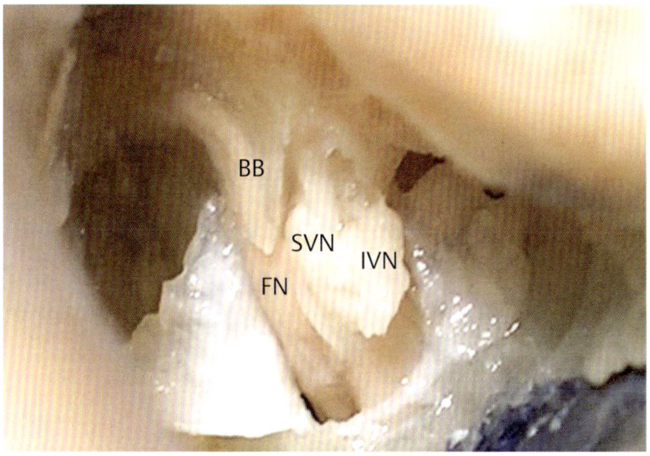

Fig. 47.13 Internal auditory meatus view via a translabyrinthine approach (dura of IAM reflected open, superior and inferior vestibular nerves cut and reflected medially).

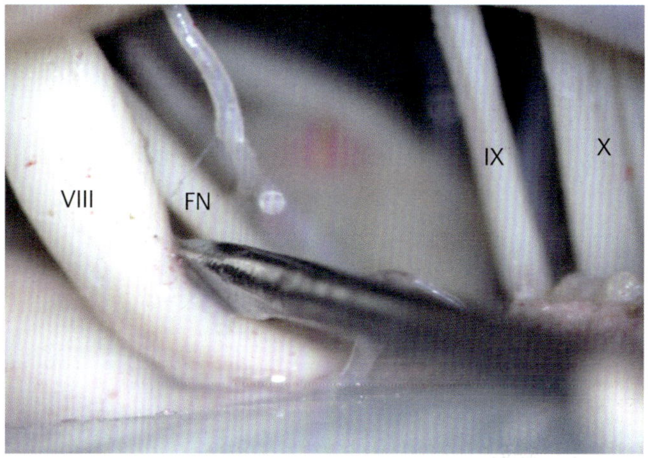

Fig. 47.14 Vestibulocochlear nerve retracted to demonstrate the anteriorly lying facial nerve close to the brainstem (retrosigmoid suboccipital approach).

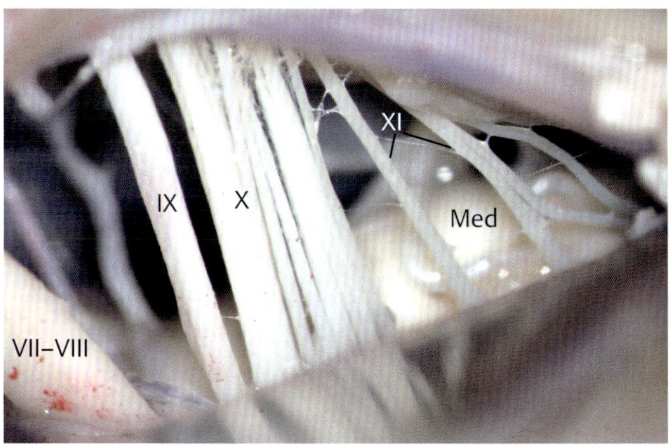

Fig. 47.15 VII–VIII nerve origin at brainstem is seen (retrosigmoid suboccipital approach).

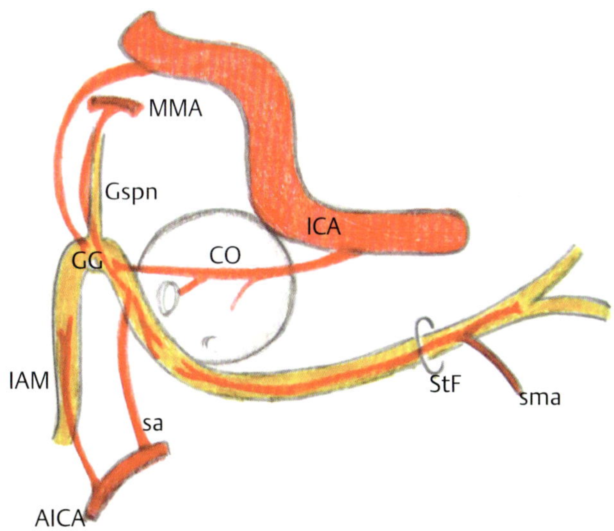

Fig. 47.16 Vascular supply to the facial nerve. (Courtesy Dr Madhuri Mehta.

off just after the entry of the MMA into the foramen spinosum, runs along with the greater superficial petrosal nerve, and gives off multiple fine twigs to the geniculate ganglion, part of labyrinthine segment as also part of tympanic segment of the facial nerve. It anastomoses with the stylomastoid artery. The stylomastoid artery arises from the posterior auricular artery or the occipital artery and forms a loop at the stylomastoid foramen on the medial side of the facial nerve. The returning limb of the loop leaves the canal together with the posterior auricular nerve. The convexity of the stylomastoid artery loop gives off two branches. One of them breaks up into fine twigs and supplies the facial nerve along the fallopian canal. The main ascending branch lies on the medial aspect of the facial nerve in the fallopian canal and also gives off twigs to the mastoidal segment along the medial aspect (floor) of the fallopian canal. At the second genu of facial nerve, this stylomastoid artery branch loops around the nerve to reach the lateral aspect of the tympanic segment and then to supply the tympanic segment. It anastomoses with the superficial petrosal artery to form an arterial arcade around the mastoidal and tympanic segments of the facial nerve. In the extratemporal course (beyond stylomastoid foramen), the facial nerve is supplied by the main returning limb of the stylomastoid artery described above. It also receives branches from the posterior auricular, occipital, superficial temporal and transverse facial arteries extracranially.

Section XVIII

Translabyrinthine Approach

Chapter 48 The Enlarged Translabyrinthine Approach

Narayan Jayashankar, Suresh Sankhla, and Rajan Shah

Introduction

The translabyrinthine approach was described by Prof William House in 1961. He revolutionized excision of vestibular schwannomas by using the microscope. This led to better outcomes resulting in a decrease in intraoperative mortality to less than 10% (mortality rates at that time ranged from 68 to 86%). Prof House also described methods that improved rates of tumor removal as also the preservation of facial nerve. The translabyrinthine approach described was, however, limited to 180-degree exposure of the internal auditory meatus (IAM). As refinements to the approach were described by various authors, the most significant contribution in my mind is the development of the enlarged translabyrinthine approach and its transapical extension described by Prof Mario Sanna. This approach is being routinely performed by the authors at their institution and is described below.

Indications

- Vestibular schwannomas of any size with unserviceable hearing.
- Vestibular schwannomas exceeding 2 cm in extrameatal diameter irrespective of the preoperative hearing thresholds. It has been found to be extremely difficult to retain serviceable hearing in this class of subjects if a hearing preservation approach (retrosigmoid approach) is used.
- Vestibular schwannoma less than 2 cm in extrameatal diameter if the hearing is worse than Grade C as per modified Sanna classification (worse than 40-dB hearing threshold and speech discrimination score is less than 60%) (**Fig. 48.1**).
- Vestibular schwannoma wherein the tumor is extending far into the fundus of the IAM, since it is very difficult to preserve serviceable hearing in these cases.
- Some cases of cerebellopontine angle epidermoids.

Surgical Steps

1. A C-shaped postaural incision is taken around 3 to 4 cm behind the postaural groove. It starts superior to the helix, traverses behind the posterior border of the mastoid, and terminates at the mastoid tip area (**Fig. 48.2**). It includes the skin and subcutaneous tissue (**Fig. 48.3**).
2. The musculoperiosteal layer is incised in a T-shaped manner (**Fig. 48.4**). The horizontal incision is taken at the level of the supramastoid crest. The vertical limb is taken from the horizontal incision to the mastoid tip, between the posterior wall of the external ear and the skin incision. This is done so that the incisions of skin

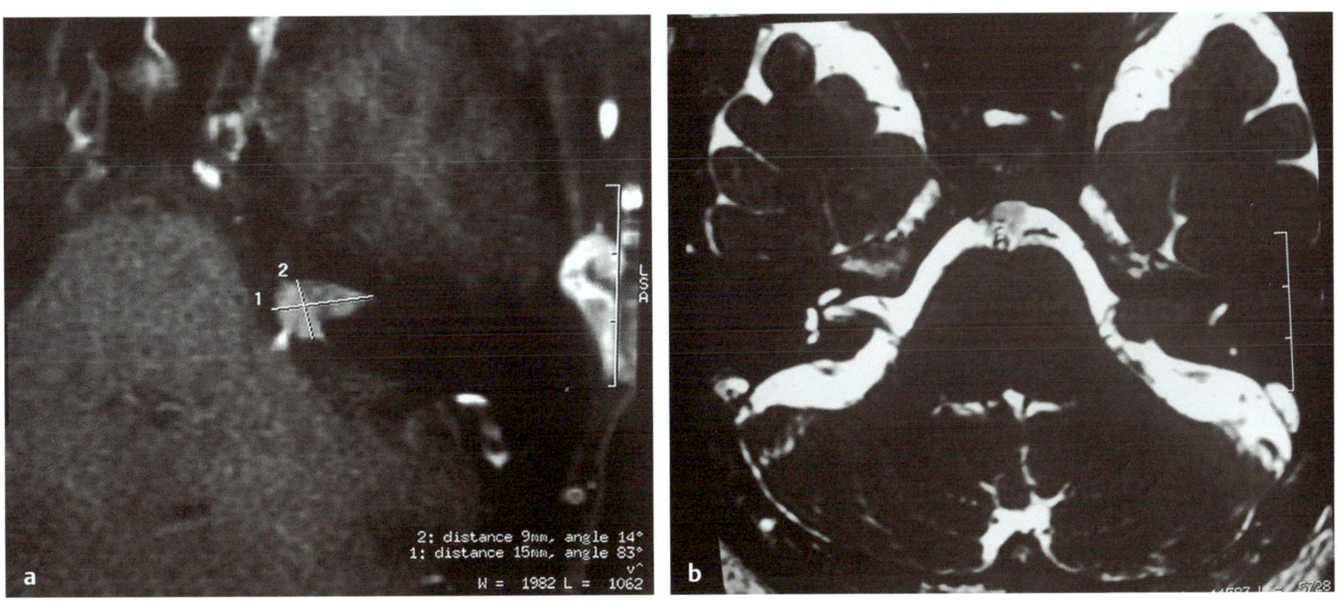

Fig. 48.1 **(a, b)** MRI scans of a subject with a left-sided vestibular schwannoma.

and musculoperiosteal layer do not overlap thereby minimizing the risk of cerebrospinal fluid leak to the outside.

3. The mastoid cortex as also the retromastoid area is exposed. The musculoperiosteal flaps are reflected and sutured (**Fig. 48.5**). Authors avoid the use of mastoid retractors for the same since retractors limit the angles for drilling.

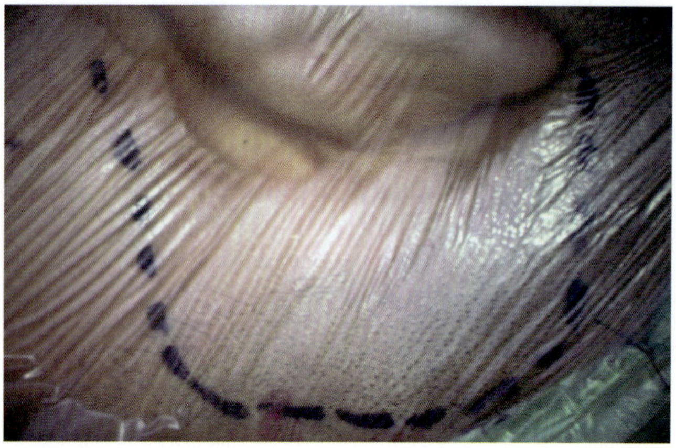

Fig. 48.2 Postaural incision—left ear.

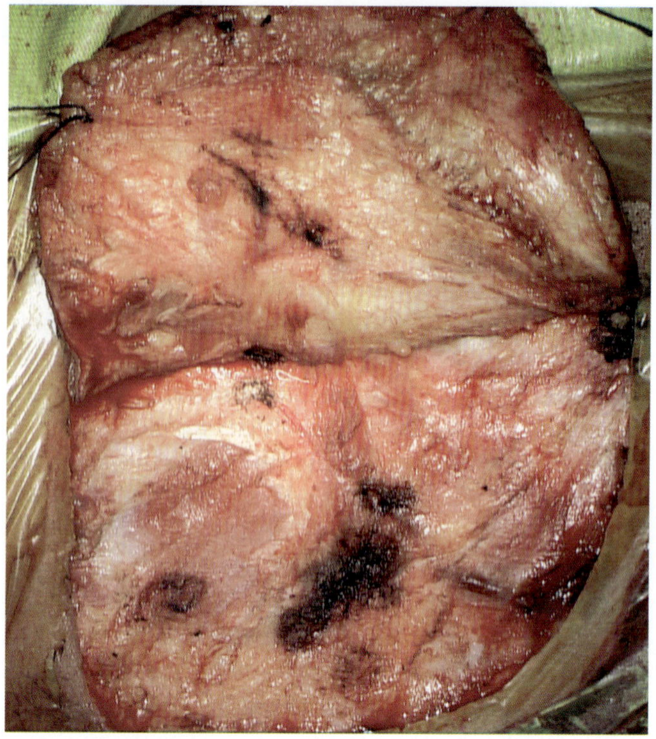

Fig. 48.3 Skin and subcutaneous flap elevated.

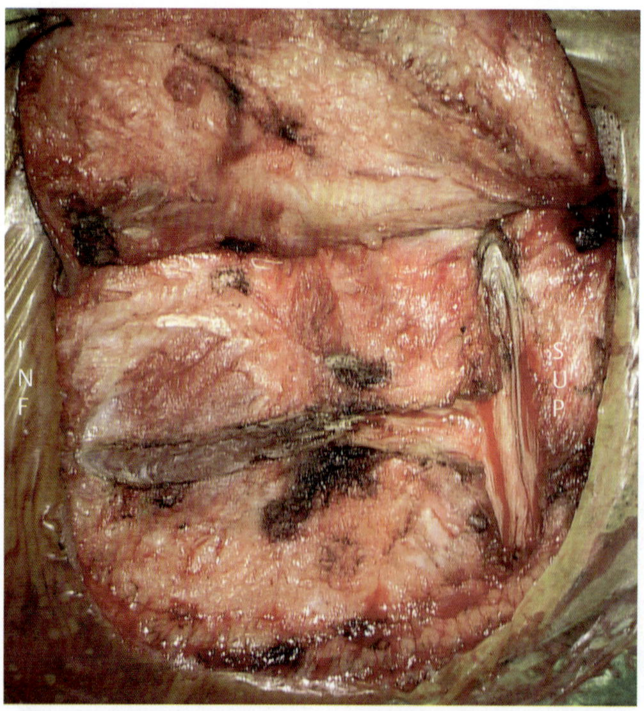

Fig. 48.4 T-shaped musculoperiosteal incision.

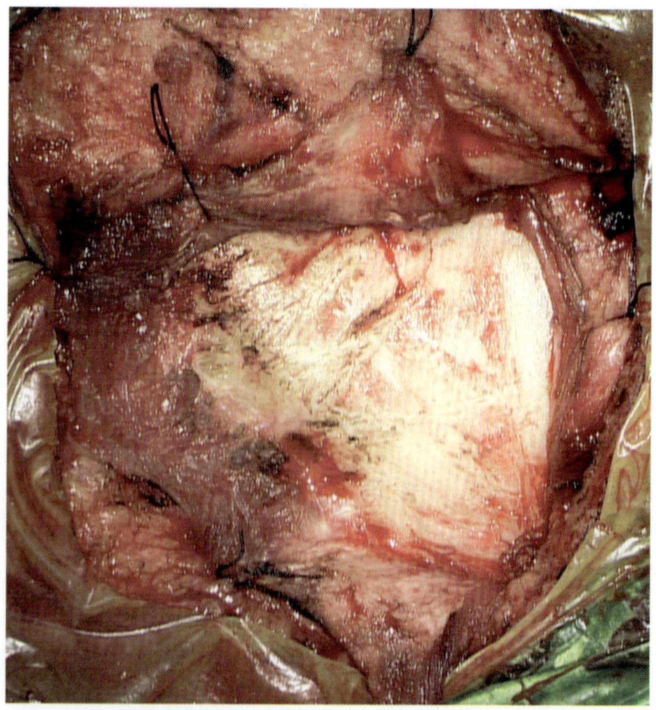

Fig. 48.5 Musculoperiosteal flaps reflected and sutured anteriorly, posteriorly, and superiorly to expose mastoid cortex.

4. A wide-based mastoidectomy is performed (**Fig. 48.6**). All the cells over the dural plate, sigmoid sinus, posterior canal wall, and mastoid tip are exenterated. Similarly, cells in the infralabyrinthine as also retrolabyrinthine areas are also exenterated. The antrum is opened, and the short process of the incus is visualized. Drilling is performed to expose about 2 cm of the retrosigmoid dura. Mastoid emissary vein in this area can be bipolarized and cut a little away from the sigmoid sinus.
5. The mastoidal segment of the facial nerve is skeletonized (**Fig. 48.7**). It is visible as an ivory white structure in the fallopian canal. It should not be decompressed. Identifying the level of the mastoidal segment of the fallopian canal helps in safe drilling in the area medial to it during exposure of the IAM.
6. A labyrinthectomy is performed next by successively drilling off the posterior, lateral, and superior semicircular canals (**Fig. 48.8**). Care is taken so that the burr doesn't slip and accidentally injure the second genu of the facial nerve. Just inferior and deep to the posterior semicircular canal is the endolymphatic duct (**Fig. 48.9**). It is important to preserve a thin shell of bone on the anterior lip of the superior and lateral semicircular canal ampullary end, so as to protect the labyrinthine and tympanic segments of the facial nerve from accidental trauma with the burr. The vestibule is opened widely and the neuroepithelium is removed (**Fig. 48.10**). The solid bone medial to the vestibule needs to be drilled to approach the IAM (**Fig. 48.11**).
7. The bone over the sigmoid sinus is thinned adequately and then taken off. In case of a forward lying sigmoid

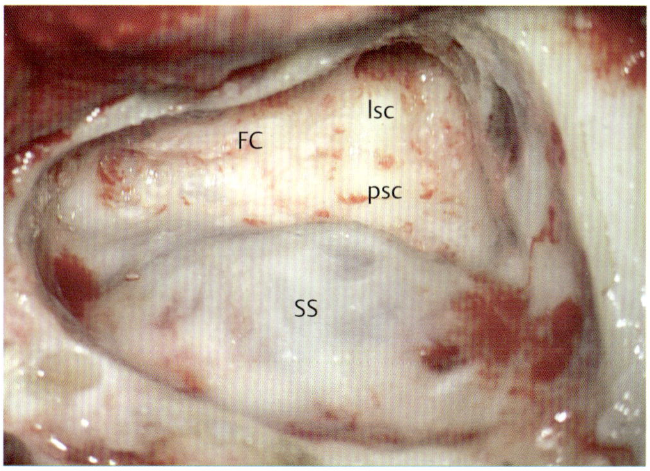

Fig. 48.6 Cortical mastoidectomy is performed.

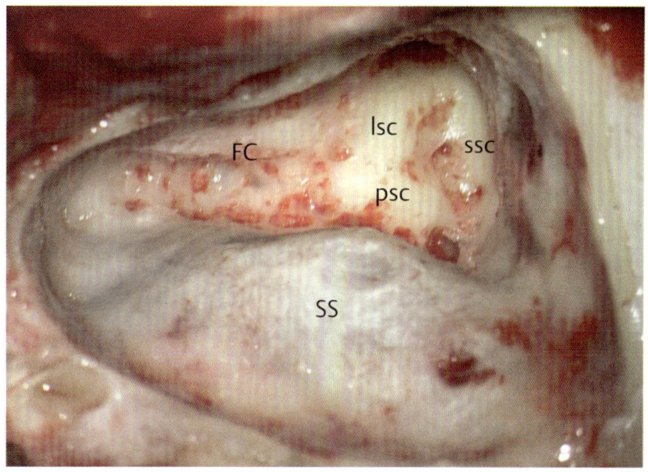

Fig. 48.7 Delineation of semicircular canals and fallopian canal (mastoidal segment).

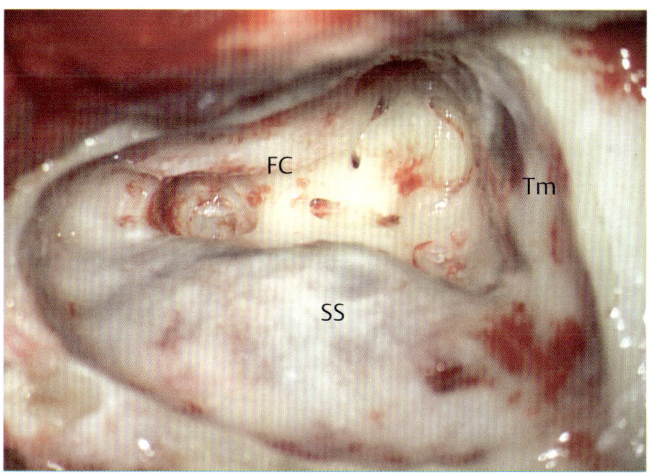

Fig. 48.8 Slits created in the semicircular canals.

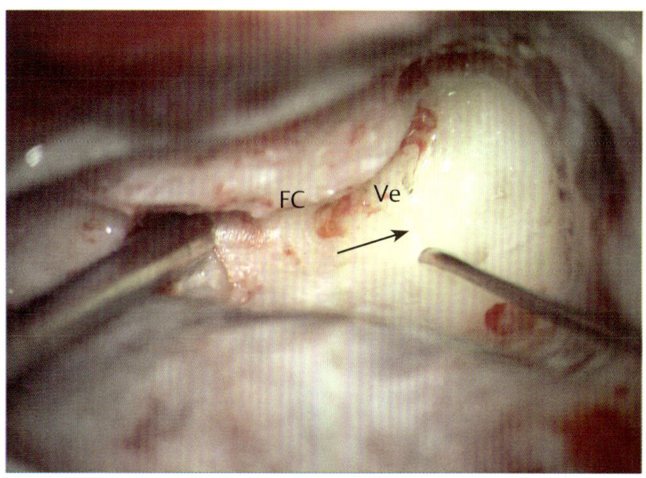

Fig. 48.9 Partial labyrinthectomy has been performed. The endolymphatic duct is seen deep to the posterior semicircular canal going toward the vestibule. *Black arrow* points to the endolymphatic duct.

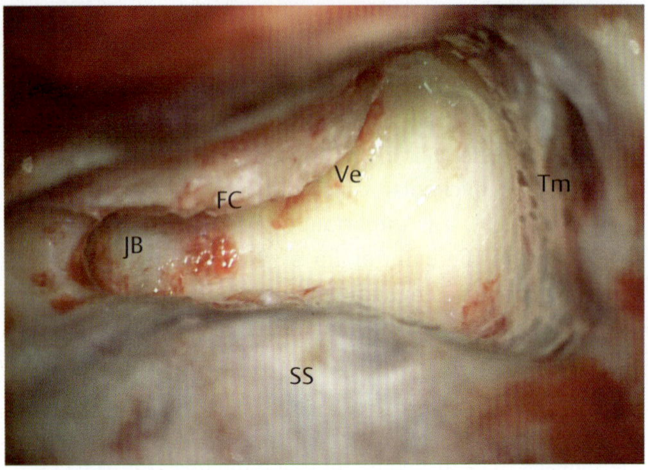

Fig. 48.10 Vestibule has been opened widely.

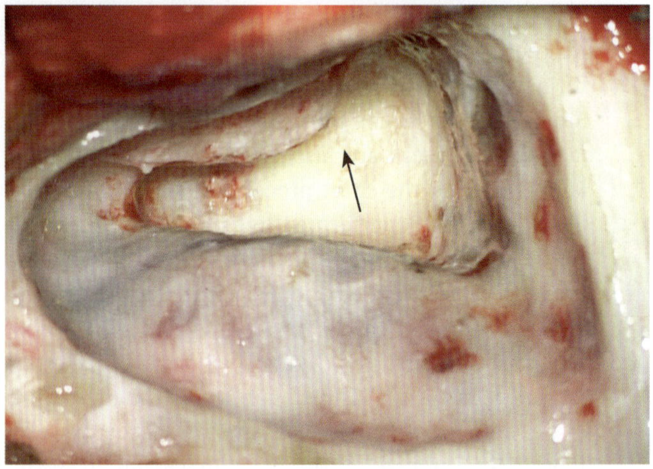

Fig. 48.11 Solid bone medial to the vestibule needs to be drilled to visualize the IAM. *Black arrow* points to the bone that needs to be drilled medial to the vestibule deeper to which lies the IAM.

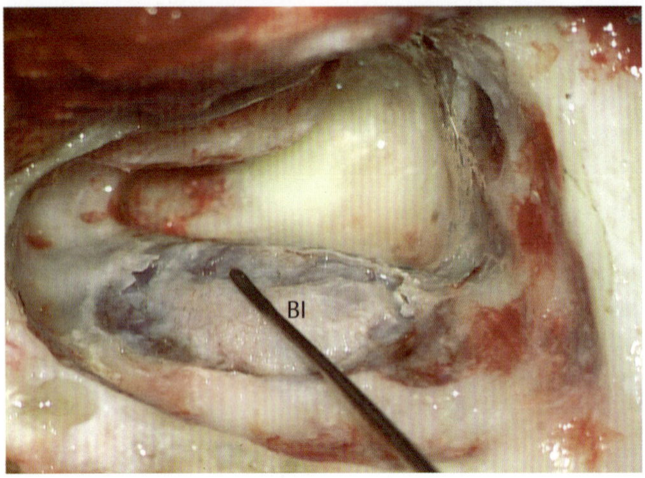

Fig. 48.12 Bill's island created and used to depress the sigmoid sinus so that more space is available for drilling toward the IAM.

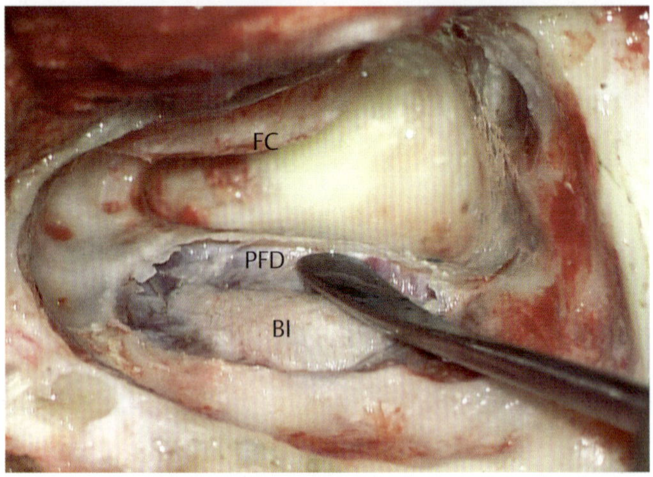

Fig. 48.13 The presigmoid posterior fossa dura is dissected off the overlying bone.

sinus, a thin island of bone is left over the area of maximum bulge of sigmoid while the rest of the sigmoid sinus is decompressed (**Fig. 48.12**). This island of bone is called Bill's island and is used to depress the sigmoid sinus while performing labyrinthectomy. Alternatively, the sigmoid sinus is decompressed completely and the bipolar is used on its surface causing the sigmoid sinus wall to shrink thereby decreasing the forward bulge of the sinus and enabling more space and better angulation for drilling the bone over the IAM.

8. To take off the bone over the presigmoid dura, the dura needs to be separated from the overlying thin bone before taking the bone off (**Fig. 48.13**). The thinned-out bone is then gently taken out (**Fig. 48.14**). The endolymphatic duct needs to be cut to release the tethering on the posterior fossa dura in that area. A coarse diamond burr is used to take off any remnant bone over the presigmoid posterior fossa dura (**Fig. 48.15**).
9. Bone over the middle fossa is also thinned out and gently lifted off the underlying dura to expose the middle fossa dura (**Fig. 48.16**).
10. Bone over the superior petrosal sinus is thinned and is taken off the sinus (**Fig. 48.17**). If bleeding occurs during this step, a bipolar is used. However, larger tears in the superior petrosal sinus necessitate the use of Surgicel to control the bleeding.
11. Drilling is performed medial to the vestibule. Care is taken not to dislocate the stapes footplate inadvertently since this can create a potential tract for cerebrospinal fluid escape postoperatively.

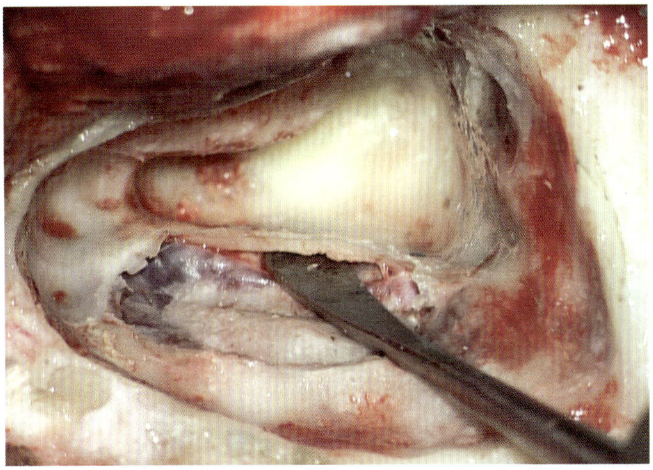

Fig. 48.14 The bone over the presigmoid posterior fossa dura is thinned and then shelled out.

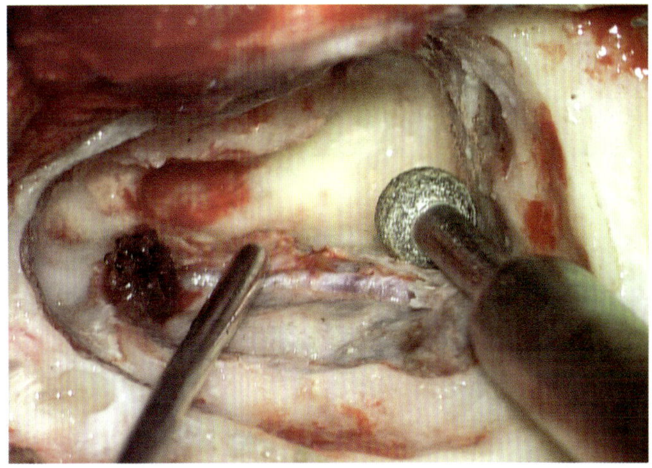

Fig. 48.15 A coarse diamond burr is used to drill off all the remnant bone over the posterior fossa dura.

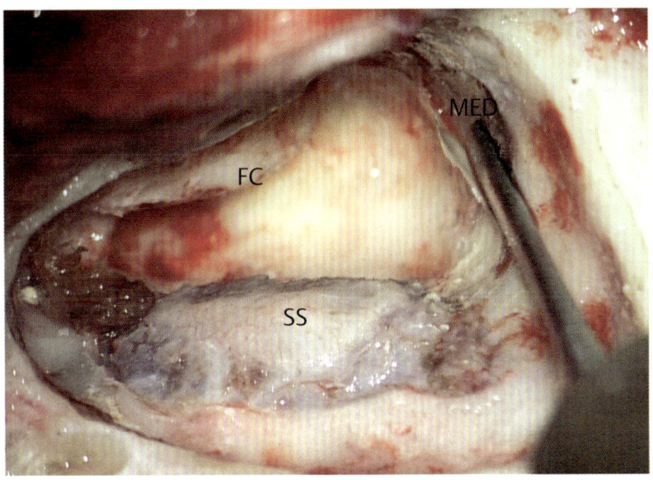

Fig. 48.16 Bone covering the middle fossa dura is thinned and then dissected off it.

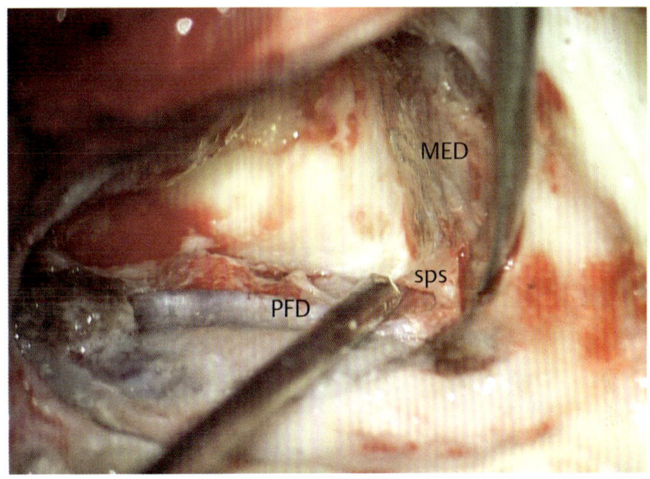

Fig. 48.17 Bone covering the superior petrosal sinus is thinned out and taken off it gently without injuring the superior petrosal sinus.

12. The bone over the IAM is ivory colored and solid. The IAM is along the same axis as that of the external auditory canal. The bone between the superior lip of IAM and the middle fossa dura contains cells. Drilling this trough helps to go around the IAM toward the area of the prepontine cistern (**Fig. 48.18**). Similarly, drilling in the trough between the inferior lip of IAM and the jugular bulb (**Fig. 48.19**) toward the petrous apex/prepontine cistern helps to gain circumferential exposure of the IAM and the anterior pole of the tumor. A 270-degree exposure around the IAM is routinely performed.
13. The middle fossa dura, the presigmoid posterior fossa dura, sigmoid sinus, and the retrosigmoid dura for about 2 cm are exposed. A circumferential control of the IAM is obtained and by drilling the superior and inferior troughs, authors gain control of the anterior pole of the tumor. This approach offers good control of the IAM and a maximally large exposure of all the poles of the tumor, and hence, was termed enlarged translabyrinthine approach. It may be extended anteriorly to 300 to 320 degrees, if required. This constitutes the transapical extension of the enlarged translabyrinthine approach described by Prof Mario Sanna.
14. In the case of a high jugular bulb, it is decompressed, a piece of Surgicel is placed on it and it is dissected and pushed inferiorly. It is held in place using bone wax.
15. The bone over the IAM is drilled parallel to its contents to make the bone eggshell thin **(Fig. 48.20**). The last shells of bone over the IAM are gently lifted off using

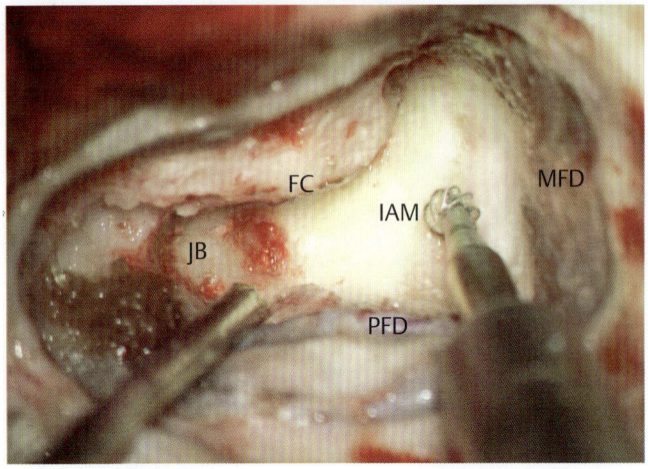

Fig. 48.18 Drilling in the superior trough between the superior lip of IAM and middle fossa dura.

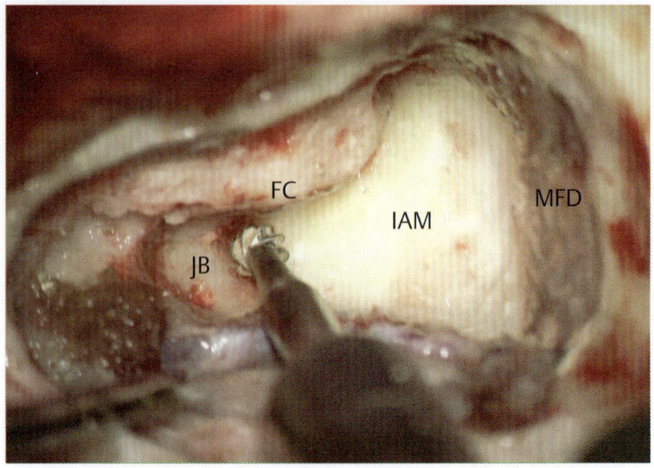

Fig. 48.19 Drilling in the inferior trough between the inferior lip of IAM and jugular bulb toward the petrous apex.

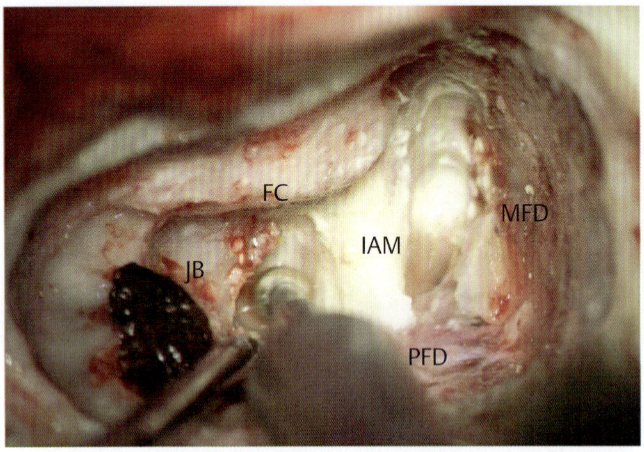

Fig. 48.20 Drilling about 270 degrees around the IAM. Lastly, bone over the IAM is drilled and thinned out.

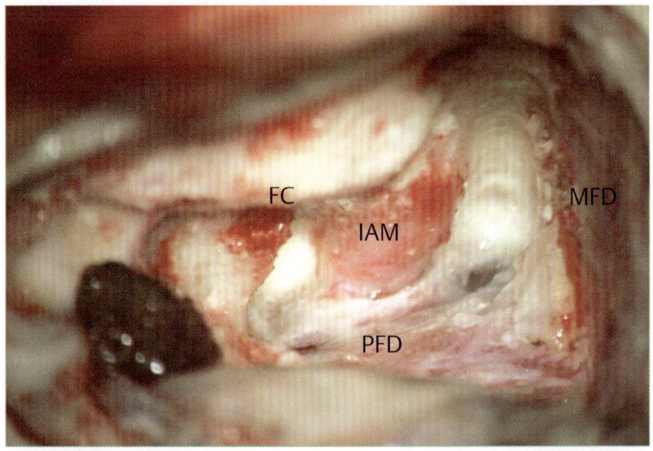

Fig. 48.21 Thin shells of bone over IAM are taken off to expose the dura covering IAM.

a raspatory. Usually tumor that has widened the IAM is immediately seen on exposing the IAM (**Fig. 48.21**).

16. Drilling is performed at the lateral end of IAM following the course of the superior and inferior vestibular nerve. Usually, a white dot called Mike's dot is seen along the lateral most end of the superior vestibular nerve. It marks the exit of the superior ampullary nerve from the superior vestibular nerve, and it innervates the ampullary end of the superior semicircular canal. A vertical crest of bone called Bill's bar separates the superior vestibular nerve from the facial nerve (**Fig. 48.22**). The facial nerve lies anteriorly and superiorly in the IAM while the cochlear nerve lies anteriorly and inferiorly. The tumor that arises from the inferior or superior vestibular nerve usually faces us in this approach with the facial and cochlear nerves lying deep to it. In our series, tumor has been found to arise most commonly from the inferior vestibular nerve. A horizontal crest of bone is seen to separate the superior and inferior vestibular nerves (**Fig. 48.23**).
17. A dural incision is taken in the presigmoid posterior fossa dura parallel to the superior petrosal sinus (**Fig. 48.24**), then circumferentially around the porus (medial end) of the IAM and then superior to the jugular bulb (**Fig. 48.25**). The dura of the IAM is incised open closer to the inferior margin of the IAM and parallel to its contents. This prevents accidental injury to the facial nerve lying along the superior margin in the IAM.
18. The superior ampullary nerve is hooked and reflected medially (**Fig. 48.26**). It immediately exposes Bill's bar more prominently with the facial nerve anterior to it (**Fig. 48.27**). The advantage of this approach is, thus, early identification of the facial nerve at the lateral

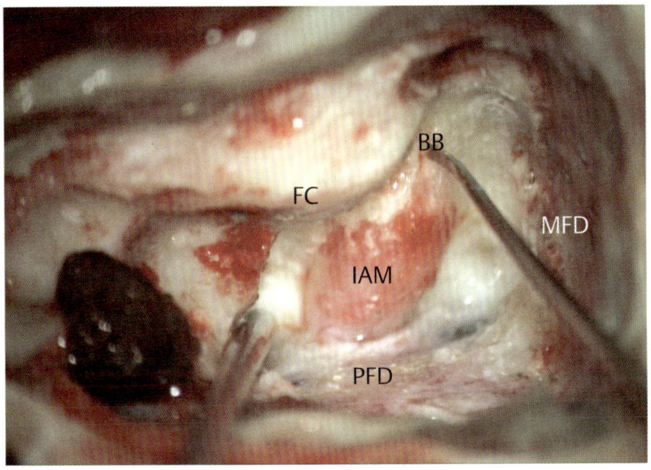

Fig. 48.22 Bill's bar separating the superior vestibular nerve from the facial nerve.

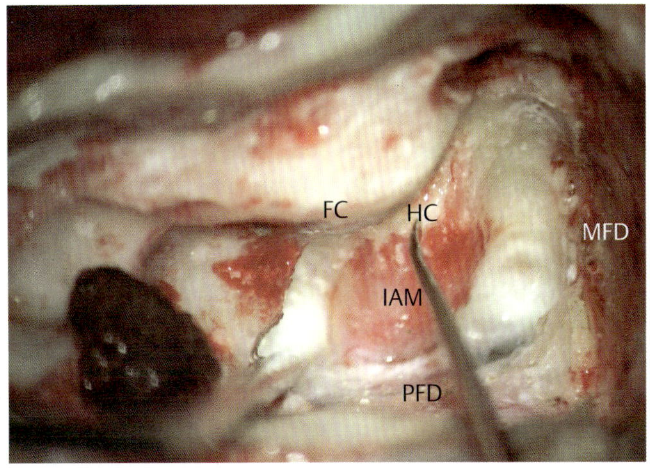

Fig. 48.23 Horizontal crest separating superior and inferior vestibular nerves.

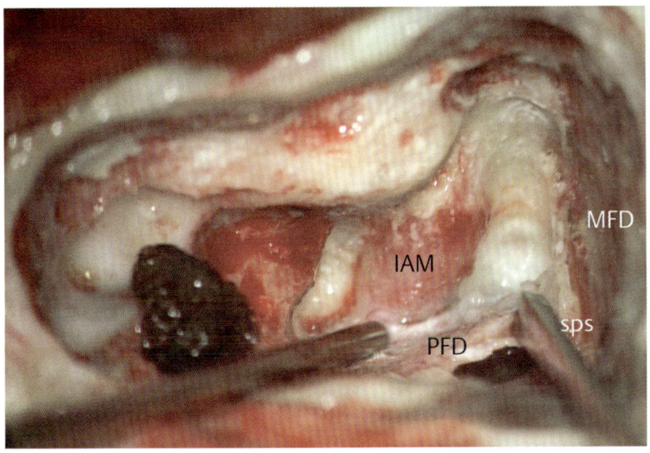

Fig. 48.24 Dural incision parallel to the superior petrosal sinus.

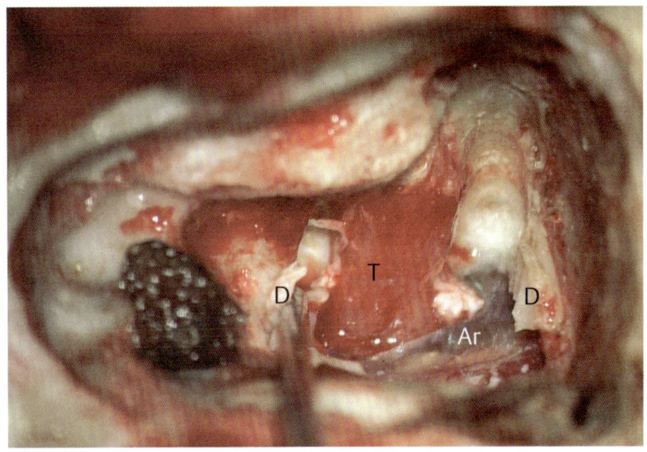

Fig. 48.25 Dura of IAM is incised along its length and reflected superiorly and inferiorly.

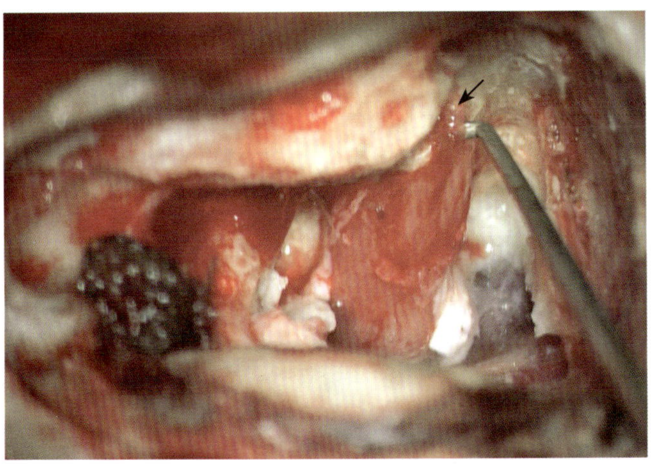

Fig. 48.26 Superior ampullary nerve is hooked and reflected medially (*black arrow*).

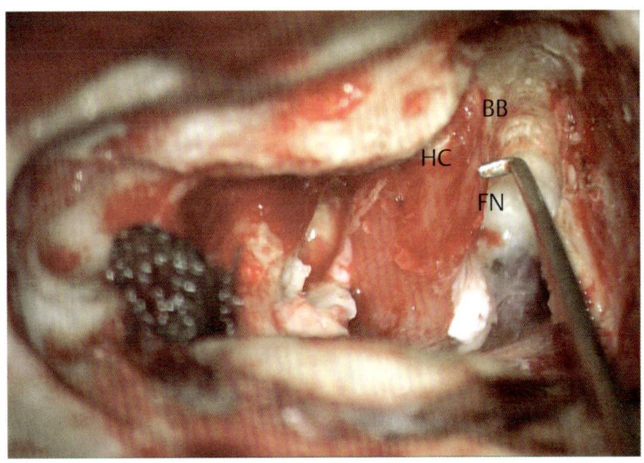

Fig. 48.27 Identification of facial nerve anterior to superior vestibular nerve (confirmed with facial nerve stimulator).

end of IAM. Similarly, the inferior vestibular nerve is reflected to expose the cochlear nerve (**Fig. 48.28**). The superior and inferior vestibular nerves are reflected toward the medial end of IAM preserving the facial and cochlear nerves. At the porus, the large cerebellopontine angle component of the tumor is seen.

19. The capsule of the vestibular schwannoma is bipolarized, opened, and sufficient internal debulking of the tumor is carried out. A CUSA is useful for this (**Fig. 48.29**).
20. The capsule of the tumor is grasped and the arachnoid is gently stripped off from the tumor capsule (**Fig. 48.30**). Preserving the arachnoid–tumor capsule plane helps preserve the medial end of the facial nerve in the cerebellopontine angle. Wherever the cleavage plane is obtained, Gelfoam is placed in the plane to prevent blood from entering the cerebellopontine angle.
21. The capsule of the tumor is gently lifted off the petrous ridge (**Fig. 48.31**) and brainstem without undue traction (**Fig. 48.32**).
22. Complete tumor excision is achieved preserving the facial (**Fig 48.33**) and cochlear nerves. In a few cases, where the tumor capsule is adherent to the facial nerve, it is prudent to leave a small capsule over the facial nerve, thereby achieving subtotal resection. Arachnoid preservation helps in the protection of critical areas.
23. Warm saline irrigations are used over patties to achieve good hemostasis.
24. Fat is harvested from the abdomen or thigh.
25. A piece of fat is used to snugly block the antrum (**Fig. 48.34**). The bone chip or bone wax is placed over it. Strips of fat are used to obliterate the cerebellopontine angle (**Fig. 48.35**). They are placed partly intradural and partly extradural. Care is taken when placing it to see that these fat strips do not prolapse completely in the cerebellopontine angle.
26. The musculoperiosteal layer is sutured in an airtight fashion.
27. Subcutaneous layer and skin are sutured separately.

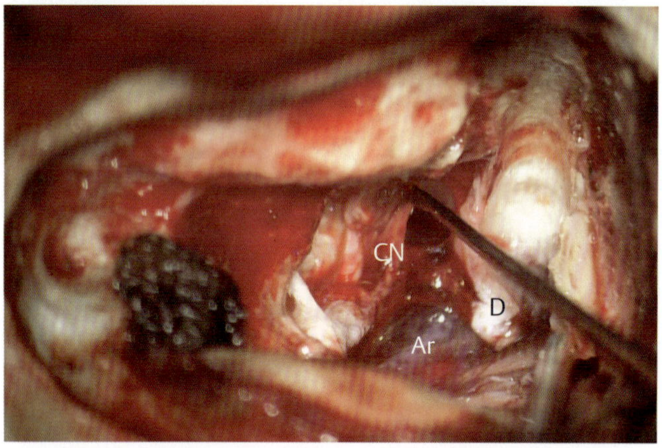

Fig. 48.28 Cochlear nerve is seen (tumor excised).

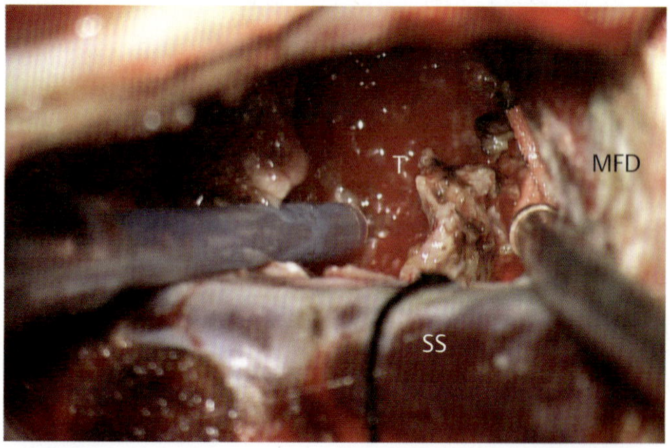

Fig. 48.29 Internal debulking of the tumor using CUSA.

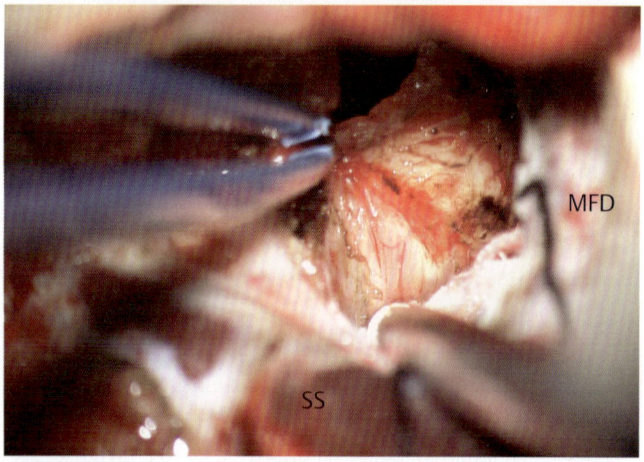

Fig. 48.30 Capsule of the tumor is grasped and the arachnoid dissected off it.

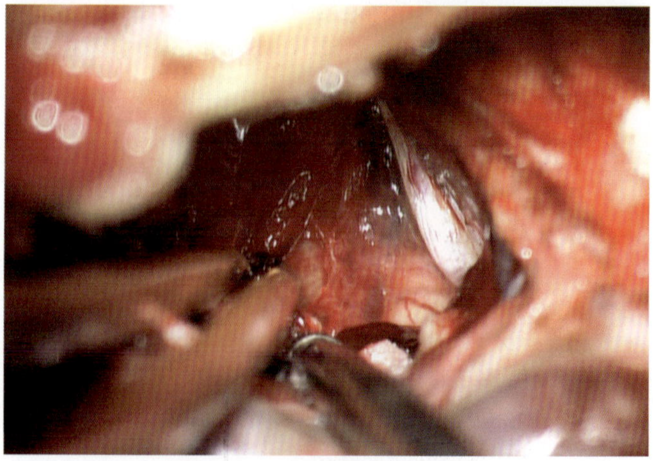

Fig. 48.31 Tumor has been dissected off the petrous ridge and tentorium (large tumor).

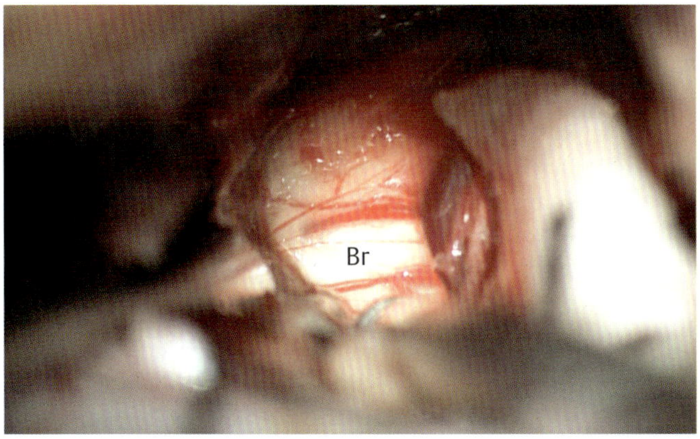

Fig. 48.32 Tumor has been dissected gently off the brainstem.

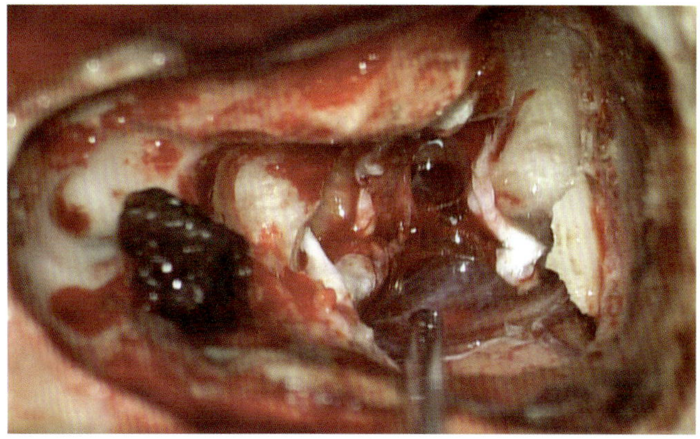

Fig. 48.33 Arachnoid plane is preserved.

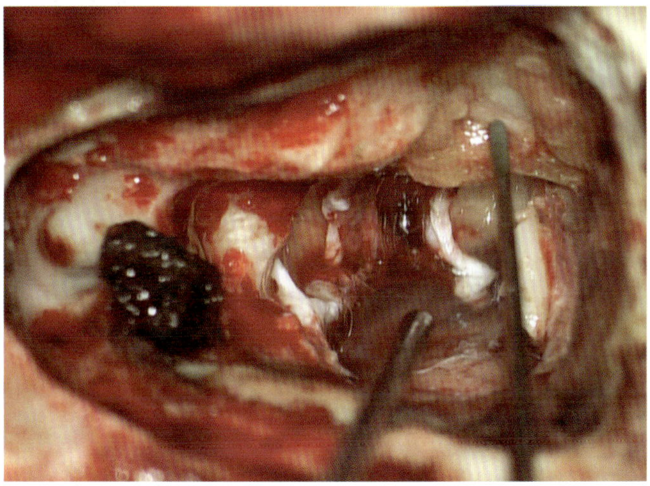

Fig. 48.34 Fat plug is used to seal the aditus to antrum. Bone chip and glue are used over it.

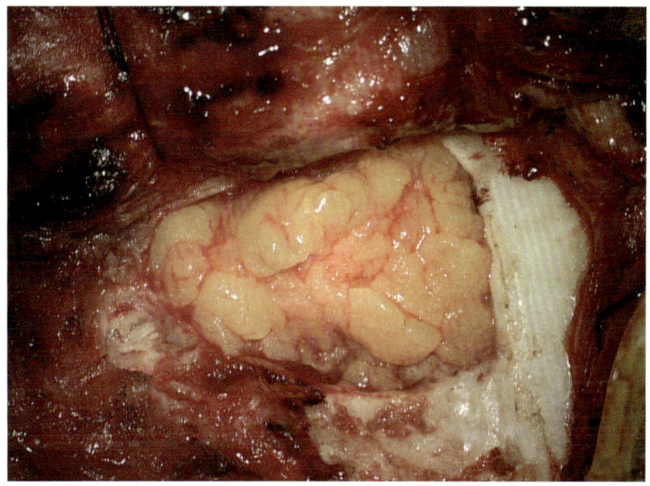

Fig. 48.35 Fat strips are used to seal the cavity.

Tips and Pearls

1. Bleeding from the sigmoid sinus or jugular bulb can occur sometimes. A suction is kept over the site of the tear so that blood does not flood the operative field and a strip of Surgicel is placed within the defect, half inside and half outside. Care is taken to see that the Surgicel does not embolize. A cotton patty is then placed over the Surgicel with gentle pressure and the patty is left in place for a few minutes for the bleeding to settle down.
2. Cystic tumors are adherent to the surrounding nerves and brainstem and are hence difficult to dissect off these structures. In such cases, it may be safer to leave the capsule attached to the facial nerve or brainstem.
3. Care is taken not to exert traction over the inferior pole of the tumor which could potentially injure the lower cranial nerves.
4. In the case of neurofibromatosis type 2 subjects with bilateral vestibular schwannomas, a cochlear implant or brainstem implant is to be considered at the same sitting as the primary surgery for the tumor.

Suggested Readings

Angeli RD, Piccirillo E, Di Trapani G, Sequino G, Taibah A, Sanna M. Enlarged translabyrinthine approach with transapical extension in the management of giant vestibular schwannomas: personal experience and review of literature. Otol Neurotol 2011;32(1):125–131

Ben Ammar M, Piccirillo E, Topsakal V, Taibah A, Sanna M. Surgical results and technical refinements in translabyrinthine excision of vestibular schwannomas: the Gruppo Otologico experience. Neurosurg 2012;70(6):1481–1491

Brackmann DE, Green JD Jr. Translabyrinthine approach for acoustic tumor removal. 1992. Neurosurg Clin N Am 2008;19(2):251–264, vi

Fagan PA, Sheehy JP, Chang P, Doust BD, Coakley D, Atlas MD. The cerebellopontine angle: does the translabyrinthine approach give adequate access? Laryngoscope 1998;108(5):679–682

Jayashankar N, Morwani KP, Sankhla SK, Agrawal R. The enlarged translabyrinthine and transapical extension type I approach for large vestibular schwannomas. Indian J Otolaryngol Head Neck Surg 2010;62(4):360–364

Lanman TH, Brackmann DE, Hitselberger WE, Subin B. Report of 190 consecutive cases of large acoustic tumors (vestibular schwannoma) removed via the translabyrinthine approach. J Neurosurg 1999;90(4):617–623

Mamikoglu B, Wiet RJ, Esquivel CR. Translabyrinthine approach for the management of large and giant vestibular schwannomas. Otol Neurotol 2002;23(2):224–227

Naguib MB, Saleh E, Cokkeser Y, et al. The enlarged translabyrinthine approach for removal of large vestibular schwannomas. J Laryngol Otol 1994;108(7):545–550

Sanna M, Russo A, Taibah A, Falcioni M, Agarwal M. Enlarged translabyrinthine approach for the management of large and giant acoustic neuromas: a report of 175 consecutive cases. Ann Otol Rhinol Laryngol 2004;113(4):319–328

Springborg JB, Fugleholm K, Poulsgaard L, Cayé-Thomasen P, Thomsen J, Stangerup SE. Outcome after translabyrinthine surgery for vestibular schwannomas: report on 1244 patients. J Neurol Surg B Skull Base 2012;73(3):168–174

Chapter 49 Translabyrinthine Approach for the Resection of a Large Vestibular Schwannoma

Adzreil Bakri, Michel Roethlisberger, Prepageran Narayanan, and Vicknes Waran

History

A 60-year-old gentleman presented with progressive left-sided hearing loss and giddiness for the last 3 months. On clinical examination, the external and middle ears were normal; however, a pure tone audiogram revealed severe to profound sensorineural hearing loss of the left ear with normal hearing on the right side. A gadolinium-enhanced magnetic resonance imaging (MRI) revealed a large vestibular schwannoma of the left cerebellopontine angle (CPA) with intracanalicular extension and evident brainstem compression (Koos Grade IV) (**Fig. 49.1**). Because of the large size of the tumor and the loss of serviceable hearing, a translabyrinthine approach was selected to provide good access and exposure to the internal acoustic meatus and CPA.

Surgical Steps

1. After general anesthesia, patients are placed in a supine position with the head rotated contralaterally, and lateroflexed downward to facilitate exposure of the inferior tentorial surface.

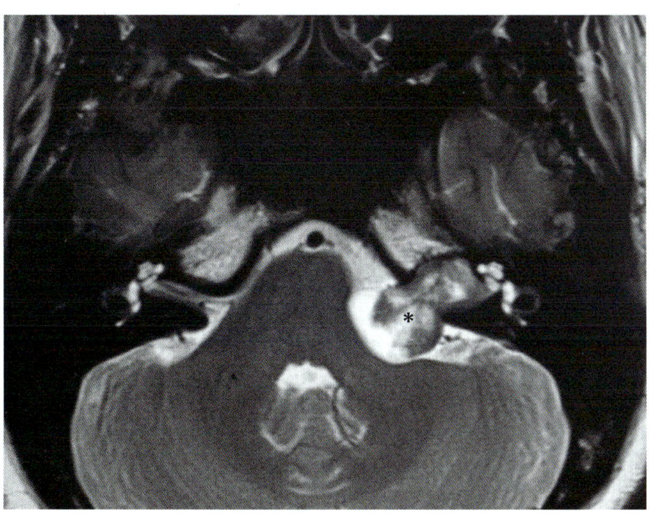

Fig. 49.1 Axial T2-weighted MRI section demonstrating a large tumor (*) at the cerebellopontine angle compressing the brainstem with relevant intracanalicular extension.

2. The patient is supported with the aid of sandbags underneath the ipsilateral shoulder and thorax.
3. The patient's head is fixed using a Mayfield clamp (**Fig. 67.1**).
4. Registration for image-guided surgery (Brainlab, Munich, Germany) follows.
5. The use of muscle relaxants should be limited to the induction phase only to allow intraoperative facial nerve monitoring.
6. Intraoperative neuromonitoring of the cranial nerves is installed by standard means described in the literature V, VI, VII, IX, X, XI, XII, acoustic evoked potentials [AEPs], motor evoked potentials [MEPs], sensory evoked potentials [SEPs]) (**Fig. 67.1**).
7. The abdomen is also prepared and draped for fat graft harvesting.
8. Head positioning should allow for the region superior to the pinna and the mastoid to be horizontal and the highest point in the surgical field. A local anesthetic with adrenaline is infiltrated along a large C-shaped incision behind the ear. This incision is approximately 4 cm posterior to the standard postauricular incision and it extends from the mastoid tip to about 2 cm above the root of the helix. This big incision facilitates adequate exposure of the sigmoid sinus and the retrosigmoid dura (**Fig. 55.1**).
9. A skin and soft tissue flap are elevated in a plane above the temporalis fascia superiorly and mastoid musculoperiosteum inferiorly. This flap is lifted anteriorly to the margins of the external ear canal.
10. Then the musculoperiosteal flap is raised from the underlying bone in a similar manner as the skin flap and is anchored anteriorly. Once the flaps are raised, two self-retaining retractors are inserted with a 90 degree angle.
11. A wide cortical mastoidectomy is performed using a combination of cutting and diamond drill burrs together with suction irrigation. This initial drilling aims to identify the middle fossa dura, sigmoid sinus, posterior fossa dura, and digastric ridge. The mastoid bowl is further drilled down to expose the mastoid antrum, lateral semicircular canal, and the long

process of incus (**Fig. 49.2**). At this point, an operating microscope is needed for optimal visualization.

12. The interlabyrinthine, retrolabyrinthine, and retrofacial air cells are all exenterated (**Fig. 49.3**). The facial canal containing the second genu and the mastoid part of the facial nerve is drilled down so that only a slight bony covering is seen lateral to the nerve.
13. The sigmoid sinus is skeletonized completely as to later facilitate mobilization of the sinus and optimize exposure of the presigmoid window. To achieve this, at least a 2-cm exposure posterior to the sigmoid sinus over the retrosigmoid and posterior fossa dura is required. Dissection near the sigmoid sinus is done with care and the remaining thin bony coverage is removed using a blunt dissector or diamond burr. Bleeding from the dural sinus can be controlled with bipolar diathermy or hemostyptic agents.
14. The middle fossa dura is also exposed up to 2 cm superiorly to facilitate drilling and wide exposure to the CPA. Bone over the middle and posterior fossa dura is thinned down gently using a cutting burr before removed using a blunt dissector or diamond burr (**Fig. 49.4**). Small bleeding areas from the dura can be controlled with bipolar diathermy or hemostatic agents such as Surgicel.
15. Once a wide exposure or extended cortical mastoidectomy has been achieved, a labyrinthectomy is then performed. Each semicircular canal is drilled and exenterated separately, and the drilling movement is parallel to each of the canal (**Fig. 49.5, Fig. 49.6,** and **Fig. 49.7**). The ampulla of the superior semicircular canal marks the superior limit of the internal auditory canal (IAC), and the ampulla of the posterior semicircular canal marks the inferior limit (**Fig. 49.8**). Care is taken around the anterior part of the lateral semicircular canal as it is in close proximity to the second genu of the facial nerve.
16. Posteriorly, the drilling of the posterior semicircular canal and common crus will lead toward the endolymphatic duct and sac. These structures are decompressed to facilitate exposure of the posterior fossa dura (**Fig. 49.6**).

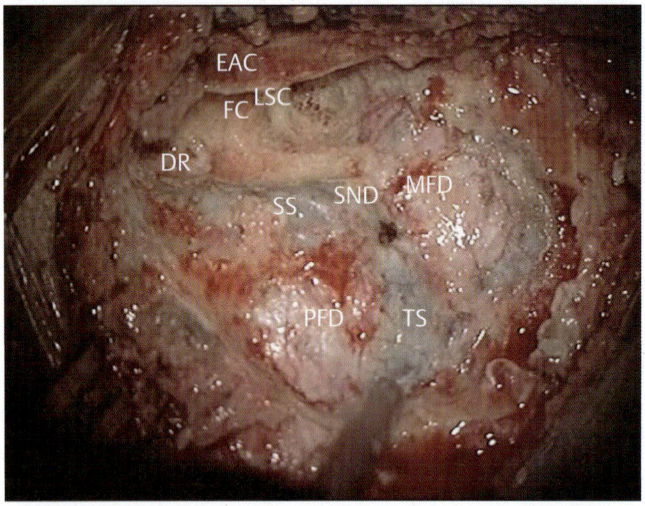

Fig. 49.2 View after an extended cortical mastoidectomy.

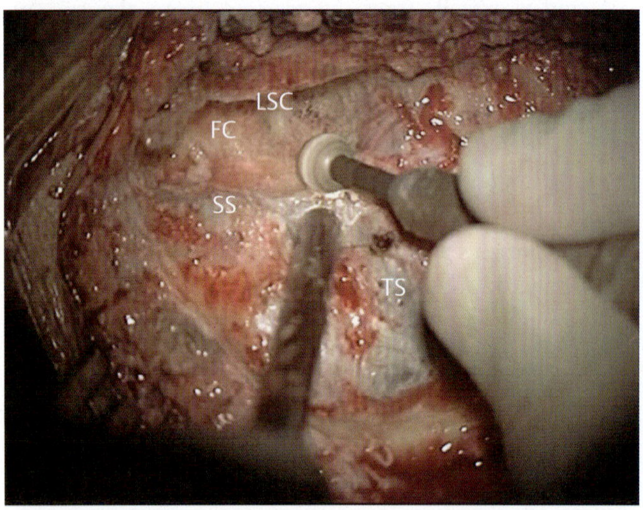

Fig. 49.3 Drilling of retrofacial and retrolabyrinthine air cells and decompressing the sigmoid sinus anteriorly.

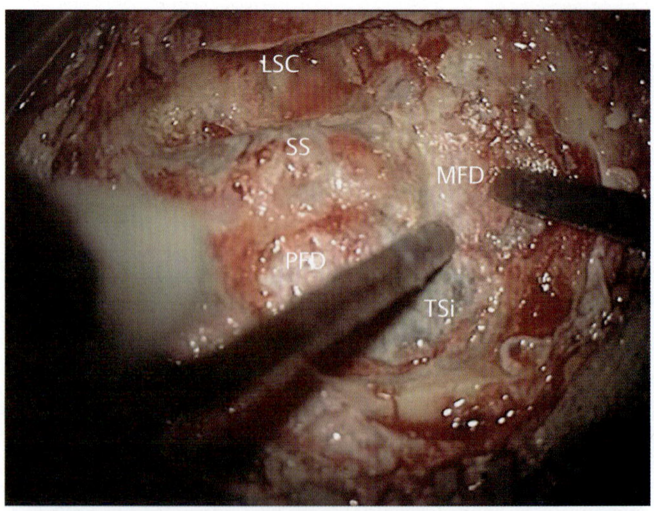

Fig. 49.4 A thin bony layer covering the middle fossa dura is removed with a blunt elevator after the bone was thinned down with a cutting and diamond drill. A similar technique can be used for decompressing the sigmoid sinus, sinodural angle, transverse sinus, and posterior fossa dura.

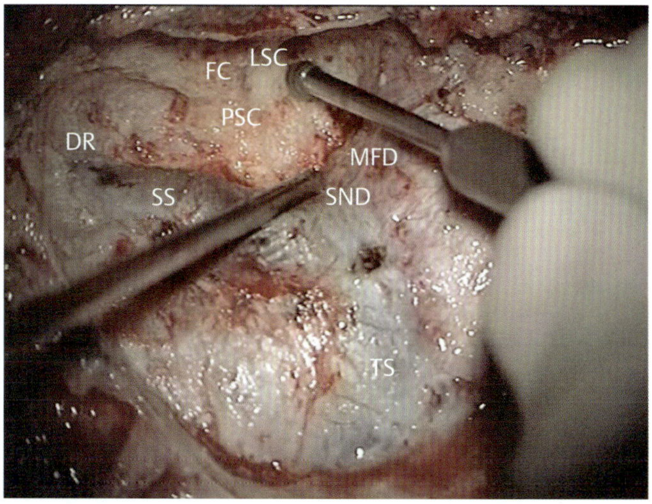

Fig. 49.5 Drilling of the lateral semicircular canal.

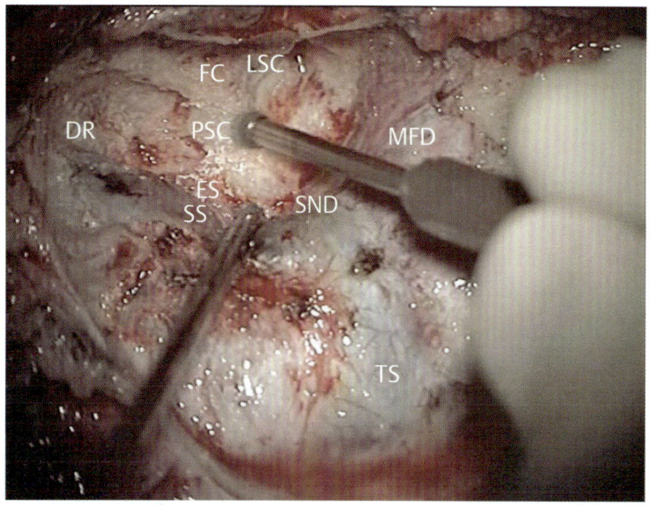

Fig. 49.6 Drilling of the posterior semicircular canal with the endolympthatic sac in view.

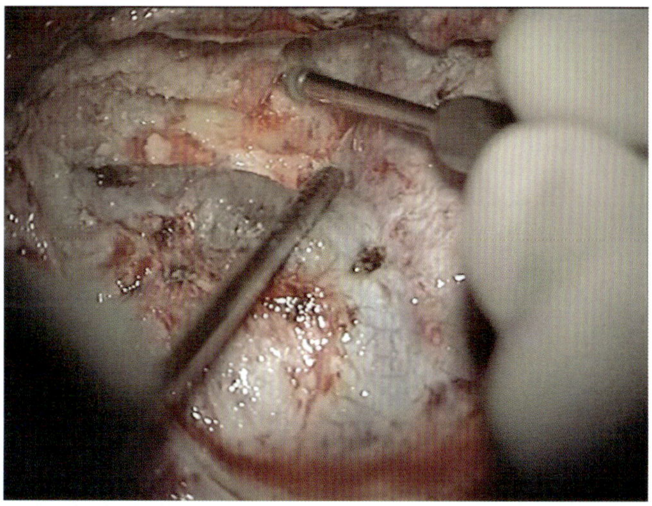

Fig. 49.7 Drilling of the superior semicircular canal.

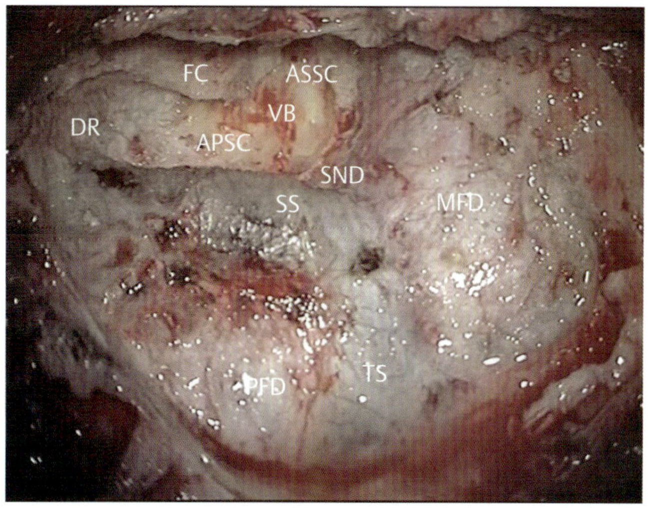

Fig. 49.8 View during labyrinthectomy.

17. Sequential drilling of the semicircular canals will eventually open into the vestibule (**Fig. 49.8**). This maneuver is performed in a wide fashion to facilitate dissection of the IAC fundus in a later stage.
18. The medial wall of the remaining bony vestibule is drilled from the middle fossa dura superiorly down to the jugular bulb inferiorly (**Fig. 49.9**). The bony IAC is exposed and decompressed 270 degrees leaving only the anterior wall intact. The jugular bulb marks the inferior limit of the IAC, the ampulla of the superior semicircular canal marks the superior limit, and the posterior fossa dura near the porus acusticus marks the posterior limit (**Fig. 49.10** and **Fig. 49.11**).
19. In this case, a relevant intracanalicular tumor extension is present up to the fundus, and the tumor is encountered immediately after decompressing the bony IAC at the porus acusticus (**Fig. 49.12**). Semicircular opening of the posterior fossa dura reflected anteriorly toward the tumor, exposes the cisternal part of the tumor within the cerebellopontine angle.

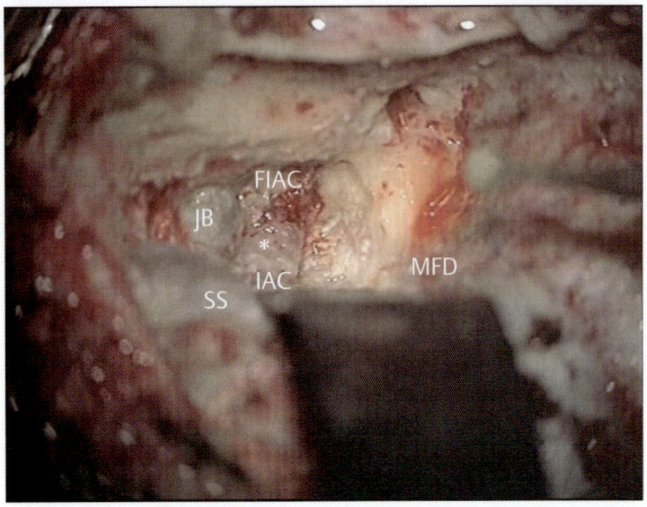

Fig. 49.9 Exposure of the IAC containing the intracanalicular tumor (*asterisk*) around the fundus of the IAC (FIAC). The sigmoid sinus is retracted posteriorly.

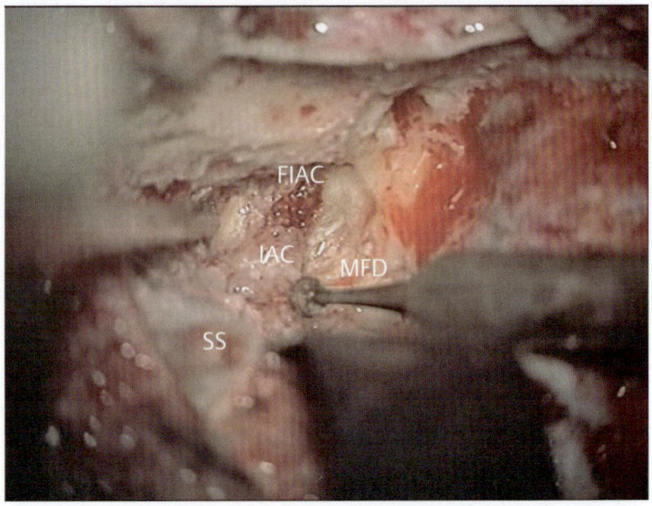

Fig. 49.10 Further exposure of the IAC superiorly, inferiorly, and at the porus acusticus. The jugular bulb is pushed inferiorly with a suction probe and the sigmoid sinus retracted posteriorly.

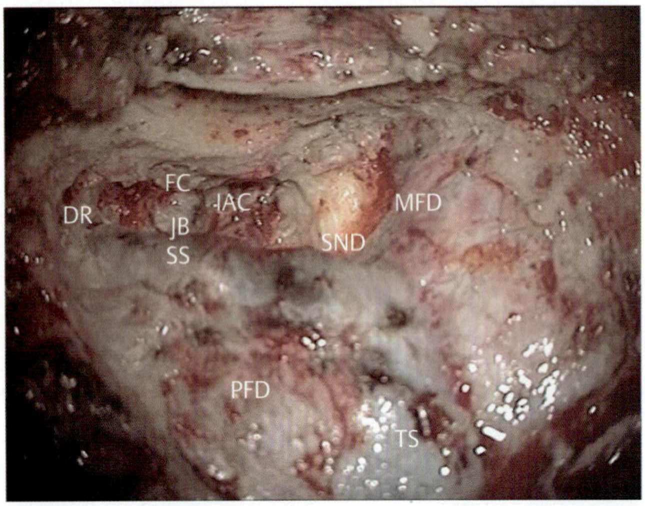

Fig. 49.11 View of the IAC and tumor after 270 degrees exposure without retraction of the jugular bulb and sigmoid sinus.

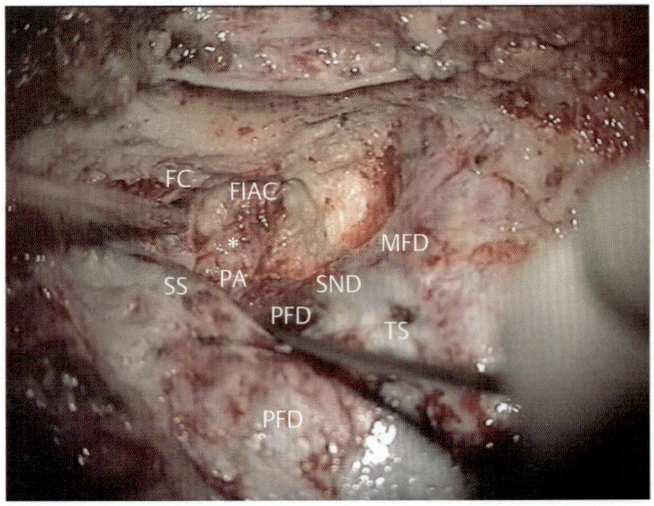

Fig. 49.12 View of the IAC and tumor after 270 degrees exposure with retraction of the jugular bulb and sigmoid sinus. Tumor in IAC (*asterisk*).

Section XIX

Approaches Through the Otic Capsule

Chapter 50 Modified Transcochlear Approach Type A

Narayan Jayashankar and K.P. Morwani

Indications

1. Extensive petrous apex cholesteatomas.
2. Extensive facial nerve schwannomas with the erosion of cochlea or labyrinth.
3. Clival chordomas and chondrosarcomas with the involvement of petrous apex.
4. Petroclival meningiomas.

Surgical Steps

Figs. 50.1 and 50.2 demonstrate CT and MRI scan showing lesions' involvement at different positions.

1. A postauricular incision is taken, starting 2 cm superior to the helix and coursing 3–4 cm behind the postaural groove till the mastoid tip. Incision includes the skin and subcutaneous tissue (**Figs. 50.3** and **50.4**).

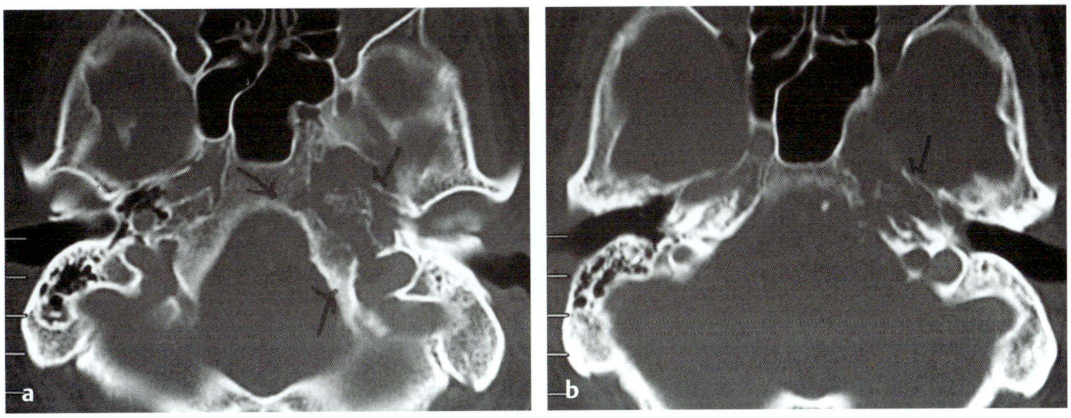

Fig. 50.1 (a, b) CT scan showing the lesion involving the left petrous apex, petroclival suture, and clivus, and involvement of the vertical infratubal and petrous segments of the internal carotid artery.

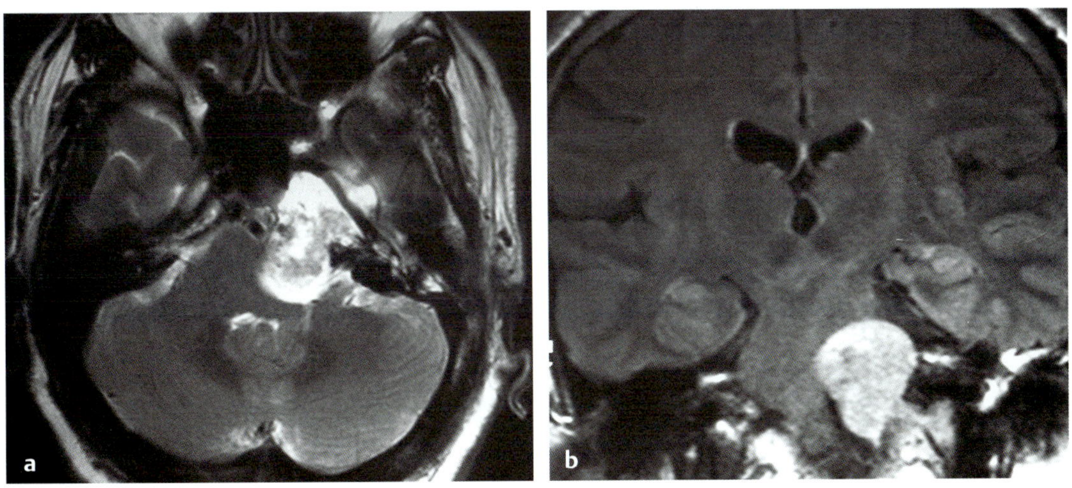

Fig. 50.2 (a, b) MRI scans showing lesion involving the petrous apex, petroclival suture and clivus, and involvement of vertical infratubal and petrous segments of the internal carotid artery. Lesion abuts the pons. It is heterogeneously hyperintense on T2W images and hypointense on T1W images.

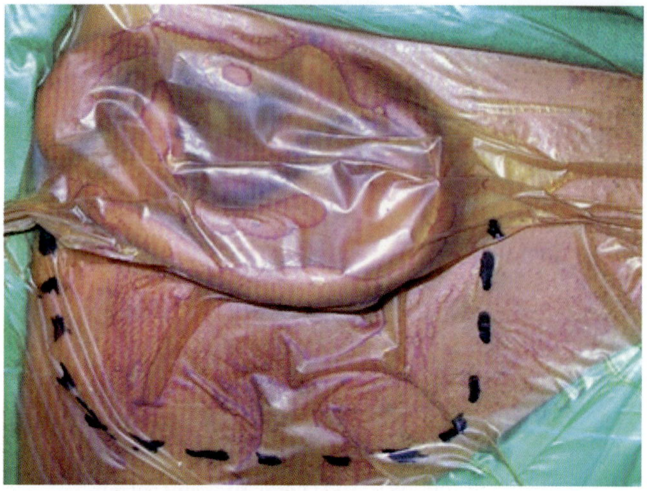

Fig. 50.3 Skin incision—left side.

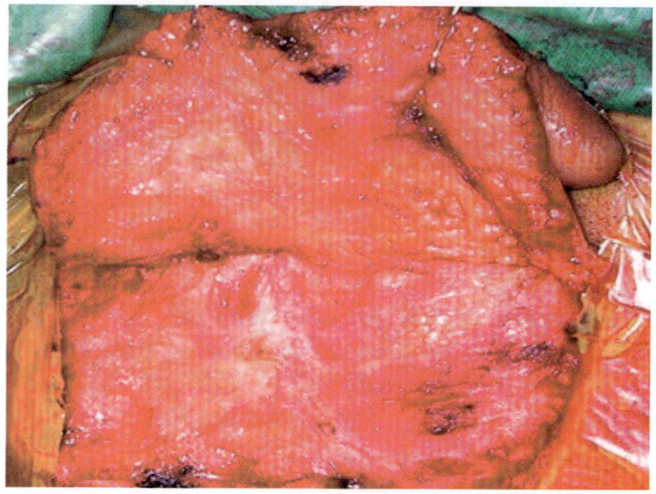

Fig. 50.4 Skin and subcutaneous tissue flap.

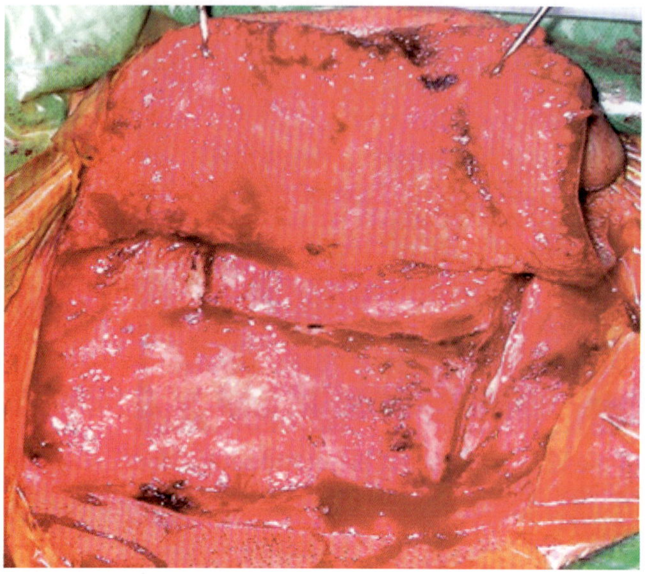

Fig. 50.5 Musculoperiosteal incisions for second layer of cul-de-sac closure of the external auditory canal.

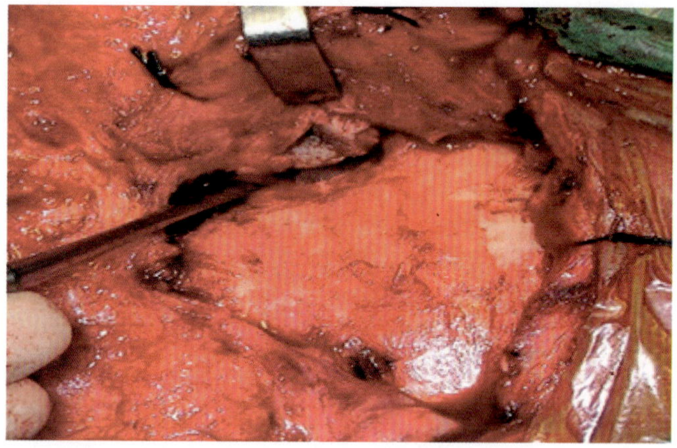

Fig. 50.6 Exposure of the mastoid cortex. Transection of the external auditory canal at the level of the spine of Henle.

2. A rectangular musculoperiosteal flap is created by incising superior, posterior, and inferiorly around the external auditory canal so that the flap is based anteriorly (**Fig. 50.5**). It is then elevated until the external auditory canal. This forms the second layer of cul-de-sac closure of the external auditory canal, as described in detail in infratemporal fossa A approach.
3. The mastoid cortex is exposed by reflecting the remaining musculoperiosteal flap posteroinferiorly. The external auditory canal is transected all around its circumference at the level of the spine of Henle (**Fig. 50.6**).
4. The skin lining the lateral part of the excised external auditory canal is separated from the cartilage to form a tube of skin. This is then everted through the external ear and sutured. It forms the first layer of cul-de-sac closure of the external auditory canal (**Fig. 50.7**).

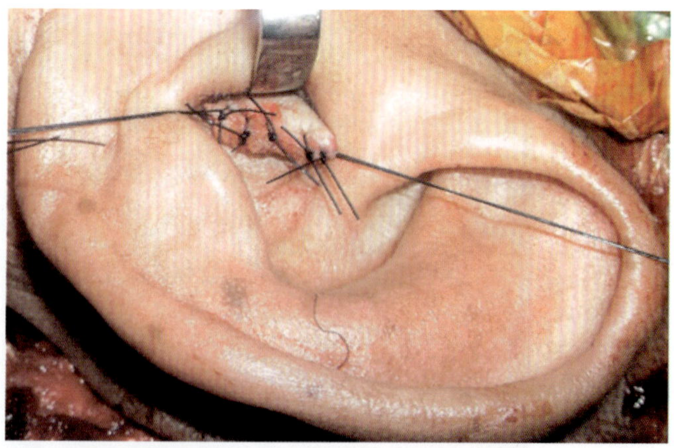

Fig. 50.7 Cul-de-sac closure of the external auditory canal.

5. The anteriorly based musculoperiosteal flap, created earlier, is then sutured to the soft tissues at the anterior canal wall. This forms the second layer of cul-de-sac closure of the external auditory canal.
6. The skin lining the medial part of the external auditory canal, along with the tympanic membrane, malleus, and incus, is excised.
7. An extended canal wall down mastoidectomy is performed. Bone removal extends for approximately 2 cm in the retrosigmoid area. The middle fossa dural plate is thinned. The superior and posterior bony external auditory canal walls are drilled out till the level of the fallopian canal. The semicircular canals are delineated. Cells are removed from the retrofacial cell area to delineate the jugular bulb. A thin shell of bone is left over the jugular bulb area to protect it during further drilling (**Fig. 50.8** and **Fig. 50.9**).
8. The facial nerve is skeletonized from the stylomastoid foramen till the geniculate ganglion, leaving an eggshell-thin bone over it. Drilling in an anteromedial direction from the geniculate ganglion exposes the greater superficial petrosal nerve adjacent to the middle fossa dura (**Fig. 50.10**).
9. Labyrinthectomy is begun by drilling the posterior, lateral, and superior semicircular canals. Utmost care is taken to prevent slippage of the burr while drilling the lateral semicircular canal, with resultant injury to the second genu of the facial nerve (**Fig. 50.11**).
10. A translabyrinthine approach is performed as described in the corresponding chapter. The sigmoid sinus and the pre- and retrosigmoid posterior fossa dura are exposed. Similarly, the tegmen mastoidale is drilled to expose the middle fossa dura deep into it. The internal auditory meatus dura is exposed in 180 to 270 degrees (**Fig. 50.12** and **Fig. 50.13**).
11. Drilling is performed till a thin shell of bone is left over the internal auditory meatus. The last shells of bone are lifted off from the internal auditory meatus with an elevator. Care is taken to retain the dura of the internal auditory meatus intact (**Fig. 50.14** and **50.15**).
12. The greater superficial petrosal nerve is lifted off from its bed and cut sharply with scissors (**Figs. 50.16 and 50.17**).
13. The eggshell bone over the facial nerve from the stylomastoid foramen till the geniculate ganglion is removed with a tympanic membrane elevator (**Fig. 50.18**).
14. The facial nerve is then lifted off from the fallopian canal bed, right from the stylomastoid foramen till the geniculate ganglion. The labyrinthine segment is also lifted off gently (**Figs. 50.19 and 50.20**).
15. At the level of the lateral end of the internal auditory meatus, the superior ampullary nerve is cut, which detaches the superior vestibular nerve. Using an angled pick, the superior vestibular, inferior vestibular, and cochlear nerves are detached at the lateral end of the internal auditory meatus. The dura of the internal auditory meatus together with its contents including the facial nerve is then rerouted posteriorly (**Figs. 50.21–50.24**).
16. The posteriorly rerouted nerves are placed in a safe area on the presigmoid posterior fossa dura to prevent it from injury while drilling the cochlea and inferior tympanic bone. Fibrin glue can be used, if needed, to keep it in place posteriorly (**Fig. 50.25**).
17. The bed of the fallopian canal, the anterior wall of the internal auditory meatus, and the cochlea are drilled anteriorly toward the petrous apex (**Figs. 50.26 and 50.27**).

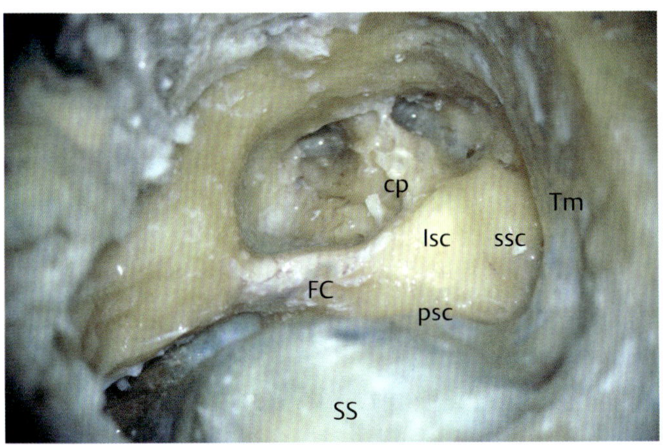

Fig. 50.8 Extended canal wall down mastoidectomy.

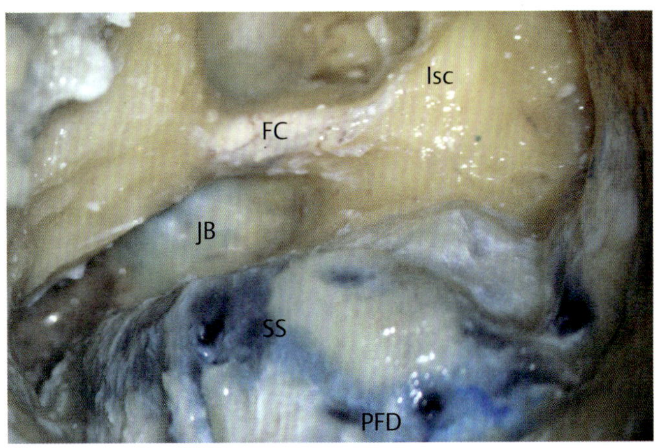

Fig. 50.9 Exposure of the retrosigmoid posterior fossa area.

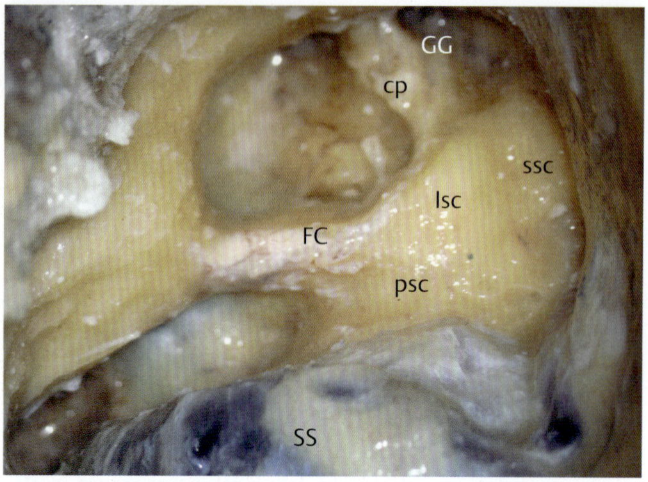

Fig. 50.10 Facial nerve skeletonized from the stylomastoid foramen till the geniculate ganglion.

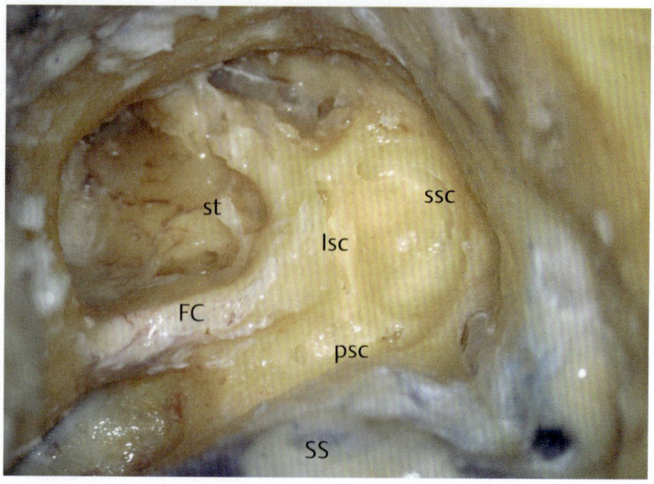

Fig. 50.11 Commencement of labyrinthectomy. Slits in the semicircular canals.

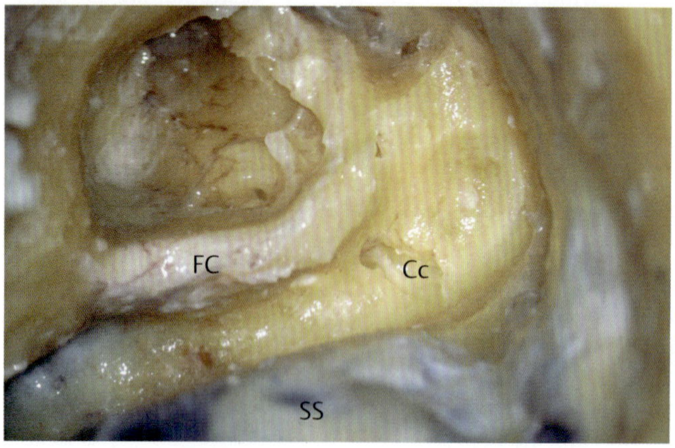

Fig. 50.12 Exposure of the crus commune.

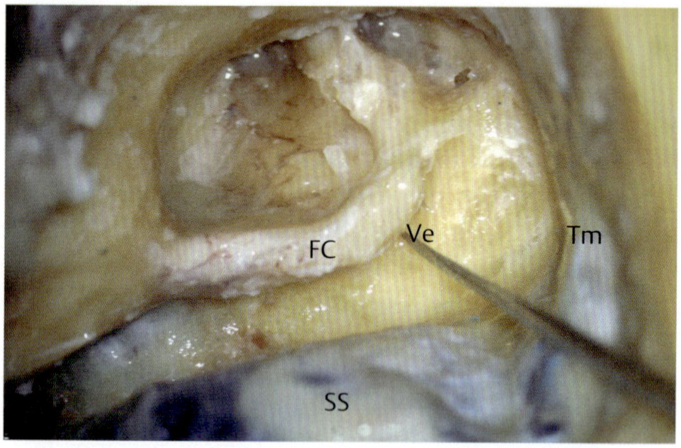

Fig. 50.13 Vestibule exposed.

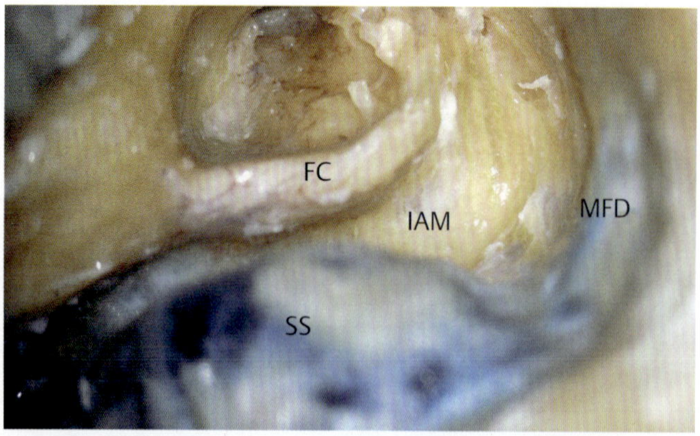

Fig. 50.14 Thin shell of bone left over the dura of internal auditory meatus.

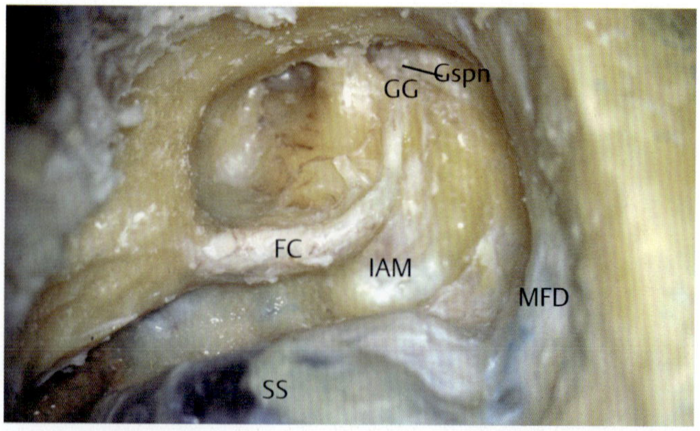

Fig. 50.15 Dura of internal auditory meatus exposed.

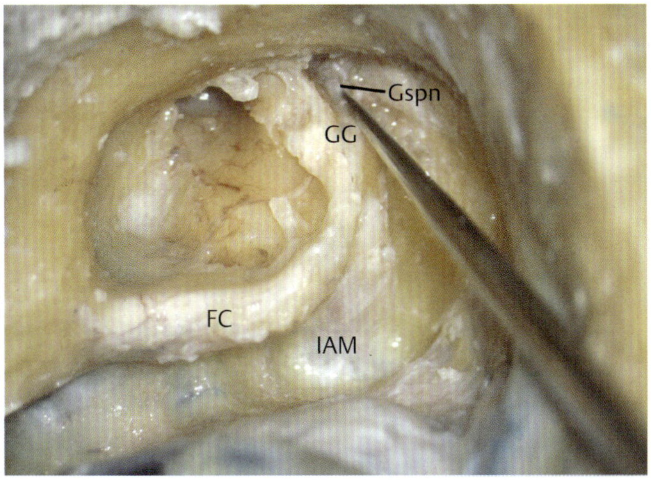

Fig. 50.16 Greater superficial petrosal nerve.

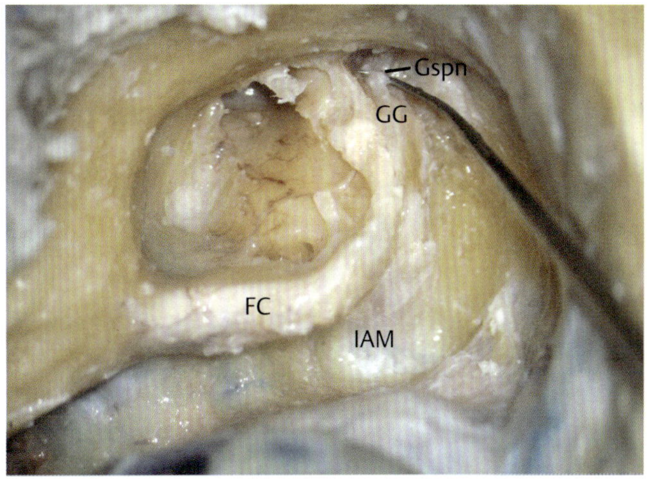

Fig. 50.17 Hooking the greater superficial petrosal nerve before transecting it.

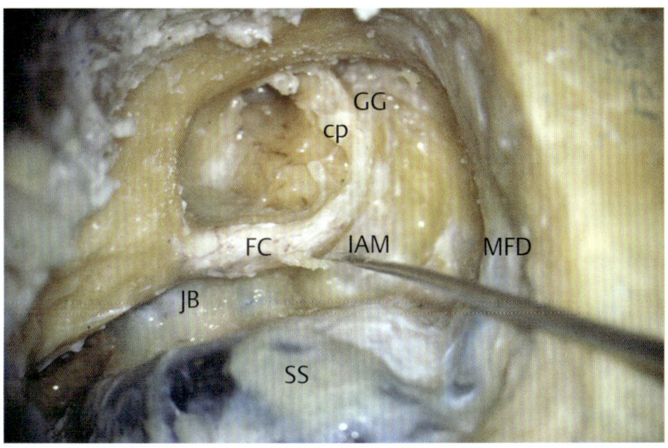

Fig. 50.18 Decompression of the facial nerve from the stylomastoid foramen till the geniculate ganglion.

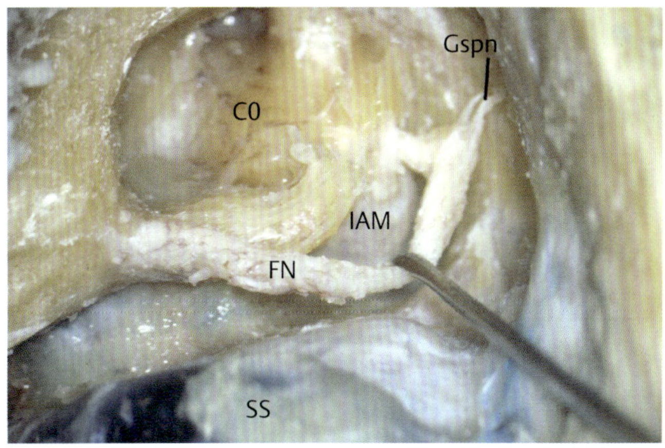

Fig. 50.19 Facial nerve lifted off its bed for posterior rerouting.

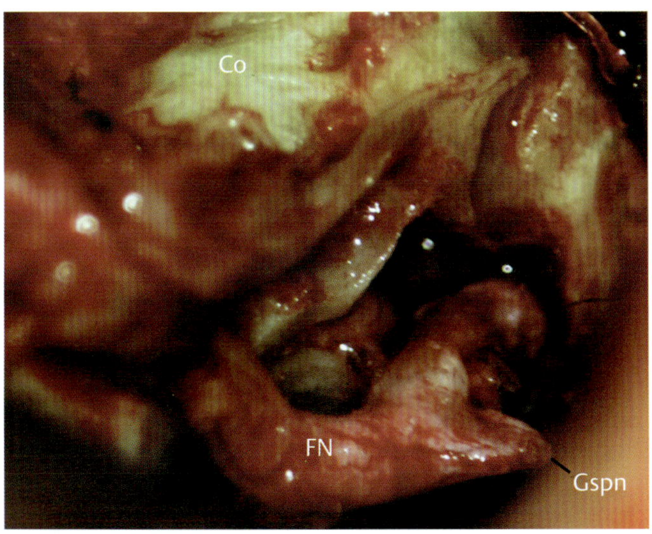

Fig. 50.20 Facial nerve mastoidal, tympanic, and labyrinthine segments reflected posteriorly after transection of the greater superficial petrosal nerve.

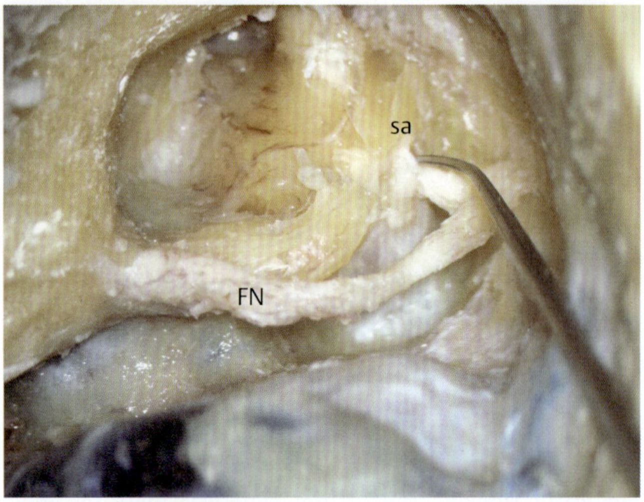

Fig. 50.21 Transection of the superior ampullary nerve at the lateral end of the internal auditory meatus.

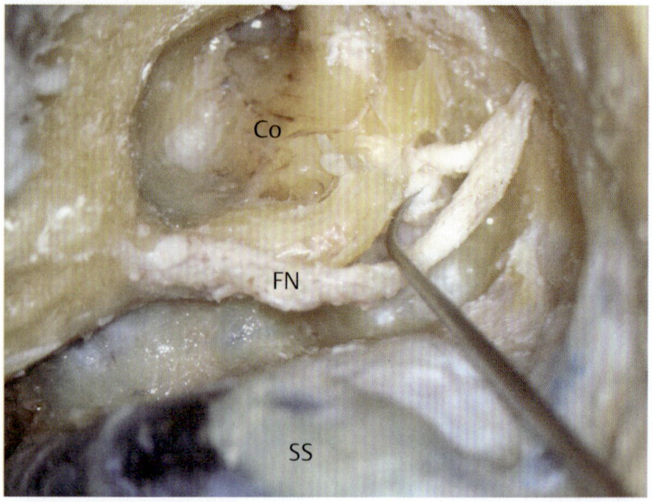

Fig. 50.22 Nerves of the internal auditory meatus with intact dura.

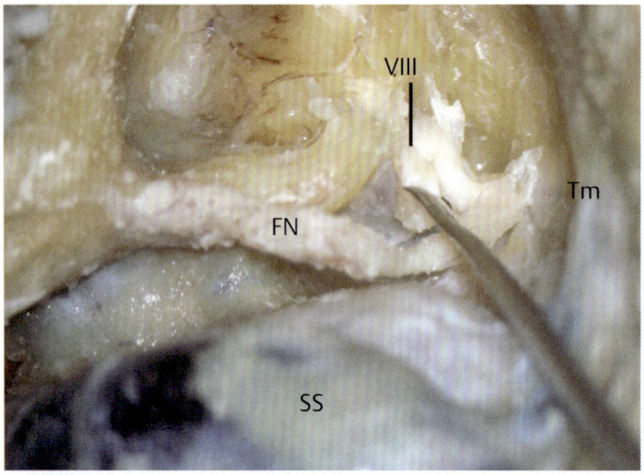

Fig. 50.23 Contents of the internal auditory meatus together with its covering dura reflected posteriorly.

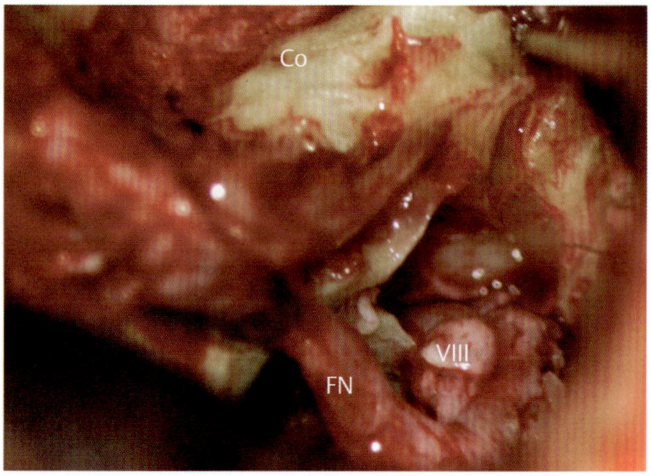

Fig. 50.24 Posterior rerouting of the facial nerve.

18. The vertical infratubal course of the internal carotid artery is exposed medial to the floor of the eustachian tube (**Figs. 50.28 and 50.29**).
19. **Fig. 50.30** shows the position of the facial nerve and internal auditory meatus contents before transposition. **Fig. 50.31** shows the improved access and angle of drilling the cochlea and petrous apex after posterior transposition of the facial nerve the and contents of the internal auditory meatus.
20. The petrous apex lying medial to the vertical internal carotid artery is drilled till the posterior fossa dura. Residual thin bone over the middle fossa is removed to expose the middle fossa dura from the region of the sinodural angle till the petrous apex. The posteriorly rerouted facial nerve and contents of internal auditory canal together with its dura are seen lying on the posterior fossa dura (**Fig. 50.32**).
21. If greater control is needed over the vertical internal carotid artery laterally, the anterior wall of the external auditory canal is drilled, mandibular condoyle is exposed and displaced anteriorly using Fisch infratemporal retractor and further bone drilled to expose around 270 degrees of the vertical internal carotid artery (**Fig. 50.33**).
22. The dura is opened to show the intracranial structures visualized through this approach. The vertical, petrous, and paraclival segments of the internal carotid artery are seen. The inferior petrosal sinus can be either extradural or intradural. Bleeding from the inferior petrosal sinus can be controlled by use of Surgicel. The abducens nerve roughly arises at the level of the vertebrobasilar junction, travels superiorly and laterally deep to the cavernous segment of the internal carotid artery and then on to the superior orbital fissure.

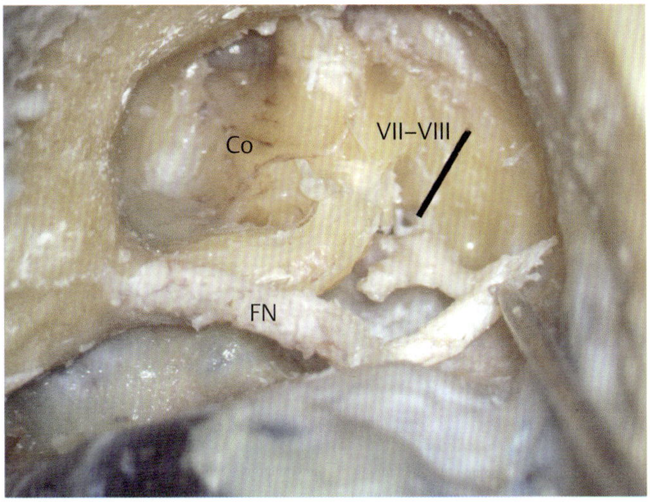

Fig. 50.25 Posteriorly rerouted facial nerve together with the nerves of the internal auditory meatus with intact dura of the internal auditory meatus.

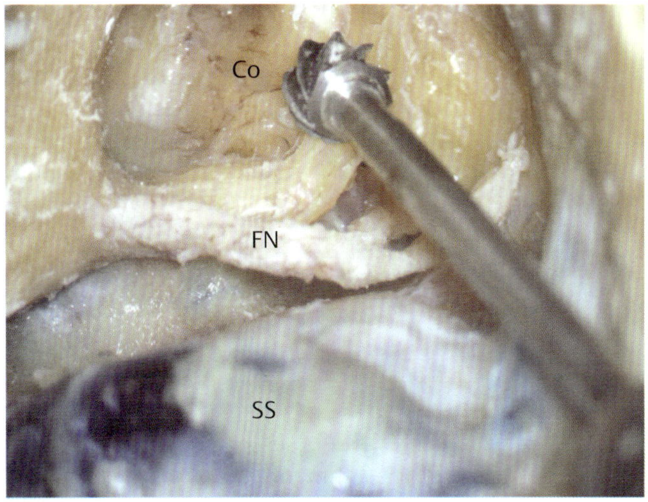

Fig. 50.26 Drilling the cochlea.

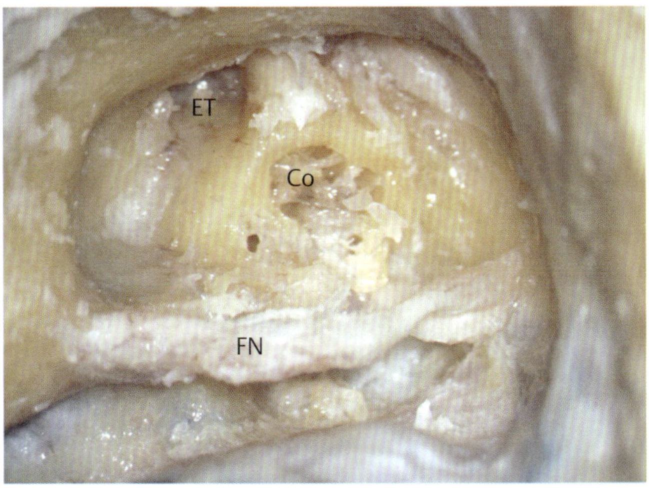

Fig. 50.27 Cochlea partially drilled out. Cochlea turns visible.

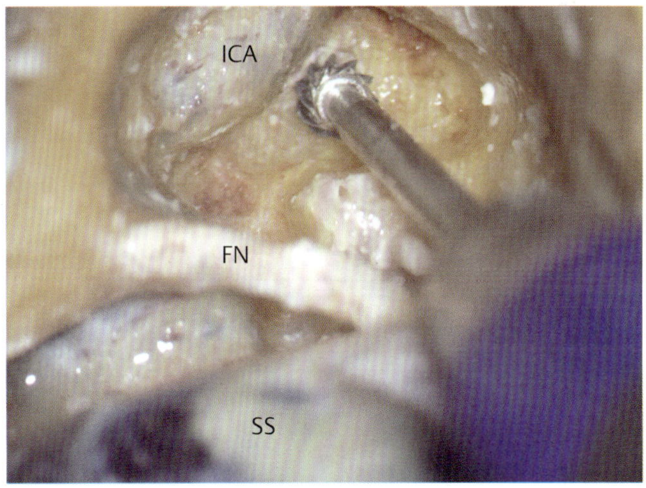

Fig. 50.28 Drilling toward the petrous apex.

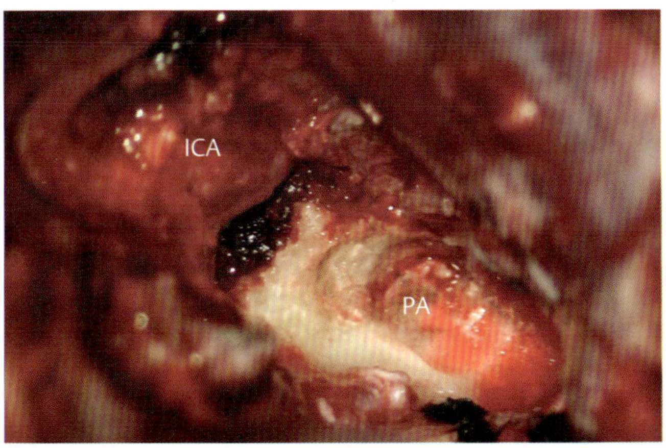

Fig. 50.29 Drilling toward the petrous apex.

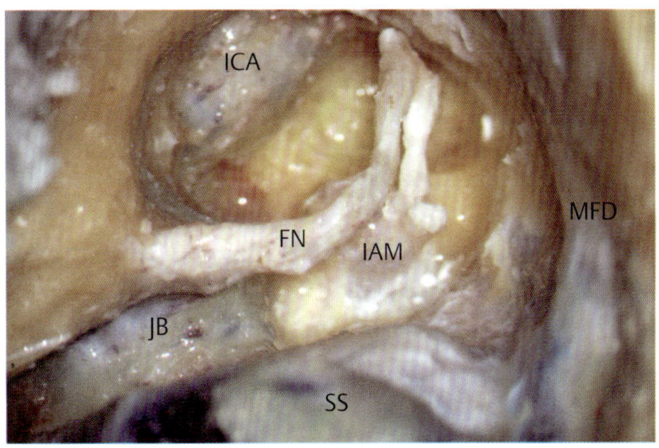

Fig. 50.30 Facial nerve placed back approximately along its usual course to demonstrate how it lies in the middle of the field of surgery.

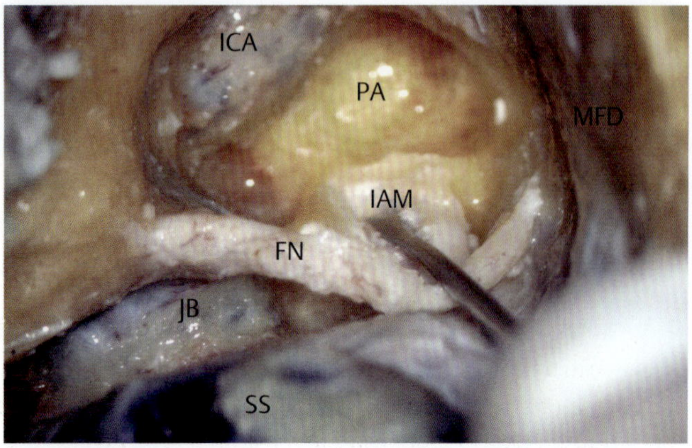

Fig. 50.31 Facial nerve transposed posteriorly. Note the improved access toward the petrous apex.

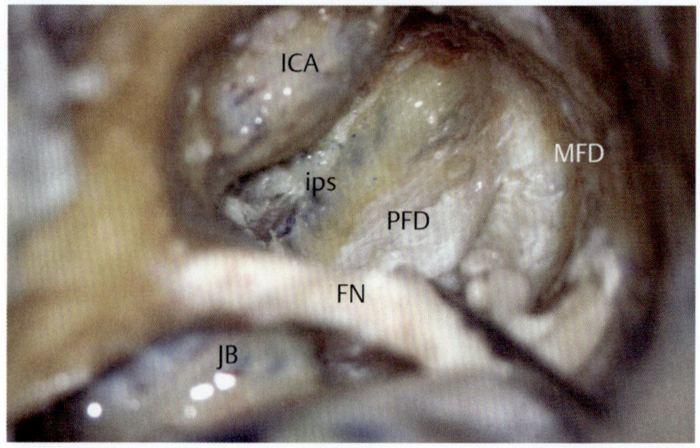

Fig. 50.32 Posterior fossa dura is decompressed from the sigmoid sinus up to the petrous apex.

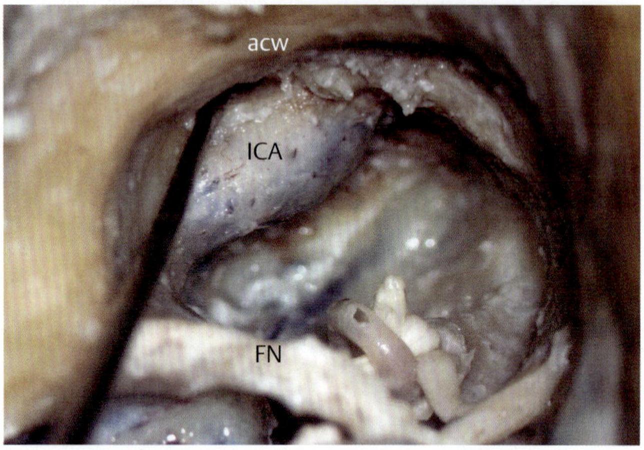

Fig. 50.33 Instrument in the eustachian tube showing the area that needs to be drilled lateral to it to gain control over the vertical infratubal internal carotid artery.

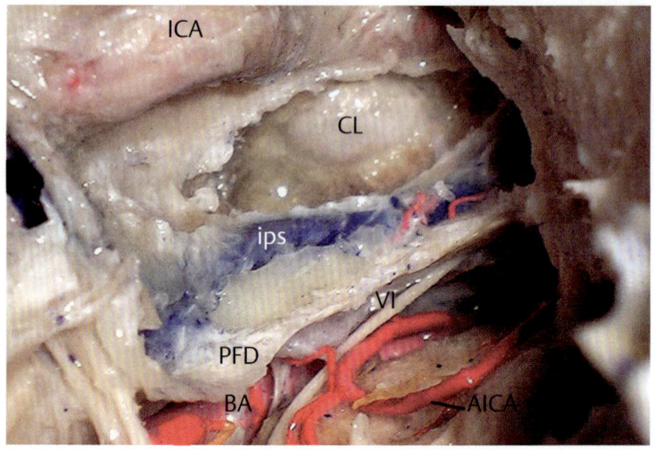

Fig. 50.34 Structures seen at the petrous apex.

Also seen are the lower cranial nerves in relation to the medial wall of the jugular bulb (**Fig. 50.34**).

23. After removal of the lesion, the eustachian tube is plugged with fat and sealed in place using bone wax.
24. A large piece of abdominal fat is used to obliterate the cavity and prevent cerebrospinal fluid leak. We use fibrin glue around the periphery of the fat.
25. The musculoperiosteal, subcutaneous, and skin layers are sutured separately.

Tips and Pearls

- The greater superficial petrosal needs to be definitely identified and sharply transected to avoid unnecessary facial nerve shearing or damage at the region of the geniculate ganglion.
- The facial nerve needs to be decompressed right up to the stylomastoid area, so that good control of the jugular bulb or lower cranial nerves is achieved.
- This approach helps achieve good clearance of lesions anterior to the internal auditory meatus, extending to the petrous apex.
- Depending on the extent of the lesion, the internal carotid artery can be further exposed along its course.
- In intradural lesions, care is taken while opening the dura of the posterior fossa, to avoid injury to the abducens nerve. Hence, it is very essential to understand the course of the abducens nerve in this area.

Suggested Readings

Sanna M, Mazzoni A, Gamoletti R. The system of the modified transcochlear approaches to the petroclival area and the prepontine cistern. Skull Base Surg 1996;6(4):237–248

Sanna M, Mazzoni A, Saleh E, Taibah A, Mancini F. The system of the modified transcochlear approach: a lateral avenue to the central skull base. Am J Otol 1998;19(1):88–97, discussion 97–98

Chapter 51 Transotic Approach

Narayan Jayashankar

Indications

1. Petrous bone cholesteatomas with the destruction of vestibular apparatus or cochlea and unserviceable hearing.
2. Giant vestibular schwannomas with extension to prepontine cistern.
3. Petrous bone tumors with normal preoperative facial nerve function.

Surgical Steps

The preoperative computed tomography (CT) scan of the subject with a right-sided congenital cholesteatoma is shown in **Fig. 51.1**. The subject had a normal facial function but had an unserviceable hearing in the right ear.

1. A C-shaped incision is taken starting from the helix, coursing about 3 cm behind the postaural groove and going up to the mastoid tip. The incision includes the skin and subcutaneous tissue.
2. A rectangular-shaped musculoperiosteal flap is created posterior to the external auditory canal (EAC). This is used as a second layer closure of the cul-de-sac that needs to be prepared (**Fig. 51.2**).
3. The EAC is transected horizontally at the level of the spine of Henle. The conchal cartilage is dissected off the skin in the lateral half of the transected EAC and a sleeve of EAC is created. Stay stitches are put on its superior and inferior edges, and the sleeve is then everted out laterally from the ear. The skin sleeve is then sutured with Vicryl. The rectangular musculoperiosteal flap previously created is then sutured as a second layer over the medial end of this blind sac closure of the EAC **(Fig. 51.3, Fig. 51.4, and Fig. 51.5).**
4. The medial half of skin lining the bony EAC is to be dissected off and excised together with the malleus and incus as the surgery proceeds.
5. The mastoid cortex is drilled. The cholesteatoma is immediately evident in the mastoid (**Fig. 51.6**).
6. A canal wall down mastoidectomy is performed. The sigmoid sinus and middle fossa dura in the roof of the mastoid are delineated leaving a thin shell of bone over them. The semicircular canals are delineated if possible, but in many cases, the canal is already destroyed by the pathology. Cells of the mastoid are drilled off completely till the mastoid tip. The posterior wall of the EAC is taken down till the mastoid segment of the fallopian canal. The cells are drilled off till a thin plate of bone is left over the presigmoid posterior fossa dura (**Fig. 51.7**).
7. The tympanic segment of the fallopian canal is traced up to the first genu, and the labyrinthine segment is tracked back to the ampullary end of the superior semicircular canal. A thin shell of bone is left over the facial nerve in its entire course unless the pathology itself has eroded the fallopian canal. In that case, the facial nerve is gently traced and preserved.
8. A labyrinthectomy is performed by successively drilling off the posterior, lateral, and superior semicircular canals. The vestibule is opened widely. Here, cholesteatoma is seen in the area (**Fig. 51.8**).
9. Drilling proceeds till the internal auditory meatus leaving thin bone over it without exposing its dura or contents. Drilling proceeds in the trough between the superior lip of internal auditory meatus and middle

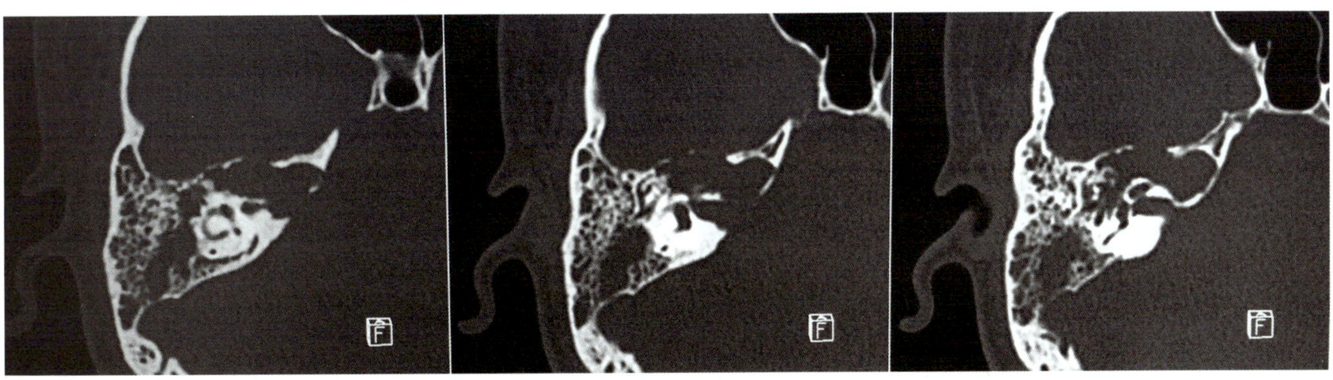

Fig. 51.1 CT scan of the subject with a congenital cholesteatoma right ear.

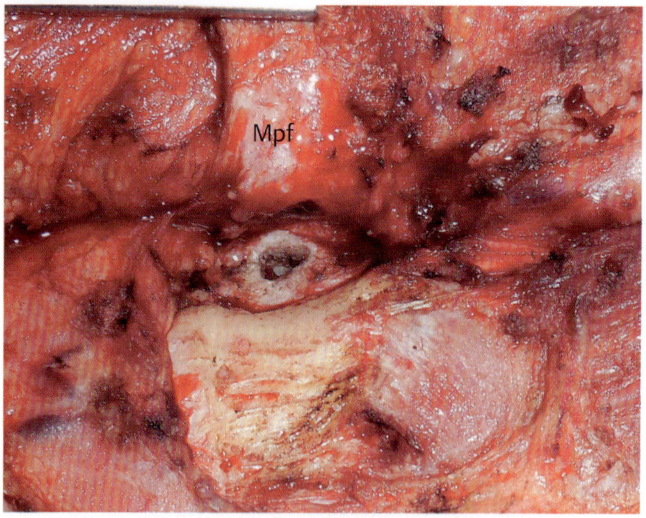

Fig. 51.2 A rectangular musculoperiosteal flap based anteriorly is created for second layer cul-de-sac closure of the external auditory canal.

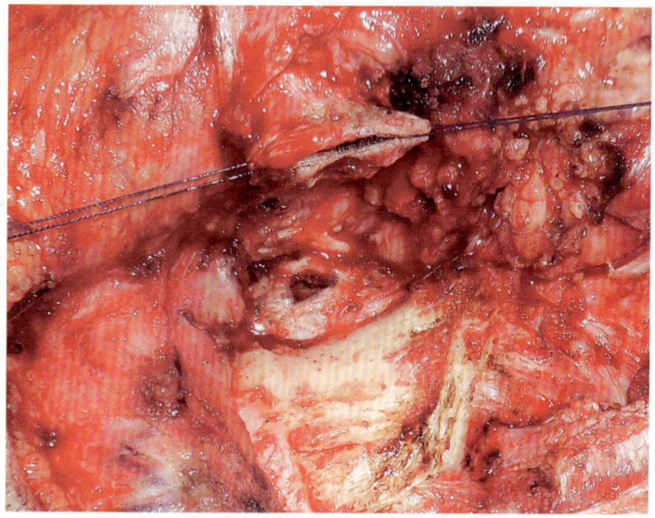

Fig. 51.3 A sleeve of skin (of the lateral part of EAC) is created by dissecting the conchal cartilage off it.

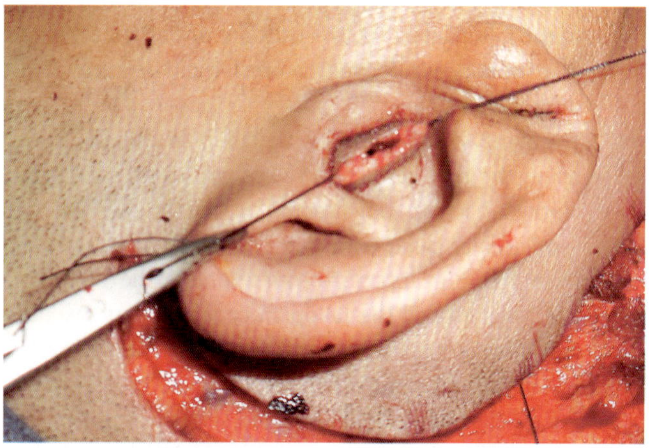

Fig. 51.4 The skin sleeve is everted out laterally and sutured.

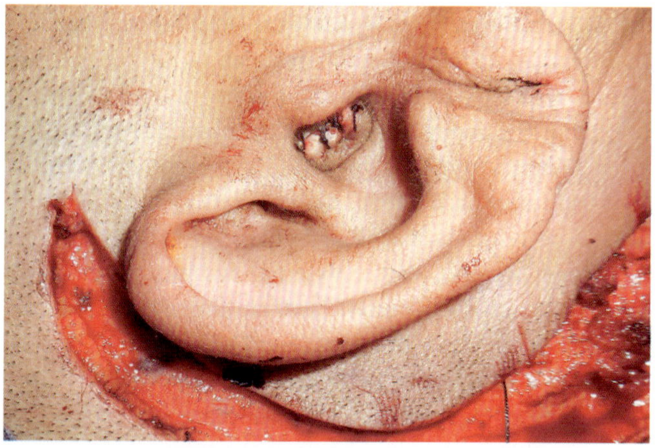

Fig. 51.5 Cul-de-sac closure of external auditory canal.

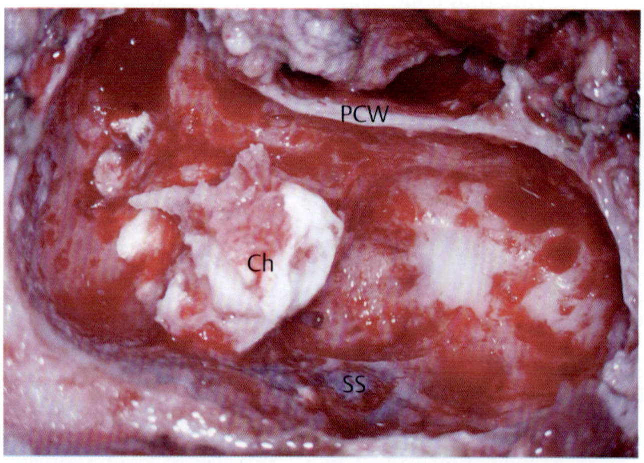

Fig. 51.6 Cholesteatoma is seen in the mastoid cavity.

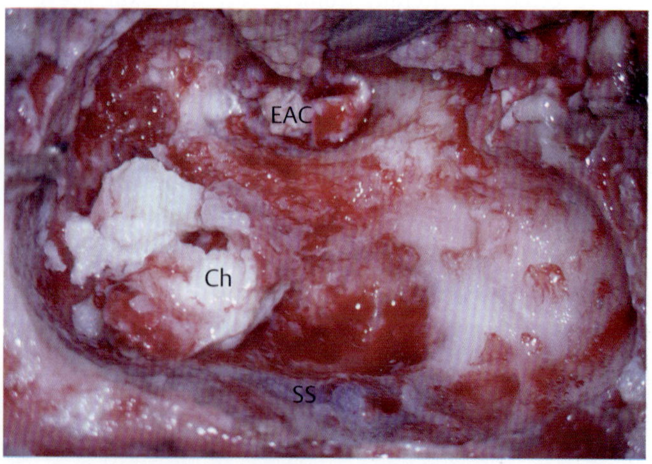

Fig. 51.7 Canal wall taken down up to the level of the fallopian canal.

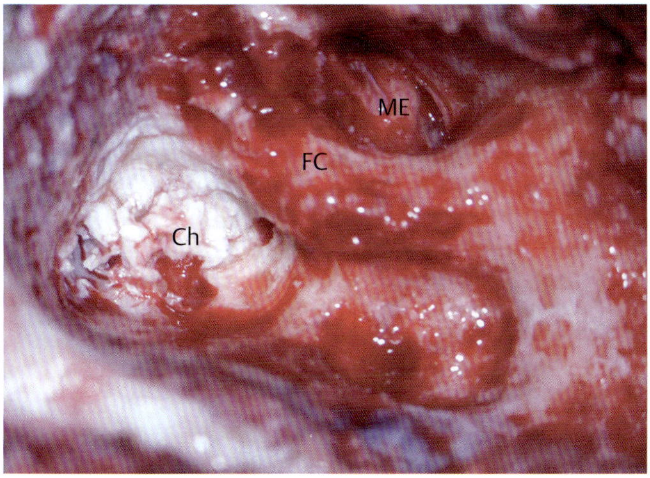

Fig. 51.8 Cholesteatoma has destroyed the labyrinth partially and is seen after drilling the labyrinth further to expose it completely.

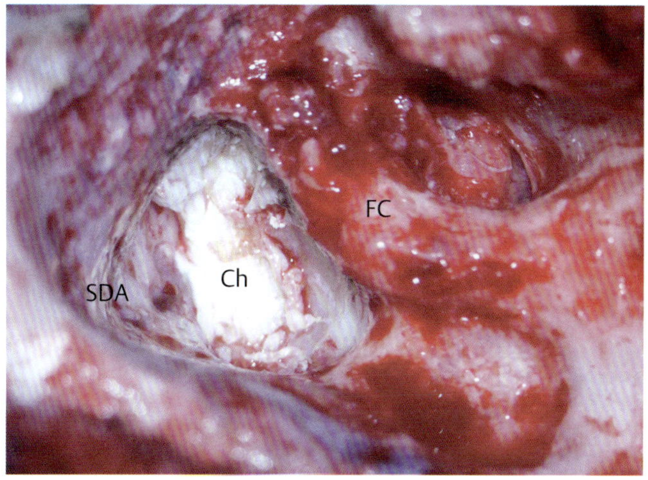

Fig. 51.9 Cholesteatoma is seen between the superior end of the internal auditory meatus and the middle fossa dura.

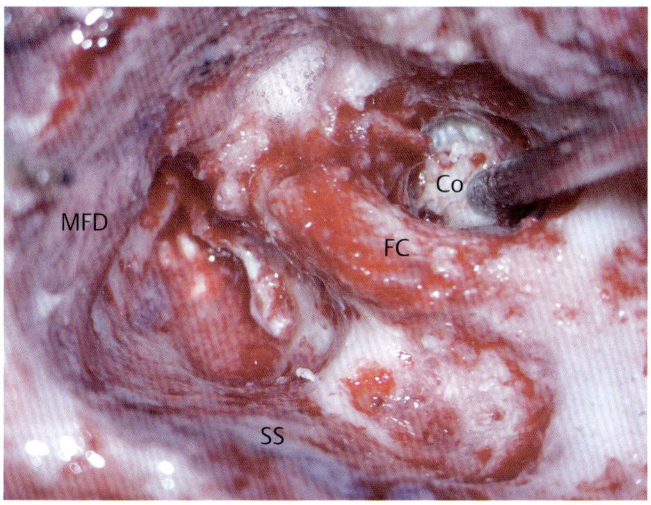

Fig. 51.10 Cochlea is drilled.

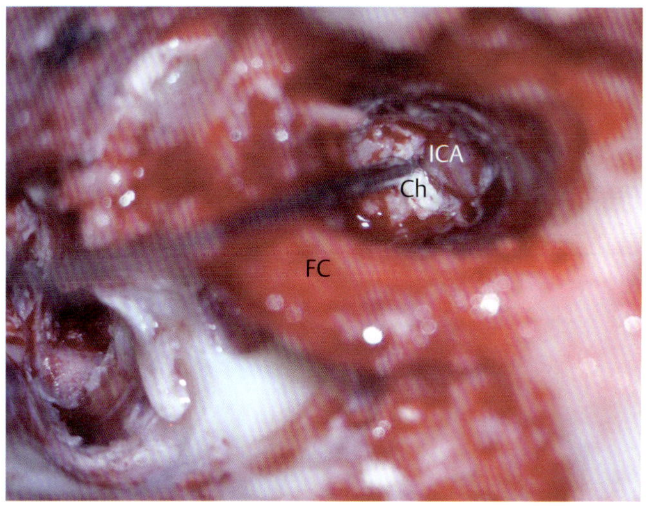

Fig. 51.11 Cholesteatoma is seen deep in the cochlea.

fossa dura toward the petrous apex. Similarly, it proceeds in the inferior trough between the inferior lip of the internal auditory meatus and the jugular bulb, again, toward the petrous apex (**Fig. 51.9**).

10. The eggshell thin tegmen mastoid bone is then removed. Taking off the bone and using the suction to push the middle fossa dura superiorly also creates additional space for drilling in the supralabyrinthine area and for better clearance of the pathology. Depending on the extent of pathology, the presigmoid posterior fossa bone can also be taken off the dura.
11. The cochlea is drilled off. The internal carotid artery lies anteroinferior to the eustachian tube. The eustachian tube is a landmark between the vertical parapharyngeal and petrous segments of the internal carotid artery. All the cells are drilled off till the petrous apex without any inadvertent damage to the internal carotid artery. The cholesteatoma is then cleared from the area (**Fig. 51.10, Fig. 51.11, and Fig. 51.12**).
12. In case of spread of pathology anterior to the first genu of the facial nerve, the greater superficial petrosal nerve (GSPN) is identified and sectioned. The bone deep to the GSPN is drilled to communicate the supratubal space to the mesotympanum (**Fig. 51.13**). This drilling also exposes the area anterior to the internal auditory meatus to clear pathology (**Fig. 51.14, Fig. 51.15, and Fig. 51.16**). The head of the subject needs to be tilted toward the surgeon to inspect this area. The major

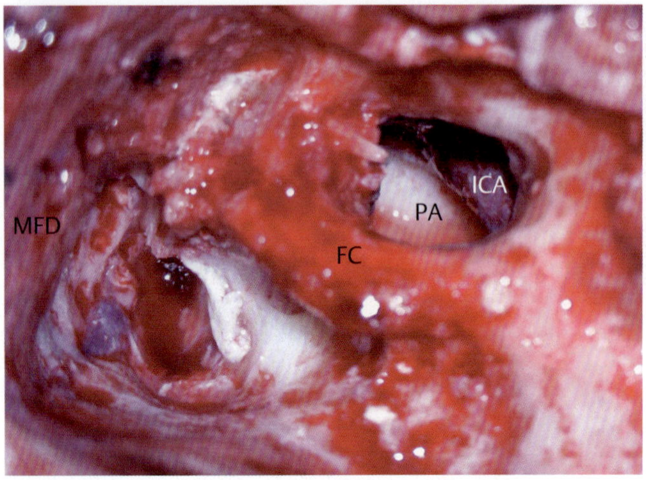

Fig. 51.12 The cholesteatoma has been cleared from the area deep to the cochlea toward the petrous apex.

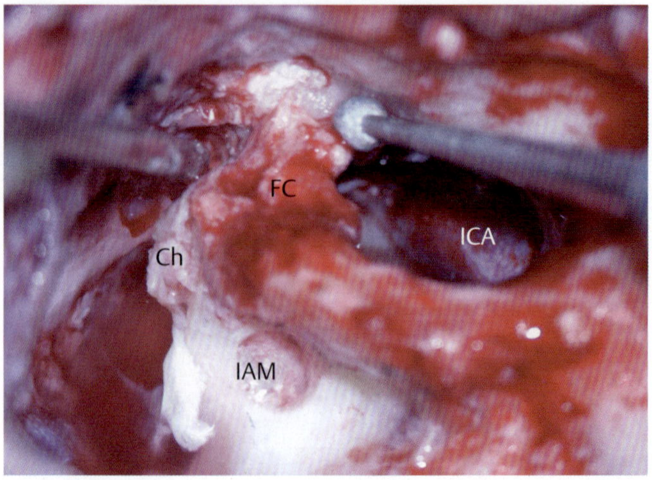

Fig. 51.13 Drilling the bone deep to GSPN to expose cholesteatoma in the region.

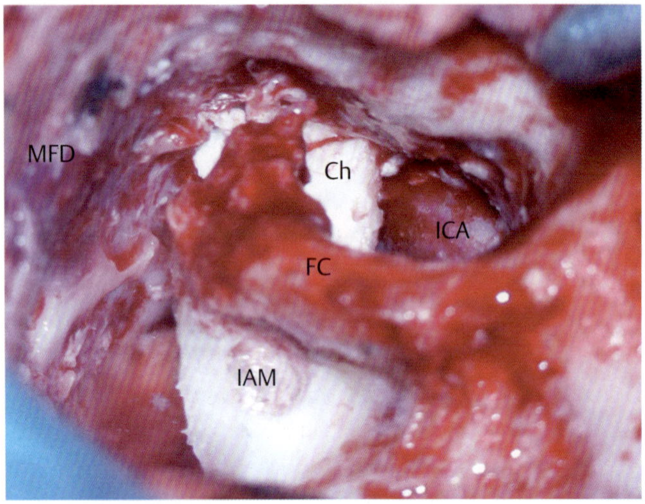

Fig. 51.14 Cholesteatoma is exposed in the region anterior to the IAM.

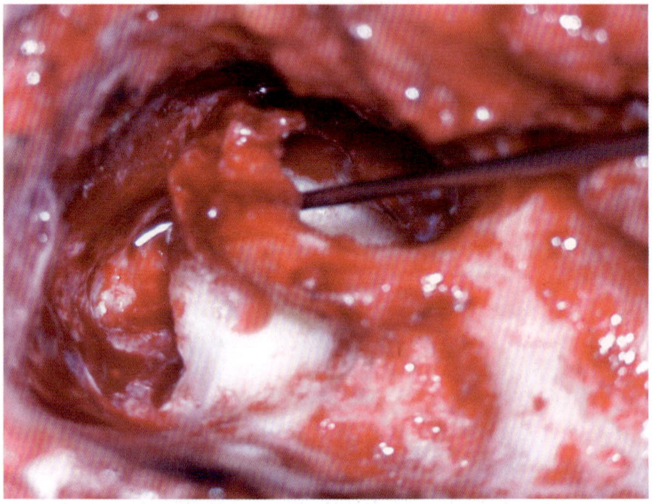

Fig. 51.15 Cholesteatoma anterior to the IAM completely removed.

limitation of the transotic approach is a limited view of this area and thereby increased incidence of residual lesion in this area. It was primarily to clear this area that posterior transposition of the facial nerve was developed. The disadvantage is nowadays limited with increasing use of endoscopes to visualize and clear this area when required.

13. Depending on the spread of the pathology, bone medial to the mastoid segment of the fallopian canal in the inferior trough can also be drilled off further, taking care not to damage the internal auditory meatus superiorly or the jugular bulb inferiorly. This drilling helps communicate the translabyrinthine space with the transcochlear space. The facial nerve in its bony tunnel is left intact from the internal auditory meatus till the stylomastoid foramen. Care is to be taken not to inadvertently fracture the fallopian canal (mastoid segment) during this step with the shaft of the burr which is the major morbidity in this step (**Fig. 51.17**).
14. After the removal of pathology, the eustachian tube is plugged with fat or periosteum. The whole cavity is filled with fat strips (**Fig. 51.18**).
15. The musculoperiosteal and skin layers are closed separately.

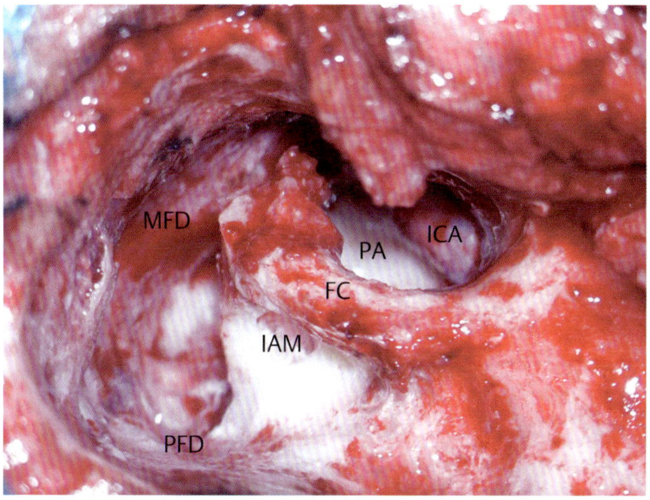

Fig. 51.16 View after clearance of the congenital cholesteatoma.

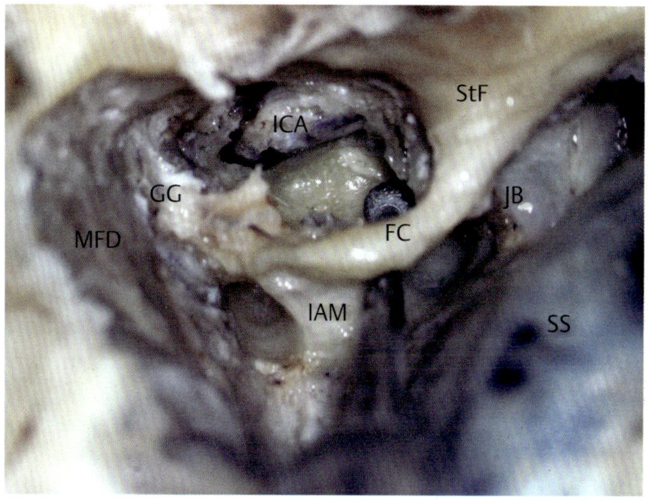

Fig. 51.17 Drilling medial to the mastoid segment of fallopian canal.

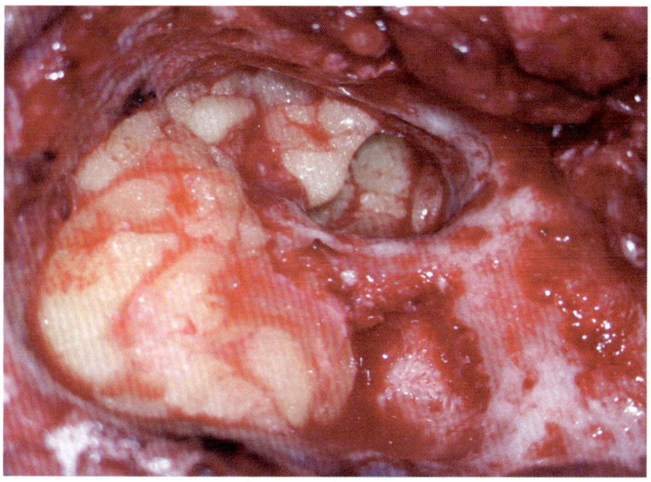

Fig. 51.18 Fat strips used to obliterate the eustachian tube as also the whole cavity.

Suggested Readings

Browne JD, Fisch U. Transotic approach to the cerebellopontine angle. Neurosurg Clin N Am 2008;19(2):265–278

Pandya Y, Piccirillo E, Mancini F, Sanna M. Management of complex cases of petrous bone cholesteatoma. Ann Otol Rhinol Laryngol 2010;119(8):514–525

Prasad SC, Piras G, Piccirillo E, et al. Surgical strategy and facial nerve outcomes in petrous bone cholesteatoma. Audiolo Neurotol 2016;21(5):275–285

Xia Y, Zhang W, Li Y, Ma X, Liu Q, Shi J. The transotic approach for vestibular schwannoma: indications and results. Eur Arch Otorhinolaryngol 2017;274(8):3041–3047

Chapter 52 Modified Transcochlear Approach Type B

Narayan Jayashankar

This approach is an anterior extension of the modified transcochlear approach type A. The steps of surgery are similar to the modified transcochlear approach type A, with additional control over the internal carotid artery anteriorly. This is achieved by performing an additional infratemporal fossa B or C approach to access lesions extending ventral to the brainstem (extradural or intradural).

Indications

1. Extensive clival chordomas or petrous apex cholesteatomas, with more anterior involvement of the internal carotid artery.
2. Petroclival meningiomas with limited extension beyond midline to the contralateral side.

Surgical Steps

1. A postauricular incision is taken, starting at the lateral margin of the orbit, and coursing 2 cm superior to the helix and 3–4 cm behind the postaural groove till the mastoid tip. Incision includes the skin and subcutaneous tissue.
2. A cul-de-sac closure of the external auditory canal is performed, as described in the modified transcochlear approach type A, steps 2 to 5.
3. The skin lining the medial part of the external auditory canal along with the tympanic membrane, malleus, and incus is excised.
4. A modified transcochlear approach type A is performed, as described in steps 7–17 (**Figs. 52.1 and 52.2**).
5. To approach the horizontal petrous internal carotid artery, the articular capsule of the mandibular condyle is excised, and the mandibular condyle is displaced inferiorly using a Fisch infratemporal retractor.
6. The glenoid fossa is drilled medially. Care is taken to remain parallel to the middle fossa dural plate, which is made eggshell thin.
7. The middle meningeal artery is identified coursing through the foramen spinosum. This is bipolarized and cut.
8. Drilling medially exposes the mandibular (V3) branch of the trigeminal nerve. This is accompanied by a rich venous network which needs to be bipolarized and cut.
9. Further drilling medially exposes the complete the horizontal course of the petrous segment of internal

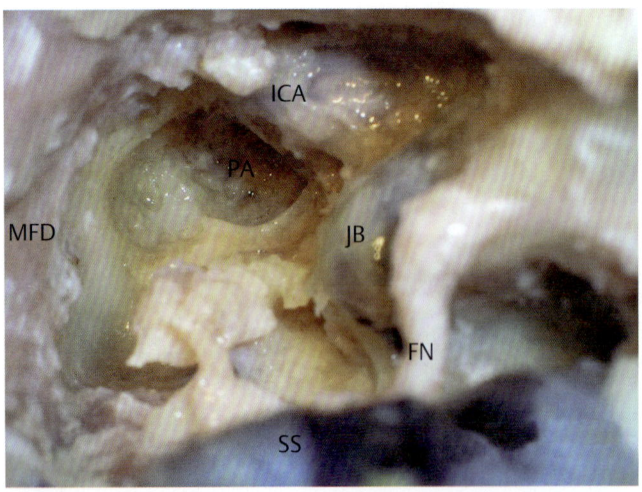

Fig. 52.1 Facial nerve rerouted posteriorly with partial drilling performed toward the petrous apex.

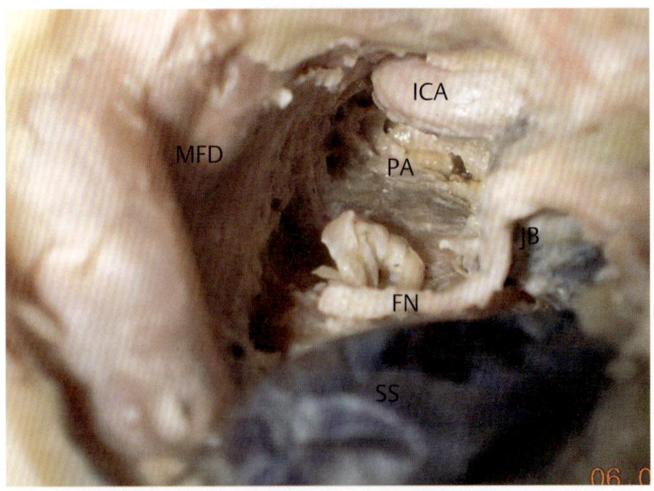

Fig. 52.2 Modified transcochlear A approach with exposure of the posterior fossa dura from the sigmoid sinus till the petrous apex, and from the middle fossa dura/superior petrosal sinus till the jugular bulb. The facial nerve is rerouted posteriorly.

carotid artery up to the foramen lacerum. All the above steps are described in detail in the chapter on the infratemporal fossa B approach (**Fig. 52.3**).

10. If a further anterior extension or more space is needed, the steps are similar to that described in detail in the infratemporal fossa C approach. The zygoma is transected after preserving the frontal branch of the facial nerve, the temporalis muscle is mobilized inferiorly, and drilling is performed of the lateral and medial pterygoid plates to access the nasopharynx or sphenoid sinus. Care must be taken not to open the nasopharynx or the sphenoid sinus if the intracranial space is opened in this approach.
11. The eustachian tube is plugged with fat may need to be sutured. In case the petroclival dura is opened, the dural defect is closed with a piece of fascia lata, which is secured in place with fibrin glue. Fat is used to obliterate the dead space in the cavity.
12. The incision is closed in musculoperiosteal, subcutaneous, and skin layers.

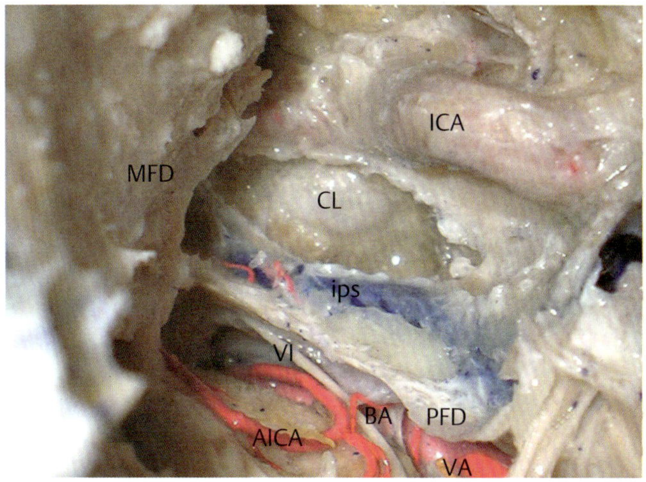

Fig. 52.3 Extradural and intradural structures at the petrous apex.

Tips and Pearls

- This approach can be extended anteriorly up to the lateral wall of the sphenoid sinus and nasopharynx. The lateral wall must not be breached, specifically when the subarachnoid space is opened. In case of such tumors that invade the sinus or nasopharynx, the procedure can be staged. This is done to prevent cerebrospinal fluid leak and subsequent complications.
- While opening the petrous dura, care is taken to avoid injuring the abducens nerve, which runs from an inferomedial position near the vertebrobasilar junction to a superolateral position behind the cavernous internal carotid artery.

Suggested Readings

Sanna M, Mazzoni A, Gamoletti R. The system of the modified transcochlear approaches to the petroclival area and the prepontine cistern. Skull Base Surg 1996;6(4):237–248

Sanna M, Mazzoni A, Saleh E, Taibah A, Mancini F. The system of the modified transcochlear approach: a lateral avenue to the central skull base. Am J Otol 1998;19(1):88–97, discussion 97–98

Chapter 53 Modified Transcochlear Approach Type C

Narayan Jayashankar

It is a superior extension of the modified transcochlear approach type A. It is used for lesions that have invaded or breached the tentorium, or extended superiorly through the tentorial notch.

Indication

1. Petroclival lesions that have breached the tentorium.

Surgical Steps

1. The initial steps are similar to those described in the modified transcochlear approach type A, that is, steps 1 to 17 (**Fig. 53.1**).
2. The bone overlying the middle fossa dura is removed completely.
3. The middle fossa dura is reflected parallel to the superior petrosal sinus to expose the temporal lobe. The superior petrosal sinus is coagulated and cut. In case bleeding persists, surgicel is packed into the superior petrosal rent, lying partly intraluminally and partly extraluminally like a cork (**Fig. 53.2**).
4. The tentorium is incised, starting from the junction of the sigmoid sinus and superior petrosal sinus, and continues parallel to the superior petrosal sinus till the tentorial notch (**Fig. 53.3**).
5. Care must be taken to not injure the vein of Labbe, which lies on the temporal lobe and drains into the transverse sinus. Injury to this vein can cause serious complications.

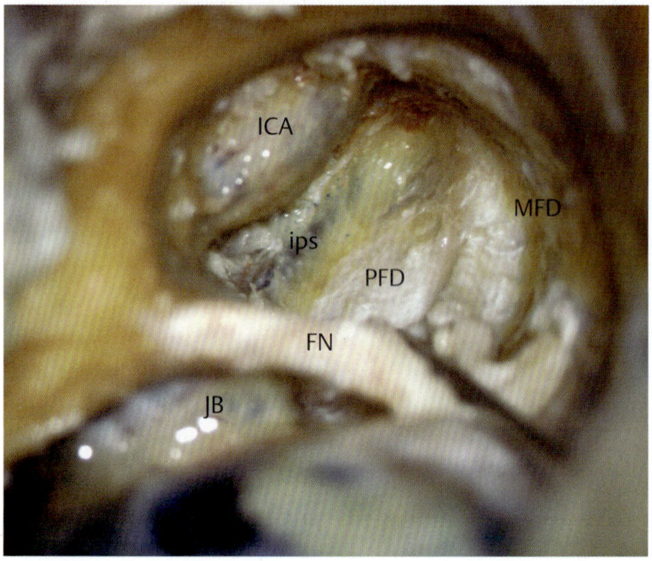

Fig. 53.1 Left side modified transcochlear type A approach.

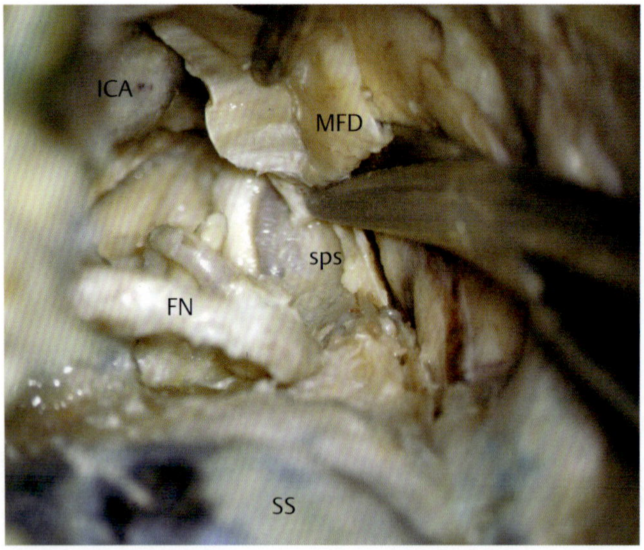

Fig. 53.2 Middle fossa dura cut parallel to the superior petrosal sinus and reflected laterally.

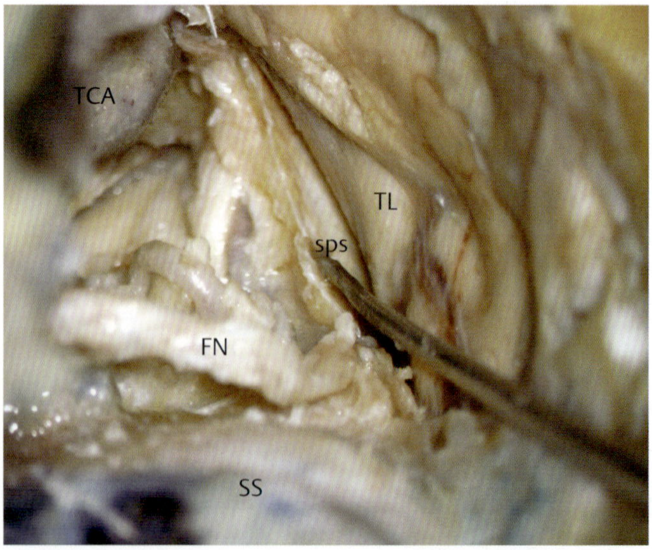

Fig. 53.3 The tentorium needs to be cut parallel to the course of the superior petrosal sinus, beginning from the sinodural junction to the tentorial notch.

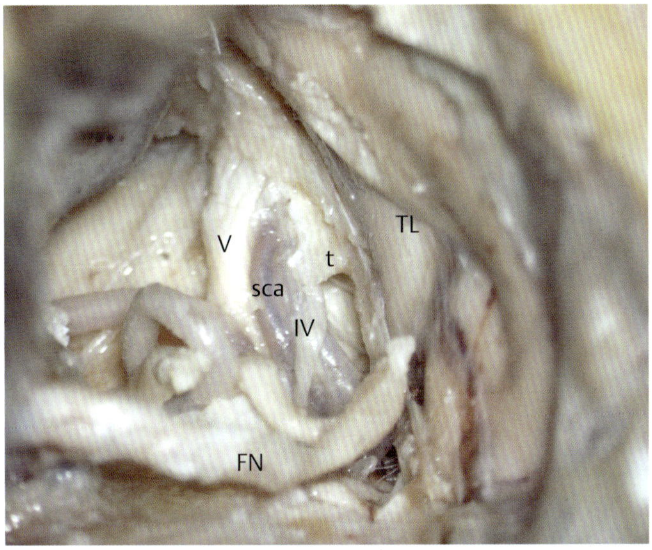

Fig. 53.4 Structures seen after incising the tentorium.

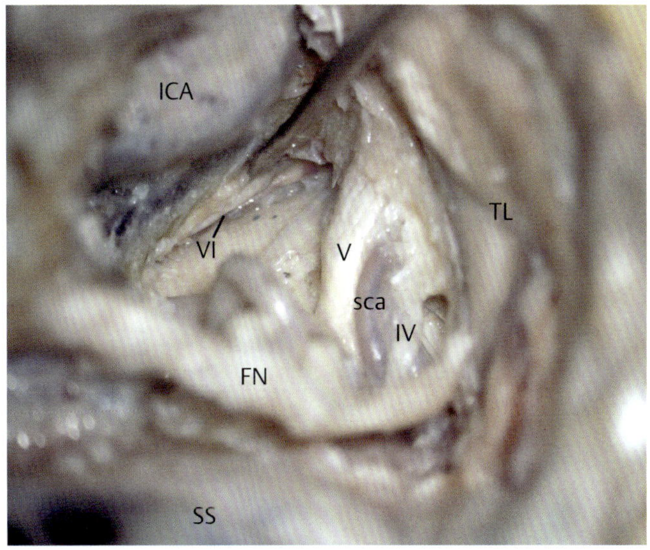

Fig. 53.5 Panoramic view of the approach.

6. The trochlear nerve lies in the infratentorial compartment, pierces the tentorium, and then courses supratentorially toward the orbit. Injury to this nerve must be avoided. The superior cerebellar artery can be seen arising from the basilar artery and coursing just inferior to the trochlear nerve (**Fig. 53.4**).
7. The posterior cerebral artery is usually seen adjacent to the oculomotor nerve. With mild temporal lobe retraction, the P1, PCom, and P2 branches can be seen.
8. With a little additional temporal lobe retraction, the middle cerebral artery, the optic nerve, and anterior cerebral artery too can be visualized, if needed.
9. At the petrous apex, the abducens nerve can be seen traversing toward the Dorello canal (**Fig. 53.5**).

Tips and Pearls

- Vein of Labbe must not be damaged while exposing the temporal lobe. Injury to the vein of Labbe causes seizures, aphasia, and can also lead to death due to massive edema of the brain.
- Superior petrosal sinus must be bipolarized and cut. Any bleeding from the end in situ can be controlled with additional use of Surgicel.
- The tentorium is always cut under direct vision to prevent injury to the trochlear nerve.

Section XX

Retrolabyrinthine Approach

Chapter 54

Petrous Apex Cholesterol Granuloma Excision—Transmastoid Retrolabyrinthine Approach

Jeyanthi Kulasegarah, Vicknes Waran, and Prepageran Narayanan

History

A 57-year-old man presented with a 6-month history of right-sided facial twitching. He denied any hearing or balance problems, and there were no other associated otological symptoms. On physical examination, both the external auditory canal and the tympanic membrane were normal. Other ENT and cranial nerve examinations were normal. Pure tone audiometry showed normal hearing bilaterally on the lower and mid-frequencies but mild high-frequency sensorineural hearing loss bilaterally. A high-resolution computed tomography scan of the temporal bone showed a soft tissue density within the right petrous apex with some expansion of the bone (**Fig. 54.1**). Magnetic resonance imaging (T2-weighted sequences) showed a hyperintense lobulated lesion involving the right petrous apex (**Fig. 54.2**). The patient underwent surgical excision of the cholesterol granuloma via a transmastoid, retrolabyrinthine approach. The surgical steps are described below.

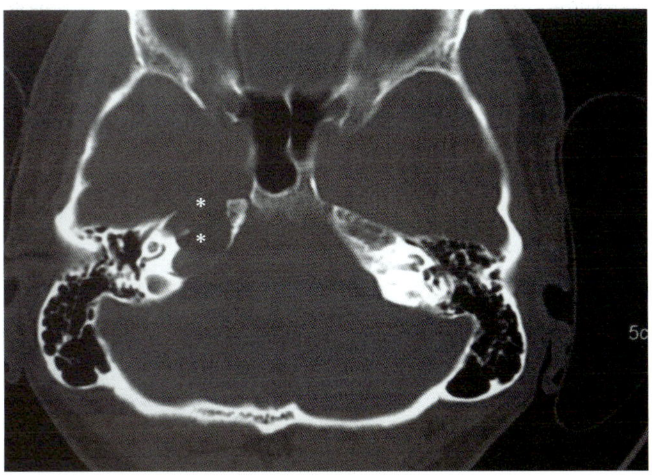

Fig. 54.1 Axial CT scan image showing a soft tissue density (*white asterisk*) with expansion of the right petrous apex abutting the petrous internal carotid artery (*black asterisk*).

Surgical Steps

1. The patient is placed under general anesthesia in the supine position with a head ring. The head is turned 70 degrees to the opposite side of the operation. Facial nerve monitor is attached, and the patient's hair around the incision site is shaved. It is important to remind the anesthetist to not use a paralytic agent to allow monitoring of facial nerve function intraoperatively.
2. Local anesthetic xylocaine 2% with epinephrine 1:200,000 is infiltrated along the skin incision site at the postauricular region. The patient's skin is then prepped and draped.
3. A "C-shaped" skin incision is made about 3 to 4 cm from the postauricular sulcus, extending from superiorly at the level of the helical crus to inferiorly to the mastoid tip.
4. Skin and subcutaneous tissue flap are elevated anteriorly to the level of the external auditory canal. Next a "T-incision" through the temporalis muscle, fascia, and periosteum is made, and the periosteum is lifted off the underlying bone with a periosteal elevator, and this exposes the mastoid cortex.
5. A cortical mastoidectomy is performed initially at the McEwan's triangle, where the mastoid bone is drilled to the tegmen superiorly, mastoid tip inferiorly, posterior canal wall anteriorly, and sigmoid sinus posteriorly using a cutting burr. The antrum, sinodural angle, lateral semicircular canal, and mastoid segment of the facial nerve were identified (**Fig. 54.3**).
6. An extended mastoidectomy is then performed with the removal of presigmoid air cells in the Trautmann's triangle using a diamond burr (**Fig. 54.3**). Bone over the posterior fossa dura between the posterior semicircular canal and sigmoid sinus is removed. The endolymphatic duct and sac are identified and preserved. The posterior semicircular canal is also carefully skeletonized (**Fig. 54.4**).

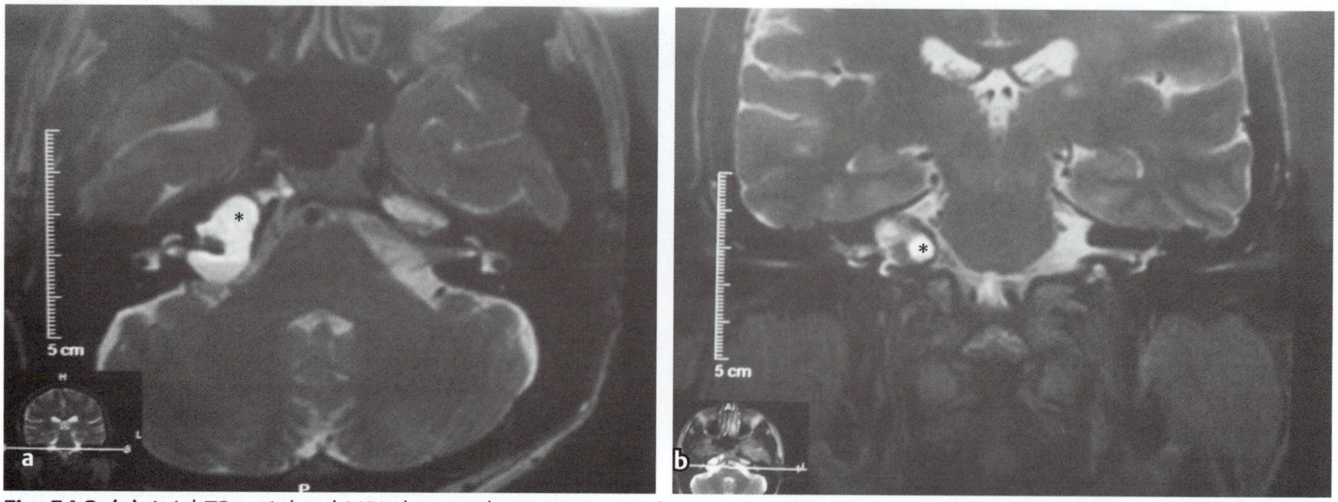

Fig. 54.2 **(a)** Axial T2-weighted MRI showing hyperintense right petrous apex lesion (*black asterisk*). **(b)** Coronal T2-weighted MRI showing hyperintense right petrous apex lesion abutting the pons (*black asterisk*).

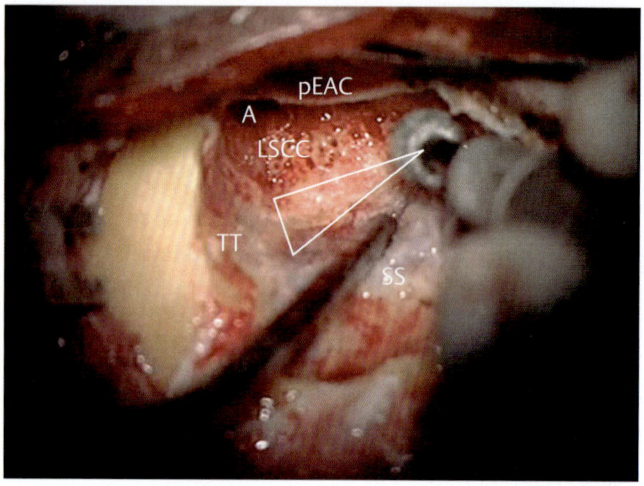

Fig. 54.3 The posterior external auditory canal wall (pEAC), tegmen tympani (TT), sigmoid sinus (SS), sinodural angle (SDA), antrum (A), and the lateral semicircular canal (LSCC) were identified. An extended mastoidectomy is then performed with the removal of presigmoid air cells in the Trautmann's triangle and using a diamond burr.

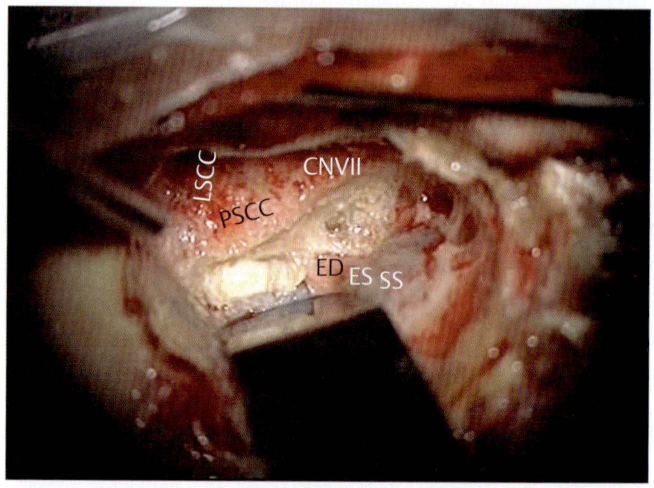

Fig. 54.4 The sigmoid sinus (SS) is compressed and the endolymphatic duct (ED) and sac (ES) are identified. The mastoid segment of the facial nerve (CNVII), lateral (LSCC) and the posterior semicircular canal (PSCC) are also skeletonized.

7. Drilling of the infralabyrinthine air cell tract is developed anteriorly using a diamond burr, which will lead to the petrous apex and the cholesterol granuloma (**Fig. 54.5**), which typically appears as a brownish cystic lesion.
8. The cholesterol granuloma cavity is opened, and the brownish liquid is removed with suction. The cavity is irrigated with warm normal saline 0.9% solution using a suction catheter (**Fig. 54.6**). Surgical drainage and aeration of the cavity are the ultimate aim of this operation to prevent the recurrence of cholesterol granuloma in this region. Therefore, in the end, the opening is enlarged, and the cavity is left open for drainage (**Fig. 54.7**).
9. Surgical site is then closed in layers and a compression mastoid dressing is placed.

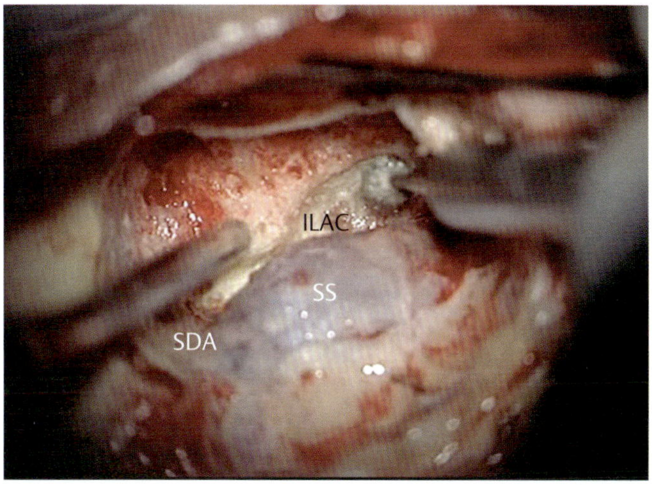

Fig. 54.5 Drilling of the infralabyrinthine air cells (ILAC), which will lead to the petrous apex and the cholesterol granuloma.

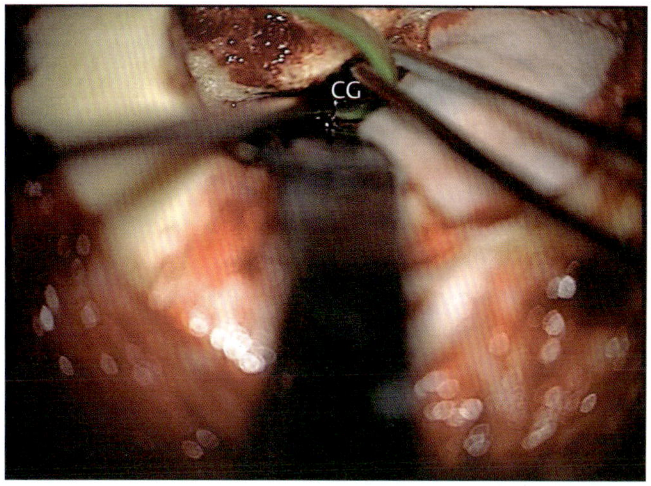

Fig. 54.6 Brownish liquid removed with suction. The cholesterol granuloma (CG) cavity is irrigated with warm normal saline 0.9% solution using a suction catheter.

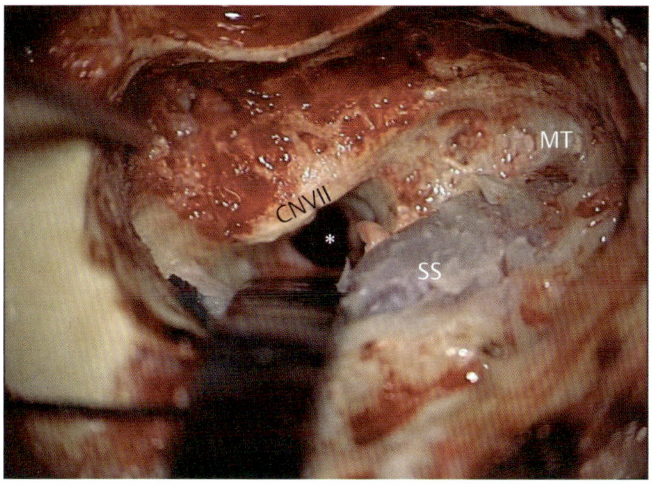

Fig. 54.7 The opening of the cavity (*white asterisk*) is enlarged and left open for drainage.

Section XXI

Presigmoid Approach

Chapter 55 Presigmoid Retrolabyrinthine Approach

Michel Roethlisberger, Vicknes Waran, and Prepageran Narayanan

Indications

The extension of the classical retrosigmoid approach is characterized by bony skeletonization of the dural sinuses to widen the dural exposure, and might even be supplemented by an additional mastoidectomy.[1]

The presigmoid retrolabyrinthine approach offers a hearing-preserving alternative by exposing the presigmoid dura of the posterior fossa behind the semicircular canals and the basal temporal fossa dura, interconnected by the superior petrosal sinus and the tentorium cerebelli.[2–8] This approach consists of three relevant steps:

1. Mastoidectomy
2. Skeletonization of the sigmoid sinus
3. Exposure of the presigmoid dura

With the division of the sinodural angle and the superior petrosal sinus, splitting of the tentorium cerebelli is possible.[1–9] With these extensions, areas ventral to the brainstem and near the tentorium cerebelli are reachable.[2–8] The posterior surface of the petrous bone and the cisternal portions of the cerebellopontine angle nerves (seventh and eighth nerve) can be exposed with a minimal degree of cerebellar retraction.[2–8,10] However, the internal auditory canal or petrous apex are without reach when using this approach, because of the preservation of the labyrinthine and cochlear structures within the petrous bone.[1–9]

Surgical Steps

1. After general anesthesia, the patient is placed in a supine position with the head rotated contralaterally and slightly elevated with minimal lateroflexion to the contralateral side.
2. The patient is supported with the aid of sandbags underneath the ipsilateral shoulder and thorax.
3. The patient's head is fixed using a Mayfield clamp with one pin placed on the forehead and two pins placed just off the midline of the occiput on each side.
4. Head positioning should allow for the region superior to the pinna and the mastoid to be horizontal and the highest point in the surgical field to be exposed (**Fig. 55.1**).
5. Intraoperative neuromonitoring of the cranial nerves is installed by standard means described in the literature (V, VI, VII, IX, X, XI, XII, acoustic evoked potentials [AEPs], motor evoked potentials [MEPs], sensory evoked potentials [SEPs]).
6. A classical C-shaped skin incision is used for this approach. The flap should allow for enough exposure of the sigmoid and transverse-sigmoid junction as well as the asterion, the confluence of the lambdoid, occipitomastoid, and parietomastoid sutures (**Fig. 55.1**).
7. A myocutaneous flap is raised in a double-layered fashion with identification of the external acoustic meatus, mastoid groove, and mastoid process (**Fig. 55.2**).
8. After identification and sufficient exposure of the relevant landmarks, a partial mastoidectomy is performed in a right triangle fashion oriented posteriorly to the external auditory canal with the aid of a large cutting burr (**Fig. 55.3**).
9. The sigmoid sinus and the transverse-sigmoid junction are consecutively skeletonized, and the presigmoidal dura is exposed (**Fig. 55.4**).
10. The dura of the middle temporal fossa is exposed and freed from the overlying bone indicating the location of the sinodural angle and the superior petrosal sinus (**Fig. 55.5**).

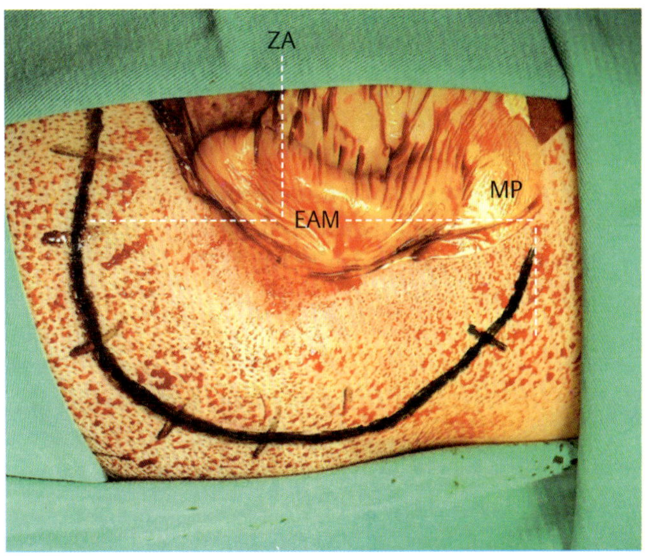

Fig. 55.1 C-shaped retroauricular skin incision. Superiorly, the incision should start at least at the level of the pinna. Inferoposteriorly, the incision should end approximately inferior to the mastoid process (MP).

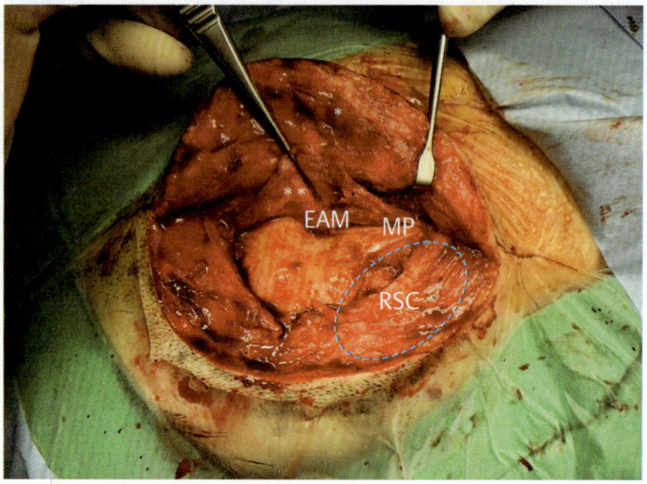

Fig. 55.2 Elevation of the myocutaneous flap in a double-layered fashion. Following skin incision, the subcutaneous flap (*) is separated from the pericranial layer using sharp dissection. The pericranial flap (**) is then elevated in a C-shaped fashion using subperiosteal dissection techniques. Tissue dissection involves exposure of the external acoustic meatus (EAM) and detachment of the sternocleidomastoid and splenius capitis muscle from the mastoid process (MP) along its posterior and lateral aspects. Both flaps are folded anteriorly and fixed. Retrosigmoid craniotomy (RSC) from a previous surgery for the staged resection of a petrous apex meningioma (*blue line*).

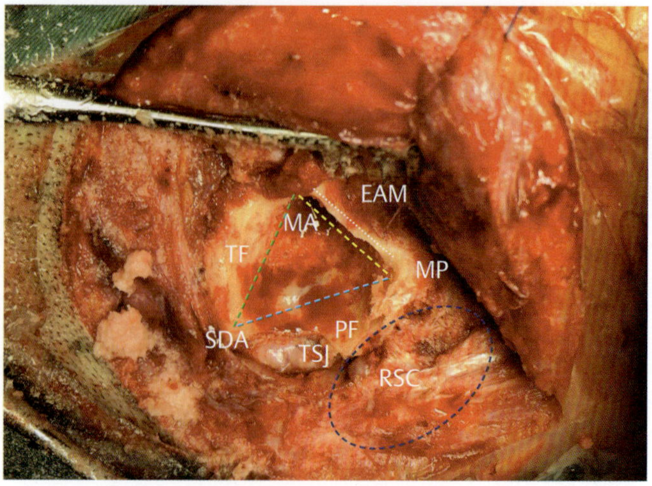

Fig. 55.3 Mastoidectomy. The bony removal is started with a large cutting burr. The anterior triangular opening (*yellow line*) is oriented toward the external acoustic meatus (EAM). The suprameatal spine (spine of Henle), running posterior and superior (*white line*), delineates the orientation of the triangular opening. This orientation allows the estimation of the mastoid antrum (MA), an air space communicating with the mastoid cells posteriorly and with the epitympanic recess anteriorly, containing the semicircular canals and the facial nerve within the fallopian canal. The superior triangular thigh (*green line*) is oriented toward the temporal fossa bone (TF) covering the middle fossa dura. The inferior triangular thigh (*light blue line*) is oriented toward the posterior fossa bone (PF) covering the presigmoid dura. The anterior triangular line (*yellow line*) hence interconnects the temporal fossa bone at its most anterior aspect of the superior triangular thigh (*yellow line*) with the most inferior aspect of the inferior triangular thigh (*light blue line*) at the mastoid process (MP). The superior and the inferior thigh of the triangle meet at the sinodural angle (SDA). Retrosigmoid craniotomy (RSC) is seen from a previous surgery for the staged resection of a petrous apex meningioma (*dark blue line*).

11. The retrolabyrinthine bone is removed completely, and the sinodural angle is defined in its lateral aspect with exposition of the middle and presigmoid dura (**Fig. 55.6**).
12. The epitympanum and the bone overlying the sinodural angle are now removed moving medially using a high-speed diamond drill (**Fig. 55.7**).
13. When the bone covering the labyrinth is removed, the semicircular canals below a protective very hard bone layer are delineated (**Fig. 55.7**).
14. With removal of the medial aspect of bony covering, the dura of the middle fossa, the sinodural angle, and the presigmoid posterior fossa are completely exposed (**Fig. 55.8** and **Fig. 55.9**).
15. The dural incision has a C-shaped form around the labyrinth.
16. The posterior fossa dura is incised, and cerebrospinal fluid (CSF) is released to relax the surgical field (**Fig. 55.10**).
17. The temporal fossa dura is incised, and CSF is released to relax the surgical field (**Fig. 55.11**).
18. The sinodural angle is clip-ligated including the superior petrosal sinus. This is a crucial step when splitting of the tentorium cerebelli is necessary (**Fig. 55.12, Fig. 55.13** and **Fig. 55.14**).
19. Lesions along the middle fossa floor, petrous apex, the posterior petrosal surface, and ventral to the brainstem can be visualized and resected accordingly (**Fig. 55.15, Fig. 55.16, Fig. 55.17, Fig. 55.18**, and **Fig. 55.19**).

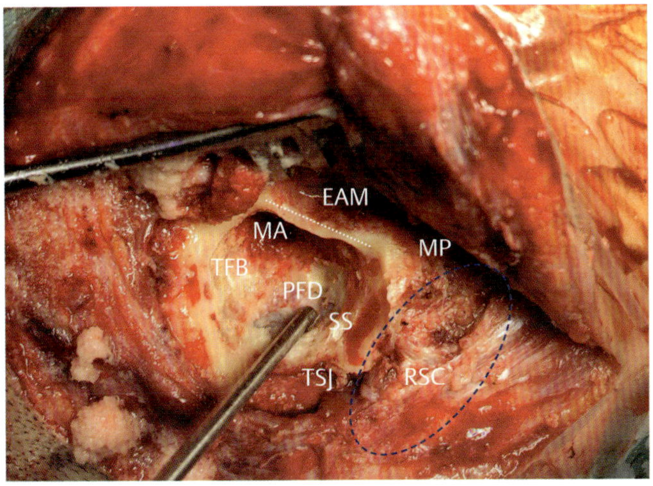

Fig. 55.4 Exposition of the presigmoidal dura after skeletonization of the sigmoid sinus (SS). Suprameatal spine (spine of Henle) (*white line*), retrosigmoid craniotomy (RSC) from a previous surgery for the staged resection of a petrous apex meningioma (*blue line*).

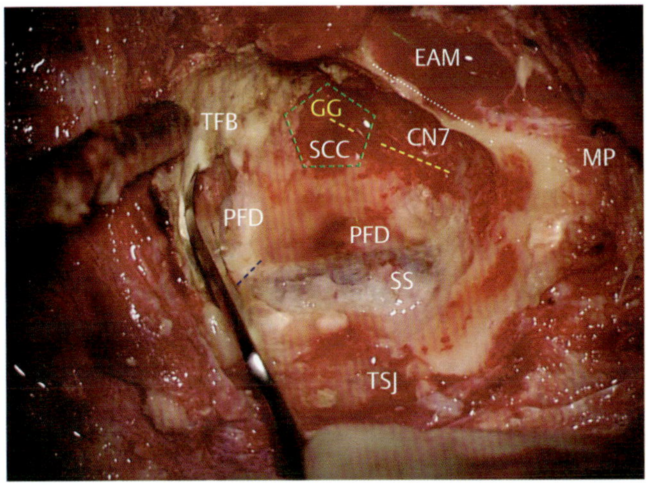

Fig. 55.5 Exposition of the middle temporal fossa dura (TFD) after drilling of the temporal fossa bone (TFB) and estimation of the sinodural angle containing the superior petrosal sinus (*blue line*), which is still covered by a thin bony layer. The suprameatal spine (spine of Henle) (*white line*), labyrinth (*green line*), facial nerve (CN 7) within the fallopian canal (*yellow line*) are seen.

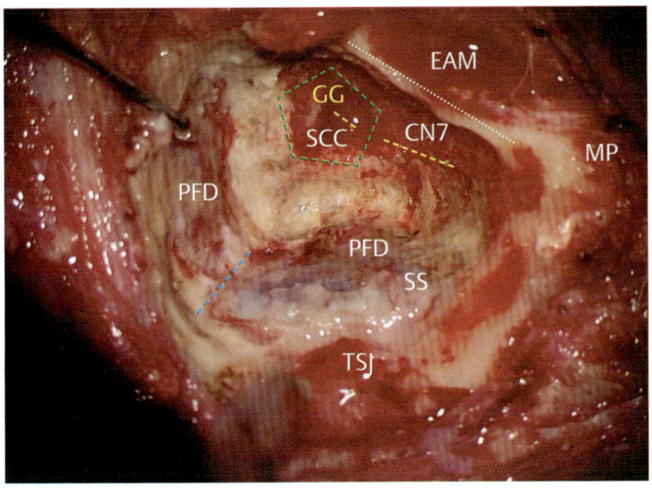

Fig. 55.6 By removing the retrolabyrinthine bone covering the presigmoid posterior fossa dura (PFD) and the bone covering the junction to the temporal fossa dura (TFD), the sinodural angle containing the superior petrosal sinus in its lateral aspect is exposed (*blue line*). The suprameatal spine (spine of Henle) (*white line*), labyrinth (*green line*), facial nerve (CN 7) within the fallopian canal (*yellow line*) are seen.

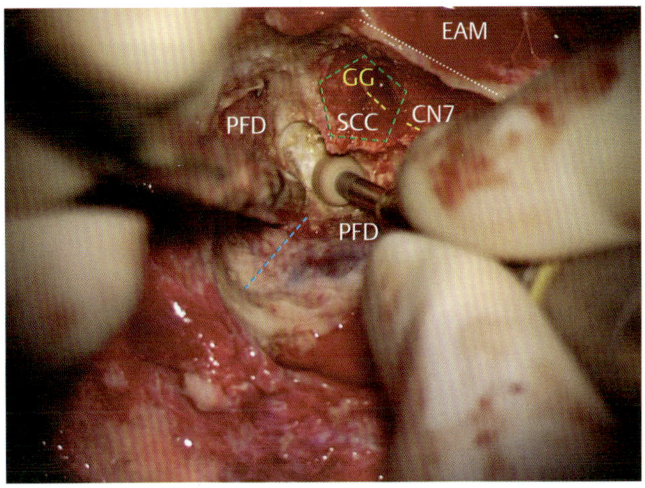

Fig. 55.7 Removal of the epitympanum and the bone overlying the medial aspect of the sinodural angle containing the superior petrosal sinus (*blue line*) using a high-speed diamond drill. The labyrinth (*green line*) and the semicircular canals (SCC) below are delineated, but the protective very hard bone is preserved. The fallopian canal is located anterior and inferior to the bony labyrinth. Suprameatal spine (spine of Henle) (*white line*), nerve (CN 7) within the fallopian canal (*yellow line*).

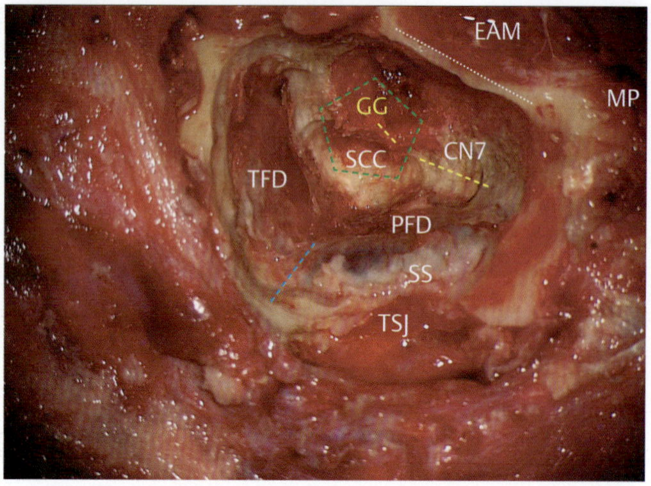

Fig. 55.8 Complete exposition of the dura covering the middle fossa (TFD) and the sinodural angle containing the superior petrosal sinus (*blue line*). The triangular shape of the mastoidectomy can be appreciated. Labyrinth (*green line*), facial nerve (CN 7) within the fallopian canal (*yellow line*).

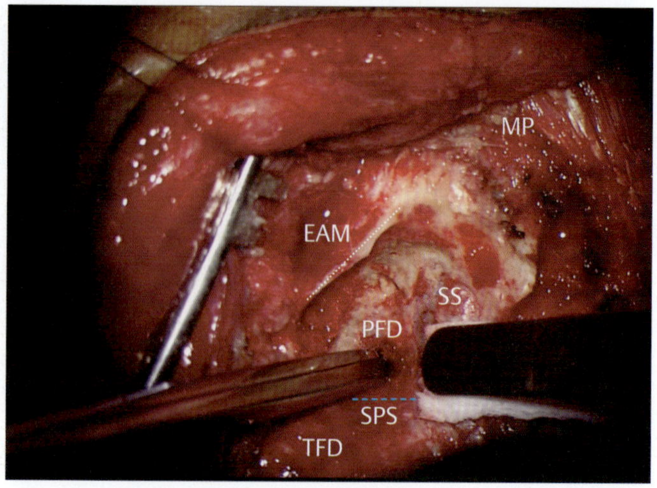

Fig. 55.9 Complete exposition of the dura covering the middle fossa (TFD) and the sinodural angle containing the superior petrosal sinus (*blue line*). The presigmoid posterior fossa dura (PFD) can be exposed down to the jugular bulb. Removal of bone can be extended below the facial nerve within the fallopian canal, which is located anterior and inferior to the bony labyrinth. Suprameatal spine (spine of Henle) (*white line*).

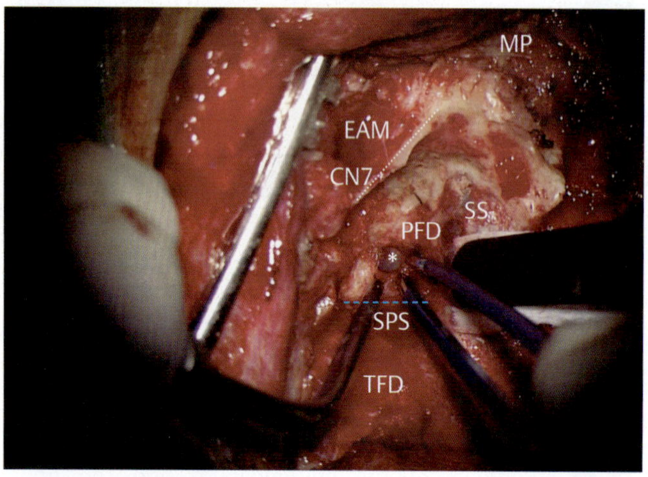

Fig. 55.10 Dural incision of the posterior fossa dura (PFD) as the first step to divide the sinodural angle (*blue line*) containing the superior petrosal sinus (SPS) and splitting the tentorium cerebelli. The arachnoid of the posterior fossa (*) is visible. Suprameatal spine (spine of Henle) (*white line*).

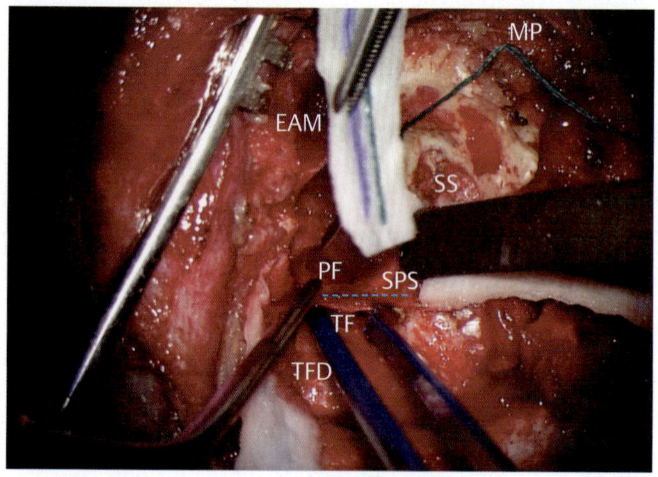

Fig. 55.11 Dural incision of the temporal fossa dura (TFD) as the second step to divide the sinodural angle (*blue line*) containing the superior petrosal sinus (SPS) and splitting the tentorium cerebelli.

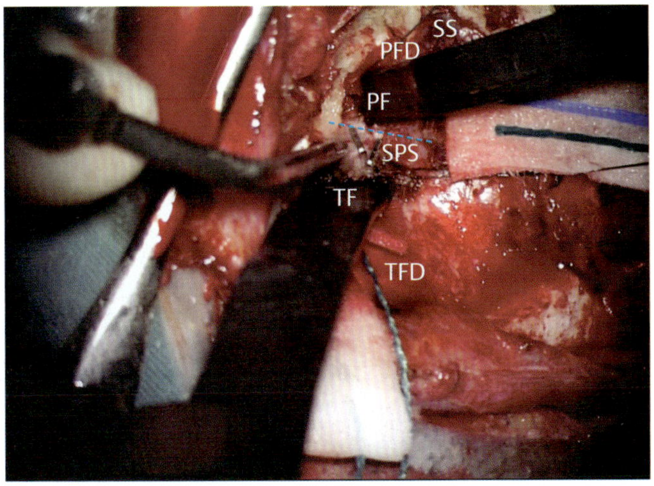

Fig. 55.12 Clip ligation of the superior petrosal sinus (SPS) prior to the division of the sinodural angle (*blue line*).

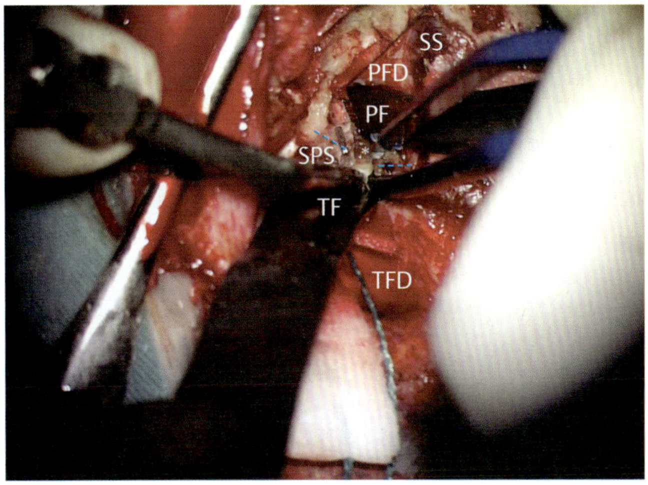

Fig. 55.13 Cauterization and division of the sinodural angle (*blue line*) and the superior petrosal sinus (SPS). The tentorium cerebelli (*asterisk*) is visible and is divided starting from a lateral to medial direction.

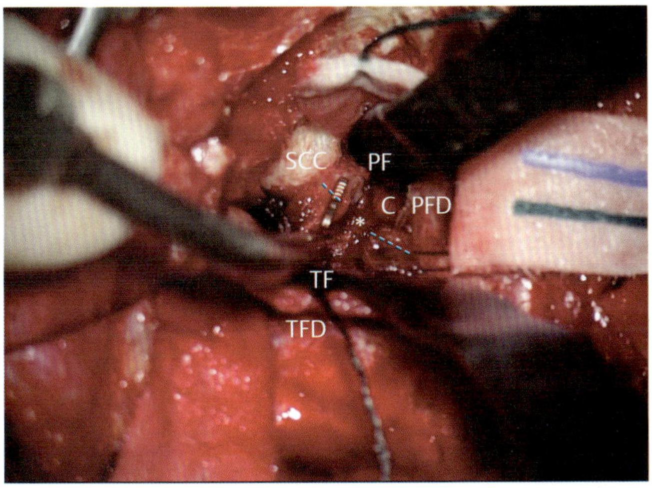

Fig. 55.14 The tentorium cerebelli (*) can be divided starting from a lateral to medial direction. Sinodural angle (*blue line*).

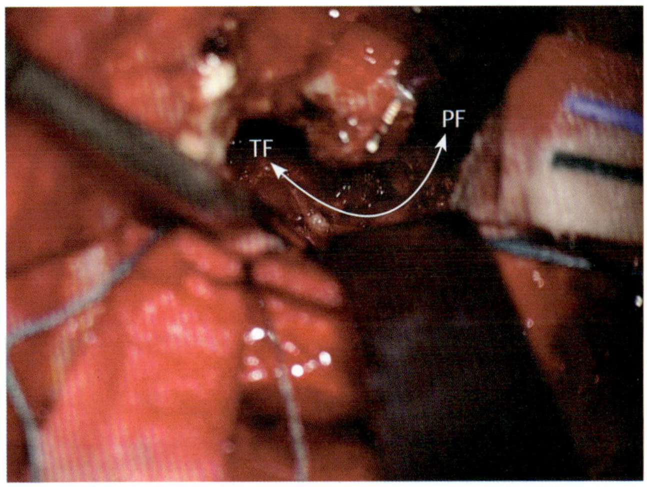

Fig. 55.15 Exposition and debulking of a petrous apex meningioma involving the middle fossa and the petroclival region. After tentorial division, the presigmoid retrolabyrinthine approach allows to expose the whole lesion within the posterior fossa (PF) and temporal fossa (TF).

References

1. Quiñones-Hinojosa A, Chang EF, Lawton MT. The extended retrosigmoid approach: an alternative to radical cranial base approaches for posterior fossa lesions. Neurosurgery 2006; 58(4, Suppl 2):ONS-208–ONS-214, discussion ONS-214
2. Alonso F, Dekker SE, Wright J, et al. The retrolabyrinthine presigmoid approach to the anterior cerebellopontine region: expanding the limits of Trautmann triangle. World Neurosurg 2017;104:180–185
3. Hao X, Li Y, Cui D, Chen B, Liu Y, Yang B. Anatomical study of presigmoid-retrolabyrinthine approach based on temporal bone high-resolution CT. Acta Otolaryngol 2019;139(2): 117–121
4. Kirazli T, Oner K, Ovül L, Bilgen C, Ogüt F. Petrosal presigmoid approach to the petro-clival and anterior cerebellopontine region (extended retrolabyrinthine, transtentorial approach). Rev Laryngol Otol Rhinol (Bord) 2001;122(3):187–190
5. Sassun TE, Ruggeri AG, Delfini R. True petroclival meningiomas: proposal of classification and role of the

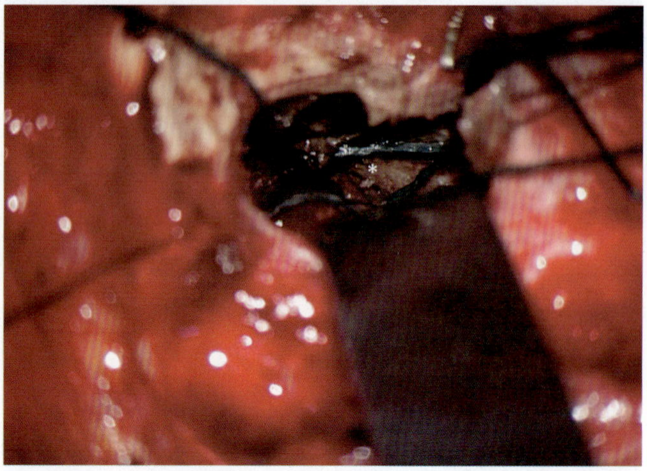

Fig. 55.16 After devascularization and resection of the middle fossa compartment of the petrous apex meningioma, the surface of the tentorium cerebelli (*) is visible.

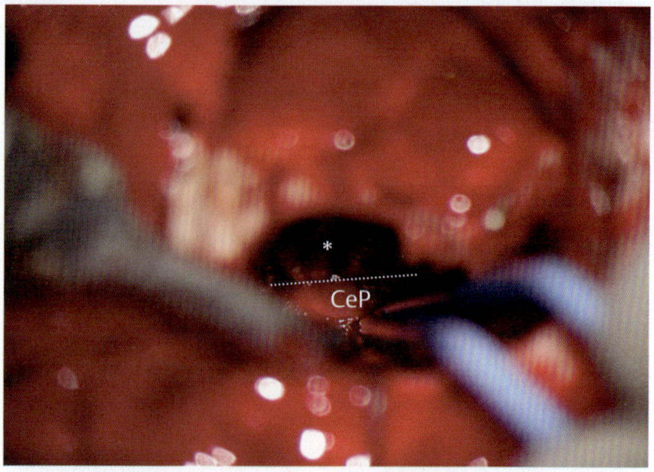

Fig. 55.17 When reaching the tentorial edge (*white line*), the cerebral peduncle (CeP) can be visualized. The temporal lobe is displaced superiorly by the tumor.

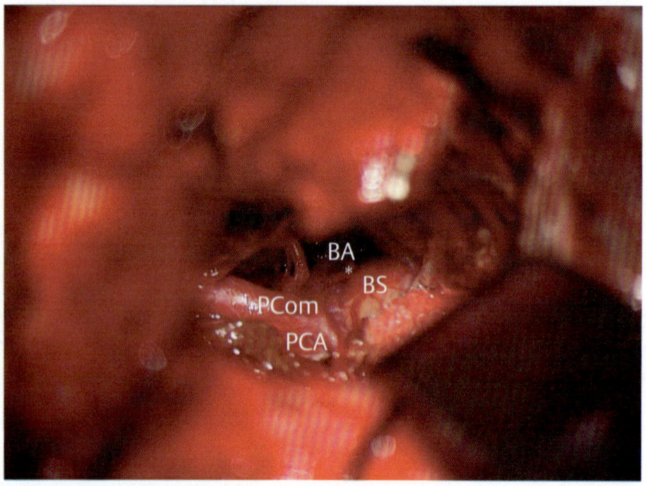

Fig. 55.18 Final view of the posterior fossa ventral to the brainstem after resection of a petrous apex meningioma using the presigmoid retrolabyrinthine approach. Brainstem perforator (*).

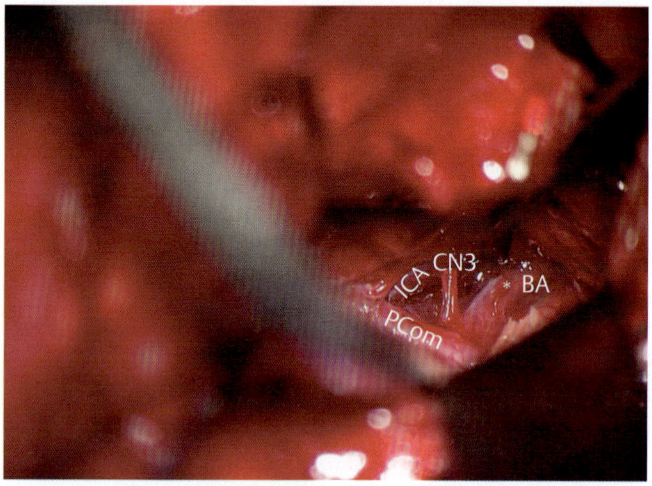

Fig. 55.19 Final view of the opened anterior ambient and carotid cistern ventral to the brainstem after resection of a petrous apex meningioma using the presigmoid retrolabyrinthine approach. Brainstem perforator (*).

combined supra-infratentorial presigmoid retrolabyrinthine approach. World Neurosurg 2016;96:111–123

6. Shelton C, Alavi S, Li JC, Hitselberger WE. Modified retrosigmoid approach: use for selected acoustic tumor removal. Am J Otol 1995;16(5):664–668
7. Goksu N, Yilmaz M, Bayramoglu I, Bayazit YA. Combined retrosigmoid retrolabyrinthine vestibular nerve section: results of our experience over 10 years. Otol Neurotol 2005;26(3):481–483
8. Russell SM, Roland JT Jr, Golfinos JG. Retrolabyrinthine craniectomy: the unsung hero of skull base surgery. Skull Base 2004;14(1):63–71, discussion 71
9. Lang J Jr, Samii A. Retrosigmoidal approach to the posterior cranial fossa. An anatomical study. Acta Neurochir (Wien) 1991;111(3-4):147–153
10. Rhoton AL Jr. The cerebellopontine angle and posterior fossa cranial nerves by the retrosigmoid approach. Neurosurgery 2000;47(3, Suppl):S93–S129

Section XXII

Management of Glomus Tumors/ Approaches to Jugular Foramen

Chapter 56 Glomus Tympanicum Tumors

Narayan Jayashankar

Indications

Glomus class A tumors (glomus tympanicum A1 and A2.)

Class A tumors: Tumors limited to middle ear cleft without invasion of hypotympanum.

Class A1: Tumor margins completely visible on otoscopic examination.

Class A2: Tumor margins are not visualized on otoscopic examination. The tumor may extend anteriorly to eustachian tube orifice or to posterior mesotympanum.

Surgical Steps

1. Class A1 tumors can be dealt with by a transcanal approach while for class A2 tumors, a postaural approach is better. Computed tomography (CT) scan of a class A2 tumor is depicted in **Fig. 56.1a, b** along with the surgical steps.
2. Postaural incision is taken from the superior pole of the helix to mastoid tip. Skin and subcutaneous tissue are elevated up to the external auditory canal leaving behind the musculoperiosteal layer.
3. A circumferential incision is taken along the bony external auditory canal including superior, posterior, and inferior canal walls.
4. A meatotomy is made just medial to the lateral end of the bony external auditory canal, that is, just medial to the spine of Henle. This is a circumferential meatotomy including all quadrants, approximately 7 to 8 mm lateral to the annulus. The red mass behind the tympanic membrane is visualized (**Fig. 56.2**).
5. The tympanomeatal flap is elevated including annulus in almost 80% circumference leaving the attachment of anterosuperior annulus intact. The tympanomeatal flap is sharply dissected over the handle of the malleus during elevation. This elevation is preferred in class A1 tumors. However, in class A2 tumors, the entire cuff of tympanomeatal flap can be excised and kept in saline to be placed back after the tumor excision. This is specifically done to avoid the skin getting shredded while widening the bony meatus for class A2 tumors (**Fig. 56.3, Fig. 56.4, Fig. 56.5, Fig. 56.6, and Fig. 56.7**).
6. A canalplasty is performed to visualize the periphery of the tumor all around (**Fig. 56.8** and **Fig. 56.9**).
7. A bipolar coagulation of the surface of the tumor is performed which helps to shrink the tumor and facilitates dissection in a relatively bloodless field (**Fig. 56.10**). Care should be taken while using bipolar in the immediate vicinity of a dehiscent tympanic segment of the facial nerve.
8. The tumor is carefully dissected off from between ossicles without disrupting the ossicles. Dissection is usually performed in superior to inferior direction (**Fig. 56.11**).

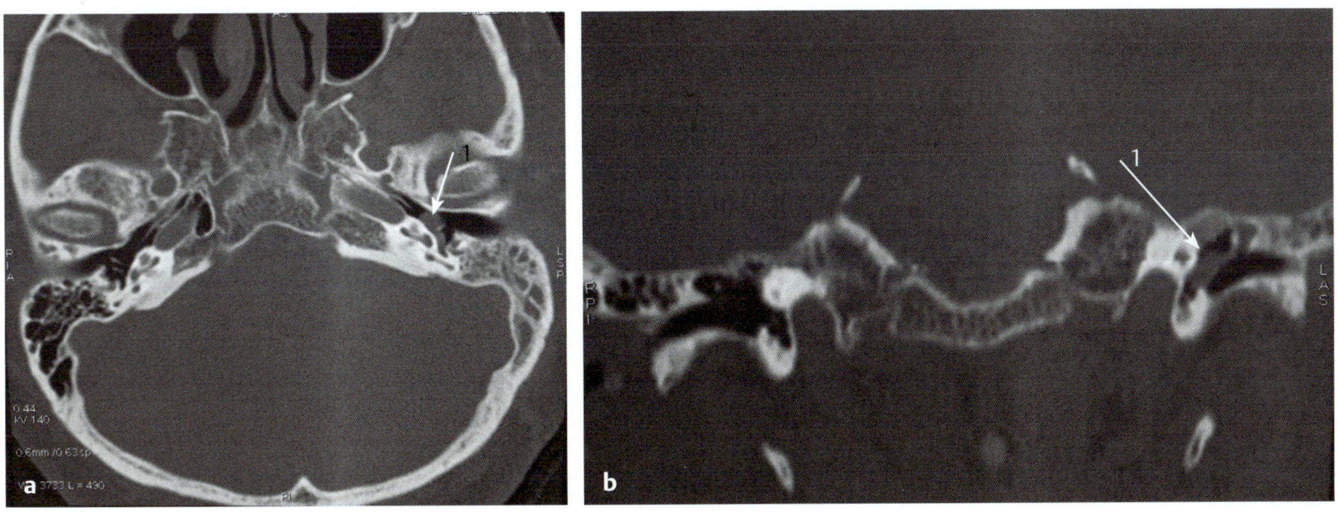

Fig. 56.1 CT scans in **(a)** axial and **(b)** coronal planes showing a left class A2 glomus tympanicum tumor for which a postaural approach is described below.

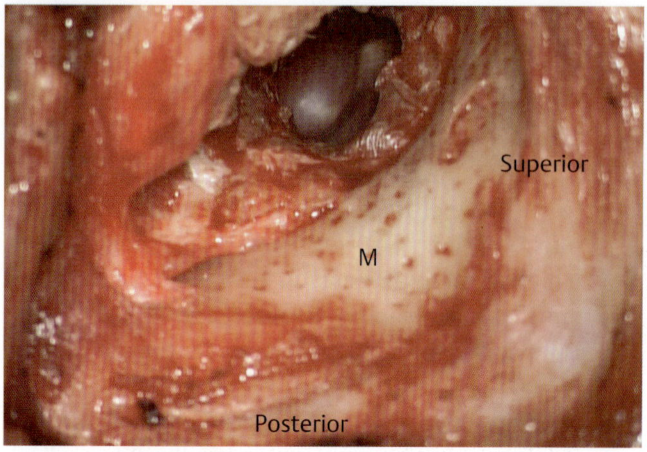

Fig. 56.2 Left ear—Meatotomy just medial to the spine of Henle level.

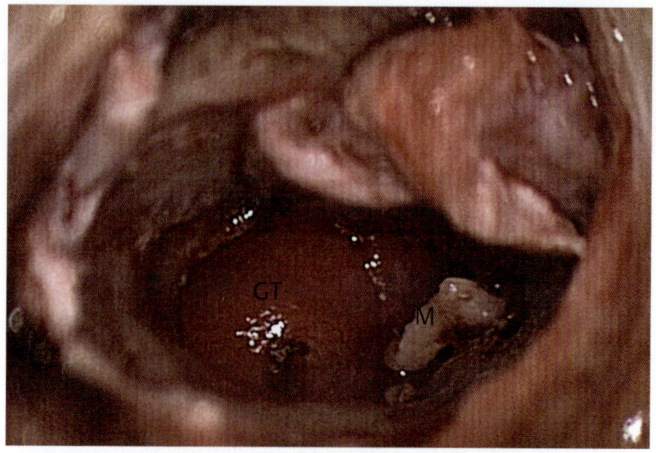

Fig. 56.3 Tympanomeatal flap elevated below annulus in around 80% circumference in class A1 tumors.

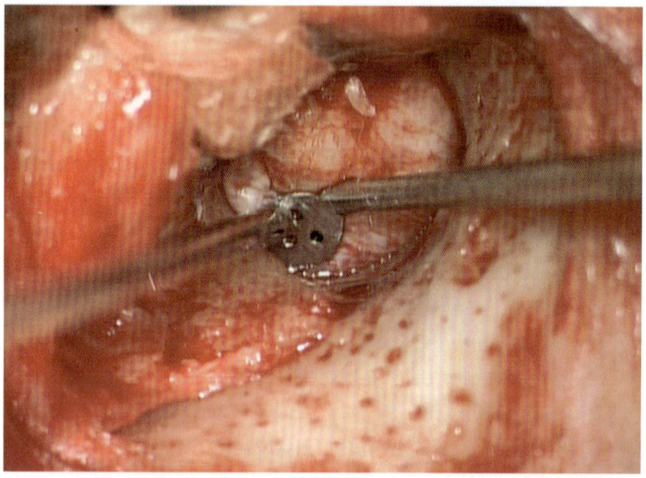

Fig. 56.4 Tympanomeatal flap elevated toward the annulus.

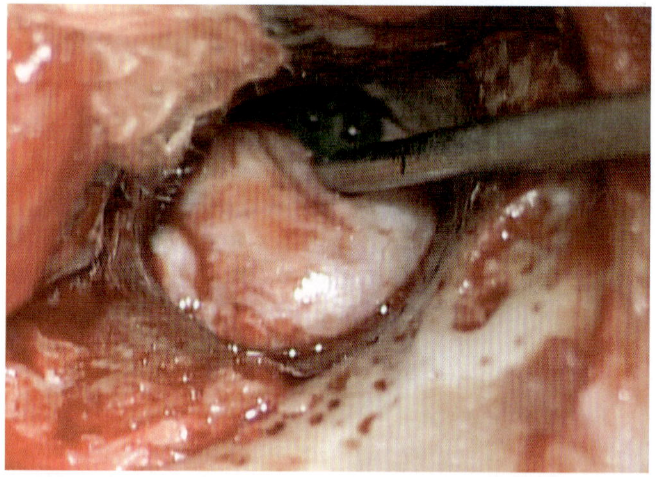

Fig. 56.5 Shows circumferential elevation of 360 degrees of the tympanomeatal flap including annulus.

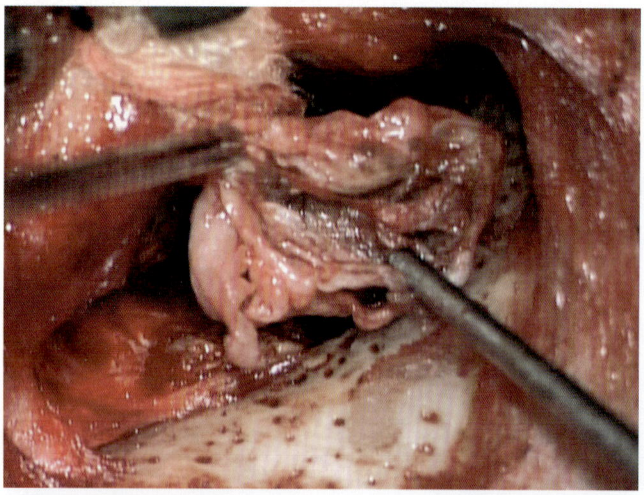

Fig. 56.6 The whole cuff of the skin of bony external auditory canal (EAC) including the annulus is taken out and placed in saline.

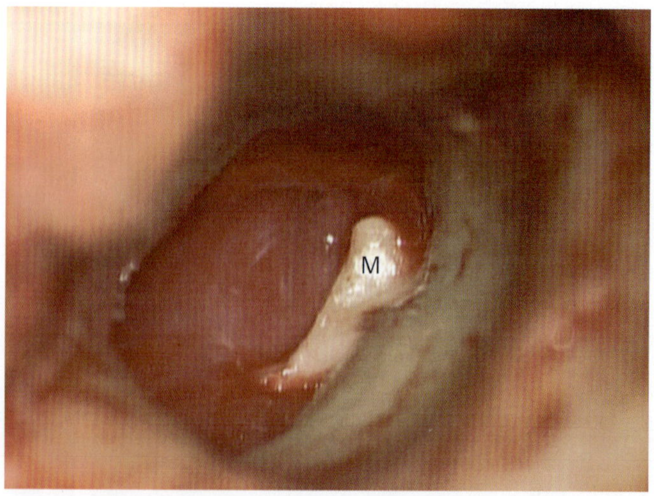

Fig. 56.7 Glomus tympanicum tumor is seen in the middle ear. Margins of tumor are not visible (class A2).

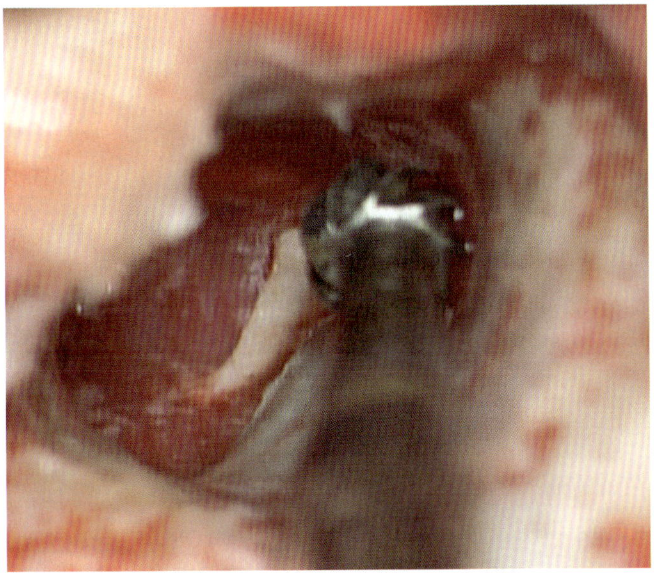

Fig. 56.8 Widening of the external auditory meatus to visualize the tumor periphery.

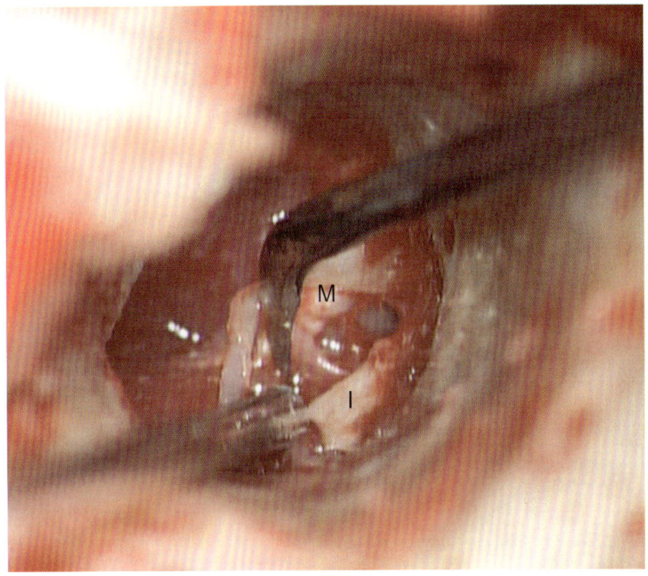

Fig. 56.9 Tumor periphery is seen in all quadrants as also the complete ossicular chain.

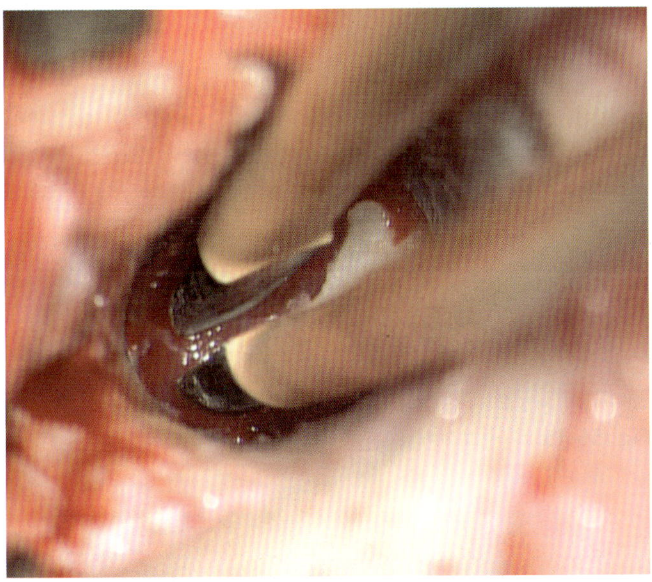

Fig. 56.10 Bipolar coagulation on the surface of the tumor.

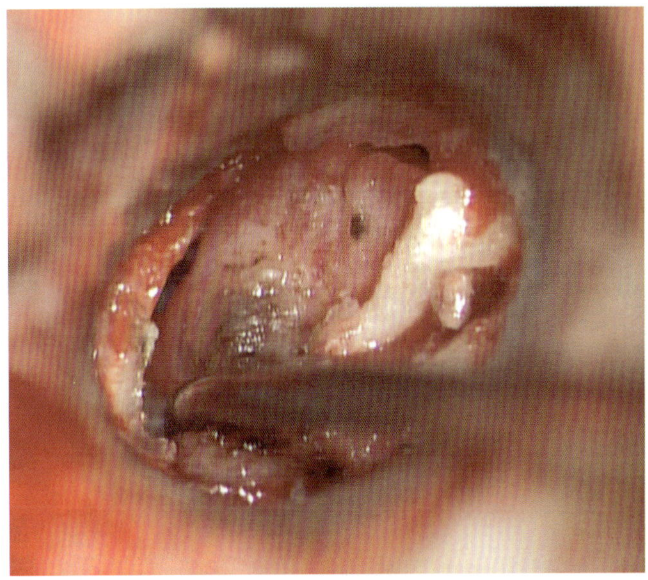

Fig. 56.11 A combination of bipolar coagulation on the surface and widening of the bony meatus helps identify the margins of the tumor.

9. The area on the promontory where the tumor arises is identified, bipolarized, and the tumor is excised (**Fig. 56.12, Fig. 56.13, Fig. 56.14, and Fig. 56.15**).
10. In cases of ossicular disruption by the tumor, an ossiculoplasty is performed.
11. A temporalis fascia graft is harvested and placed as an underlay graft. The tympanomeatal flap is replaced (**Fig. 56.16** and **Fig. 56.17**).
12. Gelfoam packing is used in the external auditory canal.
13. Postaural incision is closed.

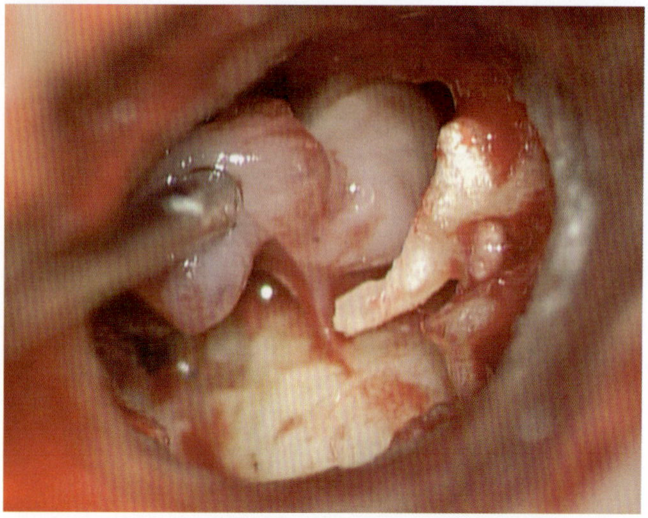

Fig. 56.12 Feeder vessels from promontory are seen.

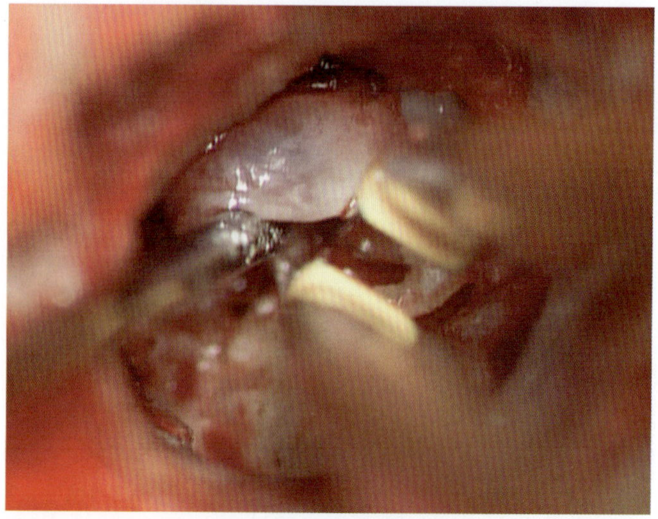

Fig. 56.13 Feeder vessels from promontory are bipolarized.

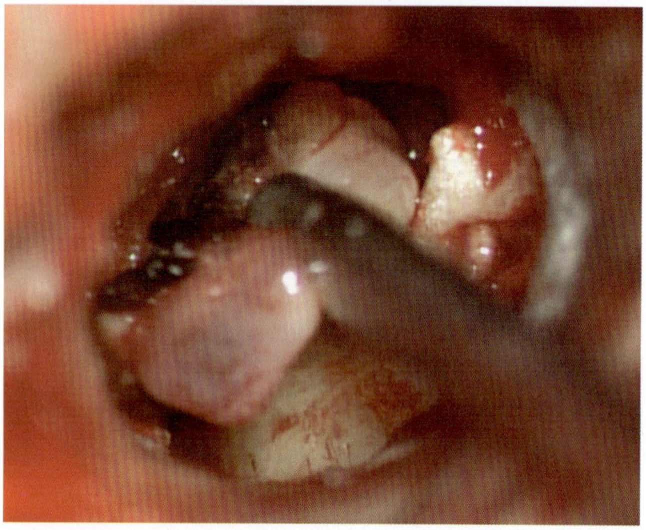

Fig. 56.14 Tumor excised in toto.

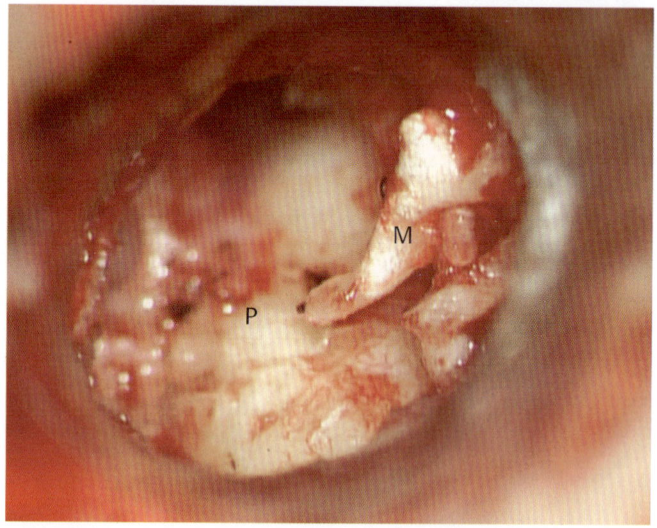

Fig. 56.15 Middle ear after tumor excision.

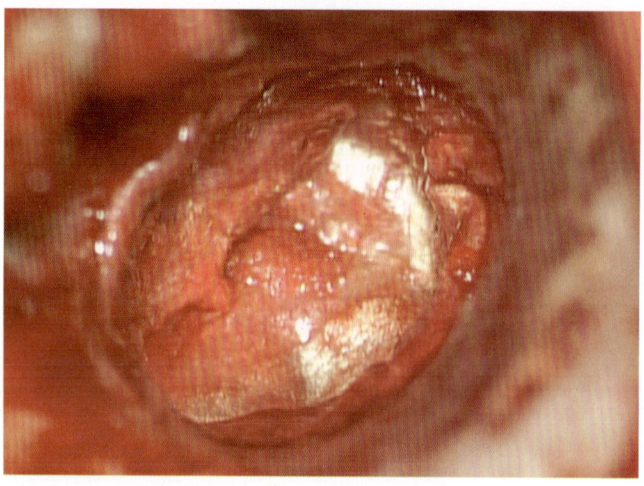

Fig. 56.16 Temporalis fascia graft is placed.

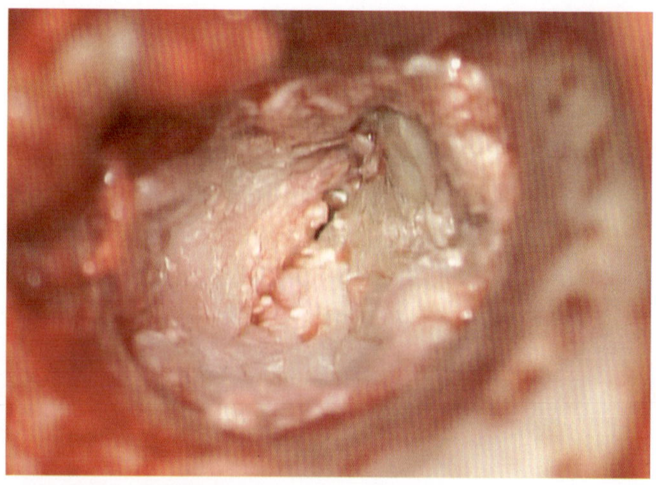

Fig. 56.17 The tympanomeatal skin cuff is replaced over the fascia graft.

Tips and Pearls

- Widening of the bony external auditory canal beyond the margins of the tumor is vital to expose and thus, excise the tumor completely.
- The tumor is preferably removed in a single piece rather than piecemeal.
- If ossicular discontinuity is present, it is addressed in the same stage.

Suggested Readings

Alaani A, Chavda SV, Irving RM. The crucial role of imaging in determining the approach to glomus tympanicum tumours. Eur Arch Otorhinolaryngol 2009;266(6): 827–831

Carlson ML, Sweeney AD, Pelosi S, Wanna GB, Glasscock ME 3rd, Haynes DS. Glomus tympanicum: a review of 115 cases over 4 decades. Otolaryngol Head Neck Surg 2015; 152(1):136–142

Rohit, Jain Y, Caruso A, Russo A, Sanna M. Glomus tympanicum tumour: an alternative surgical technique. J Laryngol Otol 2003;117(6):462–466

Sanna M, Fois P, Pasanisi E, Russo A, Bacciu A. Middle ear and mastoid glomus tumors (glomus tympanicum): an algorithm for the surgical management. Auris Nasus Larynx 2010; 37(6):661–668

Chapter 57

Management of Class B1 and B2 Temporal Bone Paragangliomas (Glomus Tumors)

Narayan Jayashankar

Introduction

Paragangliomas that arise from the tympanic canaliculus and extend into the middle ear or mastoid are classified as Class B tumors according to the modified Fisch classification. These tumors do not arise from the jugular bulb and hence the area of jugular bulb on scans appears intact in these cases. Depending on their extent of growth, they are further subclassified as follows:

- B1: Tumors confined to the middle ear cleft with extension to the hypotympanum.
- B2: Tumors involving middle ear cleft with extension to the hypotympanum and the mastoid.
- B3: Tumors confined to the tympanomastoid compartment with erosion of the carotid canal.

The surgical approach depends on the extent of spread of the tumor and approaches to the above tumors are described below.

Class B1 Glomus Tumors

1. A subject having a left-sided B1 tumor is described below. **Fig. 57.1** depicts the computed tomography (CT) scan of the subject.
2. A postaural incision is made.
3. The skin of external auditory meatus is transected circumferentially at a level just medial to the spine of Henle (**Fig. 57.2**).
4. The tympanomeatal flap is dissected medially in all quadrants toward the annulus (**Fig. 57.3**) and subsequently removed as a complete cuff. It is placed in saline for replacement at the end of the procedure.
5. The tumor is seen in the middle ear extending inferiorly toward the hypotympanum (**Fig. 57.4**).
6. An aluminum foil is placed over the tumor to avoid traumatizing it with the burr (**Fig. 57.5**) with resultant oozing that may spoil the surgical field.

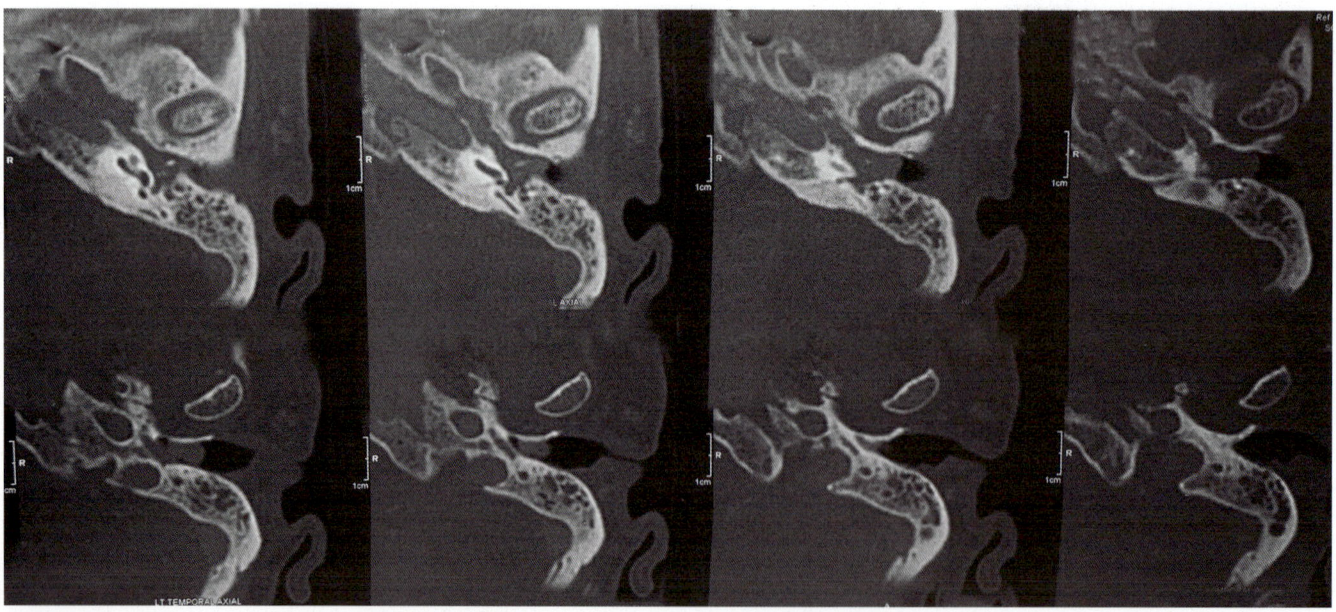

Fig. 57.1 CT scan shows tumor involving middle ear cleft with extension to the hypotympanum.

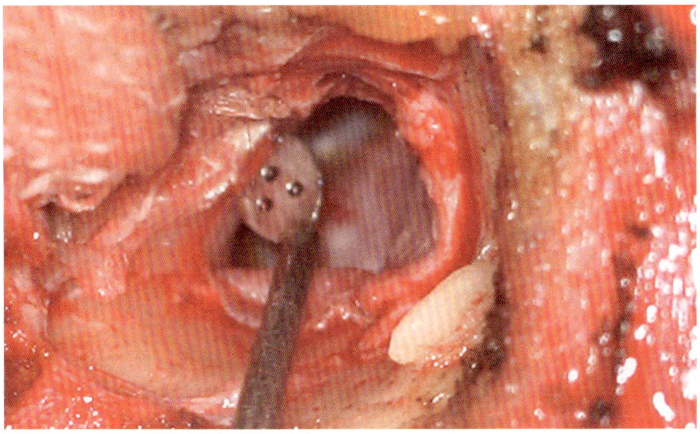

Fig. 57.2 Circumferential incision of the canal skin.

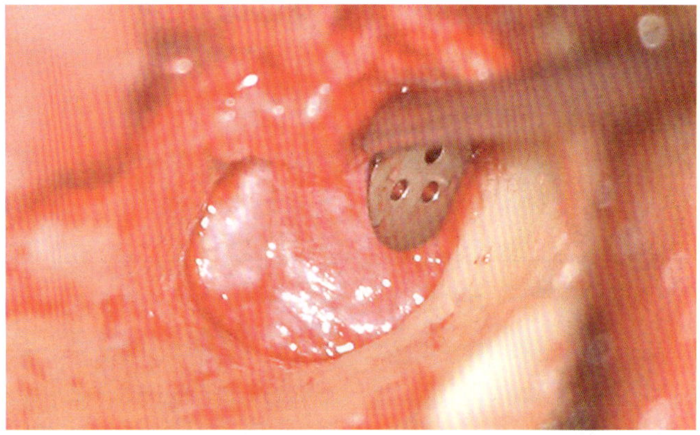

Fig. 57.3 Tympanomeatal flap elevated circumferentially from bone of external auditory canal (EAC).

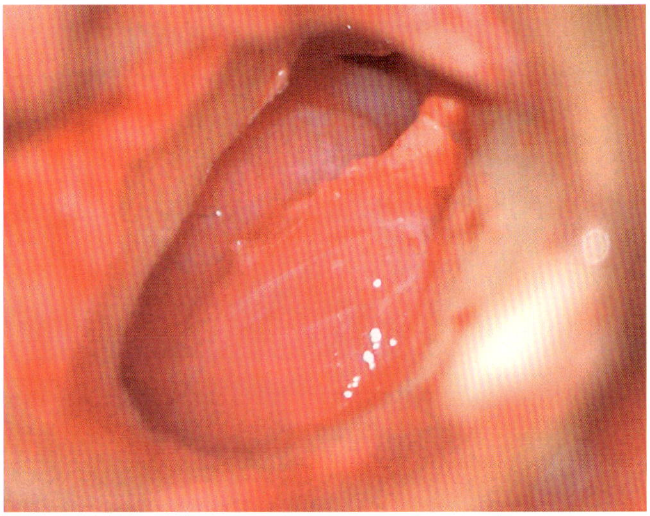

Fig. 57.4 Tumor seen in middle ear extending beyond the bony margins. Handle of malleus is visible lateral to the tumor.

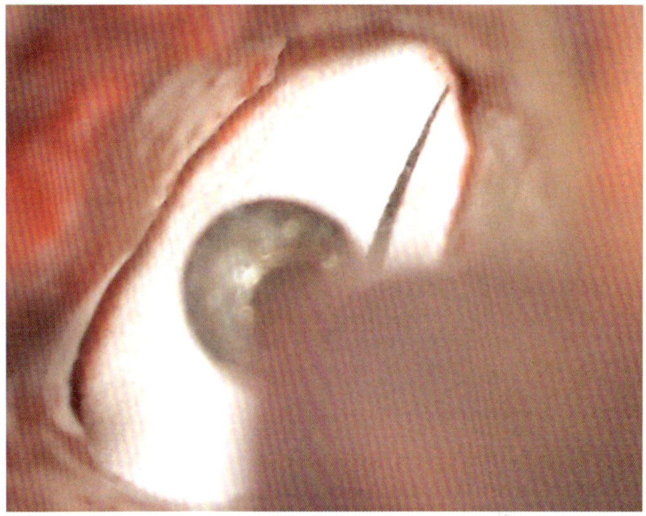

Fig. 57.5 Aluminum foil protection for drilling bony annulus.

7. The canal is widened inferiorly to expose the hypotympanum (**Fig. 57.6**). It is also widened posteriorly to expose sinus tympani, especially in cases of tumor extension in that area. Similarly, drilling the anterior canal wall exposes the tumor extension medial to the anterior bony annulus better. The usefulness of a good bony exposure to visualize the tumor cannot be overemphasized.
8. A bipolar cautery is used on the periphery of the tumor to shrink it marginally. This helps to gain access to the anterior (**Fig. 57.7**), inferior (**Fig. 57.8**), and posterior edges of the tumor.
9. The tumor is dissected off from the medial surface of the handle of malleus (**Fig. 57.9**), as also from around the incus and stapes (**Fig. 57.10**).

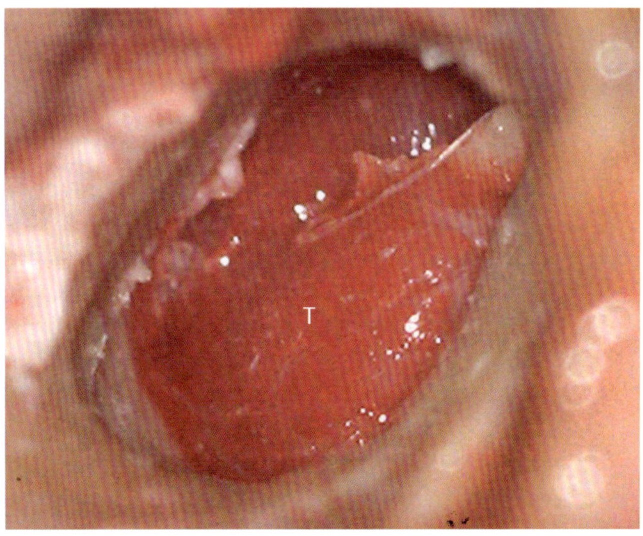

Fig. 57.6 Tumor extending to hypotympanum exposed. T, tumor.

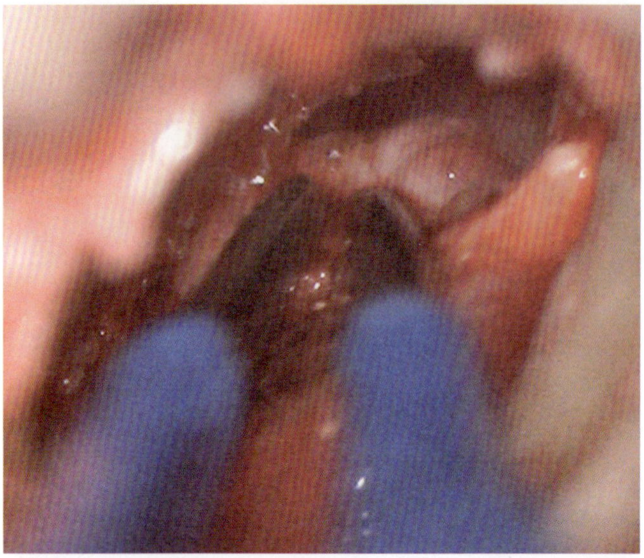

Fig. 57.7 Bipolar used on the surface of tumor. Anterior edge of tumor visualized.

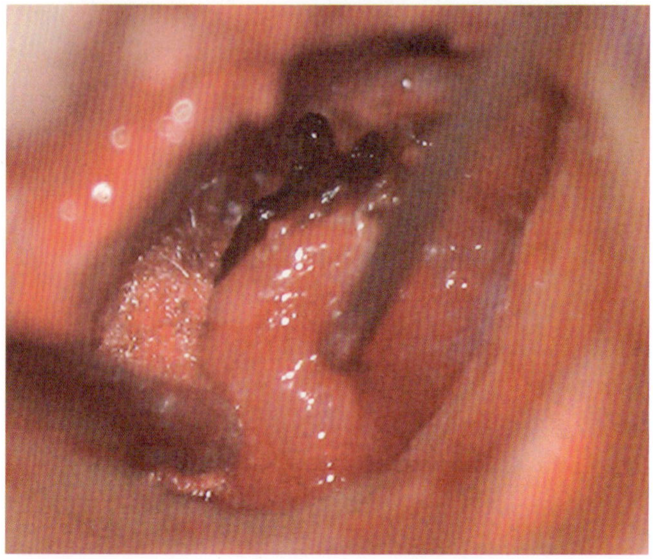

Fig. 57.8 Inferior edge of tumor in hypotympanum dissected off.

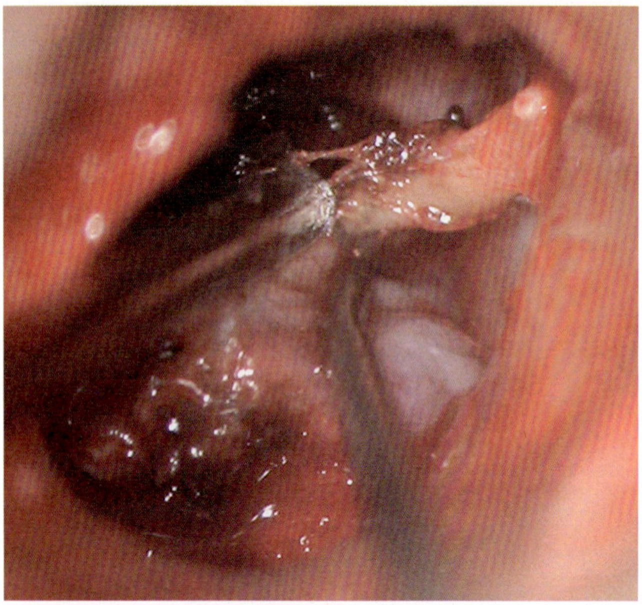

Fig. 57.9 Tumor separated from handle of malleus.

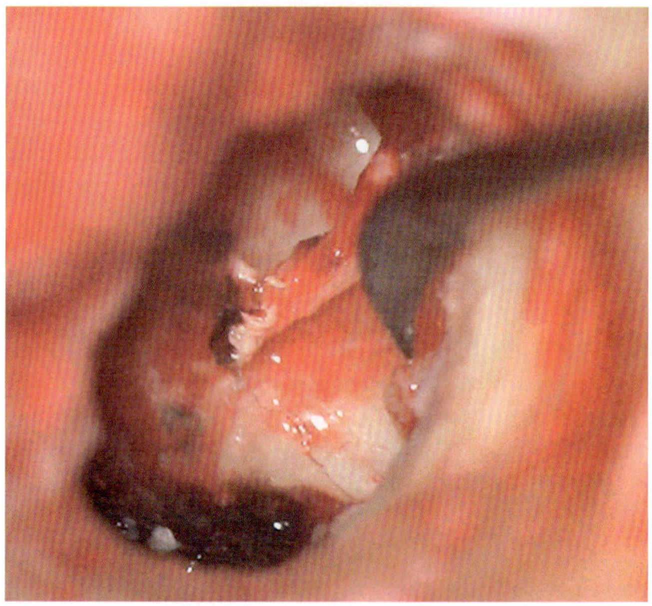

Fig. 57.10 Tumor cleared off the incudostapedial joint.

10. In case of difficulty in clearing tumor from the facial recess or sinus tympani, a posterior tympanotomy (**Fig. 57.11**) or an extended posterior tympanotomy is performed to help tumor clearance.
11. The view after complete tumor removal (**Fig. 57.12**). The bone over the promontory and infracochlear cells is gently drilled with diamond burr till white polished bone is encountered. Surgicel is placed over the hypotympanum. A thin silastic sheet is then placed over the raw middle ear.
12. A temporalis fascia is used as a graft (**Fig. 57.13**).
13. The intact cuff of tympanomeatal skin is replaced over the fascia (**Fig. 57.14**). This usually has to be slit to accommodate the extra width of the canal caused by the bony drilling of the external auditory canal (EAC). Gelfoam packing is done.

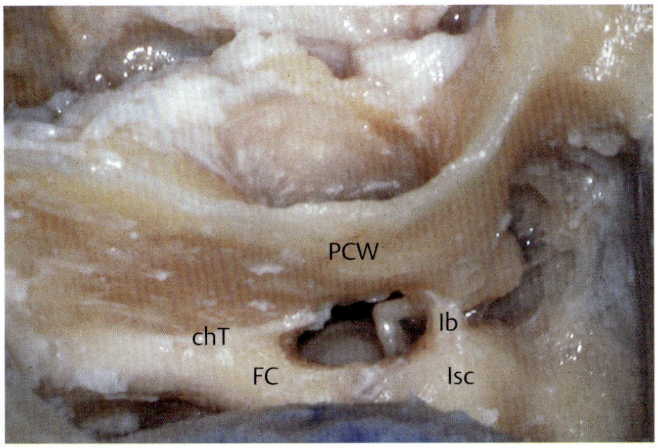

Fig. 57.11 Posterior tympanotomy (courtesy of Dr M. Shaan and Dr S. Bhatia).

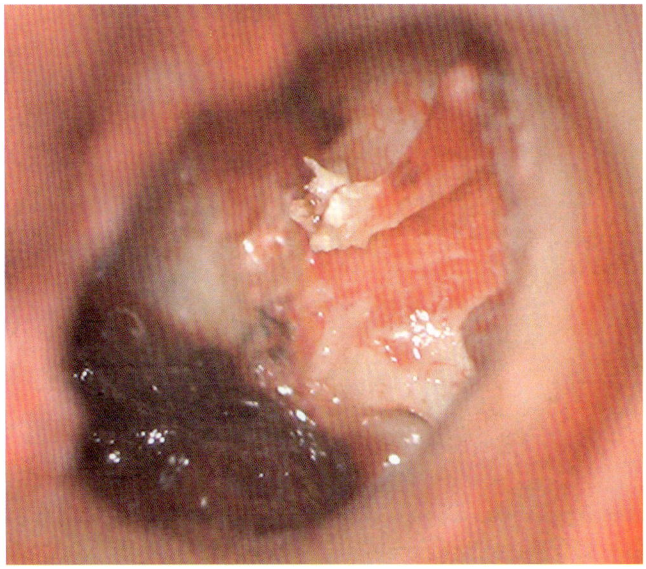

Fig. 57.12 A view of the left middle ear after tumor excision.

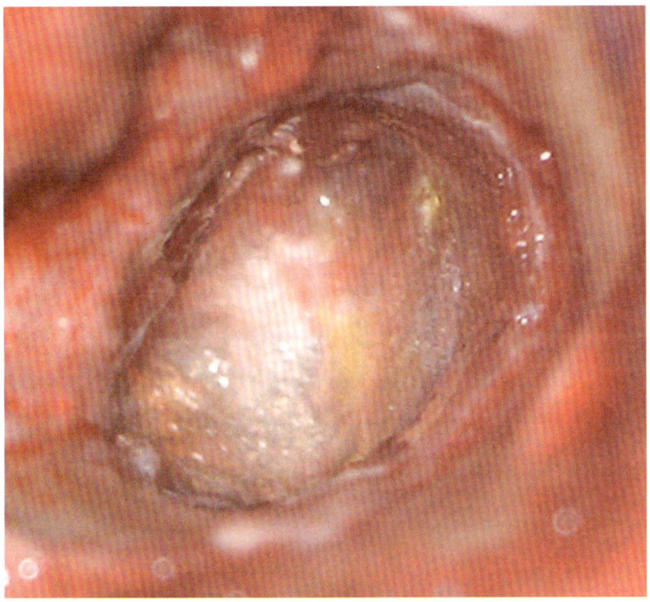

Fig. 57.13 Temporalis fascia used to graft the middle ear.

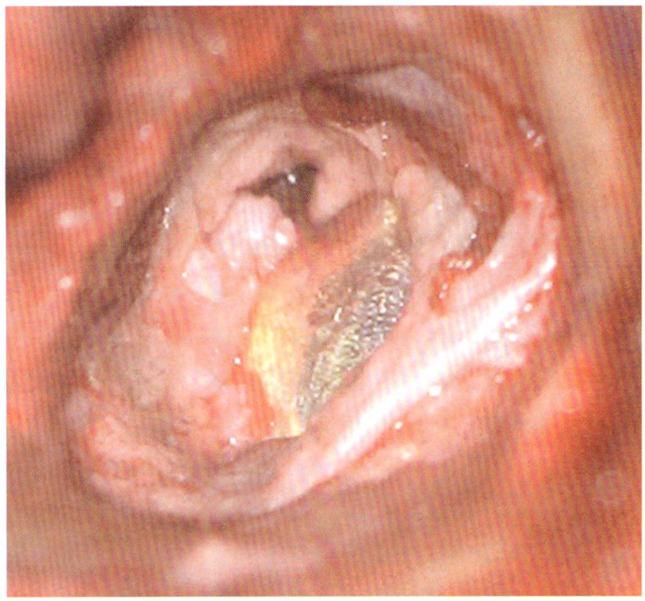

Fig. 57.14 Tympanomeatal cuff preserved earlier is placed over the fascia graft.

Class B2 Glomus Tumors

1. A surgical procedure in a subject with a right-sided B2 tumor, extending from the middle ear cleft through the mastoid antrum to the mastoid is described below. CT scan findings are seen in **Fig. 57.15**.
2. A postauricular incision is make and temporalis fascia graft is harvested (**Fig. 57.16**).
3. A circumferential meatotomy is taken involving all quadrants of the EAC (**Fig. 57.17**).
4. The tympanomeatal flap is dissected medially (**Fig. 57.18**) and the entire cuff of skin together with the annulus is removed (**Fig. 57.19**) and placed in saline for replacement at the end of the procedure.
5. A wide bony meatoplasty is performed to expose the anterior, inferior, and posterior walls of the middle ear (**Fig. 57.20**).

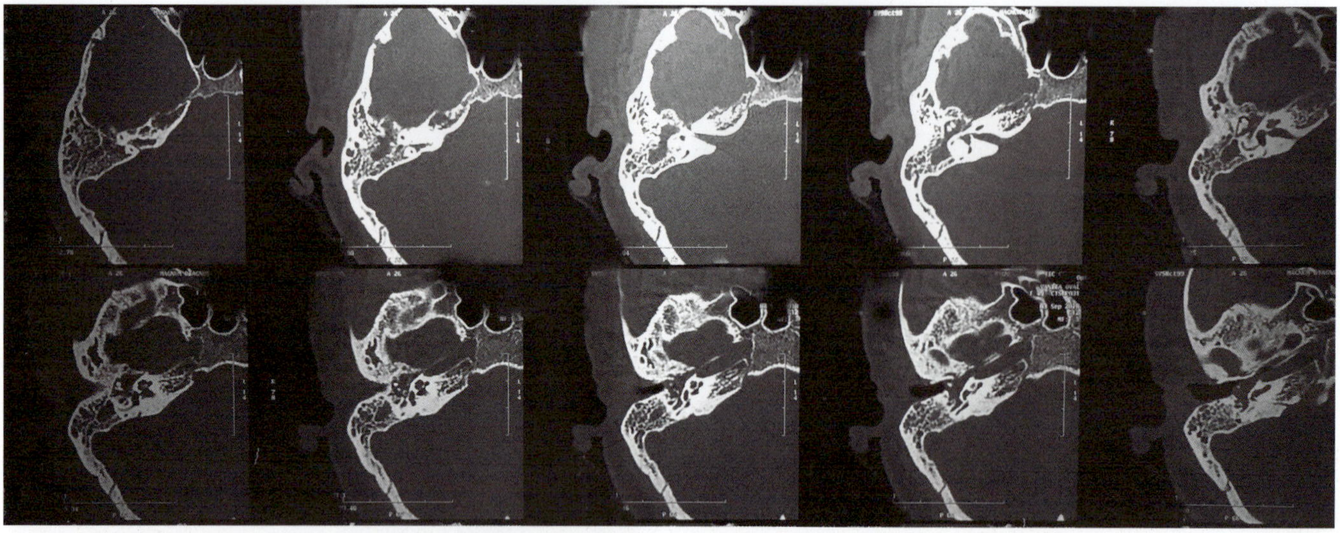

Fig. 57.15 Right-sided glomus involving middle ear with limited extension to the mastoid via the antrum.

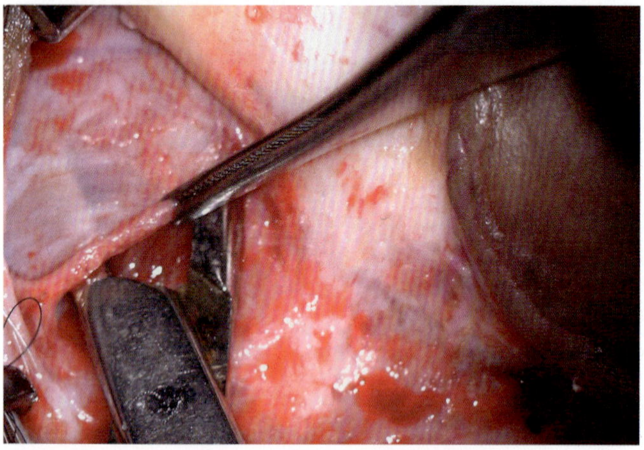

Fig. 57.16 Temporalis fascia graft harvested.

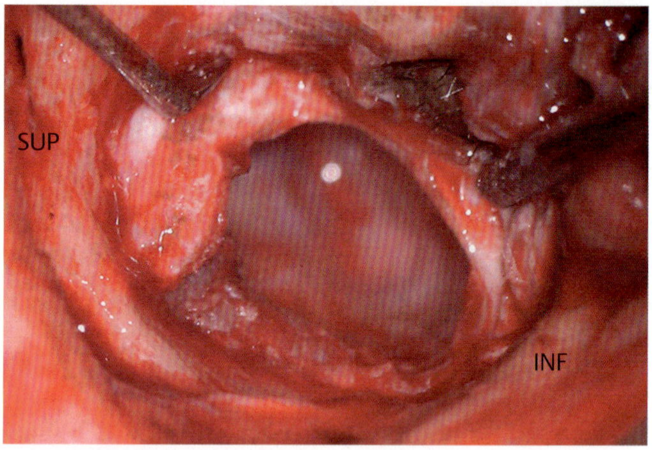

Fig. 57.17 Circumferential meatotomy.

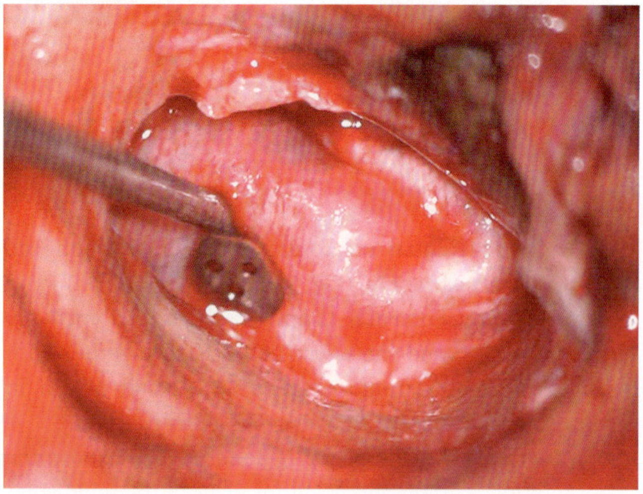

Fig. 57.18 Tympanomeatal cuff dissected medially in all quadrants.

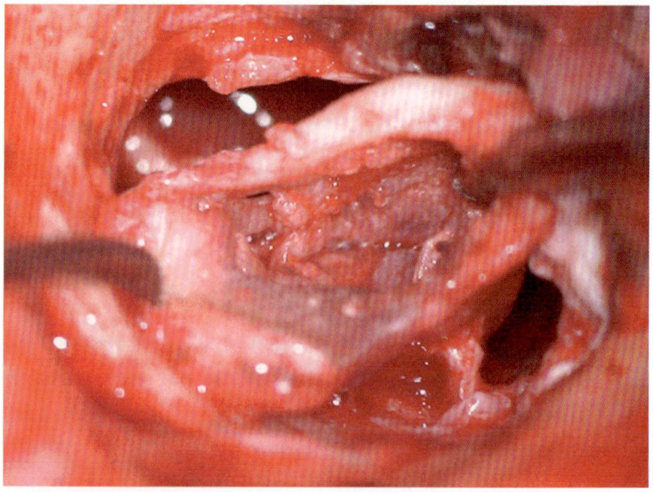

Fig. 57.19 Total cuff excised and preserved.

6. A view after bony meatoplasty giving better exposure of the tumor margins. Note that the handle of malleus lies as a necrosed, fractured fragment lateral to the tumor (**Fig. 57.21**).
7. The tumor surface is bipolarized to shrink the tumor. The tumor is then dissected off the middle ear (**Figs. 57.22 and 57.23**) with a combination of dissection and bipolarization.
8. In this particular subject, the long process of incus was necrosed. The body of incus was extracted out to open up the aditus to antrum. A limited cortical mastoidectomy was performed (**Fig. 57.24**). till the margin of the tumor was accessed in the mastoid cavity. The tumor was then dissected from the mastoid to the middle ear and excised in toto (**Fig. 57.25**).
9. However, in most instances, it is more prudent to do a wide cortical mastoidectomy and an extended posterior tympanotomy to gain good access to the tumor in its entire extent (**Fig. 57.26**). In certain cases, tumor extension may occur from middle ear to mastoid through the infrafacial cells, medial to the mastoidal fallopian canal. In these cases, we perform intact

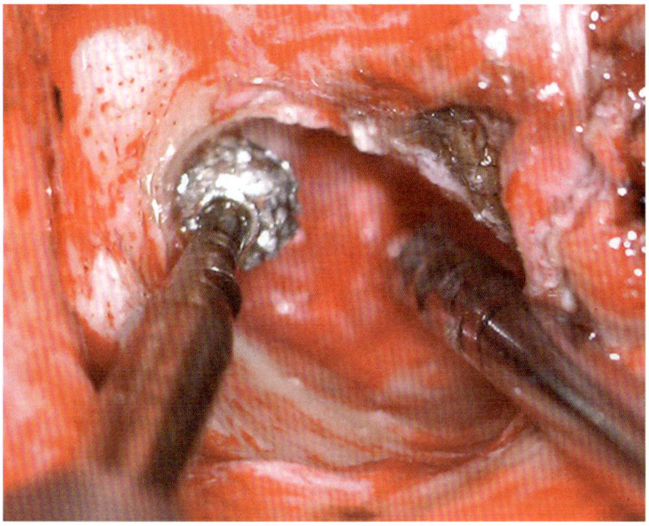

Fig. 57.20 Wide bony meatoplasty is performed.

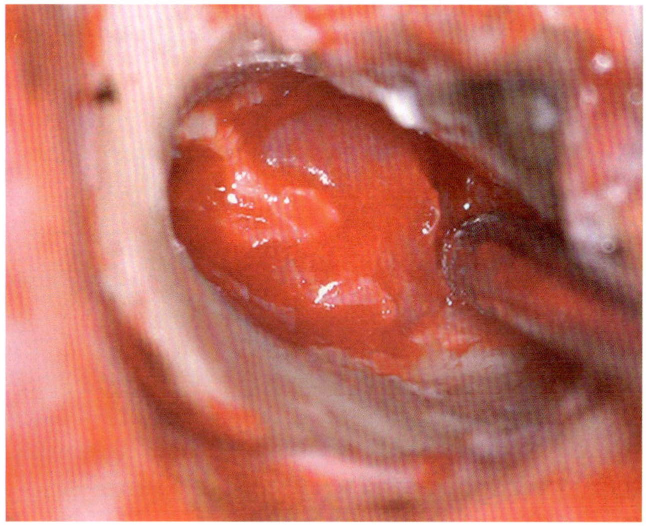

Fig. 57.21 Tumor exposed better after wide bony meatoplasty.

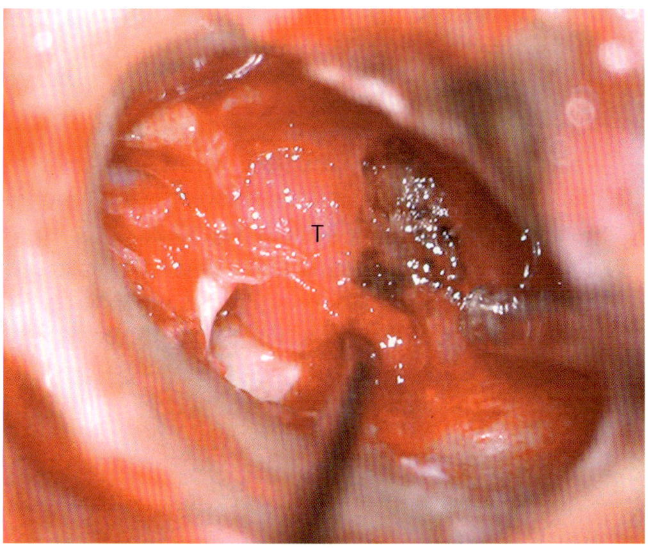

Fig. 57.22 Bipolarized tumor is dissected off from hypotympanum and promontory.

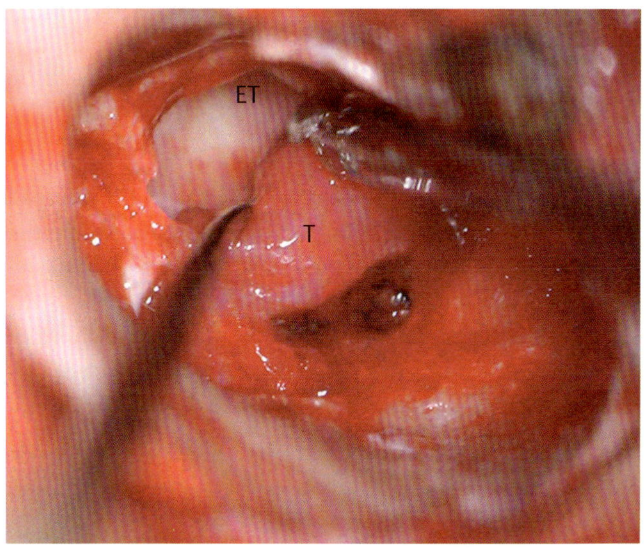

Fig. 57.23 Anterior margin of tumor cleared off the area of eustachian tube orifice.

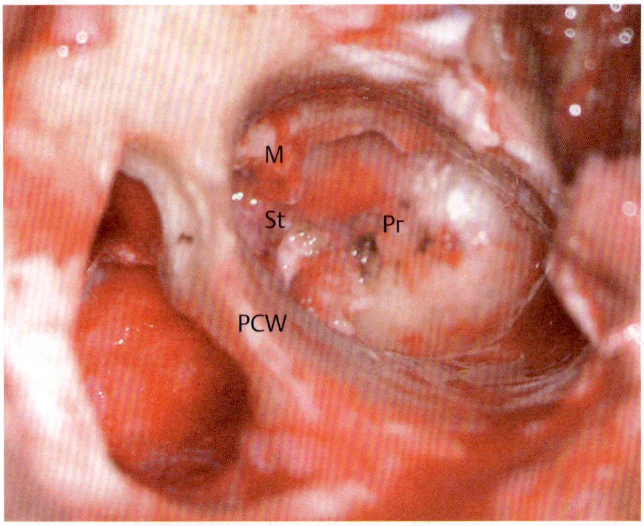

Fig. 57.24 View of the middle ear and limited cortical mastoidectomy after tumor excision.

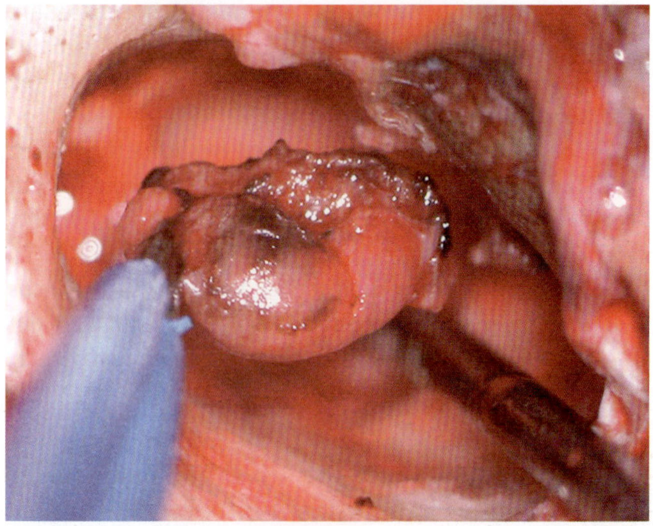

Fig. 57.25 Tumor excision in toto.

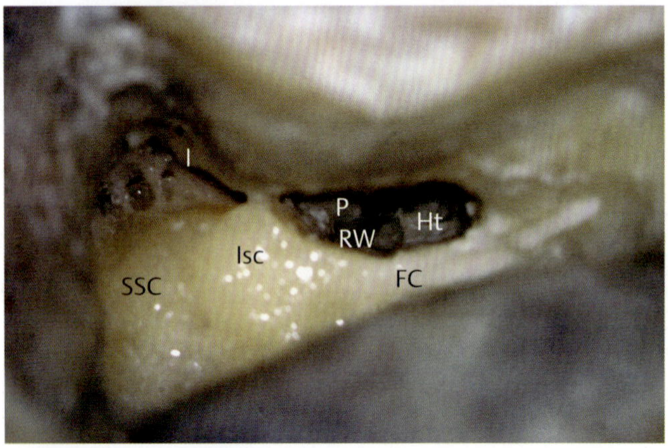

Fig. 57.26 Extended posterior tympanotomy.

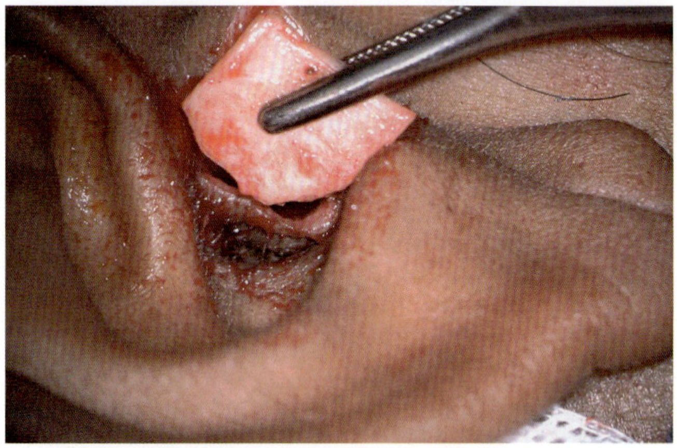

Fig. 57.27 Tragal cartilage harvested.

fallopian canal technique, wherein the facial nerve in its mastoidal segment is left intact with bone all around it while drilling is performed between the medial aspect of the mastoidal segment of fallopian canal and the jugular bulb.

10. A piece of tragal cartilage with intact perichondrium on both sides is harvested (**Fig. 57.27**). A piece of this cartilage is used to reinforce the defect in the lateral attic wall. A piece of cartilage is also used to perform interposition ossiculoplasty between the head of stapes and the neck of malleus (**Fig. 57.28**).
11. The harvested temporalis fascia is used to graft the middle ear (**Fig. 57.29**). The cuff of skin of EAC is split and placed over the fascia (**Fig. 57.30**). Gelfoam packing in the EAC is performed.
12. Postaural incision is closed.

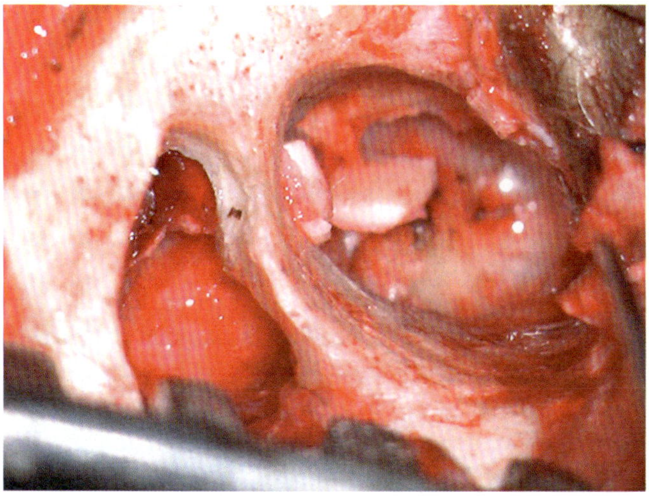

Fig. 57.28 Reinforcement of lateral attic wall with cartilage and cartilage interposition ossiculoplasty between stapes head and malleus neck.

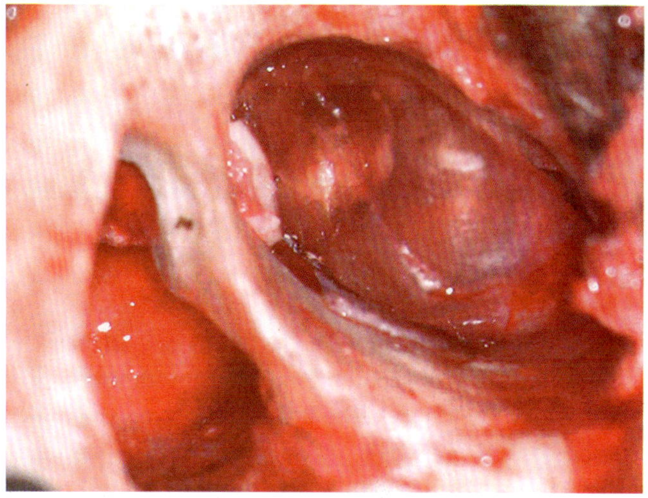

Fig. 57.29 Temporalis fascia grafting.

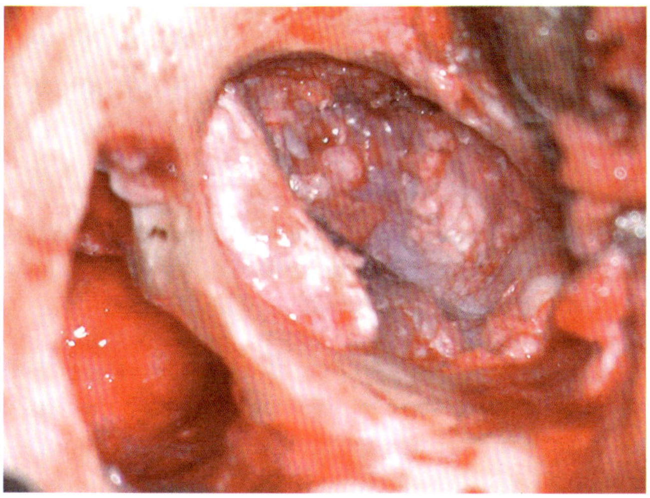

Fig. 57.30 Skin cuff replaced over the fascia.

Suggested Readings

Alaani A, Chavda SV, Irving RM. The crucial role of imaging in determining the approach to glomus tympanicum tumours. Eur Arch Otorhinolaryngol 2009;266(6):827–831

Fisch U, Mattox D. Paragangliomas of the temporal bone. In: Microsurgery of the Skull Base. New York: Thieme;1988: 148–281

Sanna M, Fois P, Pasanisi E, Russo A, Bacciu A. Middle ear and mastoid glomus tumors (glomus tympanicum): an algorithm for the surgical management. Auris Nasus Larynx 2010; 37(6):661–668

O'Leary MJ, Shelton C, Giddings NA, Kwartler J, Brackmann DE. Glomus tympanicum tumors: a clinical perspective. Laryngoscope 1991;101(10):1038–1043

Chapter 58 Management of Class B3 Temporal Bone Paragangliomas (Glomus Tumors)

Madhuri Mehta

Introduction

Class B3 tumors, like the rest of Class B tumors, originate in canalis tympanicus of hypotympanum and invade middle ear and mastoid. They invade the bone of the hypotympanum but the cortical bone over jugular bulb and the carotico-jugular crest remains intact.

The difference from Class B2 tumors is that in addition to filling the middle ear with extension into the mastoid, there is an erosion of the vertical carotid canal.

Surgical Steps

1. A postaural incision is made. A rectangular musculoperiosteal flap is created just posterior to the external auditory canal (EAC) to be used as a second layer in the blind sac closure of the EAC. The EAC is then transected circumferentially at the level of the spine of Henle. The skin of the lateral (cartilagenous) half of the transected EAC is separated off the conchal and tragal cartilages (**Fig. 58.1a**). The skin sleeve is then everted to the outside (**Fig. 58.1b**) and sutured with 3-0 Vicryl. The previously created musculoperiosteal flap as described above is used as a second layer to create a blind sac closure of the EAC (**Fig. 58.2**).
2. The epithelium lining the bony EAC is then excised. The malleus and the incus are also excised. Care is taken to disarticulate the incudostapedial joint if intact. In many cases, the lenticular process of incus is necrosed and the incus can be easily extracted out. In cases of tumor completely obliterating the middle and external ear (**Fig. 58.3**) as in the present case example depicted, the tumor is bipolarized on the surface (**Fig. 58.4**) and drilling is performed around it in all quadrants to expose complete tumor in EAC and middle ear (**Figs. 58.5, 58.6, and 58.7**). The tumor in the middle and external ear is then bipolarized at the base and debulked partially (**Fig. 58.8**).
3. A subtotal petrosectomy is performed (**Fig. 58.9**). The tegmen plate, sinus plate, sinodural angle, and mastoid tip cells are exenterated. Similarly, the infrafacial and perilabyrinthine cells are cleared completely. The posterior canal wall is taken down up to the level of the Fallopian canal in its vertical course. There was a dehiscence in the tegmen mastoidale with the tumor adherent to the middle fossa dura in the same area. The tumor in this area was meticulously bipolarized and excised from the middle fossa dura (**Fig. 58.10**). The remnant tegmen mastoidale deeper to the tumor needs to be thoroughly drilled to achieve good tumor clearance (**Fig. 58.11**).

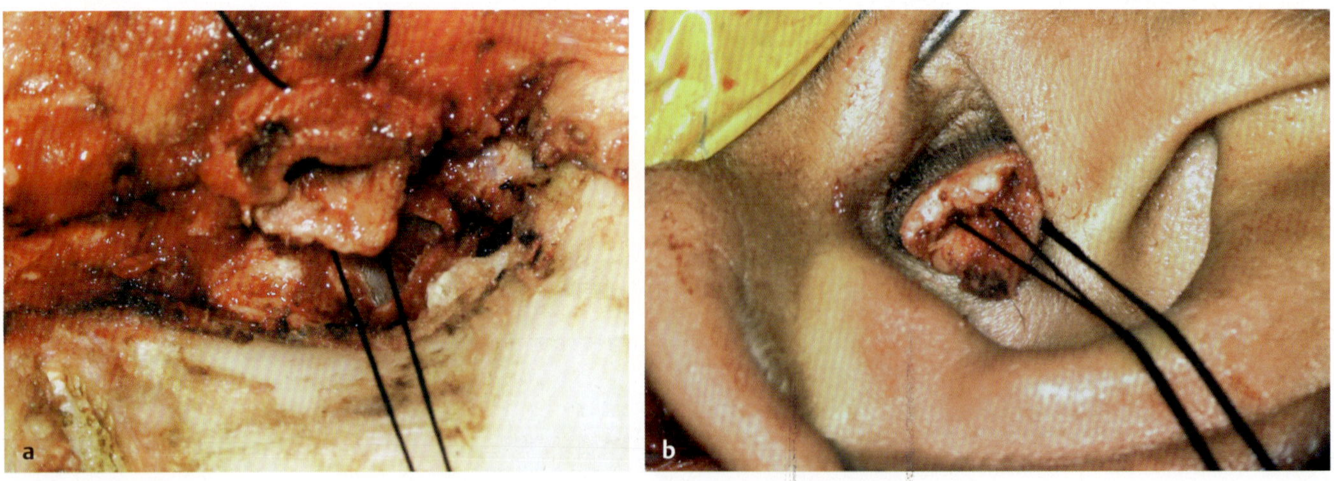

Fig. 58.1 **(a)** Skin of lateral external auditory canal (EAC) separated from surrounding conchal and tragal cartilages and soft tissue. Stay sutures placed on two sides to evert the complete circumference of skin flap out of EAC. **(b)** Everted skin of cartilagenous EAC to be sutured with 4.0 Vicryl as first layer of blind sac closure.

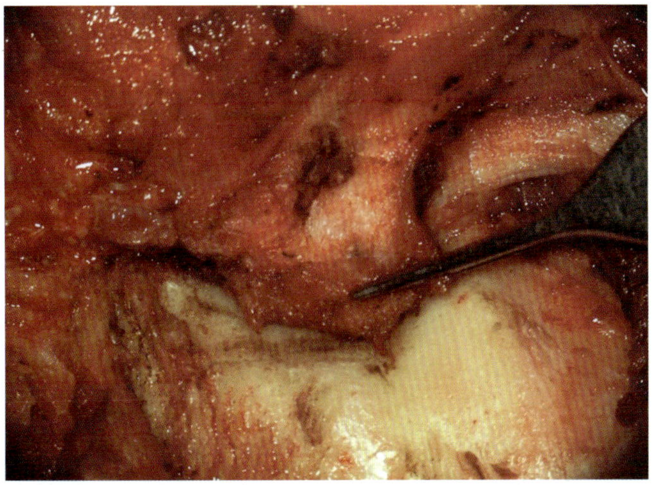

Fig. 58.2 Anteriorly based musculoperiosteal flap for second layer of blind sac closure.

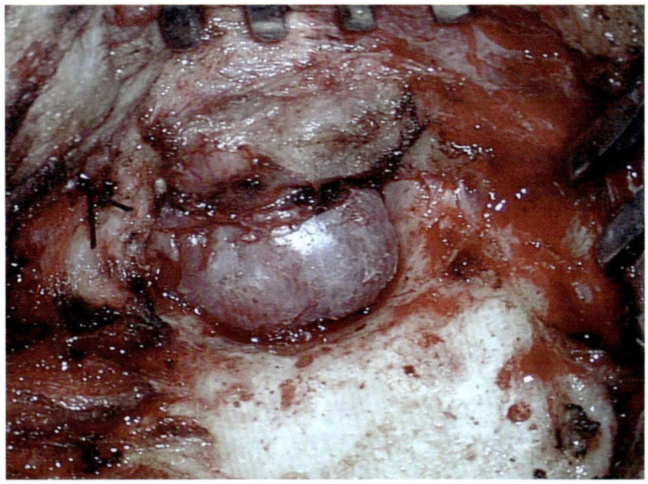

Fig. 58.3 Tumor seen completely occupying the middle ear and external auditory canal.

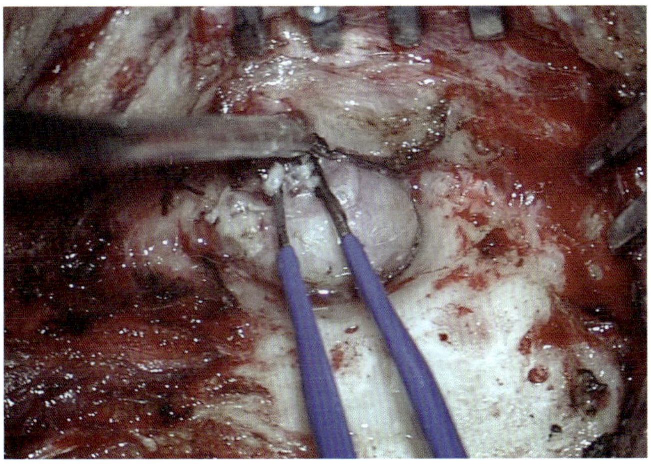

Fig. 58.4 Tumor is bipolarized to shrink it marginally and create space for drilling.

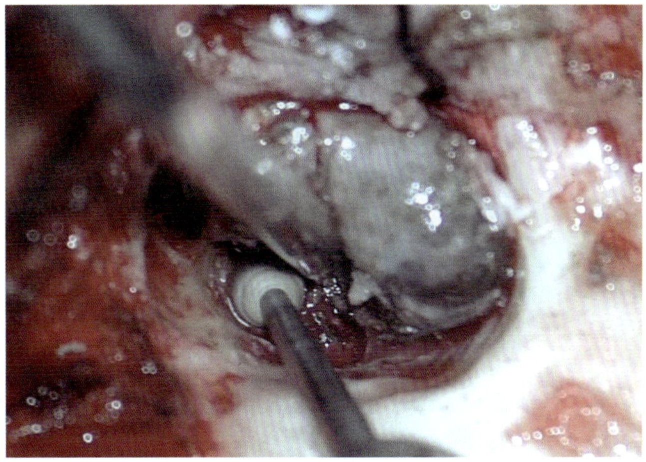

Fig. 58.5 Drilling of the inferior margin to expose the hypotympanum.

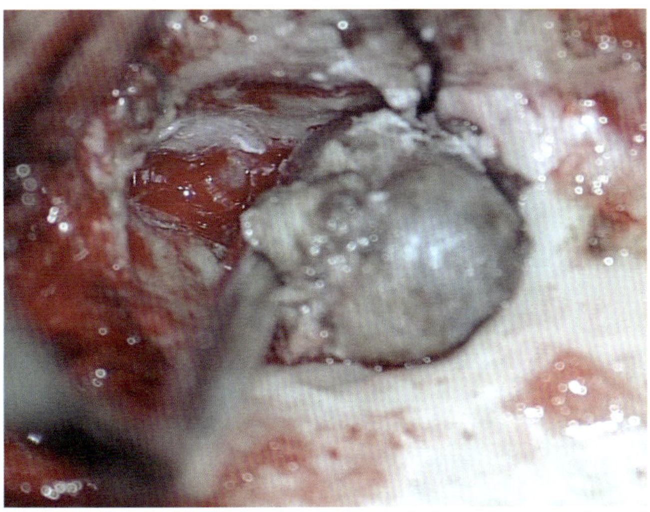

Fig. 58.6 The hypotympanum is exposed beyond the tumor margin inferiorly.

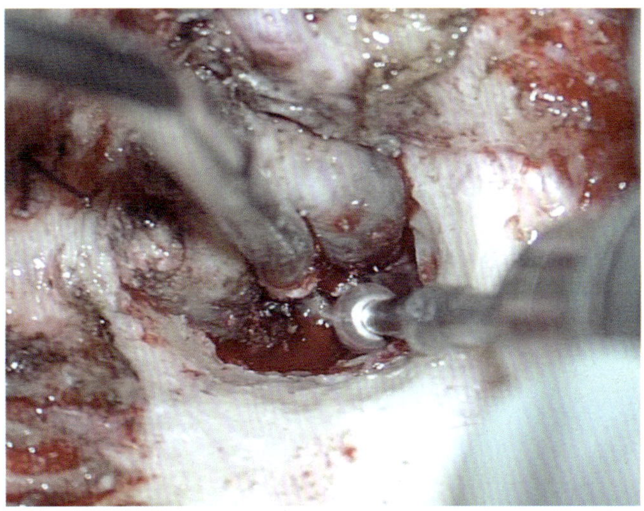

Fig. 58.7 Drilling the posterior and posterosuperior canal wall.

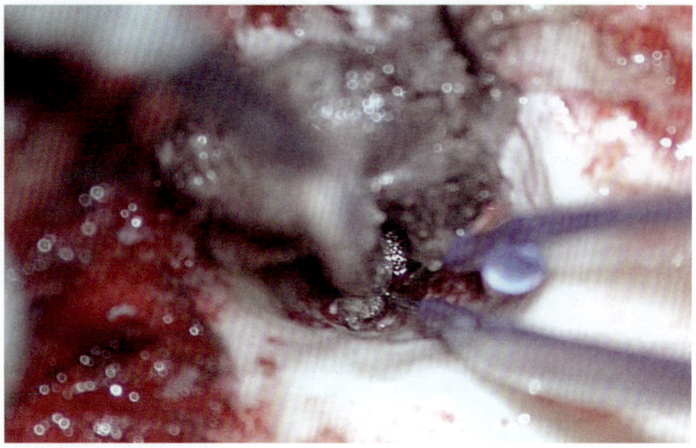

Fig. 58.8 Tumor is bipolarized at the promontory and debulked partially.

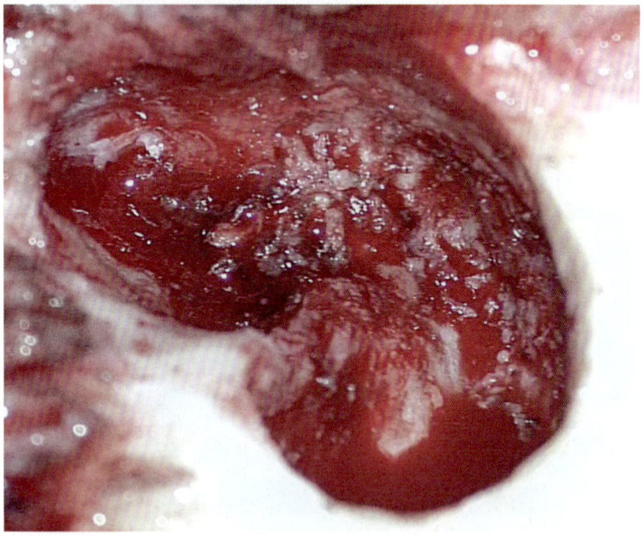

Fig. 58.9 A subtotal petrosectomy in progress. Plenty of remnant tumor is seen.

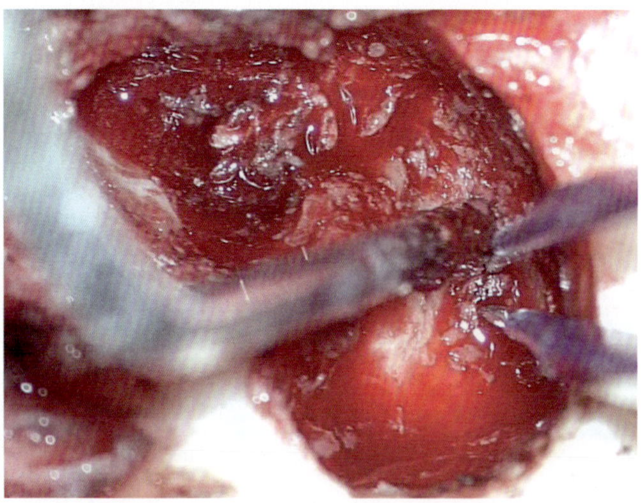

Fig. 58.10 Tumor bipolarized and excised from the sinodural angle and tegmen plate.

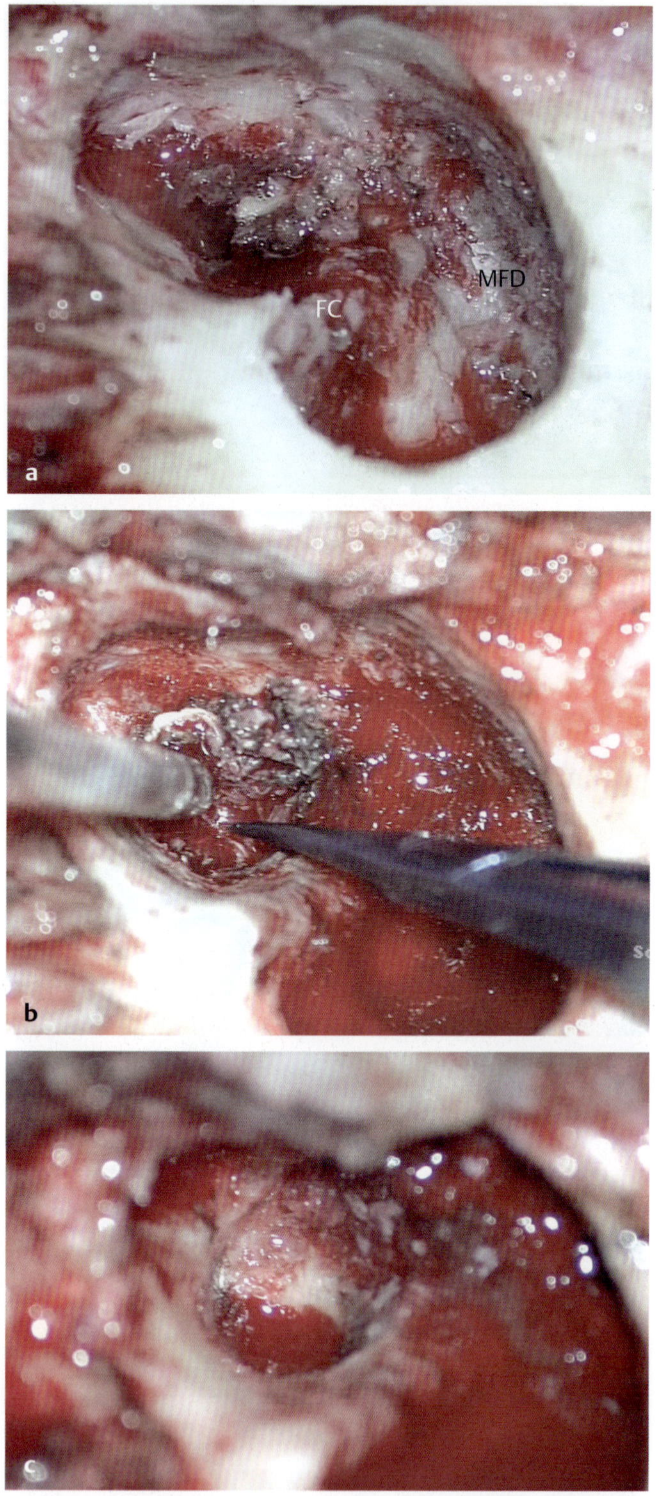

Fig. 58.11 **(a)** Cleared middle fossa dura is seen. **(b)** Residual tumor in middle ear being cleared by removing the cauterized tumor with iris scissors. **(c)** Clearance of tumor in hypotympanum. Carotid artery exposed in vertical part. Anterior tympanic plate also drilled to expose and clear the tumor in infratubal part.

4. The tumor in the mastoid or middle ear is bipolarized and is removed piecemeal. In this case, the tumor had involved the tympanic segment of facial nerve. Hence, the facial nerve segment from the second genu up to the geniculate ganglion area was excised to achieve good tumor clearance (**Fig. 58.12**). A sural nerve graft was harvested later and used as an interposition graft between the cut ends of the facial nerve. This was covered with fibrin glue and the anastomotic sites protected with a small piece of fascia. The bone deeper to the tumor is drilled to exenterate all cells and achieve white polished bone.

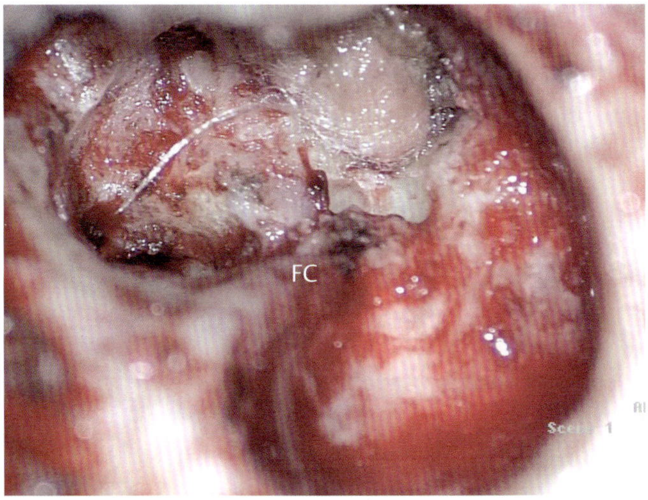

Fig. 58.12 Glomus tumor involved tympanic segment of facial nerve and hence tympanic segment of facial nerve is excised. Bone deeper to the tumor in the entire middle ear cleft is drilled till white polished bone is seen all around.

5. In these tumors, it is imperative to drill the anterior wall of the EAC to access the infratubal vertical course of carotid, which is eroded due to the tumor (**Fig. 58.13**). Tumor is bipolarized and excised. If necessary, the periosteum around the internal carotid in the area is excised to improve tumor clearance. Cells medial to the vertical segment of internal carotid artery (ICA) can also be exenterated to excise tumor in cases of tumor extension to that area. The bone over the carotid canal is drilled with a large sized diamond burr to exenterate any remnant tumor or cells.
6. The eustachian tube is plugged with periosteum or fat. Fat strips are also used to obliterate the entire cavity. Alternatively, pedicled musculoperiosteal flaps are rotated into the cavity to obliterate it (**Fig. 58.14**).
7. Incision is closed in layers.

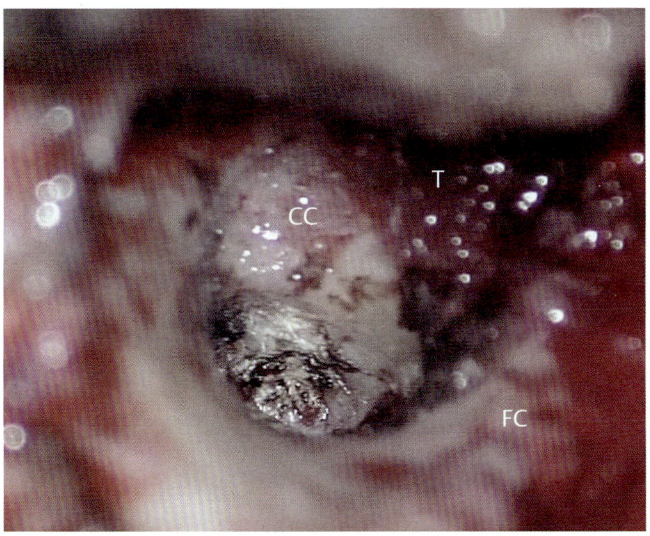

Fig. 58.13 Tumor seen eroding the infratubal carotid canal. The drilled area of hypotympanum and infracochlear cells medial to carotid canal are seen.

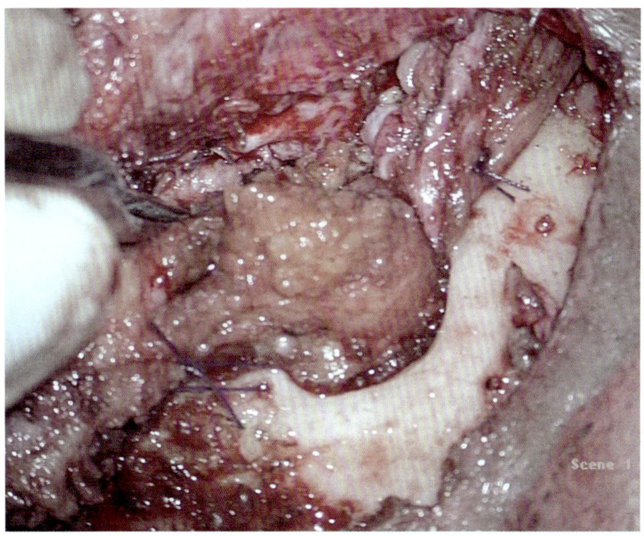

Fig. 58.14 Pedicled musculoperiosteal flap used to obliterate the cavity.

Chapter 59 Management of Type C Glomus Tumors: Infratemporal Fossa Type A Approach for Glomus Jugulare Tumors

Satish Jain and Narayan Jayashankar

Indications

- Glomus jugulare tumors types C and D according to the modified Fisch classification
- Jugular foramen meningiomas
- Some cases of jugular foramen neuromas; however, these cases are most often managed by the petro-occipital transsigmoid approach (POTS)
- Clival chordomas of lower clivus

Imaging

HRCT Scan with Contrast

It is important to study the axial and coronal images on high-resolution computed tomography (HRCT) with contrast to determine involvement of structures and extent of spread of the lesion. The pathognomic feature is an irregular widening of the jugular foramen on the involved side with a typical "moth eaten" appearance with destruction of the carotico-jugular spine (**Fig. 59.1**). The tumor grows along planes of least resistance and hence, involvement of infralabyrinthine and infracochlear cells is common. The tumors arising from the jugular bulb grow along the internal carotid artery (ICA) and are classified according to the modified Fisch[1,2] classification as Class C tumors with subdivisions as follows:

- C1: Tumors destroying the jugular bulb with limited involvement of the vertical portion of the carotid canal (**Infratemporal Type A approach**)
- C2: Tumors involving the vertical portion of the carotid canal (**Infratemporal Type A approach**)
- C3: Tumors growing along the horizontal petrous segment of the carotid canal (**Infratemporal Type B approach**)
- C4: Tumors reaching the anterior foramen lacerum (**Infratemporal Type C approach**)

Very large tumors may destroy the jugular tubercle, hypoglossal canal, or invade the foramen magnum or clivus and need to be dealt accordingly with extensions of the approach.

Computed tomography (CT) angiogram is of specific value in identifying the arterial supply to the tumor and also the status of the venous sinuses and jugular bulb on the involved side as also the opposite side (especially a hypoplastic sinus system on the opposite side that could lead to modification of the surgical strategy).

Magnetic Resonance Imaging (MRI) Scan

MRI is necessary for differential diagnosis and to confirm the extent of tumor growth. MRI shows a characteristic salt and pepper appearance on T1- and T2-weighted images[3] due to the hypervascularity of the tumor. It enhances brightly on postcontrast images (**Fig. 59.2a, b**). MRI also helps to identify dural involvement/intracranial spread. Tumors are subclassified accordingly as:

- De: Intracranial spread of tumor but extradural
- Di: Intradural extension of tumor

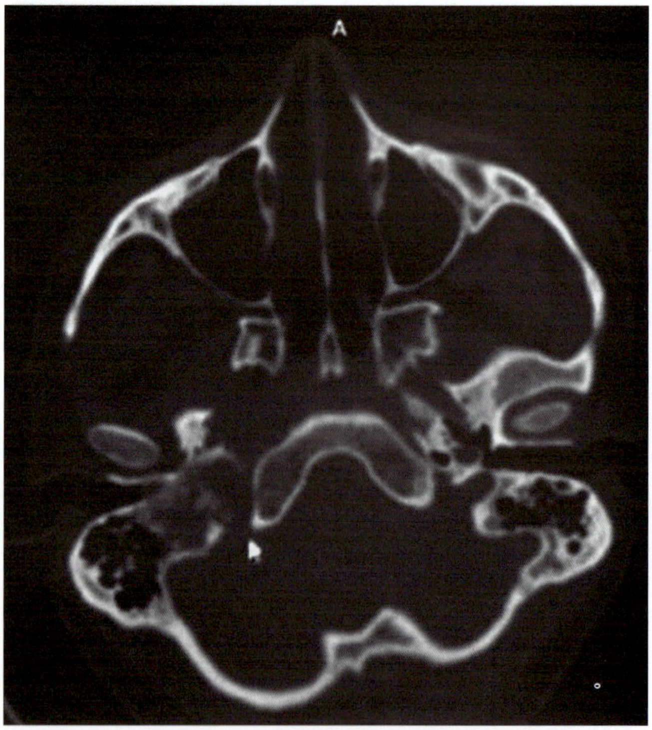

Fig. 59.1 Computed tomography (CT) scan showing destruction of the carotico-jugular spine and a moth eaten appearance of bone in the right jugular foramen.

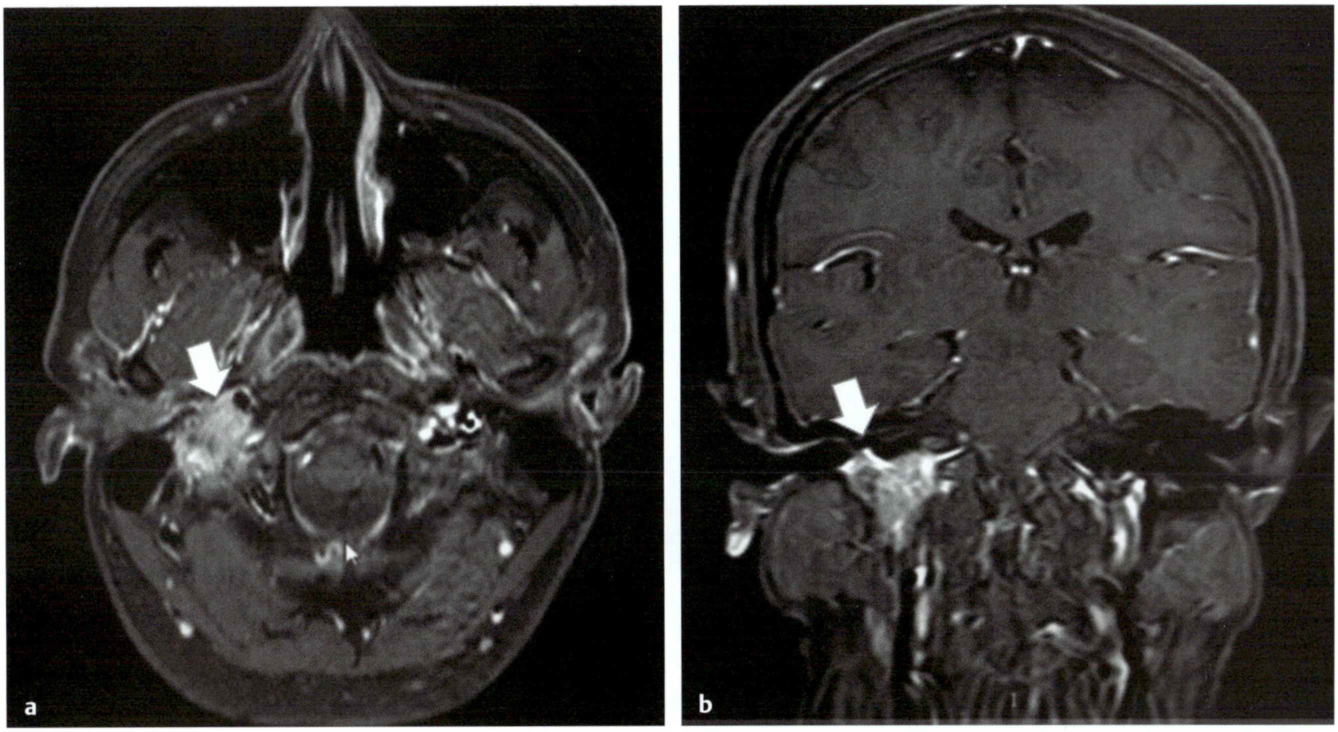

Fig. 59.2 (a) Axial and (b) coronal postcontrast T1-weighted images depicting heterogeneously intensely enhancing ill-defined mass lesion (*white solid arrows*) seen in the region of right jugular foramen with resultant widening of the same. The right internal carotid artery is seen along its anteromedial aspect and is flushed with the same.

Vertebral artery involvement is classified as:

- Ve: Tumors engulfing the extradural vertebral artery
- Vi: Tumors involving the intradural vertebral artery

Concept of No Embolization

Satish Jain performs CT angiogram (**Fig. 59.3a, b**) and uses the information to identify the arterial feeders to the tumor. This is done by studying the CT angiogram in detail on the radiology software and tracing the branches from the external or internal carotid system supplying the tumor (**Fig. 59.3c**). He intraoperatively ligates the arterial feeders to the tumor from the external carotid artery as an alternative to preoperative embolization of these feeder vessels. Good superior and inferior control of the ICA is ascertained. The tumor is dissected off the ICA and any feeder vessels are bipolarized to devascularize the tumor. Dr Satish Jain uses embolization only if there is intracranial extension with feeders to the tumor from intracranial segment of ICA where superselective embolization of these feeders are performed.

Embolization

Narayan Jayashankar does embolization of glomus jugulare tumors preoperatively. An example of tumor embolization is shown (**Fig. 59.4a–f**). Advantages of embolization include decreased blood loss, improvement in tumor consistency, and mild reduction in size. It facilitates better tumor mobilization and dissection from vital neurovascular structures. Angiography and selective/superselective embolization are performed using polyvinyl alcohol (PVA) and is performed 48 hours prior to the procedure by an experienced neuroradiologist.

Surgical Steps

1. A cranio-temporo-cervical incision is made (**Fig. 59.5**), starting 1 cm above the superior pole of the helix in the temporal area, curving postaurally just beyond the posterior border of mastoid and further continuing in the neck toward the greater cornu of hyoid bone. This incision includes the skin and subcutaneous tissue. In the neck, the flap is elevated in the subplatysmal plane. Care is taken to preserve the greater auricular nerve, which runs perpendicular to a line drawn from the mastoid tip to the angle of mandible over the sternocleidomastoid muscle (**Fig. 59.6**).
2. The external auditory canal (EAC) is transected circumferentially at the level of the spine of Henle. The skin lining the lateral half of EAC is separated from the

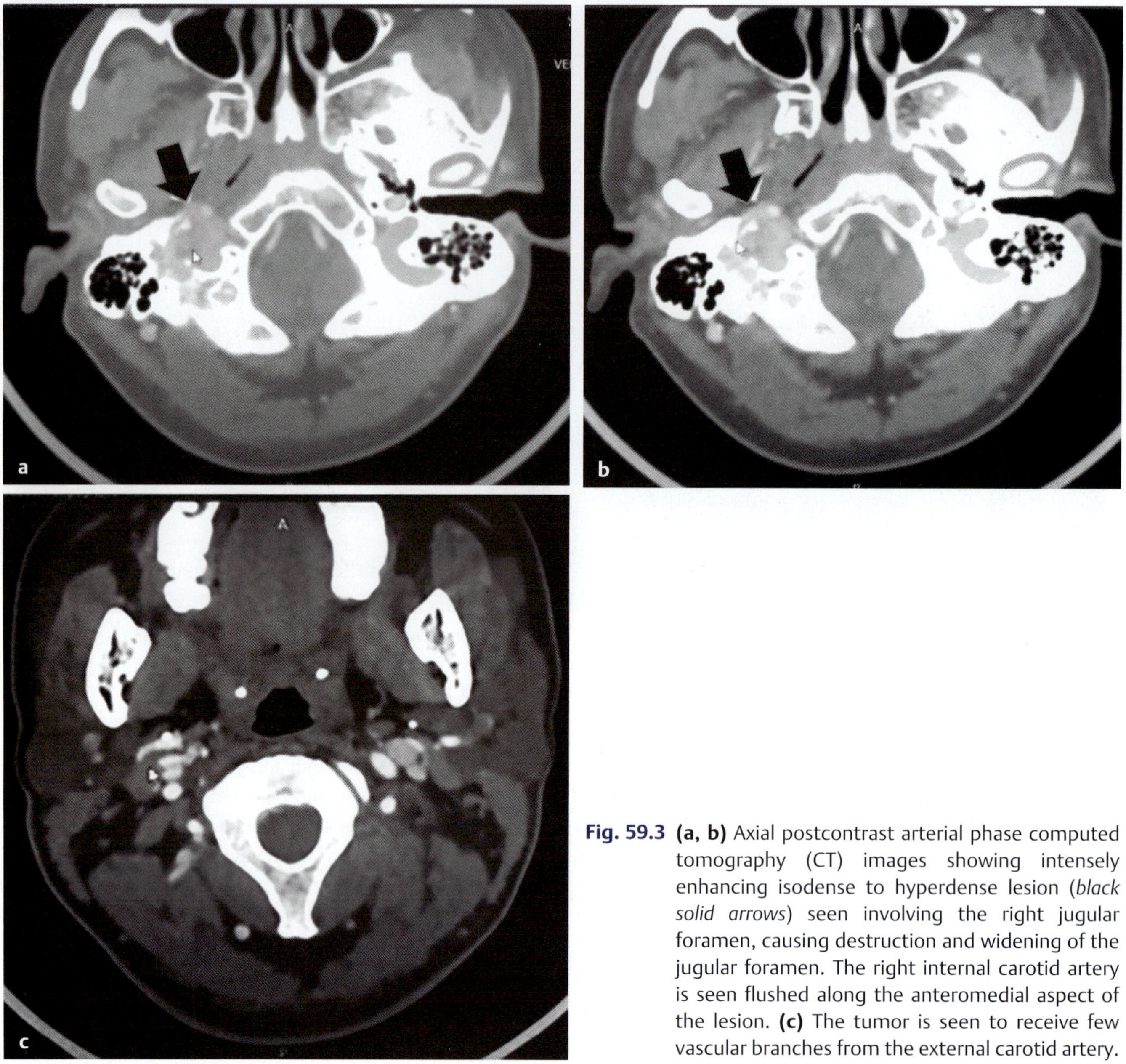

Fig. 59.3 **(a, b)** Axial postcontrast arterial phase computed tomography (CT) images showing intensely enhancing isodense to hyperdense lesion (*black solid arrows*) seen involving the right jugular foramen, causing destruction and widening of the jugular foramen. The right internal carotid artery is seen flushed along the anteromedial aspect of the lesion. **(c)** The tumor is seen to receive few vascular branches from the external carotid artery.

conchal and tragal cartilages to form a sleeve of skin (**Fig. 59.7**). Stay sutures are put on the superior and inferior ends of the skin tube which helps in everting the sleeve of skin through the EAC (**Fig. 59.8**). The everted skin is sutured with 4-0 vicryl (**Fig. 59.9**).

3. The separated conchal cartilage can be sutured to the tragal cartilage as a second layer of cul-de-sac closure of the EAC (**Fig. 59.10**).
4. A posteroinferiorly based musculoperiosteal flap is created. An incision is made from the base of zygoma along the temporal line. At the mastoid tip, fibers of sternocleidomastoid are separated from their attachment and retracted posteriorly.
5. The external carotid artery (ECA) and ICA and the internal jugular vein (IJV) are identified and exposed in the neck (**Fig. 59.11a, b**). The IJV is located immediately anterior to the transverse process of atlas. Plastic tubings of the scalp vein set (the needle end and the syringe end are cut) are looped loosely around these great vessels for establishing control over them during the surgery.
6. Cranial nerves IX, X, XI, and XII are identified in the neck (**Fig. 59.11a, b**). The hypoglossal nerve lies medial to the jugular bulb in its intracranial to extracranial course, positioning itself between the IJV and ICA first, and traverses lateral to the ICA and ECA just inferior

AQ

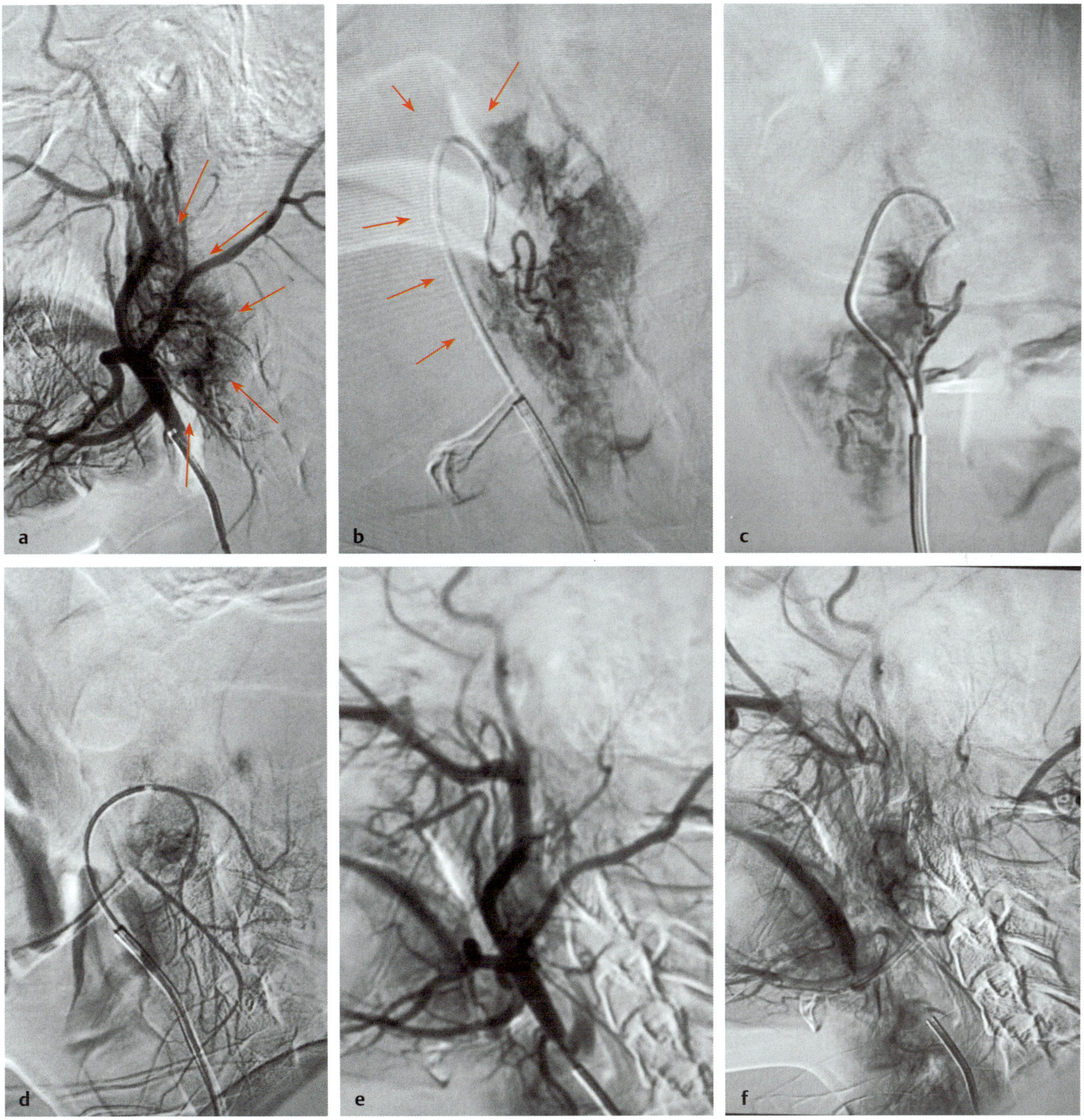

Fig. 59.4 **(a)** Abnormal hypervascular blush on external carotid angiogram. **(b)** Microcatheter in ascending pharyngeal artery showing pre-embolization dense blush. **(c)** Feeders from branches of superficial temporal artery. **(d)** Feeders from branches of posterior auricular artery. **(e)** Postembolization arterial phase—no blush seen. **(f)** Postembolization delayed arterial phase—no blush seen.

to the digastric tendon to go past the submandibular space toward the tongue. The descendens hypoglossi branch of hypoglossal nerve is also preserved. The glossopharyngeal nerve lies medial to the jugular bulb in its intracranial to extracranial course, and traverses lateral to the ICA, first deep to the styloid process and its attached muscles, and then superior and anterior to the hypoglossal nerve and digastric tendon to go deep to hyoglossus muscle toward the oropharynx. The vagus nerve lies medial to the jugular bulb and then courses between the ICA and the IJV in the neck. Accessory nerve lies deep to the jugular bulb in its

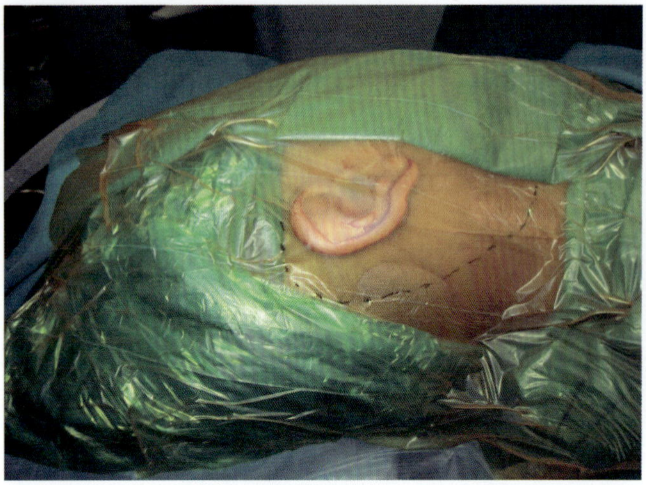

Fig. 59.5 Incision.

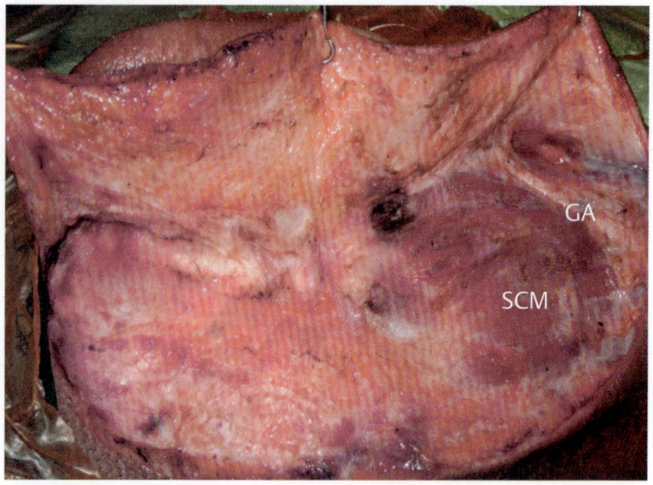

Fig. 59.6 Skin flap elevation.

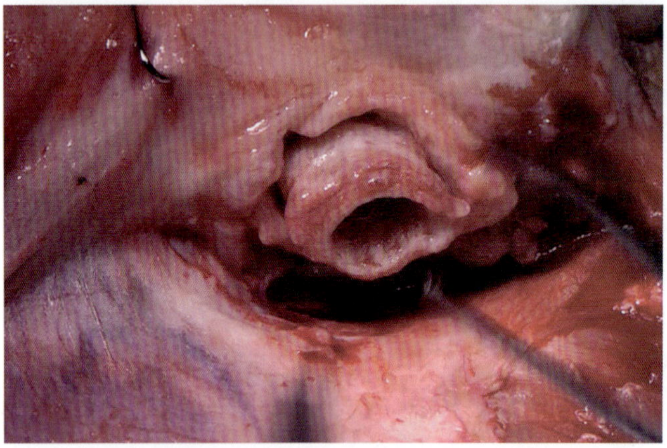

Fig. 59.7 Skin sleeve of external auditory canal (EAC) separated from the conchal and tragal cartilage.

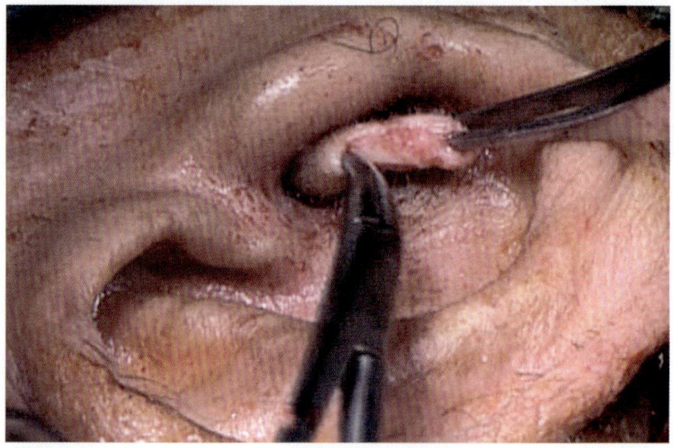

Fig. 59.8 Skin sleeve everted out of the external auditory canal (EAC).

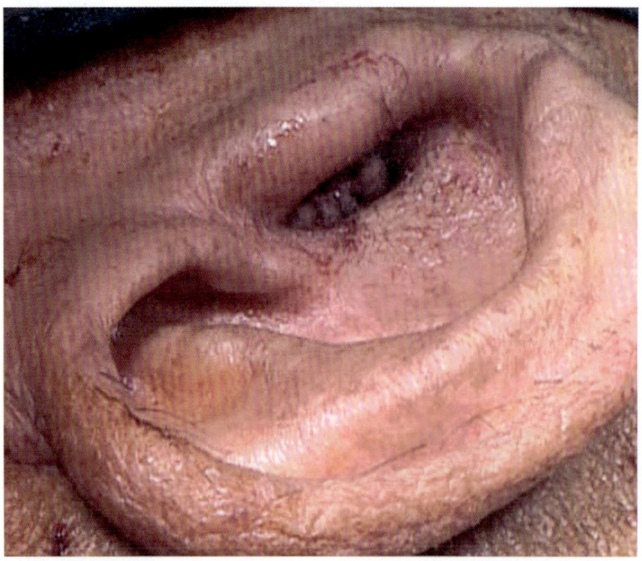

Fig. 59.9 Cul-de-sac closure of external auditory canal (EAC).

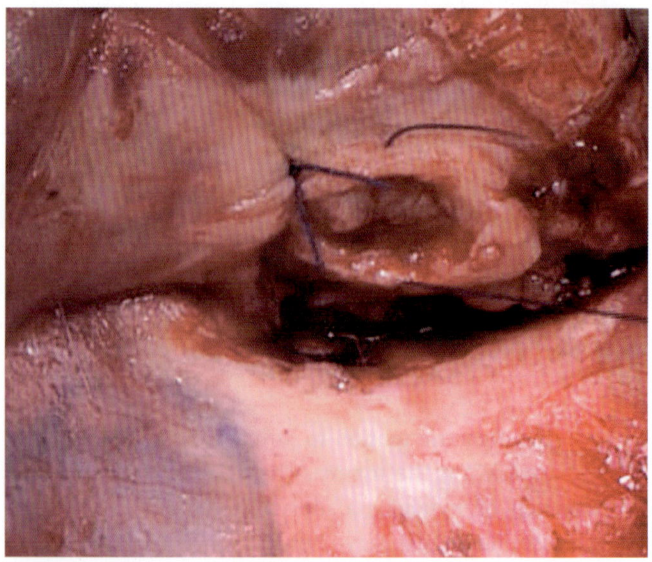

Fig. 59.10 Second layer closure of the external auditory canal (EAC)—suturing conchal to tragal cartilage.

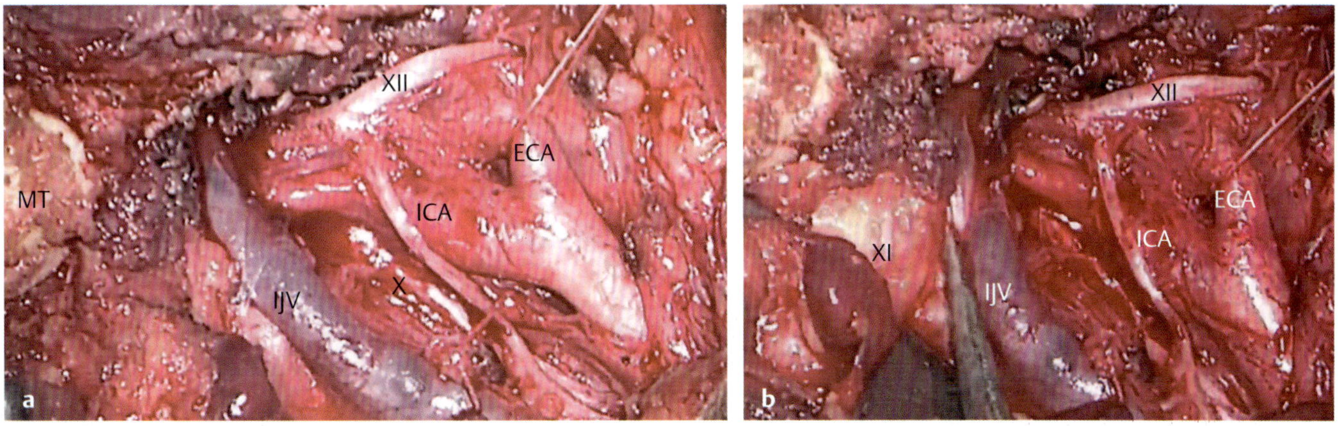

Fig. 59.11 **(a, b)** Exposure and control over the great vessels and lower cranial nerves in the neck.

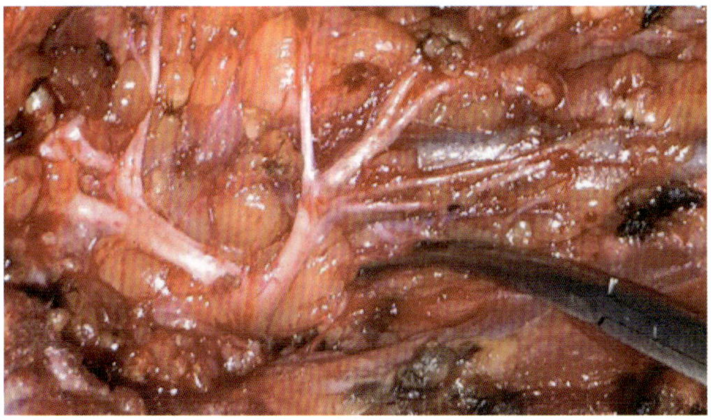

Fig. 59.12 Identification and mobilization of facial nerve in parotid.

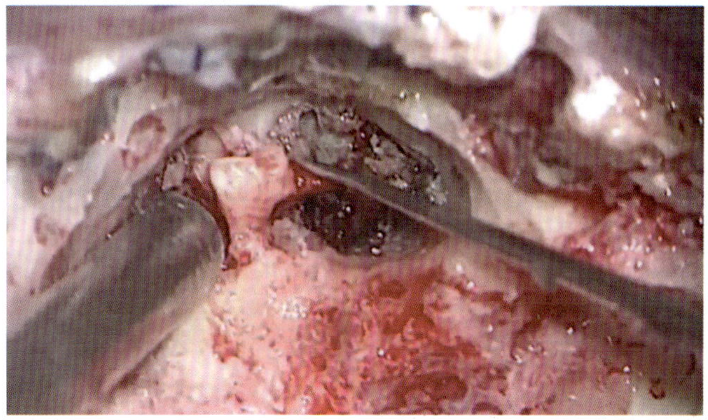

Fig. 59.13 Incus and malleus are taken out.

intracranial to extracranial course, traverses superficial to the IJV in a posterior direction deep to the sternocleidomastoid muscle, pierces it, and supplies it at the junction of the upper one-third and lower two-thirds to go to the posterior triangle of neck en route to supplying the trapezius muscle.

7. The facial nerve is identified in its extratemporal course similar to parotid surgery (**Fig. 59.12**). The main trunk is located at the perpendicular bisection of a line joining the cartilaginous pointer to the mastoid tip at its exit from the stylomastoid foramen. The nerve lies approximately 1 cm deep to the tragal pointer. The anterior border of posterior belly of digastric muscle is delineated and the facial nerve main trunk lies just anterior and deep to these fibers. The upper and lower divisions of the facial nerve in parotid is traced and surrounding tissues are dissected off to free the nerve.
8. The skin lining the medial half of the EAC is dissected off together with the malleus and incus after dislocation of the incudostapedial joint (**Fig. 59.13**). If needed for tumor clearance, the suprastructure of stapes can also be excised.
9. A subtotal petrosectomy is performed. All cells over the tegmen dura and sigmoid sinus are exenterated. The facial nerve is skeletonized in its mastoidal and tympanic segments leaving egg shell thin bone over it.
10. The mastoid tip is excised by drilling over the digastric ridge to expose the muscle fibers of posterior belly of digastric (**Fig. 59.14a**). Vertical cuts are made over the anterior and posterior walls of the mastoid tip up to the digastric muscle fibers. The tip is held with stout forceps or rongeur (**Fig. 59.14b**) and sharp dissection on its undersurface releases remnant muscles attached to it. The mastoid tip is thus excised. The posterior belly of digastric muscle is excised.
11. The facial nerve is traced in continuity from the mastoidal course to its main trunk in parotid (**Fig. 59.15**). A sleeve of periosteum is left around the facial nerve at this zone where it exits the temporal bone.
12. The facial nerve is decompressed in 270 degrees along its mastoidal and tympanic segments till the geniculate ganglion by taking off the eggshell bone over the facial nerve (**Fig. 59.16**). A groove is drilled on the anterior canal wall at the base of the zygoma to receive

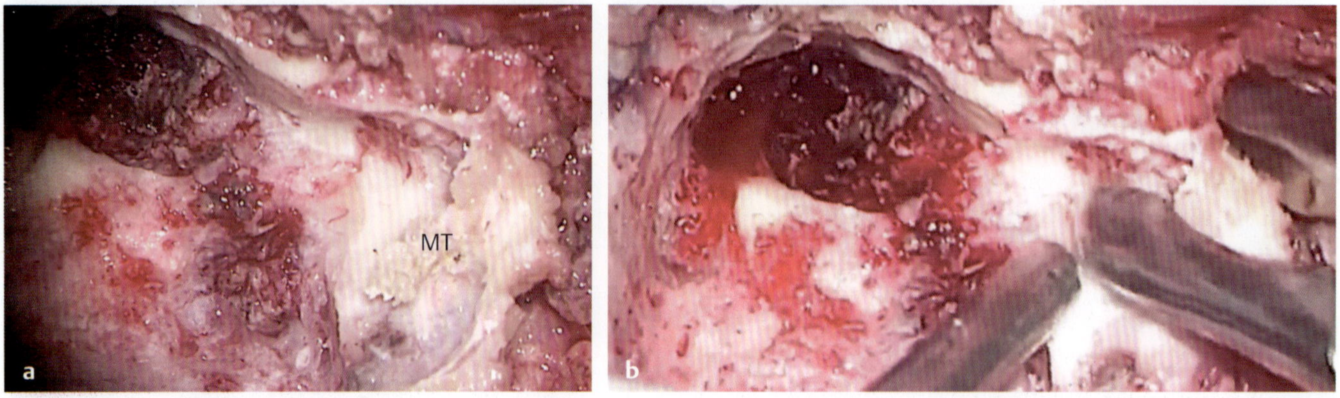

Fig. 59.14 (a, b) Mastoid tip excision.

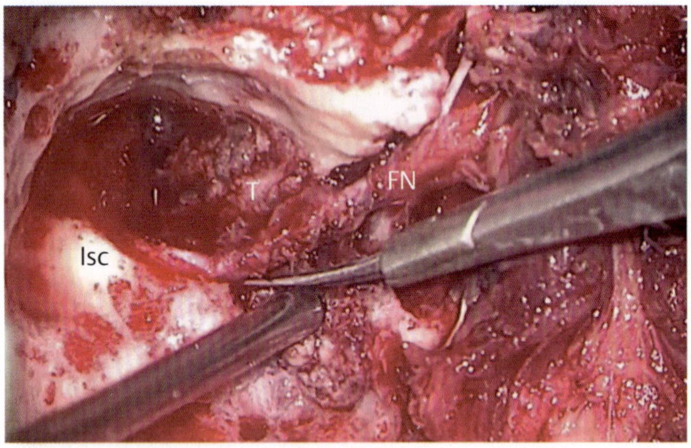

Fig. 59.15 Facial nerve mobilization from mastoidal segment to parotid.

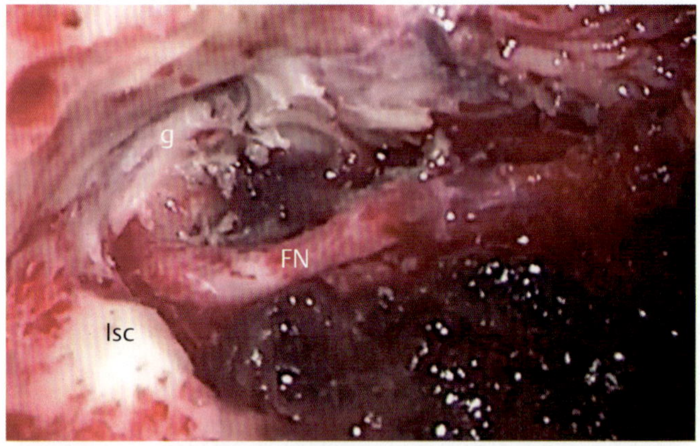

Fig. 59.16 Facial nerve decompressed and lifted out of the fallopian canal till geniculate ganglion.

an anteriorly transposed facial nerve. The facial nerve is lifted off its bed from the geniculate ganglion till its exit from the temporal bone and mobilized up to the distal ends of the upper and lower divisions of the facial nerve in parotid. It is then transposed anteriorly (**Fig. 59.17**). The tympanic segment is placed securely in the groove previously created at the base of zygoma and held in place with fibrin glue. The periosteum around the nerve at stylomastoid foramen is sutured to the parotid tissue to help keep the nerve anteriorly transposed.

13. The infracochlear and infralabyrinthine cells are drilled to expose the inferior end of sigmoid sinus, as also the jugular bulb. Tumor is generally encountered in this area. The tympanic plate of bone that was medial to the mastoidal segment of facial nerve is now drilled off completely to expose the base of styloid process.
14. The styloid process and its attached muscles separate the ICA medially from the external carotid artery laterally. The muscular attachments are taken off the styloid process with an electrocautery and the styloid process is excised (**Fig. 59.18**). This exposes the ICA at the skull base.
15. All the bone at the anterior end of the tympanic plate and the anterior canal wall is drilled off till the temporomandibular joint. The ICA is then traced starting from the neck (**Fig. 59.19**), going superiorly toward the vertical infratubal segment till its bend medial to the

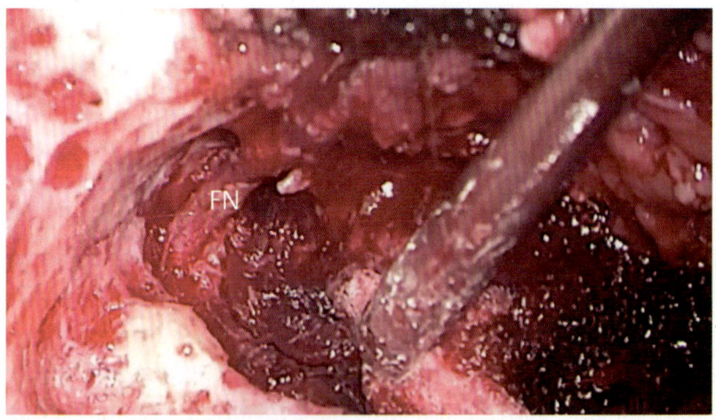

Fig. 59.17 Facial nerve anteriorly transposed.

eustachian tube orifice. At the junction between the cervical course and the vertical carotid canal course, there usually occurs a loop of the ICA and care must be taken here to identify the same.

16. The tumor most often adheres to the fibroperiosteal layer covering the ICA. A healthy subperiosteal plane is identified over the ICA at the carotid foramen (**Fig. 59.20**) and is followed superiorly toward the vertical segment of ICA to dissect the tumor off the ICA. This step cannot be performed if there is invasion of the ICA wall itself, in which case, the treatment strategy should include a prior carotid stenting,[4,5] or in cases of good collateral circulation, a decision of carotid resection. These decisions along with testing for collateral circulation are made preoperatively when surgical strategy is discussed with the subject.
17. The sigmoid sinus in its inferior half and the jugular bulb are uncovered. A wedge of bone is left intact on the superior half of the sigmoid sinus to perform extraluminal packing of the sigmoid. The lateral wall of the sigmoid sinus is dissected off from the overlying bone (**Fig. 59.21**) and strips of surgicel are placed between the lateral wall of the sigmoid and the overlying bone to obliterate the upper end of the sinus (**Fig. 59.22**). IJV is double ligated in the neck and cut (**Fig. 59.23**).
18. The IJV is then lifted superiorly and resected together with the lateral wall of the jugular bulb and the lateral wall of sigmoid sinus (**Fig. 59.24**). The medial wall of the jugular bulb is left intact, deep to which run the lower cranial nerves from their intracranial to extracranial course. At this point, there occurs brisk bleeding from the openings of the inferior petrosal sinus in the medial wall of the jugular bulb. Occasionally, a condylar emissary vein also opens into the jugular bulb (**Fig. 59.25**). The openings are gently packed with surgicel strips till bleeding settles. Too tight packing of these openings is avoided to prevent compression injury to the lower cranial nerves. The tumor is meticulously bipolarized and excised from involved areas.
19. In case of extradural extension to the posterior fossa dura, the tumor is dissected off the dura and excised. Any remnant tumor bits or suspicious areas over the dura are bipolarized. In cases of limited intradural extension, the dura is opened, the tumor is excised,

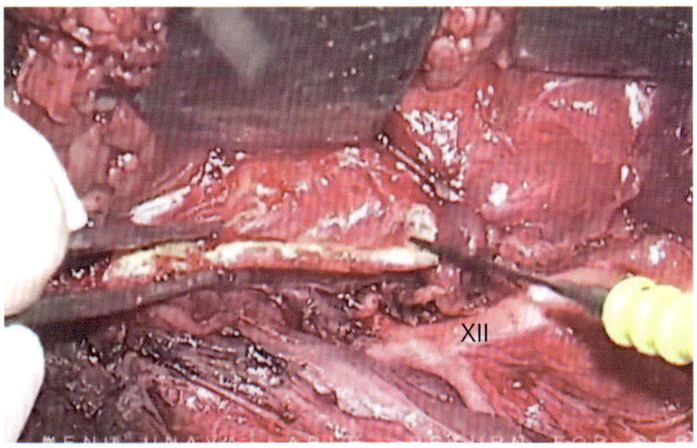

Fig. 59.18 Styloid process excision.

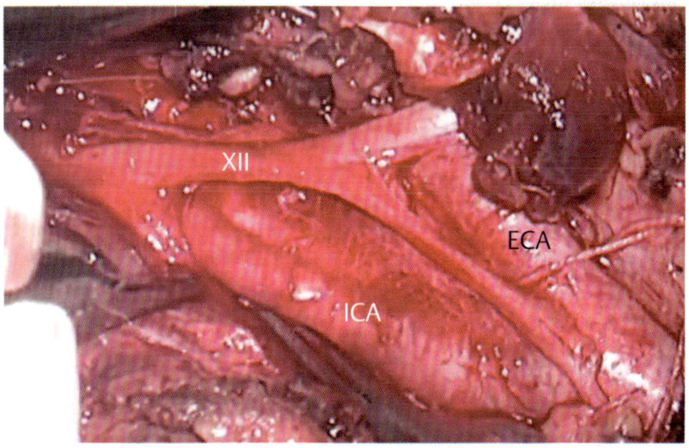

Fig. 59.19 Internal carotid artery (ICA) is traced in continuity from the cervical segment going superiorly.

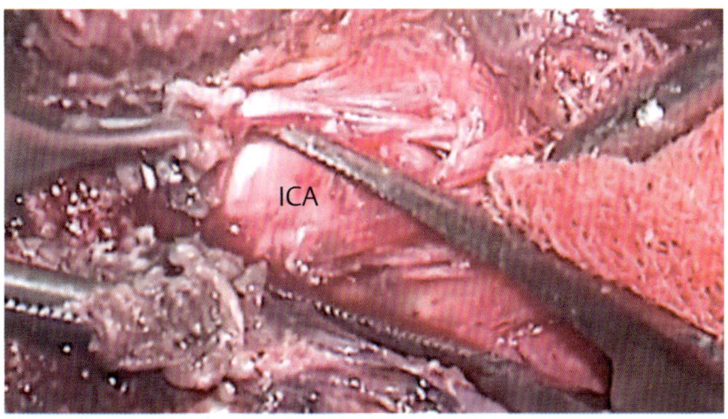

Fig. 59.20 Tumor dissected off the internal carotid artery (ICA) in subperiosteal plane.

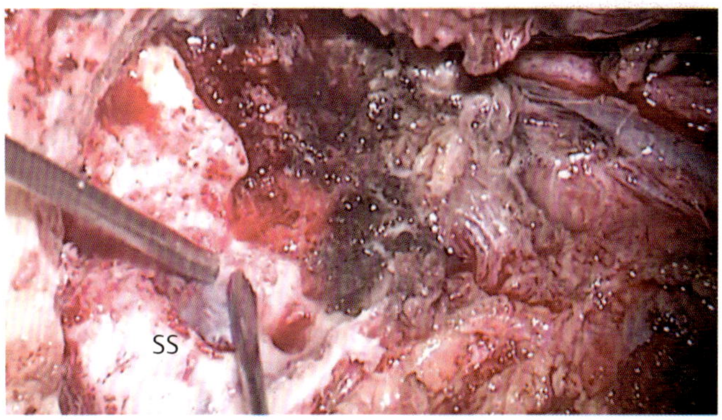

Fig. 59.21 Dissection in plane between the sigmoid sinus and overlying bone.

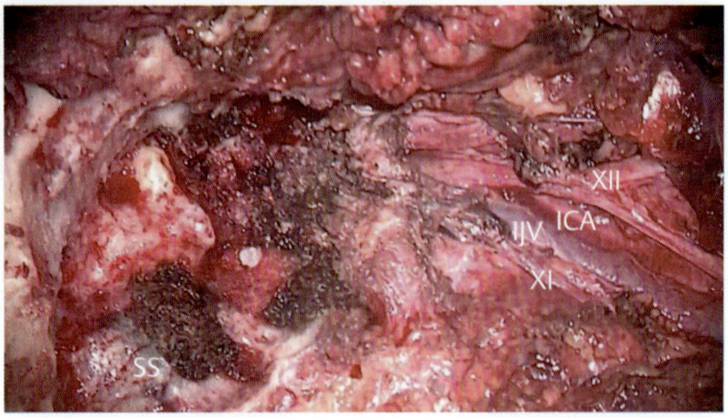

Fig. 59.22 Extraluminal compression of sigmoid sinus performed with surgicel.

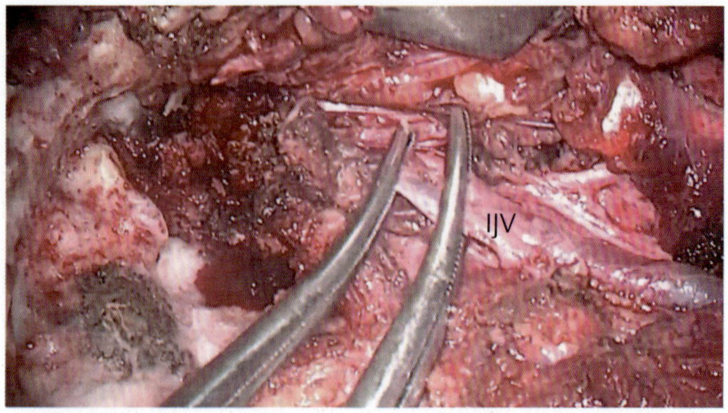

Fig. 59.23 Internal jugular vein (IJV) ligated in neck.

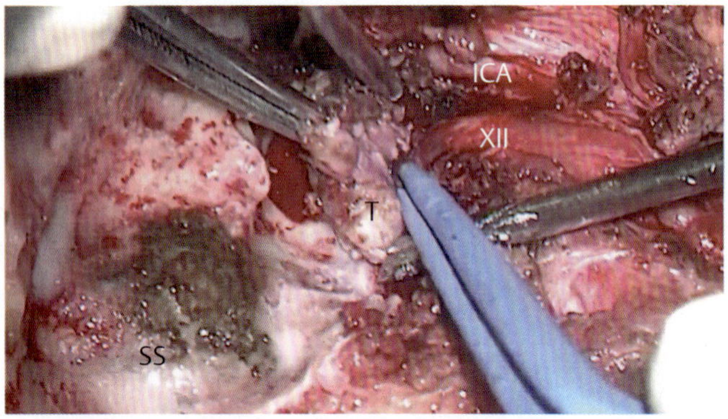

Fig. 59.24 Tumor with the lateral wall of jugular bulb is being resected.

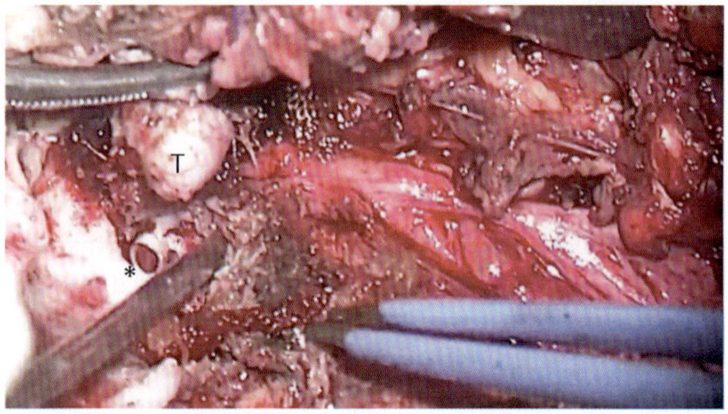

Fig. 59.25 Condylar emissary vein opening on the medial wall of jugular bulb (*) seen.

and the dural defect is plugged with fat. It must be noted that large intracranial extensions are excised in a second stage.[6]

20. In cases where the facial nerve is found invaded with tumor, the surgical strategy involves a resection of the involved segment with nerve grafting.[7,8] A case example of a glomus tumor in another subject involving the facial nerve on left side is shown (**Fig. 59.26**). The cut end of tympanic segment close to the geniculate ganglion is seen (**Fig. 59.27**). A sural nerve graft is harvested. The epineurium is stripped back from the edges (**Fig. 59.28**) and the nerve graft is then sutured to the main trunk in the parotid (**Fig. 59.29a**). The other end of the nerve graft is then approximated to the tympanic segment (**Fig. 59.29b**). Fibrin glue is used over the anastomosis.
21. In case of extension of the tumor to the occipital condyle posteriorly, a transcondylar transtubercular extension of the infratemporal fossa approach is performed.[8]
22. Strategies for vertebral artery involvement[9] is a broad subject and is not discussed here.
23. After tumor removal, all the bone deep to the tumor is drilled till healthy white polished bone is seen all around. The remnant middle ear mucosa is excised and bone over the promontory drilled (**Fig. 59.30**).

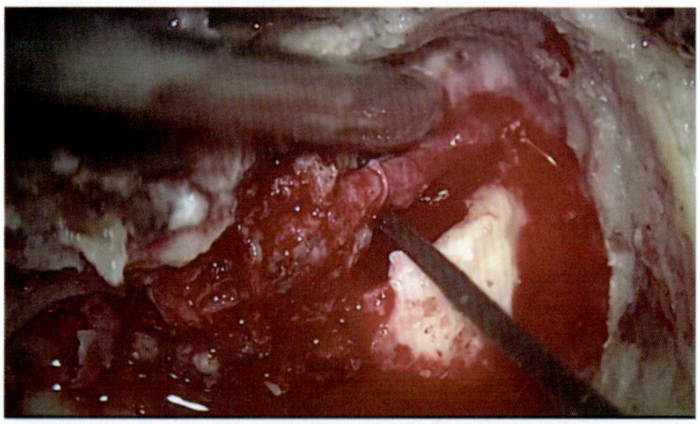

Fig. 59.26 Left-sided glomus—facial nerve mastoidal segment invaded by tumor.

24. Periosteum or fat is used to block the eustachian tube orifice. The entire operative cavity is obliterated with fat strips taken from the abdomen or thigh (**Fig. 59.31**).
25. The musculoperiosteal layer is reflected back and sutured. Subcutaneous and skin layers are sutured separately.

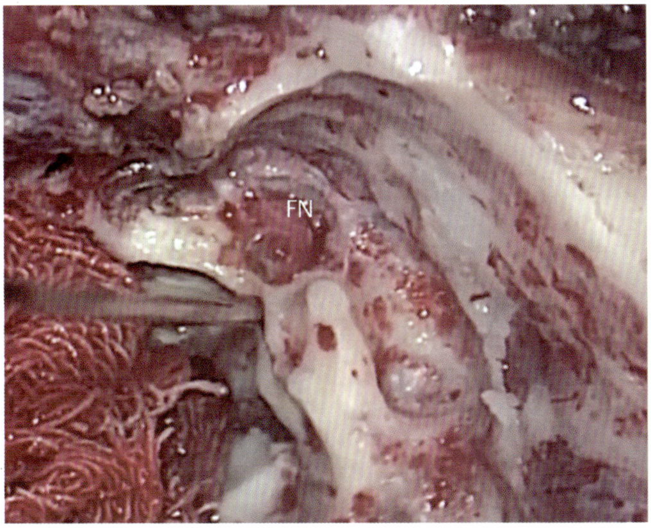

Fig. 59.27 Resected end of facial nerve (tympanic segment seen).

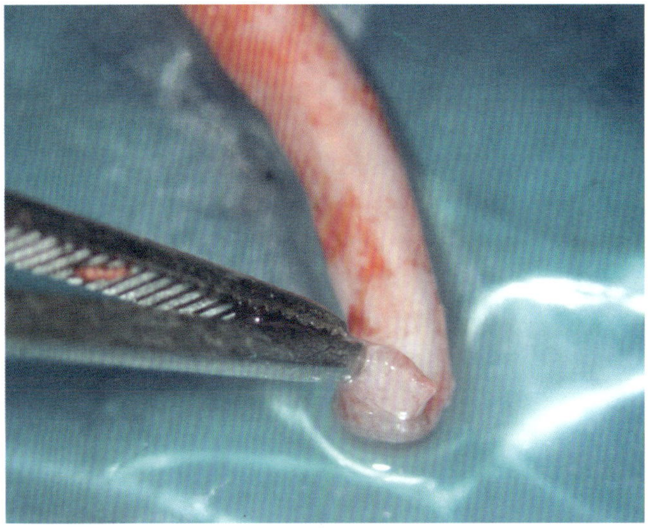

Fig. 59.28 Sural nerve graft harvested and epineurium stripped back.

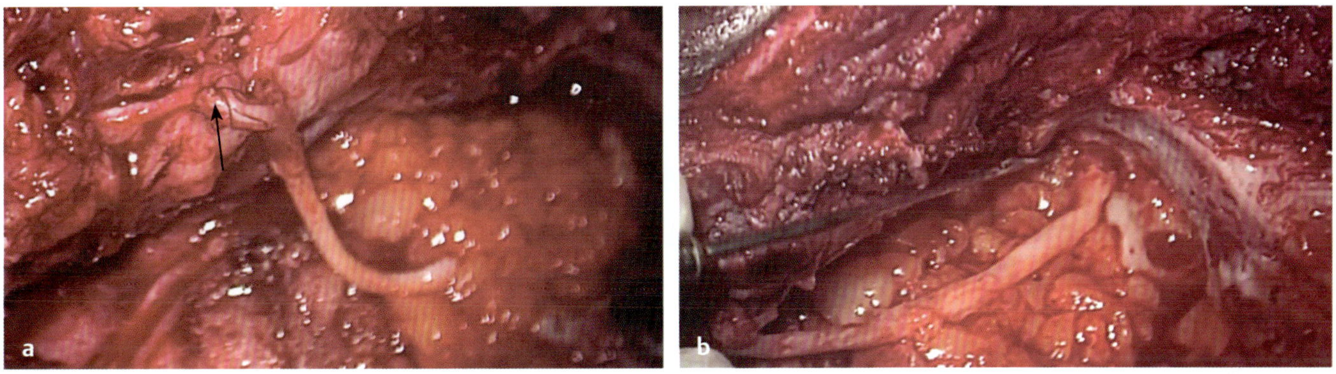

Fig. 59.29 **(a)** Nerve graft sutured to main trunk (*black arrow*) of facial nerve with 8-0 ethilon. **(b)** Nerve graft between cut end of tympanic segment and main trunk in parotid.

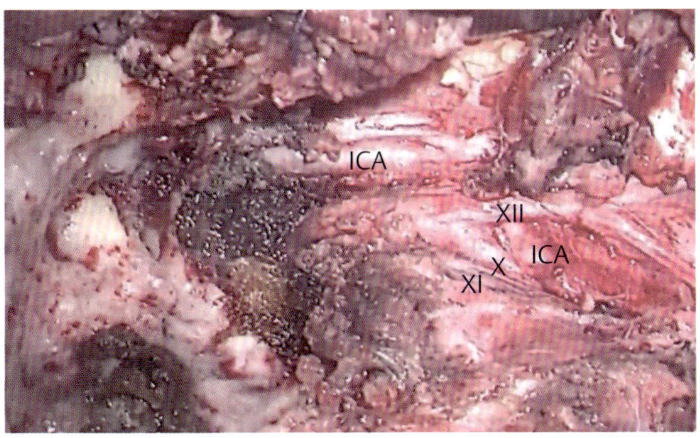

Fig. 59.30 View after complete tumor excision.

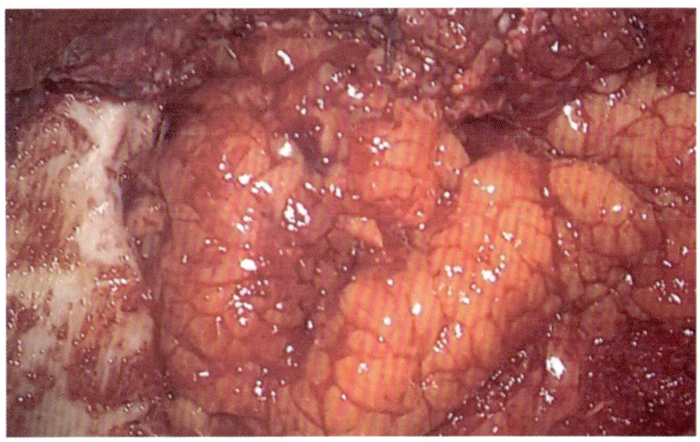

Fig. 59.31 Fat packed in the cavity.

References

1. Moe KS, Li D, Linder TE, Schmid S, Fisch U. An update on the surgical treatment of temporal bone paraganglioma. Skull Base Surg 1999;9(3):185–194
2. Sanna M, Mancini T, Russo F, Taibah A. The Facial Nerve in Temporal Bone and Lateral Skull Base Surgery. Stuttgart: Thieme; 2006
3. Olsen WL, Dillon WP, Kelly WM, Norman D, Brant-Zawadzki M, Newton TH. MR imaging of paragangliomas. AJR Am J Roentgenol 1987;148(1):201–204
4. Piazza P, Di Lella F, Bacciu A, Di Trapani G, Ait Mimoune H, Sanna M. Preoperative protective stenting of the internal carotid artery in the management of complex head and neck paragangliomas: long-term results. Audiol Neurotol 2013;18(6):345–352
5. Sanna M, Shin SH, De Donato G, et al. Management of complex tympanojugular paragangliomas including endovascular intervention. Laryngoscope 2011;121(7):1372–1382
6. Sanna M, Jain Y, De Donato G, Rohit, Lauda L, Taibah A. Management of jugular paragangliomas: the Gruppo Otologico experience. Otol Neurotol 2004;25(5):797–804
7. Leonetti JP, Anderson DE, Marzo SJ, Origitano TC, Vandevender D, Quinonez R. Facial paralysis associated with glomus jugulare tumors. Otol Neurotol 2007;28(1):104–106
8. Sanna M, Shin SH, Piazza P, et al. Infratemporal fossa approach type a with transcondylar-transtubercular extension for Fisch type C2 to C4 tympanojugular paragangliomas. Head Neck 2014;36(11):1581–1588
9. Prasad SC, Mimoune HA, Khardaly M, Piazza P, Russo A, Sanna M. Strategies and long-term outcomes in the surgical management of tympanojugular paragangliomas. Head Neck 2016;38(6):871–885

Chapter 60 Petro-Occipital Transsigmoid Approach

Narayan Jayashankar and R. Chandra Shekar Reddy

Introduction

Tumors of the jugular foramen region present a surgical challenge owing to the close association with surrounding neurovascular structures. The infratemporal fossa type A approach allows access to the jugular foramen. However, in this approach, the subject is left with a conductive hearing loss because of the obliteration of the cavity and cul-de-sac closure of the external auditory canal. The subject could also have a sensorineural hearing loss depending on the extent of the tumor. Additionally, it also involves the transposition of the facial nerve with resultant facial paresis eventually recovering to grade 3 or 2 (House–Brackmann grading) in most cases. The main aim of the petro-occipital transsigmoid (POTS) approach is to excise tumors of the jugular foramen without causing facial weakness or audiological deficit.

The POTS approach provides good access to the jugular foramen which is directed posterolaterally compared to the infratemporal fossa approach which is directed laterally.

Indications

- Benign nonvascular tumors (schwannoma, meningioma, chordoma) of the jugular bulb, located posteroinferiorly at the jugular foramen.
- Glomus jugulare type C1 tumors, which are predominantly posteriorly located.

Surgical Steps

A case example is given below. The preoperative magnetic resonance imaging (MRI) scans showing a cystic lesion in the left jugular foramen is shown (**Fig. 60.1a–f**).

1. A curvilinear C-shaped postauricular incision is made 4 to 5 cm behind the postaural groove. It begins superiorly approximately 1 cm above the superior pole of the helix going into the retromastoid area posteriorly and inferiorly extending into the neck approximately 2 cm below the level of the mandible (**Fig. 60.2**). Extension

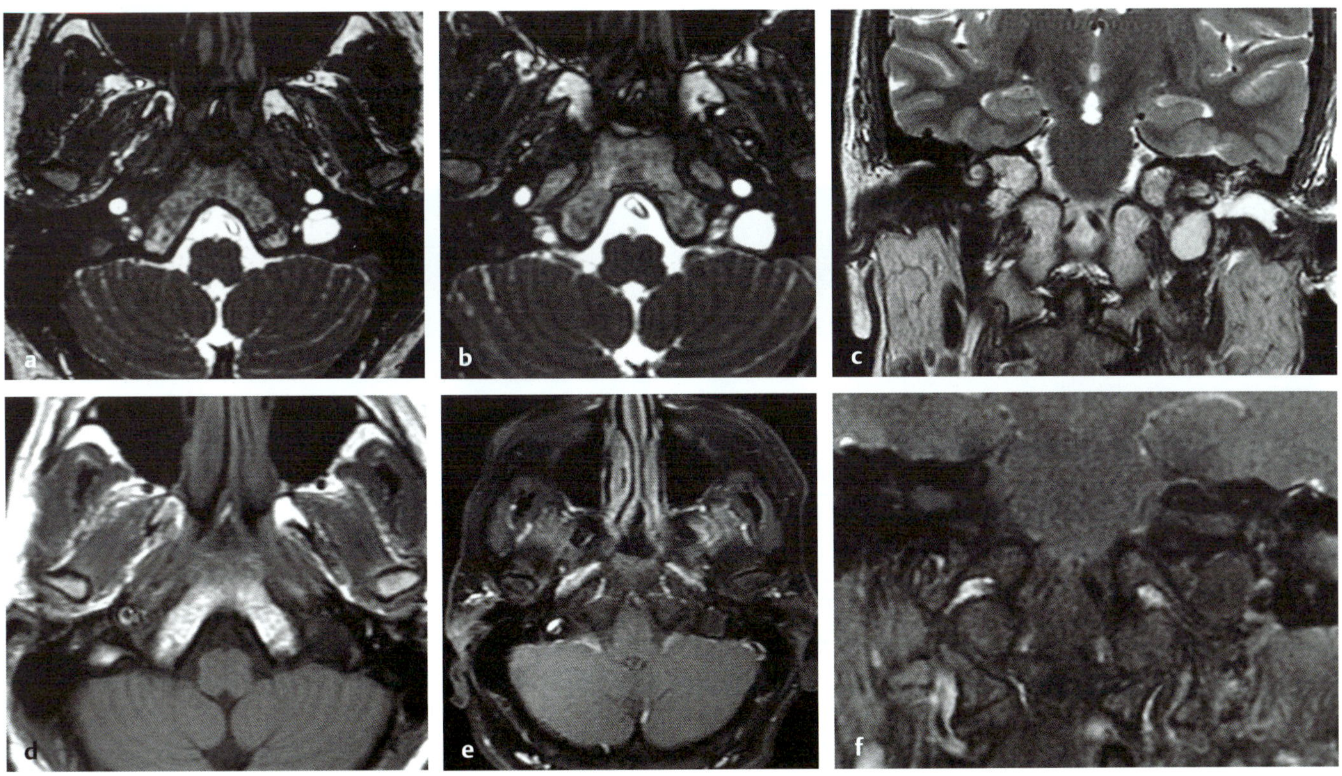

Fig. 60.1 **(a, b)** Axial T2-weighted images showing a hyperintense well-defined cystic lesion in left jugular foramen. **(c)** Coronal T2, **(d)** axial T1, **(e, f)** axial T1 and coronal T1 postcontrast images show no significant enhancement.

into the neck is very limited since we avoid opening neck spaces extensively for achieving control of postoperative cerebrospinal fluid (CSF) leakage.

2. The skin and subcutaneous tissue are elevated, leaving the musculoperiosteal layer behind (**Fig. 60.3**). This cutaneous flap is reflected anteriorly and sutured to hold it in place.
3. Using monopolar cautery, an inverted U-shaped musculoperiosteal flap is made pedicled inferiorly (**Fig. 60.4**). An incision is made starting from the anterior border of the sternocleidomastoid going adjacent to the cuff of the external auditory canal superiorly including the temporalis muscle curving around the superior temporal line and posteriorly involving the retromastoid muscle area. All the muscles are reflected inferiorly in a single layer.
4. After retracting the sternocleidomastoid muscle posteriorly in the neck, the lateral process of the atlas is palpated (**Fig. 60.5**). Blunt dissection just in front of this exposes the internal jugular vein (IJV). A silicone rubber tube (from a scalp vein set with its ends cut) is looped around the IJV for control.
5. Cortical mastoidectomy is performed. The semicircular canals and the mastoidal segment of the facial nerve are delineated. The infralabyrinthine cells are cleared completely (**Fig. 60.6**). Care is taken to clearly delineate

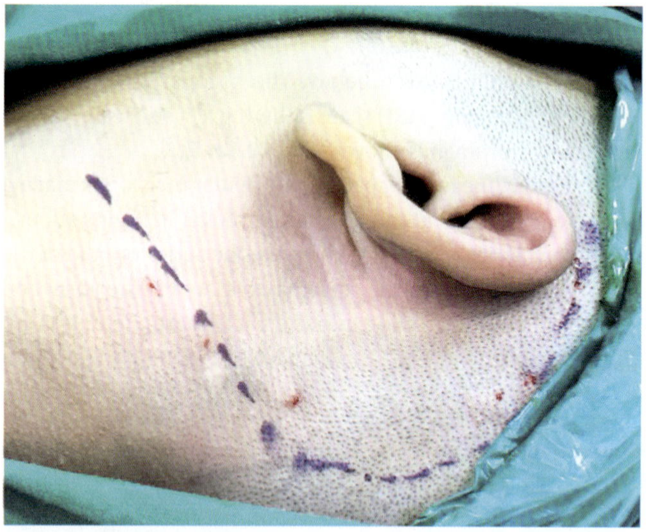

Fig. 60.2 Incision.

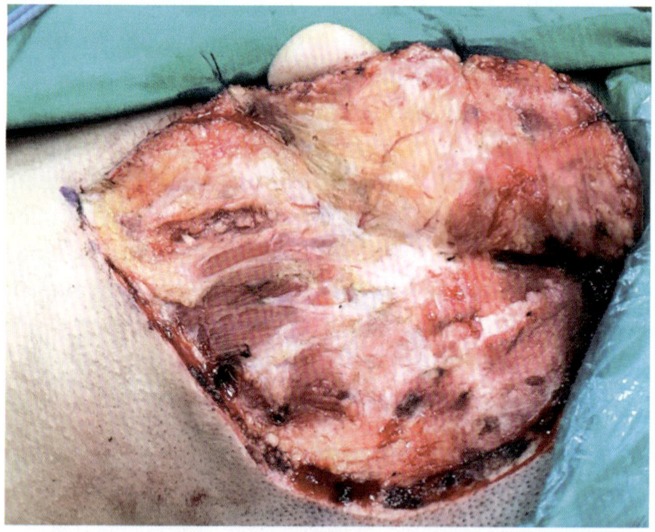

Fig. 60.3 Cutaneous flap elevation.

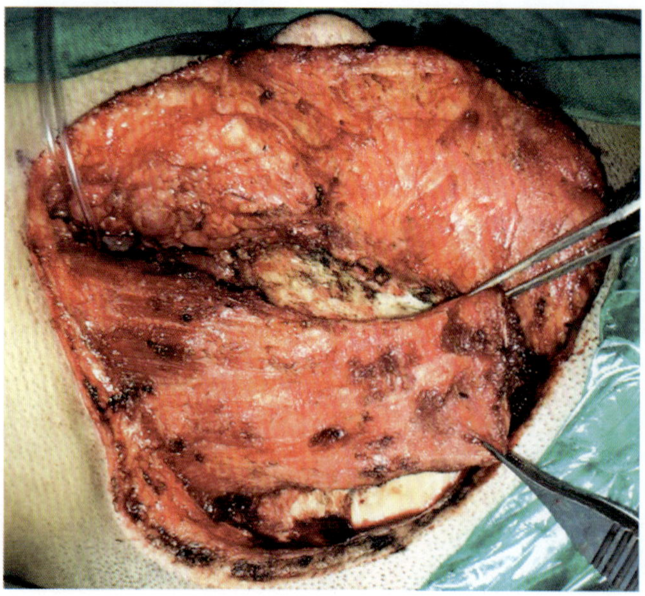

Fig. 60.4 Musculoperiosteal flap.

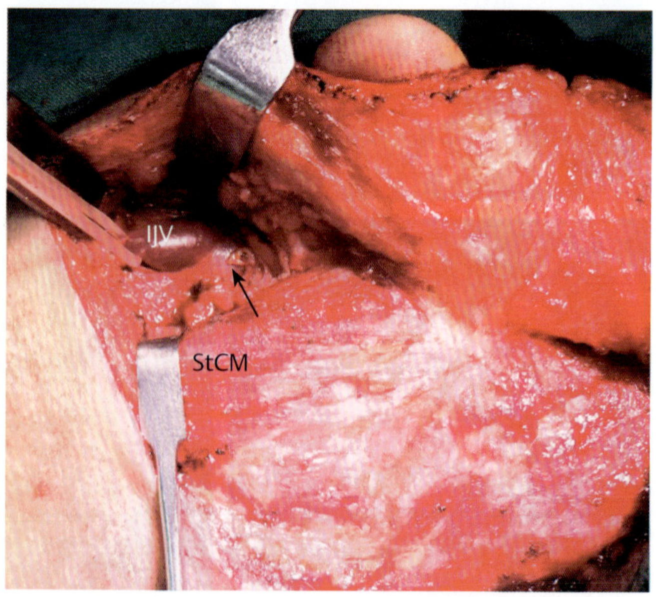

Fig. 60.5 Identification and control of IJV. *Black arrow* shows transverse process of atlas.

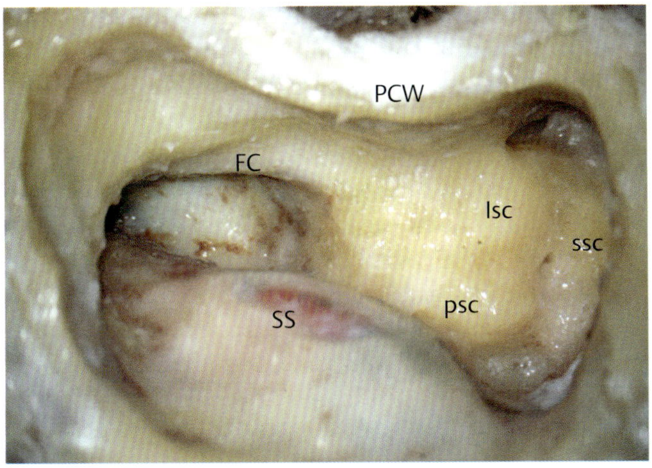

Fig. 60.6 Cortical mastoidectomy.

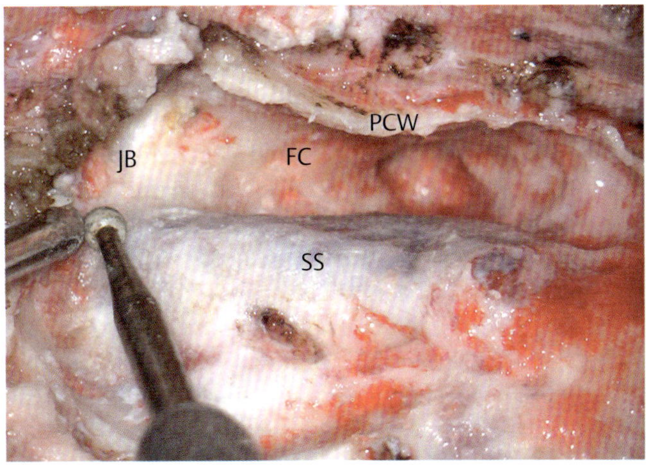

Fig. 60.7 Delineation of sigmoid sinus and jugular bulb.

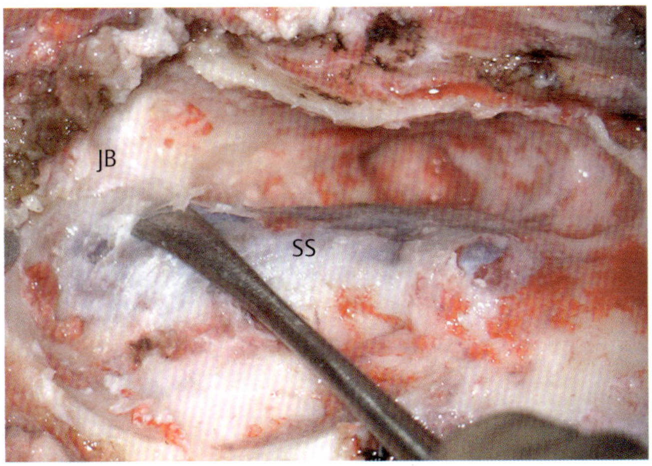

Fig. 60.8 Decompression of lower third of sigmoid sinus.

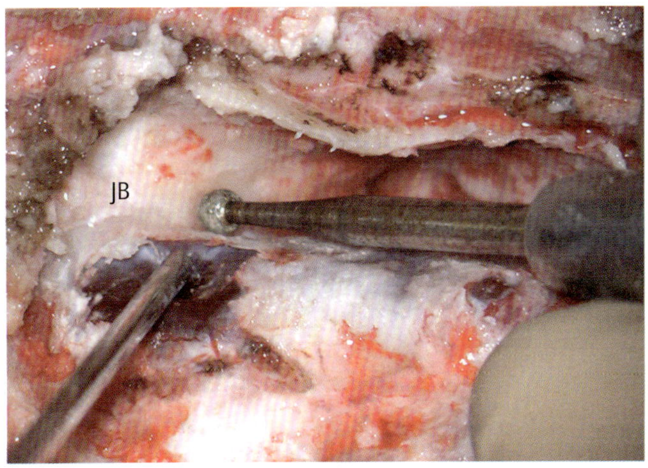

Fig. 60.9 Drilling to decompress jugular bulb.

the posterior semicircular canal without blue lining it, since this exposure will be useful to get the additional space for the approach toward the infratubal segment of the internal carotid artery deep to the mastoidal segment of the facial nerve. The tegmen plate is left intact as a thin bone covering the middle fossa dura. The sigmoid sinus and jugular bulb are delineated, and the bone covering these structures is drilled eggshell thin (**Fig. 60.7**).

6. Presigmoid posterior fossa bone is drilled. Eggshell thin bone over the sigmoid sinus in its lower two-thirds, jugular bulb, and presigmoid posterior fossa dura can be elevated off using a Freer elevator (**Fig. 60.8, Fig. 60.9,** and **Fig. 60.10**).
7. The endolymphatic sac is identified just inferior to the Donaldson line, and it can be seen over the presigmoid

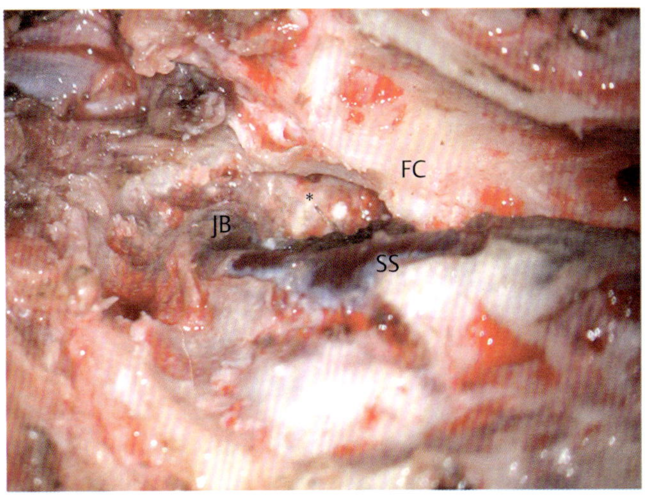

Fig. 60.10 Decompressed sigmoid sinus, jugular bulb. *Black star* shows infrafacial area to be drilled.

posterior fossa as a shiny white double-layered dural sheath (**Fig. 60.11**).

8. Retrofacial cells are drilled in a direction parallel to the facial nerve. Drilling is continued in the area deeper to the mastoid segment of the facial nerve and the jugular bulb toward the vertical, infratubal internal carotid artery (**Fig. 60.12**). This segment of the internal carotid artery is decompressed (**Fig. 60.13a, b**). The decompressed jugular bulb can be depressed with the suction tip to create additional space for drilling.
9. The occipital condyle is partially drilled to improve the exposure of the posteroinferior part of the jugular foramen (**Fig. 60.14**).
10. For glomus jugulare tumors that are posteriorly based, extraluminal compression of the sigmoid sinus is now performed at the upper third using Surgicel inserted between the upper third of the sigmoid sinus and the overlying bone. Similarly, the IJV is ligated in the neck. The sigmoid sinus is opened at its inferior end and the dome of the jugular bulb (**Fig. 60.15**) can now be resected along with the lesion (**Fig. 60.16**). On opening the jugular bulb, there occurs brisk bleeding from the openings of the inferior petrosal sinus. These openings of inferior petrosal sinus on the medial wall of the sigmoid sinus need to be packed with Surgicel strips, which lie partly intraluminal and partly extraluminal.

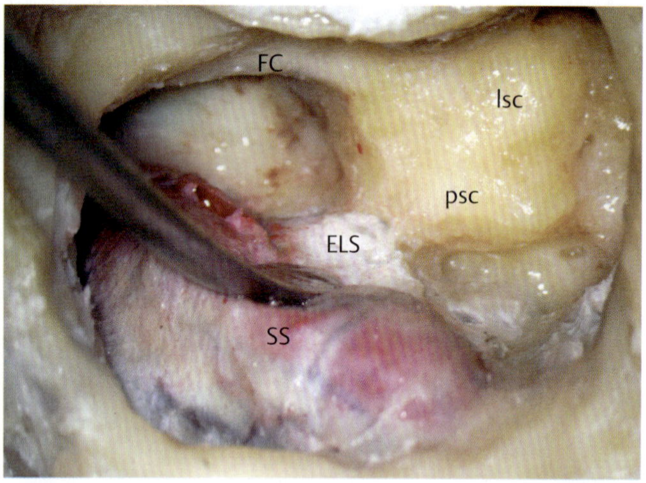

Fig. 60.11 Exposure of endolymphatic sac and presigmoid posterior fossa dura.

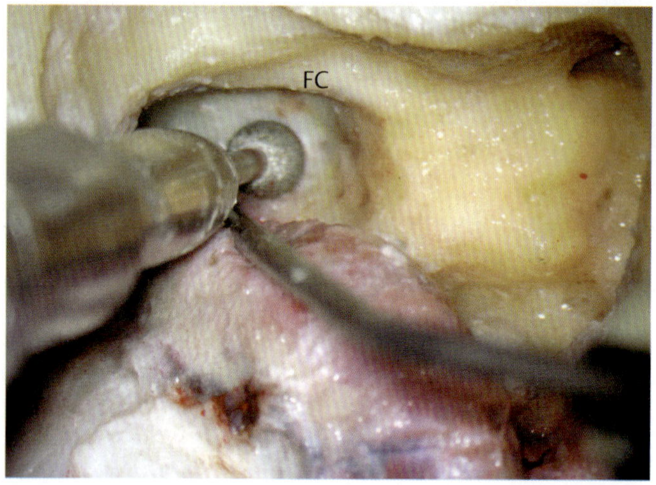

Fig. 60.12 Drilling deep to facial nerve toward the infratubal internal carotid artery.

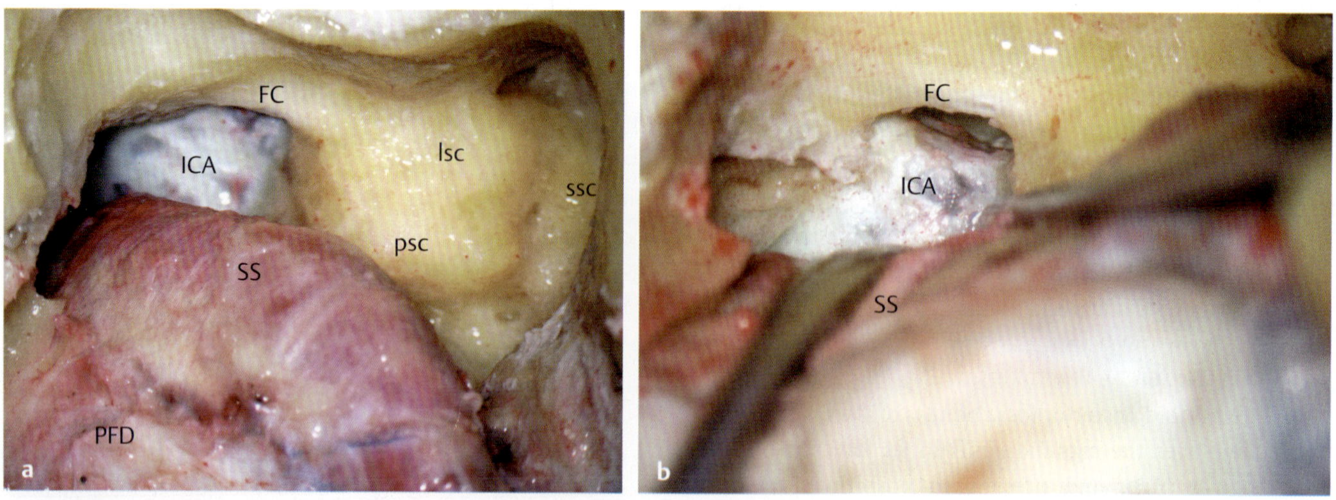

Fig. 60.13 **(a)** Decompressed internal carotid artery (ICA) (infratubal segment). **(b)** Magnified view of decompressed ICA.

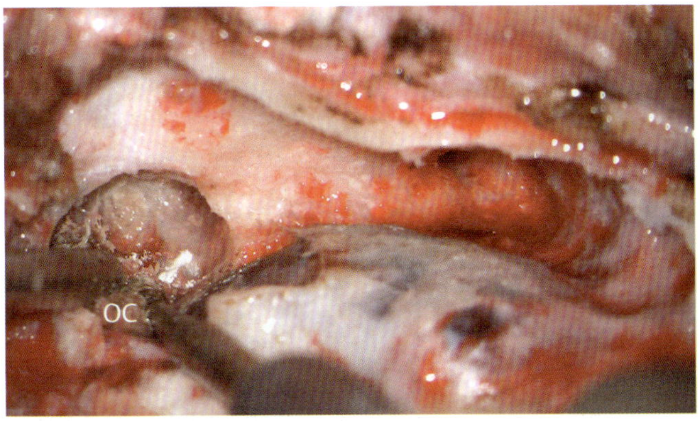

Fig. 60.14 Drilling of the occipital condyle.

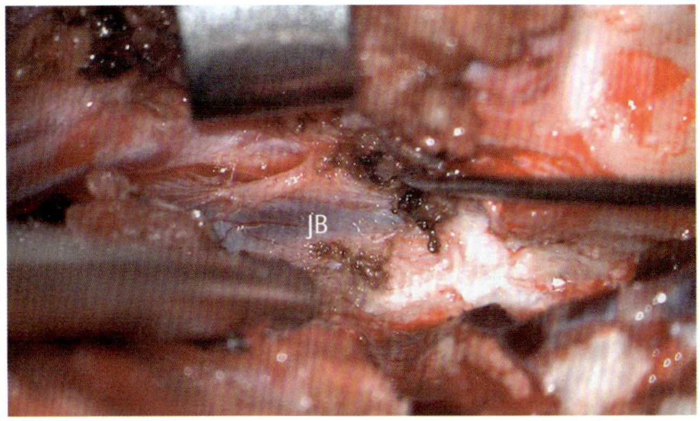

Fig. 60.15 Jugular bulb is completely exposed.

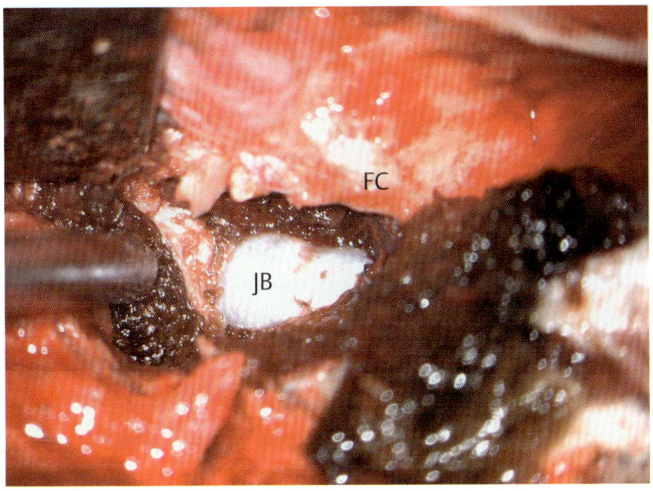

Fig. 60.16 Lateral wall of jugular bulb is excised. Medial wall of jugular bulb is seen.

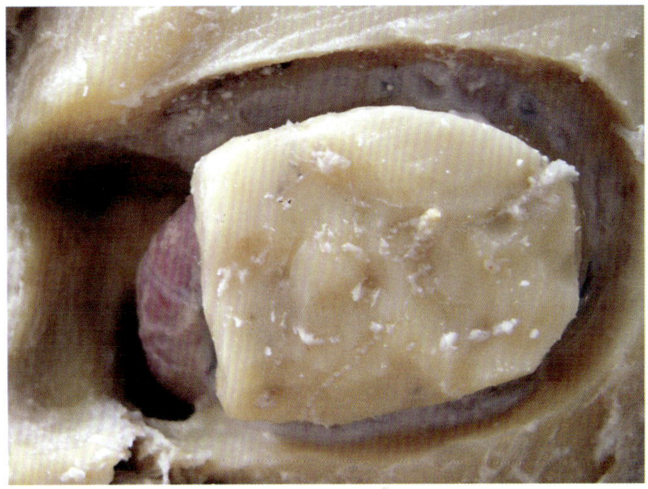

Fig. 60.17 Retrosigmoid craniotomy.

Care is to be taken to prevent embolization of the Surgicel strips. The Surgicel strips must not be jammed into the medial wall of the jugular bulb since the lower cranial nerves run deep to the medial wall of the jugular bulb.

11. It is hereby again emphasized that in case of glomus going anteriorly or involving the anterior wall of internal carotid artery, this approach is contraindicated since we cannot achieve adequate control of the desired areas.
12. **For schwannoma:** Initially, the tumor capsule in the infralabyrinthine compartment is opened and the tumor is debulked. The remnant tumor is dissected along with the lateral wall of the jugular bulb.
13. **Intracranial extent of tumor:** If there is an intracranial component of the tumor, access is gained using a 3 × 3 cm retrosigmoid craniotomy (**Fig. 60.17**). Craniotomy is limited anteriorly by the sigmoid sinus and superiorly by the transverse sinus. Bone is preserved for replacement at the end of the procedure, if needed.
14. The posterior fossa dura is incised in a posterior to anterior direction, starting retrosigmoid and passing through the walls of the sigmoid sinus and ending inferior to the endolymphatic sac (**Fig. 60.18**).
15. Dural cuts can be extended as desired, and the dural flaps are elevated superiorly and inferiorly to expose the intracranial extent of the tumor (**Fig. 60.19**). The tumor capsule is opened and the tumor is debulked using standard principles of tumor excision. The capsule of the tumor is then gently dissected off.
16. At the end of the procedure, the retrosigmoid dura is sutured and reinforced with DuraGen (bovine dura). The mastoid aditus is blocked with periosteum. The cavity is obliterated with fat strips taken from the thigh or abdomen. The external auditory canal is not opened in this procedure.
17. The musculoperiosteal, subcutaneous, and skin layers are sutured separately in an airtight fashion.

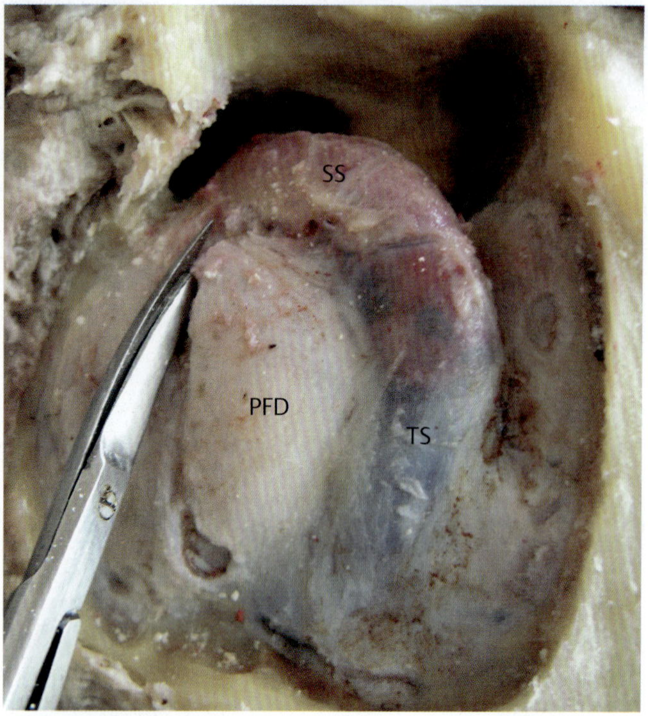

Fig. 60.18 Dural incision.

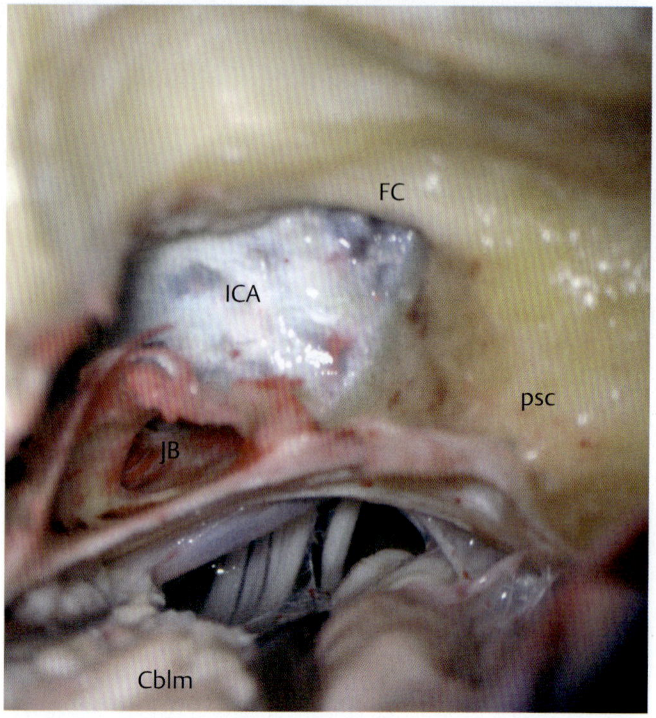

Fig. 60.19 Lower cranial nerves are exposed. Note the relationship of the medial wall of the jugular bulb to the lower cranial nerves as they course extracranially from their intracranial course.

Tips and Pearls

- Preservation of function in POTS also depends on the underlying pathology. Jugular foramen schwannomas usually have the best prognosis among the lesions of this area.
- Benign lesions like infralabyrinthine cholesterol granuloma, and cystic masses usually have a good outcome with this approach.
- Subjects with meningioma may present a difficult case as the jugular fossa is usually filled by the tumor, and both soft tissue and bone infiltration are usually seen.
- This approach is unfavorable for paraganglioma excision and has a high chance of residual disease. The POTS approach can occasionally be used for C1 class paragangliomas that extend posteriorly into the jugular fossa and cerebellopontine angle (CPA) but has minimal anterior extension into the tympanic cavity.

Suggested Readings

Mazzoni A. The petro-occipital trans-sigmoid approach for lesions of the jugular foramen. Skull Base 2009;19(1):48–56

Mazzoni A, Sanna M. A posterolateral approach to the skull base: the petro-occipital transsigmoid approach. Skull Base Surg 1995;5(3):157–167

Section XXIII

Approach to Foramen Magnum Tumors

Chapter 61

Far and Extreme Lateral Transcondylar Approach to the Foramen Magnum

Sanjay Behari, Ashish R. Sharma, Kuntal Kanti Das, and Kamlesh Singh Bhaisora

Indications

Accessing the ventral foramen magnum lesions situated just anterior to the foramen magnum becomes difficult with a pure posterior suboccipital approach as a more lateral corridor to the region anterior to the brainstem is required. Defining the vertical extent of the lesion, these approaches are appropriate for anteriorly placed lesions, posterior to the clivus and ventral to the brainstem, located below the level of the jugular foramen, extending to the foramen magnum and the atlas and axis vertebrae. Defining the horizontal extent to the lesion, this approach is most appropriate for a lesion that extends along the ventral foramen magnum reaching up to or encasing either one or both vertebral arteries, where no part of the tumor capsule comes in contact with the posterior dural surface. Thus, the brainstem intervenes between the lesion and the posterior dural covering along the entire length of the posterior tumor capsule.

Principle

The extreme lateral transcondylar (ELTC) approach utilizes a lateral corridor at the foramen magnum with the drilling of posterior one-third of the occipital condyle for accessing ventral foramen magnum lesions. The visualization of the tumor–cord interface from a lateral aspect significantly decreases the morbidity of tumor removal.

- This is often required for anterior foramen magnum meningiomas with a wide dural attachment to the anterior inner surface of dura. It is difficult to mobilize and slide off these lesions from the ventral brainstem surface and its arachnoidal plane because of their attachment to the anterior clival dura.
- In recurrent tumors in this location, the tumor–brainstem interface and the arachnoidal plane are compromised. This approach helps to visualize the tumor from an entirely lateral perspective and helps to preserve the tumor–brainstem interface and the neurovascular structures.
- In the cases of extensive extradural bony tumors of the foramen magnum that have encased one or both vertebral arteries, this approach is very suitable.
- A very large intradural–extramedullary tumor that has caused significant cervicomedullary compression and may endanger the vertebral or anterior spinal artery during its dissection may also be resected using this approach with vertebral artery mobilization.
- In the case of a large tumor, located ventral to the brainstem and upper cervical cord with a very firm consistency (appearing isointense on T2-weighted imaging), tumor debulking becomes extremely difficult without resulting in significant cord traction. The tumor has to be removed piecemeal with microscissors, and the ultrasonic suction aspirator also does not work in these cases. Having an adequate lateral corridor helps in these circumstances (**Fig. 61.1**).

The far lateral approach utilizes a similar corridor of approach as the ELTC approach. However, drilling of lateral one-third of the occipital condyle for mobilization of the V3 segment of the vertebral artery is not done in the far lateral approach. Thus, a more restricted access to the ventral aspect of the thecal sac is obtained in the latter case, and condylar drilling as well as vertebral artery mobilization are not performed. The indications for a far lateral approach include the following:

- An intra- or extradural ventral foramen magnum tumor with the tumor capsule reaching up to the posterior dura, so that by debulking the tumor from a posterolateral approach, an appropriate corridor is created for further access to the ventrally situated part of the lesion.
- Large neurofibromas (especially the dumbbell ones, with both intra- and extraspinal canalicular extent) that are soft in consistency (and, therefore, easier to debulk even if a small operative corridor is available) and may slide out of the tumor cavity, maintaining the arachnoidal plane between the brainstem and the tumor (**Fig. 61.2**).
- Significant and extensive bony tumors of the area that have compromised the ipsilateral vertebral artery, where the tumor shifts the brainstem and provides an adequate corridor.
- Vertebrobasilar artery aneurysms and arteriovenous malformations at the anterior aspect of cervicomedullary junction, where a proximal control of the vertebral artery is required without its mobilization.

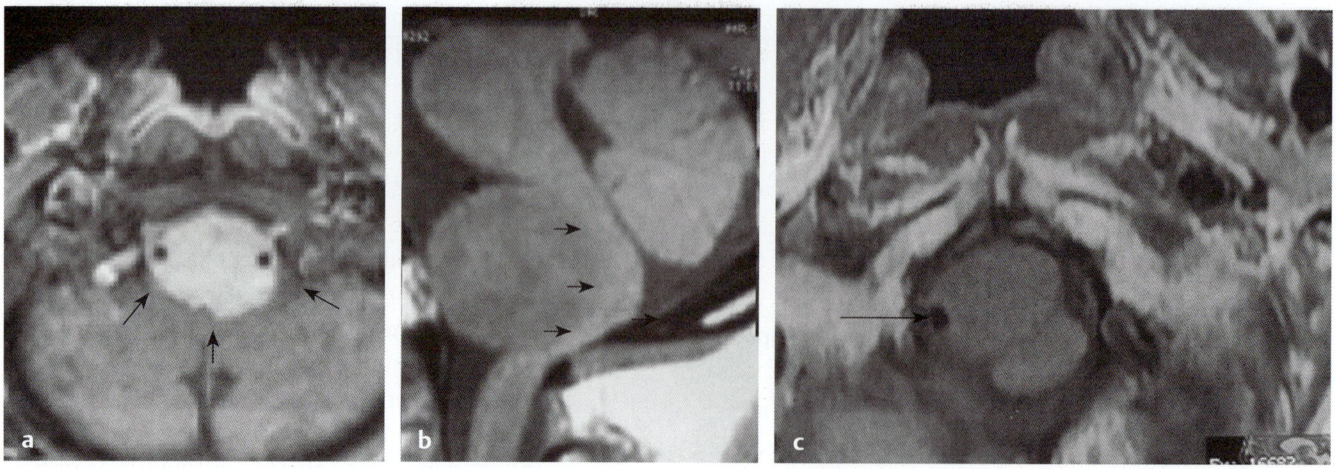

Fig. 61.1 **(a)** Contrast MRI axial image showing an anterior foramen magnum meningioma with a wide dural attachment to the anterior inner surface of dura. It is difficult to mobilize and slide off this lesion from the ventral brainstem surface and its arachnoidal plane using a posterior approach since the entire posterior tumor capsule stretches the brainstem (*arrows*) and prevents the tumor contact with the posterior dural surface (any contact between the posterior tumor capsule and the dural surface would have provided a corridor to the tumor). **(b)** A T1-weighted sagittal MR image showing a significant cervicomedullary kink. Tumor removal utilizing the conventional posterior or posterolateral approach may endanger the vertebral or anterior spinal artery during its dissection and requires the visualization of the cord–tumor interface (*arrows*) from a lateral aspect. **(c)** A T1-weighted axial image showing an anteriorly based meningioma that has encased the dominant vertebral artery (*arrow*). In all three instances, the lateral trajectory provided by condylar drilling and vertebral artery mobilization proved to be extremely useful.

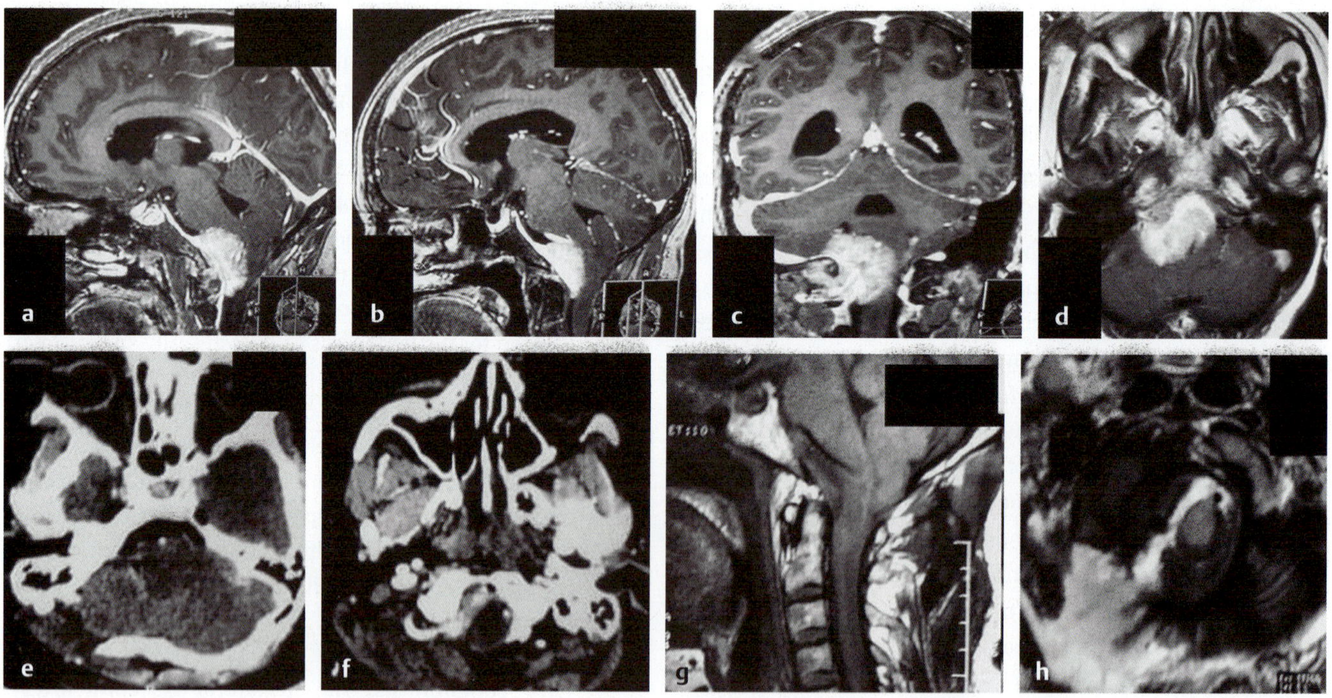

Fig. 61.2 **(a, b)** T1-weighted contrast sagittal image. **(c)** T1-weighted contrast coronal image. **(d)** T1-weighted contrast axial image showing an anteriorly placed meningioma at the cervicomedullary junction. The dumbbell shape and lateral extent of the meningioma with both extra- and intradural components provided the corridor for excision of the anteriorly situated component of the lesion. Hence, a far lateral approach without vertebral artery mobilization sufficed in this situation. **(e, f)** Postoperative axial CT scan showing total excision of the lesion using a far lateral approach. **(g)** T1-weighted contrast sagittal MR scan. **(h)** T2-weighted axial MR scan showing total tumor excision. Neither condylar drilling nor vertebral artery mobilization was done.

- Ventral developmental craniovertebral junction anomalies, such as a high basilar invagination, causing ventral cervicomedullary compression.
- Ventrally located cystic lesions of the foramen magnum, where decompression of the cyst through the lateral corridor between the spinal nerves collapses the tumor capsule, facilitating the capsular removal using this posterolateral corridor.

These two approaches have an advantage over the conventional transoral and the posterior approaches to the foramen magnum in accessing ventral lesions located in this area. This is because in addition to the provision of a very limited working space, the transoral approach, particularly in excising intradural pathologies, is often complicated by cerebrospinal fluid (CSF) leak, meningitis, and iatrogenic instability. With the posterior approach, visualization of tumor–cord interface is not possible. The far lateral and ELTC approaches not only help in providing an adequate corridor to the ventral foramen structures but also working through a sterile field, help to visualize both the ipsilateral and contralateral vertebral artery as well as the ventral brainstem surface, and occasionally also the anterior spinal artery (**Fig. 61.3** and **Fig. 61.4**).

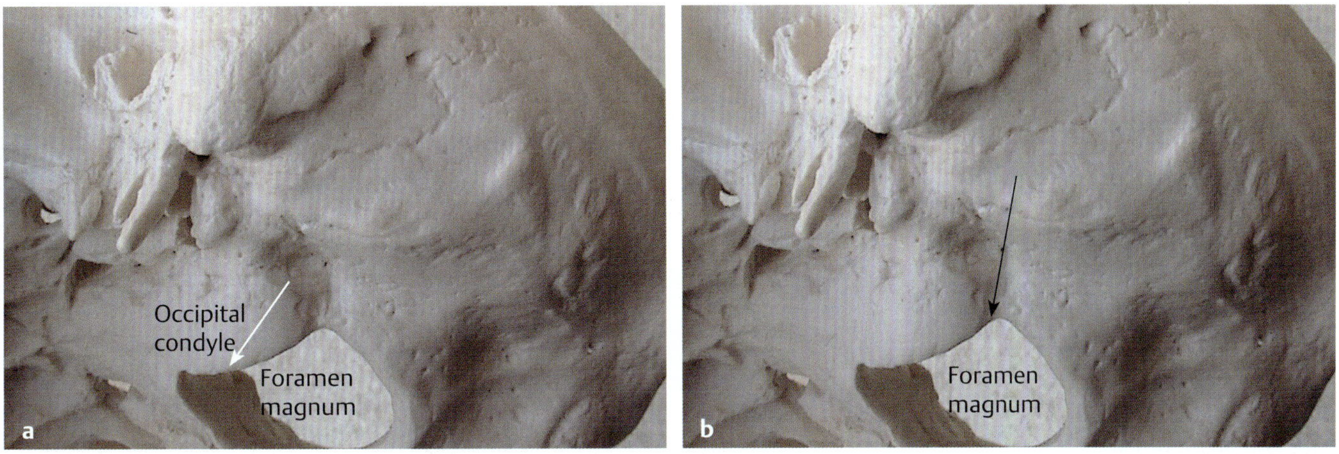

Fig. 61.3 **(a)** Trajectory of the extreme lateral transcondylar approach (*arrow*) that drills the posterior one-third of the occipital condyle to permit an anterolateral approach to the anterior margin of foramen magnum and the clivus. Drilling of only the lateral one-third of the occipital condyle until the cortical bone covering the hypoglossal canal preserves most of the condylar weight-bearing area and maintains occipitoatlantal stability. **(b)** Trajectory of the far lateral approach (*arrow*) without condylar drilling. The approach accesses the anterior clival region to a much lesser extent than the extreme lateral transcondylar approach.

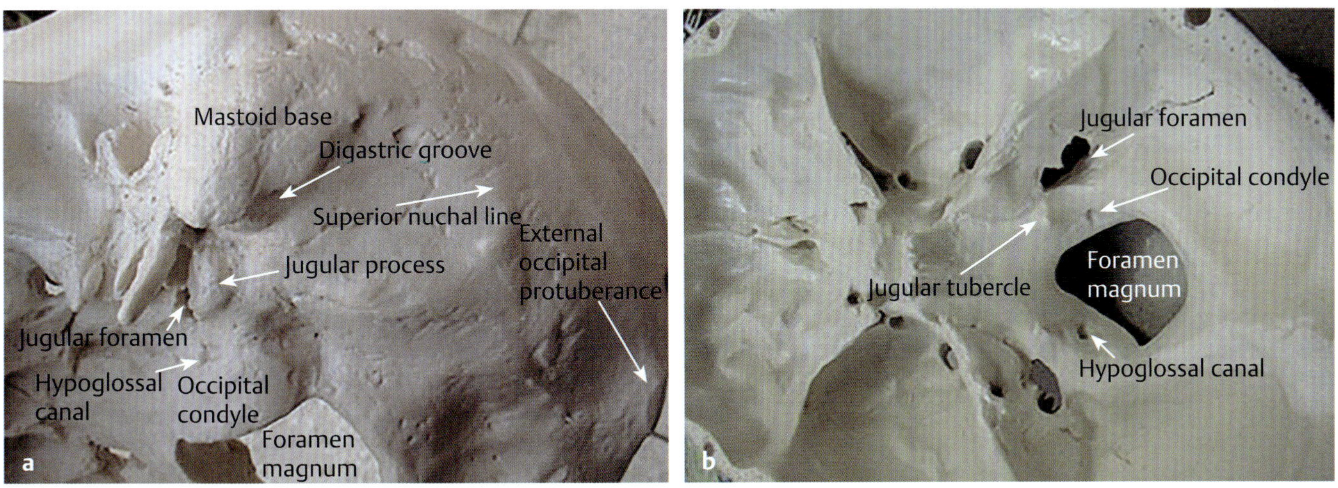

Fig. 61.4 **(a)** The major anatomical landmarks. The hypoglossal canal is obliquely oriented dividing the occipital condyle into the anterior two-thirds and the posterior one-third. Drilling of the occipital bone lateral to the occipital condyle up to the jugular process leads to the jugular foramen. **(b)** The posterior fossa showing the inner aspect of the occipital condyle and the inner opening of the hypoglossal canal. The jugular tubercle, a bony prominence situated just anterolateral to the hypoglossal canal, obstructs approach to the lower clivus and requires drilling. The jugular foramen is also visible.

Preoperative Assessment

A comprehensive imaging workup with computed tomography (CT) and magnetic resonance imaging (MRI) with an angiogram is essential before undertaking this procedure. An MRI with contrast shows the tumor extent in multiple planes. The direction of tumor growth and side shift of the neuraxis in the axial plane is the crucial information required for choosing the side of the approach. An angiogram, usually done with MRI, not only shows the vertebral artery (VA) encasement by a lesion but also illustrates the side of dominance of the vessels. In the case of a lesion that is strictly situated in the midline, the side having the nondominant VA should be chosen for approach. A venogram helps to determine the anatomy of the transverse and sigmoid sinuses, including the side of dominance and position of the jugular bulb. Thus, this approach is undertaken from the side from which the tumor is surfacing laterally and contralateral to the side where the cord has shifted. In strict midline tumors ventral to the foramen magnum, the side of the nondominant VA and jugular bulb are chosen. This ensures that in case of injury, dissection, or thrombosis of the VA during its mobilization, the dominant VA remains intact.

Assessment of the MR and CT images also helps in determining the size of the surgical corridor, that is, the distance between posteromedial margin of occipital condyle and the outer margin of cord in the axial plane.

Surgical Steps

Patient Positioning

A lateral position of the head without any rotation or tilt, that is fixed on a head clamp, with the torso also in a lateral position supported by padded supports on sides is the ideal position, as it has two advantages: one, it provides a lateral surgical corridor that facilitates visualization of the tumor–cord interface; and two, the position of the vertebral artery emerging from the foramen transversarium of the atlas and axis remains constant facilitating its early localization during surgery. Various other positions have been described including a supine position with contralateral head rotation by approximately 45 degrees or, a park bench position with lateral rotation and tilt of the head to make the head oriented in a lateral position.

Skin Incision

Three skin incisions are useful for this approach, each with its specific indications:

Horseshoe Incision

The medial vertical limb extends from just below the external occipital protuberance to C4 spinous process, while the lateral vertical limb extends from the base of the mastoid to just below the parietal eminence. The horizontal limb joins the vertical limbs from just below the external occipital protuberance to a point just below the parietal eminence. This incision facilitates exposure of the cerebellum, the cervicomedullary junction, and the upper part of the cervical cord. This horseshoe-shaped incision has several advantages: the midline vertical limb passes through the avascular midline ligamentum nuchae; an orientation of the midline is constantly maintained by palpating the spinous processes of the cervical vertebrae; the lateral limb remains above the mastoid process and does not endanger the facial nerve emerging from the stylomastoid foramen or the VA traversing the upper border of the lateral one-third of the posterior arch of the atlas vertebra; and, a wide exposure is obtained that may also be useful in facilitating an occipitocervical fusion in case greater than one-third of the occipital condyle is drilled (**Fig. 61.5a**).

Inverted "J-Shaped" Incision

The medial vertical limb extends from the external occipital protuberance to C4 spinous process. Its upper end gently curves laterally along the superior nuchal line to end at the base of the mastoid. This incision is preferable for anteriorly located tumors that are extending from the foramen magnum to the C5 level and not reaching up to the medulla oblongata.

A Curvilinear "C-Shaped" Incision behind the Pinna

This incision runs approximately 2 cm behind the pinna with the upper end curved toward the temporal region and the lower end anteriorly toward the neck. This incision facilitates the combination of the ELTC approach with posterior petrosectomy and presigmoid approaches. It helps in tracing the sigmoid sinus to its continuation as the jugular bulb in the mastoid region and the internal jugular vein in the carotid sheath in the neck.

Reflection of the Suboccipital Muscle Layers

After elevation of the skin flap, muscle layers of the posterior triangle of the neck come into view. The first layer consists of the sternocleidomastoid and trapezius muscle. The next layer is formed by the splenius capitis, semispinalis capitis, and longissimus capitis. These muscles are detached from their attachment at the mastoid base and nuchal lines, leaving a musculofascial cuff for later reapproximation, and reflected inferiorly. The occipital artery and vein traversing the muscular plane in the suboccipital region close to the nuchal lines have to be coagulated and divided (**Fig. 61.5b–d**). The accessory nerve, supplying the middle third of the sternocleidomastoid and entering the posterior triangle of the neck, should be preserved. Usually, the two muscular layers are reflected in a single flap (rather than attempting individual muscle reflection) as it avoids muscle atrophy in the region. This muscle reflection in a single flap with its base toward the neck exposes the suboccipital triangle formed by the third layer of muscles in the suboccipital region.

Palpation of Bony Landmarks for Orientation

In the suboccipital region, palpation of three important bony landmarks gives a good orientation of the small muscles of the suboccipital triangle: the bifid spinous process of the axis in the midline; the posterior tubercle of the atlas in the midline; and, the lateral mass of the atlas with its small transverse process situated laterally (**Fig. 61.5e, f**).

Exposure of the Suboccipital Triangle

The suboccipital triangle is horizontally oriented with its apex situated laterally on the transverse process of atlas and its base located medially. The upper and lower borders are formed by superior and inferior oblique muscles which have a common attachment at the transverse process of C1. The other end of the superior oblique attaches superiorly to the occipital bone and the inferior oblique attaches to the spinous process of axis. The medial border is constituted by rectus capitis posterior major and minor, which attach to the inferior nuchal line superiorly and the posterior arch of atlas and the spinous process of axis, inferiorly. The contents of this triangle are the horizontal portion of the V3 segment of the vertebral artery that crosses behind the atlanto-occipital joint and across the upper surface of the posterior arch of atlas; and, the C1 root that traverses laterally in close proximity to the vertebral artery. A venous plexus surrounds the vertebral artery in the suboccipital triangle and may lead to troublesome bleeding. The rectus capitis posterior major and minor are reflected downwards and medially and the superior and inferior oblique muscles reflected downwards (**Fig. 61.5g**).

Exposure and Control of the Vertebral Artery

The vertebral artery can be exposed either at the superior border of C1 or between the C1/2 foramen transversarium. At the lateral one-thirds of the superior border of the posterior arch of atlas, the vertebral artery is present in a fascial canal and is usually quite superficial. The vertebral artery, after it emerges from the foramen transversarium of the atlas, is crossed by the C1 nerve root, passes distally behind the atlantal lateral mass, gives rise to a posterior meningeal branch (and in 5% of patients, also a low lying posterior inferior cerebellar artery), and passes deep to the posterior atlanto-occipital membrane to enter the dura. Here, the constant location of the vertebral artery in its fibrous canal above the posterior arch of atlas, the C1 nerve root as well as the rectus capitis lateralis muscle (situated lateral to the vertebral artery extending from the transverse process of C1 to the occipital bone behind the jugular foramen) help in identifying the vertebral artery. The vertebral artery may also be identified between the foramen transversarium of C1 and C2. The loose areolar tissue between C1/2 is dissected along the inferior border of inferior oblique muscle till the C2 ganglion and the C2 nerve root is identified. The C2 ganglion usually overlies the vertical portion of the V3 segment of the vertebral artery between the C1 and C2 foramen transversarium. The posterior arch of the atlas and the lamina of the axis are exposed using a subperiosteal dissection. Laterally, the curving of the horizontal portion of the distal third part of the vertebral artery into its vertical segment that traverses the foramen transversarium of the atlas can be exposed after detaching the oblique muscles.

The foramen transversarium of the atlas (and occasionally also the axis) may be drilled to release the vertebral artery. The subperiosteal dissection of the horizontal portion of the vertebral artery on sulcus arteriosus on the superior border of the lateral one-third of the posterior arch of the atlas mobilizes the vertebral artery (**Fig. 61.5h–k**). The gentle medial retraction of the mobilized vertebral artery permits drilling of the occipital condyle and the lateral mass of the atlas up to the dura and provides a more ventral exposure to the thecal sac at the foramen magnum.

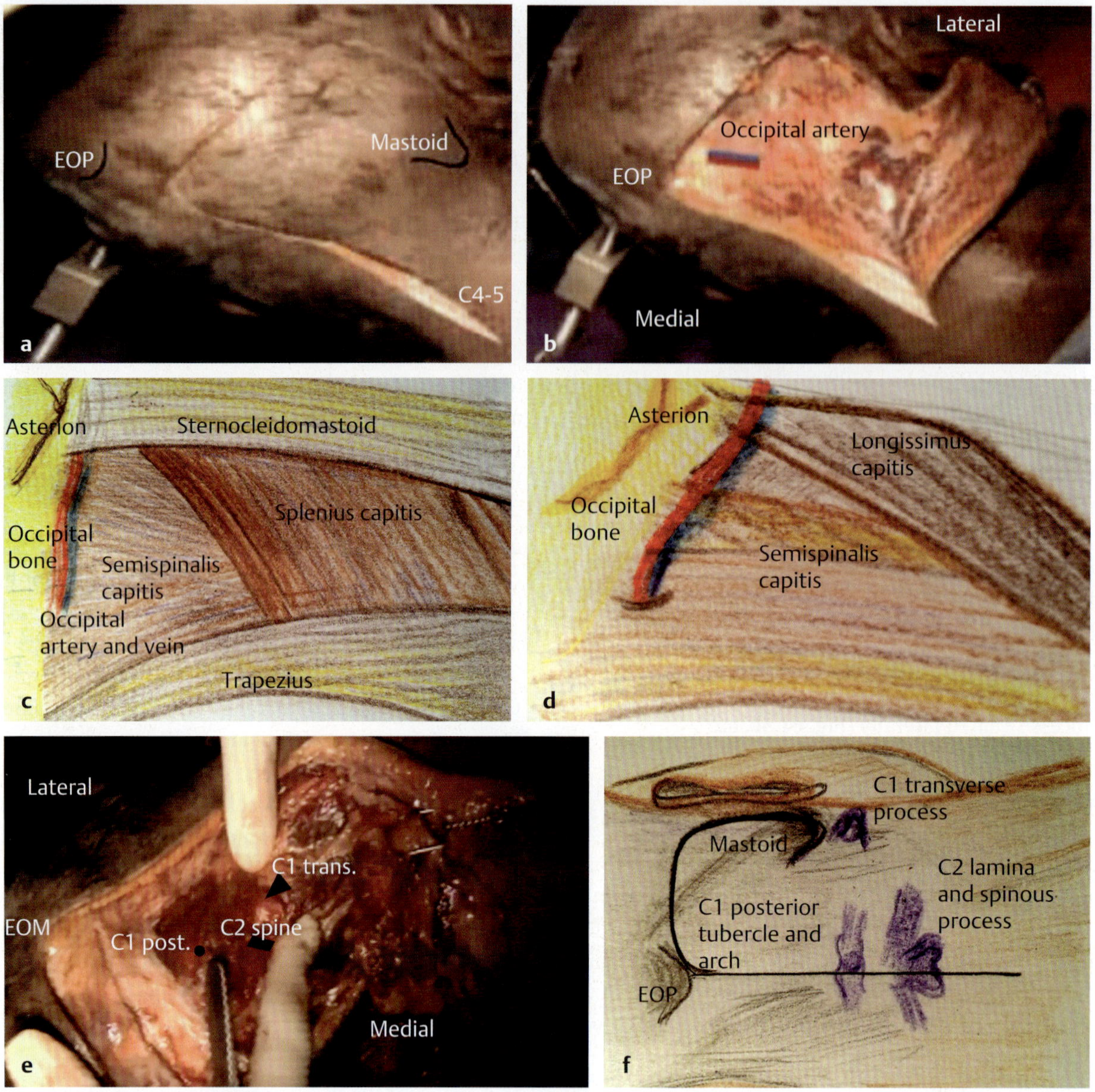

Fig. 61.5 **(a)** The horseshoe-shaped skin incision in which the medial vertical limb extends from just below the external occipital protuberance (EOP) to C4 spinous process, while the lateral vertical limb extends from the base of the mastoid process to just below the parietal eminence. The horizontal limb joins the vertical limbs, traversing just below the external occipital protuberance to a point just below the parietal eminence. **(b)** After elevation of the skin flap, muscle layers of the posterior aspect of the neck come into view. The first layer consists of the sternocleidomastoid and trapezius muscle. The next layer is formed by the splenius capitis, semispinalis capitis, and longissimus capitis. These muscles are detached from their attachment at the mastoid base and nuchal lines, leaving a musculofascial cuff for later reapproximation, and reflected inferiorly. The occipital artery and vein (*red and blue lines* in the figure, respectively) traversing the muscular plane in the suboccipital region close to the nuchal lines have to be coagulated and divided. **(c)** The superficial layer of muscles includes the sternocleidomastoid laterally and the trapezius medially covering the splenius capitis and the semispinalis capitis. The occipital artery and vein may be encountered while a tendinous cuff of the muscles is being left on the occipital bone. **(d)** Once the sternocleidomastoid, the trapezius, and the splenius capitis muscles are reflected, the semispinalis capitis medially and the longissimus capitis muscles laterally are encountered. **(e)** Palpation of three important bony landmarks gives a good orientation of the suboccipital triangle: the bifid spinous process of the axis in the midline (C2 spine), the posterior tubercle of the atlas in the midline (C1 post.), and, the lateral mass of the atlas with its small transverse process (C1 trans.) situated laterally. **(f)** Schematic diagram showing the horseshoe-shaped incision from the midline extending from the C4 spine to the external occipital protuberance and the base of the mastoid process laterally. It also shows the anatomy of the three palpable bony landmarks: the posterior tubercle of the atlas, the transverse process of the atlas, and the spinous process of axis.

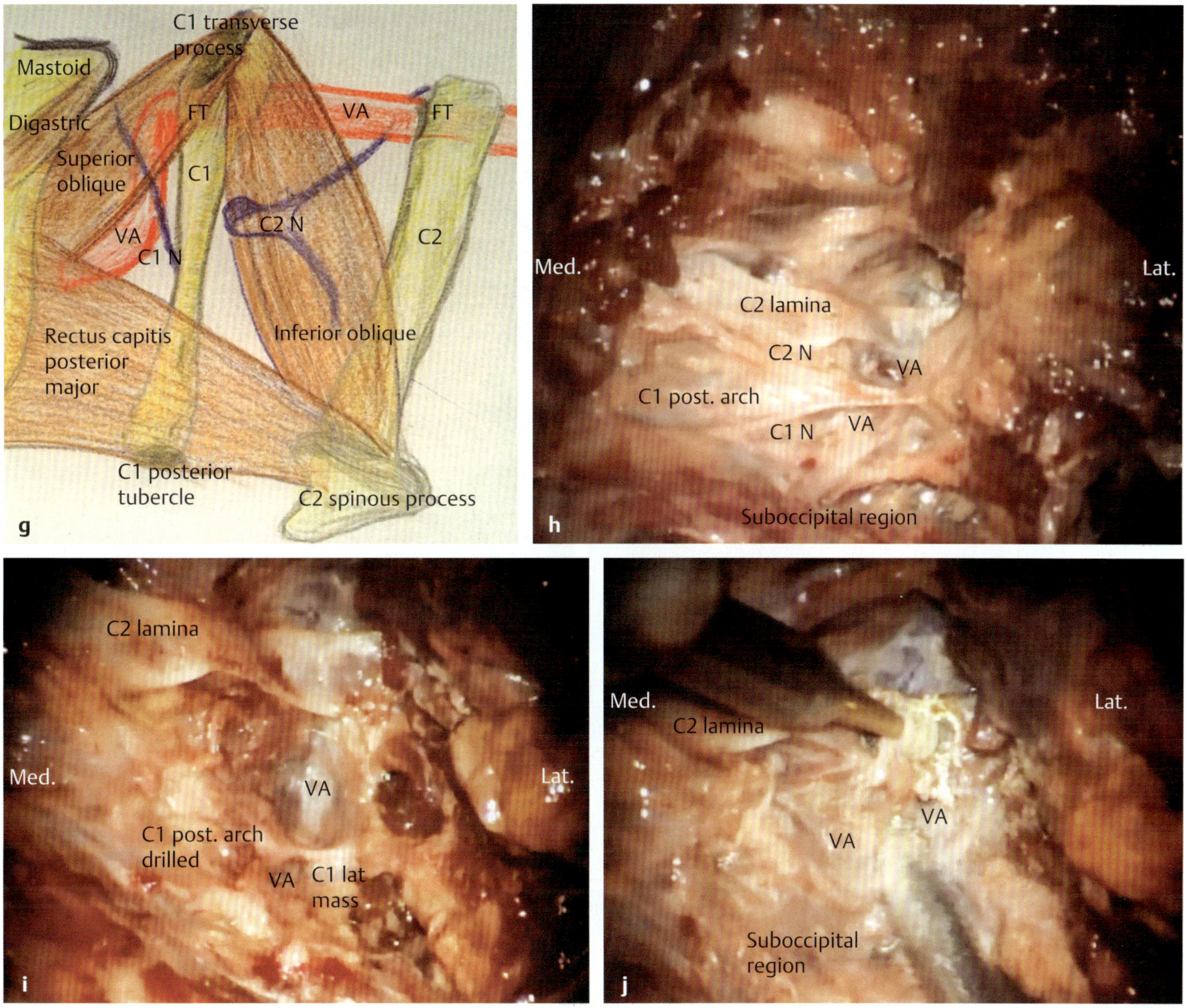

Fig. 61.5 *(Continued)* **(g)** Reflection of the major muscles of the posterior triangle in the neck exposes the suboccipital triangle formed by the superior and inferior oblique laterally, and the rectus capitis posterior major and minor muscles (medially). The contents of the suboccipital triangle include the vertebral artery (VA) after its emergence from the foramen transversarium (FT) of the atlas, lying in its fascial covering on the lateral one-third of the posterior arch of the atlas. The C1 nerve root (C1N) between the occiput and the atlas and the C2 nerve root (C2N) between the atlas and the axis may be traced to the location of the vertebral artery. **(h)** The vertebral artery (VA), after it emerges from the foramen transversarium of the atlas, is lying in a shallow groove on the superior surface of the lateral one-third of the C1 posterior arch (C1 post. arch). It is crossed by the C1 nerve root (C1 N). The vertebral artery may also be identified between the foramen transversarium of C1 and C2. The loose areolar tissue between C1/2 is dissected along the inferior border of inferior oblique muscle till the C2 ganglion and C2 nerve root are identified. The C2 nerve root and ganglion lead to the vertebral artery laterally located between C1 and C2. **(i)** Following the drilling of the C1 foramen transversarium and C1 posterior arch (C1 post. arch), the vertebral artery (VA) can be seen traversing through the C1 foramen transversarium and may also be located between the C1 and C2 foramen transversarium. The remaining C1 lateral mass (C1 lat mass) is also seen. **(j)** Drilling of the foramen transversarium of the axis exposes the vertebral artery (VA) traversing through it.

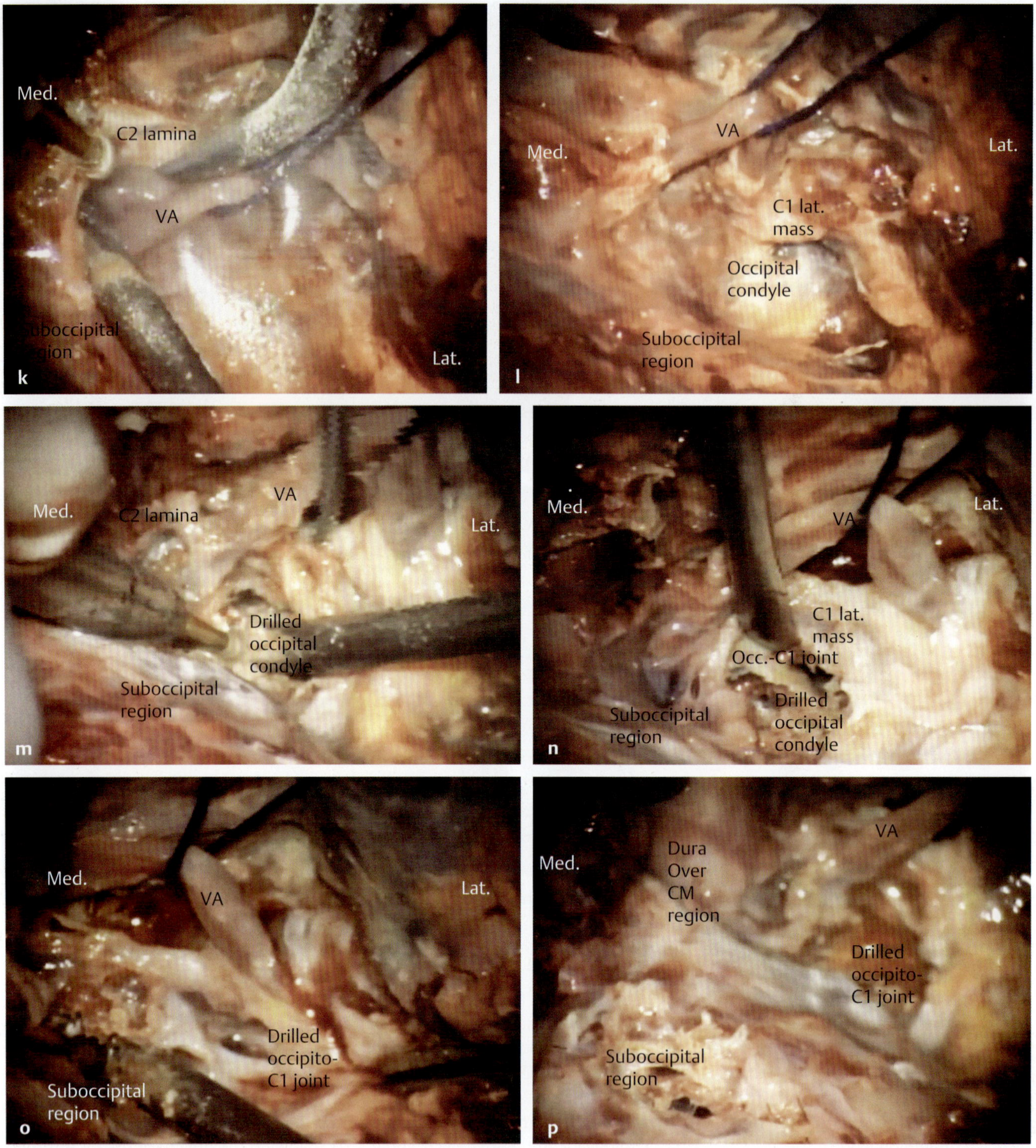

Fig. 61.5 *(Continued)* **(k)** The vertebral artery (VA) has been mobilized and shifted medially and downwards. The C2 laminectomy is being performed. **(l)** The medial and inferior mobilization of the vertebral artery (VA) exposes the occipital condyle and C1 lateral mass (C1 lat. mass) and the occipito-axial joint in between. **(m)** The drilling of medial one-third of the occipital condyle provides an access to the anterior cervicomedullary dura. **(n)** The partially drilled occipital condyle and the C1 lateral mass with the exposed occipito-C1 facet joint (occ.-C1 joint) is seen. The vertebral artery (VA) has been mobilized medially and inferiorly. **(o)** Drilled medial one-third of the occipito-cervical joint exposes the anterolateral aspect of the cervicomedullary dura. **(p)** The exposed dura over the cervicomedullary region and the anterolateral space provided by the drilled medial one-third of the occipito-C1 joint is visualized.

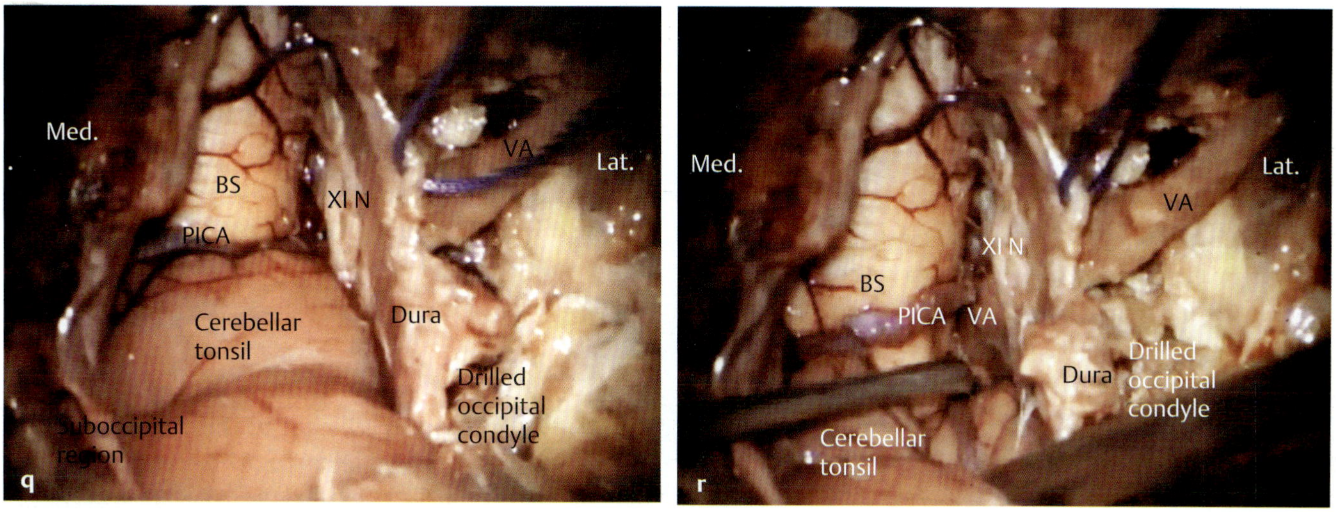

Fig. 61.5 *(Continued)* **(q)** Opening of the dura exposes the cerebellar tonsil, the posterior inferior cerebellar artery (PICA) and the spinal accessory nerve (XI N). The mobilized extradural component of the vertebral artery (VA) is also seen. **(r)** On opening the dura, the posterior inferior cerebellar artery (PICA), just prior to its junction with the vertebral artery, is visible within the roots of the glossopharyngeal and vagus nerves (the latter are entering the jugular foramen; XI, X N). The spinal accessory nerve (XI) N ascends through the foramen magnum. The superior attachment of the dentate ligament lies at the level of the foramen magnum. The rootlets of the hypoglossal nerve are enmeshed around the posterior surface of the intradural part of the vertebral artery. Dividing the first ligamentum denticulatum provides an anterolateral trajectory to dura over the clivus and the anterior cervicomedullary region. The intradural ipsilateral vertebral artery (VA) which forms the intradural continuation of the extradural vertebral artery is also seen. The anterior surface of the brain stem is well seen.

Bone Drilling

The transcondylar exposure permits drilling of the posterior one-third of the occipital condyle and/or the superior articular process of the atlas to provide a more ventral access to the lower clivus and the premedullary area. A more extensive removal of the occipital condyle and the superior articular process of the atlas gives access to ventrolateral extradural lesions at the foramen magnum. A variation in the drilling that involves an upward trajectory through the occipital condyle above the atlanto-occipital joint sparing the hypoglossal canal provides a wider access to the lower clivus and the premedullary region (**Fig. 61.5l–p**).

The paracondylar approach involves drilling of the jugular process of the occipital bone lateral to the occipital condyle, and if required, the mastoid bone. It thus exposes the posterior part of the jugular foramen, and if required, the presigmoid area up to the stylomastoid foramen (by drilling the mastoid bone).

The supracondylar approach involves drilling the part of the occipital bone superior to the occipital condyle thus providing access to the region medial to the jugular tubercle, hypoglossal canal and the lateral one-third of the clivus. The prominent jugular tubercle that obstructs the view to the clivus and the medulla anterior to the glossopharyngeal, vagus and accessory nerves may be drilled to increase the exposure.

The extent of bone removal is thus dictated by the extent of the tumor. Retromastoid craniectomy/craniotomy may also be performed for tumors of the posterior fossa extending into the ventral foramen magnum region. Drilling of the posterior one-third of the occipital condyle and lateral mass of C1 facilitates exposure of at least 1 cm of dura lateral to the vertebral artery. Additional occipital condylar drilling beyond its lateral one-third must be supplemented by an occipito-cervical fusion.

Removal of the middle two-thirds of the posterior arch of atlas and the spinous process and lamina of axis provides access to the lesions situated anterior to the cervicomedullary junction and the upper cervical cord.

Dural Opening

The dura can be opened in a longitudinal or a curvilinear fashion, the extent of which largely depends on the limits imposed by the tumor. A cuff of the dura may be left around the point of intradural penetration of the vertebral artery, which allows for a watertight dural closure following tumor excision. Adequate bone work allows the dural leaf to be reflected laterally while the vertebral artery and its dural cuff are reflected downwards and medially. Additionally, division of the dentate ligaments (attached medially to the lateral aspect of the cord between the points of emergence of the anterior and posterior nerve roots and laterally to the dura) widens the corridor further.

Tumor Removal

Meticulous dissection of the arachnoid separating the tumor from the neurovascular structures is essential for the success of the surgery. Coagulation of the arachnoid vitiates this interface and must be avoided. Piecemeal internal tumor decompression permits the separation of the tumor capsule from the neural structures. On opening the dura, the posterior inferior cerebellar artery, just prior to its junction with the vertebral artery, is visible within the roots of the glossopharyngeal and vagal nerves (the latter are entering the jugular foramen). The spinal accessory nerve ascends through the foramen magnum. The superior attachment of the dentate ligament lies at the level of the foramen magnum. The rootlets of the hypoglossal nerves are enmeshed around the posterior surface of the intradural part of the vertebral artery. During dissection along the cord-tumor interface, it is important to protect the anterior spinal artery arising at the ventral cord surface from the vertebral artery by preserving the arachnoidal plane. The dural point of attachment in meningiomas needs to be completely coagulated after excision of the tumor to achieve a better Simpson's grade of excision (**Fig. 61.5 q–r**).

Dural Closure

The dura has to be closed in a watertight manner in order to prevent cerebrospinal fluid leak. Leaving a cuff of dura around the vertebral artery entry allows for a watertight dural approximation in this critical area where cerebrospinal fluid leak is fairly common. If watertight dural closure cannot be done primarily, a fascia lata/fat patch, with or without augmentation with fibrin glue should be done.

Limits of the Approach

Anteriorly, the approach is limited by the nasopharynx, posteriorly by the dura over the cervico- medullary junction and, superiorly by the jugular bulb and the hypoglossal nerve.

Occipito-Cervical Fusion

If more than one-third of the occipital condyle is removed, especially if it is combined with drilling of the lateral mass of the atlas, the occipito-cervical junction becomes unstable and requires fusion. Fusion can be done by sublaminar wires, screw and rod technique or by the simpler contoured rod with stainless steel wires.

Postoperative Management

Postoperatively, prevention of aspiration pneumonitis, bed sores and deep vein thrombosis are of paramount importance. In case an extensive condylar drilling had been performed, a hard cervical collar is advised for at least 3 months.

Four Different Stages of Anterolateral Approach to the Cervicomedullary Junction

1. **ELTC approach with vertebral artery mobilization from foramen transversarium of both atlas and axis:** This approach is utilized for accessing an anteriorly placed cervicomedullary lesion extending from the lower clivus (the region between the jugular foramen to foramen magnum) to the atlas and axis vertebrae. It also includes lesions involving the occipital condyle (**Fig. 61.6a–g**).

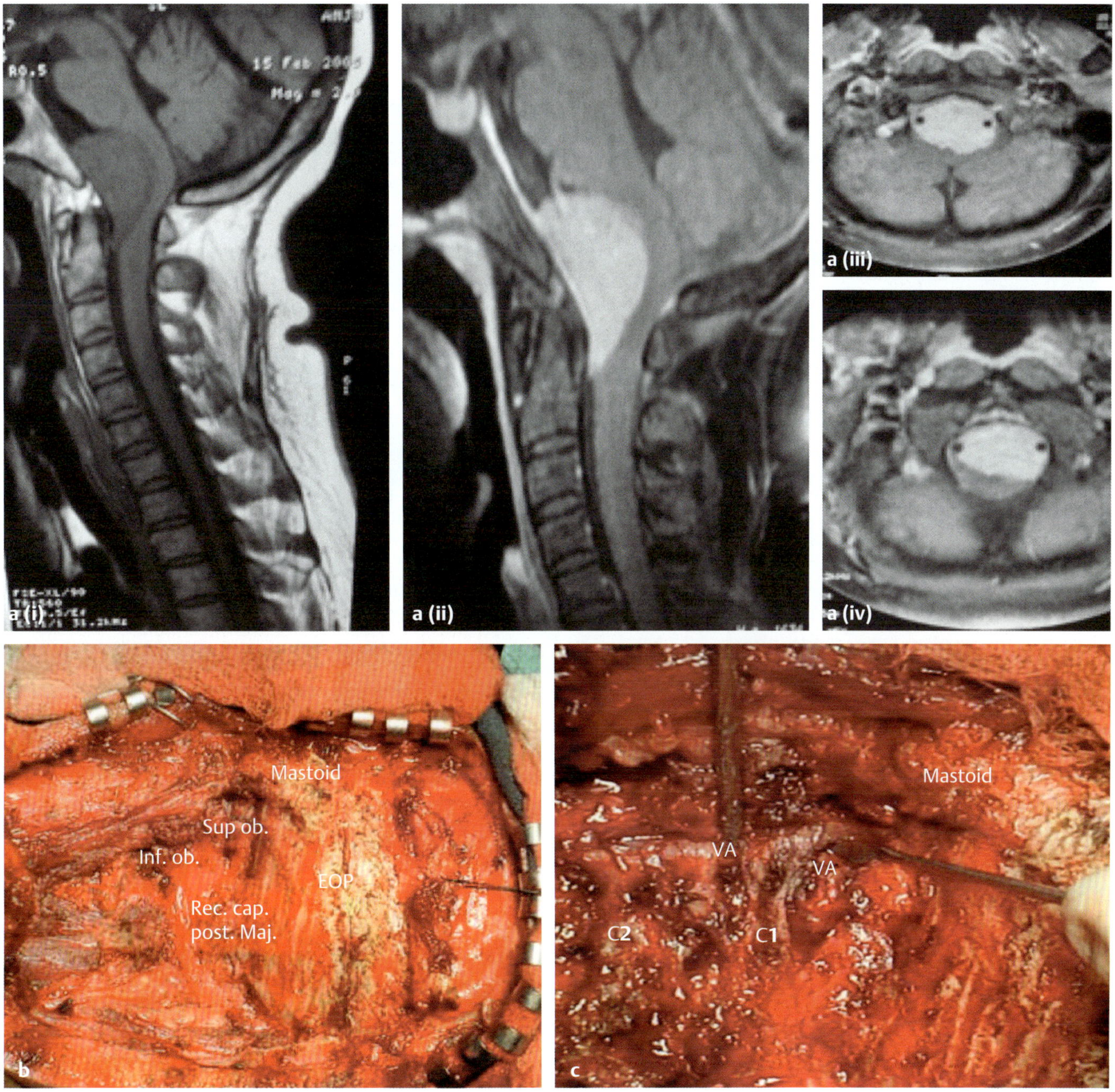

Fig. 61.6 **(a)** This 56-year old woman presented with progressive spastic quadriparesis of grade II in all four limbs, and respiratory distress. **(i)** T1 weighted sagittal image showing a cervicomedullary isointense meningioma with a broad dural attachment extending from the lower clivus to the axis vertebra. **(ii)** On T1 weighted contrast image, the lesion was uniformly enhancing and had a dural tail sign. (**iii** and **iv**) Axial T1 contrast images showing the mass attached to the anterior dura extending to both vertebral arteries. The brain stem is compressed by the lesion. **(b)** After a horse-shoe incision in the suboccipital region below the external occipital protuberance (EOP), and extending up to the mastoid base laterally, the entire muscle bulk of the two layers was lifted exposing the muscles of the suboccipital triangle, superior oblique (sup. ob) and inferior oblique (inf. ob) laterally and rectus capitis posterior major (rec. cap. post. maj.) medially. The C1 posterior arch with the vertebral artery and the C1 nerve root lies in the center of this triangle. **(c)** The muscles of the suboccipital triangle have been removed exposing the atlantal (C1) posterior arch and the lamina of the axis (C2) up to the lateral masses of the two respective vertebrae. The vertebral artery (VA) is seen traversing through the foramen transversarium of C1 and C2 and then on the lateral one-third of the superior surface of the atlas vertebra.

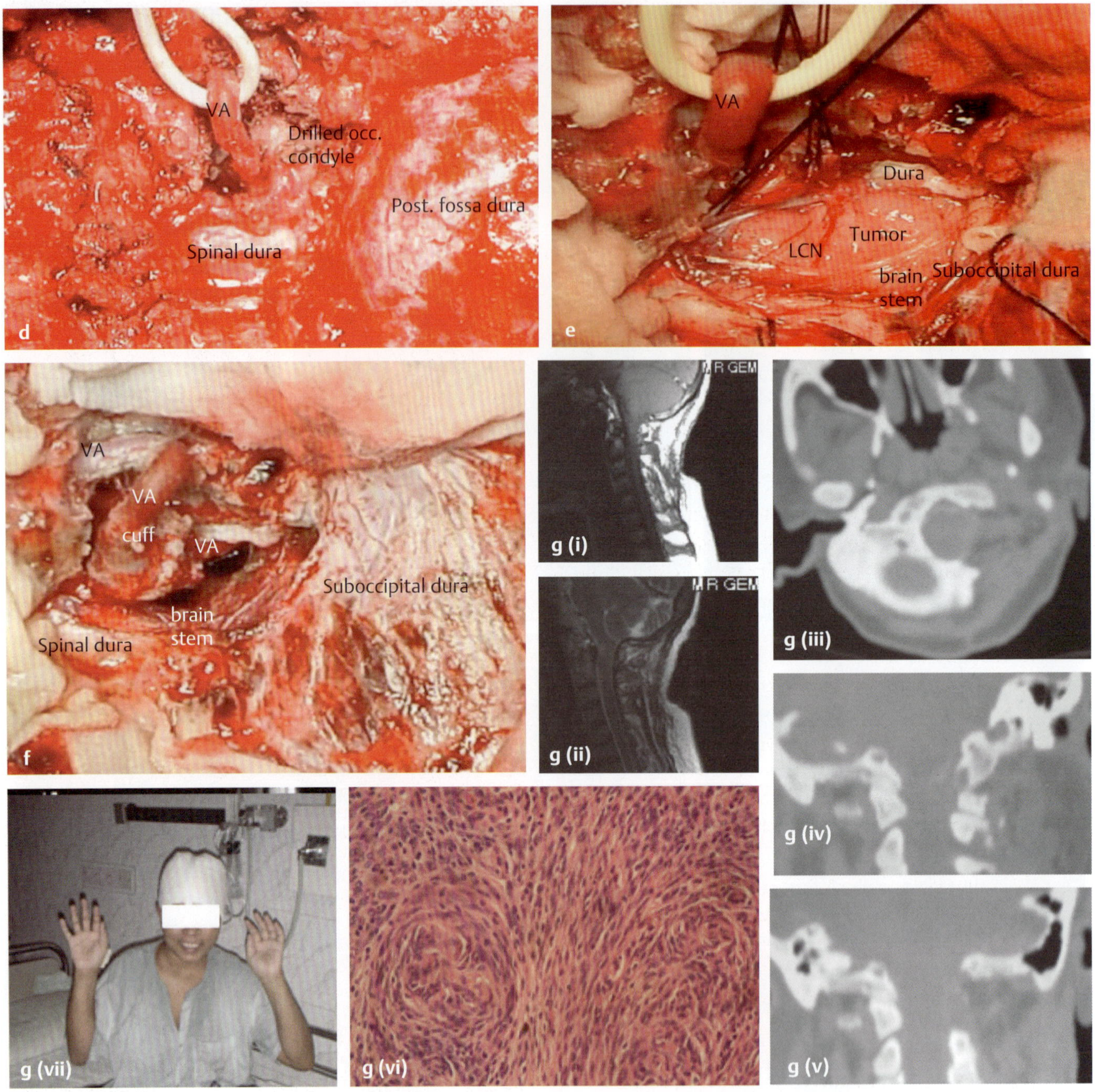

Fig. 61.6 *(Continued)* **(d)** A suboccipital craniectomy and C1-2 laminectomy exposes the posterior fossa (post. fossa) and spinal dura. The drilled occipital condyle (drilled occ. condyle)and the medially and downward mobilized vertebral artery (VA) provide a significant area to expose the dura anterolateral to the cervicomedullary region. **(e)** Opening of the suboccipital and upper cervical dura and working between the lower cranial nerves (LCN) gives direct access to the tumor and the ability to observe the brainstem-tumor interface from a lateral aspect. **(f)** The anterolateral brain stem (BS) surface after total tumor removal is seen. A cuff of dura is left surrounding the vertebral artery (VA). The extradural vertebral artery can be traced to its intradural segment. The change in color of the extradural vertebral artery from its vertical course between the foramen transversarium of C1 and C2 (pink color) and its horizontal course along the superior border of the lateral one-third of the C1posterior arch is evident. **(g)** Postoperative sagittal **(i)** T1 and **(ii)** T2 weighted MRI of the patient showing total excision of the tumor with mild cord intensity changes at the cervicomedullary junction. **(iii)** axial and (**iv** and **v**) coronal images of bone windows of postoperative CT scan showing the partial excision of the occipital condyle and the C1 facet joint. **(vi)** Hematoxylin and eosin stain of the tumor specimens showing a meningothelial meningioma. **(vii)** The patient made an uneventful recovery and regained her limb power. Her respiration also normalized.

2. **ELTC approach with vertebral artery mobilization from the foramen transversarium of atlas:** If the tumor is located at the level of the lower clivus and foramen magnum, reaching up to atlas but not the axis vertebra, then a condylar lateral one-third resection with vertebral artery mobilization from the foramen transversarium of the atlas may suffice (**Fig. 61.7a–m**).
3. **Far lateral approach with vertebral artery visualization:** In the cases where the tumor has encased the distal vertebral artery; or, in the cases where a proximal control of the vertebral artery is being sought for clipping a posterior inferior cerebellar artery aneurysm situated more distally, the proximal vertebral artery is exposed at its third segment traversing over the superior surface of lateral one-third of the posterior arch of atlas. The artery is, however, not mobilized from the foramen transversarium of atlas or axis (**Fig. 61.8a, b**).
4. **Far lateral approach (without vertebral artery visualization or mobilization):** The far lateral approach also involves reflection of the suboccipital muscles and exposure of the occipital bone, the C1 arch and the suboccipital triangle. The vertebral artery is identified traversing above the posterior arch of the atlas. A suboccipital craniotomy/craniectomy with upper cervical laminectomy (usually limited to the drilling of lateral one-third of the posterior arch of the atlas) without drilling of the occipital condyles or mobilization of the vertebral artery is performed. Thus, this approach provides a more limited exposure of the ventrolateral aspect of the cervicomedullary region when compared with the extreme lateral transcondylar approach. This approach is especially useful in the circumstances when a large ventral exposure at the foramen magnum is not required, such as when there is a significant extradural or lateral component of a lesion or when there is a neurofibroma that may be easily mobilized due to the sliding out of the tumor capsule along its arachnoidal plane (**Fig. 61.9a–l**); when there is an extensive extradural anterolateral bony tumor involving the clivus or the occipital condyle and occluding the ipsilateral vertebral artery (**Fig. 61.10**); or, when there is a predominantly cystic lesion like a neurentric cyst that, when decompressed, permits removal of the tumor capsule from a posterolateral aspect without brain stem/upper cervical cord manipulation (**Fig. 61.11**).

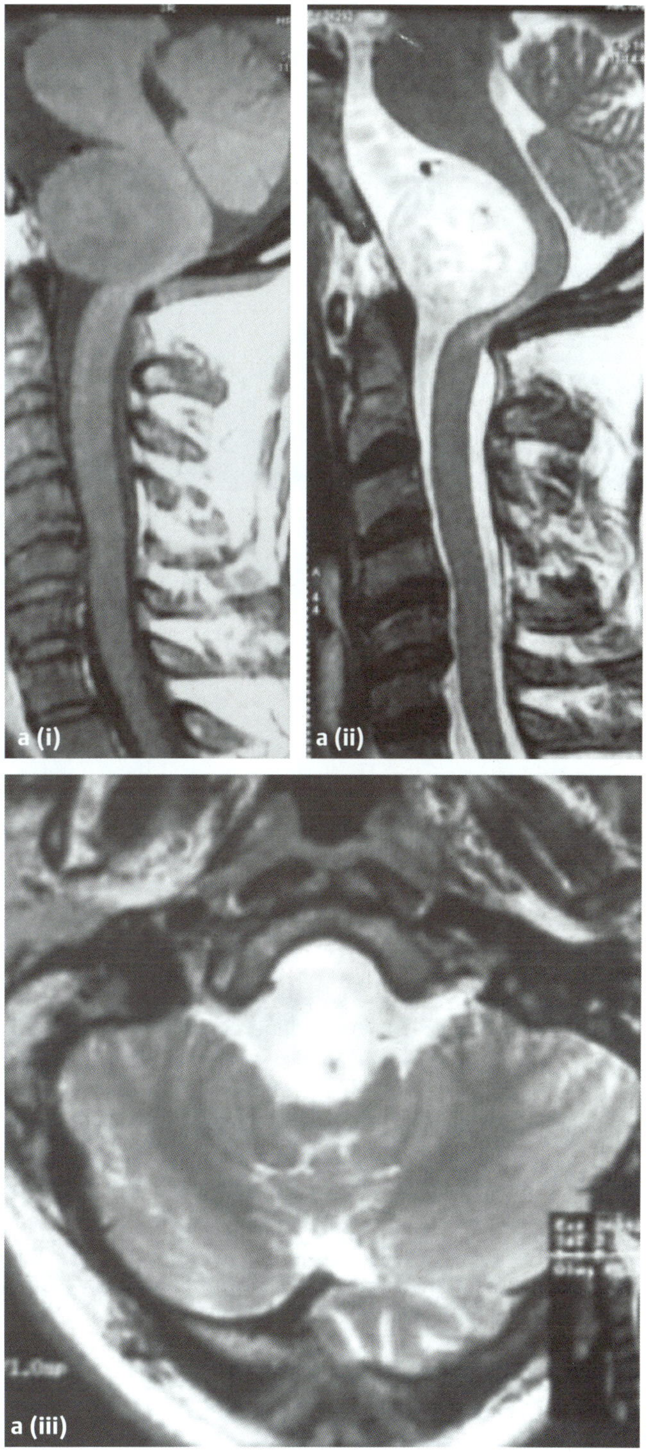

Fig. 61.7 Sagittal T1 **(a[i])** T2 **(a[ii])**, and axial T2 **(a[iii])** weighted MR scan showing a large anteriorly situated foramen magnum meningioma causing significant cervicomedullary compression.

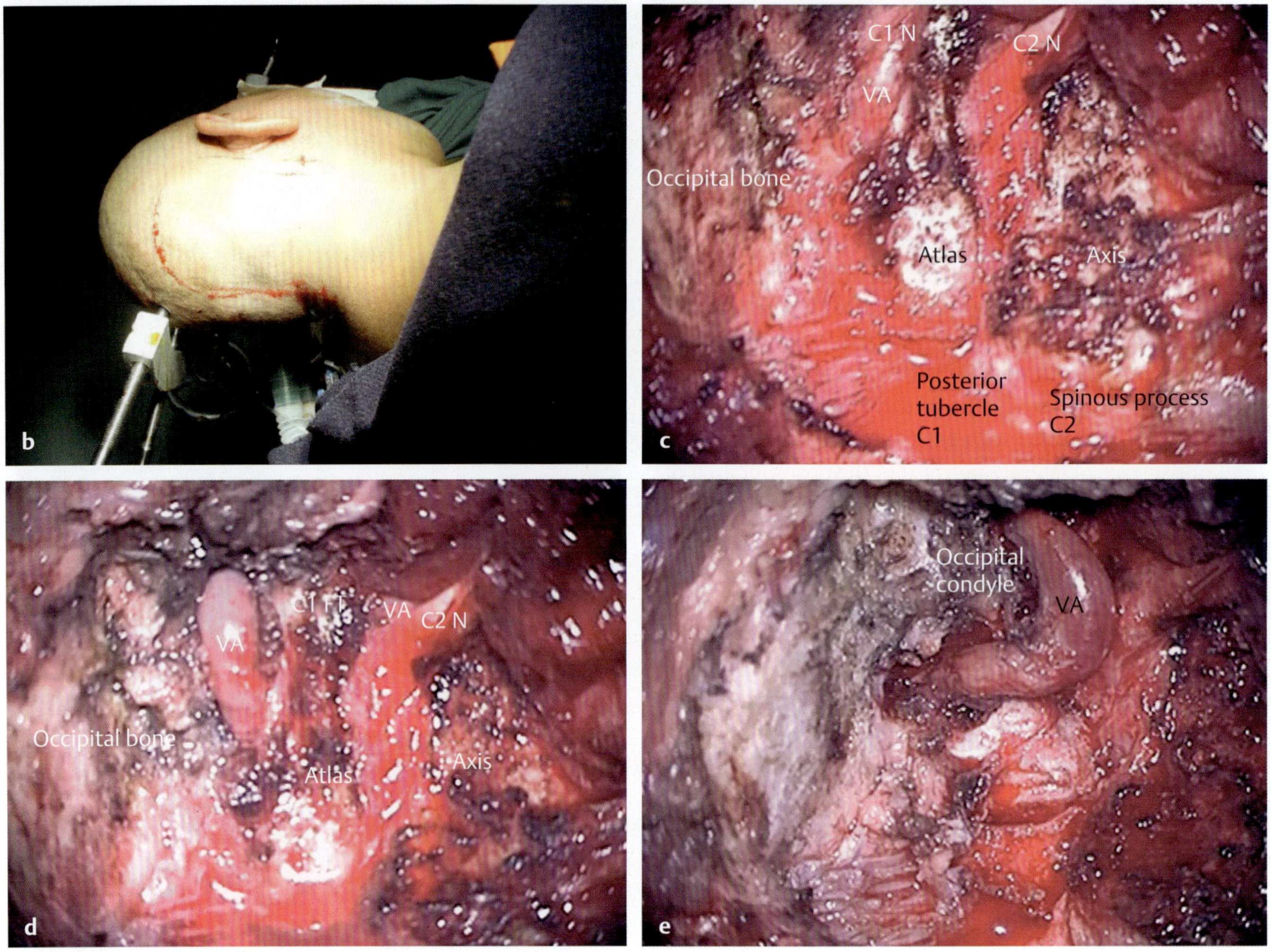

Fig. 61.7 *(Continued)* **(b)** The patient's head is fixed in a strict lateral position without head rotation or tilt to maintain the position of the vertebral artery relative to the foramen transversarium (FT) of C1 and C2. A horse-shoe shaped incision has been given. **(c)** The vertebral artery (VA) may be localized on the superior border of the lateral one-third of the posterior arch of the atlas (C1). The C1 nerve root (C1 N) is in close proximity to it and leads upto the fascial canal housing the vertebral artery. Alternatively, the vertebral artery may also be located in the space between the foramen transversarium of the atlas (C1) and axis (C2). Following the C2 nerve root (C2 N) between the atlas and axis leads to this part of the vertebral artery. **(d)** A subperiosteal dissection along the posterior arch of the atlas and the lamina of the axis avoids troublesome venous plexus bleeding. The vertebral artery (VA) has been exposed by dissecting it from its fascial tunnel at the lateral one-third of the superior border of the atlas. The entire third part of the vertebral artery at its emergence from the foramen transversarium of the atlas (C1 FT) to the point where it becomes intradural has been exposed. The foramen transversarium of the atlas is drilled to mobilize the vertebral artery. The C2 nerve root (C2 N) is leading to the part of the vertebral artery between the foramen transversarium of the atlas and axis. **(e)** Drilling of the foramen transversarium of the atlas mobilizes the vertebral artery that is then displaced posteromedially to expose the occipital condyle.

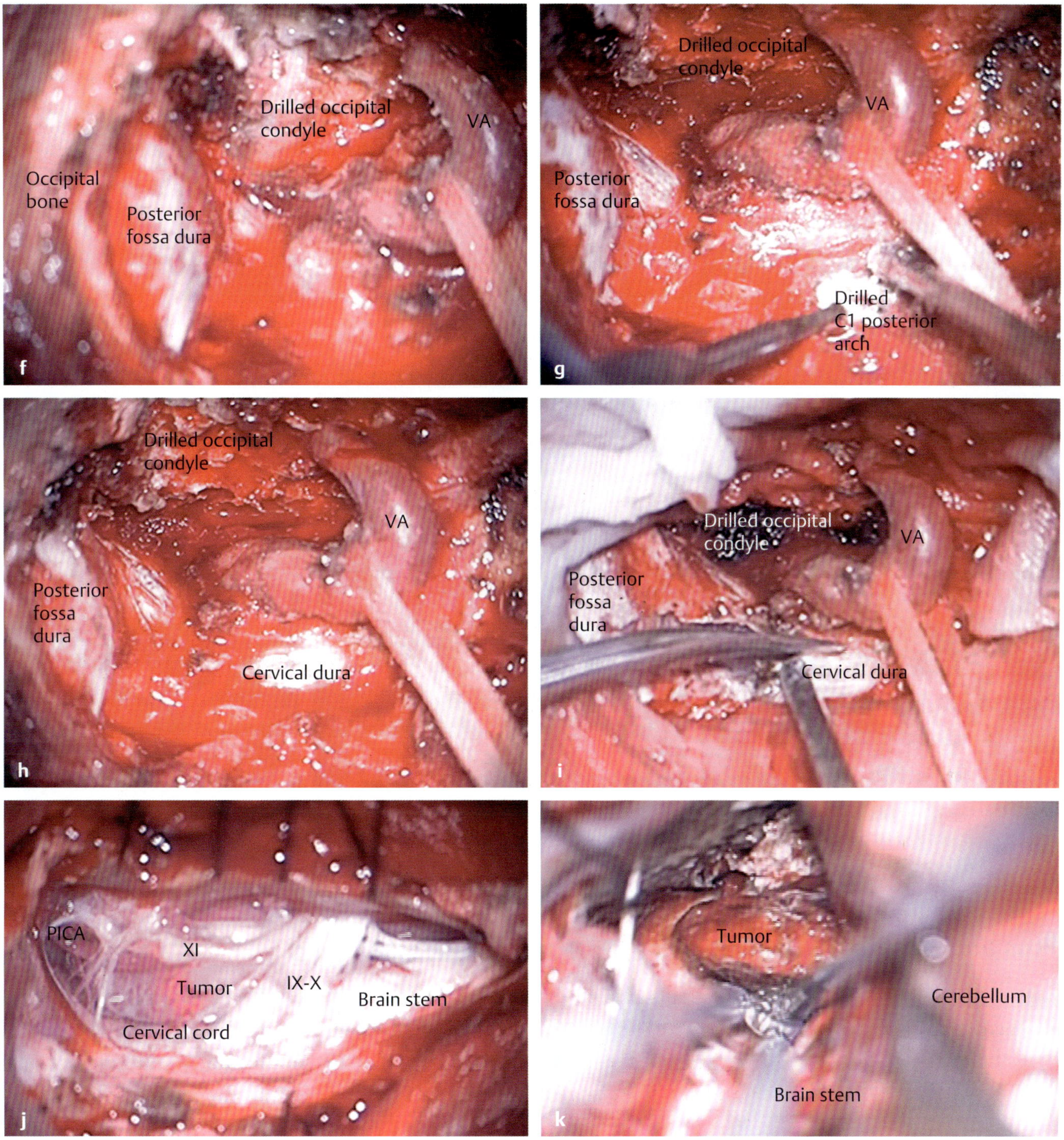

Fig. 61.7 *(Continued)* **(f)** Drilling of lateral one-third of the occipital condyle provides access to the anterolateral part of the thecal sac at the cervicomedullary junction. Suboccipital craniectomy has been performed exposing the posterior fossa dura. **(g)** Drilling of the posterior arch of the atlas is being carried out. **(h)** The final dural exposure obtained after a suboccipital craniectomy, C1 posterior arch removal and drilling of the occipital condyle after downward and medial mobilization of the vertebral artery is seen. **(i)** Suboccipital and upper cervical dural opening is carried out. The annular sinus between the dural leaves at the foramen magnum needs to be coagulated and divided. **(j)** On opening the dura, the tumor-brain stem/upper cervical cord interface is well seen. The layer of arachnoid covering the tumor and the brain stem has to be meticulously opened. The lower cranial nerves (IX–X), the spinal accessory nerve (XI) and the posterior inferior cerebellar artery (PICA) are seen overlying the tumor. **(k)** Intracapsular decompression while maintaining the arachnoidal plane helps in the dissection of the tumor from the brain stem and upper cervical cord.

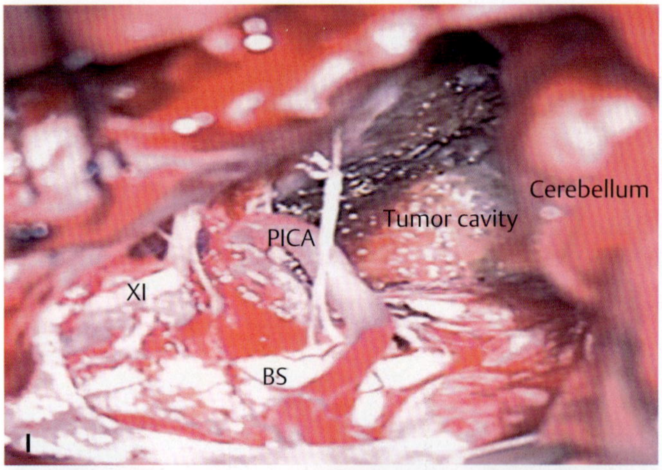

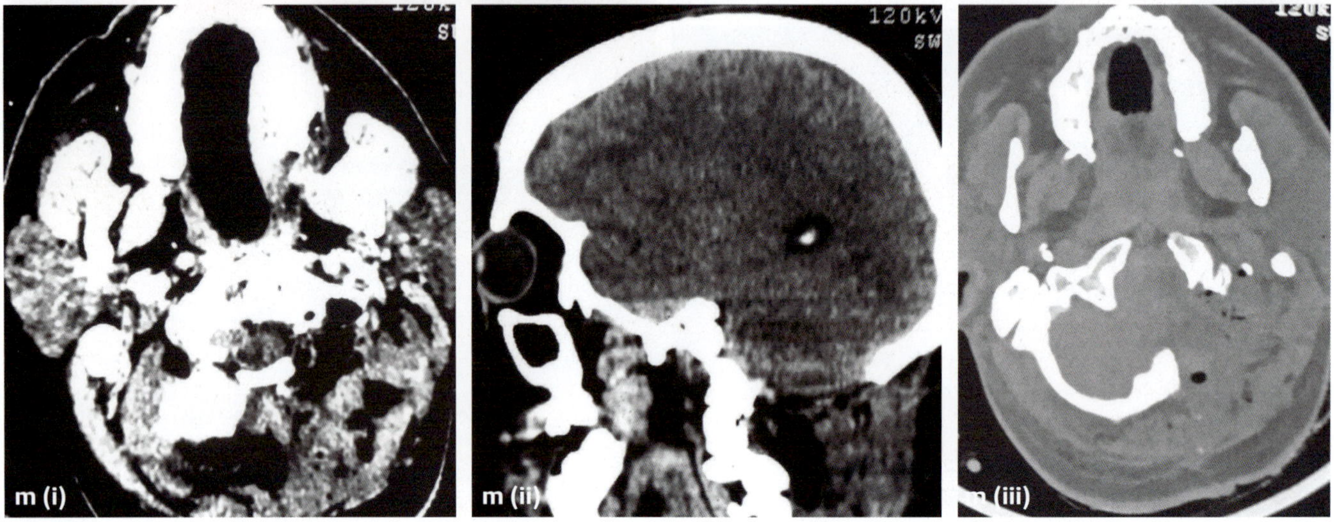

Fig. 61.7 *(Continued)* **(l)** The anterior dural attachment has been coagulated and the tumor cavity after total tumor removal is lined with Surgicel. **(m)** Postoperative **(i)** axial, **(ii)** sagittal reconstructed, and **(iii)** axial bone windows of CT scan shows the bony resection and tumor removal.

Pros and Cons

The approach has several advantages. It provides a wide surgical corridor with a relatively short trajectory. The tumor-neuraxis interface is under direct parallel vision facilitating better dissection. Ventral intradural extramedullary lesions from the foramen magnum to the upper cervical vertebrae may be accessed by a single approach. Both intra- and extradural components of the tumor may be accessed at the same time. Early control of the vertebral artery and the origin of the posterior inferior cerebellar artery facilitate interruption of the blood supply to the tumor and also help in providing adequate proximal control for aneurysms in this region. Unlike the transoral exposure, the surgical trajectory is through a sterile corridor. Its combination with the suboccipital, upper cervical, presigmoid or subtemporal-infratemporal approach significantly increases the field of view and exposure.

The disadvantages include a longer operative time through relatively unfamiliar anatomy; precipitation of additional neurological deficits or worsening of preexisting deficits; cerebrospinal fluid leak and infection; precipitation of instability; vertebral artery injury or spontaneous thrombosis/dissection of the vertebral artery during its dissection; lower cranial nerve paresis leading to aspiration pneumonitis, rhinolalia and nasal regurgitation.

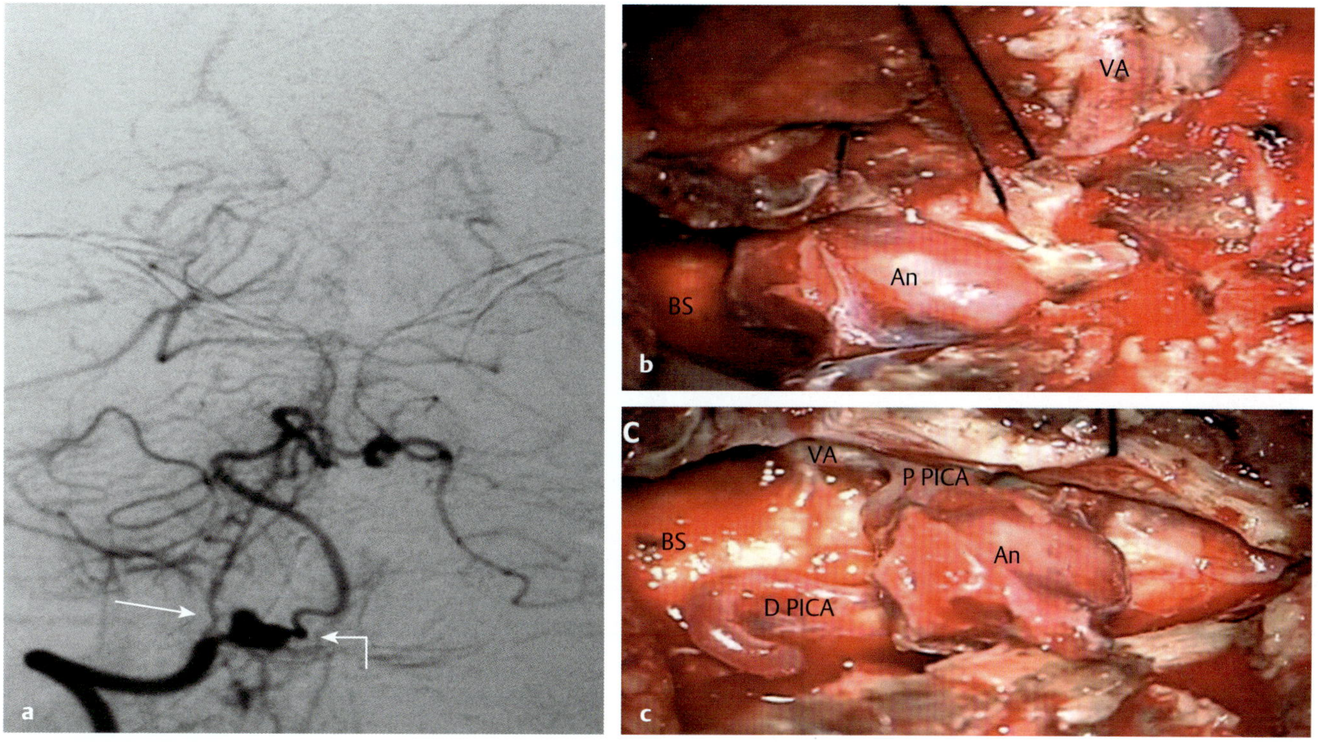

Fig. 61.8 **(a)** A posterior circulation digital subtraction angiogram showing the vertebral artery dissection with a fusiform aneurysm of the dominant posterior inferior cerebellar artery. The posterior inferior cerebellar artery is dominant and supplying both cerebellar surfaces (*curved arrow*). The thin basilar artery (straight arrow) with both posterior cerebral arteries are also visible. **(b)** Intraoperative view of the aneurysm (An) and brain stem (BS) after dural opening at the cervicomedullary junction in the far lateral approach. Proximal control of the ipsilateral vertebral artery is taken at the level of the posterior arch of atlas (VA) by its in situ visualization at the level of the C1 arch (without its mobilization). **(c)** Intraoperative view of the aneurysm (An) and the underlying brain stem (BS). The dominant posterior inferior cerebellar artery is seen both proximal (P PICA) and distal (D PICA) to the aneurysm (An). The PICA is arising from the ipsilateral intradural vertebral artery (VA).

Tips and Pearls

- Keeping the head and torso in lateral position without any rotation or tilt prevents displacement of the vertebral artery relative to the atlas and the axis vertebrae and facilitates its early localization.
- Reflecting the muscle layers in a single flap prevents postoperative muscle atrophy in the suboccipital region.
- The venous plexus in the suboccipital triangle bleeds profusely. Bipolar coagulation, subperiosteal dissection, sugicel and fibrin glue help in controlling the persistent venous ooze.
- In the cases with a ventral midline tumor, the approach to the tumor should be from the side of the non-dominant vertebral artery. This helps in preventing vertebrobasilar insufficiency in case the vertebral artery is compromised during the surgical procedure.
- Leaving a fascial sheath surrounding the mobilized vertebral artery and continuous irrigation of the surgical field helps in protecting it from spontaneous thrombosis or dissection.
- Drilling of lateral one-third of the occipital condyle is not associated with instability and does not require any additional stabilization. This is usually adequate to get a proper ventral exposure.

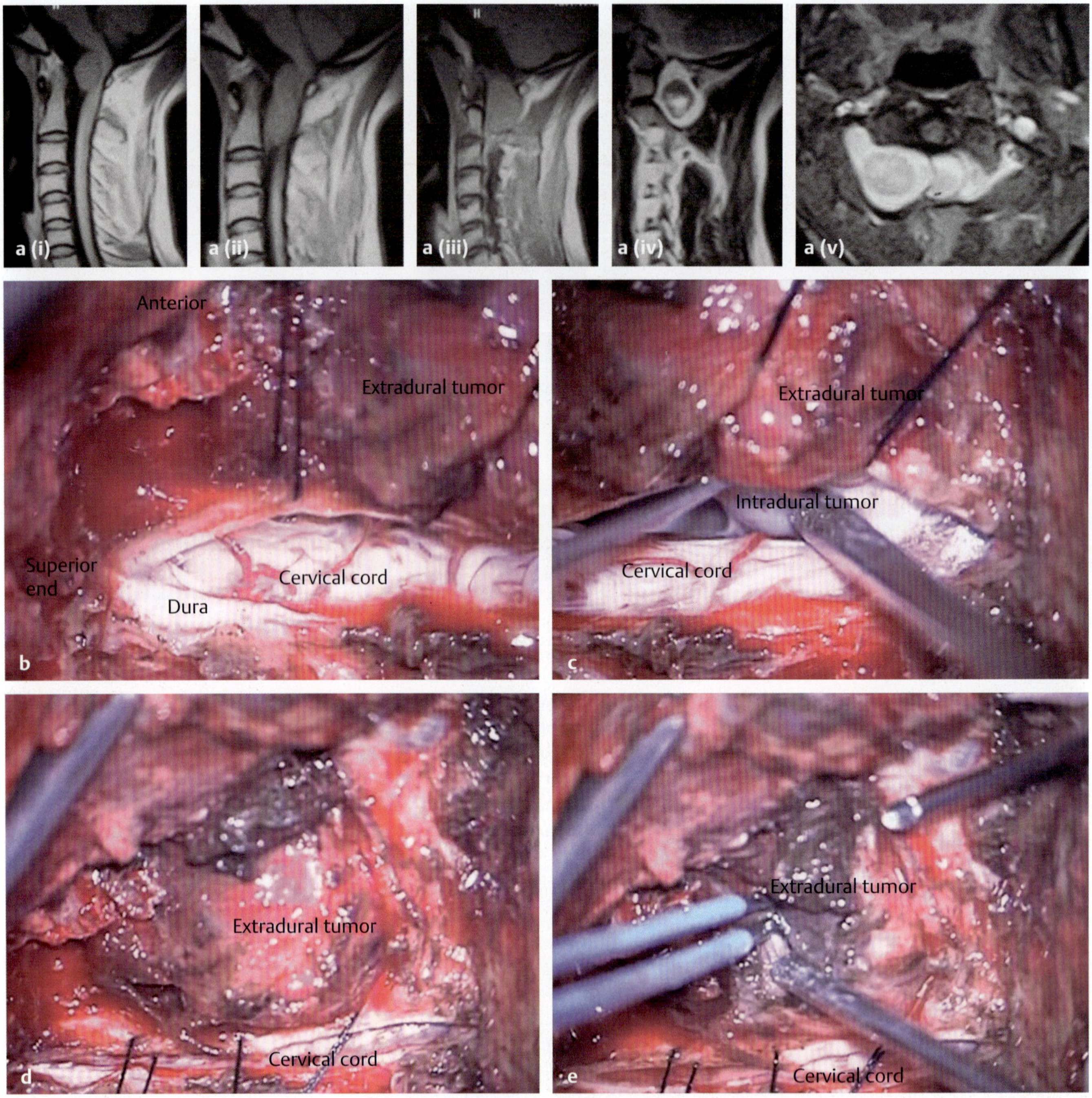

Fig. 61.9 **(a) (i, ii, iii,** and **iv)** Sagittal and parasagittal and **(v)** axial MR images showing an anteriorly placed dumb-bell neurofibroma at the foramen magnum with significant intra- and extradural components. The laterally placed tumor causes shifting of the cord to the opposite side giving adequate field of view for the surgical approach so that vertebral artery mobilization and condylar drilling are not required. **(b)** The extradural part of the tumor is seen. The dural opening exposes the upper cervical cord. **(c)** The intradural component of the tumor is also visualized. **(d)** The dural retraction reveals the entire extradural tumor. **(e)** Intratumoral decompression using bipolar cautery is performed before mobilizing the tumor capsule.

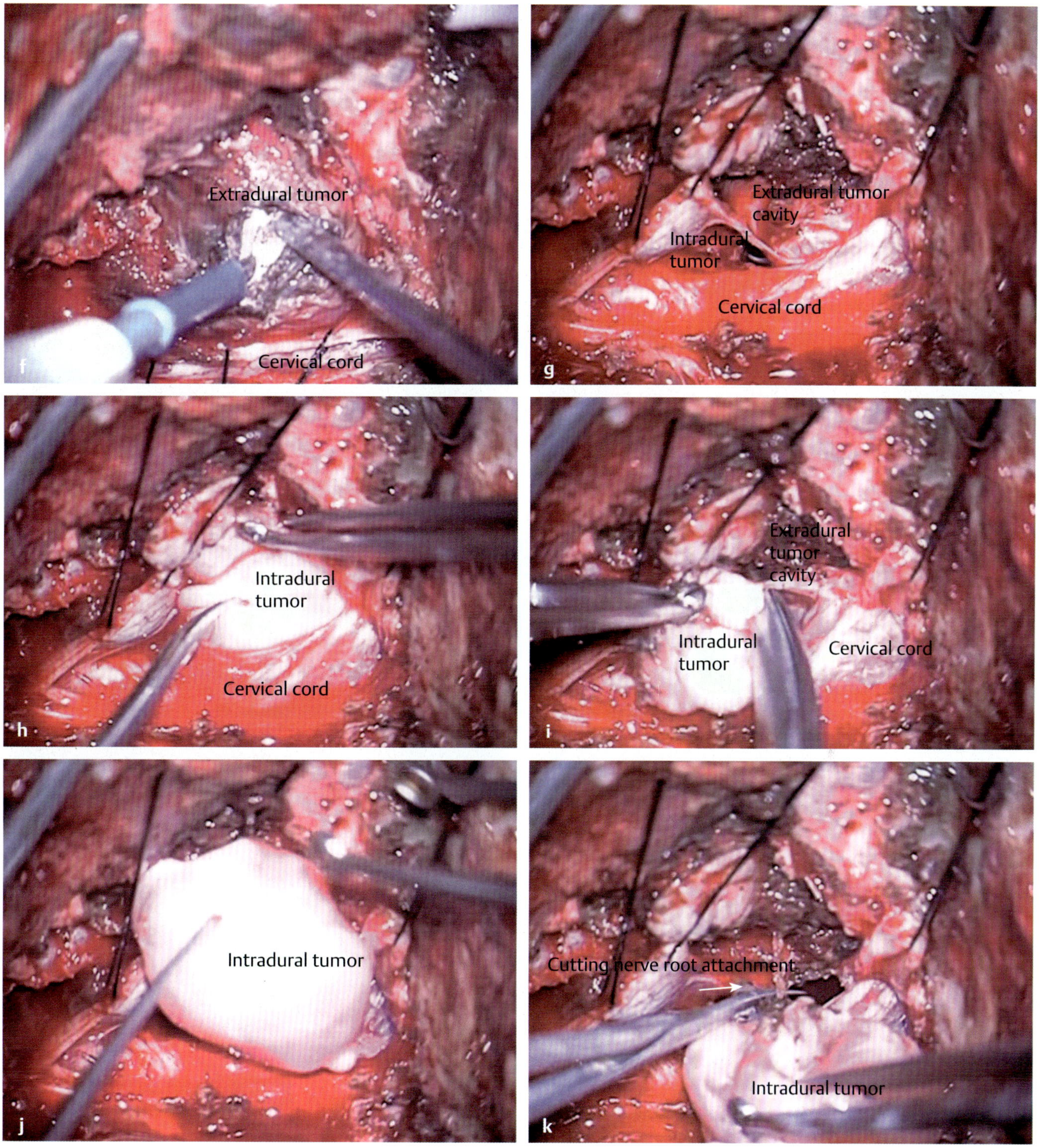

Fig. 61.9 *(Continued)* **(f)** The firm tumor may also be decompressed using monopolar coagulation and ultrasonic suction aspirator. **(g)** Total extradural tumor removal is performed. **(h)** It is possible to slide off the intradural part of the tumor along the arachnoidal plane without complete visualization of the anterior part of the brain stem. The tumor can be moblilized as it is not attached to the dural surface. Thus, vertebral artery mobilization and condylar resection are not required. **(i)** The intradural part of the tumor that emerges is decompressed facilitating further intradural tumor mobilization from the anterior aspect of the upper cervical cord. **(j)** The entire intradural component of the tumor has been delivered out. **(k)** The nerve rootlet from which the tumor arose is being divided to remove the tumor.

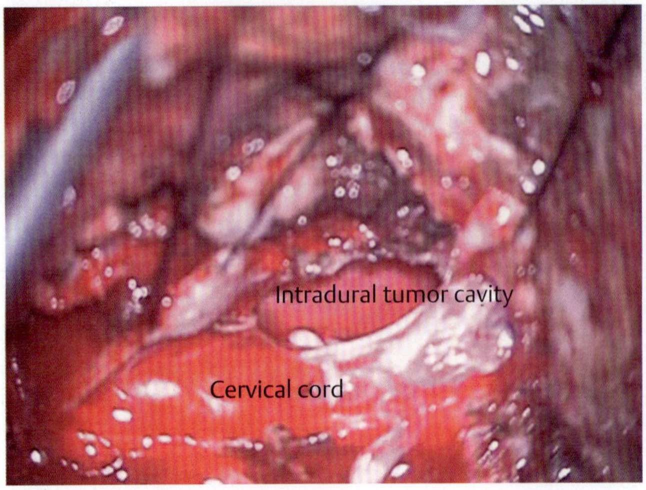

Fig. 61.9 *(Continued)* **(l)** The final tumor cavity with the decompressed upper cervical cord.

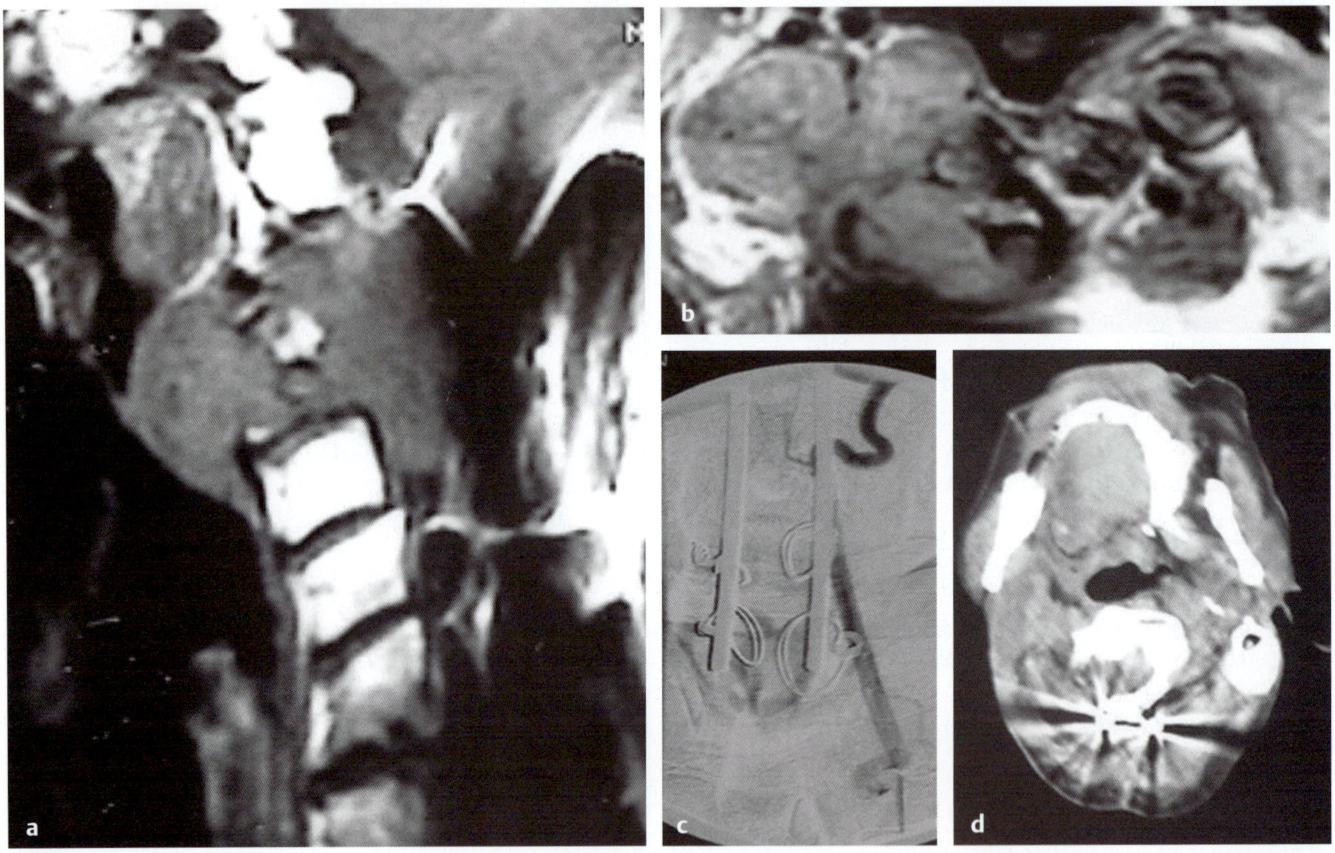

Fig. 61.10 **(a)** Cervical sagittal reconstructed CT image showing a recurrent clival chordoma destroying the anterior arch of atlas and the odontoid process and body of the axis. **(b)** The axial CT image shows an extensive lateral extent of the lesion with ipsilateral vertebral artery occlusion. **(c)** The angiogram shows non-visualization of the ipsilateral vertebral artery and the contoured rod occipitocervical stabilization procedure that had already been performed in the previous surgery. **(d)** Postoperative bone windows of axial CT scan showing total tumor removal utilizing the far lateral approach. The ipsilateral C1 lateral mass and facet are preserved.

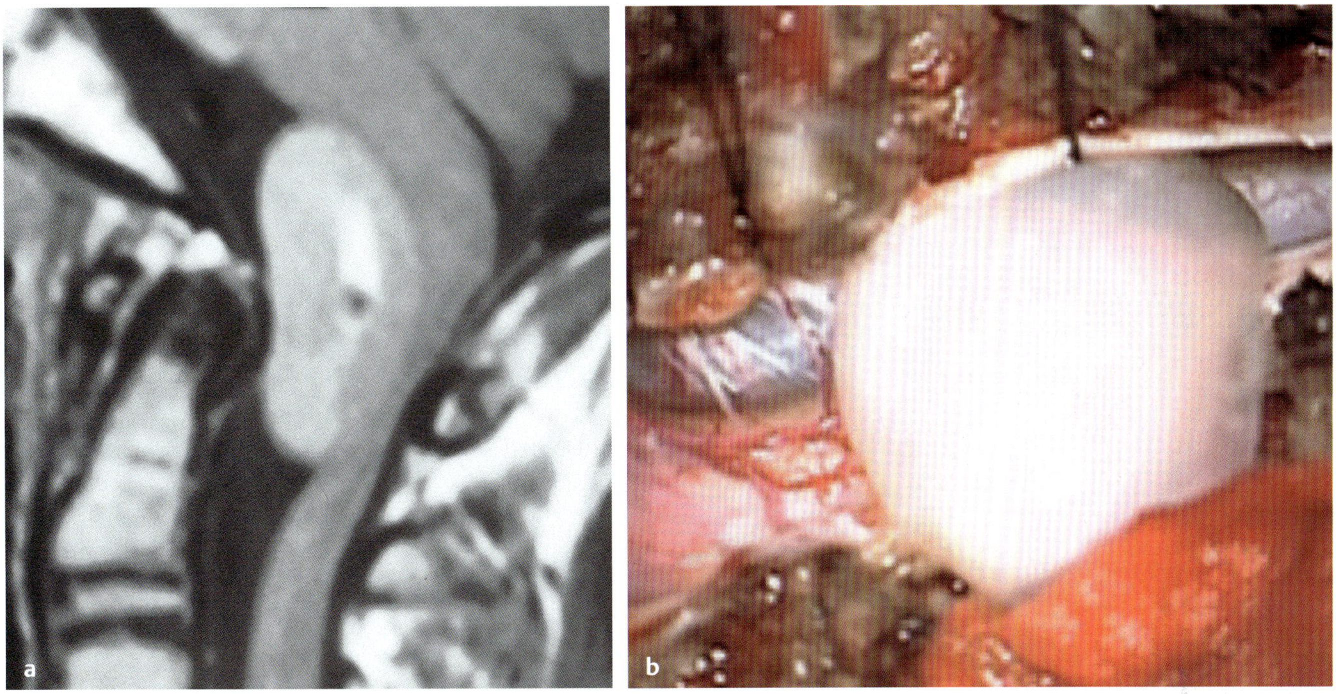

Fig. 61.11 **(a)** T1-weighted sagittal image showing the intradural extramedullary cystic neurenteric cyst. **(b)** The intraoperative image showing delivery of cyst using the far lateral approach in lateral position without vertebral artery visualization or mobilization.

- The anterior limit of condylar drilling is the cortical bony hypoglossal canal traversing the occipital condyle along the junction between its medial two-thirds and lateral one-thirds.
- Leaving a dural sheath around the vertebral artery at the point of its entry into the dura helps in meticulous dural closure following tumor excision.
- Following dural opening, starting the arachnoidal dissection at a distance from the tumor-neurovascular interface helps in sliding the arachnoid from the tumor. In the case of bleeding from the tumor, the plane is still maintained and not compromised by bipolar coagulation.
- Adequate intratumoral decompression is mandatory before attempting to mobilize the tumor from the brain stem. This also helps in preserving the arachnoidal plane since the tumor capsule falls away from the brain stem, the cervical cord, the vertebrobasilar complex and the anterior spinal arteries. In the case of a ventrally situated meningioma, excising its ventral dural attachment helps in both restricting the intratumoral bleeding and in mobilizing the tumor.
- A piece-meal removal, working between the corridors provided by the lower cranial nerves, helps in preserving the latter and significantly assists in improving the postoperative outcome.
- The vertical extent of the exposure is determined by the location of the tumor. An unnecessarily wide exposure should be avoided.
- Despite adequate dural closure, packing the extradural operative cavity with fat/fascia harvested from the abdomen or thigh and applying fibrin glue to reinforce and maintain the padding helps in preventing a cerebrospinal leak through the operative wound in the postoperative period. A prophylactic intrathecal closed lumbar drain maintained for three days also helps in preventing cerebrospinal fluid leak.

Section XXIV

Surgeries for Vertigo

Chapter 62 Endolymphatic Sac Decompression

Narayan Jayashankar

Indications

- Meniere's disease unresponsive to medical therapy with serviceable hearing.

It must be specified here that endolymphatic sac decompression is not a preferred surgery at our center. Treatment of Meniere's disease is medical in a vast majority of cases. However, in cases of intractable vertigo, a vestibular neurectomy is the most preferred surgical option. In cases of poor hearing (unserviceable) in the affected ear, a transmastoid labyrinthectomy can be offered to the subject as an alternative procedure. Endolymphatic sac decompression is offered only if the other surgical options are not acceptable to the subject. If offered, the inconsistent long-term result of endolymphatic sac decompression is explained to the subject preoperatively.

Surgical Steps

1. A postaural incision is taken 2 cm behind the postaural groove from the superior pole of helix till the mastoid tip. The skin and subcutaneous tissues are elevated anteriorly till the posterior canal wall.
2. A posteroinferiorly-based musculoperiosteal flap is created (**Fig. 62.1**). The horizontal limb of the incision is taken along the temporal line from the root of the zygoma till the junction of the temporal line with the posterior border of the mastoid. A circumferential incision is made along the bony canal wall including the superior, posterior, and inferior circumferences. The musculoperiosteal flap is retracted and sutured to expose the mastoid cortex.
3. A cortical mastoidectomy is performed (**Fig. 62.2**). The semicircular canals are delineated. A thin shell of the bone is left over the sigmoid sinus and jugular bulb. It is very important to remove the cells inferior as also posterior to the posterior semicircular canal. Similarly, the bone over the presigmoid posterior fossa dura is drilled with a diamond burr to make it eggshell thin.
4. The endolymphatic sac is located inferior to Donaldson's line (**Fig. 62.3**). This line passes along the axis of the lateral semicircular canal and bisects the posterior semicircular canal as it courses toward the presigmoid posterior fossa dura. In our view, it is not essential to blue-line the posterior semicircular canal to identify the endolymphatic sac.
5. The eggshell thin bone over the presigmoid posterior fossa dura is removed (**Fig. 62.4** and **Fig. 62.5**). The presigmoid posterior fossa dura is also first depressed medially to separate it from the overlying bone before taking off the eggshell thin bone over it using a Freer elevator. The posterior fossa dura is widely exposed posterior and inferior to the posterior semicircular canal up to the jugular bulb.

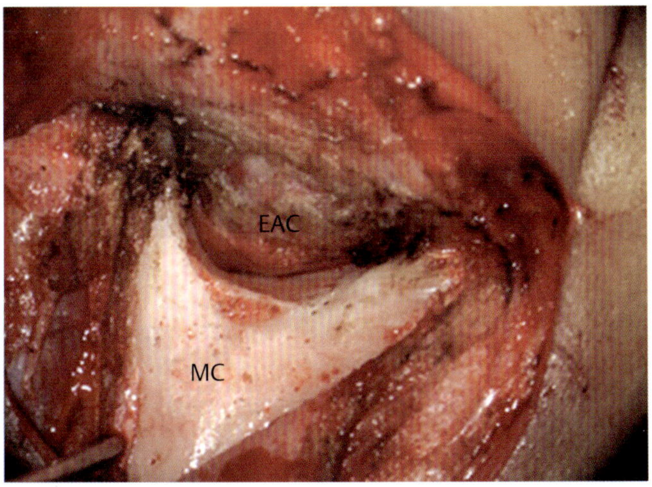

Fig. 62.1 Musculoperiosteal incisions to create a posteroinferiorly based musculoperiosteal flap.

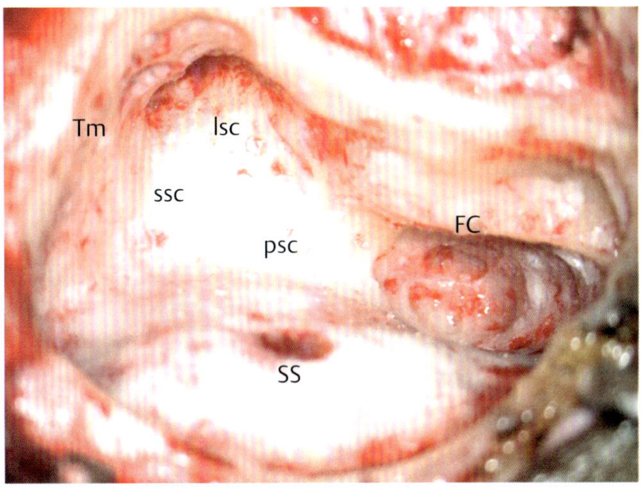

Fig. 62.2 Cortical mastoidectomy.

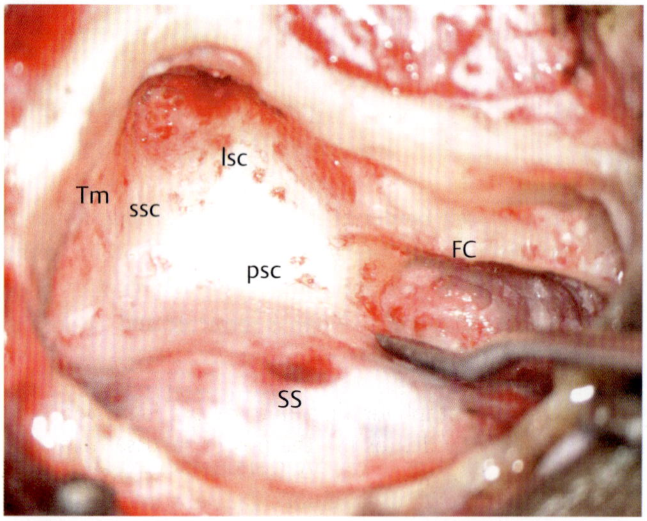

Fig. 62.3 Surface landmark of endolymphatic sac.

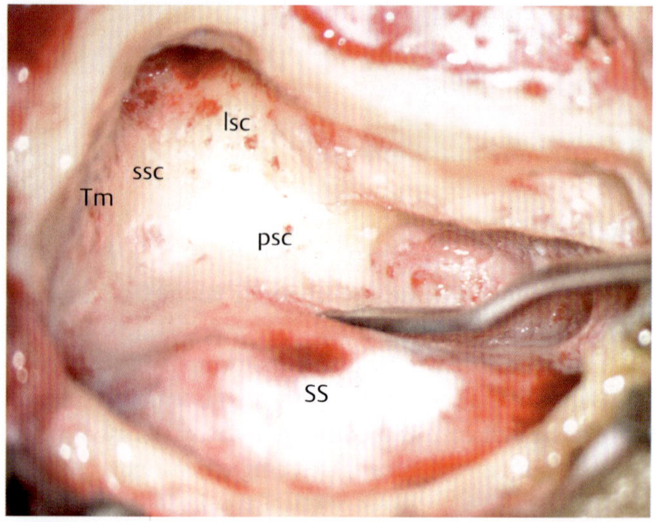

Fig. 62.4 Eggshell thin bone lifted off the presigmoid posterior fossa dura.

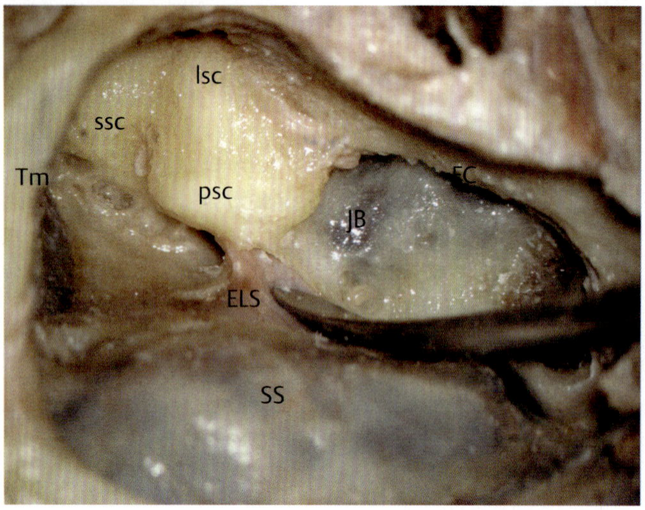

Fig. 62.5 Exposure of the presigmoid dura posterior and inferior to area of endolymphatic sac using Freer's elevator.

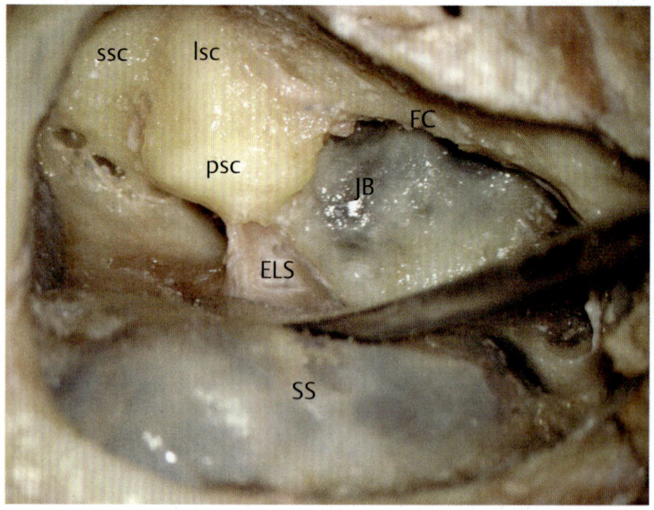

Fig. 62.6 Endolymphatic sac and duct are exposed.

6. In case the jugular bulb is very high, it needs to be decompressed. Gentle retraction of the high jugular bulb with side of suction gives the required visualization of the presigmoid posterior fossa dura.
7. The endolymphatic sac appears white compared to the bluish hue of the posterior fossa dura. On depressing it medially, the endolymphatic duct is seen to get prominent as it traverses medial to the posterior semicircular canal on its course toward the vestibule (**Fig. 62.6** and **Fig. 62.7**). A Freer elevator, if moved from superior to the inferior direction along the presigmoid posterior fossa dura, fails to move freely since it gets obstructed by the double fold of dura that constitutes the endolymphatic sac. It is very important to definitely identify the endolymphatic sac and duct to prevent incising the posterior fossa dura and inadvertently causing cerebrospinal fluid leak.
8. The outer wall of endolymphatic sac is incised with a sickle or Beaver knife (**Fig. 62.8a, b**). A ball point probe is passed into its lumen to open it up widely (**Fig. 62.9, Fig. 62.10** and **Fig. 62.11**).
9. A T-shaped thin silastic sheet is prepared. The horizontal limb of this silastic sheet is placed within the lumen of the sac and duct, and the vertical limb comes out from the lumen into the mastoid cavity (**Fig. 62.12** and **Fig. 62.13**). This effectively creates an endolymphatic mastoid shunt.
10. The musculoperiosteal and skin incisions are closed in separate layers.

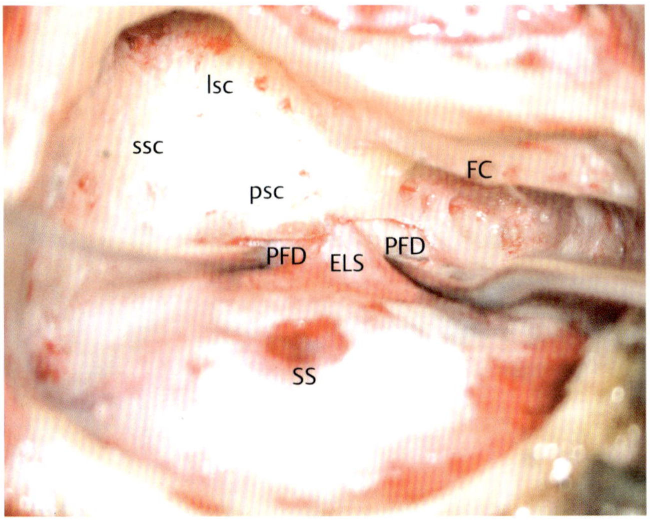

Fig. 62.7 The endolymphatic duct and sac are identified conclusively by depressing the posterior fossa dura. The duct gets lifted off from the posterior fossa dura and is seen going medial to the posterior semicircular canal.

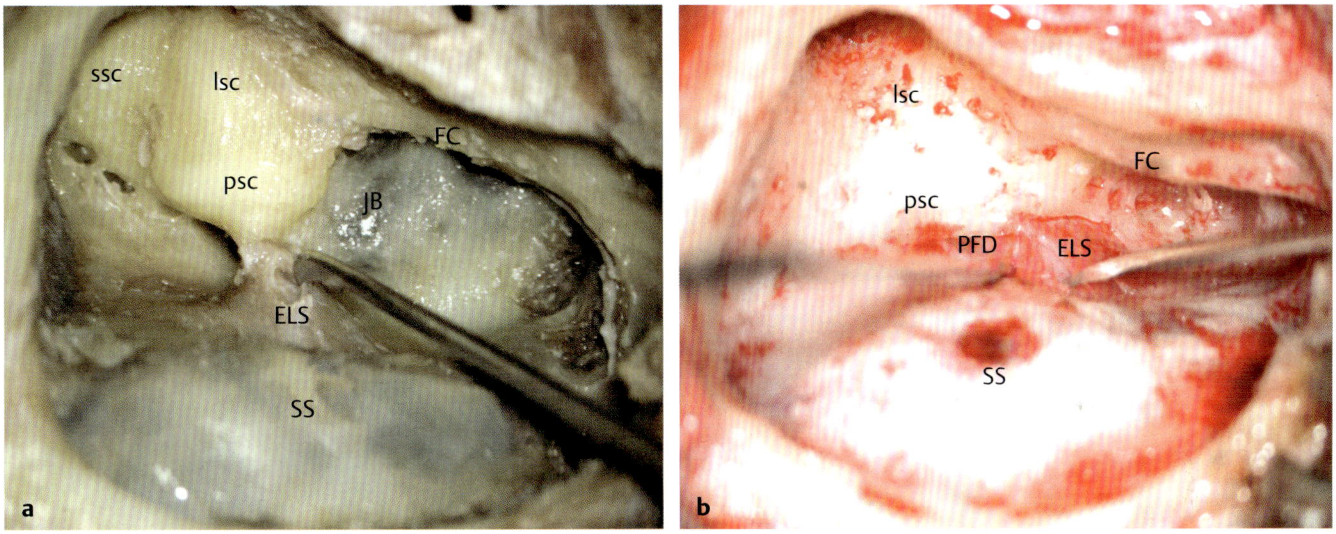

Fig. 62.8 **(a, b)** Endolymphatic sac outer wall incised.

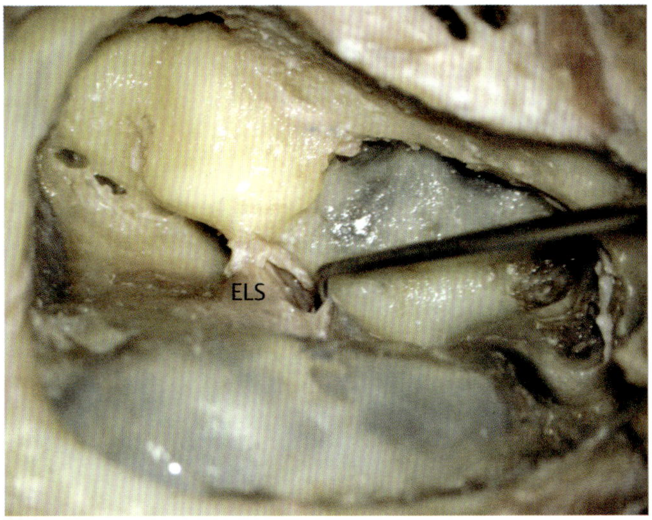

Fig. 62.9 Ball point probe in the lumen of endolymphatic sac.

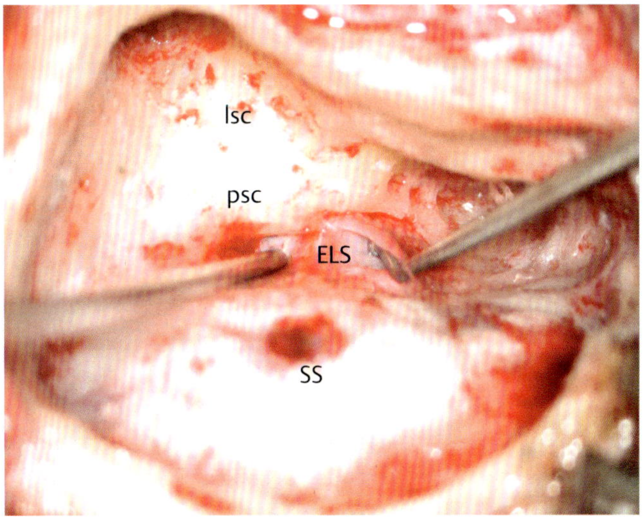

Fig. 62.10 Ball point probe in the lumen of endolymphatic sac.

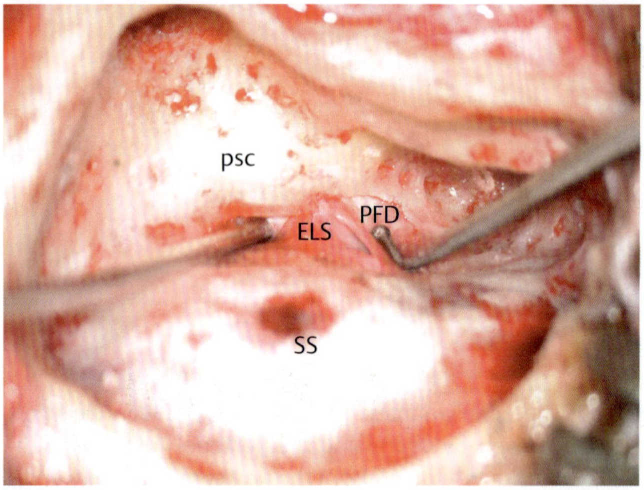

Fig. 62.11 Open lumen of the endolymphatic sac is visualized.

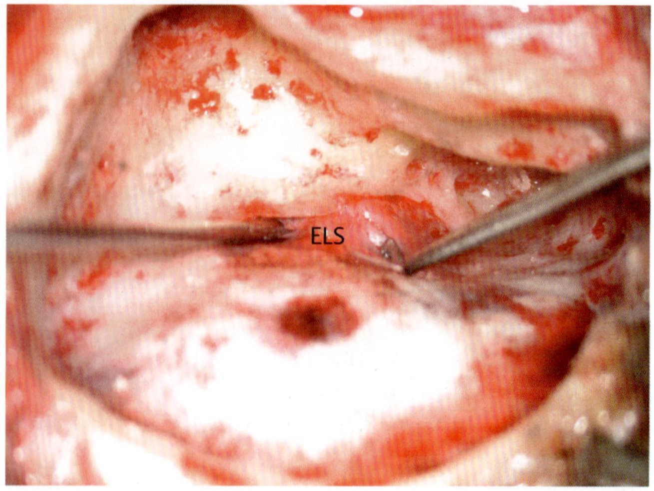

Fig. 62.12 Silastic sheet is inserted in the lumen of endolymphatic sac.

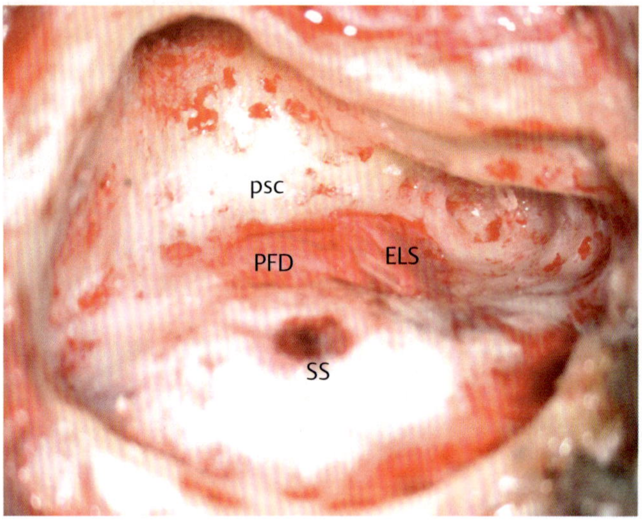

Fig. 62.13 Vertical limb of silastic sheet is seen outside the lumen of endolymphatic sac creating an endolymphatic mastoid shunt.

Tips and Pearls

- Do not incise the endolymphatic sac unless confirmed that it is indeed the endolymphatic sac. Accidental incision over the posterior fossa dura will result in a cerebrospinal fluid leak.
- The elevation of the endolymphatic duct from the posterior fossa dura helps to identify the endolymphatic sac.
- A silastic sheet in the shape of "T" is used to maintain the patency of the endolymphatic mastoid shunt.

Suggested Readings

Kato BM, LaRouere MJ, Bojrab DI, Michaelides EM. Evaluating quality of life after endolymphatic sac surgery: The Ménière's disease outcomes questionnaire. Otol Neurotol 2004; 25(3): 339–344

Sood AJ, Lambert PR, Nguyen SA, Meyer TA. Endolymphatic sac surgery for Ménière's disease: a systematic review and meta-analysis. Otol Neurotol 2014;35(6):1033–1045

Chapter 63 Transmastoid Labyrinthectomy

Narayan Jayashankar

Indications

- Unilateral peripheral vestibular disease with unserviceable hearing.
- As a route to translabyrinthine vestibular nerve section or eighth nerve section.
- Intralabyrinthine schwannomas with unserviceable hearing (rare).

Surgical Steps

1. A postaural incision is taken along the posterior border of the mastoid, approximately 1.5 cm behind the postaural groove. The incision includes the skin and subcutaneous tissue (**Fig. 63.1**).
2. A T-shaped musculoperiosteal incision is made. The horizontal limb extends along the temporal line. A vertical incision is made perpendicular to the horizontal limb midway between the postaural groove and the skin incision. The musculoperiosteal flaps are retracted and sutured anteriorly, posteriorly, and superiorly to expose the mastoid cortex (**Fig. 63.2**).
3. A cortical mastoidectomy is performed with exenteration of cells from over the sigmoid sinus, middle fossa dural plate, posterior canal wall, and mastoid tip. Similarly, cells are also exenterated from the lateral, posterior, and superior semicircular canals. The fallopian canal is identified in its mastoidal course. The retrofacial and infralabyrinthine cells are cleared, and a shell of bone is left over the jugular bulb (**Fig. 63.3**).
4. Drilling is done along the direction of the posterior, lateral, and superior semicircular canals, respectively. The slits in the canal denote the direction of the semicircular canals (**Fig. 63.4**).
5. Bleeding occurs from the center of the curve formed by the superior semicircular canal. This is the subarcuate artery, and bleeding from it is controlled by the use of bipolar or drilling over it with a diamond burr to crush it.
6. The ampullary ends of the semicircular canals are drilled to open up the same (**Fig. 63.5**). The cristae of the three canals are removed.

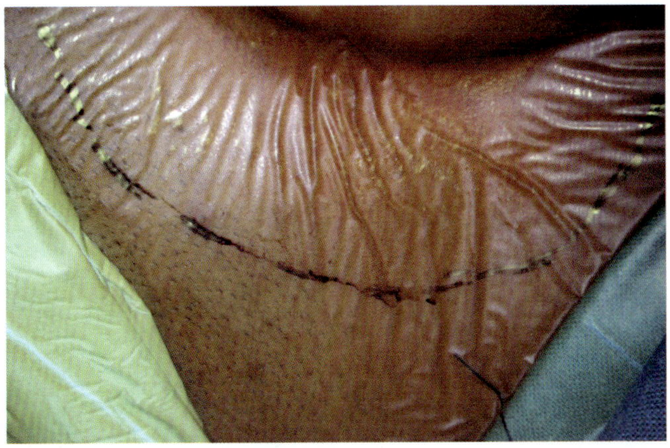

Fig. 63.1 Incision—right side.

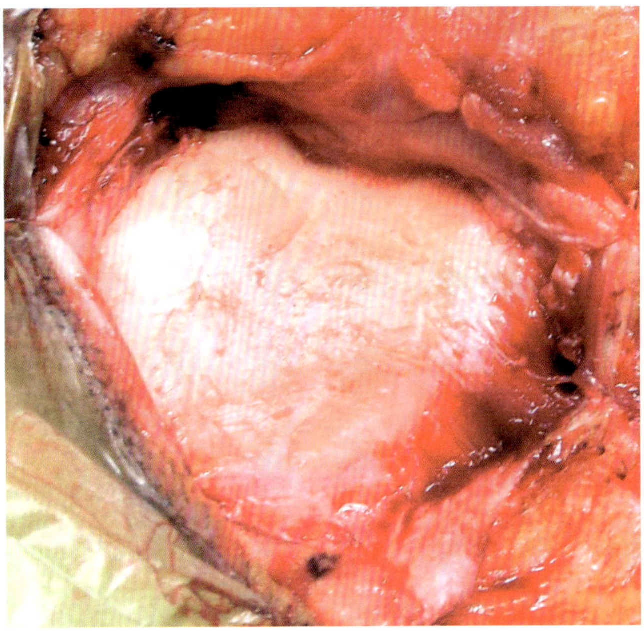

Fig. 63.2 Exposure of mastoid cortex.

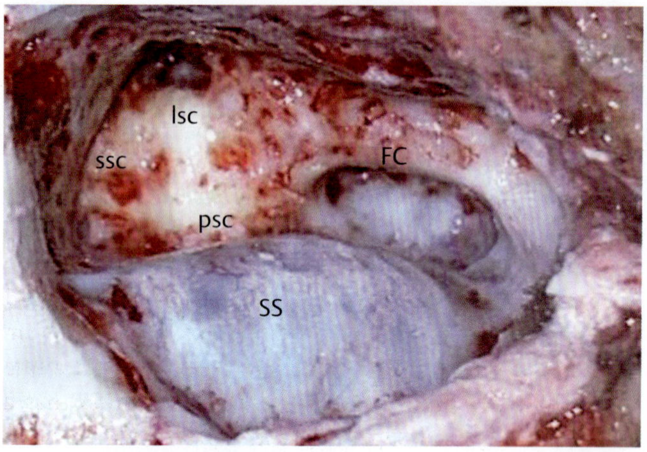

Fig. 63.3 Cortical mastoidectomy.

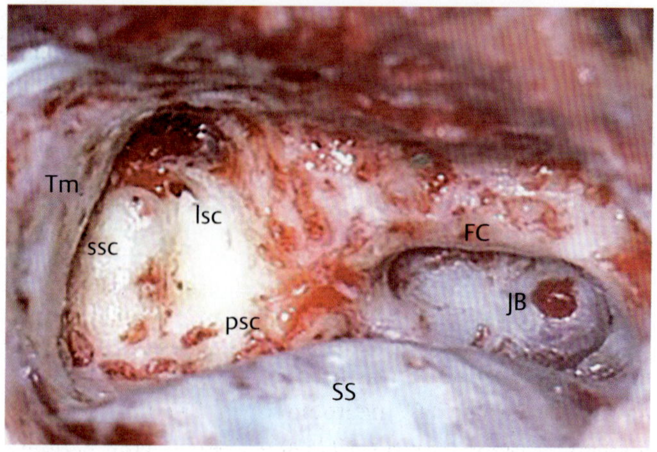

Fig. 63.4 Slits in the semicircular canals.

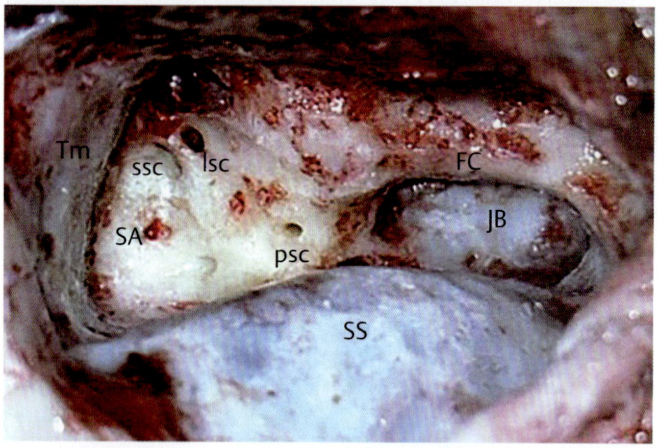

Fig. 63.5 Ampullary ends of semicircular canals are seen.

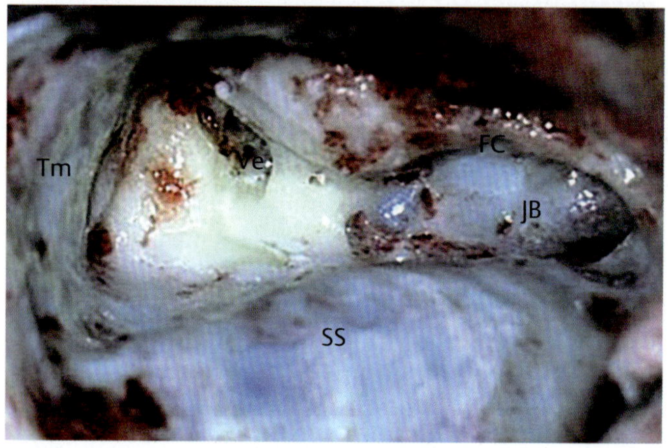

Fig. 63.6 Vestibule is opened and neuroepithelium is removed.

7. The vestibule is widely opened and the neuroepithelium is removed (**Fig. 63.6**). Care is taken not to injure the second genu of the facial nerve that lies immediately lateral to the vestibule.
8. The musculoperiosteal layer is closed.
9. The skin and subcutaneous tissue are sutured in a single layer.

Tips and Pearls

- This procedure is only used when hearing is unserviceable.
- It is essential to clear the neuroepithelium from the vestibule as also the ampullated ends of the three semicircular canals.

Chapter 64

Vestibular Neurotomy by Retrosigmoid Approach

Jacques Magnan

Introduction

It was Dandy[1] who first recognized that selective neurotomy of the vestibular nerve was possible via the posterior fossa, and he performed 607 neurotomies in 587 patients with Ménière's disease between 1924 and 1946.[2] In France, Aubry and Ombredanne[3] used the same suboccipital craniotomy. However, the morbidity and mortality associated with this surgery prevented it from gaining widespread acceptance. Vestibular neurotomy fell into obscurity until being resurrected by the new microsurgical procedures popularized by House[4] in the 1960s.

After Fluur and Tovi,[5] who published the microsurgical intracranial technique to cut the vestibular nerve, Bremond et al[6,7] described in 1974 an *à minima* approach through a keyhole retrosigmoid craniotomy.

However, the operation was not much publicized until Millen and Meyer,[8] then Silverstein and Haberkamp[9] stressed the advantages of this surgical procedure, and gave up the useless intracanalicular dissection proposed firstly.

It is now confirmed that retrosigmoid vestibular neurotomy provided certain and safe access to the eighth cranial nerve in the cerebellopontine angle,[10] and led to the concept of minimally invasive otoneurosurgery.[11–13]

Surgical Steps

1. The patient is placed in a supine position on the operating table with his or her head turned so that the involved side is facing upward.[13] Under general anesthesia, a 7-cm incision is made from the level of the transverse sinus at the midline occiput to the posterior margin of the tip of the mastoid process. The skin and soft tissues are retracted from the mastoid and adjacent suboccipital region and held in place with a self-retaining retractor. The mastoid emissary vein centers the retromastoid craniotomy.
2. A 15-mm circular craniotomy is performed with an electric cutting drill, behind and close to the sigmoid sinus. The dura is opened. At this time, the cerebellum retracts spontaneously, thanks to the combined effects of profound anesthesia (including a narcotic agent [Diprivan] and an analgesic [Sulfenta]), with assisted hyperventilation, resulting in hypocapnia (pCO_2 < 25 mm Hg). The cerebellum surface is protected from injury by a strip of cottonoid in order to obtain a safe corridor within which to operate. The corridor has a safe bony wall superiorly and a protected cerebellar surface inferiorly, which is maintained spontaneously without the need for retractors to provide this.
3. Under the operating microscope with 250-mm focus, author starts by opening the arachnoid surrounding the acousticofacial nerve bundle. The cerebrospinal fluid (CSF) escapes, and the cerebellum spontaneously falls away without the need for retraction. Specially adapted microinstrumentation is useful. Conventional otologic instruments are too short, and the usual neurosurgical instruments are too bulky. A specific set offers instruments with a bayonet handle, which facilitates visualization with the keyhole approach.
4. The acousticofacial nerve bundle is visualized 55-mm deep, and the entrance of nerves into the porus acousticus provides unquestionable identification (**Fig. 64.1a, b**).

   The key point of the procedure is to know that there is always an intervestibulocochlear cleavage plane when the arachnoid wrapping is dissected away from the nerve bundle, and a groove along the eighth nerve is visible and well-marked near the porus. A small dissector inserted into this partition line divides the acoustic nerve into its two parts (**Fig. 64.2a, b**).
5. The vestibular nerve appears grayish as compared with the cochlear nerve (**Fig. 64.2a, b**).

   The vestibular fibers are more superior (rostral) and closest to the fifth cranial nerve. The cochlear nerve is inferior (caudal) and closest to the ninth nerve. Vestibular neurotomy is performed with microsurgical scissors (**Fig. 64.3a, b**).

   After complete neurotomy, the ends of the nerve retract spontaneously so that the surgeon does not need to perform neurectomy. The facial nerve, which is much deeper, is safe from injury (**Fig. 64.4a, b**).
6. The per-operatory cochleovestibular monitoring and mapping is an effective electrophysiological procedure to achieve a safe and perfect vestibular section when

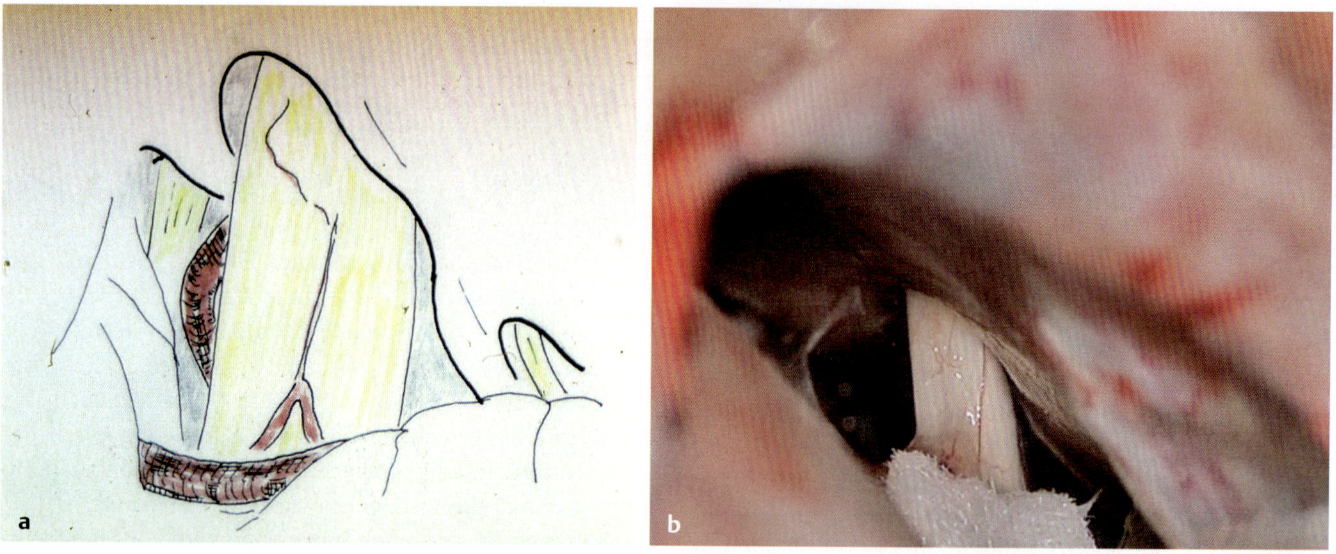

Fig. 64.1 **(a, b)** The acousticofacial nerve bundle crosses through the middle of the cerebellopontine angle and its entry into the internal auditory canal provides a sure identification.

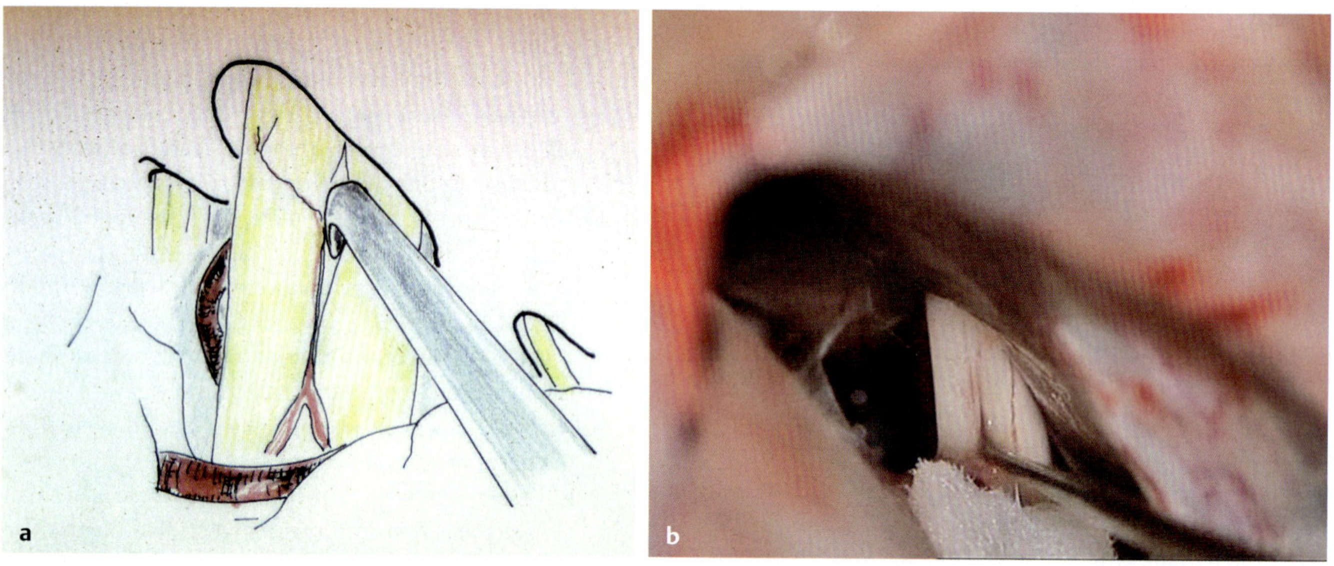

Fig. 64.2 **(a, b)** A small dissector is inserted in the intervestibulocochlear cleavage plane and isolates the vestibular from the cochlear.

the cleavage line between vestibular and cochlear components of the auditory nerve doesn't seem to be clearly identified.

7. At the end, the dura and soft tissue are closed in the usual way. The average time for this procedure is 1.5 hours.
8. The patient returns to the ward on the same day postoperatively, is mobilized as soon as possible the next day, and is usually discharged after 1 week. The patient is able to go back to work after 1 to 3 months of recovery. An early physiotherapy helps the vestibular compensation.
9. The most common side effect was the CSF leak in 3% of patients. Nowadays, a postoperative chronic headache is unusual after the retrosigmoid approach.

Some patients complained of pain in the field of Arnold's nerve which was solved using a local treatment. Neither postoperative facial paralysis nor total hearing loss occurred in our series.

Indications

The goal of vestibular neurotomy is to control disabling vertigo while preserving hearing in patients with Ménière's

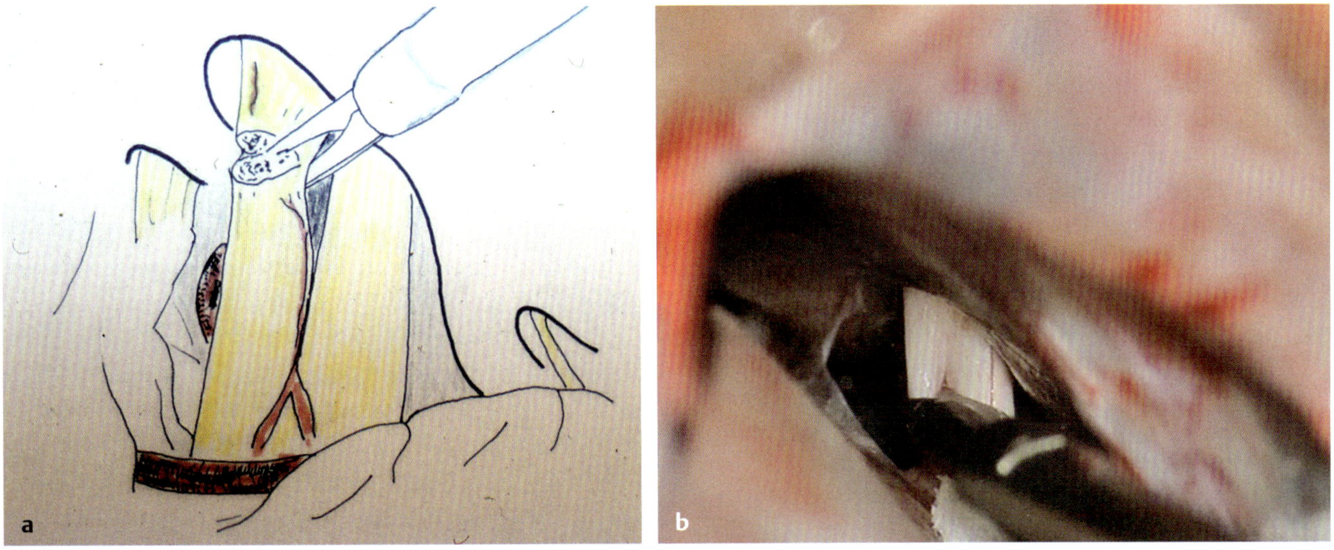

Fig. 64.3 **(a, b)** Vestibular neurotomy is performed with microscissors.

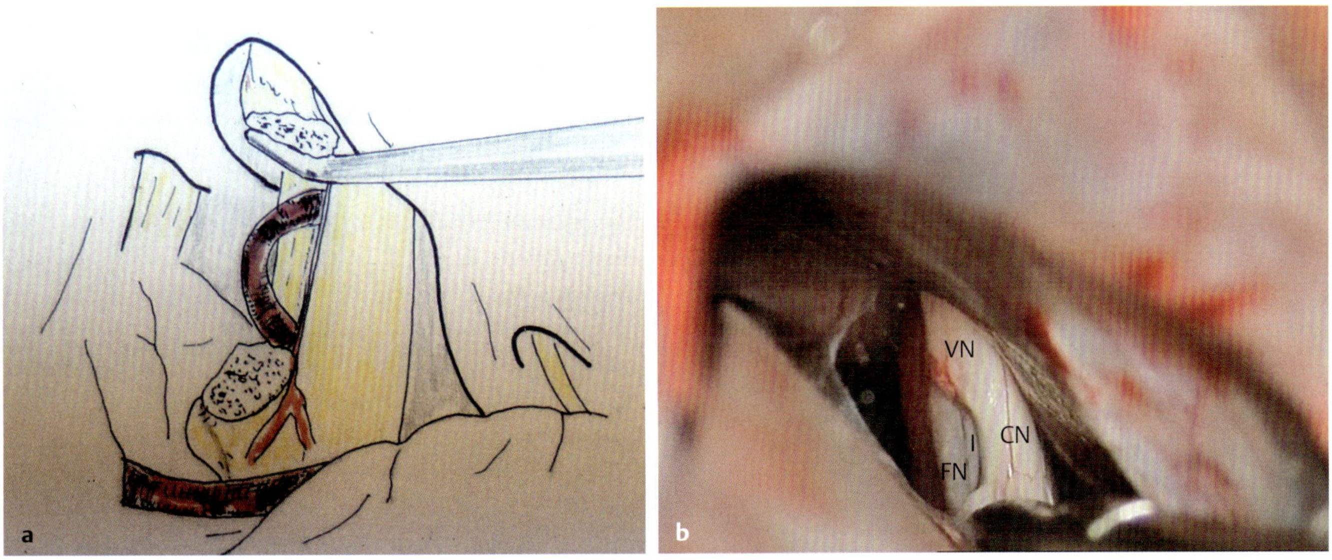

Fig. 64.4 **(a, b)** After sectioning, the ends of the vestibular nerve retract spontaneously. CN, cochlear nerve; FN, facial nerve; I, intermedius nerve; VN, vestibular nerve.

disease who were unresponsive to medical treatment or in whom an endolymphatic sac procedure had failed. The principle of vestibular neurotomy is to produce a total loss of afferent input from the offending vestibular periphery in Ménière's disease, which as a consequence leads to a vestibular compensation.

Vestibular compensation can be defined as a central complex process involving multiple sensory substitution mechanisms leading to the restoration of posture and equilibrium. Recent fundamental research dealing with experimental model of neuroplasticity has carefully described the vestibular compensation process occurring after unilateral lesion of the peripheral labyrinth or the vestibular nerve. The process of vestibular compensation is considered to be slower in elderly patients because of associated visual and proprioceptive dysfunctions. This has not been confirmed in our experience.

Although, vestibular neurotomy can be summarized as surgery of Ménière's disease, such a surgical procedure can be offered to any patient with recurrent and incapacitating vertigo of certain peripheral origin (traumatic labyrinthitis).

Material

Since 1974, the author has performed more than 500 vestibular neurotomies in Ménière's disease patients.[14, 15]

The criteria for deciding on surgery depend on several factors, including the following:

- **Medical failure:** The mean duration between the onset of the disorder and surgery was 6 years.
- **Frequency of attacks:** Prior to surgery, the patients complained of daily crisis in 38% of cases, weekly crisis in 44% of cases, and monthly crisis in 18% of cases.
- Impairment of hearing in the affected ear as well as on the other side.
- Professional status.

Finally, the decision is made to proceed with surgery by the patients themselves, when their vertigo has produced sufficient disability in their lifestyle (57% stop to work among them, 18% lose their job, 45% stop to drive) to outweigh the surgical reluctances and miss information spread by the non-surgical trained specialists.

Results

Vertigo

Out of 283 patients followed from 1974 to 1998, 270 were relieved of their vertigo (95.5%). The recurrence of vertigo in 13 patients included five cases of bilateral disease, four incomplete vestibular sections, two benign paroxysmal positional vertigo (BPPV) in the opposite site, and two wrong indications. Ice water caloric stimulation revealed no response in all cases but four. Some patients continued to mention an occasional feeling of unsteadiness but were able to carry on a normal life.

The assessment of "patient's point of view" was stressed by Reid et al[16] and studied by chart review and by sending out a questionnaire. Patient satisfaction with unilateral retrosigmoid vestibular neurotomy was recorded as follows:

- Vertigo was cured and the patient came back to normal activities in 62% of cases (165 patients).
- Vertigo was cured and imbalance remained only in specific circumstances, as in the dark or with fast movement of the head in 21.5% of cases (61 patients).
- Vertigo was cured but significant walking unsteadiness felt in 9.5% of cases (36 cases).
- Vertigo was cured but there was dissatisfaction in eight patients (2.5% of cases) for various reasons (tinnitus, fullness in the ear, visual problem).
- Further vertigo was seen in 4.5% of cases (13 cases: five bilateral, four incomplete sections, two BPPV in opposite ear, and two wrong indications).
- Worse than before surgery: No patients.

Lastly, 83% of patients expressed a high level of satisfaction.

The 36 cases with a chronic feeling of being off-balance were interpreted as incomplete vestibular compensation and required complementary vestibular rehabilitation.

A second study from 2000 to 2009 on 114 patients demonstrated that there was a relevant correlation between anxiety score and postoperative disequilibrium handicap. In other words, a high level of anxiety or stress in a Ménière patient modified his or her pure peripheral vestibulopathy and induced a partial central dysfunction which interfered in the quality of the vestibular compensation.

Hearing

Most of the patients undergoing vestibular neurotomy had serviceable hearing in the involved ear at the time of surgery. The preoperative hearing loss average was 49 dB, after 1 year of follow-up it was 46 dB, after 5 years of follow-up it was 53 dB.

The variance of posttraumatic amnesia (PTA) scores in patients with hearing improvement (40%) and in those with worsened hearing (29%) shows a similar average for the pre- and postoperative hearing thresholds. These data do not mean improving or worsening because of surgery, but only the inability of the surgical procedure to retain the fluctuating hearing of the patient at the best level.

There was particular interest in studying the outcome of patients with good preoperative hearing (between 10 and 20 dB). Out of 19 patients selected according to this criterion, after 5 years postoperatively, hearing was unchanged in 11 patients, decreased by less than 20 dB in 3 patients, decreased more than 20 dB in 5 patients, so a long-term hearing preservation in 73%. These data are of particular interest for patients with good or serviceable hearing and suggest that surgery should be performed at an early stage of Ménière's disease, in order to preserve the hearing in the affected ear and not at the last stage of the evolution of the disease. In long-term follow-up studies of successful hearing preservation cases, contradictory results have been published with deterioration over time[17,18] or stability.[19,20] Authors found that hearing was stable in the long term in 70% of vestibular neurotomy patients.

Tinnitus, Aural fullness

They are not arguments in decision-making. Tinnitus usually only stabilizes after several months, and 55% of patients graded their tinnitus at the same level as prior to the surgery while 22% of patients did not mention it, and 4% of patients experienced worsened aural fullness.

Bilateral

The natural history of Ménière's disease shows the development of contralateral symptoms in one-third of cases. In our study group, bilateralization of the disorder occurred in 2% of cases (four cases within 5 years, and one case after 10 years).

Conclusion

The infrequency of complications and the efficiency of the vestibular compensation allow considering retrosigmoid vestibular neurotomy as the procedure of choice for incapacitating Ménière's disease when residual hearing still exists, until authors found the etiopathogenical and medical treatment of such a disease.

References

1. Dandy W. Menière's disease: diagnosis and treatment of thirty cases. Am J Surg 1933;20:693–698
2. Green R, Douglas C. Intracranial division of the eighth nerve for Menière's disease: a follow-up study of patients operated on by Dr Walter Dandy. Ann Otol Rhinol Laryngol 1951;60:610–621
3. Aubry M, Ombredanne M: Deux cas de section partielle du nerf auditif avec guérison des vertiges et conservation de l'audition. Ann Otolaryngol (Paris) 1935:52:535–539
4. House W. Surgical exposure of the internal auditory canal and its contents through the middle cranial fossa. Laryngoscope 1961;71:1363–1365
5. Fluur E, Tovi D. Microscopic intracranial section of vestibular nerve. Acta Otolaryngol (Stokh) 1965;59: 604–606
6. Bremond G, Garcin M, Magnan J, Bonnaud G. L'abord à minima de l'angle ponto-cérébelleux. Cah ORL 1974;9: 443–460
7. Bremond G, Garcin M. Microsurgical approach to the cerebellopontine angle. J Laryngol Otol 1975;89:237–248
8. Millen S, Meyer G. Retrosigmoid intracanicular vestibular nerve section: an alternative surgical approach for Meniere's disease. Am J Otol 1986;7:330–332
9. Silverstein H, Haberkamp T. A comparison of retrosigmoid IAC, retrolabyrinthine, and middle fossa vestibular neurectomy for treatment of vertigo. Laryngoscope 1987;97: 165–173
10. Silverstein H, Wanamaker H, Flanzer J, Rosenbergs. Vestibular neurectomy in the United States 1990. Am J Otol 1992;13: 23–30
11. Magnan J, Sanna M. Endoscopy in Neuro-Otology. New York, NY, Stuttgart: Thieme; 1999
12. Jackler R, Whinney D. A century of eight nerve surgery. Otol Neurotol 2001;23:401–416
13. Magnan J, Bremond G, Chays A. Vestibular neurotomy by retrosigmoid approach: technic, indications and results. Am J Otol 1991;12:101
14. Magnan J, Parikh B, Miyazaki H. Functional surgery of cerebellopontine angle by minimally invasive retrosigmoid approach. Jaypee Brothers Medical Publishers; 2013
15. Magnan J. Vestibular neurotomy by retrosigmoid approach Menière's disease 1999. The Hague: Kugler Publications; 2000: 65–69
16. Reid C, Eisenberg R, Halmagyi M, Fagan P. The outcome of vestibular nerve section for intractable vertigo: the patient's point of view. Laryngoscope 1996;106:1553–1556
17. Papas D, Pappas D. Vestibular nerve section: long-term follow up. Laryngoscope 1997;107:1203–1209
18. Wazen J, Spitzer J, Kasper C, Anderson B. Long-term hearing results following vestibular surgery in Meniere's disease. Laryngoscope 1998;108:1470–1473
19. Rosenberg S, Silverstein H, Hoffer M, Thaler E. Hearing results after posterior fossa vestibular neurectomy. Otolaryngol Head Neck Surg 1996;114:32–37
20. Goksu N, Bayazit Y, Beder L. Posterior fossa vestibular nerve. Section for the management of peripheral vertigo. Eur Arch. Otorinolaryngol 1999;256:230–232

Section XXV

Microvascular Decompression

Chapter 65 Endoscope-Assisted Retrosigmoid Approach in Neurovascular Decompression

Jacques Magnan

Introduction

Cranial nerves in the cerebellopontine angle (CPA) share a common pathology: the neurovascular compression syndrome induced by an offending contact of vascular structure to the related cranial nerve, which has been definitively proved by the surgical decompression of the cross-compression and the resolution of the patient's symptoms.

By 1934, Dandy[1] had found during operative treatment for tic douloureux that adjacent vessels were in contact with the nerve in 45% of 215 cases and postulated that such vascular compression could be the cause of trigeminal neuralgia.

Gardner[2,3] carried Dandy's idea a step further, extending the concept to hemifacial spasm.

Since 1967, Jannetta[4–6] has accumulated a vast experience in posterior fossa cranial nerves dysfunction syndromes and popularized microvascular decompression (MVD) in trigeminal neuralgia, hemifacial spasm, glossopharyngeal neuralgia, certain vestibulocochlear nerve dysfunctions, and even some cases of essential hypertension.

Whatever the additional experience, in 1980, Jannetta[7] noted the poor acceptance of the concept of neurovascular compression of the cranial nerves and summarized the reasons as following:

- Few surgeons ventured safely and comfortably in the CPA.
- Magnification techniques were not routinely used as in ear surgery.
- Inadequate documentation of the findings.

These arguments have been vanished, thanks to the improvements in technology, instrumentation, and anesthesia.

- The development of minimally invasive techniques, first described by Bremond et al,[8–10] has drastically reduced the risk of morbidity, the need of intensive care, and extend the surgery whatever may be the age of the patient.
- Endoscope-assisted procedure introduced in 1993 by Magnan et al[11–15] offers an unobstructed panoramic view on all neurovascular components crossing the CPA without the need of excessive retraction or drainage offering a safe and accurate identification of the course of the offending vessel(s).
- Magnetic resonance imaging (MRI) assessment in T2 sequence shows with a high sensitivity the site and the offending vessel(s) compressing the nerve and distorting the neural structures.[16–19]

While the knowledge about the pathophysiology of the vascular compression is still limited, it is indisputable that the MVD operation is effective in curing trigeminal neuralgia and hemifacial spasm.[20–22]

Nowadays endoscope-assisted MVD represents the best and most logical functional surgical treatment for cases resulting from a neurovascular conflict of the trigeminal, facial, auditory, and glossopharyngeal nerves. It gives excellent long-term results with a very low rate of morbidity. The minimally invasive retrosigmoid approach provides a direct and easy access to the involved cranial nerve.[23–26]

Material

Instrumentation in Endoscope-Assisted Retrosigmoid Approach

Microscopic Setup

Until recently the operating microscope represents the prime and single most important equipment for any surgery in CPA. Regarding the keyhole retrosigmoid approach, the operating microscope must not be too bulky to allow adequate freedom movements of both the microscope itself and the surgeon's hand maneuvers.

Video-Endoscopic Equipment and Setup

Major companies (by alphabetical order Karl Storz, Olympus, Wolff, Xion) are offering a large choice of endoscopic technology. The video-endoscopic setup includes endoscopes, autoclavable fiber cable, cold light source (halogen or xenon light), high-resolution endoscopic camera, video monitoring with video recording system.

Rigid and autoclavable Hopkins rod lens endoscopes are used.

The most helpful is the 30-degree endoscope, 4 mm in diameter and 18 cm in length. Rotating the 30-degree endoscope around its longitudinal axis changes the field of vision in contrast to the 0-degree endoscope and allows the surgeon to "look around the corner."[19]

- The 30-degree, 2.7-mm in diameter endoscope becomes useful when the space is limited.
- The 0- or 30-degree endoscopes with shorter length (6 or 11 cm) are recommended when the operator is not familiar with endoscopic procedure to prevent from injury of the deeper neurovascular structures.
- More angled endoscope 45 and 70 degrees, 18 cm in length allows a more lateral view, but the exact position of the tip is not so easy to appreciate and could cause injury to the surrounding structures during introduction or when maneuvering the scope for side vision.
- A new multifunctional endoscope, 4 mm in diameter changes the viewing angle in five steps from 15 to 90 degrees.

Whatever the endoscope and the video camera used, the endoscopic device is held with both hands not to make contact with the surrounding nerves and vessels in the CPA while inserting it and to be safer and more accurate during insertion. One hand holds the camera while the other, in contact with the craniotomy, controls and guides the insertion of the endoscope. The endoscopic mapping of the CPA combined with microsurgery represents a significant help in the vascular decompression procedure.

The lens of the endoscope is soaked with sterile antifog solution, or in warm saline or betadine. The best cleaning solution is the cerebrospinal fluid (CSF) itself. So a long piece of cottonoid is placed inferiorly between the cerebellum and the petrous bone. Touching the cottonoid with the tip of the endoscope defogs the lens without the need to withdraw the endoscope to clean it.

Endoscopic maneuvers in one-hand manipulation as suction of CSF, dissection of the arachnoid covering, and adhesions as well as mobilization of the arteries require training. Bimanual operating requires the use of articulated endoscope holder or commitment of the cosurgeon to hold the endoscope. Until now a fully endoscopic procedure was only tried in very favorable conditions but never as a routine or recommendable procedure to properly manage the various aspects of vascular compression of the cranial nerve. The advantage of the two-hand manipulation offers by the operating microscope is not questionable.

Instruments

Specific suitable microinstruments are required because both otologic microinstruments are too short and neurosurgical ones are too long and too cumbersome. Bayonet-shaped instruments with the length of 19 cm and the working distance of 9.5 cm have been adapted to the keyhole retrosigmoid approach.

Neurophysiological Monitoring

Facial nerve monitoring during MVD for hemifacial spasm can be used as an indicator of the effectiveness of the procedure. The cessation of the spontaneous firing activity of the facial nerve detected at the beginning of the intervention may indicate an effective decompression of the nerve.

Cochlear nerve monitoring is mandatory in decompression of the auditory nerve for tinnitus or disabling positional vertigo. First, it can help to prevent cochlear nerve injury, second, the return to normal intraoperative auditory brainstem response (ABR) objectifies the efficiency of the decompression. Unfortunately, the return to normal is not constant.

Surgical Technique

Endoscope-assisted keyhole retrosigmoid approach provides a direct and safe access to the CPA through a protected corridor to reach the acousticofacial nerve bundle, the lower cranial nerve inferiorly and the trigeminal nerve superiorly in the CPA, and allows easy handling of all the structures occupying this area.

Positioning

The patient is placed in the dorsal decubitus position, with the head nonfixed, flexed, and turned to the contralateral side.

Anesthesia

General endotracheal anesthesia is administered with the complementary use of analgesics, hypnotics, or neuroleptics (propofol, sufentanil). Before opening the dura, the patient is hyperventilated to obtain hypocapnia (PCO_2 inferior to 25) and so as to diminish the intracranial pressure that helps spontaneous cerebellar retraction. This step allows an easy penetration in the posterior fossa without the use of a cerebellar retractor. This type of anesthesia makes it unnecessary to use lumbar of CSF drainage or mannitol IV.

Landmarks, Incision, Craniotomy

The landmarks of the approach are the posterior border of the mastoid, which demarcates the sigmoid sinus as the anterior limit, the occipital line, or Frankfurt line that corresponds to the posterior extension of the line joining the outer canthus of the eye to the superior border of the external auditory canal.

The skin incision is curvilinear, 6 to 8 cm long, passing over the posterior part of the craniotomy area, about two fingerbreadths behind the pinna. The cutaneous flap is anteriorly based, whereas the underlying musculoperiosteal flap is fashioned posteriorly based (**Fig. 65.1**).

The mastoid emissary vein is identified and coagulated and blocked with bone wax. Burring for the craniotomy is centered on this vein using a cutting burr head. Bone dust is collected to make a bone pâté that will be used during closure. A circular bone flap may be removed in one piece to be put back in place at the end of the procedure. The retromastoid craniotomy is usually 15- to 20 mm in diameter, slightly extended inferiorly toward the digastric groove, which gives it an elliptical shape.

After the posterior fossa dura (white in color) and the posterior border of the sigmoid sinus (blue in color) have been exposed, the surgeon uses the operating microscope. The craniotomy must reach the posterior border of the sigmoid sinus anteriorly, but it is not necessary to entirely skeletonize it.

All opened mastoid air cells should be obliterated using Horsley's bone wax to avoid CSF leakage through these cells to the middle ear cavities.

Opening of the Dura Mater and Cerebellopontine Angle

The best moment to open the dura is when transmitted CSF pulsations are clearly seen, which is a sign of spontaneous cerebellar retraction. The opening of the dura is a U-shaped incision so as to form an anteriorly based dural flap. This flap is suspended anteriorly using stitch or fibrin glue (**Fig. 65.2**).

A fine cottonoid or synthetic dura substitute is introduced to protect the cerebellum, then following the posterior surface of the petrous bone in an anteroinferior direction to reach the lower cranial nerve area, the posterior cistern is opened. The CSF escapes, and the cerebellum falls away without any pressure on it.

After dissecting the arachnoid wrapping the cranial nerves using the operative microscope, an endoscopic look of the CPA is made with a 4-mm, 30-degree-angled rigid endoscope.

Cerebellopontine Endoscopy

The CPA is endoscopically divided into two zones separated by the acousticofacial bundle (**Fig. 65.3a–c**).

The superior zone corresponds to the trigeminal nerve which is visualized from the Meckel cave to the pons. The most common compressing vessel of the trigeminal nerve is the superior cerebellar artery (SCA). The inferior zone corresponds to the lower cranial nerves zone that is inspected in case of hemifacial spasm. A high vertebral artery and the posterior inferior cerebellar artery (PICA) are the most common offending vessels at the root exit zone (REZ) of the facial nerve. The auditory nerve is the most exposed in the middle of the CPA. The anterior inferior cerebellar artery (AICA) is commonly in contact with the acousticofacial nerve bundle. So, its role as offending vessel is less obvious, and its decompression is more delicate. The surgeon must be aware

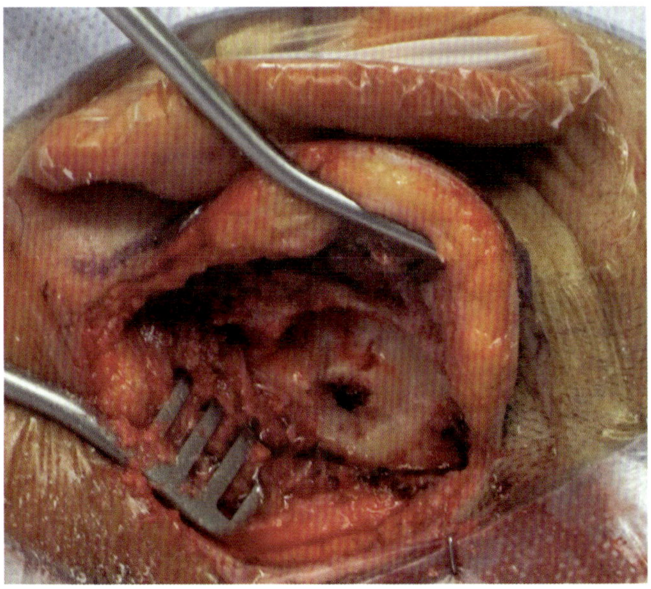

Fig. 65.1 Left minimally invasive retrosigmoid approach, the craniotomy is centered on the emissary vein.

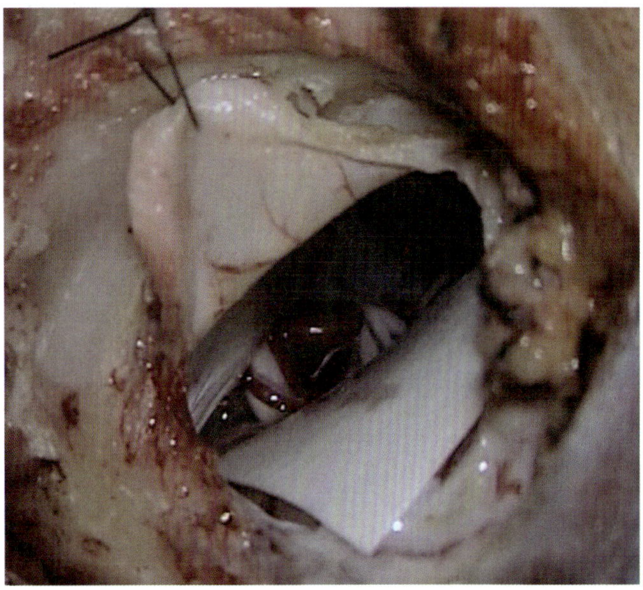

Fig. 65.2 Left minimally invasive retrosigmoid approach, the "protected" surgical corridor to access the cerebellopontine angle.

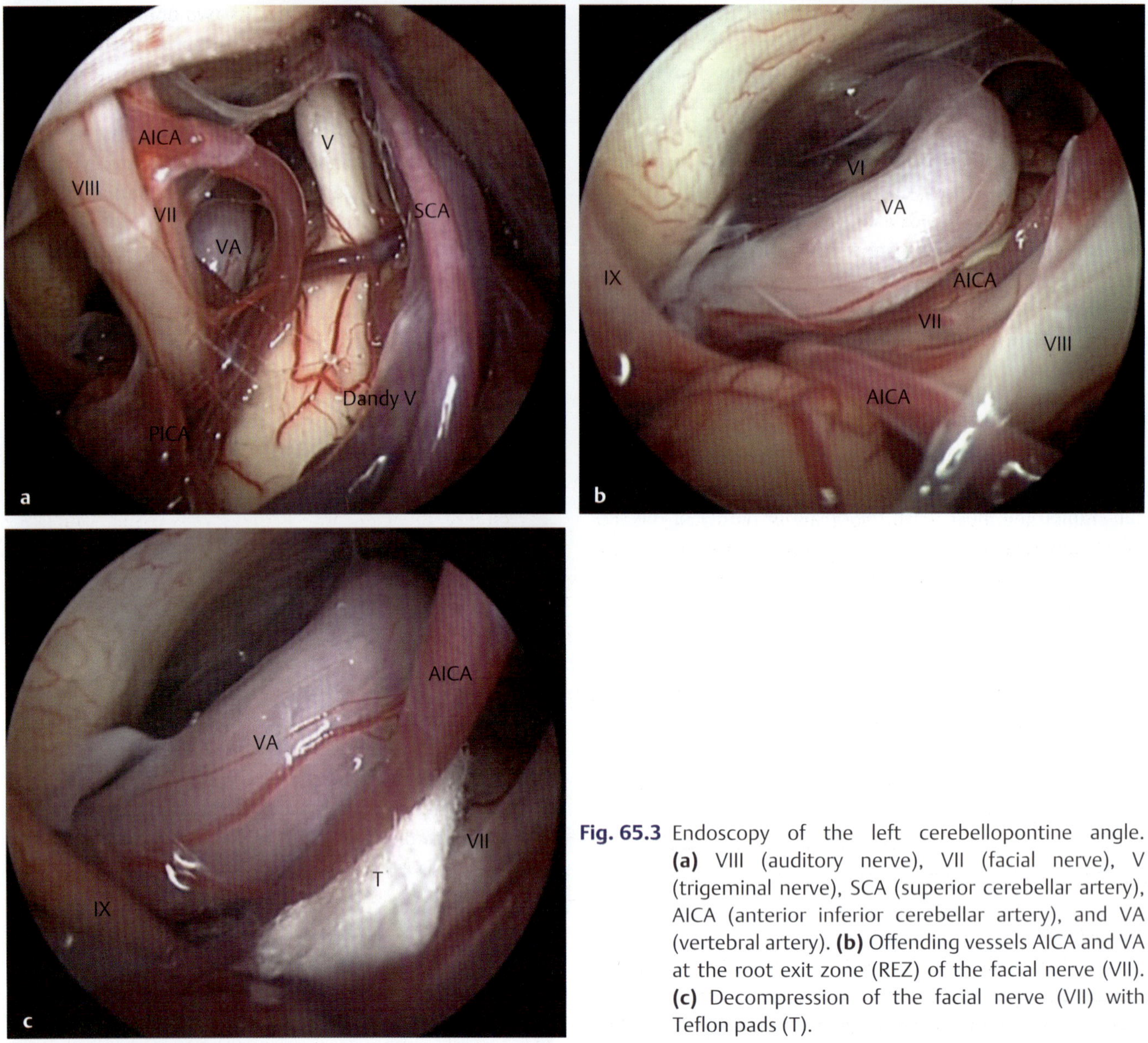

Fig. 65.3 Endoscopy of the left cerebellopontine angle. **(a)** VIII (auditory nerve), VII (facial nerve), V (trigeminal nerve), SCA (superior cerebellar artery), AICA (anterior inferior cerebellar artery), and VA (vertebral artery). **(b)** Offending vessels AICA and VA at the root exit zone (REZ) of the facial nerve (VII). **(c)** Decompression of the facial nerve (VII) with Teflon pads (T).

of potential thermal injury to the auditory nerve by the heat of the endoscope tip. Consequently, close and prolonged contact between cranial nerves and endoscope tip should be avoided.

Vascular Decompression

Whatever the site of the neurovascular compression, MVD aims to change the offending vessel axis and to keep it away from the offended cranial nerve. This surgical procedure is done under the operating microscope. The offending vessel is carefully mobilized using a microelevator or a microhook. Further, meticulous and careful dissections allow the artery axis of direction to change. By inserting one or more small Teflon pads (2 to 3 mm) between the artery and the nerve and adjusting it or them with a microinstrument, the decompression is completed. Teflon is an inert material well tolerated in the CPA. The operation ends with another endoscopic look to assess the correct positioning of the Teflon pad and to check the absence of contact between the decompressed nerve and all adjacent vascular structures that could maintain the hyperactivity of the nerve. The surgery must perform both decompression and an insolation of the nerve from any vessels that could maintain its hyperactivity.

Closure

Before closure, the operative field should be bloodless and is filled with physiological saline at body temperature to extrude air, which could cause postoperative headaches.

The dura is sutured using 5–0 silk sutures. Because of the small size of the dura flap opening, a watertight closure is not always easy to achieve (**Fig. 65.4**). For bridging the defect, a synthetic absorbable dural substitute is used. The gaps between sutures are filled by pieces of subcutaneous fat and a fibrin glue layer, then the dura is covered by another piece of dural substitute, Surgicel, and fibrin glue. The craniotomy is then filled with a mixture of bone pâté and fibrin glue, and bone is put back. The musculoaponeurotic flap is sutured in place; finally, the subcutaneous and skin layers are sutured. Duration of the intervention is usually between 1.5 and 2.5 hours.

Indications and Results

Trigeminal Nerve

Trigeminal neuralgia or "tic douloureux" is a recognizable facial pain, which occurs suddenly in the sensory trigeminal distribution (V3 most commonly) and lasts a few seconds.[27,28] The pain is unilateral, shooting, electrical with trigger zone, and pain-free intervals. There is predominance for women (60%). Idiopathic trigeminal neuralgia does not exist; there is always a cause highlighting with MRI: tumors and multiple sclerosis represent around 5% of cases, the great majority is a vascular compression: the SCA alone in 46% associated in 30%, a venous structure alone in 11% or associated to artery in 18%, other arteries alone (AICA, dolichovertebral artery, basilar artery) in 4% but multiple combination in 34%.

The vascular decompression is performed in a deep but relatively wide area on a large and resistant cranial nerve (**Fig. 65.5a–f**).

The SCA is detached from the nerve and pons by dissecting the pial-arachnoid wrapping that maintains the artery adherent to the nerve with microscissors or sharp microinstrument. The SCA with its two branches is further kept apart the trigeminal nerve in a horizontal position toward the tentorium by fibrin glue and Teflon.

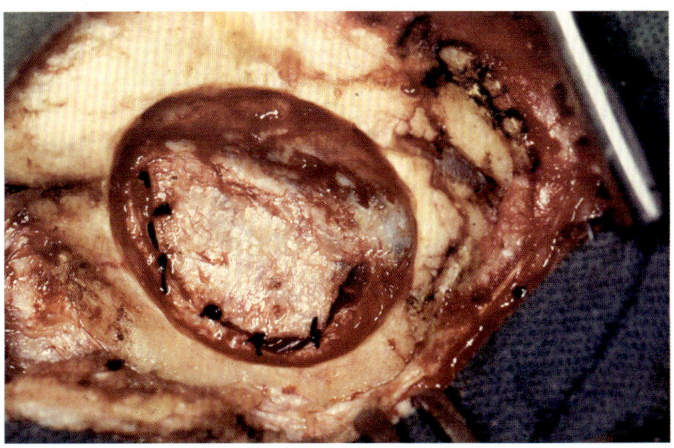

Fig. 65.4 Closure of the dura flap with 5–0 silk sutures.

When a vein is involved (**Fig. 65.6a, b**), usually aberrant trigeminal vein, which is rarely mobilized and must be coagulated with bipolar coagulation after verifying that this vein does not represent the predominant venous drainage.

In the literature, the success of the procedure varies from 73 to 97%.

Since 1994, we have performed MVD on 301 patients suffering from trigeminal neuralgia resistant to medical treatment. The oldest patient was 87 years old. The complete resolution of the pain is immediate in 86% and required revision surgery to increase the overall successful result at 91%. The recurrence after immediate postoperative relief is mentioned in all MVD series. The recurrence occurred in 14% in our patients, between 3 months and 2 years after initial surgery. Its main cause is the fibrous tissue around the trigeminal nerve inducing a new neurovascular conflict or embedding the Teflon in the nerve. Postoperative complications were limited in CSF leak in 2%. There was no facial paralysis, no hearing loss.

Facial Nerve

Hemifacial spasm is a clear clinical entity with sudden involuntary contraction of the muscles of hemiface. The contractions begin as unilateral blepharospasm, which gradually spreads the face and the neck without the history of facial palsy. There is predominance of women (65%). The cause is a vascular compression at the REZ of the facial nerve in 98% of cases.[29–32]

The most common offending vessel in hemifacial spasm is PICA alone in 37% (**Fig. 65.7**) or rising from a dolichovertebral artery just below the REZ of the facial nerve and distorting it in 32% (**Fig. 65.8**). The endoscope-assisted procedure allows to not missing multiple offending vessels: a pica with an obvious offending vertebral artery (11%) obstructing the view (**Fig. 65.9a**), a second loop of PICA at the medullopontine junction (**Fig. 65.9b, c**), or an AICA along the brainstem underlying the other vessels (9%). The bifurcation of a dominant PICA or AICA occurs in contact with the root of the facial nerve and the vascular angle formed by this division embedding the nerve (8%). The AICA can be responsible for a facial compression in 13%, on the cisternal course of the nerve or at the porus. If AICA is not the most common offending vessel, its pulsatile contact to a "hyperfunctioning" facial nerve can maintain hyperactivity on it and abnormal muscle responses.

The success of the procedures varies from 83 to 97% in the literature.

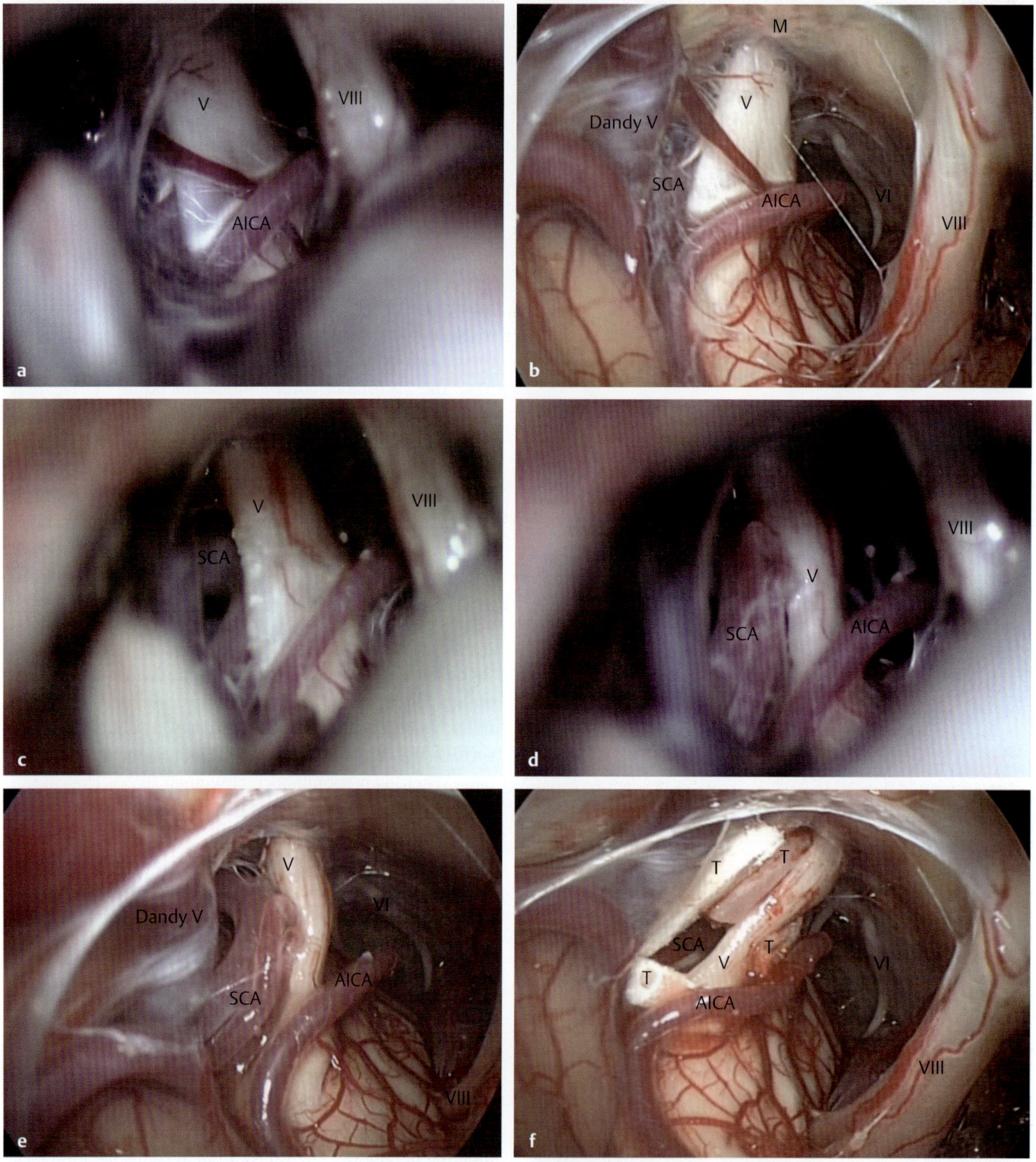

Fig. 65.5 Right trigeminal neuralgia. **(a)** Operative microscope view, trigeminal nerve (V) with AICA posteriorly, the SCA from anterior distorted the V. **(b)** Same view with endoscope giving a panoramic view from the Meckel entrance (M) to the pons. **(c, d)** Microdecompression of the trigeminal nerve (V) from the superior cerebellar artery (SCA) elevated superiorly. **(e)** Endoscopic view of the decompression of the caudal and cranial branches of the SCA are mobilized superior to the V. **(f)** Teflon pads (T) insulating V from SCA and AICA.

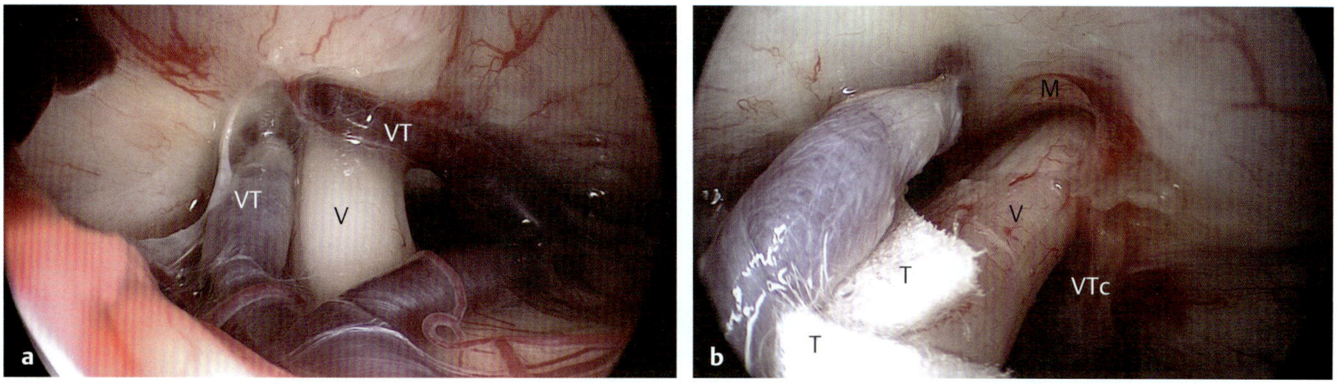

Fig. 65.6 Right trigeminal neuralgia. **(a)** Aberrant trigeminal vein (VT) as offending vessel. **(b)** Decompression with Teflon pads (T) without coagulation of the vein. VT and coagulation of the vein VTc.

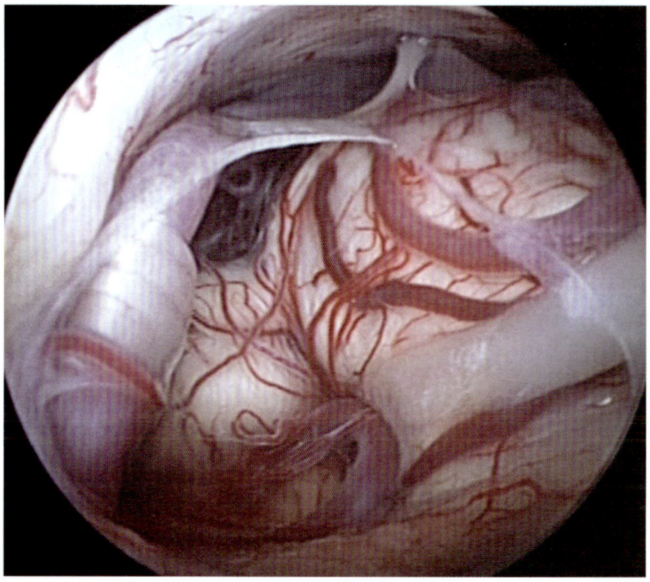

Fig. 65.7 Endoscopy of a left hemifacial spasm with PICA loop distorting the REZ of the facial nerve.

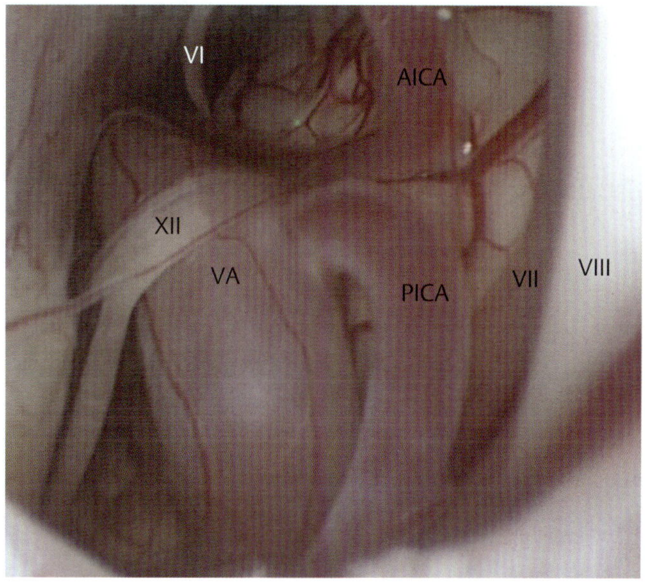

Fig. 65.8 Endoscopy of a left hemifacial spasm with PICA and vertebral artery as offending vessels.

Since 1990, 705 patients suffering from hemifacial spasm were operated on. The complete relief of spasm is achieved in 94% but 11% after an additional revision surgery. The complete resolution of spasm is immediate within 1 week of surgery in 75% and delayed in 25% of patients up to several weeks or months, with two successful results after a long period of 12 and 18 months. The explanation for this delay is not clear and evokes the hypothesis of a residual hyperactivity of the facial nucleus.

About 17% of our patients had no resolution of the disorders after a primary surgery and underwent reoperation. The main cause of unsuccessful MVD was "a missed arterial loop." The percentage of success rate at the revision surgery was the same as the primary surgery without additional side effects. The result of MVD is stable over time, only two patients developed a distant recurrence, 5 and 11 years later.

The complications are low, essentially CSF leak in 3%. The incidence of hearing impairment to deafness has been decreasing over the time from 5 to 1%. Only one postoperative facial paralysis occurred in a revision surgery of patient operated previously somewhere else.

Auditory Nerve

Unilateral tinnitus or equilibrium disorders (so-called disabling positional vertigo or vestibular paroxysmia) have no specificity. During the assessment of patients with cochleovestibular complaints MR images show a vascular loop

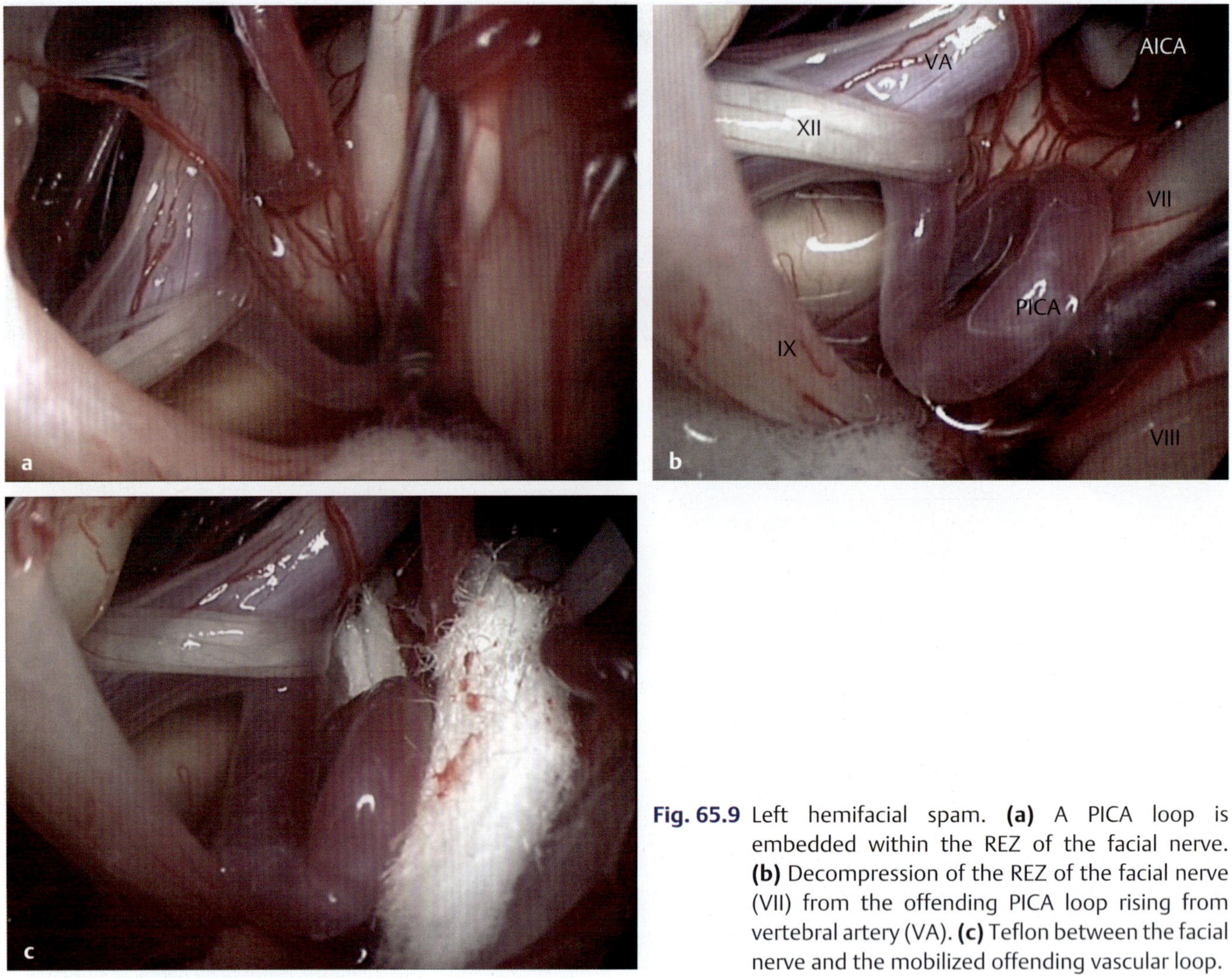

Fig. 65.9 Left hemifacial spam. **(a)** A PICA loop is embedded within the REZ of the facial nerve. **(b)** Decompression of the REZ of the facial nerve (VII) from the offending PICA loop rising from vertebral artery (VA). **(c)** Teflon between the facial nerve and the mobilized offending vascular loop.

(most commonly AICA) in contact with the auditory nerve in its cisterna or intracanalicular course. The relationship between the vascular compression and the symptoms is a "thorny issue" because of the lack of specificity of clinical signs and the frequency of AICA loop in contact with the acousticofacial nerve bundle.[33–36]

- The MRI must be done with thin slices, 0.4 mm, to show the distortion of the nerve (**Fig. 65.10a, b**). An artery adjacent or in contact with the acousticofacial nerve bundle is common and without value.
- Complementary tests must confirm the involvement of the cochlear nerve in tinnitus with ABR abnormality (I–III interpeak prolonged latency of >0.2 ms to opposite side or I–III interpeak absolute interval superior to 2.3 ms) or of the vestibular nerve with a hyporeflexia that is relatively insensitive but at least points to the affected side.

AICA, alone in 40% (**Fig. 65.11a**) or associated with PICA in 10%, is the more delicate vessel to manipulate because the complexity of 50% of its course between the seventh and eight nerve, which prevents a fully efficient and complete vascular decompression. An intracanalicular loop requires drilling of the internal auditory canal (**Fig. 65.11b**). The labyrinthine artery rising from the most lateral loop limits the displacement of the vessel.

Consequently preoperative cochlear monitoring is mandatory. By placing the recording electrode in the foramen de Luschka ABR, cochlear compound action potential (CCAP) and dorsal nucleus action potential (DNAP) can be recorded.

The other offending vessels can be the PICA in 28% (**Fig. 65.12**), a subarcuate artery "hugging" the auditory nerve in 12% (**Fig. 65.13** and **Fig. 65.14**) and vein in 5%.

The surgical results are not comparable to those got for trigeminal or facial nerves; vascular compression–induced

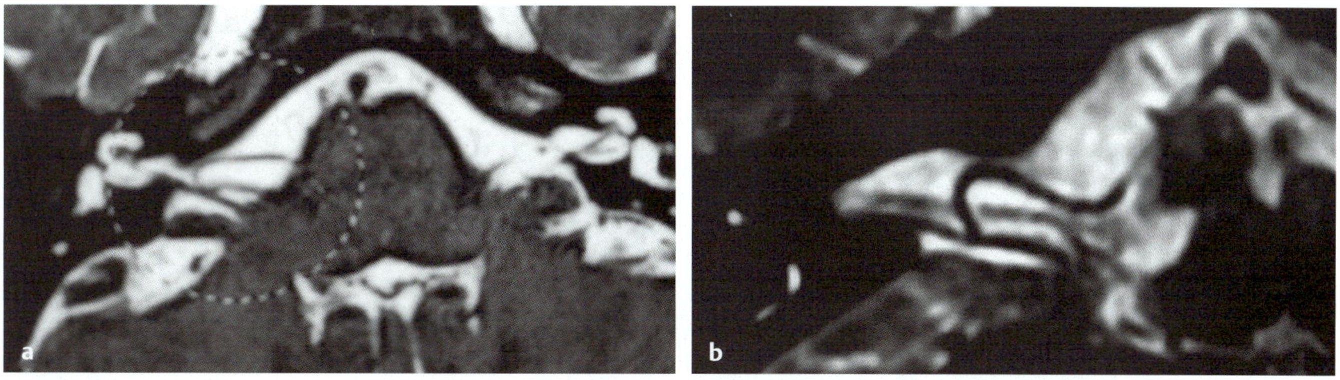

Fig. 65.10 (a, b) MRI T2 sequence, thin slices 0.4 mm, axial view, showing clearly the relationship between vessel and acousticofacial nerve bundle showing not only a contact but a distortion of the auditory nerve.

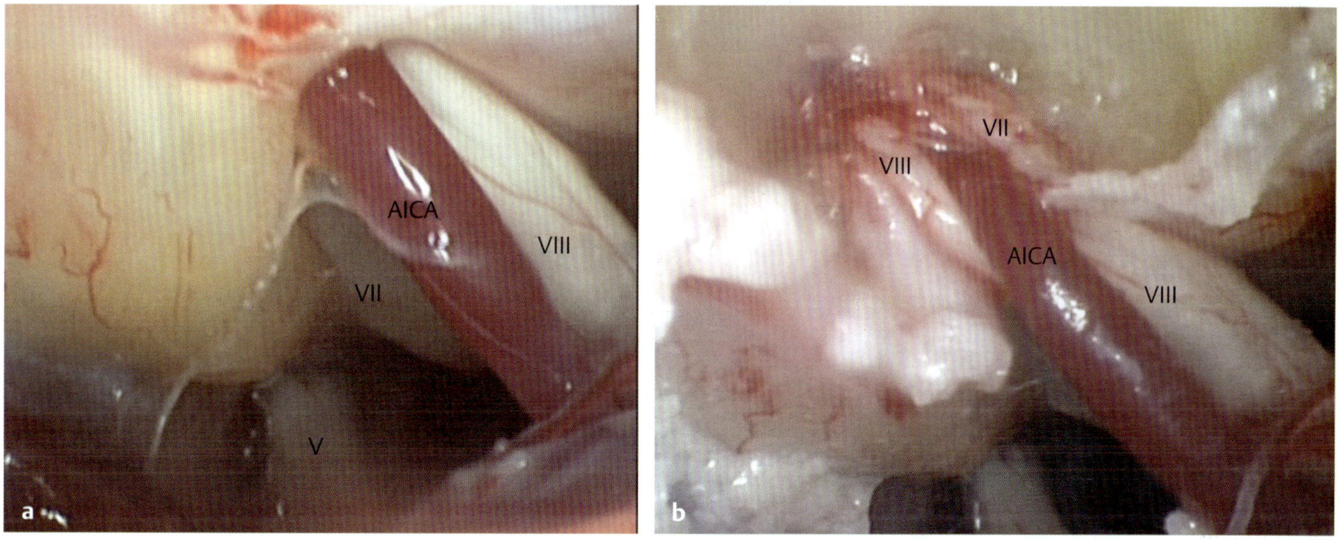

Fig. 65.11 Left incapacitating tinnitus. **(a)** Intracanalicular loop of the AICA. **(b)** Drilling the internal auditory canal to expose the cross-compression between AICA and auditory nerve (VIII).

cochleovestibular neuropathy is still a controversial diagnosis with an uncertain vascular decompression.

In the literature, the success rate varies from 33 to 77% with a large range of interpretation.

Since 1993, we performed 64 MVD of the auditory nerve in 62 cases mainly for unilateral incapacitating tinnitus alone or associated with vestibular symptoms in 40% and two cases of disabling vertigo without tinnitus (all other cochleovestibular diseases other than vascular compression of the auditory nerve were eliminated).

At 2 years follow-up, tinnitus symptom was absent in 21%, decreased significantly for the patient in 31%, similar in 44%, and worsening in 4%. The best results were in cases of subarcuate artery "hugging" the auditory nerve (seven cases), no result was achieved in cases of intracanalicular AICA loop. Interestingly, the hearing thresholds were slightly improved and ABR (I–III < 0.2 ms relative to nonoperated side) returned to normal in patients with successful results. Postoperative hearing was unchanged in 37%, 5 to 10 dB worsening in 15%, and one case of hearing loss. In the follow-up, one sudden, one progressive hearing loss occurred.

The vestibular disorders disappeared without recurrence in 56%, and MVD was ineffective in 44%.

The failure as well as the success of the eight cranial nerve MVD require a critical analysis with respect to the complex process of patient selection, the surgical findings, which can limit the efficacy of the procedure and the duration of the trouble with a central component.

Conclusion

Surgery of trigeminal and facial nerves based on neurovascular decompression is the only curative treatment of patient suffering from trigeminal neuralgia and hemifacial spasm.

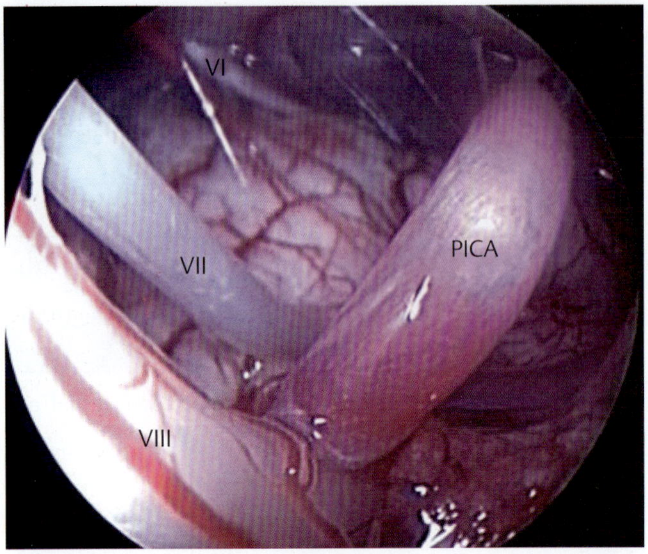

Fig. 65.12 Right incapacitating tinnitus with PICA as offending vessel. The endoscope identified clearly both the site of the cross-compression and the course of the vessel involved.

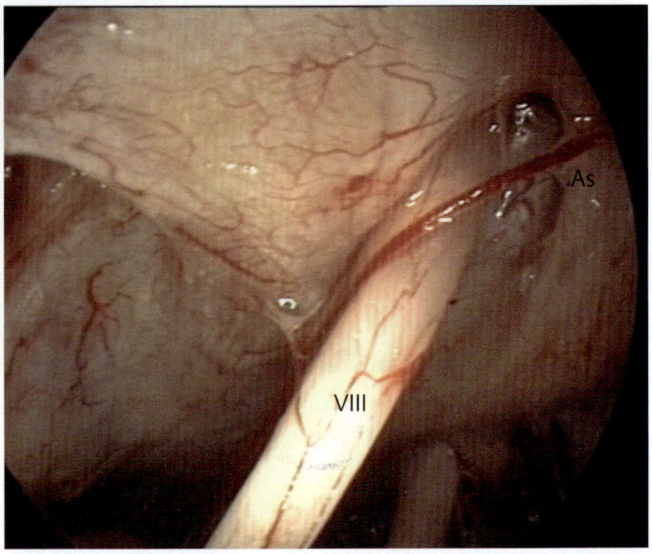

Fig. 65.13 Left incapacitating tinnitus, subarcuate artery (As) "hugging" the auditory nerve (VIII).

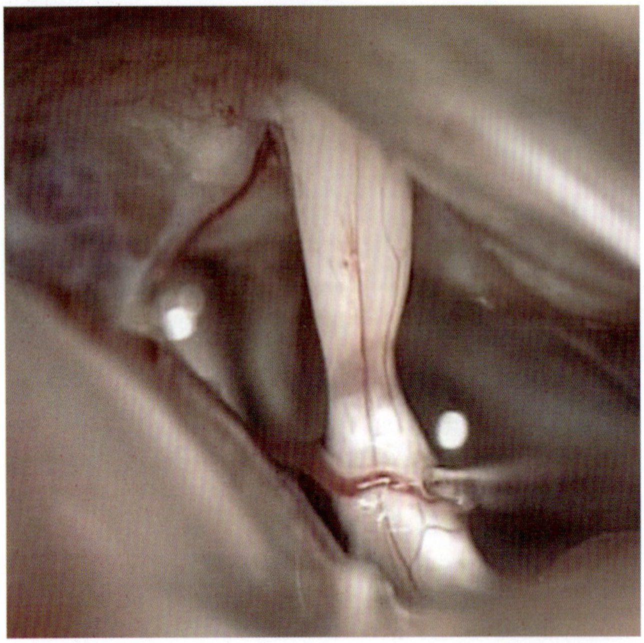

Fig. 65.14 Right incapacitating tinnitus with unsteadiness, AICA loop compressing the auditory nerve is displaced medially. The artery spasm is noticed which is resorbed using in situ papaverine.

Combining the use of both microscope and endoscope increases the efficiency of the procedure and decreases drastically the potential morbidity of the surgical procedure.

Surgery of auditory nerve is more challenging, and the results are not comparable with that of trigeminal neuralgia and hemifacial spasm. Once the selection of the patients with vascular compression–induced tinnitus or vertigo will be clarified, the MVD of the auditory nerve should get a full acceptance.

References

1. Dandy W. Concerning the cause of trigeminal neuralgia. Am J Surg 1934;24:447–455
2. Gardner J, Sava G. Hemifacial spasm—a reversible pathophysiologic state. J Neurosurg 1962;19:240–247
3. Gardner WJ. Concerning the mechanism of trigeminal neuralgia and hemifacial spasm. J Neurosurg 1962;19: 947–958
4. Jannetta PJ. Arterial compression of the trigeminal nerve at the pons in patients with trigeminal neuralgia. J Neurosurg 1967;26(1):159–162
5. Jannetta PJ. Trigeminal neuralgia and hemifacial spasm—etiology and definitive treatment. Trans Am Neurol Assoc 1975;100:89–91
6. Jannetta P, Abbasy M, Maroon J, Ramos FM, Albin MS. Etiology and definitive microsurgical treatment of hemifacial spasm. Operative techniques and results in 47 patients. J Neurosurg 1977;47:321–328
7. Jannetta PJ. Neurovascular compression in cranial nerve and systemic disease. Ann Surg 1980;192(4):518–525
8. Bremond G, Garcin M, Magnan J, Bonnaud G. L'abord à minima de l'espace pontocérébelleux. Cah ORL 1974;9: 443–460

9. Bremond G, Garcin M. Microsurgical approach to the cerebellopontine angle. J Laryngol Otol 1975;89(3):237–248

10. Bremond G, Garcin M, Magnan J. Progrès en oto-neurochirurgie: l'abord à minima de l'angle ponto-cérébelleux par la voie rétro-sinusale. Acta ORL (Belg) 1976;30:127–144

11. Magnan J, Chays A, Caces F, et al. Apport de l'endoscopie de l'angle pontocerebelleux par voie retrosigmoide: neurinomes et conflits vasculo-nerveux. Ann Otolaryngol Chir Cervicofac (Paris) 1993;110:259–265

12. Magnan J, Chays A, Caces F, et al. Place de l'endoscopie et de la decompression vasculaire dans le traitement du spasme de l'hemiface. Ann Otolaryngol Chir Cervicofac (Paris) 1994;111:153–160

13. Magnan J, Chays A, Lepetre C, Pencroffi E, Locatelli P. Surgical perspectives of endoscopy of the cerebellopontine angle. Am J Otol 1994;15(3):366–370

14. Magnan J, Sanna M. Endoscopy in neuro-otology. New York, Stuttgart: Thieme; 1999

15. Magnan J. The value of endoscopy in otology and neuro-otology. Otol Jpn 2003;13:165–167

16. Girard N, Poncet N., Tallon Y, et al. Neurovascular conflict of the CP angle: 3D-FT high definition MR analysis. Rivista di Neuroradiologia 1994;7:485–490

17. Girard N, Poncet M, Chays A, et al. Neurovascular compression in the CP angle. Revista di Neuroradiologia 1995;8: 981–989

18. Girard N, Poncet M, Caces F, et al. Three-dimensional MRI of hemifacial spasm with surgical correlation. Neuroradiology 1997;39(1):46–51

19. Elaini S, Miyazaki H, Rameh C, Deveze A, Magnan J. Correlations between MRI and surgical findings in vasculo-neural compression syndrome. Int Adv Otol 2009; 5(Suppl 3):1–23

20. Barrow D. Surgery of the cranial nerves of the posterior fossa. AANS Publications; 1993

21. Møller AR. Vascular compression of cranial nerves. I. History of the microvascular decompression operation. Neurol Res 1998;20(8):727–731

22. Møller AR. Vascular compression of cranial nerves: II: pathophysiology. Neurol Res 1999;21(5):439–443

23. Miyazaki H, Deveze A, Magnan J. Neuro-otologic surgery through minimally invasive retrosigmoid approach: endoscope assisted microvascular decompression, vestibular neurotomy, and tumor removal. Laryngoscope 2005;115(9): 1612–1617

24. Magnan J, Miyazaki H, Elaini S, Deveze A. Endoscope-assisted retrosigmoid keyhole approach. Tuttlingen: Endo Press; 2010

25. Magnan J, Parikh B, Miyazaki H. Functional Surgery of CPA by Minimally Invasive Retrosigmoid Approach. Jaypee Brothers; 2013

26. Magnan J, El Garem H, Miyazaki H, Caces F. Endoscope-assisted microvascular decompression. In: Sekkar L, Fessler R, eds. Atlas of Neurosurgical Techniques. Thieme; 2016;2: 675–683

27. El-Garem HF, Badr-El-Dine M, Talaat AM, Magnan J. Endoscopy as a tool in minimally invasive trigeminal neuralgia surgery. Otol Neurotol 2002;23(2):132–135

28. Balansard ChF, Meller R, Bruzzo M, Chays A, Girard N, Magnan J. [Trigeminal neuralgia: results of microsurgical and endoscopic-assisted vascular decompression]. Ann Otolaryngol Chir Cervicofac 2003;120(6):330–337

29. Caces F, Chays A, Locatelli P, et al. [Neuro-vascular decompression in hemifacial spasm: anatomical, electrophysiological and therapeutic results apropos of 100 cases]. Rev Laryngol Otol Rhinol (Bord) 1996;117(5):347–351

30. Magnan J, Caces F, Locatelli P, Chays A. Hemifacial spasm: endoscopic vascular decompression. Otolaryngol Head Neck Surg 1997;117(4):308–314

31. Magnan J, Curto CL. Hemifacial spasm. In: Slattery W, Azzizaadeh B, eds. The Facial Nerve. Thieme; 2014:137–145

32. Badr-El-Dine M, El-Garem HF, Talaat AM, Magnan J. Endoscopically assisted minimally invasive microvascular decompression of hemifacial spasm. Otol Neurotol 2002; 23(2):122–128

33. Møller MB, Møller AR, Jannetta PJ, Jho HD. Vascular decompression surgery for severe tinnitus: selection criteria and results. Laryngoscope 1993;103(4 Pt 1):421–427

34. Magnan J, El Garem H, Deveze A. et al. The value of endoscopy in the surgical management of vertigo. Mediterr J Otol 2006; 2:1–8

35. Guevara N, Deveze A, Busa V, et al. Microvascular decompression of cochlear nerve for tinnitus incapacity: pre-surgical data, surgical analyses and long-term follow up of 15 patients. Eur Arch Otorhinolaryngol 2008;265:397–401

36. Magnan J, Lafont B, Rameh C. Long-term follow-up of MVD for tinnitus. In: Møller AR, ed. Textbook of Tinnitus. Springer; 2011:669–679

Section XXVI

Retrosigmoid Approach

Chapter 66 Retrosigmoid Approach

Suresh Sankhla and Narayan Jayashankar

Introduction

The retrosigmoid approach is a variant of the lateral suboccipital approach in which the cranial opening extends up to or over the posterior edge of the sigmoid sinus. It is most commonly selected for approaching lesions in the cerebellopontine angle (CPA).

By strictly adhering to the area below the transverse sinus and behind the sigmoid sinus, this surgical approach offers an advantage of providing an excellent exposure of the CPA with no or minimal cerebellar retraction. The retrosigmoid approach is commonly selected for CPA lesions like meningiomas, vestibular and other cranial nerve schwannomas, epidermoid cysts, exophytic pontine masses, and certain vascular lesions, as well as the microvascular decompression procedures. It can be combined with a far-lateral exposure for lesions that involve both the cervicomedullary junction and CPA, or with a presigmoid approach directed through the mastoid and labyrinth to reach lesions involving the petrous apex, clivus, and cavernous sinus. A temporo-occipital craniotomy can be added to this approach to get a combined supra- and infratentorial approach for lesions involving both posterior and middle fossae.

Surgical Steps

Patient Positioning

The patient can be positioned supine, lateral (park bench) or in the sitting position, with the head flexed and turned to the contralateral side. The head is secured in the three-point Mayfield clamp, and the foot end of the table is raised above the heart level (**Fig. 66.1a**). Each position has its own advantages and disadvantages, and the best position is the one that the surgeon and the anesthesiologist are familiar with. The sitting position helps draining the cerebrospinal fluid (CSF), blood, and irrigation fluid by gravity, and the surgeon's both hands are free for tumor dissection. This position also accelerates spontaneous descent of the larger tumors after initial debulking. The disadvantages include hypotension during positioning, especially in elderly patients, high risk of air embolism and pneumocephalus, and uncomfortable for the surgeon during prolonged surgery.

Head elevation is used to minimize bleeding and reduce intracranial hypertension. An arterial PCO_2 is monitored around 30 mm Hg and the electrodes of the facial nerve stimulator are placed on the orbicularis oculi and oris.

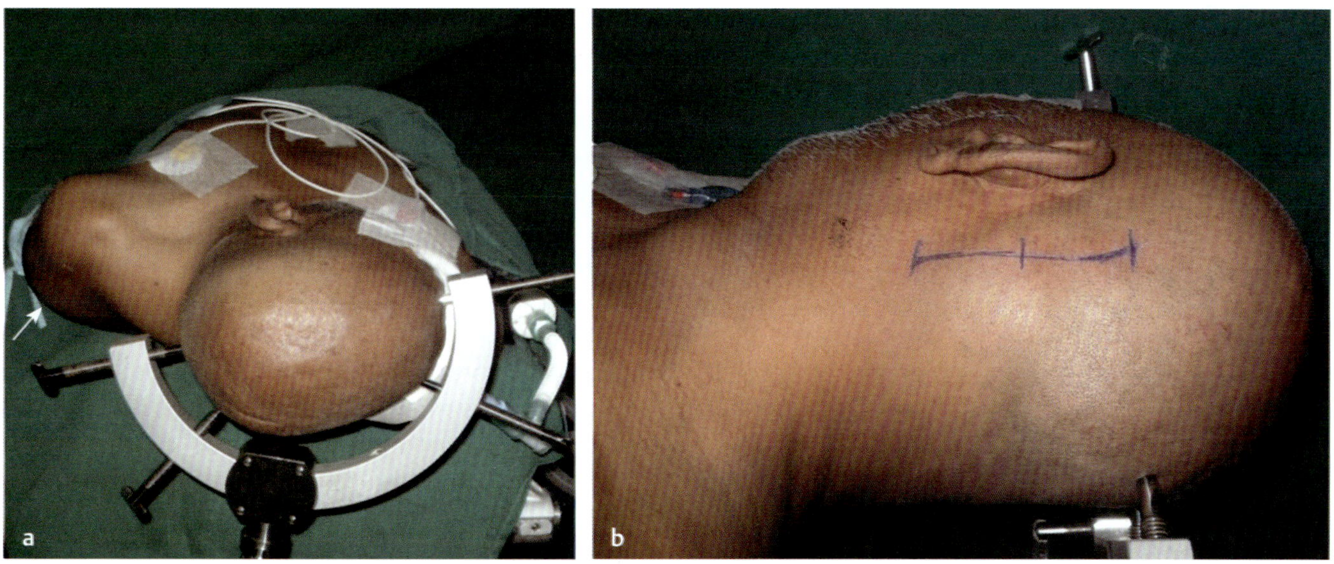

Fig. 66.1 **(a)** Patient position. The patient is placed supine with the ipsilateral shoulder lifted up by a soft cotton roll (*arrow*), and the head is fixed in a flexed and contralaterally rotated position in such a way that its midsagittal plane is roughly parallel to the floor. Note, the ipsilateral ear remains the highest point in this position. **(b)** Skin incision. A linear skin incision is marked in a *blue line*, 2 cm medial to the base of the mastoid (*dotted line*), begins from a point 2 cm above the superior nuchal line and is extended straight down in the suboccipital region beyond the tip of the mastoid process.

The monitoring equipment for brainstem auditory evoked response (BAER) should be positioned and checked before the patient is draped.

Incision and Exposure

A linear skin incision, 2 cm medial to the base of the mastoid, is begun 2 cm above the superior nuchal line and extended below in the suboccipital region beyond the tip of the mastoid process, which corresponds to the C1–C2 space (**Fig. 66.1b**). The skin, subcutaneous tissue, and the suboccipital muscles are divided. The occipital bone exposure extends superiorly to the superior nuchal line, inferiorly to the foramen magnum, laterally to the mastoid groove, and medially about 3 to 4 cm (**Fig. 66.2a**). The lateral margin of the craniotomy exposure should be in line with the petrous bone to avoid or minimize cerebellar retraction.

A burr hole is drilled in the medial part of the exposed occipital bone, and the underlying dura is separated with a blunt dissector. A bone flap (3–5 cm) is then raised using a cutting blade attachment with a footplate. A drill burr is subsequently used to extend the craniotomy exposure superiorly up to the edge of the transverse sinus, laterally up to the medial margin of the sigmoid sinus, and inferiorly up to the superior part of the rim of the foramen magnum (**Fig. 66.2b**). The mastoid air cells, opened inadvertently during the lateral extension of the exposure, should be packed immediately with bone wax. A watertight covering with muscle or pericranium and tissue glue is essential at the time of wound closer to avoid postoperative CSF leakage. An additional burr hole may be made at Keen's point in the parietal bone, in case temporary external drainage of CSF for hydrocephalus is required.

Dural Opening

Dura is opened with an inverted T-shaped incision (**Fig. 66.2c**). The long horizontal limb of the incision extends from the medial and superior corner, toward the lateral and inferior corner of the dural exposure. This incision divides the dural exposure in the lateral and medial halves. The vertical limb of the incision begins from the center point of the horizontal incision, divides the dura of the lateral half, and extends superiorly up to the transverse-sigmoid junction. The dural opening in this manner helps providing exposure of the superior most part of the CPA to its maximum and also protects the cerebellar lobe from prolapsing out (**Fig. 66.2d**). The cerebellum is retracted superomedially to expose the lateral cerebellomedullary cistern (**Fig. 66.3a**). It is very important to open the cistern and drain the CSF in order to bring about complete cerebellar relaxation and minimize retraction injury (**Fig. 66.3b**).

Tumor Exposure

All of the intradural part of the procedure is done using the operating microscope. The intradural anatomical orientation varies with the nature and growth pattern of the tumors. In the case of a vestibular schwannoma (**Fig. 66.4a, b**), the lower cranial nerves are immediately visualized when the arachnoid of the lower pole of the tumor is mobilized (**Fig. 66.4c**). Care should be taken to avoid any breach in the continuity of arachnoid covering of the lower cranial nerves. The cerebellum is gently retracted superomedially to expose the arachnoid covering of the tumor (**Fig. 66.4d**). It is important to remember that a double layer of arachnoid exists in the cerebellum–tumor interface. The first layer of arachnoid covers the posterior surface of the cerebellum, and the second layer covers the tumor capsule. The arachnoid should be carefully removed from the tumor capsule using sharp dissection techniques. The use of bipolar coagulation at this stage should be discouraged as it causes blunting of the arachnoid plane. The arachnoid dissection frequently releases more CSF which causes further relaxation of the cerebellum leading to wider tumor exposure without any retraction. No attempt is made to see the whole tumor initially.

Tumor Decompression

Once the arachnoid from the posterior surface of the tumor has been separated, the tumor capsule is incised and tumor debulking is performed to decrease tumor size and thereby facilitating safe capsular mobilization (**Fig. 66.5a, b**). Generally, the facial nerve courses in the anteroinferior pole of the tumor, and tumor decompression from the posterior part is usually safe. However, the facial nerve fibers may occasionally be present on the posterior aspect of the tumor surface. It is therefore safer to use facial nerve stimulation to identify the presence and the course of the nerve before tumor debulking is started. Various techniques for tumor decompression using suction, curettes, scissors, and ultrasonic aspirator have been described and can be used alone or in combination. One has to be extremely careful to avoid an inadvertent breach in the tumor capsule during the process of debulking, particularly in cases of tumors with a soft consistency and friable capsule, as it may lead to injury to the vital blood vessels, nerves, or brainstem. Tumor debulking should be done uniformly in all directions to avoid asymmetrical capsular relaxation.

Care needs to be taken to avoid excessive manipulations during tumor decompression which may produce undue stress or traction on delicate cranial nerves (seventh and eighth) or brainstem. Intraoperative electrophysiological monitoring of the facial nerve helps early identification

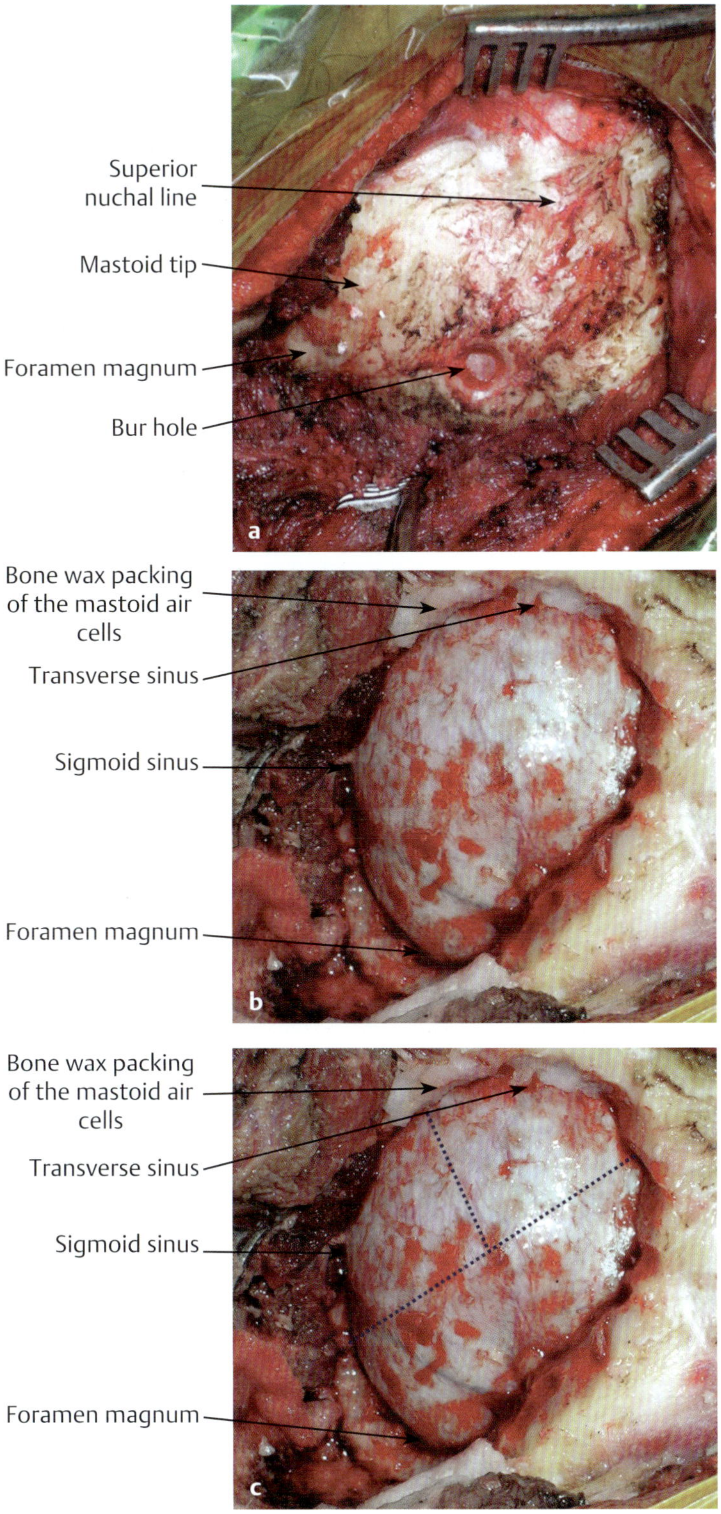

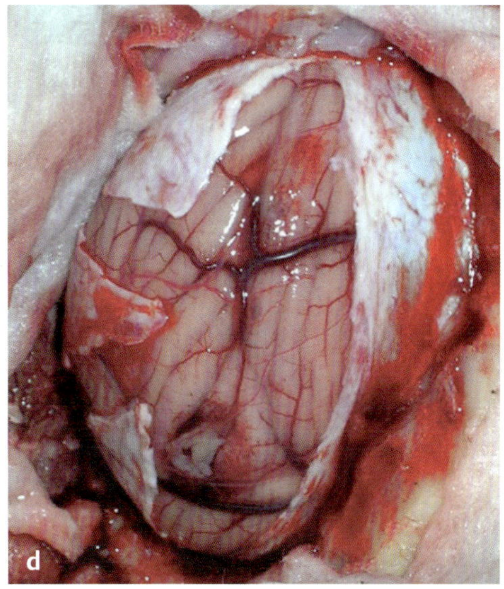

Fig. 66.2 Craniotomy and exposure. **(a)** The occipital bone is exposed up to the superior nuchal line superiorly, foramen magnum inferiorly, mastoid groove laterally, and medially about 3 to 4 cm. Note the position of the burr hole from where the craniotomy is begun using a cutting saw. The lateral margin of the craniotomy exposure should be in line with the petrous bone to avoid or minimize cerebellar retraction. Opened mastoid air cells are immediately packed with bone wax and are covered meticulously at the time of wound closure. **(b)** Dural exposure extends from the transverse sinus superiorly, the transverse-sigmoid junction and the sigmoid sinus laterally, and the foramen magnum region inferiorly. Approximately 3- to 4-cm wider exposure of the dura is generally adequate. **(c)** Dura is opened with an inverted T-shaped incision (*dotted line*). The long horizontal limb of the incision extends from the medial and superior corner, toward the lateral and inferior corner of the dural exposure. This incision divides the dural exposure in the lateral and medial halves. The vertical limb of the incision begins from the center point of the horizontal incision, divides the dura of the lateral half, and extends superiorly up to the transverse-sigmoid junction. The dural opening in this manner helps providing exposure of the superior most part of the cerebellopontine angle to its maximum and also protects the cerebellar lobe from prolapsing out. **(d)** Note bulged out cerebellar lobe immediately after the opening of the dura. The medial half of the exposed dura protects the cerebellum to prolapse out of the dural opening.

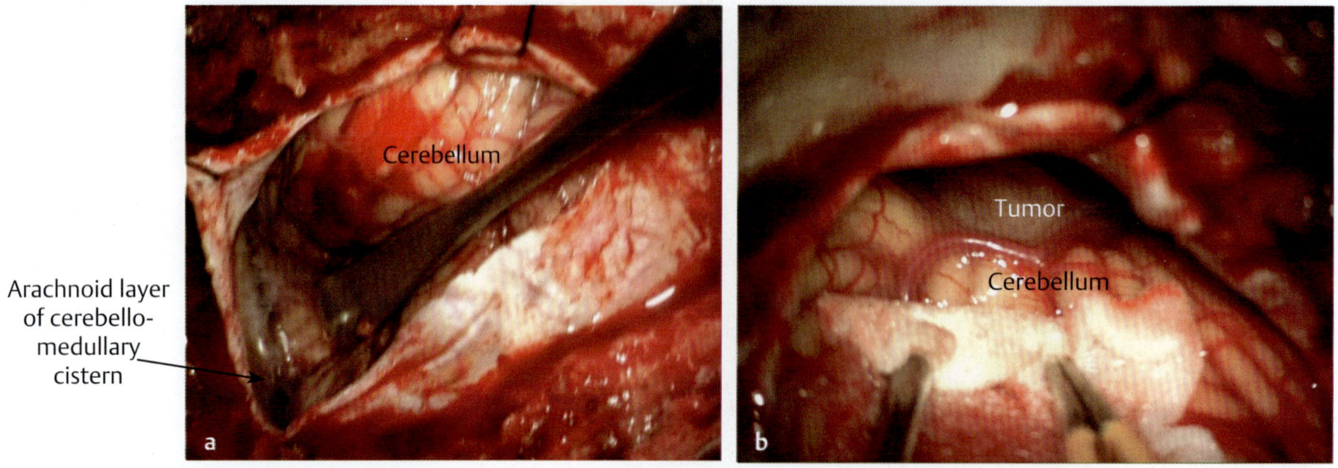

Fig. 66.3 Intradural microscopic view. **(a)** The arachnoid membrane over the cerebellomedullary cistern is opened in the beginning to allow drainage of cerebrospinal fluid (CSF). This maneuver results in immediate relaxation of the cerebellum. **(b)** The relaxed cerebellum often does not require any retraction. Note, the tumor is visible through the arachnoid covering of the CPA.

and avoidance of serious traction injury to the nerve (**Fig. 66.6a–c**). Internal decompression of the tumor can at times be a tedious exercise, particularly in cases when the tumor is firm or vascular. Overzealous use of bipolar coagulation is harmful and should not be used.

Capsular Dissection

Once adequate tumor debulking has been performed, the relaxed tumor capsule can be mobilized safely and relatively easily. In large tumors, decompression and capsule mobilization should be done alternatively. The capsule can be held firmly by a tumor-holding forceps and the overlying arachnoid can be pushed away gently. The dissection should be restricted to the plane between the arachnoid and tumor capsule. The capsule separation should be done uniformly in all directions to avoid losing the plane of cleavage. Intermittent careful low-degree bipolar coagulation of the capsule is useful as it reduces the tumor vascularity and shrinks the capsule significantly.

Facial and Vestibulocochlear Nerves

Sometimes, particularly when the tumor is small, the facial nerve can be identified inferomedially at the root exit zone. However, the most definite area to identify the seventh nerve is the internal auditory meatus (IAM) after opening the porus acusticus (**Fig. 66.7a–c**). This can be done at the beginning of tumor removal in smaller or predominantly intracanalicular tumors and after adequate tumor decompression in larger tumors. The porus is identified by following the tumor to its entry into the meatus. The dura over the posterior wall of the IAM is coagulated, incised, and reflected anteriorly in a flap manner (**Fig. 66.7b**). Using a high-speed diamond drill, the posterior wall of the meatus is drilled up to 1 cm laterally on the petrous bone. More lateral drilling has the risk of exposing and injuring the posterior semicircular canal and labyrinth or a high placed jugular bulb. The intracanalicular dura is incised, and the tumor is gently removed using sharp dissection (**Fig. 66.7c**). The vertical Bill's bar is identified, which divides the canal into the anterior and posterior parts. The facial nerve is situated superiorly and the cochlear nerve inferiorly in the anterior part, while the vestibular nerves are located posteriorly. The labyrinthine artery, a branch of anterior inferior cerebellar artery (AICA), courses through the IAM and an attempt should be made to preserve it. An endoscope can be very useful for early identification of the facial nerve, either behind the tumor, at the root exit zone, or in the IAM without drilling. It also helps to check for the residual tumor in the meatus.

The facial nerve can be traced carefully along with its arachnoid covering from the IAM laterally to its root exit zone medially. The position of the facial nerve in relation to the tumor capsule in the CPA can vary and may need facial nerve stimulation to identify. The nerve is most vulnerable close to the meatus where it takes a right-angle turn anteriorly over the anterior margin of the IAM. This is usually the tightest junction between the tumor and the nerve–vessel bundle. Extreme care should be taken to avoid any traction on the nerve during tumor dissection in this region. In small tumors, the nerve is well visualized as a bundle, but in larger tumors, the fascicles of the nerve may be displayed out over the capsule of the tumor, making it extremely difficult to preserve the nerve anatomically. It is therefore advisable in this situation to leave small bits of the tumor behind in order to preserve facial nerve function.

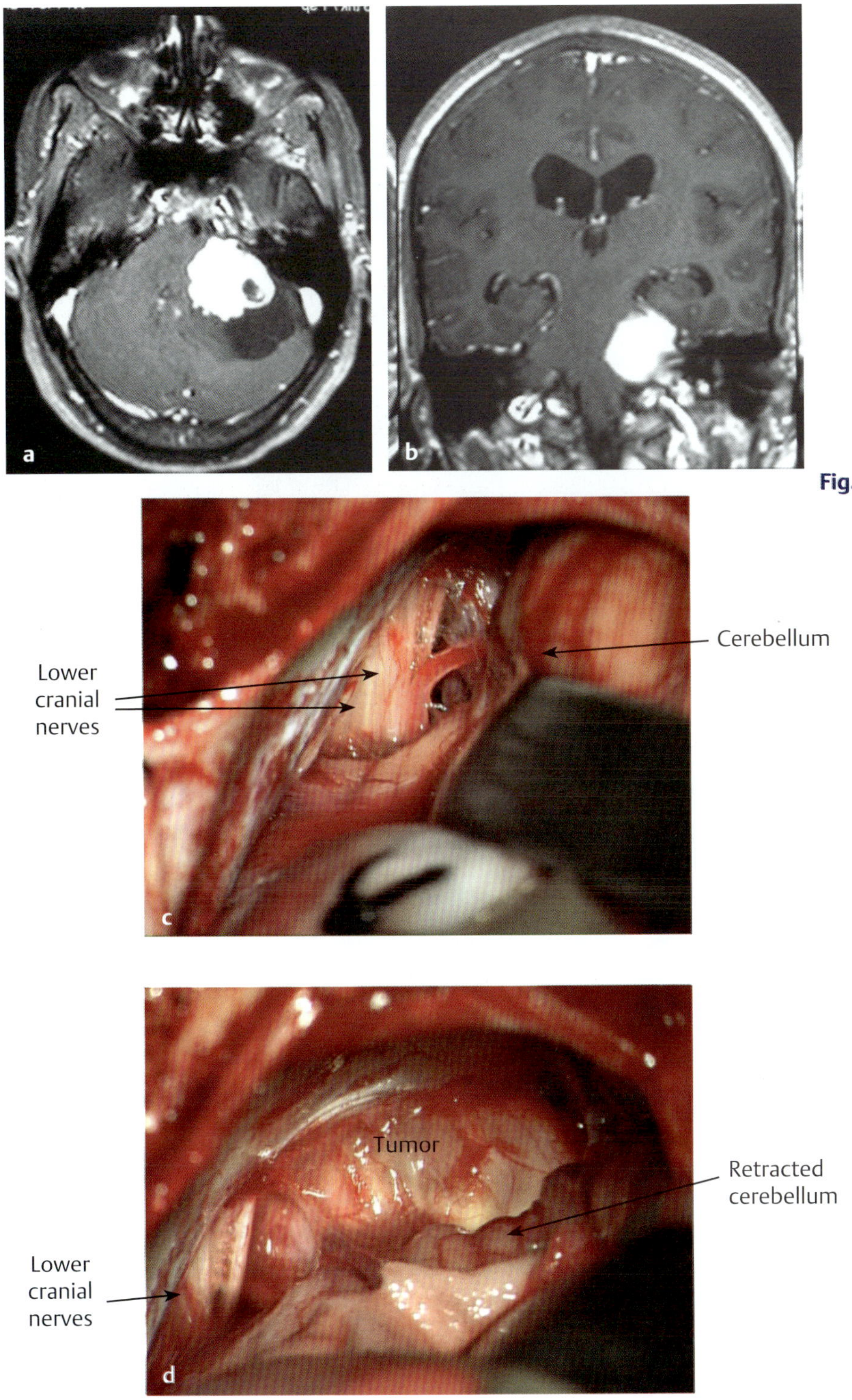

Fig. 66.4 T-1 contrast **(a)** axial and **(b)** coronal MR images of a 57-year-old man, who presented with headaches, left-sided tinnitus, and progressive hearing loss, demonstrate a large well-enhancing vestibular schwannoma with mass effect. Note the tumor extending into the internal auditory meatus. **(c)** Intraoperative photograph. The inferolateral part of the cerebellum is slowly retracted and more CSF is drained by opening the arachnoid coverings of the CPA, resulting in a further relaxation of the cerebellum. Note the cisternal course of the lower cranial nerves. **(d)** The cerebellum is gently retracted superomedially to expose the tumor covered by arachnoid layers. It is important to remember that a double layer of arachnoid exists in the cerebellum–tumor interface. The first layer of arachnoid covers the posterior surface of the cerebellum, and the second layer covers the tumor capsule. The arachnoid should be carefully dissected away from the tumor capsule using sharp dissection techniques.

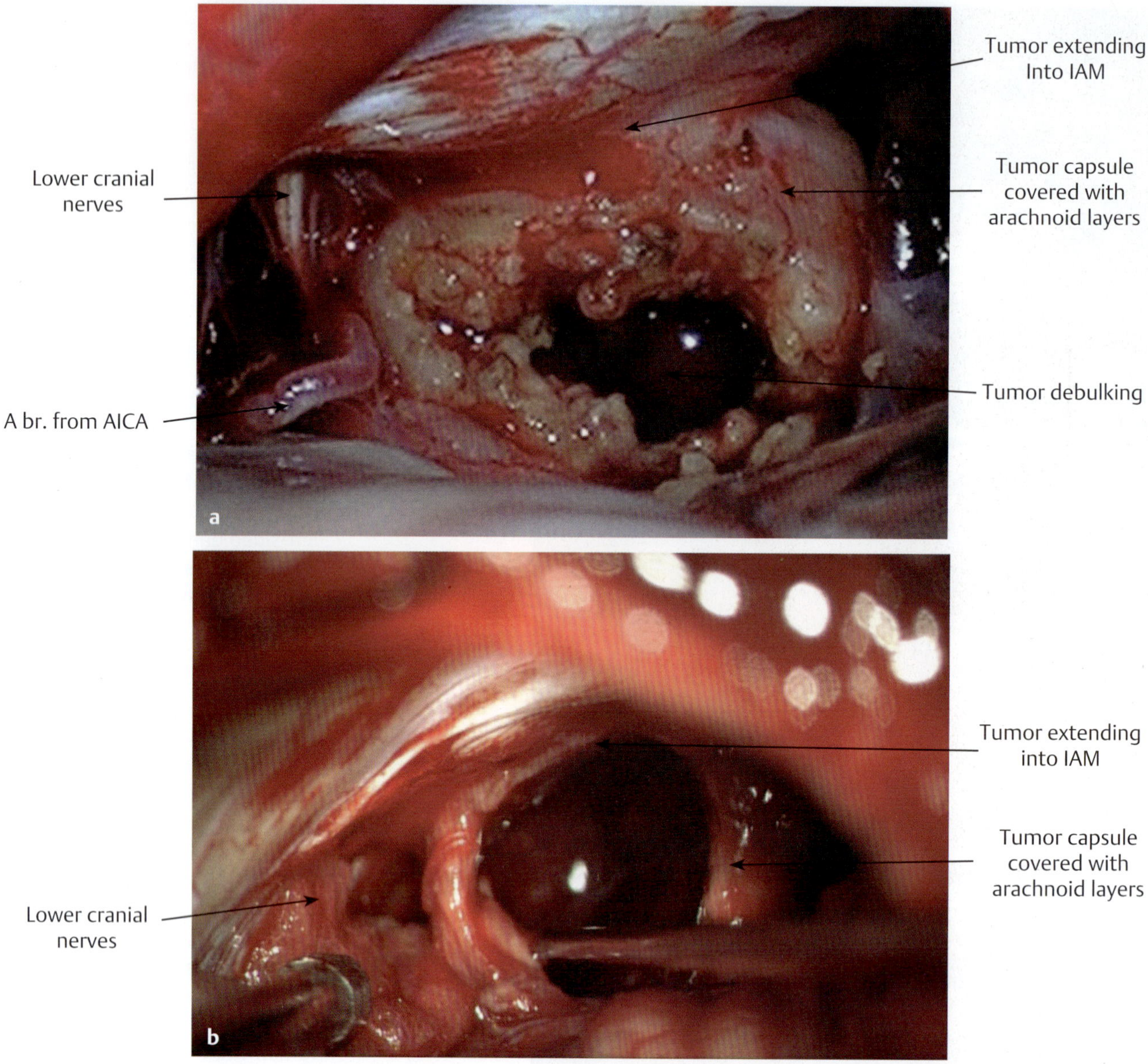

Fig. 66.5 Microsurgical tumor removal. **(a, b)** Internal decompression of the tumor, generally done by suction, cavitational ultrasonic aspirator (CUSA), or piecemeal removal using sharp instruments, is an important step of surgery. Tumor decompression relaxes the tumor capsule and relieves pressure on the cranial nerves, cerebellum, and brainstem. The redundant capsule can then be gradually dissected away more easily from the surrounding arachnoid without causing any significant traction on the cranial nerves and brainstem. Note, tumor extending into the IAM is visualized better after sufficient tumor decompression.

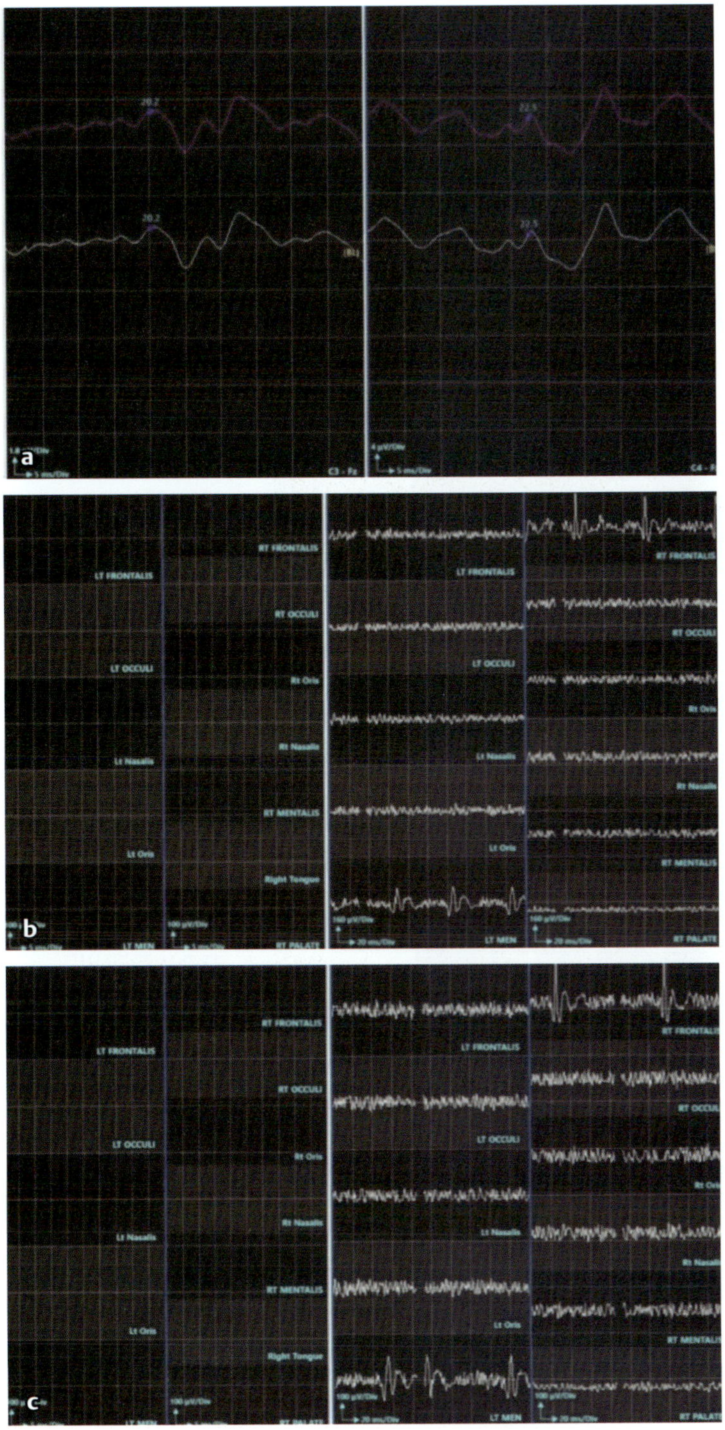

Fig. 66.6 Electrophysiological facial nerve monitoring. **(a)** Baseline facial nerve stimulation. **(b)** Facial nerve–frontalis irritation during traction on the tumor capsule. **(c)** Facial nerve irritation and disturbances during surgery.

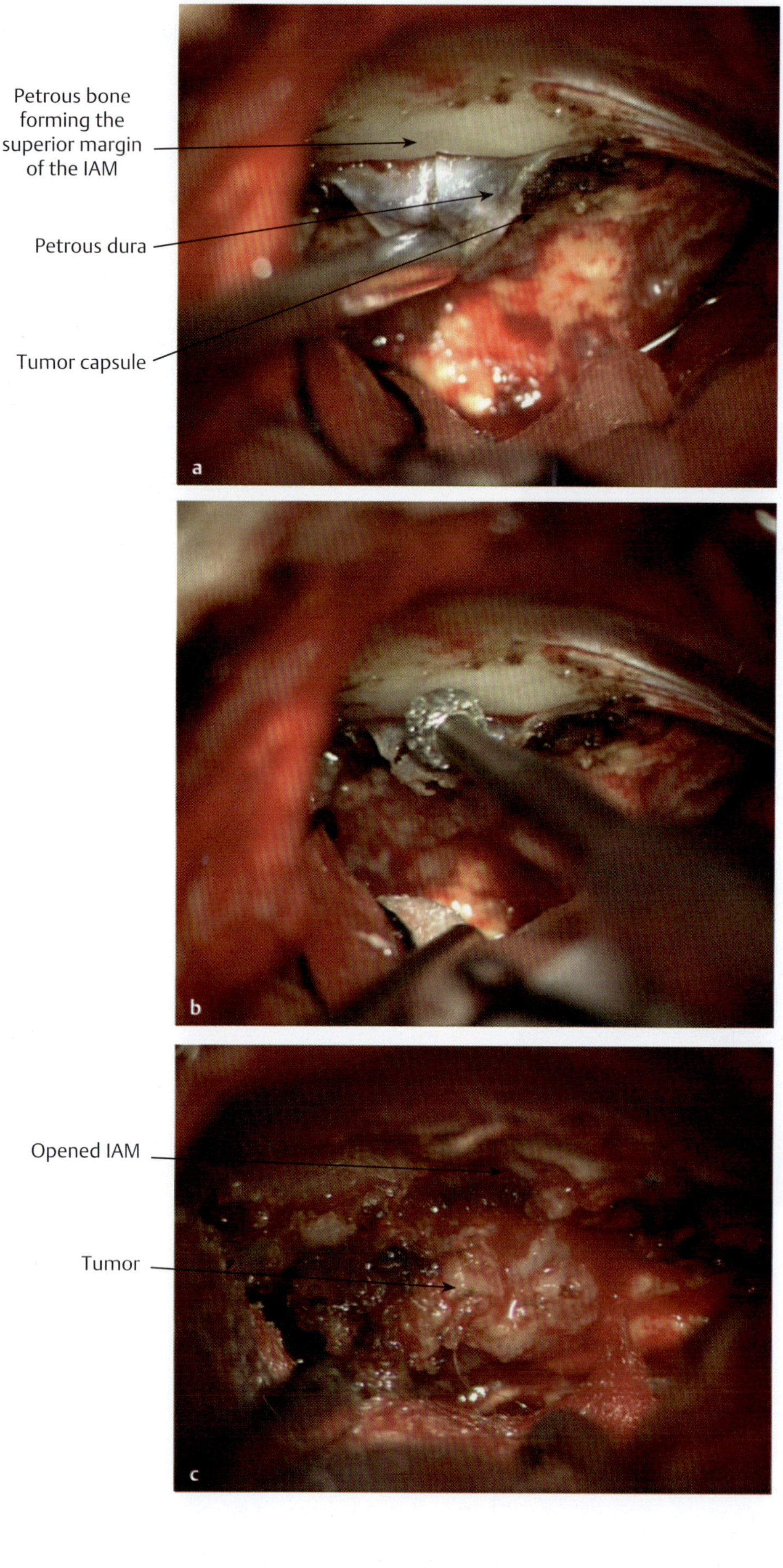

Fig. 66.7 Opening the IAM. **(a)** The IAM is first exposed by elevating the petrous dural layer in a flap manner. **(b)** A high-speed diamond drill is then used to open the meatus, first from the posterior and then the superior margins, until it is wide enough to expose and mobilize the **(c)** intracanalicular tumor.

The cochlear nerve usually fans out near the anterior part of the capsule. In small tumors (< 3 cm), it may be possible to preserve the cochlear nerve and hearing, but the nerve is difficult to identify in most cases with larger tumors. Care should be taken to protect the labyrinthine artery and avoid injury to the semicircular canal and the labyrinth because of overzealous drilling of the porus acusticus.

Lower Cranial Nerves

The lower cranial nerves are usually compressed by the lower pole of the tumor and are almost always protected by their own arachnoid covering (**Fig. 66.4c, Fig. 66.5a, b**). The arachnoid over the tumor capsule is incised and mobilized inferiorly by retracting the decompressed tumor capsule upward. Any unnecessary coagulation and traction during the dissection in this region should be avoided. The AICA often courses in close proximity to the lower pole and its branches supplying the tumor should be coagulated and incised close to the capsule.

Trigeminal Nerve

The upper pole of the tumor is closely related to the trigeminal nerve and petrosal vein. In large tumors, the upper pole may even extend rostrally through the tentorial hiatus. However, the identification and separation of the nerve from the tumor capsule usually do not pose great difficulty (**Fig. 66.8a**). The petrosal vein, on the other hand, may at times be difficult to identify and requires a careful dissection to separate it from the tumor. Excessive traction on the vein during dissection may cause its avulsion from the petrosal sinus. Coagulation of the petrosal vein should be avoided as it may be the only draining vein from that area. Frequently, one or two smaller venous channels may also be seen running along the capsule, probably representing the venous drainage of the tumor which can be divided. The abducens nerve can be seen as a thin cord anterior to the tumor, and the trochlear nerve lies in close proximity to the tentorium superior to the tumor.

Brainstem

The arachnoid–capsule interface always separates the tumor from the brainstem and cerebellum (**Fig. 66.8b**). However, in cases of large tumors, the arachnoid plane is difficult to find because of tumor compression or adherence. The difficulty is increased further with anatomical rotation and distortion of the brainstem. In these circumstances, it is often helpful to change the area of dissection and follow the well-defined plane from a different angle toward the brainstem. Occasionally, a few small branches arising from the basilar artery supplying the tumor may be recognized, coagulated, and divided close to the capsule. Smaller venous channels closer to the brainstem, when injured, tend to retract into the brainstem and cause small hemorrhages and ischemia/edema of the brainstem. At the end of the tumor removal, intact and shining arachnoid of the CPA as well as a completely relaxed cerebellum can be visualized (**Fig. 66.8b, c**).

In the case of a CPA meningioma (**Fig. 66.9**), the cranial nerves are pushed posteriorly and inferiorly by the tumor, which can be removed through the corridors between the cranial nerves.

Closure

Brainstem surface hemostasis should be achieved by surgical and gentle cotton patty pressure, and bipolar coagulation should be avoided. The drilled IAM should be meticulously sealed with fat and fibrin glue to avoid postoperative CSF leak. The tumor bed is irrigated with copious warm saline, and the dura is closed in a watertight fashion using a pericranial or fascial graft, if necessary. The opened mastoid air cells are sealed with bone wax, or by using muscle/fat graft and fibrin glue. The suboccipital muscles, fascial sheath, subcutaneous tissue, and skin are closed in separate layers.

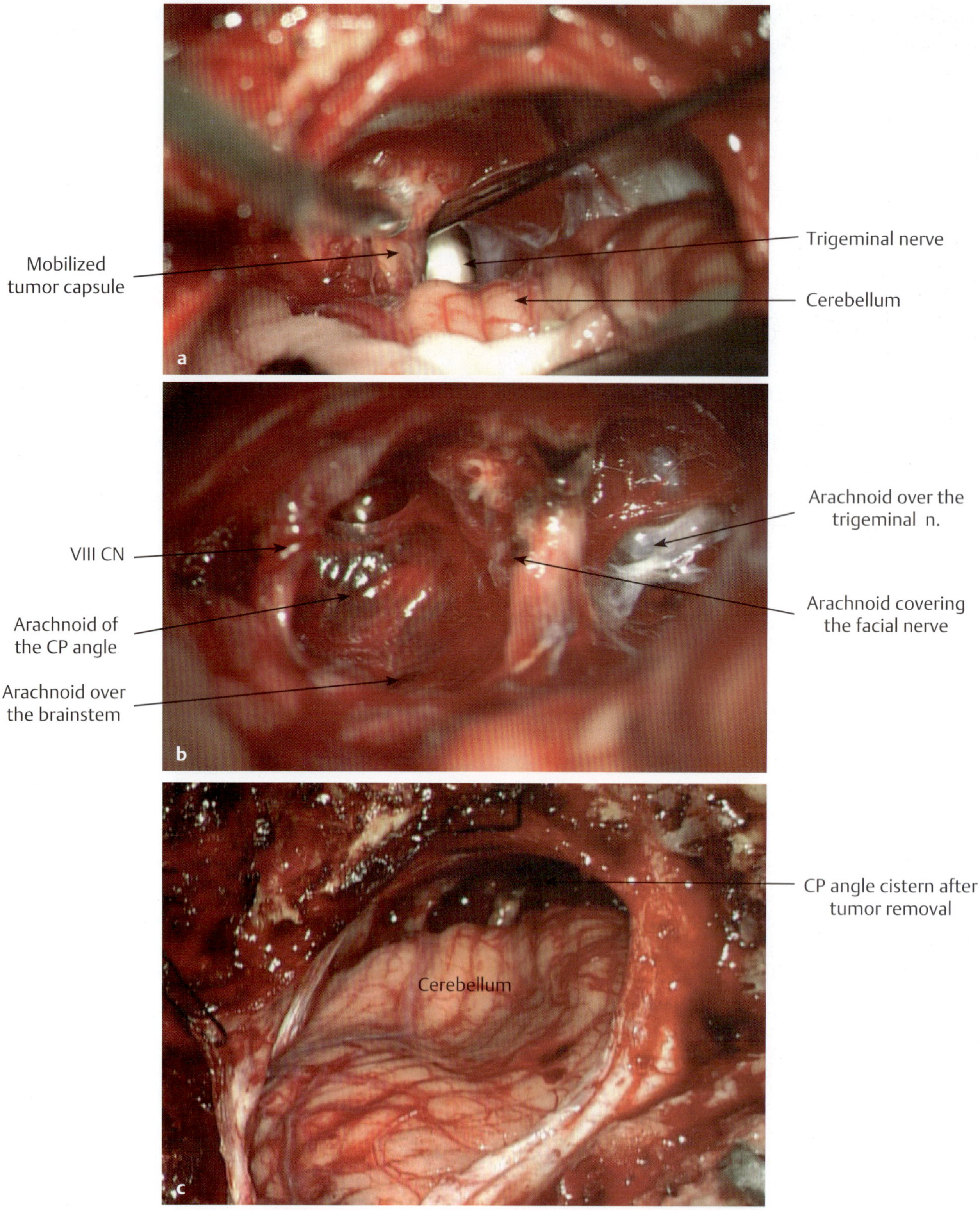

Fig. 66.8 Capsule dissection. **(a)** Mobilization of the relaxed tumor capsule can be commenced after sufficient tumor decompression has been achieved. The capsule can be held firmly by tumor-holding forceps and the overlying arachnoid can be pushed away gently. The dissection should be restricted to the plane between the arachnoid and tumor capsule. The capsule separation should be done uniformly in all directions to avoid losing the plane of cleavage. Note, the trigeminal nerve is frequently visible after separating the capsule of the superior pole. **(b)** Total removal of the tumor with intact arachnoid of the CPA, trigeminal nerve, VII–VIII nerves, and lower cranial nerves. **(c)** Completely relaxed cerebellum at the end of the procedure.

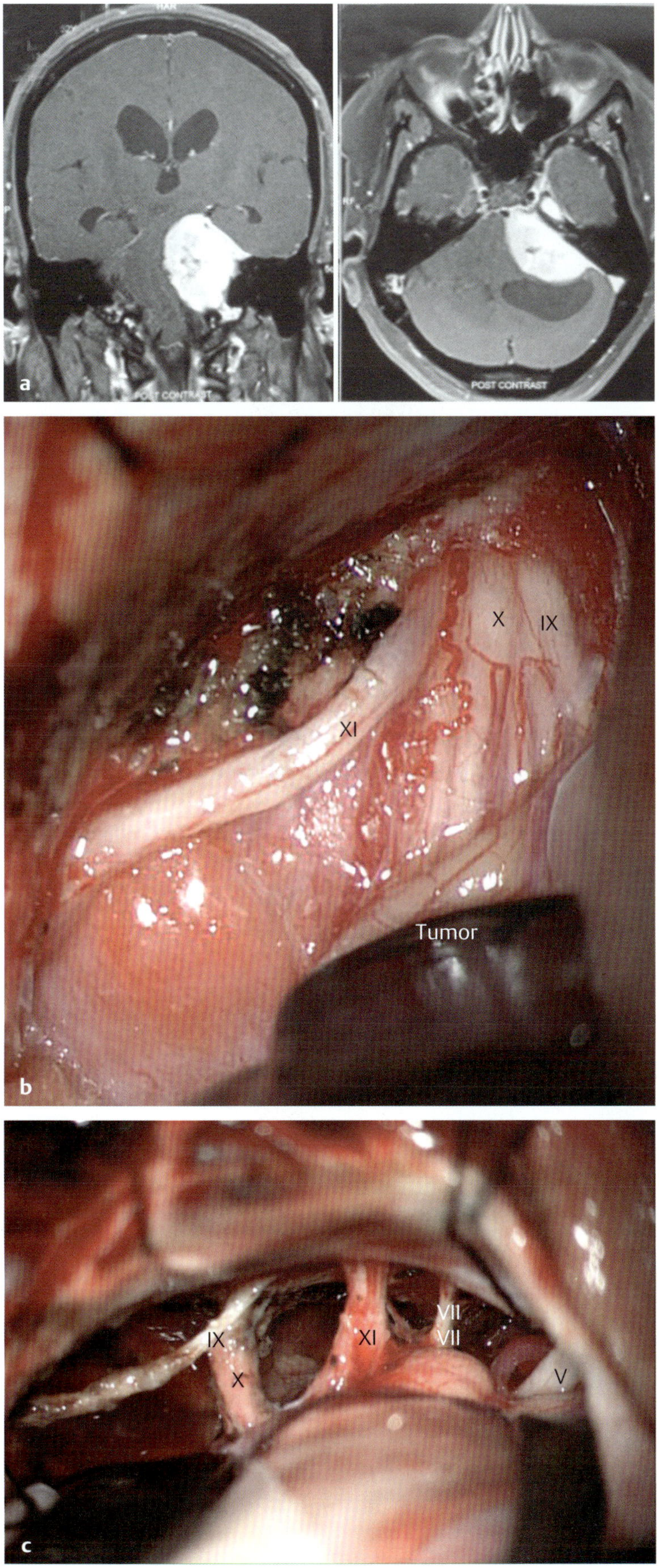

Fig. 66.9 CPA meningioma. **(a)** Contrast coronal and axial MR images of a 48-year-old lady showing a large uniformly enhancing dural base mass (meningioma) in the left CPA. **(b)** Intraoperative photograph shows a large meningioma in the left CPA pushing the cranial nerves posteriorly and inferiorly. **(c)** Approaches to meningioma of the CPA. Surgical removal can be performed between the cranial nerves—above the trigeminal nerve (V), between the trigeminal nerve and facial (VII) and vestibulocochlear nerves (VIII), between the facial and vestibulocochlear nerves and glossopharyngeal nerve (IX), between the glossopharyngeal and vagus nerves (X), between the vagus nerve and accessory rootlets (XI), and between the rootlets of the accessory nerve.

Chapter 67

Retrosigmoid Craniotomy with Stereotactic Supratentorial Cerebrospinal Fluid Diversion

Michel Roethlisberger, Prepageran Narayanan, and Vicknes Waran

Indications

The retrosigmoid approach is a commonly employed procedure for conditions involving the cerebellopontine angle (CPA) and brainstem areas.[1-6] Various surgical approaches, including the translabyrinthine, transcochlear, and presigmoid retrolabyrinthine, have extensively been described in the literature.[1-6] The retrosigmoid craniotomy is the most commonly used craniotomy allowing for easy and rapid access to this eloquent anatomical area.[1-6] Lesions located within the CPA and the petroclival region are surgically challenging to resect because of surrounding neurovascular structures, and especially the cranial nerves passing from their origin to enter into the base of skull.[4] The close topoanatomical relationship to the brainstem and the cranial nerves provides zero tolerance for retraction.[4]

Besides being technically difficult from patient positioning to good surgical clearance of the pathology at hand, the surgeon would commonly encounter cerebellar herniation through the dural defect upon durotomy.[7] This herniation most likely develops due to raised pressure within the posterior fossa owing to the presence of a mass lesion or neck flexion during the procedure causing impedance to the venous drainage. Cerebellar herniation in turn causes cerebellar trauma, contusions, and cortical bleeding.[7] Standard methods of obtaining adequate cerebellar relaxation are the use of osmotic diuretics, steroids, and mild hyperventilation. For moderate to large lesions, the placement of a lumbar subarachnoid drain for temporary cerebrospinal fluid (CSF) diversion during surgery has been recommended.[1-6] The microsurgical release of CSF from the subarachnoid spaces and cisterns is commonly done to achieve a relaxed surgical field.[2,4,6] However, this maneuver is performed after the dural opening and carries no role in preventing cerebellar herniation during the dural opening in cases where conservative measures have been baled out.[8] The retrosigmoid approach can be used for many different entities of extra-axial lesions in the CPA and intra-axial lesions arising along the petrosal surface of the cerebellum, cerebellar peduncles, or brainstem.[2,4,9] The insertion of a stereotactically guided supratentorial external ventricular drain with controlled temporary CSF diversion provides a possibility to avoid cerebellar herniation through the dural opening in larger lesions.

Preoperative magnetic resonance imaging (MRI) venography (MRV) is helpful to confirm the patency of the venous sinuses contralaterally to the approach.

Surgical Steps

1. After general anesthesia, patients are placed in a supine position with the head rotated contralaterally, and lateroflexed downward to facilitate exposure of the inferior tentorial surface (**Fig. 67.1**).
2. The patient is supported with the aid of sandbags underneath the ipsilateral shoulder and thorax.
3. The patient's head is fixed using a Mayfield clamp (**Fig. 67.1**).
4. Intraoperative neuromonitoring of the cranial nerves is installed by standard means described in the literature [V, VI, VII, IX, X, XI, XII, acoustic evoked potentials (AEPs), motor evoked potentials (MEPs), sensory evoked potentials (SEPs); **Fig. 67.1**].
5. A classical postauricular "C-shaped" incision is marked after delineating the transverse sinus using image guidance (**Fig. 67.2**).
6. The myocutaneous skin incision is raised in a double layer fashion.
7. Using a cutting burr, the course of the transverse and the sigmoid sinus is defined superficially along the bony surface and slowly skeletonized (**Fig. 67.3**).
8. The transverse-sigmoid junction can be assumed where the "asterion" is located, the confluence of the lambdoid, occipitomastoid, and parietomastoid sutures.
9. The image-guided external ventricular drainage (EVD) insertion is performed prior to opening the posterior fossa dura. The EVD entry point is planned within the exposed skull through the same incision, above the transverse sinus (**Fig. 67.3**).

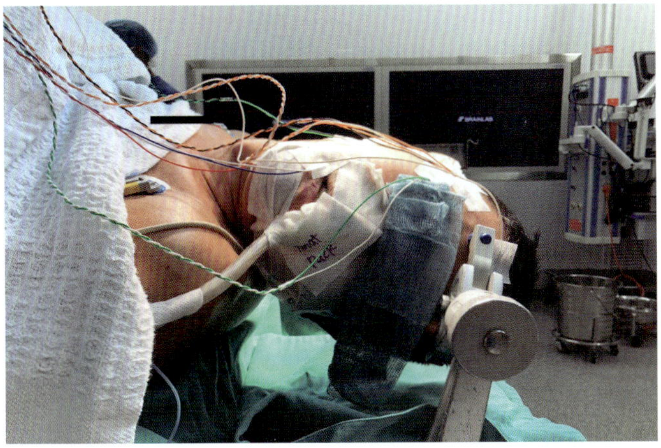

Fig. 67.1 Installation of the neuronavigation is dictated by the extension of the pathology and cranial nerve involvement. Motor- and sensory evoked potentials are part of the intraoperative neuromonitoring when relevant brainstem compression is present.

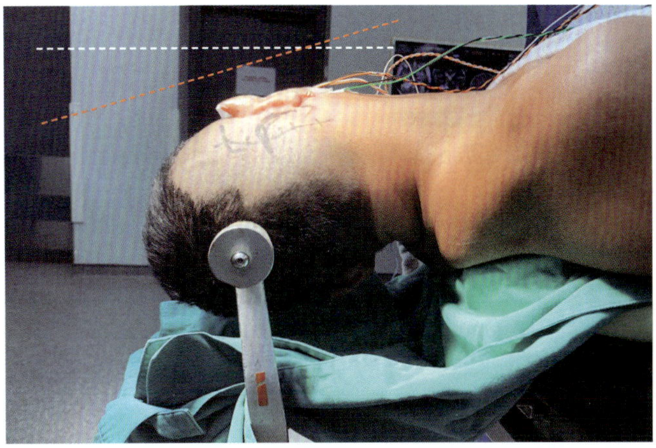

Fig. 67.2 Patient's head fixation with rotation and latero-flexion (*white* and *orange line*) to the contralateral side to expose the inferior surface of the tentorium cerebelli in large CPA lesions. Postauricular "C-shaped" incision and delineation of the dural sinuses using image-guided surgery are seen.

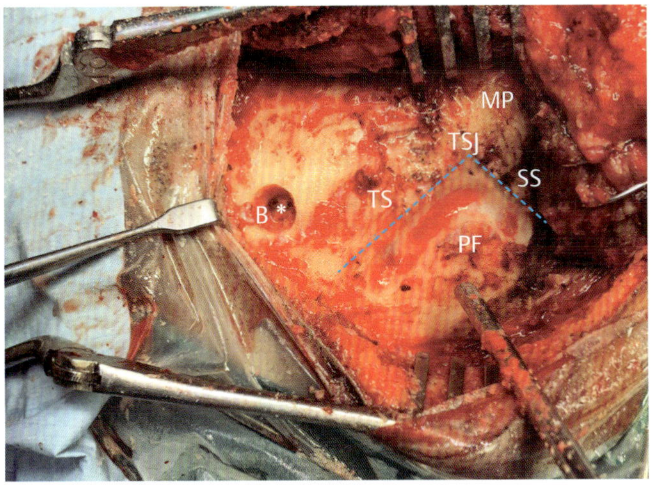

Fig. 67.3 After myocutaneous skin incision, the course (*blue line*) of the transverse (TS) and the sigmoid sinus (SS) and the transverse-sigmoid junction (TSJ) is defined superficially along the bony surface using image-guided surgery. A burr hole (B) for the stereotactically navigated EVD is placed with the trajectory aimed toward ipsilateral occipital horns of the lateral ventricle; the dura is opened, and a small corticotomy is performed (*asterisk*).

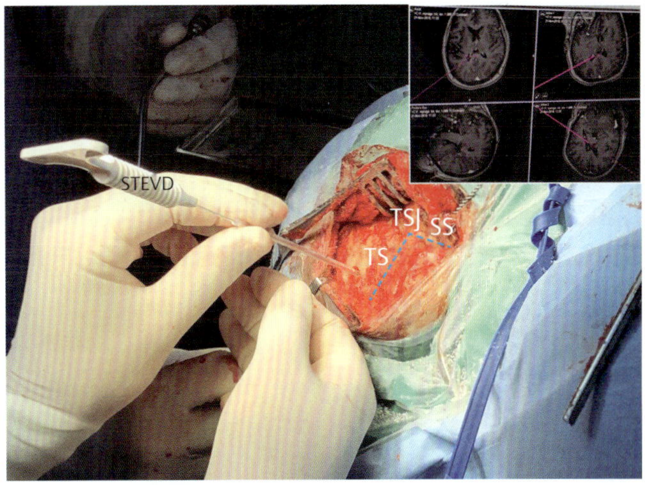

Fig. 67.4 A sterile image guidance probe replacing the supply trocar of the external ventricular drain is inserted into the ipsilateral occipital horn of the lateral ventricle. The anatomical course of the dural venous sinuses (*blue line*).

10. A burr hole is placed at the entry point with the trajectory aimed toward the ipsilateral occipital horn of the lateral ventricle (**Fig. 67.3**).
11. Once the burr hole is done, the dura is opened in a cruciate manner, and a small corticotomy is performed (**Fig. 67.3**).
12. A sterile image guidance probe replacing the supply trocar of the external ventricular drain is inserted via the corticotomy into the ipsilateral occipital horn of the lateral ventricle. (**Fig. 67.4**).
13. Minimal egress of CSF confirms optimal placement (**Fig. 67.4**).
14. The EVD is then tunneled out about 5 cm away from the scalp wound and left clamped (**Fig. 67.5a**).
15. While skeletonizing of the sigmoid sinus, mastoid air cells are commonly opened in most cases and have to be thoroughly waxed to prevent CSF fistula.

16. After the dural sinuses are delineated and skeletonized, a circumferential craniotomy over the posterior fossa is performed, adapted to the size of the targeted lesion (**Fig. 67.5b**).
17. The bone flap is then raised and the dura is visualized (**Fig. 67.5c**).
18. Subsequently, the CSF is judiciously released until the dura is visibly pulsatile and not tense.
19. The EVD is then clamped again until further CSF release is necessitated to facilitate cerebellar retraction.
20. The dura is incised along the posterior aspect of the sigmoid sinus in a C-shaped manner.
21. With the aid of the EVD, no cerebellar herniation through the durotomy is appreciated.
22. CSF can be released from the subarachnoid spaces and cisterns and the pathology can be microsurgically exposed with a relaxed surgical field (**Fig. 67.6a–e** and **Fig. 67.7**).
23. Postoperatively, the EVD is removed within 48 hours after surgery.

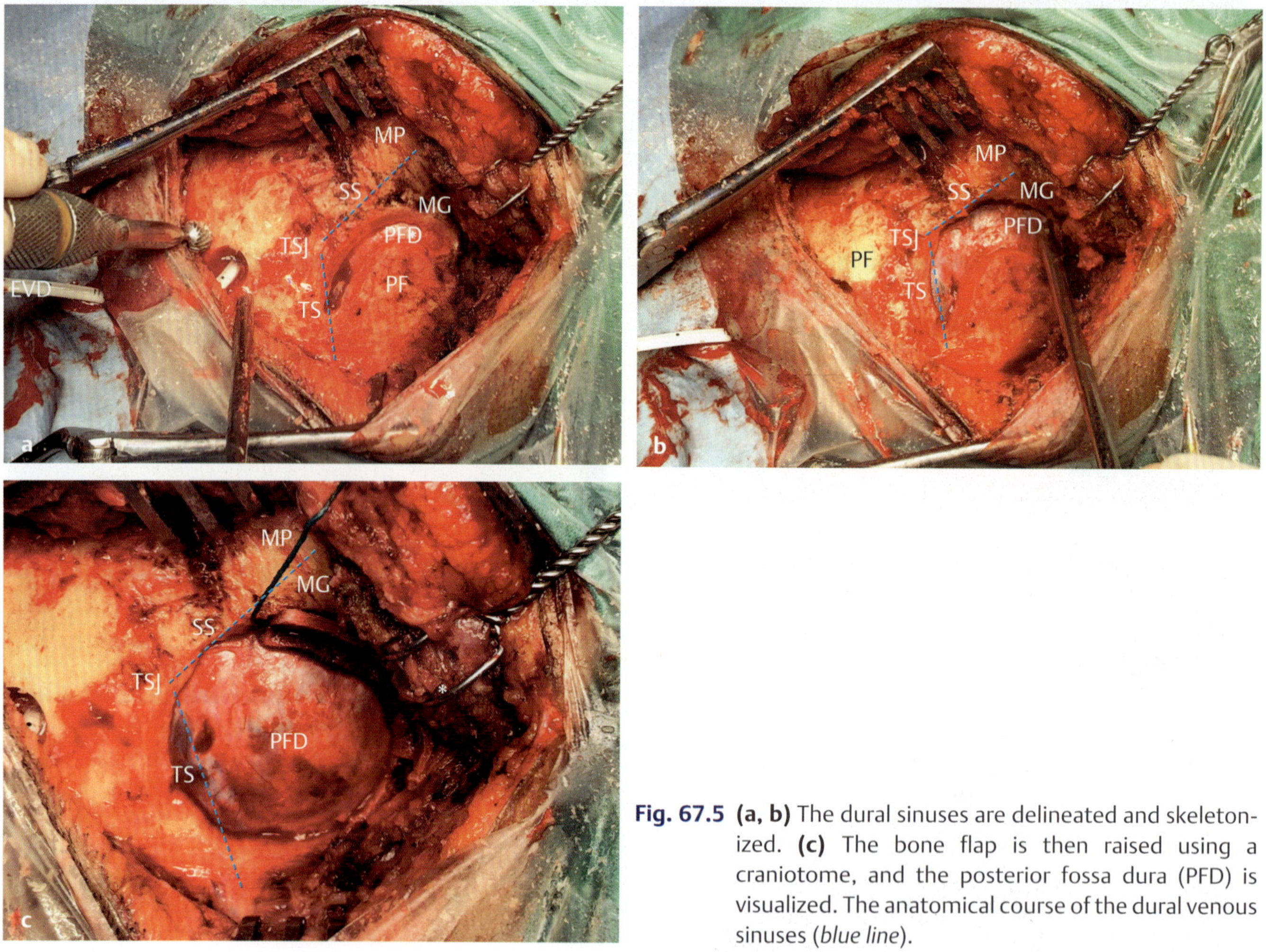

Fig. 67.5 **(a, b)** The dural sinuses are delineated and skeletonized. **(c)** The bone flap is then raised using a craniotome, and the posterior fossa dura (PFD) is visualized. The anatomical course of the dural venous sinuses (*blue line*).

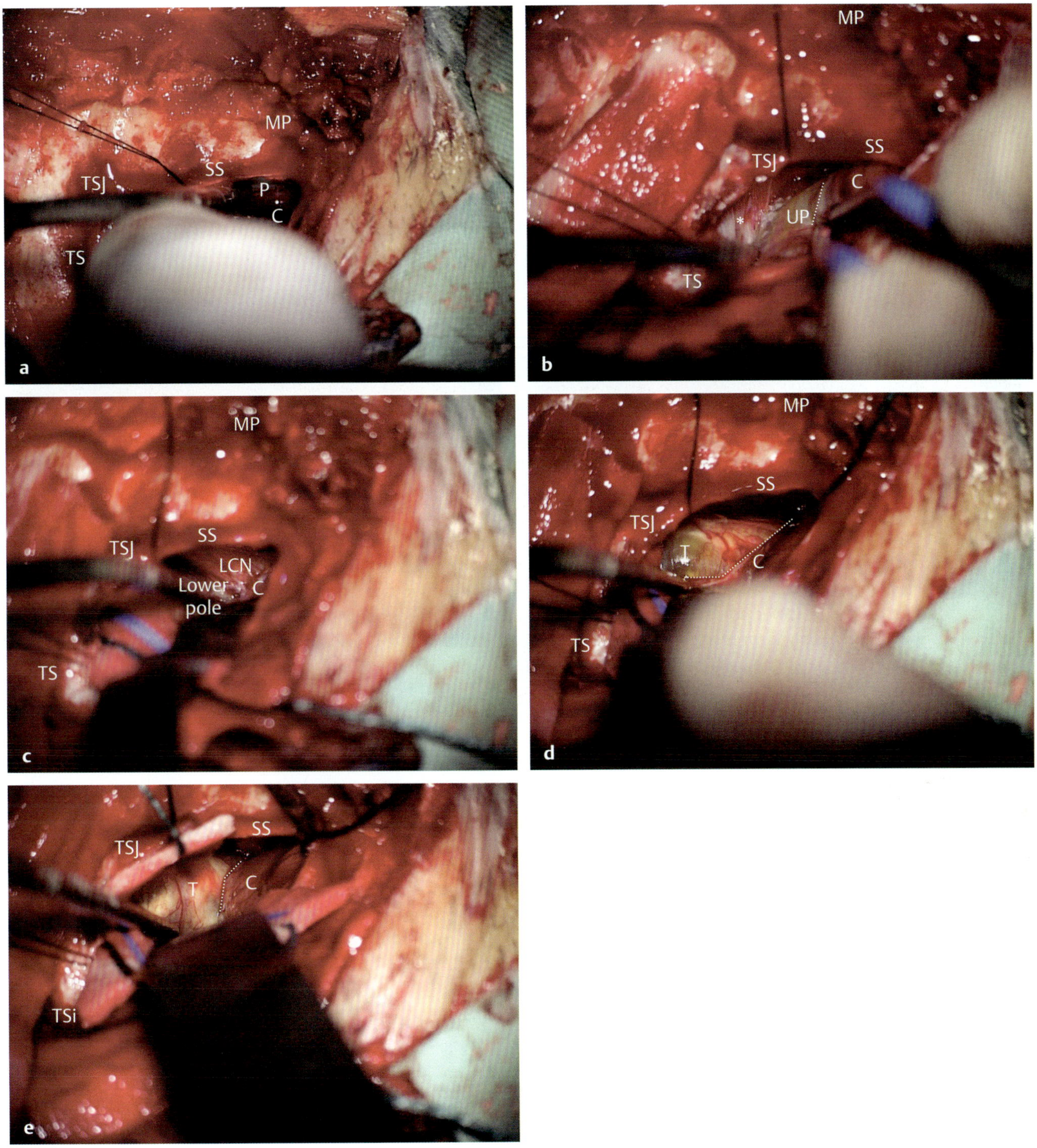

Fig. 67.6 Intradural microsurgical resection of a large cystic vestibular schwannoma KOOS grade IV. **(a)** After dural opening along the course of the transverse sinus (TSi), the transverse-sigmoid junction (TSJ) and the sigmoid sinus (SS), the cerebellum (C) can be retracted away from the petrosal wall (P) without relevant cerebellar swelling, and the subarachnoid spaces and cisterns can be dissected to release more CSF for a relaxed surgical field. **(b)** The upper pole of the lesion is identified along the tentorium cerebelli (*), and the arachnoid plane between the tumor and the cerebellum (*white line*) is identified. **(c)** The lower pole of the lesion is identified, in close contact with the lower cranial nerves (LCNs), in particular IX (glossopharyngeal) and X (vagal), entering into the jugular foramen. **(d, e)** Definition of the brain–tumor interface (*white line*) while freeing the tumor surface (T) from the arachnoid layer with adjacent cortical vessels of the cerebellum (C). Meticulous electrophysiological stimulation of the tumor capsule is mandatory prior to cauterization, incision, and debulking of the tumor.

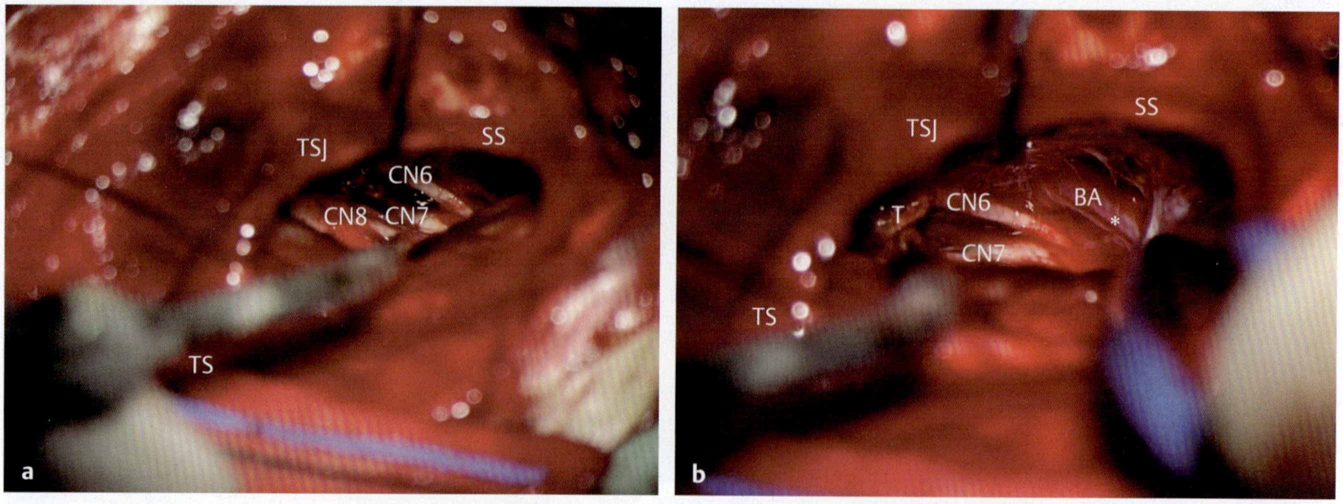

Fig. 67.7 Intraoperative view of the cerebellopontine angle through the retrosigmoid approach after near-total excision of a vestibular schwannoma KOOS grade IV. **(a)** The vestibulocochlear nerve (CN8) is flattened out in the superior aspect of the operative field and in close relationship with the facial nerve (CN7). The facial nerve (or seventh cranial nerve) in this particular case is nicely "bundle shaped" and not flattened out, and dissection from the root exit zone of the nerve along the brainstem and in the cisternal portion was possible. The abducent nerve (CN6) is visualized at the same depth as the seventh cranial nerve indicating the dislocation of the seventh nerve towards the midline. **(b)** Remnant tumor (T) is seen along the seventh and eighth nerve near the cisternal portion where the nerves enter the internal auditory canal. In this region, the seventh nerve usually is flattened out, and the tumor capsule is very adherent to the perineurium. The lower pole of the tumor widened up the subarachnoid space and dislocated the brainstem and the root exit zone of the seventh nerve medially. Hence, the sixth nerve is visualized at the same level together with the basilar artery (BA) and a perforating artery (*asterisk*).

References

1. Katsuta T, Rhoton AL Jr, Matsushima T. The jugular foramen: microsurgical anatomy and operative approaches. Neurosurgery 1997;41(1):149–201, discussion 201–202
2. Lang J Jr, Samii A. Retrosigmoidal approach to the posterior cranial fossa. An anatomical study. Acta Neurochir (Wien) 1991;111(3-4):147–153
3. Quiñones-Hinojosa A, Chang EF, Lawton MT. The extended retrosigmoid approach: an alternative to radical cranial base approaches for posterior fossa lesions. Neurosurgery 2006; 58(4, Suppl 2):ONS-208–ONS-214, discussion ONS-214
4. Rhoton AL Jr. The cerebellopontine angle and posterior fossa cranial nerves by the retrosigmoid approach. Neurosurgery 2000;47(3, Suppl):S93–S129
5. Samii M, Gerganov V, Samii A. Improved preservation of hearing and facial nerve function in vestibular schwannoma surgery via the retrosigmoid approach in a series of 200 patients. J Neurosurg 2006;105(4):527–535
6. Van Rompaey J, Bush C, McKinnon B, Solares AC. Minimally invasive access to the posterior cranial fossa: an anatomical study comparing a retrosigmoidal endoscopic approach to a microscopic approach. J Neurol Surg A Cent Eur Neurosurg 2013;74(1):1–6
7. Dubey A, Sung WS, Shaya M, et al. Complications of posterior cranial fossa surgery—an institutional experience of 500 patients. Surg Neurol 2009;72(4):369–375
8. Li J, Gelb AW, Flexman AM, Ji F, Meng L. Definition, evaluation, and management of brain relaxation during craniotomy. Br J Anaesth 2016;116(6):759–769
9. Zuccaro G, Sosa F. Cerebellopontine angle lesions in children. Childs Nerv Syst 2007;23:177–183

Section XXVII

Middle Cranial Fossa

Chapter 68 Middle Cranial Fossa Approach

Narayan Jayashankar and K.P. Morwani

Indications

- Vestibular neurectomy for intractable vertigo.[1,2]
- Intracanalicular vestibular schwannoma.[3,4,5,6]
- Facial nerve trauma.[7]
- Meningoencephalocele.[8]

Surgical Steps

Magnetic resonance imaging (MRI) of a subject with a right-sided intracanalicular vestibular schwannoma with preserved hearing is shown (**Fig. 68.1**), and surgical steps of the subject are described below:

1. An incision is made starting just anterior to the helix coursing superiorly, with a gentle curve first posteriorly and then anteriorly at its superior limit. This incision is about 6 to 7 cm in length and extends till about the temporoparietal suture line (**Fig. 68.2**). The incision includes the skin and subcutaneous tissue (**Fig. 68.3**).
2. An inferiorly based pedicled musculoperiosteal flap is created next (**Fig. 68.4**). It is based on the superficial temporal artery. The musculoperiosteal cuts are taken along the line of insertion of temporalis muscle, and the pedicled flap is reflected inferiorly over the zygomatic arch to expose the temporal craniotomy site.
3. A craniotomy is performed 4 cm in length and 4 cm in height. It is based approximately one-third posterior and two-thirds anterior to the perpendicular line drawn superiorly along the external auditory canal (**Fig. 68.5**). The inferior craniotomy cut should be as close to the zygoma as possible. This helps to prevent an overhanging ledge of bone inferiorly which obscures vision and instrument manipulation in depth. Care should be taken to avoid injury to the vascular pedicle of temporalis musculoperiosteal flap while drilling inferiorly. The initial cuts are made with a cutting burr, and on seeing the color change as one approaches dura, one must change to a diamond burr to prevent inadvertent injury to the temporal dura. On completing the cuts, the temporal dura is separated from the overlying bone by dissecting it off with a Freer elevator. The bone flap excised is placed in saline for replacement at the end of the procedure. The edges of the craniotomy are smoothened out using a diamond burr. The temporal dura is seen (**Fig. 68.6**).
4. The middle fossa dura is elevated from posterior to anterior (**Fig. 68.7**).

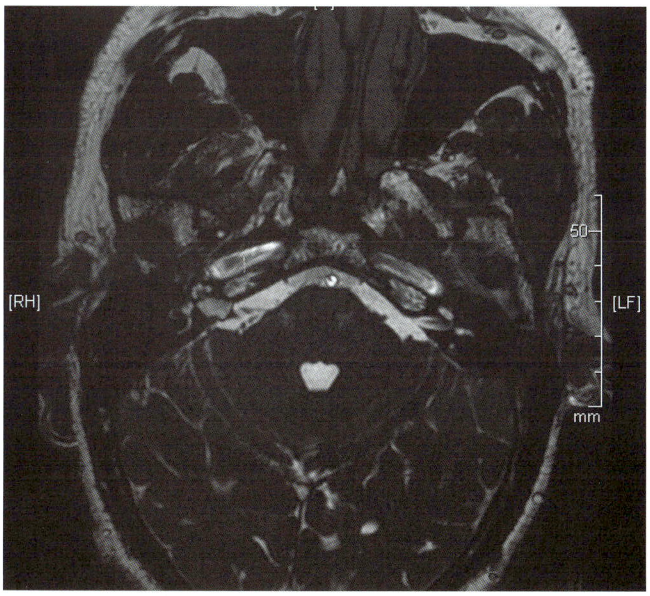

Fig. 68.1 MRI showing a right-sided intracanalicular vestibular schwannoma.

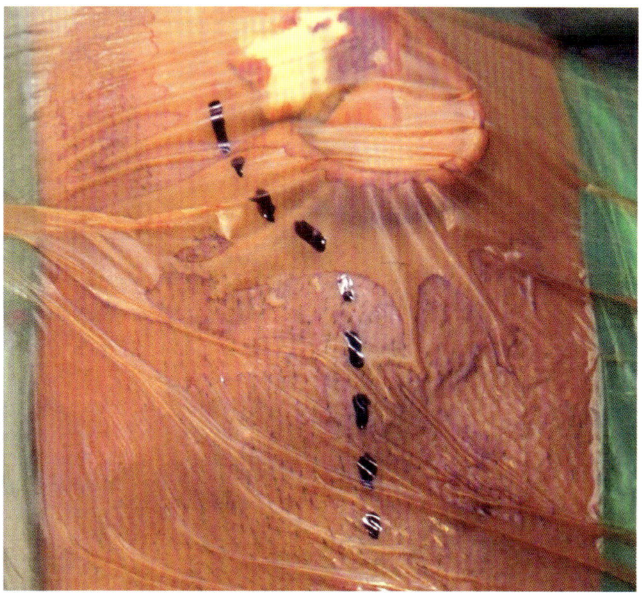

Fig. 68.2 Incision for middle cranial fossa approach.

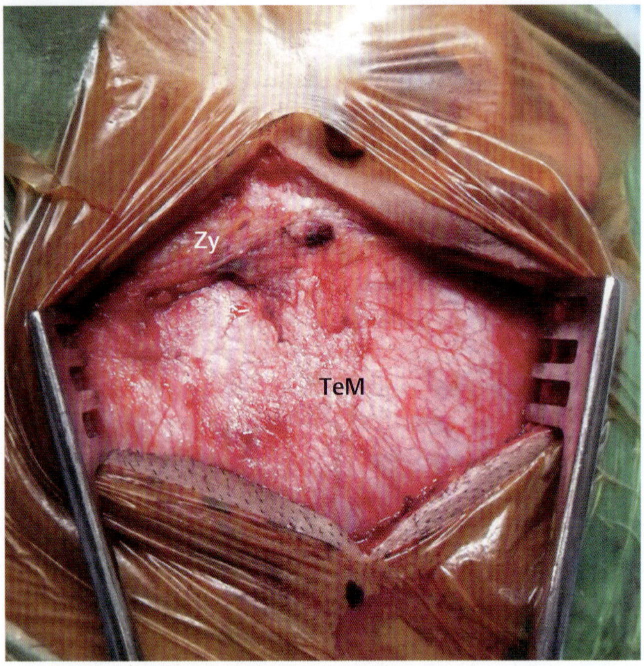

Fig. 68.3 The temporalis muscle with its fascia is exposed.

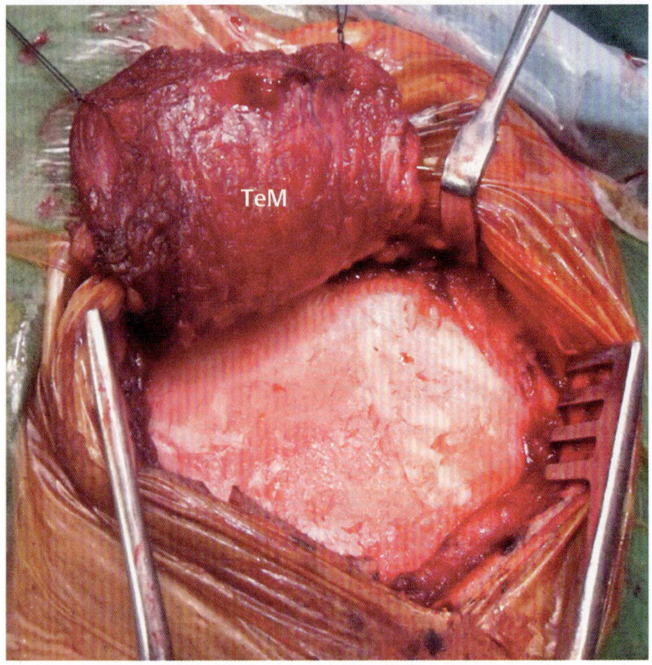

Fig. 68.4 Inferiorly based temporalis muscle flap.

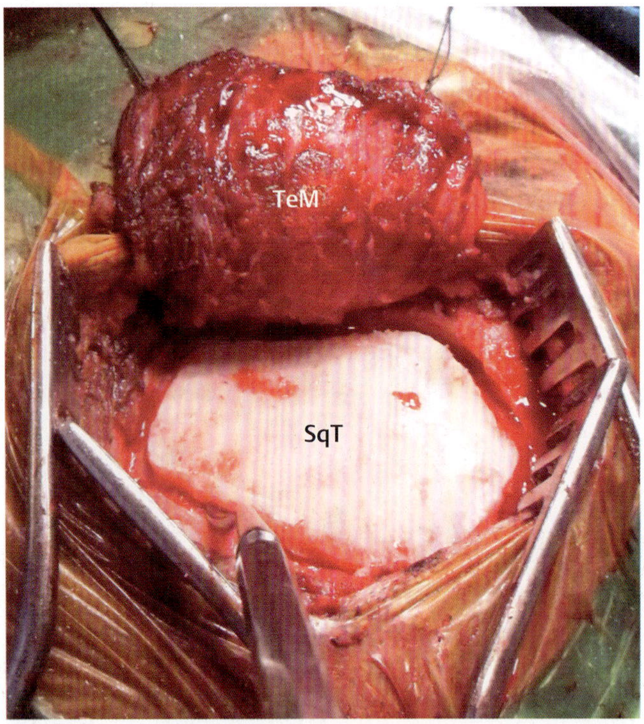

Fig. 68.5 A craniotomy is made as described.

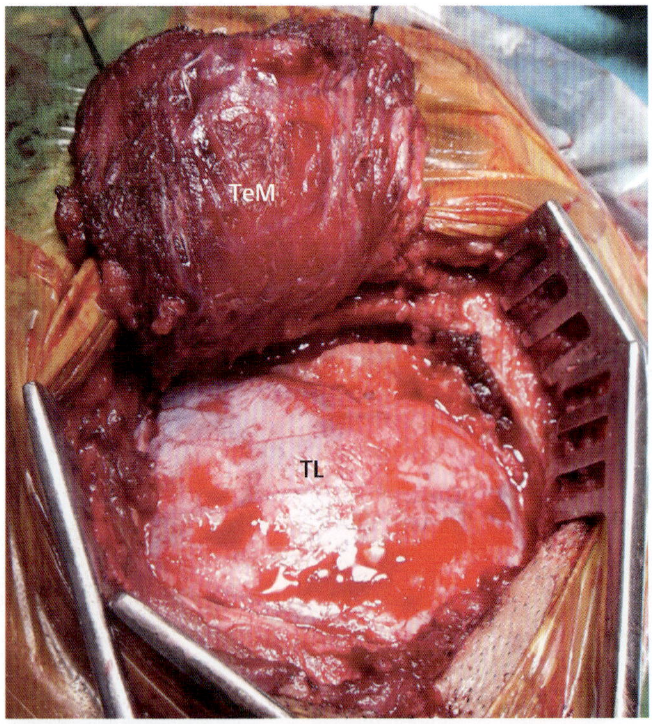

Fig. 68.6 Craniotomy bone flap is removed to expose the temporal lobe.

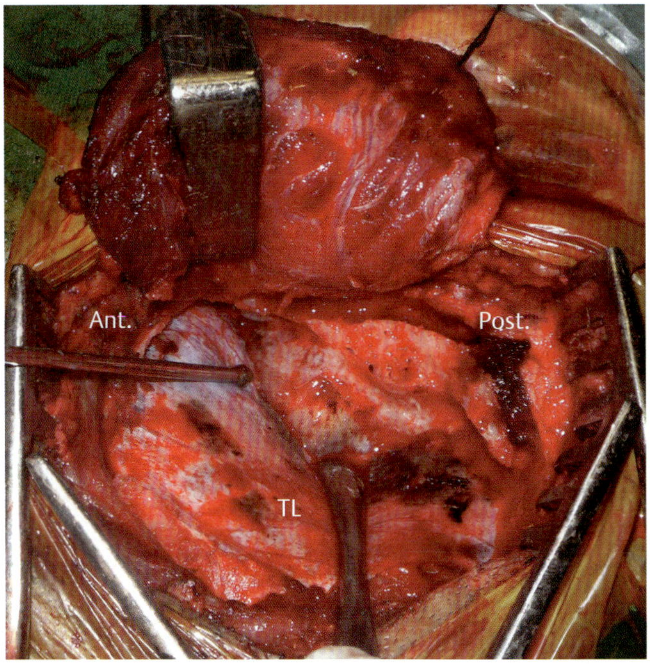

Fig. 68.7 Temporal lobe is dissected off the floor of the middle cranial fossa.

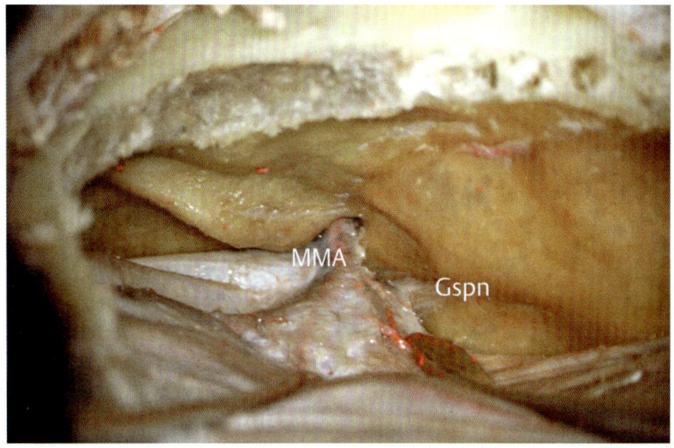

Fig. 68.8 Middle meningeal artery is seen at the foramen spinosum.

5. During the elevation of the dura, the arcuate eminence and greater superficial petrosal nerve are identified on the surface of the middle fossa bone. At the anterior end, the middle meningeal artery is seen, which is then bipolarized and cut, if required (**Fig. 68.8**). This offers the advantage in certain cases that the temporal lobe dura gets retracted nicely toward the petrous ridge giving adequate space for the approach. Dural elevation proceeds up to the petrous ridge (**Fig. 68.9**), where the superior petrosal sinus is identified. The middle fossa retractor is applied.
6. It must be remembered that in approximately 50% cases, the arcuate eminence does not correspond to the superior semicircular canal. In **Figs. 68.10, 68.11, and 68.12**, the tegmen has been uncovered to understand the anatomy of the middle fossa and the location of internal auditory meatus (IAM) more explicitly.
7. House's method (**Fig. 68.10**): Trace the greater superficial nerve retrograde to identify the geniculate ganglion, labyrinthine segment, and then follow it to the fundus of the IAM. Drilling then proceeds to uncover the whole IAM. As seen in **Fig. 68.10**, the cochlea and also the vestibule are in very close proximity to the labyrinthine segment, so, accidental injury to cochlea or labyrinth can occur easily during drilling. Since this is essentially a hearing preservation surgery, this approach is not preferred since it risks hearing.
8. Fisch's Method (**Fig. 68.11**): The superior semicircular canal is identified and blue-lined. Drilling then proceeds at a 60-degree angle from the ampullated end of the blue-lined superior semicircular canal to avoid injury to the cochlea. Drilling in this approach is again from the fundus of IAM toward the porus, similar to House's method.
9. Garcia–Ibanez method (**Fig. 68.12**): The IAM corresponds approximately to a line bisecting the angle formed between the greater superficial petrosal nerve and the arcuate eminence. Drilling is commenced from the area of the superior petrosal sinus over the internal auditory meatus, specifically from the porus toward the fundus (**Fig. 68.13**). This method decreases the risk of injury to hearing.
10. The fundus of IAM is intimately related to the cochlea anteriorly and the superior semicircular canal and vestibule posteriorly (**Fig. 68.14**). On the other hand, the medial end of the IAM does not have any vital structures crowding it. It roughly makes an angle of 35 to 55 degrees with the superior petrosal sinus. Drilling can start slightly posterior or anterior to the porus of the internal auditory canal, which is the safe area, and then progresses over the porus end of the IAM. Once the color change at porus end of IAM is identified, indicating the presence of the underlying dura of IAM, we drill with a wide base medially, that is, from the porus

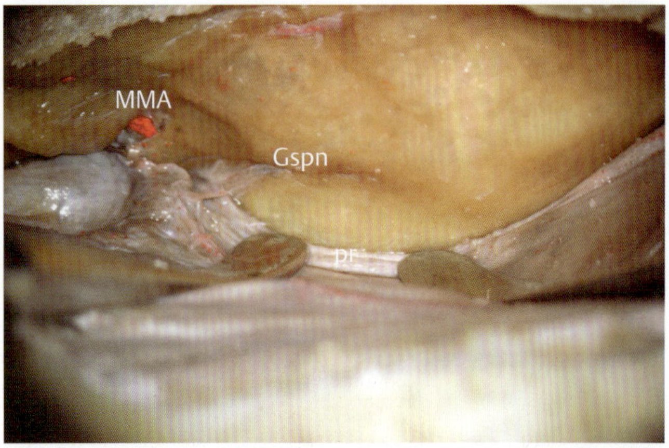

Fig. 68.9 Temporal lobe dura reflected off the floor of the middle cranial fossa up to the petrous ridge where bluish tinge of superior petrosal sinus is evident.

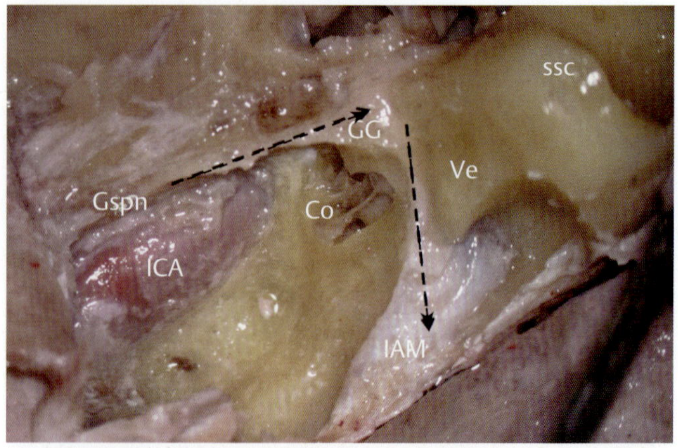

Fig. 68.10 House's method to identify IAM.

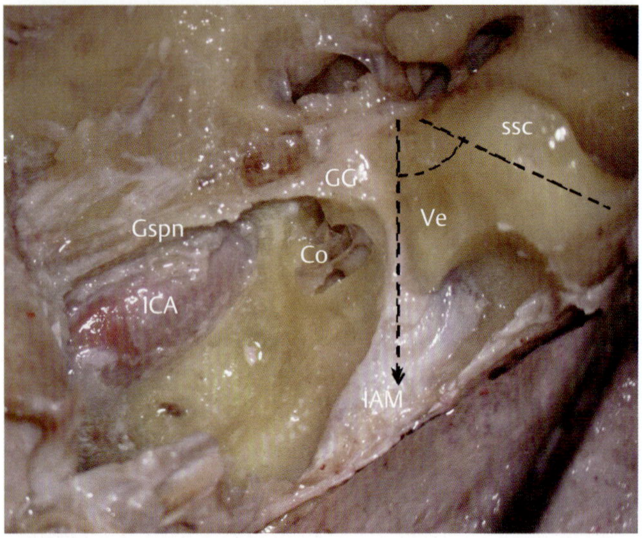

Fig. 68.11 Fisch's method to identify IAM.

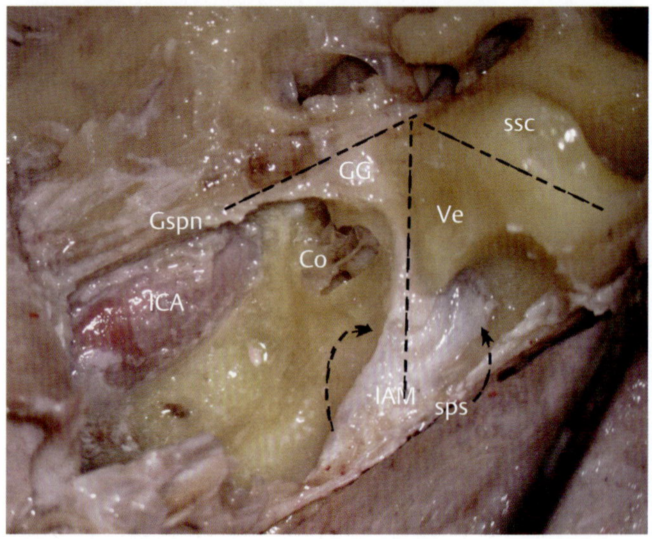

Fig. 68.12 Ibanez's method to identify IAM.

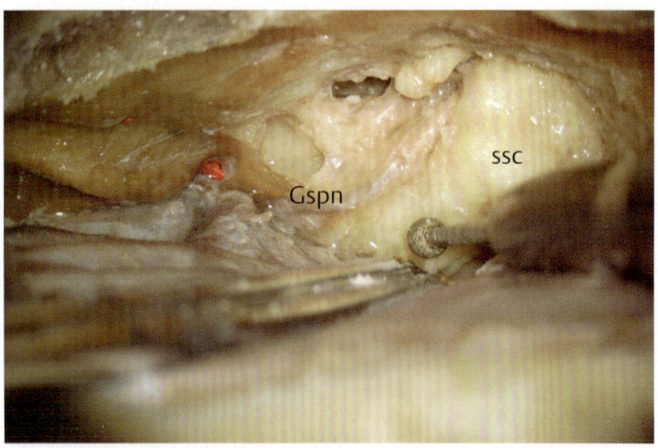

Fig. 68.13 Area of drilling for internal auditory meatus.

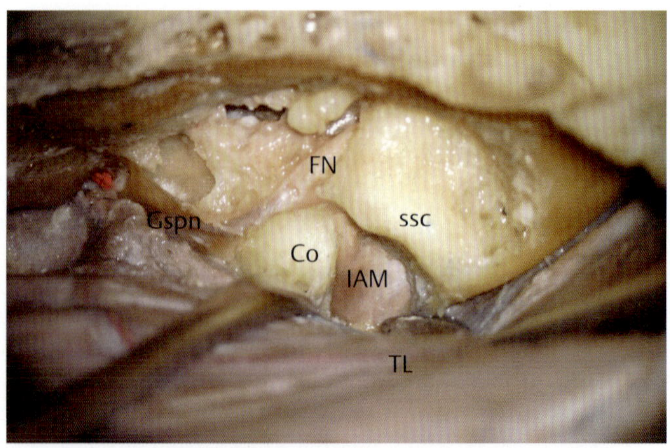

Fig. 68.14 Internal auditory meatus is seen via middle cranial fossa approach.

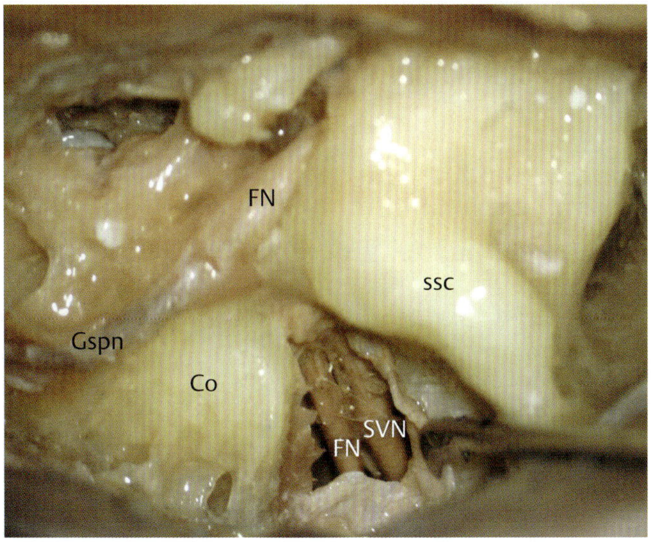

Fig. 68.15 Dura of internal auditory meatus is opened.

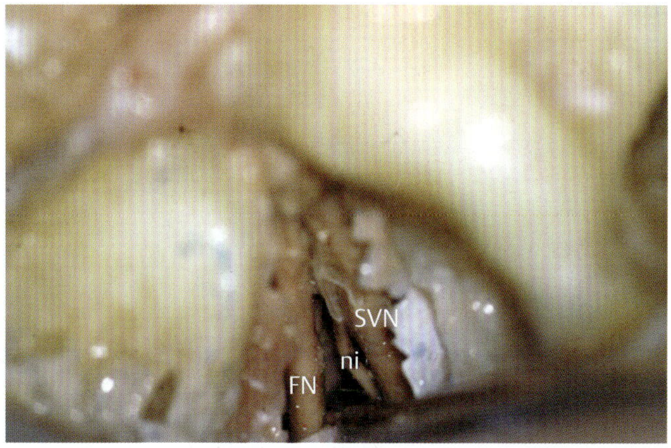

Fig. 68.16 Nervus intermedius is seen in the middle.

end of IAM narrowing toward the lateral end to expose 180-degree circumference of the IAM. The bone over the IAM is made eggshell thin, and the last shells of the bone are lifted off with an elevator.

11. Bill's bar is seen at the lateral end of the IAM separating facial nerve anteriorly from the superior vestibular nerve posteriorly.
12. The dura of the IAM is incised along its length over the superior vestibular nerve (**Fig. 68.15**). This is to prevent any inadvertent injury to the facial nerve.
13. The nervus intermedius is identified in the center (**Fig. 68.16**).
14. The cochlear nerve lies deeper to the facial nerve, while the inferior vestibular nerve lies deeper to the superior vestibular nerve in this approach.
15. The tumor is excised taking care to use sharp dissection (**Fig. 68.17**). There should be no traction on the other nerves.
16. A plug of fat is used to seal the opening at the end of the procedure (**Fig. 68.18**). Fibrin glue is put on its edges.
17. The craniotomy flap is replaced and sutured in place using 1–0 Vicryl (**Fig. 68.19**).
18. The pedicled temporalis musculoperiosteal flap is replaced and sutured using 2–0 Vicryl (**Fig. 68.20**).
19. The subcutaneous and skin layers are sutured together (**Fig. 68.21**).

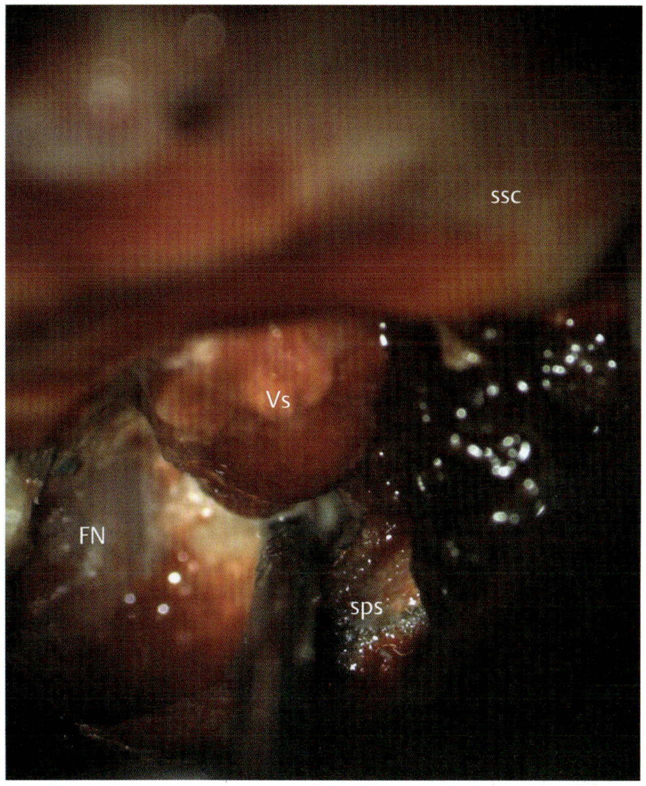

Fig. 68.17 Vestibular schwannoma is excised.

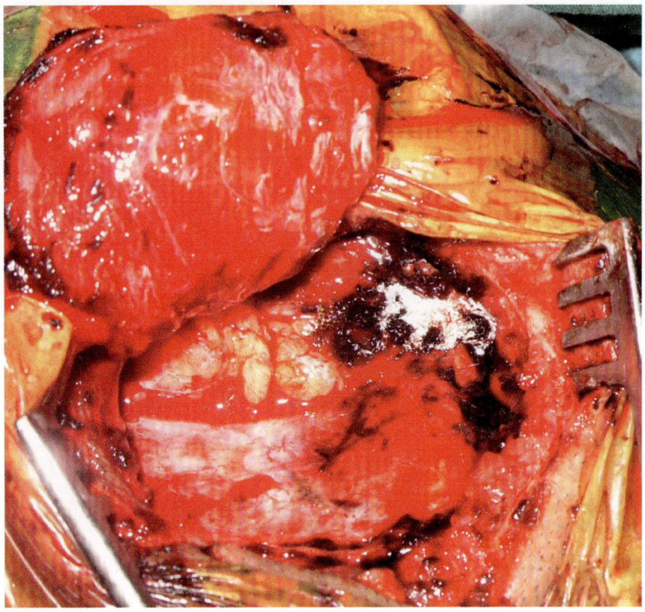

Fig. 68.18 Fat placed over the internal auditory meatus.

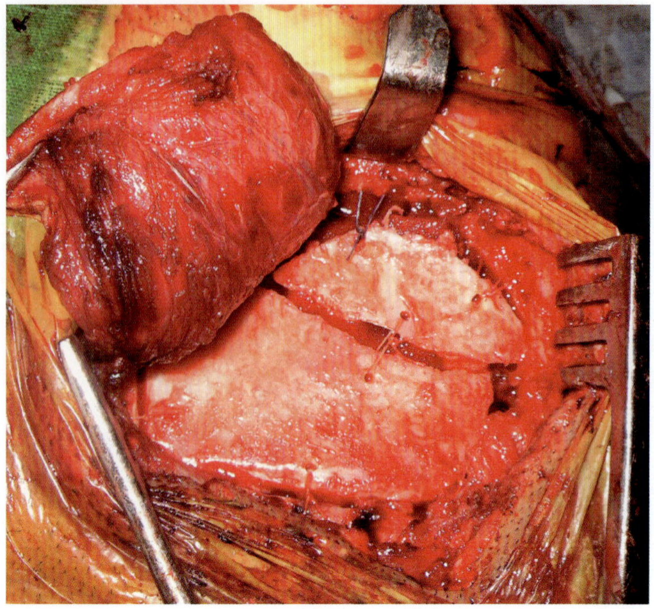

Fig. 68.19 Craniotomy flap replaced and sutured in place.

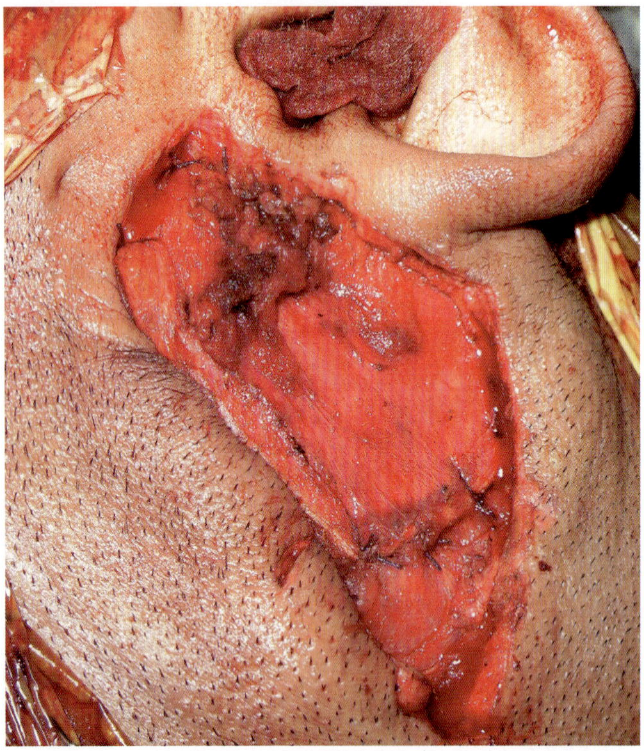

Fig. 68.20 Temporalis muscle is sutured back in place.

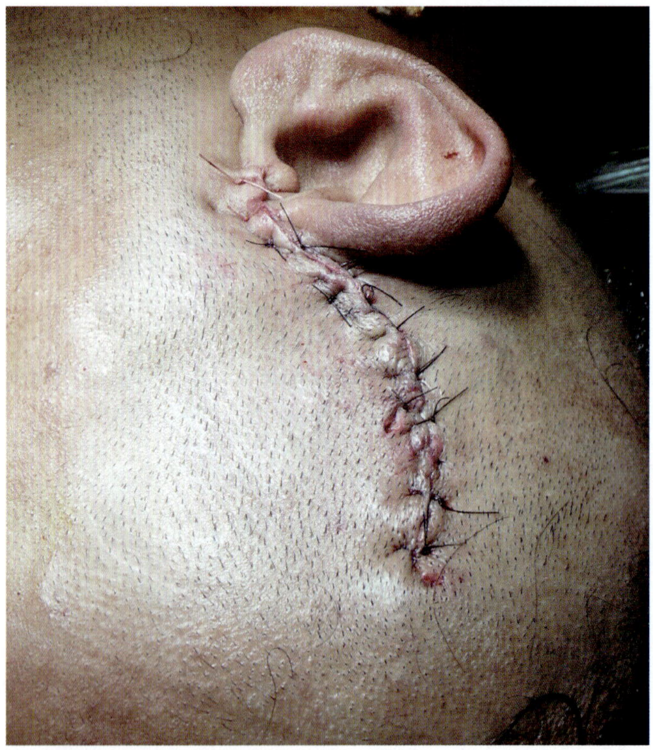

Fig. 68.21 Skin is sutured.

Tips and Pearls

- Bone removal for craniotomy should be as close to zygoma at the base as possible else visualization is hampered.
- Dissection of the temporal lobe is always from posterior to anterior to prevent traction on greater superficial petrosal nerve or a dehiscent geniculate ganglion.
- The IAM is deeper at the medial end as compared to the fundus end, so that the dura of IAM is encountered with lesser drilling at the fundus.

References

1. Fisch U. Transtemporal supralabyrinthine (middle cranial fossa) vestibular neurectomy: a review of the last 100 cases. Skull Base Surg. 1996;6(4):221-5
2. Green JD Jr, Shelton C, Brackmann DE. Middle fossa vestibular neurectomy in retrolabyrinthine neurectomy failures. Arch Otolaryngol Head Neck Surg. 1992;118(10):1058-60
3. Raheja A, et al. Middle fossa approach for vestibular schwannoma: good hearing and facial nerve outcomes with low morbidity. World Neurosurg. 2016;92:37-46
4. Rabelo de Freitas M, Russo A, Sequino G, Piccirillo E, Sanna M. Analysis of hearing preservation and facial nerve function for patients undergoing vestibular schwannoma surgery: the middle cranial fossa approach versus the retrosigmoid approach--personal experience and literature review. Audiol Neurootol. 2012;17(2):71-81
5. Kosty JA, et al. Middle fossa approach for resection of vestibular schwannomas: a decade of experience. Oper Neurosurg (Hagerstown). 2019;16(2):147-158
6. Gantz BJ, Parnes LS, Harker LA, McCabe BF. Middle cranial fossa acoustic neuroma excision: results and complications. *The Annals of otology, rhinology, and laryngology.* 1986; 95(5 Pt 1):454-459
7. da Franca Pereira MA, Bittencourt AG, de Andrade EM, Bento RF, de Brito R. Decompression of the tympanic and labyrinthine segments of the facial nerve by middle cranial fossa approach: an anatomic study. Acta Neurochir (Wien). 2016;158(6):1205-1211
8. Gupta A, Sikka K, Irugu DVK, Verma H, Bhalla AS, Thakar A. Temporal bone meningoencephaloceles and cerebrospinal fluid leaks: experience in a tertiary care hospital. J Laryngol Otol. 2019;133(3):192-200

Chapter 69 Extended Middle Cranial Fossa Approach

Narayan Jayashankar, K.P. Morwani, and Suresh Sankhla

Indications

1. Vestibular schwannoma or facial nerve schwannoma of the internal auditory canal with less than 1 cm extension into the cerebellopontine angle with preserved hearing.
2. Cases of petrous bone cholesteatomas located superior or anterior to the cochlea.

Surgical Steps

1. Steps 1 to 5 are the same as mentioned in the middle cranial fossa approach.
2. The extended middle fossa approach offers increased access to the posterior fossa by drilling posterior and anterior to the internal auditory meatus.
3. By drilling posterior to the internal auditory meatus, the middle fossa dural plate is uncovered. As mentioned earlier, the arcuate eminence does not correspond to the superior semicircular canal in approximately 50 percent of cases. Hence, the arcuate eminence has to be carefully drilled off till the color change indicates that the superior semicircular canal is seen. We never blue line the superior semicircular canal. This area is triangular and is bound by the internal auditory meatus anteriorly, the dome of the superior semicircular canal posteriorly, and the superior petrosal sinus medially. Drilling further lateral to the superior semicircular canal, the lateral and posterior semicircular canals, as well as the junctional zone, where the superior petrosal sinus meets the sigmoid sinus is encountered (**Fig. 69.1**).
4. Drilling lateral to the labyrinthine segment of the facial nerve uncovers the tegmen tympani, forming the roof of the middle ear. Thus, the head of the malleus and the body of the incus along with its short process is seen in the attic. The Prussak space, the anterior epitympanum, and the cochleariform process are all easily identified. The short process of incus lateral to the dome of the lateral semicircular canal is appreciated in **Fig. 69.1**.
5. As mentioned earlier, the middle meningeal artery is bipolarized and cut for anterior extensions (**Fig. 69.2**). This exposes the dura covering the gasserian ganglion. On opening the dura, fibers of the gasserian ganglion are exposed (**Figs. 69.3 and 69.4**).
6. The cochlea is intimately related anteriorly to the lateral end of the internal auditory meatus. Drilling is performed anterior to the internal auditory meatus in an area bounded anterolaterally by the cochlea, anteromedially by the petrous segment of the internal carotid artery, anteriorly by the Gasserian ganglion, medially by the superior petrosal sinus, and posteriorly by the internal auditory meatus. This area is roughly quadrilateral and exposes the posterior fossa dura at the petrous apex (**Fig. 69.5**).
7. The authors here describe a surgical case of right-sided facial nerve schwannoma using the extended middle cranial fossa approach (**Fig. 69.6**).
8. On retracting the temporal lobe, much of the tumor was found abutting the temporal lobe and cleared to get the landmarks on the middle fossa (**Fig. 69.7**).

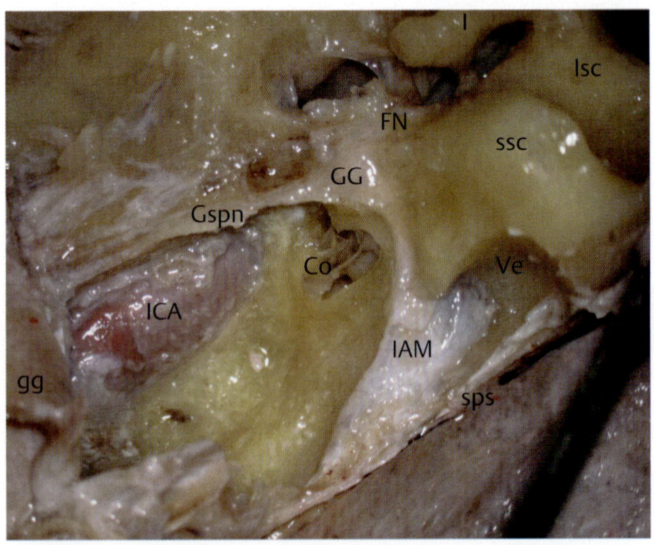

Fig. 69.1 Triangular area posterior to the internal auditory meatus. (Picture courtesy Dr Yash Pandya)

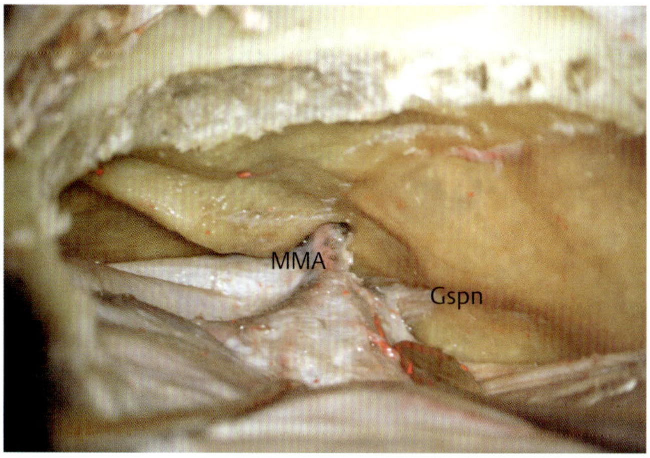

Fig. 69.2 Middle meningeal artery at the foramen spinosum.

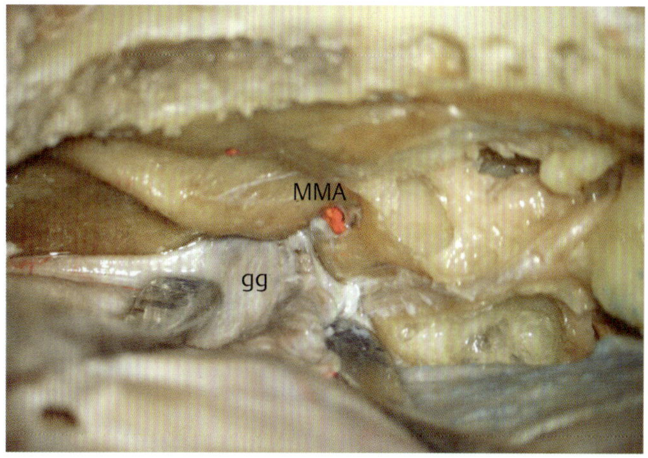

Fig. 69.3 The dura covering the gasserian ganglion is seen anterior to the cut middle meningeal artery. gg, gasserian ganglion; MMA, middle meningeal artery.

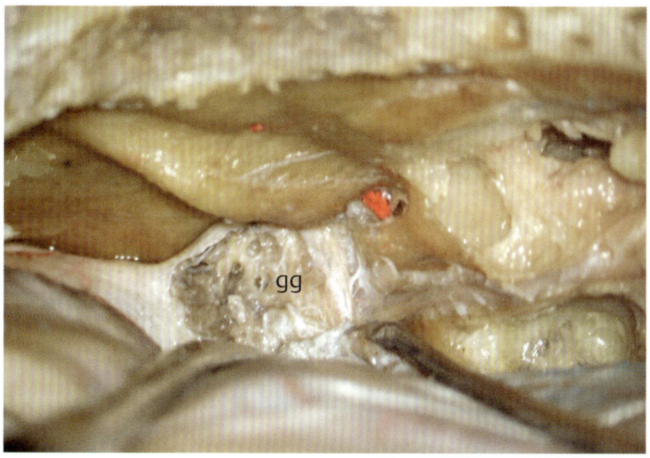

Fig. 69.4 Gasserian ganglion exposed.

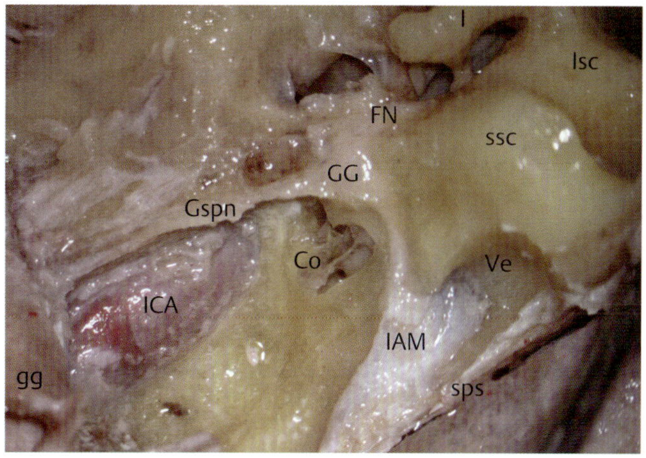

Fig. 69.5 Quadrilateral area anterior to the internal auditory meatus.

9. As seen on the scans, the tumor had caused a lot of widening of the internal auditory meatus and eroded the wall to extend into the middle fossa (**Figs. 69.8 and 16.9**).
10. The internal auditory meatus is drilled to expose the remnant tumor up to the fundus (**Fig. 69.10**).
11. Tumor extends from the internal auditory meatus into the posterior fossa as well (**Figs. 69.11 and 69.12**).
12. The facial nerve schwannoma was cleared from the posterior fossa as well. The facial nerve was transected beyond the tumor. After obtaining histopathological confirmation that the cut edge of the facial nerve was clear, it was decided to do a grafting of the facial nerve from near the brainstem to the geniculate ganglion segment (**Figs. 69.13 and 69.14**).
13. Fat harvested from the abdomen or thigh is used to obliterate the defects.
14. The temporal lobe retractor is removed, allowing the temporal lobe to take its normal position.
15. The craniotomy flap is sutured back in place with 1–0 Vicryl.
16. The temporalis musculoperiosteal pedicled flap is sutured back in place.
17. Subcutaneous and skin layers are sutured together.

Tips and Pearls

- Anatomical knowledge of the structures, as seen in the middle fossa, is very important to extend the drilling beyond the internal auditory meatus. The triangular area posterior to the internal auditory meatus leads to the posterior fossa dura at the cerebellopontine angle. The quadrilateral area anterior to the internal auditory meatus leads to the posterior fossa dura at the petrous apex.

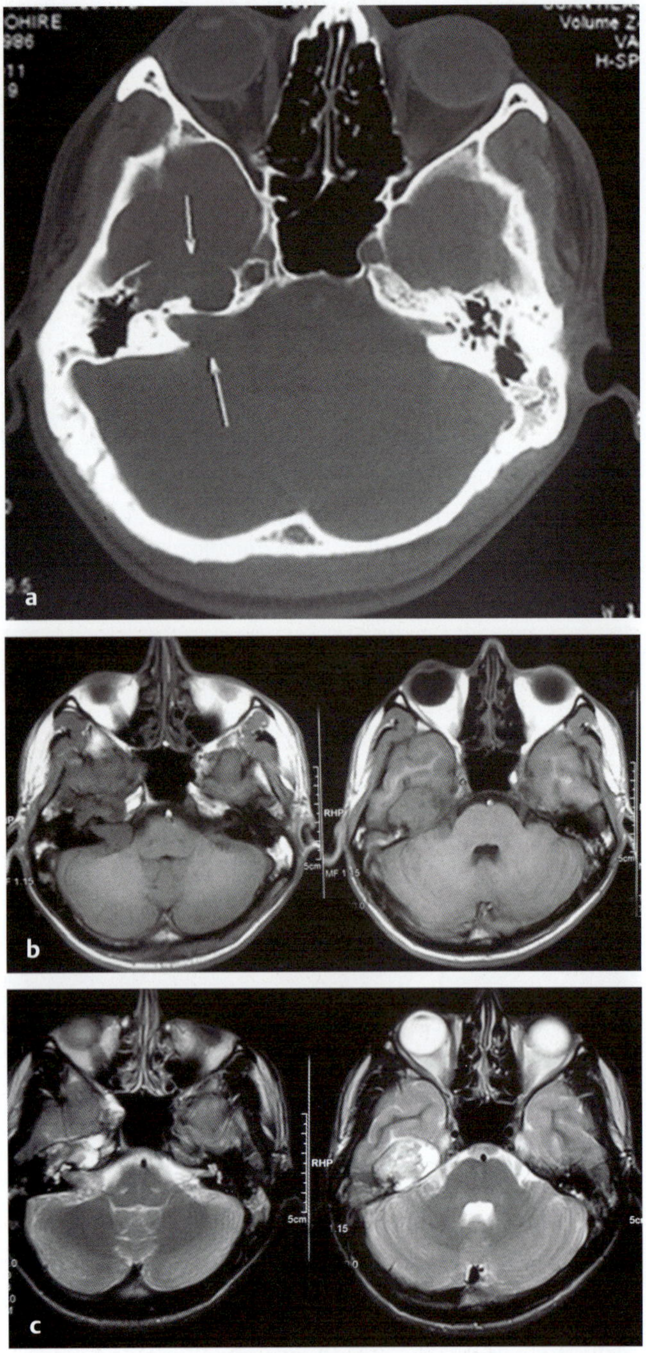

Fig. 69.6 **(a)** CT scan showing widening of the right internal auditory meatus and erosion of the floor of the middle cranial fossa. **(b)** T1-weighted MRI showing lesion in the right internal auditory meatus, with extension to the middle cranial fossa and a small component in the posterior cranial fossa. **(c)** MRI showing a lesion in the right internal auditory meatus, with extension to the middle cranial fossa and a small component in the posterior cranial fossa.

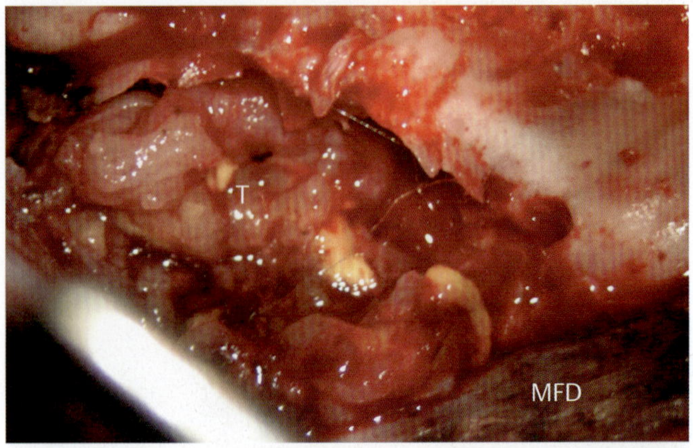

Fig. 69.7 Tumor seen abutting the middle cranial fossa floor anterior to the internal auditory meatus.

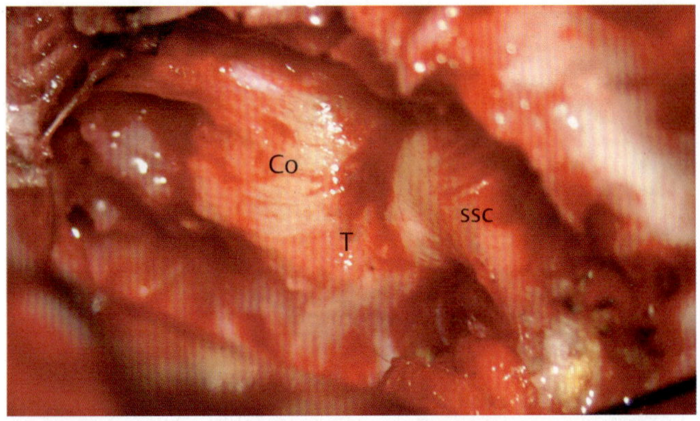

Fig. 69.8 On removing the tumor from the middle fossa, tumor widening the internal auditory meatus is noted. Tumor is also seen posterior to the internal auditory meatus.

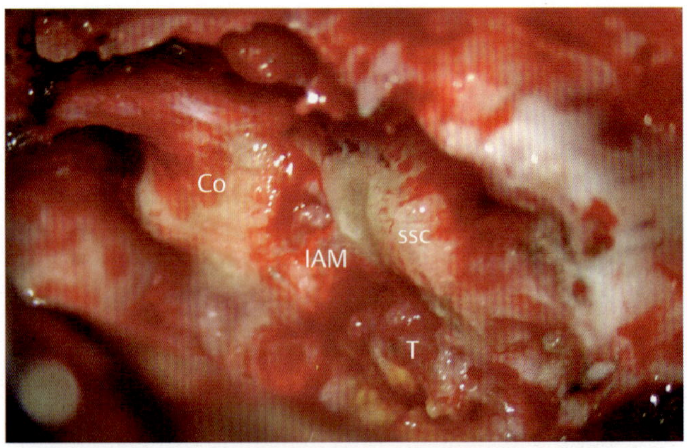

Fig. 69.9 Tumor widening, and eroding the internal auditory meatus, is also present posterior to the internal auditory meatus (IAM; filled with the tumor).

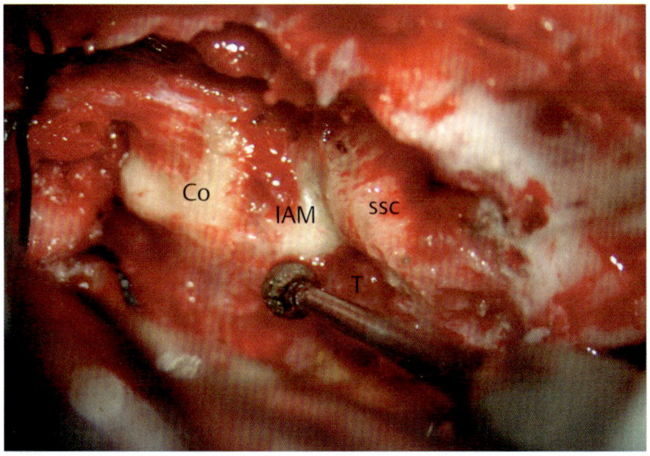

Fig. 69.10 Drilling toward the fundus to expose the tumor completely in the internal auditory meatus (IAM; filled with the tumor).

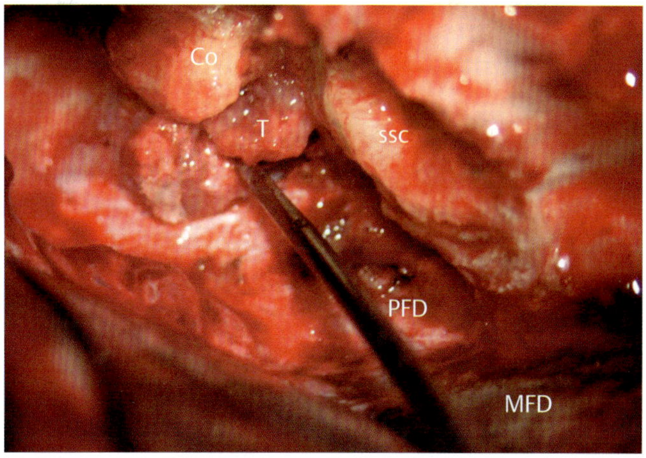

Fig. 69.11 Tumor at the fundus of the internal auditory meatus (IAM; filled with the tumor).

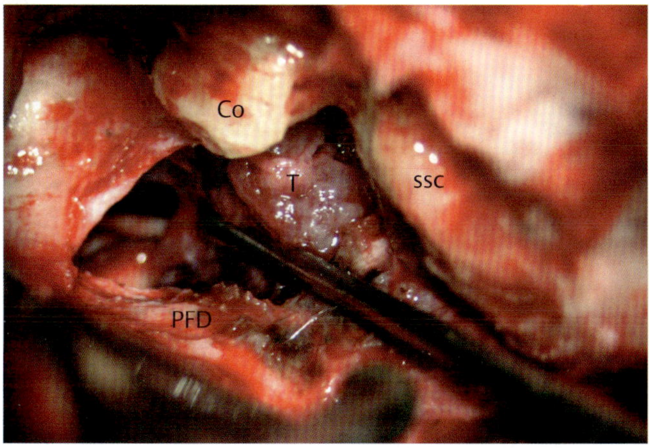

Fig. 69.12 Tumor extension into the posterior fossa.

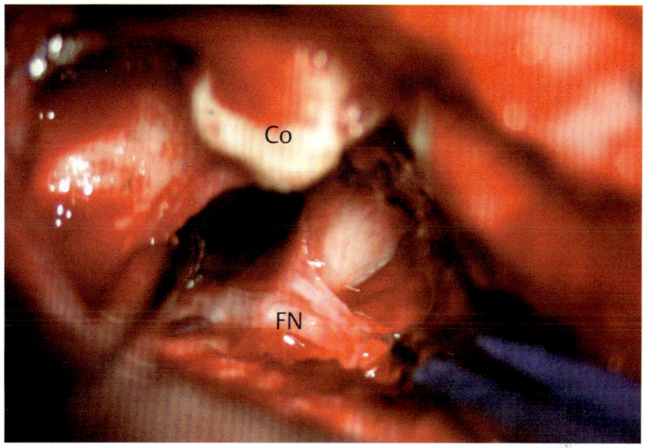

Fig. 69.13 Being a facial nerve schwannoma, facial nerve transected is close to the brainstem.

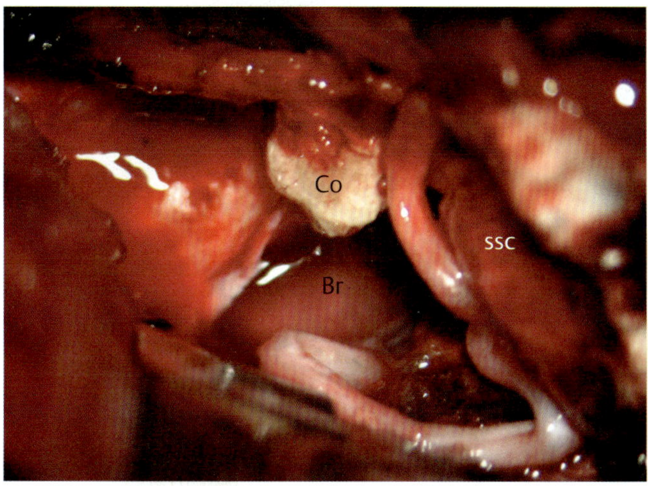

Fig. 69.14 Grafting from the facial nerve at the brainstem to the geniculate ganglion using a sural nerve graft.

- The dural defects are sealed with fat strips, taking care to see that fat obliterates the defect but does not prolapse into the intracranial spaces.
- In case the tegmen is eroded, at the end of the procedure, the roof of the middle ear is reconstructed using cartilage, superior to which a piece of fascia is placed followed by fat.

Suggested Readings

1. Arìstegui M, et al. Surgical anatomy of the extended middle cranial fossa approach. Skull Base Surg. 1994;4(4):181-8
2. Lipschitz N, Kohlberg GD, Zuccarello M, Samy RN. Comprehensive review of the extended middle cranial fossa approach. Curr Opin Otolaryngol Head Neck Surg. 2018; 26(5):286-292

Section XXVIII

Otogenic Infections and Tumors

Chapter 70

Single-Stage Transmastoid Drainage of Otogenic Intracranial Abscess

K.P. Morwani, Madhuri Mehta, and Narayan Jayashankar

Introduction

The commonest cause of abscesses in the temporal lobe and the cerebellum is a chronic ear infection. Incidence of intracranial abscess, whether extradural, subdural, or brain abscess, is 41% in cholesteatomatous ears and 59% in noncholesteatomatous ears, that is, ears with granulation tissue disease. A high-resolution computed tomography scan is useful to study complications because of the otogenic focus of disease. In most cases, authors can clearly delineate the erosion of some part of temporal bone leading to abscesses in adjacent locations like perisinus area, posterior cranial fossa, or temporoparietal lobe area.

Morbidity and mortality of otogenic intracranial abscesses will be least when both the pathologies are dealt with simultaneously, preferably at the same time and under the same anesthesia. In cases where the neurosurgeon has drained the abscess in an emergency state to save the life of the patient or in a situation where the otogenic intracranial abscess is not in continuity with the mastoid disease site, the otogenic focus is dealt with as early as possible, preferably within 12 to 24 hours of the neurosurgical drainage procedure.

Indications

- Cerebritis secondary to an ear infection.
- Intracranial abscess which can be extradural, subdural, or brain abscess associated with the otogenic focus.

It is hereby highlighted that in noncholesteatomatous ears, a canal wall up mastoidectomy is performed followed by delineating the tract leading to the abscess. However, in cholesteatomatous ears, a canal wall down mastoidectomy is performed, followed by removal of cholesteatoma and then delineating the tract leading to the abscess. A suitable cavity obliteration procedure as also ossicular reconstruction with cartilage is performed during the primary otogenic surgery.

Case examples of both situations are as follows.

Surgical Steps

Case 1

Right-sided cholesteatoma with right temporal lobe abscess. Relevant images of the scans are shown in **Fig. 70.1a–c**.

1. On the right side, a postaural C-shaped incision is given 2 to 3 mm behind postaural groove starting from temporal region to 1 cm below the mastoid tip.
2. Temporalis fascia graft of at least 3 × 3 cm dimension is harvested (**Fig. 70.2**).
3. A posteroinferiorly based musculoperiosteal flap is developed (**Fig. 70.3**). For this, one horizontal incision is taken from the base of the zygoma to the junction of the transverse sinus with the upper end of the sigmoid sinus. A second curvilinear incision is taken along the bony margin of the external auditory meatus. The musculoperiosteal flaps are elevated and the cortex of the mastoid is exposed (**Fig. 70.4** and **Fig. 70.5**).
4. Skin of external auditory meatus (tympanomeatal flap) is separated from the bony meatus in three-fourth circumference, that is, posteriorly, superiorly, and inferiorly (**Fig. 70.6**).
5. Tympanomeatal flap is elevated below annulus and reflected anteriorly to expose the bony meatus and bony annulus in over three-fourth circumference (**Fig. 70.7**).
6. Canalplasty is performed if needed (**Fig. 70.8**). It can be performed in a single quadrant or along the whole circumference depending on the narrowing in bony external auditory meatus. It is important to preserve the integrity of meatal skin which is reflected anteriorly while doing canalplasty. An aluminum foil is used when required to protect the skin from the burr.
7. Canal wall down mastoidectomy is performed for extensive cholesteatomas by drilling around and lateral to cholesteatoma till we reach the end of cholesteatoma (**Fig. 70.9, Fig. 70.10** and **Fig. 70.11**), which is then removed in continuity toward the middle ear (**Fig. 70.12**). The posterior canal wall is lowered to the level of the fallopian canal. The facial ridge is thinned, which essentially means drilling the bone between the annulus and the mastoidal segment of the fallopian canal to expose the sinus tympani completely. All cells beneath the excised cholesteatoma sac and in the mastoid cavity (sinodural, perilabyrinthine, retrolabyrinthine, infralabyrinthine, and mastoid tip cells) are drilled off to polish the cavity. A smooth dural plate and the sigmoid plate of bone is left over the

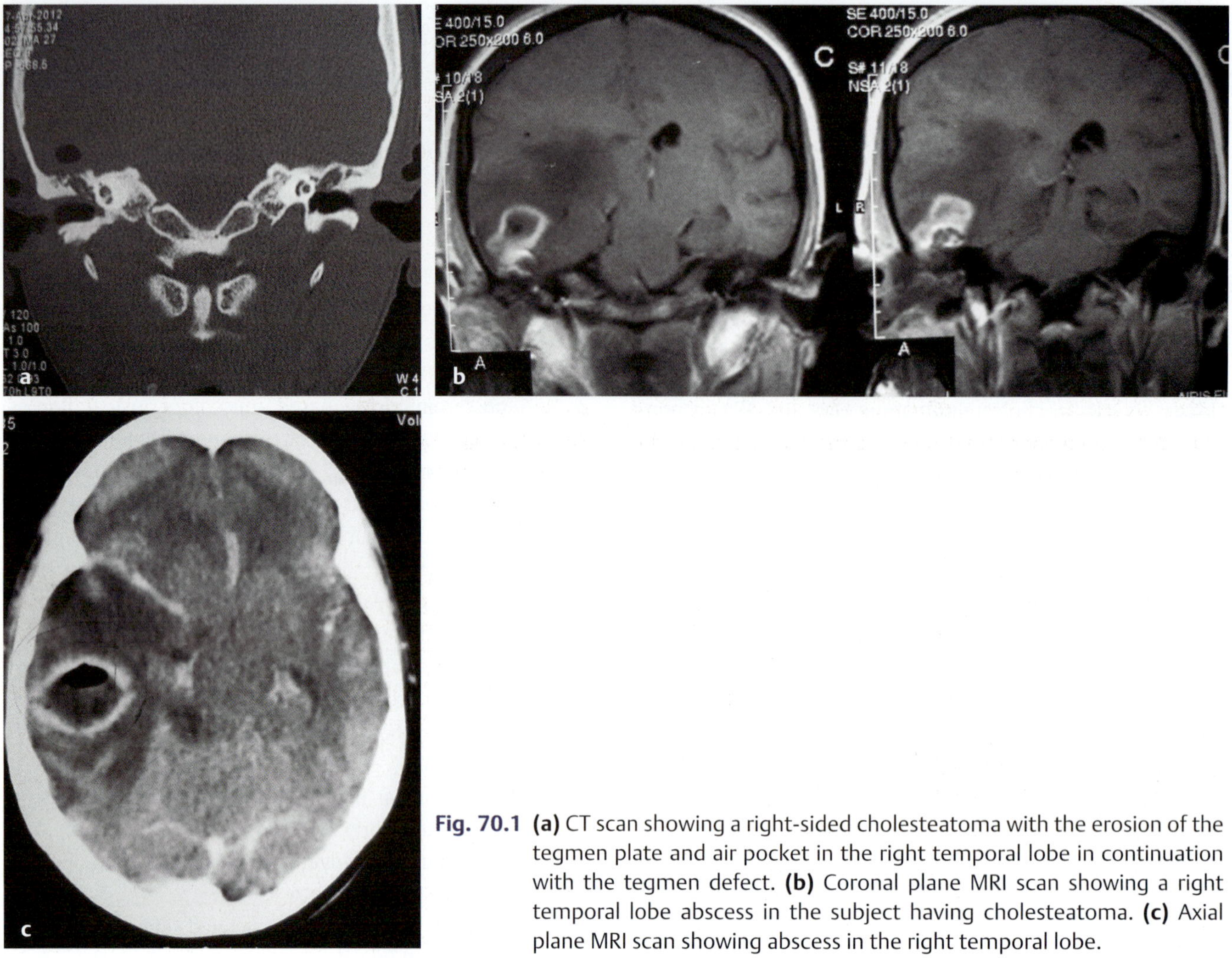

Fig. 70.1 **(a)** CT scan showing a right-sided cholesteatoma with the erosion of the tegmen plate and air pocket in the right temporal lobe in continuation with the tegmen defect. **(b)** Coronal plane MRI scan showing a right temporal lobe abscess in the subject having cholesteatoma. **(c)** Axial plane MRI scan showing abscess in the right temporal lobe.

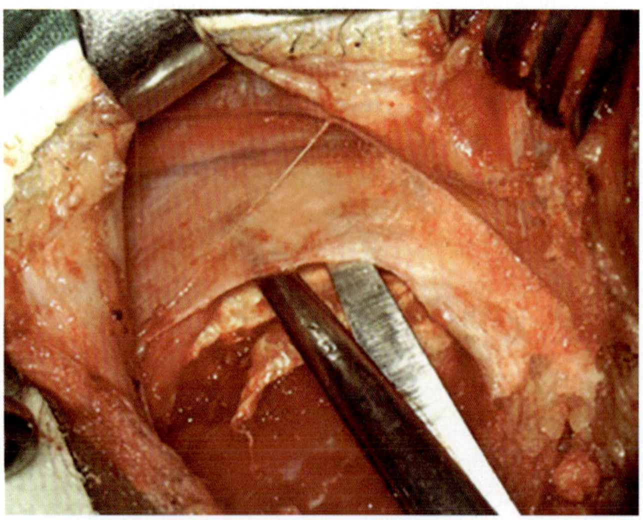

Fig. 70.2 Temporalis fascia graft is harvested.

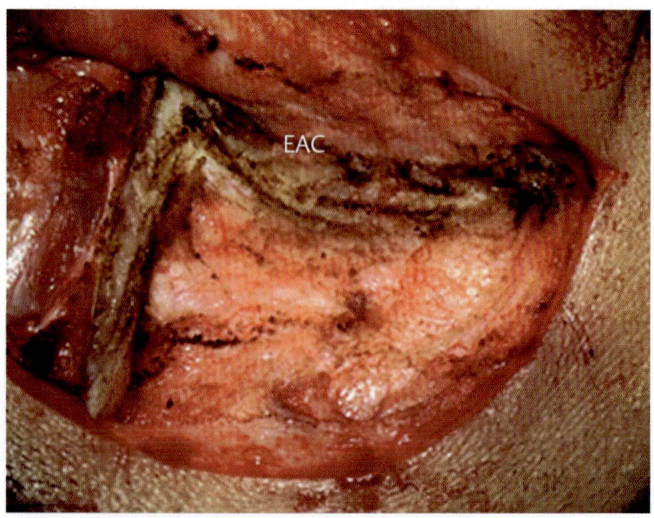

Fig. 70.3 Posteroinferiorly based musculoperiosteal flap is developed.

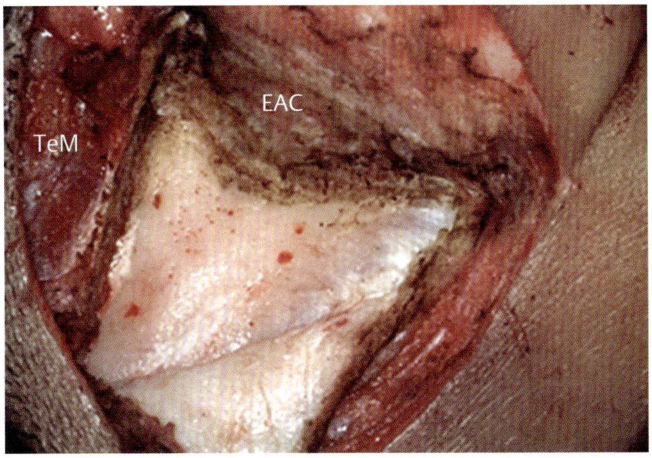

Fig. 70.4 Musculoperiosteal flap is elevated to expose the mastoid cortex widely.

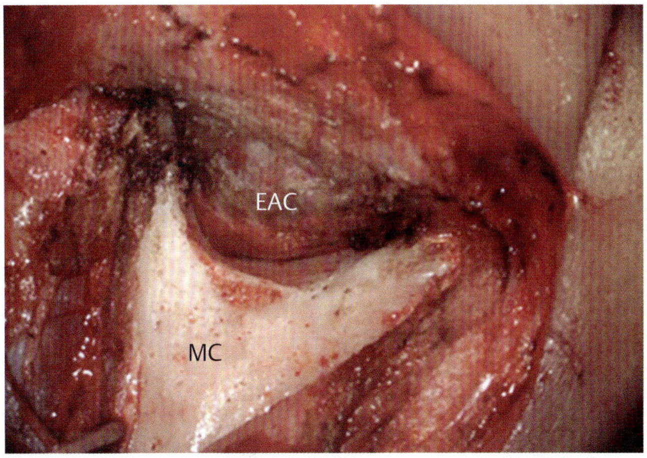

Fig. 70.5 Flaps are sutured to expose the mastoid cortex completely.

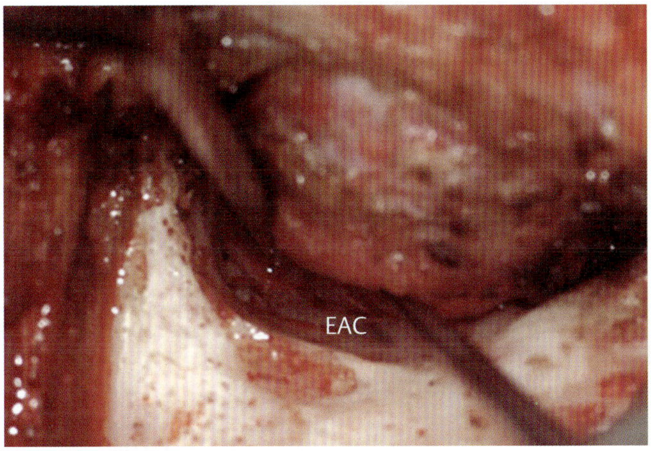

Fig. 70.6 Elevation of the tympanomeatal flap in three-fourths of its circumference.

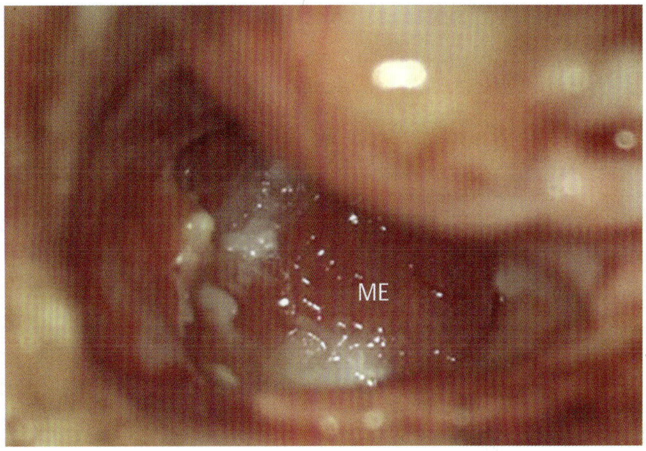

Fig. 70.7 Tympanomeatal flap is elevated below the annulus and is reflected anteriorly.

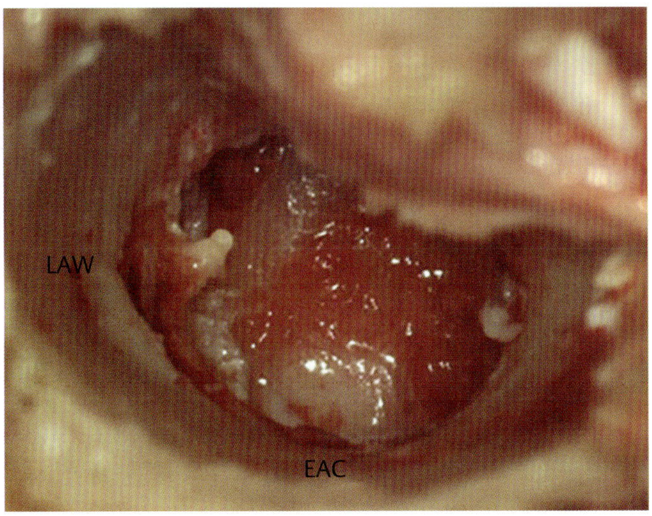

Fig. 70.8 Widening of the external auditory canal from lateral to medial.

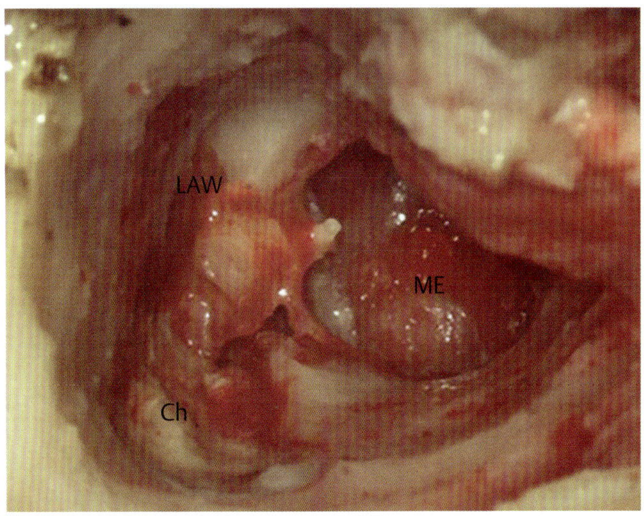

Fig. 70.9 Drilling has been started from the attic (inside out approach).

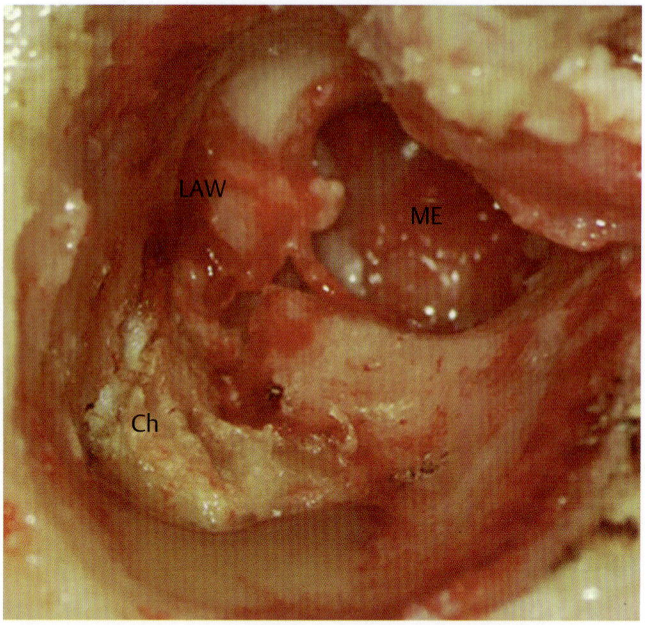

Fig. 70.10 Drilling is performed around and lateral to the cholesteatoma matrix.

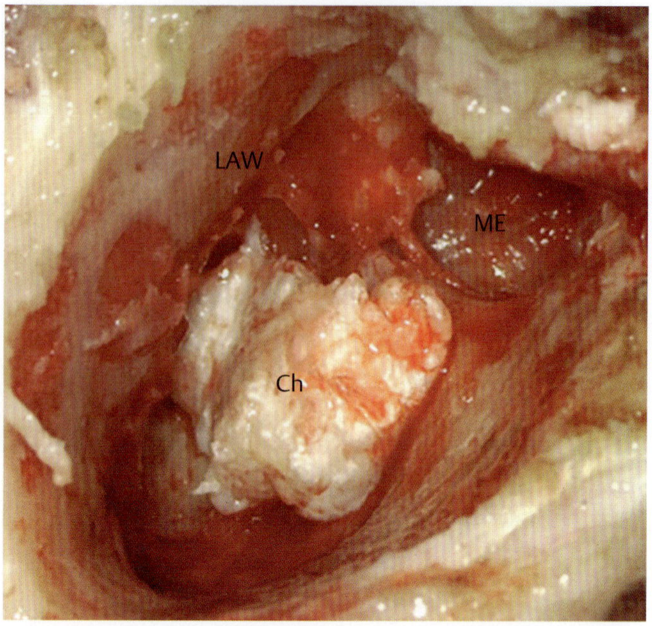

Fig. 70.11 Cholesteatoma matrix is extending in the mastoid. Cholesteatoma is exposed in all areas before removal in continuity.

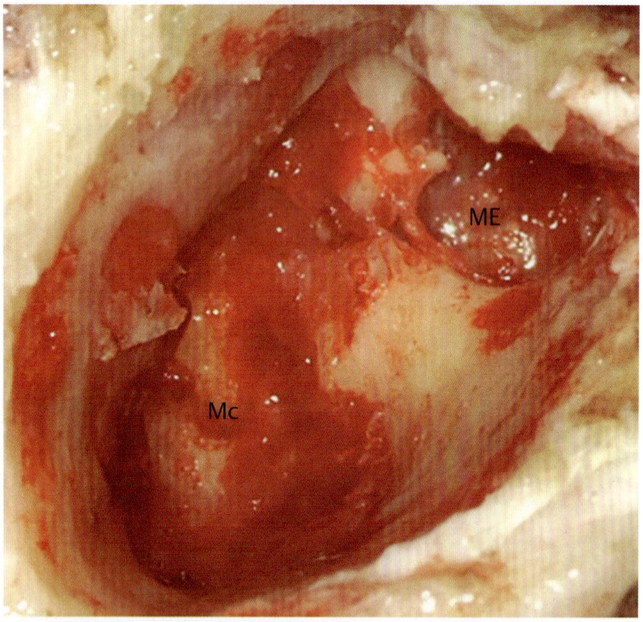

Fig. 70.12 Cholesteatoma sac is excised completely from the mastoid to the middle ear.

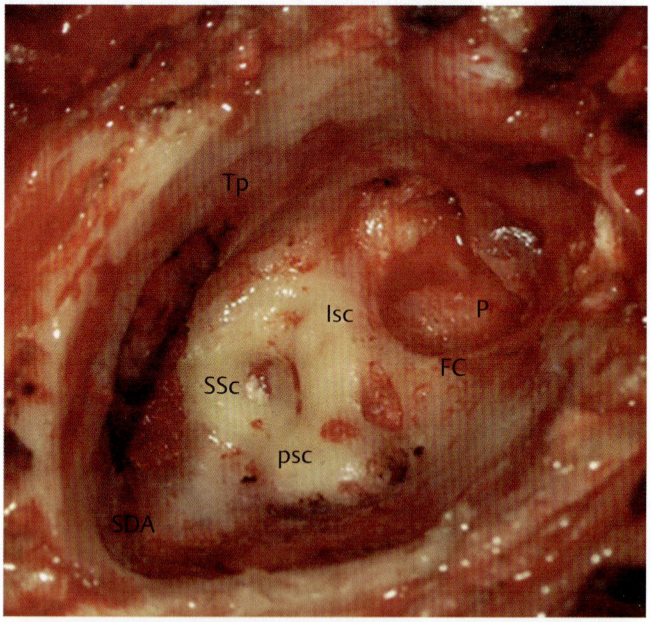

Fig. 70.13 Mastoid cavity is polished by drilling off cells deep to excised cholesteatoma.

respective structures. Cavity is saucerized and smooth, a single cavity is created (**Fig. 70.13**).

8. The thin plate over the tegmen dura, posterior fossa dura, or sigmoid sinus is inspected for erosion in correlation with computed tomography (CT) scan findings, depending on the site of the abscess.
9. During removal of the unhealthy mucosa from the dural plate in this case, the infective tract in continuation with the abscess capsule is identified (**Fig. 70.14**).
10. On teasing the disease tract, the abscess capsule opens up and the purulent material gushes into the operative field. The mouth of the abscess facing the mastoid

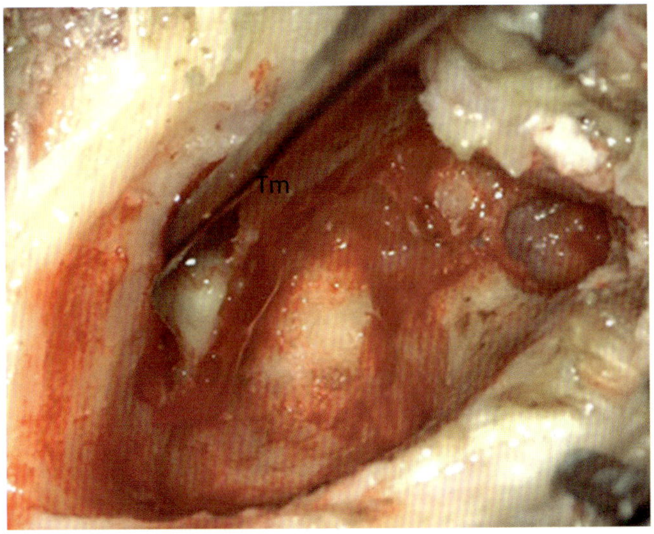

Fig. 70.14 Abscess site is located in the tegmen mastoidale.

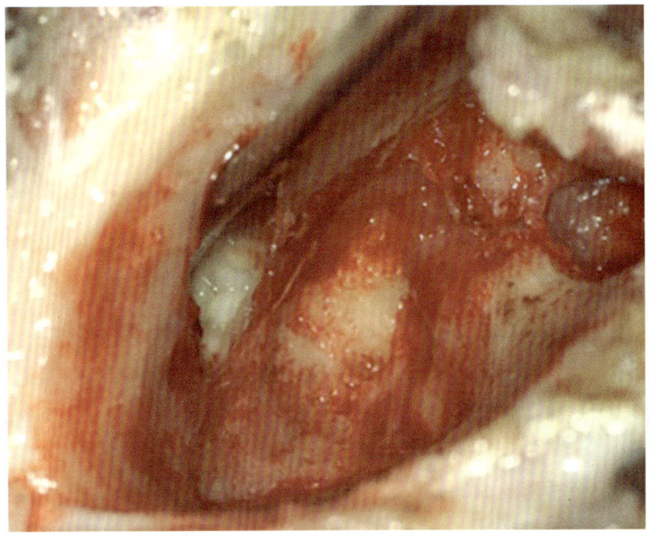

Fig. 70.15 Wall of abscess facing the mastoid cavity is removed and pus evacuated.

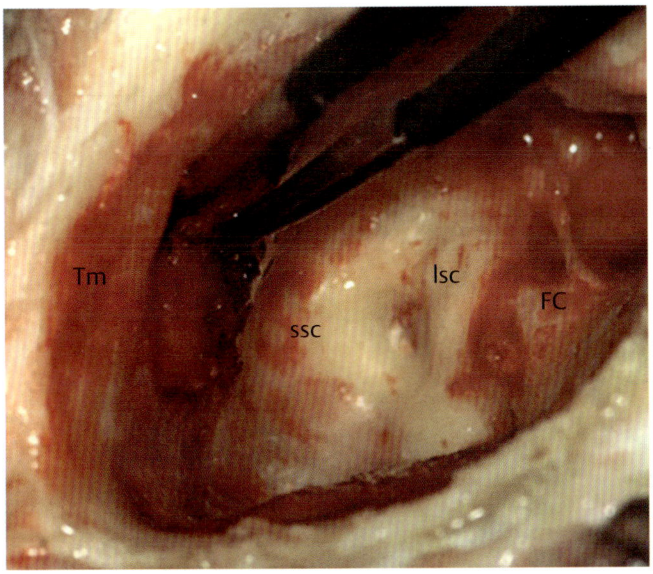

Fig. 70.16 Bipolar cauterization of the infective tissue around the mouth of the abscess cavity.

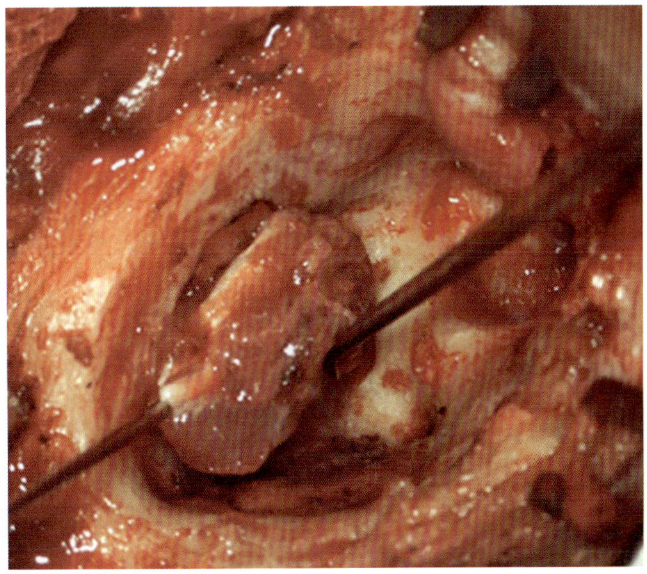

Fig. 70.17 Muscle graft to plug the dural defect.

cavity is opened widely to open up the abscess completely (**Fig. 70.15**).

11. The abscess cavity is then repeatedly washed with dilute hydrogen peroxide and povidone-iodine (1:10). The lavage is discontinued only after the returning fluid is clear. In cases where possible, a 0-degree endoscope is used to visualize inside the abscess cavity to ensure complete evacuation of pus and infective debris.
12. Unhealthy tissue around the mouth of the abscess cavity is cauterized (**Fig. 70.16**).
13. The mouth of the abscess cavity/dural defect is then plugged with a free muscle graft harvested from the local site. The muscle graft is pushed into the defect in all directions up to two-thirds of its length, and the remaining one-third lies outside the mouth of the abscess cavity so that the opening is plugged like a cork (**Fig. 70.17** and **Fig. 70.18**).
14. Second layer of graft is the temporalis fascia graft which is spread over the plugged dural defect extending to the healthy dura, thereby reinforcing the primary repair. The temporalis fascia is placed between

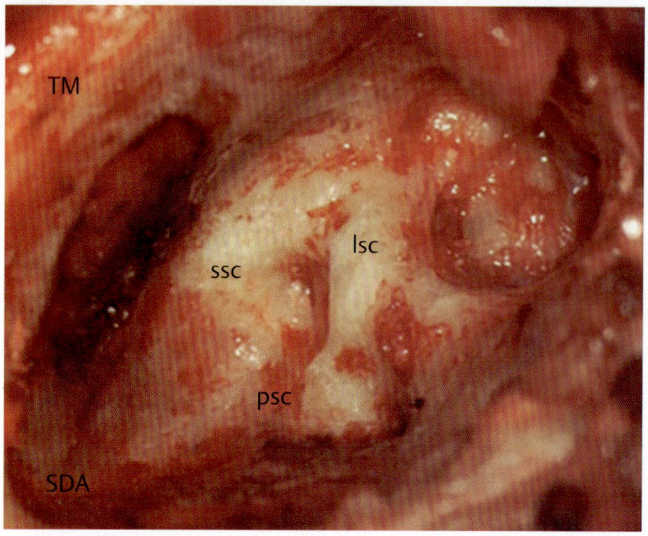

Fig. 70.18 Muscle graft is plugged into the defect in the tegmen mastoidale.

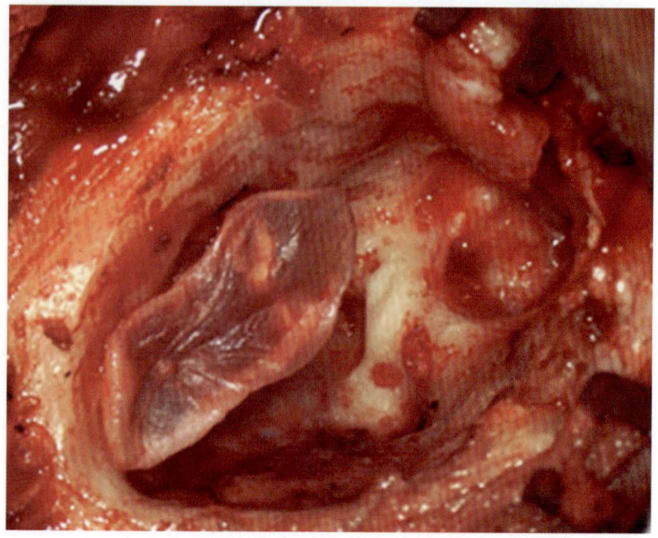

Fig. 70.19 Temporalis fascia graft is used as a second layer of grafting (to be placed on the intracranial side of the dural plate).

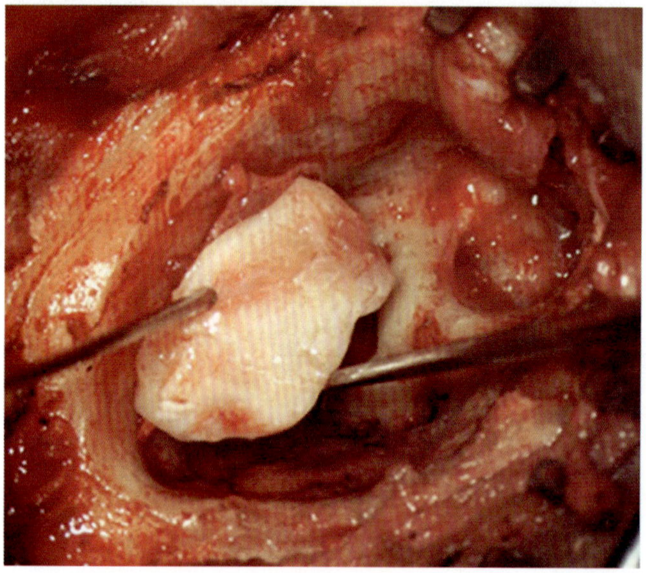

Fig. 70.20 Cartilage is harvested to be used to repair the tegmen bony defect.

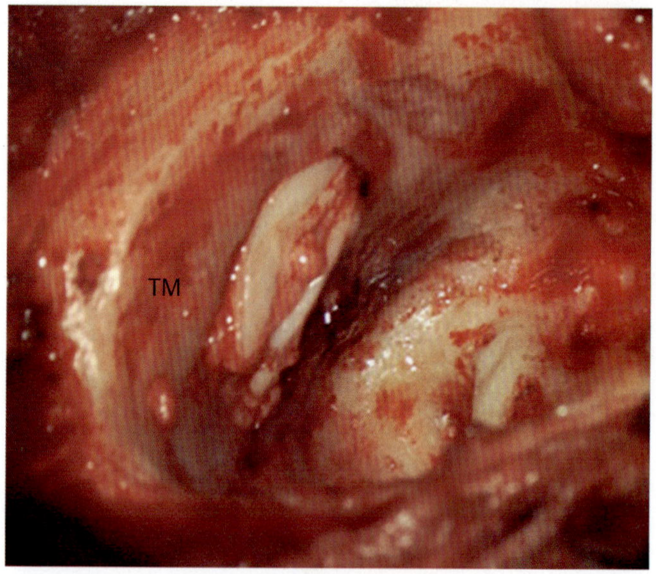

Fig. 70.21 Cartilage is used as a third layer of reinforcement.

the muscle plug and the intracranial surface of the dural plate (**Fig. 70.19**).

15. A piece of harvested cartilage (usually tragal cartilage) is used as the third layer for the closure of bony defect of tegmen or posterior fossa dura (**Fig. 70.20**). This piece of cartilage is placed on the intracranial side of the dural plate wedged under the bony edges of the defect (**Fig. 70.21**).
16. Once the repair of the bony defect is complete, reconstructive procedures for hearing are taken up in the form of ossiculoplasty (depending on the residual ossicles left with us). We prefer cartilage ossiculoplasty (**Fig. 70.22**) in these cases (first stage). If hearing augmentation is needed, a second stage ossiculoplasty is performed with the desired ossicular prosthesis.
17. Obliteration of the cavity can be achieved using bone dust (**Fig. 70.23**) or cartilage, and if the cavity is big, we use pedicled muscle flap. A fascia graft lines the whole mastoid cavity (**Fig. 70.24**).
18. Adequate meatoplasty is done. The aim should be to line the exposed mastoid cavity with temporalis fascia graft or skin (**Fig. 70.25** and **Fig. 70.26**).

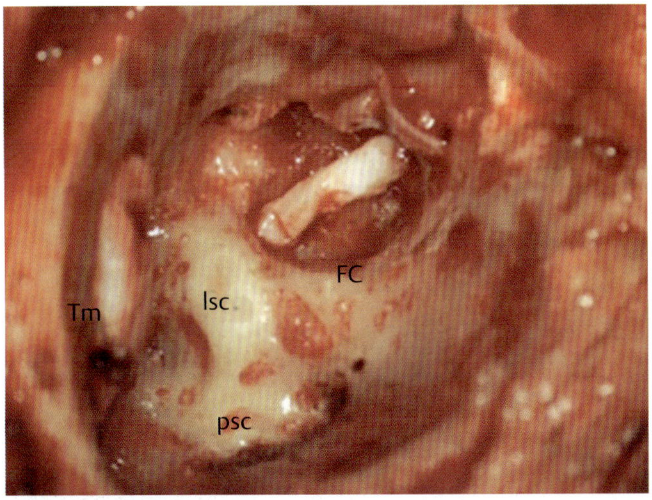

Fig. 70.22 Cartilage ossiculoplasty is performed from the head of stapes to the anteroinferior annulus.

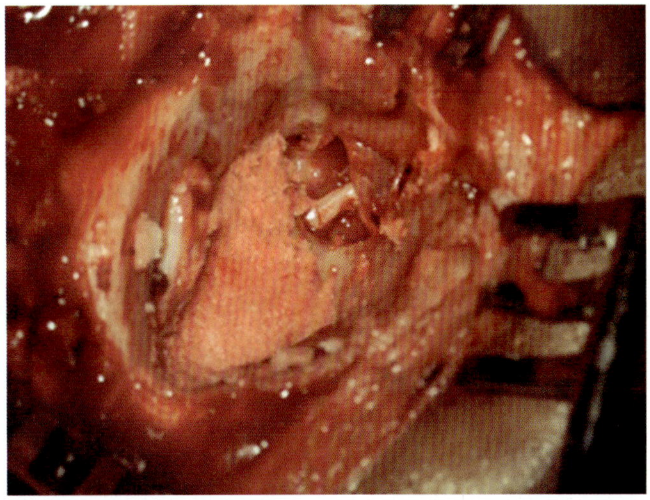

Fig. 70.23 Bone dust is collected from the healthy cortical bone that is used to obliterate cavity.

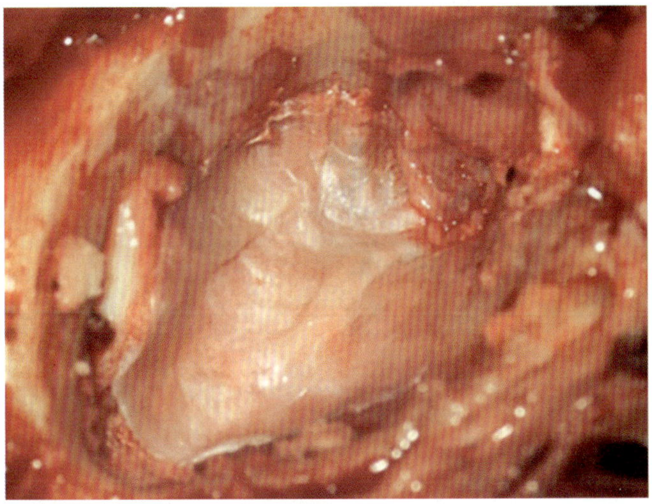

Fig. 70.24 Temporalis fascia graft is used to line the obliterated cavity.

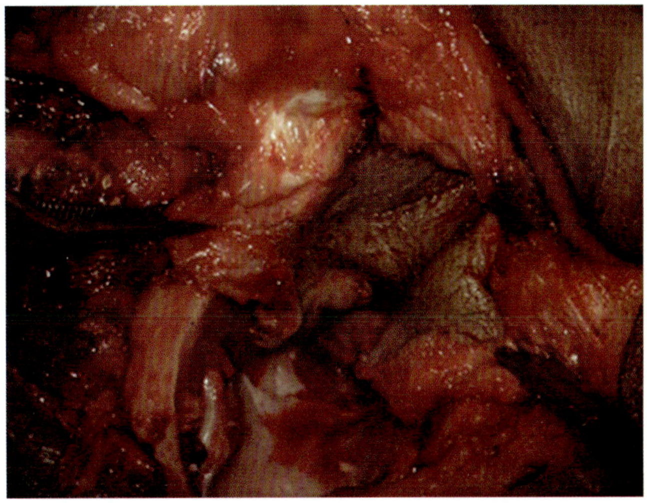

Fig. 70.25 Skin of the external auditory canal has been opened up.

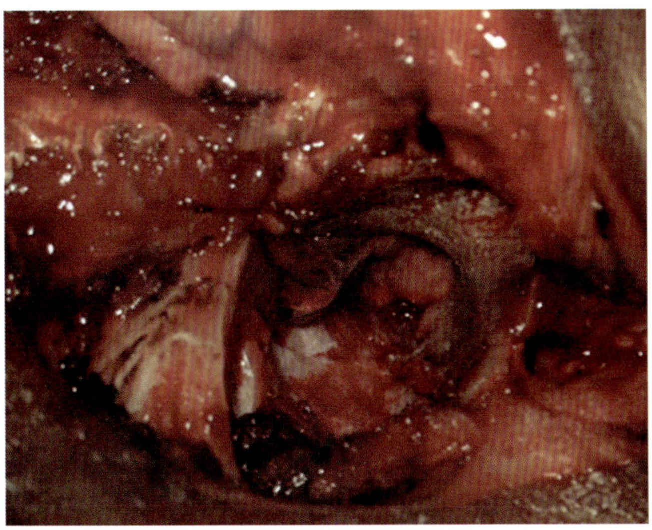

Fig. 70.26 Meatoplasty flaps are sutured superiorly and inferiorly.

Case 2

Right-sided cholesteatoma with a right perisinus abscess (**Fig. 70.27a, b**). The initial steps of surgery remain the same and only the main steps are shown in **Fig. 70.28, Fig. 70.29, Fig. 70.30,** and **Fig. 70.31**.

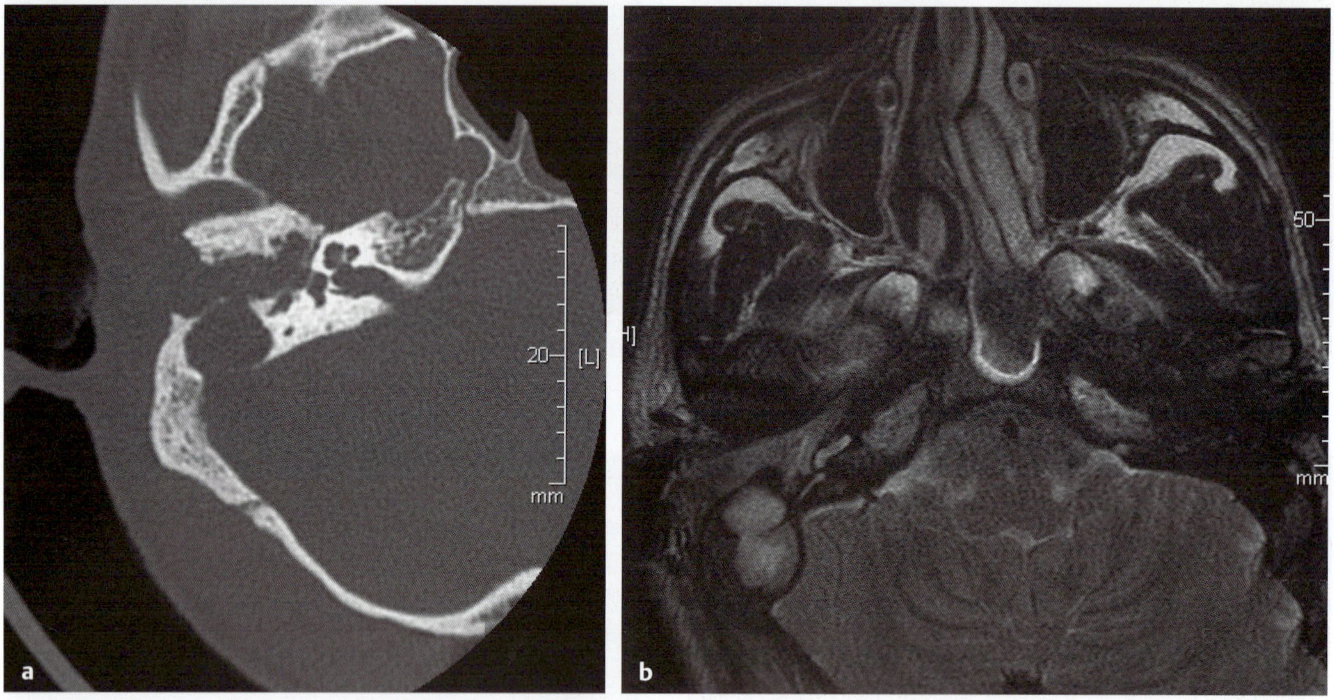

Fig. 70.27 **(a)** CT scan showing a right-sided cholesteatoma with the erosion of the bone around the sigmoid sinus and presigmoid posterior fossa dura. **(b)** MRI scan showing a right-sided perisinus abscess.

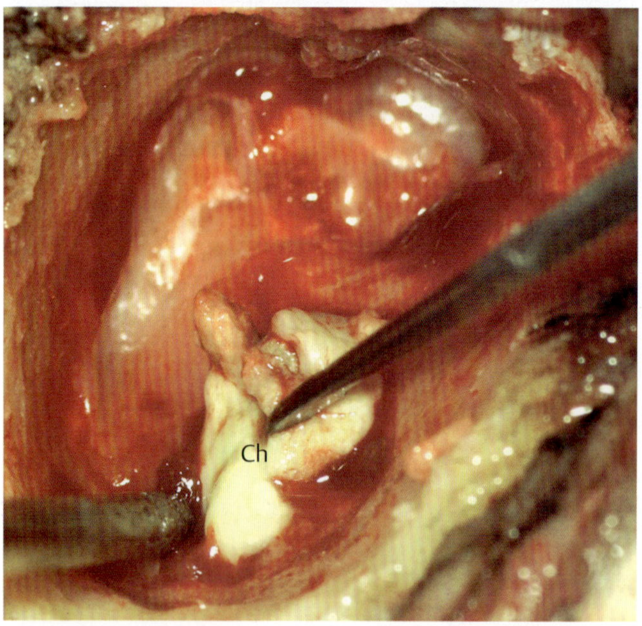

Fig. 70.28 Cholesteatoma that caused perisinus abscess, which extended to the presigmoid posterior fossa dura, is being excised.

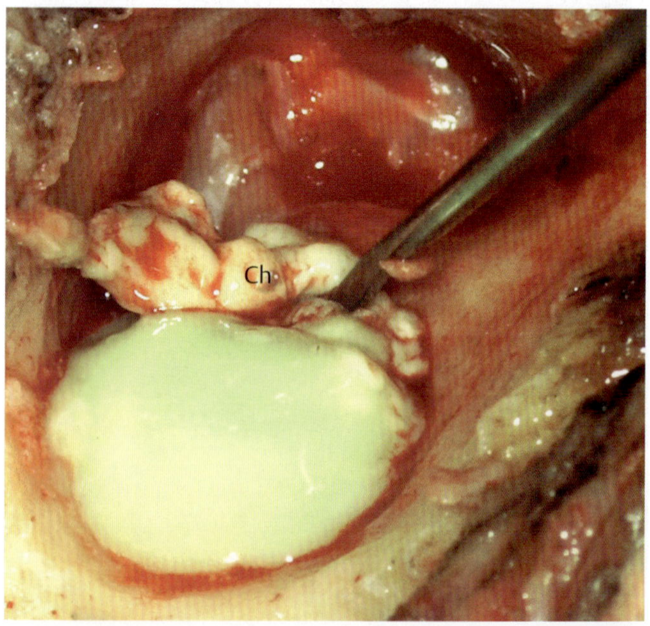

Fig. 70.29 Perisinus abscess is draining into the mastoid cavity.

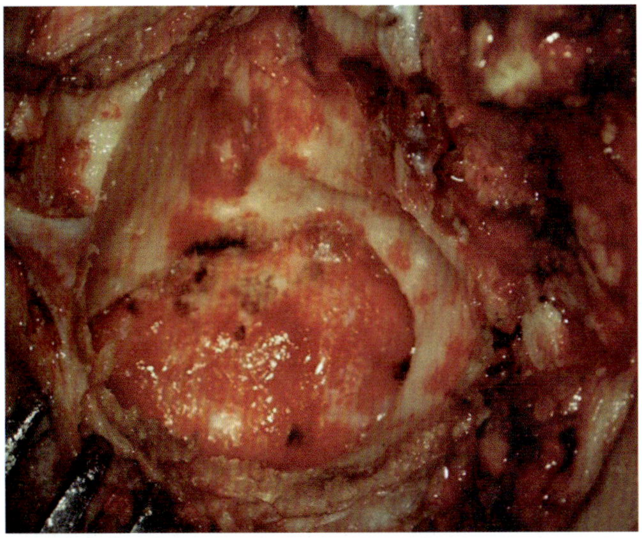

Fig. 70.30 Following removal of cholesteatoma and drainage of abscess, the healthy sigmoid sinus and presigmoid posterior fossa dura are seen.

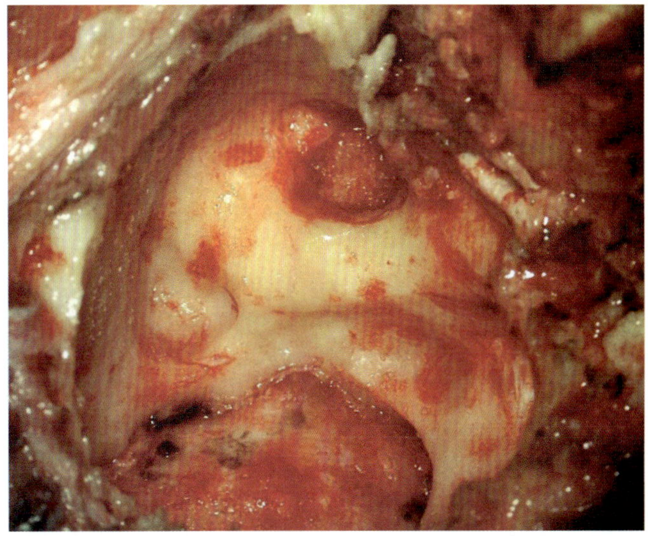

Fig. 70.31 Cellular tracts in mastoid cavity are cleared to achieve a smooth, well-saucerized cavity.

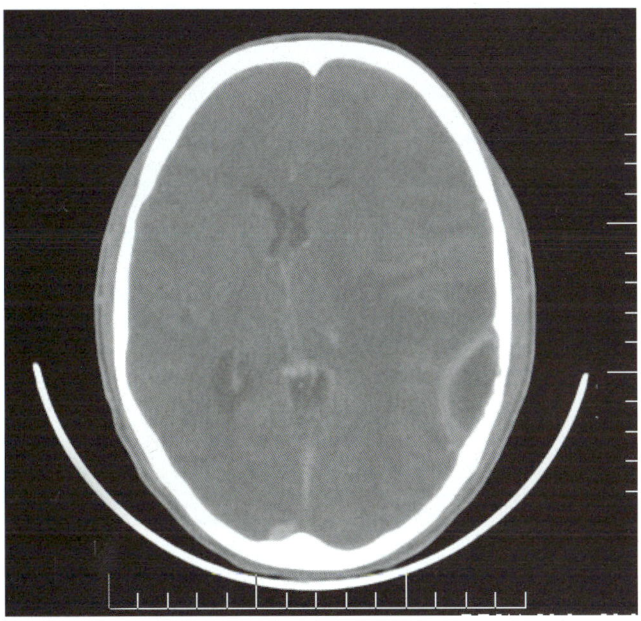

Fig. 70.32 Temporal lobe abscess, left side.

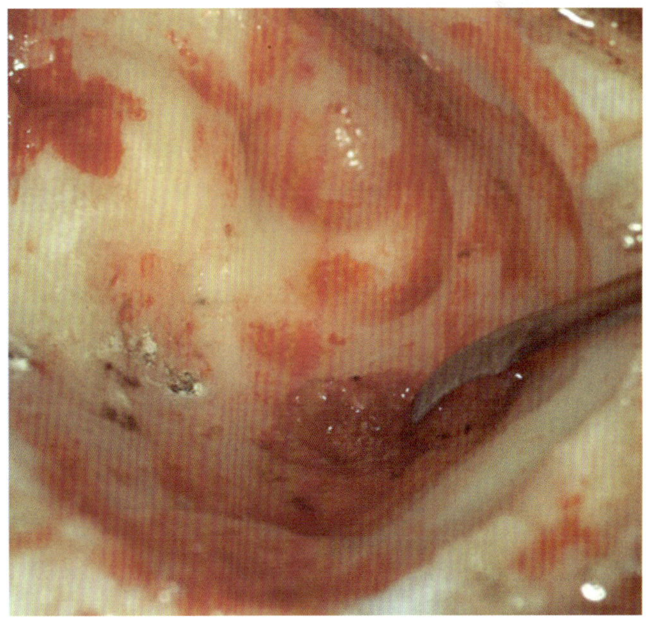

Fig. 70.33 Left side—Granulation tissue is seen at the junction of the upper end of sigmoid sinus and tegmen mastoidale at the sinodural angle area.

Case 3

A right-sided temporal lobe abscess is seen adjacent to tegmen mastoidale at the sinodural angle area with no evidence of cholesteatoma (**Fig. 70.32**).

1. Since there is no associated cholesteatoma, a cortical mastoidectomy is performed on the left side.
2. On clearing the cells in the mastoid cavity, usually an area of granulation tissue is seen (**Fig. 70.33**). Drilling over this granulation exposes more and more granulation than was evident in the initial view. The granulation tissue is bipolarized and excised (**Fig. 70.34** and **Fig. 70.35**). The granulation tissue tract is followed by removing more bone over it till a healthy area is reached.

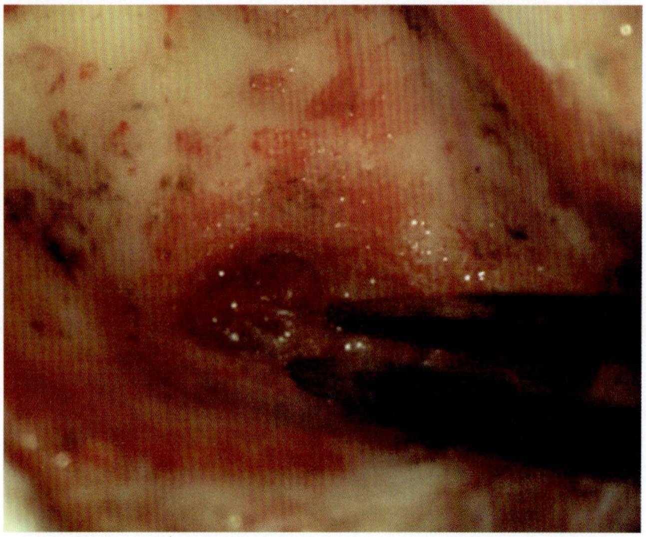

Fig. 70.34 Granulation tissue is bipolarized and excised.

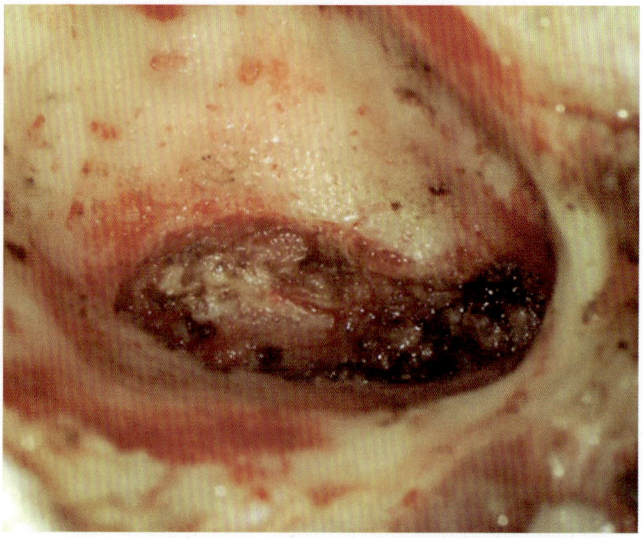

Fig. 70.35 Granulation tissue is seen bipolarized at sinodural angle area. Note how much more granulation tissue is exposed as compared to **Fig. 70.34**.

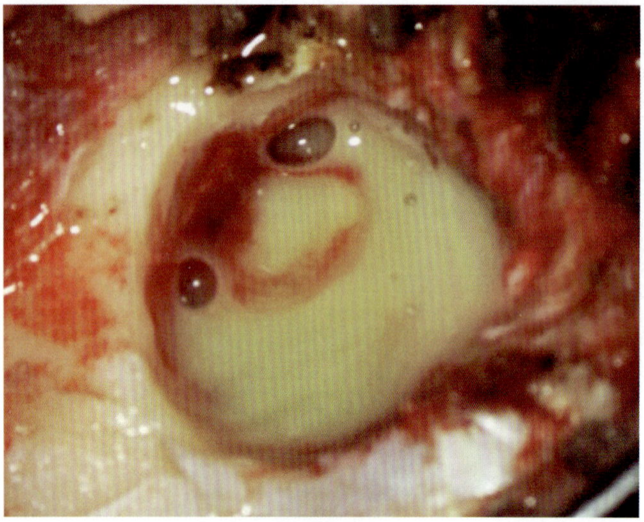

Fig. 70.36 Pus in the mastoid cavity.

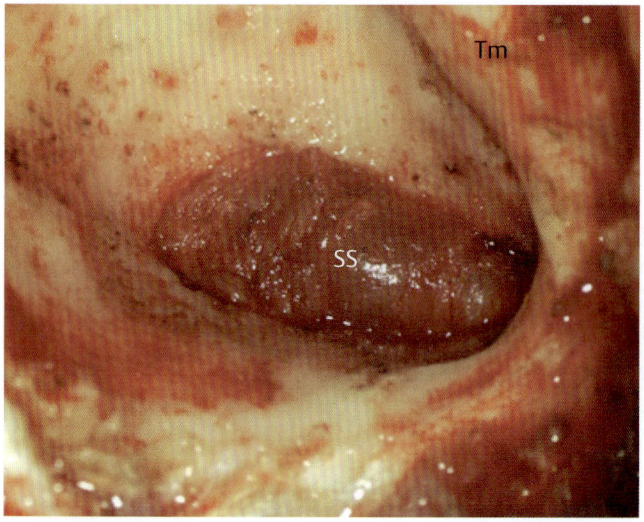

Fig. 70.37 Healthy sigmoid sinus.

3. On teasing the granulation tissue, a pus tract is seen and on probing this tract, a sudden gush of pus is seen in the cavity (**Fig. 70.36**).
4. The tract is lavaged with a diluted mixture of betadine and hydrogen peroxide. All infected granulation tissue around the area is excised after bipolarization to have healthy tissue all around (**Fig. 70.37**).
5. Closure of musculoperiosteal and skin layers is performed as for any cortical mastoidectomy.

Tips and Pearls

- Extradural, subdural, brain, and perisinus abscesses with an otogenic focus are associated more often in noncholesteatomatous ears compared to cholesteatomatous ears.
- Every otogenic brain abscess need not be in continuity with temporal bone pathology. It has to be addressed conventionally. However, we prefer that the brain

abscess and the temporal pathology be dealt with in the same anesthesia, wherever possible.

- If the subject is drowsy or comatose because of the pathology and the abscess, the abscess and the pathology must be dealt with as early as possible. If the abscess is in continuity with the middle ear cleft, a single-stage transmastoid route can still be performed.
- The procedure offers the advantage that the dural or tegmen defect is repaired, thus preventing the possibility of a persistent source of infection.
- In cases of cholesteatoma with surrounding abscess, we recommend that after eradication of the cholesteatoma, a partial obliteration of cavity or reduction in size of the cavity is to be performed along with tympanoplasty, similar to routine management of cholesteatoma. Additionally, although the subject is always informed about a second stage ossiculoplasty, we perform ossiculoplasty in the first stage itself. A small percentage of cases do benefit significantly in hearing and this obviates the need for a second stage ossiculoplasty in those cases. We use only cartilage for these cases and no prosthesis for first stage ossicular reconstruction.
- In case of a big dural defect, recurrent brain abscess, or dead ear, authors recommend cul-de-sac closure of the ear.

Suggested Readings

Kurien M, Job A, Mathew J, Chandy M. Otogenic intracranial abscess: concurrent craniotomy and mastoidectomy—changing trends in a developing country. Arch Otolaryngol Head Neck Surg 1998;124(12):1353–1356

Morwani KP, Jayashankar N. Single stage, transmastoid approach for otogenic intracranial abscess. J Laryngol Otol 2009;123(11):1216–1220

Mukherjee D, Das C, Paul D. Single-stage trans-mastoid drainage of otogenic brain abscess: a single-institution experience. Indian J Otolaryngol Head Neck Surg 2016;68(2):179–184

Chapter 71

Subtotal Petrosectomy for Cochlear Implantation

Sampath Chandra Prasad Rao, Ananth Chintapalli, and Kanu Lal Saha

Introduction

Subtotal petrosectomy is an effective procedure in cases of chronic and recurrent middle ear conditions as it obliterates the middle ear, eustachian tube, and the mastoid cavity with a blind sac closure of the external auditory meatus. The procedure can hence be employed for extensive middle ear diseases with significant dural exposure, exposed petrous carotid, and more importantly, where a realistic reconstruction of the conductive hearing mechanism practically stands no chance. The procedure also reduces the dangers of the inner ear fluids getting exposed to the outer environment to a bare minimum.

Subtotal petrosectomy was defined and introduced by Ugo Fisch in 1965 albeit the technique was followed since late 1950s and 1960s.[1,2] Rambo[3] reported the early description of the origins of the procedure as musculoplasty technique for suppurative middle ear disease, where he used the pedicled temporalis muscle flap to obliterate the mastoid cavity but left the external auditory canal open. He later described in another study wherein he obliterated the external auditory canal in a blind sac fashion using an endaural incision without obliterating the eustachian tube.[4] Fritz and Crawford[5] and Tschopp, in 1960, published a large series based on this technique. Gacek, in 1976, obliterated the eustachian tube, the external auditory canal in a blind sac fashion and obliterated the cavity with abdominal fat harvest using postauricular approach in complicated cases with dural exposure and cerebrospinal fluid (CSF) leak.[6-9] Although several terms such as middle ear obliteration and total obliteration of the mastoid, middle ear cleft, and the external auditory canal had been used, Ugo Fisch distinguished subtotal petrosectomy from other lateral skull base procedures. Fisch described the procedure as complete exenteration of all the air cell tracts of the temporal bone including the retrofacial, retrolabyrinthine, pre- and postsigmoid air cells, the supralabyrinthine, infralabyrinthine, peritubal, and the pericarotid air cells.[2]

Subtotal petrosectomy is distinct from the other lateral skull base approaches in a way that it is a more conservative procedure than other procedures as most of the air cell tracts are exenterated leaving behind the cortical bony plates over the middle cranial fossa, posterior cranial fossa, sigmoid sinus, facial nerve, and the otic capsule. Other lateral skull base approaches such as the translabyrinthine and transotic approaches require drilling the labyrinthine block and the bony cover over the middle and the posterior cranial fossae. Subtotal petrosectomy differs from subtotal temporal bone resection in a way that the later involves removing of the entire tympanic bone en bloc along with the anterior canal wall, retroparotid soft tissue, and varying degree of parotid gland and neck node dissection as done in cases of malignancies of the external auditory canal. Subtotal petrosectomy, on the other hand, does not involve drilling of the anterior bony meatal wall and parotid or neck node dissection. Subtotal petrosectomy varies from infratemporal fossa approaches, as the anterior bony meatal wall is drilled and the facial nerve is anteriorly rerouted to reach more deeper structures such as the petrous internal carotid, the jugular bulb, and further anteriorly to gain access into the infratemporal fossa in the later approaches, while, it is not the case with the former. It is erroneous to term any lateral skull base procedure with blind sac closure as subtotal petrosectomy albeit subtotal petrosectomy could be the initial step in many of these procedures.[10]

Indications of Subtotal Petrosectomy for Cochlear Implantation

Indications of subtotal petrosectomy is to eliminate the disease from the tympanomastoid cleft, which essentially do not extend deep into the petrous apex or the internal auditory canal, by exteriorizing multiple air cell tracts and thereby preventing recurrence of the disease. It is a logical option to remove large tumors without intradural extension and in cases which require to eliminate the chance of spreading infection intracranially because of exposure of the dura and the inner ear fluids. A newer philosophy which is gaining much acceptance is cochlear implantation as an indication for subtotal petrosectomy as a surgical option.[11-13] Reported in 1990s as a means to look for residual disease clearance for cases where the cochlear implantation was performed in a staged manner, subtotal petrosectomy when well performed enhances the feasibility of cochlear implantation in the same procedure.

- Chronic otitis media with or without cholesteatoma.
- Osteoradionecrosis of the temporal bone.

- In a preexisting radical cavity or a canal wall down the mastoid cavity.
- Cochlear ossification/obliteration.
- Congenital inner ear malformations.
- Temporal bone fractures disrupting the otic capsule.
- Unfavorable middle ear anatomy.
- Disease in the only hearing ear.
- Extensive skull base lesion with functioning cochlea and cochlear nerve.

Chronic Otitis Media

Approach to the cochlear implant in chronic ear involves ensuring disease clearance before device implantation.[14] The surgical approach varies depending on the clinical scenario. Tympanoplasty alone would suffice in an ear with good eustachian tube function. Intractable chronic otitis media warrants mastoid exploration with an intact canal wall. Nevertheless, these cases do not assure complete disease clearance, in which case subtotal petrosectomy provides a safe option, given the rationale of thorough removal of all the middle ear mucosa as the substrate of chronic inflammation by a radical mastoidectomy and a multilayer blind sac closure of the external auditory canal.

A chronic ear despite several previous surgeries is a prompt indication for a subtotal petrosectomy, where all the air cell tracts of the tympanomastoid cleft are exenterated and the cavity closed in a blind sac after being obliterated with abdominal fat harvest. Chronic otitis media without realistic chance of reconstructing the middle ear air conduction mechanism and the cases with profound hearing loss secondary to the disease itself or by its treatment benefit from a cochlear implant. In the case of chronic otitis media with cholesteatoma where the disease has to be removed completely, cochlear implant is planned in the same sitting, provided a complete disease clearance is assured, or is planned after 6 to 12 months.[15,16]

In severe atelectatic ear, particularly after failed surgical attempts to strengthen the tympanic membrane, subtotal petrosectomy should be the preferred choice as it removes beyond doubt any chances of developing a cholesteatoma at a later stage, or, a possibility of electrode extrusion.

Canal Wall Down Mastoid Cavity

Subtotal petrosectomy is a logical option when cochlear implant is contemplated in an already performed canal wall down mastoid cavity as these cavities have only a thin lining of squamous epithelium, and an attempt to implant the device in them not only renders the electrode array vulnerable for extrusion but also the potential risk of the inner ear fluid getting infected is relatively high. Subtotal petrosectomy minimizes these risks significantly.[17–19]

Cochlear Ossification/Obliteration

Several conditions such as meningogenic labyrinthitis, autoimmune ear disease, chronic middle ear cleft infection, labyrinthine fracture, intracochlear hemorrhage, and persistent perilymphatic fistula leave the cochlea partially or totally obliterated. Cochlear implant in these cases warrants a cochlear drill-out procedure. Performing the cochlear drill-out procedure through the posterior tympanotomy significantly hampers the maneuverability of the instruments and puts several of vital structures like the petrous carotid, the jugular bulb, and the facial nerve at much risk. Subtotal petrosectomy in these cases offers a wide exposure and much control over these structures.[20–23]

Inner Ear Malformations

Subtotal petrosectomy offers a viable option for cochlear implant in cases with inner ear malformations. The degree of aberrations of anatomical landmarks in these cases is relatively high, and an expanded surgical exposure as offered by subtotal petrosectomy significantly reduces the associated complications in such cases while performing cochlear implant. Also, the possibility of CSF gusher/leak is high particularly in IP I and III deformities, and the general incidence of contracting meningitis among these patients even without undergoing cochlear implant is significant when compared with the normal population. Subtotal petrosectomy addresses these aspects as the tympanomastoid cavity is obliterated from the external environment.[24–28]

Temporal Bone Fractures Involving the Otic Capsule

Head trauma leads to temporal bone fracture with disruption of the otic capsule; when not addressed immediately leaves behind not only sensorineural hearing loss but also fibrosis of the labyrinth. Hence, the cochlear implant is a solution to affirm hearing in these patients with patent lumen and an intact cochlear nerve.[29–32] These fractures heal by fibrosis, and cochlear ossification ensues later on. A cochlear drill-out procedure could be the only option at times for inserting the implant. The incidence of meningitis in these cases is high as the risk of infection spreading from the tympanomastoid cavity into the subarachnoid space along these fracture lines exists, and device insertion further increases this potential risk.[33] Subtotal petrosectomy in these cases with a combination of cochlear implantation significantly reduces the incidence of meningitis. Subtotal petrosectomy as a surgical option for cochlear implantation is a newer philosophy gaining much acceptance.

Unfavorable Middle Ear Anatomy

Unfavorable anatomy as extremely forward-lying sigmoid sinus, high jugular bulb, in cases of meningocele makes viewing the round window and electrode insertion difficult through posterior tympanotomy.[34] Subtotal petrosectomy in anatomically challenging cases gives a better view, control over these structures, and electrode array insertion.

Disease in the Only Hearing Ear

It is often encountered where pathologies such as intractable chronic otitis media, with or without cholesteatoma, paragangliomas, and many such tumors involving the only the hearing ear and the individual ends in a severe to profound hearing loss. Simultaneous cochlear implantation after disease clearance by subtotal petrosectomy is a viable option in such cases.

Contraindications

The presence of residual hearing on the operating side is an absolute contraindication for a subtotal petrosectomy as the spared hearing can be utilized by electroacoustic stimulation,[35] which can be augmented with an intrameatal hearing device, for which a patent external auditory canal is required. The other relative contraindications of the procedure include the presence of active infection, particularly of purulent nature, osteomyelitis of the temporal bone, despite prolonged antibiotic therapy, cholesteatoma of the tympanomastoid cleft after multiple surgeries, and where the surgeon is not sure of complete disease clearance. Subtotal petrosectomy in these cases is performed in a staged manner, 3 to 6 months after the initial disease clearance procedure.

Procedure

The procedure and steps of subtotal petrosectomy for cochlear implantation is described below as performed in a patient with significant chronic otitis and hearing loss in the only hearing ear with long-standing total deafness on the opposite side.

A wide retroauricular incision (**Fig. 71.1**) is usually required, but varies depending on the pathology that is being addressed. A cervical extension if required is added to the incision for the exposure as done for ITFA-A.

The subcutaneous tissue is raised as an anteriorly based flap after giving a "T-shaped" incision (**Fig. 71.2** and **Fig. 71.3**). The external auditory meatal skin is incised at the bony cartilaginous junction as lateral as possible considering the fact that the meatal skin is thicker laterally. The meatal skin is freed all along its attachments, and from the tragal cartilage anteriorly, it is then everted exteriorly and sutured tightly with 3–0 resorbable sutures. The conchal and the tragal cartilages are sutured together, thus forming a second inner layer of the blind sac closure (**Fig. 71.4**). The anteriorly based subcutaneous flap is then inverted and reposed over this cartilaginous second layer and sutured to the surrounding soft tissue thereby further reinforcing the blind sac closure. The meatal skin medial to the blind sac is then meticulously elevated from the bony meatus, taking utmost care not to leave behind any traces of squamous epithelium to avoid entrapped cholesteatoma at a later stage. The elevated meatal skin along with the fibrous tympanic annulus and the ossicular chain except for the stapes infrastructure is removed.

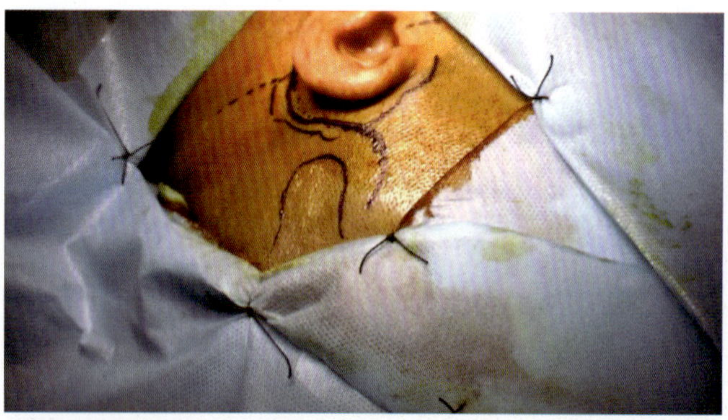

Fig. 71.1 Incision marking for subtotal petrosectomy with simultaneous cochlear implantation on the left ear in a case of intractable chronic otitis media with extensive granulations.

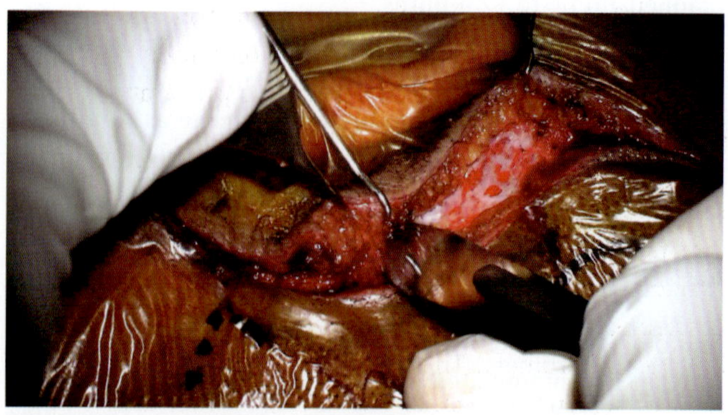

Fig. 71.2 Skin incision and subcutaneous dissection.

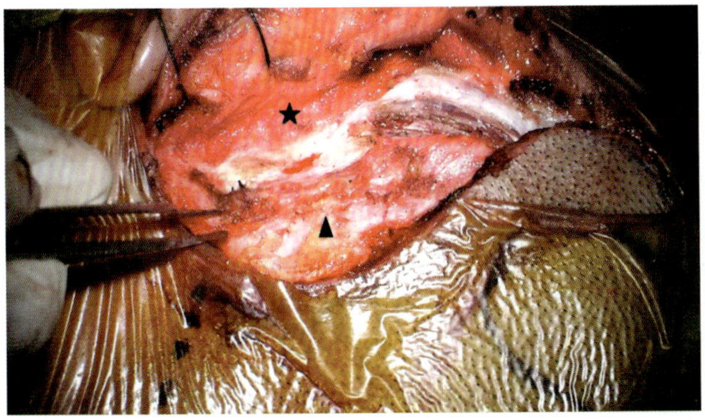

Fig. 71.3 The musculoperiosteal flaps developed. (*solid black star*, anteriorly based flap; *solid black arrow head*, posteroinferiorly based flap).

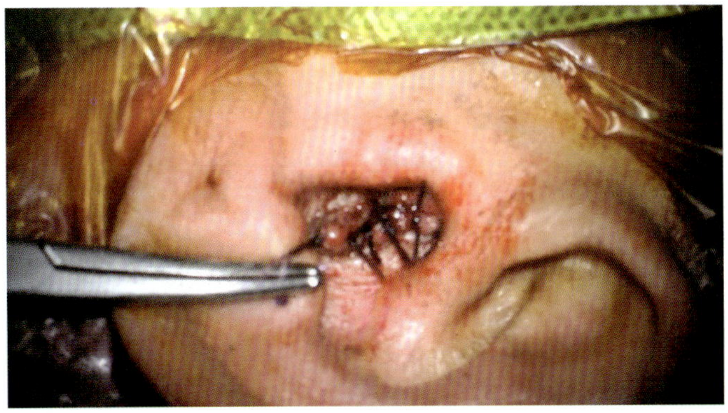

Fig. 71.4 The blind sac closure of the external auditory canal.

Cortical bone is drilled out performing a cortical mastoidectomy. The canal wall is then lowered, and all the bony meatus is meticulously drilled to make sure there are no squamous remnants. Each group of the tympanomastoid air cell tracts is meticulously exenterated (**Fig. 71.5** and **Fig. 71.6**). The eustachian tube mucosa is stripped and obliterated either with the periosteum, fascia, or muscle plugs and finally reinforced with bone wax (**Fig. 71.7**). The peritubal air cell tracts around the eustachian tube are drilled out as they form a potential route for CSF communication to the nasopharynx, and a cavity completely cleared of disease is achieved (**Fig. 71.8**). The receiver well is created over the flat surface of the squamous portion of the temporal bone after marking with the template (**Fig. 71.9** and **Fig. 71.10**). The receiver stimulator is secured to the underlying bone either by suture material, through small holes drilled along the edges of the receiver well (**Fig. 71.11**), or with the screws fixed into the bone depending on the implant model used. The reference electrode is placed under the belly of the temporalis muscle (**Fig. 71.12**).

The abdominal fat is harvested from approximately 2 cm above the anterior iliac spine preferably on the left side to avoid confusion from the appendicectomy incision. The fat harvested is treated in antibiotic preparation, ideally in gentamicin for about 30 minutes.

The round window is now exposed adequately after reducing the bony overhangs around it. The electrode insertion is either by round window insertion in a patent cochlear lumen (**Fig. 71.13**), or, a drill-out procedure is performed depending on the stage of ossification and then inserted accordingly. The electrode array is then secured with periosteum or fascia. The cavity is then obliterated with the harvested abdominal fat which is ideally crafted into long strips, and fibrin glue is used to secure these strips in place (**Fig. 71.14**). The wound is closed in layers with nonresorbable suture material and head bandage draped.

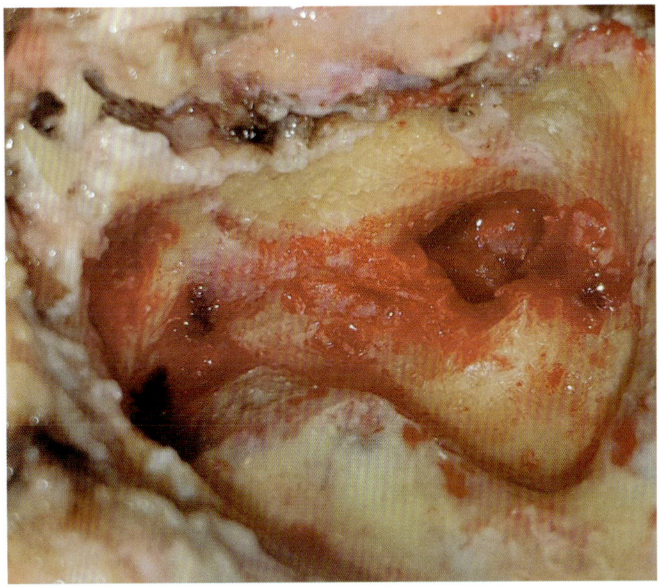

Fig. 71.5 The granulations in the tympanomastoid cavity.

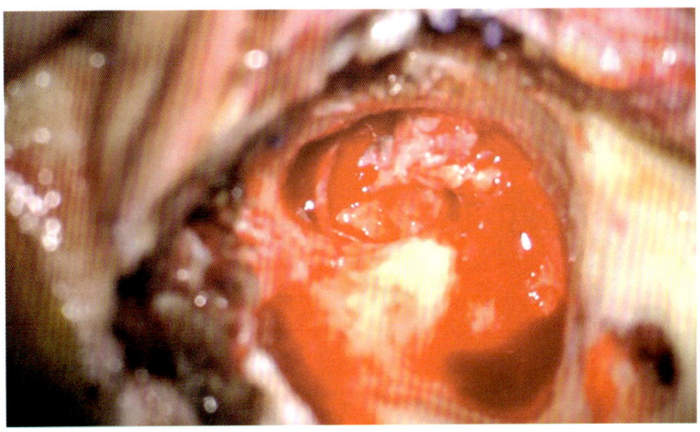

Fig. 71.6 The tympanomastoid cavity (after lowering the posterior canal wall). Note the extensive granulations in the middle ear and the mastoid cavity.

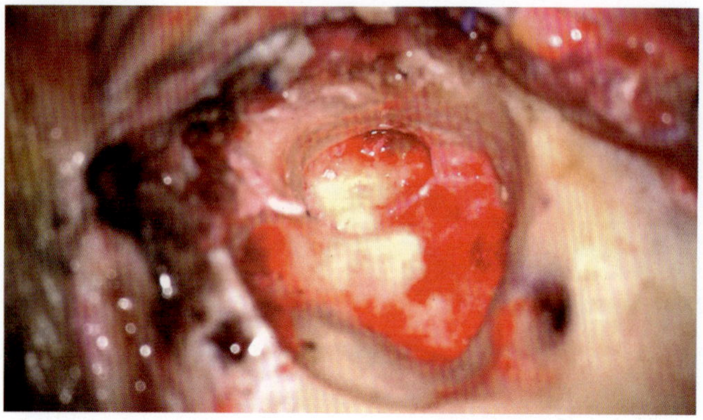

Fig. 71.7 The obliteration of the eustachian tube opening with periosteum reinforced with bone wax (*arrow*).

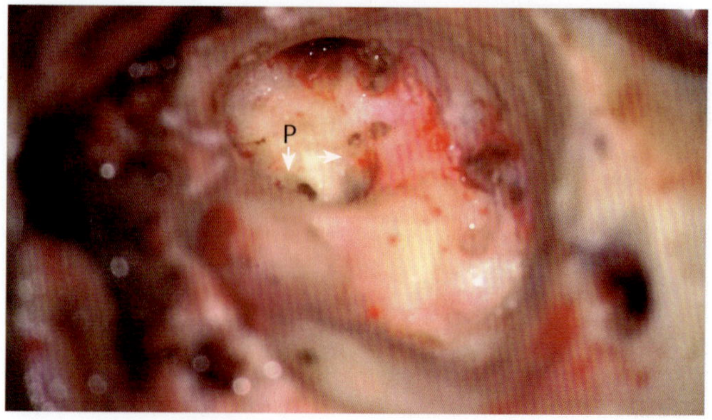

Fig. 71.8 The left tympanomastoid cavity after subtotal petrosectomy. P, promontory; round window (*down arrow*); stapes infrastructure (*right arrow*).

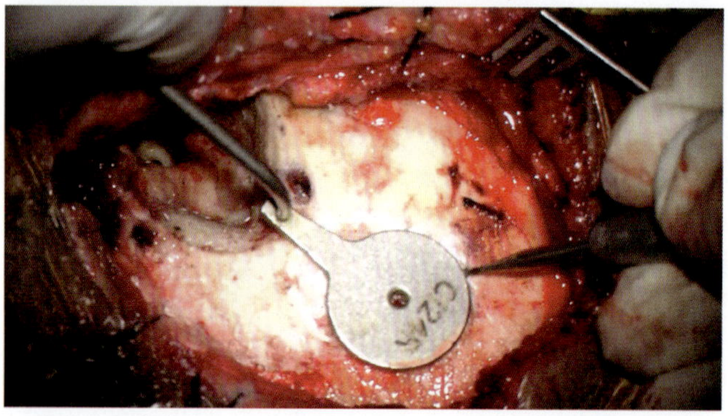

Fig. 71.9 Marking of the template for drilling well of receiver stimulator.

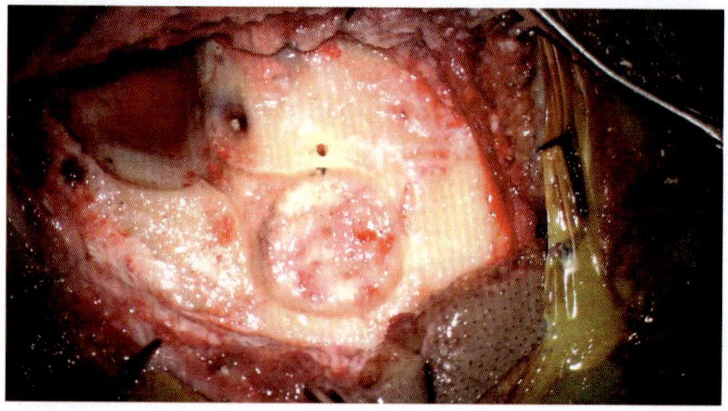

Fig. 71.10 Demonstration of the well for the receiver stimulator.

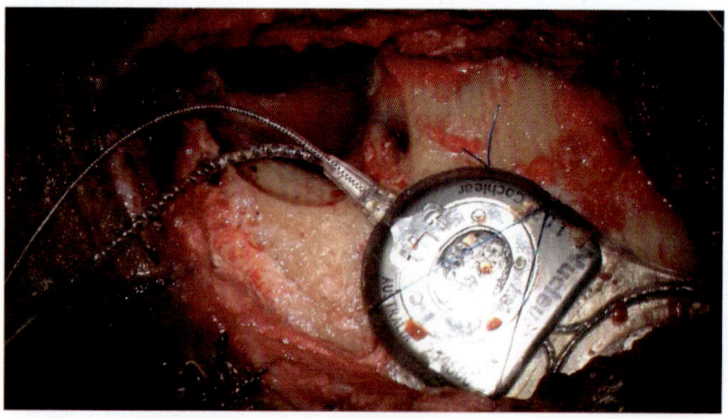

Fig. 71.11 The device positioned in the well and secured with nonresorbable suture material.

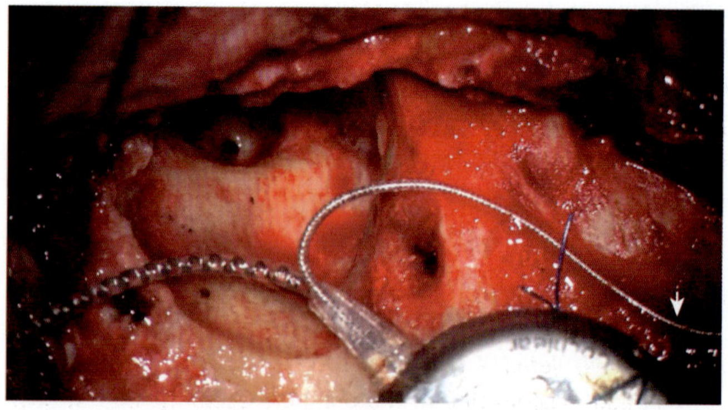

Fig. 71.12 Demonstration of the reference electrode placed under the belly of the temporalis muscle.

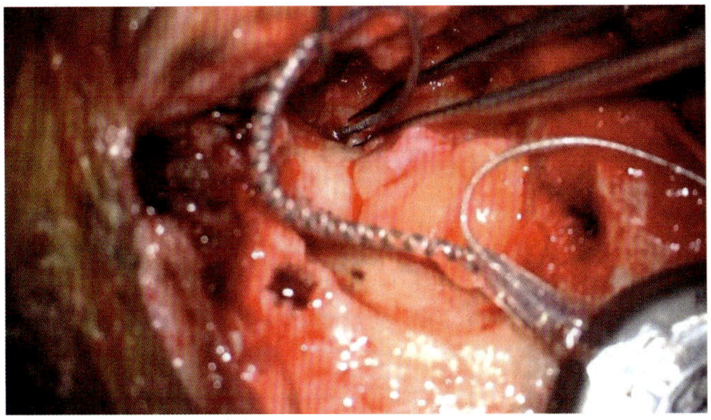

Fig. 71.13 Demonstration of the round window insertion of the electrode array into the cochlea.

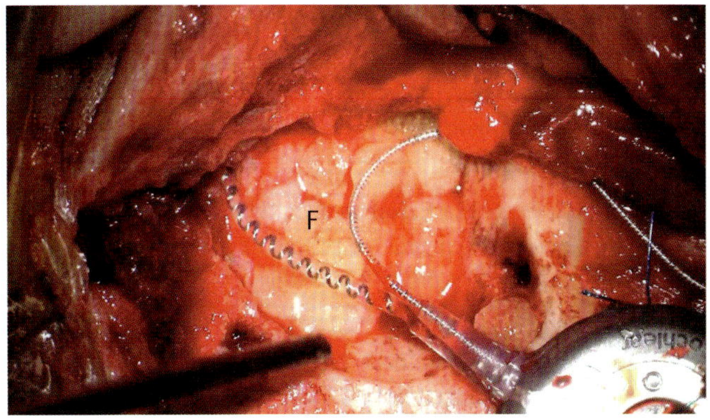

Fig. 71.14 After the cavity is obliterated with the fat **(F)**.

Complications

The complications of subtotal petrosectomy include the risk of a breakdown of the blind sac closure, or entrapment of the squamous portion of the edges developing iatrogenic cholesteatoma. Infection of the abdominal fat, particularly by the airborne infection when left exposed to the external environment for a longer duration, where the potential risk of the spread of infection to the subarachnoid space is very high with the cochlear implant in situ. Development of wound fistula occurs either secondary to the infection along the suture line or because of fat resorption leading to retraction of the site. Remnant peritubal air cells serve as a potential communication between the nasopharynx and the obliterated cavity. Possibility of inadequate disease clearance from the tympanomastoid cleft particularly cholesteatoma, or even when the meatal skin is not completely removed before the blind sac closure leading to entrapped cholesteatoma which can be significantly reduced by cottonoid dissection and thorough bone drilling.

References

1. Coker NJ, Jenkins HA, Fisch U. Obliteration of the middle ear and mastoid cleft in subtotal petrosectomy: indications, tech-nique, and results. Ann Otol Rhinol Laryngol 1986;95(1 Pt 1): 5–11
2. Fisch U, Mattox D. Microsurgery of the skull base. Thieme; 1988.
3. Rambo JH. Musculoplasty: a new operation for suppurative middle ear deafness. Trans Am Acad Ophthalmol Otolaryngol 1958;62(2):166–177
4. Rambo JH. Primary closure of the radical mastoidectomy wound: a technique to eliminate postoperative care. Laryngoscope 1958;68(7):1216–1227
5. Fritz MH, Crawford GB. An evaluation of the Rambo primary closure of the radical mastoidectomy wound. Trans Am Acad Ophthalmol 1960;64:159–167
6. Bartels LJ, Sheehy JL. Total obliteration of the mastoid, middle ear, and external auditory canal. A review of 27 cases. Laryngoscope 1981;91(7):1100–1108
7. Nadol JB Jr, Schuknecht HF. Obliteration of the mastoid in the treatment of tumors of the temporal bone. Ann Otol Rhinol Laryngol 1984;93(1 Pt 1):6–12
8. Meyerhoff WL, Stringer SP, Roland PS. Rambo procedure: modi-fication and application. Laryngoscope 1988;98(7): 795–796
9. Bendet E, Cerenko D, Linder TE, Fisch U. Cochlear implantation after subtotal petrosectomies. Eur Arch Otorhinolaryngol 1998;255(4):169–174
10. Prasad SC, Roustan V, Piras G, Caruso A, Lauda L, Sanna M. Subtotal petrosectomy: surgical technique, indications, outcomes, and comprehensive review of literature. Laryngoscope 2017; 127(12):2833–2842
11. Vincenti V, Pasanisi E, Guida M, Di Trapani G, Sanna M. Hearing rehabilitation in neurofibromatosis type 2 patients: cochlear versus auditory brainstem implantation. Audiol Neurotol 2008;13(4):273–280
12. Henseler MA, Polanski JF, Schlegel C, Linder T. Active middle ear implants in patients undergoing subtotal petrosectomy: long-term follow-up. Otol Neurotol 2014;35(3):437–441
13. Szymański M, Ataide A, Linder T. The use of subtotal petrosect-omy in cochlear implant candidates with chronic

otitis media. Eur Arch Otorhinolaryngol 2016;273(2): 363–370

14. Leung R, Briggs RJ. Indications for and outcomes of mastoid obliteration in cochlear implantation. Otol Neurotol 2007; 28(3):330–334
15. Sanna M, Dispenza F, Flanagan S, De Stefano A, Falcioni M. Management of chronic otitis by middle ear obliteration with blind sac closure of the external auditory canal. Otol Neurotol 2008;29(1):19–22
16. Sanna M, Pandya Y, Mancini F, Sequino G, Piccirillo E. Petrous bone cholesteatoma: classification, management and review of the literature. Audiol Neurotol 2011;16(2):124–136
17. Issing PR, Schönermark MP, Winkelmann S, Kempf HG, Ernst A. Cochlear implantation in patients with chronic otitis: indications for subtotal petrosectomy and obliteration of the middle ear. Skull Base Surg 1998;8(3):127–131
18. Postelmans JT, Stokroos RJ, Linmans JJ, Kremer B. Cochlear implantation in patients with chronic otitis media: 7 years' experience in Maastricht. Eur Arch Otorhinolaryngol 2009; 266(8):1159–1165
19. Pasanisi E, Vincenti V, Bacciu A, et al. Multichannel cochlear implantation in radical mastoidectomy cavities. Otolaryngol Head Neck Surg 2002;127(5):432–436
20. Lin K, Marrinan MS, Waltzman SB, Roland JT Jr. Multichannel cochlear implantation in the scala vestibuli. Otol Neurotol 2006;27(5):634–638
21. Isaacson B, Roland PS, Wright CG. Anatomy of the middle-turn cochleostomy. Laryngoscope 2008;118(12):2200–2204
22. Roland JT Jr, Coelho DH, Pantelides H, Waltzman SB. Partial and double-array implantation of the ossified cochlea. Otol Neurotol 2008;29(8):1068–1075
23. Balkany T, Bird PA, Hodges AV, Luntz M, Telischi FF, Buchman C. Surgical technique for implantation of the totally ossified cochlea. Laryngoscope 1998;108(7):988–992
24. Papsin BC. Cochlear implantation in children with anomalous cochleovestibular anatomy. Laryngoscope 2005;115(1 Pt 2, Suppl 106)1–26
25. Arndt S, Beck R, Schild C, Grauvogel TD, Laszig R, Aschendorff A. Management of cochlear implantation in patients with malformations. Clin Otolaryngol 2010;35(3):220–227
26. Kaddour HS. Recurrent meningitis due to a congenital fistula of the stapedial footplate. J Laryngol Otol 1993;107(10): 931–932
27. Graham JM, Phelps PD, Michaels L. Congenital malformations of the ear and cochlear implantation in children: review and temporal bone report of common cavity. J Laryngol Otol Suppl 2000;25(S25):1–14
28. Valencia DM, Rimell FL, Friedman BJ, Oblander MR, Helmbrecht J. Cochlear implantation in infants less than 12 months of age. Int J Pediatr Otorhinolaryngol 2008;72(6): 767–773
29. Camilleri AE, Toner JG, Howarth KL, Hampton S, Ramsden RT. Cochlear implantation following temporal bone fracture. J Laryngol Otol 1999;113(5):454–457
30. Serin GM, Derinsu U, Sari M, et al. Cochlear implantation in patients with bilateral cochlear trauma. Am J Otolaryngol 2010;31(5):350–355
31. Simons JP, Whitaker ME, Hirsch BE. Cochlear implantation in a patient with bilateral temporal bone fractures. Otolaryngol Head Neck Surg 2005;132(5):809–811
32. Greenberg SL, Shipp D, Lin VY, Chen JM, Nedzelski JM. Cochlear implantation in patients with bilateral severe sensorineural hearing loss after major blunt head trauma. Otol Neurotol 2011;32(1):48–54
33. Sudhoff H, Linthicum FH Jr. Temporal bone fracture and latent meningitis: temporal bone histopathology study of the month. Otol Neurotol 2003;24(3):521–522
34. Feenstra L, Sanna M, Zini C, Gamoletti R, Delogu P. Surgical treat-ment of brain herniation into the middle ear and mastoid. Am J Otol 1985;6(4):311–315
35. von Ilberg CA, Baumann U, Kiefer J, Tillein J, Adunka OF. Electric-acoustic stimulation of the auditory system: a review of the first decade. Audiol Neurotol 2011;16(Suppl 2): 1–30

Chapter 72 Lateral Temporal Bone Resection

Narayan Jayashankar and Swati Kodur Patil

Introduction

Malignancy of the temporal bone is a rare entity, which, in spite of much radiological and surgical advancements, remains an uncertain domain with regard to diagnosis, treatment, and prognosis. Various surgical techniques have been described in the literature for the cure or palliation of tumors involving the temporal bone. This spectrum of operative interventions starts with a simple sleeve resection of the external auditory canal (EAC) to much extensive total temporal bone resection with obvious varied indications for each. This chapter covers one of the techniques in the spectrum for early tumors of the temporal bone, lateral temporal bone resection (LTBR). A thorough description of indications and surgical steps of the same thus follow.

Indications

- A lateral temporal bone excision involves en bloc excision of the bony external auditory canal together with the tympanic membrane, malleus, and incus. T1 and T2 carcinomas of the external canal (Pittsburgh's classification) are treated with lateral temporal bone excision. It should be noted that the authors do not believe in sleeve resection and consider LTBR as the minimum surgery to be performed for T1 or T2 lesions of EAC.
- T3 and T4 stages of carcinoma of the EAC mandates subtotal or total temporal bone excision combined with superficial or total parotidectomy along with selective neck dissection plus adjuvant radiotherapy and/or chemotherapy depending on the histopathological type of carcinoma.

Surgical Steps

A tumor of the EAC which falls under T1 and T2 of Pittsburgh's staging system is treated with LTBR as definitive surgical management. **Fig. 72.1a, b** shows computed tomography (CT) scan of a patient with right-sided T2 lesion of the EAC who underwent LTBR for cure of disease.

1. Postaural incision extends from the dome of helix to mastoid tip just parallel to the postaural groove.

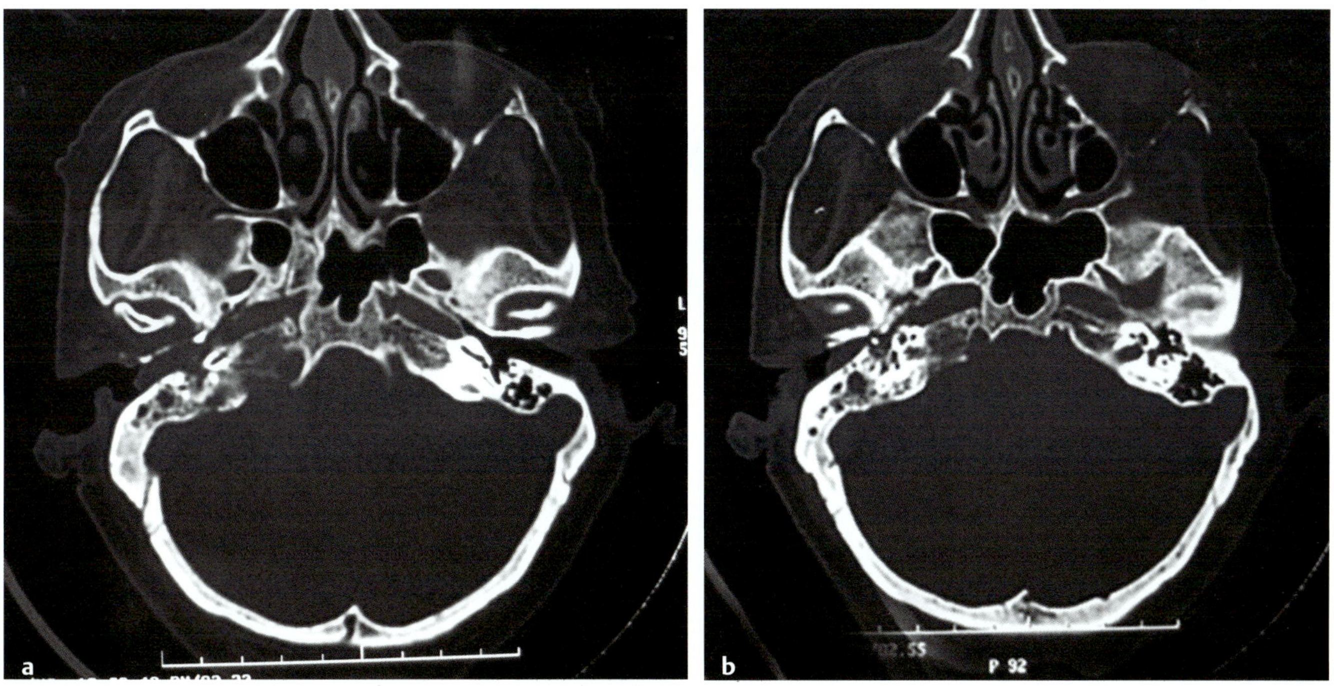

Fig. 72.1 **(a, b)** CT scan shows a lesion in the right external auditory meatus (T2 lesion as per Pittsburgh's classification).

2. A horizontal incision is then taken from the base of zygoma to the junction of the transverse sinus with the upper end of the sigmoid sinus. Followed by a second curvilinear incision is along the bony margin of EAC. This leads to developing a posteroinferiorly based musculoperiosteal flap exposing the mastoid cortex completely (**Fig. 72.2**).
3. Next step involves segregation of cartilaginous EAC from the surrounding soft tissue by a circumferential incision taken at the lateral end of EAC keeping a safe margin away from the carcinoma (**Fig. 72.3** and **Fig. 72.4**).
4. A cortical mastoidectomy then performed followed by an extended posterior tympanotomy (**Fig. 72.5a, b**) as described in Chapter 46.
5. The drilling inferiorly is extended toward the glenoid fossa, anteriorly extended from the hypotympanum along the bony inferior annular rim (of tympanic membrane) to create an inferior trough that separates the bony EAC inferiorly from the surrounding tympanic bone. Accidental exposure of the facial nerve in its mastoidal segment is avoided at this step (**Fig. 72.6a, b**).
6. Drilling is then carried out superiorly along the base of the zygoma, separating the superior wall of EAC from the tegmen tympani, thereby opening up the entire attic space. This drilling is extended toward the glenoid fossa anteriorly communicating the inferior portion of drilling (**Fig. 72.7a, b**).
7. Incudostapedial joint is dislocated (**Fig. 72.8a, b**).
8. The bony EAC is then separated from the glenoid fossa anteriorly with sharp dissection. The remnant attachments of the EAC are drilled out all around to free it from the fossa (**Fig. 72.9a, b**).
9. An en bloc excision of the entire external canal along with the tympanic membrane, malleus, and incus is done (**Fig. 72.10**).

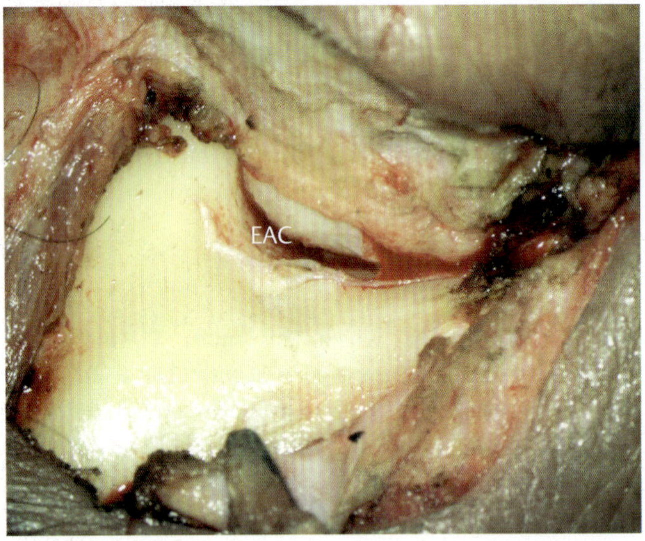

Fig. 72.2 A posteroinferiorly based musculoperiosteal flap is created.

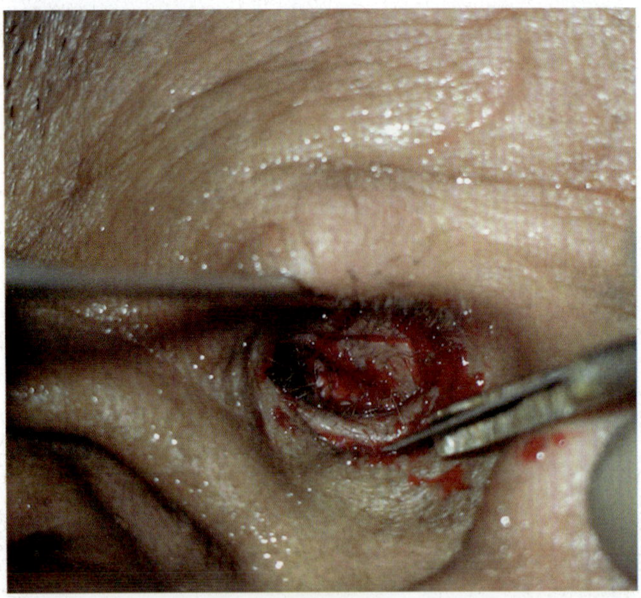

Fig. 72.3 Circumferential incision of the external auditory canal is taken with a safe margin away from the carcinoma.

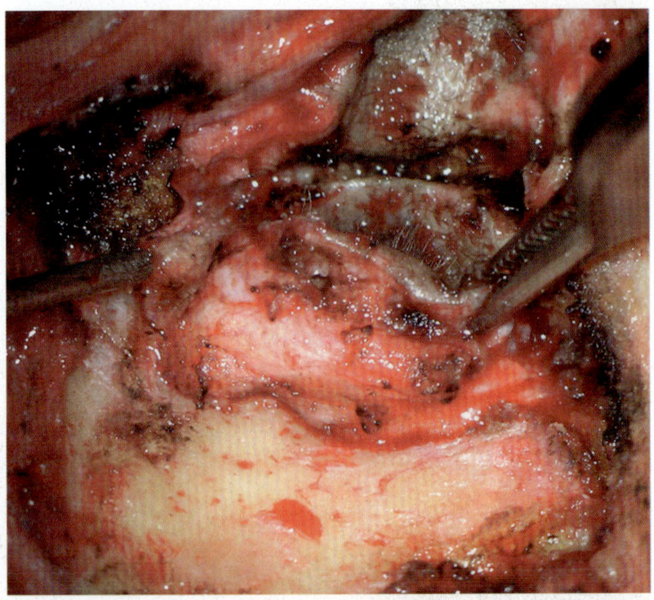

Fig. 72.4 Cartilaginous part of the involved EAC is segregated from the surrounding soft tissues.

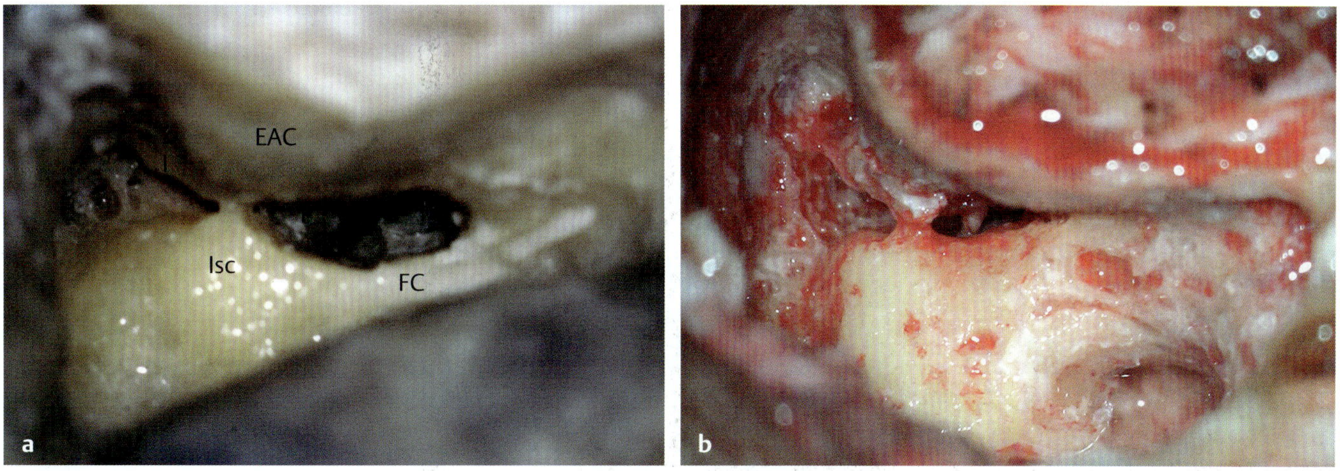

Fig. 72.5 **(a)** Cortical mastoidectomy and extended posterior tympanotomy are performed. **(b)** Extended posterior tympanotomy is performed.

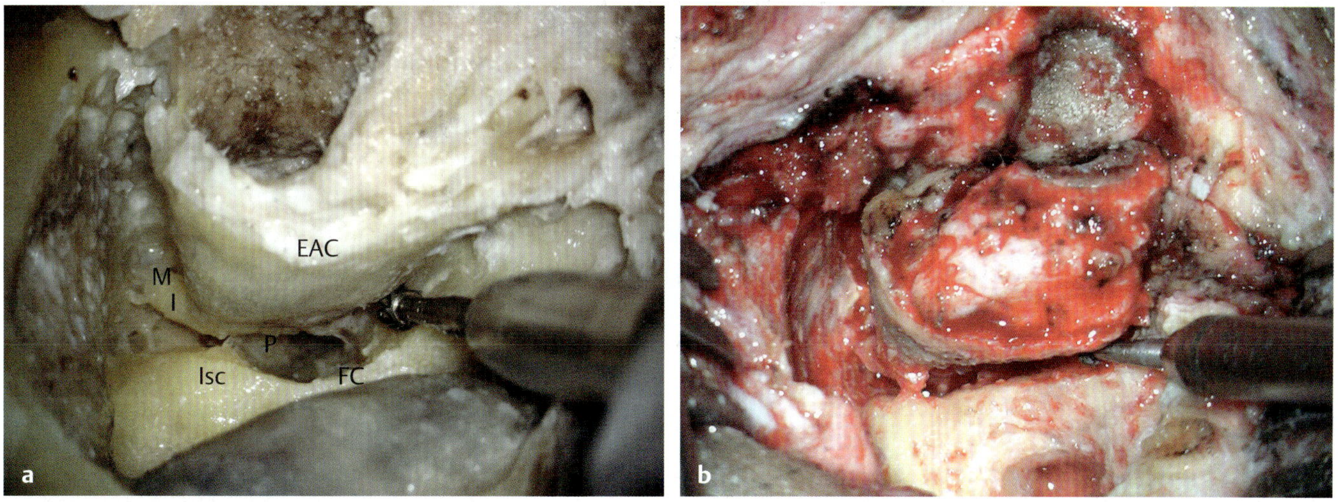

Fig. 72.6 **(a, b)** Segregation of external auditory meatus inferiorly.

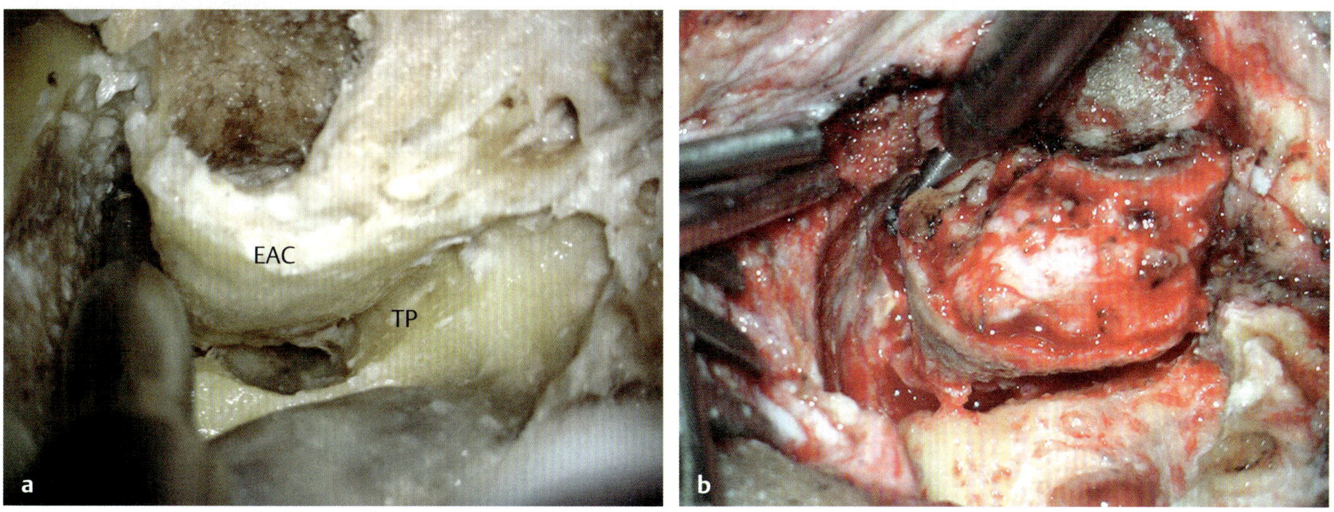

Fig. 72.7 **(a, b)** Segregation of external auditory meatus at the base of the zygoma area.

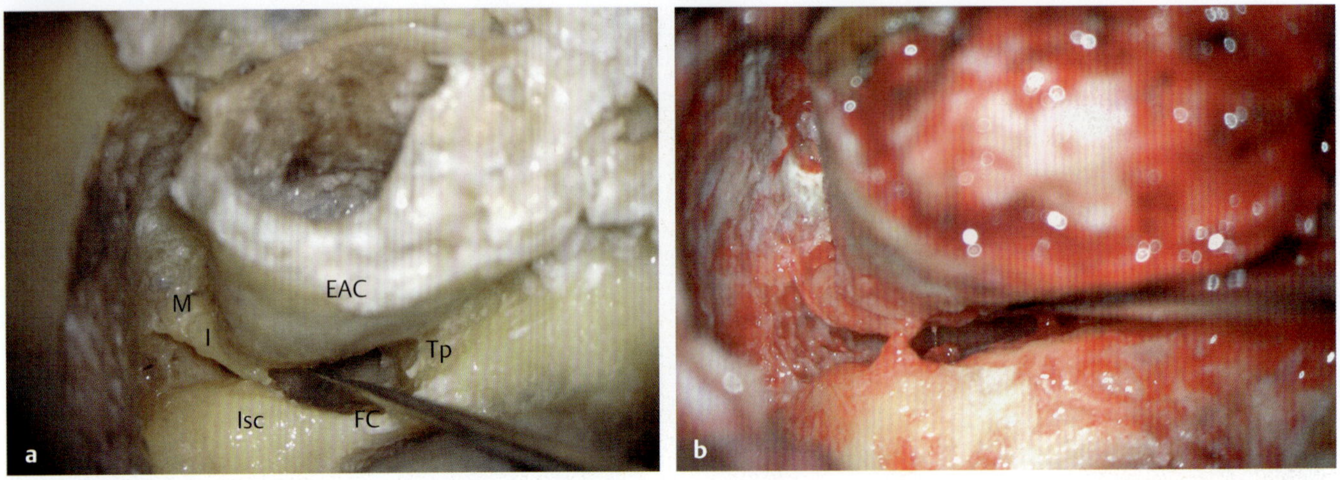

Fig. 72.8 (a, b) Dislocation of the incudostapedial joint.

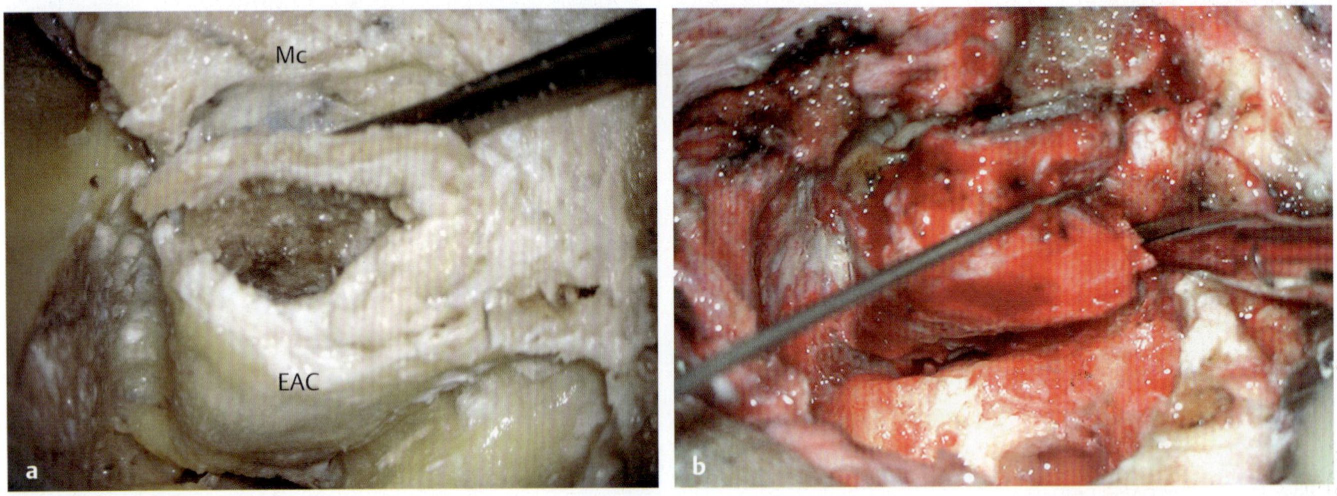

Fig. 72.9 (a, b) Separation of the external auditory meatus from the glenoid fossa.

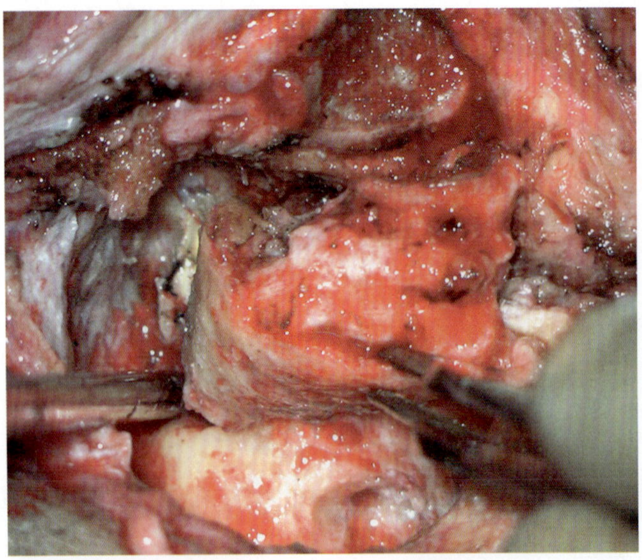

Fig. 72.10 Excision of the external auditory canal containing carcinoma.

10. The specimen is examined under the microscope for safe margins and sent for histopathological examination (**Fig. 72.11a, b**).
11. The middle ear cleft is seen after resection of the EAC (**Fig. 72.12a, b**).
12. A thorough inspection of the middle ear and the mastoid cavity is done for any remnant carcinoma. If any area is found suspicious, it is then separately removed piecemeal and any remnant cells exenterated.
13. Wherever feasible, cartilage ossiculoplasty (**Fig. 72.13**) and grafting of the cavity are performed (**Fig. 72.14**). The objective of ossiculoplasty, apart from some improvement in hearing, is to retain a middle ear space. A very wide meatoplasty will eventually ensue.
14. A split-thickness skin graft is harvested from the thigh of the subject. This is then used to line the cavity (**Fig. 72.15**) to promote early epithelization and healing of the entire cavity.

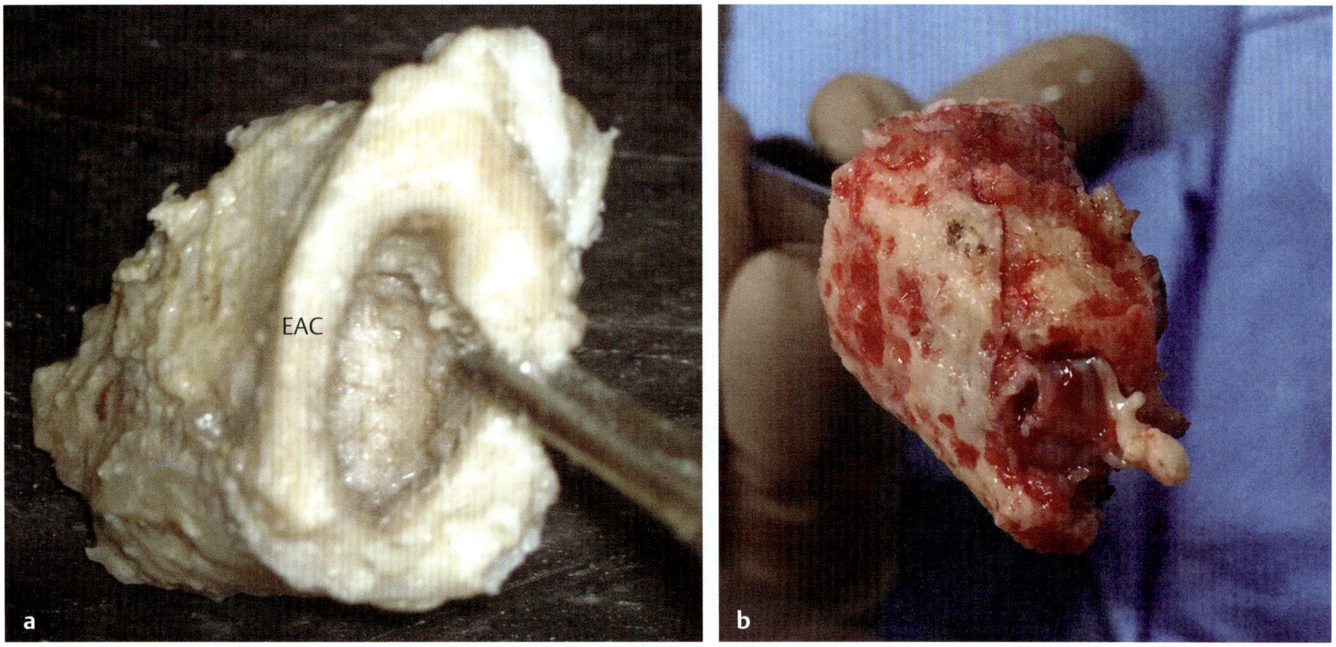

Fig. 72.11 (a, b) Excision of the external auditory canal en bloc with tympanic membrane, malleus, and incus.

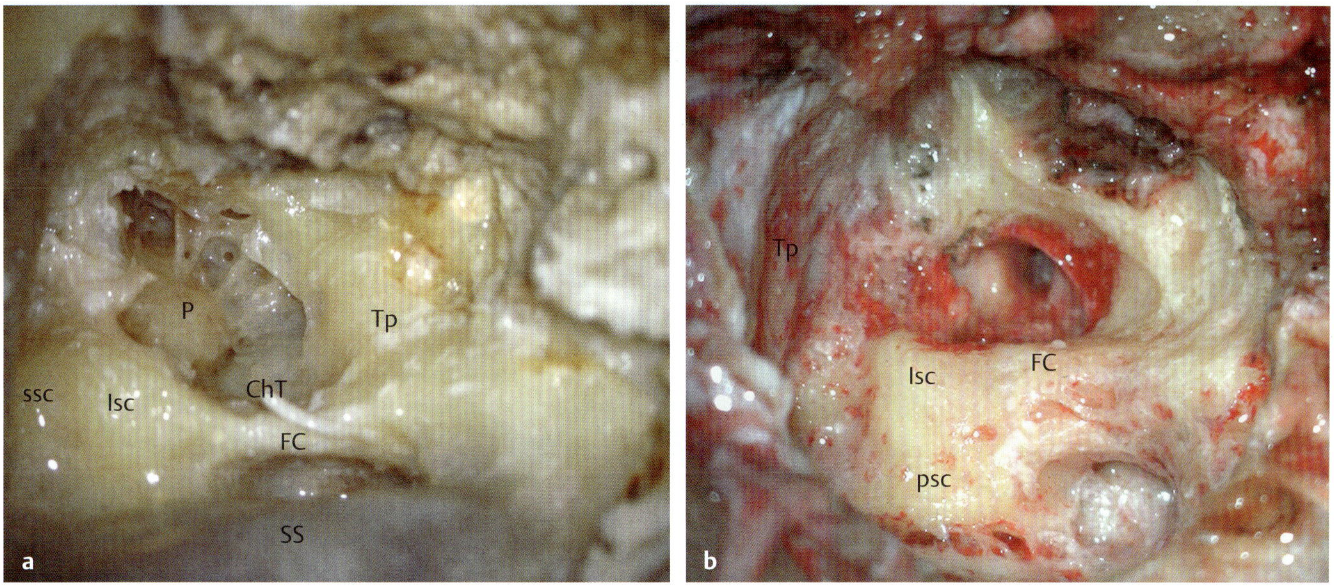

Fig. 72.12 (a, b) The structures visualized after lateral temporal bone resection.

15. LTBR with minimal erosion of anterior canal wall can additionally be combined with superficial parotidectomy, whenever considered necessary.

Tips and Pearls

- Although there is no perfect classification, Pittsburgh's classification is followed. T1 carcinomas are treated with LTBR. We do not advocate sleeve resection.
- Treatment strategies for T2 lesions are tailored depending on the location and possible spread of the carcinoma.
- In some T2 lesions, occasionally, the anterior wall of EAC is marginally eroded. Depending on the proximity of the carcinoma to the parotid, a decision is made to perform a superficial parotidectomy to improve clearance and prognosis.

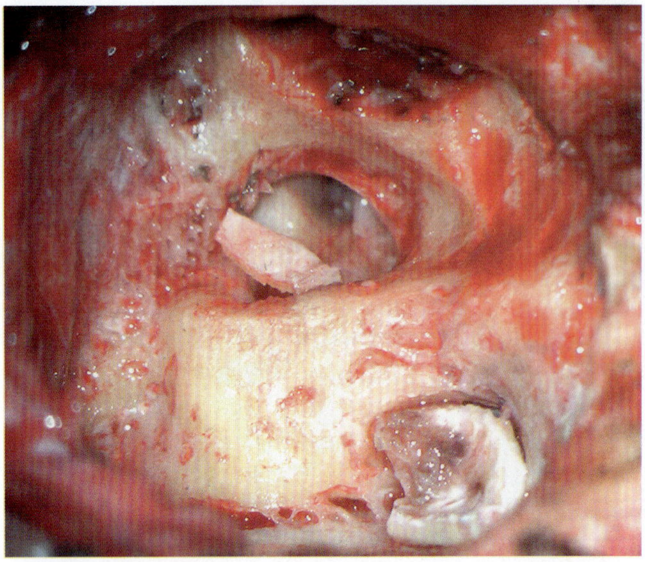

Fig. 72.13 Cartilage is placed on the head of stapes. A piece of cartilage is also used to obliterate the infralabyrinthine area.

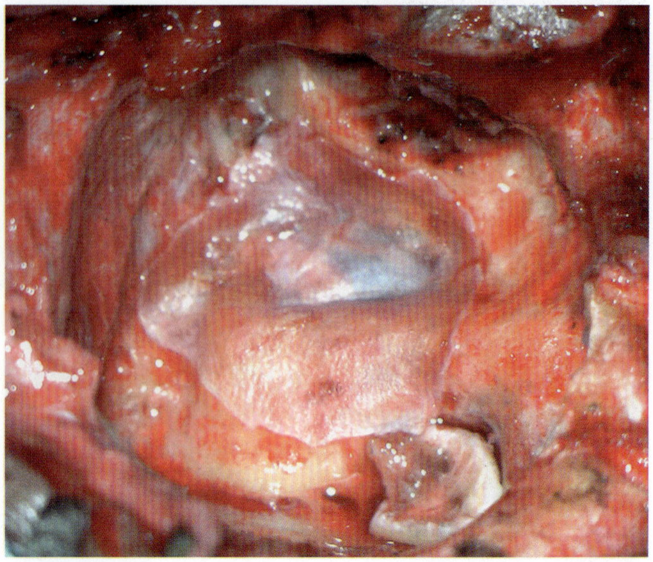

Fig. 72.14 Temporalis facia is used as a graft.

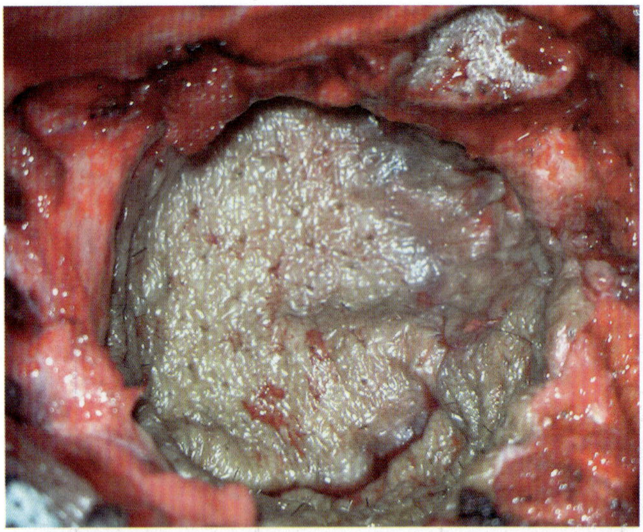

Fig. 72.15 Split-thickness skin graft is lining the whole mastoid cavity.

- In T2 lesions, a level II neck node sampling is performed. If found involved, a modified neck dissection is performed.
- If parotid or neck nodes are found involved in histopathology, postoperative radiotherapy is indicated.
- Carcinomas that have breached the tympanic membrane to reach the middle ear, mastoid, or further beyond (T3 and T4) are treated by a subtotal or total temporal bone resection. In these cases, a cul-de-sac closure of the canal is to be performed. A superficial or total parotidectomy with modified neck dissection and postoperative radiotherapy is also indicated in these cases.
- Carcinomas that have involved the internal carotid artery or sigmoid sinus, those that have spread to the jugular foramen or hypoglossal canal, intradural extensions are all considered unresectable since it is not possible to obtain safe margins.

Suggested Readings

Bacciu A, Clemente IA, Piccirillo E, Ferrari S, Sanna M. Guidelines for treating temporal bone carcinoma based on long-term outcomes. Otol Neurotol 2013;34(5):898–907

Higgins TS, Antonio SA. The role of facial palsy in staging squamous cell carcinoma of the temporal bone and external auditory canal: a comparative survival analysis. Otol Neurotol 2010;31(9):1473–1479

Mazzoni A, Zanoletti E, Marioni G, Martini A. En bloc temporal bone resections in squamous cell carcinoma of the ear. Technique, principles, and limits. Acta Otolaryngol 2016;136(5):425–432

Morris LG, Mehra S, Shah JP, Bilsky MH, Selesnick SH, Kraus DH. Predictors of survival and recurrence after temporal bone resection for cancer. Head Neck 2012;34(9):1231–1239

Prasad SC, D'Orazio F, Medina M, Bacciu A, Sanna M. State of the art in temporal bone malignancies. Curr Opin Otolaryngol Head Neck Surg 2014;22(2):154–165

Zhang T, Li W, Dai C, Chi F, Wang S, Wang Z. Evidence-based surgical management of T1 or T2 temporal bone malignancies. Laryngoscope 2013;123(1):244–248

Chapter 73 Facial Neuroma

K.P. Morwani, Madhuri Mehta, and Amol Patil

Introduction

Neuromas are benign tumors that arise from the nerve sheath.[1] Facial nerve is devoid of the sheath at its root entry zone or cerebellopontine angle (CPA).[2] Neuromas do not arise here, on the contrary, they may arise from the internal auditory canal and may fall onto the CP angle. A neuroma can be present in any location from the internal auditory meatus (IAM) to its extratemporal bifurcation in the parotid.

We believe that the facial nerve neuroma arises commonly from the thickened portion of the nerve than the thinner portion. The nerve sheath is thinner in the IAM and in the portion beyond the bifurcation in the parotid. Hence, the incidence of facial nerve neuromas is much lesser in these portions in comparison to the incidence at the stylomastoid foramen and the vertical portion as the nerve sheath is thick at this portion.

A large number of facial nerve neuroma patients are misdiagnosed or diagnosed late, as to begin with, these patients may not have any localized symptom or sign neither facial paresis nor palsy. Every case of an idiopathic facial nerve palsy lasting more than 2 months despite adequate medical management must be investigated with a computed tomography (CT) scan bone window complete study in thinnest possible slices in all the three planes, at times complemented with magnetic resonance imaging (MRI).

Occasionally, patients of facial nerve neuroma presenting with paresis can have a complete recovery with medical line of management in spite of having a small neuroma. Hence, every case of recurrent facial paresis or palsy diagnosed as Bell's palsy should undergo CT and/or MRI as mentioned above.

Facial nerve palsy can also be secondary to vascular tumors, compressing the nerve at the IAM or at the geniculate ganglion.[3] In the IAM, it is the cavernous vascular malformation, whereas, capillary hemangioma is common in the geniculate ganglion. These patients may present with facial nerve paresis or palsy associated with hearing loss, occasionally, tinnitus and dizziness mimicking the symptoms of acoustic neuroma, but the clinical differentiating feature is that a small-sized acoustic neuroma arising in the IAM would not cause facial paresis or palsy. At times, in these cases, it is possible to peel off the tumor with negligible damage to the nerve.[3] Capillary hemangioma is the commonest tumor located in the first genu area, which on high-resolution CT scan shows a honeycomb appearance; these findings are usually missed if the CT scan is not of thin slices and high resolution. The facial nerve paresis secondary to these tumors occasionally does subside with high doses of steroids. These cases are often misdiagnosed as a case of recurrent Bell's palsy. Both these pathologies are very rare in Asian community. Until now, we have seen only one case of hemangioma at the first genu area; unfortunately, the patient refused to continue treatment as the fellow colleagues diagnosed him with Bell's palsy and was lost to follow up (**Fig. 73.1**).

In recurrent cases of Bell's palsy with residual deficit, we believe in decompressing the facial nerve at the labyrinthine portion; further decompression along its course is dependent on the edema over the nerve. At times, hemangiomas can be an incidental finding during the decompression of the first genu in cases of recurrent Bell's palsy.

In the past, literature suggested to avoid surgery in cases of neuromas if the patient had anything lesser than grade 3 paresis (House–Brackmann classification). The belief was that every case of facial nerve neuroma would require excision of the tumor along with the nerve with few millimeters of safe margins followed by grafting, as the best results following grafting would be grade 3 (House–Brackmann

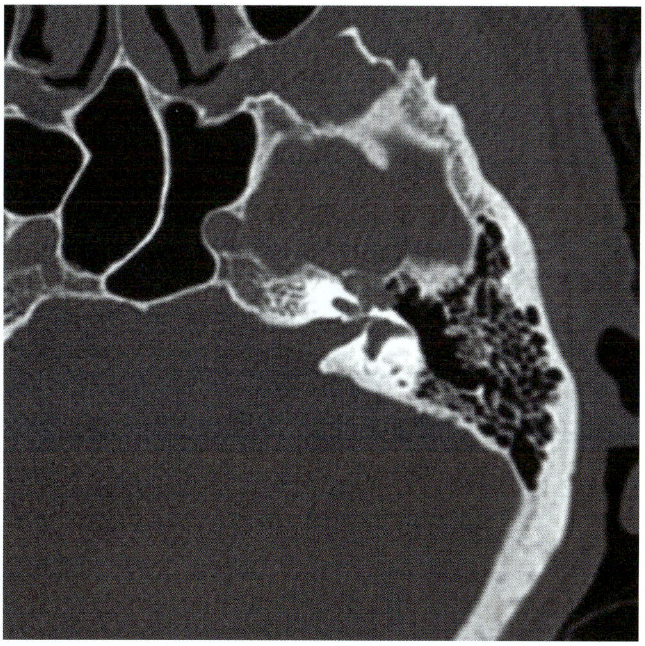

Fig. 73.1 Honeycomb appearance in CT scan capillary hemangioma over the left geniculate ganglion.

classification) in most of the cases. Thus, surgery deferred if the patient did not have any other associated symptoms demanding surgical interference.[4]

Facial nerve neuroma was diagnosed earlier in cases with associated symptoms or clinical signs that demand CT scan or MRI and one can pick up the neuroma preoperatively even when the patient had no paresis or palsy. Any infra-aural swelling or angle of mandible or beyond the angle of the mandible or in the parotid region can routinely be diagnosed by fine-needle aspiration cytology (FNAC), and further size and extent confirmed by necessary investigation.

At times, patients may present without any paresis with swelling in the external canal, visible swelling in the middle ear under the tympanic membrane with conductive hearing loss, tinnitus, or vertigo depending on the location and the extent of the tumor. The radiological investigation gives the suspicion/confirmation of the neuroma owing to the destruction of the bone of the fallopian canal with smooth widening. In these situations, one can confirm the diagnosis by performing FNAC of the mass seen in the external canal or by transtympanic FNAC of the mass in the middle ear.

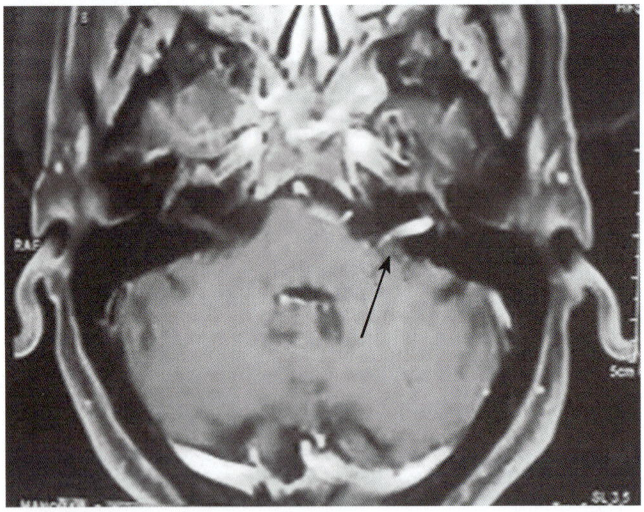

Fig. 73.2 Neuroma in the left internal auditory canal (*arrow*).

As per CT scan bone window is concerned, every neuroma causes bone destruction, in the horizontal portion as the bone overlying is thin and as it may not be easy to identify the destruction of the bone, but from the second genu to stylomastoid foramen, it is much easier to diagnose because of the smooth expansion of the neuroma. Similarly, it is much easier to diagnose at the first genu and labyrinthine portion because of the typical bony destruction.

The tumor may present in the IAM at times extending into the CP angle. The CT scan and MRI findings will be the same as that of acoustic neuroma, but if the presenting symptom is facial nerve paresis or palsy, one should clinically diagnose it as facial nerve neuroma and not as acoustic neuroma, as small-sized acoustic neuroma would never give palsy or paresis of the facial nerve (**Fig. 73.2**).

We have seen facial nerve neuroma causing extensive destruction or widening of IAM or labyrinthine portion extending into the middle cranial fossa also into the posterior cranial fossa. Similarly, the patient can have a dumbbell-shaped extending in the intra- and extratemporal part because of constriction at the stylomastoid foramen.[5] At times, one can have multiple skipped neuromas in its course (**Fig. 73.3a, b**).

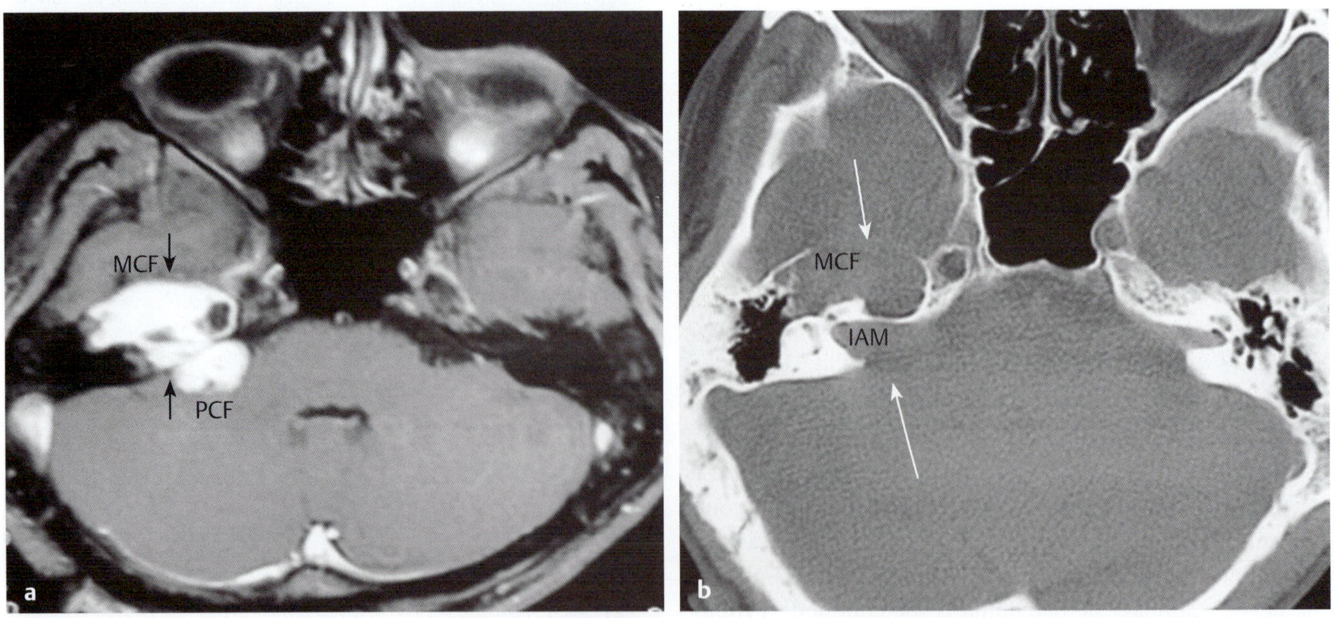

Fig. 73.3 **(a)** MRI showing neuroma extending into middle cranial fossa and into posterior cranial fossa. **(b)** CT scan showing widening of internal auditory meatus and tumor extending in middle cranial fossa.

Rarely, one may encounter perineural infiltration of the facial nerve at the parotid region extending along its complete vertical course to IAM. The widening of the canal will be minimal and may mimic as a skipped lesion, as the destruction of the bone varies with the type of bone in various portions of the fallopian canal. For example, the thinnest bone is in the horizontal portion, around the first genu, and under the (medial) surface of the vertical course to the otic capsule. The thickest bony part in the middle ear is the otic capsule, that is, labyrinthine block and cochlea, which can occasionally thin out or may get eroded completely presenting as fistula of the cochlea or labyrinthine block, which is rare to be seen in facial nerve neuroma.

Investigation

An investigation is required to confirm the diagnosis of the neuroma, to find the extent of the tumor and management of associated symptoms, if any.

CT scan temporal bone thinnest possible slice bone window is the investigation of choice, complemented with MRI from time to time. Most often, the diagnosis of facial nerve neuroma is from symptom sign and radiological finding. Occasionally, FNAC is done to confirm the diagnosis for tumor in the intraparotid region, infratemporal region, tumor extending into the external canal, and occasionally tumor present in the middle ear lying under the tympanic membrane; these are the situation where you can have diagnosis preoperatively, in the rest of the location, the frozen section is performed to obtain the diagnosis.

Management

The mainstay of treatment of facial nerve neuroma is surgical excision. Occasionally, gamma knife is used for small residual or recurrent tumors if the lesion is in the IAM or CP angle. Gamma knife has a role in elderly patients or in medical unfit patients. The approach for the surgical excision will vary from the location of the tumor and associated symptoms, if any.

Patients of facial nerve neuroma without any paresis, or patient with grade 3 facial nerve palsy (House–Brackman classification) are managed by peeling off the tumor from facial nerve whenever possible without causing any further damage to the facial nerve.[6] At times, one may see only nerve sheath lose without any damage to nerve fibers. In cases with damage to few fibers, one should attempt to peel off the tumor from the nerve without disturbing the continuity of the rest of the fibers, as this does not require any repair of deficit of nerve fibers. In cases with 50% damaged fibers, we believe in preserving the remaining 50% fibers and in performing partial-thickness grafting with the greater auricular nerve, the graft ends depending on the location are either glued (in the intracranial portion), sutured (in the neck), or kept in the tunnel of the fallopian canal with just good approximation.

While using the glue, the prerequisite is to have perfect approximation of the nerve endings, and the glue should be going around the ends of the nerve rather than between them. One may use fascia graft to wrap around in complete circumference around the nerve and the graft and glue used around the ends rather going between the two ends.

As far as suturing is concerned, we use 8-0, 9-0 monofilament sutures; suturing is performed approximating the perineurium or epineurium of both ends. This can additionally be reinforced with tissue glue over the anastomosis.

While performing the surgical excision, it is important to make sure to have tumor-free margins, and confirmation is obtained by sending a small bit of the nerve ends after complete excision of the tumor for the frozen section.

Philosophy of Preservation of Nerves in Cases of Neuromas (Lower Cranial Neuroma and Facial Nerve Neuroma)

In the last two decades, the management of cases of lower cranial neuroma and facial nerve neuroma has changed when patients present without any respective nerve paresis or even with nerve paresis. In such situations, even if the tumor is firmly adherent to the nerve or if the nerve is entering the tumor, one has to make every effort to peel out the tumor from the nerve. These cases, if one could preserve the nerve completely, or with damage only to the nerve sheath or damage to minimum fibers of the nerve, one will be surprised in most of the situation that the paresis of the nerve will recover completely or substantially. The recovery time and extent of recovery depend on duration of the preoperative nerve paresis, age of the patient, and extent of damage of the nerve while peeling off the tumor.

Approaches

Approaches will depend on the location of the tumor and associated symptoms and signs.

1. **Tumor arising in the internal auditory meatus:** In this case, the approach depends on the hearing loss.
   If serviceable hearing, middle cranial fossa or the retrosigmoid approach is used with excision of tumor with safe margin.
   If nonserviceable hearing, transmastoid translabyrinthine approach is used with excision of the tumor with safe margin.

Both were followed by nerve grafting with glue used at the approximated nerve ends (**Fig. 73.4** and **Fig. 73.5**).

2. **Tumor arising in the internal auditory meatus extending into cerebellopontine angle:** In this case, the approach depends on the hearing loss. If serviceable hearing, the retrosigmoid approach is used with excision of the tumor with a safe margin.
   If nonserviceable hearing, the translabyrinthine approach is used.
   The advantage of the translabyrinthine approach is one can reroute the facial nerve from the labyrinthine portion and horizontal portion and may be able to do primary approximation without any use of graft.
   The disadvantage of this is to sacrifice the greater superficial petrosal nerve with its blood supply at the geniculate ganglion from the middle meningeal artery (**Fig. 73.6**).

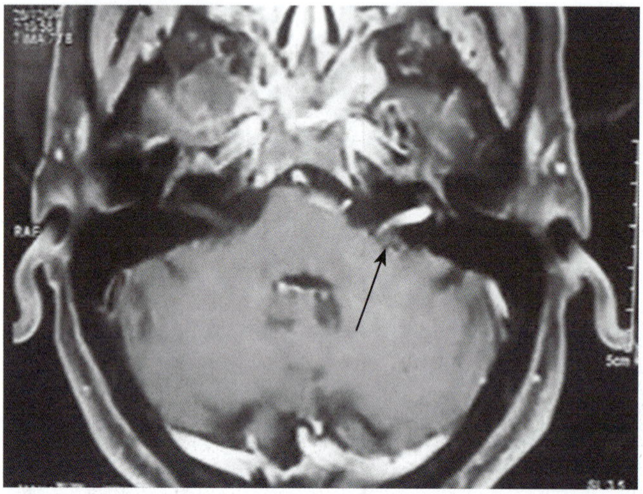

Fig. 73.4 Facial nerve neuroma in the left internal auditory canal.

3. **Tumor eroding the roof of petrous bone presenting into the middle cranial fossa and extending to posterior cranial fossa:** This facial nerve neuroma was removed by extended middle cranial fossa approach as the tumor was extending into the posterior cranial fossa (**Fig. 73.7a, b** and **Fig. 73.8**).
   The tumor was extending from the first genu involving the IAM portion and part of CP angle portion and was excised with safe margins. The margin of the healthy nerve on both sides was sent for frozen section after confirming nerve ends free of tumor, cable graft was placed from the horizontal portion of the facial nerve to CP angle. The CP angle part of the nerve was wrapped with temporalis fascia graft and glued, whereas in the horizontal part the ends of the nerve glued after approximating the nerve end and the graft in the tunnel.
   In cases when there is no improvement after 9 months to 1 year of postgrafting, or when the distal end of the nerve is not seen, one can opt for the faciohypoglossal anastomosis or faciomasseteric anastomosis, and if these grafting procedures fail, one can always go for reanimation procedures.
4. **Tumor involving the first genu and extending in the horizontal portion:** This tumor is removed by the transzygomatic anterior attic approach.
   - Patient is in lateral position.
   - Surgeon sits in front of patient.
   - Endaural/postaural incision is done.
   - External ear canal (EAC) skin is reflected in complete circumference and retracted laterally.
   - Tympanic membrane with handle of malleus and bony canal skin is retracted inferiorly from 3- to 9 o'clock position.

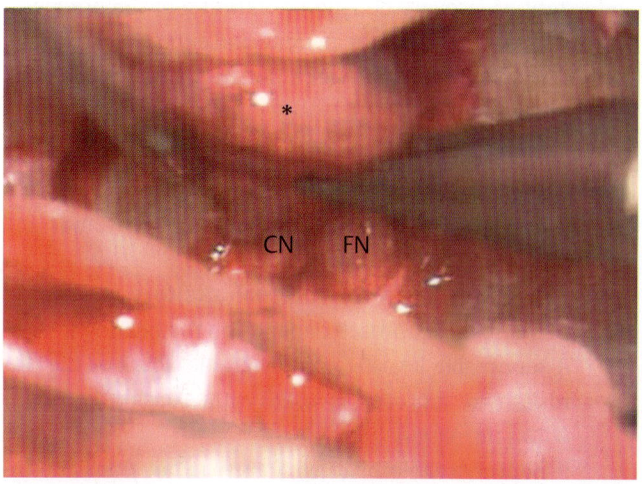

Fig. 73.5 Intraoperative image of facial nerve neuroma in the left internal auditory canal.

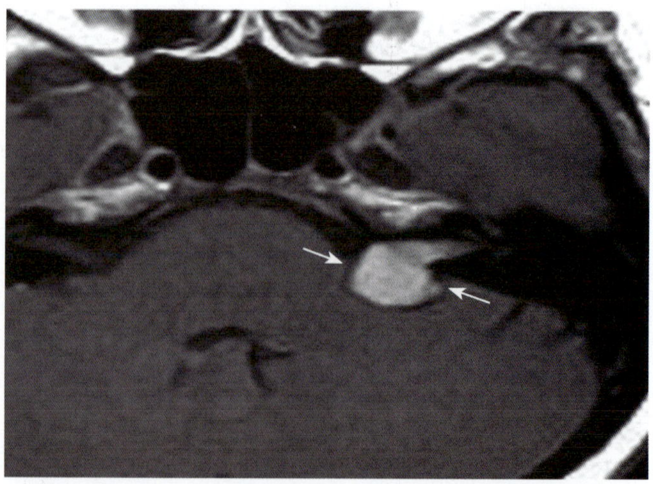

Fig. 73.6 Tumor in the left IAM extending in the CP angle.

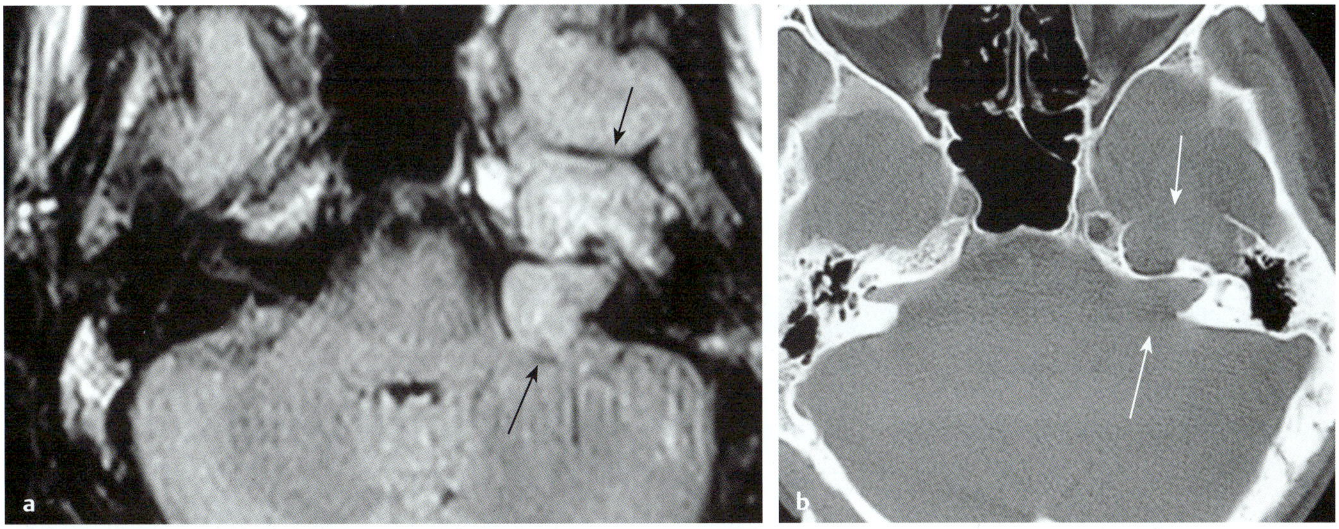

Fig. 73.7 **(a)** MRI showing neuroma extending into middle cranial fossa and into posterior cranial fossa. **(b)** CT scan showing widening of IAM and tumor extending in middle cranial fossa.

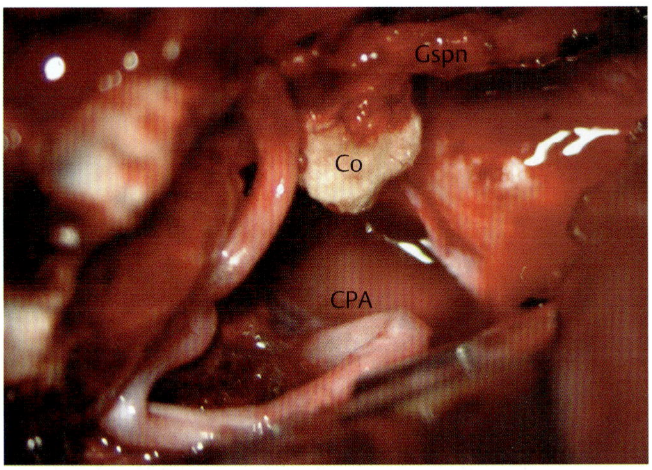

Fig. 73.8 Nerve grafting from CP angle to horizontal portion of facial nerve.

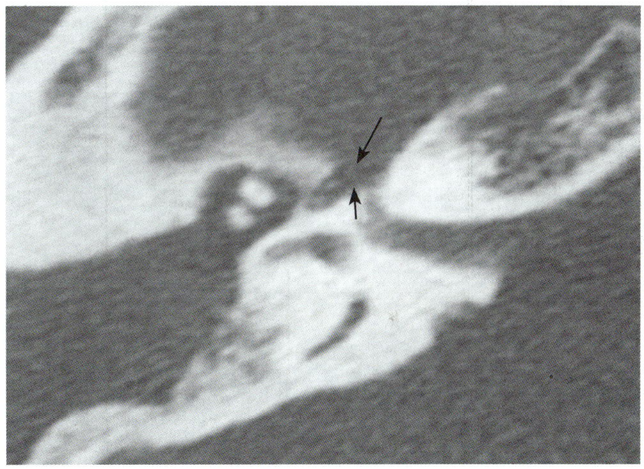

Fig. 73.9 Tumor in the first genu area.

- Head of the malleus and incus removed later is used for ossiculoplasty.
- Drilling is started in the base of the zygoma, and atticotomy performed is extended further anteriorly.
- Removal of cells and bone between the processes cochleariformis and tegmen to expose the first genu—zygomatic, supratubal, attic, supralabyrinthine, and suprafacial cells removed.
- All the cells superior to the horizontal part of fallopian canal (dissection to be done anterior to the ampulla of lateral semicircular canal [LSCC] and superior semicircular canal [SSCC]), superior to genu, and superior to labyrinthine portion are removed.
- Removal of the tumor with safe margins is done followed by nerve grafting.
- Attic defect is reconstructed with a piece of cartilage.
- Underlay temporalis fascia graft is placed and ossiculoplasty performed (**Fig. 73.9, Fig. 73.10, Fig. 73.11,** and **Fig. 73.12**).

5. Neuroma of the horizontal portion of facial nerve extending up to the first genu and extending beyond the second genu. Tumor is excised by transcanal transattic approach; tumor excision performed with safe margins is confirmed with the frozen section. Greater auricular nerve is used for grafting; at the first genu area, it is kept in place with the aid of glue; at the second genu, the graft end and the nerve are approximated in the tunnel of the fallopian canal without any suture or glue (**Fig. 73.13** and **Fig. 73.14a, b**).

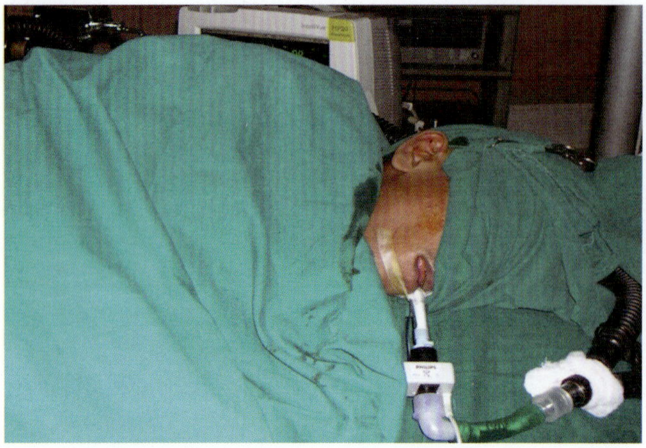

Fig. 73.10 Lateral position of the patient.

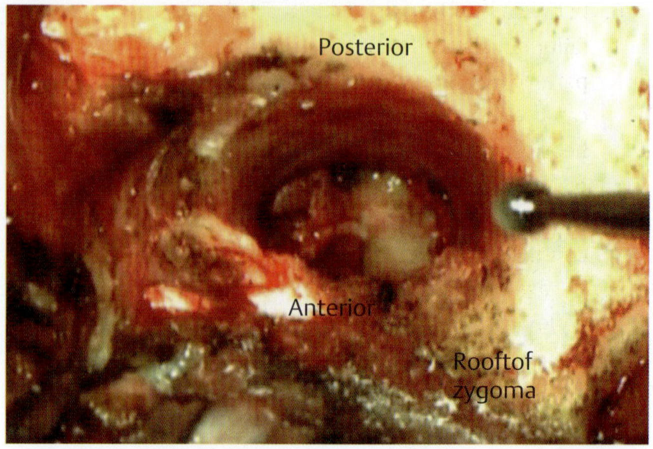

Fig. 73.11 Drilling of right ear root of zygoma.

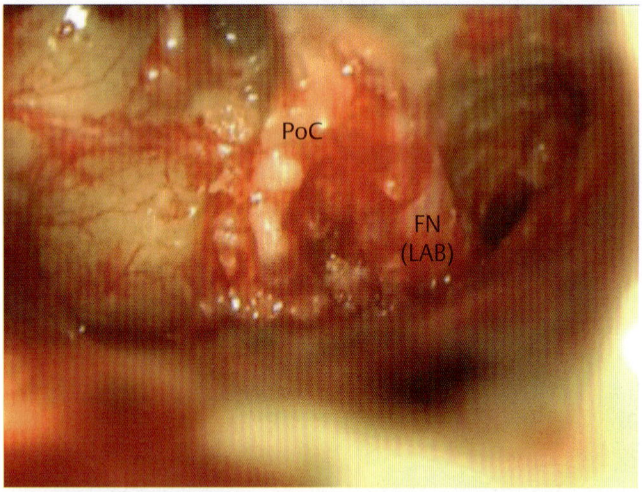

Fig. 73.12 Labyrinthine portion of the facial nerve is exposed by transzygomatic transattic approach.

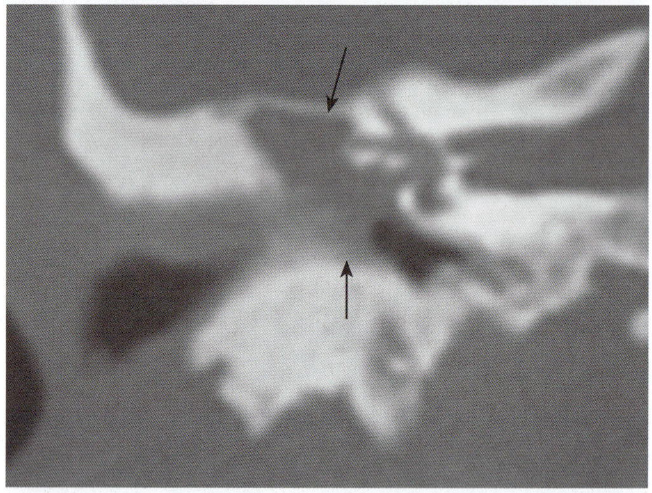

Fig. 73.13 Tumor filling the middle ear.

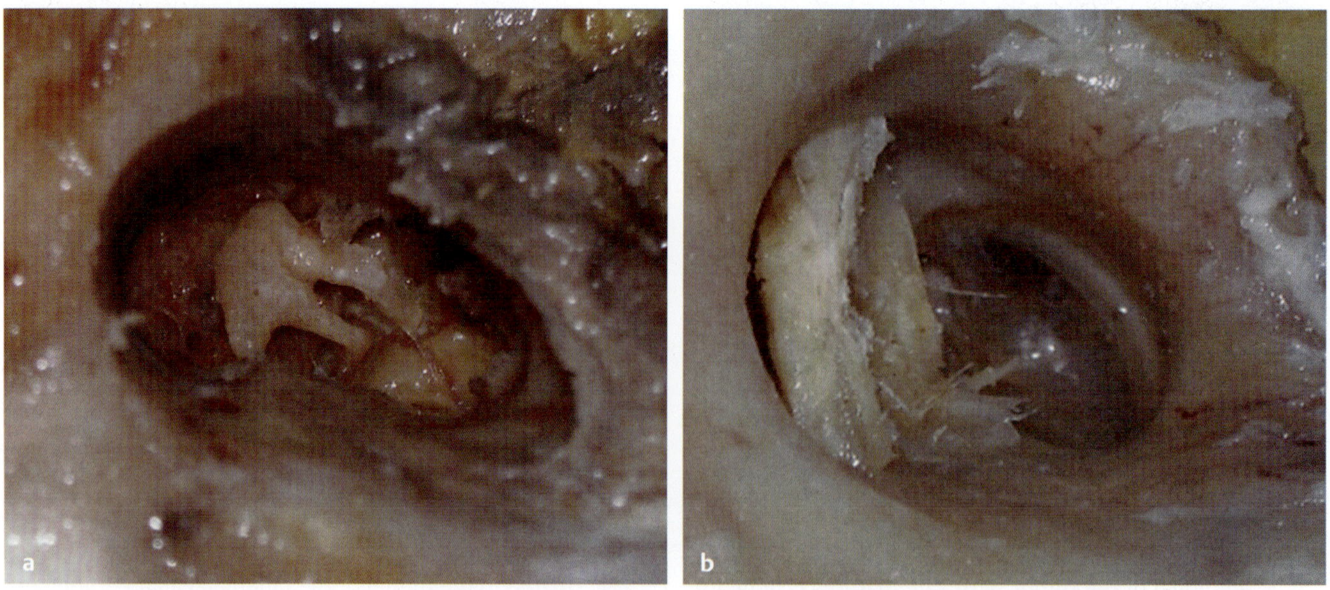

Fig. 73.14 (a) Cadaver dissection specimen showing transcanal atticotomy. (b) Attic is reconstructed with a piece of cartilage.

6. In the case of tumor arising from the vertical portion of fallopian canal, the approach depends on the extension pattern of the tumor; it can present as a growth in the canal with intact tympanic membrane and conductive hearing loss; in this situation, surgery is performed by the transcanal approach, and necessary grafting is performed after excising the tumor with free margins confirmed on the frozen section (**Fig. 73.15**).
7. In case of the tumor in the vertical part just above the stylomastoid portion, which doesn't extend toward the external canal, and on clinical examination there is no positive finding, these cases are almost always misdiagnosed as cases of Bell's palsy (**Fig. 73.16**).
8. Patients presenting with facial nerve neuroma without any facial nerve paresis.
   At times patients present with a mass in the external canal with conductive hearing loss. In such cases, the tumor is diagnosed as facial nerve neuroma owing to the destruction of the fallopian canal seen in the CT scan and diagnosis confirmed by FNAC.
   In this case, the tumor is in the vertical course inferior to LSCC just short of the stylomastoid foramen (**Fig. 73.17a–c, Fig. 73.18, Fig. 73.19,** and **Fig. 73.20a, b**). This patient in the immediate postoperative period had grade 6 palsy and 3 months postoperation improved to grade 2 weakness with complete recovery at the end of 6 months.
9. At times patients with facial nerve neuroma may not present in the external canal, and there is no possibility of doing FNAC as the tumor is inaccessible.
   These patients are operated by a transmastoid approach, and the specimen sent for frozen section confirms the diagnosis followed by which complete excision of the tumor is done. The cases where preoperatively there were no facial nerve paresis or palsy, one will be able to peel out the tumor from the facial nerve fibers without any damage or negligible damage to nerve fiber.
   These patients on immediate postoperative period will have some grade of paresis, which most often eventually improves completely.
10. **Tumor involving the vertical part extending into stylomastoid foramen extending into the infratemporal fossa (Fig. 73.21):** If the CT scan shows the adequate bone over the jugular bulb deeper to the neuroma, then these tumors can be removed by transmastoid, infralabyrinthine, and infracochlear approach. The dissection will be extended toward the infratemporal fossa to identify the free margin of the tumor in the parotid region. The upper limit of the tumor

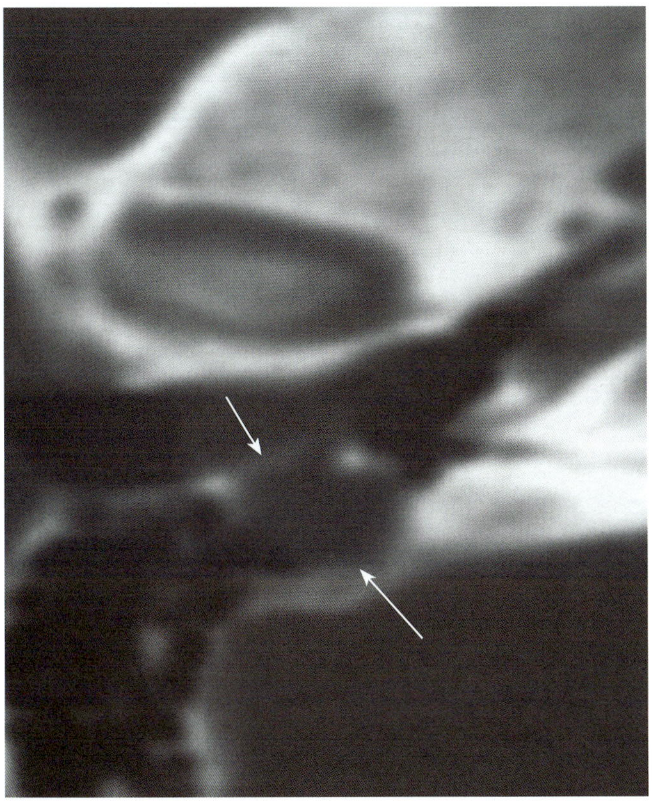

Fig. 73.15 Facial nerve neuroma of the vertical segment of the facial nerve.

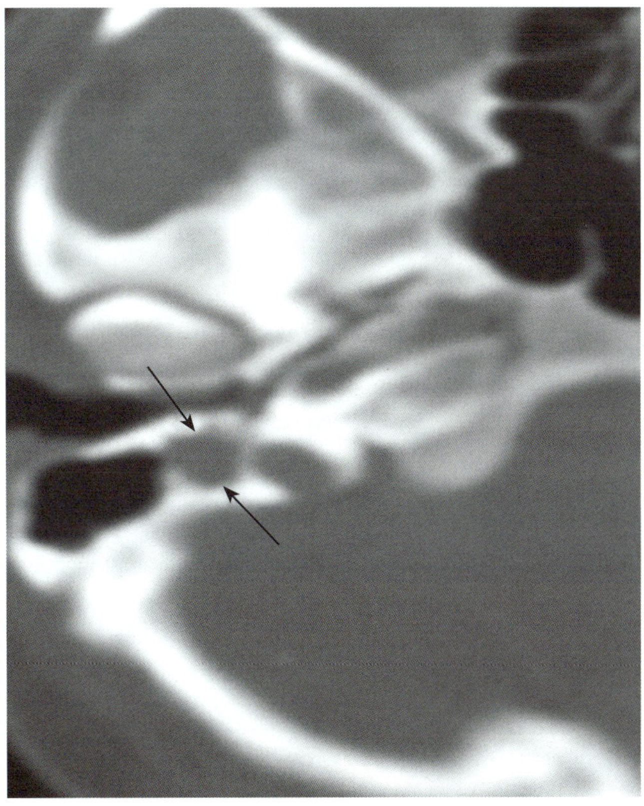

Fig. 73.16 Neuroma at the stylomastoid foramen level.

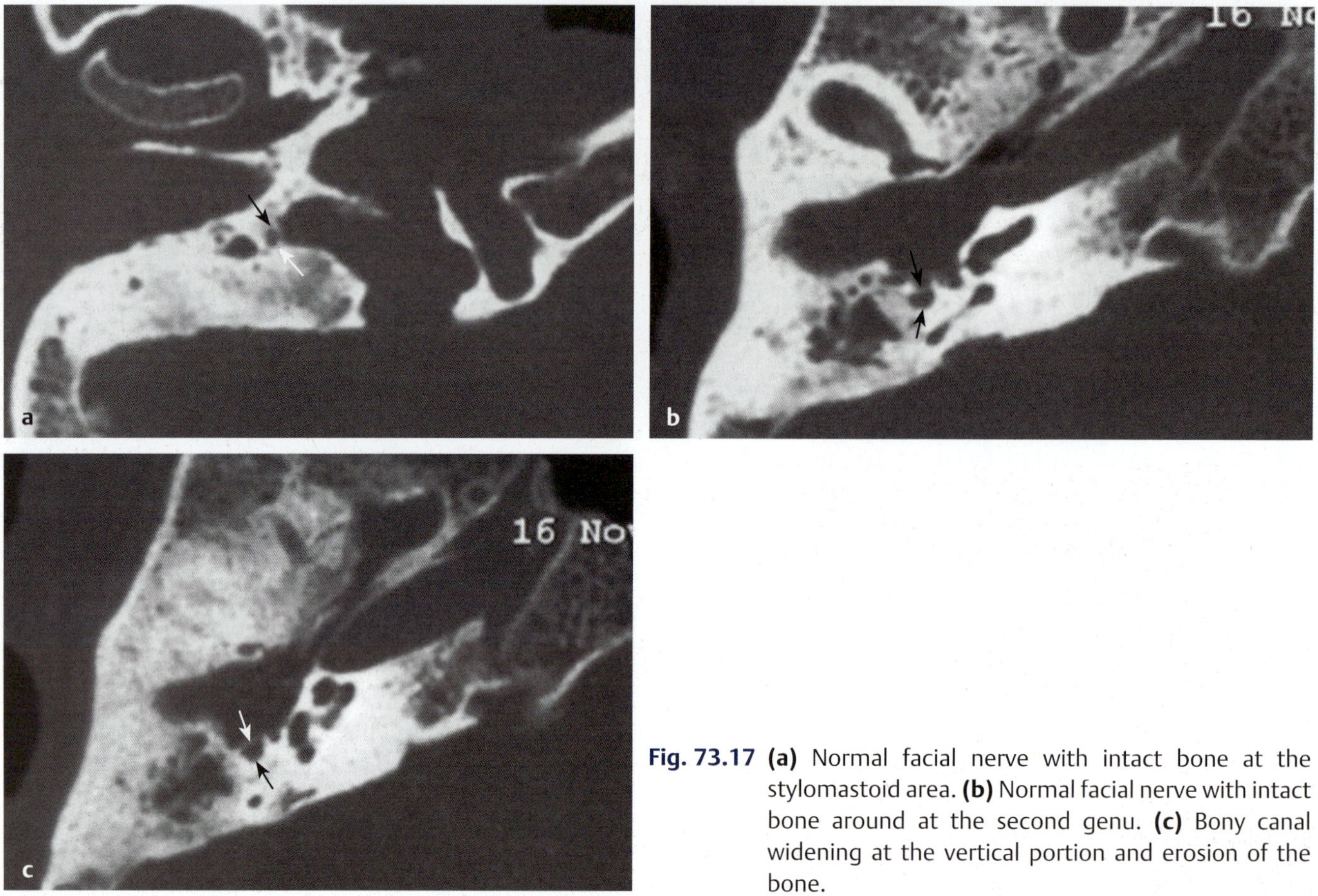

Fig. 73.17 **(a)** Normal facial nerve with intact bone at the stylomastoid area. **(b)** Normal facial nerve with intact bone around at the second genu. **(c)** Bony canal widening at the vertical portion and erosion of the bone.

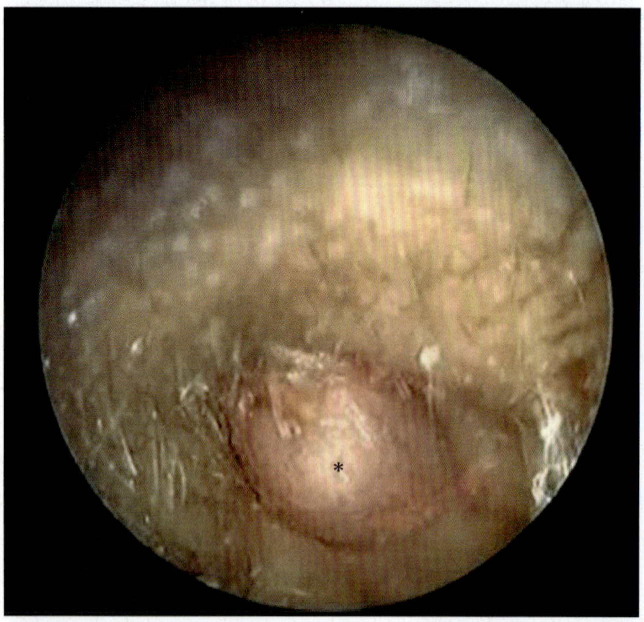

Fig. 73.18 Tumor mass (*) is filling the external auditory canal.

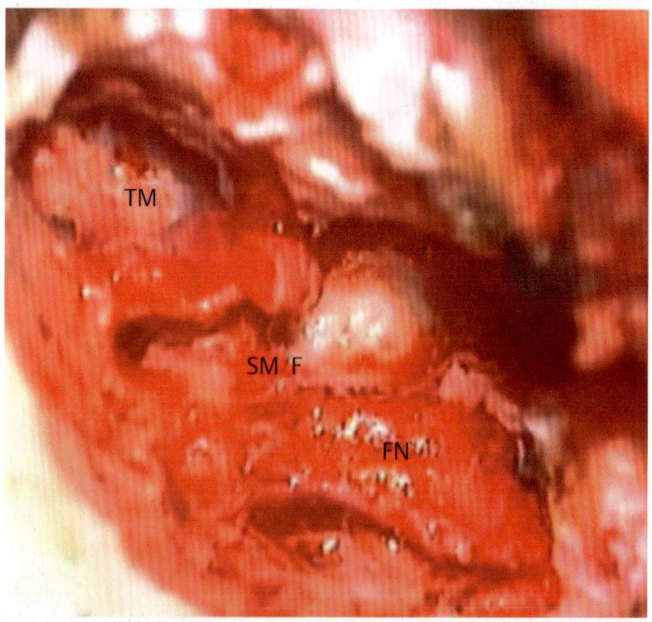

Fig. 73.19 Intraoperative image of the intact facial nerve after complete excision of the tumor with minimal damage to the sheath.

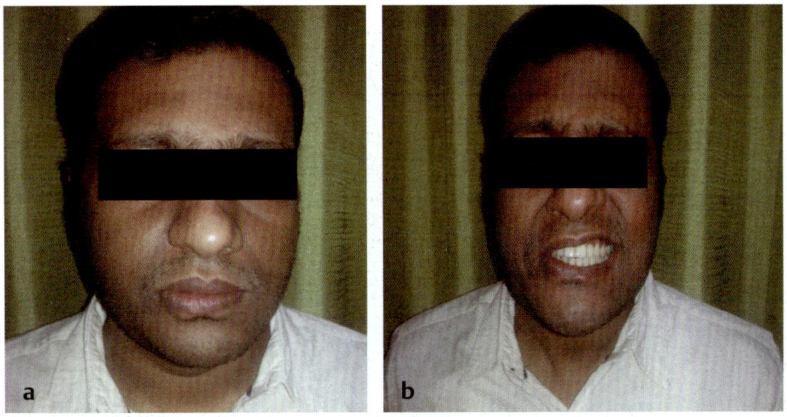

Fig. 73.20 **(a, b)** Three months' postoperative grade 2 weakness.

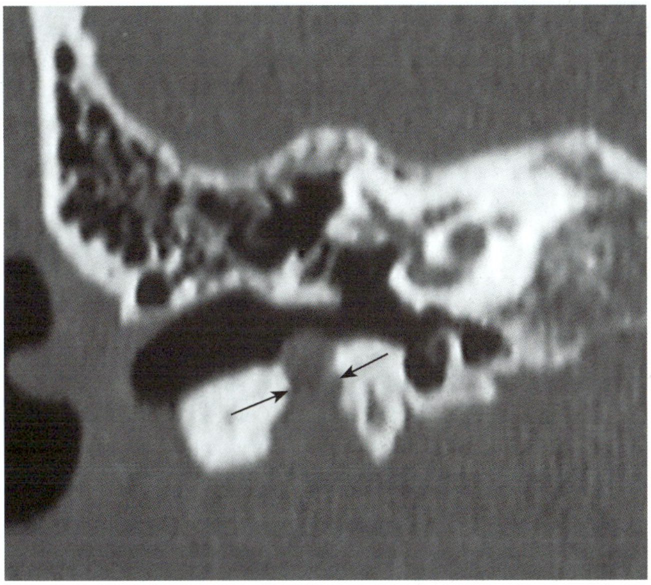

Fig. 73.21 Tumor in the vertical part extending into the stylomastoid foramen extending into the infratemporal fossa.

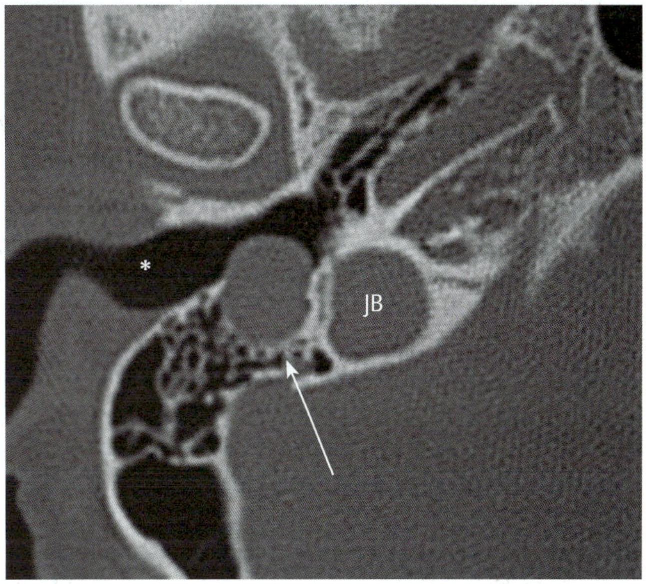

Fig. 73.22 Tumor over the stylomastoid area with thinning out the bone over the jugular bulb. *Denotes the external auditory canal. Thinned out bone between the facial neuroma and the jugular bulb is also visible (*arrow*).

is most often few millimeters inferior to the second genu, that is inferior LSCC; after excision of the tumor, the nerve graft is sutured with 9–0 monofilament at least three sutures in the parotid region. Along the vertical course, in the infracochlear infralabyrinthine dissection, the obliteration of the depth with the pedicle postaural muscle flap is vital to create a vascular bed for the nerve graft to rest. In situation, when the tumor at this location has been there for a long duration, then there is erosion of jugular bulb and subsequently, the possibility of damaging the jugular bulb. One such case was referred to us as glomus jugulare as the operating surgeon while manipulating the tumor at the jugular bulb area led to profuse bleeding; in such situations, it is always wise to keep blood reserved with cross match readily available. The incision and surgery for the tumor in this location will be similar to the tumors of jugular foramen, and as in glomus jugulare, we may obliterate the sigmoid sinus extraluminally that aids in decompressing the jugular bulb from the tumor. Obliteration of the sigmoid sinus is rarely required if the preoperative diagnosis is made and the procedure is planned properly (**Fig. 73.22** and **Fig. 73.23**).

11. **Facial nerve neuroma in the infratemporal fossa or parotid gland area:** This case is approached by parotid incision, that is, modified Blair's incision (**Fig. 73.24**). The size of the incision is modified depending on the location of the tumor. As discussed, earlier one must

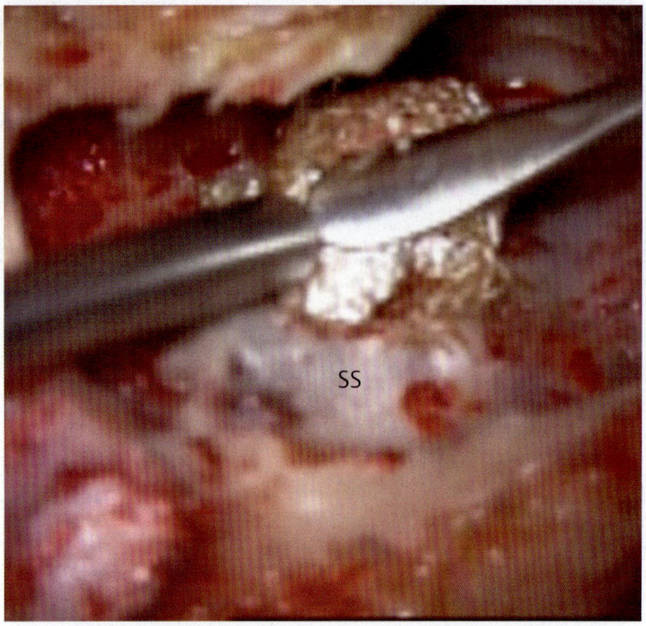

Fig. 73.23 Extraluminal packing of the sigmoid sinus.

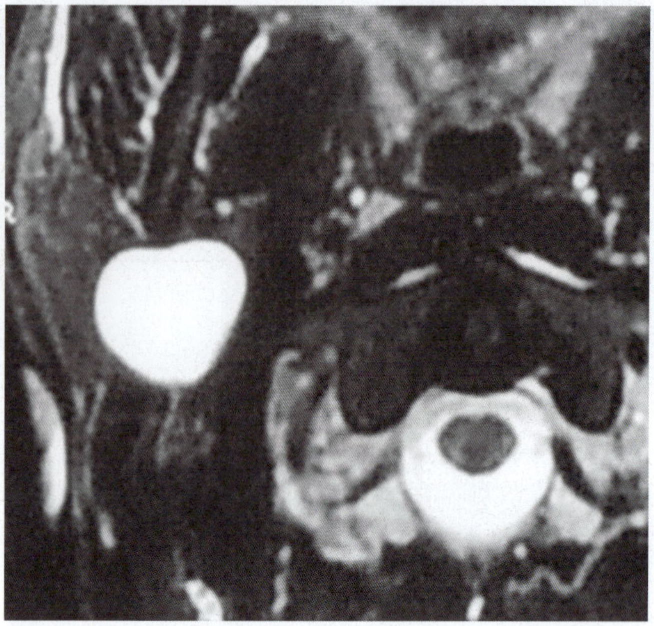

Fig. 73.24 Tumor in the the parotid area.

make every effort to peel off the tumor from the nerve whenever possible. In situations with minimal damage to the fibers, that is, 10 to 15% of fibers, there is no role of grafting. If around 50% of fibers are damaged, one can preserve the rest 50% fibers and perform split-thickness grafting. In a situation where substantial nerve fiber is damaged and/or tumor has involved the main trunk and/or part of the bifurcation after excision, one can perform grafting of the main trunk and the bifurcation with greater auricular nerve with its two branches.

References

1. Schmid C. Neurinom des N. facialis. Jahresz Gersellschaft Schweiz Halsund Ohrenarte. 1930;16:329
2. Sataloff RT, Frattali MA, Myers DL. Intracranial facial neuromas: total tumor removal with facial nerve preservation: a new surgical technique. Ear Nose Throat J 1995;74(4):244–246, 248–256
3. Shelton C, Brackmann DE, Lo WW, Carberry JN. Intratemporal facial nerve hemangiomas. Otolaryngol Head Neck Surg 1991;104(1):116–121
4. Liu R, Fagan P. Facial nerve schwannoma: surgical excision versus conservative management. Ann Otol Rhinol Laryngol 2001;110(11):1025–1029
5. Shambaugh GE Jr, Arenberg IK, Barney PL, Valvassori GE. Facial neurilemmomas: a study of four diverse cases. Arch Otolaryngol 1969;90(6):742–755
6. Pulec JL. Facial nerve neuroma. Laryngoscope 1972;82(7): 1160–1176

Section XXIX

Rehabilitative Surgery

Chapter 74

Hearing Restoration in Skull Base Surgery

Raghu Nandhan and Mohan Kameswaran

Introduction

The lateral skull base encompasses the organ of hearing and balance which may be afflicted in a variety of ways and to different extents, because of involvement by the pathology per se or because of surgical approaches to lesions in its vicinity which warrant a destructive surgical approach toward this special sensory organ. With technological advancements in the auditory neural prosthesis, today there are a number of ways in which hearing can be restored in such scenarios whereby the integrity and function of the inner ear have been compromised in the realm of skull base surgery. This chapter highlights the various options available for hearing rehabilitation in individuals who have undergone skull base surgery involving the inner ear, the salient among these are the contralateral routing of signal (CROS) aids and various implantable hearing solutions including bone conduction implants (BCIs), cochlear implants (CIs), and auditory brainstem implants (ABIs).

Hearing Restoration in Single-sided Deafness and Asymmetrical Hearing Loss Scenarios

If a skull base lesion involves the otic capsule/eighth cranial nerve complex/ cerebellopontine angle (CPA) or if a transotic/transcochlear/translabyrinthine approach is undertaken toward the petrous apex and CPA, hearing loss is profound in that ear. In individuals whose cochlear thresholds are preserved, the onus in skull base dissection is to achieve complete disease clearance while maximally preserving the integrity of the inner ear if possible unless the surgical approach warrants taking down the inner ear. In other inner ear preserving approaches also, surgery can still lead to cochlear insult because of mechanical, thermal, vibratory, or ischemic trauma. Hence, it is paramount that the risk of total hearing loss is always explained to patients while counseling for lateral skull base surgery.

Total hearing loss may be present while the contralateral ear is disease free and holds normal cochlear thresholds (aka single-sided deafness [SSD]) or when the contralateral ear has hearing compromised to a lesser extent (aka asymmetrical hearing loss [AHL]). SSD can result from a variety of etiologies including vestibular schwannoma, Ménière's disease, meningitis, temporal bone trauma, extensive cholesteatoma, radical ear surgery, and other CPA tumors. Rarely, congenital malformations of the inner ear or the seventh cranial nerve complex may also manifest with SSD.[1]

Individuals suffering from SSD/AHL have hearing loss in the affected ear to such a degree that speech discrimination is less than 50% in the worse ear, and the hearing loss asymmetry is to such an extent that there is a speech discrimination differential of approximately 50% between ears, distorting acoustic signal perception (**Fig. 74.1**). They describe a pronounced "head shadow effect" which requires the individual to constantly adjust their head position in an attempt to hear on the affected side. This effect is more pronounced for high-frequency sounds, and affected individuals experience particular difficulty in speech processing and sound localization. In AHL, higher-order binaural sound processing is also lost resulting in impairment of summation and squelch, producing additional difficulties for speech discrimination in noise. Some affected individuals are so profoundly disabled that their hearing loss leads to social isolation and depression.[2]

The traditional approach to auditory rehabilitation in SSD and AHL involves routing the sound signal to the good side with either CROS/BiCROS aids or BCIs. These do not restore a binaural signal but can overcome some of the associated disabilities by placing a sound sensor on the deaf side.

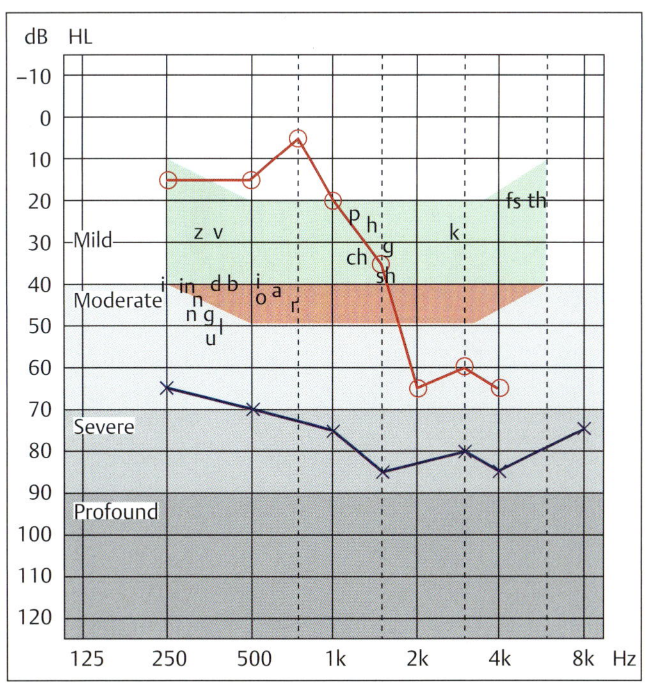

Fig. 74.1 Representative audiogram showing AHL.

Today, this principle of bone conduction is used in implantable hearing devices which use advanced technology to bypass the affected ear and provide precise sound impulses for normal hearing via the contralateral ear, as interaural attenuation for bone conduction across the skull is zero.[3]

Nonsurgical Solution with CROS Hearing Aids

The first hearing solution for SSD/AHL was the CROS or BiCROS hearing aid device, a hearing aid system that consisted of a wired system that connected a transmitter on the poorer ear to the hearing receiver on the better hearing ear. Both the transmitter and receiver hearing aid units could be fitted wirelessly in-the-ear (ITE) or over-the-ear/behind-the-ear (OTE/BTE) models. Traditionally, the CROS system is used when the better ear is ear normal or near-normal, and directional amplification to the better ear is unnecessary for good speech discrimination. The BiCROS system is used when the better ear has some hearing loss as in AHL individuals.[1,2] As a result, directional amplification is necessary for good speech discrimination as well as for receiving the transmission from the offside mike (**Fig. 74.2**).

Technological advancements in wireless transmission via FM lead to the WiFi CROS system which was more cosmetically appealing and user friendly. The small-time delay associated with the transmission gives the user the necessary temporal cues to help determine from which side the sound originated. The minor problems faced with this system were the pressure effects over the skull with vibration-induced discomfort in the ears.[1]

The main advantages of CROS technology are (1) sounds coming from the deaf side can be heard better (even though hearing in the better ear) and (2) can get some cues about the location of the sound. Primary disadvantages are (1) the extra sound from the bad side may, at times, interfere with the ability to understand what is being heard from the good side, and (2) CROS technology certainly cannot restore natural localization and sound reduction, as that requires two ears, and CROS only inserts sound into one ear. These issues have encouraged the use of implantable hearing solutions postsurgery in recent times.[2]

Pseudobinaural Solution with Bone Conduction Implants

This is a popular implantable solution available for hearing rehabilitation post skull base surgery, whereby the BCI may be placed simultaneously along with the completion of disease clearance or as a staged procedure after the primary wound healing for individuals who have the maximal conductive loss because of blind sac closure with middle ear and mastoid cavity obliteration, wherein the inner ear is preserved or a dead ear as in the translabyrinthine approaches to CPA lesions.[3]

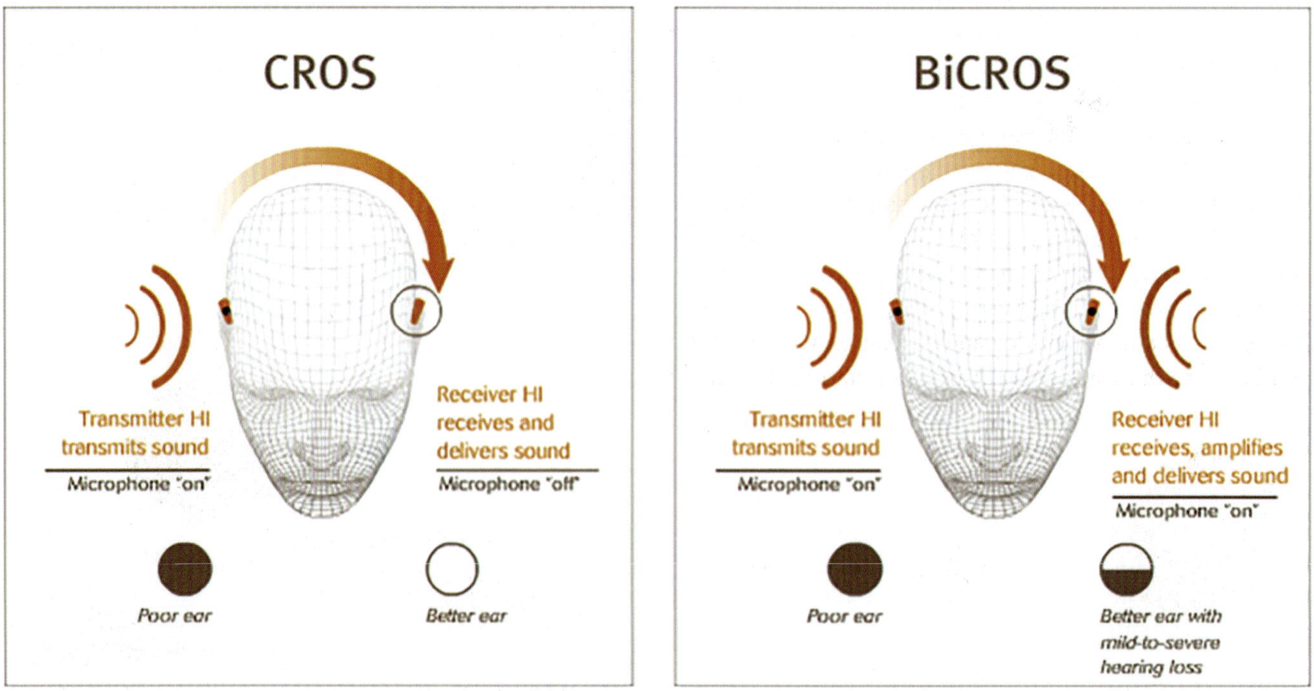

Fig. 74.2 CROS and BiCROS aid technology.

The implantable bone-anchored hearing aid (BAHA) system (Cochlear Inc, Melbourne, Australia) is the most popular among the BCI, and it uses the unique principle of osseointegration for coupling the hearing aid to the skull of the patient using an abutment and titanium fixture (**Fig. 74.3**). The BAHA was cleared to treat SSD/AHL when patients cannot use (as in total pinnectomy for pinna/ear canal malignancy) or for any reason will not use a CROS aid. BAHA candidacy includes SSD candidates with bone conduction thresholds better than 35 dB in the good ear and AHL candidates whose better ear has thresholds better than 55 dB.[3]

The BAHA device works by transferring sound directly into the ipsilateral cochlea or from the deaf side to the cochlea of the hearing ear using bone conduction. The device has three main parts: an external sound processor, an abutment, and a small titanium implant or fixture, which is placed in the skull bone, behind the deaf ear. The abutment is then attached and the sound processor clipped onto the abutment. The sound processor transmits sound waves to the titanium fixture, which in turn causes the sound waves to travel through the skull and ultimately to the cochlea of the hearing ear, resulting in the sensation of hearing from the deaf side. A subtle difference in sound combined with a minimal time delay associated with transmission gives the user the necessary temporal cues to help determine from which side the sound originated.

The BAHA device placement requires a precise surgery which can also be performed under local anesthesia and is especially staged in children allowing time for wound healing and osseointegration (**Fig. 74.4**). The procedure involves precise surface marking on the temporal cortex at an angle of 45 degrees above the Frankfurt plane and 55 mm behind the ear. A small linear incision is given to expose the bony cortex. After eversion of the periosteum with a cruciate incision, a 3-mm and then a 4-mm guided sinkhole is made with the drill system at a perpendicular angle to the cortex. A countersink of 4 mm is performed around the sinkhole with sharp bony margins after confirming the base with a respiratory to avoid dural exposure. Diathermy is best avoided and drilling needs to be done with copious irrigation to avoid thermal injury to the bone. A BAHA titanium fixture is carefully anchored into this well with a torque of 45 Ncm rotation to promote osseointegration. The abutment which comes preloaded is of different lengths based on scalp thickness. Postoperative wound site care is routine and simple. Loading of the sound processor happens 6 to 8 weeks allowing time for complete osseointegration and wound healing. Problems with wound are managed based on the Holger's grading.[3]

Although BAHA is a highly effective treatment option after skull base surgery, its major drawback has been the percutaneous transmission technique, which may lead to wound infection and noncompliance among patients. BCI technology has further advanced today, with newer devices becoming sophisticated and surgery done by minimal access technique (as in the MIPS technique for Ponto, Oticon medical, Nijmegen, The Netherlands). The biggest breakthrough came with the introduction of implants like the BAHA Attract (Cochlear Ltd, Australia) and the vibrant BoneBridge implant (MedEL Inc, Innsbruck, Austria) both of which use transcutaneous technology similar to the radiofrequency conduction across two magnets as in CI (**Fig. 74.5**). The only difference

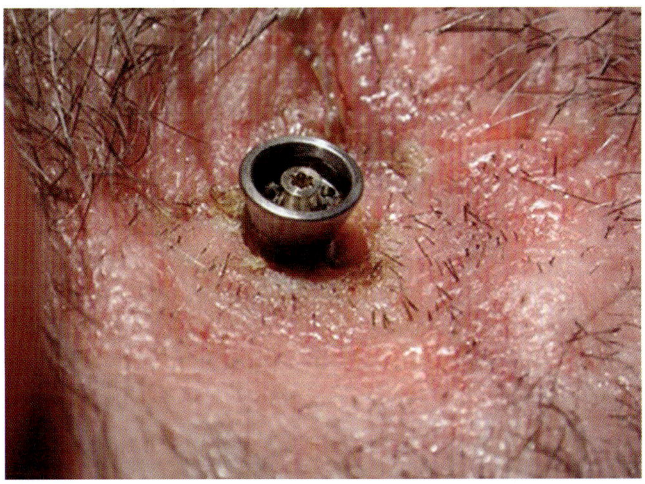

Fig. 74.4 BAHA fixture with abutment in situ in a skull base surgery patient.

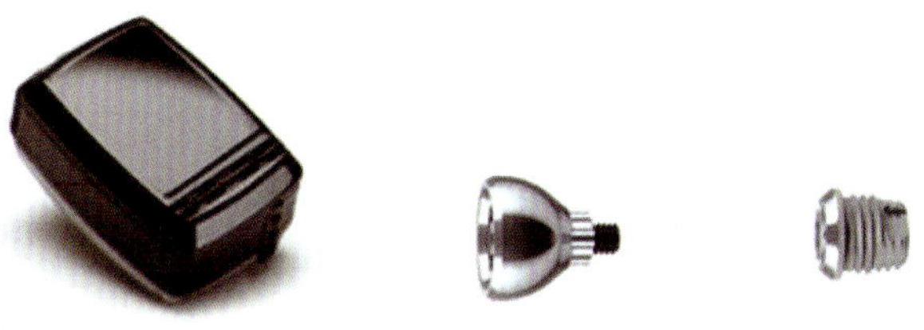

Fig. 74.3 BAHA (Cochlear Ltd, Australia) bone conduction implant system.

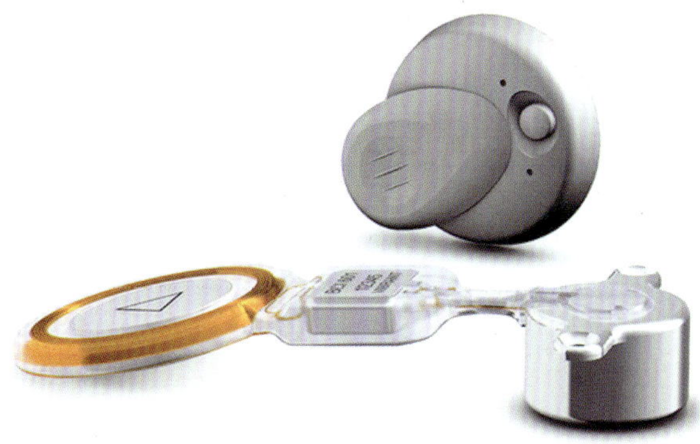

Fig. 74.5 The MedEL BoneBridge system, Innsbruck, Austria.

being the BoneBridge has an actively vibrating floating mass transducer in the internal package, unlike the BAHA Attract system, which just transmits sound vibrations via the magnets across the surface.

The BoneBridge includes an external part, the audio processor, and an implanted part, the BCI. The surgery is very similar to BAHA but requires a larger incision and bed drilling to fit in the implant as per company specifications. The audio processor is worn on the head and contains two microphones, a digital signal processor and a battery. The BCI consists of a receiver coil, a demodulator, and a transducer. Information from the audio processor is sent transcutaneously to the BCI so that the transducer (the bone conduction floating mass transducer [BC-FMT]) actively vibrates in a controlled manner, specific to each patient's hearing needs. The BC-FMT is about 10 mm in height (with a drill depth of 8.7 mm), 15.8 mm in diameter, and weighs about 10 g. The BCI is implanted in the mastoid and temporal region of the ear (**Fig. 74.6**). When the implant is in position and is stimulated from the externally worn audio processor, it causes the bone to vibrate and stimulates the auditory system.

It is highly recommended to do a preoperative high-resolution computed tomography (HRCT) scan that needs to be thoroughly analyzed for cortical bone thickness (should be at least 10 mm at the implant bed site) and consistency of the mastoid bone, the placement of sigmoid sinus and the dura. The BC-FMT is installed into the sinodural angle of the mastoid bone, and the receiver coil of the BCI is installed under the skin in the postauricular area not more than 7 mm below the external surface of the skin (**Fig. 74.7**).

Since osseointegration of the screws is not needed after implantation, the processor can be programmed as soon as the swelling of the skin has reduced. The BoneBridge ensures optimal daily hearing performance while remaining discreet and unobtrusive, but it has encountered complications like postsurgery displacement of the implant, postsurgical translocation of the BC-FMT because of trauma or inferior surgical positioning, extrusion of the implant, and the potential risk of meningitis in case the dura or sigmoid sinus is damaged during the operation. Hence, at present, this BoneBridge implant is not approved for children younger than 5 years, in whom the skull thickness is not adequate for implantation.

MedEL Inc, Austria has recently launched a novel nonsurgical alternative to BCI, the MedEL ADHEAR system which has a BCI processor clipped onto the mastoid area with an adhesive pad to transmit signals transcutaneously into the skull bone (**Fig. 74.8**). This is a viable option for those who do not like percutaneous devices and for those whose bony cortex is not amenable for implanting a BoneBridge or BAHA Attract.

True Bimodal Binaural Solution with Cochlear Implants

CIs have the potential to restore true binaural hearing, not possible with other technologies, but require the brain to integrate electric and acoustic stimuli. CI in SSD provides binaural–bimodal hearing, which is acoustic in the normal ear and CI-aided electrical stimuli on the side of SSD. On the other hand, CI in AHL candidates provides acoustically amplified hearing aid signals in one ear to match up with electrical hearing in the implanted ear. Recent literature has produced evidence to support tangible benefits of CI in SSD and AHL including improved spatial orientation, squelch, temporal summation, and music appreciation[5]

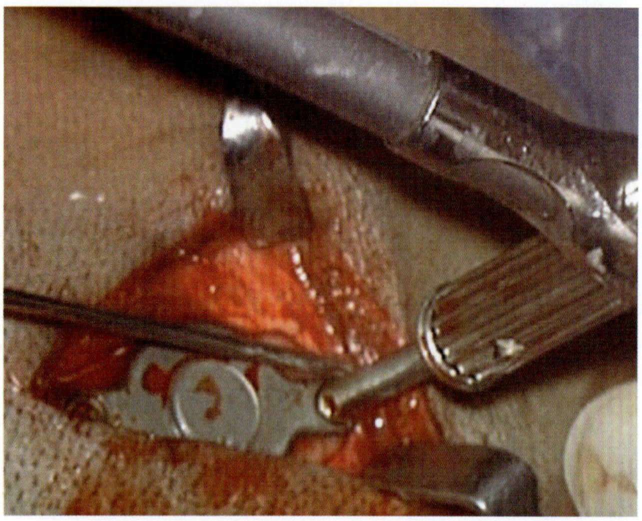

Fig. 74.6 MedEL BoneBridge BC-FMT being anchored in situ with titanium screws.

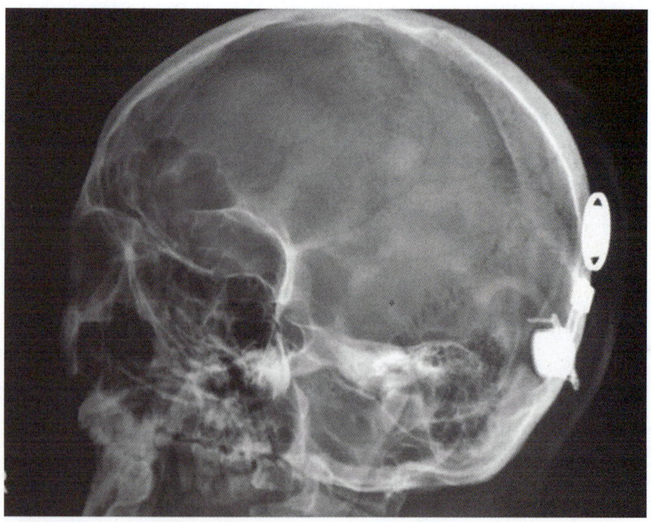

Fig. 74.7 Postoperative X-ray skull lateral view showing BoneBridge in situ.

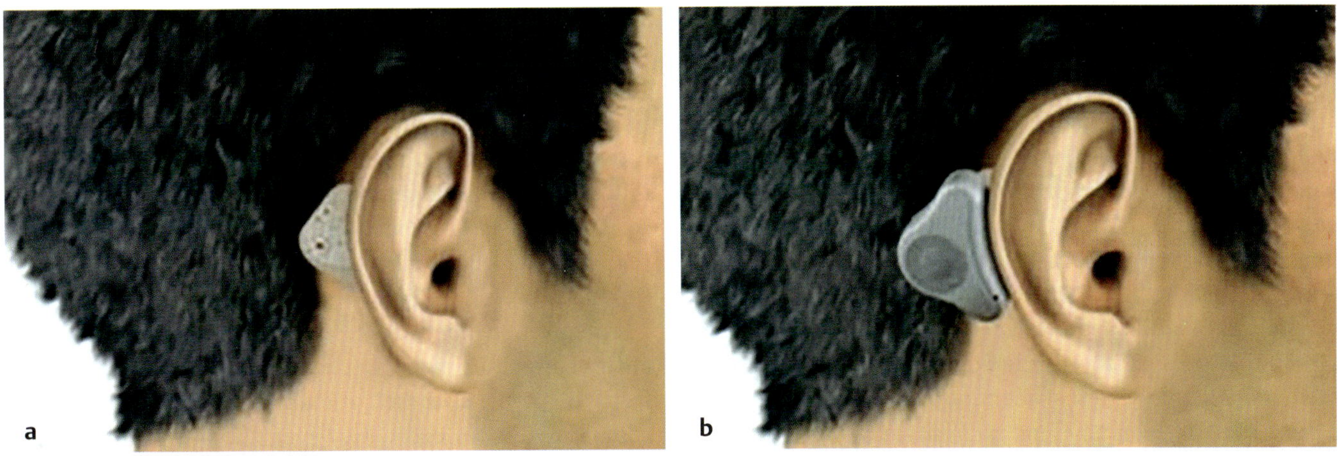

Fig. 74.8 Adhesive test device: **(a)** adhesive adaptor, **(b)** audio processor (MED-EL, Innsbruck, Austria).

AHL individuals, who have profound loss due to skull base pathology/surgery on one side and age-related progressive hearing loss on the other ear, may suffer from cochlear dead regions which are more common with thresholds above 70 dB HL.[6] Also, the high levels required to render high-frequency speech audible with hearing aid in their precious ear, may in fact degrade the acoustic signals in these individuals. Such individuals experience significant difficulty in everyday communication, particularly in noisy backgrounds, where low-frequency amplification alone is not sufficient to allow high levels of speech understanding.

By receiving a CI in their profoundly deaf ear (provided the integrity of the cochlea and the eighth cranial nerve complex is preserved postsurgery), these candidates can perceive sounds through bimodal–binaural hearing using both CI and hearing aid synchronized together. This method of bimodal (electrical + acoustic) binaural stimulation provides better sound localization and speech discrimination in noise improving the patients' communication skills and quality of life. Unlike in the SSD group, the benefits in AHL have been observed largely because of the CI input which predominated when compared with the hearing aid. It is, however, often a challenge especially in children to program the implant synchronously to match the contralateral hearing aid use. There are issues with defining optimal habilitation techniques and predicting outcomes for such candidates, as they need to get accustomed to receiving the bimodal combined psychophysical signals in their auditory cortex.[7,8]

An evidence base is emerging to support the use of CI in skull base disease/surgery for individuals with SSD and AHL. Reported benefits include improvement in auditory capacity, tinnitus suppression, and improved quality of life. Thereby, many skull base centers across the world have now adopted CI as a standard measure of hearing rehabilitation post skull base surgery.[9] Author's institution follows this norm as a simultaneous and staged procedure as indicated when dealing with situations like osseous labyrinthectomy done for burnt-out Ménière's disease, repair of meningoencephaloceles affecting the inner ear, subtotal petrosectomy done for cholesteatoma, glomus tumor surgery while preserving the inner ear, translabyrinthine vestibular schwannoma excision with cochlear nerve preservation, etc.[10,11,12]

CI in patients with chronic tympanomastoid disease is complicated and challenging. Subtotal petrosectomy with CI is indicated in previous chronic otitis media/mastoid cavities/healed dry ears as a single stage and in those in quiescent phase. This procedure is also undertaken in atelectatic ears, burnt-out Ménière's disease, recalcitrant otitis externa, or extensive tympanosclerosis. Patients with unfavorable anatomical conditions like contracted sclerotic mastoid with anteriorly placed sigmoid sinus may also need this approach to gain access for CI. Inner ear malformations are associated with an abnormally positioned facial nerve, or cerebrospinal fluid (CSF) or perilymph "gusher." Easy identification and better exposure of anatomical landmarks like facial nerve trajectory, high chances of CSF or perilymph gusher, sealing off eustachian tube, and isolating cavity to reduce the possibility of CSF leak and meningitis are the reasons to consider subtotal petrosectomy with CI in patients with inner ear malformations. Subtotal petrosectomy with CI has also been proposed for fractures of temporal bone with intact cochlear nerve, as fractures of otic capsule heal just by fibrous union rather than new bone formation, which carries a lifelong risk of meningitis with or without CI. Some authors recommend this as a standard approach in skull base disease in order to avoid damage to critical structures like facial nerve, jugular bulb, and internal carotid artery.[13,14,15]

This procedure helps in isolating the middle ear/mastoid cavity from external environment after removal of disease, improves the exposure and access, reduces risk of infection and CSF leaks, and facilitates CI within a secure aseptic space. Additionally, it improves the access and visibility of round window and promontory in difficult situations requiring drill out. Meticulous surgical technique will reduce the complications, and long-term follow-up is needed to detect any recurrence of cholesteatoma. The technique was first described by Fisch and Mattox and involves drilling and eradication of all mastoid cells, removal of middle ear mucosa, tympanic membrane, skin of external auditory canal (EAC) along with closure of eustachian tube, and external ear canal with obliteration of cavity with fat or muscle.[16]

The surgical procedure is akin to any tympanomastoid approach and is performed by the postauricular route. An anteriorly based Palva pedicled flap or superiorly based temporal flap is raised. The EAC is completely transected, and the skin is everted to perform a blind sac closure. The subcutaneous tissue and tragal cartilage are used to reinforce the blind sac with a second layer. The skin of EAC is elevated up to the annulus and removed along with tympanic membrane, incus, and malleus. Canal wall down mastoidectomy is performed to remove as many pneumatized cells as possible to eradicate the disease. The eustachian tube is packed with muscle after inverting the mucosa (**Fig. 74.9**). The bed is drilled for receiver–stimulator of implant. The electrode is then inserted through round window if present or drill out is done in ossification cases. The cavity is packed with abdominal fat and temporalis muscle flap, and the wound is closed in layers.

In cases of previous cavity, meticulous elevation of cavity lining should be done to avoid leaving any remnant debris which would leave a potential risk of cholesteatoma in an obliterated cavity. In patients with cholesteatoma, complete removal of disease should be confirmed before inserting the implant or else the implant should be staged after at least 6 months when disease-free status is confirmed on repeat diffusion-weighted imaging (DWI) and magnetic resonance imaging (MRI) scans (**Fig. 74.10**). Blind sac closure and mastoid cavity obliteration with muscle/fat need to be done at the end of procedure (**Fig. 74.11**).

Fat infection, blind sac closure breakdown, and entrapped cholesteatoma are risks associated with this technique. Long-term follow-up of these patients is recommended, as late complications can occur. However, the detection of recurrent cholesteatoma is limited clinically and radiologically by the blind sac closure of the EAC and the artefact caused by the cochlear implant making MRI redundant. Soft tissue expansion or bony erosion in sequential CT scanning has been advocated as an indicator of recurrent cholesteatoma, but distinguishing between soft tissue and cholesteatoma reliably remains a challenge. Long-term follow-up is recommended in view of late complications.[17,18,19]

Incidence of severe to profound sensorineural hearing loss in Ménière's disease is reported to be 1 to 6% in literature.[19,20,21] CI has proved to be an effective management option for profound hearing loss in patients with unilateral or bilateral Ménière's disease. CI also helps with reduction in tinnitus. Osseous three-canal labyrinthectomy is required in patients who have disabling vertigo to alleviate their symptom and this can be staged or done simultaneously with CI (**Fig. 74.12**). The benefits of simultaneous labyrinthectomy and CI include prevention of implantation of a fibrosed or ossified cochlea, a decrease in the duration of deafness, and a single operative procedure. During simultaneous

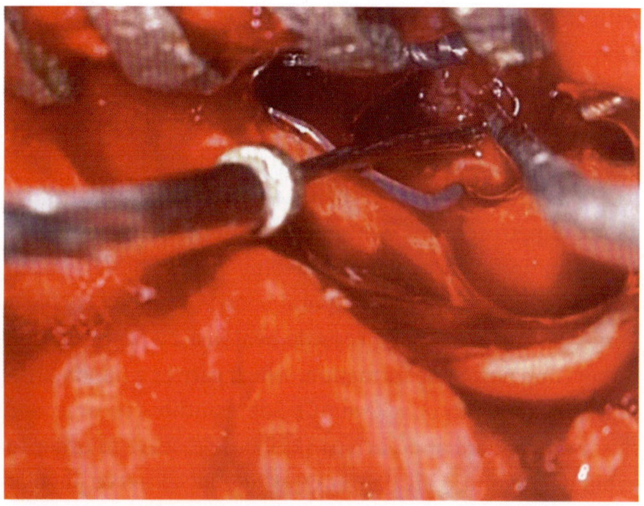

Fig. 74.9 ET plugging post-CI electrode placement.

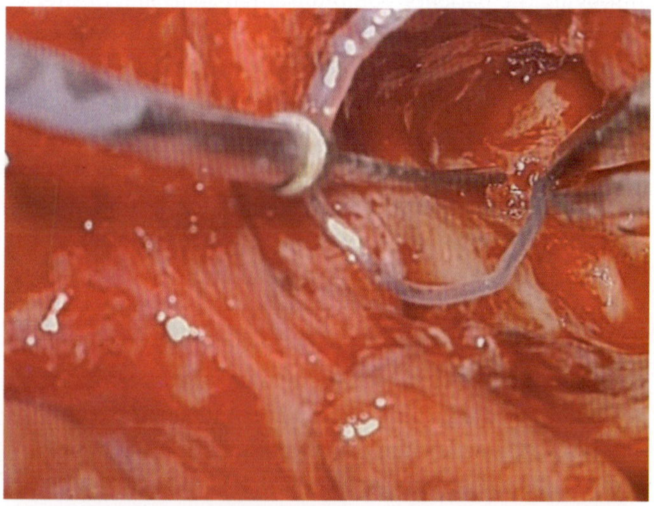

Fig. 74.10 CI electrode insertion staged after subtotal petrosectomy.

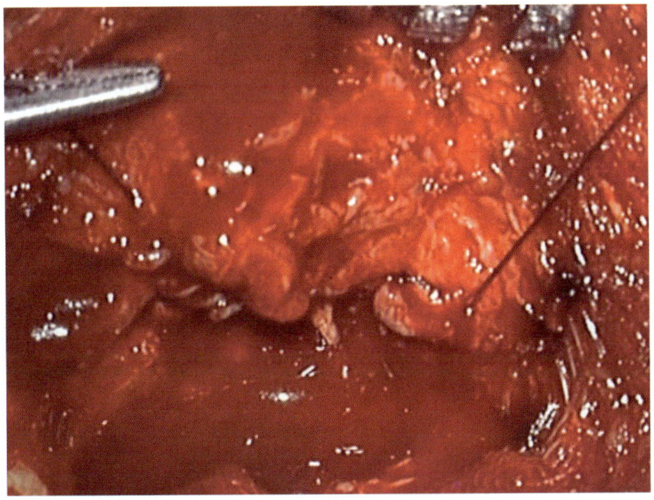

Fig. 74.11 Post-CI blind sac closure performed with mastoid cavity obliteration.

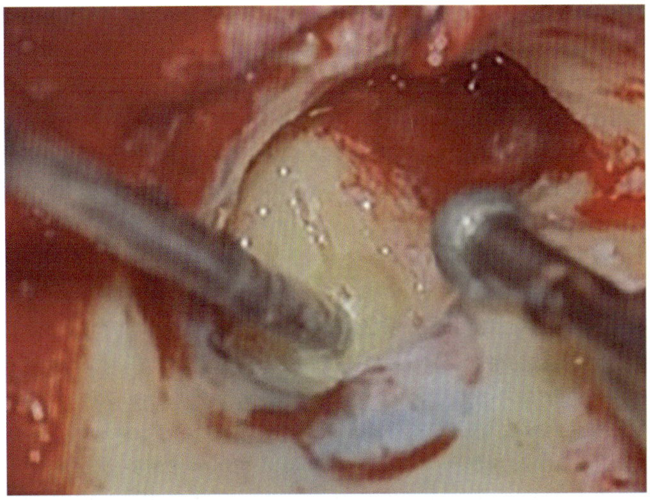

Fig. 74.12 Three canal osseous labyrinthectomy in progress with preservation of cochlea.

labyrinthectomy and CI, the round window is identified and exposed through a posterior tympanotomy before undertaking labyrinthectomy (**Fig. 74.13**).[22] CI has proved to be effective in hearing restoration, control of vertigo, and reduction of tinnitus in patients with advanced Ménière's disease.[23,24] Proper selection criteria for CI and good preoperative counseling are vital for achieving the anticipated outcomes.

Postoperative complications of this approach may be vertigo, tinnitus, facial paresis, and inadvertent facial stimulation at "switch-on" of the implant similar to CI in advanced otosclerosis because of dissipation of current beyond the confines of the bony cochlea.[24,25] Significant hearing improvement occurs with CI, and implantation does not seem to adversely alter the natural history of vestibular function. Beneficial effect of CI on tinnitus has been noted in most patients because CI addresses the changes in neural activity caused by reduced auditory input, thought to be responsible for tinnitus. Fluctuation in hearing performance during acute attacks has been reported and is seen in approximately one-third of patients.[26] Fluctuation in hearing during an acute attack is because of physical changes relative to the implant array with the spiral ganglion neurons or changes in spiral ganglion neurons because of the hydropic state. During an acute attack, the ability to hear with a cochlear implant may decrease, sound may become very high pitched, there may be intolerance to sound, distortion of sound, or tinnitus. The hearing returns to the baseline following resolution of acute attacks. Fluctuations in hearing can be overcome by CI reprogramming. Timely and appropriate audiological expertise with habilitationist's inputs are necessary to achieve optimal CI performance in such cases.[26,27]

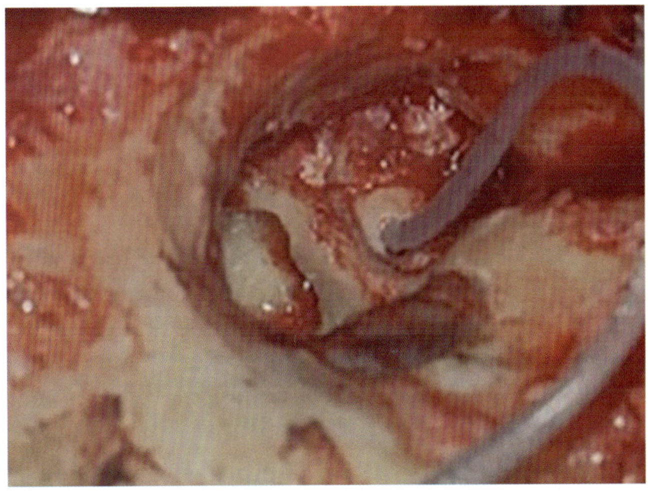

Fig. 74.13 Single-stage CI insertion postlabyrinthectomy.

Hearing Restoration with Auditory Brainstem Implantation

When the cochlea/cochlear nerve is damaged by skull base pathology or through surgery, the only viable option left for hearing restoration is performing an ABI.[28] Multidisciplinary collaboration between neurotologist, neurosurgeon, implant audiologist, and neuroanesthetist is required in order to perform this intricate and sophisticated surgery. ABIs are indicated for patients with neurofibromatosis type 2 (NF2) tumors involving both vestibulocochlear nerves. The ABI helps bypass the damaged cochlear nerves and stimulates the cochlear nucleus in the brainstem directly thereby restoring auditory sensation. The implant is placed in the lateral recess of the fourth ventricle abutting the dorsal and ventral cochlear nuclei after tumor resection.[27,28] The indications for ABI have recently expanded from CPA tumors onto even nontumoral cases, such as congenital bilateral cochlear nerve aplasia/hypoplasia. In such cases, the ABI helps bypass the nonfunctioning hypoplastic or absent cochlear nerves and stimulates the cochlear nucleus directly thereby restoring auditory sensation.[29]

Researchers at the House Ear Institute (HEI), in USA where the ABI was initially developed, agree that most patients with the implant have good auditory awareness with appreciation of environmental sounds but obtain more modest benefit with regard to speech perception.[28] Majority of ABI patients use the implant in order to facilitate lip reading, while some can, in varying degrees, comprehend speech directly. It has been demonstrated that the ABI with surface electrodes may provide sufficient stimulation of the central auditory system in adults for open-set speech recognition.[29] These favorable results motivated the clinicians to extend ABI indications onto children with profound hearing loss because of labyrinthitis ossificans or cochlear nerve aplasia who were not candidates for CI. ABI system consists of a receiver–stimulator, electrode array and electrode plate internally and a speech processor, microphone, and transmitter coil externally (**Fig. 74.14**).[28,30]

A meticulous work-up is mandatory, prior to selection of ideal cases for ABI. High-resolution radioimaging with CT/MRI of the brain and inner ear often provides valuable clues to the operating team for planning the side of implantation and the surgical approach. Especially, serial MRI imaging for surveillance of residual pathology in the CPA may be an issue with a magnet in situ.[31] If warranted, the magnet alone may need to be removed prior to imaging. Newer cochlear implants have packages which are MRI friendly withstanding up to a dose of 1.2 Tesla and this may be a way forward in the future of ABI as well. Advanced objective electrophysiological hearing tests need to be performed in order to assess the functions of the brainstem and higher auditory centers. Extensive counseling for the patients and their families regarding the details of surgery, habilitation process, and the expected outcomes of the ABI is vital.[31]

The operative procedure is a joint venture reminiscent of any skull base surgery involving the neurosurgeons and ENT skull base surgeons approaching the CPA.[32] ABI is more challenging than CI because of the involvement of surgery at the level of brainstem and CSF in the posterior fossa in the background of a pulsatile field for implantation. Knowledge of the anatomical landmarks and variants in anatomy of the brainstem is vital for ABI surgery.[33]

Under intensive neuroanesthesia with intraoperative cranial nerve monitoring, the patient is positioned head and neck flexed in order to gain good exposure of the occipital and retromastoid regions. A reverse hockey stick incision or extended curvilinear incision is made in the retromastoid region in order to expose the squamous part of occipital bone and temporal bone (**Fig. 74.15**). A burrow is made at the asterion using the craniotome. Craniotomy exposes the transverse sinus superiorly and sigmoid sinus laterally. Dura needs to be opened by a vertical incision 1 cm away from the sigmoid sinus and is reflected laterally. CSF is let out from the basal cisterns to make the cerebellum lax. Cerebellum is retracted medially to reach the CPA where the seventh and eighth nerve complex is identified (**Fig. 74.16**). Inferiorly, the lower cranial nerves are seen and followed medially onto the foramen of Luschka where the choroid plexus is identified. Further dissection is done to reach the floor of the fourth ventricle, where a constant vein called the straight vein is present, which leads to the site of the cochlear nucleus.[34]

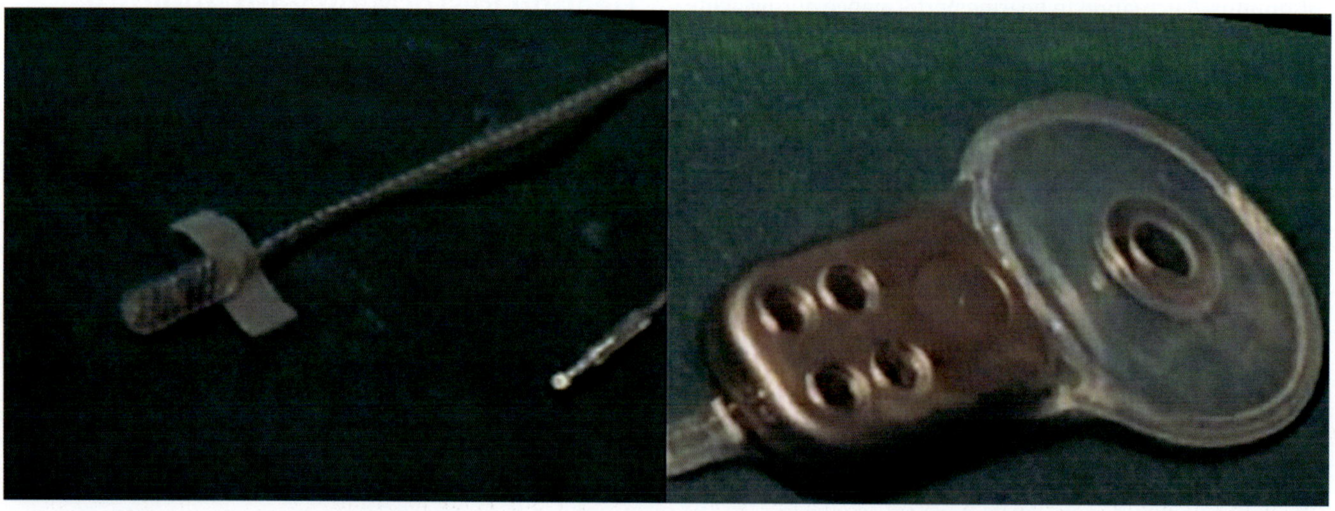

Fig. 74.14 Two ends of auditory brainstem implant.

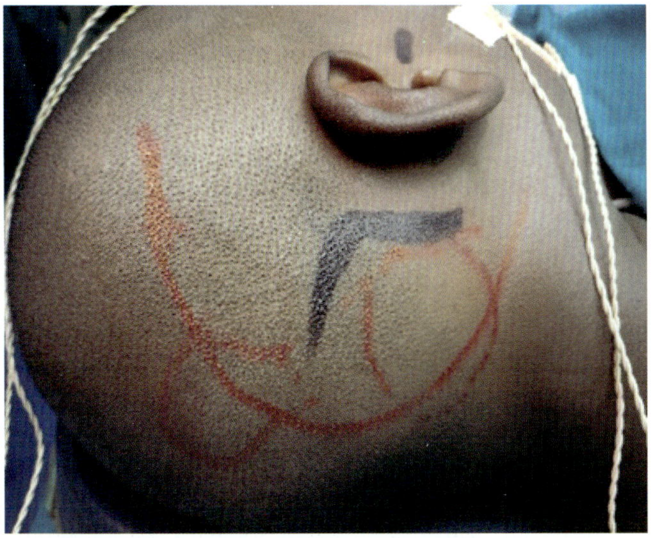

Fig. 74.15 Showing the markings for incision, placement of receiver stimulator complex and craniotomy in *red*. Junction of transverse and sigmoid sinus in *blue*.

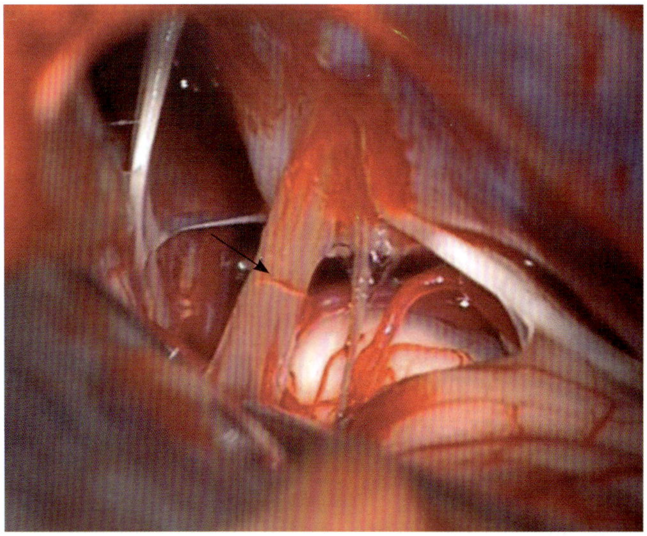

Fig. 74.16 CP angle showing facial nerve with hypoplastic vestibulocochlear nerve bundle.

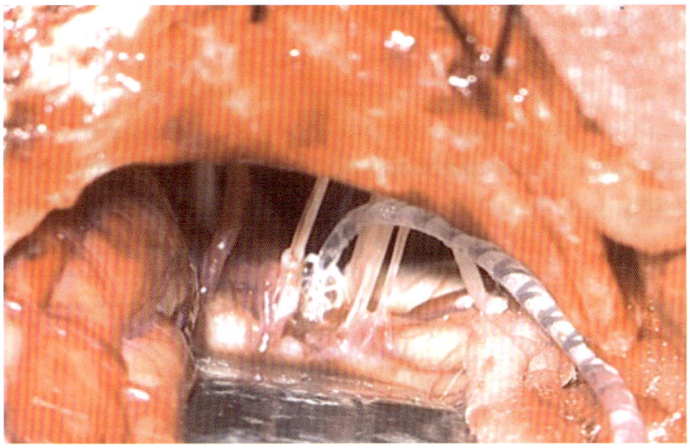

Fig. 74.17 Optimal placement of ABI electrode in the lateral recess abutting the cochlear nucleus.

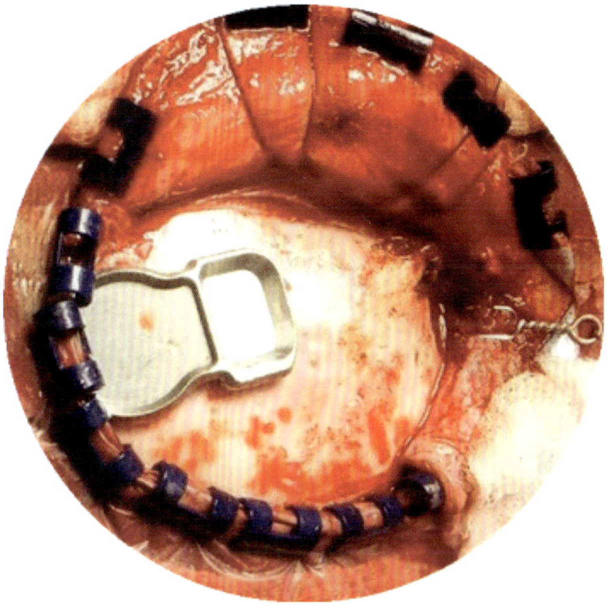

Fig. 74.18 Showing the placement for receiver stimulator complex and craniotomy site inferiorly.

In tumoral cases as in NF2, tumor excision via the same approach precedes the implantation. After tumor excision, the landmarks (seventh, eighth, and ninth cranial nerves, choroid plexus) for the foramen of Luschka are identified. Location of the lateral recess can be confirmed by noting the egress of CSF during the Valsalva maneuver. Initially, a dummy electrode is negotiated through the foramen of Luschka to the floor of the fourth ventricle to check optimal positioning of electrodes, followed by placing the permanent electrode through the same route.[34,35]

The true electrode array is snuggly inserted into the lateral recess and positioned once the cochlear nucleus is well delineated. Initially, temporary electrodes are placed on it and electrically evoked auditory brainstem responses early midlatency responses (EMLRs), and device telemetry are performed to check the optimal positioning and functioning of the electrodes (**Fig. 74.17**). Once integrity is confirmed, the permanent electrodes are then placed onto the cochlear nucleus and positioned with fibrin glue and Surgicel.[34]

The receiver–stimulator coil is placed in a bed created in the area posterosuperior to the craniotomy. It is placed at least 10 mm behind the edge of the auricle and above the canthomeatal line and is angled 30 to 45 degrees posterosuperiorly. Tie-down holes are made on either side of the receiver–stimulator for securing the implant (**Fig. 74.18**).[35]

During the surgery, the following anatomical landmarks are very helpful in guiding the electrode toward the cochlear nucleus, which is not under direct vision:[33]

- Choroid plexus marks the entrance of the lateral recess and the taenia traverses the roof of the lateral recess.
- Flocculus of cerebellum which forms an operculum covering the entry to lateral recess of the fourth ventricle.
- Exits of cranial nerves VI, VIII, and IX form a triangle which helps in identification of the entrance of the lateral recess of the fourth ventricle (~ 5 × 6 mm).
- Straight vein, running from ninth/tenth/eleventh cranial nerve complex to seventh/eighth cranial nerve complex forming floor of lateral recess and heading to the entrance of the foramen of Luschka.

A subjective grading of cerebellar flocculus and electrode insertion difficulty for different grades of flocculus has been described by our institution as below. This helps to judge the ease of insertion and correct positioning of the electrode pad (**Fig. 74.19**).[33]

- Grade 1 is nonvisualization of cerebellar flocculus with a prominent choroid plexus.
- Grade 2 cerebellar flocculus is hypoplastic and lying rostrally with a prominent choroid plexus.
- Grade 3 cerebellar flocculus is small and more central with a small choroid plexus.
- Grade 4 cerebellar flocculus is large and central with a small choroid plexus.
- Grades 1 and 2 flocculus cover the root entry zone of seventh, eighth and lower cranial nerves (ninth, tenth, eleventh).

Reconfirmation of implant function is done with electrophysiological tests. The stimulus to ABI is delivered by an external component comprising a microphone, a signal processor, and a transmitter coil very similar to the cochlear implant. Dura is closed primarily in a watertight fashion. Postoperative neuro-ICU care is necessary with cranial nerve monitoring. Suture removal is recommended on the 10th postoperative day, except for cases with complications, like wound dehiscence or pseudomeningocele.[35]

There are several other approaches described for tumor removal and placement of ABI. The translabyrinthine approach provides optimal access for both removal of the tumor and placement of the electrode array. A translabyrinthine approach is used by ENT surgeons and has the advantage of offering the best lateral angle to the exit of the cochlear nerve, allows the early identification of the facial nerve, and does not require cerebellar retraction. Disadvantages with translabyrinthine approach are limited exposure of cranial nerves and vessels in the posterior fossa. The lateral suboccipital approach is preferred by neurosurgeons. It is fast, safe, and offers very good exposure of the

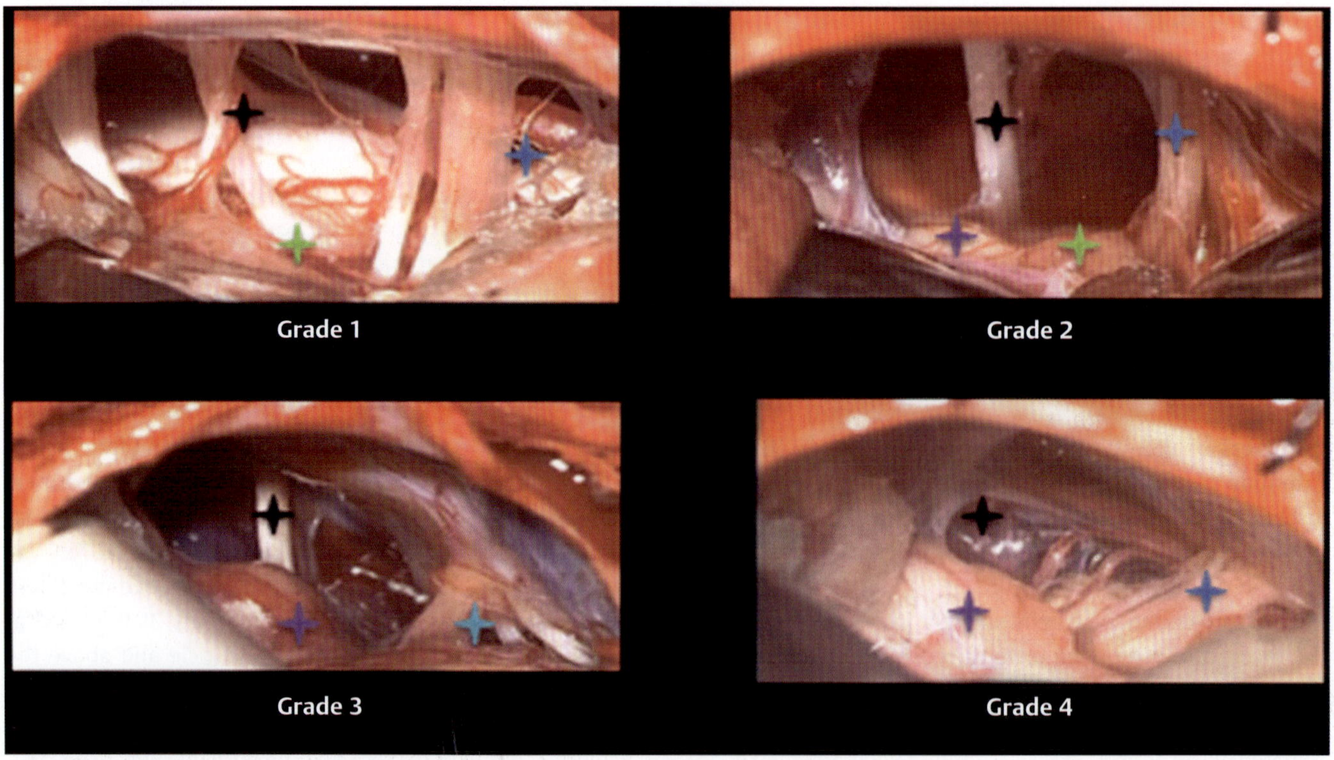

Fig. 74.19 Grading of cerebellar flocculus.

lateral posterior fossa. The problems are cerebellar retraction and late identification of facial nerve. The angle to the lateral recess, the direct vision of the entrance is more difficult than in the translabyrinthine approach. The middle cranial fossa approach is only possible with angled endoscopes; however, it is technically the most difficult and places the facial nerve at greatest risk. Penetrating electrodes have also been tried on the cochlear nucleus. This implant has the potential of offering improved performance because of better access to the complex tonotopic organization of the cochlear nucleus. Endoscopic guided placement of electrodes through retrosigmoid approach may also be of help in reducing the morbidity of surgery.[34,35]

A CT scan is to be done to postoperatively confirm the position of device. Activation of device is usually done 6 to 8 weeks later with monitoring of vital signs and nonauditory effects (**Fig. 74.20**). "Switch-on" is done under neurological monitoring of seventh, eighth, and lower cranial nerve in an ICU setup. Adequate preparation for active cardiopulmonary resuscitation (CPR) is mandatory, as there may be inadvertent stimulation of other brainstem nuclei and the possibility of nonauditory stimulation of vital centers. If there is a side effect, the current level is lowered until hearing sensation without any side effects is achieved. If this is not possible, the channel leading to the side effect is closed. Common side effects include stimulation of facial nerve, nystagmus, vagal stimulation, dizziness, change in gait, which should resolve over time.[31,34]

Intensive auditory verbal habilitation therapy (AVHT) is to be given, and evoked auditory brainstem response (EABR) is done regularly during the follow-up period for confirming the device integrity and assessment of the optimal performance. The auditory outcomes are measured with the help of categories of auditory performance (CAP) scores and Speech Intelligibility Rating (SIR) scores at 3, 6, 9, and 12 months of implant age similar to CI. CAP measures supraliminal performance, which reflects everyday auditory performance in a more realistic way. The SIR scores are used to measure the speech intelligibility of the implantees by quantifying their everyday spontaneous speech. Most implantees develop very good sound awareness and good gross auditory discrimination with appropriate habilitation over a period of implant use. Achievement of lucid environmental sound perception with pitch discrimination for closed-set speech is often the culmination of the habilitation process.[34,35]

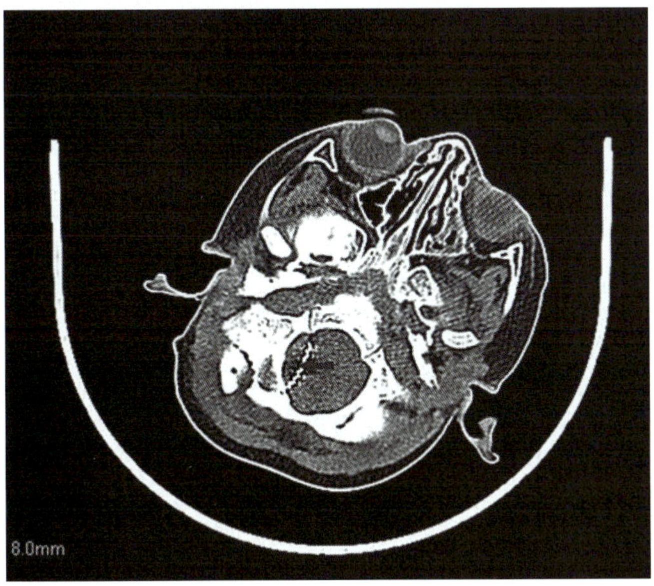

Fig. 74.20 CT scan (axial) showing ABI in situ.

In the near future, it may be used in bilateral–temporal bone fractures and demyelinating diseases affecting the eighth cranial nerves but sparing at least one cochlear nucleus. Auditory brainstem implantation has also been recommended for use in cases of bilateral totally ossified cochleae in which a CI cannot be used. Contraindications to ABI include previous stereotactic radiotherapy which has the risk of radiation necrosis of the cochlear nucleus region and anatomical distortion and fibrosis. ABI may not be possible in very large tumors which cause distortion of the brainstem.[35]

Conclusion

Today with the rapid technological developments in the field of implantable hearing devices, there is a variety of hearing restoration options available for individuals with skull base lesions involving the cochlea and cochlear nerve. It is prudent to counsel patients appropriately regarding all these possible options while proceeding to treat their disease. The peripheral auditory system is known to be conducive to electroneural integration and hence can be replaced by electronic circuitry unlike any other special sense. Research is being done to establish near-natural hearing function using this circuitry with precise speech processing technology. Outcomes are being monitored with objective tests like positron emission tomography computed tomography (PET-CT)/PET-MRI, functional MRI, near-infrared spectroscopy (NIRS), and cortical auditory evoked potentials (CAEP). Neuronavigation and CPA endoscopy have further helped appreciate the 3D surgical anatomy and proper placement of electrodes. Optogenetic stimulation of cochlear nucleus and the use of light-based neuronal stimulation also offers the promise to increase spatial resolution of current CI/ABI electrode arrays.

The journey through implantation in skull base surgery is an exciting but challenging one. Very few centers across the world have successfully established this comprehensive but sophisticated service till date. Initial results have been gratifying but outcomes are variable because of the spectrum of primary pathology, coexistent morbidities, and type of hearing restoration chosen. In case of recurrence of skull base disease, hearing options remain limited. Long-term clinical and audiological outcomes from these centers have been long awaited. More centers are now emerging in the horizon signaling the evolution of auditory neural implantation as a standard of care for hearing restoration in individuals who have lost their inner ear function to skull base pathology and surgery.

References

1. Harford E, Barry J. A rehabilitative approach to the problem of unilateral hearing impairment: contralateral routing of signals (CROS). J Speech Hear Disord 1965; 30:121–138
2. Nolan M, Lyon DJ. Transcranial attenuation in bone conduction audiometry. J Laryngol Otol 1981;95:597-608
3. Vaneecloo FM, Ruzza I, Hanson JN, et al. Single sided deafness. Rev Laryngol Otol Rhinol 2001;122(5):343–350
4. van der Pouw CT, Snik AF, Cremers CW. The BAHA HC200/300 in comparison with conventional bone conduction hearing aids. Clin Otolaryngol Allied Sci 1999; 24(3):171–176
5. Kitterick PT, Lucas L. Predicting speech perception outcomes following cochlear implantation in adults with unilateral deafness or highly asymmetric hearing loss. Cochlear Implants Int 2016;17(Suppl 1):51–54
6. Arndt S, Aschendorf A, Laszig R, et al. Comparison of pseudobinaural hearing to real binaural hearing rehabilitation after cochlear implantation in patients with unilateral deafness and tinnitus. Otol Neurotol 2011;32(1):39–47
7. Vlastarakos PV, Nazos K, Tavoulari EF, Nikolopoulos TP. Cochlear implantation for single sided deafness: the outcomes. An evidence based approach. Eur Arch Otorhinnolaryngol 2014;271(8):2119–2126
8. Ramos Macias A, Borkoski-Barreiro SA, Falcon Gonzalez JC, Ramos de Miguel A. AHL, SSD and bimodal CI results in children. Eur Ann Otorhinolaryngol Head Neck Dis 2016;133(Suppl 1):S15–S20.
9. Van Zon A, Peters JP, Stegeman I, Smit AL, Grolman W. Cochlear implantation for patients with single-sided deafness or asymmetrical hearing loss: a systematic review of the evidence. Otol Neurotol 2015;36(2):209–219
10. Balkany T, Bird PA, Hodges AV, Luntz M, Telischi FF, Buchman C. Surgical technique for implantation of the totally ossified cochlea. Laryngoscope 1998;108(7):988–992
11. Bendet E, Cerenko D, Linder TE, Fisch U. Cochlear implantation after subtotal petrosectomies. Eur Arch Otorhinolaryngol 1998;255(4):169–174
12. El-Kashlan HK, Arts HA, Telian SA. External auditory canal closure in cochlear implant surgery. Otol Neurotol 2003; 51(2):221–225
13. Free RH, Falcioni M, Di Trapani G, Giannuzzi AL, Russo A, Sanna M. The role of subtotal petrosectomy in cochlear implant surgery—a report of 32 cases and review on indications. Otol Neurotol 2013;34(6):1033–1040
14. Green KMJ, Bhatt YM, Saeed SR, Ramsden RT. Complications following adult cochlear implantation: experience in Manchester. J Laryngol Otol 2004;118(6):417–420
15. Incesulu A, Kocaturk S, Vural M. Cochlear implantation in chronic otitis media. J Laryngol Otol 2004;118(1):3–7
16. Issing P R, Schönermark MP, Winkelmann S, Kempf HG, Ernst A, Lenarz T. Cochlear implantation in patients with chronic otitis: indications for subtotal petrosectomy and obliteration of the middle ear. Skull Base Surg 1998;8(3):127–131
17. Leung R, Briggs RJ. Indications for and outcomes of mastoid obliteration in cochlear implantation. Otol Neurotol 2007; 28(3):330–334
18. Postelmans JT, Stokroos RJ, Linmans JJ, Kremer B. Cochlear implantation in patients with chronic otitis media: 7 years experience in Maastricht. Eur Arch Otorhinolaryngol 2009;266(8):1159–1165
19. Vincenti V, Pasanisi E, Bacciu A, Bacciu S. Long-term results of external auditory canal closure and mastoid obliteration in cochlear implantation after radical mastoidectomy: a clinical and radiological study. Eur Arch Otorhinolaryngol 2014;271(8):2127–2130
20. Fife TA, Lewis MP, May JS, Oliver ER. Cochlear implantation in Ménière's disease. JAMA Otolaryngol Head Neck Surg 2014; 140(6):535–539
21. Perkins E, Rooth M, Dillon M, Brown K. Simultaneous labyrinthectomy and cochlear implantation in unilateral Meniere's disease. Laryngoscope 2018;3(3):225–230
22. Samy RN, Houston L, Scott M, Choo DI, Meinzen-Derr J. Cochlear implantation in patients with Meniere's disease. Cochlear Implants Int 2015;16(4):208–212
23. Heywood RL, Atlas MD. Simultaneous cochlear implantation and labyrinthectomy for advanced Meniere's disease. J Laryngol Otol 2016;130(2):204–206
24. Mukherjee P, Eykamp K, Brown D, et al. Cochlear implantation in Meniere's disease with and without labyrinthectomy. Otol Neurotol 2017;38(2):192–198
25. Hansen MR, Gantz BJ, Dunn C. Outcomes after cochlear implantation for patients with single-sided deafness, including those with recalcitrant Meniere's disease. Otol Neurotol 2013;34:1681–1687
26. MacKeith SA, Bottrill LD, Ramsden JD. Simultaneous labyrinthectomy with cochlear implantation in patients

with bilateral Meniere's disease. Ann Otol Rhinol Laryngol 2014;123(7):485–489

27. Manrique-Huarte R, Calavia D, Alvarez-Gomez L, Huarte A, Perez-Fernández N, Manrique M. Vestibulo-cochlear function after cochlear implantation in patients with Meniere's disease. J Int Adv Otol 2018;14(1):18–22
28. Otto SR, Brackmann DE, Hitselberger W. Auditory brainstem implantation in 12- to 18-year- olds. Arch Otolaryngol Head Neck Surg 2004;130(5):656–659
29. Kanowitz SJ, Shapiro WH, Golfinos JG, Cohen NL, Roland JT Jr. Auditory brainstem implantation in patients with neurofibromatosis type 2. Laryngoscope 2004;114(12): 2135–2146
30. Sollmann WP, Laszig R, Marangos N. Surgical experiences in 58 cases using the Nucleus 22 multichannel auditory brainstem implant. J Laryngol Otol Suppl 2000;(27): 23–26
31. Colletti V. Auditory outcomes in tumor vs. non-tumor patients fitted with auditory brainstem implants. Adv Otorhinolaryngol 2006;64:167–185
32. Sennaroglu L, Colletti V, Manrique M, et al. Auditory brainstem implantation in children and non-neurofibromatosis type 2 patients: a consensus statement. Otol Neurotol 2011; 32(2): 187–191
33. Goyal S, Krishnan SK, Kameswaran M, Vasudevan MC, Ranjith R, Natarajan K. Does cerebellar flocculus size affect subjective outcomes in pediatric auditory brainstem implantation. Int J Pediatr Otorhinolaryngol 2017;97:30–34
34. Kameswaran M, Vasudevan MC, Kumar RS, Nagasundaram J, Natarajan K, Raghunandhan S. Auditory brainstem implantation: the first Indian experience. Indian J Otolaryngol Head Neck Surg 2005;57(1):58–63
35. Raghunandhan S, Kameswaran M. Auditory brainstem implants. Otorhinolaryngol Clin 2010;2(2):151–155

Chapter 75 Reanimation of the Paralyzed Face

Part A

Facial Reanimation

Narayan Jayashankar and K.P. Morwani

Introduction

Facial paresis and palsy have been better understood with improved knowledge of nerve degeneration and regeneration. It is now possible to offer various techniques to improve the cosmesis in these patients. A thorough understanding of nerve physiology helps to offer the correct technique with the best possibility of a positive outcome in these patients. The technique of reanimation offered depends on the degree of nerve injury, duration of paresis or palsy, and correct assessment by the treating surgeon.

In this chapter, we discuss reanimation techniques like facial nerve decompression, facial nerve suturing, grafting, gold implant in the upper eyelid, facial hypoglossal anastomosis, and temporalis muscle sling with their indications and results.

Facial Nerve Decompression

Indications

- Nerve decompression suffices if intraoperatively there is edema of the nerve, nerve sheath is lacerated, or when less than 25% nerve fibers are damaged.
- Fracture line along the fallopian canal seen on high-resolution computed tomography (CT) scan with facial paresis or palsy.

The approach taken for surgery depends on site of injury of facial nerve and hearing status of the patient.

- Serviceable hearing
  - *Middle cranial fossa*: When injury is at internal auditory canal, labyrinthine segment of facial nerve, or geniculate ganglion.
  - *Transzygomatic, transattic*: When injury is anywhere along labyrinthine segment, geniculate ganglion, or tympanic segment of facial nerve.
  - *Transmastoid*: When injury occurs at geniculate ganglion, tympanic segment, or mastoidal segment of facial nerve up to stylomastoid foramen.
  - *Transmastoid transcervical*: For injuries going from stylomastoid foramen to the extratemporal facial nerve.
- Nonserviceable hearing
  - Transmastoid: When the injury occurs at geniculate ganglion, tympanic segment, or mastoidal segment of facial nerve up to stylomastoid foramen.
  - Translabyrinthine: When the injury is in labyrinthine segment or in internal auditory meatus.

Surgical Steps

1. The bone over the facial nerve in the area of trauma is made eggshell thin, using a cutting burr at first and gradually shifting to a diamond burr closer to the facial nerve. The last shells of bone over the facial nerve are lifted off using a flat raspatory or elevator (**Fig. 75A.1**). Decompression of the facial nerve proceeds on either

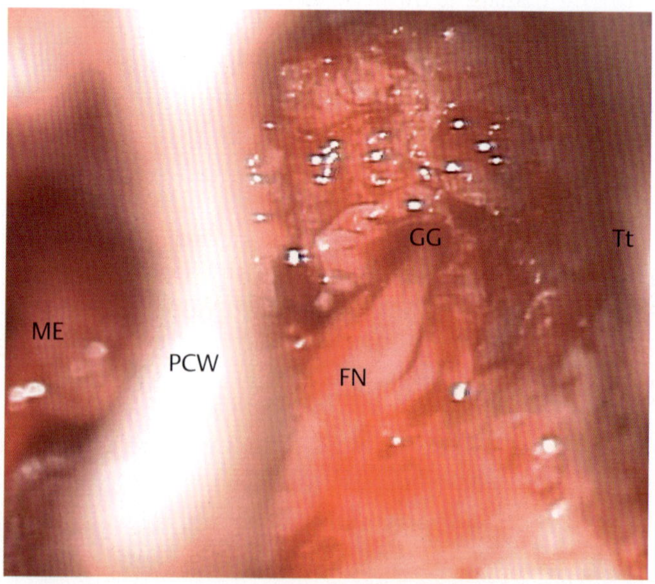

Fig. 75A.1 Decompressed tympanic segment of the facial nerve up to the geniculate ganglion—left side. (Photo provided courtesy of Dr Rahul Agrawal).

side of the trauma till healthy facial nerve is visualized. Decompression is done for 180 degrees around the nerve without lifting it off the bed. A sickle knife is used to incise the epineurial sheath of the facial nerve to release the tension on the nerve fibers because of edema. Care is taken not to damage the neural filaments during this step. In a few cases, it is possible to incise the sheath on both sides of the site of trauma but not at the site of trauma itself because of poor differentiation between nerve sheath and nerve fibers. In these cases, incising the sheath at the site of trauma is deferred to prevent the risk of damaging nerve fibers at the site.

The preoperative and postoperative photographs of a subject of facial nerve decompression are shown in **Fig. 75A.2a, b**.

Results

Results are better when nerve decompression is performed earlier rather than later after the injury. Over 90% of subjects improve to grade II or I (House–Brackmann grading) if surgery is performed within 2 weeks of trauma. Few cases that do not improve at all after decompression could, in our mind, possibly have additional concussion injury to the facial nerve in the intracranial part which may have gone undetected.

Facial Nerve Grafting

Indications

When the damage to the nerve is such that the two cut ends of the nerve can be reapproximated without tension, then an end-to-end anastomosis is performed. However, when the two cut ends of the facial nerve do not approximate well or have a gap between the cut ends, nerve grafting is performed. A general guideline is given below:

- If only 20 to 25% thickness of nerve fibers are damaged, then no grafting is required. Decompression of the nerve may suffice.
- Partial-thickness grafting is required when 25 to 50% of the thickness of nerve fibers is damaged.
- Full-thickness grafting should be done when damage is above 50% of nerve thickness.

Selecting and Harvesting the Nerve Graft

The two main considerations in selection of nerve graft are length of the defect and axon volume. The greater auricular nerve and sural nerve are two most easily available nerve grafts with adequate axon volume and length and hence are preferred over other nerve grafts. The greater auricular nerve graft can be harvested up to a length of around 7 cm whereas the sural nerve can be harvested of length up to 20 cm or more.

The greater auricular nerve graft is traced by first drawing a line between the angle of the mandible and the mastoid tip. The greater auricular nerve lies along a perpendicular line bisecting the above line as it courses from the posterior border of the sternocleidomastoid muscle, lies superficial to the sternocleidomastoid muscle and courses toward the parotid gland (**Fig. 75A.3**).

The sural nerve is located between the lateral malleolus and the Achilles tendon posterior to the saphenous vein (**Fig. 75A.4**). It can be traced superiorly where it is seen between the two heads of gastrocnemius muscle. It is very important to bear in mind that the length of the nerve graft is at least 1 cm longer than the estimated defect so that the nerve graft is not sutured under tension.

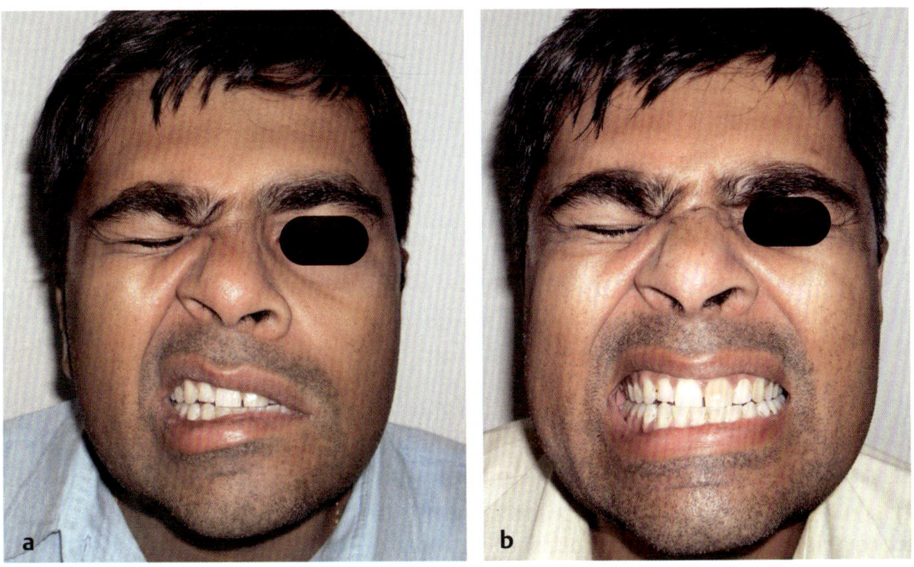

Fig. 75A.2 **(a)** Preoperative image showing left-sided grade III weakness. **(b)** Post facial nerve decompression image showing left side grade II facial function at 2 months' post decompression.

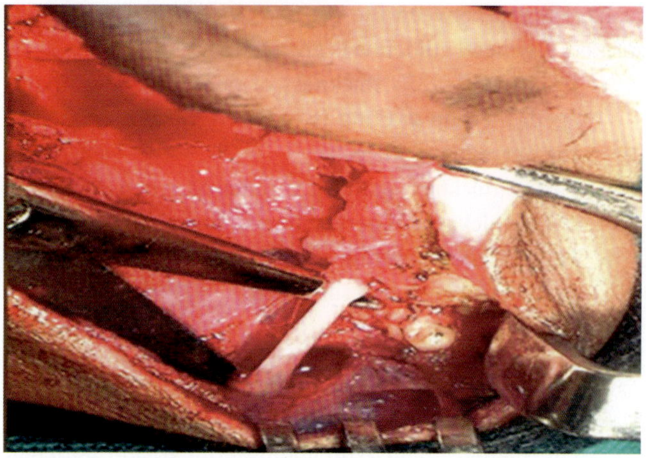

Fig. 75A.3 Greater auricular nerve graft.

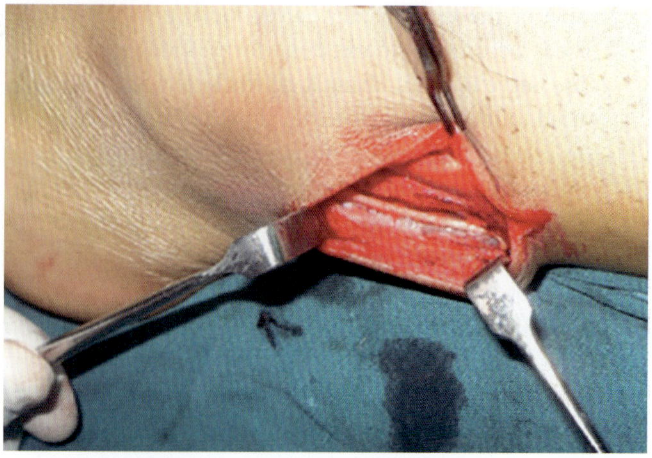

Fig. 75A.4 Sural nerve graft (from left leg).

Once harvested, the loose areolar tissue over the nerve is cleared. The two cut ends of the nerve graft should be clean cuts with no crushing of axons. The epineurium over the two ends of the nerve graft is stripped back for about 1 to 2 mm to expose the perineurium for suturing.

Surgical Steps

The two ends of the facial nerve that were damaged are identified. The two ends of the nerve may have ischemia, necrosis, neuroma, or fibrous degeneration. This must be resected to expose healthy facial nerve for grafting. The freshening of edges is done with a sharp knife without crushing the nerve ends. Facial nerve and nerve graft are cut obliquely at times to obtain good apposition with the nerve graft in case the nerve graft is of a different diameter than the facial nerve. This increases the contact surface area used for anastomosis. The epineurium of the cut ends of the facial nerve is stripped back for 1 to 2 mm to aid suturing. The nerve graft is placed on a bed of healthy tissue and not kept hanging like a bridge between two cut ends of the facial nerve (**Fig. 75A.5**). Under high magnification of microscope, using 8.0 monofilament, perineurium of the cut end of the facial nerve is sutured to the perineurium of the nerve graft. Usually, two to three sutures suffice to gain a very good approximation. Alternatively, fibrin glue can be used at the approximated ends. It should, however, be noted that in the parotid, the nerve graft is sutured, and fibrin glue alone should not be used. Once grafting is complete, the sutured nerve ends can be covered with temporalis fascia or fascia lata.

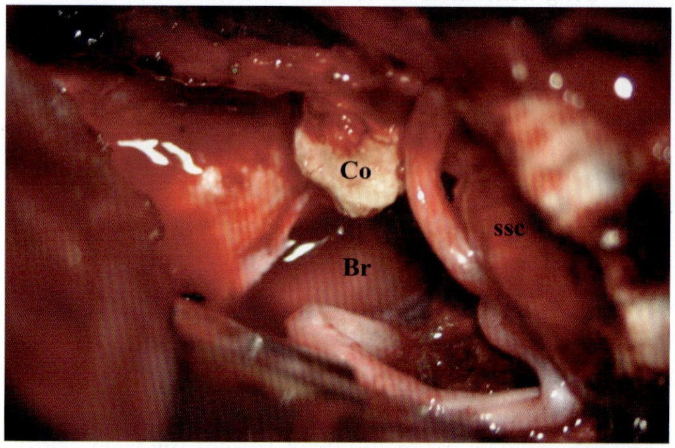

Fig. 75A.5 Grafting between the facial nerve at brainstem and labyrinthine segment—extended middle cranial fossa approach.

Results

In 55 to 70% of subjects, the result of facial nerve grafting expected is grade III or less frequently grade II (House–Brackmann grading). It has been established that results of nerve grafting are better when performed within the first 1 month after injury rather than later, and results are very poor when performed more than 1 year after injury. In fact, the duration of a preoperative deficit was found to be the most significant prognostic factor for good results. The preoperative (**Fig. 75A.6a**) and postoperative images (**Fig. 75A.6b**) of a subject are shown.

Gold Upper Eyelid Implant for Paralytic Lagophthalmos

Indications

- Paralytic lagophthalmos of any etiology to prevent corneal complications.
- Facial paresis with eye symptoms where conservative eye drops, ointments, and taping of eyelid are not beneficial.

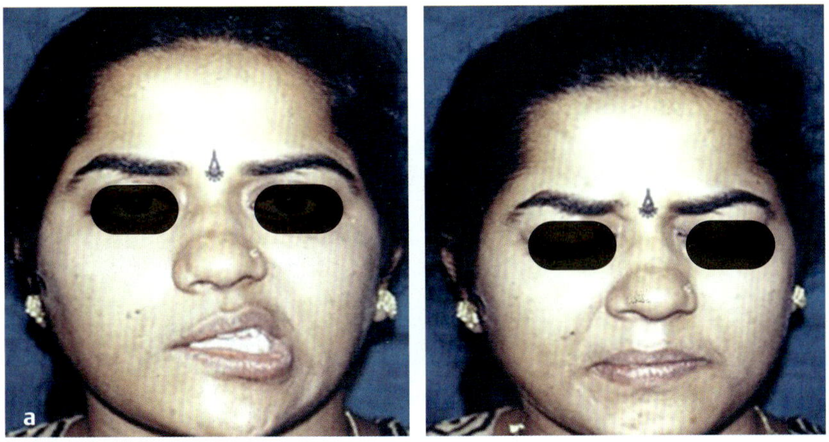

Fig. 75A.6 (a) Preoperative image of a different patient showing grade V facial nerve function on right side (iatrogenic injury). **(b)** One year after nerve grafting showing recovery to grade III facial nerve function on right side. A gold implant was implanted on the right upper eyelid for eye symptoms.

- Along with facial nerve end-to-end anastomosis, grafting, facial–hypoglossal anastomosis, and facial nerve rerouting procedures where recovery of the facial nerve function is expected over a reasonably long period.

Principle

It is the procedure of choice for reanimation of the eye in paralytic lagophthalmos. Early reanimation of the upper eyelid is necessary to prevent corneal abrasions and ulcerations with eventual deep corneal ulcers that can lead to blindness. It is essential to understand the concept behind the use of the gold implant. The orbicularis oculi is innervated by the facial nerve and helps to shut the eyelid close. The levator palpebrae superioris is innervated by the oculomotor nerve and it helps to elevate the upper eyelid resulting in eye opening. Thus, when the levator palpebrae superioris relaxes, the orbicularis oculi contracts and helps to close the eye. The principle of surgery is to substitute the action of the orbicularis oculi on the paralytic side by implantation of a suitable gold weight over the tarsal plate. Thus, when the levator palpebrae superioris relaxes, the weight of the gold implant coupled with the effect of gravity helps to close the eye. This simulates normal eye closure on the paralyzed side.

Customized Gold Implant for Upper Eyelid

Preoperatively, the weight of the gold implant needs to be determined. Internationally, prefabricated implants are available. However, these implants take time to import as also are fairly expensive. We have devised a method wherein these implants are custom-made to the required dimensions and weight suited for the subject.[1] The weight of the gold implants is measured preoperatively (sitting position) by taping implants of different weights from a measuring set (**Fig. 75A.7**) to the upper eyelid and confirming the weight that completely closes the upper eyelid (**Fig. 75A.8**). A 0.05 g

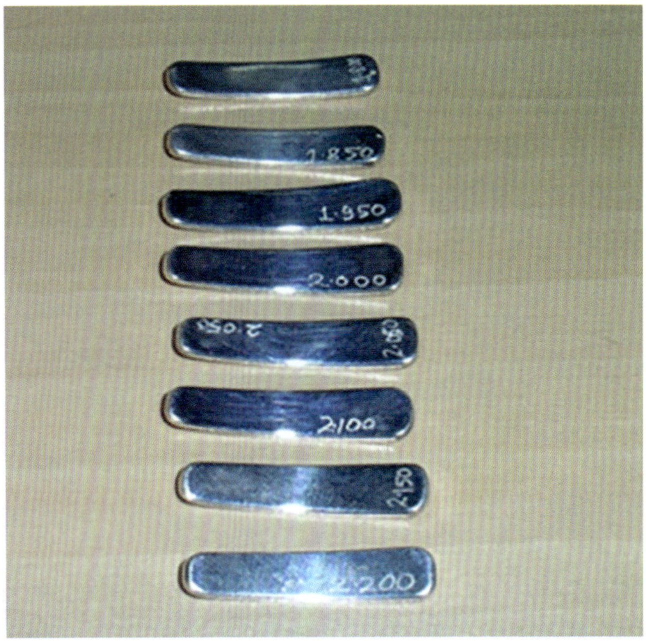

Fig. 75A.7 Implant weight measuring set.

is added to this measured weight to abolish any marginal error. The gold implant is prepared of 24-carat gold or 99.9% purity (**Fig. 75A.9**). The length of the implant measures two-thirds the length of the affected upper eyelid as measured from medial to the lateral canthus. The breadth on the medial end measures 5 mm while that on the lateral end measures 4 mm in adults. However, the breadth is proportionately decreased as needed in the younger age group. This is based on the observation that slightly greater weight is used to close the medial end of the eye as compared to the lateral end. The implant edges are smoothened, and it is provided with three holes for fixation to the tarsal plate. The implant is made with a local trained goldsmith. It is autoclaved prior to use. In our subjects, the weights required in adults ranged from 1.8 to 2.1 g. The advantages of implant prepared in this

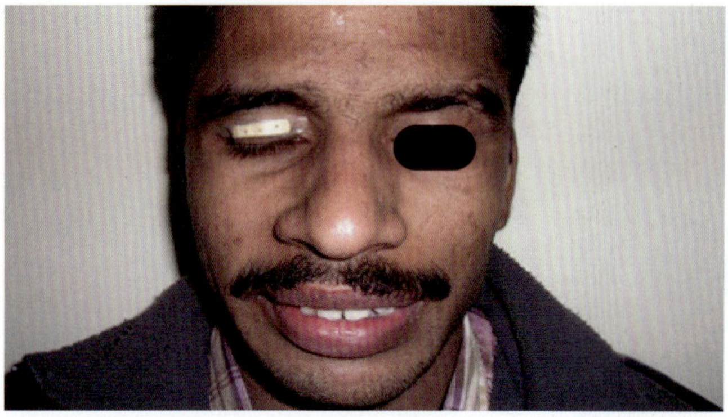

Fig. 75A.8 Implant from measuring set taped to the affected upper eyelid to determine the weight of the implant that closes the eye.

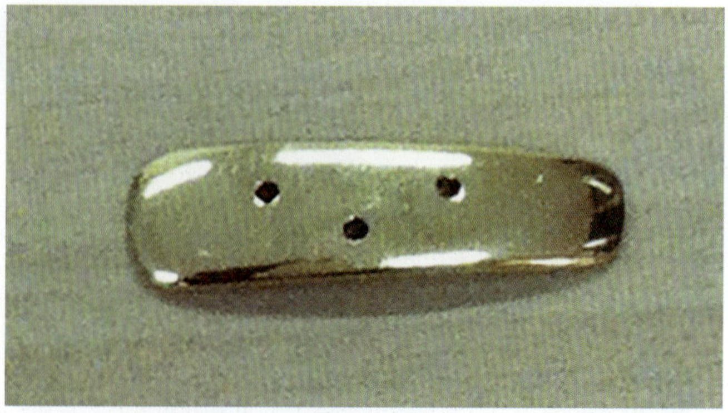

Fig. 75A.9 Gold upper eyelid implant.

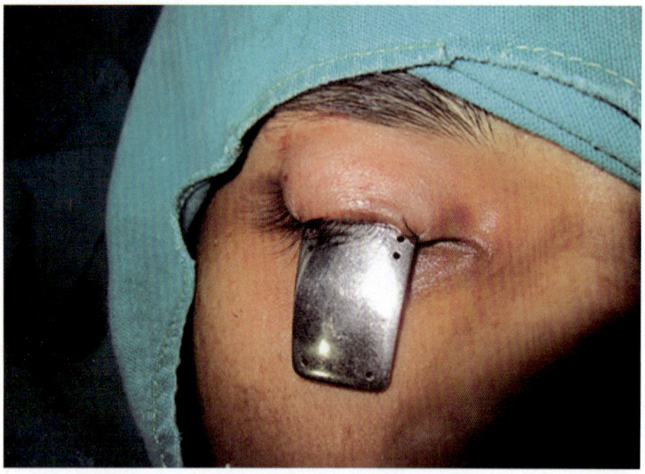

Fig. 75A.10 Corneal guard in place.

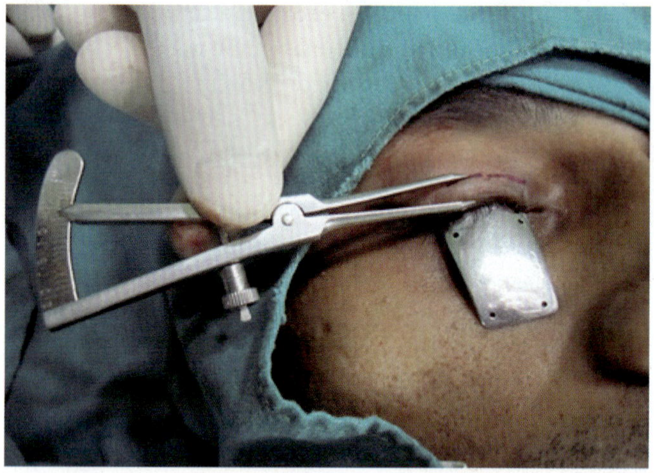

Fig. 75A.11 Incision 6 mm from upper lid margin.

way are easy availability in even remote areas, economical cost, and, most importantly, perfect dimensions and weight for the subject.

Surgical Steps

1. The procedure is performed under local anesthesia. Two drops of 4% xylocaine are instilled over the cornea. A corneal guard is placed and fixed to the margin of the eyelid (**Fig. 75A.10**). About 2 mL of xylocaine with adrenaline 1:200,000 is infiltrated over the tarsal–supratarsal crease on the upper eyelid.
2. The incision is taken in the tarsal–supratarsal fold and involves the middle one-third of the upper eyelid, approximately 6 mm away from the lid margin (**Fig. 75A.11**).
3. Incision involves the skin and the orbicularis oculi superficial to the tarsal plate. A pocket is created in the plane between the orbicularis oculi and the tarsal plate (**Fig. 75A.12**).

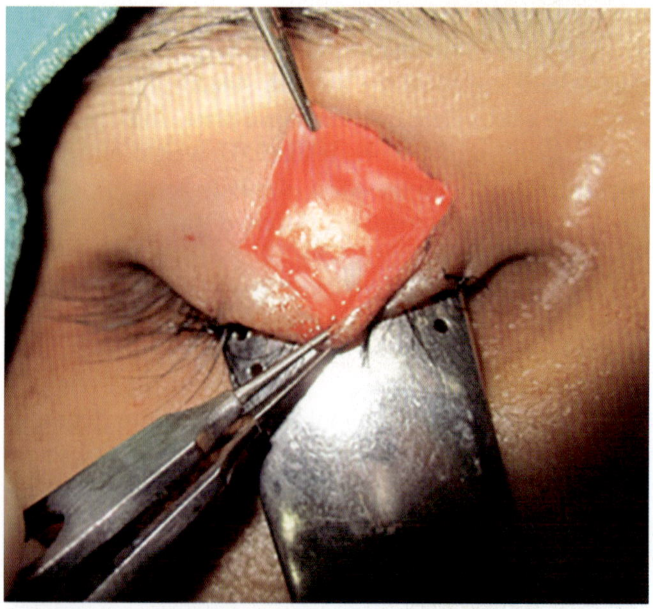

Fig. 75A.12 Pocket created between the orbicularis oculi and tarsal plate.

4. The implant is placed in this pocket, the lower edge of the implant about 3 mm from the lid margin (**Fig. 75A.13**).
5. The implant is then sutured to the partial thickness of the tarsal plate with 6–0 Ethilon passed through each of the three holes in the prosthesis (**Fig. 75A.14**).
6. The orbicularis is sutured with 5–0 Vicryl (**Fig. 75A.15**).
7. Skin is closed with 6–0 Ethilon (**Fig. 75A.16**).
8. The preoperative and postoperative photographs are shown (**Fig. 75A.17a, b**).
9. In the case of lower lid droop, a lid tightening procedure is performed for the lower eyelid.

Results

Of the 130 subjects in our series with follow-up of minimum 1 year, we have had four extrusions. Extrusion causes were implant in contact with skin incision because of inadequate orbicularis oculi cover (in one elderly subject), improper fixation or loosening of the ligatures that fix the implant to the tarsal plate (three subjects). We have not encountered any complications because of the procedure. There has been healing of superficial corneal ulcers with significant improvement in visual acuity in about 86.6% of subjects having the above-mentioned findings.

Facial–Hypoglossal Anastomosis

Indications

- Proximal facial nerve stump damaged or not of reasonable length near brainstem for anastomosis as can occur, for example, after vestibular schwannoma or other cerebellopontine angle surgery.
- Long-standing, that is, more than 12 months but less than 18 months facial palsy. However, in the younger

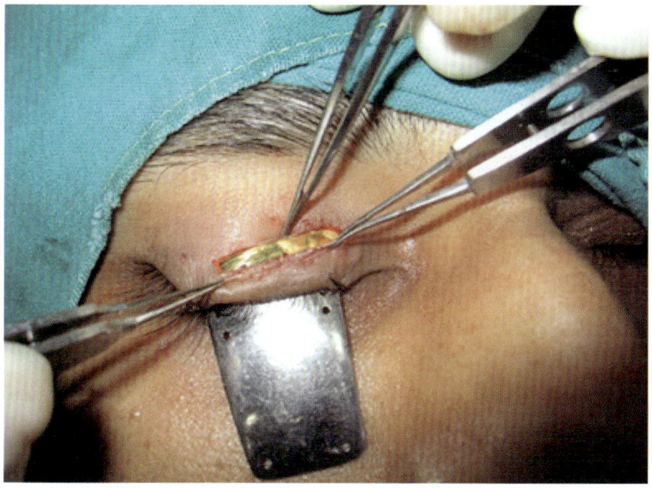

Fig. 75A.13 Implant placed in the pocket.

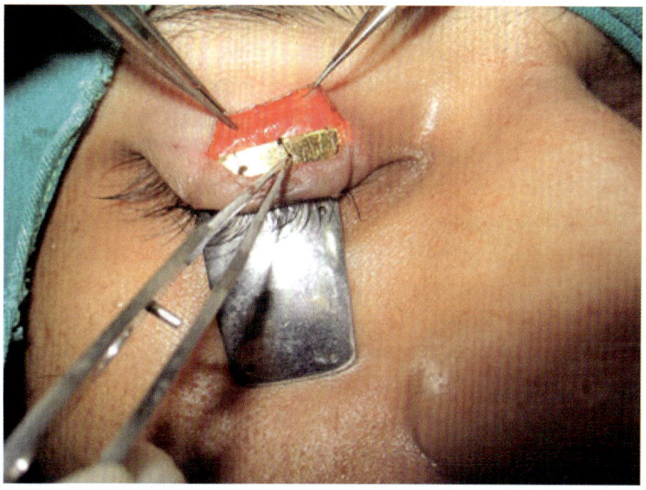

Fig. 75A.14 Implant sutured to the partial thickness of tarsal plate.

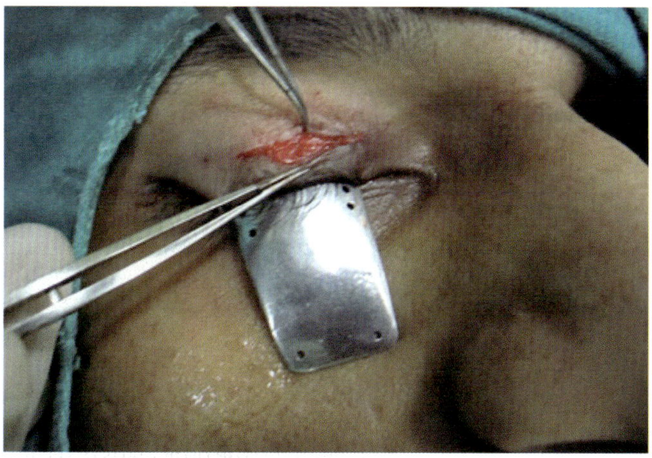

Fig. 75A.15 Suturing of orbicularis oculi muscle.

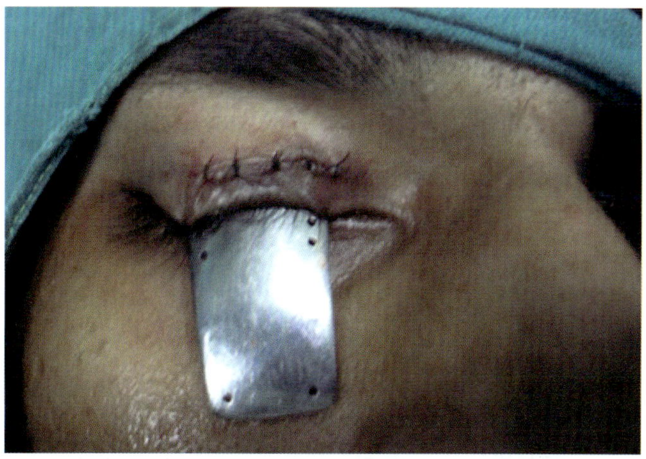

Fig. 75A.16 Skin incision sutured.

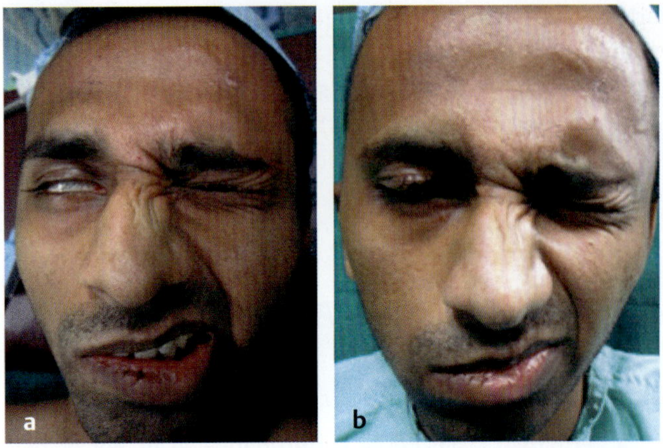

Fig. 75A.17 (a) Preoperative image showing paralytic lagophthalmos on right side. (b) Postoperative image showing complete closure of eye palpebral aperture on right side.

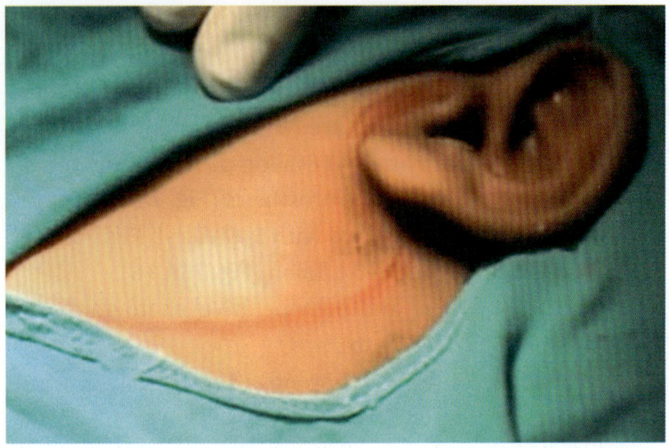

Fig. 75A.18 Incision—left side.

subjects where muscle atrophy takes longer, we have successfully performed facial–hypoglossal anastomosis up to 26 months. These cases have to be selected carefully and extending the outer limit beyond 18 months in elderly adults will in most instances not give the expected results.
- Failure of facial nerve anastomosis or grafting performed earlier.

Contraindications

- Type 2 neurofibromatosis, where multiple cranial nerves could be potentially involved.
- Vagal palsy, since additional hypoglossal paresis can aggravate speech and swallowing problems.
- Loss of the tone of facial muscles as occurs between 2 and 3 years after the onset of facial palsy.

Hypoglossal nerve (cranial nerve [CN] XII) is generally chosen for the reinnervation of the facial nerve because of the anatomical proximity, the similarity in size, and the functional relationship in that both are motor nerves with some degree of interactive function, especially during swallowing. What started as a facial nerve to complete-thickness hypoglossal nerve anastomosis was modified to a partial hypoglossal neurectomy to serve as means to reduce tongue weakness in facial reconstructive surgery. As the surgery has evolved, a jump graft is now used to anastomose the distal facial nerve trunk to one-third thickness of hypoglossal nerve.

Surgical Steps

1. An incision similar to the parotid incision is created; the skin flap is elevated (**Fig. 75A.18**).

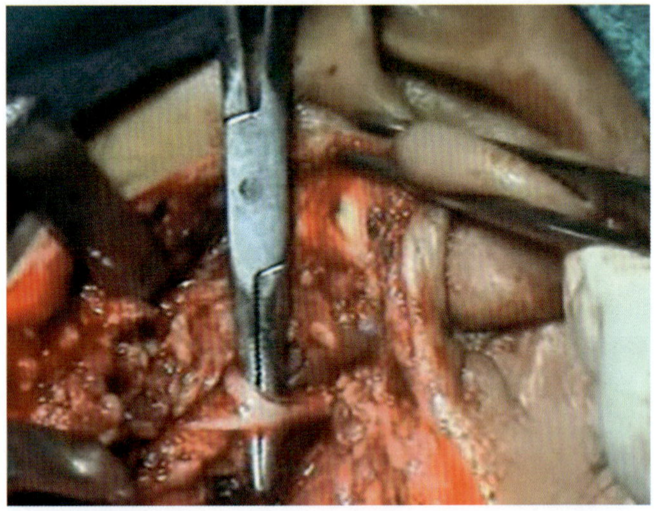

Fig. 75A.19 Facial nerve main trunk identified distal to stylomastoid foramen.

2. The facial nerve is identified at its exit from the stylomastoid foramen and followed into the parotid gland until the bifurcation. The main trunk of the facial nerve is identified by using the tragal pointer as a landmark. Alternatively, the upper end of the posterior belly of digastric muscle is identified and facial nerve lies anteromedial to it. The facial nerve is cut close to its exit from the stylomastoid foramen and the main trunk reflected inferiorly (**Fig. 75A.19**).
3. The hypoglossal nerve is identified in its vertical and horizontal course until it passes deep to the tendon of the posterior belly of the digastric muscle. The occipital artery crossing the genu of the nerve posteriorly should be preserved if possible. Hypoglossal nerve is

identified in the neck, and a wedge is created involving one-third of the thickness of the nerve. This partial neurectomy helps to preserve the partial function of hypoglossal nerve (**Fig. 75A.20**).

4. Most often a relaxed approximation of the facial and hypoglossal nerve ends cannot be achieved, hence a jump nerve graft (sural or greater auricular nerve) is used. The polarity of the jump graft needs to be reversed, that is, distal end to be sutured proximally to facial nerve's main trunk.
5. The perineurial covering of both nerve ends is retracted for a couple of millimeters to expose the endoneurial surfaces. Over a large piece of Gelfoam or rectangular piece of glove, the nerve ends are sutured together using a monofilament suture of size 8.0 with a cutting needle. Generally, three or four sutures are sufficient on each end of the jump graft to secure the graft between the main trunk of the facial nerve and one-third thickness of hypoglossal nerve (**Fig. 75A.21**). Microscope is required for these steps. A piece of fascia collected at the beginning of the approach is used to wrap around the anastomosis.
6. The closure of the wound is done in two layers. If needed, a small drain can be placed away from the anastomosis between the muscular layer and the skin.

Results

This is most rewarding for reanimation of the lower face. Grade III results have been possible in around 50 to 62.5% of the cases. Partial symmetry and voluntary smile may be achieved in 6 to 12 months and further improvement may be seen till around 24 months. Of course, these cases are combined with a gold weight upper eyelid implantation of the affected eyelid.

Sling Surgery

Indications

- Facial palsy of more than 3 years' duration (when facial muscle atrophy sets in).
- Failure of any nerve anastomosis performed earlier.

Types of Slings

- Static slings
  - Fascia lata.
  - Barbed proline wire.
- Dynamic sling
  - Temporalis muscle transfer.

Static Slings

Static techniques are used in patients who are unwilling for muscle transposition and/or are unable to undergo muscle transposition because of poor follow-up or postoperative rehabilitation facilities. Fascia lata is most often used for the same. One end of the fascia lata is fixed to the periosteum of the zygomatic arch as the suspension point. The other end is split into three divisions. One division is anchored to the upper end of the nasolabial fold, lateral to nasal ala. The second division is anchored to the lateral angle of the upper lip while the third division is anchored to the lateral angle of the lower lip. The suturing is done to the submucosa of the upper and lower lips.

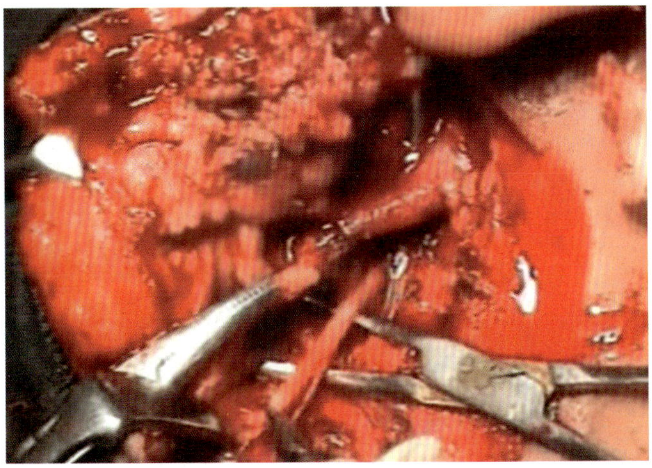

Fig. 75A.20 Hypoglossal nerve identified in neck coursing just inferior to the digastric tendon.

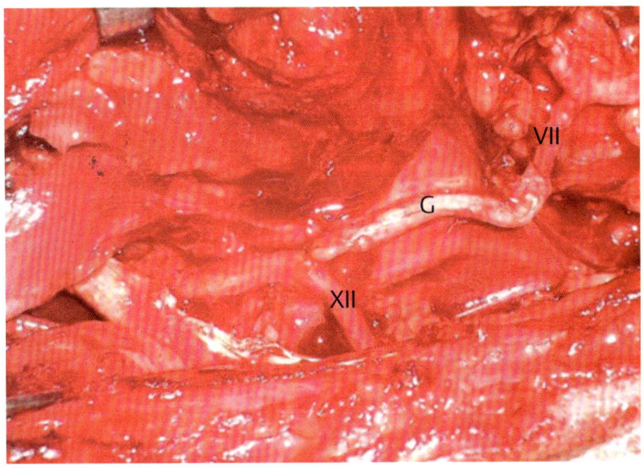

Fig. 75A.21 Greater auricular nerve graft sutured to main trunk of the facial nerve and one-third thickness of hypoglossal nerve.

The disadvantage of this procedure is that although facial symmetry is observed at rest, no voluntary facial movement is possible on that side, thereby retaining facial asymmetry during various facial expressions.

Dynamic Slings

Temporalis Muscle Sling

Muscle transposition technique was devised to achieve symmetry of the face at rest and also to obtain dynamic movement of the paralyzed side of the face on voluntary effort. Temporalis muscle sling is the most widely accepted technique of facial reanimation for the lower face. When combined with gold weight implant for the upper eyelid, excellent overall results can be obtained for dynamic movement on the paralyzed side of the face.

Indications

Same as that mentioned under sling surgery.

Contraindications

- Atrophic temporalis muscle as in edentulous patient.
- Temporalis muscle is involved as a part of any surgical procedure.

Surgical Steps

1. A vertical incision is taken from anterior to helix up to the parietal area involving skin and subcutaneous tissue. Loose tissue over the temporalis fascia is cleared and the pocket is extended to expose the temporalis muscle with fascia all around. The middle two-thirds of the muscle along with the fascia and periosteum is then mobilized toward the zygomatic arch (**Fig. 75A.22**).
2. The zygomatic arch, if retained, gives a bulky appearance when the temporalis muscle is reflected toward the lower face. Hence, to improve the cosmesis, we now prefer to excise the zygomatic arch.
3. In case the muscle strip is short, the temporalis fascia or the periosteum is lifted off from the muscle retaining its attachment to the cut edge of the temporalis muscle which gives it additional length. At this cut edge, it can be strengthened by suturing the fascia or periosteum to the cut edge of the temporalis muscle (**Fig. 75A.23**).
4. Subcutaneous tunnels are created from the pedicle of temporalis muscle toward the nasolabial fold and lower lip. The mobilized temporalis muscle is then divided into two strips, each strip passed through the relevant subcutaneous tunnel toward the nasolabial fold and lower lip (**Fig. 75A.24a, b**).
5. The strips of muscle are sutured to orbicularis oris muscle or the submucosa in a way such that the pull creates a good nasolabial fold and the lateral commissure of the mouth is also similar to the opposite side. It must be noted that this suturing must overcorrect the pull on the affected side since it eventually loosens as time progresses.
6. The skin incisions around the nasolabial and lower lips are sutured. A drain is kept in the temporal area, and the wound there is closed in subcutaneous and skin layers.

The preoperative and postoperative photographs are shown (**Fig. 75A.25a, b**).

Results

It was successful in restoring a smile to 80% of the 219 patients and provided overall improvement in mouth function in 96% according to one of the largest series of 224 subjects by May M. Our series is small in comparison but results are similar.

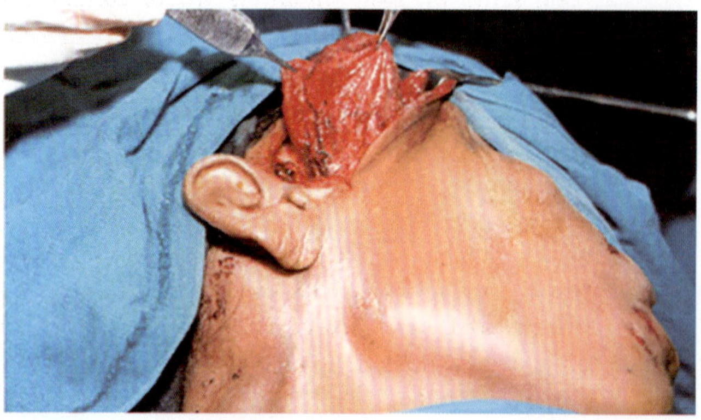

Fig. 75A.22 The middle two-thirds of the temporalis muscle is mobilized with the temporalis fascia and periosteum.

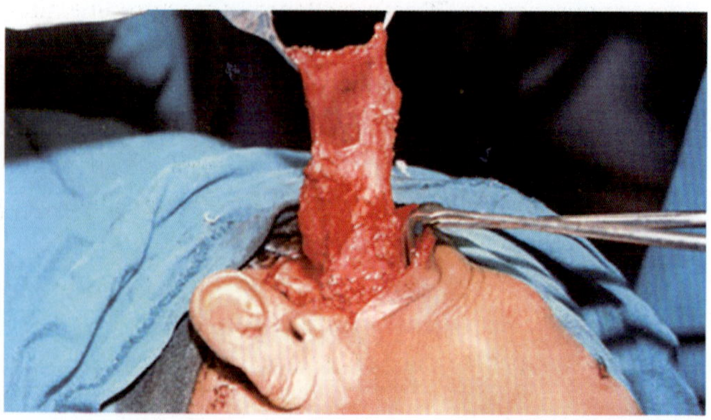

Fig. 75A.23 The temporalis fascia is lifted off the muscle except at its distal end to gain additional length for transposition.

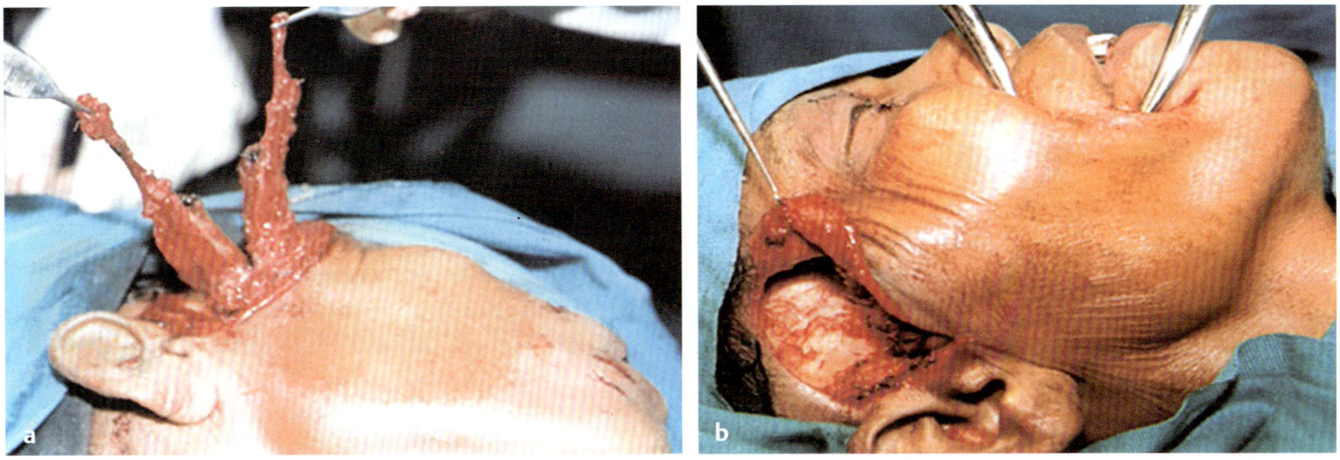

Fig. 75A.24 **(a)** Two strips are created: one for the nasolabial/upper lip and the other for the lower lip. **(b)** The muscle strips are transposed via subcutaneous tunnels to the nasolabial and lower lip areas.

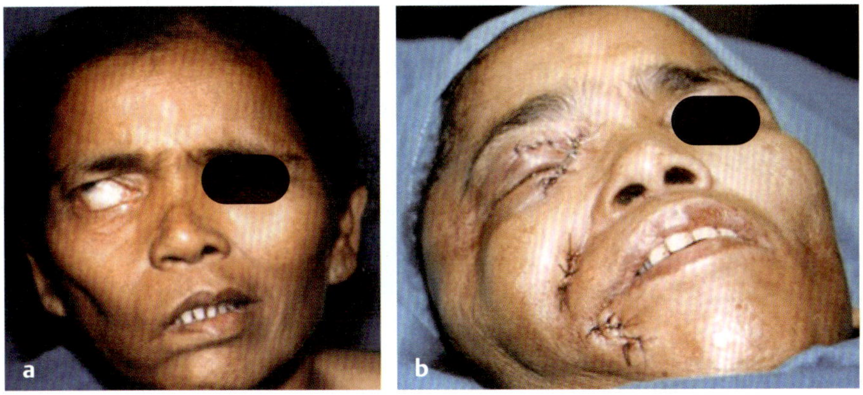

Fig. 75A.25 **(a)** Preoperative image showing right-sided facial palsy. **(b)** Right-sided gold upper eyelid implant, lower lid tightening, and temporalis muscle transposition to nasolabial and lower lip areas.

Tips and Pearls

- Although literature describes ideal time periods for the relevant reanimation surgery, it is additionally based on clinical parameters, age of the subject, and also the personal experience of the surgeon.
- In our view, a CT scan evidence of fracture line along the fallopian canal with facial paresis or palsy is a definite indication for decompression. However, if otological surgery is indicated in the posttrauma situation for conductive hearing loss or persistent cerebrospinal fluid (CSF) otorrhea without any fracture line along the fallopian canal, then, in the same surgery, a facial nerve decompression can be performed (in experienced hands) via a transmastoid route for the mastoidal, tympanic, and if possible, labyrinthine segment of the facial nerve. This is performed without causing any untoward damage to the facial nerve which could negate the beneficial effect of decompression. This decompression could possibly accelerate recovery period of the nerve.
- Customized gold implants can be prepared in even a rural setup in many countries where commercial implants are not easily available. The correct method to fashion these implants has been explained above and additionally has been published by us for interested readers.[1]

References

1. Jayashankar N, Morwani KP, Shaan MJ, Bhatia SR, Patil KT. Customized gold weight eyelid implantation in paralytic lagophthalmos. J Laryngol Otol 2008;122(10):1088–1091

Part B

Facio-Masseteric Anastomosis for Management of Facial Nerve Palsy

Madhuri Mehta

Introduction

The masseter nerve lately has become the first choice for nerve transfer because of its comparable size, easy dissection as it lies in the same surgical field, close proximity, so early recovery, and least effect on the masticatory function of the masseter nerve (as alternative muscles for mastication are available), though the length may not be sufficient in certain situations.

Use of masseter nerve can be in the form of direct end-to-end anastomosis with facial nerve stump if the length of both nerve stumps is sufficient. In case the length of the masseter nerve or the distal facial nerve stump is not sufficient, (as seen in cases of facial nerve neuroma involving nerve till the extratemporal segment, leaving smaller stump for coaptation), interposition cable graft has to be used in between, which delays the recovery a bit.

Use of masseter nerve can be in the form of the following:

- Direct neurotization with facial nerve stump.
- As "babysitter" techniques, in association with neuromuscular free tissue transfer in cases of long-term facial nerve palsy.

Advantage over Facio-Hypoglossal Anastomosis

- Anatomically, it is located in the vicinity of the facial nerve in the same surgical field, so relative ease of dissection.
- Nerve recovery is better that facio-hypoglossal anastomosis with low morbidity and a high potential for motor neural output.
- In faciohypoglossal anastomosis, the main limitation is that the patient has difficulty in the first stage of deglutition and articulation for a very long time. Whereas in faciomasseteric anastomosis, there is no such restriction of function. The donor deficit is very minimal as there are other muscles for mastication available.
- Better nerve for producing spontaneous smile as it is the natural function of the masseter muscle, which is supplied by the masseter nerve.
- Reinnervation takes lesser time.
- Its use is not contraindicated in patients with lower cranial nerve deficits or palsies or in patients susceptible to develop multiple cranial nerve deficits.

Disadvantages

- It is quite close to temporal and zygomatic branches of the facial nerve which can get injured while locating the masseter nerve. So, the dissection has to be very meticulous and accurate.
- Unless the surgeon is well versed with the surgical anatomy of the masseter nerve, it may take long time and at times difficult to locate the nerve.
- Loss of sensitivity of earlobe and preauricular region.

Anatomy of Masseter Nerve

Originates as a branch from anterior division of mandibular branch of trigeminal nerve (V3). It leaves the mandibular nerve shortly after its entrance into the infratemporal fossa. The nerve passes over the lateral pterygoid muscle and leaves the infratemporal fossa through the sigmoid notch, accompanied by the masseteric artery. It is located in the plane between the middle and deep lobes of the masseter muscle and enters the muscle from its medial surface. Distance from the notch to the entrance into the muscle is an average of 32 mm, which means that approximately 3 cm length of the nerve can be made available for anastomosis if dissected well. While descending, it lies in close proximity to the zygomatic branch of the facial nerve.

Surface Marking of Masseter Nerve

See **Fig. 75B.1**.

- Approximately 3.16 cm anterior to tragus.
- Approximately 1.06 cm inferior to zygomatic arch inferior margin.
- Around 1.5 cm deep to superficial musculoaponeurotic system (SMAS).
- Bisects the subzygomatic triangle.
- It is in close proximity to the zygomatic branch of the facial nerve, forming an angle of 50 degrees with it while descending.

The subzygomatic triangle is an important landmark to locate masseter nerve (**Fig. 75B.2**). It is formed by the following: Superior—Zygomatic arch inferior margin. Posterior—Vertical line through temporomandibular joint anterior margin. Inferoanterior—Frontal branch of the facial nerve.

The masseter nerve bisects this triangle.

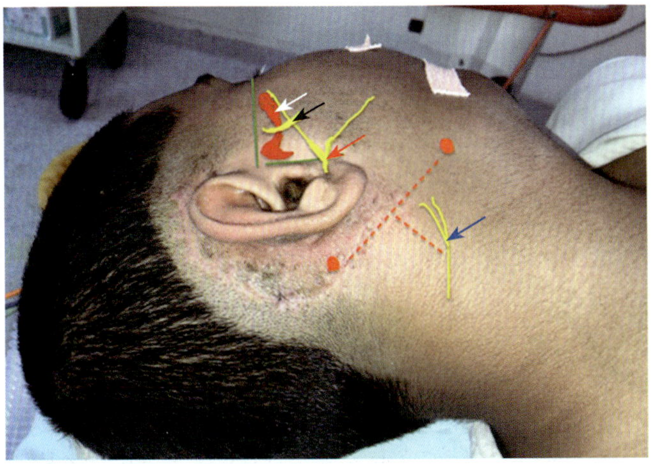

Fig. 75B.1 Image showing the surface marking for locating the masseter nerve. *Blue arrow*, great auricular nerve (GAN); *red arrow*, facial nerve; *black arrow*, masseter nerve; *white arrow*, sigmoid notch; *green outlines* are for demarcating the two limbs of subzygomatic triangle (lower border of zygomatic arch and line along the anterior margin of temporomandibular joint). The third limb of the triangle is formed by frontal branch of facial nerve.

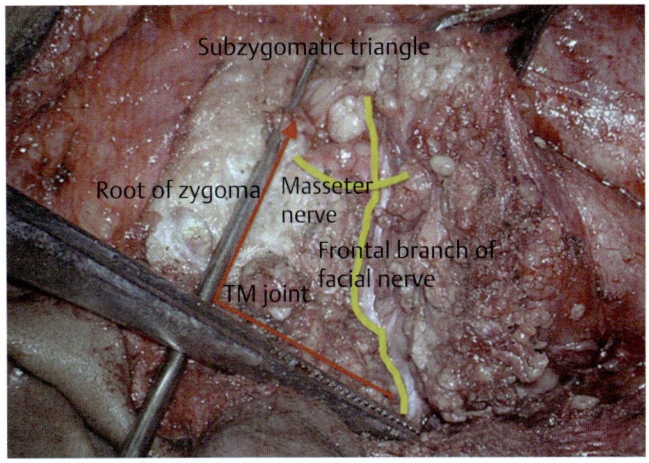

Fig. 75B.2 Diagrammatic depiction of the masseter nerve bisecting the subzygomatic triangle.

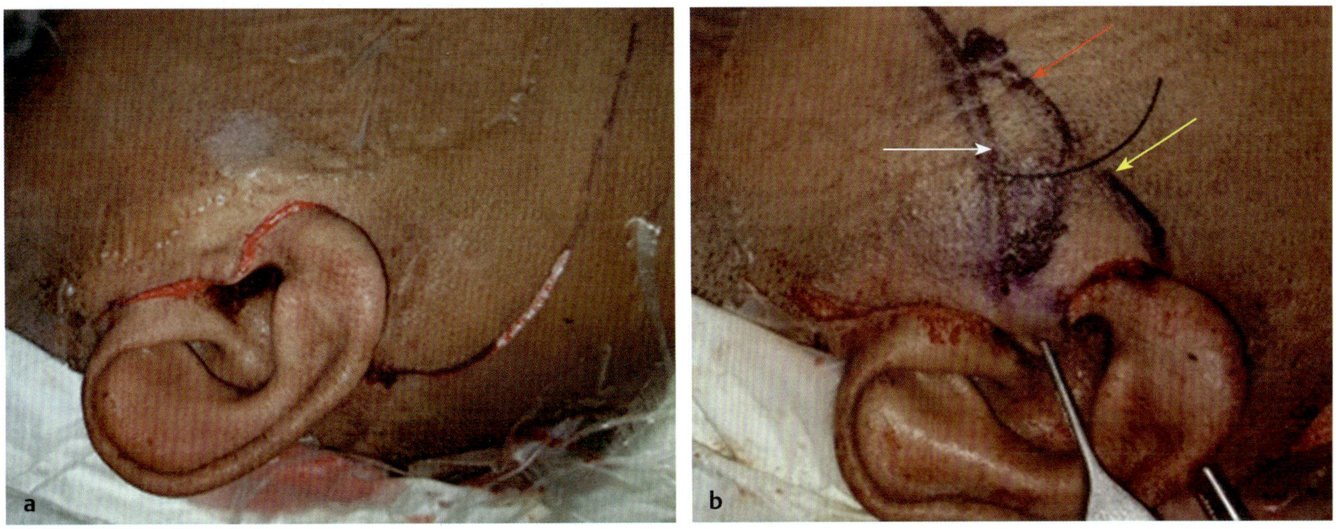

Fig. 75B.3 **(a, b)** Modified Blair's incision is given. Surface marking for important structures like zygomatic arch inferior border (*white arrow*), anterior margin of the tragus (tip of the forceps), sigmoid notch (*red arrow*), frontal the branch of the facial nerve (*yellow arrow*), and the masseter nerve (*black thread*) are shown with a blue marker.

Surgical Steps (Right Side)

- Modified Blair's incision with submandibular extension is made (**Fig. 75B.3**).
- Lift skin and SMAS flap (part of subcutaneous tissue, parotid capsule, and platysma) up to the anterior border of the masseter muscle (**Fig. 75B.4a**).
- Identify parotid gland and masseter muscle (**Fig. 75B.4**).
- Identify the GAN in the neck (**Fig. 75B.4b**).
- Identify facial nerve at its exit at the stylomandibular foramen and dissect it from surrounding parotid tissue following it up to its frontal branch (**Fig. 75B.5**). For identifying facial nerve, the different markers are as follows:

  Tragal pointer: The anterior part of the tragus points anterior and inferior and just deep to superficial

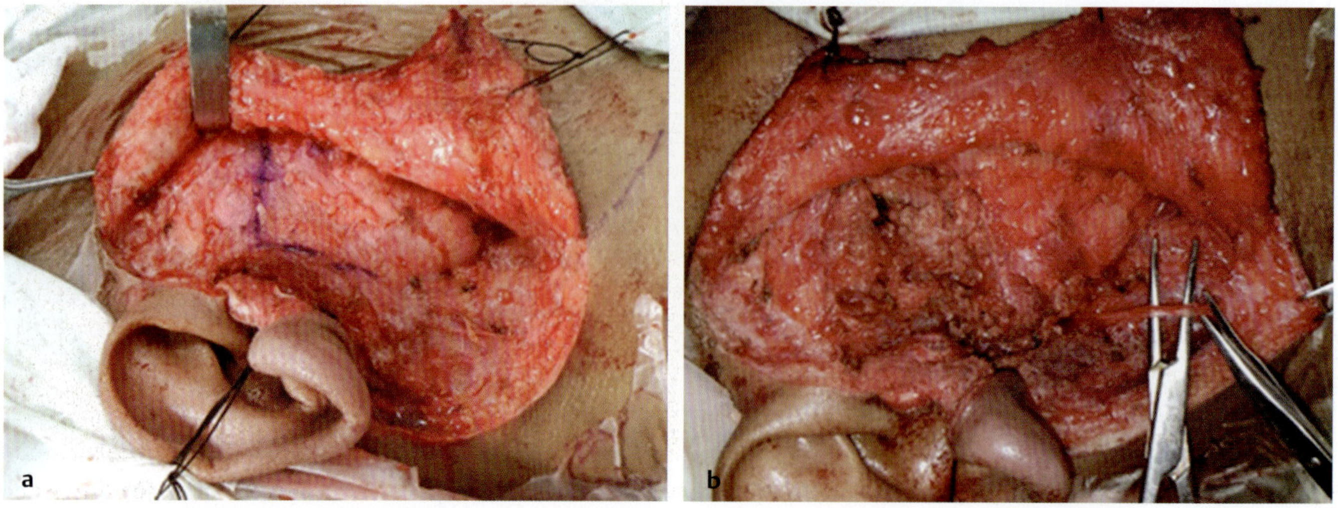

Fig. 75B.4 (a, b) Skin flap with SMAS lifted and great auricular nerve (GAN) exposed in the neck and harvested.

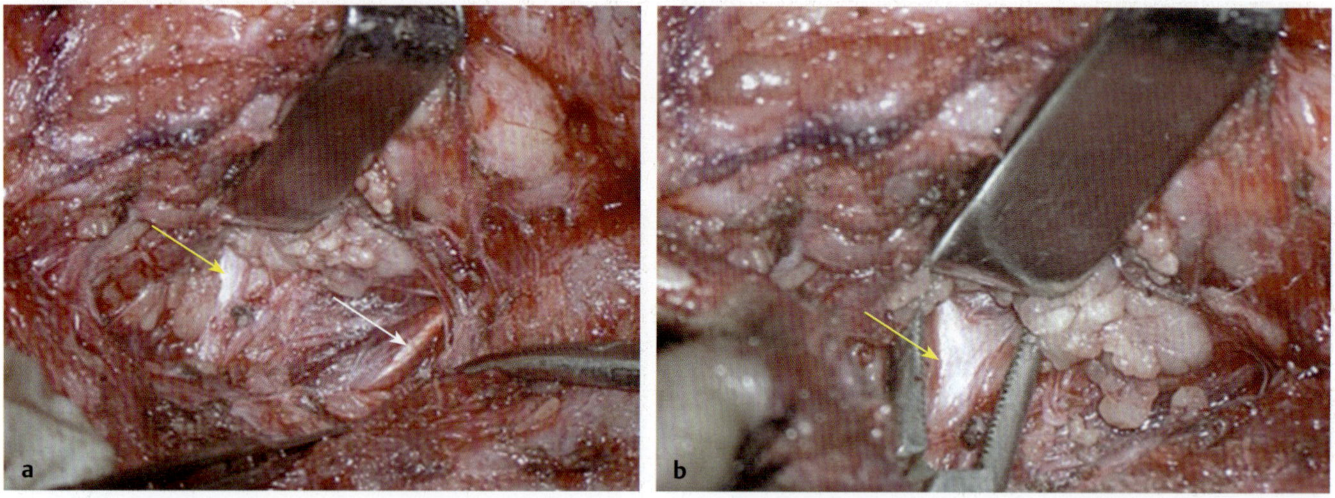

Fig. 75B.5 (a) For identification of the facial nerve, the posterior belly of the digastric muscle (*white arrow*) has been exposed. The facial nerve (*yellow arrow*) at its exit from the stylomastoid foramen lies 1 cm superior to the superior border of the posterior belly of the digastric muscle (*white arrow*). **(b)** Facial nerve with bifurcation identified. The artery forceps is inserted in the plane between the facial nerve and the parotid tissue and lifted, and the parotid tissue dissected away for further exposure of facial nerve branches.

surface of the preauricular region. Its anterior end starts narrowing and takes a pointed shape on its medial aspect and thus called "pointer." The facial nerve at its exit at stylomastoid foramen lies approximately 1 cm inferior and deeper to the tragal pointer.

Tympanomastoid suture: It is palpable as a hard ridge deep to the cartilaginous part of external auditory canal in its posteroinferior quadrant. The facial nerve emerges a few millimeters deep to its outer edge. Mean distance of the tympanomastoid suture line from the facial nerve trunk is 3.5 mm (2.5–4.5 mm).

Posterior belly of digastric muscle: It is the most consistent landmark for facial nerve dissection. After exposure and lateral retraction of the sternocleidomastoid muscle, the posterior belly of the digastric muscle is identified as it inserts on the mastoid ridge. The facial nerve trunk lies approximately 1 cm above and parallel to the upper border of the digastric muscle near its insertion.

- Expose subzygomatic triangle between zygomatic arch lower margin, vertical line along the anterior margin of the temporomandibular joint, and the frontal branch of the facial nerve (**Fig. 75B.1** and **Fig. 75B.5**).
- Also, identify the sigmoid or mandibular notch, which lies between the condylar and coronoid process of the mandible (**Fig. 75B.6**).
- Make a transverse incision in the parotid capsule.

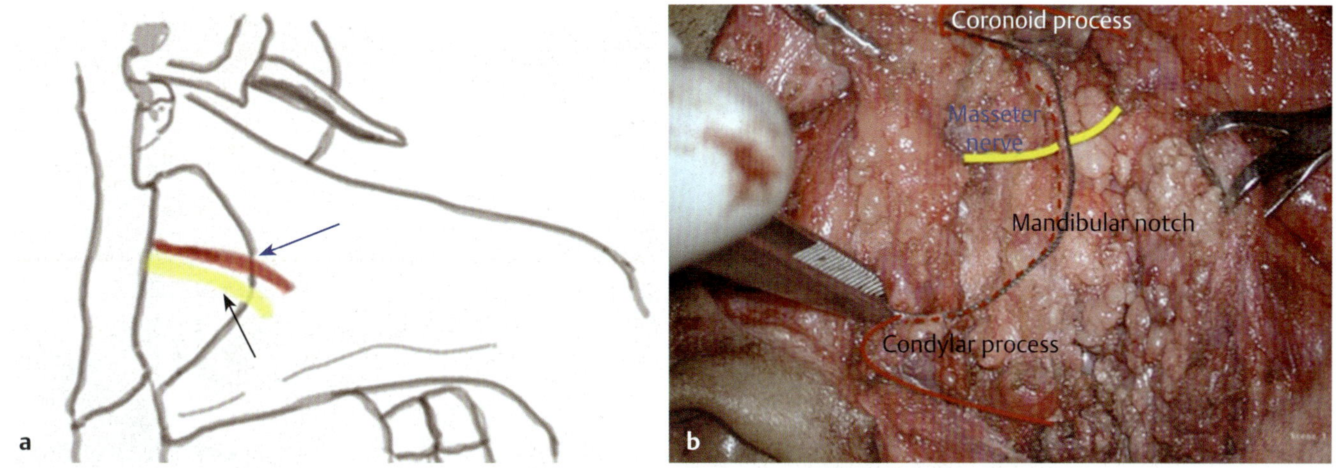

Fig. 75B.6 **(a)** Diagram depicting sigmoid notch (*blue arrow*) and exit of masseter nerve and artery (*black arrow*). **(b)** The same structures depicted in live surgery.

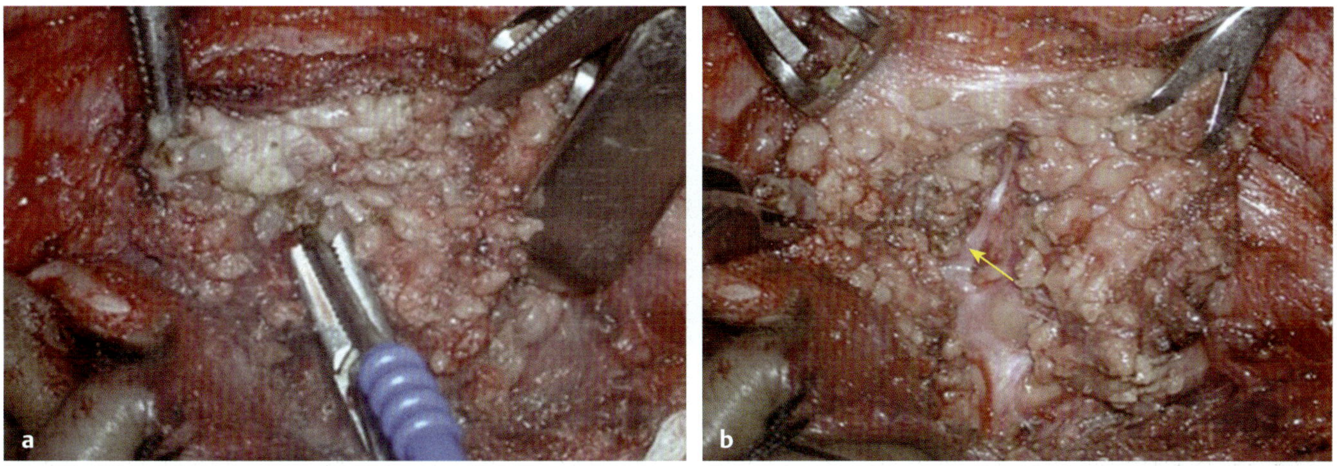

Fig. 75B.7 **(a)** Insertion followed by lifting and spreading of artery forceps in the plane between the facial nerve and parotid tissue which is further followed by cutting the parotid tissue lateral to the facial nerve. **(b)** Identifying and exposing the upper division of the facial nerve (*yellow arrow*).

- Bluntly dissect through the parotid tissue up to the surface of the masseter muscle, keeping in plane with the temporozygomatic branch of the facial nerve, so as to avoid transecting it accidentally (**Fig. 75B.7**).
- The masseter nerve can be located approximately 3.06 cm anterior to anterior border of tragus, 1.16 cm inferior to the inferior border of the zygomatic arch, and approximately 1.5 cm deep to the SMAS (**Fig. 75B.8** and **Fig. 75B.9**).
- The important point to remember is that the nerve courses vertically downward at the posterior margin of the muscle just below the zygomatic arch and then enters the masseter muscle from its medial, deeper surface (**Fig. 75B.10**).
- As the masseter nerve is located on the undersurface of the masseter muscle, the transmuscular identification of masseter nerve is performed.
- The dissection is always in the direction of the masseter nerve so as to avoid injuring the nerve while locating it.
- For locating the nerve, the overlying fascia and the origin of the masseter muscle are cleared from the zygomatic arch, and the dissection is carried downward through the whole depth of muscle till its undersurface. The muscle fibers are carefully retracted and transected till its undersurface. Once the nerve is identified, distal dissection of the nerve is carried out for achieving maximum length.
- The distance from the origin of the masseter nerve to its ramification in masseter muscle is around 3.5 cm, which means approximately, 3 cm length of branch-free segment of the nerve can be dissected for direct end-to-end anastomosis.

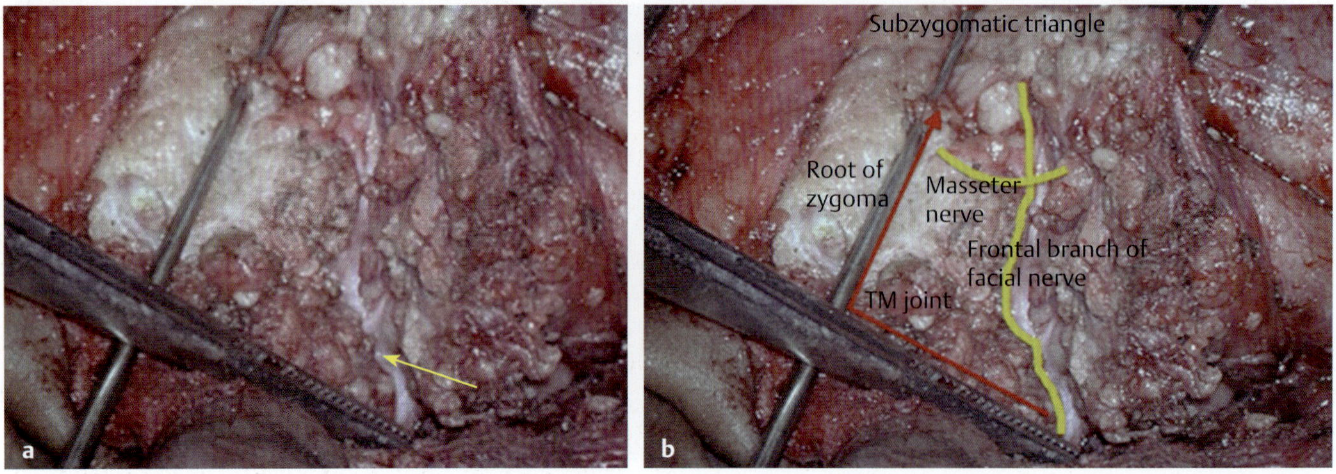

Fig. 75B.8 **(a)** Zygomatic arch and temporomandibular joint identified for the subzygomatic triangle. The frontal branch of the facial nerve is visible (*yellow arrow*). **(b)** The three sides of subzygomatic triangle are depicted: first line shows the inferior border of the zygomatic arch (*horizontal red line)*; second line is drawn along the anterior border of temporomandibular joint (*vertical red line*); and third line is drawn along the frontal branch of the facial nerve (*slanting yellow line*). The masseter nerve bisects this triangle (*vertical yellow line*).

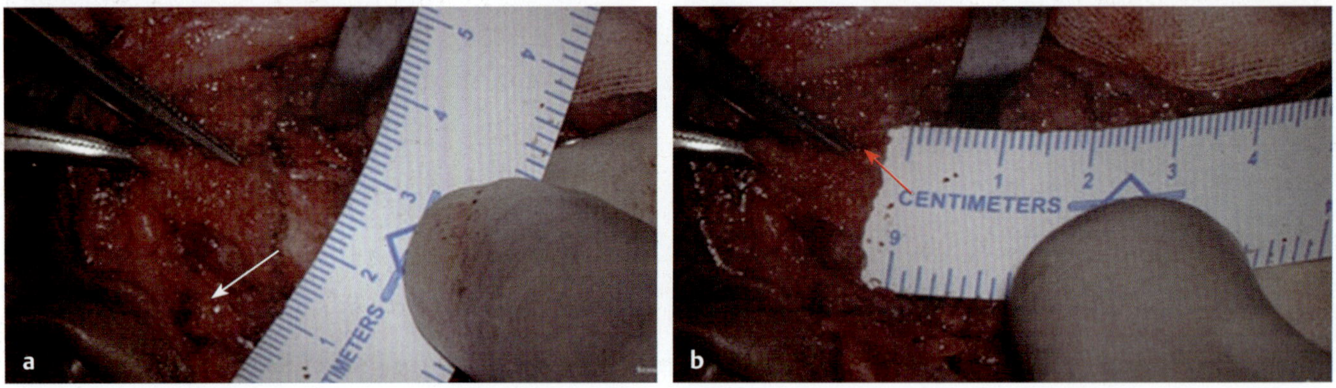

Fig. 75B.9 **(a, b)** Scale is used to measure point 3.06 cm from the anterior margin of the tragus (*white arrow*) and 1.16 cm from inferior border of the zygomatic arch (*red arrow*) for identifying the masseter nerve.

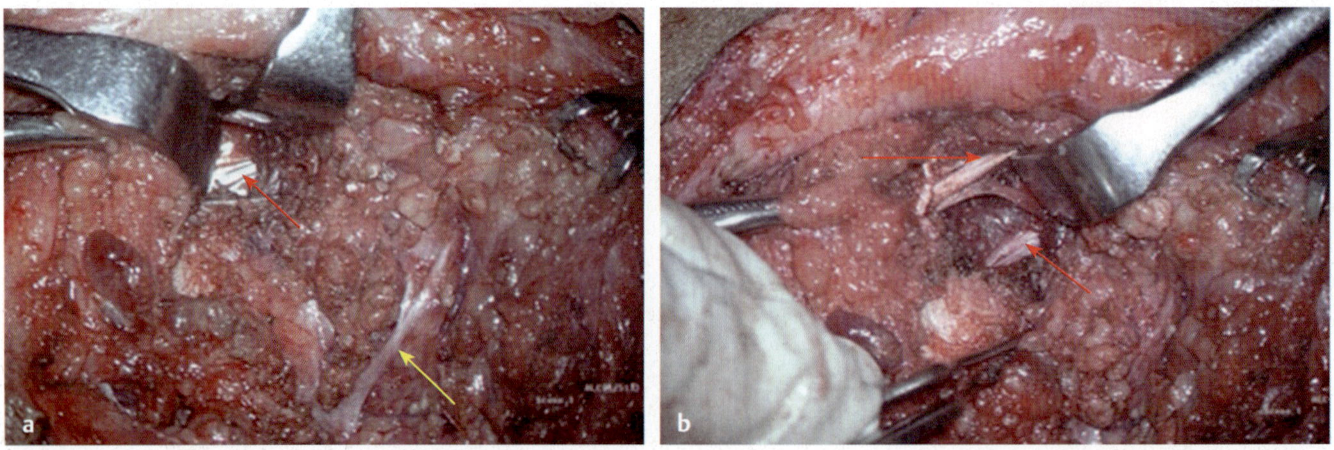

Fig. 75B.10 **(a)** Transmuscular dissection for identification of masseter nerve. The superficial part of the masseter muscle is dissected to expose deeper glistening white fibers of the tendon of the masseter muscle (*red arrow*). The zygomatic branch of the facial nerve (*yellow arrow*) is visible. **(b)** The deeper part of the masseter muscle is being dissected. The white fibers of the tendon of the muscle though look like masseter nerve, but they can be differentiated by their flatter and broader shape (*red arrows*).

- The nerve is transected at its distal end after complete exposure and reflected out, into the wound (**Fig. 75B.11**).
- Now prepare facial nerve stump by transecting it at stylomastoid foramen (**Fig. 75B.12**).
- In situations where the length of the masseter nerve is not sufficient, extra length can be achieved by transecting the facial nerve at the second genu rather than at stylomastoid foramen.
- In cases of facial nerve tumor where the nerve is involved distally till stylomastoid foramen or beyond, after complete resection of the tumor, the facial nerve stump may not be long enough to be directly coapted with the masseter nerve. In that situation, a great auricular cable nerve graft is interposed between the masseter and facial nerve (**Fig. 75B.13**).

There is a gap of almost 1.5 cm between the lower end of the masseter nerve and facial nerve stump, as this is a case of facial nerve neuroma where first stage surgery involved total excision of neuroma extending from internal auditory meatus to stylomastoid foramen. The mastoid portion and second genu of the facial nerve have already been in surgery for tumor removal. So, the length of the distal stump cannot be increased. A cable graft (GAN) is needed as the interposition graft between the cut ends of facial and masseter nerves (**Fig. 75B.14**). When the cable graft is used, the suture line

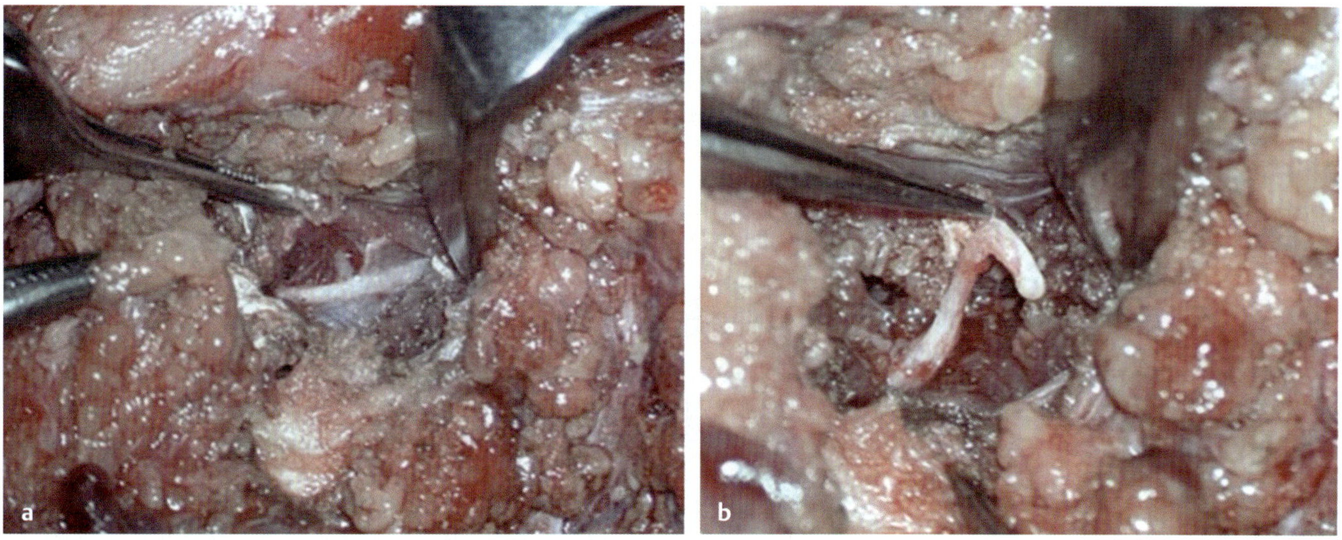

Fig. 75B.11 **(a)** Masseter nerve is identified almost 1 cm deep to deeper part of masseter muscle. **(b)** Maximum length of masseter nerve is exposed and transected at its entry into masseter muscle and lifted.

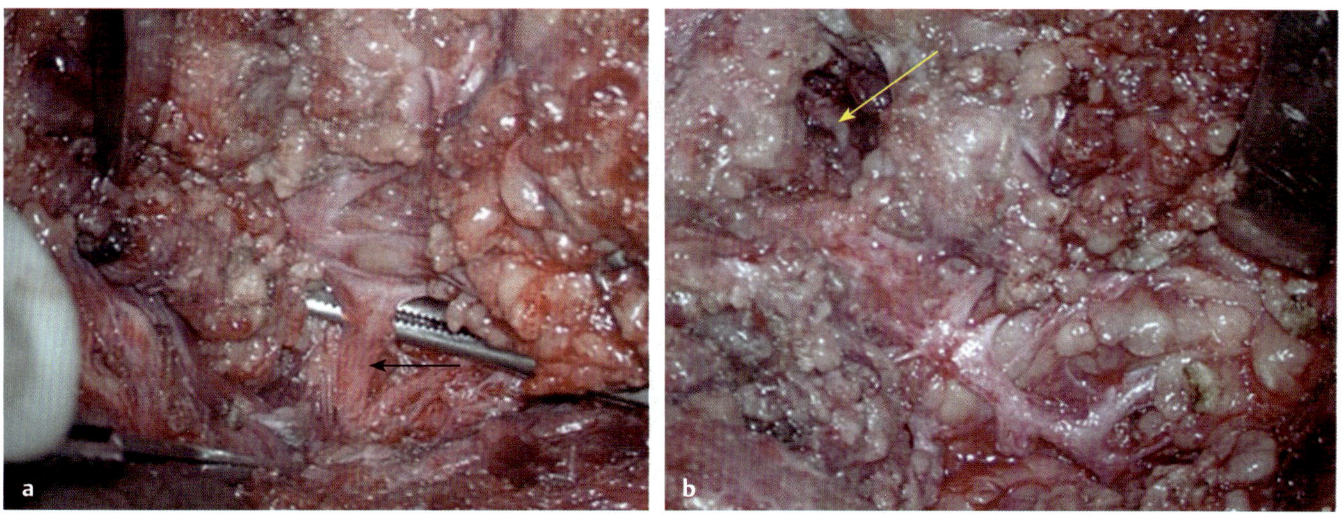

Fig. 75B.12 **(a)** Artery forceps lifting the facial nerve to be cut at its exit in stylomastoid (SM) foramen (*black arrow*). **(b)** Facial nerve stump (*black arrow*) prepared by transecting the nerve at SM foramen. Both upper and lower divisions of the facial nerve are exposed, to release the facial nerve in its maximum length. The masseter nerve is also visible in the vicinity (*yellow arrow*).

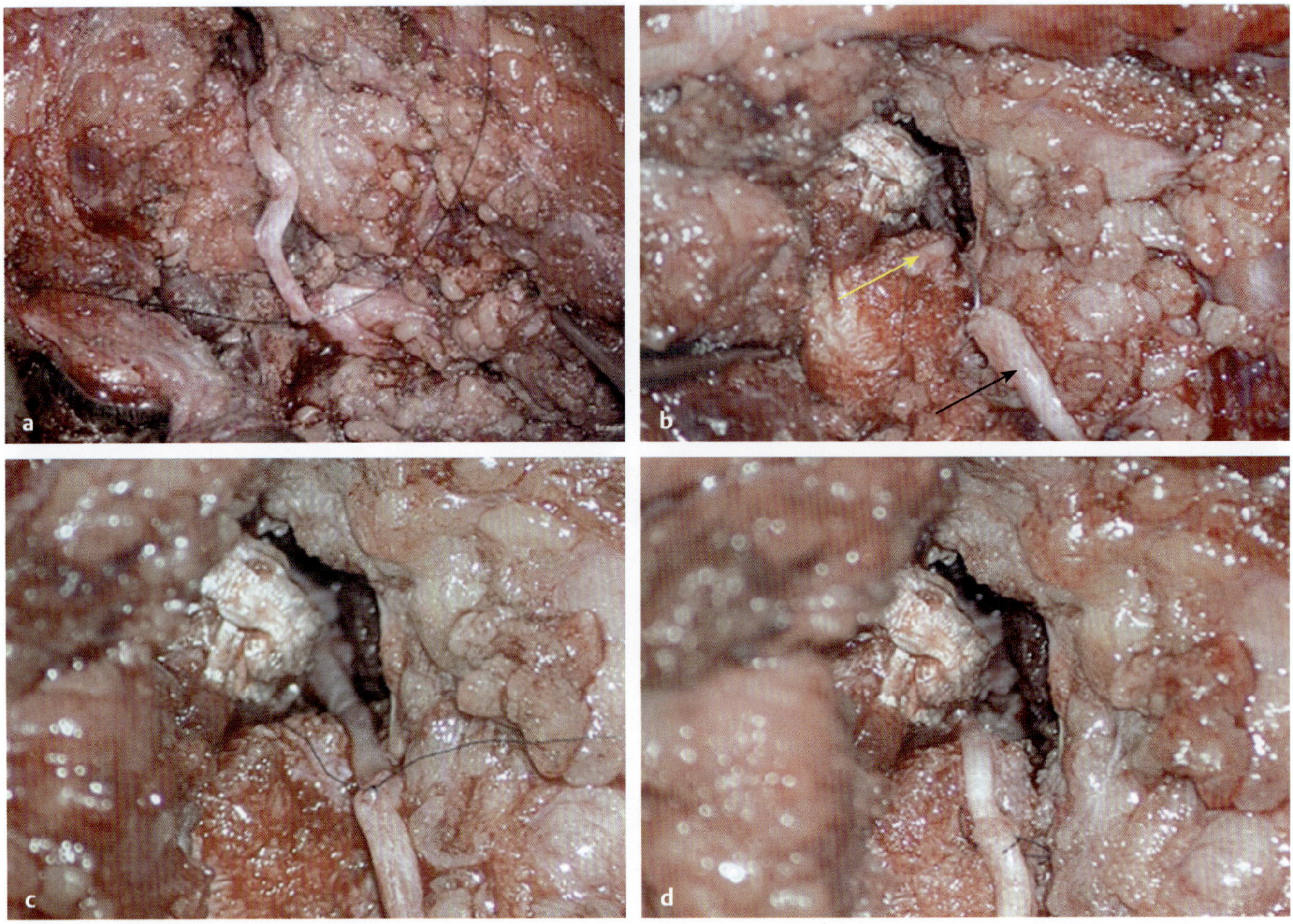

Fig. 75B.13 **(a)** Great auricular nerve is used as the cable graft between the two motor nerves. Polarity of the great auricular nerve is reversed. **(b, c)** The cut end of masseter nerve is being sutured to the great auricular nerve in an end-to-end manner. The suture is passed from the epineurium of the masseter nerve (*yellow arrow*) stump to the epineurium of the cut end of the great auricular nerve (*black arrow*). First suture is placed. **(d)** Two sutures are visible.

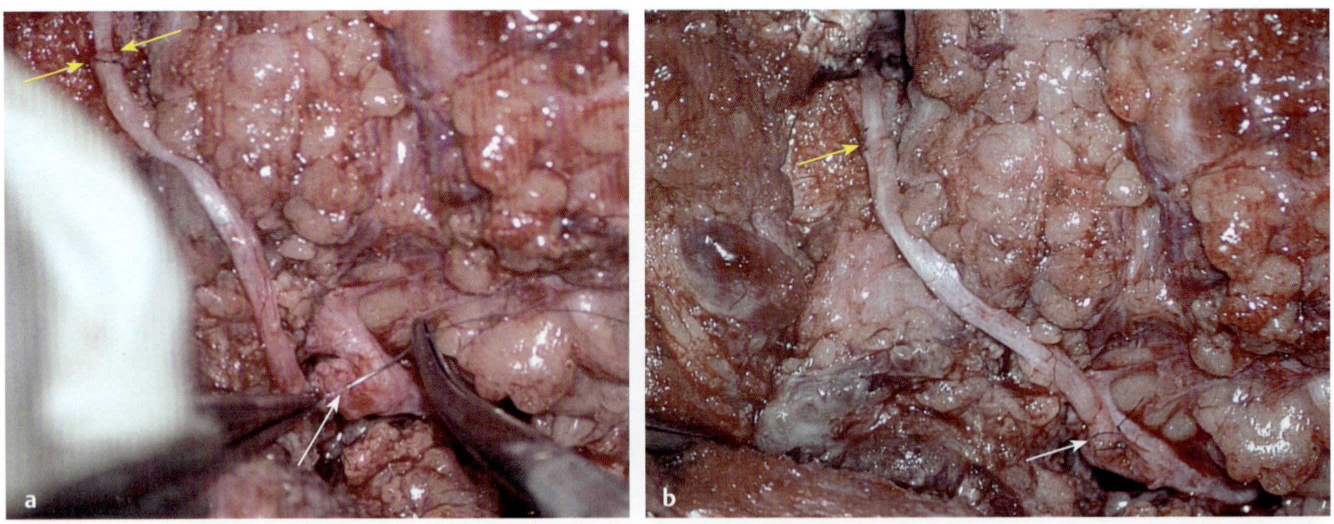

Fig. 75B.14 **(a)** Suture is being applied between distal facial nerve stump and the other end of the great auricular nerve (*white arrow*). Anastomosis between the masseter nerve and the cable graft is visible (*yellow arrows*). **(b)** Two sutures are placed between the facial nerve stump and the cable graft lower end (*white arrows*). Both anastomotic sites between facial nerve and masseter nerve through cable graft are visualized in one frame (*white and yellow arrows*).

should not be under any undue tension, and the length of the cable graft should be longer than the gap. In the immediate postoperative days, the blood supply to the grafted nerve comes from the surrounding tissue, so the anastomotic sites should be covered well by vascularized tissue around.

Postoperative Care and Physiotherapy Training

The patient is discharged 48 hours after surgery after the removal of dressing. First follow-up is 10 days after surgery when the sutures are removed.

At six weeks postsurgery, on the first rehabilitative visit, the patient is taught to activate the reinnervated facial muscles through teeth clenching, which means bite and smile together. Slowly, over time, the patient is taught to decrease bite and increase facial function. With regular physiotherapy training, facial muscles showed signs of recovery within 2 to 9 months. Around 18 months after the surgery, the patient displays dramatic improvement of voluntary control on facial symmetry and smile and remarkable reduction of disability, and finally the patient gets an independent facial function. However, none of the patients are able to achieve an effortless spontaneous smile.

Chapter 76 Rehabilitation of Lower Cranial Palsies after Skull Base Surgeries

Anagha Joshi

Introduction

The complications associated with skull base surgeries are because of the involvement of the lower cranial nerves (LCNs) IX to XI. Injury can occur via interruption of nerve continuity or impairment of neural functional integrity and can result in dysphagia, hoarseness, articulation deficits, and aspiration. However, with the advancements in microsurgical techniques, these complications have markedly reduced.

Functional Anatomy of the Lower Cranial Nerves

Glossopharyngeal Nerve (Cranial Nerve IX)

This is a mixed nerve carrying both motor efferents and sensory afferents. The nerve mediates five distinct functions:

- **Branchial motor:** Voluntary control of the stylopharyngeus muscle which dilates and elevates the pharynx during swallowing and speech.
  - ➢ Isolated loss of motor fibers to this muscle results in little swallowing dysfunction; however, when combined with the loss of general sensory fibers of the glossopharyngeal plexus and vagal motor fibers, severe swallowing deficits result.
- **Visceral motor:** Innervates the parotid gland.
  - ➢ Injury to these fibers may occur at many levels and lead to decreased parotid salivary flow; rarely, this leads to chronic parotitis.
- **Visceral sensory:** From the carotid sinus and carotid bodies.
- **General somatic afferent:**
  - ➢ Sensation from the skin of the external ear, the internal surface of the tympanic membrane.
  - ➢ The sensory fibers to the base of tongue and pharynx form glossopharyngeal plexus.
    - Disruption of the glossopharyngeal plexus causes a significant delay in the oropharyngeal phase of swallowing on the ipsilateral side.
  - ➢ Afferent limb of the gag reflex.
  - ➢ Afferent limb of the cough reflex.
- **Special sensory:** Taste sensation from the posterior third of the tongue.

Vagus Nerve (Cranial Nerve X)

It is most crucial in the control of the airway and swallowing function. The functions are as follows:

- **General sensory:** Afferent signals from the external auditory canal, tympanic membrane, supraglottic larynx, and lateral pharyngeal wall.
- **Visceral sensory:** Afferent sensory function to the pharynx, larynx, trachea, esophagus, thoracic viscera, and abdominal viscera distally to the level of the splenic flexure of the colon.
- **Branchial motor:**
  - ➢ **The pharyngeal branch:** Motor function to the pharynx and palate with the exception of the tensor veli palatini.
    - Damage to this branch results in unilateral palatal and pharyngeal paralysis, which causes a loss of lateral wall motion on the affected side and an ineffective sphincter for closing the nasopharyngeal port; this leads to nasal regurgitation and hypernasal speech.
  - ➢ **Superior laryngeal nerve:** It has both internal and external branches.
    - **The internal branch:** Supplies sensory and parasympathetic fibers to the epiglottis, tongue base, aryepiglottic folds, and the larynx to the level of the glottis.
    - **The external branch:** It is a motor branch, innervating the cricothyroid muscle and inferior pharyngeal constrictors and participating significantly in pitch control and swallowing.
    - Loss of this nerve results in decreased vocal range, which is usually a problem only for professional voice patients. Because the vagus is usually resected or injured at the skull base, patients have both superior and recurrent laryngeal nerve (RLN) paralyses.
  - ➢ **Recurrent laryngeal nerve:** It provides innervation to the intrinsic laryngeal musculature and the cricopharyngeus muscle.

- True vocal fold paralysis and lack of cricopharyngeal relaxation result from resection or neural injury at the time of surgery.
- The resultant glottal incompetence leads to a weak, breathy voice and an inefficient cough.
- Combined sensory and motor deficits result in a higher likelihood of aspiration and more complex phonatory problems.

➢ **Parasympathetic function:** To the pharynx, larynx, trachea, esophagus, thoracic viscera, and abdominal viscera distally to the level of the splenic flexure of the colon.

- Unilateral loss of vagal function may cause decreased gastroesophageal motility, loss of lower esophageal sphincter tone, and delayed gastric emptying owing to inadequate pyloric sphincter function.

Spinal Accessory Nerve (Cranial Nerve XI)

Branchial motor component: Its lower motor neuron cell bodies arise in the spinal cord, and its motor fibers ascend into the cranium and then descend through the pars nervosa of the jugular foramen to innervate the sternocleidomastoid and trapezius muscles.

- Loss of sternocleidomastoid function results in weakness when turning the head away from the operated side, although this is rarely noticed by most patients.
- Loss of trapezius function results in downward and lateral rotation of the scapula with a shoulder droop.

Hypoglossal Nerve (Cranial Nerve XII)

It provides somatic motor control to all the intrinsic and extrinsic muscles of the tongue except the palatoglossus. The nerve exits the skull base through the hypoglossal canal medial to the jugular foramen. As it passes laterally, it shares fibers with the vagus nerve near the inferior (nodose) ganglion. Separation of these fibers leads to vocal fold paresis or paralysis and should be avoided.

- Affection of this nerve causes unilateral tongue paralysis. The deficit is characterized by difficulty in positioning the bolus during the oral phase of swallowing. Often the bolus becomes lodged beneath the tongue on the paralyzed side.

Cervical Sympathetic Chain

Superior cervical ganglion: Damage to the superior cervical ganglion or the internal carotid plexus results in Horner's syndrome, consisting of ptosis, miosis, and anhidrosis.

Sympathetic innervation to the parotid gland

- Injury to the cervical sympathetic nerves at the skull base causes loss of sympathetic innervation to the parotid gland.
- **"First bite syndrome":** Spasmodic pain over the parotid region that begins with the first bite and subsides within the next several bites.[1]

Physiology of Swallowing

There are four stages of swallowing:

1. **Oral preparatory stage:** Mastication and bolus formation.
2. **Oral stage:** Tongue and hard palate transport the bolus to the posterior portion of the oral cavity.
3. **Pharyngeal stage:** This reflex involves a group of precise actions. There is elevation and retraction of the soft palate and closure of the nasopharynx, upper esophageal sphincter relaxation, laryngeal closure, tongue loading and propulsion, and pharyngeal contraction. This complex and coordinated pattern of events serves not only to guide the bolus through the pharynx into the esophagus but also to protect the larynx and airways.
4. **Esophageal stage:** During the fourth stage, the bolus progresses at a rate of 3 to 4 cms per, driven by a peristaltic wave beginning at the upper third of the esophagus and progressing to the stomach.

This entire process, although complex, is completed in about 1 second. Neural control of these stages primarily involves three areas of the medulla: the nucleus solitaries, the adjacent reticular formation, and the nucleus ambiguus. Cranial nerves V, VII, IX, X, and XII are also intimately involved in the swallowing process.

Clinical Evaluation

Assessment should be done by the skull base surgeon, laryngologist, and speech pathologist early in the course of diagnosis and should be dealt with by a comprehensive, coordinated approach. The patient should be mainly assessed with regard to voice-related symptoms and dysphagia. Dysphagia is a complication that if not handled properly can lead to malnutrition and psychological consequences as well as aspiration.

Bed Side Head and Neck Examination

It involves assessing oral motor and vocal functions.

1. **The face and jaw:** Observations of the facial muscles at rest and during movement, jaw muscle strength, and mobility.

2. Lingual functions.
3. **The palate and pharynx:** Palatal weakness and asymmetry.
4. Gag reflex.
5. Palpating the larynx and assessing laryngeal elevation during a dry swallow.
6. Clinical measures for laryngeal function (CN X).
   - **Volitional cough.**
   - **Voice quality:** Subjective ratings of voice quality are made during the sustained /a/, reading, and conversation.
   - **Maximum phonation time (MPT):** It is measured with the patient in a sitting or standing position, sustaining a vowel sound at a comfortable pitch and loudness level, for as long as possible on one breath. Depending on the position of the vocal folds, MPT may range from less than 4 seconds, indicating vocal fold vibration for a short period of time, to an almost normal length of 20 seconds, indicating vibration throughout most of the expiratory cycle.
   - **The S/Z ratio:** It provides the clinician with an idea of phonatory function. The duration of a sustained voiceless S phoneme is compared with the duration of a voiced Z phoneme. If glottal closure is adequate, the ratio of S to Z should be around 1; with adequate glottal closure, voiced and voiceless sounds should be of approximately equal duration. If there are difficulties in glottal valving, the "s" will be phonated longer as compared "z," and will be reflected by ratios greater than 1. Generally, ratios greater than 1.4 are considered abnormal.
   - **GRABS scale:** This is a subjective acoustic evaluation based on the patient's and physician's rating of the dysphonia. The following parameters are measured on a scale of 0 (absent) to 3 (severe): G is the degree of global dysphonia; R is roughness; B is breathiness; A is an asthenic or weak voice; and S is a strained or forced voice.[2]
   - **Voice handicap index (VHI):** VHI consists of patients' self-ratings on three subscales: functional (VHI-F), emotional (VHI-E), and physical (VHI-P). Each subscale has 10 questions. Pretreatment scales are helpful as a baseline for future comparison.[3]
   - **Computerized voice analysis:** It involves measurements of various parameters of voice such as fundamental frequency, intensity, perturbation measures, etc. It is an objective measure of voice.

Videolaryngoscopy/Videostroboscopy

A 70 or 90-degree rigid Hopkins laryngoscope is used to assess the vocal cord mobility, glottic closure, mucosal lesions, pooling, and any vocal fold asymmetry. The position of the vocal processes and motion with pitch change is determined. Phonation can be assessed more physiologically with a flexible nasopharyngoscope.

Flexible Fiberoptic Evaluation of Swallowing

This is done if the patient complaints of dysphagia. This allows direct visualization of the larynx and pharynx before and after the swallow.

- In the first level, the anatomy and the sensation of the laryngopharynx are assessed.
  - ➢ Velopharyngeal closure.
  - ➢ Pooling of secretions in the pharynx.
  - ➢ **Laryngeal elevation:** Passage of the bolus and movement of the pharyngeal structures cannot be observed during the swallow because of reflected light from pharyngeal and laryngeal tissues into the endoscope, causing a brief condition referred to as "white-out."
  - ➢ Vocal fold function.
    - Eee-sniff maneuver.
    - **Breath-holding maneuver:** Patient's ability to close supraglottis and protect airway.
    - Vocal fold position.
  - ➢ **Pharyngeal squeeze maneuver (PSM):** The patient says a forceful "eee" sound, and the degree of pharyngeal muscular contraction and narrowing of the pyriform sinus during voluntary forceful adduction of the vocal folds is noted.
  - ➢ Ability to clear secretions by coughing.
  - ➢ **Laryngeal adductor response (LAR):** The sensation of the larynx is tested with the tip of the laryngoscope. The LAR is a brainstem-mediated airway protective reflex; the afferent component is internal branch of the superior laryngeal nerve, and the efferent arc is the RLN.
- In the second level, food is administered and the laryngopharynx is visualized through the scope during the act of swallowing.
  - ➢ If LAR is present and PSM is absent, then only water is given for testing.
  - ➢ If PSM is present and LAR is absent, then only semi-solids are given for testing.

- If both are absent, then ice chips which will enhance the sensory information to the patient and will cause lesser harm if aspirated are given to the patient.[4]
- The presence of abundant secretion in the laryngeal vestibule or a nonprotective cough can be contraindications to an examination with a bolus.
- The tip of the scope is kept at the level of the base of tongue and observation of swallowing is done for the following:
  - **Premature spillage:** Loss of bolus into the pharynx before the initiation of swallowing.
  - **Swallowing white out:** The oropharyngeal stage is not visible endoscopically when the swallowing reflex starts, because the endoscope will be in contact with the base of the tongue, with the epiglottis and the bolus itself.
  - **Penetration:** Passage of material into the laryngeal inlet.
  - **Aspiration:** Passage of material below the vocal cord (**Fig. 76.1a**).
  - Pooling of food.

At the end of the swallow, if the remains of the bolus are abundant, (in cases of cricopharyngeal spasm) (**Fig. 76.1b**), they might penetrate the larynx and cause later inhalation (postswallowing inhalation).

Dynamic endoscopic examination with boluses of different consistency not only reveals eventual inhalation but also reveals the efficacy of the various postures and maneuvers that facilitate swallowing and which are either spontaneous in the patient or acquired after specific rehabilitation therapy.

Modified Barium Swallow—Videofluoroscopy

For details see **Fig. 76.2a, b**.

The videofluroscopic swallowing study (VFSS), also known as the modified barium swallow study (MBSS) is a radiographic procedure that provides a direct, dynamic view of oral, pharyngeal, and upper esophageal function.[5] Sensory deficits and nasopharyngeal reflux may be more apparent on an MBS than on visual inspection alone. The MBS examines oral, pharyngeal, and esophageal function. It identifies the cause of aspiration (i.e., when and how the event occurs during the different phases of swallowing) and also allows assessment of the efficacy of treatment and management strategies. Rosenbek et al[6] described an eight-point penetration–aspiration scale based on videofluoroscopic data that fulfills this purpose (**Table 76.1**).

Treatment

Treatment primarily involves the management of aspiration and improvement of voice. Management of aspiration, particularly in the acute setting immediately following nerve injury, always takes precedence as aspiration can lead to life-threatening pneumonia. If aspiration is not an issue, treatment of vocal quality can be tailored to the patient's needs.

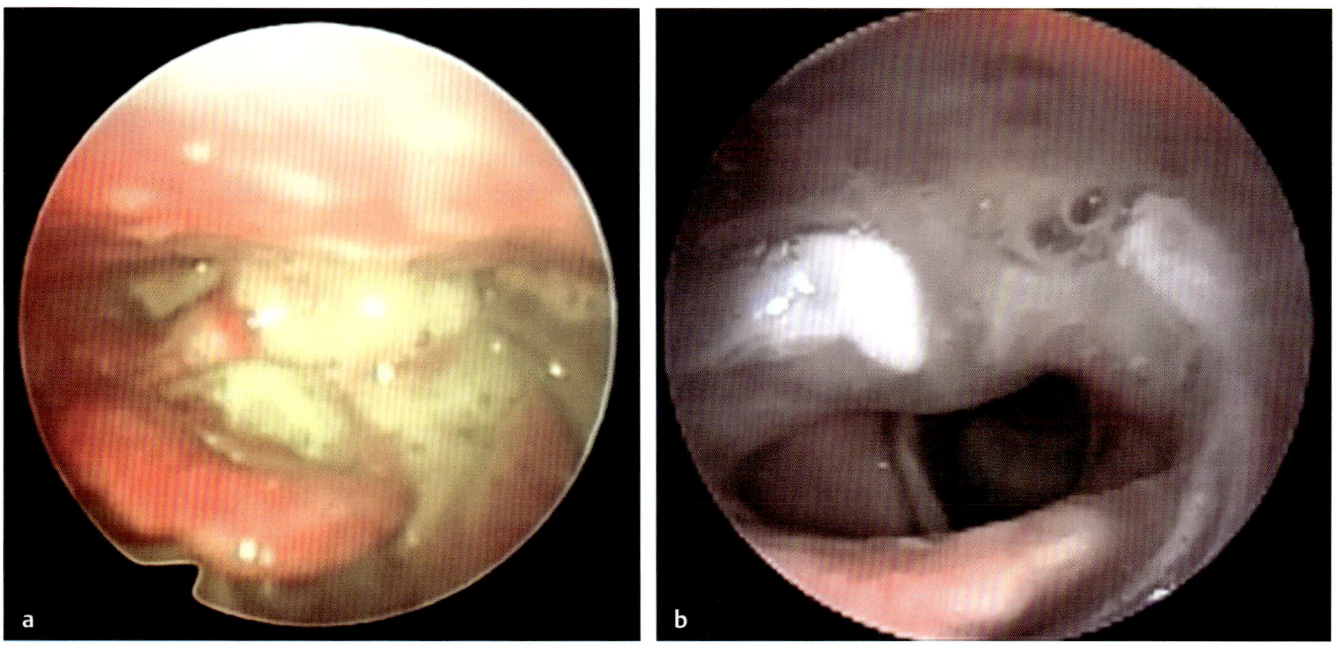

Fig. 76.1 Fiberoptic evaluation of swallowing (FEES). **(a)** Aspiration and passage of ingested material into the larynx, and **(b)** abundant bolus still remaining at the end of the swallow, in cases of cricopharyngeal spasm.

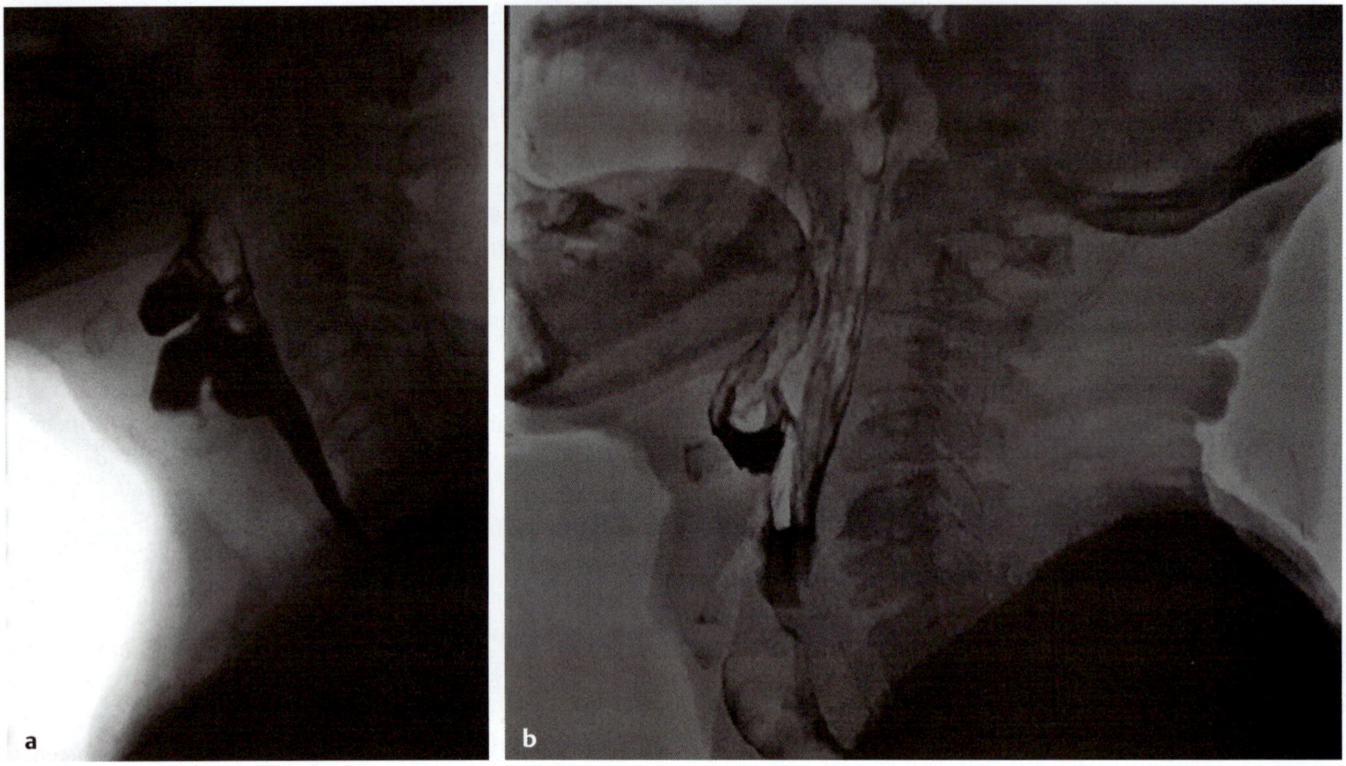

Fig. 76.2 Video fluoroscopy. **(a)** Laryngeal penetration, and **(b)** aspiration and lining of the trachea with radiopaque dye.

Table 76.1 Eight-point penetration–aspiration scale

1.	Material does not enter the airway
2.	Material enters the airway, remains above the vocal folds, and is ejected from the airway
3.	Material enters the airway, remains above the vocal folds, and is not ejected from the airway
4.	Material enters the airway, contacts the vocal folds, and is ejected from the airway
5.	Material enters the airway, contacts the vocal folds, and is not ejected from the airway
6.	Material enters the airway, passes below the vocal folds, and is ejected into the larynx or out of the airway
7.	Material enters the airway, passes below the vocal folds, and is not ejected from the trachea despite effort
8.	Material enters the airway, passes below the vocal folds, and no effort is made to eject

Glossopharyngeal Nerve (Cranial Nerve IX)

- **Disruption of the glossopharyngeal plexus:** Isolated, unilateral CN IX deficits are well compensated for with swallowing therapy that focuses on maintaining passage of the food bolus adjacent to the contralateral sensate side of the pharynx using a chin-tuck and head-turn maneuver toward the side of the deficit. When this deficit is combined with the loss of CNs X and XII at the skull base, the dysfunction becomes severe. Rehabilitation of this combined loss involves correction of glottal incompetence with thyroplasty and intensive swallowing therapy.
- **Loss of the carotid sinus reflex**[7]
  - Unilateral loss does not interfere with the control of blood pressure and pulse, presumably because of the presence of an intact reflex on the contralateral side.
  - Bilateral alteration of this system can occur rarely when CN IX fibers of the contralateral neck may have been disrupted because of previous surgery, such as carotid endarterectomy. It causes acute elevation of blood pressure to greater than 220 mm Hg within a 60-second period. Consultation with an intensivist in the preoperative period is strongly recommended if a bilateral loss is anticipated.

Vagus Nerve (Cranial Nerve X)

Of the LCNs, the vagus is most intimately involved in the control of the phonation, airway, and swallowing function. Simultaneous injury to cranial nerve IX (glossopharyngeal nerve) causes far greater morbidity, including vocal cord paralysis, hoarseness, inability to cough, and pharyngeal weakness and hypesthesia, that results in severe dysphagia and aspiration.

Treatment of Paralytic Dysphonia

Vocal fold paralysis leads to insufficient closure of the vocal folds causing symptoms such as hoarseness, breathiness or aphonia, and aspiration. The main goal in the management is to achieve better glottic closure during phonation.

Speech Therapy

A team approach between an otolaryngologist and speech language pathologist for the management of a patient with vocal fold immobility is recommended. After the initial work-up and diagnosis by the otolaryngologist, the patient is referred to a speech pathologist for objective voice analysis, assessment, and voice therapy. It is important to document the degree of vocal dysfunction prior to further intervention in order to objectively evaluate the progress of the voice. Voice therapy aims to improve glottal closure without causing supraglottic hyperfunction while developing abdominal support for breathing and improving intrinsic muscle strength and agility. Vocal exercises include hard glottal attacks, pushing, half-swallow boom, and abdominal breathing.

Vocal Cord Medialization

Injection Augmentation

In this procedure, a material is injected into the true vocal fold in an attempt to add bulk and medialize the edge of the vocal fold. After a period of weeks to months, the injected substance is typically resorbed. It can provide immediate functional improvement while the patient awaits RLN recovery and does not preclude further intervention with other injectables or laryngeal framework surgery. Previously, it was accepted that waiting several months before intervention would allow time for spontaneous recovery to occur. However, because of its ease of use and low risk and complication rate, early injection laryngoplasty (IL) under topical anesthetic provides an excellent therapeutic option for both patient and physician. Friedman et al hypothesized that with early intervention (< 6 months from the time of injury), the implant material allows the vocal fold to be in a more favorable final vocal fold position, during the time window of synkinetic reinnervation, as compared to those who were not injected or injected late. Functional recovery of the injured vocal fold may be influenced by vibrotactile stimulation from contact with the contralateral cord which would otherwise have not occurred during the recovery period without injection augmentation. It could also be postulated that medial position of the vocal fold can prevent poorly reversible compensatory hyperfunction, which may result in better long-term voice outcomes.[8,9] There might be a greater degree of benefit to an even earlier acute intervention in terms of decreasing the likelihood of requiring a subsequent permanent laryngeal framework procedure.[10]

The ideal vocal fold injection material would be readily available, inexpensive, inert, easy to use, and completely biocompatible.

Temporary Injection Substances

- **Bovine Gelatin (Gelfoam, Surgifoam):** Gelfoam is a material made of bovine gelatin that comes in a powder form or foam sheet and can be mixed with saline to be used as an injectable paste. One gram of Gelfoam is mixed with 4 mL of saline while stirring it continuously.[11] This produces a thick paste of 5 mL which is then fed into a syringe for transoral or percutaneous injection. However, its higher viscosity requires use of a large-gauge needle (18 or 19), which can make awake injection more uncomfortable for the patient. Injections are made laterally into the muscle of the vocal fold and the paraglottic space. It is inexpensive and readily available in most surgical centers. The duration of benefit lasts for 4 to 6 weeks, which is often an adequate amount of time to allow spontaneous recovery or determination of prognosis after RLN injury.
- **Collagen, Alloderm, and Fascia-** (Zyplast, Cosmoplast/Cosmoderm, Cymetra): Zyplast is derived from bovine collagen and the effect lasts for up to 4 months. There is a 2% risk of an allergic reaction, allergy testing is recommended prior to usage of bovine collagen injection products.[12] Collagen is available in liquid form, and hence it can be injected transcutaneously through a 27-gauge needle. The use of human collagen (Dermalogen, Collagenesis, Beverly, MA) eliminates the severe reactions encountered with bovine collagen. Cymetra micronized Alloderm (Lifecell Corporation, Branchburg, NJ) is an acellular human tissue material that includes collagen, elastin proteoglycans, and like collagen; it too can be injected transcutaneously.
- **Carboxymethylcellulose (Radiesse Voice Gel):** Carboxymethylcellulose (CMC) gel can be easily injected percutaneously or transorally through a 25-gauge needle. It is well tolerated by patients and produces excellent voice results. The duration of effectiveness is around 2 to 3 months depending on the amount injected.
- **Hyaluronic Acid Gel (Restylane TM, Hyalaform):** Hyaluronic acid (HA) is a polysaccharide that is a primary component of the extracellular matrix and is found within the superficial lamina propria. Animal

and laboratory studies suggest that when injected, HA products closely resemble the native viscoelastic properties of the vocal folds.[13] This property of HA has made it a popular option for otolaryngologists. There is an absence of animal products in the HA gel material, which reduces the risk of an allergic reaction. Superficial injections are also much better tolerated than with any other injection material. The duration of the beneficial effects may last anywhere between 3 to 6 months. We prefer to use this material for injection.

Lasting Injection Substances

- **Autologous fat:** Fat is available in abundant quantity, is relatively easy to harvest, and its viscoelastic properties are similar to the vocal fold lamina propria. The disadvantages are donor site morbidity, unpredictable degree of resorption and duration of effect, and the need to inject through a large (18- to 19-gauge) needle to limit trauma to adipocytes. It works best for small glottal gaps, especially correction of persistent hoarseness after thyroplasty. Fat is harvested from the abdomen or thigh, and prepared by washing, drying, and cutting into small pieces for injection. It can also be obtained by aspiration through a liposuction cannula and is then centrifuged in sterile conditions for 3 minutes by a handheld centrifuge, which separates the fat from red blood cells (**Fig. 76.3**). The fat is then

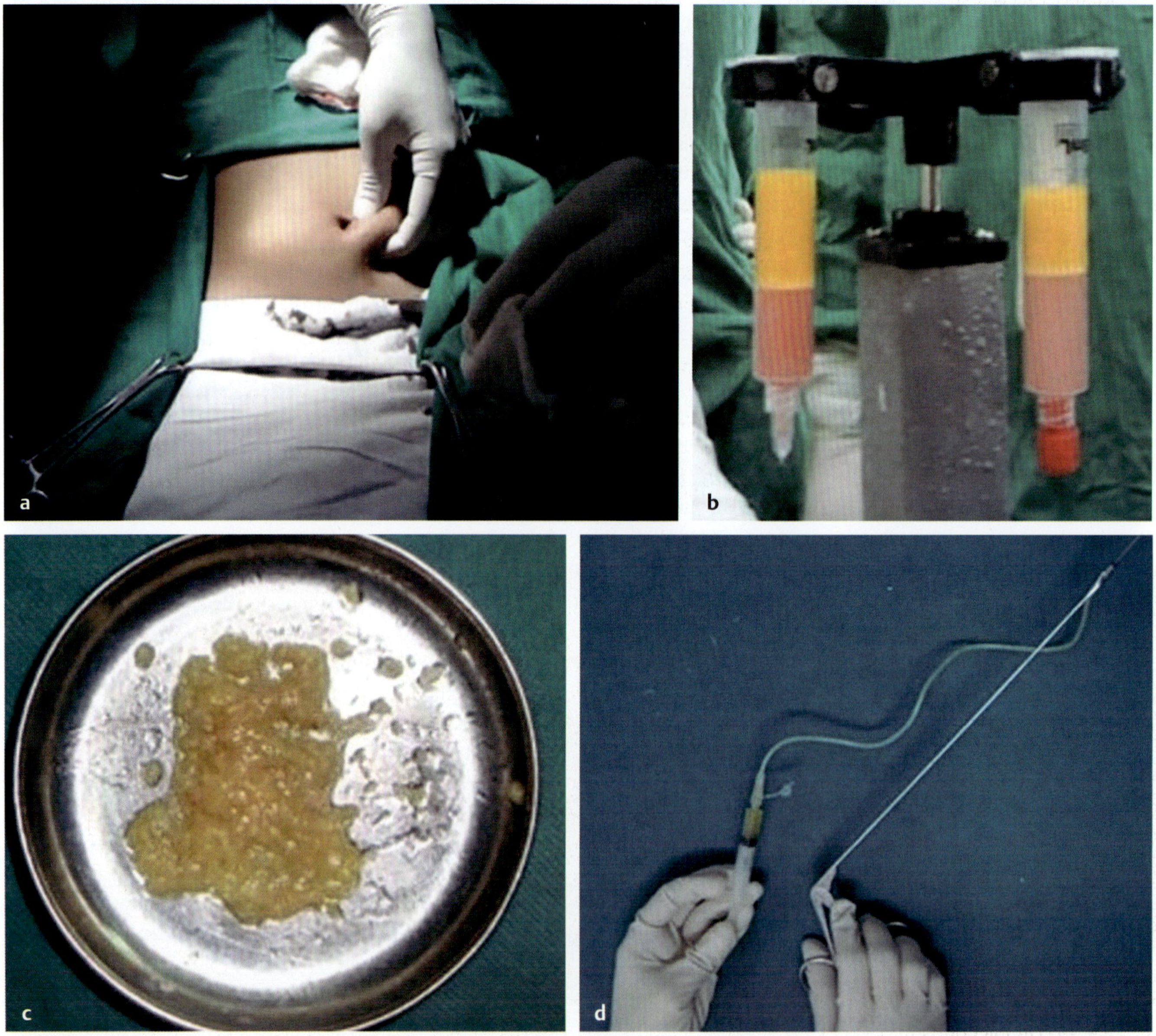

Fig. 76.3 Harvesting fat for injection. **(a)** Aspiration of fat with liposuction, **(b)** separation of fat from blood with a hand -held centrifuge, **(c)** harvested fat minced into small pieces, **(d)** fat-filled into the syringe for injection.

transferred to syringes to which an 18-gauge butterfly syringe is fitted for injection. The small plastic wings around the needle are cut off almost completely so that the needle can be held with a Kleinsasser microforceps inside the laryngoscope. Under direct microlaryngoscopy, up to 3 mL of the purified fat is injected into the middle third of the vocal fold. Because of the inconsistent survival of the adipocytes, over-injection of the vocal fold by 50% is recommended (**Fig. 76.4**). The need for graft harvest and preparation along with the large injection needle limits fat injection procedures to the operating room under general anesthesia.

- **Calcium hydroxylapatite (Radiesse):** Calcium hydroxylapatite (CaHA) (Radiesse, Bioform Medical, Inc., San Mateo, CA) is a suspension of CaHA microspherules in a glycerin-carboxymethyl cellulose-water gel and has the minimal inflammatory response and no evidence of toxicity. It is a Food and Drug Administration (FDA)-approved substance for vocal cord injection. Because of its viscosity, it needs to be injected with a 25-gauge needle. A 10% over-injection is recommended to compensate for the absorption of the carrier gel. Beneficial effects achieved from CaHA injection generally last for 1.5 to 3 years. When injected superficially, Radiesse leads to increased stiffness of the vocal folds, increased resistance to airflow, and worsened mucosal wave.[14] Though it can be injected in the office, the need for its precise placement leads one to opt for its injection under controlled settings of the operation theater.
- **Teflon:** The use of Teflon (Dupont, Wilmington, NC) has been virtually abandoned since mid-1980s because of occurrence of severe foreign body reaction and granuloma formation at the injection site.

General Principles of Vocal Fold Injection Augmentation

- It is done under local anesthesia in most cases to monitor the patients' voice during the procedure. Fat injection is performed under general anesthesia to facilitate fat harvesting and preparation.
- Injection techniques include the following:
  - ➢ Peroral:
    - Curved injection device in the clinic setting. This approach affords the surgeon an excellent visualization of the injection needle during the procedure. With the patient in a sitting position, the oropharynx and base tongue are anesthetized with a topical 10% lidocaine spray. After anesthetizing the nasal mucosa, a flexible laryngoscope is passed through the nasal cavity and advanced to visualize the vocal cords. "Laryngeal gargle" is then given by dripping 4% lidocaine directly onto the arytenoids and vocal folds during phonation through an Abraham-type catheter. The injection needle is then passed orally into the oropharynx. Once the needle tip is in view, the tip is rotated inferiorly toward the vocal cords and inserted lateral to the vocal process in the thyroarytenoid muscle. The transoral approach can also be done by a 70-degree telescope. The patient or an assistant can hold the patient's tongue. The surgeon holds the telescope in the nondominant hand and the injection needle in the other (**Fig. 76.5**).

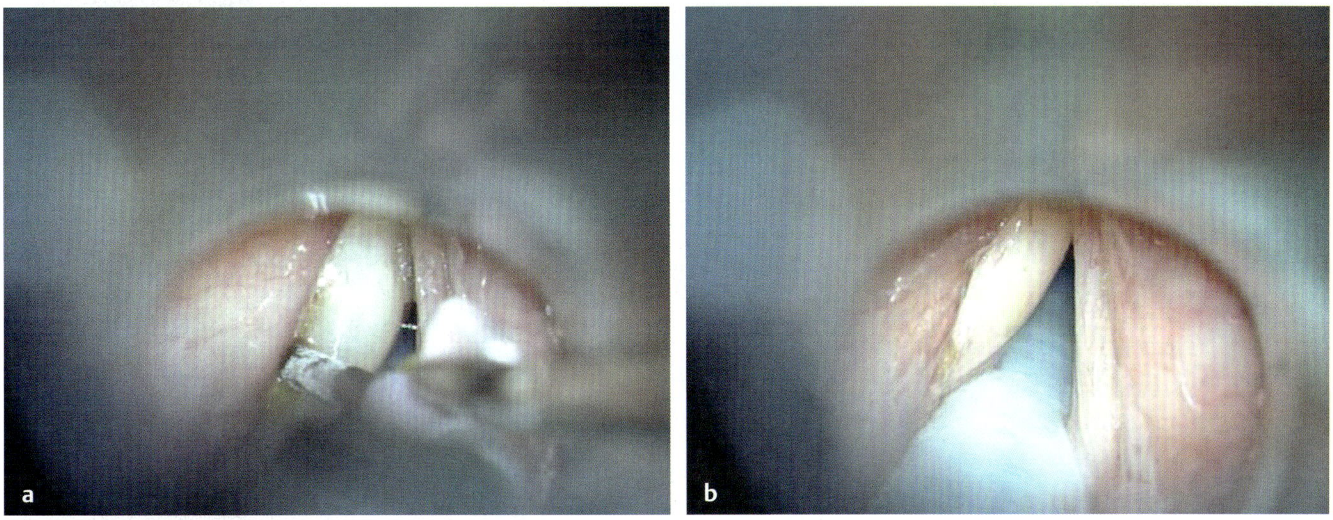

Fig. 76.4 (a) Fat injection into the left vocal fold through microlaryngoscopy, and **(b)** medialised left vocal fold after injection.

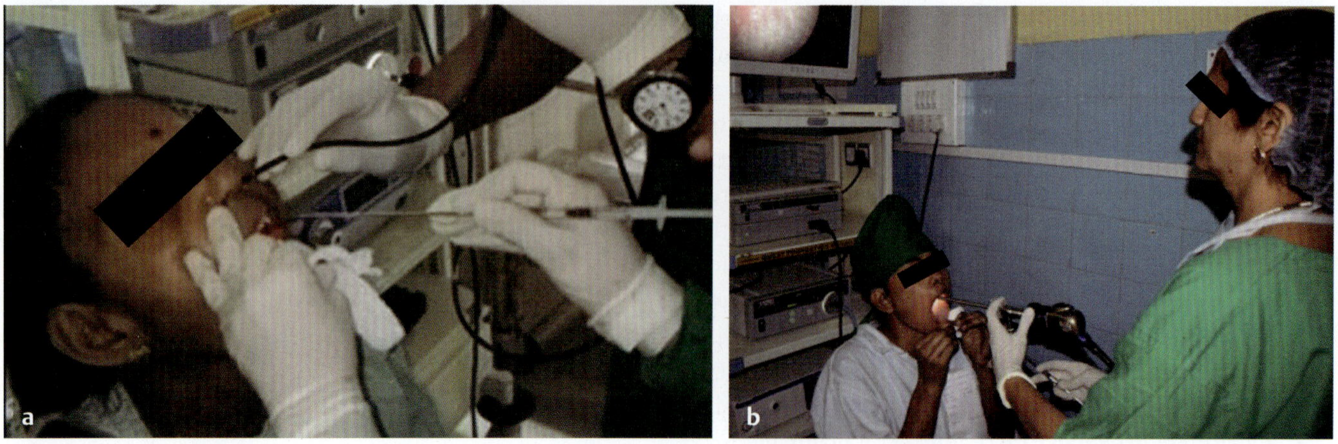

Fig. 76.5 Trans oral laryngeal injection with the use of fiberoptic laryngoscope **(a)** and with the use of rigid 70° Hopkins laryngoscope **(b)**.

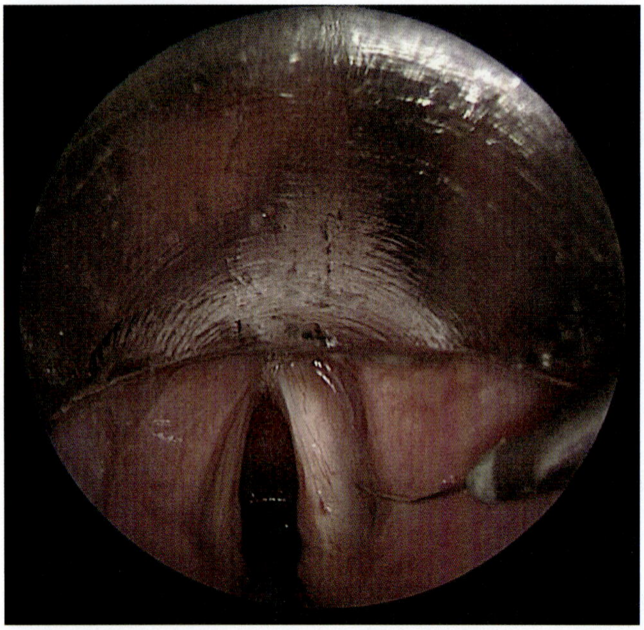

Fig. 76.6 Laryngeal injection through the microlaryngoscope.

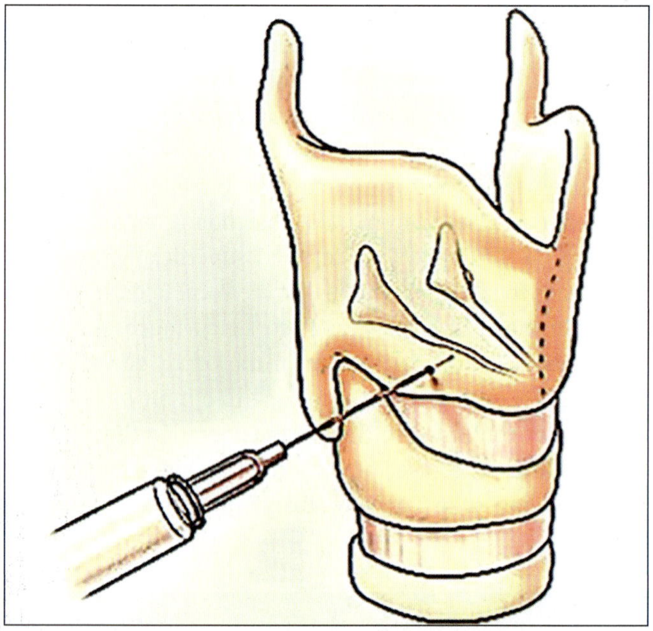

Fig. 76.7 Transthyroid laryngeal injection technique. The needle is introduced perpendicular to the thyroid ala, 4 to 5 mm from the midline and 2 to 3 mm from the lower border of the thyroid cartilage.

  - With a straight injection device via direct laryngoscopy or suspension microlaryngoscopy in the operating room (**Fig. 76.6**).
- Percutaneous:
  - Transthyroid (through the thyroid cartilage) (**Fig. 76.7**). The patient is in the sitting position with the neck extended. The skin and soft tissue immediately overlying the thyroid cartilage are anesthetized with 1:200,000 adrenaline. A flexible laryngoscope is passed transnasally and subsequently held by the assistant to get a good close view of the vocal folds. Larynx can be anesthetized by laryngeal gargle with 4% lidocaine given through the side channel of the laryngoscope, or by percutaneous transtracheal injection of 4 mL of 4% lidocaine with a 23-gauge needle just inferior to the cricoid cartilage. For transthyroid IL, a 20/21-gauge needle is used, as a thinner needle tends to get blocked. The needle is introduced perpendicular to the thyroid ala, 4 to 5 mm from the midline and 2 to 3 mm from the lower border of the thyroid cartilage with a boring action. A give way sensation is felt twice with the piercing of the outer and the inner

laminae. The position of the needle can be confirmed by observing the "tenting up" and movement of the membranous vocal fold. Around 0.3 to 0.6 cc of material is injected into the paraglottic space causing ballooning and medialization of the vocal fold. This procedure may be difficult or impossible in older patients because of the calcification of the thyroid cartilage.

- Transcricothyroid (**Fig. 76.8**): The skin and soft tissue immediately overlying the cricothyroid membrane are anesthetized with 1:200,000 adrenaline. The larynx is anesthetized with any of the above-mentioned methods. With the flexible laryngoscope in position, a 27-gauge needle loaded with the injection material is inserted below the inferior margin of the thyroid cartilage on the ipsilateral side as the target vocal fold and angled superolaterally toward the midportion of the vocal fold. The needle is maintained submucosally throughout the procedure, and its position can be confirmed by moving the tip from side to side.

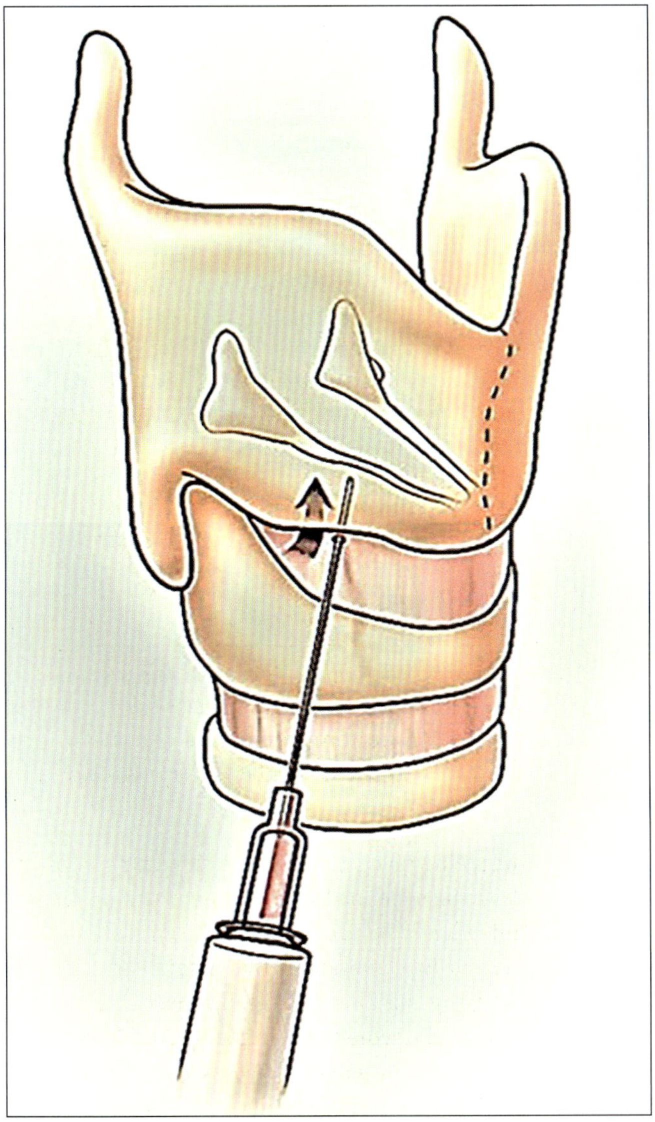

Fig. 76.8 Transcricothyroid injection technique—the needle is inserted below the inferior margin of the thyroid cartilage.

- Transthyrohyoid (**Fig. 76.9a–c**). This approach gives the best visualization and precision, while allowing the tongue and larynx to remain in its natural position. Using a 25-gauge needle, the skin and soft tissue immediately overlying the thyrohyoid notch are anesthetized with 1:200,000 adrenaline. The nasal cavity is anesthetized and decongested with 2% lidocaine and 0.025% oxymetazoline spray, followed by percutaneous transtracheal injection of 4 mL of 4% lidocaine with a 23-gauge needle just inferior to the cricoid cartilage. At this point, a 1.5-inch 25-gauge needle is bent in two locations, with the needle bevel directed caudally. Two separate 45-degree angle bends are created at the hub and 1.5 cm from the needle tip as shown in **Fig. 76.10**. The needle is passed through the thyrohyoid membrane just superior to the thyroid notch, perpendicular to the skin of the neck. As the needle is advanced inferior to the epiglottis, the needle tip is visualized through the mucosa below the petiole in the midline. The double bend achieves a 90-degree angle between the syringe and the needle tip, and therefore with the syringe perpendicular to the skin, the tip points downward onto the superior surface of the vocal folds.[15] Our preference is to inject via this approach using a 25-gauge needle bent at 45-degree angles (**Fig. 76.10**). Limitations may include bleeding from the injection site, insufficient needle length in tall patients, and the potential difficulty of passing a needle through a calcified thyrohyoid membrane.

- Ideal injection location is at a point where a transverse line from the tip of the vocal process laterally intersects the superior arcuate line. A second injection site is sometimes needed at the midmembranous vocal fold along the superior arcuate line (**Fig. 76.11**).
- The depth of injection is generally 3 to 5 mm, slightly inferior or at the level of the inferior lip of the free edge of the vocal fold (**Fig. 76.12**).
- Injection into the superficial layer of the lamina propria (Reinke's space) should be avoided, as this will

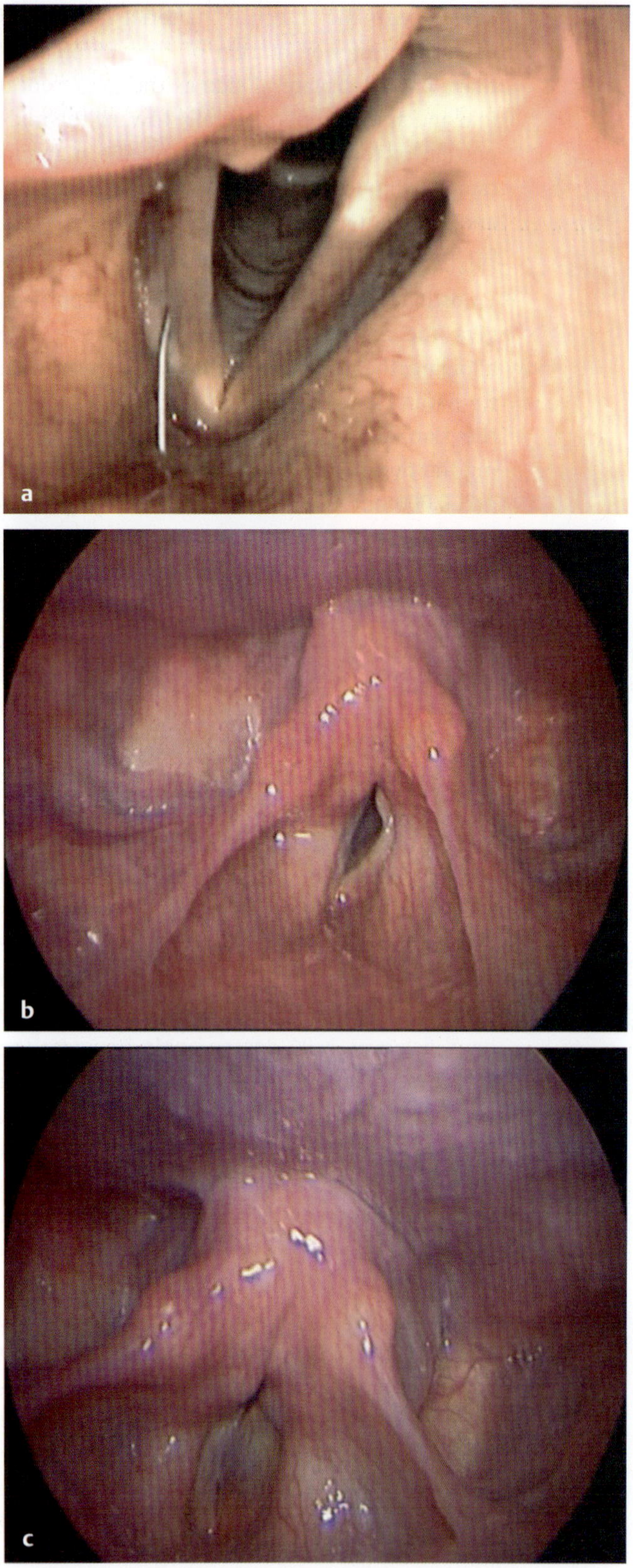

Fig. 76.9 Transthyrohyoid injection technique. **(a)** The needle tip is visualized through the mucosa below the petiole in the midline, **(b)** left vocal fold paralysis with a large phonatory gap, and **(c)** medialized left vocal fold with the closure of the phonatory gap.

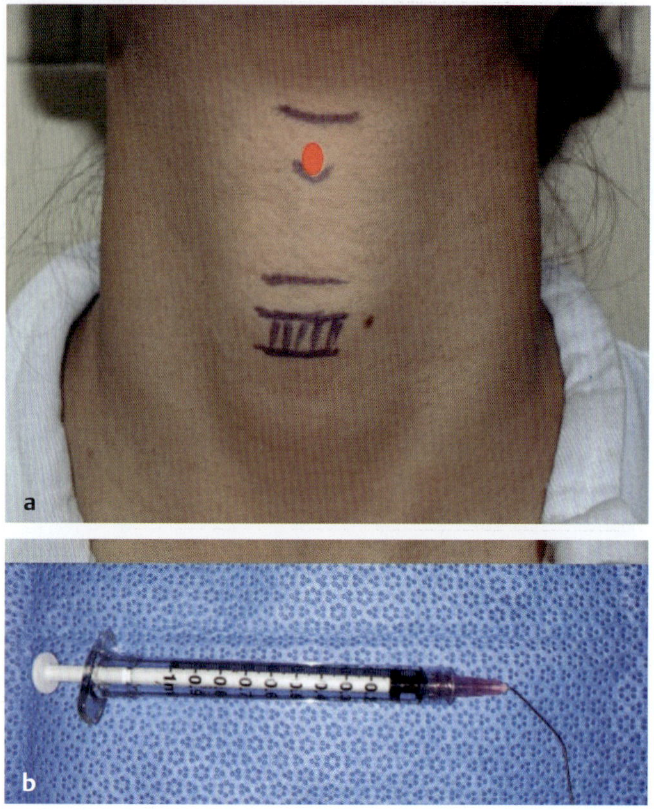

Fig. 76.10 **(a)** Surface marking over the neck showing thyroid notch marked with a *red dot*, cricoid cartilage is marked as the *shaded area*. **(b)** 1.5-inch 25-gauge needle is bent at an angle of 45° at 2 sites, one at the hub and the other at 1.5 cm from the needle tip.

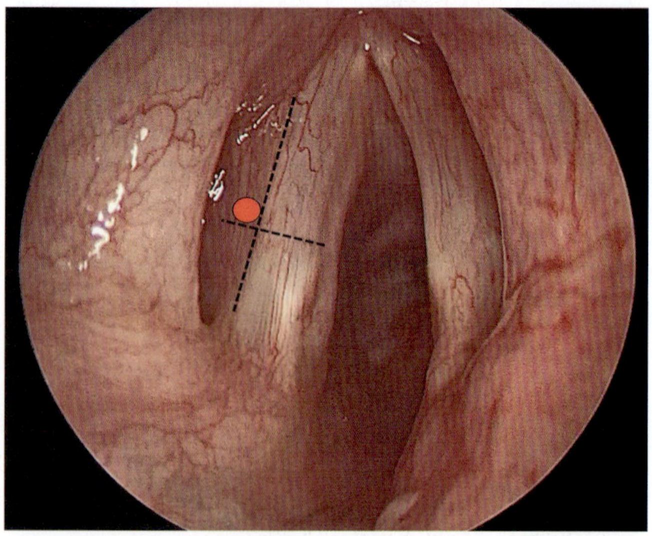

Fig. 76.11 The injection is given at a point just lateral to the point where the transverse line from the tip of the vocal process intersects the superior arcuate line.

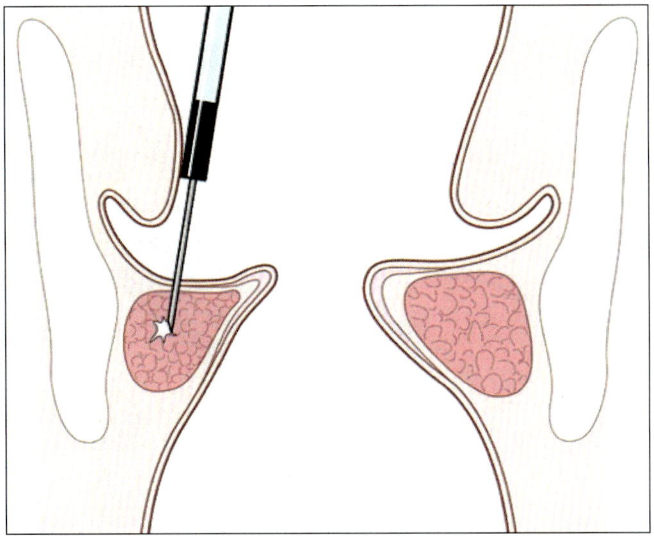

Fig. 76.12 Diagrammatic representation of the coronal section of the larynx, showing the depth of injection of 3 to 5 mm.

result in loss of mucosal pliability and poor vocal quality.

- Over-injection up to 15 to 30% is recommended in order to compensate for resorption of the water-based component present in the injectables. This overcorrection usually results in a slightly rounded, convex contour to the injected vocal fold. Aggressive overcorrection (100%) is recommended in cases of autologous fat injection to account for the substantial resorption of fat that generally occurs within the first 6 to 8 weeks after lipoinjection.

Medialization Thyroplasty (Type I Thyroplasty)

It is a surgical technique for vocal cord medialization by alteration of the laryngeal framework by insertion of an implant into the paraglottic space. It is considered to be the long-term solution for glottic insufficiency that caused unilateral vocal fold paralysis or paresis. A variety of implants and implant materials are available, these materials include silastic, hydroxylapatite, polytetrafluoroethylene ribbon (Gore-Tex), and titanium. Silastic is well tolerated with minimal tissue reactivity over time. A silastic block can be hand-carved to the desired shape as required, depending on the patient's laryngeal anatomy and the cartilaginous window. Preformed silastic blocks are also available (Montgomery Thyroplasty Implant System). Some surgeons prefer to use Gore-Tex ribbon implants, which does not require any carving, and where the degree of medialization can be adjusted easily. Implant selection largely depends on the surgeon's preference, as none of the implants has been proven to be superior to others. Arytenoid adduction can be combined with a type I thyroplasty if sufficient posterior closure is not obtained with an implant alone. An arytenoid adduction is done by placing a suture in the arytenoid, rotating the muscular process posteromedially, allowing for glottic closure and improving posterior closure.

Surgical Technique

It is best done in the operation theater under local anesthesia to allow assessment of the voice during surgery to optimize results. A small amount of sedation is recommended to alleviate the anxiety. Skin and soft tissue are infiltrated with 1:200,000 lidocaine adrenaline solution. The underlying soft tissues are infiltrated with the solution, including injecting directly onto the thyroid lamina, along the posterior border of the thyroid lamina and into the inferior pharyngeal constrictor muscles. Following proper preparation, a horizontal skin crease incision is taken at about the lower border of the thyroid cartilage. Skin, subcutaneous tissue, and platysma are cut, and strap muscles are identified and separated in the midline. The muscles are retracted to allow for full exposure of the thyroid cartilage on the involved side, while they are retracted to a lesser extent on the other side. Once the cartilage is exposed, the outer perichondrium is incised in the midline from the thyroid notch to its lower border and then laterally along the superior and inferior borders. The perichondrium is then elevated with a Freer elevator. The distance from the thyroid notch to the inferior border is measured, and the midpoint is marked. The upper edge of the thyroplasty window is marked lateral to this point, which is 5 mm for females, and 7 mm for males. From this point, a line is drawn vertically down for 5 mm and posteriorly for 10 to 12 mm. The final location and size of the window depend on the chosen implant. The lower edge should be at least 3 mm from the lower border of thyroid cartilage to prevent the cartilage from breaking as the prosthesis is placed. (**Fig. 76.13**). After the window has been created, the inner perichondrium is elevated from undersurface of the thyroid cartilage on all sides except anteriorly. The superior, posterior, and inferior margins of the perichondrium are incised without injuring the lateral fascia of the thyroarytenoid muscle just deep to this (**Fig. 76.14**). A depth gauge is used to medialize the cord, and voice quality and cord position are assessed (**Fig. 76.15**). An implant is carved to appropriate dimensions from a preformed silastic block based on these visual and auditory inputs. Its inferior border is thicker than the superior border, and the posterior border is thicker than the anterior border. This creates an even medialization of the vocal fold with the point of maximum medialization at the lower edge of the window. All edges of the silastic block are beveled to allow ease of insertion through the window. The average size of the block that is used is 2 to 3 mm thick anteriorly and 5 to 7 mm thick at the point of maximal medialization with an overall length of 13 to 18 mm (**Fig. 76.16a, b**). The implant is then secured with a nonabsorbable suture, and closure of all layers including the outer perichondrium, strap muscles, platysma, and skin is performed. A drain may be placed if necessary.

Postoperatively, the patient is observed for any airway compromise, and voice rest is advised for a week.

Complications

- **Vocal fold edema and hematoma:** Postoperative systemic steroids are recommended to prevent or treat airway compromise because of vocal cord edema or hematoma.
- **Implant extrusion:** This can happen if the laryngeal mucosa is violated. It can be checked intraoperatively before insertion of the implant by irrigating the surgical field and asking the patient to do the Valsalva maneuver. The presence of bubbles indicates mucosal penetration.
- **Persistent hoarseness:**
  - ➢ Undermedialization: When the procedure is prolonged, vocal fold edema sets in, which misleads the surgeon to believe the vocal fold was sufficiently medialized. This can be prevented by giving intravenous dexamethasone preoperatively, and if

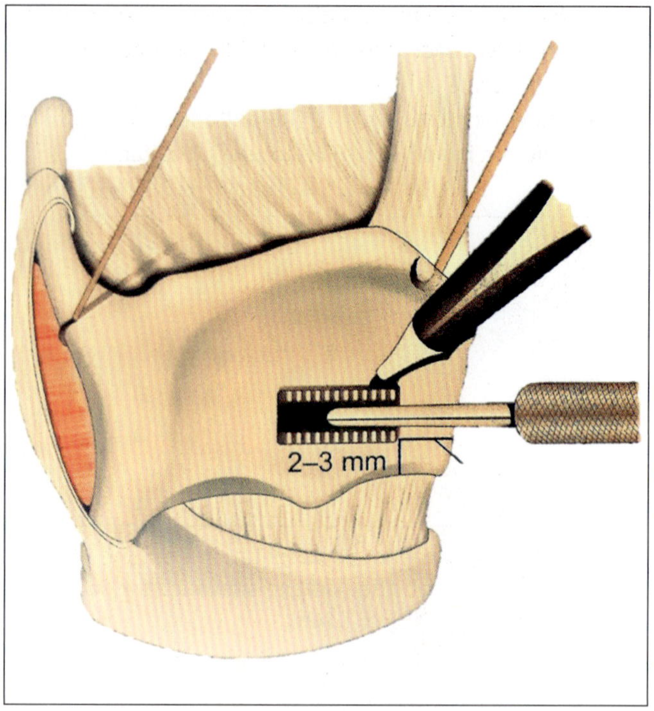

Fig. 76.13 Marking of the thyroplasty window. The anterior end of the upper edge of the window is 5 mm (in females) to 7 mm (in males) lateral to the midline. The window is approximately 10 to 12 mm by 5 mm. The lower edge should be at least 3 mm from the lower border of the thyroid cartilage.

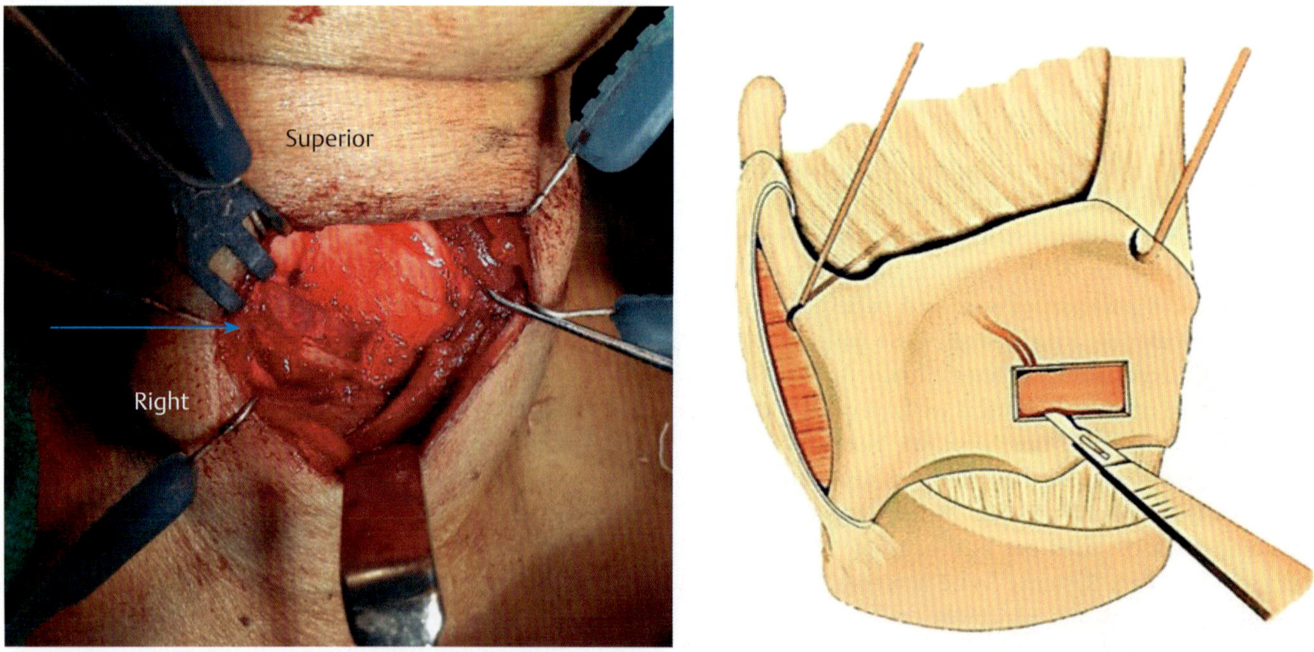

Fig. 76.14 After creating the cartilage window, the inner perichondrium is incised along the edges of the window.

vocal fold edema is suspected, then intraoperative voice feedback should be mildly strained, rather than normal.

- Posterior glottic gap: Arytenoid adduction will be required in addition to revision medialization.

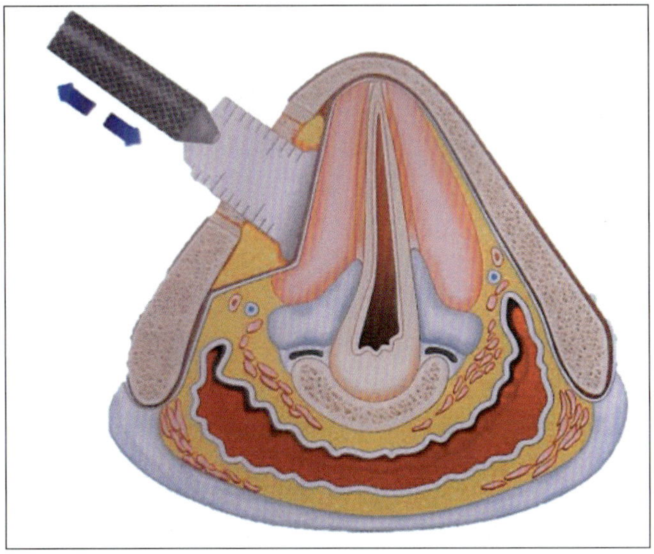

Fig. 76.15 The amount of medicalization required is measured by using a depth gauge whilst checking for patient's voice for optimum voice improvement.

- Implant malpositioning:
  - Anterior malposition would cause a strained voice.
  - Superior malposition would give rise to diplophonia because of medialization of the ventricular folds.

Arytenoid Adduction

See **Fig. 76.17 and Fig. 76.18**.

In high vagal injury with additional loss of the superior laryngeal nerve, medialization alone is not sufficient, as the vocal process remains lateralized, leaving a large posterior gap and a height mismatch. It is usually best addressed with medialization and arytenoid adduction. In arytenoid adduction, the arytenoid is rotated medially by a suture which mimics the thyroarytenoid and lateral cricoarytenoid muscle complex. Exposure of the arytenoid cartilage is achieved by first placing a hook beneath the posterior border of the thyroid cartilage and rotating the larynx forward. The perichondrium at the posterior border is divided, and the piriform sinus mucosa is elevated away from the inner surface of the thyroid cartilage. Patients are then asked to do the Valsalva maneuver to confirm the location of the piriform mucosa so that dissection may be carried out anteriorly to expose the posterior cricoarytenoid muscle. The muscular

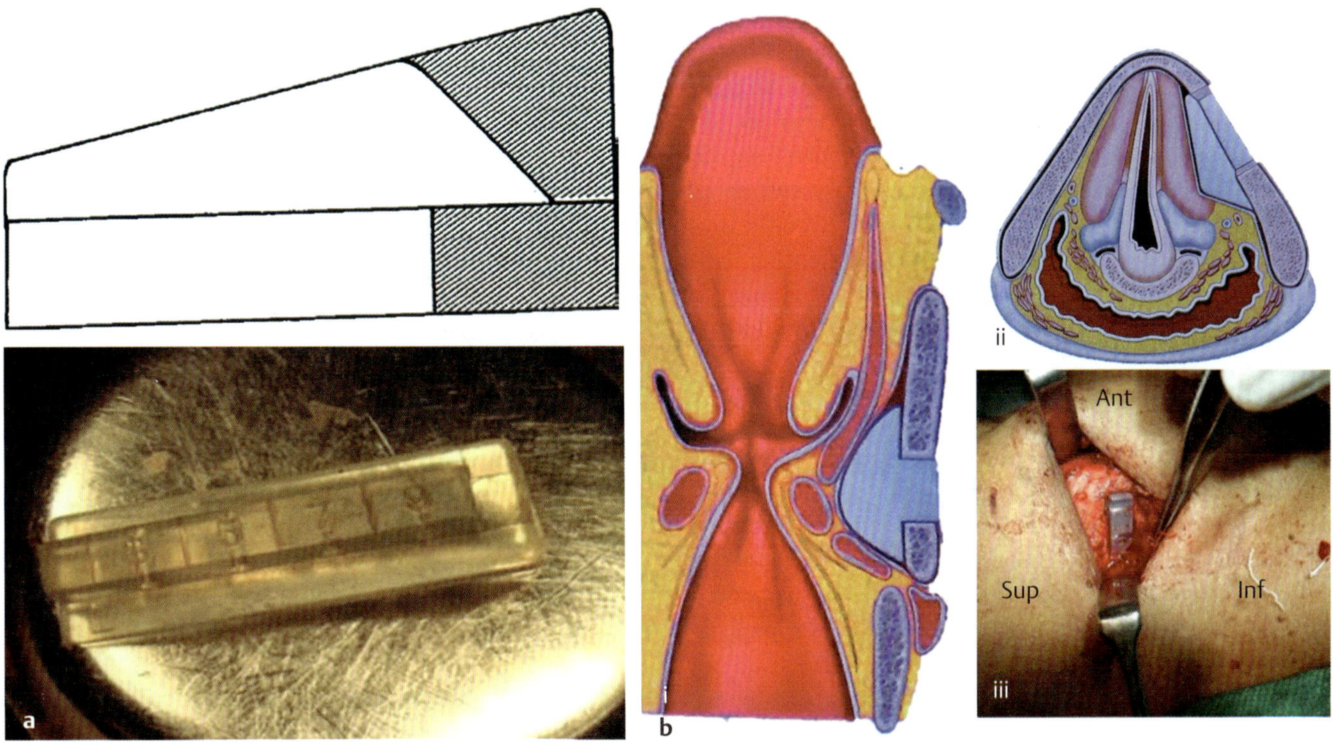

Fig. 76.16 **(a)** Implant is carved out of a preformed silastic block. **(b)** Implant after insertion: **(i)** Final position of the silastic implant in the coronal view, **(ii)** implant as seen in the axial section is placing the thyroarytenoid muscle medially, **(iii)** intraoperative view of the implant fitted on the right side.

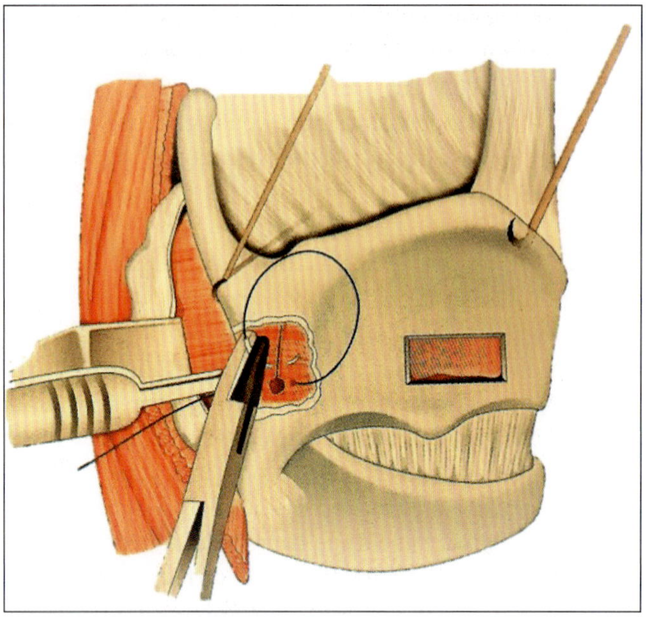

Fig. 76.17 A posterior window is created and the arytenoid is exposed. The pyriform fossa mucosa is retracted and a suture is placed through the muscular process of the arytenoid.

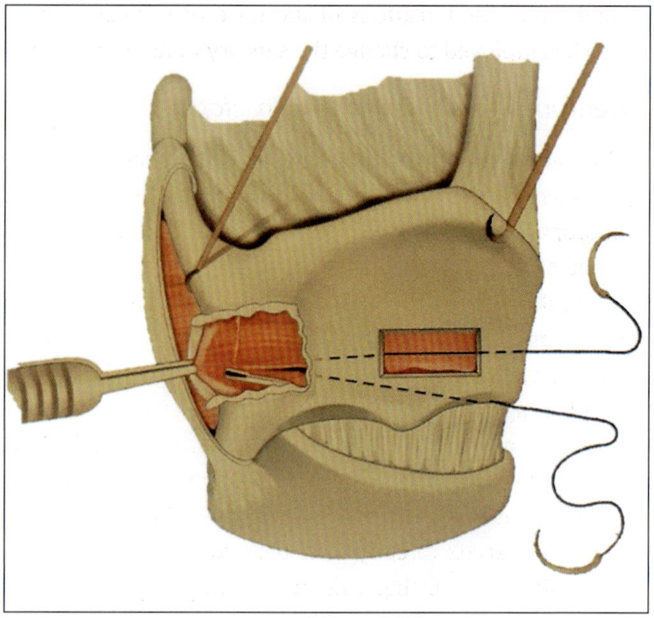

Fig. 76.18 One end of the suture is passed underneath the thyroid cartilage and brought out through it in the midline, and the other end is passed underneath the cartilage and brought out through the inferior margin of the thyroid cartilage in the midline.

process is palpated and moved in its plane of abduction and adduction while observing the monitor. A double-armed 4–0 Prolene suture is passed through the lateral edge of the muscular process in a figure eight fashion. One end of the suture is passed beneath the thyroid cartilage and brought out through the cartilage in the midline, while the other end is brought out through the cricothyroid membrane in the midline. The implant is carved and placed. Final adjustments are made to the arytenoid stitch, and it is secured on the thyroid cartilage. This procedure is surgically challenging with a higher complication rate. There is a higher risk of mucosal perforation because of the elevation of the pyriform sinus.

Treatment of Dysphagia

The effect of paralysis of the superior, middle, and inferior constrictor muscles causes severe dysphagia. As the food bolus passes into the oropharynx, the paralyzed side dilates laterally and forms a pseudopocket that collects the bolus. The normal contraction on the contralateral side pushes the bolus into this region, rather than down into the hypopharynx. This delay interrupts the normal timing of the swallowing event so that when the larynx reopens, the food bolus, which should have been in the esophagus, is still partially in the hypopharynx, where it is then aspirated.

Traditional swallowing therapy involves the following[16]:

- **Compensatory techniques:** These techniques alter the swallow, but do not create lasting functional change. The purpose of these techniques is to compensate for deficits that cannot be or are not yet rehabilitated sufficiently.
- Rehabilitative techniques, such as exercises, are designed to create lasting change in an individual's swallowing over time by improving underlying physiological function. The intent of many exercises is to improve function in the future rather than compensate for a deficit at the moment.

Swallowing Therapy

Biofeedback

It incorporates the patient's ability to sense changes and aids in the treatment of feeding or swallowing disorders.

Diet Modifications

Modifications to the texture of the food may be implemented to allow for safe oral intake. This may include changing the viscosity of liquids and/or softening, chopping, or pureeing solid foods. Modifications of the taste or temperature may also be employed to change the sensory input of the bolus.

Neuromuscular Electrical Stimulation

This can be an adjunctive therapy to the general swallowing therapy. Neuromuscular electrical stimulation (NMES) in oropharyngeal dysphagia helps by improving the sensory input of the oropharyngeal cavity, facilitating or restoring the oral or pharyngeal motor function, and achieving adequate laryngeal elevation. It can avoid the disuse of muscle dystrophy and strengthen the contraction of paralyzed oropharyngeal muscles.[17] Pharyngeal electrical stimulation (PES) is a novel rehabilitation treatment for dysphagia. PES is carried out via location-specific intraluminal catheters that are introduced transnasally that enable clinicians to stimulate the pharynx directly. This technique has demonstrated increasingly promising evidence in improving swallowing performance in patients with neurogenic dysphagia. It has been proven to be superior to traditional dysphagia therapy alone in individuals in a long-term acute care facility.[18]

Maneuvers

These are specific strategies that clinicians use to change the timing or strength of particular movements of swallowing. Examples of maneuvers include the following:

- **Effortful swallow:** It increases posterior tongue base movement to facilitate bolus clearance. The patient is instructed to swallow and push hard with the tongue against the hard palate.[19]
- **The Mendelsohn maneuver:** It is designed to elevate the larynx and open the esophagus during the swallow to prevent food/liquid from falling into the airway. The patient holds the larynx in an elevated position at the peak of hyolaryngeal elevation.
- **Supraglottic swallow:** It is designed to close the vocal folds by voluntarily holding one's breath before and during swallow in order to protect the airway. The patient is instructed to hold his or her breath just before swallowing to close the vocal folds. The swallow is followed immediately by a volitional cough.
- **Super-supraglottic swallow:** It is designed to voluntarily move the arytenoids anteriorly, closing the entrance to the laryngeal vestibule before and during the swallow.[20]

Oral-Motor Therapy/Exercises

Oral-motor treatments include stimulation to or actions of the lips, jaw, tongue, soft palate, pharynx, larynx, and respiratory muscles to improve their functions.

- **Laryngeal elevation:** The patient is asked to slide up a pitch scale and hold a high note for several seconds. This maintains the larynx in an elevated position.
- **Masako or tongue hold:** The patient holds the tongue forward between the teeth while swallowing; this is performed without food or liquid in the mouth, to prevent coughing or choking.
- **Shaker exercise, head-lifting exercises:** The patient rests in a supine position and lifts his or her head to look at the toes to facilitate an increased opening of the upper esophageal sphincter through increased hyoid and laryngeal anterior and superior excursion.
- **Lingual isometric exercises:** The patient is provided lingual resistance across exercises to increase strength.

Postural/Position Techniques

Postural techniques redirect the movement of the bolus in the oral cavity and pharynx and modify pharyngeal dimensions in a systematic way.

- **Chin-down posture:** The chin is tucked down toward the neck during the swallow, which may bring the tongue base closer to the posterior pharyngeal wall, narrow the opening to the airway, and widen the vallecular space.
- **Chin-up posture:** The chin is tilted up, which may facilitate movement of the bolus from the oral cavity.
- **Head rotation (turn to the side):** The head is turned to the weaker side, so as to close the weaker side, thus facilitating the passage of food through the opposite intact side.
- **Head tilt:** The head is tilted towards the healthy side when the food remains in the paralyzed side due to unilateral oral or pharyngeal weakness. When the head is tilted, food flows toward the direction of head tilt.

Prosthetics/Appliances

These are palatal obturator, palatal lift prosthesis.

Sensory Stimulation

Thermal-tactile stimulation (e.g., using iced lemon glycerin swab, cold laryngeal mirror) or tactile stimulation applied to the tongue, around the mouth, and/or in the oropharynx.

Surgical Treatment

Improved Glottal Closure

Medialization

In cases of persistent aspiration despite diet changes and the implementation of swallowing techniques, early vocal fold medialization procedures can be considered. It does not necessarily eliminate aspiration, but it can help the patient generate a stronger cough to protect the airway.

Protection of the Airway

- Tracheostomy.
- **Feeding tubes:** Through nasogastric tube or feeding jejunostomy.

Treatment of Velopharyngeal Incompetence

Vagal injury at or above the jugular foramen causes paralysis of not only the palate but also the pharyngeal constrictors, resulting in loss of lateral wall motion on the affected side. Nasopharyngoscopy with either a rigid or a flexible scope shows unilateral closure of the nasopharynx. Nonsurgical approaches to velopharyngeal incompetence (VPI) are speech and swallowing therapy, palatal lift prostheses, and palatal obturators. Surgically, it can be corrected by adhering the palate on the affected side to the posterior pharyngeal wall. This unilateral palatal adhesion successfully eliminates hypernasality and nasal regurgitation and has become the procedure of choice for the correction of VPI in neurotologic skull base patients. A transpalatal incision is taken in the area of the palatal crease that forms with normal palatal elevation, and the posterior pharyngeal wall is viewed through this incision. A similar incision is taken on the posterior pharyngeal wall down to the prevertebral fascia. The pharyngeal mucosa is elevated for a few millimeters all around to create an edge to which the nasopharyngeal mucosa of the palate is sutured. Multiple deep mattress sutures are taken to suture the nasopharyngeal surface of the palate to the posterior pharyngeal wall. The oral surface of the palate is closed on itself, thus creating a unilateral palatal adhesion (**Fig. 76.19**).

Treatment of Cricopharyngeal Hypertonicity or Dysfunction

Swallowing Therapy

- **The Mendelsohn maneuver:** Lifting or elevating the larynx with the muscles of the neck for a few seconds to encourage the opening of the upper esophageal sphincter.
- **Effortful swallowing:** Bearing down the neck muscles during the swallow.

Dilation

Simple dilation can afford symptomatic benefit of variable duration and can be considered in elderly patients with significant comorbidity with high operative risk.

Cricopharyngeal Myotomy

It is a surgical procedure that involves cutting the cricopharyngeus muscle, using either an external or an endoscopic approach. The endoscopic approach performed with CO_2 laser is the preferred option. Myotomy has the advantage of affecting both the muscular and the connective tissue components of the cricopharyngeus. It is indicated if patients have moderate to severe dysphagia not responding to swallowing therapy.

Botulinum Toxin Injection

It can be treated with botulinum toxin injection into the cricopharyngeus muscle, which leads to relaxation of the upper esophageal sphincter. It can be done under general anesthesia to ensure accurate drug placement, but it can also be done in an awake patient in the office aided by electromyography.

Spinal Accessory Nerve (Cranial Nerve XI)

Loss of sternocleidomastoid function results in weakness when turning the head away from the operated side, although this is rarely noticed by most patients. Loss of trapezius function results in downward and lateral rotation of

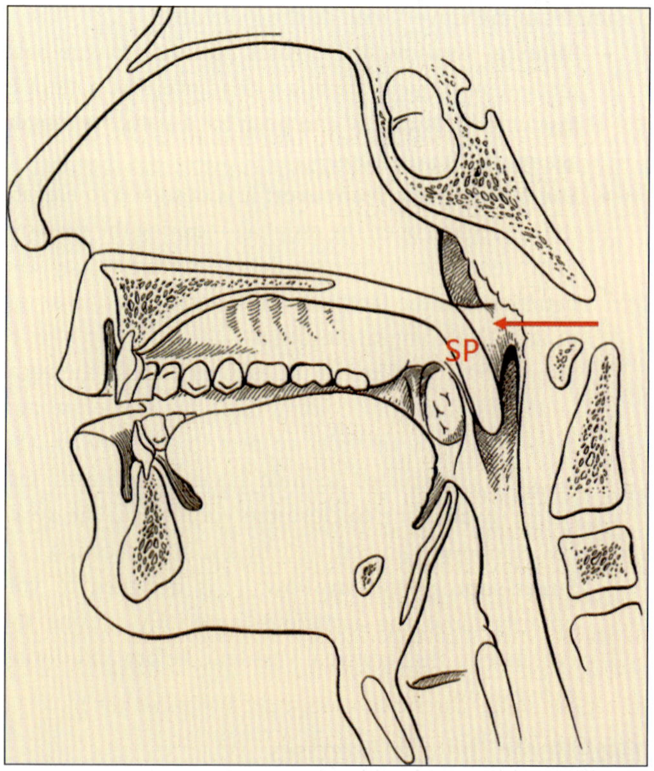

Fig. 76.19 Nasopharyngeal mucosa of the palate is sutured to the posterior pharyngeal wall creating a unilateral palatal adhesion, in cases of velopharyngeal insufficiency resistant to conservative treatment.

the scapula with a shoulder droop. This causes severe shoulder disability secondary to weakness and pain. Early postoperative rehabilitation includes aggressive physical therapy with active and passive range-of-motion exercises, particularly upper arm abduction and humoral rotation to prevent the development of impairment of shoulder function and chronic pain.[21] Failure to initiate physical therapy can result in severe disability with adhesive capsulitis, chronic pain, and shoulder dysfunction.

Hypoglossal Nerve (Cranial Nerve XII)

Hypoglossal nerve involvement by a skull base lesion results in dysarthria and oral phase dysphagia. As an isolated deficit, the hypoglossal loss may be compensated with swallowing and articulatory therapy. In combination with cranial nerves IX and X, however, hypoglossal nerve injury increases swallowing dysfunction and affects rehabilitation.

Rehabilitation consists of lingual and phonatory exercises to promote muscle strengthening, including chewing, tongue protrusion, tongue rolling, and pressing the tongue against teeth and hard palate.

Cervical Sympathetic Chain

- **Ptosis:** Elevation of the eyelid to its normal open position can be accomplished by either levator shortening or resection of Müller's muscle.[22]
- **"First bite syndrome":** Early management consists of dietary modification with bland foods and oral carbamazepine (100–200 mg twice daily). Slowly, over time, the symptoms improve.

Conclusion

Single LCN injuries result in sufficient morbidity to warrant therapy; however, most patients compensate for the isolated loss of function. Multiple cranial nerve deficits (CNs IX, IX, and XII) need the full efforts of the rehabilitative team. After procedures such as vocal cord medialization, arytenoid adduction, palatal adhesion, and speech and swallowing therapy, most patients resume adequate oral intake. However, it takes a reasonable time, often a year to return to normal meals postoperatively. Some patients, especially elderly patients, continue to struggle to maintain adequate nutrition. Hence, careful consideration should be given to the slow growth potential of certain tumors, the resulting postoperative cranial nerve deficits, and the patient's age before proceeding with aggressive surgical management of lateral skull base tumors.

References

1. Netterville JL, Reilly KM, Robertson D, Reiber ME, Armstrong WB, Childs P. Carotid body tumors: a review of 30 patients with 46 tumors. Laryngoscope 1995;105(2):115–126
2. Imaizumi S. Acoustic measures of roughness in pathological voice. J Phonetics 1986;14:457–462
3. Jacobson BH, Johnson A, Grywalski C, et al. The voice handicap index (VHI): development and validation. Am J Speech Lang Pathol 1997;6:66–70
4. Aviv JE, Spitzer J, Cohen M, Ma G, Belafsky P, Close LG. Laryngeal adductor reflex and pharyngeal squeeze as predictors of laryngeal penetration and aspiration. Laryngoscope 2002;112(2):338–341
5. Logemann JA. Manual for the videofluorographic study of swallowing. Boston, MA: Little, Brown; 1986</bok>
6. Rosenbek JC, Robbins JA, Roecker EB, Coyle JL, Wood JL. A penetration-aspiration scale. Dysphagia 1996;11(2):93–98
7. Netterville JL, Sullivan CA. Rehabilitation of Lower Cranial Nerve Deficits After Neurotologic Skull Base Surgery, In: Otologic surgery E-book, 3rd ed. Saunders Elsevier Health Sciences; 2009, Ch. 47, pg 571</bok>
8. Friedman AD, Burns JA, Heaton JT, Zeitels SM. Early versus late injection medialization for unilateral vocal cord paralysis. Laryngoscope 2010;120(10):2042–2046
9. Prendes BL, Yung KC, Likhterov I, Schneider SL, Al-Jurf SA, Courey MS. Long-term effects of injection laryngoplasty with a temporary agent on voice quality and vocal fold position. Laryngoscope 2012;122(10):2227–2233
10. Graboyes EM, Bradley JP, Meyers BF, Nussenbaum B. Efficacy and safety of acute injection laryngoplasty for vocal cord paralysis following thoracic surgery. Laryngoscope 2011;121(11):2406–2410
11. Schramm VL, May M, Lavorato AS. Gelfoam paste injection for vocal cord paralysis: temporary rehabilitation of glottic incompetence. Laryngoscope 1978;88(8 Pt 1):1268–1273 10.1288/00005537-197808000-0000
12. Mallur PS, Rosen CA. Vocal fold injection: review of indications, techniques, and materials for augmentation. Clin Exp Otorhinolaryngol 2010;3(4):177–182
13. Hertegård S, Dahlqvist A, Laurent C, Borzacchiello A, Ambrosio L. Viscoelastic properties of rabbit vocal folds after augmentation. Otolaryngol Head Neck Surg 2003;128(3): 401–406
14. Caton T, Thibeault SL, Klemuk S, Smith ME. Viscoelasticity of hyaluronan and nonhyaluronan based vocal fold injectables: implications for mucosal versus muscle use. Laryngoscope 2007;117(3):516–521

15. Amin MR. Thyrohyoid approach for vocal fold augmentation. Ann Otol Rhinol Laryngol 2006;115(9):699–702

16. Logemann JA. Treatment of oral and pharyngeal dysphagia. Phys Med Rehabil Clin N Am 2008;19(4):803–816, ix

17. Huang KL, Liu TY, Huang YC, Leong CP, Lin WC, Pong YP. Functional outcome in acute stroke patients with oropharyngeal Dysphagia after swallowing therapy. J Stroke Cerebrovasc Dis 2014;23(10):2547–2553

18. Blumenfeld L, Hahn Y, Lepage A, Leonard R, Belafsky PC. Transcutaneous electrical stimulation versus traditional dysphagia therapy: a nonconcurrent cohort study. Otolaryngol Head Neck Surg 2006;135(5):754–757

19. Huckabee ML, Steele CM. An analysis of lingual contribution to submental surface electromyographic measures and pharyngeal pressure during effortful swallow. Arch Phys Med Rehabil 2006;87(8):1067–1072

20. Donzelli J, Brady S. The effects of breath-holding on vocal fold adduction: implications for safe swallowing. Arch Otolaryngol Head Neck Surg 2004;130(2):208–210

21. Eibling DE, Boyd EM. Rehabilitation of lower cranial nerve deficits. Otolaryngol Clin North Am 1997;30(5):865–875

22. Dortzbach RK. Superior tarsal muscle resection to correct blepharoptosis. Ophthalmology 1979;86(10):1883–1891

Index

D

E